Edited by

DAVID G. NATHAN, M.D.
Physician-in-Chief
The Children's Hospital

Robert A. Stranahan Professor of Pediatrics
Harvard Medical School
Boston, Massachusetts

FRANK A. OSKI, M.D.
Pediatrician-in-Chief
The Johns Hopkins Children's Center

Given Professor of Pediatrics
Chairman, Department of Pediatrics
The Johns Hopkins University School of Medicine
Baltimore, Maryland

THIRD EDITION

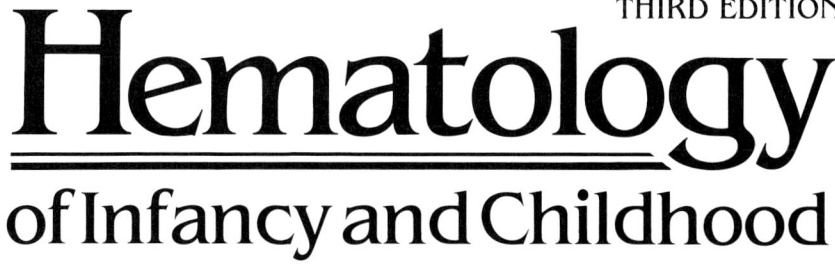

Hematology
of Infancy and Childhood

1987
W. B. SAUNDERS COMPANY
Harcourt Brace Jovanovich, Inc.

Philadelphia ☐ London ☐ Toronto
Montreal ☐ Sydney ☐ Tokyo

W. B. SAUNDERS COMPANY
Harcourt Brace Jovanovich, Inc.

West Washington Square
Philadelphia, PA 19105

Library of Congress Cataloging-in-Publication Data

Hematology of infancy and childhood.

Includes bibliographies and index.

1. Pediatric hematology. I. Nathan, David G., 1929–
II. Oski, Frank A. [DNLM: 1. Hematologic Diseases—in
infancy and childhood. WS 300 H4872]

RJ411.H46 1987   618.92'215   86–3734

ISBN 0–7216–6659–0 (set)
ISBN 0–7216–6657–4 (v. 1)
ISBN 0–7216–6658–2 (v. 2)

Editor: John Dyson
Developmental Editor: Carole Wonsiewicz
Designer: W. B. Saunders Staff
Production Manager: Peter Faber
Manuscript Editor: Erika Shapiro
Illustration Coordinator: Margaret Shaw
Indexer: Ruth Low

Hematology of Infancy and Childhood

Volume I ISBN   0–7216–6657–4
Volume II ISBN   0–7216–6658–2
Complete Set ISBN 0–7216–6659–0

© 1987 by W. B. Saunders Company. Copyright 1974 and 1981 by W. B. Saunders Company. Copyright under the Uniform Copyright Convention. Simultaneously published in Canada. All rights reserved. This book is protected by copyright. No part of it may be reproduced, stored in a retrieval system, or transmitted in any form or by any means, electronic, mechanical, photocopying, recording, or otherwise, without written permission from the publisher. Made in the United States of America. Press of W. B. Saunders Company. Library of Congress catalog card number 86–3734.

Last digit is the print number: 9   8   7   6   5   4   3   2   1

CONTRIBUTORS

HERBERT T. ABELSON, M.D. Professor and Chairman, Department of Pediatrics, University of Washington School of Medicine; Pediatrician-in-Chief, Children's Hospital and Medical Center, Seattle, Washington
Cancer Chemotherapy

CHESTER A. ALPER, M.D. Professor of Pediatrics, Harvard Medical School; Senior Associate in Hematology and Oncology, The Children's Hospital, Boston, Massachusetts
Serum Proteins and Other Genetic Markers of the Blood

BLANCHE P. ALTER, M.D. Professor of Medicine and Pediatrics, Mount Sinai School of Medicine; Attending Physician and Attending Pediatrician, Mount Sinai Medical Center, New York, New York
The Bone Marrow Failure Syndromes

ARNOLD J. ALTMAN, M.D. Professor of Pediatrics and Hartford Whalers Professor of Children's Cancer, University of Connecticut School of Medicine; Head, Division of Pediatric Hematology/Oncology, University of Connecticut Health Center, Farmington, Connecticut
Management of Malignant Solid Tumors

BERNARD M. BABIOR, M.D. Member and Head, Division of Biochemistry, Department of Basic and Clinical Research; Staff Physician, Division of Hematology/Oncology, Scripps Clinic and Research Foundation, La Jolla, California
The Megaloblastic Anemias: Folate Deficiency; Vitamin B_{12} (Cobalamin) Deficiency and Other Congenital and Acquired Disorders

JUDITH L. BADER, M.D. Senior Clinical Investigator, Radiation Oncology Branch, National Cancer Institute; Attending Physician, Bethesda Naval Hospital, NCI Clinical Center, Bethesda, Maryland
Epidemiology of Cancer in Childhood

SHELLY C. BERNSTEIN, M.D., Ph.D. Instructor in Pediatrics, Harvard Medical School; Assistant in Medicine (Hematology-Oncology), The Children's Hospital; Clinical Associate, Dana-Farber Cancer Institute, Boston, Massachusetts; Visiting Scientist, Whitehead Institute for Biomedical Research, Department of Biology, and Center for Cancer Research, Massachusetts Institute of Technology, Cambridge, Massachusetts
Oncogenes and the Molecular Biology of Cancer

ROSE-MARY BOUSTANY, M.D. Instructor in Neurology, Harvard Medical School; Assistant in Neurology, Massachusetts General Hospital, Boston, Massachusetts; Associate Director, Lysosomal Storage Diseases Laboratory, Eunice Kennedy Shriver Center for Mental Retardation, Waltham, Massachusetts
Storage Diseases of the Reticuloendothelial System

CONTRIBUTORS

LAURENCE A. BOXER, M.D.   Professor of Pediatrics, University of Michigan; Director, Section of Pediatric Hematology/Oncology, C. S. Mott Children's Hospital, Ann Arbor, Michigan
Disorders of Granulopoiesis and Granulocyte Function

MICHAEL C. BRAIN, D.M., F.R.C.P., F.R.C.P.(C)
Professor of Medicine and Pathology, McMaster University, Hamilton, Ontario, Canada
The Destruction of Red Cells by the Vasculature and Reticuloendothelial System

GEORGE R. BUCHANAN, M.D.   Professor of Pediatrics, University of Texas Health Science Center at Dallas; Director, Pediatric Hematology-Oncology, Children's Medical Center and Parkland Memorial Hospital, Dallas, Texas
Hemorrhagic Diseases; Coagulation Factors

H. FRANKLIN BUNN, M.D.   Professor of Medicine, Harvard Medical School; Senior Physician, Brigham and Women's Hospital, Boston, Massachusetts; Chief Investigator, Howard Hughes Medical Institute, Boston, Massachusetts
Human Hemoglobins: Normal and Abnormal

RITCHARD G. CABLE, M.D.   Associate Professor of Laboratory Medicine, University of Connecticut Medical School; Director of Blood Services, American Red Cross, Connecticut Region, Farmington, Connecticut
Platelet Transfusion

J. ROBERT CASSADY, M.D.   Professor and Head, Department of Radiation Oncology, University of Arizona Medical Center/Health Sciences Center, Tucson, Arizona
Radiation Therapy

HARVEY R. COLTEN, M.D.   Harriet B. Spoehrer Professor of Pediatrics, and Chairman, The Edward Mallinckrodt Department of Pediatrics, Washington University School of Medicine; Pediatrician-in-Chief, Children's Hospital at Washington University Medical Center, and Pediatrician-in-Chief, Barnes Hospital at Washington University Medical Center, St. Louis, Missouri
Primary Immunodeficiencies and Serum Complement Defects

JOHN T. CURNUTTE, M.D., Ph.D.   Assistant Member, Department of Basic and Clinical Research, Scripps Clinic and Research Foundation, La Jolla, California
Disorders of Granulopoiesis and Granulocyte Function

PETER R. DALLMAN, M.D.   Professor of Pediatrics, University of California–San Francisco; Attending Hematologist, University of California Medical Center, San Francisco, California
Iron Deficiency and Related Nutritional Anemias

BO DUPONT, M.D., D.Sc.   Professor of Immunology, Cornell University Graduate School of Medical Sciences; Member and Head, Human Immunogenetics Program, Sloan-Kettering Institute for Cancer Research; Attending Geneticist, Department of Medicine, Memorial Hospital, New York, New York
The HLA System

CONTRIBUTORS

THOMAS J. ERVIN, M.D. Clinical Assistant Professor, Harvard Medical School, Boston, Massachusetts; Clinical Associate Professor, University of Vermont School of Medicine, Burlington, Vermont
Granulocyte Transfusion

STEPHEN A. FEIG, M.D. Professor of Pediatrics, UCLA School of Medicine; Chief, Division of Pediatric Hematology-Oncology, UCLA Hospital, Los Angeles, California
Methemoglobinemia

MARTIN T. FOSBURG, M.D. Assistant Professor of Pediatrics, Harvard Medical School; Associate in Medicine, The Children's Hospital, Boston, Massachusetts
Red Cell Transfusion; Therapeutic Plasma Exchange and Cytapheresis

LAWRENCE M. GARTNER, M.D. Professor of Pediatrics, University of Chicago Pritzker School of Medicine; Chairman, Department of Pediatrics, and Director, Wyler Children's Hospital, Chicago, Illinois
Disorders of Bilirubin Metabolism

RAIF S. GEHA, M.D. Associate Professor of Pediatrics, Harvard Medical School; Chief, Division of Allergy, The Children's Hospital, Boston, Massachusetts
T Cell Control of the Immune Response

FRANCES M. GILL, M.D. Associate Professor of Pediatrics, Children's Hospital of Philadelphia, Philadelphia, Pennsylvania
Autoimmune Hemolytic Anemia

JONATHAN GLASS, M.D. Associate Professor of Medicine, Louisiana State University Medical School and Medical Center, Shreveport, Louisiana
Disorders of Heme Metabolism: Sideroblastic Anemia and the Porphyrias

HOLCOMBE E. GRIER, M.D. Instructor in Pediatrics, Harvard Medical School; Assistant in Medicine (Hematology-Oncology), The Children's Hospital; Clinical Associate, Dana-Farber Cancer Institute, Boston, Massachusetts
Chronic Myeloproliferative Disorders and Myelodysplasia

ROBERT I. HANDIN, M.D. Associate Professor of Medicine, Harvard Medical School; Staff Physician and Director, Hematology Division, Brigham and Women's Hospital, Boston, Massachusetts
Physiology of Coagulation: The Platelet

JOHN G. KELTON, M.D. Professor of Medicine and Pathology, McMaster Medical Centre, Hamilton, Ontario, Canada
The Destruction of Red Cells by the Vasculature and Reticuloendothelial System; The Platelet: Quantitative and Qualitative Abnormalities

SHERWIN V. KEVY, M.D. Associate Professor of Pediatrics, Harvard Medical School; Director of Transfusion Service, The Children's Hospital, Boston, Massachusetts
Red Cell Transfusion

CONTRIBUTORS

EDWIN H. KOLODNY, M.D. Professor of Neurology, Harvard Medical School; Associate Neurologist, Massachusetts General Hospital, Boston, Massachusetts; Director, Eunice Kennedy Shriver Center for Mental Retardation, Waltham, Massachusetts
Storage Diseases of the Reticuloendothelial System

STANLEY J. KORSMEYER, M.D. Associate Professor, Department of Medicine, Howard Hughes Medical Institute, Washington University School of Medicine; Attending Physician, Barnes Hospital at Washington University Medical Center, St. Louis, Missouri
Immunoglobulin and T Cell Receptor Genes in Human Immunodeficiency and Neoplasia

PHILIP LANZKOWSKY, M.D., F.R.C.P., D.C.H. Professor of Pediatrics, School of Medicine, Health Sciences Center of the State University of New York at Stonybrook; Chief of Pediatric Hematology-Oncology, Chairman, Department of Pediatrics, and Chief-of-Staff, Schneider Children's Hospital of Long Island Jewish Medical Center, New Hyde Park, New York
The Megaloblastic Anemias: Folate Deficiency; Vitamin B_{12} (Cobalamin) Deficiency and Other Congenital and Acquired Disorders

FREDERICK P. LI, M.D. Head, Clinical Studies Section, Clinical Epidemiology Branch, National Cancer Institute, Bethesda, Maryland; Staff Physician, Dana-Farber Cancer Institute, Boston, Massachusetts
Epidemiology of Cancer in Childhood

JEFFREY M. LIPTON, M.D., Ph.D. Associate Professor of Pediatrics, Mount Sinai School of Medicine; Chief of Pediatric Hematology/Oncology, Jack and Lucy Clark Department of Pediatrics, Mount Sinai Hospital, New York, New York
The Anatomy and Physiology of Hematopoiesis

BERTRAM H. LUBIN, M.D. Adjunct Clinical Professor of Pediatrics, University of California–San Francisco; Director of Medical Research, Children's Hospital Oakland Research Institute, Oakland, California
Appendix: Reference Values in Infancy and Childhood

JEANNE M. LUSHER, M.D. Professor of Pediatrics, Wayne State University School of Medicine; Director, Division of Hematology-Oncology, Children's Hospital of Michigan, Detroit, Michigan; Associate Medical Director, The National Hemophilia Foundation, Ann Arbor, Michigan
Diseases of Coagulation: The Fluid Phase

SAMUEL E. LUX, M.D. Professor of Pediatrics, Harvard Medical School; Chief, Division of Hematology/Oncology, The Children's Hospital, Boston, Massachusetts
Disorders of the Red Cell Membrane

W. LAURENCE MARSH, Ph.D., F.R.C.Path., F.I.Biol., F.I.M.L.S. Senior Immunohematologist, The New York Blood Center, New York, New York
Erythrocyte Blood Groups in Humans

WILLIAM C. MENTZER, JR., M.D. Professor of Pediatrics and Laboratory Medicine, University of California–San Francisco; Director, Division of

Hematology/Oncology, Department of Pediatrics, University of California–San Francisco, San Francisco, California
Pyruvate Kinase Deficiency and Disorders of Glycolysis

SHARON B. MURPHY, M.D.   Member, Department of Hematology/Oncology, St. Jude Children's Research Hospital; Professor of Pediatrics, University of Tennessee Center for the Health Sciences, Memphis, Tennessee
The Lymphomas and Lymphadenopathy

DAVID G. NATHAN, M.D.   Physician-in-Chief, The Children's Hospital; Robert A. Stranahan Professor of Pediatrics, Harvard Medical School, Boston, Massachusetts
The Anatomy and Physiology of Hematopoiesis; Sickle Cell Disease; Serum Proteins and Other Genetic Markers of the Blood

ARTHUR W. NIENHUIS, M.D.   Chief, Clinical Hematology Branch, National Heart, Lung and Blood Institute, Bethesda, Maryland
The Thalassemias

FRANK A. OSKI, M.D.   Given Professor of Pediatrics and Chairman, Department of Pediatrics, Johns Hopkins University School of Medicine; Pediatrician-in-Chief, Johns Hopkins Children's Center, Baltimore, Maryland
The Erythrocyte and Its Disorders; Differential Diagnosis of Anemia

HOWARD A. PEARSON, M.D.   Professor and Chairman, Department of Pediatrics, Yale University School of Medicine; Chief of Pediatrics, Yale New Haven Hospital, New Haven, Connecticut
The Spleen and Disturbances of Splenic Function

SERGIO PIOMELLI, M.D.   Professor of Pediatrics, Columbia University College of Physicians and Surgeons; Director, Pediatric Hematology/Oncology, The Presbyterian Hospital in the City of New York, New York, New York
Lead Poisoning; G6PD Deficiency and Related Disorders of the Pentose Pathway

ORAH S. PLATT, M.D.   Associate Professor of Pediatrics, Harvard Medical School; Associate in Medicine, The Children's Hospital; Associate in Pediatrics, Dana-Farber Cancer Institute, Boston, Massachusetts
Sickle Cell Disease

JOEL M. RAPPEPORT, M.D.   Associate Professor of Medicine, Harvard Medical School; Consultant in Hematology and Physician, Brigham and Women's Hospital and Leonard Morse Hospital, Boston, Massachusetts
Bone Marrow Transplantation

STEPHEN H. ROBINSON, M.D.   George C. Reisman Professor of Medicine, Harvard Medical School; Physician, Chief of Hematology, and Clinical Director, Department of Medicine, Beth Israel Hospital, Boston, Massachusetts
Disorders of Heme Metabolism: Sideroblastic Anemia and the Porphyrias

FRED S. ROSEN, M.D.   The James L. Gamble Professor of Pediatrics, Harvard Medical School, Boston, Massachusetts
Primary Immunodeficiencies and Serum Complement Defects

CONTRIBUTORS

ROBERT D. ROSENBERG, M.D. Professor of Medicine, Harvard Medical School; Professor of Biochemistry, Department of Biology, Massachusetts Institute of Technology; Physician, Beth Israel Hospital; Physician, Dana-Farber Cancer Institute, Boston, Massachusetts
Physiology of Coagulation: The Fluid Phase

JANET D. ROWLEY, M.D. Professor, Department of Medicine, University of Chicago School of Medicine, Chicago, Illinois
Chromosomal Abnormalities in Childhood Tumors

STEPHEN E. SALLAN, M.D. Associate Professor of Pediatrics, Harvard Medical School; Clinical Director of Jimmy Fund Clinic, Dana-Farber Cancer Institute, Boston, Massachusetts
Childhood Acute Leukemia

ALAN D. SCHREIBER, M.D. Professor of Medicine, University of Pennsylvania School of Medicine; Professor of Medicine, Hospital of the University of Pennsylvania, Philadelphia, Pennsylvania
Autoimmune Hemolytic Anemia

JERROLD F. SCHWABER, M.D. Assistant Professor, Department of Pathology, Harvard Medical School; Researcher, Division of Immunology/Cell Biology, The Children's Hospital, Boston, Massachusetts
Immunoglobulin and T Cell Receptor Genes in Human Immunodeficiency and Neoplasia

JAMES A. STOCKMAN III, M.D. Professor and Chairman, Department of Pediatrics, Northwestern University Medical School; Physician-in-Chief and Chairman, Department of Medicine, Children's Memorial Hospital, Chicago, Illinois
Hematologic Manifestations of Systemic Diseases

THOMAS P. STOSSEL, M.D., Professor of Medicine, Harvard Medical School; Chief, Hematology-Oncology Unit, Massachusetts General Hospital, Boston, Massachusetts
The Phagocyte System: Structure and Function

MARIE J. STUART, M.D. Professor of Pediatrics and Research Professor in Obstetrics-Gynecology, State University of New York Health Science Center; Director, Division of Pediatric Hematology-Oncology, and Attending Physician, State University of New York Health Science Center, Syracuse, New York
The Platelet: Quantitative and Qualitative Abnormalities

JOHN L. SULLIVAN, M.D. Professor of Pediatrics, University of Massachusetts Medical School; Attending Pediatrician, University of Massachusetts Medical Center, Boston, Massachusetts
Lymphohistiocytic Disorders

NANCY J. TARBELL, M.D. Assistant Professor, Harvard Medical School; Chief, Division of Radiation Therapy, The Children's Hospital; Staff Physician, Joint Center for Radiation Therapy, Boston, Massachusetts
Radiation Therapy

HOWARD J. WEINSTEIN, M.D.   Associate Professor of Pediatrics, Harvard Medical School; Director, Bone Marrow Transplant Service, The Children's Hospital, Boston, Massachusetts
Childhood Acute Leukemia

PETER F. WHITINGTON, M.D.   Associate Professor of Pediatrics, University of Chicago Pritzker School of Medicine; Director, Section of Gastroenterology and Hepatology, Wyler Children's Hospital, Chicago, Illinois
Disorders of Bilirubin Metabolism

BRUCE A. WODA, M.D.   Associate Professor of Pathology, University of Massachusetts Medical School; Attending Pathologist, University of Massachusetts Medical Center, Boston, Massachusetts
Lymphohistiocytic Disorders

LAWRENCE C. WOLFE, M.D.   Assistant Professor of Pediatrics, Tufts University School of Medicine; Chief, Division of Pediatric Hematology-Oncology, Boston Floating Hospital, New England Medical Center, Boston, Massachusetts
The Thalassemias

EDMOND J. YUNIS, M.D.   Professor of Pathology, Harvard Medical School; Chief, Division of Immunogenetics, Dana-Farber Cancer Institute, Boston, Massachusetts
The HLA System

ALVIN ZIPURSKY, M.D., F.R.C.P.(C)   Professor of Pediatrics, University of Toronto; Chief, Division of Hematology/Oncology, Hospital for Sick Children, Toronto, Ontario, Canada
Isoimmune Hemolytic Diseases

WOLF W. ZUELZER, M.D.   Emeritus Professor of Pediatric Research, Wayne State University School of Medicine, Detroit, Michigan; Emeritus Director of Laboratories and Hematologist-in-Chief, Children's Hospital of Michigan; Emeritus Director, Division of Blood Diseases and Resources, National Heart, Lung and Blood Institute, NIH, Bethesda, Maryland
Pediatric Hematology in Historical Perspective

PREFACE

This is the third edition of our determined effort to encompass the hematology and oncology of infancy and childhood in a multi-authored textbook essential both for those whose careers are devoted to this exciting field and, as a reference, for those who need relevant data from time to time.

When we began this effort two editions ago, we knew that the task would be monumental. Fortunately for us, our colleagues, and above all, our patients, this field has been a leading beneficiary of new knowledge in cell and molecular biology. The rapid growth in our understanding of biologic processes has created a marvelous array of new information that has been rapidly applied to extend our knowledge of the pathophysiology and treatment of blood diseases and tumors in children. However, this new information has been expressed in a flood of papers that have rendered our previous efforts almost entirely obsolete. Complete revision was required to develop a second edition of our text. This third edition barely resembles the second, with the exception that the chapter titles and their order have been generally retained.

It is difficult for us to express how exciting our careers in pediatric hematology and oncology have been. We initiated our training just as biochemistry and early aspects of membrane biology were beginning to influence the field. Today, we can transplant marrow, consider gene insertion and conduct prenatal diagnoses at the DNA level. The management of pediatric cancer, once a nightmare, has been revolutionized. The critical coagulation factors have been cloned and sequenced. Their interactions with one another are rapidly becoming understood at the molecular level. Therapy with recombinant and, hence, virus-free materials will be with us shortly on a large scale. The growth factors that regulate hematopoiesis have been cloned and produced in large amounts. Preclinical trials are already in progress.

We are grateful for the opportunity to have been able to be part of this remarkable and exciting explosion in a field to which we have devoted so much of our effort. We feel very fortunate to have been permitted the opportunity to enter the field in the beginning and to be participants in a medical revolution. We hope that those who use this book will find the facts that we and our co-authors have tried to assemble both useful and exciting. Above all, we hope that some of our readers will add to the body of knowledge in this field. Indeed, it is our students and fellows to whom this edition is fondly dedicated.

Again, we wish to express our deep thanks to our colleagues who have labored to produce the chapters set out here. It is terribly difficult to summarize this rapidly changing field with the clarity that has characterized their efforts. Where we have cavilled and criticized, deleted or adumbrated, our intent has been honorable, if sometimes irritating. We thank them for their patience and diligence.

We particularly thank Mr. Michael Banchy, without whose administrative help and editing these chapters could never have been assembled.

Again, we appreciate our editors at W. B. Saunders Company. They have been tolerant but firm and have guided this gigantic task to fruition.

As in previous editions, we wish to thank our own teachers: Louis K.

Diamond, Lewis A. Barness, Nathaniel I. Berlin, Frank H. Gardner, William B. Castle, and the late Charles A. Janeway. The quality of this book is a tribute to them.

DAVID G. NATHAN, M.D.
FRANK A. OSKI, M.D.

CONTENTS

VOLUME I

HISTORY

Chapter 1
PEDIATRIC HEMATOLOGY IN HISTORICAL PERSPECTIVE 1
Wolf W. Zuelzer

NEONATAL HEMATOLOGY

Chapter 2
THE ERYTHROCYTE AND ITS DISORDERS 16
Frank A. Oski

Chapter 3
ISOIMMUNE HEMOLYTIC DISEASES 44
Alvin Zipursky

Chapter 4
DISORDERS OF BILIRUBIN METABOLISM 74
Lawrence M. Gartner

Chapter 5
HEMORRHAGIC DISEASES 104
George R. Buchanan

BONE MARROW FAILURE

Chapter 6
THE ANATOMY AND PHYSIOLOGY OF HEMATOPOIESIS 128
Jeffrey M. Lipton ■ David G. Nathan

Chapter 7
THE BONE MARROW FAILURE SYNDROMES 159
Blanche P. Alter

Chapter 8
BONE MARROW TRANSPLANTATION 242
Joel M. Rappeport

DISORDERS OF ERYTHROCYTE PRODUCTION

Chapter 9
DIFFERENTIAL DIAGNOSIS OF ANEMIA 265
Frank A. Oski

Chapter 10
IRON DEFICIENCY AND RELATED NUTRITIONAL ANEMIAS ... 274
Peter R. Dallman

Chapter 11
THE MEGALOBLASTIC ANEMIAS: FOLATE DEFICIENCY 315

    I. Introduction to Megaloblastic Anemias 315
        Bernard M. Babior

    II. Clinical, Pathogenetic, and Diagnostic Considerations in Folate
        Deficiency 321
        Philip Lanzkowsky

Chapter 12
THE MEGALOBLASTIC ANEMIAS: VITAMIN B_{12} (COBALAMIN) DEFICIENCY AND OTHER CONGENITAL AND ACQUIRED DISORDERS 339

    I. Biochemistry of Vitamin B_{12} (Cobalamin) 339
        Bernard M. Babior

    II. Clinical, Pathogenetic, and Diagnostic Considerations of
        Vitamin B_{12} (Cobalamin) Deficiency and Other Congenital and
        Acquired Disorders 344
        Philip Lanzkowsky

Chapter 13
DISORDERS OF HEME METABOLISM: SIDEROBLASTIC ANEMIA AND THE PORPHYRIAS 363
Stephen H. Robinson ■ Jonathan Glass

Chapter 14
LEAD POISONING 389
Sergio Piomelli

HEMOLYTIC ANEMIAS

Chapter 15
AUTOIMMUNE HEMOLYTIC ANEMIA 413
Alan D. Schreiber ■ Frances M. Gill

Chapter 16
THE DESTRUCTION OF RED CELLS BY THE VASCULATURE AND RETICULOENDOTHELIAL SYSTEM 427
John G. Kelton ■ Michael C. Brain

Chapter 17
DISORDERS OF THE RED CELL MEMBRANE 443
Samuel E. Lux

Chapter 18
PYRUVATE KINASE DEFICIENCY AND DISORDERS OF
GLYCOLYSIS 545
William C. Mentzer, Jr.

Chapter 19
G6PD DEFICIENCY AND RELATED DISORDERS OF THE
PENTOSE PATHWAY 583
Sergio Piomelli

DISORDERS OF HEMOGLOBIN

Chapter 20
HUMAN HEMOGLOBINS: NORMAL AND ABNORMAL 613
H. Franklin Bunn

Chapter 21
METHEMOGLOBINEMIA 641
Stephen A. Feig

Chapter 22
SICKLE CELL DISEASE 655
Orah S. Platt ■ David G. Nathan

Chapter 23
THE THALASSEMIAS 699
Arthur W. Nienhuis ■ Lawrence C. Wolfe

THE PHAGOCYTE SYSTEM

Chapter 24
THE PHAGOCYTE SYSTEM: STRUCTURE AND FUNCTION 779
Thomas P. Stossel

Chapter 25
DISORDERS OF GRANULOPOIESIS AND GRANULOCYTE
FUNCTION 797
John T. Curnutte ■ Laurence A. Boxer

VOLUME II

THE IMMUNE SYSTEM

Chapter 26
T CELL CONTROL OF THE IMMUNE RESPONSE 848
Raif S. Geha

Chapter 27
IMMUNOGLOBULIN AND T CELL RECEPTOR GENES IN HUMAN IMMUNODEFICIENCY AND NEOPLASIA 860
Stanley J. Korsmeyer ■ Jerrold F. Schwaber

Chapter 28
PRIMARY IMMUNODEFICIENCIES AND SERUM COMPLEMENT DEFECTS 878
Fred S. Rosen ■ Harvey R. Colten

Chapter 29
THE SPLEEN AND DISTURBANCES OF SPLENIC FUNCTION 900
Howard A. Pearson

ONCOLOGY

Chapter 30
EPIDEMIOLOGY OF CANCER IN CHILDHOOD 918
Frederick P. Li ■ Judith L. Bader

Chapter 31
ONCOGENES AND THE MOLECULAR BIOLOGY OF CANCER 942
Shelly C. Bernstein

Chapter 32
CANCER CHEMOTHERAPY AND RADIATION THERAPY 981
  I. Cancer Chemotherapy 981
     Herbert T. Abelson
  II. Radiation Therapy 1019
     Nancy J. Tarbell ■ J. Robert Cassady

Chapter 33
CHILDHOOD ACUTE LEUKEMIA 1028
Stephen E. Sallan ■ Howard J. Weinstein

Chapter 34
CHRONIC MYELOPROLIFERATIVE DISORDERS AND MYELODYSPLASIA 1064
Holcombe E. Grier

Chapter 35
THE LYMPHOMAS AND LYMPHADENOPATHY 1086
Sharon B. Murphy

Chapter 36
LYMPHOHISTIOCYTIC DISORDERS 1118
John L. Sullivan ■ Bruce A. Woda

Chapter 37
MANAGEMENT OF MALIGNANT SOLID TUMORS 1136
Arnold J. Altman

STORAGE DISEASE

Chapter 38
STORAGE DISEASES OF THE RETICULOENDOTHELIAL
SYSTEM 1212
Edwin H. Kolodny ■ Rose-Mary Boustany

COAGULATION

Chapter 39
PHYSIOLOGY OF COAGULATION: THE FLUID PHASE 1248
Robert D. Rosenberg

Chapter 40
PHYSIOLOGY OF COAGULATION: THE PLATELET 1271
Robert I. Handin

Chapter 41
DISEASES OF COAGULATION: THE FLUID PHASE 1293
Jeanne M. Lusher

Chapter 42
THE PLATELET: QUANTITATIVE AND QUALITATIVE
ABNORMALITIES 1343
Marie J. Stuart ■ John G. Kelton

    I. Quantitative Abnormalities 1344
    II. Qualitative Abnormalities 1429

GENETICS

Chapter 43
CHROMOSOMAL ABNORMALITIES IN CHILDHOOD
TUMORS 1479
Janet D. Rowley

Chapter 44
ERYTHROCYTE BLOOD GROUPS IN HUMANS 1497
W. Laurence Marsh

Chapter 45
THE HLA SYSTEM 1522
Edmond J. Yunis ■ Bo Dupont

Chapter 46
SERUM PROTEINS AND OTHER GENETIC MARKERS OF
THE BLOOD 1550
Chester A. Alper ■ David G. Nathan

TRANSFUSION THERAPY

Chapter 47
RED CELL TRANSFUSION 1580
Martin T. Fosburg ■ *Sherwin V. Kevy*

Chapter 48
PLATELET TRANSFUSION 1588
Ritchard G. Cable

Chapter 49
GRANULOCYTE TRANSFUSION 1598
Thomas J. Ervin

Chapter 50
COAGULATION FACTORS 1606
George R. Buchanan

Chapter 51
THERAPEUTIC PLASMA EXCHANGE AND CYTAPHERESIS 1622
Martin T. Fosburg

HEMATOLOGIC MANIFESTATIONS OF SYSTEMIC DISEASES

Chapter 52
HEMATOLOGIC MANIFESTATIONS OF SYSTEMIC DISEASES ... 1632
James A. Stockman III

Appendix
REFERENCE VALUES IN INFANCY AND CHILDHOOD 1677
Bertram H. Lubin

GLOSSARY OF ABBREVIATIONS AND SYMBOLS i

INDEX ix

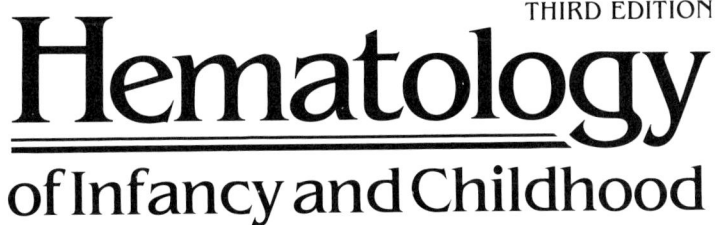

THIRD EDITION
Hematology
of Infancy and Childhood

THE IMMUNE SYSTEM

CHAPTER 26
T Cell Control of the Immune Response

RAIF S. GEHA

INTRODUCTION 848
ACTIVATION OF HELPER AND SUPPRESSOR CELLS 849
T CELL REGULATION OF B CELL ACTIVATION 851
T Cell Control of Polyclonal Immunoglobulin Synthesis
Isotype-Specific Regulation by T Cells
Antigen-Specific Regulation by T Cells
T CELL REGULATION OF OTHER IMMUNE CELLS 855
T CELL ACTIVATION BY B CELLS PRESENTING ANTIGEN 855
T CELL CONTROL OF MONOCYTE/MACROPHAGE FUNCTION 856
T CELL INTERACTION WITH NONIMMUNE CELLS 856
CONCLUSION 857

INTRODUCTION

Thymus-derived (T) lymphocytes play a key role in the control of the immune response. For the sake of clarity, this response will be divided into three phases (Fig. 26–1). These are the induction phase, the regulatory phase, and the effector phase. In the induction phase, antigen-specific T cells encounter antigen presented by accessory cells (macrophages). The recognition of antigen by T cells via their receptor leads to T cell activation. Depending on the conditions of antigen presentation, helper T cells or suppressor cells are activated. The immunoregulatory effect of T cells represents the net effect of helper and suppressor T cells. The effector phase of the immune response arises from the interaction of regulatory T cells with effector cells.

Effector cells that respond to T cell signals comprise both immune and nonimmune cells. They include both effector T cells, such as those that mediate cytotoxicity to foreign targets or vi-

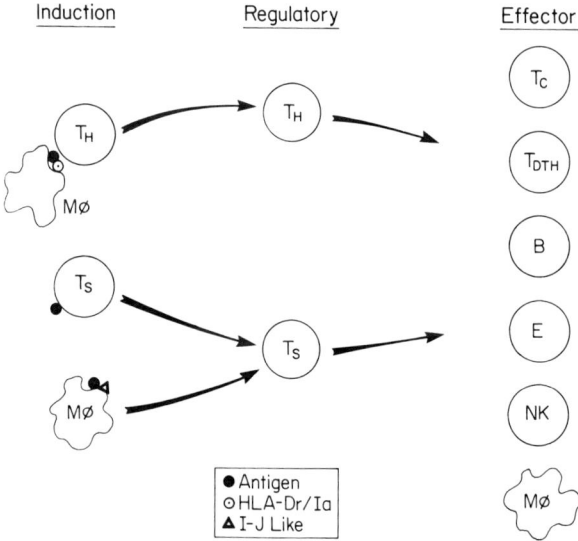

Figure 26–1. The three phases of the immune response. In the induction phase, helper T cells encounter antigen presented in the context of Ia region products by monocytes/macrophages, whereas suppressor T cells can be activated by antigen presented in the context of I-J region products or possibly by soluble antigens. In the regulatory phase helper and suppressor cells exert opposing influences on the activation of effector cells. In the effector phase, the activation and differentiation of cytotoxic T cells (T_c), T cells of delayed hypersensitivity (TDr_4), B cells (B), and nonimmune cells (red cells, precursors [E], fibroblasts, NK cells, and macrophages [Mø]) are governed by helper and suppressor cell signals.

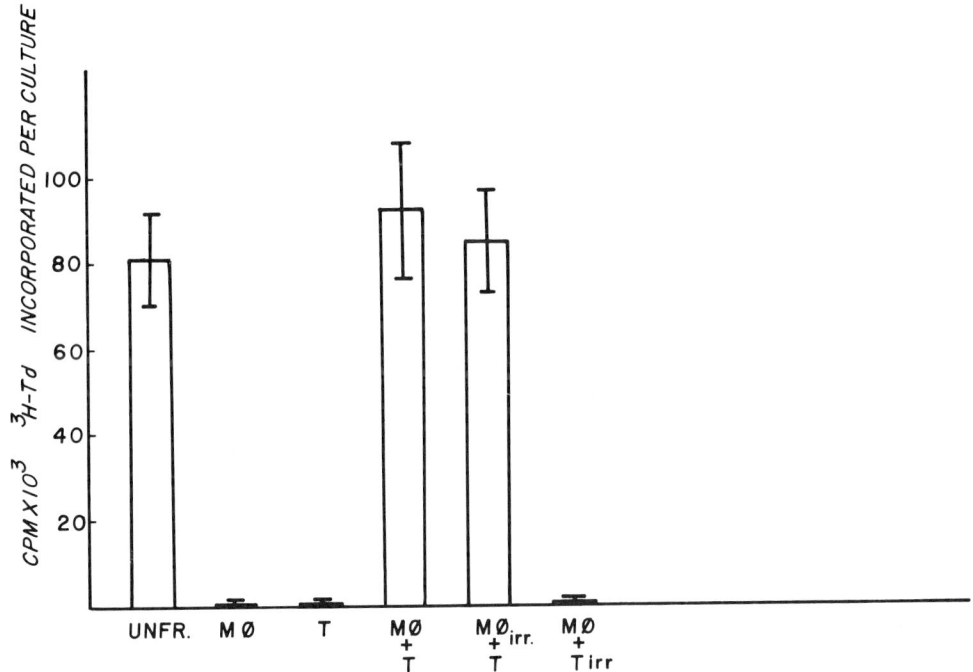

Figure 26–2. Accessory cell dependence of T cell activation. The proliferative response of peripheral blood mononuclear cells to the soluble antigen tetanus toxoid is shown as counts per minute (cpm) of ^{3}H thymidine incorporated into the DNA of 1×10^6 cultured cells. Nonirradiated T cell proliferation occurs only in the presence of added autologous monocytes, the accessory function of which is radioresistant.

rally infected targets, and B cells. They also include hematopoietic cells, such as monocytes, red cell precursors, mesenchymal cells, such as fibroblasts, endothelial cells, and others. The effect of regulatory T cells on an effector cell can be delivered directly to that cell (e.g., T cell to B cell signaling) or via another cell (e.g., T cell signaling to monocytes, which then release a product, such as interleukin 1 or prostaglandin, which in turn affects the function of effector cells, such as B cells or fibroblasts, and hepatic cell protein synthesis). Regulatory T cell–derived signals may require cell-to-cell contact or may be transduced via soluble mediators termed "lymphokines." These signals may be nonspecific, exerting their effect on neighboring effector cells without regard to the antigen specificity of the effector cells. Alternatively, the signals delivered by the regulatory T cells may be antigen-specific, exerting their effect on effector cells that bear receptors specific for the antigen recognized by the T cells. In this case, antigen may act as a bridge between regulatory T cells and effector cells (e.g., B cells).

Our understanding of T cell participation in the immune response has been greatly facilitated by two technical advances. The first is the technique of T cell cloning, which allows the isolation and propagation of monoclonal populations of T cells. The second consists of the application of molecular biology techniques to the study of T cell products, including the T cell receptor and T cell lymphokines, and the subsequent availability of these products in quantities sufficient to permit study of their physicochemical structure and their mode of action.

ACTIVATION OF HELPER AND SUPPRESSOR CELLS

T cell activation is a complex process. We will discuss the activation of helper T cells as prototype. Unlike the immunoglobulin receptor of B cells and B cell–derived serum antibody, the antigen receptor of T cells does not recognize free antigen (1). The T cell recognizes antigen only when this antigen is presented on the surface of an accessory cell, such as the monocyte/macrophage, in association with products of the major histocompatibility complex (MHC) region (Fig. 26–2). The antigenic moiety recognized by T cells is the product of "processing" of the native antigen by the accessory cells (2). This processing is an energy-dependent process that involves internalization of the antigen into lysosomes, partial digestion of the antigen (resulting in unfolding of its three-dimensional structure), and exposure of peptide sequences not usually recognized by serum antibody. The resulting antigen fragments are re-expressed on the monocyte/macrophage surface and are recognized by the helper T cells in association with self HLA-D region products, or Ia antigens (3). These Ia determinants may be the products of the HLA-DP, HLA-DQ, or HLA-DS subregions of the human HLA-D region (4). Addition of anti-Ia antibodies to cultures containing monocytes, T cells, and antigen completely inhibit recognition of antigen by T cells and the subsequent activation and proliferation of the T cells (5). Association between antigen and Ia on the accessory cell membrane is not due to a covalent link between the two moieties (6). It is not clear whether T cells use two receptors, one that binds to the antigen fragment and another that binds to self Ia (dual receptor model), or whether T cells use a single receptor to bind to a specific configuration of self Ia plus antigen (single receptor model). The T cell receptor consists of two chains, alpha and beta, which are expressed as a heterodimer on the cell surface in close linkage with the T3 molecule (7). Antibodies to T3, as well as antibodies to the T cell receptor, activate T cells and cause internalization of both T3 and the T cell receptor (8). Each of the two chains of the T cell receptor consists of a variable portion and of a constant portion (9). Recently, a third gene product, the gamma chain, has been shown to be rearranged and expressed in T cells that are usually of the suppressor or cytotoxic but rarely helper phenotype (10). Thus, there is clearly room for a dual recognition process in which one of the chains recognizes antigen and the other chain recognizes self Ia molecules. The binding of helper T cells to antigen on the accessory cell surface results in intimate contact between the two cells, evidenced in tissue cultures as cluster formation (11). This sets the stage for activation of the T cell.

T cell activation depends on two signals (Fig. 26–3). This results in opening of calcium channels in the cell membrane (13). The first signal is delivered by crosslinking of the T cell receptor for antigen and is associated with activation of the T cell membrane–associated enzyme, phosphokinase C. The second signal is provided by T cell monocyte contact and possibly involves the monocyte product termed "interleukin 1" (IL-1) (12). Monocyte-derived IL-1 is made from a 33,000-MW precursor, is secreted as a 15,000-MW peptide, and has several activities besides T cell activation. It is a pyrogen, it induces the synthesis of acute-phase reactants in liver cells, and it enhances collagen synthesis, cell division, and hematopoietic growth factor production in fibroblasts (14). Substances related to IL-1 are secreted by cells other than monocytes (e.g., keratinocytes and some B cell lines) (15). This could permit these cells to participate in T cell activation in vivo. T cells, whose receptors are crosslinked by antigen, are induced to express receptors with high affinity for interleukin 2 (IL-2) and also to synthesize IL-2 (16–18). Synthesis of IL-2 appears to require actual cell-to-cell contact between monocytes and T cells (19). Following the interaction of IL-2 (MW, 18,000) with its receptor, the T cell engages in cell division, in the secretion of a number of soluble lymphokines, e.g., gamma interferon, B cell growth factors, and interleukin 3, all of which are important in the regulation of the activity of immune and nonimmune cells, as will be discussed.

The importance of T cell–macrophage interaction in the development of the immune response is illustrated by diseases in which these interactions are deficient. Children with the bare lymphocyte syndrome fail to express HLA antigens on their cells (20). Consequently, they cannot generate effective T cell–macrophage interactions and they are severely immunodeficient. A patient with defective T cell response to IL-1 has been described (21). His T cells bound IL-1 poorly and failed to proliferate or secrete IL-2 in response to antigens

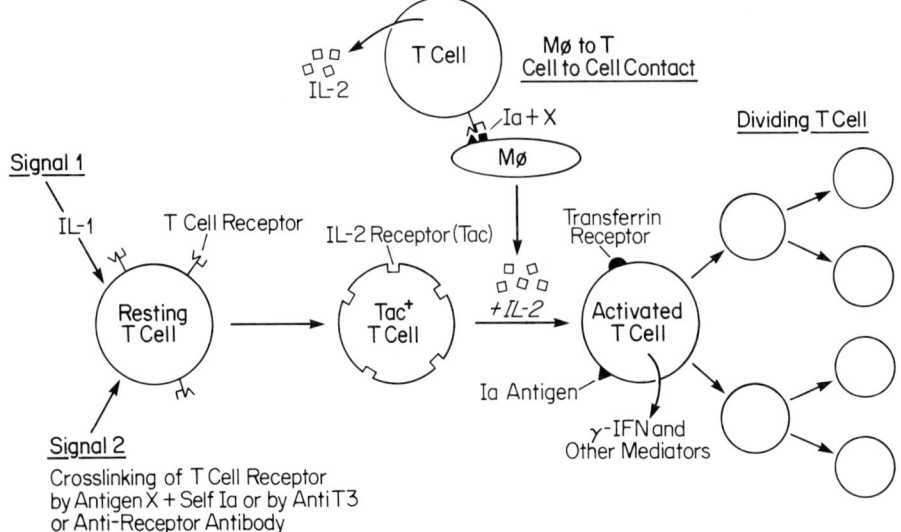

Figure 26–3. Steps involved in helper T cell activation. Resting T cells that receive two signals, IL-1 and crosslinking of their receptors, are induced to express IL-2 receptors identified as the Tac antigen. Cell-to-cell contact with antigen-presenting accessory cell is followed by IL-2 synthesis. Interaction of IL-2 with its receptor (Tac) induces T cells to express other activation antigens, to secrete soluble mediators (e.g., gamma interferon), and to divide.

and mitogens. Failure to secrete IL-2 was corrected by bypassing the IL-1 signal via the use of phorbol esters, which directly activate the membrane-associated phosphokinase C enzyme (22).

Little is known about the activation of suppressor T cells in humans. There is evidence from classic functional experiments that some suppressor T cells may recognize soluble antigen directly in the absence of monocytes or in the context of products of the J subregion of the immune response genes (23, 24). A number of murine suppressor T cell clones have been shown to have deleted their beta chain but rearranged their alpha and gamma chains (10). Bensussan and colleagues found that, unlike the case of helper T cells, crosslinking of the antigen receptors of suppressor T cell clones by antibody did not result in T cell activation as measured by expression of IL-2 receptors or synthesis of IL-2 (25). In fact it resulted in transient unresponsiveness to IL-2 by these clones. At present, the receptors and the triggering mechanisms of antigen-specific suppressor cells remain unclear.

T CELL REGULATION OF B CELL ACTIVATION

The regulation of the B cell antibody response by T cells will be discussed in detail so that the T cell regulatory influences exerted on the generation of the immune response can be illustrated. The capacity to activate B cells in vitro has been instrumental in the dissection of the activation mechanisms of normal B cells, T cell control of B cell activation, and abnormalities of antibody production. Assays that activate polyclonal and/or antigen-specific antibody synthesis by B cells in vitro have been developed. The most commonly used assays are described subsequently.

1. Pokeweed mitogen activation of B cell immunoglobulin synthesis is commonly used in vitro assay for B cell function. It depends on the production of soluble factors following PWM activation of T cells (26). These factors act on large B cells that have already been triggered by antigen or other in vivo factors to enlarge and express receptors of T cell factors (27). Thus, PWM activation is a T cell–dependent assay of the function of B cells that have already been preactivated in vivo.

2. In contrast to PWM, Epstein-Barr (EB) virus is a T cell–independent activator that activates both small resting B cells and large B cells that have been preactivated in vivo (28). EB virus activation of B cells is a T cell–independent measure of B cell function that reflects the intrinsic potential of antibody-producing B cells.

3. T cell clones with specificity for Ia antigens expressed by B cells have been used to activate B cells in vitro. These clones provide the most potent means of B cell activation because they cause the highest frequency of both small and large B cells to engage in antibody synthesis (29). With these clones, it is possible to induce substantial antibody synthesis in B cells that circulate in limited frequency, such as those B cells that make IgE or antigen-specific antibody (30).

4. Antigen in very small doses can induce T cell-dependent, antigen-specific antibody synthesis in vitro by cultured lymphocytes. This occurs in the absence of significant polyclonal immunoglobulin synthesis (31).

In vitro studies suggest that B cell activation to antibody secretion proceeds through a series of orderly steps, many of which are governed by T cells or their products (32). Figure 26–4 summarizes the steps involved. Crosslinking of the surface immunoglobulin receptors on the B cell surface by multivalent antigen or $F(ab')_2$ fragments of anti-immunoglobulin causes the B cell to enlarge, to move into the S phase of the cell cycle, and to express receptors for the T cell–derived B cell growth factor(s) (BCGF) (33). Interaction of BCGF with its receptor causes the B cells to divide and to express increased amounts of receptors for T cell–derived B cell differentiation factors (BCDF) (34). Upon interaction with BCDF, the B cell differentiates into an antibody-secreting cell.

Under normal circumstances, the progression of a B cell from the resting state to an antibody-secreting plasma cell is T cell–dependent. Thus, patients with severe combined immune deficiency who have normal numbers of B cells are unable to make antibody in the absence of functional T cells (35). T cell regulation of B cell activation can be exerted at three levels:

1. Polyclonal immunoglobulin synthesis
2. Isotype-specific immunoglobulin synthesis
3. Antigen-specific immunoglobulin synthesis

We will discuss the role of regulatory T cells in health and disease within each of these levels.

T Cell Control of Polyclonal Immunoglobulin Synthesis

The opposing influences of helper and suppressor T cells on polyclonal immunoglobulin synthesis are amenable to dissection with the PWM-driven system of B cell activation. In this system, T4 cells are the predominant source of help, whereas T8 cells exert suppressor influences on Ig synthesis (36). The T4-positive population represents 60 per cent of the total T cells. Within the T4 population, a subpopulation (25 per cent of T4 cells) that lacks the antigenic marker TQ1 accounts for the majority of T cell help in the PWM-driven system (37). Activation of T8 cells into suppression depends on a subset of T4 cells that appear to be

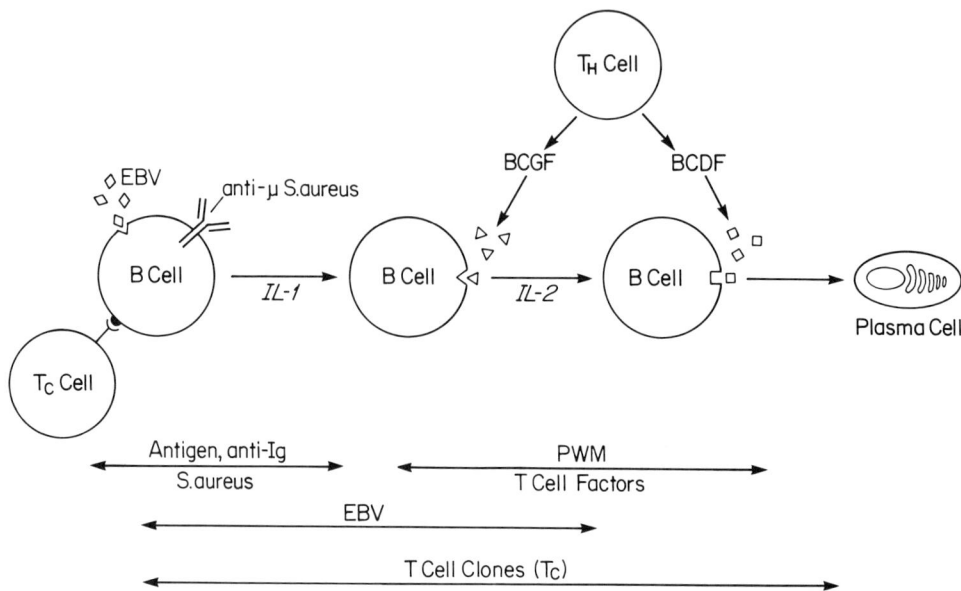

Figure 26–4. B cell activation. Small B cells are activated to enlarge and enter the G1 phase after crosslinking of their receptors by antigen, antireceptor antibodies (anti-Ig), or ligands such as the A protein of *Staphylococcus aureus*. These activated B cells express receptors for T cell–derived B cell growth factor (BCGF), which induce proliferation of the B cells. Proliferating B cells express receptors for T cell–derived B cell differentiation factors (BCDF), which drive terminal differentiation of the B cells into a plasma cell. Some of the BCDFs are isotype-specific. T cell clones that recognize Ia determinants or Ia plus antigen on the B cell surface provide all the signals necessary for the resting B cells to proliferate and to differentiate into an antibody producing cell. Epstein-Barr virus (EBV) triggers both small resting B cells and preactivated large B cells to divide and to secrete antibody. EBV-infected B cells express BCGF receptors and make their own BCGF. This autocrine pathway allows perpetual B cell proliferation. Pokeweed mitogen (PWM) induces T cells to produce soluble factors (BCDF and BCGF), which selectively cause preactivated large B cells to proliferate and to differentiate.

deficient in children with juvenile rheumatoid arthritis (JRA). These children make an autoantibody to the JRA-positive cells, which are the inducers of suppressor cells (38). Within the T8 population, suppression of Ig synthesis is mediated by cells that lack the Leu 9.3 antigen, whereas cytotoxicity is exerted by T8 (Leu 2–positive or Leu 9.3–positive) cells (39, 40). In addition to the suppressor effect exerted by T8$^+$ cells, non–T cells that express the T8 antigen but not the T3 antigen and that express markers characteristic of natural killer cells (e.g., Leu 7 and Leu 11) exert suppressor influence on B cell activation.

Simple enumeration of T4 and T8 cells does not reflect the potential helper and suppressor activity of these populations. As already discussed, there is a great deal of heterogeneity within T4 cells: One subpopulation of T4 cells is involved in B cell activation; another JRA-positive subpopulation induces suppressor T cells. Cells can be divided into those that exhibit high-density T8 and those with low-density T8. T8$^+$ cells with high T8 density include suppressor T cells and cytotoxic T cells, whereas cells with low T8 density are mostly T3-negative and represent natural killer cells and often carry the Leu 11–positive surface markers of NK cells (41). Even within a subset of T4 or T8 cells, simple enumeration does not assess the functional potential of this population.

DISORDERS OF T CELL REGULATION OF B CELL FUNCTION LEADING TO ABNORMAL POLYCLONAL IMMUNOGLOBULIN PRODUCTION

The importance of T cells in the regulation of B cell activation is illustrated in diseases in which abnormalities in immunoglobulin production are underlined by imbalances in immunoregulatory T cells. We will discuss four diseases as prototypes in which polyclonal immunoglobulin production is deranged subsequent to a derangement in immunoregulatory T cells. These diseases are listed in Table 26–1.

Transient hypogammaglobulinemia of infancy (THI) is a disease that manifests as recurrent infections, mainly respiratory, starting at 6 months of age and resolving at around 4 years of age. The hypogammaglobulinemia occurs in the face of normal numbers of B cells that are intrinsically normal because they produce normal amounts of immunoglobulins in vitro following stimulation with EB virus. The helper function of T cells in a PWM-driven system of immunoglobulin production is diminished because the patient's T cells do not support normal immunoglobulin production by normal B cells (42). This is not caused by excess suppressor T cell activity because addition of the patient's T cells to normal mixtures of T and B cells does not interfere with Ig production. The defective T cell help in THI is associated with a decreased number of circulating T4 cells. Both numerical and functional T cell abnormalities spontaneously reverse at the time of the resolution of the clinical manifestations of the disease and with the return of serum immunoglobulin levels to normal.

Failure to generate adequate T cell help, as evidenced by failure of T4 cells to express the Ia activation marker and to release soluble helper factor(s) following antigenic stimulation, has been implicated in the pathogenesis of some cases of *common variable acquired agammaglobulinemia* (43). Decreased numbers and function of helper T4 cells are observed in patients with AIDS (44) and underlie the failure of these patients to mount an effective antibody response to newly encountered antigens. This contrasts with their hypergammaglobulinemia, which may be explained by the expansion of their memory B cells by the virus HTLV-III, which is capable of infecting T4 cells (45) as well as a subset of B cells (46). This results in extremely high antibody titers to antigens that have been encountered previously by the AIDS patients and that commonly include cytomegalovirus and EB virus antigens (46).

Excessive T cell help and evidence of circulating activated T cells underlie the polyclonal B cell activation of *Kawasaki's disease*. This febrile illness is characterized by enlarged lymph nodes, inflammation of mucous membranes, and skin rash and is associated with intense polyclonal activation of B cells. As many as one third of circulating B cells have been found to be engaged in the spontaneous secretion of immunoglobulin (47). Circulating T cells express activation antigens such as the Ia antigen and spontaneously secrete B cell growth and differentiation factors that cause normal B cells to proliferate and to secrete immunoglobulins (48). The cause of the T cell activation is unknown, but the subsequent B cell activation involves the production of autoantibodies to targets such as endothelial cells, perhaps resulting in arterial wall damage with subsequent thrombus formation, which is a feature of this disease.

Increased suppressor T cell activity underlies the antibody deficiency in some cases of *common variable agammaglobulinemia (CVA)* and of *chronic graft-versus-host disease (CGVHD)*. Some CVA and CGVHD patients have an increase in suppressor T cell number or activity or both (49, 50), which, in the face of intrinsically normal B cells, is presumed to play a primary role in the antibody deficiency of these patients (52). Several patients with CVA, however, have increased suppressor T cell activity in addition to intrinsically abnormal B cells (51). In these cases, the increased suppressor T cell activity may be secondary to the recurrent infections and repetitive antigenic stimulation these patients are subjected to. In chickens rendered B cell–deficient and agammaglobulinemic by neonatal bursectomy, suppressor T cell activity increases as a consequence of the repeated antigenic and infectious stimulation (57). The rise in suppressor T cell activity is, to a large degree, prevented if these chickens are raised in a germ-free environment. The fact that powerful antigenic stimulation can cause an increase in suppressor cell number and activity is also illustrated by the observation that *several systemic viral infections (e.g., infectious mononucleosis, measles)* are associated with a transient increase in the number of circulating $T8^+$ cells, which can suppress both Ig synthesis and activation of helper T cells (53, 54). Clinically, this may contribute to the transient anergy observed in patients with these diseases. It must be noted that the suppressive effect of $T8^+$ cells in these instances may not be exclusively due to T cells, as there is a concomitant increase in T8-positive, T3-negative natural killer (NK) cells in these patients. NK cells are potent inhibitors of immune function (40). The mechanism of this inhibition by NK cells is not entirely clear but may be partly related to the generation of free hydroxyl radicals (55) and to arylsulfatase activity (56).

Decreased suppressor T cell activity has been found in several clinical situations, including *systemic lupus erythematosus, juvenile rheumatoid arthritis (JRA)*, and *severe atopic dermatitis*. In lupus, this could be a secondary event due to the formation of autoantibodies to suppressor T cells (57). Sup-

Table 26–1. PROTOTYPES OF DISEASES WITH GROSS IMMUNOREGULATORY CELL IMBALANCE

Major Immunoregulatory T Cell Defect	Disease	Remarks
Decreased T cell help	Transient hypogammaglobulinemia of infancy	Numerical and functional decrease of T4 helper cells
Increased T cell help	Kawasaki's disease	Increased number of activated Ia+ T4 cells. Increased Ig synthesis.
Decreased T cell suppression	Juvenile rheumatoid arthritis	Decreased T cell suppression associated with autoantibody to suppressor T cells; hypergammaglobulinemia
Increased T cell suppression	Selected cases of common variable agammaglobulinemia and chronic graft-versus-host disease	Increased number and activity of T8 suppressor cells; B cells are normal in number and function

pressor T cell deficiency may secondarily enhance autoantibody formation in SLE. Deficiency of the inducers of suppressor T cells in children with JRA has been discussed (38). In atopic dermatitis, a deficiency of circulating cells with high surface density of T8 antigen (cytotoxic and suppressor T cells) is associated with deficient cytotoxic T cell responses and with selective deficiency in IgE-specific suppressor T cells (58, 59). Interestingly, both the percentage of circulating low-density T8$^+$ cells and NK activity are increased in atopic dermatitis (41).

Isotype-Specific Regulation by T Cells

Some T cells have the capacity to regulate immunoglobulin synthesis in an isotype-specific fashion. Such T cells bear Fc receptors for the immunoglobulin whose synthesis they regulate (60–62). The regulatory effect can be mediated by T cell–derived factors that have affinity for the Fc portion of the specific isotype. These factors may represent the shed form of the T cell receptor. In humans, IgA- and IgE-specific B cell–differentiation factors (BCDF-α and BCDF-ε) have been extensively studied. In the case of IgE, IgE-binding factors that potentiate IgE synthesis are secreted by T4 cells bearing receptors for IgE (63). The IgE binding–enhancing factors need to be glycosylated to exert the enhancing effect (64). In their nonglycosylated form, human IgE-binding factors suppress IgE synthesis and, like rat-derived IgE suppressor factors, may be derived from Fc receptor–positive suppressor T cells. Two observations are worth noting about isotype-specific regulatory T cell–derived factors. First, their synthesis by T cells is enhanced in the presence of the isotype. Thus, IgE enhances the synthesis by T cells of IgE regulatory factors (65). Second, isotype specific T cell factors exert their effect on B cells that bear the isotype in question and that are already engaged in Ig synthesis and secretion (i.e., activated B cells) (63). These factors are generally unable to activate resting B cells. IgE-binding factors can be isolated from human serum, which suggests that they play an in vivo role in isotype-specific regulation (66). Whereas sera of normal subjects contain IgE-suppressive factors, sera from patients with *hyper-IgE states* contain IgE-enhancing factors. The malignant counterpart of IgE-specific helper T cells has been described in a child with a non-Hodgkin's lymphoma and markedly high serum IgE. The lymphoma consisted of T cells that bore receptors for IgE and that secreted IgE binding–enhancing factors (67). This further suggests the in vivo relevance of isotype-specific regulatory T cells in humans.

The role of T cells in isotype switching of B cells is poorly understood. Controversy has surrounded the existence of isotype switch T cells in experimental systems. In humans, it has been demonstrated that a malignant T cell line induces IgG and IgA synthesis in B cells from patients with the hyper-IgM syndrome, which normally make high amounts of IgM but no detectable IgG or IgA (68). Concomitantly with the induction of IgG and IgA synthesis, IgM synthesis is diminished. Cloned T cells directed against Ia antigens expressed by hyper-IgM B cells also cause these cells to make IgG (Umetsu, D., personal communication). Because hyper-IgM B cells bear no detectable surface IgG or IgA, these observations suggest that T cell–directed switching of isotype synthesis many have occurred. It remains to be established via the use of monoclonal B cell populations whether these observations indeed represent the induction of isotype switching by T cells.

Antigen-Specific Regulation by T Cells

Antigen specificity is conferred upon T and B cell interaction via two known mechanisms. First, B cells that bind antigen, in a manner similar to that shown by B cells that bind (Fab′)$_2$ fragments of anti-immunoglobulins, are activated to respond to nonspecific signals derived from the T cells, such as BCGF, BCDF, and isotype-specific BCDFs. Second, B cells that bind antigen can present this antigen in the context of their surface Ia antigens to antigen-specific activated T cells but not to resting T cells (69). Unlike resting T cells, activated T cells do not require IL-1 for their activation and thus can be readily activated by the B cells (70). In the situation of antigen presentation by B cells, T cell–B cell interaction is restricted by Ia antigens of the major histocompatibility complex (MHC). The phenomenon of antigen presentation by B cells provides for antigen specificity and for two-way T cell–B cell interactions. Once a T cell is activated by antigen presented by monocytes, it can interact with antigen-specific B cells. B cells that recognize differing determinants on an antigen molecule can interact in an antigen-specific fashion with a single antigen-specific T cell and vice versa, thus increasing the chances of successful antigen "bridging" between B and T cells.

Induction of antigen-specific antibody synthesis in vitro has been achieved with doses of antigen much lower than those required to achieve measurable T cell proliferation (31). Use of the latter doses result in polyclonal immunoglobulin synthesis, probably because of the large amounts of nonspecific B cell helper factors produced by the T cells. Antigen-specific helper T cells belong to the T4 subset. Antigen specific suppressor T cells have been difficult to identify in humans. Cloned antigen-specific suppressor T cells that fail to express IL-2 receptors and to secrete IL-2 following antigenic stimulation have been reported (25). Exposure of T cells to high doses of antigen has resulted in the generation of antigen-specific suppressor T cells, possibly via the triggering of T8 cells that share determinants with the antigen-binding portion of the B cell immunoglobulins (i.e., idiotypic determinants) and that can bind antigen or anti-idiotype (71). In animals, antigen-binding, idiotype-bearing, I-J–bearing suppressor T cells have been cloned and found to secrete I-J–restricted, antigen–specific, idiotype-positive suppressor factors (72). In humans, autoantiidiotypic antibody arises after immunization with antigen (73). This autoanti-Id may exert part of its inhibitory action on the antibody response via the activation of idiotype-positive T8 suppressor cells. One mechanism by which antigen unrespon siveness arises is seen when T cells encounter the immunogenic moiety of processed antigen in the absence of accessory cells. Thus, clones of influenza antigen–specific helper T cells exposed to high doses of the relevant immunogenic peptides of the influenza hemagglutinin become unresponsive to subsequent antigenic stimulation in the presence of monocytes (74). No suppressor cells are generated under this condition.

Some patients with *chronic mucocutaneous condidiasis* have a deficiency in *Candida* antigen–specific T lymphocyte response, which results in failure to mount cell-mediated antibody responses to *Candida* antigen (75). Antigen-specific suppressor T cells have been implicated in the unresponsiveness of T cells from patients with lepromatous leprosy and with chronic schistosomiasis to specific antigen. Failure of antigen specific T cell–B cell interaction and failure to mount antigen specific antibody response may occur in patients with severe combined immunodeficiency who are engrafted with HLA-mismatched T cells from fetal liver and whose B cells are of recipient origin (76). In haploidentical transplants, T cells restricted in their antigen recognition by nonshared recipient MHC antigens (77) may fail to cooperate with B cells of donor origin, and T cells restricted by nonshared donor MHC antigens may fail to cooperate with B cells of recipient origin in antigen-specific antibody responses (78). Organ-specific autoimmune diseases are associated with evidence of antibodies and cytotoxic T cells directed against self antigens. One reason that this selective breakdown of tolerance to self antigen may occur is that during the course of a viral infection, locally released gamma interferon induces Ia expression by tissues that normally do not express these antigens (79). Thyroid epithelium from patients with autoimmune thyroiditis has been shown to express Ia antigen and to present antigen to helper T cells (80). This antigen presentation would allow helper T cells to interact with the target tissues and provide help for B cells and cytotoxic tissue-specific T cells. It is possible that successful development of autoimmunity also involves the breakdown of suppressor T cells directed to self antigens.

T CELL REGULATION OF OTHER IMMUNE CELLS

Cytotoxic T cells play an important role in the elimination of both virally infected tissue and foreign tissue. Helper T cells and their products, IL-2 and gamma interferon, are essential to the development of cytotoxic T cells from resting precursors. Cells within the T8$^+$ subset constitute the bulk of cytotoxic activity, whereas T4$^+$ cells account for a small portion of cytolytic activity of human T cells (81). Like helper T cells, cytotoxic T cells recognize their targets in association with MHC products, HLA-A or HLA-B in the case of T8 cells and HLA-D in the case of T4 cells (82). The antigenic moiety recognized by cytotoxic T cells is, at least in some instances, similar to that recognized by serum antibody because antibodies to viral proteins can protect virally infected targets from the action of cytotoxic T cells.

Patients with severe atopic dermatitis are clinically susceptible to disseminated infection with diseases such as chickenpox (caused by the herpes zoster virus) and molluscum contagiosum. This may be due in part to the failure of these patients to generate adequate T4$^+$ cell help for the maturation of cytotoxic T8$^+$ cells (59).

Cytotoxic T cells themselves can play a role as immunoregulators when they recognize viral antigens on the surface of other lymphoid cells. Thus, cytotoxic T cells in vitro can kill virally infected B lymphoblasts. Occasionally, agammaglobulinemia with loss of circulating B cells develops after an episode of infectious mononucleosis. In this condition, cytotoxic T cells to EB virus–infected B cells could lead to B cell dysfunction.

T CELL ACTIVATION BY B CELLS PRESENTING ANTIGEN

Since 1980, it has become clear that the interaction of T and B cells is bidirectional. This finding is based on the observation that murine B lymphoma B cells (81) and human Epstein-Barr virus–transformed B cell lines (82) are capable of presenting antigen to T cells in a fashion similar to that demonstrated by monocytes/macrophages. However, activation is restricted to T cells that are already beyond the resting stage, such as antigen-specific T cell blasts and T cell clones. The reason for this is that resting T cells require additional signals, such as interleukin 1 (IL-1), that are not generated by the B cells. Indeed, antibody to IL-1 inhibits the monocyte-dependent activation of resting antigen-specific T cells but not that of cloned T cells. Addition of IL-1 reverses this inability of resting T cells (83). The capacity of B cells to present antigen to T cells is radiation-sensitive, which suggests that B cells need to be activated by T cells or that their products need to be able to process and present antigen. Thus, this bidirectional interaction between T and B cells confers exquisite specificity and sensitivity on antigen-specific interactions; in the presence of limiting amounts of antigen, only those B cells that bear surface Ig receptors for antigen can bind and take up enough antigen to enable them to present it in an immunogenic fashion to the T cells.

T CELL CONTROL OF MONOCYTE/MACROPHAGE FUNCTION

T cells and their products modulate monocyte/macrophage numbers and functions. Interleukin 3 (IL-3), released by activated T cells, enhances the maturation of the precursors of monocytes as other myeloid-derived cells (83). Activated T cells release macrophage migration inhibitory factor, which keeps macrophages in the vicinity of activated T cells. More importantly, gamma interferon released by activated T cells induces increased Ia expression by macrophages (84). The effectiveness of antigen presentation is related to the product of Ia density and antigen concentration. Thus, monocytes/macrophages that express high-density Ia are more effective in triggering T cells at low antigen doses. Other T cell–derived soluble factors activate monocytes to produce more IL-1, which enhances activation of both B and T cells. This enhancing activity of IL-1 is balanced by increased synthesis of prostaglandins, which inhibit T cell activation in part via the activation of suppressor T cells.

T CELL INTERACTION WITH NONIMMUNE CELLS

Until recently, the interaction of T cells with nonimmune cells was thought to be unidirectional. Helper T cells have been shown to influence the maturation of the red cell series as well as that of monocytes, megakaryocytes, and bone marrow–derived mast cells via the production of soluble mediators, including interleukin 3. It has now become evident that the interaction between T cells and nonimmune cells can be bidirectional, thus opening new ways for the amplification of the immune response and for the modulation of the nonimmune cells. Through their secretion of gamma interferon, T cells can induce the expression of Ia antigens on the surface of cells as diverse as fibroblasts, melanocytes, endothelial cells, and astrocytes (85–87). These Ia-positive cells can now serve as accessory antigen–presenting cells and perpetuate T cell activation and the release of T cell lymphokines. In the case of fibroblasts, T cell lymphokines can cause increased cell division and collagen synthesis (Fig. 26–5). Lymphokines can also activate other cells present in tissue, recruit B cells into division and differentiation (as already discussed), cause mast cells to release histamine (88), and cause monocytes to release IL-1 and prostaglandins. It is likely that the multicellular interaction into which T cells engage nonimmune cells plays a role in tissue injury. Thus, the skin of patients with atopic dermatitis is characterized by infiltration with Ia-bearing activated T4 cells, increased numbers of fibroblasts, increased collagen deposition, and activated macrophages. The interaction of T cells with endothelial cells activated by

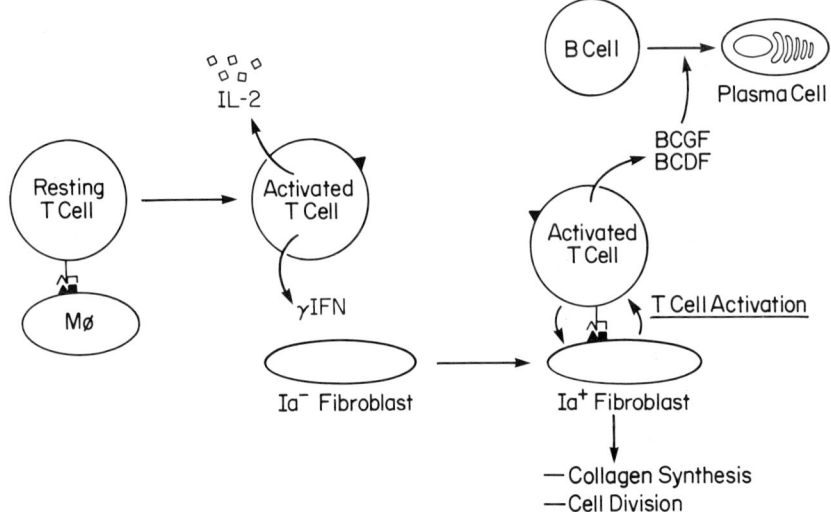

Figure 26–5. Resting T cells are activated by antigen presented by monocytes/macrophages. Activated T cells migrate into tissues. Mediators released by these T cells include factors that induce cell division and collagen synthesis in fibroblasts and gamma interferon (γIFN), which induces fibroblasts to express Ia antigen. Ia$^+$ fibroblasts can perpetuate the activation of the T cells. B cell growth factor (BCGF) and B cell differentiation factor (BCDF), released by in vitro–activated T cells, nonspecifically recruit bystander B cells into antibody synthesis. Other T cell factors cause mast cells to degranulate and release vasoactive mediator. These allow further entry of circulating lymphocytes into tissues.

gamma interferon to express Ia antigen may be important in allowing the egress of activated T cells into privileged tissues, such as the central nervous tissue. Indeed, following such interaction a decrease in size and a change in shape occur in endothelial cells, allowing the opening of intercellular junctions. Activation of T cell in tissues, (e.g., nervous tissue) can be sustained by Ia-expressing activated astrocytes (86). Soluble products of these locally activated T cells can mediate tissue injury.

The list of cell types that respond to gamma interferon by expressing Ia antigen is growing. This increases the number of tissues in which bidirectional interactions between immune and nonimmune T cells can occur, resulting in perpetuation of the inflammatory response and in tissue injury.

CONCLUSION

T cells play a key role in the regulation of the immune response. The principles that govern this regulation are as follows:

1. The activation of helper T cells is accessory T cell–dependent and occurs via the recognition of monocyte/macrophage–processed antigen in the context of Ia region antigens and via the mediation of the soluble monokine IL-1. The requirements for the activation of suppressor cells are not yet well identified.

2. The regulatory action of T cells on B cell functions can be exerted at different levels of specificity (i.e., polyclonal, isotype-specific, and antigen-specific. Each of these is mediated by specialized subsets of T cells.

3. T cells regulate the function of nonimmune cells and cause them, by the secretion of gamma interferon, to express Ia antigens. This results in bidirectional interaction, with nonimmune cells functioning as antigen-presenting cells, thus amplifying the immune response.

4. Understanding of T cell regulation of the immune response is important for the understanding of immune deficiency diseases, autoimmune diseases, and immune function in recipients of bone marrow transplants.

References

1. Benacerraf, B.: A hypothesis to relate the specificity of T lymphocytes and the activity of I region–specific Ir genes in macrophages and B lymphocytes. J. Immunol. *120*:1809, 1978.
2. Broff, M. D., Jonsen, M. E., et al.: Nature of the immunologic moiety recognized by the human T cell proliferating in response to tetanus toxoid antigen. Eur. J. Immunol. *11*:365, 1981.
3. Sørderstrup, H. G., Rubin, B., et al.: Importance of HLA-D antigens for the cooperation between human monocytes and T lymphocytes. Eur. J. Immunol. *8*:520, 1978.
4. Bodmer, J., Bodmer, W.: Histocompatibility. Immunol. Today *5*:251, 1984.
5. Geha, R. S., Milgrom, H. E., et al.: Macrophage T cell interaction in man: a subpopulation of adherent accessory cells bearing DRw antigens is required for antigen-specific human T lymphocytes proliferation. Proc. Natl. Acad. Sci. U.S.A. *76(8)*:4038, 1979.
6. Hedrick, S. M., Germain, R. N., et al.: Rearrangement and transcription of a T-cell receptor B-chain gene in different T-cell subsets. Proc. Natl. Acad. Sci. U.S.A. *82*:531, 1985.
7. Meuer, S. C., Fitzgerald, K. A., et al.: Clonotypic structures involved in antigen specific human T cell functions: relationship to the T3 molecular complex. J. Exp. Med. *157*:705, 1983.
8. Allison, J., Lanier, L.: Membrane structures associated with the murine T cell receptor. J. Cell. Biochem. Suppl. *8A*:180, 1984.
9. Yanagi, Y., Yoshikai, Y., et al.: A human T cell–specific cDNA clone encodes a protein having extensive homology to immunoglobulin chains. Nature (Lond.) *308*:145, 1984.
10. Saito, H., Kranz, D. M., et al.: A third rearranged and expressed gene in a clone of cytotoxic T lymphocytes. Nature *312*:36, 1984.
11. Inaba, K., Witmer, M. D., et al.: Clustering of dendritic cells, helper T lymphocytes, and histocompatible B cells during primary antibody responses in vitro. J. Exp. Med. *160*:858, 1984.
12. Mizel, S. B.: Interleukin 1 and T cell activation. Immunol. Rev. *63*:51, 1982.
13. Lederman, H. M., Lee, J. W. W., et al.: Monocytes are required to trigger Ca^{2+} uptake in the proliferative response of human T lymphocytes to *Staphylococcus aureus* protein A. Proc. Natl. Acad. Sci. U.S.A. *81*:6827, 1984.
14. Oppenheim, J. J., Stadler, B. M., et al.: Lymphokines: their role in lymphocyte responses: properties of interleukin 1. Fed. Proc. *41*:257, 1982.
15. Chu, E. T., Lareau, M., et al.: Antigen presentation by EBV-B cells to resting and activated T cells: role of interleukin 1. J Immunol *134*:1676, 1985.
16. Henney, C. S., Kuribayashi, K., et al.: Interleukin 2 augments natural killer cell activity. Nature (Lond.) *291*:335, 1981.
17. Uchiyama, T., Broder, S., et al.: A monoclonal antibody (anti-Tac) reactive with activated and functionally mature human T cells. J. Immunol. *126*:1393, 1981.
18. Welte, K., Andreeff, M., et al.: Interleukin 2 regulates the expression of Tac antigen on peripheral blood T lymphocytes. J. Exp. Med. *160*:1390, 1984.
19. Chu, E., Gesner, M., et al.: Role of Ia antigens and IL-1 in T cell proliferation to phytohemagglutin. Clin. Immunol. Immunopathol. *36*:70, 1985.
20. Lisowska-Grospierre, B. B., Durandy, A., et al.: *Primary Immunodeficiency Diseases*. New York, Alan R. Liss, 1983, p. 87.
21. Chu, E., Rosen, E. S., et al.: Immunodeficiency with defective T cell receptor for interleukin 1. Proc. Natl. Acad. Sci. *81*:4945, 1984.
22. Schultz, A. M., Henderson, L. E., et al.: Amino terminal myristylation of the protein kinase p60src, a retroviral transforming protein. Science *227*:427, 1985.
23. Taniguchi, M., Miller, J. E. A. P.: Enrichment of specific suppressor T cells and characterization of their surface markers. J. Exp. Med. *146*:1450, 1977.
24. Okuda, K., Mutsuhiko, M., et al.: Analysis of T cell hybridomas. II. Comparisons among three distinct types of monoclonal suppressor factors. J. Exp. Med. *154*:1838, 1981.
25. Bensussan, A., Acuto, O., et al.: T3-Ti receptor triggering of $T8^+$ suppressor T cells leads to unresponsiveness to interleukin-2. Nature *311*:565, 1984.
26. Insel, R. A., Merler, E.: The necessity for T cell help for human tonsil B cell responses to pokeweed mitogen: induction of DNA synthesis, immunoglobulin, and specific antibody production with a T cell helper factor produced with pokeweed mitogen. J. Immunol. *118*:2009, 1977.

27. Kuritani, T., Cooper, M. D.: Human B cell differentiation. II. Pokeweed mitogen–responsive B cells belong to a surface-immunoglobulin D–negative subpopulation. J. Exp. Med. *155*:1561, 1982.
28. Graham, B. A., Britton, S., et al.: Characteristics of Epstein-Barr virus activation of human B lymphocytes. J. Exp. Med. *154*:832, 1981.
29. Lanzavecchia, A.: One out of five peripheral blood lymphocytes is activated to high-rate Ig production by human alloreactive T cell clones. Eur. J. Immunol. *13*:820, 1983.
30. Umetsu, D. T., Leung, D. Y. M., et al.: Monoclonal helper T cells induce normal B cells to synthesize IgE antibody. J. Allergy Clin. Immunol. *75*:135A, 1985.
31. Volkman, D. J., Lane, H. C., et al.: Antigen induced in vitro antibody production by humans: a model for B cell activation and immunoregulation. Proc. Natl. Acad. Sci. U.S.A. *78*:2528, 1981.
32. Paul, W. E.: Regulation of B cell activation, proliferation, and immunoglobulin synthesis. Am. Acad. Allergy Immunol. 41st Annu. Meeting, 1985, p. 83.
33. Muraguchi, A., Butler, J. L., et al.: Differential sensitivity of human B cell subsets to activation signals delivered by anti-μ antibody and proliferative signals delivered by a monoclonal B cell growth factor. J. Exp. Med. *157*:530, 1983.
34. Isakson, P. C., Puri, E., et al.: T cell–derived B cell differentiation factor(s) (BCDF): effect on the isotype switch of murine B cells. J. Exp. Med. *135*:734, 1982.
35. Meeting Report on Primary Immunodeficiency Diseases in Man. Clin. Immunol. Immunopathol. *2*:415, 1974.
36. Reinherz, E., Schlossman, S.: Regulation of the immune response by inducer and suppressor T lymphocytes in man. New Engl. J. Med. *303*:370, 1978.
37. Reinherz, E. L., Morimoto, C., et al.: Heterogeneity of human T4+ inducer T cells defined by a monoclonal antibody that delineates two functional subpopulations. J. Immunol. *128*:463, 1982.
38. Morimoto, C., Reinherz, E. L., et al.: An autoantibody to an immunoregulatory inducer population in patients with juvenile rheumatoid arthritis. J. Clin. Invest. *67*:753, 1981.
39. Gatenby, P. A., Kansas, G. S., et al.: Dissection of immunoregulatory subpopulations of T lymphocytes within the helper and suppressor sublineages in man. J. Immunol. *129*:1997, 1982.
40. Damle, N. K., Engleman, E. G.: Immunoregulatory T cell circuits in man. Alloantigen-primed inducer T cells activate alloantigen-specific suppressor T cells in the absence of the initial antigenic stimulus. J. Exp. Med. *158*:159, 1983.
41. McNeil, D., Thompson, L. F., et al.: Spontaneous IgE formation in vitro by isolated B cells from patients with atopic dermatitis. J. Allergy Clin. Immunol. *75*:137A, 1985.
42. Siegel, R. L., Issekutz, T., et al.: Deficiency of T helper cells in transient hypogammaglobulinemia of infancy. New Engl. J. Med. *305*:1307, 1981.
43. Reinherz, E. L., Geha, R. S., et al.: Immunodeficiency associated with loss of T4+ inducer T cell function. New Engl. J. Med. *304*:311, 1981.
44. Rosen, E. S.: The acquired immunodeficiency syndrome (AIDS). J. Clin. Invest. *75*:1, 1985.
45. Longo, D. L., Gelmann, E. B., et al.: Isolation of HTLV-transformed B-lymphocyte clone from a patients with HTLV-associated adult T-cell leukaemia. Nature *310*:505, 1984.
46. Dalgleish, A. G., Beverley, P. C. L., et al.: The CDA (T4) antigen is an essential component of the receptor for the AIDS retrovirus. Nature *312*:763, 1984.
47. Leung, D. Y. M., Siegel, R. L., et al.: Immunoregulatory abnormalities in mucocutaneous lymph node syndrome. Clin. Immunol. Immunopathol. *23*:100, 1982.
48. Leung, D. Y. M., Chu, E. T., et al.: Immunoregulation T cell abnormalities in mucocutaneous lymph node syndrome. J. Immunol. *130(5)*:2002, 1983.
49. Reinherz, E. L., Rubenstein, A., et al.: Abnormalities of immunoregulatory T cells in disorders of immune function. New Engl. J. Med. *301(19)*:1018, 1979.
50. Reinherz, E. L., Parkman, R., et al.: Aberrations of suppressor T cells in human graft-versus-host disease. New Engl. J. Med. *300*:1061, 1979.
51. Waldmann, T. A., Broder, S.: Suppressor cells in the regulation of the immune response. Prog. Clin. Immunol. *3*:155, 1977.
52. Waldmann, T. A.: Disorders of suppressor immunoregulatory cells in the pathogenesis of immunodeficiency and autoimmunity. Ann. Intern. Med. *88*:226, 1978.
53. Tosado, T., Magrath, I.: et al.: Activation of suppressor T cells during Epstein-Barr-virus–induced infectious mononucleosis. New Engl. J. Med. *301(21)*:1133, 1979.
54. Reinherz, E. L., O'Brien, C., et al.: The cellular basis for viral-induced immunodeficiency: analysis by monoclonal antibodies. J. Immunol. *125*:1269, 1980.
55. Suthanthiran, M., Solomon, S. D., et al.: Hydroxyl radical scavengers inhibit human natural killer cell activity. Nature *307*:276, 1984.
56. Zucker-Franklin, D., Grusky, G., et al.: Arylsulfatase in natural killer cells: its possible role in cytotoxicity. Proc. Natl. Acad. Sci. U.S.A. *80*:6977, 1983.
57. Alarcon-Segovia, D., Ruiz-Arguelles, A., et al.: Antibody penetration into living cells. II. Anti-ribonucleoprotein IgE penetrates into T_γ lymphocytes causing their depletion and the abrogation of suppressor function. J. Immunol. *122(5)*:1855, 1979.
58. Leung, D. Y. M., Rhodes, A. R., et al.: Enumeration of T cell subsets in atopic dermatitis using monoclonal antibodies. J. Allergy Clin. Immunol. *67(6)*:450, 1981.
59. Leung, D. Y. M., Wood, N., et al.: Cellular basis of defective cell mediated lympholysis in atopic dermatitis. J. Immunol. *130(4)*:1678, 1983.
60. Katz, D. H.: Recent studies on the regulation of IgE antibody synthesis in experimental animals and man. Immunology *41*:1, 1980.
61. Strober, W., Hague, N. E., et al.: IgA-Fc receptors on mouse lymphoid cells. J. Immunol. *121*:2440, 1978.
62. Ishizaka, K., Suemura, M., et al.: Regulation of IgE response by IgE binding factors. Fed. Proc. *40(8)*:2162, 1981.
63. Young, M. C., Leung, D. Y. M., et al.: Production of IgE potentiating factor in man by T cell lines bearing Fc receptors for IgE. Eur. J. Immunol. *14*:871, 1984.
64. Yodoi, J., Hirashima, M., et al.: Regulatory role of IgE-binding factors from rat T lymphocytes. V. The carbohydrate moieties in IgE-potentiating factors and IgE-suppressive factors. J. Immunol. *128*:289, 1982.
65. Yodoi, J., Ishizaka, T., et al.: Lymphocytes bearing Fc-receptors for IgE. II. Induction of Fc receptor–bearing rat lymphocytes by IgE. J. Immunol. *123*:455, 1979.
66. Leung, D. Y. M., Brozek, C., et al.: IgE specific suppressor factors in normal human serum. Clin. Immunol. Immunopathol. *32*:339, 1984.
67. Young, M. C., Harfi, H., et al.: A human T cell lymphoma secreting an IgE specific helper factor. J. Clin. Invest. *75*:1977, 1985.
68. Mayer, L., Posnett, D. N., et al.: Human malignant T cells capable of inducing an immunoglobulin class switch. J. Exp. Med. *161*:134, 1985.
69. Issekutz, T., Chu, E., et al.: Antigen presentation by human B cells: T cell proliferation induced by Epstein-Barr virus B lymphoblastoid cells. J. Immunol. *129(4)*:1446, 1982.
70. Chu, E., Rosenwasser, L. J., et al.: Role of interleukin 1 in antigen specific T cell proliferation. J. Immunol. *132*:1311, 1984.
71. Geha, R. S.: Idiotypic determinants on human T cells and modulation of human T cell responses by antiidiotypic antibodies. J. Immunol. *133*:1846, 1984.
72. Taniguchi, M., Tokuhisa, T., et al.: Functional roles of two polypeptide chains that compose an antigen-specific suppressor T cell factor. J. Exp. Med. *159*:1096, 1984.
73. Geha, R. S.: Idiotypic determinants on human T cells and

modulation of human T cell responses by anti-idiotypic antibodies. J. Immunol. *133:*1846, 1984.
74. Lamb, J. R., Feldmann, M.: Essential requirement for major histocompatibility complex recognition in T-cell tolerance induction. Nature *308:*72, 1984.
75. Valdimarsson, H., Higgs, J. M., et al.: Immune abnormalities associated with chronic mucocutaneous candidiasis. Cell Immunol. *6:*348, 1973.
76. Hayward, A. R., Githens, J., et al.: *Primary Immunodeficiency Diseases.* New York, Alan R. Liss, 1983, p. 277.
77. Pober, J. S., Collins, T., et al.: Lymphocytes recognize human vascular endothelial and dermal fibroblast Ia antigens induced by recombinant immune interferon. Nature *305:*726, 1983.
78. De Villortoy, J. P., Fischer, A., et al.: Self education after mismatched HLA haploidentical bone marrow transplantation. In *Human T Cell Clones.* Feldman, M. (ed.), Oxford, Oxford University Press, in press.
79. Rosa, E., Fellous, M.: The effect of granular interaction on MHC antigens. Immunol. Today *5:*261, 1984.
80. Londei, M., Lamb, J. R., et al.: Epithelial cells expressing aberrant MHC class II determinants can present antigen to cloned human T cells. Nature *312:*639, 1984.
81. Reinherz, E. L., Kung, P. C., et al.: A monoclonal antibody reactive with the human cytotoxic/suppressor T cell subset previously defined by a heteroantiserum termed TH_2. J. Immunol. *124:*1301, 1980.
82. Moretta, L., Mingari, M. C., et al.: Surface markers of cloned human T cells with various cytolytic activities. J. Exp. Med. *154:*569, 1981.
83. Fung, M. C., Hapel, A. J., et al.: Molecular cloning of cDNA for murine interleukin-3. Nature *307:*233, 1984.
84. Steeg, P. S., Moore, R. N., et al.: Regulation of murine macrophage Ia antigen expression by a lymphokine with immune interferon activity. J. Exp. Med. *156:*1780, 1982.
85. Schultz, R. M., Kleinschmidt, W. J.: Functional identity between murine interferon and macrophage activating factor. Nature *305:*239, 1983.
86. Fontana, A., Fierz, W., et al.: Astrocytes present myelin basic protein to encephalitogenic T-cell lines. Nature *307:*273, 1984.
87. Celada, A., Gray, P. W., et al.: Evidence for a gamma-interferon receptor that regulates macrophage tumoricidal activity. J. Exp. Med. *160:*55, 1984.
88. Thueson, D. O., Speck, L. S., et al.: Histamine-releasing activity. I. Production by mitogen or antigen stimulated human mononuclear cells. J. Immunol. *123:*626, 1979.

THE IMMUNE SYSTEM

CHAPTER 27
Immunoglobulin and T Cell Receptor Genes in Human Immunodeficiency and Neoplasia

STANLEY J. KORSMEYER
JERROLD F. SCHWABER

INTRODUCTION 860
GENERATION OF A FUNCTIONAL KAPPA LIGHT
　CHAIN GENE VIA SOMATIC ASSEMBLY OF
　IMMUNOGLOBULIN GENE SEGMENTS 863
THE HUMAN LAMBDA LIGHT CHAIN GENE LOCUS
　864
LIGHT CHAIN GENE REARRANGEMENTS IN MATURE
　HUMAN B CELL LEUKEMIAS AND LYMPHOMAS 864
THE HUMAN HEAVY (H) CHAIN GENE LOCUS 865
TRANSCRIPTION AND TRANSLOCATION OF
　IMMUNOGLOBULIN GENES 866
Overview of Expression
Joining Systems
Transcription
Heavy Chain Rearrangement
MOLECULAR GENETIC BASIS OF HUMAN HEAVY
　CHAIN DISEASES 868
B CELL PRECURSORS 869
"Non T, Non B" Acute Lymphoblastic Leukemias (ALL)
The Lymphoid Blast Crises of Chronic Myelogenous
　Leukemia (CML)
IMMUNOGLOBULIN GENE REARRANGEMENTS AS
　B CELL–ASSOCIATED CLONAL MARKERS IN
　LYMPHOID NEOPLASMS 870
DNA REARRANGEMENTS IN T CELL ANTIGEN-
　SPECIFIC RECEPTOR GENES 872
MEDIATION OF CHROMOSOMAL TRANSLOCATIONS
　BY IMMUNOGLOBULIN GENE LOCI 873
ANTIBODY DEFICIENCY DISEASES 874
X-Linked Agammaglobulinemia
Common Varied Agammaglobulinemia
　"Nonsecretory" Agammaglobulinemia
Hyper-IgM Syndrome
Other Antibody Deficiency Diseases

INTRODUCTION

Humoral immunity results from the interactions of antibody molecules with the molecules of inflammation, the best understood being the complement proteins; they serve to localize and kill invading organisms, which are then eliminated by phagocytic cells. Direction of these elements of humoral immunity is provided by the specificity of the antibodies produced in response to immunologic challenge. Each antibody molecule is composed of four polypeptide chains, with two identical heavy and two identical light chains (Fig. 27–1). In turn, each heavy and light chain is divided into a constant region and a variable region. Biologic function of the molecule is determined by the constant region; antibody specificity of the molecule is determined by the variable region.

In tissues, antibodies are produced by B lymphocytes and their end stage plasma cells. Each individual is capable of producing an enormous number of different antibodies; however, the precise number of these various antibodies has not been determined. Recognition of the large number of antibodies that are produced raises two fundamental questions: (1) How is this diversity generated? and (2) How is this diversity regulated? Our understanding of the answers to these questions rests on advances in molecular and cellular biology confirming and refining two hypotheses: the clonal selection hypothesis of Burnet (1) and the combinatorial hypothesis of Dreyer and Bennett (2).

In 1959, Burnet (1) proposed that individual antibody specificities were produced by cells derived from an individual clone. Individual antibody specificities would then be regulated by expansion or reduction of individual clones of cells. Prior to the clonal selection hypothesis, individual cells were assumed to produce antibodies of many different specificities. An antibody response to antigenic stimulation would then require coordinate production of many antibodies, most of them irrelevant to the particular infection, or a mechanism by which individual cells decided which of many antibodies was to be synthesized in each infection. In the years since Burnet's proposal of his clonal selection hypothesis, antibodies have been shown to be synthesized by B lymphocytes under the direct regulation of helper and suppressor T lymphocytes. Individual B lymphocytes produce antibody molecules of a single specificity. All the B lymphocytes derived from a pre-B cell clone produce antibody of the same specificity,

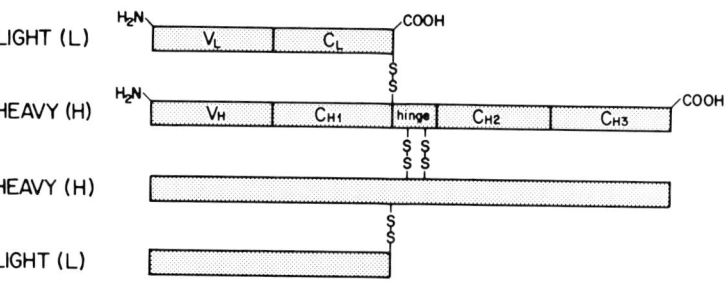

Figure 27–1. Schematic presentation of an immunoglobin molecule of IgG type. Variable (V) and constant (C) region domains of the heavy (H) and light (L) chains are demonstrated.

subject to refinement in specificity by somatic mechanisms.

There are five known classes of antibodies. They are designated IgG, IgA, IgM, IgD, and IgE in descending order of serum concentration. IgG is further subdivided into four subclasses, designated IgG1, IgG2, IgG3, and IgG4. IgA is further subdivided into two subclasses, IgA and IgA2. These various classes and subclasses of immunoglobulin are called isotypes, and the distinctiveness of each isotype can be attributed to its unique heavy chain. Two types of light chains, designated kappa and lambda, are found in all isotypes.

Each immunoglobulin is composed of two heavy chains and two light chains (Fig. 27–1), all linked covalently by disulfide bridges. IgM is a pentamer of such a structure, and some IgA is a dimer; all the other immunoglobulins are monomers. As mentioned, all immunoglobulins have two kappa or two lambda light chains (never one of each) and two heavy chains that are identical but vary from isotype to isotype. The various characteristics of these immunoglobulins are listed in Table 27–1.

In 1965, Dreyer and Bennett (2) proposed that antibody heavy and light chains were encoded as two genes in the genome. Protein sequences of myeloma proteins had shown that heavy and light chains were composed both of a highly conserved region called the constant region and of a highly divergent region termed the variable region (Fig. 27–1). Inheritance of the constant region genes for the several heavy chain isotypes and the two light chain isotypes followed the simple rules of mendelian genetics. However, widely divergent variable regions were represented with the same constant region in different myeloma proteins. Prior to the two genes/one polypeptide chain proposal of Dreyer and Bennett, immunoglobulin genes were envisioned as either (1) encoded in an uncounted number of copies, representing uncounted duplication of each of the constant regions, with each constant region associated with a different variable region (germline hypothesis) or (2) encoded as one or a few copies of each constant region gene with an unknown mechanism required to mutate randomly the variable region of the molecule to produce the diversity of antibody

Table 27–1. CHARACTERISTICS OF IMMUNOGLOBULINS

Isotype	Molecular Formula	Serum Concentration mg/ml	Cross Placenta	Fix Complement	Principal Functions
IgG1	$\gamma1_2\kappa_2$ $\gamma1_2\lambda_2$	7	+	+	Antitoxins; antibody to most bacterial antigens
IgG2	$\gamma2_2\kappa_2$ $\gamma2_2\lambda_2$	2	+	+	Antipolysaccharide antibodies to bacterial capsules
IgG3	$\gamma3_2\kappa_2$ $\gamma3_2\lambda_2$	0.7	+	+	Cytophilic antibodies, such as to Rh antigens
IgG4	$\gamma4_2\kappa_2$ $\gamma4_2\lambda_2$	0.3	+	−	Anticoagulants, such as anti–Factor VIII in hemophiliacs
IgA1	$\alpha1_2\kappa_2$ $\alpha1_2\lambda_2$	1	−	−	Virus neutralizing antibody
IgA2	$(\alpha2_2\kappa_2)_2$ $(\alpha2_2\lambda_2)_2$	0.7	−	−	Principal secretory antibody
IgM	$(\mu_2\kappa_2)_5$ $(\mu_2\lambda_2)_5$	1.5	−	+	Antibodies to lipopolysaccharides
IgD	$\delta_2\lambda_2$ $\delta_2\kappa_2$	0.3	−	−	Unknown
IgE	$\epsilon_2\lambda_2$ $\epsilon_2\kappa_2$	<0.0005*	−	−	Anaphylactic antibodies or "reagins"

*Usually expressed as international units; up to 200 IU is considered to be normal

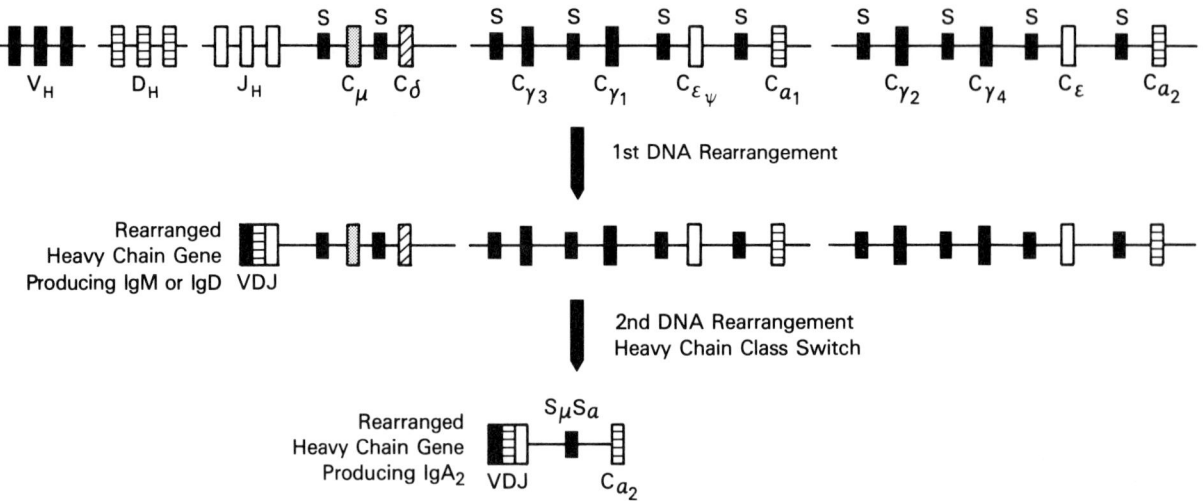

Figure 27–2. A schematic representation of the human germline heavy chain locus. The first DNA rearrangement assembles three regions—variable (V_H), diversity (D_H), and joining (J_H)—to complete the variable portion of the molecule. Later in development, a second DNA rearrangement may occur involving the homologous switch sites (S) that precede each constant (C_H) region. This results in a more distal constant region, such as C_{α_2} moving next to the rearranged VDJ as in an IgA_2-producing cell.

molecules required for host defense (somatic mutation hypothesis). Molecular studies of the immunoglobulin genes have now shown that indeed the constant regions of each heavy and light chain isotype are encoded by a single copy gene and that the variable regions are encoded by multiple copies of three (heavy chains) or two (light chains) sets of genes that further generate antibody diversity by recombination.

For a detailed discussion of these historic matters, the reader should consult the work cited in reference 3.

In summary, then, current understanding of the mechanisms for generating and regulating antibody diversity is as follows: Antibodies are produced by B lymphocytes under the direct regulatory control of T helper and suppressor lymphocytes. Ontogeny of the B lymphocytes begins with unidentified precursors of both T and B lymphocytes. An early step in commitment to B lymphoid differentiation is signalled by rearrangement of the D and J_H genes that constitute one hypervariable region of the variable region (Fig. 27–2). This rearrangement generates diversity by (1) selection from the sets of D and J_H genes, and (2) the addition of extranucleotides at the site of the juncture. Cells carrying a productive DJ_H rearrangement then undergo VH gene translocation. Antibody diversity is further enhanced by this process, which, as in the case of the DJ_H rearrangement, selects a particular variable region and joins it to the D region gene at one of several sites. Productive $V_H D$ gene rearrangement is signalled, then, by production in the cell of a complete μ heavy chain.

Pre-B cells, characterized by the expression of a cytoplasmic μ heavy chain, represent the beginning of B lymphocyte ontogeny (4–6). The μ chain may be a truncated molecule transcribed following DJ_H rearrangement or a complete μ/μ chain transcribed following $V_H DJ_H$ rearrangement. Differentiation to a B lymphocyte is accompanied by expression of light chain protein, which follows productive rearrangement of one of the light chain genes. Cells at this stage of differentiation, expressing complete antibody molecules, leave the central lymphoid organs and appear in the peripheral circulation. The earliest B lymphocytes express IgM alone (7), although their δ heavy chain gene could be transcribed without further gene rearrangement. Subsequent heavy chain isotypes are expressed on more mature, and probably more specialized, B lymphocytes, likely following deletion of the intervening heavy chain constant region genes. Resting lymphocytes circulate in blood and lymph, awaiting the appropriate stimulation to undergo terminal differentiation. Terminal differentiation includes amplification of that clone by cell division, a switch from production of predominantly membrane-bound antibody to primarily secretory antibody, a possible switch in heavy chain isotype, and production of antibody representing more than 90 per cent of total cellular protein.

The precise molecular genetic mechanisms that assemble the separated variable (V), diversity (D), joining (J), and constant (C) gene segments were determined by the experiments of Leder (8), Tonegawa (9), and other workers on human as well as murine B cell lineage malignancies. These malignancies represented clonal expansions of B cells at selected stages of development and helped reveal the elaborate system of movable gene subsegments, flexibility at the sites of recombination, somatic mutation, and alternate RNA splicing that generates messenger RNA for antibody (10–14). As a counterpoint to the B cell malignancies, examination of cells from antibody deficiency diseases has helped reveal the semihierarchical pathways of B lymphocyte ontogeny that correlate with the Ig gene rearrangements (15,16). Somatic cell genetic techniques have permitted the in vitro establishment of cellular descendants as single cell clones for molecular analysis and for dissection of the antibody deficiency diseases for possible gene complementation.

The basic rules governing DNA rearrangements and transcriptional regulation that were gleaned from the study of well-characterized B cell tumors have proved of immense importance in examinations of lymphoid neoplasms of uncertain classification. Human leukemias revealed that assembly of Ig gene subsegments occurs in an ordered sequence during early B cell development to help ensure that a mature B cell manufactures only one heavy and light chain molecule (14,17). This hierarchy of Ig gene rearrangements that occurs during the early development of a B cell has provided a new means of classifying lymphoid neoplasms and of determining their stage of differentiation (18–20). Furthermore, these rearrangements create an alteration in the size of Ig gene–containing DNA fragments and serve as unique clonal markers within B cell tumors (21, 22). Errors in Ig gene recombination and expression can now be defined that account for the truncated proteins of human heavy chain diseases and the lack of Ig products within some pre-B cells (23–25). The Ig gene loci also mediate an additional type of rearrangement in certain B cell malignancies that juxtaposes information from two nonhomologous chromosomes (26, 27). This latter rearrangement marks the site of a chromosomal translocation that introduces a cellular oncogene into an Ig gene locus (28, 29).

GENERATION OF A FUNCTIONAL KAPPA LIGHT CHAIN GENE VIA SOMATIC ASSEMBLY OF IMMUNOGLOBULIN GENE SEGMENTS

Each Ig molecule is composed of two identical heavy and two identical light chain proteins. Humans have two potential light chain classes (κ and λ) and express κ 60 per cent of the time and λ light chains 40 per cent. If a B cell is ultimately to make a κ light chain, during early stages of its development it must rearrange its κ gene locus to activate that gene. The human κ gene is located on the short arm of chromosome 2 at band 2p11 (30). Figure 27–3 schematically displays the multiple separated V_κ segments, each of which is

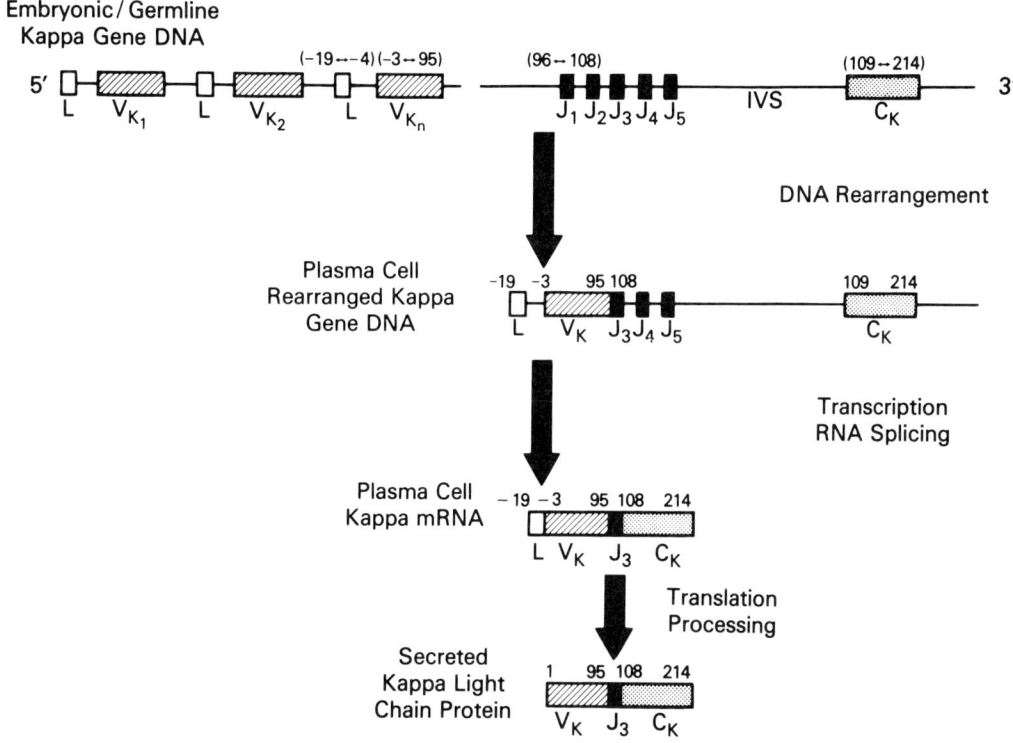

Figure 27–3. A schematic representation of the human κ gene locus reveals multiple germline variable (V_κ) regions with an accompanying leader (L) sequence. Humans have five alternative joining (J_κ) segments, each coding for amino acid positions 96 to 108. There is only one constant (C_κ) region per allele. DNA rearrangement joins a single V_κ and J_κ segment. The remaining intervening sequences (IVS) are removed after transcription by RNA splicing.

foreshortened, contributing only the N terminal 95 amino acids of the 108 that constitute the variable portion of this protein. The remaining 13 amino acids that complete the variable portion are contributed by one of five alternative joining (J_κ) gene segments. There is only one constant (C_κ) gene region on each allele, and it is separated from the strip of J_κ segments by a long intervening sequence (IVS) (31, 32). A process of DNA rearrangement activates this κ gene by bringing a single V_κ region into contiguity with one of the five alternative J_κ segments. This completes the coding sequence for the variable component of the κ light chain molecule (see Figure 27–3). An RNA transcript is then generated from this rearranged allele, and the remaining intervening sequences are removed by site-specific RNA-splicing mechanisms. The final mature mRNA is then translated into the complete κ light chain protein. The so-called leader, or signal, peptide information that is found at the 5' side of each variable region encodes a highly hydrophobic set of amino acids responsible for the transmembrane passage of this molecule.

THE HUMAN LAMBDA LIGHT CHAIN GENE LOCUS

Lambda light chain proteins are present in approximately 40 per cent of human Ig molecules and are found on a corresponding percentage of the mature B cell malignancies. The active λ gene locus is located on the long arm of human chromosome 22 at band q11 (33). This locus is organized in a different fashion than the κ gene locus, consisting of multiple, duplicated J_λ, C_λ units that are linearly arranged (34). In its simplest form this λ locus is composed of six C_λ regions (Fig. 27–4) (35). The first three C_λ regions code for three distinctly different λ chain isotypes that were known to exist from the prior analysis of Bence Jones proteins. Their differences, however, are only minimal, being confined to amino acid markers that have been termed as follows: Mcg for $C_{\lambda 1}$, Ke^-Oz^- for $C_{\lambda 2}$, and Ke^-Oz^+ for $C_{\lambda 3}$ (34). Owing to the organization of this locus, humans have at least six C_λ regions to choose from when making λ light chains. As can be seen in Figure 27–4, one can more conveniently analyze this region by subdividing it with the restriction endonuclease, EcoRI. A restriction endonuclease is an internally cleaving enzyme that reproducibly cuts DNA only when a specific set of nucleic acid bases (GAATTC for EcoRI) is aligned. In the most common form of the λ locus, this places these genes on DNA fragments that measure 14,000 base pairs (14 kb), 8 kb, and 16 kb in length (35). Much like κ genes the λ genes undergo a DNA rearrangement that joins a V_λ and a J_λ segment and produces alterations in the size of the EcoRI DNA restriction fragments. This can be detected as a DNA rearrangement within λ-producing B cell tumors (see Figure 27–4).

LIGHT CHAIN GENE REARRANGEMENTS IN MATURE HUMAN B CELL LEUKEMIAS AND LYMPHOMAS

Chronic lymphocytic leukemia, Waldenström's macroglobulinemia, many follicular and diffuse lymphomas, and Burkitt's lymphoma are clonal expansions of mature B cells representing the progeny of a single cell. Thus, every cell in that population will bear the same Ig gene recombination with the identical variable (V) and joining (J) DNA element. As can be seen in Figure 27–4, this DNA rearrangement event generates an altered-size DNA restriction fragment when it bears an Ig gene in its recombined form as compared with its germline form. As each cell in a clonal population bears the same Ig gene rearrangement, this DNA rearrangement becomes detectable by Southern blot analysis (see Figure 27–4).

Mature B cells curiously produce only one of the two available light chain isotypes (κ or λ). Furthermore, of the selected light chain class κ or λ, a B cell makes only one of the two alternative alleles, either the maternal or the paternal. These phenomena have been referred to as isotypic and allelic exclusion, respectively. However, the patterns of light chain gene rearrangement that account for these events in κ-producing cells proved different from those in λ-producing B cells (14). As can be seen in Figure 27–4, a κ-producing chronic lymphocytic leukemia displays a rearrangement corresponding to its effective $V_\kappa J_\kappa$ recombination that is responsible for the κ light chain produced by this cell. The other nonproductive, or so-called excluded, allele may be in one of three potential configurations. That is, an excluded allele may be germline, may be deleted from the genome, or may itself be rearranged but in an ineffective or aberrant fashion. Therefore, the phenomenon of allelic exclusion may reflect the fact that only one κ gene possesses an entirely effective joining of a V_κ and a J_κ segment. In terms of isotypic exclusion (the lack of λ production in a κ-producing B cell), κ-producing B cells usually retained their λ genes within the germline configuration, accounting for their inability to make the opposite light chain class.

Unexpectedly, the mechanism that ensured that λ-producing B cells did not produce the opposite κ light chain class was markedly different. As Figure 27–4 details, λ B cell leukemias possess the requisite λ gene rearrangements responsible for the λ light chain synthesized. Surprisingly, how-

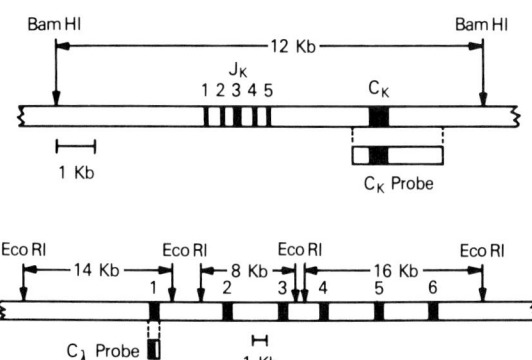

Figure 27–4. Light chain gene configurations with κ- and λ-producing B cell chronic lymphocytic leukemias (L) as compared with their matching fibroblast controls (C). A rearranged κ gene (arrow) was demonstrable with the $C_κ$ probe, whereas the $C_λ$ probe revealed the expected germline λ genes (dash marks) in the κ-producing CLL. In contrast, a λ-producing CLL with a detectable λ gene rearrangement had lost both copies of its $C_κ$ genes. The lower schematic indicates the $C_κ$ probe and $C_λ$ probes utilized.

ever, λ B cell leukemias had usually deleted both copies of their κ genes, thus preventing the production of κ chains (14). This loss of κ genes in λ B cells is a normal developmental event seen in λ B cells from normal individuals as well as in those of patients with leukemia (36). This κ gene deletion is always mediated by the same κ-deleting element, whose role is to eliminate the κ gene locus, thus preventing its expression in λ B cells (37). Furthermore, it appears that rearrangement attempts to activate a κ gene occur before λ gene rearrangement during the development of a B cell (17, 18). Any cell that fails to correctly assemble a $V_κ$ and a $J_κ$ segment can then move on to λ gene rearrangement. This ordered process of κ and λ gene rearrangements helps ensure that an individual B cell makes only one light chain.

THE HUMAN HEAVY (H) CHAIN GENE LOCUS

The heavy (H) chain gene locus also is a discontinuous gene composed of gene subsegments that must be recombined at the DNA level so that the information encoding the variable portion of the antibody protein can be assembled. In addition to multiple germline V_H genes and an alternate set of J_H gene segments, there exist several families of a third genetic component known as the diversity (D_H) element (see Figure 27–2) (13). Thus, two sites of DNA recombination are needed for correct assembly of an H chain gene. A D_H region must correctly rearrange with a J_H segment, and then a V_H region must be juxtaposed with this $D_H J_H$ unit (38, 39). Most B cells have had to rearrange both their H chain gene alleles in order to make one correct $V_H D_H J_H$ rearrangement. IgM-bearing malignancies represent the first stage of mature, surface Ig–bearing B cell development. These cells transcribe the assembled VDJ together with the nearest constant region, $C_μ$. Following this stage, some cells simultaneously produce IgM and IgD, and both these molecules bear the same VDJ information (40, 41). This is accomplished by an alternative splicing of either $C_μ$ or $C_δ$ information, with the VDJ at the level of RNA. Malignancies that represent more mature stages of B cell differentiation may have switched to producing one of the more distally located constant regions of $C_γ$, $C_α$, or $C_ε$. This phenomenon is accomplished by a second type of DNA rearrangement, known as the H chain class switch (see Figure 27–2) (42–46).

This recombination is mediated by switch sites (S) located at the 5' left hand side of each constant region. Such switch sites are composed of tandemly arrayed repetitive DNA sequences that may span several thousand nucleic acid-base pairs. Their homology facilitates a recombination within these sites and results in moving a more distally located constant region into closer proximity with the previously assembled VDJ region (see Figure 27–2). This event is an elegant conservation of genetic material in which an organism may utilize the same VDJ rearrangement in combination with multiple constant regions. This generates a large functional diversity in the Ig locus by allowing the same antigen specificity (VDJ) to be attached to multiple effector functions contributed by the constant regions.

TRANSCRIPTION AND TRANSLATION OF IMMUNOGLOBULIN GENES

Overview of Expression

Expression of immunoglobulin genes is under the control of most of the same regulatory elements described for other genes. A transcriptional promotor, composed of the sequence TATA, must be located 5' to the gene (47, 48). A transcriptional enhancer sequence is located downstream from the TATA box, between the JH sequences and the C_μ gene (49, 50). The primary RNA transcript includes both coding and noncoding sequences. The noncoding, intervening sequences must be spliced out of the RNA during processing. The 3' terminus of the gene (and thus of the RNA) encodes a sequence, specifying addition of a poly-A tail, which must be added for transport as a messenger RNA. The first element of the messenger RNA to be translated, located at the 5' end of the processed mRNA, represents a leader, or signal, sequence, which binds the RNA to the components of a ribosome for translation on the rough endoplasmic reticulum (51–53). Translated into protein, this leader sequence serves as a hydrophobic guide, permitting passage of the nascent polypeptide through the membrane of the rough endoplasmic reticulum. However, the application of these regulatory elements to immunoglobulin genes differs from that of other genes because of the process of gene rearrangement required to construct a functional immunoglobulin gene locus.

Joining Systems

Generation of antibody diversity has been described to result from the combinatorial effect of selection of the particular V_H, D, and J_H genes. In addition, there is an element of randomness added by the process of juxtaposing each gene segment to its adjacent gene. There may be as much as a 10-nucleotide variation in the particular junctures generated between V_H and D_H, and between D_H and J_H (54, 55). This permits insertion or deletion of as many as three amino acids into the sequence between the 3' terminus of the V_H and the 5' terminus of the J_H. This span of sequence represents the third complementarity-determining region (CDR3 = hypervariable region). Insertion of an amino acid at one joint position is often compensated for by deletion of an amino acid at another joint position, so that the overall length of the final heavy chain is relatively constant. This flexibility in sequence joining, however, results in the penalty that two of the three possible junctures between D and J_H, for example, result in sequences that are out of reading frame for the resulting $DJ_H C_\mu$ mRNA. The joining of V_H and D is governed by the same rules of randomness, permitting further variation in CDR3 but also carrying the penalty of RNA sequences that are out of reading frame for downstream elements. These frameshift variants do not encode immunoglobulin heavy chain molecules, and cells bearing only frameshifted immunoglobulin genes must be eliminated. It is possible that resulting gene sets that encode molecules that are too long or too short also may be produced, requiring further selection of cells to be amplified from the clones that are to be aborted.

A mechanism by which cells bearing only frameshift variant immunoglobulin genes could be eliminated has been described in pre-B cells from X-linked agammaglobulinemia and Abelson virus–transformed pre-B cell lines (53, 56). Pre-B cells from three patients with X-linked agammaglobulinemia as well as from normal human fetal liver produce a truncated μ heavy chain composed of a leader sequence and C_μ (56). In mouse Abelson virus–transformed pre-B cells, Reth and Alt (53) found that each of the D region genes had a leader sequence and promoter for transcription in their 5' sequence. Rearrangement of DJ_H would then result in transcription and translation of a truncated protein. If there is productive rearrangement (i.e., rearrangement that keeps the C_μ gene in reading frame), this truncated protein would be C_μ. The C_μ protein may serve as a signal for subsequent rearrangement of a V_H gene. Cells with nonproductive rearrangements would translate a nonsense polypeptide, which could not serve as a trigger for subsequent V_H gene rearrangement. A similar mechanism may prevail to regulate further development of pre-B cells following V_H gene rearrangement.

Discovery of the failure of pre-B cell development in X-linked agammaglobulinemia (53) suggests that V_H gene rearrangement may be under control of regulatory elements on the X chromosome. Pre-B cells from patients with X-linked agammaglobulinemia produced a truncated μ chain without an associated variable region. There is no evidence for defects in the structural genes for immunoglobulin in these patients. Additionally, this disease is linked to the X chromosome, whereas the structural genes for immunoglobulin heavy chain have been localized to chromosome 14. Other X-linked diseases have been associated with defects in humoral immunity, suggesting that there may be other regulatory genes for immunoglobulin expression on the X chromosome.

Following productive rearrangement and expression of a complete $V_H D J_H C_\mu$ gene set in a pre-B cell, a light chain gene must be rearranged. As described in another section of this chapter, first the κ light chain genes are rearranged, and then, presumably if these rearrangements fail, the λ light chain genes. We presume, without direct evidence, that the expression of a productive light chain gene set as polypeptide is necessary for progression of a pre-B cell to an early B lymphocyte. Rearrangement of light chain genes requires only integration of a V_L gene with a J_L gene. Each of the two light chain isotypes, κ and λ recombines with its own set of variable region genes. Productive rearrangement of a light chain gene is signalled by transcription of the gene and translation of the mRNA. Production of heavy and light chain yields complete IgM molecules, with insertion of the IgM into the cell membrane; the cell is then classified as an early B lymphocyte.

Transcription

Transcription of the immunoglobulin heavy chain locus starts with the 5' promoter of transcription (TATA box) and spans the following elements: leader sequence; variable region gene including V_H, D, and J_H; constant region sequence for μ heavy chain; a "membrane sequence"; and a site for addition of poly-A. The leader sequence serves, as it does for other proteins, first as an RNA sequence for attachment of the mRNA to the membrane-bound polysomes. Secondly, it serves as a protein sequence within a nascent chain to bind a signal receptor particle (SRP) in the cytoplasm. It is hypothesized that during the export process, this complex may bind to a specific docking protein that facilitates the transmembrane passage of either the secreted or membrane form of immunoglobulin. There are noncoding "intervening sequences" between the promoter and the leader sequence between the J_H gene and the constant region gene and between the constant region sequence and the membrane sequence, all of which must be removed from the primary RNA transcript to produce an mRNA to be translated.

In this processing, the membrane sequence may be spliced to the 3' end of the constant region sequence, to produce a molecule bound to the cell surface. Alternatively, the transcript may be terminated prior to the membrane (μm) exon, and the secreted (μs) information that is contiguous with the constant region (Cμ) will result in the secreted form of the molecule (57, 58).

Heavy Chain Rearrangement

Diversification of B lymphocytes is indicated by expression of the clonal heavy chain variable region with the different isotypes (C_μ–C_α) of the heavy chain constant region (see Figure 27–2). Different mechanisms have been proposed for diversification to different heavy chain isotypes. Expression of δ heavy chains occurs by differential splicing of a long RNA primary transcript. The δ heavy chain constant region gene is located only 9 kb downstream from the μ constant region gene (59). Primary RNA transcripts spanning both μ and δ constant region genes are feasible, permitting simultaneous production of IgM and IgD in the same cell by differential splicing of the long RNA transcript.

Production of the four γ, two α, and one ε heavy chain isotypes is thought to occur secondary to a deletion event (60, 61). Myeloma and lymphoid cell lines expressing one of these downstream heavy chain constant region genes have been shown to have deleted the constant region genes that intervene between that constant region gene and the $V_H D J_H$ gene locus. Highly reiterated sequences are located 5' to each of the constant region gene loci (62). By a recombination event between these reiterated "switch sequences," the $V_H D J_H$ gene locus can be inserted adjacent to a downstream heavy chain constant region gene. The mechanisms by which a particular heavy chain constant region gene is selected for recombination are not known and may be random.

The evidence for deletion of intervening constant region genes shows only that such deletion can occur in association with a class switch. That these deletions are required for isotype switching and are the only mechanism by which it occurs is less clear. Examination of IgE-bearing B cells from a selected mouse strain implies that a differential splicing mechanism might allow the expression of distally located isotypes prior to a DNA deletion process. However, studies of human B cell lines expressing γ or α heavy chains have shown (65) that intervening constant region genes are deleted (64, 65a). This would suggest that cells might produce later heavy chain isotypes by a reversible mechanism (e.g., sterically looping out of intervening constant region genes) or by production of an extremely long primary RNA transcript, and that gene deletion may serve to stabilize this isotype switch.

Detailed studies of antibodies to specific antigens have shown that there is further generation of antibody diversity beyond the combinatorial mechanisms already described. Antibodies produced after serial immunization tend to have higher affinity to the antigen used than the antibodies found in the primary response. Examination of heavy and light chain sequences has shown that this maturation of the antibody response results from single amino acid and single nucleotide changes in the antibody variable region and the genomic V, D, and J regions (66). In some cases—and the best evidence is from the λ variable region gene of mice—it has been shown that the late-appearing variable region does not represent substitution of another variable region gene into the antibody. Rather, somatic mutation of the original variable region has resulted in an antibody with higher affinity to the antigen (67). Cells producing this higher affinity antibody have an apparent selective advantage for proliferation in secondary antibody responses. The mechanism for the somatic mutation is unclear. However, the mutations observed are limited to the V, D, and J region genes and the sequences immediately surrounding these genes. This suggests that there is a specific mechanism by which these mutations are generated. Assuming that this maturation occurs secondary to random mutation in association with massive proliferation suggests that mutants should be found with mutations in the constant region and surrounding sequences as well. Such mutations are rarely observed.

B lymphocytes, as found in peripheral blood, are termed "resting lymphocytes." Implicit to this characterization is the predominance of membrane-bound immunoglobulin, serving as receptor for antigen, with little or no evidence for production of immunoglobulin for secretion. Upon appropriate stimulation, these resting B lymphocytes undergo terminal differentiation into lymphoblasts, plasma cells, and memory cells. The process of terminal differentiation may include a heavy chain isotype switch. It always includes a switch from low-level production of membrane immunoglobulin to high-level production of immunoglobulin that is secreted. In plasma cells, immunoglobulin production for secretion may represent 90 per cent of the total protein synthesized. The process of terminal differentiation, including proliferation of specific clones of B lymphocytes, selective amplification of clones with increased affinity, and termination of proliferative phase when infection has been contained, is under the direct regulation of T lymphocytes.

In light of our current understanding of the normal processes by which immunoglobulin and antibody diversity are generated and regulated, molecular rearrangement of immunoglobulin genes may be examined as markers of lymphoid malignancies and antibody deficiencies. The results of these studies are providing clues to the molecular bases for some of these diseases.

MOLECULAR GENETIC BASIS OF HUMAN HEAVY CHAIN DISEASES

The heavy chain diseases are by definition B cell lymphoproliferative disorders that bear only a surface heavy chain and lack associated light chain (68). The heavy chain proteins produced are as abnormal as they are markedly truncated. They lack all or most of the variable region information and frequently begin within the constant region at sites that closely correspond to interdomain or exon boundaries. Heavy chain diseases of all three major Ig classes—IgM, IgG, and IgA—are described (68). The molecular basis of this disease has been analyzed in cases of μ heavy chain disease (IgM) and γ heavy chain disease (IgG) (23–25). There are three broad categories of defects that could potentially result in a truncated heavy chain disease protein: (1) an extensive, postsynthetic degradation of the protein; (2) a DNA level deletional rearrangement; or (3) an RNA level defect in splicing or at the site of transcriptional initiation. Intensive examination of the synthesis of the shortened heavy chain proteins revealed that the initial synthesized products were already small and that only limited or no postsynthetic degradation occurred. This focused attention on potential DNA and RNA level defects in the Ig genes of these malignancies.

Owing to the complex process of normally activating an Ig gene, defects accounting for heavy chain disease might be expected to occur at a number of these genetic steps. Mistaken attempts at DNA rearrangements intended to assemble VDJ regions or mediate heavy chain class switches could result in abnormal heavy chains. Similarly, defects in the donor or acceptor splice sites for RNA splicing could eliminate subsegments of the variable and constant regions. Molecular analysis of such heavy chain disease cases to date have revealed multiple defects. A μ heavy chain disease had a DNA level insertion/deletion event that eliminated a normal J_H donor splice site and necessitated an aberrant RNA splice. This resulted in the hydrophobic leader sequence being spliced directly to the C_μ (constant) region (24). This eliminated all of the variable region information and resulted in a transmembrane μ chain molecule containing only constant region information. This truncated μ chain lacked the variable portion of the molecule and failed to bind any light chain (24). In contrast, two γ heavy chain disease ex-

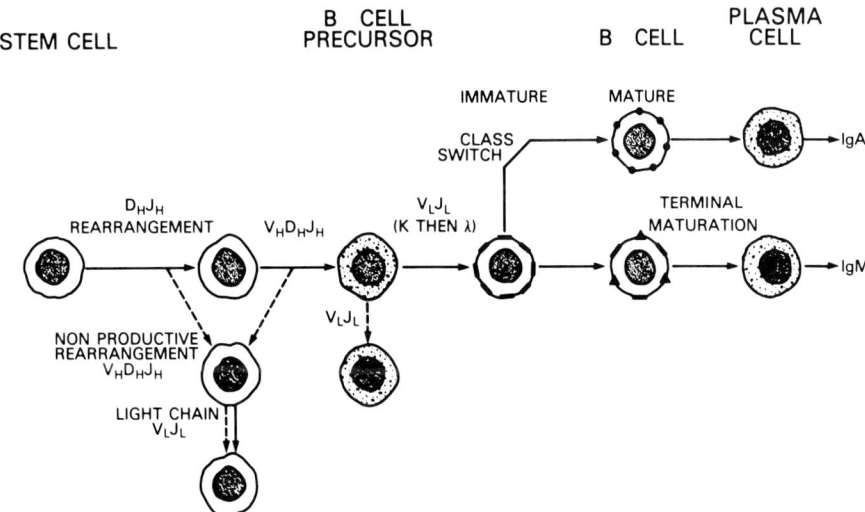

Figure 27–5. B-cell precursor leukemias reflect developmental stages in which rearrangements of a heavy chain diversity (D) segment to the joining (J) segment is followed by the addition of a variable (V) segment. Light chains subsequently rearrange in a κ before λ order. Dashed lines indicate pre B cells, which possess nonproductive, aberrantly rearranged genes. Mature B cell malignancies possess effective heavy and light chain rearrangements and display either surface IgM or another isotype such as IgA if they have undergone a switch. Multiple myeloma represents the terminally differentiated plasma cell stage.

amples have been analyzed and possess abnormal DNA rearrangements that delete portions of the variable region from their heavy chain genes (23, 25). These lost DNA segments correspond to the missing information in these truncated γ chains. Thus, multiple molecular defects representing abnormalities of the complex process that Ig genes normally undergo can account for heavy chain diseases.

B CELL PRECURSORS

"Non T, Non B" Acute Lymphoblastic Leukemias (ALL)

Previously, the majority of acute lymphoblastic leukemias (ALL) were of uncertain cellular origin because they failed to rosette with sheep red blood cells and lacked reactivity with monoclonal antibodies recognizing T cell antigens, yet also lacked the surface Ig of a mature B cell (69, 70). Despite their lack of definitive surface markers of mature T or B cells, these leukemias demonstrated the Ig gene rearrangements of serial B cell precursor stages of development (17, 19, 71). All cases of "non T, non B" acute lymphoblastic leukemia have shown Ig heavy chain gene rearrangements. Approximately 60 per cent of these leukemias retain both their light chain gene classes (κ and λ) in the germline form (Figs. 27–5 and 27–6). This subset represents the more immature B cell precursors and revealed that heavy chain rearrangements preceded light chain gene rearrangements in humans (17, 19). The 40 per cent of cases that are more mature possess light chain rearrangements that occur in κ before λ order. Those pre B cells with κ rearrangements retain germline λ genes. Those that have progressed to λ rearrangement have deleted their κ genes. Thus, the Ig gene patterns in these B cell precursor and mature B cell malignancies revealed a hierarchy of rearrangements in which heavy chain genes preceded light, and κ rearrangements preceded λ (see Figures 27–5 and 27–6).

Synchronous with this developmental cascade of Ig gene rearrangements is a coordinate sequence of cell surface antigen expression (see Figure 27–6) (19, 71). The most immature B cell precur-

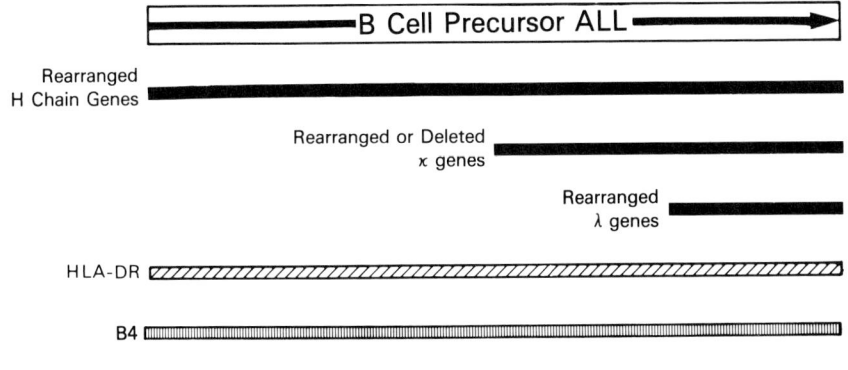

Figure 27–6. A coordinate sequence of Ig gene rearrangements and cell surface antigens in B cell precursor acute lymphoblastic leukemia (ALL). HLA-DR and B_4 antigens precede the common acute lymphoblastic leukemia antigen (CALLA) and light chain rearrangements. The B_1 antigen has a variable time of onset.

sor leukemias proved to have H chain rearrangements and HLA-DR as well as B_4, a B cell–restricted antigen described by Nadler and associates (72). Later in development, pre-B cells add the common acute lymphoblastic leukemia antigen (CALLA) and subsequently rearrange κ or λ light chain genes. The most mature B cell precursor leukemias frequently have the B cell–restricted B_1 antigen, also described by Nadler and colleagues (73).

Even though all the B cell precursor leukemias contain rearranged Ig genes, it has been noted for years that only approximately 25 per cent actually produce cytoplasmic Ig. Some of these leukemias possess an effective rearrangement correctly assembling $V_H D_H J_H$ regions yet do not produce cytoplasmic μ chain. This particular subset of leukemias can at times be induced to differentiate with such agents as phorbol esters, and once they have matured will produce cytoplasmic and occasionally surface Ig (74, 75). Thus, some aspects of the maturational arrest that retained this leukemia at a more primitive stage prevented the production of Ig. The majority of cases still fail to make Ig even after exposure to differentiating agents. Other genetic explanations exist that prevent their Ig production (19). It appears that the most frequent initial rearrangement event on the heavy chain gene results in only an intermediate form of rearrangement in which a diversity (D_H) and a joining (J_H) element are fused ($D_H J_H$). Pre-B cell leukemias that possess only these intermediate ($D_H J_H$) rearrangements while displaying a genetic commitment to B cell maturation are incapable of producing intact heavy chain (see Figure 27–5). Frequently, rearrangements fail to juxtapose gene segments properly and result in ineffective or aberrant rearrangements that also prevent the production of Ig. Such mistaken events can occur on either the heavy or light chain genes. Any cell with either a defective heavy or light chain rearrangement will be incapable of making surface Ig and will thus be retained within a pre-B cell classification (19).

This set of B cell precursor acute lymphoblastic leukemias has been extremely informative in detailing both the correct and mistaken molecular steps in the early differentiation of B cells.

The Lymphoid Blast Crises of Chronic Myelogenous Leukemia (CML)

Chronic myelogenous leukemia (CML) is known to be a clonal disorder that arises from an incredibly pluripotential cell (76). Previous studies utilizing cytogenetic and G6PD isoenzyme analysis indicated that the clonally affected cell in CML had the multipotential capacity to pursue numerous hematopoietic pathways. However, the exact lineage and stage of development of the blast crisis phases of CML had remained uncertain because of this multipotential capacity. This was particularly true for the lymphoid blast crisis phases in which the cell surface markers on the lymphoid blasts such as TdT, CALLA, and HLA-DR could be found on many different cellular lineages. The revelation that these lymphoid blasts possessed rearranged Ig H chain genes and at times light chain genes indicated that they were genetically committed B cell precursors (20, 77). Predictably, a small number of these cases have effectively rearranged and expressed Ig genes and demonstrate cytoplasmic μ chain compatible with the pre-B cell stage (20, 78).

The patterns of Ig gene rearrangements within these lymphoid blasts serve as unique clonal markers for this tumor and have enabled the clonal evolution of CML to be defined at a molecular level (20). This is schematically displayed in Figure 27–7 for one such CML patient examined serially during different phases of his disease. This example details the intact differentiative capacity of the clonally affected cells in this disease at the gene level. During this patient's chronic myelogenous phase, the clonal granulocytes bore the t(9:22) Philadelphia chromosomal marker and displayed germline heavy and light chain genes (see Figure 27–7). This individual had two temporally separated lymphoid blast crisis episodes, and both these lymphoid blasts contained a new cytogenetic marker: the loss of chromosome 7, 45XY–7t(9:22). In addition, both lymphoid crisis episodes possessed the same, identical H chain gene rearrangement pattern. However, one of these lymphoid blasts had progressed to a λ light chain rearrangement, whereas the other had totally germline light chain genes (see Figure 27–7) (20). Thus, the Ig genes have served as clonal markers in CML and indicated that the clonally affected B cell precursors are capable of sequential differentiative steps of heavy chain followed by light chain gene rearrangement. Furthermore, these genetic markers illustrate that the immediate precursor cells that give rise to the clonal expansion, recognized clinically as a lymphoid blast crisis, can indeed vary in their extent of genetic maturation.

IMMUNOGLOBULIN GENE REARRANGEMENTS AS B CELL–ASSOCIATED CLONAL MARKERS IN LYMPHOID NEOPLASMS

Any cell with an obvious commitment to the B cell lineage invariably displays a rearrangement of its Ig H chain and often its L chain genes as well. In contrast, hematopoietic cells that pursue other than the B cell pathway of development usually retain their Ig genes in the germline form. There

DIFFERENTIATION IN CHRONIC MYELOGENOUS LEUKEMIA

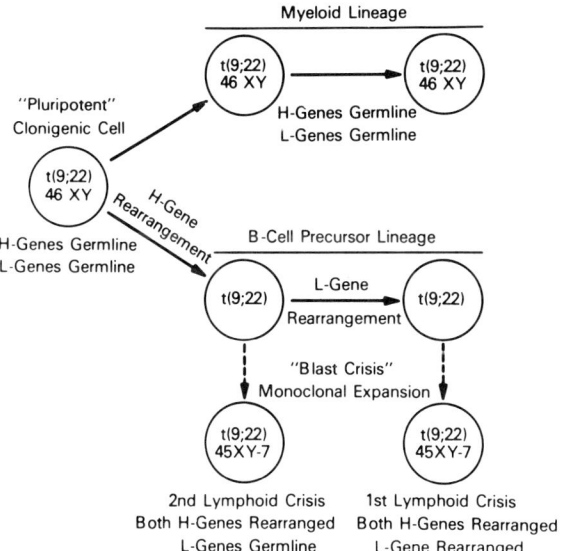

Figure 27–7. The pluripotent clonigenic cell of chronic myelogenous leukemia (CML) bears the Philadelphia chromosomal marker t(9;22). These cells retain germline Ig genes within the acute and chronic myeloid phases but are capable of sequential heavy (H) and light (L) chain gene rearrangements when they pursue the B cell pathway. In the individual whose disease is represented in this diagram, two separate lymphoid blast crisis episodes had identical heavy chain gene rearrangements and indicated loss of chromosome 7. However, the crises were genetically unique in that the first had progressed to λ light chain gene rearrangement, whereas the second involved germline genes. (Reproduced from Bakhshi, A., et al.: New Engl. J. Med. *309*:826, 1983.)

is at times a spillover of Ig H chain rearrangements into other lineages in that occasional T cells (two of 23 examined) and some myeloid cells can bear H chain rearrangements (19, 21). However, light chain genes have uniformly been retained in their germline form within T cells; myeloid, monocytic, histiocytic, and promyelocytic cell lines; and leukemias. Furthermore, the presence of germline Ig genes in most T cells indicates that the antigen-specific T cell receptor was not the product of the Ig genes. Therefore, the detection of simultaneously rearranged heavy chain plus light chain genes within a neoplasm is a strong marker for B cell lineage commitment (21).

Prior to the utilization of DNA rearrangements, the determination that a lymphoid malignancy was of clonal origin was for practical purposes restricted to B cell tumors (79, 80). Investigators accomplished this by examining surface Ig on the tumor cells and showing the exclusive presence of one Ig light chain class, either κ or λ. Occasionally, other markers associated with clonality (e.g., consistent cytogenetic abnormalities or the presence of a single G6PD allele within a heterozygous female patient) have been useful, but their application is more restricted. Quite frequently, all these conventional clonal markers may be unhelpful in evaluating even B lymphoid neoplasms, especially when large numbers of nonneoplastic cells are admixed with malignant cells. In this setting, the examination of lineage-associated DNA rearrangements is quite useful. This takes advantage of the fact that an entirely polyclonal population of normal B cells will possess numerous rearrangements of its Ig genes, and none of these will be above the threshold of detection by Southern blot analysis (36). In contrast, a monoclonal expansion of B cells represents a single cell's progeny, and all involved cells will have the same identifiable DNA rearrangement pattern specific for that tumor. These rearrangements of Ig genes, for example, are sensitive, specific markers capable of identifying even minority populations (1 to 5 per cent) of clonal B cells in tissues of mixed cellularity (21).

The detection of rearranged H and L chain Ig genes has already proved definitive in assigning a B cell lineage to tumors in which extensive characteristics of cell surface antigen, routine histology, and even electron microscopy failed to differentiate lymphomas and carcinomas (21). It has also revealed that hairy cell leukemia has the expected Ig gene rearrangement and appropriately sized mRNA of a mature B cell stage of development, even though these cells possess receptors for interleukin-2 (18). Furthermore, clonal subpopulations of B cells have been detected within known lymphomatous lesions in which T cells actually predominated. The true malignancy within some of these cases is really the minority population of B cells with an associated large number of infiltrating nonneoplastic T cells (21).

The diagnostic choice between a benign and malignant lymphoid proliferation may prove difficult on the basis of histologic grounds alone. This diagnostic dilemma arises perhaps most frequently when the lesion occurs in an immunocompromised host. In this setting, the demonstration of clonality, often based on the presence of a single surface Ig light chain (κ and λ) has served as an important piece of information favoring malignancy. However, nonneoplastic cells may frequently be present within such tissues and obscure any predominance in the κ:λ ratio. In this situation, the use of the DNA level clonal marker of Ig gene rearrangement is most helpful (22, 23). It is important to emphasize that the trait of clonality itself is not tantamount to a verdict of malignancy, nor is it necessarily a warrant for chemo- or radiotherapy. It does, however, often provide a powerful adjunctive piece of information in the diagnostic choice between an atypical hyperplasia and a lymphoma. Furthermore, the specific Ig gene rearrangement within the tissue serves as a clonal marker unique to this population of B cells and will enable such cells to be followed chronologically so that their true natural history can be determined. One example of following the clonal evolution of a tumor at the gene level was illustrated in Figure 27–7 for CML (20). Furthermore, the sensitivity of this method has enabled the detection of clonal cells in such diseases as acute lymphoblastic leukemia within remission bone marrow aspirates when routine histologic examination failed to detect a recurrence.

DNA REARRANGEMENTS IN T CELL ANTIGEN-SPECIFIC RECEPTOR GENES

T cells have been known to demonstrate specific recognition of individual antigens, which indicates that T cells must possess a cell surface receptor for antigen. The demonstration that the genes encoding Ig were retained in their germline form within most human T cells suggested that the antigen-specific receptor present on these T cells was not encoded by the Ig genes. Candidate genes for both the β and the α chains of the two-chain structure that composes the T cell receptor have been isolated (81–83). The gene that encodes the β chain of this heterodimeric receptor molecule is the best characterized to date (Fig. 27–8). It is an entirely separate gene complex located on the long arm of chromosome 7 (7q35) and bears only an evolutionary homology to the Ig locus (81–83). It has two available constant regions (C_1 and C_2), and each has associated diversity (D_1 and D_2) and joining (J_1 and J_2) regions. A set of variable (V) regions has been identified as well. Like the Ig genes, the T cell β chain gene is activated by a rearrangement that may either juxtapose a D to a J segment or make a complete VDJ rearrangement. Owing to a very clever orientation of the recombinatorial signals that flank these gene segments, the V_1 and D_1 segments of the first gene complex are able to recombine with the second cluster of J_2 regions as well as their own J_1 regions (see Figure 27–8).

This β chain locus is mandatorily rearranged in T cells bearing an antigen-specific receptor, whereas it rearranges only rarely in B cells. Thus, this DNA rearrangement offers a T cell–associated clonal marker at the DNA level. This is proving of great value in that no routinely applicable clonal markers previously existed for T cell malignancies. It has been used to demonstrate that Sézary cell leukemia and the adult T cell leukemias (human T cell leukemia/lymphoma virus–positive) are clonal disorders. Furthermore, it will permit looking for clonal T cells as well as clonal B cells within tissues of mixed cellularity. The fact that the β chain rearrangement patterns will be unique to individual malignancies will allow issues of clonal persistence, recurrence, and evolution to be addressed at last within T cell malignancies.

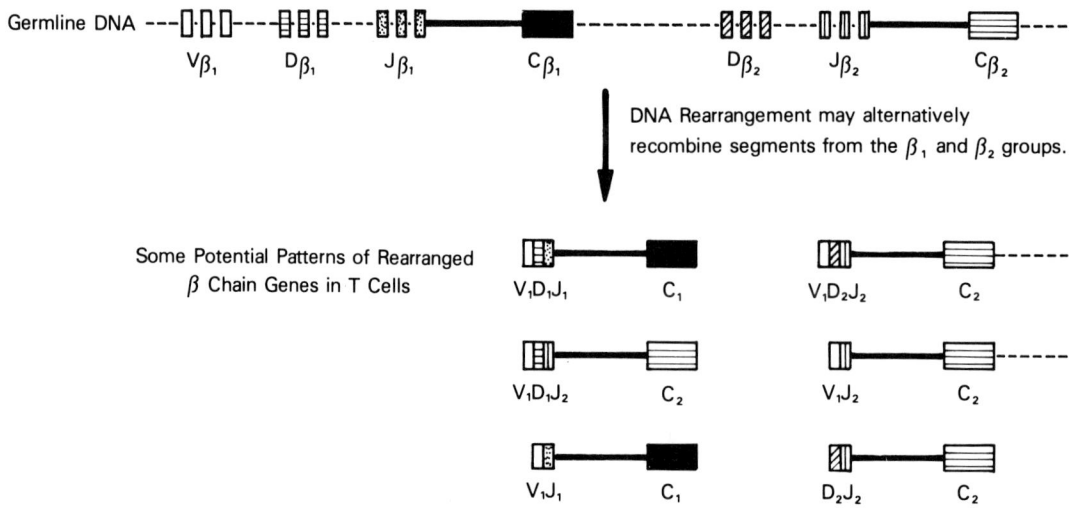

Figure 27–8. A schematic representation of the human β chain gene of the heterodimeric T cell antigen receptor. The two constant regions, C_1 and C_2, have their own associated joining (J_1 and J_2) and diversity (D_1 and D_2) segments. A set of variable (V) regions also has been identified. The spacing of the recombinant signals flanking these segments allows numerous recombinant possibilities. The flexibility during DNA rearrangement markedly augments the diversity of this receptor.

MEDIATION OF CHROMOSOMAL TRANSLOCATIONS BY IMMUNOGLOBULIN GENE LOCI

Specific chromosomal translocations are uniquely or characteristically associated with distinct neoplasms (26, 27). Perhaps the best-characterized translocations are those found in Burkitt's lymphoma. The most common of the chromosomal aberrations found in Burkitt's lymphoma is a t(8;14) reciprocal translocation of chromosome 14 at band q32 and chromosome 8 at band q24 (see Figure 27–8) (28, 29). Provocatively, somatic cell genetic studies placed the human Ig H chain genes to chromosome 14, and later chromosomal in situ hybridization put this locus at 14q32 (84). This association of Burkitt's lymphoma translocation with the Ig gene loci was considerably strengthened when variant forms of the Burkitt's translocation were noted to involve the site of the κ gene locus at 2p11 or the λ genes at 22q11 (85). Curiously, one side of this chromosomal break always occurred at a gene that was a phenotypic landmark for that stage of development, the Ig genes. However, the partner that was consistently used in all these translocations was chromosome 8 at band q24. Because these translocations occurred in malignant Burkitt's cells but not in normal B cells or even in Epstein-Barr virus–transformed B cell lines, it was compelling to think that the locus at 8q24 was actually contributing to the malignant phenotype. A set of cancer-related genes have been identified within humans and other higher eukaryotic organisms (86). These genes are referred to as cellular oncogenes (c-*onc*) and are the normal cellular predecessors of the transforming elements found in a number of retroviruses. Of interest, bursal (B cell) lymphomas of birds were shown to have activated one such oncogene, c-*myc*, by the nearby integration of avian leukosis virus (87). Given this background information, it was particularly relevant when the c-*myc* gene in humans was shown to reside on chromosome 8 at band q24 (Fig. 27–9) (28). The translocations in Burkitt's lymphoma were producing rearrangements that juxtaposed c-*myc* with an active Ig gene locus within these tumors.

Fusion of Burkitt's lymphoma cells with mouse plasmacytoma cells to create somatic cell hybrids revealed important functional details about this translocation (29). As can be seen in Figure 27–9, the normal chromosome 14 in Burkitt's cells produced the heavy chain Ig and thus possessed an effectively recombined $V_H D_H J_H$ and $C\mu$ region responsible for the IgM protein produced. The derivative $4q^+$ chromosome, however, had an aberrantly rearranged Ig locus in which part of chromosome 8 bearing the c-*myc* oncogene had been introduced. The derivative $8q^-$ reciprocally translocated chromosome had donated its c-*myc*

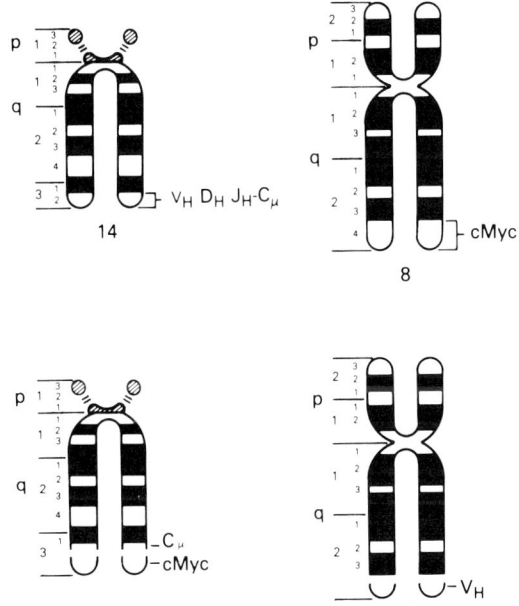

Figure 27–9. A schematic representation of the normal and reciprocally translocated chromosomes in Burkitt's lymphoma t(8;14). A normal chromosome 14 possesses an effective $V_H D_H J_H$ and C_μ responsible for the IgM produced. The normal chromosome 8 retains a nonexpressed copy of c-*myc*. The $14q^+$ chromosome has received a portion of chromosome 8 bearing the c-*myc* gene. The 8q chromosome breaks at 8q24 and receives part of chromosome 14, often including some V_H genes.

gene and had received various portions of the Ig gene locus including some V_H genes. The remaining normal chromosome 8 had a germline copy of c-*myc* present. Of considerable importance was the fact that the translocated c-*myc* gene on the $14q^+$ chromosome was transcriptionally active, whereas the normal c-*myc* gene on chromosome 8 was silent. The repositioning of c-*myc* near to an Ig gene markedly changes the regulatory control of this gene. Because Ig genes are actively transcribed at this stage of differentiation, the mechanisms that augment their expression also may influence the c-*myc* gene. The final result is not only an elevated level of c-*myc* transcription but perhaps also an altered regulation of c-*myc* during the cell cycle of such dividing tumor cells because c-*myc* has been removed from its usual negative control influences.

While the Ig to c-*myc* gene translocations are associated with Burkitt's lymphoma, there are a host of other chromosomal translocations that are uniquely or at least commonly associated with other leukemias and lymphomas. Of interest, the chromosomal breakpoint of 14q32 repeatedly appears within several histologically distinct lymphoid malignancies (Table 27–2). For example, translocations between chromosome 11q13 and 14q32 have been seen in chronic lymphocytic leukemia, small cell lymphomas, diffuse large cell lymphomas (27), and multiple myeloma. A translocation

Table 27–2. CHROMOSOMAL TRANSLOCATIONS IN HUMAN LYMPHOID NEOPLASMS

Translocation	Neoplasm
t(8;14) (q24;q32)	Burkitt's lymphoma
t(8;22) (q24;q11)	
t(2;8) (p11;q24)	
t(11;14) (q13;q32)	Chronic lymphocytic leukemia
	Small cell lymphocytic lymphoma
	Diffuse large cell lymphoma
	Multiple myeloma
t(14;18) (q32;q21)	Follicular small cleaved cell lymphoma
	Follicular mixed cell lymphoma
	Follicular large cell lymphoma
	Diffuse histiocytic lymphoma

between 18q21 and 14q32 also has been observed in follicular and some diffuse lymphomas (27). Thus, the H chain gene locus at 14q32 may be a common denominator involved in mediating translocations within a variety of B cell malignancies. By analogy with the c-*myc* event in Burkitt's lymphoma, it is likely that there are transformation-related genes being introduced by loci at 11q13 and 18q21, respectively (88, 89). Because none of the known c-*onc* genes maps to these locations, these translocations are proving useful in identifying new oncogenes (89). Chromosomal translocations may serve as a potent new gene map. One side of the chromosomal break may contain a transcriptionally active gene that is a phenotypic landmark of that particular stage of development (e.g., Ig genes). The other side of the break may contribute an oncogene that, when introduced into its new surroundings, may have a markedly altered regulation that promotes the transformed state.

ANTIBODY DEFICIENCY DISEASES

Progress in characterization of antibody deficiency diseases has been greatest in the agammaglobulinemias (89). X-linked agammaglobulinemia is the congenital form of this disease in which there is evidence for an X-linked inheritance. All other forms of agammaglobulinemia have been classified as common varied agammaglobulinemia. Detailed examination of the proteins produced by B cell lines and other in vitro analogues of B lymphocytes from patients with agammaglobulinemia have provided some molecular bases for further classification of this disease categories. These categories will be discussed subsequently.

X-Linked Agammaglobulinemia

X-linked agammaglobulinemia has been characterized by the absence of all developmental forms of B lymphocytes beyond the stage of pre-B cells (90). Schwaber and colleagues (56, 91) have found that pre B cells from three patients with X-linked agammaglobulinemia produced the constant region of μ chain without an associated variable region. Unpublished evidence shows that this truncated μ chain is produced following DJ_H gene rearrangement, similar to the intermediate products described by Reth and Alt (53). As detailed earlier, this evidence suggests that the defect in this disease is a failure of VDJ gene translocation and rearrangement. The block in VDJ gene rearrangement in these patients does not appear to be absolute, as indicated by the presence of extremely low levels of immunoglobulin in serum. Rather, the defect must be characterized by an extremely reduced rate constant for the process of rearrangement, which would result in low levels of serum immunoglobulin and the ability to clear small amounts of antigen and would be correlated with the presence of small numbers of B lymphocytes.

Common Varied Agammaglobulinemia

Common varied agammaglobulinemia is characterized in most cases by the presence of immature B lymphocytes that fail to diversify into subsequent heavy chain isotypes and fail to undergo terminal differentiation (89, 92, 93). The isotypes present on their B lymphocytes are IgD and IgM, the first two constant regions in the linear array of constant region genes. Evidence for a molecular basis for this failure to progress is lacking to date.

"NONSECRETORY" AGAMMAGLOBULINEMIA

"Nonsecretory" agammaglobulinemia is a subtype of common varied agammaglobulinemia in which patients have large numbers of circulating peripheral B lymphocytes as well as plasma cells in their bone marrow (94, 95). The antibody deficiency of these patients results from a failure of these fully differentiated cells to secrete the immunoglobulin that they produce. Electron micrographs of cells from these patients reveal extensive phagocytic vesicles surrounding the Golgi apparatus, suggestive of an autophagocytic end for the antibody molecules (Schwaber and Schwaber, unpublished data). Schwaber and associates (95) have reported that the failure to secrete immunoglobulin is correlated with production of an undersized heavy chain. Molecular studies in progress suggest that there is a deletion of the 5' or variable region terminus of the heavy chains from "nonsecretory" agammaglobulinemia (Schwaber, unpublished results).

Hyper-IgM Syndrome

Hyper-IgM syndrome, formerly termed dysgammaglobulinemia, is associated with a failure of heavy chain isotype switching (93). Peripheral lymphocytes circulate in normal numbers in these patients, but they are limited to production of IgM and, in some cases, IgD (96). Serum levels of IgM and IgD can reach ten times normal. However, the antibody present in these patients seems not to be protective, even against the polysaccharide antigens of bacteria. McLane and colleagues described the product of a T cell hybrid that induced production of IgG by B lymphocytes from these patients, suggesting that this disease may result from a defect in the T cell regulation of B lymphocyte isotype diversification (97).

Other Antibody Deficiency Diseases

Molecular characterization of other antibody deficiency states, especially of the severe combined immunodeficiencies, has not yet been reported. Because of the complexity of the gene rearrangements necessary to produce the diversity of antibody specificities, it seems likely that other steps in gene rearrangement will be identified with antibody deficiency diseases in the near future.

References

1. Burnet, F. M.: *The Clonal Selection Theory of Acquired Immunity.* Nashville, Vanderbilt University Press, 1959.
2. Dreyer, W., and Bennett, J. C., : The molecular basis of antibody formation: a paradox. Proc. Natl. Acad. Sci. U.S.A. *54*:864, 1965.
3. Kindt, T., Capra, J.: *The Antibody Enigma.* New York, Plenum Press, 1984.
4. Osmond, D., and Nossal, G.: Differentiation of lymphocytes in mouse bone marrow. Cell. Immunol. *13*:132, 1974.
5. Raff, M., Megson, M., et al.: Early production of intracellular IgM by B lymphocyte precursors in mouse. Nature. *259*:224, 1976.
6. Cooper, M.: Pre-B cells; normal and abnormal development. J. Clin. Immunol. *1*:81, 1981.
7. Abney, E., Cooper, M., et al.: Sequential expression of immunoglobulin in developing mouse B lymphocytes. J. Immunol. *120*:2041, 1978.
8. Leder, P.: The genetics of antibody diversity. Sci. Amer. *246*:102, 1982.
9. Tonegawa, S.: Somatic generation of antibody diversity. Nature *302*:575, 1983.
10. Hozumi, N., and Tonegawa, S.: Evidence for somatic rearrangement of immunoglobulin genes coding for variable and constant regions. Proc. Natl. Acad. Sci. U.S.A. *73*:3628, 1976.
11. Brack, G., Hirama, M., et al.: A complete immunoglobulin gene is created by somatic recombination. Cell *15*:1, 1978.
12. Seidman, J. G., and Leder, P.: The arrangement and rearrangement of antibody genes. Nature *276*:790, 1978.
13. Early, P., Huang, H., et al.: An immunoglobulin heavy chain variable region gene is generated from three segments of DNA V_H, D, and J_H. Cell *22*:918, 1980.
14. Hieter, P. A., Korsmeyer, S. J., et al.: Human immunoglobulin kappa light chain genes are deleted or rearranged in lambda producing B cells. Nature *290*:368, 1981.
15. Cooper, M.: B cell differentiation. In *Primary Immunodeficiency Diseases.* Wedgwood, R., Rosen, F., et al. (eds.), New York, A. R. Liss, 1983, pp. 25–29.
16. Schwaher, J.: Agammaglobulinemia in vitro: lymphoid cell lines and somatic cell hybrids. In *Primary Immunodeficiencies.* Seligmann, M., Hitzig, W. (eds.), Amsterdam, Elsevier/North Holland, 1980, pp. 49–57.
17. Korsmeyer, S. J., Hieter, P. A., et al.: A developmental hierarchy of immunoglobulin gene rearrangements in human leukemic pre-B cells. Proc. Natl. Acad. Sci. U.S.A. *78*:7096, 1981.
18. Korsmeyer, S. J., Greene, W. C., et al.: Rearrangement and expression of immunoglobulin genes and expression of Tac antigen in hairy cell leukemia. Proc. Natl. Acad. Sci. U.S.A. *80*:4522, 1983.
19. Korsmeyer, S. J., Arnold, A., et al.: Immunoglobulin gene rearrangement and cell surface antigen expression in acute lymphocytic leukemias of T-cell and B-cell precursor origins. J. Clin. Invest. *71*:30, 1983.
20. Bakhshi, A., Minowada, J., et al.: Lymphoid blast crisis of chronic myelogenous leukemia represents stages in the development of B-cell precursors. New Engl. J. Med. *309*:826, 1983.
21. Arnold, A., Cossman, J., et al.: Immunoglobulin gene rearrangements as unique clonal markers in human lymphoid neoplasms. New Engl. J. Med. *309*:1593, 1983.
22. Cleary, M. I., Warnke, R., et al.: Monoclonality of lymphoproliferative lesions in cardiac transplant recipients. New Engl. J. Med. *310*:477, 1984.
23. Alexander, A., Steinmetz, M., et al.: γ heavy chain disease in man: cDNA sequence supports partial gene deletion model. Proc. Natl. Acad. Sci. U.S.A. *79*:3260, 1982.
24. Bakhshi, A., Guglielmi, P., et al.: A DNA insertion/deletion necessitates an aberrant RNA splice accounting for a human μ heavy chain disease protein. Proc. Natl. Acad. Sci. USA *83*:2689, 1986.
25. Guglielmi, P., Bakhshi, A., et al.: DNA deletion in human gamma heavy chain disease. Clin. Res. *32*:348A, 1984.
26. Rowley, J. D., and Testa, J. R.: Chromosome abnormalities in malignant hematologic diseases. Adv. Cancer Res. *36*:103, 1982.
27. Yunis, J. J.: The chromosomal basis of human neoplasia. Science *221*:227, 1983.
28. Taub, R., Kirsch, I., et al.: Translocation of the c-myc gene into the immunoglobulin heavy chain locus in human Burkitt's lymphoma and murine plasmacytoma cells. Proc. Natl. Acad. Sci. U.S.A. *79*:7837, 1982.
29. Nishikura, K., Ar-Rushdi, A., et al.; Differential expression of the normal and of the translocated human c-myc oncogenes in B cells. Proc. Natl. Acad. Sci. U.S.A. *80*:4822, 1983.
30. Malcolm, S., Barton, P., et al.: Localization of human immunoglobulin light chain variable region genes to the short arm of chromosome 2 by *in situ* hybridization. Proc. Natl. Acad. Sci. U.S.A. *79*:4957, 1982.
31. Hieter, P. A., Max, E. E., et al.: Cloned human and mouse kappa immunoglobulin constant and J region genes conserve homology in functional segments. Cell *22*:197, 1980.
32. Hieter, P. A., Jr., Maizel, J. V., et al.: Evolution of human immunoglobulin J region genes. J. Biol. Chem. *257*:1516, 1982.
33. McBride, O. W., Hieter, P. A., et al.: Chromosomal location of human kappa and lambda immunoglobulin light chain constant region genes. J. Exp. Med. *155*:1480, 1982.
34. Hieter, P. A., Hollis, G. R., et al.: The clustered arrangement of immunoglobulin lambda constant region genes in man. Nature *294*:536, 1981.
35. Taub, R. A., Hollis, G. F., et al.: The variable amplification of immunoglobulin lambda light chain genes in human populations. Nature *304*:172, 1983.
36. Korsmeyer, S. J., Hieter, P. A., et al.: Normal human B-cells display ordered light-chain gene rearrangements and deletions. J. Exp. Med. *156*:975, 1982.
37. Siminovitch, K. A., Bakhshi, A., et al.: A uniform deleting element mediates the loss of κ genes in human B cells. Nature *316*:260, 1985.

38. Siebenlist, U., Ravetch, J. V., et al.: Human immunoglobulin D segments encoded in tandem multigenic families. Nature 294:631, 1981.
39. Ravetch, J. V., Siebenlist, U., et al.: The structure of the human immunoglobulin μ locus: characterization of embryonic and rearranged J and D genes. Cell 27:583, 1981.
40. Knap, M. R., Liu, C.-P., et al.: Simultaneous expression of immunoglobulin μ and δ heavy chains by a clonal B-cell lymphoma: a single copy of the V_H gene is shared by two adjacent C_H genes. Proc. Natl. Acad. Sci. U.S.A. 79:2996, 1982.
41. Moore, K. W., Rogers, J., et al.: Expression of IgD may use both DNA rearrangement and RNA splicing mechanisms. Proc. Natl. Acad. Sci. U.S.A. 78:1800, 1981.
42. Davis, M. M., Kim, S. K., et al.: DNA sequences mediating class switching in α-immunoglobulins. Science 209:1360, 1980.
43. Kataoka, T., Miyata, T., et al.: Repetitive sequences in class switch recombination regions of immunoglobulin heavy chain genes. Cell 23:357, 1981.
44. Marcu, K. B., Lang, R. B., et al.: A model for the molecular requirements of immunoglobulin heavy chain class switching. Nature 298:87, 1982.
45. Ravetch, J. V., Kirsch, I. R., et al.: Evolutionary approach to the question of immunoglobulin heavy chain switching: evidence from cloned human and mouse genes. Proc. Natl. Acad. Sci. U.S.A. 77:6734, 1980.
46. Flanagan, J. G., and Rabbitts, T. H.: Arrangement of human immunoglobulin heavy chain constant region genes implies evolutionary duplication of a segment containing γ, ε, α genes. Nature 300:709, 1982.
47. Kelley, D., Coleclough, C., et al.: Functional significance and evolutionary development of the 5' terminal regions of immunoglobulin variable-region genes. Cell 29:681, 1982.
48. Kataoka, T., Nikaido, T., et al.: The nucleotide sequences of rearranged and germ line immungloulin VH genes of a mouse myeloma MC101 and evolution of VH genes in mouse. J. Biol. Chem 257:277, 1982.
49. Clarke, C., Berenson, J., et al.: An immunoglobulin promoter region is unaltered by DNA rearrangement and somatic mutation during B-cell development. Nucl. Acids Res. 10:7731, 1982.
50. Gillies, S., Morrison, S., et al.: A tissue-specific transcription enhancer element is located in the major intron of a rearranged immunoglobulin heavy chain gene. Cell 33:717, 1983.
51. Blobel, G., and Dobberstein, B.: Transfer to proteins across membranes. II. Reconstitution of functional rough microsomes from heterologous components. J. Cell Biol. 67:852, 1975.
52. von Heijne, G.: How signal sequences maintain cleavage specificity. J. Mol. Biol. 173:243, 1984.
53. Reth, M., and Alt, F.: Novel immunoglobulin heavy chains are produced from DJh gene segment rearrangements in lymphoid cells. Nature 312:418, 1984.
54. Sakano, H., Maki, R., et al.: Two types of somatic recombination are necessary for the generation of complete immunoglobulin heavy chain genes. Nature 286:676, 1980.
55. Kurosawa, Y., von Boehmer, H., et al.: Identification of D segments of immunoglobulin heavy chain genes and their rearrangement in T lymphocytes. Nature 290:565, 1981.
56. Schwaber, J., Molgaard, H., et al.: Early pre-B cells from normal and X-linked agammaglobulinemia produce Cμ without associated VH region. Nature 304:355, 1983.
57. Early, P., Rogers, J., et al.: Two mRNAs can be produced from a single immunoglobulin μ gene by alternative RNA processing pathways. Cell 20:313, 1980.
58. Alt, F., Bothwell, A., et al.: Synthesis of secreted and membrane bound μ heavy chains is directed by mRNAs that differ at their 3' ends. Cell 20:293, 1980.
59. Liu, C., Tucker, P., et al.: Mapping of heavy chain genes for mouse immunoglobulin M and D. Science 209:1348, 1980.
60. Kataoka, T., Kawakami, T., et al.: Rearrangement of immunoglobulin gamma-1 gene and mechanism for heavy chain class switch. Proc. Natl. Acad. Sci. U.S.A. 77:919, 1980.
61. Obata, M., Kataoka, T., et al.: Structure of a rearranged gamma-1 chain gene and its implication to immunoglobulin class switch mechanism. Proc. Natl. Acad. Sci. 78:2437, 1981.
62. Ravetch, J., Kirsch, I., et al.: Evolutionary approach to the question of immunoglobulin heavy chain switching: evidence from cloned human and mouse genes. Proc Natl. Acad. Sci. 77:6734, 1980.
63. Yaoita, Y., Kumagai, Y.,. et al.: Expression of lymphocytes surface IgE does not require switch recombination. Nature 297:697, 1982.
64. Brown, N., Liu, C., et al.: Immunoglobulin JH, Cμ, and C-gamma gene rearrangements in human B lymphocytes clonally transformed by Epstein-Barr virus. Proc. Natl. Acad. Sci. U.S.A., 1985, 82:556, 1985.
65. Webb, C. F., Cooper, M. D., et al.: Immunoglobulin gene rearrangement and deleting in human Epstein-Barr virus–transformed cell lines producing different IgG and IgA subclasses. Proc. Natl. Acad. Sci. USA 82:5495, 1982.
66. Bothwell, A., Paskind, M., et al.: Heavy chain variable region contribution to the NPb family of antibodies: somatic mutation evident in a gamma-2a variable region. Cell 24:625, 1981.
67. Griffiths, G., Berek, C., et al.: Somatic mutation and the maturation of immune response to 2-phenyl oxazolone. Nature 312:271, 1984.
68. Seligmann, M., Mihaesco, E., et al.: Heavy chain disease: Current findings and concepts. Immunol. Rev. 48:145, 1979.
69. Chessells, J. M., Hardisty, R. M., et al.: Acute lymphoblastic leukemia in children: classification and prognosis. Lancet 2:1307, 1977.
70. Brouet, J. C., Valensi, F., et al.: Immunological classification of acute lymphoblastic leukemias: evaluation of its clinical significance in a hundred patients. Br. J. Haematol. 33:319, 1976.
71. Nadler, L. M., Korsmeyer, S. J., et al.: The B-cell origin of non-T-cell acute lymphoblastic leukemia: a model for discrete stages of neoplastic and normal pre-B-cell differentiation. J. Clin. Invest. 74:332, 1984.
72. Nadler, L. M., Anderson, K. C., et al.: B_4, a human B-lymphocyte associated antigen expressed on normal, mitogen-activated, and malignant B lymphocytes. J. Immunol. 131:244, 1983.
73. Nadler, L. M., Ritz, J., et al.: A unique cell surface antigen identifying lymphoid malignancies of B-cell origin. J. Clin. Invest. 67:134, 1981.
74. Cossman, J., Neckers, L. M., et al.: Induction of differentiation in the primitive B cell of common, acute lymphoblastic leukemia. New Engl. J. Med. 307:1251, 1982.
75. Nadler, L. M., Ritz, J., et al.: Induction of human B-cell antigens in non-T cell acute lymphoblastic leukemia. J. Clin. Invest. 70:433, 1982.
76. Barr, R. D., and Fialkow, P. J.: Clonal origin of chronic myelocytic leukemia. New Engl. J. Med. 289:307, 1973.
77. Ford, A. M., Molgaard, H. V., et al.: Immunoglobulin gene organization and expression in hematopoietic stem cell leukemia. Embo. J. 2:997, 1983.
78. LeBien, T. W., Hozier, H., et al.: Origin of chronic myelocytic leukemia in a precursor of pre-B lymphocytes. New Engl. J. Med. 301:144, 1979.
79. Aisenberg, A. C.: Cell surface markers in lymphoproliferative disease. New Engl. J. Med. 304:331, 1978.
80. Levy, R., Warnke, R., et al.: The monoclonality of human B-cell lymphomas. J. Exp. Med. 145:1014, 1977.
81. Yanagi, Y., Yoshikai, Y., et al.: A human T-cell specific

cDNA clone encodes a protein having extensive homology to immunoglobulin chains. Nature 308:145, 1984.
82. Hedrick, S. M., Cohen, D. I., et al.: Isolation of cDNA clones encoding T-cell specific membrane-associated proteins. Nature 308:149, 1984.
83. Saito, H., Kranz, D. M., et al.: Complete primary structure of a heterodimeric T-cell receptor deduced from cDNA sequences. Nature 309:757, 1984.
84. Kirsch, I. R., Morton, C. C., et al.: Human immunoglobulin heavy chain genes map to a region of translocation in malignant B lymphocytes. Science 216:301, 1982.
85. Lenoir, G. M., Preud'homme, J. L., et al.: Correlation between immunoglobulin light chain expression and variant translocation in Burkitt's lymphoma. Nature 298:474, 1982.
86. Bishop, J. M.: Cancer genes come of age. Cell 32:1018, 1983.
87. Hayward, W. S., Nell, B. G., et al.: Activation of a cellular onc gene by promoter insertion in ALV-induced lymphoid leukosis. Nature 290:475, 1981.
88. Tsujimato, Y., Yunis, J., et al.: Molecular cloning of the chromosomal breakpoint of B-cell lymphomas and leukemias with the t(11;14) chromosome translocation. Science 224:1403, 1984.
89. Rosen, F., Cooper, M., et al.: The primary immunodeficiencies. New Engl. J. Med. 311:235, 1984.
90. Pearl, E., Vogler, L., et al.: B lymphocyte precursors in human bone marrow: an analysis of normal individuals and patients with antibody deficient states. J. Immunol. 120:1169, 1978.
91. Schwaber, J.: Pre-B cells in X-linked agammaglobulinemia, Birth Defects 19:177, 1983.
92. Schwaber, J., Lazarus, H., et al.: Bone marrow derived lymphoid cell lines from patients with agammaglobulinemia. J. Clin. Invest. 62:302, 1978.
93. Schwaber, J., and Rosen, F.: Isotypes of surface immunoglobulin from patients with immune deficiency, J. Clin. Immunol. 2:30, 1982.
94. Schwaber, J., and Rosen, F.: Somatic cell hybrid of mouse myeloma cells and B lymphocytes from a patient with agammaglobulinemia: failure to secrete human immunoglobulin. J. Immunol. 122:1849, 1978.
95. Schwaber, J., and Rosen F.: Altered heavy chain produced by lymphoid cell lines from patients with "non-secretory" agammaglobulinemia. J. Mol. Cell Immunol. 1:279, 1984.
96. Schwaber, J., Lazarus, H., et al.: IgM restricted production of immunoglobulin by lymphoid cell lines from patients with immunodeficiency with hyper-IgM (dysgammaglobulinemia). Clin. Immunol. Immunopathol. 19:91, 1981.
97. Mayer, L., Posnett, D., et al.: Human malignant T-cells capable of inducing an immunoglobulin class switch. J. Exp. Med. 161:134, 1985.

THE IMMUNE SYSTEM

CHAPTER 28
Primary Immunodeficiencies and Serum Complement Defects

FRED S. ROSEN
HARVEY R. COLTEN

INTRODUCTION 878
PRIMARY B CELL DEFICIENCIES 878
Transient Hypogammaglobulinemia of Infancy
X-Linked Agammaglobulinemia (Congenital Agammaglobulinemia, Bruton's Disease)
X-Linked Immunodeficiency With Increased IgM Concentration
Selective Immunoglobulin Deficiencies (Dysgammaglobulinemia)
Transcobalamin II (TCII) Deficiency
Varied Unclassified Immunodeficiency Disorders (Acquired Hypogammaglobulinemia)
PRIMARY T CELL DEFICIENCIES 884
Severe Combined Immunodeficiency
Immunodeficiency With Ataxia Telangiectasia
Immunodeficiency With Thrombocytopenia and Eczema (Wiskott-Aldrich Syndrome)
Congenital Thymic Aplasia (DiGeorge's Syndrome)
Immunodeficiency With Unusual Response to Epstein-Barr Virus
SECONDARY IMMUNODEFICIENCY INFECTION FOLLOWING SPLENECTOMY 890
SECONDARY HYPOGAMMAGLOBULINEMIA 890
PEDIATRIC AIDS 890
THE COMPLEMENT SYSTEM 892
The Activation Phase
  Down-Regulation
The Terminal Phase
Complement and Inflammation
Complement Receptors
Genetics and Biosynthesis
Genetic Deficiencies
  Hereditary Angioneurotic Edema
  Acquired C1 INH Deficiency
  Early Complement Component Deficiencies
  Deficiencies of C3 and the C3 Control Proteins
  Late Complement Component Deficiencies
Acquired Defects

INTRODUCTION

Five classes of antibodies are known: IgG, IgM, IgD, IgA, and IgE. Four subclasses of IgG have been described—IgG1, IgG2, IgG3, and IgG4—and two subclasses of IgA are known—IgA1 and IgA2. IgM is found principally in the vascular compartment. Most of the antibodies to the lipopolysaccharide antigens belong to the IgM class. They fix complement efficiently and may be important in protection against gram-negative sepsis, but they may also cause rapid in vivo hemolytic anemia. IgG is distributed equally in the vascular and extravascular spaces. IgG antibodies are most important in defense against pyogenic organisms. Macrophages and monocytes have receptors only for IgG1 and IgG3. Because anti-Rh antibodies belong exclusively to these two subclasses and do not fix complement, this IgG receptor is of importance in the erythrophagocytosis of red cells coated with anti-Rh antibodies. IgG1, IgG2, and IgG3, but not IgG4, fix complement. Most of the antibody to the linear polysaccharides of bacterial capsules belong to the IgG2 subclass.

IgA is found principally in all the body secretions. It is usually secreted as a dimer, and the monomers are joined together by a J chain. As IgA passes through epithelial cells, another polypeptide chain, secretory piece, is added to IgA to facilitate secretion. IgM is pentameric, and its five monomers also are held together by J chain.

IgE is the principal anaphylactic antibody in humans. Mast cells have receptors for IgE, and when cell-bound IgE molecules are cross-linked by antigen, mediators of anaphylaxis are released from mast cells. IgD is found mostly as a surface immunoglobulin of immature B lymphocytes. Its function is not entirely clear.

Only two types of light chains are known—κ and λ. The heavy chains also are designated by Greek letters—γ for IgG, α for IgA, δ for IgD, μ for IgM, and ϵ for IgE. Thus, a molecular formula can be written for all antibodies, for example: $\gamma 1_2 \kappa_2$, $(\mu_2 \lambda_2)_5$, $(\alpha 2_2 \kappa_2)_2$.

PRIMARY B CELL DEFICIENCIES

The outstanding clinical manifestation of patients with quantitative or qualitative defects of B cell function is recurrent, invasive infection with pyogenic bacteria. These infections are not different from those observed in normal individuals of the same age (pyoderma, pharyngitis, sinusitis, otitis media, pneumonia, sepsis, and meningitis).

They respond normally to antimicrobial therapy but are notable for their frequency and often for their severity. There is a diminished or absent antibody response to injected antigens or to infection, which has given rise to the term introduced by Swiss workers—the antibody deficiency syndrome. Because this basic pathogenic defect results in failure of opsonization, an essential step in the control of invasion by pyogenic bacteria, it is not surprising that an indistinguishable clinical picture has been observed in patients with deficiency of the third component of complement (C3). Because cellular immune responses of the T cells are preserved, these patients respond normally to most viral, fungal, and mycobacterial infections. A number of different primary disorders can give rise to the antibody deficiency syndrome (Table 28–1) (1).

Transient Hypogammaglobulinemia of Infancy

Normally, the synthesis of immunoglobulins in response to infection and other antigenic stimuli begins after birth. However, if the fetus is infected in utero after the twentieth week of gestation by rubella virus, cytomegalovirus, *Toxoplasma,* or syphilis, it can mount an impressive antibody response to the invasive pathogen. This antibody response, consisting primarily of IgM and to a lesser extent of IgA and IgG antibodies, can be helpful in the diagnosis of prenatal infection. A cord or neonatal serum level of IgM in excess of 20 mg per 100 ml is considered presumptive evidence of intrauterine infection. The level of IgG globulin, which is passively acquired by transplacental passage, falls rapidly during the first

Table 28–1. CLASSIFICATION OF PRIMARY IMMUNODEFICIENCY DISEASES*

	Predominantly Antibody Defects				
Designation	Serum Ig and Antibodies	Circulating B Cells	Presumed Pathogenesis	Inheritance	Associated Features
X-Linked agammaglobulinemia	All isotypes decreased	Usually absent	Intrinsic defect pre- B- to B-cell differentiation	XL[a]	—
X-Linked hypogammaglobulinemia with growth hormone deficiency	All isotypes descreased	Usually absent	Unknown	XL	Short stature
Autosomal recessive agammaglobulinemia	All isotypes decreased	Decreased	Unknown	AR[a]	—
Ig deficiency with increased IgM (and IgD) ("hyper-IgM syndrome")	IgM and IgD increased or normal, other isotypes decreased	IgM- and IgD-bearing cells normal, others absent	Isotype switch defect	Various: XL, AR, unknown	—
IgA deficiency	IgA$_1$ and IgA$_2$ decreased, with or without IgG$_2$, IgG$_3$, or IgG$_4$ decrease	Normal	Failure of terminal differentiation	Various: AR, unknown	Frequent in families with CVID
	IgA$_1$ or IgA$_2$ decreased	Normal	Chromosomal deletion at 14q32 in some patients	AR	—
Selective deficiency of other Ig isotypes	Decrease in one or more isotype, other isotypes normal or increased	Unknown	Defects of isotype differentiation	Unknown	—
κ-Chain deficiency	Ig(κ) decreased; antibody response normal or decreased	Normal or κ$^+$ decreased	In some patients point mutations at chromosome 2p11	Unknown	—
ID with thymoma	All isotypes decreased	Absent or very low	Unknown	Unknown	Thymoma, anemia, eosinopenia
Transient hypogammaglobulinemia of infancy	IgG and IgA decreased	Normal	Terminal differentiation maturation defect; delayed maturation of helper function in some	Unknown	Frequent in families with other IDs

*Report of a WHO Scientific Group.
[a]XL—X linked; AR—autosomal recessive.

Table continued on following page

Table 28–1. CLASSIFICATION OF PRIMARY IMMUNODEFICIENCY DISEASES (Continued)

Designation	Serum Ig and Antibodies	Circulating B Cells	Circulating T Cells	Presumed Pathogenesis	Inheritance	Associated Features
Combined Immunodeficiency						
Common variable immunodeficiency						
Predominant antibody deficiency	Various decreases of multiple isotypes	Normal or decreased	Usually normal	Intrinsic B-cell defect; low B-cell number; defective helper function; antibodies to B cells	AR, AD,[a] or unknown	
Predominant CMI defect	Various decreases of multiple isotypes	Normal	Normal or decreased	Activated suppressor-T-cell function; markedly reduced T-cell numbers; autoantibodies to T cells	Unknown, AR	Autoimmune phenomena
Severe combined immunodeficiency						
Reticular dysgenesis	Decreased	Decreased	Decreased	Defective differentiation of T and B cells; lymphomyeloid maturation defect	AR	Pancytopenia
Low T- and B-cell numbers	Decreased	Decreased	Decreased	Maturation defect of both T and B cells	AR or XL	—
Low T-, normal B-cell numbers	Normal or decreased	Normal	Decreased	Lymphoid maturation defect of both T and B cells	AR or XL	—
Adenosine deaminase deficiency	Progressive decrease	Decreased	Decreased	T-Cell (and B-cell) defects from toxic metabolites due to enzyme deficiency	AR	Dysostosis in some
Purine nucleoside phosphorylase deficiency	Progressive decrease	Normal	Progressive decrease	T-Cell defect from metabolites due to enzyme deficiency	AR	Anemia, mental retardation
MHC class I deficiency ("bare lymphocyte syndrome")	Normal or decreased	Normal	Normal (CMI defective)	Defect of gene transcription	AR	—
MHC class II deficiency	Decreased or normal	Normal	Normal (CMI defective)	Defect of gene transcription	AR	Intestinal malabsorption

[a] AD—autosomal dominant.

month of life, levels off during the second month, and then soon begins to rise. Rarely, there is delay in the maturation of B cells and their immunologic function; the level of IgG globulins received by passive transfer from the mother continues to fall and is not adequately raised by immunoglobulins synthesized by the infant, so that within a few months the total gamma globulin level is much lower than usual for that age. The infants have overt infections, unexplained episodes of fever, and often bronchitis with wheezing. The disease probably results from a failure of adequate T cell activity that ordinarily helps B cell function. Regular injections of gamma globulin (to be discussed) will protect these infants from severe, invasive infections. The injections may be discontinued when the IgG globulin levels begin to rise toward normal levels, usually before the age of 3 years. The cause of this transient hypogammaglobulinemia is not known. Normal numbers of B cells are present in the circulation of affected infants (2) (see also Chapter 25).

X-Linked Agammaglobulinemia (Congenital Agammaglobulinemia, Bruton's Disease)

X-linked agammaglobulinemia usually manifests itself in the second year of life, although the onset of the characteristically severe, recurrent infections may begin at any age from 8 months to 3 years. The infections are those caused by the common pyogenic organisms—*Staphylococcus aureus, Diplococcus pneumoniae, Neisseria meningitidis, Hemophilus influenzae*, and, less often, *beta-hemolytic Streptococcus* or *Pseudomonas*. They differ from infections in normal children only in their frequency, severity, and tendency for infection with the same organism to occur more than once. Pyoderma, purulent conjunctivitis, pharyngitis, otitis media, sinusitis, bronchitis, pneumonia, empyema, purulent arthritis, meningitis, and sepsis occur with surprising frequency and may be associated with unusually high fever and unexpected elevation or depression of the leukocyte count. A

Table 28–1. CLASSIFICATION OF PRIMARY IMMUNODEFICIENCY DISEASES (*Continued*)

		ID Associated with Other Major Defects				
Designation	*Serum Ig and Antibodies*	*Circulating B Cells*	*Circulating T Cells*	*Presumed Pathogenesis*	*Inheritance*	*Associated Features*
Wiskott-Aldrich syndrome	Decreased IgM: antibody to polysaccharides particularly decreased	Normal	Progressive decrease	Cell membrane defect affecting hematopoietic stem cell derivatives	XL	Thrombocytopenia; small defective platelets; eczema; lymphoreticular malignancy
Ataxia telangiectasia	Often decreased IgA, IgE, and IgG; increased IgM (monomers); antibodies variably decreased	Normal	Decreased	Unknown; defective T-cell maturation	AR	Ataxia; telangiectasia; defective chromosomal repair; raised α fetoprotein; lymphoreticular malignancy
3rd and 4th pouch/arch syndrome (DiGeorge)	Normal or decreased		Decreased	Embryopathy: abnormal thymus with resultant T-cell defects	None or unknown	Hypoparathyroidism: cardiac outflow tract malformation; abnormal facies; mental defect (some); GI tract malformation (some)
Transcobalamin 2 deficiency	All isotypes decreased	Normal	Normal	Defect in B12 transport resulting in defective cell proliferation, B cell to plasma cell differentiation	AR	Megaloblastic anemia; intestinal villous atrophy; defective granulocyte bactericidal activity
ID with partial albinism	Decreased	Normal	Decreased or normal	Unknown	AR	Cerebral atrophy; pigment clumping in melanocytes; defective NK cells
ID following hereditary defective response to EBV	Decreased only after EBV infection	Decreased only after EBV infection	Decreased only after EBV infection; NK cells increased	Unknown	XL, AR	Fatal EBV infection; aplastic anemia, lymphoproliferative disease in some

rather indolent rheumatoid arthritis with sterile effusion into one of the large joints develops in about one third of patients and may be the presenting complaint. The children usually, but not always, handle most viral infections normally (1).

There should be a high index of suspicion about this diagnosis based on the history of repeated severe bacterial infections. A careful family history may uncover instances of death from overwhelming infection or multiple severe infections in other male siblings, maternal uncles, or male offspring of maternal aunts. Examination reveals little except the signs of infection, evidence of joint involvement, and unusually small, smooth tonsils. Lateral films of the pharynx fail to reveal an adenoid shadow. Lymph nodes are small but palpable, and regional nodes may be swollen and tender during episodes of infection. Immunochemical assay reveals a marked diminution of IgM, IgA, and IgG globulins in the serum. It is important to remember that because of individual variations and the low levels of immunoglobulins normally found in the early months of life, the diagnosis cannot be firmly established by immunoelectrophoresis until 6 to 8 months of age (Fig. 28–1). However, failure of IgM or IgA to appear in significant concentration and a steady fall in IgG levels during the first 3 to 4 months of life should suggest the diagnosis, especially in the presence of a positive family history. Isohemagglutinins are usually absent or in very low titer. Injection of vaccines is not followed by an adequate antibody rise, and removal of a stimulated regional lymph node discloses absence of the expected germinal centers, secondary follicles, and plasma cells.

The thymus is normal, but the lymph nodes and spleen lack the usual follicular architecture. Germinal centers are absent, and there are few, if any, plasma cells in the medullary cores or red pulp.

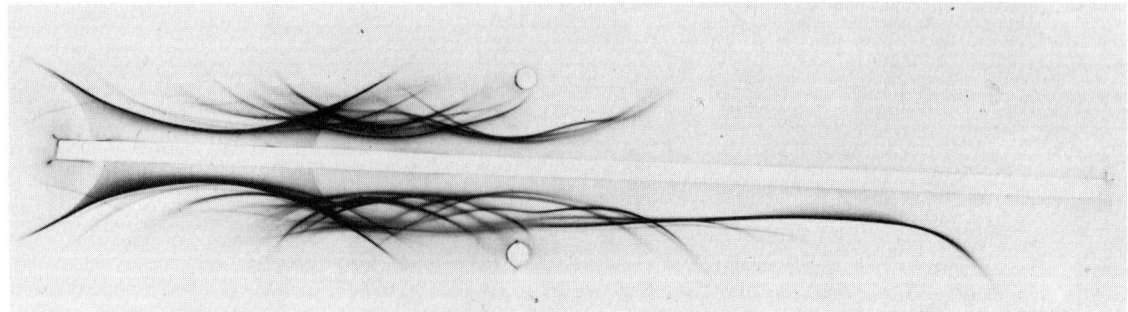

Figure 28–1. Immunoelectrophoresis of normal (bottom) and agammaglobulinemic (top) sera. The anode is to the left. The pattern was developed with horse antihuman serum.

Although the number of lymphocytes in the tissues appears diminished, these cells are present in the thymus-dependent areas of lymphoid tissue, and normal numbers are found in the blood. Plasma cells are absent from the bone marrow; however, plasma cells may be normally absent from the bone marrow in children under 5 years of age, so this is not a helpful finding. Study of the circulating lymphocytes has revealed normal numbers of T cells but complete absence of B cells. A detailed discussion of the B cell defect can be found in Chapter 25.

Provided the diagnosis is made before repeated infections have produced serious anatomic damage (e.g., bronchiectasis, pulmonary insufficiency, middle ear deafness), the immediate prognosis for these children is excellent, and they gain and grow normally. However, in later childhood, adolescence, or early adult life, complications may develop in some of these patients. Slowly progressive neurologic disease, suggesting a "slow virus" infection, accompanies a dermatomyositis-like syndrome with brawny edema, perivascular mononuclear infiltrates, and, terminally, severe systemic symptoms and death. Echo virus has been found in all the viscera (3, 4).

Vigorous antimicrobial therapy is indicated for individual infections that respond to treatment as do infections in normal individuals. Regular injections of gamma globulin, which is almost pure IgG, in doses adequate to maintain a plasma concentration of IgG globulin above 200 mg per 100 ml, are essential. Maintenance therapy is initiated with a loading dose of 0.3g (1.8 ml) per kg of IgG globulin. This may be given in divided doses over a period of 1 week in order to minimize discomfort. Thereafter, an average dose of 0.1 g (0.6 ml) per kg per month is required to maintain a protective level of antibody (the volume of the injection may be scaled down if injections are given every 2 or 3 weeks). Intramuscular administration is necessary to avoid reactions when the standard preparation is being used. Preparations satisfactory for intravenous administration also have been shown to be effective in preventing infections in these patients. The feasibility of giving larger doses of immunoglobulins by the intravenous route has revealed that these patients were not being adequately treated in the past (5, 6). At present, the optimal dose of replacement therapy is not known, and it may well vary from patient to patient. Prophylaxis with gamma globulin is usually effective in preventing invasive bacterial infection and communicable disease, and its institution generally cures hydrarthrosis. In a few instances, antimicrobial drugs also may have to be given to control chronic sinusitis, most frequently due to *H. influenzae*. Infections may be prevented for considerable periods by the administration of broad-spectrum antibiotics without gamma globulin.

Once a case of X-linked agammaglobulinemia has been identified in a family, each subsequent male sibling or male offspring of a maternal aunt should be followed carefully, with clinical examination and serial immunoelectrophoretic analyses of the serum at intervals of 2 months from birth through the first year. Infants so detected and given prophylactic gamma globulin before severe infections have occurred seem to thrive particularly well.

X-Linked Immunodeficiency With Increased IgM Concentration

In a few instances, patients are observed with manifestations similar to those in X-linked agammaglobulinemia but with higher levels of immunoglobulins, which, when analyzed, turn out to reflect a marked deficiency of serum IgA and IgG but an elevation in the concentration of IgM. The congenital form of this disease seems to occur almost entirely in males and has a suggestive X-linked pattern of inheritance. Almost all patients with this disease have an "autoimmune" hematologic disorder (neutropenia, hemolytic anemia, thrombocytopenia); the clinical course in these patients otherwise resembles that of X-linked agammaglobulinemia. Histologically, there is disorganization of the follicular architecture of the lymphoid tissues. However, PAS-positive plasmacytoid cells containing IgM are present, and even tonsillar hypertrophy due to these cells has been observed. Only B cells with IgM and IgD surface fluorescence are found. No B cells with surface IgA or IgG are present. IgM-secreting plasmacytoid cells are evident in the peripheral blood, a finding unique to this immunodeficiency. When established in long-term culture, the B cell lines manifest the abnormality in that they secrete only IgM. Similar disturbances of the immunoglobulin picture associated with the antibody deficiency syndrome have been seen in adults with frequent respiratory tract infections and bronchiectasis and in some infants with congenital rubella (7, 8).

Selective Immunoglobulin Deficiencies (Dysgammaglobulinemia)

This term is used to describe consistent deficiencies of one or more of the recognizable plasma immunoglobulins. Although often associated with the clinical manifestations of the antibody deficiency syndrome, some instances of selective immunoglobulin deficiency may be chance laboratory findings in otherwise apparently normal individuals.

Selective deficiency of IgG subclasses may occur, in which the patient is unable to synthesize one or more of the IgG subclasses and thus fails to produce antibodies in one or more of the four presently identified IgG subclasses. This results in failure to respond to particular types of antigens, increased susceptibility to a limited spectrum of bacterial infections, and a reduction in total serum IgG concentration proportional to the percentage of the total IgG pool accounted for by the deficient IgG subclass. Of course, a deficiency in IgG1 is most severe because this subclass constitutes more than 70 per cent of the IgG (9, 10).

Selective IgA deficiency is observed with considerable frequency (3 to 7 per 1000 population). In a few patients, this may portend the development of ataxia telangiectasia, but an appreciable number of such individuals remain healthy throughout life. However, high incidences of rheumatoid arthritis, systemic lupus erythematosus, and malabsorption syndrome have been observed among this group of patients. A significant number of IgA-deficient individuals have circulating antibodies to IgA and undergo anaphylactic reactions when receiving whole blood or plasma (11, 12).

Deficiency of secretory IgA may well play a role in undue susceptibility to certain infections, particularly viral, or the respiratory and gastrointestinal tracts. Secretory IgA is the form of antibody synthesized in plasma cells that are closely related to the mucous membranes. It is secreted into colostrum, saliva, and respiratory and intestinal secretions as two subunits of IgA in combinations with a "secretory piece" synthesized by the epithelial cells. Rare cases of deficiency of secretory component have been described, and these patients appear to have difficulty in tropical settings with diarrhea (13). The efficacy of certain respiratory viral vaccines when administered intranasally or of oral poliomyelitis vaccine may depend more on the establishment of local immunity than on the stimulation of systemic antibody formation.

Rare cases of *immunodeficiency with normal or increased immunoglobulins* have been observed. In these cases, the classic picture of the antibody deficiency syndrome was accompanied by a normal or even an increased level of immunoglobulins and the presence of plasma cells in the tissues, but a failure to form specific antibodies to a variety of antigens was noted. These disorders have not been adequately studied with modern methods to provide a satisfactory explanation.

Transcobalamin II (TCII) Deficiency

The rare genetic deficiency of TCII results in the very early onset of profound megaloblastic anemia. Most infants with this disease develop agammaglobulinemia as well. In affected infants, B cell numbers are normal, but they will not mature to plasma cells without vitamin B_{12}. TCII deficiency also gives rise to a defect in phagocytosis because the mobility of leukocytes also is vitamin B_{12}–dependent. The anemia, agammaglobulinemia, and phagocyte defects all are corrected by administration of vitamin B_{12} (14).

Varied Unclassified Immunodeficiency Disorders (Acquired Hypogammaglobulinemia)

This is the most common form of immunodeficiency, having serious clinical consequences and probably including a number of entities. It occurs in either sex at any age without any known causative factor, either genetic or acquired. However, a predisposition may be inherited because development of this syndrome has been reported in siblings and among other relatives.

The picture is that of the antibody deficiency syndrome associated with immunoglobulin deficiency, which may be somewhat less severe than in the X-linked form of gammaglobulinemia. Pathologically, there is necrobiotic change in the follicular architecture of the lymph nodes and spleen or lymphadenopathy and splenomegaly due to reticulum cell hyperplasia. B cell hyperplasia may give rise to intestinal nodular lymphoid hyperplasia (15). The predominant infections are sinusitis and pneumonia, often leading to bronchiectasis unless intensively treated. Although rheumatoid arthritis–like complications are occasionally seen, a spruelike malabsorption syndrome and pernicious anemia are more common. About 30 per cent of patients with this disease develop pernicious anemia with obvious megaloblastic changes in the bone marrow and macrocytic anemia (16). This complication should be suspected when an agammaglobulinemic patient who is receiving adequate replacement therapy develops a severe infection that is refractory to antibiotic therapy and ISG therapy. Vitamin B_{12} administration will promptly reverse a disastrous clinical course. It has been demonstrated that the malabsorption syndrome is often due to Giardia lamblia, demonstrated either in the aspirates of duodenal fluid or in biopsy specimens of duodenal mucosa (17).

Management is the same as for X-linked agammaglobulinemia, that is, substitution therapy with regular injections of large doses of immune serum globulin for prophylaxis and intensive antimicrobial therapy for acute infections. The chronic diarrhea and malabsorption due to giardiasis, which may give a picture of protein-losing enteropathy, usually respond promptly to quinacrine hydrochloride (Atabrine).

Common variable immunodeficiency can result from three different immunologic causes: intrinsic B cell defects, immunoregulatory T cell imbalances, and autoantibodies to T or B cells. In contrast to X-linked agammaglobulinemia, common variable immunodeficiency is characterized by the presence of low or high numbers of B cells (18). These cells are clonally diverse, appear to be relatively immature, and fail to respond to most antigens and mitogens by differentiating into plasma cells. Yet, some patients have B cells that synthesize but do not secrete immunoglobulin (19, 20). In any of these groups of patients, the helper: suppressor T cell ratio may be reversed, and this has been thought to be pathogenetic—that is, suppressor T cells prevent terminal B cell differentiation (21). However, subsequent observations suggest that this reversal is not a primary factor but rather a secondary reflection of repeated infections (22). Nonetheless, some patients with common variable immunodeficiency have perfectly normal B lymphocytes that cannot function in vivo because of the absence of helper T cells or the presence of activated suppressor T cells (23–25). Such patients constitute a rare subgroup of those with common variable immunodeficiency. Even rarer are patients in whom the disorder results from autoantibodies to T or B cells (26, 27). T cell function in common variable immunodeficiency tends to deteriorate with time and complicates the therapy of this disease.

PRIMARY T CELL DEFICIENCIES

Patients with T cell deficiency have much more serious susceptibility to infection than do patients with complete or partial B cell defects. In its most severe forms, T cell deficiency results in an inability to terminate opportunistic infections caused by organisms that are ordinarily innocuous. Consequently, varicella, vaccinia, and herpes and measles viruses can be fatal infections. The enterobacilli are invasive, and infection with monilial organisms is common. Malignancy of both the lymphoreticular organs and other viscera also is a common complication of the T cell disorders (see Table 28–1) (1).

Severe Combined Immunodeficiency

Severe combined immunodeficiency (Swiss-type agammaglobulinemia, alymphocytosis, thymic alymphoplasia) is the most profound of the cellular defects. Affected patients usually have no T or B cells; the disease is invariably fatal. It is genetically determined, and there is clear evidence of autosomal recessive and X-linked recessive transmission of the disease. The clinical and laboratory findings may be quite variable from patient to patient, even among affected members of a single family.

Despite all attempts at routine therapy, persistent infection of the lungs; monilial infection of the oropharynx, esophagus, and skin; chronic diarrhea; and wasting and runting begin in the early months of life and progress with monotonous regularity to a fatal termination. Affected infants usually do not survive the first 1 or 2 years of life. Examination usually reveals absence of tonsils, very small or absent lymph nodes despite chronic infection, chronic pneumonitis evidenced by a pertussis-like cough, a somewhat distended abdomen with wasting, and oral thrush.

Roentgenographic signs include pulmonary infiltration and absence of a thymic shadow. There is usually an absolute decrease in the number of circulating lymphocytes, and occasionally neutropenia is found. In typical cases, the immunoglobulins are markedly decreased, but variants have been described in which circulating immunoglobulins are normal or there is selective immunoglobulin deficiency. M components may be present in the circulation. Plasma cells have been found in the tissues of such patients, but antibody formation is almost always impaired or absent. Tests of delayed hypersensitivity give negative results—sensitization cannot be induced with dinitrochlorobenzene, cultured lymphocytes do not respond to phytohemagglutinin, and skin allografts are not rejected. T cells are almost always absent from the circulation, and the few lymphocytes present in the blood usually have the characteristics of B cells or null cells or may prove to be natural killer cells. The thymus morphology is fetal and is pathognomonic of the disease (Fig. 28–2).

In one study, 50 per cent of infants with the autosomal recessive form of the disease were found to lack the enzyme adenosine deaminase

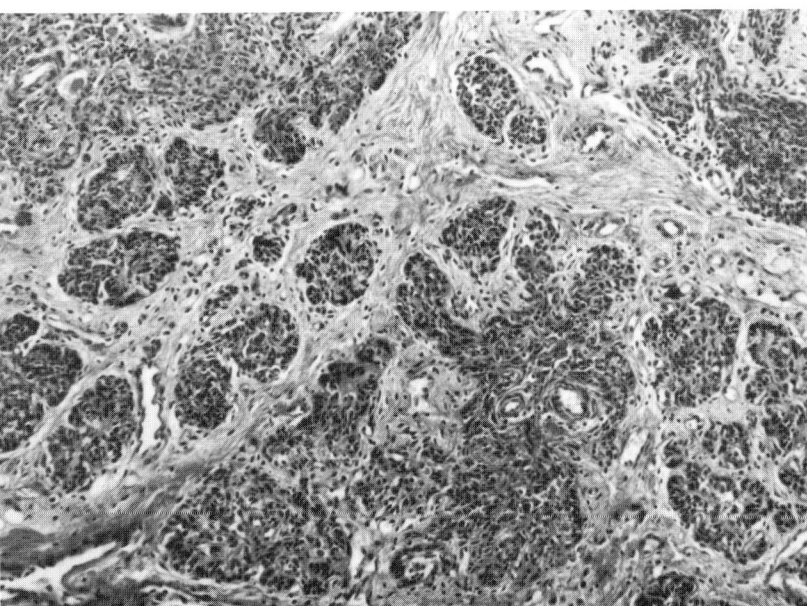

Figure 28–2. Photomicrograph of thymus from a patient with severe combined immunodeficiency (×400). No Hassall bodies are present, the blood vessels are small, and islets of fetal spindle cells are seen without lymphoidal elements.

(ADA) in their red cells and other tissues (28). Heterozygosity was detectable in the parents by their half-normal levels of ADA, the structural gene for which is on chromosome 20 (29). ADA has a common polymorphism, so that the inheritance of a silent gene has been documented in a few informative families. Furthermore, a mutant enzyme has been found in the fibroblasts of affected children. This mutant enzyme is abnormal with regard to its electrophoretic mobility, molecular weight, heat stability, and Km. Its detection has enabled the prenatal diagnosis of ADA deficiency (30). Several children with erythrocyte ADA deficiency have been found. They are completely normal, and their lymphocytes contain normal or suboptimal ADA (31, 32).

ADA is universally distributed in all mammalian cells, yet its deficiency results in a profound perturbation of the lymphoid system but of no other organ system. Although the enzyme deficiency is causally related to the immunodeficiency, the reasons for this are not entirely clear. Another enzyme defect, purine nucleoside phosphorylase deficiency (NP), has been found to result in profound T cell deficiency (33). Its gene is on chromosome 14, and it is not very polymorphic (34). The disease is also inherited as an autosomal recessive trait and may result from a deficiency of nucleoside phosphorylase or an inactive mutant of this enzyme (35).

Children with nucleoside phosphorylase deficiency excrete large quantities of deoxyguanosine triphosphate (deoxy-GTP) in the urine (36). This prompted an examination of ADA-deficient children for deoxy-ATP, which was found in very elevated concentrations in their lymphocytes (Fig. 28–3). Deoxy-GTP and deoxy-ATP inhibit DNA synthesis by blocking the enzyme ribonucleotide reductase (Fig. 28–4) (37, 38).

Murine and human T cell lines have been studied in vitro. They have a very active dA and dG kinase and relatively little 5′ ribonucleotidase (39, 40) (Fig. 28–3). Thus, they preferentially accumulate dATP and dGTP. T cell lines that are deficient in adenosine deaminase or nucleoside phosphorylase are rapidly killed in vitro by adenosine or guanosine and can be rescued by cytidine, which restores ribonucleotide reductase activity (Fig. 28–4). The disease results from a failure of null cell maturation into T cells. Null cells have high levels of ADA but not of NP. Their in vitro maturation into T cells, but not B cells, is completely inhibited by the ADA inhibitor, coformycin (41). ADA-deficient children have very high levels of deoxy-ADA in their lymphocytes (null cells), but this abnormality improves following bone marrow transplantation or infusions of frozen red cells as a source of ADA (42).

These factors taken together suggest, but do not prove, that deoxy-ATP is the pathogenetic metabolic event in severe combined immunodeficiency with ADA deficiency. Further complicating factors are coming to light. For instance, the hydrolase of S-adenosylhomocysteine is blocked by high levels of adenosine. This results in accumulation of S-adenosylmethionine and S-adenosylhomocysteine, thus blocking DNA methylation (Fig. 28–5) (43). The relevance of this and other metabolic abnormalities to the failure of normal ontogeny of lymphocytes remains to be resolved. Certainly, the same metabolic abnormalities are found in other tissues, such as erythroblasts, of ADA-deficient children, yet the maturation of these tissues is not impaired.

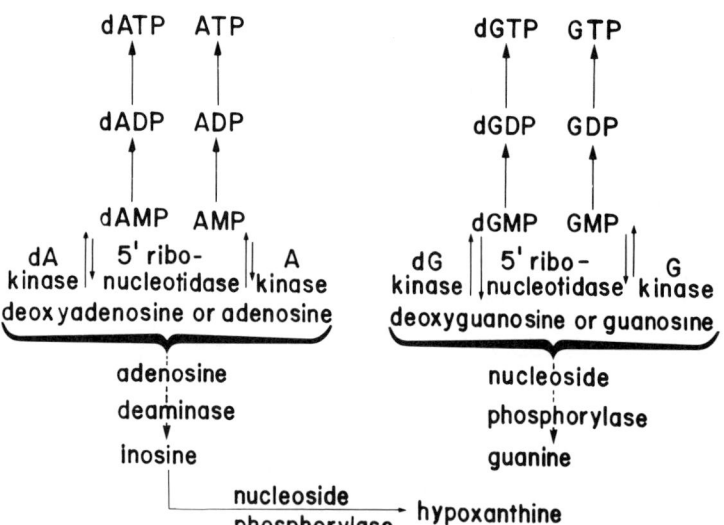

Figure 28–3. Purine degradation pathways.

Treatment of the infections in these patients must be specific. Pulmonary infection is frequently due to *Pneumocystis carinii*, requiring administration of (1) sulfadiazine with pentamidine or pyrimethamine or (2) trimethoprim and sulfamethoxazole (Bactrim). Routine antimicrobial therapy, fungistatic drugs, or human gamma globulin is only temporarily effective and does not prevent the inexorably fatal course of the disease if the immunologic deficiency is not overcome. The use of attenuated viral or BCG vaccines must be avoided because the attenuated viruses or mycobacteria can produce fatal generalized disease, and natural infection with herpes, varicella, or measles virus is uniformly and progressively fatal.

The establishment of immunologic competence with transplants of bone marrow in these infants is still experimental and should be carried out only in those centers with adequate personnel, clinical and laboratory experience, and physical facilities for what is an exacting ordeal for the patient, family, nurses, and physicians. Success depends on attention to a number of complex factors (Fig. 28–6).

For an index case in a family, the diagnosis is seldom made until infection is already established. Every subsequent sibling should be carefully watched for early signs of the disease—absence of clinically demonstrable thymic tissue at birth, low peripheral lymphocyte count, absence of serum IgM, and failure of cultured lymphocytes from cord blood or subsequent blood samples to respond to phytohemagglutinin. Affected infants can be maintained in a sterile environment or laminar flow apparatus. They require exquisite care in the administration of systemic and topical antibiotics.

A bone marrow donor should be found whose cells are HLA-identical and can be shown to be histocompatible in vitro by mixed lymphocyte culture (MLC). In practice, this almost always means a sibling. However, a successful transplant from an MLC-identical unrelated donor has been accomplished (44). Administration of a suitable dose of bone marrow cells from the donor when the infant is as free of infection as possible is accomplished with 50×10^6 nucleated cells per kg of body weight intravenously. More cells are optimal for intraperitoneal injection, perhaps 50×10^7 per kg. Evidence that the graft has become established and that immunologic reconstitution has occurred (T cell function as shown by phytohemagglutinin responses; B cell function as demonstrated by immunoglobulin synthesis) usually requires 3 to 8 weeks (Fig. 28–7). Success has been achieved with the use of haploidentical parental bone marrow that has been depleted of T cells by treatment with monoclonal antibodies or passage over lectin columns. These successes have greatly expanded the scope of bone marrow transplants as a therapeutic modality (45, 46).

In skilled hands, patients with this hitherto fatal disease have been cured and appear normal. Nevertheless, success is not universal, there is much to learn, and the treatment is heroic. Intrauterine diagnosis of this disorder has been accomplished.

Individuals have been reported with variant forms of severe combined immunodeficiency.

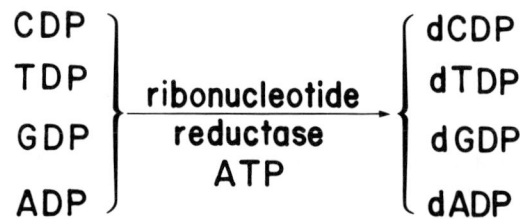

Figure 28–4. Substrates of ribonucleotide reductase.

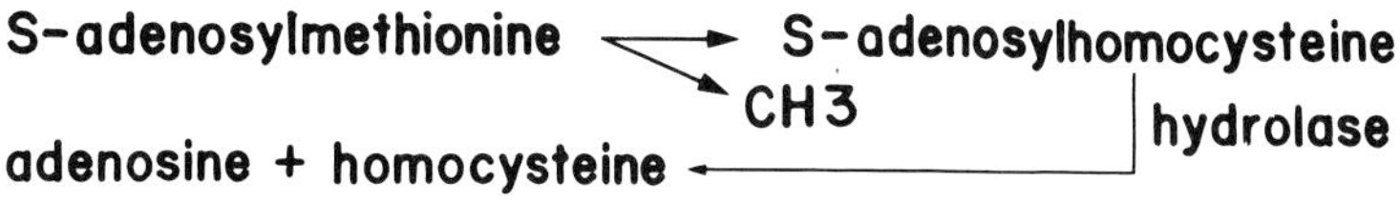

Figure 28-5. The methyl donation pathway.

$$\text{S-adenosylmethionine} \rightleftarrows \underset{CH3}{\overset{}{\text{S-adenosylhomocysteine}}}$$
$$\text{adenosine + homocysteine} \longleftarrow \quad \bigg| \text{hydrolase}$$

These include patients with dysostosis (short-limbed dwarfism) and rare patients with generalized hematopoietic hypoplasia. The latter disorder has been called reticular dysgenesis; infants with this type of immunodeficiency also lack granulocytic precursors in the bone marrow and granulocytes in the peripheral blood and survive for only a short time after birth. Nezelof's syndrome, which is combined immunodeficiency with normal immunoglobulin, is better called combined immunodeficiency with predominant T cell deficiency.

Immunodeficiency With Ataxia Telangiectasia

This is an autosomal recessive disease in which abnormalities of the thymus have been found at postmortem examination. Progressive cerebellar ataxia begins in early childhood. This is associated with increasing telangiectasia, which first becomes apparent as a rather inconspicuous dilatation of small blood vessels in the bulbar conjunctivae and ultimately is visible in the skin at about 5 years of age. Gonadal dysgenesis and failure of sexual maturation may be present in those who survive into the second decade. In late childhood, recurrent sinobronchial infections begin in many patients, often leading to bronchiectasis. There also is a tendency to the development of malignant tumors, particularly of the lymphoid system. These reflect an immunologic disturbance affecting T cell function, as shown by blunting of delayed hypersensitivity reactions, failure to reject allografts normally, and reduced response of the lymphocytes to phytohemagglutinin. At postmortem examination late in the disease, the thymus is abnormally small and has a decreased number of lymphocytes, and there is a poor differentiation between the cortex and medulla and decided diminution in Hassall's corpuscles. The number of circulating lymphocytes and the architecture of the lymph nodes vary considerably and do not always correlate well with the patient's history.

The most consistent B cell defect is a low level or absence of IgA globulin in the serum, which occurs in about 70 per cent of affected persons and may precede clinical evidence of immunologic deficiency by a number of years. The alpha-fetoprotein level is always elevated.

Untoward sensitivity of patients with ataxia telangiectasia to radiotherapy of tumors has opened a Pandora's box (47); the syndrome appears to be causally related to a basic repair defect in the DNA of ataxia telangiectasia cells. Numerous chromosomal breaks and translocations have been reported (48), the majority of which have been clustered at chromosome 14q12 with translocations to chromosomes 6, 7, and X. Ring formation of chromosome 14 also has been seen. In culture, ataxia telangiectasia fibroblasts are three times more sensitive to killing by ionizing radiation and radiomimetic chemicals but not to ultraviolet light—a characteristic that distinguishes such cells from those of xeroderma pigmentosum (49, 50). It has been postulated that defective DNA repair after irradiation may reflect a defect in tissue differentiation during rapid cell division or the failure of repression of a DNA repair gene (51–53). That ataxia telangiectasia is a model of aberrant gene control is supported by the persistence of elevated levels of serum alpha$_1$-fetoprotein (54) and carcinoembryonic antigen (55). These measurements are useful in early establishment of the diagnosis. It has been postulated that a low-molecular-weight peptide that is a clastogenic factor may be responsible for the DNA repair defects, and the presence of the factor in amniotic fluid can be used in prenatal diagnosis (56). Ataxia telangiectasia appears, however, to be a heterogeneous disease. Fibroblasts from different patients have been fused and found to cross-correct the defects in x-ray sensitivity. With the use of such heterokaryons, at least five complementation groups have been found (57, 58). This suggests that the ataxia telangiectasia gene is relatively frequent in the normal population and poses the question of whether heterozygotes are more susceptible to

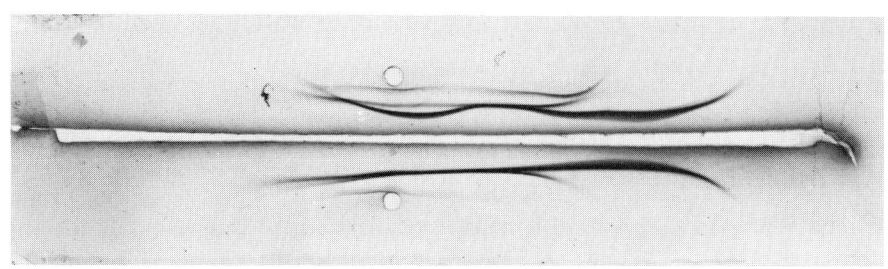

Figure 28–6. Immunoelectrophoresis of serum from a normal individual (bottom) and from a patient with severe combined immunodeficiency (top) following bone marrow transplantation. A number of M components are visible. The anode is to the left.

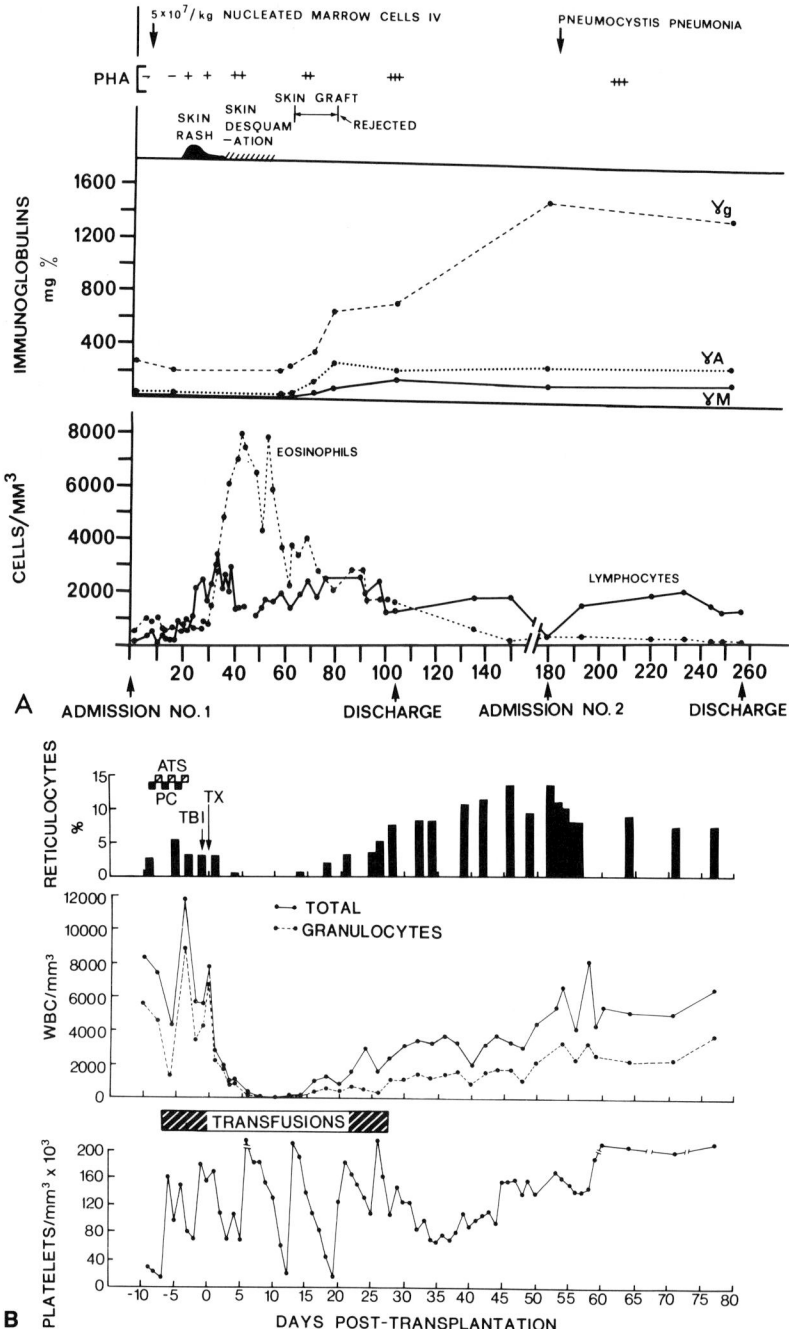

Figure 28–7. *A*, The course of immunologic reconstitution by bone marrow cells from an HLA-, MLC-identical donor in a patient with severe combined immunodeficiency. *B*, The course of hematopoietic reconstitution by bone marrow cells from an HLA-, MLC-identical donor in a patient with Wiskott-Aldrich syndrome.

tumors. Indeed, a survey of relatives of patients with ataxia telangiectasia revealed an increased incidence of neoplasms, with a fivefold higher risk for assumed heterozygotes under 45 years of age (59).

Immunodeficiency With Thrombocytopenia and Eczema (Wiskott-Aldrich Syndrome)

The Wiskott-Aldrich syndrome is characterized by severe eczema, thrombocytopenia, and suscep- tibility to opportunistic infections (60, 61). The signs and symptoms of the disease appear in the first few months of life. The syndrome is inherited as an X-linked recessive trait, and it has been estimated that there are four affected male infants per million male births (62). In a retrospective survey of 301 cases, it was found that the median survival was 5.7 years and that 59 per cent of affected boys died of infection, 27 per cent of a hemorrhagic episode, and 5 per cent of tumors. Almost all the tumors are of the lymphoreticular system—leukemia or Hodgkin's disease (62).

Obligate female heterozygotes cannot be identified by any known test. Early reports that platelets of such persons have a defect in mitochondrial adenosine triphosphate resynthesis could not be confirmed (63). The reason for this failure to identify female carriers apparently results from preferential inactivation of the affected X chromosome in marrow precursors of platelets and T cells but not of red cells, polymorphonuclear leukocytes, macrophages, and B cells (64). These interesting results were found in mothers of affected boys who had informative glucose-6-phosphate dehydrogenase variants (65).

The serum of affected boys contains elevated concentrations of IgA and IgE, whereas the IgM level is decreased and the IgG level is usually normal. Paraproteins or monoclonal IgG may occur in the blood—a rare finding in the pediatric age group (66). Despite these diverse serum immunoglobulin changes, the fractional catabolic rate is markedly increased for all the immunoglobulins, and it has been attributed to reticuloendothelial hyperplasia. One very peculiar aspect of the immunodeficiency in boys is their lack of response to polysaccharide antigens (67, 68); thus, their serum lacks isohemagglutinins.

The T cells in this syndrome exhibit a progressive decline in number and function, so that profound lymphopenia does not usually become apparent until 6 years of age (69). The T cell–dependent areas of lymph nodes and spleen are depleted of cells. The mixed lymphocyte responses are more depressed than the response to nonspecific mitogens. Platelets are half the normal size and turn over rapidly, and there is decreased thrombopoiesis.

All these defects can be corrected by bone marrow transplantation after ablation of the recipient's marrow by busulfan or total body irradiation, with subsequent establishment of total bone marrow chimerism (Fig. 28–7) (70). In patients with advanced lymphoid depletion, it is relatively easy to establish T cell chimerism by bone marrow transplantation without the aforementioned drastic preparation. In such cases in which mixed T cell chimerism is established, eczema disappears, B cell and immunoglobulin defects are corrected, and T cell function becomes normal. However, thrombocytopenia persists.

Early reports that transfer factor improved affected boys have not been confirmed by further observation. However, splenectomy has proved useful; after the procedure had been performed in 16 boys, the mean platelet count rose from 19,000 to 262,000, and the platelet volume rose from 3μ to 5.1 μm^3 (71). In many cases splenectomy is only a stop gap measure, thrombocytopenia recurs, and a transplant is advised.

Lactoperoxidase surface labeling of T cells and platelets reveals the absence of a 115,000-dalton glycoprotein from T cell membranes and of glycoprotein Ib from platelets (72). It is likely that an instability of cell membrane glycoproteins is present in these patients' T cells and platelets, but the precise nature of the defect has yet to be elucidated.

Congenital Thymic Aplasia (DiGeorge's Syndrome)

Congenital thymic aplasia (DiGeorge's syndrome; third and fourth pharyngeal pouch syndrome) results from a failure of the normal embryogenesis of the thymus and parathyroid glands, which are derived from the third and fourth pharyngeal clefts. The syndrome is not genetically determined but appears rather to result from some intrauterine accident before the eighth week of gestation. Affected infants invariably have neonatal tetany. Anomalies of the great blood vessels, usually right-sided aortic arch defects, are very frequently encountered, as is tetralogy of Fallot. These cardiac complications are the cause of death in late childhood. Mental subnormality also accompanies this syndrome.

The T cell defect in children with congenital thymic aplasia varies from the most profound to the barely discernible. In any case, T cell function improves in these children with age, so that by 5 years of age no T cell deficit can be ascertained. It is not clear how this grossly retarded T cell maturation occurs in the absence of a thymus gland. Some children may have a small thymic remnant, but T cell maturation may occur at sites other than the thymus.

Transplants of fetal thymus into these infants result in a rapid acquisition of T cell function.

Immunodeficiency With Unusual Response to Epstein-Barr Virus

A group of patients has been described in whom Epstein-Barr virus infection had an untoward outcome in the form of B cell lymphomas, marrow aplasia, fatal infectious mononucleosis, or agammaglobulinemia (73, 74). Before the disastrous encounter with Epstein-Barr virus, these patients appeared to be immunologically normal (75). However, after the infection their B cells and immunoglobulins were decreased, and the predominant T cells in the circulation were natural killer cells. Although at first this susceptibility to Epstein-Barr virus appeared to be transmitted as an X-linked recessive trait, several cases have subsequently been reported in female patients. The precondition for acquisition of this usually fatal disease remains to be elucidated.

SECONDARY IMMUNODEFICIENCY INFECTION FOLLOWING SPLENECTOMY

The risk of death from overwhelming sepsis following splenectomy is well established. The young are more at risk than those who have been splenectomized at a later age (*i.e.*, after 5 years of age). Children with congenital asplenia and Ivemark's syndrome (asplenia and partial situs inversus) have the greatest mortality from septic infection. Fatal blood-stream infection results presumably from bacteria to which the splenectomized child has no pre-existent antibody.

The pathophysiology of this immunologic deficit may be multifactorial but is quite straightforward. The spleen has two important roles. First, it is the lymph node of the blood stream and is the site of antibody response to antigens presented via that route. Second, it has an important phagocytic function in the absence of antibody. That is, the granulopectic activity of the liver is adequate for clearing immune complexes, but in the absence of antibody the accessory phagocytic function of the spleen is required to clear the blood stream of foreign or bacterial particles. When mice were injected intravenously with small doses of killed *Diplococcus pneumoniae* and then splenectomized 8 or more hours later, they were resistant to a challenge of the same type of live *D. pneumoniae* that was fatal to a control group of mice that were simply splenectomized. In other words, the opportunity to synthesize some antibody to the challenging bacteria was absolutely protective. Splenectomized children should be given prophylactic antibiotics and immunized against *D. pneumoniae* and *Hemophilus influenzae* type B.

SECONDARY HYPOGAMMAGLOBULINEMIA

Serum levels of immunoglobulins may be decreased because of loss, as through the gut, or because of hypercatabolism, as in the nephrotic syndrome. In any case, hypoalbuminemia also is almost always present. It is futile to replace gamma globulin in these clinical settings because it is not feasible to keep up with the losses that are occurring. In patients with intestinal lymphangiectasia with or without Milroy's disease, lymphocytes may also be lost in the gut, further complicating the patient's problems with T cell immunodeficiency.

PEDIATRIC AIDS

The acquired immunodeficiency syndrome (AIDS) is caused by a lymphocytotropic retrovirus called human immunodeficiency virus (HIV) (76, 76a).* The T4 antigen, a surface glycoprotein of helper T lymphocytes, is the receptor for HIV. T4 is also expressed in smaller amounts on a subpopulation of B lymphocytes and brain cells. The latter accounts for the high incidence of cerebritis in AIDS. Absolute T4 lymphopenia is required for the diagnosis of full-blown AIDS, because HIV causes a lytic infection of these cells (97). Certain non-T, non-B large granular lymphocytes responsible for the production of interferon-α are also depressed by infection with HIV (77a). As a consequence of this, patients with AIDS have extreme susceptibility to opportunistic infections, mainly with *Pneumocystis carinii, Mycobacterium avium intracellulare, Cryptosporidia, Toxoplasma,* herpes simplex virus, and *Candida*. In addition, AIDS patients have certain bizarre malignancies such as Kaposi's sarcoma and Burkitt's lymphoma. In adults, AIDS has been recognized almost exclusively in "at-risk" groups, including homosexually active males, intravenous drug abusers, and recipients of blood and some blood products. Heterosexual partners of individuals in "at-risk" groups have also acquired AIDS.

An HIV-associated disease called AIDS-related complex (ARC), is observed in infected individuals who have fever, night sweats, weight loss, and lymphadenopathy but no opportunistic infections and no bizarre malignancies. There are probably 300 HIV-infected individuals with no symptoms for every case of AIDS or ARC. AIDS is, at present, fatal. Ten per cent of patients with ARC progress to full-blown AIDS.

A form of AIDS has been observed in infants of HIV-infected mothers and has been designated pediatric AIDS (92, 93). This form of the disease is different in many respects from the disease observed in adults and therefore cannot be defined by the criteria used to define AIDS in adults. Over 90 per cent of mothers who transmit the disease to the fetus are asymptomatic; the remainder have ARC. HIV traverses the placenta in the first trimester. About 35 per cent of HIV-infected mothers transmit the disease to the fetus. The occurrence rises to approximately 65 per cent in offspring who have a sibling with pediatric AIDS. Thus, pediatric AIDS can be acquired only in utero; no child with pediatric AIDS has yet been known to transmit the disease to another person.

Infected infants manifest the first symptoms of AIDS between 3 weeks and 23 months (mean 5½ months). Rubinstein has proposed that the cases be defined by the major and minor criteria listed in Table 28–2 (94). Table 28–3 lists the clinical and laboratory findings in order of decreasing frequency, based on a study of 92 cases observed by Rubinstein at the Albert Einstein College of Medicine.

The most frequently associated complication of pediatric AIDS is a chronic pneumonitis with pulmonary lymphoid hyperplasia. This appears to be

---

*Formerly called AIDS-related virus (ARV), human T cell lymphocytotropic virus III (HTLV-III), or lymphadenopathy virus (LAV).

Table 28–2. PEDIATRIC AIDS-RELATED COMPLEX (PROPOSED CASE DEFINITION)*

(Two major and two minor criteria and two laboratory criteria persisting for more than three months)
Major criteria
   Pulmonary lymphoid hyperplasia (PLH) or lymphocytic interstitial pneumonitis (LIP)
   Oral thrush—persistent or recurrent on appropriate therapy
   Salivary gland enlargement
   Bacterial sepsis or meningitis
   Documented AIDS or ARC in the mother or in a sibling
Minor criteria
   Recurrent bacterial infections
   Lymphadenopathy at two or more sites (bilateral adenopathy counts as one site)
   Hepatomegaly +/− splenomegaly
   Diarrhea—chronic or recurrent
   Failure to thrive
   Progressive developmental delay and/or encephalopathy
Laboratory criteria
   Positive serologic findings for HTLV-III or virus detection
   Elevated serum IgG, IgD, or IgA levels
   Low T4/T8 ratio
   Low in vitro lymphocyte mitogenic responses to PWM; SAC
   Low FTS/elevated thymosin α1
   Elevated circulating B cells
   Elevated serum β2 microglobulin
   Cutaneous anergy to recall antigens

*From Rubinstein, A.: Pediatric AIDS. In Lockhart, J. (ed.): *Current Problems in Pediatrics*. Chicago, Year Book Medical Publishers, 1986.

Table 28–3. PEDIATRIC HTLV-III INFECTION—MAJOR FINDINGS (IN ORDER OF FREQUENCY)*

Chronic pneumonitis (PLH; LIP)
Recurrent bacterial infections/sepsis
Oral thrush—persistent or recurrent
Diarrhea—chronic or recurrent
Lymphadenopathy (two or more sites)
Hepatosplenomegaly
Failure to thrive
Developmental delay
Encephalopathy
Small for gestational age
Thrombocytopenia
Salivary gland enlargement
Opportunistic infections
Kaposi's sarcoma
B-cell lymphoma

*From Rubinstein, A.: Pediatric AIDS. In Lockhart, J. (ed.): *Current Problems in Pediatrics*. Chicago, Year Book Medical Publishers, 1986.
Based on a study of 92 HTLV-III serologically positive infants.

the result of infection with Epstein-Barr virus (EBV) (Fig. 28–8). EBV also is associated with parotitis and persistent salivary gland enlargement, a peculiar manifestation of pediatric AIDS that is readily confused with lymphadenopathy. Septicemia with pneumococci or with *Haemophilus influenzae* type b is also a distinctive feature of the pediatric disease entity. Infected infants fail to thrive, are small for their age, gain weight poorly, and show delayed development. Opportunistic infections occur late in the course of pediatric AIDS, and Kaposi's sarcoma and B cell lymphomas are very rare.

The diagnosis is established by the presence of serum antibodies to HIV. Like adults with AIDS, children develop polyclonal B cell activation, with even more remarkable elevations of serum IgG, IgM, and IgD. We observed one infant with 11 g per dl of IgG (90). This finding differentiates pediatric AIDS from primary immunodeficiency diseases. Thrombocytopenia is frequently observed. However, lymphopenia occurs in infants only in the late stages of the disease. This absence of absolute T4 lymphopenia is an important distinction between the adult and pediatric forms of AIDS. Lymph node biopsies reveal striking follicular lymphoid hyperplasia caused by the exuberant proliferation of B lymphocytes. Despite this B cell hyperactivity, affected infants cannot respond to new antigenic stimuli. Their cell-mediated immunity is also severely compromised as determined by in vitro lymphocyte responses to mitogens or delayed-type hypersensitivity skin responses.

There is no satisfactory therapy for AIDS. Infections should be treated with appropriate antibiotics. Prednisone reduces the lymphocytic hypertrophy of the pneumonitis and has proved useful in reducing cough and tachypnea and improving the chest x-ray findings. Intravenous gamma globulin (200 mg per kg per month) has prevented many bacterial complications of AIDS and improved survival of these infants.

Children have been infected with HIV and acquired ARC and AIDS from blood transfusions

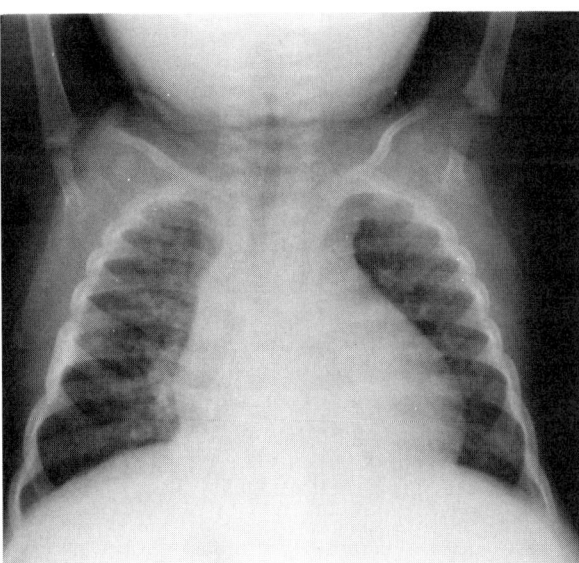

Figure 28–8. The most frequently associated complication of pediatric AIDS is chronic pneumonitis with pulmonary lymphoid hyperplasia. It apppears to be due to infection with Epstein-Barr virus (EBV).

and blood products. This has been a particular problem with hemophiliac males. These children do not have pediatric AIDS but rather the adult form of the syndrome.

THE COMPLEMENT SYSTEM

When bacteria or cells have interacted with antibody, they can be killed or lysed in fresh serum by complement. During this process, complement is activated and consumed; these events are called complement fixation. Complement fixation can readily be divided into two phases: (1) the activation phase and (2) the terminal phase. During the first phase, limited proteolytic interactions occur in sequence and activate the system. During the second phase, five proteins are assembled to form the macromolecular attack complex that becomes inserted into the cell membrane and causes the target to lose intracellular K^+, imbibe Na^+ and water, and lyse.

The Activation Phase

The activation phase of complement fixation can occur by two different pathways. The first of these requires antibody and is called the classical pathway. The second of these does not require antibody and is called the alternative pathway.

The classical pathway is activated by antibody molecules of either the IgM or the IgG class. Only 50 per cent of the IgM molecules are active in this system, and IgG1, IgG2, and IgG3 but not IgG4 have this capacity. Other immunoglobulin molecules are incapable of initiating complement fixation. Although a single IgM molecule bound to antigen is effective in starting complement fixation, at least two IgG molecules bound to adjacent antigenic sites are required for this. The IgG antibodies bound to Rh antigens on the human red cell do not fix complement because the Rh antigenic sites are so widely spaced on the red cell surface. Consequently, the IgG anti-Rh antibodies can never be in sufficiently close juxtaposition to initiate complement fixation.

The activation of the classical pathway begins by the activation of the first component of complement—C1, a large macromolecule composed of three subcomponents, C1q, C1r, and C1s, held together by Ca^{++} ligands. The C1q subcomponent consists of six globular heads joined together in a collagen-like stalk. It resembles a cluster of tulips. To each C1q stalk are attached two molecules of C1r and two molecules of C1s. Each globular head of C1q can fix to a CH2 domain of a complement-fixing immunoglobulin. When this occurs, C1r is activated by an unknown process, and activated C1r then activates C1s. Both C1r and C1s are trypsin-like serine esteratic proteases. They both cleave artificial substrates of arginine esters. The natural substrates of C1s are sequentially the fourth component of complement (C4) and the second component of complement (C2). The interaction of C1s with C4 and C2 causes both these molecules to be cleaved, and the resultant larger fragments are joined together to form another proteolytic enzyme, C4,2. C4 is a β globulin composed of three polypeptide chains. C1s splits a small peptide from the N-terminus of the heaviest of these polypeptide chains, or α chain. This fragment is designated C4a, and the larger fragment is called C4b. The α chain of C4 contains an internal thiol ester that is hydrolyzed during the activation phase and causes C4b to bind covalently to immunoglobulin CH1 domain by a transacylation reaction. C2 is composed of a single polypeptide chain. It is split into a smaller N-terminal fragment C2b and a larger C-terminal fragment C2a that binds to C4b. Thus, the enzyme formed by C4 and C2 is properly designated C4b2a. The active enzymatic site for the next interaction resides in the C2a moiety. C4b2a now activates the third component of complement, C3, and is designated the classical pathway C3 convertase. C4b2a requires Mg^{++} to function. C3 is composed of two polypeptide chains, and the classical pathway C3 convertase, C4b2a, cleaves a small peptide from the N-terminus of the heavy, or α, chain of C3; this peptide is called C3a. The resultant large fragment is designated C3b. In analogy to C4, the α chain of C3 also contains an internal thiol ester, and it also is hydrolyzed upon C3 activation. During this activation, C3 binds to cellular or bacterial surfaces, thereby facilitating their ingestion by phagocytic cells that have receptors for C3b. The activation of C3 to C3b is an amplication step in the process of complement fixation because one molecule of C4b2a may result in the binding of 1000 C3b molecules. In addition, C3b can activate the alternative pathway of the activation phase.

As has already been stated, the alternative pathway does not require antibody for activation. It functions by a positive feedback mechanism for which C3b is required (78). Under physiologic conditions, small amounts of C3b are generated at all times. C3b binds another protein, Factor B, to form the alternative pathway C3 convertase, C3bB. Factor B, composed of a single polypeptide chain, like C2, is cleaved by another serum protease, Factor D, into a smaller N-terminal fragment, Ba, and an active larger C-terminal fragment, Bb, that contains the enzymatically active site of the alternative pathway convertase, C3bBb. It also requires Mg^{++}. Thus, the alternative pathway and the classical pathway are analogous in their component parts.

$$C1q + r + s \longrightarrow C4 + C2 \longrightarrow C4b2a$$
$$\searrow$$
$$C3 \longrightarrow C3b$$
$$\nearrow$$
$$D \longrightarrow C3b + B \longrightarrow C3bBb$$

DOWN-REGULATION

A number of proteins impede the activation of the C3 convertases for both the classical and the alternative pathways. They act to control the potential unregulated activation of the system. An α glycoprotein of the blood, called the C1 inhibitor (C1 INH), covalently binds to C1r and C1s. One molecule of C1 INH can bind one molecule of activated C1r and C1s. When this complex of C1r-C1s-C1 INH forms, the C1r and C1s are dissociated from C1q. The enzymatic activation of C4 and C2 are thereby inhibited.

The C4b2a enzyme has a defined decay rate; the enzyme splits into its two component parts C4b and C2a. A membrane protein of the red cell, the decay-accelerating factor (DAF), hastens the process (79). Another blood protein, the C4b-binding protein, also accelerates this decay and renders C4b susceptible to cleavage by an inactivator, called Factor I. Factor I cleaves the α chain of C4 at two sites, excising a peptide C4d, thereby rendering C4b inactive. C4d contains the thiol ester site and remains bound to the immune complex, thus liberating the larger part of the molecule, C4c, where α, β, and γ chains are still held intact by disulfide bonds.

Another blood protein, the C3-binding protein (also called Factor H), accelerates the decay of C3bBb so that C3b can be rapidly inactivated by Factor I. Factor I cleaves the α chain of C3b at three sites. The first two cleavages result in the excision of a small peptide of 3000 daltons from the α chain (C3f), and the remaining molecule—C3bi, iC3b, or inactivated C3b—can no longer sustain its role in the alternative pathway C3 convertase (Fig. 28–9). Factor I splits the α chain again, excising a peptide, C3d, that also contains the internal thiol ester of C3, thus leaving C3d bound to cell surfaces. The remainder of the molecule C3c is thus liberated into the fluid phase. The peptide that induces leukocytosis is cleaved from C3d (80).

Another blood protein, called properdin, stabilizes C3bBb and counteracts the action of factors H and I. Because properdin was the first protein discovered in this pathway, the alternative pathway is also known as the properdin system. The regulatory events in the activation phase of complement fixation are important in determining the rate at which the reaction proceeds and in impeding the useless consumption of complement proteins, except on the antigen-antibody surface, where the reaction is proceeding at great speed.

The Terminal Phase

With one exception—the activation of C5—the terminal phase of complement fixation is not an enzymatic process. Like C3, C5 is composed of two chains, and a small peptide, C5a, is split from the N terminal of the α chain during activation. C5 can be activated by both the alternative pathway and the classical pathway, and the enzymatically active sites are in Bb or C2a, respectively. The alternative pathway C5 convertase is $(C3b)_2Bb$, and the classical pathway C5 convertase is C4b2a3b.

C5b, now fixed to an immune complex, binds C6 and C7, and the trimolecular complex, C5b, 6, 7, overcomes the charge barrier of the cell membrane and becomes firmly anchored in the lipid bilayer. Unlike C6 and C7, which are single polypeptide chains, C8 is composed of three polypeptide chains: α, β, and γ. The α and γ chains are joined by disulfide bonds, but the β chain is joined to C8α,γ by loose bonds. C8β has an affinity for the C5b,6,7 complex, and, when it binds, the C8α,γ is inserted into the cell membrane. The complex, C5b-8, causes C9 to bind to the complex and to polymerize. As many as 18 molecules of C9 may polymerize into a cylindrical structure 120 Å tall with an internal diameter of 100 Å surmounted by a ringlike cap 210 Å in diameter. These structures form transmembrane channels. The normally ordered bilayer lipids reorient into micellar domains around the C5b-9 complexes. The cell membrane permeability barrier is broken, and leaky patches form and become confluent. The cells lose intracellular potassium, imbibe sodium and water, and lyse.

Complement and Inflammation

It has been pointed out that the activation of C3, C4, and C5 results in the generation of peptides from the N-terminal end of the heavy chains of each of these proteins. These peptides are called

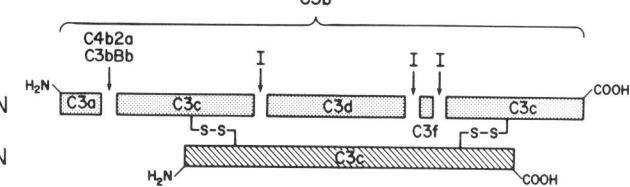

Figure 28–9. Cleavage of C3 α-chains by Factor I and the classic pathway C3 convertase C4b2a or the alternative C3bBb.

C3a, C4a, and C5a, respectively, and they are collectively known as anaphylatoxins. Human C3a and C4a are approximately 9000 daltons in molecular weight; C5a is 11,000 daltons. They are highly basic peptides. Minute amounts release histamine from mast cells and contract smooth muscle. C3a and C5a are 500 times more potent than C4a, which probably has little physiologic relevance. C5a is most potent in provoking chemotaxis. All the anaphylatoxins have a C-terminal arginine residue that is rapidly cleaved by a blood enzyme, carboxypeptidase. After the arginine is removed, anaphylatoxins lose their ability to contract smooth muscle and release histamine. However, C5a, inactivated by carboxypeptidase and called $C5a_{desarg}$, retains its chemotactic properties and is physiologically the most important of these substances. Another peptide is cleaved from C2b. It enhances vascular permeability and is involved in the generation of symptoms in hereditary angioedema and will be discussed later.

Complement Receptors

Receptors on cells have been identified for C3b and C3d. The C3b receptor is called CR1 and is found on red cells and all leukocytes. It is the so-called immune adherence receptor. A receptor for C3d is found on B lymphocytes and is designated CR2. Phagocytic cells have a receptor for C3bi, designated CR3. The importance of CR3 in phagocytosis has been shown in studies of genetic deficiency of CR3 (see Chapter 24).

Genetics and Biosynthesis

Genetically determined polymorphisms have been described for C4, C2, C3, C6, C7, C8α, γ, C8β, and Factor B. With these markers, it has been determined that the genes for C4, C2, and Factor B are linked to the major histocompatibility complex on the short arm of human chromosome 6. The C4 gene is duplicated, and the two allelic pairs are designated C4A and C4B. The order of the genes is Factor B, C4A, and C4B, and they are located between HLA-B and HLA-D (81).

The complement components are synthesized principally in the liver (82). However C4, C2, Factor B and C1 inhibitor synthesis by monocytes has proved most useful in studies of the control of complement biosynthesis and genetic defects in complement (83). Multichain structures such as C3, C4, and C5 are synthesized as a single chain and cleaved posttranslationally in two- or three-chain structures.

Genetic Deficiencies

Genetically determined deficiencies of almost all the complement components are known. With two exceptions, these deficiencies are inherited as autosomal recessive traits. One exception is the genetic deficiency of the C1 INH; the defect is inherited as an autosomal dominant and results in hereditary angioneurotic edema (HANE). The other exception is the deficiency of properdin that is inherited as an X-linked recessive trait. The genetic deficiencies of the complement system may be grouped into four categories according to the symptoms to which they predispose:

1. Angioedema: C1 INH
2. Immune complex disease: C1q, C1r, C1s, C2, C4
3. Susceptibility to recurrent pyogenic infections: C3, Factor H, Factor I
4. Susceptibility to recurrent or overwhelming *Neisseria* infection: C5, C6, C7, C8, properdin

C9 deficiency appears to be without clinical consequences. The deficiency is very common in Japan, where one in 40 people are heterozygous carriers of the deficient gene. Antibody-sensitized bacteria or red cells will lyse in C9-deficient serum, albeit slowly. C9 accelerates the damaging effects of the terminal phase macromolecular attack complex but is not required for the formation of transmembrane channels.

HEREDITARY ANGIONEUROTIC EDEMA

Hereditary angioneurotic edema results from a genetically determined deficiency of the C1 inhibitor, which is transmitted as an autosomal dominant trait. The serum of affected patients contains from 5 to 30 per cent of the normal concentration of C1 inhibitor (18 mg per 100 ml) (84).

Patients with this disease are prone to recurrent episodes of swelling (Fig. 28–10). The edema fluid accumulates rapidly in the affected part, which becomes tense but not discolored. Itching, pain, and redness are not associated with the edema. Laryngeal edema may be fatal because of airway obstruction and consequent pulmonary edema. If the intestinal tract is involved (most often the jejunum), severe abdominal cramps and bilious vomiting ensue. Clear, watery diarrhea occurs when the colon is affected. The attacks last from 48 to 72 hours. Although they are often unheralded, they may occur subsequent to trauma, menses, excessive fatigue, and mental stress. Attacks of angioedema are infrequent in early childhood; the disease exacerbates at adolescence and tends to subside in the sixth decade of life. In children especially, a mottling of the skin, reminiscent of erythema marginatum, may be frequently noticed; this is not necessarily associated with the angioedema (85).

Attacks of angioedema are associated with the generation of activated C1 in the plasma, an event that cannot be measured in normal plasma (86). The natural substrates of C1, C4 and C2, are consumed so that their serum concentration falls

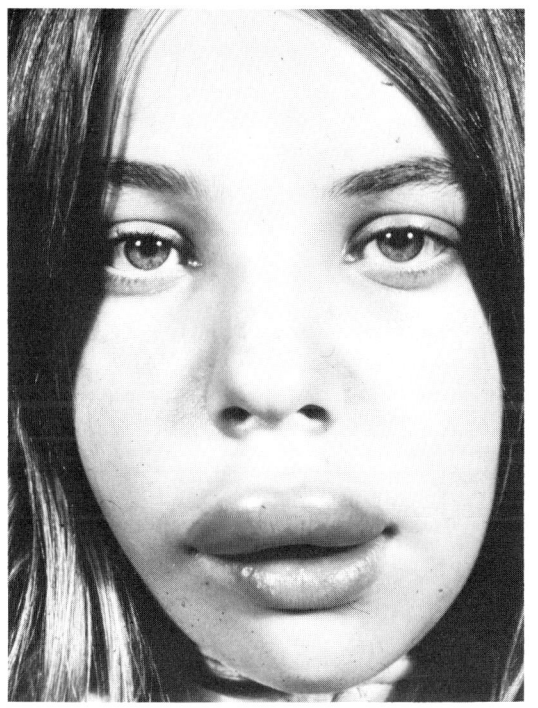

Figure 28–10. Face of a girl with hereditary angioneurotic edema during an attack. (From Rosen, F. S., and Alper, C. A.: Disorders of the complement system. In *Immunologic Disorders in Infants and Children.* Stiehm, E. R., and Fulginiti. V. A. [eds.], Philadelphia, W. B. Saunders Company, 1973, p. 291.)

precipitously as the attack progresses. The terminal components of the complement system remain unaffected. Highly purified C1 or C1s, when injected intradermally, induces angioedema, regardless of whether the skin is normal or abnormal. This reaction does not occur in humans genetically deficient in C2 or in guinea pigs genetically deficient in C2, suggesting that the interaction of C1 with C4 and C2 generates one or more factors that enhance vascular permeability—the effect is on the postcapillary venule. A polypeptide kinin–like substance that has vasopermeability-inducing properties also has been generated in the plasma of these patients (86).

The activation of C1 in hereditary angioneurotic edema may occur via fibrinolysin, the intrinsic clotting mechanism, or the kallikrein system. In any case, the fibrinolytic inhibitors, ϵ-aminocaproic acid and its cyclic analogue, tranexamic acid, provide effective prophylaxis against recurrent episodes of angioedema. Impeded (nonvirilizing) androgens are very effective in preventing angioedema. Danazol, 150 to 200 mg daily, or stanozolol, 2 to 4 mg daily, provides excellent prophylaxis against attacks of angioedema. Their mechanism of action is not understood.

Two genetic variants of HANE are recognized. In Type I, the serum contains very little C1 inhibitor (average, 17 per cent of normal). In 15 per cent of affected kindred, sera of patients contain normal or elevated amounts of a cross-reacting, immunologically nonfunctional protein (cross-reacting material, CRM). This is called Type II angioedema. There is no difference in the clinical picture of CRM+ patients and that of CRM− patients (84).

ACQUIRED C1 INH DEFICIENCY

A rare complication of monoclonal B cell expressions is the acquisition of C1 INH deficiency. Patients with this deficiency are found to have anti-idiotypic antibodies to the surface immunoglobulin idiotypes on their abnormal B cells. The idiotype–anti-idiotype results in fixation of C1 and rapid consumption of C4, C2, and C1 INH. C3 and late C components are normal. It is not known why idiotypic–anti-idiotypic reactions lead to this aberrant complement fixation (87).

EARLY COMPLEMENT COMPONENT DEFICIENCIES

Genetic deficiencies of C1q, C1r, C1r and C1s, and C4 and C2 have been described. Genetic deficiencies of the alternative pathway proteins, factor B and Factor D, have not yet been discovered. C2 deficiency is the most common genetic deficiency of complement in humans. One in 100 persons carries this gene defect, and one in 10,000 is homozygous for the deficiency (88). Deficiency of C1q, C1r, C1s, and C4 are rare.

It was originally anticipated that people with early complement component deficiencies would be very susceptible to infections, which surprisingly turned out to be untrue. Some of these patients do indeed have more infections than normal, but the major problem sustained by these patients is immune complex disease. For the present, it is important to note that the early-acting complement components, as revealed by their genetic deficiency, appear to play an important role in dissolving immune complexes. This can be shown in vitro when the dissolution of immune complexes or aggregates in normal serum is compared with the same phenomenon in serum that is deficient in one of the early-acting complement components. The mechanism whereby complement dissolves immune complexes is not known.

DEFICIENCIES OF C3 AND THE C3 CONTROL PROTEINS

It has already been pointed out that the principal opsonin of the blood is C3 and that phagocytic cells have receptors for C3b and iC3b, so that bacteria and other microorganisms coated with C3b or iC3b are rapidly ingested and killed (89). Patients who are genetically deficient in C3 have recurrent bacterial infections. Their clinical problems resemble those seen in boys with X-linked agammaglobulinemia. This fact illustrates the importance of the whole opsonic system in protection against bacterial infection. As can be predicted, a defect in the phagocytic cells will also predispose to recurrent bacterial infections. As already discussed, patients with genetic defects in the classical pathway complement proteins do not primarily have susceptibility to infection because the alternative pathway is intact and this "rescues" them from a failure to activate C3.

The six proteins of the alternative pathway—C3, Factor H, Factor I, Factor D, Factor B, and properdin—are present in the serum in a constant concentration. If Factor H or Factor I is removed from serum, the whole alternative pathway spontaneously activates. Similarly, if the six proteins are mixed together in vitro in concentrations as they exist in serum, nothing happens. If, however, the concentration of Factor H or Factor I is reduced, the system will spontaneously activate. Individuals who are genetically deficient in Factor H or Factor I sustain constant in vivo alternative pathway activation. They have C3bBb in their blood and are thus continuously destroying C3 in vivo. Consequently, they have a very low level of C3 in their blood and they cannot effectively opsonize bacteria. Because they produce large amounts of C3a, their histamine excretion is very elevated and they sustain repeated attacks of hives, or urticaria.

LATE COMPLEMENT COMPONENT DEFICIENCIES

Deficiencies of C5, C6, C7, and C8 result in extraordinary susceptibility to severe infections with bacteria of the *Neisseria* genus. There are two common human pathogens in this genus: (1) *N. gonorrhoeae*, which causes gonorrhea; and (2) *N. meningitidis*, which causes one form of meningitis. Obviously, a deficiency of any one of these components causes a failure of the bactericidal mechanism of serum, and the clinical observation of recurrent *Neisseria* infection in these deficient individuals points to the importance of this mechanism in protection against *Neisseria* in contrast to all other bacteria.

All late-acting component deficiencies are inherited as autosomal recessive traits. It is interesting that the genes for C8α,γ and for C8β are not linked. Consequently, C8-deficient patients are either C8α,γ-deficient or C8β-deficient. C8β deficiency has been found only in whites, whereas C8α,γ deficiency occurs predominantly in blacks.

Acquired Defects

It is generally considered that a decrease in serum complement results from in vivo "complement fixation." On further reflection, this is a naive notion, for the serum level of any one of or all the complement components reflects the rate of synthesis as well as the rate of catabolism of these proteins. It has been most convenient to assay for the serum concentration of C3 or the β_{1c} globulin. This measurement is readily available in most clinical laboratories. C3 levels in serum may decrease to very low concentrations in the presence of hepatocellular damage because the hepatic parenchymal cell is the site of C3 synthesis. However, decreased serum C3 levels in lupus erythematosus reflect in vivo consumption of this protein by antigen-antibody interaction. One can confirm this by studying the catabolic rate of ^{125}I-labeled C3 in patients with systemic lupus erythematosus or mixed cryoglobulinemia.

C3 levels are very low in sera of children with acute poststreptococcal glomerulonephritis or membranoproliferative glomerulonephritis. In both instances, the lowered C3 level is due to a combination of decreased synthesis and increased catabolism. In acute poststreptococcal glomerulonephritis, there is initially a marked fall in all classic complement components, but within 2 or 3 days of the onset of symptoms most of the components return to normal. The concentrations of C3 and C5, however, remain low for 3 or 4 weeks. Evidence from metabolic studies with purified ^{125}I-labeled C3 suggests that, in the initial phase, the C3 concentration is lowered as part of the activation of the complement system, presumably by antigen-antibody complexes. Circulating conversion products of C3 can sometimes be demonstrated during this initial phase. Studies performed 2 or 3 days after the onset of symptoms suggest that depressed C3 synthesis is responsible for the prolonged lowering of the level of C3 (and perhaps of C5 as well) after the initial activation phase.

The situation in membranoproliferative glomerulonephritis is far less clear. In this disorder, particularly as it occurs in children and adolescents, lowered hemolytic complement is a usual finding. This is almost always the result of markedly reduced levels of C3 and C5, with normal levels of most other complement components. Serum concentrations of properdin Factor B are usually normal in these patients, or at most slightly reduced. By immunofluorescent techniques involving antibodies to immunoglobulins and C3, the proteins are demonstrable on the glomeruli in most patients. The sera of some patients with membranoproliferative glomerulonephritis contain circulating C3d and may also contain nephritic factor. Depressed synthesis of C3 in vitro by liver cells obtained from such patients also has been demonstrated. However, an infant who acquired nephritic factor from his mother via the placenta had a low serum C3 for 2 weeks postnatally.

There is some evidence that complement activation may occur in severe disseminated intravascular coagulation with fibrinolysis. In this clinical situation, it may be that the generated plasmin and possibly thrombin attack C3 directly. Serum levels of the C3 serum concentrations observed in patients with advanced hepatic cirrhosis or other hepatocellular disease may result from associated disseminated intravascular coagulation and fibrinolysis or from interference with C3 synthesis in the liver, which is its site of synthesis. We have observed marked elevations of C3 serum concentration in patients with severe biliary obstruction. The mechanisms for this elevation are unknown.

In certain cases of acquired hemolytic anemia, C3 is detected on erythrocytes by a Coombs' antiglobulin reagent specific for this protein. General Coombs' reagents vary in their content of anti-C3 and for the most part are anti-IgG. The presence of C3 on patients' red cells may indicate an antierythrocyte antibody that has "fixed complement," activation of C3 by other means with C3 deposition as part of the "innocent bystander" reaction, or an unusual abnormality of the red cell membrane, making it more "susceptible" to C3 uptake, as in paroxysmal nocturnal hemoglobinuria.

Total serum hemolytic complement and the levels of individual complement proteins are normal or elevated in patients with rheumatoid arthritis, and there is no evidence of complement activation in serum. However, the joint space is relatively sequestered from the circulating plasma, and there is now considerable evidence that complement participates locally in rheumatoid joint inflammation. Hemolytic complement is reduced in joint fluid from patients with rheumatoid arthritis, particularly those with rheumatoid factor and nodules, when compared with joint effusions from patients with other diseases. There is a reduction in the relative concentrations in the rheumatoid joint effusions of several complement proteins, including C4, C2, C3, and Factor B, and conversion products of the latter two proteins are often found. Chemotactic factors, thought to consist of C5a, are found in the majority of rheumatoid joint effusions. By immunofluorescence, C3 and C4 have been identified in the lining cells, blood vessels, and intercellular connective tissue of rheumatoid synovial membranes. Incubation of normal leukocytes with joint fluid from patients with seropositive rheumatoid arthritis caused the development of intracellular inclusions containing IgG, IgM, and C3. It is not clear whether complement activation in joints affected by rheumatoid arthritis results from the presence of complexes of IgG antibody with an unknown, possibly viral, antigen; of complexes of IgM rheumatoid factor with aggregated gamma globulin; of proteolytic enzymes from leukocytes; or of some combination of these factors.

Tests for paroxysmal nocturnal hemoglobinuria (PNH) depend on the unusual susceptibility of red cells in this disease to complement lysis. In the Ham test, the test red cells are incubated in acidified (pH 6.7) fresh serum from an ABO-compatible person or from the patient. The minimal complement activation that occurs at somewhat acid pH will produce lysis of PNH cells but not normal erythrocytes. An important control consists of incubating the patient's red cells with serum heated at 56°C prior to acidification. With destruction of total hemolytic complement, such serum will not lyse PNH cells. The sugar-water test for PNH depends on minimal complement activation, probably attendant on euglobulin precipitation. In this test, the patient's whole blood is mixed with nine volumes of a 10 per cent solution and incubated. All tests for PNH lysis depend on the integrity of the properdin system in the lytic reagent. PNH cells, for unknown reasons, take up much more C3 than do normal erythrocytes.

As pointed out previously, PNH cells lack the decay-accelerating factor (DAF) that prevents the formation of C3 convertase in the cell membrane.

References

1. Rosen, F. S., Cooper, M.D., and Wedgwood, R. J. P.: The primary immunodeficiencies. New Engl. J. Med. *311*:235; 300, 1984.
2. Siegel, R. L., Issekutz, T., et al.: Deficiency of T helper cells in transient hypogammaglobulinemia of infancy. New Engl. J. Med. *305*:1307, 1981.
3. Mease, P. J., Ochs, H. D., and Wedgwood, R. J.: Successful treatment of echovirus meningoencephalitis and myositis-fasciitis with intravenous gamma globulin therapy in a patient with X-linked agammaglobulinemia. New Engl. J. Med. *304*:1278, 1981.
4. Wilfert, C. M., Buckley, R. H., et al.: Persistent and fatal central-nervous-system echovirus infections in patients with agammaglobulinemia. New Engl. J. Med. *296*:1485, 1977.
5. Ammann, A. J., Ashman, R. F., et al.: Use of intravenous gamma globulin in antibody immunodeficiency: results of a multicenter controlled trial. Clin. Immunol. Immunopathol. *22*:60, 1982.
6. Eibl, M., Cairns, L., and Rosen, F. S.: Safety and efficacy of a monomeric functionally intact intravenous IgG preparation in patients with primary immunodeficiency syndromes. Clin. Immunol. Immunopathol. *31*:151, 1984.
7. Geha, R. S., Hyslop, N., et al.: Hyper–immunoglobulin M immunodeficiency (dysgammaglobulinemia): presence of immunoglobulin M–secreting plasmacytoid cells in peripheral blood and failure of immunoglobulin M–immunoglobulin G switch in B-cell differentiation. J. Clin. Invest. *64*:385, 1979.
8. Schwaber, J. F., Lazarus, H., and Rosen, F. S.: IgM-restricted production of immunoglobulin by lymphoid cell lines from patients with immunodeficiency with hyper-IgM (dysgammaglobulinemia). Clin. Immunol. Immunopathol. *19*:91, 1981.
9. Schur, P. H., Borel, H., et al.: Selective gamma-G globulin deficiencies in patients with recurrent pyogenic infections. New Engl. J. Med. *283*:631, 1970.
10. Oxelius, V.-A.: Chronic infections in a family with hereditary deficiency of IgG2 and IgG4. Clin. Exp. Immunol. *17*:19, 1974.
11. Oxelius, V.-A., Laurell, A.-B., et al.: IgA subclasses is in selective IgA deficiency: importance of IgG2-IgA deficiency. New Engl. J. Med. *304*:1476, 1981.
12. Cunningham-Rundles, C., Oxelius, V.-A., and Good, R. A.: IgG2 and IgG3 subclass deficiencies in selective IgA deficiency in the United States. Birth Defects *19*:173, 1983.
13. Strober, W., Krakauer, R., et al.: Secretory component

deficiency: a disorder of the IgA immune system. New Engl. J. Med. *294:*351, 1976.
14. Hitzig, W. H., Dohmann, U., et al.: Hereditary transcobalamin II deficiency: clinical findings in a new family. J. Pediatr. *85:*622, 1974.
15. Johnson, B. L., Jr., Goldberg, L. S., et al.: Clinical and immunological studies in a case of nodular lymphoid hyperplasia of the small bowel. Gastroenterology *61:*369, 1971.
16. Gelfand, E. W., Berkel, A. I., et al.: Pernicious anemia, hypogammaglobulinemia and altered lymphocyte reactivity. A family study. Clin. Exp. Immunol. *11:*187, 1972.
17. Ochs, H. D., Ament, M. E., and Davis, S. D.: Giardiasis with malabsorption in X-linked agammaglobulinemia. New Engl. J. Med. *287:*341, 1972.
18. Cooper, M. D., Lawton, A. B., and Backman, D. E.: Agammaglobulinemia with B lymphocytes: specific defect of plasma-cell differentiation. Lancet *2:*791, 1971.
19. Geha, R. S., Schneeberger, E., et al.: Heterogeneity of "acquired" or common variable agammaglobulinemia. New Engl. J. Med. *291:*1, 1974.
20. Schwaber, J., and Rosen, F. S.: Somatic cell hybrids of mouse myeloma cells and B lymphocytes from a patient with agammaglobulinemia: failure to secrete human immunoglobulin. J. Immunol. *122:*1849, 1979.
21. Waldmann, T. A., Durm, M., et al.: Role of suppressor T cells in pathogenesis of common variable hypogammaglobulinemia. Lancet *2:*609, 1974.
22. Siegal, F. P., Siegal, M., and Good, R. A.: Suppression of B-cell differentiation by leukocytes from hypogammaglobulinemic patients. J. Clin. Invest. *58:*109, 1976.
23. Reinherz, E. L., Rubinstein, A. J., et al.: Abnormalities of immunoregulatory T cells in disorders of immune function. New Engl. J. Med. *301:*1018, 1979.
24. Reinherz, E. L., Geha, R., et al.: Immunodeficiency associated with loss of T4+ inducer T-cell function. New Engl. J. Med. *304:*811, 1981.
25. Reinherz, E. L., Cooper, M. D., et al.: Abnormalities of T cell maturation and regulation in human beings with immunodeficiency disorders. J. Clin. Invest. *68:*699, 1981.
26. Gelfand, E. W., Borel, H., et al.: Autoimmunosuppression: recurrent infections associated with immunologic unresponsiveness in the presence of an auto-antibody to IgG. Clin. Immunol. Immunopathol. *1:*155, 1972.
27. Tursz, R., Preud'homme, J.-L., et al.: Autoantibodies to B lymphocytes in a patient with hypogammaglobulinemia: characterization and pathogenic role. J. Clin. Invest. *60:*405, 1977.
28. Hirschhorn, R., Vawter, G. F., et al.: Adenosine deaminase deficiency: frequency and comparative pathology in autosomally recessive severe combined immunodeficiency. Clin. Immunol. Immunopathol. *14:*107, 1979.
29. Tischfield, J. A., Creagan, R. P., et al.: Assignment of a gene for adenosine deaminase to human chromosome 20. Hum. Hered. *24:*1, 1974.
30. Hirschhorn, R., Beratis, N., et al.: Characterization of residual enzyme activity in fibroblasts from patients with adenosine deaminase deficiency and combined immunodeficiency: evidence for a mutant enzyme. Proc. Natl. Acad. Sci. U.S.A. *73:*213, 1976.
31. Reem, G. H., Borkowsky, W., and Hirschhorn, R.: Purine and phosphoribosyl-pyrophosphate metabolism of lymphocytes and erythrocytes of an adenosine deaminase–deficient immunocompetent child. Pediatr. Res. *13:*649, 1979.
32. Hirschhorn, R., Martiniuk, F., et al: Genetic heterogeneity in partial adenosine-deaminase deficiency. J. Clin. Invest. *71:*1887, 1983.
33. Giblett, E. R., Ammann, A. J., et al.: Nucleoside-phosphorylase deficiency in a child with severely defective T-cell immunity and normal B-cell immunity. Lancet *1:*1010, 1975.
34. Ricciuti, F., and Ruddle, F. H.: Assignment of nucleoside phosphorylase to D-14 and localization of X-linked loci in man by somatic cell genetics. Nature (New Biol.) *241:*180, 1973.
35. Gelfand, E. W., Dosch, H.-M., et al.: Partial purine nucleoside phosphorylase deficiency: studies of lymphocyte function. J. Clin. Invest. *61:*1071, 1978.
36. Cohen, A., Coyle, D., et al.: Abnormal purine metabolism and purine overproduction in a patient deficient in purine nucleoside phosphorylase. New Engl. J. Med. *295:*1449, 1976.
37. Cohen, A., Gudas, L. J., et al.: Deoxyguanosine triphosphate as a possible toxic metabolite in the immunodeficiency associated with purine nucleoside phosphorylase deficiency. J. Clin. Invest. *61:*1405, 1978.
38. Carson, D. A., Wasson, D. B., et al.: Possible metabolic basis for the different immunodeficient state associated with genetic deficiencies of adenosine deaminase and purine nucleoside phosphorylase. Proc. Natl. Acad. Sci. U.S.A. *79:*3848, 1982.
39. Gudas, L. J., Ullman, B., et al.: Deoxyguanosine toxicity in a mouse T lymphoma: relationship to purine–nucleoside phosphorylase–associated immune dysfunction. Cell *14:*531, 1978.
40. Ullman, B., Gudas, L. J., et al.: Isolation and characterization of purine–nucleoside phosphorylase–deficient T-lymphoma cells and secondary mutants with altered ribonucleotide reductase: genetic model for immunodeficiency disease. Proc. Natl. Acad. Sci. U.S.A. *76:*1074, 1979.
41. Ballet, J., Insel, R., et al.: Inhibition of maturation of human precursor lymphocytes by coformycin: an inhibitor of the enzyme adenosine deaminase. J. Exp. Med. *143:*1271, 1976.
42. Hirschhorn, R., Roegner-Maniscalco, V., et al.: Bone marrow transplantation only partially restores purine metabolites to normal in adenosine deaminase–deficient patients. J. Clin. Invest. *68:*1387, 1981.
43. Hershfield, M. S., and Kredich, N. M.: Resistance of an adenosine kinase–deficient human lymphoblastoid cell line to effects of deoxyadenosine on growth, S-adenosylhomocysteine hydrolase inactivation, and dATP accumulation. Proc. Natl. Acad. Sci. U.S.A. *77:*4292, 1980.
44. O'Reilly, R. J., Dupont, B., et al.: Reconstitution in severe combined immunodeficiency by transplantation of marrow from an unrelated donor. New Engl. J. Med. *297:*1311, 1971.
45. Reinherz, E. L., Geha, R., et al.: Reconstitution after transplantation with T-lymphocyte–depleted HLA haplotype–mismatched bone marrow for severe combined immunodeficiency. Proc. Natl. Acad. Sci. U.S.A. *79:*6047, 1982.
46. Reisner, Y., Kapoor, N., et al.: Transplantation for severe combined immunodeficiency with HLA-A,B,D,Dr incompatible parental marrow cells fractionated by soybean agglutinin and sheep red blood cells. Blood *61:*341, 1983.
47. Gotoff, S. P., Amirmokri, E., et al.: Ataxia telangiectasia: neoplasia, untoward response to X-irradiation and tuberous sclerosis. Am. J. Dis. Child. *114:*617, 1967.
48. McCaw, B. K., Hecht, F., et al.: Somatic rearrangement of chromosome 14 in human lymphocytes. Proc. Natl. Acad. Sci. U.S.A. *72:*2071, 1975.
49. Taylor, A. M. R., Harnden, D. G., et al.: Ataxia telangiectasia: a human mutation with abnormal radiation sensitivity. Nature *258:*427, 1975.
50. Povirk, L. F., and Goldberg, I. H.: Inhibition of mammalian deoxyribonucleic acid synthesis by neocarzinostatin: selective effect to replicon initiation in CHO cells and resistant synthesis in ataxis telangiectasia. Biochemistry *21:*5857, 1982.
51. Patersen, M. D., and Smith, P. J.: Ataxia telangiectasia: an inherited human disorder involving hypersensitivity to ionizing radiation and related DNA-damaging chemicals. Annu. Rev. Genet. *13:*291, 1979.

52. Taylor, A. M. R., Metcalfe, J. A., et al.: Is chromatid-type damage in ataxia telangiectasia after irradiation at G_0 a consequence of defective repair? Nature 260:441, 1976.
53. Paterson, M. C., Smith, B. P., et al.: Defective excision repair of gamma-ray damaged DNA in human (ataxia telangiectasia) fibroblasts. Nature 260:444, 1976.
54. Waldmann, T. A., and McIntire, K. R.: Serum-alpha-fetoprotein levels in patients with ataxia-telangiectasia. Lancet 2:1112, 1972.
55. Sugimoto, T., Sawada, T., et al.: Plasma levels of carinoembryonic antigen in patients with ataxia-telangiectasia. J. Pediatr. 92:436, 1978.
56. Shaham, M., Voss, R., et al.: Prenatal diagnosis of ataxia telangiectasia. J. Pediatr. 100:134, 1982.
57. Murnane, J. P., and Painter, R. B.: Complementation of the defects in DNA synthesis in irradiated and unirradiated ataxia-telangiectasia cells. Proc. Natl. Acad. Sci. U.S.A. 79:1960, 1982.
58. Jaspers, N. G. J., and Bootsma, D.: Genetic heterogeneity in ataxia-telangiectasia studied by cell fusion. Proc. Natl. Acad. Sci. U.S.A. 79:2641, 1982.
59. Swift, M., Sholman, L., et al.: Malignant neoplasms in the families of patients with ataxia-telangiectasia. Cancer Res. 36:209, 1976.
60. St. Geme, J. W., Jr., Prince, J. T., et al.: Impaired cellular resistance to herpes-simplex virus in Wiskott-Aldrich syndrome. New Engl. J. Med. 273:229, 1965.
61. Takemoto, K. K., Rabson, A. S., et al.: Isolation of papovavirus from brain tumor and urine of a patient with Wiskott-Aldrich syndrome. J. Natl. Cancer Inst. 53:1205, 1974.
62. Perry, G. S., III, Spector, B. D., et al.: The Wiskott-Aldrich syndrome in the United States and Canada (1892–1979). J. Pediatr. 97:72, 1980.
63. Akkerman, J. W. N., van Brederode, W., et al.: The Wiskott-Aldrich syndrome: studies on a possible defect in mitochondrial ATP resynthesis in platelets. Br. J. Haematol. 51:561, 1982.
64. Gealy, W. J., Dwyer, J. M., and Harley, J. B.: Allelic exclusion of glucose-6-phosphate dehydrogenase in platelets and T lymphocytes from a Wiskott-Aldrich carrier. Lancet 1:63, 1980.
65. Prchal, J. T., Carroll, A. J., et al.: Wiskott-Aldrich syndrome: cellular impairments and their implications for carrier detection. Blood 56:1048, 1980.
66. Bruce, R. M., and Blaese, R. M.: Monoclonal gammopathy in the Wiskott-Aldrich syndrome. J. Pediatr. 85:204, 1974.
67. Cooper, M. D., Chase, H. P., et al.: Wiskott-Aldrich syndrome: immunologic deficiency disease involving the efferent limb of immunity. Am. J. Med. 44:499, 1968.
68. Blaese, R. M., Strober, W., et al.: The Wiskott-Aldrich syndrome: a disorder with a possible defect in antigen processing or recognition. Lancet 1:1056, 1968.
69. Ochs, H. D., Slichter, S. J., et al.: The Wiskott-Aldrich syndrome: studies of lymphocytes, granulocytes and platelets. Blood 55:243, 1980.
70. Parkman, R., Rappeport, J., et al.: Complete correction of the Wiskott-Aldrich syndrome by allogeneic bone-marrow transplantation. New Engl. J. Med. 298:921, 1978.
71. Lam, L. G., Tubergen, D. G., et al.: Splenectomy in the management of the thrombocytopenia of the Wiskott-Aldrich syndrome. New Engl. J. Med. 302:892, 1980.
72. Remold-O'Donnell, E., Kenney, D. M., et al.: Characterization of a human lymphocyte surface sialoglycoprotein that is defective in Wiskott-Aldrich syndrome. J. Exp. Med. 159:1705, 1984.
73. Purtilo, D. T., DeFlorio, D., Jr., et al.: Variable phenotypic expression of an X-linked recessive lymphoproliferative syndrome. New Engl. J. Med. 297:1077, 1977.
74. Provisor, A. J., Iacuone, J. J., et al.: Acquired agammaglobulinemia after a life-threatening illness with clinical and laboratory features of infectious mononucleosis in three related male children. New Engl. J. Med. 293:62, 1985.
75. Sullivan, J. L., Byron, K. S., et al.: X-linked lymphoproliferative syndrome: natural history of the immunodeficiency. J. Clin. Invest. 71:1765, 1983.
76. Coffin, J., Haase, A., et al.: What to call the AIDS virus? Nature 321:10, 1986.
76a. Wong-Stahl, F., and Gallo, R. C.: The family of human T-lymphotropic leukemia viruses: HTLV-I as the cause of adult T cell leukemia and HTLV-III as the cause of acquired immune deficiency syndrome. Blood 65:253, 1985.
77. Seligmann, M., Chess, L., et al.: AIDS—an immunologic reevaluation. New Engl. J. Med. 311:1286, 1984.
77a. Siegal, F. P., Lopez, C., et al.: Opportunistic infections in AIDS result from synergistic defects of both the natural and adaptive components of cellular immunity. J. Clin. Invest. 78:115, 1986.
77b. Rubinstein A., Sicklick, M., et al.: Acquired immunodeficiency with reversed T4/T8 ratios in infants born to promiscuous and drug-addicted mothers. J.A.M.A. 249:2350, 1983.
77c. Oleske, J., Minnefor, A., et al.: Immune deficiency syndrome in children. J.A.M.A. 249:2345, 1983.
77d. Rubinstein, A.: Pediatric AIDS. In Year Book/Current Problems in Pediatrics. Lockhart, J. (ed.): Chicago, Year Book Medical Publishers, 1986.
78. Pangburn, M. K., and Müller-Eberhard, A. J.: The alternative pathway of complement. Springer Semin. Immunopathol. 7:163; 1984.
79. Nicholson-Weller, A., Burge, J., et al.: Isolation of a human erythrocyte membrane glycoprotein with decay-accelerating activity for C3 convertase of the complement system. J. Immunol. 129:184, 1982.
80. Holprich, P. D., Dahinden, C. A., et al.: A synthetic monopeptide corresponding to the NH_2-terminal sequence of C3d-K causes leukocytosis in rabbits. J. Biol. Chem. 260:2597, 1985.
81. Carrol, M. C., Campbell, R. D., et al.: A molecular map of the human major histocompatibility complex class III region linking complement genes C4, C2 and factor B. Nature 307:237, 1984.
82. Morris, K. M., Aden, D. P., et al.: Complement biosynthesis by the human hepatoma-derived cell line Hep G2. J. Clin Invest 70:906, 1982.
83. Cole, F. S., Whitehead, A. S., et al.: The molecular basis for genetic deficiency of the second component of human complement. New Engl. J. Med. 313:11, 1985.
84. Rosen, F. S., Alper, C. A., et al.: Genetically determined heterogeneity of the C1 esterase inhibitor in patients with hereditary angioneurotic edema. J. Clin. Invest. 50:2143, 1971.
85. Donaldson, V. H., and Rosen, F. S.: Hereditary angioneurotic edema: a clinical survey. Pediatrics 37:1017, 1966.
86. Donaldson, V. H., and Rosen, F. S.: Action of complement in hereditary angioneurotic edema. The role of C'1-esterase. J. Clin. Invest. 43:2204, 1964.
87. Geha, R. S., Quinti, I., et al.: Acquired C1-inhibitor deficiency associated with antiidiotypic antibody to monoclonal immunoglobulins. New Engl. J. Med. 312:534, 1985.
88. Klemperer, M. R., Woodworth, H. C., et al.: Hereditary deficiency of the second component of complement (C'2) in man. J. Clin. Invest. 45:880, 1966.
89. Alper, C. A., Colten, H. R., et al.: Homozygous deficiency of the third component of complement (C3) in a patient with repeated infections. Lancet 2:1179, 1972.

THE SPLEEN

CHAPTER 29
The Spleen and Disturbances of Splenic Function

HOWARD A. PEARSON

HISTORY 900
EMBRYOLOGY AND ANATOMY 901
HISTOLOGY AND CIRCULATION 901
ASPLENIA-POLYSPLENIA SYNDROMES 901
Congenital Asplenia
Congenital Polysplenia Syndrome
Accessory Spleens
SPLENIC CYSTS 903
SPLENIC TUMORS 903
SPLENOSIS 903
SPLENIC HYPOPLASIA OR ATROPHY 904
SPLENIC FUNCTION 905
Normal Function
Developmental Aspects of Splenic Function
FUNCTIONAL HYPOSPLENIA 909
Sickle Cell Disease
Hyposplenism in "Autoimmune" Disease
SPLENOMEGALY 909
SPLENECTOMY 910
Postsplenectomy Infection

HISTORY

The spleen and its functions have excited the imagination of physicians since the beginnings of medical history. Both Hippocrates and Aristotle commented on the form and anatomic relationships of the spleen. Galen described it as "misterii organum plenum," an organ full of mystery. It was believed that the spleen extracted the melancholic humors from the blood and thus was associated with merriment and laughter ("great laughers have great spleens"—Pliny the Elder, 150 A.D.). Sometime during the sixteenth or seventeenth century, however, the word "spleen" underwent a change in meaning to its present connotation of spite and testiness. Early investigators recognized that the spleen was not indispensable because normal life continued after its removal (1).

During the seventeenth century, investigators including Harvey, Glisson, Bartholin, and Wharton described the detailed structure of the spleen. The great Italian anatomist Malpighi first described the malpighian bodies, which he erroneously assumed to be secreting glands, and this belief persisted for more than a century. William Hewson, in 1777, wrote that the spleen was concerned with converting the lymph into blood elements and assigned the organ to the lymphatic system. In 1846, Virchow demonstrated that the malpighian follicles were concerned with the formation of white blood cells (2). In 1885, Ponfick recognized that the spleen could remove various particles, including erythrocytes, from the blood and thus was involved in blood destruction (3).

Possible instances of splenectomy were described as early as the sixteenth century, and a number of definite splenectomies were reported during the seventeenth and eighteenth centuries. The usual indications were trauma and splenomegaly secondary to leukemia; not surprisingly, mortality was high. In 1888, Sir T. Spencer Wells, a prominent Victorian surgeon, reported performing a splenectomy for "abdominal tumor" in a 22-year-old woman who had a lifelong history of dark urine and frequent attacks of jaundice. After removal of an enlarged spleen, the patient was restored to complete health (4). Twenty-six years later, the same woman, when studied by Lord Dawson, had the increased red cell osmotic fragility characteristic of congenital spherocytosis (5).

A medical student, Kasnelson, suggested that the spleen played an important role in purpura hemorrhagica (ITP). He persuaded his professor of surgery to perform a splenectomy in a patient with this disorder, and the operation induced a remission (6).

For most of medical history, the spleen was considered nonessential to life. This concept was seriously challenged in 1952 by King and Shumacher, who reported five infants who developed fulminating bacterial infections shortly after splenectomy for congenital hemolytic anemia (7). Their observations formed an impetus for extensive studies of the spleen, including investigations of its functions and its surgery, which are continuing today.

EMBRYOLOGY AND ANATOMY

The primordium of the spleen can be recognized in the left dorsal mesogastrium at about 5 weeks' gestational age (crown–rump length, 8 to 10 mm). By 4 months it is an active center of hematopoiesis; however, the germinal centers are not fully developed during fetal life.

At birth, the dimensions of the human spleen average $4.6 \times 2.7 \times 1.3$ cm. The mean weight at birth is 11 g (7); at 6 years the spleen weighs about 55 g and at puberty approximately 125 g (8–10). During growth, splenic weight is an almost linear function of body weight, as indicated by the allometric relationship, $S = (3.5 \times 10^{-3})B^{0.97}$, in which S and B are the weights of the spleen and body, respectively (11). The maximal splenic weight is reached at puberty and decreases thereafter, and the spleen of the adult male is somewhat larger than that of the adult female. The average length of the adult spleen is 10.7 cm. Spleen size is usually estimated by physical examination. Recently, radionuclide imaging has been extensively used to define the size, anatomy, and location as well as some functions of the spleen (1, 12).

HISTOLOGY AND CIRCULATION

The spleen is a complex organ made up of several distinct but anatomically related components. The white pulp consists of germinal centers, which are dense collections of lymphocytes, plasma cells, and macrophages grouped about a central artery. T cells are found predominantly in the periarteriolar sheaths, whereas B cells occur in the germinal center of the white pulp. The red pulp, which makes up the largest part of the organ, consists of the endothelial cords of Billroth, which interdigitate between the macrophage-lined splenic sinusoids (Fig. 29–1). The splenic capsule and fibrous trabeculae form a basic supporting skeleton through which the larger blood vessels of the organ pass.

The pattern of circulation of blood within the spleen has anatomic arrangements that are consistent with some important splenic functions. Blood enters the spleen through the splenic artery and its major branches in the hilus. A number of collateral arterial connections to the gastric arteries occur through the splenic capsule, so that ligation of the splenic artery does not result in infarction of the organ (13). Splenic blood flow in the adult has been estimated to be approximately 150 ml per minute (14). The major splenic arteries branch into trabecular arteries, and after several bifurcations, distal small arteries enter the white pulp, where they constitute the central arteries of the germinal centers. A number of acute arterial branches from the central artery are observed. The arrangement results in a "skimming off" of plasma, and many of these arteries contain only plasma. Suspended particulate material would also be delivered directly into the substance of the white pulp, an arrangement believed to facilitate preferential antibody formation in response to particulate intravenous antigenic stimulation (15, 16).

The terminal splenic arteries, carrying blood that is now somewhat concentrated, enter the marginal zone of the red pulp and are directly contiguous with the cords of Billroth. There has been considerable controversy over the years concerning the nature of the splenic blood circulation at this point, which has revolved around the issue of whether blood flow occurs exclusively within channels lined with endothelial cells ("closed" circulation) versus an "open" circulation in which blood reaches the sinuses outside defined blood vessels. The preponderance of opinion, based on careful electron microscopic and dynamic studies, favors the "open" view (17–21a).

The blood is carried intravascularly to the red pulp. Only 10 per cent of the blood is emptied directly into sinusoids; the rest is forced into the cords of Billroth (22, 23). The cords, which lie between and share a basement membrane with adjacent sinuses, are bound by reticular cells and can be considered to be blood vessels lined with endothelial cells. Blood cells and other particulate material must circulate within the cords until they squeeze between the small apertures between epithelial cells lining the sinus. Arteriovenous connections have been demonstrated that may permit a bypassing of the sinusoids (24). Weiss has suggested that the reticular material that is present between the arterial vessels and venous channels is contractile and that the action may facilitate either rapid or slow passage of blood (23).

ASPLENIA-POLYSPLENIA SYNDROMES

The syndromes of congenital asplenia and polysplenia have many similar features, including a tendency for symmetric development of normally asymmetric organs and isomerism of paired organs. The embryologic fact that the spleen is the only organ that arises entirely from the left side

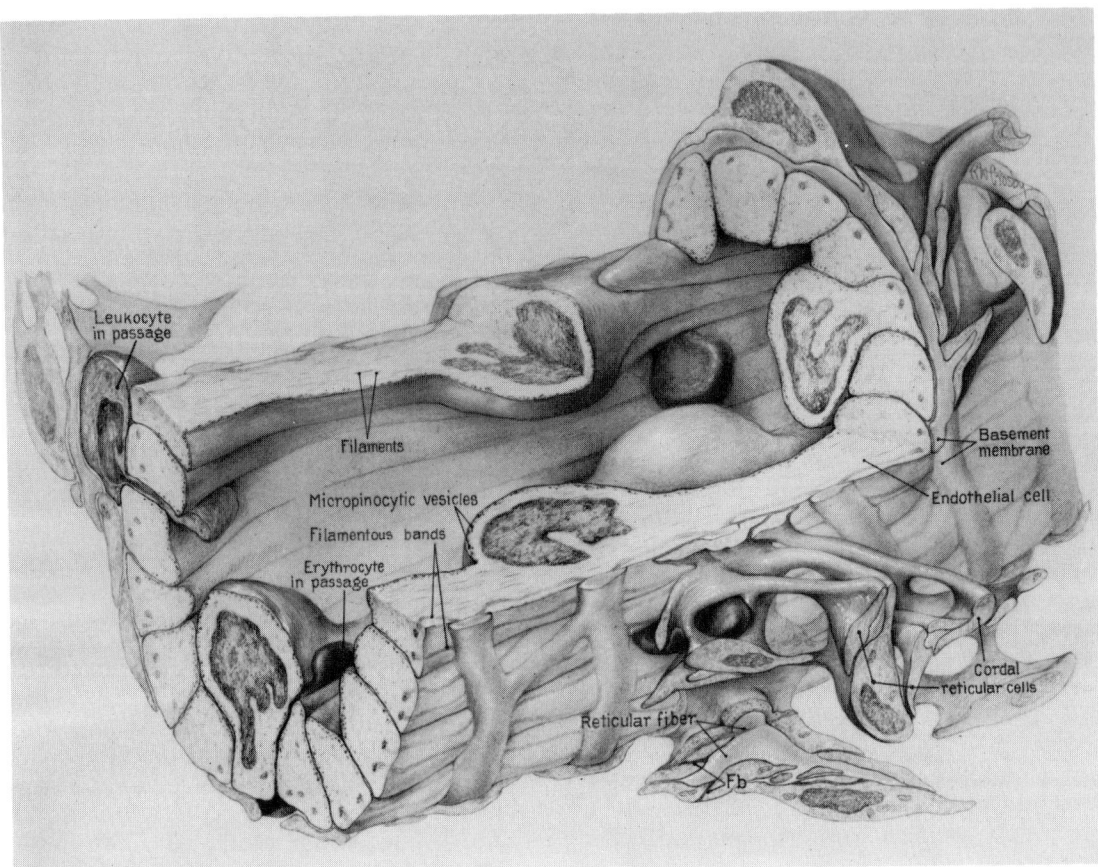

Figure 29–1. Diagram of splenic sinus, which represents the structure of a sinus in the red pulp based on electron microscopic observations. The sinus wall consists of a single layer of endothelial cells, a basement membrane, and adventitial cells that partially cover the cordal surface of both the basement membrane and the endothelium. The sinus is cut transversely and longitudinally. The endothelial cells running parallel to the longitudinal axis of the sinus are partially covered by ring and longitudinal components of basement membranes and by the adventitial cells. The adventitial cells branch into the cords and are part of the cordal reticulum. Most of the adventitial cells are omitted in this diagram in order to depict the basement membrane and filamentous bands in the basal portions of the endothelial cells. In reality, the basement membrane is completely covered by the endothelial cells and adventitial cells, and the reticular fibers by the reticular cells. The basement membrane is continuous with the reticular fibers of the cords. The endothelial cells contain three distinctive structures: micropinocytotic vesicles and two types of cytoplasmic filaments loosely organized and tightly aligned into arching bands. The filamentous bands depicted through the plasmalemma and in cross and longitudinal sections lie in the basal portions of the endothelial cells. The bands arch between the ring components of basement membrane, running perpendicular to the ring and, therefore, parallel to the long axis of the sinuses and their endothelial cells. The filaments of the filamentous bands are inserted into the plasmalemma. Blood cells are frequently present in passage through the slits of the sinus wall. They are tightly constricted. Filamentous bands (Fb) also are present in cordal reticular cells. Here, however, the bands do not have the orientation or arrangement they have in the sinus endothelium. (From Chen, L.-T., and Weiss, L.: Am. J. Anat. *134*:425, 1972.)

of the body provides a basis for some of the anatomic observations in these syndromes (25).

Congenital Asplenia

Multiple anatomic visceral abnormalities are noted in this rare syndrome of bilateral "right-sidedness," including bilateral trilobed lungs and a symmetric, centrally located liver (Ivemark syndrome) (26). The stomach is on the right side of the abdomen in about half the cases. The most important anomalies involve the cardiovascular system. In about one third of cases, the heart is in the right chest (dextrocardia). Abnormalities of the venae cavae and pulmonary venous connections, transposition of the great arteries, pulmonary stenosis, and absence of the coronary sinus are frequently found. In about half the cases there is a single functioning ventricle. Because of the complex nature of the cardiac anomalies, surgical correction may be difficult, and death often occurs in infancy.

Characteristic morphologic abnormalities of the blood such as Howell-Jolly (HJ) bodies and siderocytes permit a diagnosis of asplenia to be made noninvasively (27, 28). However, the red blood cells of newborn infants with intact spleens, particularly those of neonates with cyanotic heart disease, may contain HJ bodies and show substantial numbers of "pocked" red cells (29, 30). We have studied a full-term newborn with angiographically proven asplenia. The proportion of pocked RBCs was 14.2 per cent, which considerably exceeds that seen in normal term infants (3.9 ± 0.4) (31). In children who survive beyond infancy with the congenital asplenia syndrome, severe bacterial infections are frequent (32).

Congenital Polysplenia Syndrome

In this syndrome of bilateral "left-sidedness," multiple spleens are found along the greater curvature of the stomach. There are usually two large main spleens and a number of small splenules. Both lungs are bilobed, resembling left lungs. Isomerism of the liver is present in about one fourth of these syndromes, and the stomach is on the right side of the abdomen in two thirds of cases (33).

Cardiac anomalies are generally stated to be less frequent than in the asplenia syndromes. In 25 per cent of cases, the heart is entirely normal, and in others only simple, relatively benign cardiac anomalies are noted (33). However, other series describe a higher percentage of serious cardiac lesions (34). A frequent association between polysplenia and biliary atresia also has been described (35). Although splenic activities in the polysplenic state are generally thought to be normal, one patient has been described with HJ bodies in the blood (36).

Accessory Spleens

Accessory spleens occur with considerable frequency. In a multi-institutional survey of nearly 1500 splenectomies performed for a variety of indications, more than one spleen was noted in 16 per cent of cases (37).

Most accessory spleens are located in the hilus of the spleen or in the adjacent tail of the pancreas. However, they may be widely located, and instances of scrotal ectopic spleens have been described (38). They are usually small, 1 to 2 cm in length, but may hypertrophy under stimulation. Instances of recurrent autoimmune blood disease have been reported to be caused by hypertrophied accessory spleens (39–42).

SPLENIC CYSTS

Splenic cysts are relatively uncommon abdominal tumors (43, 44). Two general types of splenic cysts have been described. So-called "true" epidermoid cysts have a lining of stratified squamous epithelium; however, this may be present only in discontinuous plaques. The interior surface may be smooth or densely trabeculated. These cysts tend to be large and contain clear or turbid fluid with suspended cholesterol crystals or fat (45, 46). Lymphangiomatous cysts that are lined with endothelial tissues also have been described.

The second variety, called pseudocysts, result from intrasplenic infarction or hemorrhage with subsequent degeneration and liquefaction of tissue within a fibrotic capsule (47). Pseudocysts contain brown, turbid fluid made up of decomposed blood and tissue. Microscopic examination of the inner surfaces reveals no epithelial or endothelial lining.

Splenic cysts are usually noted as nontender, smooth, left upper quadrant masses that displace and indent the greater curvature of the stomach. Radionuclide scanning with ^{99m}Tc-sulfur colloid is useful for diagnosis and outlines cysts as rounded areas having no reticuloendothelial (RE) activity that are surrounded by relatively normal splenic tissue, giving the appearance of two small spleens (48). Angiographic studies are rarely necessary for diagnosis (49). Sonography also is valuable in establishing the cystic nature of intrasplenic masses (Fig. 29–2). CT scans also provide definitive identification of splenic cysts. Splenectomy is usually indicated for large splenic cysts because they may rupture or bleed following trauma or may become infected, but surgical excision with preservation of normal splenic tissue has been advocated (49).

SPLENIC TUMORS

Reticuloendothelial malignancies such as leukemia, lymphoma, reticulum cell sarcoma, and Hodgkin's disease frequently involve the spleen. This involvement may be diffuse or occur in a nodular pattern. In adults with non-RE malignancies other than multiple melanoma, splenic metastases are found in only 2 to 4 per cent of cases, even when the disease is very widespread (50). The spleen lacks efferent lymphatic vessels; thus, lymphatic metastases to the spleen are unusual (51). Except for neuroblastoma, the common non-RE childhood solid tumors infrequently metastasize to the spleen. Studies in experimental animals have demonstrated that the growth of metastatic tumors is suppressed by the splenic milieu (52). Large hemangiomatous tumors of the spleen have been described and are occasionally associated with similar tumors in the skin and bone (53).

SPLENOSIS

Heterotopic autotransplantation of splenic tissue, or splenosis, occurs when cells spilled from the pulp of the damaged spleen become implanted on peritoneal surfaces and grow into visible nodules of splenic tissue. Splenic tissue can be shown to exert a number of splenic functions, including phagocytosis and antibody formation (54). Splenosis has usually been a coincidental finding either at autopsy or at subsequent laparotomy in persons who have had previous splenic injury requiring

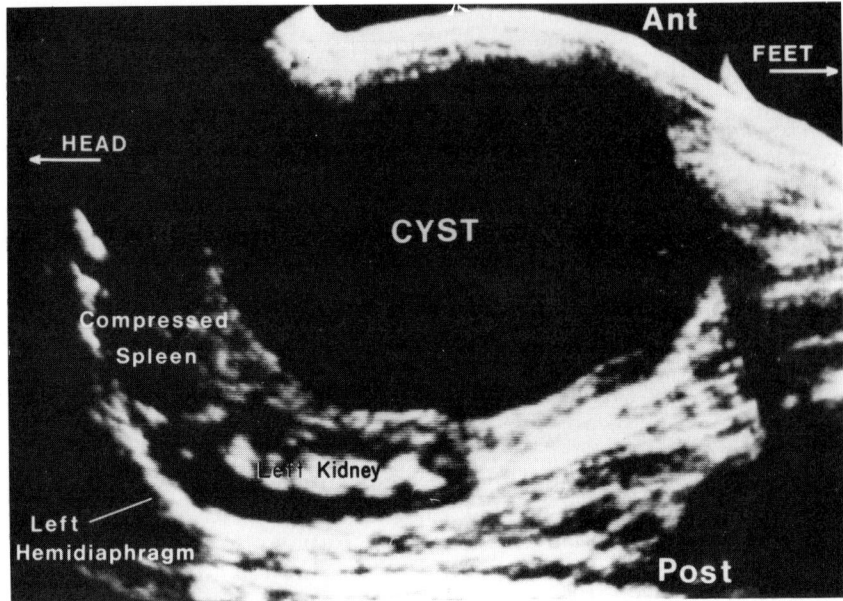

Figure 29–2. Sonography of large splenic pseudocyst.

splenectomy (55). Although splenosis has generally been regarded as an infrequent phenomenon, interference phase contrast microscopic examination of the blood cells of persons who have had splenectomy for traumatic rupture has revealed evidence of recurrent splenic function in about half the cases (55–57). ^{99m}Tc-sulfur colloid scans have shown multiple splenotic nodules in these cases (Fig. 29–3). The use of ^{99m}Tc-tagged heated RBCs provides even more specific imaging of splenic tissue (58). The regrowth of the splenic tissue following splenectomy has been attributed to "work hypertrophy" (59–61). Experimental work suggests that immature animals develop splenosis more frequently than adults do (61a).

Splenosis has been associated with recurrent idiopathic thrombocytopenic purpura, indicating hyperactivity of the tissue (62). It is possible that recurrent splenic tissue, due to splenosis, may offer some degree of protection (although probably not absolute protection) against bacterial infection and may in part account for the low frequency of sepsis after splenectomy for trauma (63). However, infections have occurred in individuals with proven splenosis (64–66). Whether a critical mass of splenic tissue is necessary for protection has not been determined. Experimental studies in animals have yielded conflicting results concerning protective activity of splenic tissue against infection (67–69). Studies involving induced transepithelial infection, perhaps more analogous to naturally acquired disease, have indicated that transplanted splenic tissue does reduce mortality (70–72).

SPLENIC HYPOPLASIA OR ATROPHY

A number of conditions are associated with a small or atrophic spleen. Familial splenic hypoplasia has been described in three offspring of consanguineous parents (73). These children had recurrent severe bacterial infections. A small spleen is also frequently found in children with Fanconi's aplastic anemia and in some children with an unusual sideroblastic anemia with vacuolated marrow precursors and pancreatic insufficiency (74, 75). Splenic atrophy has been reported in adults with a variety of diseases and is indicated by morphologic changes in the circulating blood (Table 29–1) (75a–81). This phenomenon has not been systematically defined in pediatric patients with the same diseases and requires further study.

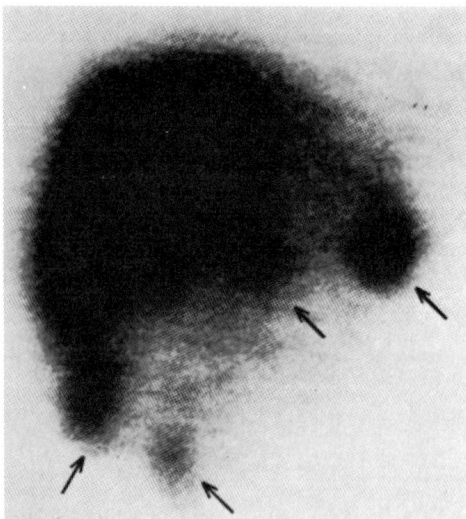

Figure 29–3. Multiple splenotic nodules (arrows) under surface of liver demonstrated by ^{99m}Tc colloid scan in a patient splenectomized 5 years previously because of splenic trauma. (From Pearson, H. A., et al.: New Engl. J. Med. *298*:1391, 1978.)

Table 29–1. REPORTED CAUSES OF ACQUIRED SPLENIC HYPOFUNCTION AND ATROPHY

Adult celiac disease and sprue
Ulcerative colitis
Dermatitis herpetiformis
Thyrotoxicosis
Thorotrast administration
HbS disorders (SS, SC, S. thal, etc.)
Fanconi's anemia

Using a technique measuring clearance of autologous-labeled antibody-coated or heat-damaged red blood cells, investigators have shown decreased splenic function in patients with nephritis or vasculitis. Splenic reticuloendothelial blockade was reversed by plasma exchange (82).

SPLENIC FUNCTION

Normal Functions

A number of distinct, normal functions of the spleen have been described (Table 29–2) (83–85).

SITE OF HEMATOPOIESIS

The spleen is a normal hematopoietic organ during fetal life. At midgestation, active blood formation is centered in the liver and spleen. After this time, the bone marrow becomes progressively more important for blood formation, and at term only occasional small nests of hematopoietic cells are found in the spleen. Infants with severe intrauterine hematologic stress such as erythroblastosis fetalis often have massive splenomegaly due to extramedullary hematopoiesis that rapidly recedes after birth. However, the potential for splenic hematopoiesis remains, and under certain severe hematologic stresses, such as imposed by thalassemia and osteopetrosis, splenic blood formation persists postnatally. The stimulus that maintains or reinitiates extramedullary hematopoiesis is not clear, and in other hemolytic states, such as sickle cell anemia and hereditary spherocytosis, it does not regularly occur.

Agnogenic myeloid metaplasia is a myeloproliferative disorder of adult life characterized by extramedullary hematopoiesis and fibrosis of the marrow (86).

Radioactive iron (^{59}Fe) can be used to determine the sites and effectiveness of extramedullary erythropoiesis. Because the normal spleen cannot remove iron bound to serum transferrin, an accumulation of radioactivity within the spleen after intravenous injection of ^{59}Fe-transferrin indicates splenic erythropoiesis. In subsequent days, the degree of fall in splenic radioactivity indicates whether the splenic erythropoiesis is effective or not (87, 88).

ERYTHROCYTE DESTRUCTION

In normal individuals, senescent red cells are destroyed within the spleen and bone marrow at the end of their life span because these effete cells have lost activity of many enzymes as well as membrane elasticity (89–91). This custodial function can also be assumed by other parts of the reticuloendothelial system, and red cell survival in the asplenic, but otherwise normal, individual is not prolonged. In pathologic states, intrasplenic red cell destruction may be prodigious ("the graveyard becomes an abattoir") (92). This may be due to hyperactivity of splenic phagocytic elements, sequestration of antibody-coated cells (particularly those coated with IgG), the unfavorable biochemical milieu of the spleen for red cells with metabolic abnormalities such as hereditary spherocytosis, or the cellular rigidity induced by abnormal hemoglobins such as Hb S or Hb C (93–95).

PHAGOCYTOSIS

The spleen removes particulate material from the blood. However, this filtering capacity is somewhat discriminating. In part, filtration by the spleen depends on the size of particle presented to it (1). ^{198}Au-colloid (radiogold) has a particle size of 0.001 to 0.01 μ. When this material is injected intravenously, most is cleared by the liver and very little is taken up by the normal spleen. However, when active hepatic disease is present, a reversal of this pattern may occur. Because of this inconsistent localization, ^{198}Au-colloid is infrequently used for examination of the spleen (1).

^{99m}Tc-gelatin sulfur colloid has become the predominant radiopharmaceutical for spleen studies. The colloidal particles of this material are usually made about 1 μ in diameter. A small amount of the administered dose accumulates in the spleen, permitting clear visualization by scintigraphy. The RE elements of liver and bone marrow also take up the isotope, permitting scintigraphic imaging of these structures.

Substantially larger particles are preferentially cleared by the spleen. Heat-denatured (50°C for 30 minutes) human red blood cells, which are about 7 μ in diameter, are cleared almost exclusively by the spleen, probably as a result of their surface rigidity. When these heated cells are tagged with ^{51}Cr or ^{99m}Tc, preferential visualization of splenic tissue is possible. However, further heating also results in hepatic uptake (96). Splenic

Table 29–2. FUNCTIONS OF THE SPLEEN

Site of hematopoiesis
Phagocytosis
Erythrocyte destruction
Reservoir (platelets, Factor VIII)
"Culling" and "pitting"
Control of hematopoiesis
Platelet and leukocyte destruction
Immunologic and host defense mechanisms

uptake of particles such as red cells and bacteria also is affected by immune interactions, which will be discussed later in this chapter.

RESERVOIR

The spleen serves as a reservoir for blood-borne elements. This reservoir function is marked in animals such as the dog. The canine splenic capsule and trabeculae contain smooth muscle that can contract and force intrasplenic blood into the circulation in response to physiologic stress. The effect is considerably less in humans, whose spleen has no capsular muscle and contains only about 50 ml of blood. A functional splenic reservoir does exist for some platelets and plasma proteins (97–99). The splenic reservoir is indicated by the rise in the platelet count and Factor VIII (antihemophilic factor) level that follows intravenous epinephrine administration. This response is not observed in splenectomized individuals (100).

"CULLING AND PITTING"

These apt terms were coined and extensively discussed by Crosby (83). "Culling" indicates a selective removal of morphologically abnormal erythrocytes such as spherocytes and poikilocytes from the circulation of the spleen. Following splenectomy, increased numbers of these abnormally shaped cells are noted in the blood. Closely related to culling is the ability of the spleen to retain reticulocytes preferentially, probably because of their excessive membrane and weak negative surface changes (83, 101). The lack of splenic detention of reticulocytes is responsible for the prodigious reticulocytosis (up to 60 per cent) seen in some patients with pyruvate kinase deficiency after splenectomy (102).

The "pitting" function refers to the fact that the spleen has the ability to remove a variety of intraerythrocytic inclusions, such as Howell-Jolly (HJ) bodies, Heinz bodies, and siderocytic inclusions ("intercellular rubbish"), without destroying the red cells that contain them (103). Crosby provided an elegant demonstration of this function. In his experiment, blood containing large numbers of siderocytes (erythrocytes with iron-staining inclusions) from a donor with a refractory sideroblastic anemia was labeled with ^{51}Cr and was then transfused into a normal recipient. The number of inclusions in the recipient's circulation rapidly decreased, and the siderocytes were not demonstrable after 4 hours. However, when ^{51}Cr-tagged siderocytes were transfused into a splenectomized recipient, both the ^{51}Cr activity in the circulation and the number of siderocytes decreased very slowly and in a parallel fashion. Crosby compared the spleen to a housewife making a cherry pie, who plucks the pit without crushing the fruit! (104).

Observation of HJ bodies, which are unextruded nuclear remnants in circulating erythrocytes, provides an important morphologic indicator of defective splenic function. Circulating HJ bodies can be found in all asplenic individuals (105). However, their numbers are usually small (1 to 5 per 1000 RBCs), and therefore their presence may be a relatively subtle and nonquantitative indicator of defective splenic function.

More recently, autophagic vacuoles, which appear as craters, or "pocks," on the red cell membrane when examined by interference phase contrast microscopy (Nomarski optics), have been shown to reflect splenic function (30, 106). Twelve to 40 per cent of the circulating erythrocytes of splenectomized individuals bear one or more of these surface indentations, or "pocks," but they are found in fewer than 1 to 2 per cent of circulating red blood cells of persons with intact spleens. This technique has also permitted semiquantitative assessment of degrees of splenic function, ranging from eusplenia to hyposplenia to asplenia (107). When blood that contained a substantial number of "pocked" RBCs was taken from an asplenic individual, tagged with ^{51}Cr, and transfused into a normal individual, the "pocks" disappeared rapidly, but ^{51}Cr activity persisted, indicating that removal of these surface "pocks" was a function of the spleen (108).

The mechanism of splenic "pitting" can be demonstrated in sections from excised splenic tissue (109, 110). As they percolate between the splenic cords and sinuses, the red cells must insinuate themselves through the minute apertures between the endothelial cells of the splenic cords and their fenestrated basement membranes. Because normal red cells are plastic and deformable, they easily make this passage. However, when red cells contain noncompressible inclusions such as HJ or Heinz bodies, their passage is obstructed. The membrane is stretched progressively until a small portion of the red cell with the contained inclusion is pinched off. The membrane then reconstitutes, and the red cell is released into the sinusoid without inclusions (Fig. 29–4).

SPLENIC CONTROL OF HEMATOPOIESIS

Pluripotential stem cells occur in the murine spleen, and the organ contains a significant proportion of the marginal blood pool (111, 112). Destruction of these progenitors may explain why splenic radiation has a more suppressive effect on the circulating white blood cell count than does a comparable dose applied to other organs (113).

In occasional cases of aplastic anemia, splenectomy is followed by an increase in the circulating blood count, and these observations have been cited as evidence of a splenic hormonal effect on hematopoiesis. Montz and Schneider reported a change in bone marrow volume after splenectomy (114). Oral administration of spleen extracts has been associated with increases in blood counts, but the response has been inconstant (115). *All* these findings lend themselves to alternative explanations, and at present there is little substantial evidence for splenic "hormonal" activity or control of blood formation, although the spleen may be a limited site of erythropoietin production (116, 117).

PLATELET AND LEUKOCYTE DESTRUCTION

Following splenectomy, thrombocytosis and leukocytosis usually occur in humans. This change is usually attributed to elimination of the splenic reservoir, since platelet survival is similar in normal and asplenic individuals. Postsplenectomy thrombocytosis has been suggested as a possible factor in an increased rate of atherosclerotic complications noted in veterans splenectomized for trauma during World War II (118). The spleen probably has a role in normal destruction of lymphocytes and monocytes (23). In immunohematologic disorders involving leukocytes or platelets, the spleen may be a major site of destruction of these elements, and splenectomy may induce a remission.

IMMUNOLOGIC AND HOST RESISTANCE MECHANISMS

The spleen has been identified as having a number of roles that affect host resistance. When immunization is performed with soluble antigens that are delivered by the subcutaneous or intramuscular routes, most investigators have demonstrated no significant differences between the antibody responses of the asplenic compared with the normal animal or human (119, 120). However, in a study of the immune response to polyvalent pneumococcal vaccine in which an enzyme-linked immunosorbent assay for pneumococcal antibodies was used, Hosea described impaired responses in splenectomized patients. This affected both IgG and IgM responses (121a). Whether these differences significantly affect clinical responses is not clear, but they suggest that, when possible, polysaccharide immunization should be administered before elective splenectomy. In contrast to the foregoing findings, the IgM, IgA, and IgG responses of asplenic individuals to meningococcal polysaccharide antigens were described as "nearly" normal (121a). In addition, under certain specific conditions a unique splenic role can be identified. When the antigen is particulate and is given intravenously in small amounts, the spleen is almost the exclusive site of antibody formation. In 1950, Rowley administered small numbers of heterologous red cells to rats and humans and subsequently measured the changes in serum heterophile hemolysins as an indicator of antibody response to this antigenic stimulus. Recipients with normal spleens responded rapidly, with significant increases in

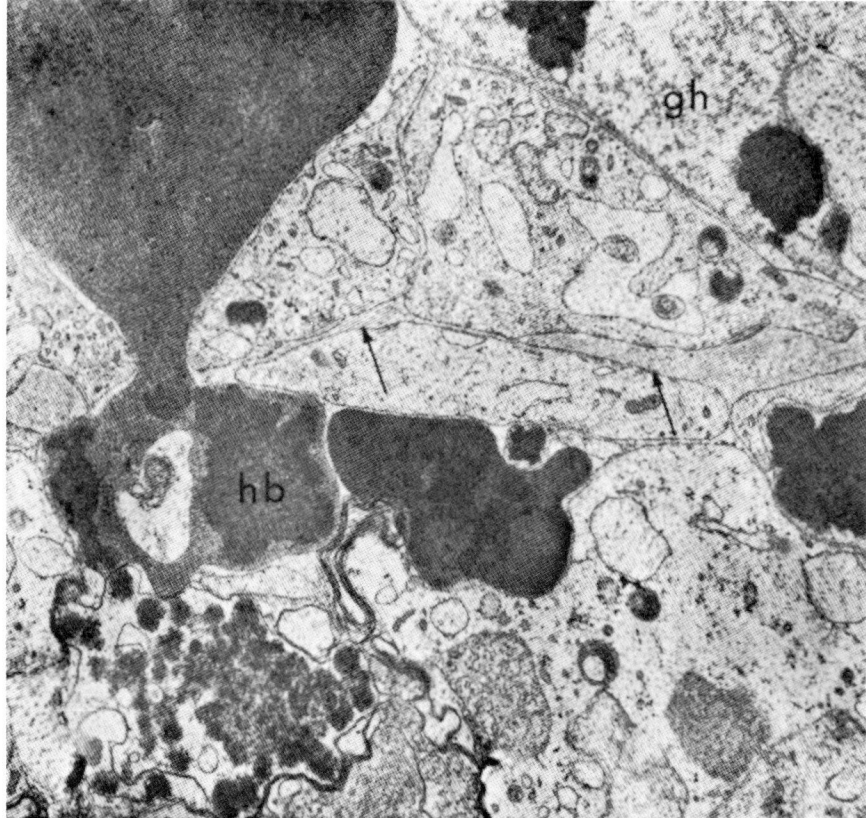

Figure 29–4. Electron micrograph of a portion of a red cell burdened by a Heinz body (hb) entrapped within the spleen. The red cell appears to be impeded in its passage through a slit in the basement membrane (arrows) separating a splenic cord (below) from an adjacent sinusoid (above). A Heinz body containing ghost (gh) lies in the splenic sinusoid. (From Rifkind, R. A.: Blood 26:433–448, 1965.)

serum hemolysin titer, but recipients who had been splenectomized showed either no response or only an insignificant change (15, 121, 121b). The same findings can be demonstrated in patients with the splenic dysfunction of sickle cell anemia (122).

Splenic antibody production in response to intravenous immunization may be very rapid. "Early antibodies" may be detected soon after antigenic challenge, and immunization, in which killed organisms are used as early as 8 hours before challenge with virulent pneumococci, decreases mortality (123, 124).

The spleen produces a notable percentage of IgM, and levels of this class of immunoglobulin are lower in hyposplenic people than in eusplenic individuals (125–128). The spleen also produces properdin, for this activity is decreased in the blood of splenectomized individuals compared with that in controls (129). Constantopoulos and Najjar described a circulating phagocytosis-promoting tetrapeptide that they designated "tuftsin." Tuftsin is believed to originate from the Fc fragment of IgG and is released in vivo as the free tetrapeptide after enzymatic cleavage (130, 131). This material is reduced in the blood of asplenic and hyposplenic individuals, and low levels may increase susceptibility to infection (132).

In adults and children with chronic idiopathic thrombocytopenic purpura (ITP), splenic synthesis of a considerable amount of antiplatelet antibody has been demonstrated (133, 134). Removal of this source of antibody production may, in considerable part, be responsible for the beneficial hematologic effects of splenectomy in this disease.

A final aspect of splenic function contributing to host resistance involves the spleen as a biologic filter. When particulate material in the form of bacteria enters the circulation, it is cleared by reticuloendothelial elements in the liver, spleen, and bone marrow, and the rate and anatomic sites of clearance can be determined by various radioactive isotopic labels.

In immune animals, circulating bacteria such as pneumococci become heavily coated with specific complement-fixing antibodies. In these animals the liver, because of its large mass of reticuloendothelial tissue, is the most important primary site for clearance of ^{125}I-labeled pneumococci. However, in nonimmune animals, in which little antibody is available for opsonization, the spleen assumes a much greater importance. On a weight-by-weight basis, the spleen is 10 to 60 times more efficient than the liver in phagocytic activity (124).

Jandl and Jones demonstrated selective splenic activity using ^{51}Cr-tagged RBCs reacted in vitro with specific antibody. These were injected by surface counting. When the ratio of antibody to RBC antigen was low, the spleen removed most of the red cells and was 20 times more active than the liver on a gram-for-gram basis. However, when RBCs were strongly coated with antibody, the liver was the primary site of red cell sequestration (135). The difference may be due to the fact that the sluggish splenic blood flow increases the chance that the macrophage receptors will contact the Fc moiety of the IgG antibody on the surface of the sensitized red cell (136, 137).

These experimental data indicate that the spleen appears to be the crucial first line of defense in clearing small numbers of bacteria such as pneumococci and *Haemophilus influenzae* from the circulation in infants who lack specific immunity as a developmental phenomenon (138, 139). This is probably the most important basis for the age-related and bacterial specificities of the syndrome of postsplenectomy overwhelming sepsis (to be discussed subsequently).

In both humans and animals, the spleen plays a role in host resistance to infections caused by the intraerythrocytic parasites *Bartonella*, *Plasmodium*, and *Babesia* by removing such parasites from the red cell (141). Splenectomy may result in an accelerated clinical course and greater degrees of parasitemia (142–144). Most reported cases of human babesiasis have occurred in individuals who have been splenectomized (145).

Developmental Aspects of Splenic Function

There is a body of clinical and experimental data that indicates that the spleen may be relatively inactive during the early weeks and months of life. In the blood of newborns, especially premature infants, morphologic abnormalities such as HJ bodies and siderocytes are often observed, suggesting decreased splenic function. Premature infants were shown to have a decreased capacity to remove red cells containing Heinz bodies when compared with normal adults. The rate of clearance of these inclusion-bearing cells was comparably retarded in premature infants and splenectomized adults (146). Holroyd and associates demonstrated an increased number of "pocked" red cells in term newborns and even greater numbers in premature infants, indicating splenic hypofunction. By 2 months of age, the proportion of "pocked" red cells had substantially decreased, approaching the normal range (30). These studies have been extended into midgestation and in postmature infants (31).

Ozsoylu and associates studied splenic phagocytic function in rats and showed the spleen to have markedly reduced activity at birth. Phagocytic function increased to normal adult levels by 2 to 4 weeks (147). Whether this developmental delay in splenic function has pathophysiologic correlates has not been established. However, it is possible that this could contribute to the propensity to severe bacterial infections characteristic of the newborn period.

FUNCTIONAL HYPOSPLENIA

Sickle Cell Disease

The concept that anatomically enlarged spleens might have defective function was suggested by studies of children with sickle cell anemia (148). Children with palpably enlarged spleens had HJ bodies in their circulating RBCs, and ^{99m}Tc-sulfur colloid scans showed no uptake of radiocolloid. It was shown later that the functional hyposplenia in sickle cell anemia was not congenital but rather was a defect acquired during the first 2 to 3 years of life (range, 5 to 36 months of age) and that the defect could be reversed by transfusion of normal RBCs (149, 150). Studies with interference phase contrast microscopy demonstrating increasing numbers of red cells having "pocks" (PkRBC) have shown that the loss of splenic function is a gradual phenomenon during the first 5 years of life in these children (107). An important goal of the National Comprehensive Clinical Study of Sickle Cell Diseases was to define the pattern and timing of splenic dysfunction in the various sickling disorders (143). It was noted that a PkRBC greater than 3.5 per cent correlated strongly with nonvisualization of the spleen by ^{99m}Tc scanning. The pattern of splenic dysfunction showed considerable differences in the various disorders (Fig. 29–5). In HbSS and HbS β⁰ thalassemia, the PkRBC exceeded 3.5 per cent early in life. In contrast, in HbSC disease the mean PkRBC did not exceed 3.5 per cent until after the age of 5 or 6 years, the period of greatest risk for severe bacterial infections in hyposplenic individuals. This study also confirmed a relationship between the level of HbF and splenic dysfunction. At a level of 15 to 20 per cent, splenic function regularly occurred (151). The finding of normal splenic function in many sickle cell patients from the Eastern Province of Saudi Arabia, who characteristically have high levels of HbF greater than 20 per cent, confirms the relationship (152). In addition to these hematologic changes, children with sickle cell anemia and functional hyposplenia have the same type of susceptibility to overwhelming bacterial infection that occurs in splenectomized infants and children. Bacterial meningitis is some 300 times more frequent in children with sickle cell anemia than in controls, and this propensity is most striking during the first 5 years of life (153–156). A number of humoral defects of immunity have been described in patients with sickle cell disease, including decreased serum pneumococcal opsonins (149) and low properdin activity (157–160). These could well interact with functional hyposplenism.

Various functions of the spleen may be affected

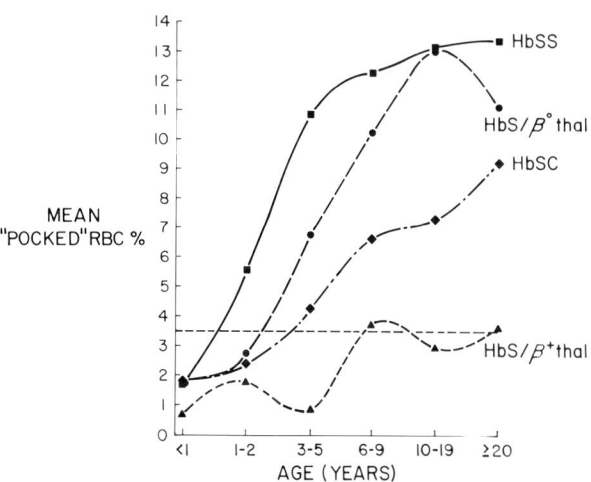

Figure 29–5. Determination of percentage of pocked red cells in more than 3000 patients with sickle cell anemia studied by the Cooperative Study of Sickle Cell Diseases of the NHLBI. PkRBC greater than 3.5 per cent indicates functional hyposplenism.

to a different degree. Those young children with sickle cell anemia whose spleens cannot take up radiocolloids and who are susceptible to serious infections demonstrate a rise in platelet count following epinephrine infusions, indicating preservation of the splenic reservoir function (161).

After 6 to 8 years of age, a state of anatomic asplenia develops, as repetitive episodes of infarction reduce the spleen to a siderofibrotic nubbin, a phenomenon designated "autosplenectomy."

Hyposplenism in "Autoimmune" Disease

Recent studies of the clearance of antibody-coated or heat-damaged red cells have revealed that the phagocytic capacity of the spleen may be impaired in a wide variety of so-called "autoimmune" diseases, including various forms of acute nephritis, lupus erythematosus, vasculitis, and Wegener's granulomatosis (82). The hypofunction may be reversed in some cases by plasmapheresis.

SPLENOMEGALY

The spleen cannot usually be felt by physical examination; however, 2.9 per cent of presumably healthy college freshmen were found to have palpable spleens. Only one third of these organs were enlarged on subsequent examination (162). In adults, the spleen must be 1½ to 2 times increased in size to be palpable. In children, palpable spleens are much more frequently encountered, owing to the thinness of the abdominal musculature, and in as many as 10 per cent of children the spleen tip can be palpated.

There are many different reasons for splenic enlargement, some of which are listed in Table 29–3.

Table 29–3. SOME CAUSES OF SPLENOMEGALY

Hemolytic anemias ("work hypertrophy"): hereditary spherocytosis, nonspherocytic hemolytic anemias, hemoglobinopathies, thalassemia major

Extramedullary hematopoiesis: thalassemia major, osteopetrosis, myelofibrosis

Neoplasms: leukemia, Hodgkin's disease, lymphoma, metastatic malignancy, hemangioma, hamartomas

Strong and infiltrative processes: lipidoses, histiocytosis, mucopolysaccharidoses

Congestive disorders: cirrhosis, hepatic fibrosis, cystic fibrosis, portal or splenic venous obstruction (Banti's syndrome), chronic congestive heart failure

Infections and inflammatory responses: bacterial (subacute bacterial endocarditis), protozoal (malaria), viral infections (mononucleosis and others), SLE and sarcoid

Cysts: true cysts, pseudocysts

Hemolytic states are frequently associated with splenomegaly resulting from engorgement of the splenic sinusoids by red cells as well as by "work hypertrophy" of the RE elements (60, 61). Extramedullary hematopoiesis resulting in splenic enlargement occurs in Cooley's anemia and in obliterative processes involving the bone marrow, such as osteopetrosis. A variety of benign and malignant lymphoreticular neoplasms and leukemias are frequently associated with large spleens. Obstruction of venous drainage due to cirrhosis, congestive heart failure, or thrombosis of splenic or portal veins results in congestive splenomegaly (Banti's syndrome). Although depression of the formed elements of the blood is frequently observed, overt infection and bleeding are unusual, suggesting that the cytopenia and anemia may be a consequence of excessive pooling and dilution rather than of cell destruction (163).

In the lipidoses such as Niemann-Pick and Gaucher's diseases, the phagocytic RE elements may accumulate large amounts of lipid because of abnormal lysosomal function.

In mucopolysaccharidoses such as Hurler's and Hunter's syndromes, large amounts of mucopolysaccharide accumulate in the spleen, and in a variety of inflammatory or infectious processes, splenomegaly is frequent, owing primarily to hypertrophy of lymphatic and reticuloendothelial elements.

SPLENECTOMY

There are many indications for splenectomy, which, in general, can be divided into medical (hematologic) and surgical categories (Table 29–4).

Medical indications such as congenital and acquired hemolytic anemias, thrombocytopenic purpura, Cooley's anemia, lipidosis, and others are discussed throughout this book in their respective chapters and sections.

A prime surgical indication has been traumatic rupture. However, this is now being questioned, and nonoperative management of splenic injury (164–168) and techniques for direct surgical repair of the lacerated spleen with preservation of splenic tissue and function (169, 170) are being increasingly reported.

Splenectomy as part of a staging procedure in Hodgkin's disease and lymphoma is generally recognized as important for prognostication and direction of therapy. Incidental splenectomy may also be performed for the purpose of surgical exposure or as part of a shunting procedure for portal hypertension. In humans as well as animals, changes in the formed elements of the blood occur after splenectomy (171). The morphologic changes in the red cells have previously been described. Quantitative alterations of the leukocytes and platelets regularly occur. Leukocytosis resulting from an increase in neutrophils occurs in the first few postoperative weeks, but leukocyte numbers return to normal after about 3 months. A slight, persistent lymphocytosis also has been described (172).

Thrombocytosis occurs to a varying degree in about half of splenectomized patients. The increase begins within the first postoperative week, reaching a maximum at 2 to 3 weeks (173). In general, the highest platelet counts occur in patients who have persistent hemolysis after splenectomy, and platelet counts exceeding 2×10^6 cells per mm^3 may occur in patients with Cooley's anemia. Thrombotic problems have been rare despite high platelet counts, and most authorities do not recommend anticoagulation therapy. If therapy is deemed necessary, drugs that inhibit aggregation such as aspirin or dipyridamole (Persantine) should be considered.

Persistent elevation of platelets in the splenectomized patient has been suggested as a predisposing factor for ischemic heart disease (118).

Postsplenectomy Infection

The 1952 report of King and Shumacher describing severe bacterial infections in five infants who had been splenectomized for hereditary spherocytosis focused attention on the importance of the spleen in host defense mechanisms (7). During the years following their report, a number of studies appeared in the literature, some apparently refuting, but most confirming, the existence of a definite syndrome of severe postsplenectomy bacterial infection. Today, there is little controversy about the reality of this syndrome, but questions do remain about its relative frequency and pathophysiologic basis and the therapeutic strategies to prevent it.

The syndrome has distinct clinical, bacteriologic, and age-related features. It is manifested as septicemia that is frequently associated with meningitis. There is usually no obvious focus of infection. It has been suggested that a synergistic viral infection may be a triggering event (65). The syndrome has an abrupt onset and rapid progression. Death occurs in about two thirds of patients, often within 12 to 24 hours of onset. There is an enormous proliferation of bacteria in the blood stream, and the organisms are often demonstrable by Gram stains of buffy-coated preparations of blood. A purpuric rash, disseminated intravascular coagulation, and adrenal hemorrhage due to accumulation of capsular polysaccharides in the circulation are often present (174–177).

Relatively few species of bacteria are responsible for most postsplenectomy infections. Pneumococci of varying serotypes cause about 6 per cent, and *Haemophilus influenzae* type B and *Neisseria meningitidis* account for about 25 per cent of the cases. The rest are due to a variety of organisms, including *Escherichia coli, Staphylococcus,* and *Streptococcus* (63).

The syndrome has a certain degree of age specificity, being more frequent in younger patients. Horan and Colebatch noted a frequency of severe infections in 50 per cent of splenectomized patients less than 1 year old, compared with 1.8 per cent in children over 1 year of age (178). Eraklis and Filler reported that infection occurred twice as frequently in children under 4 years of age as in those over 4 years (37). Two thirds of cases occur within 2 years after operation, but remote occurrences, decades after the operation, have been reported (179). The frequency of the syndrome varies, depending on the reason for which splenectomy was performed. In general, the risk is greatest when the underlying condition, in itself, is associated with increased susceptibility to infection. The relative risks in various conditions, as determined from Singer's review of the literature (63), are illustrated in Figure 29–6. The risk of death from bacterial infection for "normal" infants less than 1 year of age was estimated to be 0.3 per cent; for children 1 to 7 years, 0.07 per cent; and for children 5 to 14 years, 0.02 per cent. The risk of death in splenectomized children was greatly increased over these background rates, ranging from 58 times greater when splenectomy was carried out for traumatic rupture to 1000 times greater when the procedure was performed in children with thalassemia major (63). Not included in Singer's analysis was the Wiskott-Aldrich syndrome (180, 181), in which the risk of sepsis after splenectomy is extraordinarily high. Splenectomy is regularly followed by an increase in the platelet count. However, special precautions are essential if death is to be prevented. In one report, five of seven patients not receiving prophylactic antibiotics died of sepsis within 33 months of surgery. None of nine patients treated with prophylactic antibiotics developed this complication (182). There may be an atypical form of Wiskott-Aldrich syndrome, manifested primarily by thrombocytopenia. A definite male prevalence has been noted in young children dying after splenectomy for presumed ITP, suggesting that some of these patients may have had the Wiskott-Aldrich syndrome or another inherited thrombocytopenia rather than ITP (183). Splenectomy as a staging procedure in Hodgkin's disease also imposes a relatively high risk (184, 185).

As previously mentioned, the spleen is very important in clearing bacteria from the blood when there are absent or low levels of circulating specific antibodies against that bacterial species. When circulating antibody is present, the liver is able to perform this function. However, if there are absent or very low levels of antibody in an asplenic individual, simple bacteremia may progress to an overwhelming septicemia.

It has long been known that there are important developmental changes in circulating antibodies

Table 29–4. SOME INDICATIONS FOR SPLENECTOMY

Surgical
Traumatic rupture (not absolute)
Splenorenal shunting
Exposure
Splenic cysts
Mechanical size

Medical
Congenital hemolytic anemias: hereditary spherocytosis, elliptocytosis, some nonspherocytic disorders (pyruvate kinase deficiency)
Acquired immunohematologic disorders (autoimmune hemolytic anemia and idiopathic thrombocytopenia)
Staging for Hodgkin's disease
Hypersplenic cytopenias in Cooley's anemia, congestive splenomegaly, Gaucher's disease

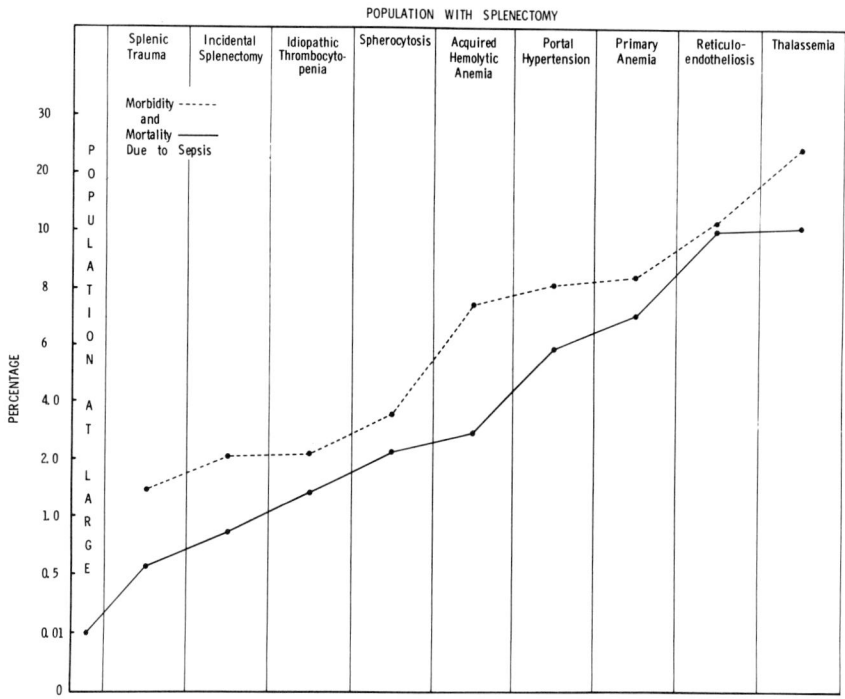

Figure 29–6. Relative risks of infection after splenectomy for various reasons. (From Singer, D. B.: Perspect. Pediatr. Pathol. *1*:285, 1973.)

against various strains of *Diplococcus pneumoniae* and *H. influenzae* type B (138, 139). At birth, the infant has circulating antibodies due to transplacentally acquired IgG from the mother. These IgG antibodies disappear during the first 6 months of life, and for the next 2 years most infants lack circulating antibodies. This reflects a lack of exposure and also a relative inability of young infants to form antibodies to the polysaccharide capsular antigens of these bacteria (140, 186).

An individual adult also may lack circulating antibodies to certain strains of bacteria. If such a person is also asplenic and experiences bacteremia due to an organism to which he has no immunity, fulminating sepsis may develop.

Consideration of these factors provides the basis for an approach to splenectomy in children. Splenectomy should not be performed unless it is necessary and unless the benefits can be expected to exceed the immediate and long-term risks. When possible, as in selected cases of traumatic splenic rupture, it may be possible to preserve or repair the spleen. More and more, the ruptured spleen is being treated "conservatively" (164–168, 187). Thus far, the risk of late hemorrhage or splenic pseudocysts appears to be small. The possibility of inducing splenosis or attempting autotransplantation of splenic tissue has also been suggested in order to preserve some degree of splenic function when splenectomy is necessary (61). Splenectomy for hematologic indications should be deferred as long as possible, ideally until after 6 or 7 years of age. In recognition of the fact that most cases of postsplenectomy sepsis are caused by *Diplococcus pneumoniae*, administration of prophylactic penicillin has been advocated. Until recently, there have been no large controlled studies to prove the effectiveness of this practice; small series have demonstrated a degree of protection, and results in experimental animals have also demonstrated protection (188). Recent studies of prophylaxis in sickle cell disease confirm the efficacy of prophylaxis (188a). In addition, the apparent excellent protection of prophylactic antibiotics in the Wiskott-Aldrich syndrome supports their efficacy (189). However, patient compliance may be unpredictable. In a careful study of prophylactic antibiotics in sickle cell patients, only 60 per cent compliance was attained despite strenuous education and supportive efforts (191). In addition, fatal pneumococcal infections have been reported in patients receiving parenteral penicillin prophylaxis (190). Furthermore, strains of *Diplococcus pneumoniae* that are resistant to penicillin are being reported, and penicillin would not be expected to be effective against *H. influenzae* type B or *Neisseria meningitidis*. An effective polysaccharide vaccine against 24 serotypes of *Streptococcus pneumoniae* is currently available. In addition, vaccines for *H. influenzae* and *Neisseria meningitidis* types A and C have been developed and are available, although only on an investigational basis at present. These vaccines evoke antibodies that should be protective against postsplenectomy sepsis (185).

However, clinical studies proving effectiveness have not been reported. Overwhelming sepsis has occurred in children vaccinated against the offending capsular type (192), and nonincluded types also have caused sepsis after vaccination. The vaccines are reported to be of unpredictable value in children less than 2 years of age. Immunosuppressed individuals, such as those receiving radiation therapy and chemotherapy for Hodgkin's disease, respond poorly to pneumococcal vaccines (193, 194). However, one report describes antibody response to certain serotypes in children as young as 3 to 6 months of age (195). These findings have led to a recommendation for immunization of asplenic patients at 6 months of age, followed by reimmunization at 2 years.

In addition to receiving penicillin and immunization, splenectomized patients need to be appropriately educated about their condition without being terrified of it. They and their parents should understand that a shaking chill, unusual lethargy, or fever in excess of 38.8°C (102°F) may indicate a life-threatening infection that should be treated promptly. Ideally, the patient should be brought to a physician for immediate diagnosis and therapy. If circumstances or distances preclude such an approach, the patient or the parents should have an antibiotic such as amoxicillin in their possession that can be taken orally. The newer cephalosporins, which are active against both *Diplococcus pneumoniae* and *H. influenzae*, may emerge as the drugs of choice. Such an approach may create some confusion, but it is apt to save lives. The problem of antibiotic-resistant *Diplococcus pneumoniae* (196) poses yet another difficulty. Whether sufficient antibody titers to these strains are generated by current pneumococcal vaccines is not well established. Splenectomized patients who live in areas in which such organisms are prevalent should be treated with amoxicillin or chloramphenicol.

Regardless of the age of the patient or the time that has elapsed after splenectomy and regardless of the indication, the asplenic person has a finite risk of developing and dying from infection (197). The risk is appreciably higher in those who are not rendered hematologically normal by the procedure. If an asplenic individual develops notable fever (greater than 38.8°C) or toxicity, diagnostic and therapeutic measures should be instituted on the premise that life-threatening infection may be present. If no cause for the fever is obvious, blood culture studies should be obtained, and therapy with intravenous antibiotics such as ampicillin or a combination of penicillin and chloramphenicol should be given. If toxicity is extreme, intensive monitoring and supportive measures are indicated. In sickle cell anemia, exchange transfusions also may be beneficial.

References

1. Spencer, R. P., and Pearson, H. A.: *Radionuclide Studies of the Spleen.* Cleveland, CRC Press, 1975, p. 1.
2. Virchow, R.: Weisses Blut und Milztumoren. Med. Zeit. *15:*157, 1846.
3. Ponfick, E.: Über Haemoglobinamie und ihre Folge. Berl. Klin. Wochenschr. *20:*389, 1885.
4. Wells, T. S.: Remarks on splenectomy with a report of a successful case. Med. Chiur. Trans. *71:*255, 1888.
5. Dawson, B.: In discussion of paper by Thursfield, H.: Splenectomy for congenital acholuric jaundice. Proc. R. Soc. Med. *7:*84, 1913–1914.
6. Kasnelson, P.: Verschwinden der hämorrhagischen Diathese bei einem Falle von essentieller Thrombopenie (Frank) nach Milzextirpation. Wein Klin. Wochenschr. *29:*1451, 1916.
7. King, H., and Shumacher, H. B.: Splenic studies. I. Susceptibility to infection after splenectomy performed in infancy. Ann. Surg. *136:*239, 1952.
8. Schulz, D. M., Giordano, D. A., et al.: Weights of organs of fetuses and infants. Arch. Pathol. *71:*244, 1962.
9. DeLand, F. H.: Normal spleen size. Radiology. *97:*589, 1970.
10. Krumbhaar, E. B., and Lippincott, S. W.: The postmortem weight of the "normal" spleen at different ages. Am. J. Med. Sci. *197:*344, 1939.
11. Spencer, R. P., and Chaundhuri, T. K.: Quantitative estimates of changes in splenic size during life. Yale J. Biol. Med. *41:*333, 1969.
12. Spencer, R. P.: Spleen scanning as a diagnostic tool. J.A.M.A. *273:*1473, 1977.
13. Nuland, S. B., Cornelius, E. A., et al.: Scan evidence of organ involution and improvement in Hodgkin's disease following splenic artery ligation. J. Nucl. Med. *11:*693, 1970.
14. Blendis, L. M., Ramboer, C., et al.: Studies on the haemodilution anaemia of splenomegaly. Eur. J. Clin. Invest. *1:*54, 1970.
15. Rowley, D.: The formation of circulating antibody in the splenectomized human being following injection of heterologous erythrocytes. J. Immunol. *65:*515, 1950.
16. Nossal, G. J. V., Austin, C. M., et al.: Antigens in immunity. XII. Antigen trapping in the spleen. Int. Arch. Allergy *29:*368, 1966.
17. Burke, J. S., and Simon, G. T.: Electron microscopy of the spleen. I. Anatomy and microcirculation. Am. J. Pathol. *58:*127, 1970.
18. Hirassawa, Y., and Tokuhiro, H.: Electron microscopic studies on the normal human spleen, especially on the red pulp and the reticuloendothelial cells. Blood *35:*201, 1970.
19. Weiss, L., and Javassoli, M.: Anatomical hazards to the passage of erythrocytes through the spleen. Semin. Hematol. *7:*372, 1970.
20. Sliwinski, A. J., and Lilienfield, L. S.: Evidence for a functional closed circulation in the spleen. Clin. Res. *10:*28, 1962.
21. Weiss, L.: Spleen. In *Histology*, 2nd ed. Greep, R. O. (ed.) New York, McGraw-Hill Book Company, 1966, p. 394.
21a. Weiss, L.: The red pulp of the spleen: structural basis of blood flow. Clin. Haematol. *12:*375, 1983.
22. Chen, L. T.: Microcirculation of the spleen: an open or closed circulation? Science *201:*157, 1978.
23. Weiss, L.: A scanning electron microscopic study of the spleen. Blood *43:*665, 1974.
24. Barnhart, M. I., Baechler, C. A., et al.: Arteriovenous shunts in the human spleen. Am. J. Hematol. *1:*105, 1976.
25. Van Mierop, L. H. S., Gessner, I. H., et al.: Asplenia and polysplenia syndromes. Birth Defects *8:*36, 1972.
26. Ivemark, B. I.: Implications of agenesis of the spleen on

the pathogenesis of cono-truncus anomalies in childhood: analysis of the heart malformations of the splenic agenesis syndrome with fourteen new cases. Acta Paediatr. 44(Suppl. 104):1, 1955.
27. Gasser, C., and Willi, H.: Spontane innenkörperbildung bei Milzagenesie. Helv. Paediatr. Acta 7:369, 1952.
28. Polhemus, D. W., and Schaefer, W. B.: Absent spleen syndrome. Hematologic findings as an aid to diagnosis. Pediatrics 24:254, 1959.
29. Pearson, H. A., Shieber, G. L., et al.: Functional hyposplenia in cyanotic congenital heart disease. Pediatrics 48:277, 1971.
30. Holroyd, C. P., Oski, F. A., et al.: The "pocked erythrocyte": red cell alterations in reticuloendothelial immaturity of the neonate. New Engl. J. Med. 281:516, 1960.
31. Freedman, R. M., Johnston, D., et al.: Development of splenic reticuloendothelial dysfunction in neonates. J. Pediatr. 96:466, 1980.
32. Waldman, J. D., Rosenthal, A., et al.: Sepsis and congenital asplenia. J. Pediatr. 90:555, 1977.
33. Moller, J. H., Nakih, A., et al.: Congenital cardiac disease associated with polysplenia: a developmental complex of bilateral "left-sidedness." Circulation 36:789, 1967.
34. Muir, C. S.: Splenic agenesis and multilobulate spleens. Arch. Dis. Child. 34:431, 1959.
35. Dimmick, J. E., Bove, K. E., et al.: Extrahepatic biliary atresia and the polysplenia syndrome. J. Pediatr. 86:644, 1975.
36. Rodin, A. E., Sloane, J. A., et al.: Polysplenia with severe congenital heart disease and Howell-Jolly bodies. Am. J. Clin. Pathol. 55:127, 1972.
37. Eraklis, A. J., and Filler, R. M.: Splenectomy in childhood: a review of 1413 cases. J. Pediatr. Surg. 7:382, 1972.
38. May, J. E., and Bourne, C. W.: Ectopic spleen in the scrotum. Report of 2 cases. J. Urol. 111:120, 1974.
39. Aspnes, G. T., Pearson, H. A., et al.: Recurrent idiopathic thrombocytopenic purpura with "accessory" splenic tissue. Pediatrics 55:131, 1975.
40. Hann, I. M., and Wainscoat, J. S.: Recurrent thrombocytopenic purpura associated with accessory spleen. Arch. Dis. Child. 51:154, 1976.
41. Bast, J. B., and Appel, M. F.: Recurrent hemolytic anemia secondary to accessory spleens. South. Med. J. 71:608, 1978.
42. Verheyden, C. N., Beart, R. W., et al.: Accessory splenectomy in management of recurrent idiopathic thrombocytopenic purpura. Mayo Clin. Proc. 53:442, 1978.
43. Qureshi, M. A., Hafner, C. D., et al.: Nonparasitic cysts of the spleen. Arch. Surg. 89:570, 1964.
44. McNamara, J. J., Murphy, L. J., et al.: Splenic cysts in children. Surgery 64:487, 1968.
45. Davis, C. E., Jr., Montero, J. M., et al.: Large splenic cysts. Am. Surg. 173:686, 1971.
46. Blank, E., and Campbell, J. R.: Epidermoid cysts of the spleen. Pediatrics 51:75, 1973.
47. Schecter, D. C., Owens, J. C., et al.: Hemorrhagic cysts of the spleen. Am. J. Surg. 104:777, 1962.
48. Pearson, H. A., Touloukian, R. J., et al.: The binary spleen: a radioisotopic scan sign of splenic pseudocyst. J. Pediatr. 77:216, 1970.
49. Bron, K. M., and Hoffman, W. J.: Preoperative diagnosis of splenic cysts. Arch. Surg. 102:459, 1971.
50. Gould, H. R., Clemitt, A. R., et al.: Radiologic diagnosis of splenic metastasis. Am. J. Roentgenol. 109:755, 1970.
51. Goldberg, G. M.: Metastatic carcinoma of the spleen resulting from lymphatic spread. Lab. Invest. 6:383, 1957.
52. Miller, J. M., and Milton, G. W.: An experimental comparison between tumor growth in the spleen and liver. J. Pathol. Bacteriol. 90:515, 1965.
53. Sammis, A. F., Jr., Weitzman, S., et al.: Hemangiolymphangioma of spleen and bone. N. Y. State J. Med. 71:1762, 1971.
54. Schwartz, A. D., Dadash, Z. M., et al.: Antibody response to intravenous immunization following splenic tissue autotransplantation in Sprague Dowley rats. Blood 51:475, 1978.
55. Brewster, D. C.: Splenosis: report of two cases and review of the literature. Am. J. Surg. 126:14, 1973.
55a. Pearson, H. A., Johnston, D., et al.: The born-again spleen: return of splenic function after splenectomy for trauma. New Engl. J. Med. 298:1389, 1978.
56. Ritchey, K., Pearson, H. A., et al.: Splenosis following splenectomy for trauma in adults. Blood 52(Suppl. 1):88, 1978.
57. Messmore, H. L. Quoted in Medical News: Autotransplantation of spleen tissue after trauma: encouraging evidence. J.A.M.A. 241:437, 1979.
58. Bowering, C. S.: *Radionuclide Tracer Techniques in Haematology.* London, Buttersworth, 1981.
59. Jacob, H. S., MacDonald, R. A. et al.: Regulation of spleen growth and sequestering function. J. Clin. Invest. 42:1476, 1963.
60. Jandl, J. H., Files, N. M., et al.: Proliferative response of the spleen and liver to hemolysis. J. Exp. Med. 122:299, 1965.
61. Jacob, H. S.: Born-again to work again. New Engl. J. Med. 298:1415, 1978.
61a. Kovacs, K. F., Caride, V. J., and Touloukian, R. J.: Regeneration of splenic autotransplants in suckling and adult rats. Arch. Surg. 116:335, 1981.
62. Mazure, E. M., Field, W. W., et al.: Idiopathic thrombocytopenic purpura occurring in a subject previously splenectomized for traumatic splenic rupture: role of splenosis in the pathogenesis of thrombocytopenia. Am. J. Med. 65:843, 1978.
63. Singer, D. B.: Postsplenectomy sepsis. Perspect. Pediatr. Pathol. 1:285, 1973.
64. Price, H. M., and James, D. D.: Ectopic splenic tissue failed to prevent pneumococcal septicemia after splenectomy for trauma. Lancet 1:565, 1980.
65. Hyslop, M. E., Jr.: Fever and circulatory collapse in an asplenic man. New Engl. J. Med. 293:547, 1975.
66. Rice, H. M., and James, P. D.: Ectopic splenic tissue failed to prevent fatal pneumococcal septicemia after splenectomy for trauma. Lancet 1:565, 1980.
67. Crosby, W. H., and Benjamin, N. R.: Frozen spleen reimplanted and challenged with *Bartonella.* Am. J. Pathol. 39:119, 1961.
68. Perla, D., and Marmoiston-Gollesman, J.: Studies on *Bartonella muris* anemia of albino rats. III. The protective effects of autoplastic splenic transplants on *Bartonella muris* anemia of splenectomized rats. J. Exp. Med. 52:131, 1930.
69. Schwartz, A. D., Goldthorn, J. F., et al.: Lack of protective effect of autotransplanted splenic tissue to pneumococcal challenge. Blood 51:475, 1978.
70. Dickerman, J. D., Horner, S. R., et al.: The protective effect of intraperitoneal splenic autotransplants in mice exposed to an aerosolized suspension of Type III *Streptococcus pneumoniae.* Blood 54:354, 1979.
71. Moxon, E. R., and Schwartz, A. D.: Heterotopic splenic autotransplantation in the prevention of H. influenzae meningitis and sepsis in Sprague-Dowley rats. Blood 55:842, 1980.
72. Livingston, C. D., Levine, A. A., et al.: Site of splenic autotransplantation affects protection from sepsis. Am. J. Surg. 146:734, 1983.
73. Kevy, S. V., Tifft, M., et al.: Hereditary splenic hypoplasia. Pediatrics 42:752, 1968.
74. Garega, S., and Crosby, W. H.: The incidence of leukemia in families of patients with hypoplasia of the marrow. Blood 14:1008, 1959.
75. Pearson, H. A., Lobel, J. S., et al.: A new syndrome of refractory sideroblastic anemia with vacuolization of mar-

row precursors and exocrine pancreatic dysfunction. J. Pediatr. 95:976, 1984.
75a. Marsh, G. W., and Stewart, J. S.: Splenic function in adult coeliac disease. Br. J. Haematol. 19:445, 1970.
76. Martin, J. B., and Bell, H. E.: The association of splenic atrophy and intestinal malabsorption: report of a case and review of the literature. Can. Med. Assoc. J. 92:875, 1965.
77. Ryan, R. P., Smart, R. C., et al.: Hyposplenism in inflammatory bowel disease. Gut 19:50, 1978.
78. Pettit, J. E., Hoffbrand, A. V., et al.: Splenic atrophy in dermatitis herpetiformis. Br. Med. J. 2:438, 1972.
79. Brownlie, B. E., Hammer, J. W., et al.: Thyrotoxicosis associated with splenic atrophy. Lancet 2:1046, 1975.
80. Marsh, G. W., Lewis, S. M., et al.: The use of ^{51}Cr-labeled heat-damaged red cells to study splenic function. II. Splenic atrophy in thrombocythaemia. Br. J. Haematol. 12:167, 1966.
81. Bensinger, T. A., Keller, A. R., et al.: Thorotrast-induced reticuloendothelial blockage in man. Am. J. Med. 51:663, 1971.
82. Lockwood, C. M., Worlledge, S., et al.: Reversal of impaired splenic function in patients with nephritis or vasculitis (or both) by plasma exchange. New Engl. J. Med. 300:524, 1979.
83. Crosby, W. H.: Normal function of the spleen relative to the red blood cells. Blood 14:399, 1959.
84. Crosby, W. H.: Splenic remodeling of red cell surfaces. Blood 50:643, 1977.
85. Eichner, E. R.: Splenic function: normal, too much and too little. Am. J. Med. 66:311, 1979.
86. Ward, H. P., and Block, M. H.: The natural history of agnogenic myeloid metaplasia (AMM) and a critical evaluation of its relationship with the myeloproliferative syndrome. Medicine 50:357, 1971.
87. Finch, C. A., Duebelbeiss, K., et al.: Ferrokinetics in man. Medicine 49:17, 1970.
88. Pettit, J. E.: Splenic function. Clin. Hematol. 6:639, 1977.
89. Weiss, L.: The role of the spleen in the removal of normal aged red cells. Am. J. Anat. 111:175, 1962.
90. Ehrenstein, G. V., and Lockner, D.: Sites of the physiological breakdown of the red blood corpuscles. Nature (Lond.) 181:911, 1958.
91. Bowning, C. S., Ferrant, A. E., et al.: Quantitative measurement of splenic and hepatic red-cell destruction. Br. J. Haematol. 31:467, 1975.
92. Rous, P.: Destruction of the red blood corpuscle in health and disease. Physical Rev. 3:75, 1923.
93. Prankerd, T. A. J.: Studies on the pathogenesis of haemolysis in hereditary spherocytosis. Q. J. Med. 29:199, 1960.
94. Jandl, J. H., Greenberg, M. S., et al.: Clinical determination of the sites of red cell destruction in the hemolytic anemias. J. Clin. Invest. 35:842, 1956.
95. Ferrant, A.: The role of the spleen in haemolysis. Clin. Haematol. 12:489, 1983.
96. Levesque, M. J.: Sequestration of the heat-treated autologous red cells in the spleen. J. Lab. Clin. Med. 90:606, 1977.
97. Aster, R. H.: Pooling of platelets in the spleen: role of the pathogenesis of "hypersplenic" thrombocytopenia. J. Clin. Invest. 45:645, 1966.
98. Penny, R., Rozenberg, M. C., et al.: The splenic platelet pool. Blood 27:1, 1966.
99. Peters, A. M.: Splenic blood flow and blood cell kinetics. Clin. Haematol. 12:421, 1983.
100. Libre, E. B., Cowan, D. H., et al.: Relationship between spleen, platelets, and Factor VIII levels. Blood 31:358, 1968.
101. Lux, S. E., and John, K. M.: Isolation and partial characterization of a high molecular weight protein complex normally removed by the spleen. Blood 50:643, 1977.
102. Tanaka, K. R., and Paglia, D. E.: Pyruvate kinase deficiency. Semin. Hematol. 8:367, 1971.
103. Nathan, D. G.: Rubbish in the red cell. New Engl. J. Med. 281:588, 1969.
104. Crosby, W. H.: Siderocytes and the spleen. Blood 12:165, 1956.
105. Lipson, R. I., Bayrd, E. D., et al.: The post-splenectomy blood picture. Am. J. Clin. Pathol. 32:526, 1959.
106. Nathan, D. G., and Gunn, R. B.: Thalassemia: consequences of unbalanced hemoglobin synthesis. Am. J. Med. 41:815, 1966.
107. Pearson, H. A., McIntosh, S., et al.: Developmental aspects of splenic function in sickle cell diseases. Blood 53:358, 1979.
108. Holroyd, C. P., and Gardner, F. H.: Acquisition of autophagic vacuoles by human erythrocytes: Physiological role of the spleen. Blood 36:566, 1970.
109. Rifkind, R. A.: Heinz body anemia: an ultrastudy. II. Red cell sequestration and destruction. Blood 26:433, 1965.
110. Koyama, S.: Electron microscopic observations of the splenic red pulp with special reference to the pitting function. Mie. Med. J. 14:143, 1964.
111. Schofield, I. R.: The pluripotential stem cell. Clin. Haematol. 8:221, 1978.
112. Mona, L., Ponassi, A., et al.: Influence of the spleen on the blood distribution of the colony-forming cells (CFU-c) in man. Acta Haematol. 66:81, 1981.
113. Koeffler, H. P., Cline, M. J., et al.: Splenic irradiation in myelofibrosis. Br. J. Haematol. 43:69, 1979.
114. Montz, R., and Schneider, C.: Eine Methodo Zur: Bestimmung der Gosse des erythropoetischer Knochenmarks beim Menschen, aus der Radioeisenkinet k. Blut 21:283, 1978.
115. Cooper, M., Buggs, R. S., et al.: Therapy of refractory idiopathic thrombocytopenic purpura. Conn. Med. 32:509, 1968.
116. Fried, N., and Anagnostou, A.: Extrarenal erythropoietin production. In Kidney Hormones. II. Erythropoietin. Fisher, J. (ed.), New York, Academic Press, 1977, p. 231.
117. Lewis, S. M.: The spleen—mysteries solved and unresolved. Clin. Haematol. 12:363, 1983.
118. Robinette, C. D., and Fraumini, J.: Splenectomy and subsequent mortality in veterans of the 1939–45 war. Lancet 2:127, 1977.
119. Saslaw, S., Bournocle, B. A., et al.: Studies on the antibody response in splenectomized persons. New Engl. J. Med. 261:120, 1959.
120. McFadzean, A. J., and Tsang, K. C.: Antibody formation in cryptogenic splenomegaly. II. Response to antigen injected subcutaneously. Trans. R. Soc. Trop. Med. Hyg. 50:438, 1956.
121. Motohashi, S. J.: The effect of splenectomy on the production of antibodies. J. Med. Res. 43:473, 1972.
121a. Hosea, S. W., Burch, C. G., et al.: Impaired immune response of splenectomized patients to polyvalent pneumococcal vaccine. Lancet 1:804, 1981.
121b. Ruben, F. L., Hankins, W. A., et al.: Antibody responses to meningococcal polysaccharide vaccines in adults without a spleen. Am. J. Med. 76:115, 1984.
122. Schwartz, A. D., and Pearson, H. A.: Impaired antibody response to intravenous immunizations in sickle-cell anemia. Pediatr. Res. 6:145, 1972.
123. Taliaferro, W. H., and Taliaferro, L. G.: The dynamics of hemolysin formation in intact and splenectomized rabbits. J. Infect. Dis. 87:37, 1950.
124. Shulkind, M., Ellis, E. F., et al.: Effect of antibody upon clearance of 125 I labeled pneumococci by the spleen and liver. Pediatr. Res. 1:178, 1967.
125. Shumacher, M. J.: Serum immunoglobulin and transferrin levels after childhood splenectomy. Arch. Dis. Child. 45:114, 1970.

126. Gavrilis, P., Rothenberg, S. P., et al.: Correlation of low serum IgM levels with absence of functional splenic tissue in sickle cell disease syndromes. Am. J. Med. 57:542, 1972.
127. Mondorf, W., Lennert, K. A., et al.: Zur Immunglobulinbildung in der menschlichen Milz. In Die Milz (The Spleen). Lennert, K., and Harms, D. (eds.), Berlin and New York, Springer-Verlag, 1970, p. 162.
128. Walzer, P. D., Armstrong, D., et al.: Serum immunoglobulin levels in childhood Hodgkin's disease. Cancer 45:2084, 1980.
129. Carlisle, H. N., and Saslaw, S.: Properdin levels in splenectomized persons. Proc. Soc. Exp. Biol. Med. 102:150, 1959.
130. Najjar, V. A., and Nishioka, K.: Tuftsin, a physiologic phagocytosis stimulating peptide. Nature 228:672, 1970.
131. Constantopoulos, A., Najjar, V. A., et al.: Defective phagocytosis due to tuftsin deficiency in splenectomized subjects. Am. J. Dis. Child. 125:663, 1973.
132. Spirer, Z., Zakuth, V., et al.: Decreased tuftsin concentrations in patients who have undergone splenectomy. Br. Med. J. 2:1574, 1977.
133. McMillan, R., Longmire, R. L., et al.: Quantitation of platelet binding IgG produced in vitro by spleens of patients with idiopathic thrombocytopenic purpura. New Engl. J. Med. 291:812, 1974.
134. Lightsey, A. L., McMillan, R., et al.: In vitro production of platelet binding IgG in childhood idiopathic thrombocytopenic purpura. J. Pediatr. 88:414, 1976.
135. Jandl, J. H., Jones, A. R., et al.: The destruction of red cells by antibodies in man. I. Observations on the sequestration and lysis of red cells altered by immune mechanisms. J. Clin. Invest. 36:1428, 1957.
136. Lo Buglio, A. F., Cotran, R. S., et al.: Red cells coated with immunoglobulin G. Binding and sphering by mononuclear cells in man. Science 158:1582, 1967.
137. Frank, M. M., Schreiber, A. D., et al.: Pathophysiology of immune hemolytic anemia. Ann. Intern. Med. 87:210, 1977.
138. Sutliff, W. D., and Finland, M.: Antipneumococcal immunity reactions in individuals of different ages. J. Exp. Med. 55:837, 1932.
139. Fothergill, L. D., and Wright, J.: Influenzal meningitis: the relationship of age incidence to the bactericidal power of blood against the causal organism. J. Immunol. 24:273, 1933.
140. Hoyle, L.: Influenza Viruses. New York, Springer-Verlag, 1968.
141. Schnitzer, B., Sodeman, T. M., et al.: An ultrastructural study of the red pulp of the spleen in malaria. Blood 44:207, 1973.
142. Stiffel, C., Mouton, D., et al.: Influence de la splenectomie sur l'immunite specifique et a specifique au couis de l'infection paludeene du rat par "Plasmodium berghei." Ann. Inst. Pasteur 123:55, 1972.
143. Finch, S. C., and Jonas, A. M.: Ethyl palmitate-induced bartonellosis as an index of functional splenic ablation. J. Reticuloendothel. Soc. 13:20, 1973.
144. Perla, D., and Marmorstein-Gottesman, J.: Studies on Bartonella muris anemia in albino rats. The protective effect of autoplastic splenic transplants on the Bartonella muris anemia of splenectomized rats. J. Exp. Med. 52:131, 1930.
145. Western, K. A., Benson, G. D., et al.: Babesiosis in a Massachusetts resident. New Engl. J. Med. 283:854, 1970.
146. Acevedo, G., and Mauer, A. M.: The capacity for removal of erythrocytes containing Heinz bodies in premature infants and patients following splenectomy. J. Pediatr. 63:61, 1963.
147. Ozsoylu, S., Hosain, F., et al.: Functional development of phagocytic activity of the spleen. J. Pediatr. 90:560, 1977.

148. Pearson, H. A., Spencer, R. P., et al.: Functional asplenia in sickle-cell anemia. New Engl. J. Med. 281:923, 1969.
149. O'Brien, R. T., McIntosh, S., et al.: Prospective studies of sickle-cell anemia in infancy. J. Pediatr. 89:205, 1976.
150. Pearson, H. A., Cornelius, E. A., et al.: Transfusion reversible functional asplenia in young children with sickle-cell anemia. New Engl. J. Med. 283:334, 1970.
151. Pearson, H. A., Gallagher, D., et al.: Developmental patterns of splenic dysfunction in sickle cell disorders. Pediatrics 76:392, 1985.
152. Al-Alwamy, B., Wilson, W., et al.: Splenic function in sickle cell disease in the Eastern Province of Saudi Arabia. J. Pediatr. 104:714, 1984.
153. Robinson, M. G., and Watson, R. J.: Pneumococcal meningitis in sickle-cell anemia. New Engl. J. Med. 274:1006, 1966.
154. Kabins, S. A., and Lerner, C.: Fulminant pneumococcemia and sickle-cell anemia. J.A.M.A. 211:467, 1970.
155. Barrett-Connor, E.: Bacterial infections in sickle-cell anemia: an analysis of 250 infections in 166 patients and a review of the literature. Medicine 50:96, 1971.
156. Powars, D. R.: Natural history of sickle-cell disease—the first ten years. Semin. Hematol. 12:267, 1975.
157. Winkelstein, J. A., and Drachman, R. H.: Deficiency of pneumococcal serum opsonizing activity in sickle-cell disease. New Engl. J. Med. 279:459, 1968.
158. Johnston, R. B., Jr., Newman, S. L., et al.: An abnormality of the alternate pathway of complement activation in sickle-cell disease. New Engl. J. Med. 288:803, 1973.
159. Wilson, W. A., Hughes, G. R. V., et al.: Deficiency of Factor B of the complement system in sickle-cell anemia. Br. Med. J. 1:367, 1976.
160. Bjornson, A. B., Gaston, M. H., et al.: Decreased opsonization for streptococcus pneumonia in sickle-cell disease: studies on selected components and immunoglobulins. J. Pediatr. 91:371, 1977.
161. Schwartz, A. D.: The splenic platelet reservoir in sickle-cell anemia. Blood 40:678, 1972.
162. McIntyre, O. R., and Ebaugh, F. G., Jr.: Palpable spleens in college freshman. Ann. Intern. Med. 66:301, 1967.
163. Bowdler, A. J.: Dilution anemia corrected by splenectomy in Gaucher's disease. Ann. Intern. Med. 58:664, 1963.
164. Howman-Giles, R., Gilday, D. L., et al.: Splenic trauma: non-operative management and long-term follow-up by scintiscan. J. Pediatr. Surg. 13:121, 1978.
165. Solheim, K.: Non-operative management of splenic rupture. Acta Clin. Scand. 145:55, 1979.
166. Traub, A. C., and Perry, J. F., Jr.: Splenic preservation following splenic trauma. J. Trauma 22:496, 1982.
167. Hebler, R. F., Ward, R. E., et al.: The management of splenic injury. J. Trauma 22:492, 1982.
168. La Mura, J., Chung-Fat, S. P., et al.: Splenorrhaphy for treatment of splenic rupture in infants and children. Surgery 81:497, 1977.
169. Morgenstern, I., and Shapiro, S. J.: Techniques of splenic conservation. Arch. Surg. 114:449, 1979.
170. Buntain, W. L., and Lynn, H. B.: Splenorrhaphy: changing concepts for the traumatized spleen. Surgery 86:748, 1979.
171. Krumbhaar, E. B.: The changes produced in the blood picture by removal of the normal mammalian spleen. Am. J. Med. Sci. 184:215, 1932.
172. McBride, J. A.: The effect of splenectomy on the leucocyte count. Br. J. Haematol. 14:225, 1968.
173. Wallstein, M., and Kreidel, K. V.: Blood picture after splenectomy in children. Am. J. Dis. Child. 51:765, 1936.
174. McCracken, E. H., Jr., and Dickerman, J. D.: Septicemia and disseminated intravascular coagulation occurrence in four asplenic children. Am. J. Dis. Child. 118:431, 1969.
175. Whitaker, A. N.: Infection and the spleen. Association

between hyposplenism, pneumococcal sepsis, and disseminated intravascular coagulation. Med. J. Aust. *1:*1213, 1969.
176. Bisno, A. L., and Freeman, J. C.: The syndrome of asplenia, pneumococcal sepsis and disseminated intravascular coagulation. Ann. Intern. Med. *72:*389, 1970.
177. Rytel, M. W., Dee, T. H., et al.: Possible pathogenetic role of capsular antigens in fulminant pneumococcal disease with disseminated intravascular coagulation. (DIC). Am. J. Med. *57:*889, 1974.
178. Horan, M., and Colebatch, J. H.: Relation between splenectomy and subsequent infection: a clinical study. Arch. Dis. Child. *37:*398, 1962.
179. Grinblat, J., and Billoa, Y.: Overwhelming pneumococcal sepsis 25 years after splenectomy. Am. J. Med. Sci. *270:*523, 1975.
180. Pearson, H. A., Shulman, N. R., et al.: Platelet survival in Wiskott-Aldrich syndrome. J. Pediatr. *68:*754, 1966.
181. Wolff, J. A.: Wiskott-Aldrich syndrome: clinical, immunological and pathologic observations. J. Pediatr. *70:*221, 1967.
182. Lum, L. G., Tubergen, D. G., et al.: Splenectomy in the management of the thrombocytopenia of Wiskott-Aldrich syndrome. N. Engl. J. Med. *302:*892, 1980.
183. Weiden, P. L., and Blaise, R. M.: Hereditary thrombocytopenia: relation to Wiskott-Aldrich syndrome with special reference to splenectomy. J. Pediatr. *80:*226, 1972.
184. Donaldson, S. S., Glatstein, E., et al.: Bacterial infections in pediatric Hodgkin's disease. Cancer *41:*1949, 1978.
185. Donaldson, S. S., Moore, M. R., et al.: Characterization of postsplenectomy bacteremia among patients with and without lymphoma. New Engl. J. Med. *287:*69, 1972.
186. Smith, D. H., Peter, G., et al.: Responses of children immunized with the capsular polysaccharide of *Hemophilus influenzae* Type B. Pediatrics *52:*637, 1973.
187. Grosfeld, J. L., and Ranochak, J. E.: Are hemisplenectomy and/or splenic repair feasible? J. Pediatr. Surg. *11:*419, 1976.
188. Lanzkowsky, P., Shienden, A., et al.: Staging laparotomy and splenectomy: treatment and complications of Hodgkin's disease in children. Am. J. Hematol. *1:*393, 1976.
188a. Gaston, M. H., Verter, J. I., et al.: Prophylaxis with oral penicillin in children with sickle cell anemia. A randomized trial. New Engl. J. Med. *314:*1593, 1986.
189. Dickerman, J., Bolton, E., et al.: Protective effect of prophylactic penicillin on splenectomized mice exposed to an aerosolized suspension of Type III *Streptococcus pneumoniae*. Blood *53:*498, 1979.
190. Ertel, I. J., Bobes, E. T., Jr., et al.: Infection after splenectomy. New Engl. J. Med. *296:*1174, 1977.
191. Buchanan, G. R., Siegel, J. D., et al.: Oral penicillin prophylaxis in children with impaired splenic function: a study of compliance. Pediatrics *70:*926, 1982.
192. Overturf, G. D., Field, R., et al.: Death from type 6 pneumococcal septicemia in a vaccinated child with sickle cell disease. New Engl. J. Med. *300:*143, 1979.
193. Amman, A. J., Addiego, J., et al.: Polyvalent pneumococcal-polysaccharide immunization of patients with sickle cell anemia and patients with splenectomy. New Engl. J. Med. *297:*897, 1977.
194. Siber, G. R., Weitzman, S. A., et al.: Impaired antibody response after treatment for Hodgkin's disease. New Engl. J. Med. *299:*442, 1978.
195. Cowan, M. J., Amman, A. J., et al.: Pneumococcal polysaccharide immunization in infants and children. Pediatrics *62:*721, 1978.
196. Jacobs, M. R., Kornhoff, H. K., et al.: Emergence of multiple resistant pneumococci. New Engl. J. Med. *299:*735, 1978.
197. Likhite, V. V.: Immunological impairment and susceptibility to infection after splenectomy. J.A.M.A. *236:*1376, 1976.

ONCOLOGY

CHAPTER 30
Epidemiology of Cancer in Childhood

FREDERICK P. LI
JUDITH L. BADER

DEMOGRAPHIC CHARACTERISTICS OF CANCER PATIENTS 918
CANCER RATES 920
CANCER RISK FACTORS 921
Environmental Carcinogens
Host Susceptibility
EPIDEMIOLOGY OF SELECTED CHILDHOOD CANCERS 927
Leukemia
Lymphomas
Central Nervous System Tumors
Neuroblastoma
Soft Tissue Sarcomas
Skeletal Sarcomas
Wilms' Tumor
Retinoblastoma
Liver Tumors
Testicular Cancer
Ovarian Cancer
Epidemiology of Other Childhood Neoplasms
SURVIVORS OF CANCER IN CHILDHOOD 934

Research in cancer epidemiology has provided knowledge of both basic biology and clinical behavior of neoplastic diseases. These studies have identified host and environmental factors in the development of human cancers and have clarified the natural history of these disorders. The findings are applicable to cancer prevention, early detection, and analysis of treatment effects (1–4).

This chapter summarizes current knowledge of the epidemiology of childhood cancers and suggests directions for future investigations. The etiology and epidemiology of common cancers in adults have been examined in recent textbooks (5–9) and are therefore excluded from detailed consideration, even though prenatal and childhood events may predispose to cancer in later life.

DEMOGRAPHIC CHARACTERISTICS OF CANCER PATIENTS (Table 30–1)

In epidemiologic studies of cancer, demographic variables—characteristics of person, place, and time—are analyzed to identify population subgroups at unusually high or low risk for malignancy. The most commonly studied variables are age, sex, and race; others of interest in pediatric cancer epidemiology include birthplace, birth order, sibship size, parental occupation and age at conception, religion, ethnicity, and socioeconomic status.

Age. Variations in rates of cancer with age are shown in graphs of age-specific incidence or mortality data. Etiologic hypotheses can be generated by analyzing the slopes, peaks, and troughs for individual tumors (10). For example, neoplasms with a prominent peak in the first years of life may have developed prenatally by the action of prezygotic or intrauterine influences (11). These malignancies rarely develop as metastases from a maternal neoplasm (12). Data from the Third National Cancer Survey, a 3-year study (1969 to 1971) of cancer incidence in approximately 10 per cent of the United States population, show that 9 per cent of cancers in children under 15 years of age were diagnosed in the first year of life (13, 14). The most common cancers of infancy were neuroblastoma, leukemia, sarcomas, Wilms' tumor, retinoblastoma, neural tumors, and liver tumors (14, 15). Thereafter, several cancers have more than one prominent age peak, e.g., Hodgkin's disease (16), osteosarcoma (17), testicular cancer (18), and certain brain tumors (19). Bimodal or multimodal age peaks may indicate heterogeneous etiologies for the same neoplasm (16).

Race and Sex. Rates of several childhood cancers vary by sex and ethnicity. Lymphomas have the highest male:female ratio, 2:1 (20), suggesting that X-linked immunodeficiency disorders may partly account for the higher frequency in males (20, 21). Other variations in host susceptibility are suggested by the lower than expected frequency of Ewing's sarcoma among blacks in Africa and the United States, and the higher frequency of leukemia among Jews (22, 23).

Clusters. In the last two decades, attention has focused on reported clusters of acute leukemia, which may indicate the action of an infectious agent (24). Patients within a cluster have developed leukemia over a short period of time and in a small geographic area. When appropriate statistical methods were used to analyze such aggregations, many "clusters" seemed to be explainable by chance (25). However, a recently completed retrospective study of Woburn, Massachusetts, showed a two-fold excess of childhood leukemias in the community from 1969 to 1979. Prospective observation during 1980–83 showed that childhood leukemias were still developing in excess in the community (25A).

A second model of aggregation of cancer cases is based on linkage networks of patients who have had a history of personal contact with each other, despite dissimilar times and geographic locations at diagnosis of cancer (26). This second model, which postulates person-to-person transmission of a hypothetical infectious agent (27), will be discussed in detail in the section on Hodgkin's disease.

Maps. Another analytic approach to the distribution of cancer in the United States involves the use of computer-generated maps to depict geographic patterns of cancer mortality (28, 29). Maps by county or state economic area have been constructed from official death certificate information obtained from the United States Department of Vital Statistics. The maps show geographic patterns of mortality that can be analyzed by age, sex, race, site, and histology. By correlating high and low rate areas with cities, industries, population characteristics, water supply, climate, and other factors, hypotheses have been generated regarding environmental influences on cancer incidence in adults (30, 31). Figure 30–1 is a map of cancer mortality rates by county for white male children in the United States under age 15 from 1950 to 1975 (prepared by F. W. McKay). Aside from concentrations in a few scattered regions, no remarkable distributions appear on this map or on those depicting specific tumors of childhood (32). The usefulness of this tool in studies of childhood cancer may be limited by low rates and possibly by the absence of major differences in environmental influences among geographic regions.

Clinical Observations. Demographic data can stimulate etiologic studies of cancer by identification of patients who are far outside the demographic norm for a particular neoplasm. These individuals may have developed their tumor through unusual etiologic mechanisms, such as genetic predisposition or intense carcinogenic exposures. The initial evaluation of such patients involves obtaining a detailed medical, occupational, and family history and performing a complete physical examination to uncover evidence of host or environmental influences. Etiologic hypotheses derived from clinical investigations pro-

Table 30–1. INCIDENCE OF MALIGNANT NEOPLASMS AMONG CHILDREN UNDER 15 YEARS OF AGE IN THE UNITED STATES

Tumor Type	White Children			Black Children			White and Black Children
	Rate*	% of Total Cancers	Male:Female Ratio†	Rate*	% of Total Cancers	Male:Female Ratio†	U.S. Incidence‡ (New Cases/yr)
Leukemia	42.1	33.8	1.4	24.3	24.9	1.0	2357
Central nervous system	23.9	19.2	1.2	23.9	24.4	0.3	1417
Lymphoma	13.2	10.6	2.0	13.9	14.2	-	787
Neuroblastoma	9.4	7.7	1.3	7.0	7.1	-	540
Soft tissue sarcoma	8.4	6.8	1.2	3.9§	4.0	-	463
Wilms' tumor	7.6	6.1	1.1	7.8	8.0	-	450
Bone tumor	5.6	4.5	1.2	4.8	4.9	-	323
Retinoblastoma	3.4	2.7	0.9	3.0§	3.1	-	197
Liver tumor	1.9	1.5	-	0.4§	0.4	-	100
Ovarian tumor	1.2	0.9	-	2.1§	2.2	-	77
Testicular tumor	1.0	0.8	-	0.4§	0.4	-	57
Other	6.8	5.4	-	6.3	6.4	-	400
Total	124.5	100	1.3	97.8	100	1.0	7168

*Rate per million per year based from the Third National Cancer Survey (1969–1971), as reported by Young and Miller (20).
†Computed for tumor types with more than 50 cases.
‡Number of new cases in the United States in 1970, as calculated from Young and Miller (20).
§Rate based on fewer than 10 cases.

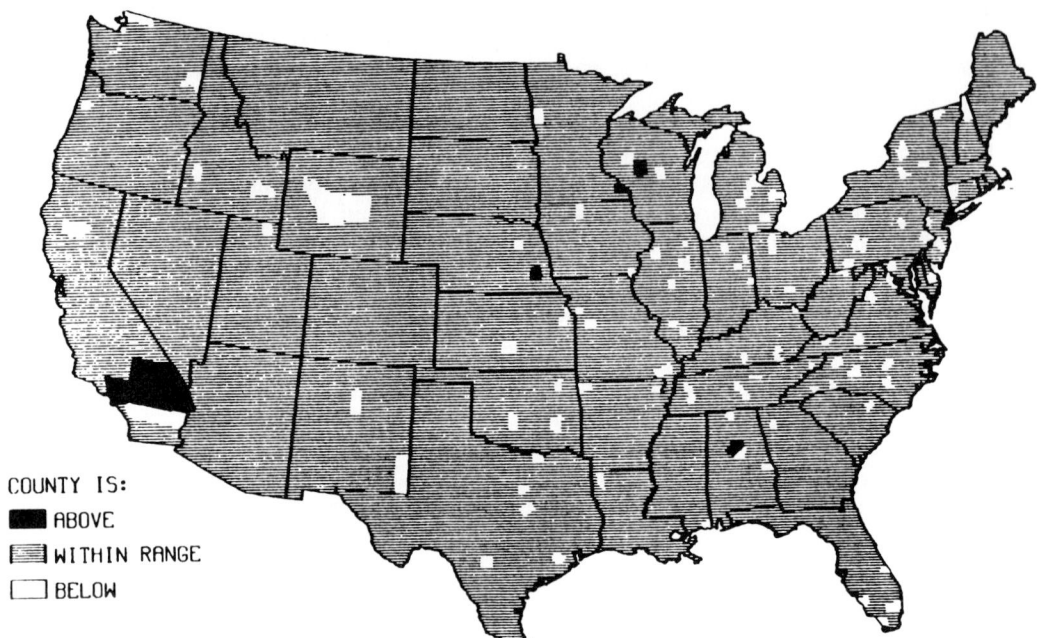

Figure 30–1. Cancer mortality rates by county, 1950–1975. Rate for each county is significantly above (shown in black), significantly below (in white), or within the 0.95 confidence interval (in gray) of the national rate.

vide new leads both for laboratory studies and for more classic epidemiologic investigations. These clinical case studies have produced the initial discovery of many of the known risk factors in childhood cancer (33). From seemingly isolated case reports and small series, biologic mechanisms of susceptibility to a neoplasm can be recognized, e.g., chromosomal abnormality as a feature is common among diverse constitutional diseases with high risk of acute leukemia (34).

CANCER RATES

Cancer accounts for approximately 10 per cent of deaths among children in the United States from ages 1 to 14 years and is second only to accidents as the leading cause of death in this age group. Between 1960 and 1966, the cancer mortality rate among United States children, from birth to 14 years, was approximately 70 per million per year (35). With improvements in treatment, cancer mortality rates for children have declined and no longer reflect disease incidence (36).

No nationwide system exists to register each new cancer and to report cancer incidence for the entire United States population. However, several states, such as Connecticut, have developed population-based registries to monitor cancer statistics. These registries are linked by the SEER (Surveillance, Epidemiology, and End Results) Program of the National Cancer Institute and provide data on approximately 10 per cent of the United States population (37). In addition, United States cancer incidence figures can be estimated from data of the Third National Cancer Survey, which show that the incidence of cancer in children under 15 years of age was approximately 124 per million per year among United States whites and 98 per million per year among United States blacks (Table 30–1) (20). The difference resulted primarily from a lower rate of acute lymphocytic leukemia among black children.

Rates for specific cancers in the United States and elsewhere are usually derived from data in pathology files, hospital discharge records, death certificates, and other official documents. Cancers are usually coded according to the primary site, e.g., malignant neoplasm of the stomach (38). The system of classification by site was devised primarily for cancers in adults and is less useful for studying childhood tumors that can arise at diverse sites. For example, neuroblastoma can be classified with neoplasms of the adrenal gland or the nervous system; therefore, neuroblastoma rates cannot be determined from site-specific data (39). Other coding schemes are now based on tumor site, morphology, or both (40, 41). Further division of individual diagnostic categories becomes necessary when distinct subsets of patients are recognized, e.g., those with acute lymphocytic leukemia of T or B cells (42).

Rates of cancer for children in a few geographic areas worldwide are summarized in *Cancer Incidence in Five Continents* (43). Comparisons of national rates should be made with caution because of the variability in medical services, diagnostic practices, methods of ascertainment and reporting of cancers, and accuracy of baseline demographic data (44–46). Available data indicate that overall childhood cancer incidence rates are generally similar in the United States, Denmark, New Zealand, and Finland (22, 43, 47). The rates are higher in Israel and Ibadan (Nigeria) and lower in Miyagi (Japan), Manchester (England), and Bombay (India) (22, 47, 48). Age- and sex-specific rates of individual forms of childhood cancer show more striking differences that are not readily explained by inadequacies of the data, e.g., high rates of Burkitt's lymphoma in tropical Africa (49). The frequency patterns may be due to population differences in genetic susceptibility or exposure to environmental carcinogens (23). Variations in rate can be further examined by studies of migrant populations and by comparisons of cancer rates among heterogeneous populations in one geographic area, e.g., Arabs; Asiatic, European, and native-born Jews in Israel; and Caucasians, Japanese, Chinese, and native Hawaiians in Hawaii (44, 50). Changes in cancer rates over time can also provide support for etiologic associations: increased cigarette smoking was followed by rises in lung cancer rates (51).

The low rates and diversity of cancers in children hinder certain classic types of epidemiologic investigations (35). Large, stable study populations are required for cohort studies, which compare the cancer rates in a group of persons exposed to a specific risk factor with rates in a nonexposed group (46). Costs are also high for case-control studies, which compare the frequency of exposure to a risk factor in cancer patients with the frequency in an appropriate control group. These studies of cancer in childhood usually require the patient resources of a large cancer center, cooperative group, or special childhood cancer registration system. When patients are gathered for therapeutic trials, consideration should be given to the potential for concurrent etiologic studies.

CANCER RISK FACTORS

Studies of carcinogenic agents in the environment have examined the etiologic role of radiation, drugs, chemicals, and viruses (6). Susceptibility to these agents may be modified by certain demographic characteristics or by genetic constitution (7). For clarity, each of the major risk factors for the development of cancer is examined individually in the following section, even though host and environmental factors may interact. Identification of high-risk individuals aids early cancer diagnosis and prevention, by elimination of carcinogens and by genetic counseling.

Environmental Carcinogens

IONIZING RADIATION

Studies of survivors of nuclear bombing, workers exposed to radiation, and patients irradiated for diverse medical conditions show that ionizing radiation can induce human cancers (52–55). The irradiated tissues are the sites of development of diverse benign and malignant neoplasms, e.g., carcinomas of the skin, thyroid, breast, and salivary glands; sarcomas of bones and soft tissues; brain tumors; meningiomas; lymphomas; and leukemias other than chronic lymphocytic leukemia (53). The latent period after exposure may be as brief as several years, or as long as a lifetime (52).

The relation of radiation dose to the development of cancer is complex (55). Frequency of cancer induction is influenced by quality of the radiation, total dose, fraction size, dose rate, and other exposure variables. Because complete details of radiation exposures in humans are seldom available, laboratory studies have been used to help study the dose-response relationship and the biologic mechanisms of radiation carcinogenesis (56). In one dose-response model used to set radiation safety standards for humans, the relationship is assumed to be linear and without threshold (52, 57). Thus a doubling of the dose doubles the number of induced cancers, whereas dose reduction lowers, but does not eliminate, the cancer risk. This model appears to be applicable within an intermediate range of radiation exposure of several tissues, but the effects of doses in the very high or very low ranges remain uncertain (52, 58).

It is uncertain whether the developing fetus is unusually susceptible to radiation carcinogenesis. Several investigators have reported that prenatal exposure to approximately 1 rad of diagnostic x-ray was associated with a 50 per cent increase in the risk of acute leukemia and perhaps other cancers during the first years of life (59, 60). However, parental radiation exposure before conception reportedly has the same carcinogenic effect (60a). Furthermore, Diamond and co-workers (61) found that prenatal radiography was associated with an excess of childhood leukemia in whites, a corresponding deficit of leukemia in blacks, and an overall rate that was in accord with expectation. The exposed white children also showed increased mortality from all noncancerous conditions, but not from cancers other than leukemia (61). Studies of atomic bomb survivors show that in utero exposure to much higher doses of radiation has not produced an excess of any cancer (62). One explanation for the discordant findings is that low dose prenatal diagnostic radiography produces neoplastic transformation, whereas the higher doses of atomic bombing are lethal to cells (62). Alternatively, the apparent cancer excess associated with diagnostic radiography is due to ascertainment bias in selecting pregnant women who have characteristics that predispose to cancer in the offspring (53, 63). The issue is not resolved. However, practitioners should recognize that the question is whether exposure of thousands of fetuses to low dose diagnostic radiography produces even one excess cancer in early childhood. A risk of this magnitude should be weighed against the expected benefits from the x-ray studies, and unnecessary exposures should be avoided.

Factors such as age, sex, and genetic constitution can modify the risk of developing radiogenic cancers. For example, radiation-associated breast cancers develop primarily in females (64, 65). The influence of age is suggested by the higher relative risk of acute leukemia among atomic bomb survivors exposed before 10 years of age, as compared with exposed adults (52). Also, rates of thyroid cancers after partial or whole-body radiation are higher among persons exposed in childhood (52). Increased susceptibility to radiogenic malignancy may be due to genetic susceptibility in patients treated for bilateral retinoblastoma and medulloblastoma associated with the basal cell nevus syndrome. After unusually short latent periods, these patients have developed a greater than expected number of sarcomas following treatment for the eye tumor, and skin cancers in the field of radiation for medulloblastoma (66). Host factors also predispose patients with xeroderma pigmentosum to develop skin cancers at sites exposed to sunlight; these cancers may result from an inherited defect in repair of ultraviolet-radiation-induced DNA damage (67). Patients with ataxia-telangiectasia have a corresponding defect in repair of ionizing radiation injury and are susceptible to lymphoreticular neoplasms and acute radiation toxicity (68).

DRUGS

Diverse drugs have carcinogenic activity in animals, but the causal role of many of these agents in the development of human cancer has not been established (69). The few medications implicated as carcinogens in humans are listed in Table 30–2 (70). The risk of cancer associated with most of these drugs is small, and for many diseases acceptable treatment alternatives are not available. Thus, alkylating agent therapy may be indicated for selected patients with life-threatening childhood disorders such as cancer, chronic hepatitis, rheumatoid arthritis, and renal failure, even though a few patients may subsequently develop leukemia (71). Alkylating agents with a leukemogenic potential include cyclophosphamide, melphalan, chlorambucil, nitrogen mustard, procarbazine, and nitrosoureas (71–75). Bladder cancers have also been reported after cyclophosphamide-associated cystitis (76). Bladder cancer after administration of chlornaphazine, a now discarded alkylating agent, may be the result of biotransformation to the carcinogen betanaphthylamine (77). The current use of combination chemotherapy for diverse cancers has created a need for information about possible oncogenic interactions of drugs (78, 79). Drugs used for non-neoplastic diseases, such as hormones, radioactive agents, immunosuppressants, and other agents, have also been linked to the development of malignancies (80–83). Some of these drugs, e.g., inorganic arsenicals and thorium dioxide (Thorotrast), have little or no current utility but may continue to produce cancers because their latency period for carcinogenesis may be decades (69).

Transplacental chemical carcinogenesis in humans was first demonstrated when seven young women developed clear cell adenocarcinoma of the vagina and cervix after maternal ingestion of the drug diethylstilbestrol (DES) during early gestation (84). Among prenatally exposed women, the risk of developing this cancer in early adulthood is approximately 1 per 1000 (85, 86). Longer follow-up will determine whether these patients will develop other forms of DES-associated neoplasia in later life. DES is also a teratogen and has been implicated in vaginal adenosis and other minor anomalies in up to 80 per cent of exposed daughters, and epididymal cysts in approximately 10 per cent of sons (87). The DES studies have raised the possibility that other agents may also act as transplacental carcinogens. In isolated reports, other childhood cancers have developed in patients whose mothers used estrogens during early pregnancy (88, 89), and neuroblastoma has developed in at least four patients with fetal hydantoin syndrome (90, 91). Both cancer chemotherapy with folic acid antagonists and abdominal radiotherapy during pregnancy have been associated with fetal loss and congenital anomalies (92).

CHEMICAL CARCINOGENS AND OTHER PRODUCTS

Occupational exposures to carcinogens are associated with high risk of certain cancers, particularly neoplasms of the lung, bladder, skin, and hematopoietic system (93). Children can be exposed by contamination of the air, soil, food, and other articles in their environment (94, 94a). Mesotheliomas, for example, have developed in adults who lived near asbestos mines during childhood or who were exposed to asbestos carried home on a parent's workclothes (95). Working mothers may transmit occupational carcinogens by breastfeeding, but no proof of cancer induction by this route of exposure has been demonstrated (96). One study has reported a high risk of cancer associated with employment of the father in hydrocarbon-related industries at the time of conception; the observation was not confirmed in a second study (97, 98).

Exposures during childhood may have a role in

the development of diverse neoplasms in later life (94). Personal habits, such as cigarette smoking, are often formed in childhood and adolescence (51). In the United States, up to one cancer in four is attributable to cigarette smoking, and reduced smoking among the young can prevent a substantial number of future cancers of the lung and other sites (99). Although maternal cigarette smoking during gestation is associated with fetal respiratory depression, low birthweight, and perhaps respiratory tract infections during infancy, a direct carcinogenic effect on offspring has not been identified (100).

Human and animal studies have implicated dietary factors during childhood in later development of cancers of the colon, breast, stomach, and other sites (101). Exposure during childhood to contaminants in drinking water, food additives, pesticides, and other ingredients in the diet (e.g., nitrosamines, aflatoxin) may have carcinogenic effects, but the evidence is circumstantial and controversial at present (94, 102, 103).

Patients often report physical trauma at the site of a cancer, but there is no clear evidence that acute injury per se causes cancer in humans (104). It is more likely that the presence of a neoplasm, particularly a bone tumor, makes the site more vulnerable to injury and brings the patient to medical attention. However, chronic injury from mechanical irritation of the skin, esophageal stricture after lye ingestion, burn scars, and unhealed osteomyelitis has been associated with the development of cancer in the damaged tissues (69, 104–106). In mice, tumors have also developed at the site at which certain foreign bodies were implanted (107). Psychologic trauma has also been suggested as a factor in carcinogenesis in humans, but no definitive data are available (108).

INFECTIOUS AGENTS

Although several viruses have been shown to induce cancers in animals, a similar oncogenic effect in humans has been difficult to demonstrate (109, 110). Methods traditionally used to study epidemics of infectious disease have limited applicability to studies of viral oncogenesis. Some candidate viruses in humans are ubiquitous and rarely produce neoplastic transformation after infection (111). The latent period for cancer induction can be many years or even generations after insertion of the virus into the genome of the host. Thus, several human cancers have been associated with specific viral infections, but a causal relationship remains uncertain (109, 110). African Burkitt's lymphoma may in part result from infection with the Epstein-Barr virus (EBV); the agent also causes infectious mononucleosis and has been implicated in the development of nasopharyngeal carcinoma

Table 30–2. DRUGS WITH CARCINOGENIC POTENTIAL

Medication	Associated Neoplasms*
Cancer chemotherapeutic agents:	
Cyclophosphamide	Acute leukemia, bladder cancer†
Melphalan	Acute leukemia†
Chlornaphazine	Bladder cancer†
Busulfan	Acute leukemia†
Nitrosoureas	Acute leukemia†
Chlorambucil	Acute leukemia†
Radioisotopes:	
Radium	Osteogenic sarcoma and other cancers†
Thorium dioxide	Liver tumors and others†
Radioactive iodine	Thyroid cancer‡
Hormones:	
Prenatal diethylstilbestrol	Vaginal adenocarcinoma†
Androgenic steroids, oral contraceptive	Liver tumors†
Estrogen compounds	Endometrial carcinoma†
Others:	
Immunosuppressive therapy for organ transplantation	Lymphomas and occasional carcinomas†
Phenacetin	Renal pelvis cancer‡
Inorganic arsenicals	Skin cancer, perhaps other cancers‡
Coal tar ointments	Skin cancer‡
Phenytoin	Lymphomas
Chloramphenicol	Acute leukemia
Intramuscular iron	Sarcoma at injection site
Phenylbutazone	Leukemia
Prenatal hydantoin	Neuroblastoma

*See text for references.
†Causal association considered to be established.
‡Causal association suspected; remaining associations have been reported in isolated caases, but require additional study.

(111). Rearrangement of a human proto-oncogene (c-*myc*) to sites of immunoglobulin genes, and *Blym* gene activation may also have a role in the development of Burkitt's lymphoma (112, 113). Another candidate for a human oncogenic virus is hepatitis B virus (114). Studies show that chronic hepatitis B antigenemia is associated with a high risk of hepatocellular carcinoma in several geographic areas (114, 115). In addition, recent studies have implicated a T cell leukemia virus in a rare form of T leukemia in adults, and a variant virus in the development of acquired immune deficiency syndrome (AIDS) (116, 117, 117a). Other suspected oncogenic viruses in humans include herpesvirus type 2 in cervical cancer, herpesvirus type 1 in certain head and neck cancers, RNA virus type C in acute leukemia, and RNA virus type B in breast cancer (109). Animal models of viral oncogenesis have been proposed for many of the cancers that develop with high frequency in children, e.g., acute leukemia, certain lymphomas, neural tumors, sarcomas, and renal tumors. Although none of the tumors of children are known to have a viral etiology, studies of oncogenes and tumorigenic viruses have yielded new knowledge of the biology of cancer (110, 118).

Nonviral infectious agents with reported carcinogenic potential include *Clonorchis sinensis* in biliary tract cancer in China and *Schistosoma haematobium* in bladder cancer in North Africa (119). Reports of reduced incidence of acute leukemia in childhood after vaccination with the bacteria bacillus Calmette-Guérin (BCG) have not been substantiated (120).

In several recipients of bone marrow transplantation therapy for leukemia, the donor cells have become leukemic (121). Possible explanations include transformation of donor cells by a leukemogenic virus present in the recipient and a virus-independent defect in regulation of donor cells by the recipient. Recipients of peripheral blood transfusions from donors who later developed leukemia or lymphoma have shown no tendency to develop the same diseases (122).

Host Susceptibility

Clinical observations have identified unusual susceptibility to cancer in children with certain heritable diseases, chromosomal disorders or constitutional syndromes (123). Table 30–3 summarizes the host factors that have been linked to development of the common cancers in childhood (124–169). Each factor is characteristically associated with development of only one or a few specific types of cancer, indicating different etiologies among the diverse cancers in children. Table 30–3 can be used to identify appropriate patients for screening and additional etiologic studies. The strength of each association has been estimated, and care is needed in interpretation of the table. Some associations, designated by an asterisk, are well-documented indicators of high cancer risk. Patients with these risk factors may be candidates for periodic screening for cancer. Entries designated by a dagger are suspected relationships for which further confirmation is needed. The remaining associations, reported in a few patients, may represent coincidence but are shown primarily to stimulate additional studies. Deliberately omitted are conditions associated with benign tumors or with malignancies that appear to develop exclusively in adults.

SINGLE-GENE DISEASES

Mulvihill (170) has compiled a list of 200 single-gene diseases in which a benign or malignant tumor has been a concomitant finding. Table 30–3 is shorter and includes only conditions associated with cancers in childhood. Most of the genetic disorders have diagnostic clinical or laboratory features that are identifiable prior to development of the associated cancer. However, in a few conditions, such as hereditary retinoblastoma, cancer is the earliest manifestation (154). Familial cancers not known to be inherited through a single gene are listed in Table 30–3 as constitutional or familial conditions.

Patients with genetic forms of cancer have several features in common: earlier than usual age at diagnosis, multifocal lesions within one organ, bilateral lesions in paired organs, and development of multiple primary cancers. To explain these findings, Knudson (171) has proposed a model of carcinogenesis based on at least two mutational events. In hereditary cancers, the first (germinal) mutation is prezygotic and therefore is present in all somatic cells. Cancer arises in the one or few somatic cells that undergo a second (somatic) mutation. In the nonhereditary cases, the same type of cancer arises in the rare single cell that undergoes two somatic mutations. The model has been found to fit the laterality and age patterns of retinoblastoma (172), Wilms' tumor (173), and neuroblastoma (151). The model predicts that approximately 40 per cent of retinoblastomas, and smaller percentages of Wilms' tumors and neuroblastomas, are heritable. From data in the literature, penetrance is estimated to be 95 per cent for the retinoblastoma gene and considerably lower for the Wilms' tumor and neuroblastoma genes. Patients with bilateral, and therefore heritable, lesions may have a poorer prognosis and often die before bearing offspring. Those who survive hereditary retinoblastoma tend to develop second primary neoplasms, which may be one of the pleiotropic effects of the cancer gene (174).

Table 30–3. SINGLE-GENE TRAITS, CONSTITUTIONAL DEFECTS, AND FAMILIAL CONDITIONS ASSOCIATED WITH CANCER IN CHILDHOOD

Type of Malignancy	Associated Single-Gene-Trait (Ref)	Associated Constitutional and Familial Conditions (Ref)
Acute leukemia, lymphocytic (L) and nonlymphocytic (NL), if known	Fanconi's anemia (NL) (34)* Bloom's syndrome (34)* von Recklinghausen's neurofibromatosis (NL) (124)* Congenital X-linked agammaglobulinemia (125)* Ataxia-telangiectasia (L) (125)* Severe combined system immunodeficiency (125)† Wiskott-Aldrich syndrome (125)† Schwachman's syndrome (L and NL) (129) Osteogenesis imperfecta (126) Marfan's syndrome (126) Kostmann's infantile genetic agranulocytosis (128) Glutathione reductase deficiency (128) WT syndrome (130) Ellis-van Creveld syndrome (NL) (126) Osteochondromatosis (NL) (127) Achondroplasia (L) (126) Hereditary brachydactyly, type C (L) (126) Xeroderma pigmentosum, De Sanctis-Cacchione type (L) (127) Incontinentia pigmenti (NL) (132) Phenylketonuria (NL) (127)	Down's syndrome (L and NL) (34)* Acute leukemia in identical twins under 6 years of age (34)* D- and F-trisomy (34) Turner's syndrome (34) XXY and XYY chromosome disorders (34) Parental consanguinity (134, 135) Familial leukemia (34) Treacher Collins syndrome (127) Rubenstein-Taybi syndrome (136) Poland's syndrome (126) Klippel-Feil syndrome (NL) (126) Blackfan-Diamond syndrome (131) Familial cellular folate uptake defect (133) Ataxia-pancytopenia (136a)
Brain Tumors	von Recklinghausen's neurofibromatosis (137)* Tuberous sclerosis (glial tumors) (137)* von-Hippel-Lindau syndrome (cerebellar hemangioblastoma) (137)† Wiskott-Aldrich syndrome (125) Nevoid basal cell carcinoma syndrome (medulloblastoma)(137)* Glioma-polyposis syndrome (138) Ataxia-telangiectasia (125) Cleidocranial dysplasia (127) Common variable immunodeficiency (125) IgA deficiency (125) Beckwith-Wiedemann syndrome (139)	Familial brain tumors (141)* Brain tumor associated with adrenocortical carcinoma, sarcomas, and breast cancer (142)† Down's syndrome (143) Turner's syndrome (144) DiGeorge's syndrome (glioma) (140) Aneuploidy of chromosome 18 (140a) Turcot's syndrome (140b)
Hodgkin's disease (HD) and non-Hodgkin's lymphomas (NHL)	Ataxia-telangiectasia (NHL and HD) (125)* Wiskott-Aldrich syndrome (NHL) (125)* Severe combined immunodeficiency (NHL) (125)* X-linked lymphoproliferative syndrome (NHL) (21)† Common variable immunodeficiency (125)† Chédiak-Higashi syndrome (127, 145) Congenital X-linked agammaglobulinemia (125) Achondroplasia (146) IgA deficiency (NHL) (125) Phenylketonuria (NHL) (127)	Familial HD and NHL (147, 149)* Aggregation with childhood colon cancer (NHL) (148)* Familial immunodeficiency (146)† Familial vitiligo (NHL) (146)
Neuroblastoma ganglioneuroblastoma	von Recklinghausen's neurofibromatosis (150)† Tuberous sclerosis (232a)†	Familial neuroblastoma (151)* Hirschsprung's disease (150) Heterochromia iritis (152) D-trisomy and other chromosomal disorders (153)
Soft tissue sarcomas	von Recklinghausen's neurofibromatosis (238)* Hereditary retinoblastoma (154)† Beckwith-Wiedemann syndrome (139) Hereditary lymphedema (127) Tuberous sclerosis (127) Wiskott-Aldrich syndrome (125)	Familial sarcomas, associated in some with breast cancer, brain tumor, adrenocortical carcinoma, and other tumors (142)*

*Association considered to be established.
†Association probable; remaining associations based primarily on case study and may represent coincidence.

Table continued on following page

Table 30–3. SINGLE-GENE TRAITS, CONSTITUTIONAL DEFECTS, AND FAMILIAL CONDITIONS ASSOCIATED WITH CANCER IN CHILDHOOD (*Continued*)

Type of Malignancy	Associated Single-Gene Trait (Ref)	Associated Constitutional and Familial Conditions (Ref)
Wilms' tumor	Beckwith-Wiedemann syndrome (139)* von Recklinghausen's neurofibromatosis (155)†	Genitourinary malformations (156)* Familial Wilms' tumor (141)* Sporadic aniridia (156)* Hemihypertrophy (156)* 11 p 13 chromosome deletion (157)* Pseudohermaphroditism and nephron defect (246)† Hamartomas, skin and other organs (156)† Diverse chromosomal defects (157)† Klippel-Trenaunay syndrome (156)
Skeletal sarcomas	Hereditary retinoblastoma (osteosarcoma) (154)* Multiple exostosis (chondrosarcoma) (17)† Osteogenesis imperfecta (17) Beckwith-Wiedemann syndrome (Ewing's sarcoma) (17)	Osteochondromatosis (chondrosarcoma) (17)† Maffucci's syndrome (chondrosarcoma) (17)† Familial osteogenic sarcoma and macrocytosis (158) Familial bone sarcoma with breast cancer, brain tumors, and adrenocortical carcinoma (142)
Ovarian tumors	Peutz-Jeghers syndrome (159)† Ataxia-telangiectasia (125)	Gonadal dysgenesis with Y chromosome (gonadoblastoma, dysgerminomas) (160)* Familial arrhenoblastoma-thyroid adenoma (161)
Testicular cancer		Undescended testis and other genitourinary anomalies (18)* Down's syndrome (18)
Primary liver cancer	Chronic hereditary tyrosinemia (162)* Fanconi's anemia (163) de Toni-Fanconi syndrome (164) Beckwith-Wiedemann syndrome (139) Glycogen storage disease 1 (von Gierke's disease) (127) Alpha$_1$-antitrypsin deficiency (165)	Familial hepatoma (166) Hemihypertrophy (164) Skin hemangiomas (hepatic hemangioendothelioma) (167) Congenital biliary atresia (164) Cerebral gigantism (168) Neonatal hepatitis or cirrhosis (164)
Retinoblastoma	Hereditary retinoblastoma (154)*	13q14 chromosome deletion (154, 169)* Down's syndrome, and sex chromosomal defects (169) Pierre-Robin syndrome (127)

*Association considered to be established.
†Association probable; remaining associations based primarily on case studies and may represent coincidence.

CHROMOSOMAL DISORDERS

Chromosomes bear the genetic material and can be studied for changes associated with human cancers. Recent advances in cytogenetic techniques, particularly chromosome banding and prophase analysis, permit identification of individual chromosomes and detection of previously unrecognizable abnormalities (169, 175, 176). Some chromosome defects are present in nonmalignant cell lines and are associated with a high risk of developing cancer. These chromosome abnormalities can be either inborn, as in Down's syndrome, or acquired through exposure to environmental agents such as radiation and alkylating agents (34). Other nonrandom chromosome abnormalities are found in the neoplastic cells of some forms of cancer. For example, the Philadelphia chromosome, usually a translocation between the long arm of chromosome 22 and chromosome 9 or other sites, is present in approximately 85 per cent of patients with chronic myelogenous leukemia (175, 176). Although the chromosome changes within cancer cells may have a role in disease development, their precise role as initiators and promoters of neoplastic growth remains uncertain. One hypothesis, based mainly on animal data, suggests that a specific chromosome change within tumors results from a specific oncogenic agent (176, 177). The recent findings of oncogenes at sites of nonrandom tumor chromosomal rearrangement suggest that oncogene activation may have a pathogenetic role, e.g., translocation of c-*abl* from chromosome 9 to chromosome 22 in chronic myelocytic leukemia (169, 176, 177) (see Chapter 34). Other studies have reported associations between human cancer and specific HLA histocompatibility antigens on chromosome 6 (178), but additional investigations are needed to substantiate these observations.

Chromosomal disorders are discussed in greater detail in Chapter 43.

FAMILIAL CANCERS

Most forms of childhood cancer have been reported to aggregate within families. These aggregates may result from a single gene defect, polygenic inheritance, common source exposure to carcinogens, or a combination of factors. For many human cancers, close relatives of an affected patient are reported to have a two- to threefold increase in risk for that neoplasm (179). Recent data for children are consistent with this risk estimate, e.g., sibs of a child with cancer have approximately twice the usual risk of a childhood neoplasm, often of the same type (141). If two siblings develop cancer during childhood, the risk to other sibs may be even higher (180), perhaps because of underlying genetic disease. Certain dissimilar types of cancer also tend to aggregate in young siblings (Table 30–3). One of these familial patterns involves childhood sarcomas of soft tissues associated with breast cancers in young women and with brain tumors, acute leukemia, adrenocortical carcinoma, and other neoplasms in related children (142, 148).

CANCER AND BIRTH DEFECTS

Certain childhood neoplasms develop with high frequency among patients with specific malformation syndromes (Table 30–3) (128, 181). The neoplasm may arise within the malformed organ, such as dysgerminoma and gonadoblastoma in those with gonadal dysgenesis (160), or in another organ, such as Wilms' tumor of the kidney in patients with sporadic aniridia or hemihypertrophy (156).

Cancers associated with birth defects may have prenatal origins that are either inherited or acquired in utero. In laboratory animals, several environmental agents have been reported to possess both carcinogenic and teratogenic properties (182). However, Miller (183) states that diethylstilbestrol, androgens, ionizing radiation, phenytoin, and alcohol possess both carcinogenic and teratogenic effects in humans; many more agents demonstrate only one of these two properties in humans. A closer correlation apparently exists between mutagenic and carcinogenic properties of chemicals. Some laboratory screening tests for carcinogens in humans, such as the Ames test (184), assay the frequency of mutations produced by the agent. An advantage of bacterial assays is the low cost of screening numerous agents to help identify priorities for epidemiologic studies in humans. However, bacterial data may not be fully predictive of risk in humans, whose cells can differ in metabolic transport and activation systems, repair mechanisms, and other biologic properties (185).

EPIDEMIOLOGY OF SELECTED CHILDHOOD CANCERS

This section reviews the epidemiology of 11 forms of childhood cancer. For most neoplasms, a discussion of general epidemiologic features is followed by a review of specific host and environmental risk factors.

Leukemia

In the United States the frequency of leukemia in patients under 15 years of age increases rapidly after birth, peaks before 5 years of age, and subsequently declines (186). Acute lymphocytic leukemia (ALL) in whites accounts for this early age peak, which emerged in the 1920's in England, in the 1940's in the United States, and in the 1960's in Japan (23). Populations without this peak (e.g., black children in the United States and Africa) may be nonsusceptible to or not exposed to environmental carcinogens that became prevalent during this century.

In contrast to ALL, acute nonlymphocytic leukemia (ANLL) in the United States shows no marked age peak. The ALL/ANLL case ratio in children under 15 years old is 4:1, approximately the reverse of the ratio in adults (187). Acute myelocytic leukemia (AML) is the most common subtype of childhood ANLL, followed by myelomonocytic, promyelocytic, monocytic, and erythrocytic leukemia (187). Chronic myelocytic leukemias (CML) of the juvenile or adult subtypes account for less than 5 per cent of childhood leukemias. Chronic lymphocytic leukemia rarely occurs in children.

Geographic variations in leukemia incidence rates and distribution by subtype have been observed. In Turkey, acute myelomonocytic leukemia (often with ocular chloroma) accounts for approximately 35 per cent of cases, in contrast to 5 per cent in the United States (188). Among children diagnosed with leukemia in Shanghai, China, nearly one half are reported to have acute nonlymphocytic leukemia (188a).

Persons with certain constitutional or acquired chromosomal aberrations have a greater than normal risk of acute leukemia (34). Genetic diseases associated with chromosomal instability and predisposition to acute leukemia include three autosomal recessive disorders: Bloom's syndrome, Fanconi's anemia, and ataxia-telangiectasia (132). The chromosomes of patients with Bloom's syndrome also uniquely display quadriradial formation and an increased rate of spontaneous sister-chromatid exchanges (189). Children with Fanconi's anemia have short stature, hyperpigmentation, limb defects, and fragile chromosomes, and their cells are sensitive in vitro to several chemical mutagens (189a). Ataxia-telangiectasia is commonly accompanied by rearrangement of the long arm of chromosome 14 and is one of the inborn immunodeficiency syndromes that predispose to lymphoreticular neoplasms, including ALL (125, 190). Patients with ataxia-telangiectasia display increased toxicity to therapeutic doses of ionizing radiation, and their cells are unusually sensitive to in vitro radiation (68). Isolated instances of leukemia have been reported with glutathione reductase deficiency, incontinentia pigmenti, and Kostmann's infantile agranulocytosis, which are other disorders reported to be associated with chromosomal breaks (125, 191). The predisposing influence of constitutional chromosomal fragility has gained increasing attention with the recent finding of chromosomal rearrangements in leukemic cells of nearly all patients (169).

Down's syndrome (trisomy 21) is a constitutional chromosomal abnormality associated with at least a 10-fold increased risk of leukemia during the first decade of life (143). The cell types of leukemia follow the usual distribution, but the age peak is nearly 3 years earlier than expected (143, 192). Other constitutional aneuploid syndromes have been reported less frequently in association with leukemia (Table 30–3).

Von Recklinghausen's neurofibromatosis has been reported in more than 20 patients with childhood nonlymphocytic leukemia, especially acute myelomonocytic leukemia and juvenile CML (124, 193). Neurofibromatosis is an uncommon example of a genetic predisposition to childhood leukemia occurring without either known chromosomal abnormalities or immunodeficiency.

When a patient with an identical twin develops acute leukemia before 6 years of age, the risk of disease in the other twin is 20 per cent (34). Leukemia usually develops in the co-twin within months of the first case. Risk for the *second* twin diminishes with the age at which the *first* twin is affected and is the highest, nearly 100 per cent, in the first year of life (134). Concordant leukemia in monozygotic infant twins may reflect a common prezygotic determinant, shared intrauterine insult, or blood-borne metastases, from one twin to the other (194).

For fraternal twins and siblings, the risk of developing leukemia is approximately fourfold higher than that for children in the general population (34). This increase in risk from 4 per 100,000 per year to 16 per 100,000 annually is slight. Among families with more than one case of leukemia, parental consanguinity is uncommon, and shared environmental exposures to leukemogens have rarely been found (134). Although no clear evidence has been presented for a viral etiology of childhood leukemia, a virus is suspected as the cause of a rare T cell leukemia in adults (195). Other epidemiologic studies show no significantly increased frequency of leukemia in children of leukemic parents, in children breastfed by mothers who subsequently developed leukemia, in owners of pets with leukemia, or in recipients of blood from donors who later developed leukemia (122, 196).

Children exposed to *whole-body* radiation from the atomic bombs in Japan had nearly a sixfold increased incidence of leukemia compared with the expected rate for Japanese children, with the peak occurring 4 to 6 years after the event (197). The usual distribution of acute leukemia subtypes was observed (198). Children exposed under 10 years of age were two to three times more susceptible to radiogenic leukemia than were older persons exposed to the same dose (52). The magnitude of the leukemia excess declined after a decade following the exposure but did not disappear entirely after more than 20 years (198). AML accounted for the excess of late-occurring leukemias. *Partial-body radiation* in high doses for therapy of cancer and benign conditions in childhood such as tinea capitis can also induce tumors (52, 54, 55).

Following the use of bone marrow transplantation as therapy for leukemia, at least 8 patients have been reported to develop recurrent leukemia in transplanted donor cells (199, 200). Most of these patients had lymphoblastic leukemia, and the same morphology in the original and the donor cells. Explanations for this finding include infection of donor cells by a leukemia virus and persistence of a regulatory defect in the host after transplantation.

Both bone marrow hypoplasia and leukemia have followed exposure to various drugs and environmental chemicals (201). Benzene is a suspected leukemogen that primarily affects exposed workers, although children may be exposed in different settings.

Lymphomas

The Third National Cancer Survey showed a 2:1 male:female sex ratio for all childhood lymphomas in youngsters under 15 years of age, the highest ratio for any nongonadal tumor of childhood (20). Several classic morphologic categories of lymphoma show distinct age distribution curves (146), but these will need review after reclassification by newer and more precise immunologic and histochemical markers.

BURKITT'S LYMPHOMA

Studies reveal geographic differences in disease rates and clinical features of childhood lymphomas, particularly Burkitt's lymphoma (202, 203). In certain areas of tropical Africa, this tumor is the most common malignant neoplasm in children (204). Within these regions, Burkitt's lymphoma develops primarily in children between 5 and 9 years of age and has a predilection for the jaw

(204); outside endemic areas, the median age at diagnosis is generally several years older, and jaw involvement is not a characteristic feature (205). High-risk populations in Africa have diverse ethnic and tribal backgrounds and dissimilarities in diet. These areas appear to share three environmental features in common: ambient temperature above 60°F, annual rainfall of at least 20 inches, and altitude below 5000 feet, conditions that favor endemic malaria. The finding has suggested the possibility of an etiologic interaction between malaria infection and other etiologic influences such as an oncogenic virus (206).

At present it is uncertain whether Epstein-Barr virus (EBV) is an etiologic factor in some cases of Burkitt's lymphoma or is merely a passenger virus (111, 207). Infection with EBV has been found in almost all African patients, but in only some American patients with Burkitt's lymphoma (112). Patients harboring the virus have multiple copies of EBV genome in specimens of their tumor and a characteristic serologic profile of EBV antigen and antibody titers (208). Burkitt's lymphoma is a monoclonal B cell malignancy, and selective EBV infection and transformation of B lymphocytes in cell culture enhance the possibility of an etiologic relationship. Time-space clustering of cases in Africa has been reported, but could not be verified in more recent studies (209). A prospective seroepidemiologic study in Uganda has found high EBV titers prior to development of Burkitt's lymphoma in 14 children, but the study was terminated prematurely (210).

Cytogenetic studies of Burkitt's lymphoma cells have shown non-random translocations between chromosome 8 and chromosomes 2, 14, or 22 (167). Analysis of the breakpoints shows that the rearrangements of chromosomes 2, 14, and 22 involved immunoglobulin gene loci (211). Furthermore, the breakpoint on chromosome 8 is near the oncogene, c-*myc*, suggesting that translocation of the oncogene to an immunoglobulin locus in B cells predisposes to cancer. In most instances, the karyotypic change is predictive of the immunoglobulin expression of the Burkitt's tumor (211). A second oncogene, *Blym*-1, has also been detected in Burkitt's lymphoma cells, indicating that more than one oncogene may be involved (113).

HODGKIN'S DISEASE

In the United States, Hodgkin's disease is rare before age 5 years and increases in frequency thereafter (212, 213). The neoplasm exhibits a bimodal age curve in adults, with the first peak occurring in persons from 15 to 34 years of age and the second in adults over 50 (16).

International studies of Hodgkin's disease have identified four distinct epidemiologic patterns that correlate with the regional level of socioeconomic development (214). In general, progressively better socioeconomic conditions are associated with progressively decreasing Hodgkin's disease rates in children, a corresponding rise among young adults, and a shift of histologic subtypes. Why socioeconomic status influences the development of Hodgkin's disease remains unclear. Factors associated with socioeconomic status, such as hygiene and sibship size, may influence the age and other conditions under which a person encounters an etiologic agent in the environment (215). The influence of social class on the use of medical services may explain the finding in some studies that appendectomy or tonsillectomy is associated with a slightly elevated risk of Hodgkin's disease (215).

Another model of the etiology of Hodgkin's disease postulates that an infectious agent is transmitted from person to person, usually before clinical diagnosis of the disease (26). Some studies show that Hodgkin's disease patients can be linked with each other through direct or indirect (via an intermediary) personal contacts several years prior to diagnosis; high schools are reported to be the setting of many of these contacts (27). Other investigators have not found *excessive* linkages among Hodgkin's disease patients and have questioned whether the linkage networks resulted from chance or a nonviral environmental carcinogen (215-216a).

Familial aggregation of Hodgkin's disease has been described in more than 100 instances (147). In one study the risk for Hodgkin's disease was found to be higher among like-sex siblings of probands, compared with those of the opposite sex (149). Familial cases of the neoplasm in the inbred Amish population and in a consanguineous Newfoundland family have suggested the role of genetic factors (147, 217). Childhood non-Hodgkin's lymphoma (see following section) has also aggregated in families (146).

NON-HODGKIN'S LYMPHOMA (NHL)

Constitutional and acquired aberrations in the immune system have been linked to increased risk of lymphomas (125, 218). Lymphoreticular tumors in childhood constitute more than half the neoplasms associated with inborn immune deficiency disorders; B cell lymphomas account for most of these tumors (219). The inherited immunodeficiency states associated with lymphoid malignancy include ataxia-telangiectasia, Wiskott-Aldrich syndrome, common variable hypoglobulinemia, severe combined immunodeficiency, isolated deficiencies of IgA and IgM, X-linked lymphoproliferative syndrome, and other less-well-defined familial immunodeficiency states (125). In the X-linked lymphoproliferative syndrome, neoplasms of B cells are postulated to result from a defect in B cell capacity to respond to EBV infection (21). Acquired immune suppression after renal transplantation is also associated with 30 to 40 times the expected risk of lymphoma (80). Autoimmune phenomena, particularly thrombocytopenic purpura, hemolytic anemia, and nephropathy, have been described in lymphoma patients, but the findings may be secondary to the neoplasm (220, 221). Several models for the role of immune defects in the pathogenesis of human lymphomas have been proposed (222, 223).

It has been suggested that structural rearrangements of the long arm of chromosome 14 may promote abnormal growth of lymphocytes and possibly lead to the development of lymphoid malignancies (190). Abnormalities of 14q have been found in the malignant cell line in NHL, Hodgkin's disease, Burkitt's lymphoma, and multiple myeloma (224). The abnormality has also been reported in peripheral blood lymphocytes of patients with ataxia-telangiectasia, which predisposes to lymphoma (225).

Central Nervous System Tumors

In the Third National Cancer Survey central nervous system (CNS) tumors constituted about 20 per cent of malignant neoplasms in patients through 14 years of age, but only 1 per cent among older patients (20). The four most common CNS neoplasms in childhood are astrocytoma, glioblastoma, medulloblastoma, and ependymoma; other brain tumors in children include meningioma, teratoma, pinealoma, and pituitary tumors (226). Each of the four most common neoplasms has an age peak during the first decade of life; medulloblastoma, unlike the other three, has no major peak in adulthood (227). About 60 per cent of pediatric CNS neoplasms occur infratentorially, compared with 10 per cent in adults.

Autosomal dominant single-gene disorders that predispose to malignant neural tumors in children include neurofibromatosis, tuberous sclerosis, and nevoid basal cell carcinoma syndrome (Table 30–3) (137). These single-gene disorders have characteristic features that usually appear before development of the neoplasm. Other anomalies have been observed in individual patients with CNS tumors (228).

Familial aggregation of certain types of CNS tumors also occurs in persons lacking any of the well-described single-gene disorders. Some of these familial cases of brain tumor, particularly gliomas and medulloblastomas, may be manifestations of an autosomal dominant single-gene disorder (229). Tumors of the CNS also occur in families with increased susceptibility to cancer of several other sites (142).

Histiocytic lymphoma of the brain is associated with several immune disorders, including Waldenström's macroglobulinemia, Wiskott-Aldrich syndrome, and certain immunoglobulin defects (230). Immunosuppressed transplant patients also develop lymphomas in the brain (and other sites) at an excessive rate (218). Some of these lymphoid lesions in the brain have been shown by analysis of immunoglobulin-gene rearrangements to be monoclonal and most likely neoplastic (230).

Neuroblastoma

Nearly 50 per cent of all neuroblastomas are diagnosed in patients under 2 years of age and almost 90 per cent before 10 years of age (39). The most frequent location for the primary tumor is the adrenal medulla, followed by sympathetic nervous tissue in the chest, pelvis, and other sites. Boys are affected slightly more often than girls (1.3:1.0), and the prognosis is generally better in girls (231).

Adrenal neuroblastoma in situ has been found incidentally in about 1 in 250 infants dying in the first few months of life, and in many fetuses of 10 to 30 weeks' gestation (231a). Thus, primitive neuroblasts apparently represent a normal finding in the developing adrenal gland. These neuroblasts appear to either regress or mature spontaneously with development, since they are not found in adrenals of normal older infants and children.

Approximately 50 instances of familial neuroblastoma, including affected tumors, have been reported (232). Based on reported clinical associations, there may be a common etiologic link between neuroblastoma and neural-crest-derived disorders such as neurofibromatosis, tuberous sclerosis, and aganglionosis of the colon (Hirschsprung's disease), and heterochromia of the iris (150, 232a).

Elongated chromosomal homogeneous-staining regions and double-minute chromosomes have been found in cytogenetic studies of human neuroblastoma (233). These regions contain an amplified gene, N-*myc*, with DNA sequence similarities to c-*myc*. Also, a deletion of the short arm of chromosome 1 has been found in several primary neuroblastoma tumor explants and established cell culture lines (234). Isolated neuroblastoma patients with constitutional chromosomal disorders of diverse types have been reported, but no consistent pattern has been found (153).

There are greater differences in the geographic distribution of neuroblastoma than of Wilms' tumor or retinoblastoma—most notably a substantial deficiency of neuroblastoma in the "Burkitt's lymphoma belt" of Africa (23). Such findings suggest that regional factors may influence tumor development. The recent case reports of neuroblastoma after exposure to phenytoin during gestation provide an etiologic hypothesis for further study (89).

Soft Tissue Sarcomas

Rhabdomyosarcoma accounts for 50 per cent of soft tissue sarcomas in children in the United States. It has two distinct age peaks—the first before the fifth year of life and the second in the teens (235). The first peak derives mainly from rhabdomyosarcomas of the head, neck, and genitourinary system, and the second peak derives from tumors of more diverse sites (236). The embryonal and botryoid subtypes of rhabdomyosarcoma tend to develop in younger children, whereas the alveolar and embryonal subtypes predominate in adolescents. Less common forms of soft tissue sarcomas in childhood include fibrosarcoma, neurofibrosarcoma, liposarcoma, undifferentiated sarcoma, mesenchymoma, synovial sarcoma, and lieomyosarcoma (35, 237). In adults, both fibrosarcoma and liposarcoma exceed rhabdomyosarcoma in frequency by about 2:1.

Some soft tissue sarcomas are diagnosed at birth or during the first few months of life and may have prenatal origins. Two reviews of large numbers of patients dying of childhood sarcoma found no excessive association with specific forms of congenital anomalies (235, 237), although isolated patients have been described with a variety of inborn defects (237a).

Both benign and malignant soft tissue tumors can have a familial or genetic origin. Neurofibromatosis and hereditary retinoblastoma, which are single-gene disorders with autosomal dominant transmission, predispose to the development of childhood sarcomas (154, 238). Sarcomas also occur as part of several family cancer syndromes, particularly one involving sarcoma in childhood, breast cancer, and, in some instances, osteosarcomas and brain tumors (142, 238a).

Skeletal Sarcomas

The two major malignant bone tumors of children in the United States are osteosarcoma, which accounts for more than 60 per cent of cases, and Ewing's sarcoma, which accounts for about 30 per cent of cases (20). The first age peak for osteosarcoma begins during adolescence and early adulthood (32). A second peak occurs after age 50 and is often associated with pre-existing Paget's disease of bone. Ewing's sarcoma has a single smaller age peak in adolescence. The age peak for white boys extends further into early adulthood than that for white girls. A marked deficiency of Ewing's sarcoma, but not of osteosarcoma, has been found among blacks in both the United States and Africa (17). Chondrosarcoma and other neoplasms of skeletal origin are uncommon in children (20).

Recent cytogenetic studies of Ewing's sarcoma cells have shown translocations involving chromosome 22q12 (239). However, this nonrandom rearrangement is not at the c-*sis* oncogene locus, and this gene does not appear to be abnormally activated (240). Relationship between this chromosome abnormality and the tendency of Ewing's sarcoma patients to secondary osteosarcomas merits additional study (240a).

Skeletal sarcomas, particularly osteosarcomas, have been reported to aggregate in families (148, 158). Therapeutic external-beam irradiation and bone-seeking radioisotopes such as radium and thorium have induced human osteosarcomas (see Table 30–2 (52, 241).

Wilms' Tumor

Wilms' tumor, the most common malignant kidney tumor of childhood, usually occurs in patients between 1 and 3 years of age (156). Seventy-five per cent of cases present before age 5 years (156). Although congenital Wilms' tumor does occur, kidney tumors diagnosed in infancy are usually one of several recently identified variant neoplasms, such as mesoblastic nephroma (242). These lesions tend to be less aggressive clinically than classic Wilms' tumor.

About 15 per cent of patients with Wilms' tumor have congenital anomalies (156), including sporadic aniridia, genitourinary malformation accompanied in some patients by a nephron disorder, hamartomas of the skin, hemihypertrophy, and the Beckwith-Wiedemann syndrome (omphalocele, macroglossia, and visceral cytomegaly) (156, 243). Some individuals have several of these features.

Sporadic bilateral aniridia (absence or hypoplasia of the iris) occurs in 1 per cent of Wilms' tumor patients, compared with 0.01 per cent frequency in the general population (156). Conversely, in a series of 20 children with sporadic (nonfamilial) aniridia, 7 developed Wilms' tumor (244). Sporadic aniridia can be accompanied by other ocular defects, mental retardation, and malformations of the central nervous system, craniofacial bones, ears, and genitourinary tract (157, 245). *Familial* aniridia is more common than *sporadic* aniridia but is rarely associated with Wilms' tumor (245).

Congenital overgrowth of a limb, an organ, or half the body (hemihypertrophy) is seen in about 3 per cent of reported patients with Wilms' tumor (156). Hemihypertrophy also occurs with liver tumors and adrenocortical carcinoma, as well as the Beckwith-Wiedemann syndrome (139). The neoplasm does not always develop on the hypertrophied side.

Genitourinary anomalies associated with Wilms' tumor include male pseudohermaphroditism, hypospadias, cryptorchidism, diverse upper and lower urinary tract malformations, and a severe nephron disorder (246). Wilms' tumors associated with most genitourinary anomalies or with hemihypertrophy are typically unifocal and are diagnosed in the usual age range (173). In one exceptional pedigree the mother had hemihypertrophy, three children had Wilms' tumor (bilateral in one), and a fourth child had a double collecting system of one kidney (247).

Aniridia, genitourinary abnormalities, mental retardation, and an interstitial deletion of band p13 of chromosome 11 have been described in the peripheral blood of patients with Wilms' tumor (157, 247a). It is possible that the deleted segment contains a gene that inhibits the formation of Wilms' tumor (247a). The cellular oncogene Harvey-*ras* has been assigned to chromosome 11p, but is outside the deleted region (247a). However, the importance of this deletion to the pathogenesis of Wilms' tumor is revealed by molecular studies showing homozygosity of the region in tumors of patients who are heterozygotes in somatic cells (247a).

Several cases of neurofibromatosis with Wilms' tumor have been described (155). Embryologic and clinical arguments support a genetic link between the two conditions when they occur together.

Retinoblastoma

Collected clinical series report that approximately 5 to 10 per cent of retinoblastoma patients have a family history of the disease (172). These patients can transmit retinoblastoma to their progeny through a highly penetrant autosomal dominant gene. Approximately 30 per cent of patients without this family history may also have hereditary retinoblastoma as the consequence of new germinal mutations (172). A substantial proportion of these patients have bilateral lesions.

In the United States, black and white children of both sexes develop retinoblastoma with almost equal frequency (20). More advanced disease at presentation may account for the higher mortality reported among blacks (248). The incidence of retinoblastoma in several areas of the world appears to be increasing (249), perhaps in part because of more successful treatment of hereditary retinoblastoma.

A small fraction of patients with retinoblastoma have been shown to have a 13q14 chromosomal deletion (154). Some of these patients also have developmental defects, usually of the eye, skeleton, face, genitourinary tract, and central nervous system, including mental retardation (249a). The pattern of birth defects and retinoblastoma in an individual appears related to the site and size of the chromosome deletion. By enzymatic (esterase D) and restriction length polymorphism studies of chromosome 13, retinoblastoma cells have been shown in heterozygotes to become homozygous in this region of a presumed retinoblastoma inhibitory gene (154, 250). At the cellular level, retinoblastoma appears to be a recessive disorder in these patients (251).

Second primary tumors, predominantly sarcomas, were found in 10 per cent of almost 600 survivors of *bilateral* retinoblastoma, with an average latent interval of about 11 years (252). The second tumors develop both within and outside the field of radiation, and some may represent a pleiotropic effect of the retinoblastoma gene (174). The same neoplasms that occur as second primaries in survivors of bilateral retinoblastoma have also occurred in the close relatives of these patients (253, 254). Genetic counseling in these families may need to consider risk for other cancers as well as for retinoblastoma. Patients with nonheritable retinoblastoma have a smaller risk of other cancers than patients with the heritable form (174).

Liver Tumors

Hepatoblastoma and hepatocellular carcinoma are, respectively, the two most common malignant primary neoplasms of the liver in childhood (164). Hepatoblastoma occurs most often in the first 2 years of life, declines sharply in frequency thereafter, and rarely presents after 5 years of age. Hepatocellular carcinoma is usually diagnosed *after* 5 years of age, although one case series derived from multiple institutions found two childhood age peaks for this neoplasm—the first under 4 years of age and the second between 12 and 15 years of age (255).

In children, primary hepatic malignancies have been described with several antecedent hepatic disorders (Table 30–3) (164). The risk of developing liver cancer following hepatic cirrhosis of childhood is unequal for different causes of cirrhosis. The highest risk, about 37 per cent, is seen with chronic hereditary tyrosinemia (162). As supportive techniques permit survival of children with previously fatal liver diseases, these patients may develop hepatic malignancy later in life.

Although infection with hepatitis B virus (HBV) seldom leads to liver cancer, the frequency of HBV antigenemia (HBsAg) is very high in patients with hepatocellular carcinoma in Southeast Asia and Africa (114). The recent findings of hepatitis B virus in primary liver cancer in humans and the development of animal models of hepatitis virus–associated liver cancers provide additional evidence for an etiologic role of this agent (115). Availability of a vaccine against hepatitis B infection raises the possibility of primary prevention of hepatocellular carcinoma, but logistical problems remain (256).

Diverse chemicals induce liver cancer in experimental animals, and some of these agents can be carcinogenic in humans (257), e.g., angiosarcoma of the liver in vinyl chloride workers (258). Epidemiologic data also show a correlation between aflatoxin contamination of the food supply and regional incidence rates of liver cancer (257).

Both hepatocellular carcinoma and benign liver tumors have developed in women using oral contraceptives and in patients treated with anabolic-androgenic steroids for bone marrow hypoplasia (259, 260). In some instances the neoplasms regressed after the medication was stopped. Factors other than steroid effect, e.g., host predisposition, may also have an oncogenic influence. Hepatoblastoma was diagnosed in an infant whose mother took contraceptive pills during the first trimester of pregnancy (88).

Malignant liver tumors of early childhood are associated with several anomalies that also occur extensively with Wilms' tumor and adrenocortical carcinoma, i.e., hemihypertrophy, Beckwith-Wiedemann syndrome, and hamartomas (139, 164). These associations suggest that the three neoplasms have etiologic mechanisms in common.

Testicular Cancer

Malignant tumors of germ cell origin account for the majority of primary testicular cancers in males of all ages, whereas tumors of gonadal stroma (e.g., Sertoli and Leydig cell tumors) are uncommon (18). In children, intrascrotal neoplasms of nontesticular origin are well described, e.g., paratesticular rhabdomyosarcoma and leukemia or lymphoma metastatic to the testis. A small, limited age peak for primary testicular cancer occurs about 2 years of age, during which embryonal carcinoma is by far the most common histologic type found. A second and much larger peak begins near puberty, extends through early adulthood, and includes a wider variety of pure and mixed forms of germ cell neoplasms. A third peak for testicular cancer appears after age 50 (261). There is a relative deficiency of malignant testicular cancer among young adult blacks in the United States and Africa (262). Incidence of testis cancer has risen among young adults in the United States and several European areas in recent decades, for unknown reasons (261).

Malignancy in an undescended testis has developed in a few children (18). In adults, the neoplasm is at least 10 times more frequent in cryptorchid patients than in those with a normally descended gonad (263). Orchiopexy, if performed *after* 6 years of age, may not substantially reduce the high risk of cancer (264). The unilaterally maldescended testis is at higher risk than the opposite gonad, but both are susceptible (264a). Atrophic or hypoplastic descended testes are also at increased risk, although a relationship between mumps orchitis and subsequent testicular cancer is uncertain (264b).

In children, inguinal hernia and urinary tract malformations are found excessively in patients having testes with cryptorchidism, malignancy, or both (18). Although in utero exposure to diethylstibestrol is associated with cryptorchidism, development of testis cancer in these males has rarely been reported (89). These anomalies and testicular cancer may have common prenatal determinants and be part of the same complex of malformations and cancer. Testis cancer has also been reported in siblings and twins (265). Patients with Klinefelter's syndrome (XXY) are prone to develop germ cell tumors in extragonadal sites, particularly the mediastinum (265a).

Ovarian Cancer

In females from birth to 19 years of age, approximately 60 per cent of ovarian cancers have germ cell origin, e.g., dysgerminoma, embryonal carcinoma, teratoma, endodermal sinus tumor (yolk sac tumor), gonadoblastoma, choriocarcinoma, and tumors of mixed histology (266). Tumors derived from ovarian germinal epithelium develop infrequently in children but make up more than 80 per cent of gonadal cancers in older women (267). Malignancies derived from the gonadal stroma (e.g., granulosa cell tumors) are rare at any age. Although cancer of the female gonad shows no marked age peak in childhood, such neoplasms are slightly more common in the second decade of life than the first (266).

Hormonal factors probably influence the development of ovarian cancers of both epithelial and germ cell origin (268). Tumors of the latter type increase in frequency after ovarian function becomes established at puberty and peak in the third decade of life, when reproductive activity is highest.

Persons with Peutz-Jeghers syndrome have increased susceptibility to granulosa cell tumors (159). Gonadal dysgenesis predisposes to gonadoblastoma only in patients who have a Y chromosome in at least some of their germ cells (160). Most reported cases of familial ovarian neoplasms involve adults with cancers of epithelial origin (269). An association between familial arrhenoblastoma and thyroid adenoma has also been reported (161).

There are reports of thecomas occurring in ovaries of epileptic children receiving chronic anticonvulsant medication (270).

Epidemiology of Other Childhood Neoplasms

Carcinomas, i.e., tumors of epithelial cell origin, are rare in the first two decades of life but are common in adults. Because environmental exposures have been implicated in the etiology of many adult carcinomas, similar influences have been sought when these neoplasms develop in younger people. Carcinomas of early life probably induced by environmental factors include the following:

1. Thyroid carcinoma following neck irradiation (52).
2. Vaginal and cervical clear cell adenocarcinoma among adolescent girls exposed transplacentally to diethylstilbestrol (84).
3. Liver carcinoma associated with hepatitis infection and with the use of anabolic steroids (114, 259).
4. Skin cancer following ultraviolet (sun) light exposure in genetically susceptible individuals (66).

Like Wilms' tumors and liver tumors, adrenocortical carcinomas have also been described with various conditions involving growth excess: congenital hemihypertrophy, Beckwith-Wiedemann syndrome, and hamartomas (271). Rare reports have linked adrenocortical carcinoma in childhood to neurofibromatosis (272).

Mortality from teratomas is bimodal, with a peak under 3 years of age, primarily from sacrococcygeal tumors in girls (273). An increasing trend in mortality develops after age 6 for primary ovarian neoplasms and after age 14 years for testicular primaries. Patients with sacrococcygeal tumors often have congenital anomalies of the genitourinary tract. Cytogenetic and biochemical data indicate that benign cystic teratomas of the ovary are parthenogenic tumors that arise from a single germ cell after the first meiotic division (274). In patients with these neoplasms, tumor tissue was shown to be uniformly homozygous for chromosomal and electrophoretic markers, whereas normal tissues were heterogeneous for the same markers. Mouse teratoma cells have also been implanted experimentally into developing blastocysts with the surprising result that full-grown mouse "offspring" showed genetic characteristics clearly derived from both the neoplastic implant and the blastocyst cells (275). Such experiments have major implications regarding control mechanisms for both normal and neoplastic growth and development.

SURVIVORS OF CANCER IN CHILDHOOD

Advances in the treatment of childhood cancers have improved survival and produced increasing numbers of successfully treated patients. U.S. mortality data for 1950–1980 show that deaths from childhood cancer declined by 50 per cent or more for leukemia, Hodgkin's disease, kidney cancer, and other neoplasms (36). Among surviving patients, second primary cancers are a major cause of late morbidity and mortality. Some of these second cancers are associated with radiotherapy or alkylating agent chemotherapy (276, 277). Constitutional susceptibility may be an additional influence in the development of second primary cancers (276). In a study of 102 children with multiple malignancies, a genetic or familial factor was identified in 27 (276).

Survivors of childhood cancer may have permanent deficits produced by the malignancy or by treatments with surgery, radiotherapy, and chemotherapy (278, 279). Treatments such as amputation of a limb produce immediate losses, whereas the effects of other therapies may develop later (279, 280). Attention has focused on neurologic and intellectual function among children treated for acute leukemia, the largest group of childhood cancer survivors. Data suggest that early age at treatment and high doses of radiation to the brain are risk factors for neurologic dysfunction, though additional studies are needed (281, 282). Abnormalities of the heart, lungs, kidneys, liver, and bone have also been associated with specific treatment modalities (280). In endocrine tissues, hypopituitarism after brain tumor irradiation, hypothyroidism after neck irradiation, and gonadal failure after chemotherapy or radiotherapy have been reported (283–285). Sterility or amenorrhea is more common after treatment involving irradiation of both ovaries (285). Infertility has been reversible in a few patients who generally received less intense treatments.

Radiation and certain cancer chemotherapeutic drugs have mutagenic properties in laboratory systems, but several small studies of the offspring of patients treated for cancer in childhood have not demonstrated genetic transmission of treatment effects (286). However, one study of offspring of Wilms' tumor patients showed low birthweight when the affected mother had received abdominal radiotherapy (287). Low birthweight was not observed when the father had treatment for Wilms' tumor, suggesting that abdominal radiation might damage the reproductive apparatus in females (287).

Preliminary findings suggest that survivors of childhood cancer can experience long-term psychologic and social effects of their disease (288). Within their physical limitations, most patients appear to live productive lives. They have been able to complete school, work, raise a family, and function in society. However, residual psychologic as well as physical scars undoubtedly remain, and research is needed to define approaches to patient management that will minimize these and other sequelae.

References

1. Newell, G. R. (ed.).: *Cancer Prevention in Clinical Medicine.* New York, Raven Press, 1983.
2. Peto, R., Pike, M. C., et al.: Design and analysis of

randomized clinical trials requiring prolonged observation of each patient: I. Introduction and design. Br. J. Cancer 34:585, 1976.
3. Peto, R., Pike, M. C., et al.: Design and analysis of randomized clinical trials requiring prolonged observation of each patient: II. Analysis and examples. Br. J. Cancer 35:1, 1977.
4. Feinstein, A. R.: *Clinical Biostatistics*. St. Louis, The C. V. Mosby Company, 1977.
5. Schottenfeld, D., and Fraumeni, J. F., Jr. (eds.).: *Cancer Epidemiology and Prevention*. Philadelphia, W. B. Saunders Company, 1982.
6. Fraumeni, J. F., Jr.: *Persons at High Risk of Cancer: An Approach to Cancer Etiology and Control*. New York, Academic Press, 1975.
7. Mulvihill, J. J., Miller, R. W., et al.: *Genetics of Human Cancer*. New York, Raven Press, 1977.
8. Lynch, H. T.: *Cancer Genetics*. Springfield, Ill., Charles C. Thomas, Publisher, 1976.
9. Bergsma, D.:*Cancer and Genetics*. Birth Defects: Original Article Series Vol. XII, The National Foundation–March of Dimes, 1976.
10. McKay, F. W., Hanson, M. R., et al.: *Cancer Mortality in the United States: 1950–1977*. National Cancer Institute Monograph No. 59. Washington, D.C., U.S. Government Printing Office, 1982.
11. Miller, R. W.: Prenatal origins of cancer in man: epidemiological evidence. In *Transplacental carcinogenesis*. Tomatis, L., and Mohr, U. (eds.), Lyon, International Agency for Research on Cancer, 1973, p. 175.
12. Potter, J. F., and Schoeneman, M.: Metastasis of maternal cancer to the placenta and fetus. Cancer 25:380, 1970.
13. Bader, J. L., and Miller, R. W.: U.S. cancer incidence and mortality in the first year of life. Am. J. Dis. Child. 133:157, 1979.
14. Cutler, S. J., and Young, J. L., Jr.: *Third National Cancer Survey: Incidence Data*. National Cancer Institute Monograph No. 41. Washington, D.C., U.S. Government Printing Office, 1975.
15. Bertelone, S.: Neonatal oncology. Pediatr. Clin. North Am. 24:585, 1977.
16. Gutensohn, N. M.: Social class and age at diagnosis of Hodgkin's disease. Cancer Treat. Rep. 66:689, 1982.
17. Glass, A. G., and Fraumeni, J. F., Jr.: Epidemiology of bone cancer in children. J. Natl. Cancer Inst. 44:187, 1970.
18. Li, F. P., and Fraumeni, J. F., Jr.: Testicular cancers in children: epidemiological characteristics. J. Natl. Cancer Inst. 48:1575, 1972.
19. Schoenberg, B. S., Christine, B. W., et al.: The descriptive epidemiology of primary intracranial neoplasms: the Connecticut experience. Am. J. Epidemiol. 101:499, 1976.
20. Young, J. L., and Miller, R. W.: Incidence of malignant tumors in U.S. children. J. Pediatr. 86:254, 1975.
21. Purtilo, D. T.: Pathogenesis and phenotypes of an X-linked recessive lymphoproliferative syndrome. Lancet 2:882, 1976.
22. Munoz, N.: Geographical distribution of pediatric tumors. Tumor 62:145, 1976.
23. Miller, R. W.: Ethnic differences in cancer occurrence: genetic and environmental influences with particular reference to neuroblastoma. In *Genetics of Human Cancer*. Mulvihill, J. J., Miller, R. W., et al. (eds.), New York, Raven Press, 1977, pp. 1-39.
24. Caldwell, G. G., and Heath, C. W.: Case clustering in cancer. South. Med. J. 69:1598, 1976.
25. Glass, A. G., and Mantel, N.: Lack of time-space clustering of childhood leukemia in Los Angeles County, 1960-1964. Cancer Res. 29:1995, 1969.
25a. Lagakos, S. W., Wessen, B., et al.: The Woburn Health Study. (unpublished data).
26. Vianna, N. J., Greenwald, P., et al.: Hodgkin's disease: cases with features of a community outbreak. Ann. Intern. Med. 77:169, 1972.
27. Vianna, N. J.: Epidemiologic evidence for transmission of Hodgkin's disease. New Engl. J. Med. 289:499, 1973.
28. Mason, T. J., McKay, F. W., et al.: *Atlas of Cancer Mortality for U.S. Counties:* 1950-1969. Washington, D.C., U.S. Government Printing Office, 1975.
29. Mason, T. J., McKay, F. W., et al.: *Atlas of Cancer Mortality Among U.S. Nonwhites:* 1950-1969. Washington, D.C., U.S. Government Printing Office, 1976.
30. Hoover, R., Mason, T. J., et al.: Cancer by county: new resource for etiologic clues. Science 189:1005, 1975.
31. Hoover, R., and Fraumeni, J. F., Jr.: Cancer mortality in U.S. counties with chemical industries. Environ. Res. 9:196, 1975.
32. Miller, R. W.: Etiology of childhood bone cancer: epidemiologic observations. In *Recent Results in Cancer Research*, Vol. 54. Grundmann, E. (ed.), Berlin, Springer-Verlag, 1976, p. 50.
33. Miller, R. W.: The discovery of human teratogens, carcinogens, and mutagens: lessons for the future. In *Chemical Mutagens*. V. Hollander, A., and deSerres, F. (eds.), New York, Plenum Press, 1978, p. 101.
34. Miller, R. W.: Persons with exceptionally high risk of leukemia. Cancer Res. 27:2420, 1967.
35. Miller, R. W.: Fifty-two forms of childhood cancer: United States mortality experience, 1960–1966. J. Pediatr. 75:685, 1969.
36. Miller, R. W., and McKay, F. W.: Decline in US childhood cancer mortality 1950 through 1980. J.A.M.A. 251:1567, 1984.
37. Young, J. L., Percy, C. L., et al.: *Incidence and mortality data: 1973–1977*. National Cancer Institute Monograph No. 57. Washington, D.C., U.S. Government Printing Office, 1981.
38. *Eighth Revision International Classification of Diseases*. Adapted for use in the U.S. (ICDA), Washington, D.C., U.S. Government Printing Office, 1968.
39. Miller, R. W., Fraumeni, J. F., et al.: Neuroblastoma: epidemiologic approach to its origin. Am. J. Dis. Child 115:253, 1968.
40. Percy, L. P., Berg, J. W., et al.: *Manual of Tumor Nomenclature and Coding*, 1968 Ed. New York, American Cancer Society, 1968.
41. *International Classification of Diseases for Oncology*, 1st Ed. Geneva, World Health Organization, 1976.
42. Chessells, J. M., Hardisty, R. M., et al.: Acute lymphoblastic leukemia in children: classification and prognosis. Lancet 1:1307, 1977.
43. Waterhouse, J., Muir, C., et al.: *Cancer Incidence in Five Continents*, Vol. III. Lyon, International Agency for Research on Cancer, 1976.
44. Davies, J. N. P.: Some variations in childhood cancers throughout the world. In *Tumors in Children, Recent Results in Cancer Research*, Vol. 13. Marsden, H. B., and Steward, J. K. (eds.), Berlin, Springer-Verlag, 1976, p. 28.
45. Devesa, S. S., and Schneiderman, M. A.: Increase in the number of cancer deaths in the United States. Am. J. Epidemiol. 106:1, 1977.
46. MacMahon, B., and Pugh, T. F.: *Epidemiology: Principles and Methods*. Boston, Little, Brown and Company, 1970.
47. Teppo, L., Salonen, T., et al.: Incidence of childhood cancer in Finland. J. Natl. Cancer Inst. 55:1065, 1975.
48. Leck, I.: Congenital malformations and childhood neoplasms. J. Med. Genet 14:321, 1977.
49. Morrow, R. H., Pike, M. C., et al.: Further studies of space-time clustering of Burkitt's lymphoma in Uganda. Br. J. Cancer 35:668, 1977.
50. Wronkowski, Z., Stemmerman, G., et al.: Stomach carcinoma among Hawaiians and Caucasians in Hawaii. Cancer 39:2310, 1977.

51. *Smoking and Health:* Report of the Advisory Committee to the Surgeon General of the Public Health Service. Washington, D.C., U.S. Government Printing Office, 1964.
52. *The Effects on Populations of Exposure to Low Levels of Ionizing Radiation.* Report of the Advisory Committee on the Biological Effects of Ionizing Radiations. Washington, D.C., U.S. Government Printing Office, 1972.
53. Boice, J. D., and Fraumeni, J. F., Jr. (eds.).: Radiation Carcinogenesis. New York, Raven Press, 1984.
54. Hutchison, G. B.: Late neoplastic changes following medical irradiation. Cancer 37:1102, 1976.
55. Kohn, H. I., and Fry, R. J. M.: Radiation carcinogenesis. New Engl. J. Med. 301:504, 1984.
56. Shellabarger, C. L.: Radiation carcinogenesis: laboratory studies. Cancer 37:1090, 1976.
57. Upton, A. C., Beebe, G. W., et al.: Report of the NCI ad hoc working group on the risks associated with mammography in mass screening for the detection of breast cancer. J. Natl. Cancer Inst. 59:481, 1977.
58. Gregg, E. C.: Radiation risks with diagnostic x-rays. Radiology 123:447, 1977.
59. Stewart, A.: The carcinogenic effects of low level radiation. A reappraisal of epidemiologists' methods and observations. Health Phys. 24:223, 1973.
60. MacMahon, B., and Hutchison, G. B.: Prenatal x-ray and childhood cancer. Acta Un. Int. Cancer 20:1172, 1964.
60a. Graham, S., Levin, M. L., et al.: Preconception, intrauterine and postnatal irradiation as related to leukemia. Natl. Cancer Inst. Monogr. 19:347, 1966.
61. Diamond, E. I., Schmerler, H., et al.: The relationship of intrauterine radiation to subsequent mortality and development of leukemia in children. Am. J. Epidemiol. 97:283, 1973.
62. Jablon, S., and Kato, H.: Childhood cancer in relation to prenatal exposure to atomic-bomb radiation. Lancet 2:1000, 1970.
63. Monson, R. R., and MacMahon, B.: Prenatal x-ray exposure and cancer in children. In *Radiation Carcinogenesis.* Boice, J. D., and Fraumeni, J. F., Jr. (eds.), New York, Raven Press, 1984, p. 97.
64. McGregor, D. H., Land, C. E., et al.: Breast cancer incidence among atomic bomb survivors, Hiroshima and Nagasaki, 1950–69. J. Natl. Cancer Inst. 59:799, 1977.
65. Boice, J. D., and Monson, R. R.: Breast cancer in women after repeated fluoroscopic examinations of the chest. J. Natl. Cancer Inst. 59:823, 1977.
66. Strong, L. C.: Genetic and environmental interactions. Cancer 40:1861, 1977.
67. Cleaver, J. E., and Bootsma, D.: Xeroderma pigmentosum: biochemical and genetic characteristics. Ann. Rev. Genet. 9:19, 1975.
68. Paterson, M. C., Smith, B. P., et al.: Defective excision repair of x-ray-damaged DNA in human (ataxia-telangiectasia) fibroblasts. Nature 260:444, 1976.
69. Schmahl, D., Thomas, C., et al.: *Iatrogenic Carcinogenesis.* Berlin, Springer-Verlag, 1977.
70. Stolley, P. D., and Hibberd, P. L.: Drugs. In *Cancer Epidemiology and Prevention.* Schottenfeld, D., and Fraumeni, J. F., Jr. (eds.), Philadelphia, W. B. Saunders Company, 1982, p. 304.
71. Casciato, D. A., and Scott, J. L.: Acute leukemia following prolonged cytotoxic agent therapy. Medicine 58:32, 1979.
72. Greene, M. H., Boice, J. D., et al.: Acute nonlymphocytic leukemia after therapy with alkylating agents for ovarian cancer. New Engl. J. Med. 307:1416, 1982.
73. Berk, P. D., Goldberg, J. D., et al.: Increased incidence of acute leukemia in polycythemia vera associated with chlorambucil therapy. New Engl. J. Med. 304:441, 1981.
74. Boice, J. D., Greene, M. H., et al.: Leukemia and preleukemia after adjuvant treatment of gastrointestinal cancer with Semustine (methyl-CCNU). New Engl. J. Med. 309:1079; 1983.
75. Reimer, R. R., Hoover, R., et al.: Acute leukemia after alkylating-agent therapy of ovarian cancer. New Engl. J. Med. 297:177, 1977.
76. Wall, R. W., and Clausen, K. P.: Carcinoma of the urinary bladder in patients receiving cyclophosphamide. New Engl. J. Med. 293:271, 1975.
77. Clayson, D. B., and Shubik, P.: The carcinogenic action of drugs. Cancer Det. Prev. 1:43, 1976.
78. Pedersen-Bjergaard, J., and Larsen, S. O.: Incidence of acute nonlymphocytic leukemia, preleukemia, and acute myeloproliferative syndrome up to 10 years after treatment of Hodgkin's disease. New Engl. J. Med. 307:965, 1982.
79. Harris, C. C.: The carcinogenicity of anticancer drugs. Cancer 37:1014, 1976.
80. Hoover, R., and Fraumeni, J. F., Jr.: Risk of cancer in renal-transplant recipients. Lancet 2:55, 1973.
81. Meadows, A. T., Naiman, J. L., et al.: Hepatoma associated with androgen therapy for aplastic anemia. J. Pediatr. 84:109, 1974.
82. Cutler, B. S., Forbes, A. P., et al.: Endometrial carcinoma after stilbestrol therapy in gonadal dysgenesis. New Engl. J. Med. 287:628, 1972.
83. Berlin, N. I., and Wasserman, L. R.: The association between systemically administered radioisotopes and subsequent malignant disease. Cancer 37:1097, 1976.
84. Herbst, A. L., Ulfelder, H., et al.: Adenocarcinoma of the vagina. New Engl. J. Med. 284:878, 1971.
85. Ulfelder, H.: Stilbestrol, adenosis, and adenocarcinoma. Am. J. Obstet. Gynecol. 117:794, 1973.
86. Lanier, A. P., and Noller, K. L.: Cancer and stilbestrol: a follow-up of 1,719 persons exposed to estrogens in utero and born 1943–1959. Mayo Clin. Proc. 48:793, 1973.
87. Bibbo, M., Maysoon, A., et al.: Follow-up study of male and female offspring of DES-treated mothers. J. Reprod. Med. 15:29, 1976.
88. Melamed, I., Bujanover, Y., et al.: Hepatoblastoma in an infant born to a mother after hormonal treatment for sterility. New Engl. J. Med. 307:820, 1982.
89. Conley, G. R., Sant, G. R., et al.: Seminoma and epididymal cysts in a young man with known diethylstilbestrol exposure in utero. J.A.M.A. 249:1325,1983.
90. Pendergrass, T. W.: Fetal hydantoin syndrome and neuroblastoma. Lancet 2:150, 1976.
91. Allen, R. W., and Buehler, B.: Fetal hydantoin syndrome, neuroblastoma, and hemorrhagic disease. Pediatr. Res. 14 (Part 2):530, 1980.
92. Sieber, S., and Adamson, R.: Toxicity of antineoplastic agents in man, chromosomal aberrations, antifertility effects, congenital malformations, and carcinogenic potential. Adv. Cancer Res. 22:57, 1975.
93. Cole, P., and Goldman, M. B.: Occupation. In *Persons at High Risk of Cancer: An Approach to Cancer Etiology and Control.* Fraumeni, J. F., Jr. (ed.), New York, Academic Press, 1975, p. 167.
94. Miller, R. W.: Environmental causes of cancer in childhood. Adv. Pediatr. 25:97, 1978.
94a. Janerich, D. T., Burnett, W. S., et al.: Cancer incidence in the Love Canal area. Science 212:1404, 1981.
95. Anderson, H. A., Lilis, R., et al.: Household contact asbestos neoplastic risk. Ann. N.Y. Acad. Sci. 271:311, 1976.
96. Miller, R. W.: Pollutants in breast milk. J. Pediatr. 90:510, 1977.
97. Hakulinen, T., Salonen, T., et al.: Cancer in the offspring of fathers in hydrocarbon-related occupations. Br. J. Prev. Soc. Med. 30:138, 1976.
98. Terracini, B., Pastore, G., et al.: Association of father's occupation and cancer in children. Biol. Res. Preg. Perinat. 4:40, 1983.
99. Reif, A. E.: Public information on smoking: an urgent

responsibility for cancer research workers. J. Natl. Cancer Inst. 57:1207, 1976.
100. Miller, R. W.: Effects of cigarette smoking on the fetus and child. Pediatrics 57:411, 1976.
101. Willett, W. C., and MacMahon, B.: Diet and cancer—an overview. New Engl. J. Med. 310:633, 1984.
102. Shubik, P.: Potential carcinogenicity of food additives and contaminants. Cancer Res. 35:3475, 1975.
103. Miller, R. W.: Carcinogens in drinking water. Pediatrics 57:462, 1976.
104. Monkman, G. R., Orwoll, G., et al.: Trauma and oncogenesis. Mayo Clin. Proc. 49:157, 1974.
105. Li, F. P., Miller, R. W., et al.: Cotton as a cause of cancer. Lancet 1:1014, 1972.
106. Fitzgerald, R. H., Brewer, N. S., et al.: Squamous-cell carcinoma complicating chronic osteomyelitis. J. Bone Joint Surg. 58:1146, 1976.
107. Brand, G. K.: Diversity and complexity of carcinogenic process: conceptual inferences from foreign-body tumorigenesis. J. Natl. Cancer Inst. 57:973, 1976.
108. Miller, T. R.: Psychophysiologic aspects of cancer: the James Ewing lecture. Cancer 39:413, 1977.
109. Rapp, F., and Reed, C. L.: The viral etiology of cancer: a realistic approach. Cancer 40:419, 1977.
110. Allen, D. W., and Cole, P.: Viruses and human cancer. New Engl. J. Med. 286:70, 1972.
111. Klein, G.: The Epstein-Barr virus and neoplasia. New Engl. J. Med. 293:1353, 1975.
112. ar-Rushdi, A., Nishikura, K., et al.: Differential expression of the translocated and the untranslocated c-*myc* oncogene in Burkitt lymphoma. Science 222:390, 1983.
113. Diamond, A., Cooper, G. M., et al.: Identification and molecular cloning of the human *Blym* transforming gene activated in Burkitt's lymphomas. Nature 305:112, 1983.
114. Beasley, R. P., Lin, C. C., et al.: Hepatocellular carcinoma and hepatitis B virus. Lancet 2:1129, 1981.
115. Blumberg, B. S., and London, W. T.: Hepatitis B virus and the prevention of primary hepatocellular carcinoma. New Engl. J. Med. 304:782, 1981.
116. Robert-Guroff, M., Nakao, Y., et al.: Natural antibodies to human retrovirus HTLV in a cluster of Japanese patients with adult T cell leukemia. Science 215:975, 1982.
117. Gallo, R. C., Salahuddin, S. Z., et al.: Frequent detection and isolation of cytopathic retroviruses (HTLV-III) from patients with AIDS and at risk for AIDS. Science 224:500, 1984.
117a. Wong-Staal, F., and Gallo, R. C.: Human T-lymphocytic retroviruses. Nature 317:395, 1985.
118. Perutz, M. F.: Fundamental research in molecular biology: relevance to medicine. Nature 262:449, 1976.
119. Templeton, A. C.: Acquired diseases. In *Persons at High Risk of Cancer: An Approach to Cancer Etiology and Control.* Fraumeni, J. F., Jr. (ed.), New York, Academic Press, 1975, p. 69.
120. Comstock, G. W.: Leukemia and B.C.G.: A controlled trial. Lancet 2:1062, 1971.
121. Thomas, E. D., Buckner, C. D., et al.: Leukemic transformation of engrafted human marrow cells in vivo. Lancet 1:1310, 1972.
122. Greenwald, P., Woodard, E., et al.: Morbidity and mortality among recipients of blood from preleukemic and prelymphomatous donors. Cancer 38:324, 1976.
123. Li, F. P.: Host factors in the development of childhood cancers. Semin. Oncol. 5:17, 1978.
124. Bader, J. L., and Miller, R. W.: Neurofibromatosis and childhood leukemia. J. Pediatr. 92:925, 1978.
125. Filipovich, A. H., Spector, B. D., et al.: Immunodeficiency in humans as a risk factor in the development of malignancy. Prev. Med. 9:252, 1980.
126. Hananian, J., Koch, K., et al.: Leukemia in a twin with multiple congenital limb abnormalities. In *Birth Defects: Original Article Series,* Vol. XII. Bergsma, D. (ed.), The National Foundation-March of Dimes, 1976, p. 171.
127. Miller, R. W.: Childhood cancer and congenital defects: a study of U.S. death certificates during the period 1960–1966. Pediatr. Res. 3:389, 1969.
128. Mulvihill, J. J.: Congenital and genetic diseases. In *Persons at High Risk of Cancer: An Approach to Cancer Etiology and Control.* Fraumeni, J. F., Jr. (ed.), New York, Academic Press, 1975, p. 3.
129. Woods, W. G., Roloff, J. S., et al.: The occurrence of leukemia in patients with the Schwachman syndrome. J. Pediatr. 99:425, 1981.
130. Gonzalez, C. H., Stamm, M. V., et al.: The WT syndrome—A "new" autosomal dominant pleiotropic trait of radial-ulnar hypoplasia with high risk of bone marrow failure and/or leukemia. In *Birth Defects: Original Article Series,* Vol. XIII, 3B. Bergsma, D. (ed.), National Foundation-March of Dimes, 1977, p. 31.
131. Krishnan, E., Wegner, K., et al.: Congenital hypoplastic anemia terminating in acute promyelocytic leukemia. Pediatrics 61:898, 1978.
132. Hecht, F., and McCaw, B. K.: Chromosome instability syndromes. In *Genetics of Human Cancer.* Mulvihill, J. J., Miller, R. W., et al. (eds.), New York, Raven Press, 1977, p. 105.
133. Branda, R. F., Moldow, C. F., et al.: Folate-induced remission in aplastic anemia with familial defect of cellular folate uptake. New Engl. J. Med. 298:469, 1978.
134. Zuelzer, W. W., and Cox, D. E.: Genetic aspects of leukemia. Semin. Hematol. 6:228, 1969.
135. Kurita, S., Yoshitaka, K., et al.: Genetic studies on familial leukemia. Cancer 34:1098, 1974.
136. Jonas, D. M., Heilbron, D. C., et al.: Rubenstein-Taybi syndrome and acute leukemia. J. Pediatr. 92:851, 1978.
136a. Li, F. P., Hecht, F., et al.: Ataxia–Pancytopenia. Cancer Genet. Cytogenet. 4:189, 1981.
137. Horton, W. A.: Genetics of central nervous system tumors. In *Birth Defects: Original Article Series,* Vol. XII, No. 1. Bergsma, D. (ed.), National Foundation-March of Dimes, 1976, p. 91.
138. Baughman, F. A., List, C. F., et al.: The gliomapolyposis syndrome. New Engl. J. Med. 281:1345, 1969.
139. Sotelo-Avila, C., and Gooch, W. M., III: Neoplasms associated with the Beckwith-Wiedemann syndrome. In *Perspectives in Pediatric Pathology,* Vol. 3. Rosenberg, H. S., and Bolande, R. P. (eds.), Chicago, Yearbook Medical Publishers, Inc., 1976, p. 255.
140. Asamoto, H., Furuta, M., et al.: DiGeorge syndrome associated with glioma and two kinds of viral infection. New Engl. J. Med. 296:1235, 1977.
140a. Robinson, M. G., and McCorquodale, M. M.: Trisomy 18 and neurogenic neoplasia. J. Pediatr. 99:428, 1981.
140b. Li, F. P., Little, J. B., et al.: Acute leukemia after radiotherapy in a patient with Turcot's syndrome. Am. J. Med. 74:343, 1983.
141. Draper, G. J., Heaf, M. M., et al.: Occurrence of childhood cancers among sibs and estimation of familial risks. J. Med. Genet. 14:81, 1977.
142. Li, F. P., and Fraumeni, J. F., Jr.: Prospective study of a family cancer syndrome. J.A.M.A. 247:2692, 1982.
143. Miller, R. W.: Neoplasia and Down's syndrome. Ann. N.Y. Acad. Sci. 171:637, 1970.
144. Wertelecki, W., Fraumeni, J. F., Jr., et al.: Nongonadal neoplasia in Turner's syndrome. Cancer 26:485, 1970.
145. Blume, R. S., and Wolff, S. M.: The Chediak-Higashi syndrome: studies in four patients and a review of the literature. Medicine 51:217, 1972.
146. Grundy, G. W., Creagan, E. T., et al.: Non-Hodgkin's lymphoma in childhood: epidemiologic features. J. Natl. Cancer Inst. 51:767, 1973.
147. Fraumeni, J. F., Jr.: Family studies in Hodgkin's disease. Cancer Res. 34:1164, 1974.

148. Miller, R. W.: Deaths from childhood leukemia and solid tumors among twins and other sibs in the United States, 1960–67. J. Natl. Cancer Inst. 46:203, 1971.
149. Grufferman, S., Cole, P., et al.: Hodgkin's disease in siblings. New Engl. J. Med. 296:248, 1977.
150. Knudson, A. G., and Meadows, A. T.: Developmental genetics of neuroblastoma. J. Natl. Cancer Inst. 57:675, 1976.
151. Knudson, A. G., Jr., and Strong, L.: Mutation and cancer: neuroblastoma and pheochromocytoma. Am. J. Hum. Genet. 24:514, 1972.
152. Meadows, A. T., and Knudson, A. G.: Heterochromia and neuroblastoma. J. Pediatr. 88:168, 1976.
153. Nevin, N. C., Dodge, J. A., et al.: Two cases of trisomy D associated with adrenal tumors. J. Med. Genet. 9:119, 1972.
154. Cavenee, W. K., Dryja, T. P., et al.: Expression of recessive alleles by chromosomal mechanisms in retinoblastoma. Nature 305:779, 1983.
155. Stay, E. J., and Vawter, G.: The relationship between nephroblastoma and neurofibromatosis (von Recklinghausen's disease). Cancer 39:2550, 1977.
156. Pendergrass, T. W.: Congenital anomalies in children with Wilms' tumor. Cancer 37:403, 1976.
157. de Martinville, B., and Francke, U.: The c-Ha-*ras*1, insulin and B-globin loci map outside the deletion associated with aniridia–Wilms' tumor. Nature 305:641, 1983.
157a. Editorial: Genes and cancer: the story of Wilm's Tumor. Science 207:970, 1980.
158. Mulvihill, J. J., Gralnick, H. R., et al.: Multiple childhood osteosarcomas in an American Indian family with erythroid macrocytoses and skeletal anomalies. Cancer 40:3115, 1977.
159. Christian, C. D.: Ovarian tumors; an extension of the Peutz-Jeghers syndrome. Am. J. Obstet. Gynecol. 111:529, 1971.
160. Segall, M., Shapiro, L. R., et al.: XO/XY gonadal dysgenesis and gonadoblastoma in childhood. Obstet. Gynecol. 41:536, 1973.
161. Jensen, R. D., Norris, H. J., et al.: Familial arrhenoblastoma and thyroid adenoma. Cancer 33:218, 1974.
162. Weinberg, A. G., Mize, C. E., et al.: The occurrence of hepatoma in the chronic form of hereditary tyrosinemia. J. Pediatr. 88:434, 1976.
163. Shapiro, P., Ideda, R. M., et al.: Multiple hepatic tumors and peliosis hepatis in Fanconi's anemia treated with androgens. Am. J. Dis. Child. 131:1104, 1977.
164. Fraumeni, J. F., Jr., Miller, R. W., et al.: Primary carcinoma of the liver in childhood. J. Natl. Cancer Inst. 40:1087, 1968.
165. Lieberman, J., Silton, R. M., et al.: Hepatocellular carcinoma and intermediate alpha-1-antitrypsin deficiency (MZ phenotype). Am. J. Clin. Pathol. 64:304, 1975.
166. Fraumeni, J. F., Jr., Rosen, P. J., et al.: Hepatoblastoma in infant sisters. Cancer 24:1086, 1969.
167. Chabalko, J. J., and Fraumeni, J. F., Jr.: Blood vessel neoplasms in children: epidemiologic aspects. Med. Pediatr. Oncol. 1:135, 1975.
168. Sugarman, G. I., Heuser, E. T., et al.: A case of cerebral gigantism and hepatocarcinoma. Am. J. Dis. Child, 131:631, 1977.
169. Yunis, J. J.: The chromosomal basis of human neoplasia. Science 221:227, 1983.
170. Mulvihill, J. J.: Genetic repertory of human neoplasia. In *Genetics of Human Cancer*. Mulvihill, J. J., Miller, R. W., et al. (eds.), New York, Raven Press, 1977, p. 137.
171. Knudson, A. G.: Hereditary cancers of man. Cancer Investigation 1:187, 1983.
172. Knudson, A. G., Jr.: Mutation and cancer: statistical study of retinoblastoma. Proc. Natl. Acad. Sci., 68:820, 1971.
173. Knudson, A. G., Jr., and Strong, L.: Mutation and cancer: a model for Wilms' tumor of the kidney. J. Natl. Cancer Inst. 48:313, 1972.
174. Kitchin, F. D., and Ellsworth, R. M.: Pleiotropic effects of the gene for retinoblastoma. J. Med. Genet. 11:244, 1974.
175. Lawler, S. D., and Reeves, B. R.: Chromosome studies in man: past achievements and recent advances. J. Clin. Pathol. 29:569, 1976.
176. Heisterkamp, N., Stephenson, J. R., et al.: Localization of the c-*abl* oncogene adjacent to a translocation break point in chronic myelocytic leukaemia. Nature 306:239, 1983.
177. Canaani, E., Steiner-Saltz, D., et al.: Altered transcription of an oncogene in chronic myeloid leukaemia. Lancet 1:593, 1984.
178. Schaller, J. G., and Omenn, G. S.: The histocompatibility system and human disease. J. Pediatr. 88:913, 1976.
179. Anderson, D. E.: Familial susceptibility. In *Persons at High Risk of Cancer: An Approach to Cancer Etiology and Control*. Fraumeni, J. F., Jr. (ed.), New York, Academic Press, 1975, p. 39.
180. Li, F. P., Tucker, M. A., et al.: Childhood cancer in sibs. J. Pediatr. 88:419, 1976.
181. Miller, R. W.: Relation between cancer and congenital defects in man. New Engl. J. Med. 275:87, 1966.
182. DiPaolo, J. A., and Kotin, P.: Teratogenesis-oncogenesis: a study of possible relationships. Arch. Pathol. 81:3, 1966.
183. Miller, R. W.: Relationship between human teratogens and carcinogens. J. Natl. Cancer Inst. 58:471, 1977.
184. Ames, B. N., Durston, W. E., et al.: Carcinogens are mutagens: a simple test system combining liver homogenates for activation and bacteria for detection. Proc. Natl. Acad. Sci. 70:2281, 1973.
185. Miller, E. C.: Some current perspectives on chemical carcinogenesis in humans and experimental animals: presidential address. Cancer Res. 38:1479, 1978.
186. Fraumeni, J. F., Jr., and Manning, M. D.: Acute leukemia: epidemiologic study by cell type of 1,263 cases at the Children's Cancer Research Foundation in Boston, 1947–1965. J. Natl. Cancer Inst. 46:461, 1971.
187. Choi, S. I., and Simone, J. V.: Acute nonlymphocytic leukemia in 171 children. Med. Pediatr. Oncol. 2:119, 1976.
188. Cavdar, A. O., Arcasoy, A., et al.: Ocular granulocytic sarcoma (chloroma) with acute myelomonocytic leukemia in Turkish children. Cancer 41:1606, 1978.
188a. Li, F. P., Jin, F., et al.: Incidence of childhood leukemia in Shanghai. Int. J. Cancer 25:701, 1980.
189. German, J., Bloom, D., et al.: Bloom's syndrome. V. Surveillance for cancer in affected families. Clin. Genet. 12:162, 1977.
189a. Ishida, R., and Buchwald, M.: Susceptibility of Fanconi's anemia lymphoblasts to DNA-cross-linking and alkylating agents. Cancer Res. 42:4000, 1982.
190. McCaw, B. K., Hecht, F., et al.: Somatic rearrangement of chromosome 14 in human lymphocytes. Proc. Natl. Acad. Sci. 72:2071, 1975.
191. Schroeder, T. M., and Kurth, R.: Spontaneous chromosomal breakage and high incidence of leukemia in inherited disease. Blood 37:96, 1971.
192. Rosner, F., and Lee, S. L.: Down's syndrome and acute leukemia: myeloblastic or lymphoblastic? Am. J. Med. 53:203, 1972.
193. Clark, R. D., and Hutter, J. J.: Familial neurofibromatosis and juvenile chronic myelogenous leukemia. Hum. Genet. 60:230, 1982.
194. Clarkson, B. D., and Boyse, E. A.: Possible explanation of the high concordance for acute leukemia in monozygotic twins. Lancet 1:699, 1971.
195. Blattner, W. A., Takatsuki, K., et al.: Human T-cell leukemia-lymphoma virus and adult T-cell leukemia. J.A.M.A. 250:1074, 1983.
196. Krakower, J. M., and Aaronson, S. A.: Seroepidemiologic assessment of feline leukaemia virus infection risk for man. Nature 273:463, 1978.

197. Bizzozero, O. J., Johnson, K. G., et al.: Radiation-related leukemia in Hiroshima and Nagasaki 1946–1964: observations of type-specific leukemia, survivorship, and clinical behavior. Ann. Intern. Med. 66:522, 1957.
198. Brill, A. B., Tomonaga, M., et al.: Leukemia in man following exposure to ionizing radiation: summary of findings in Hiroshima and Nagasaki, and a comparison with other human experience. Ann. Intern. Med. 56:590, 1962.
199. Marmont, A., Frassoni, F., et al.: Recurrence of Ph'-positive leukemia in donor cells after marrow transplantation for chronic granulocytic leukemia. New Engl. J. Med. 310:903, 1984.
200. Newburger, P. E., Latt, S. A., et al.: Leukemia relapse in donor cells after allogeneic bone-marrow transplantation. New Engl. J. Med. 304:712, 1981.
201. Bloomfield, C. D., and Brunning, R. D.: Acute leukemia as a terminal event in nonleukemic hematopoietic disorders. Semin. Oncol. 3:297, 1976.
202. Correa, P., and O'Conor, G. T.: Geographic pathology of lymphoreticular tumors: summary of survey from the Geographic Pathology Committee of the International Union Against Cancer. J. Natl. Cancer Inst. 50:1609, 1973.
203. Wright, D. H.: The epidemiology of Burkitt's tumor. Cancer Res. 27:2424, 1967.
204. Magrath, I. T., Ziegler, J. L., et al.: A comparison of clinical and histopathologic features of childhood malignant lymphoma in Uganda. Cancer 33:285, 1974.
205. Levine, P. H., Kamaraju, L. S., et al.: The American Burkitt's lymphoma registry. Cancer 49:1016, 1982.
206. Burkitt, D. P.: Etiology of Burkitt's lymphoma—an alternative hypothesis to a vectored virus. J. Natl. Cancer Inst. 42:19, 1969.
207. de-The, G., Geser, A., et al.: Epidemiology of the Epstein-Barr virus infection and associated tumors in man: a tool for etiology and control. Bibl. Haematol. 43:216, 1975.
208. Gravelle, M., Levine, P. H., et al.: Epstein-Barr virus in an American patient with Burkitt's lymphoma: detection of viral genome in tumor tissue and establishment of a tumor-derived cell line (NAB). J. Natl. Cancer Inst. 56:701, 1976.
209. Siemiatycki, J., Brubaker, G., et al.: Space-time clustering of Burkitt's lymphoma in East Africa: analysis of recent data and a new look at old data. Int. J. Cancer 25:197, 1980.
210. de-The, G., Geser, A., et al.: Epidemiological evidence for causal relationship between Epstein-Barr virus and Burkitt's lymphoma from Ugandan prospective study. Nature 274:756, 1978.
211. Bernheim, A., Berger, R., et al.: Cytogenetic studies on African Burkitt's lymphoma cell lines: t(8;14), t(2;8) and t(8;22) translocations. Cancer Genet. Cytogenet. 3:307, 1981.
212. Chaves, E.: Hodgkin's disease in the first decade. Cancer 31:925, 1973.
213. Fraumeni, J. F., Jr., and Li, F. P.: Hodgkin's disease in childhood: an epidemiologic study. J. Natl. Cancer Inst. 42:681, 1969.
214. Schottenfeld, D.: Epidemiology of Hodgkin's disease. In Hodgkin's Disease. Lacher, M. G. (ed.), New York, John Wiley and Sons, Inc., 1976, p. 5.
215. Gutensohn, N., and Cole, P.: Epidemiology of Hodgkin's disease in the young. Int. J. Cancer 19:595, 1977.
216. Smith, P. G., and Kinlen, L. J.: Contacts between young patients with Hodgkin's disease. Lancet 2:59, 1977.
216a. Grufferman, S., Cole, P., et al.: Evidence against transmission of Hodgkin's disease in high schools. New Engl. J. Med. 300:1006, 1979.
217. Buehler, S. K., Fodor, G., et al.: Common variable immunodeficiency Hodgkin's disease, and other malignancies in a Newfoundland family. Lancet 1:195, 1975.
218. Fraumeni, J. F., Jr., and Hoover, R.: Immunosurveillance and cancer: epidemiologic observations. Natl. Cancer Inst. Monogr. 47:121, 1977.
219. Editorial. Immunological deficiency and the risk of cancer. Br. Med. J. 2:654, 1977.
220. Jones, S. E.: Autoimmune disorders and malignant lymphoma. Cancer 31:1092, 1973.
221. Hymans, L. R., Burkholder, P. M., et al.: Malignant lymphoma and nephrotic syndrome: a clinicopathologic analysis with light, immunofluorescence and electron microscopy of renal lesions. J. Pediatr. 82:207, 1973.
222. Order, S. E., and Hellman, S.: Pathogenesis of Hodgkin's disease. Lancet 1:571, 1972.
223. Kaplan, H. S.: Hodgkin's disease and other human malignant lymphomas: advances and prospects—G.H.A. Clowes Memorial Lecture. Cancer Res. 36:3863, 1976.
224. San Roman, C., Ferro, M. T., et al.: Translocation (11;14) in B-cell lymphoproliferative disorders. Cancer Genet. Cytogenet. 7:279, 1982.
225. Oxford, J. M., Harnden, D. G., et al.: Specific chromosome aberrations in ataxia telangiectasia. J. Med. Genet. 12:251, 1975.
226. Schoenberg, B., Schoenberg, D., et al.: The epidemiology of primary intracranial neoplasms of childhood. Mayo Clin. Proc. 51:51, 1976.
227. Schoenberg, B. S., Christine, B. W., et al.: The descriptive epidemiology of primary intracranial neoplasms: the Connecticut experience. Am. J. Epidemiol. 101:499, 1976.
228. Mulcahy, G. M., and Harlan, W. L.: Occurrences of central nervous system tumors, with special reference to relative genetic factors. In Cancer Genetics. Lynch, H. (ed.), Springfield, Ill., Charles C Thomas, Publisher, 1976, p. 263.
229. Knudson, A. G., Jr.: Genetics and etiology of human cancer. In Advances in Human Genetics, Vol. 18. Harris, H., and Hirschorn, K. (eds.), New York, Plenum Press, 1970, p. 1.
230. Cleary, M. L., Warnke, R., et al.: Monoclonality of lymphoproliferative lesions in cardiac-transplant recipients. New Engl. J. Med. 310:477, 1984.
231. Wilson, L. M. K., and Draper, G. J.: Neuroblastoma, its natural history and prognosis: a study of 487 cases. Br. Med. J. 3:301, 1974.
231a. Turkel, S. B., and Itabashi, H. H.: The natural history of neuroblastic cells in the fetal adrenal gland. Am. J. Pathol. 76:225, 1974.
232. Mancini, A. F., Rosito, P., et al.: Neuroblastoma in a pair of identical twins. Med. Pediatr. Oncol. 10:45, 1982.
232a. Miller, D. R., Patel, K., et al.: Neuroblastoma, tuberous sclerosis, and subependymal giant cell astrocytoma. Am. J. Pediatr. Hematol. Oncol. 5:213, 1983.
233. Schwab, M., Varmus, H. E., et al.: Chromosome localization in normal human cells and neuroblastomas of a gene related to c-myc. Nature 308:288, 1984.
234. Brodeur, G. M., Sekhon, G. S., et al.: Chromosomal aberrations in human neuroblastomas. Cancer 40:2256, 1977.
235. Li, F. P., and Fraumeni, J. F., Jr.: Rhabdomyosarcoma in children: Epidemiologic study and identification of a familial cancer syndrome. J. Natl. Cancer Inst. 43:1365, 1969.
236. Miller, R. W., and Dalager, N. A.: Fatal rhabdomyosarcoma among children in the United States, 1960–69. Cancer 34:1897, 1974.
237. Chabalko, J. J., Creagan, E. T., et al.: Epidemiology of selected sarcomas in children. J. Natl. Cancer Inst. 53:675, 1974.
237a. Sloane, J. A., and Hubbell, M. M.: Soft tissue sarcomas in children associated with congenital anomalies. Cancer 23:175, 1968.
238. McKeen, E. A., Bodurtha, J., et al.: Rhabdomyosarcoma

complicating multiple neurofibromatosis. J. Pediatr. 93:992, 1978.
238a. Birch, J. M., Hartley, A. L., et al.: Excess risk of breast cancer in the mothers of children with soft tissue sarcomas. Br. J. Cancer 49:325, 1984.
239. Becher, R., Wake, N., et al.: Chromosome changes in soft tissue sarcomas. J. Natl. Cancer Inst. 72:823, 1984.
240. Bechet, J. M., Bornkamm, G., et al.: The c-sis oncogene is not activated in Ewing's sarcoma. New Engl. J. Med. 310:393, 1984.
240a. Strong, L. C., Herson, J., et al.: Risk of radiation-related subsequent malignant tumors in survivors of Ewing's sarcoma. J. Natl. Cancer Inst. 62:1401, 1979.
241. Speiss, H., and Mays, C. W.: Bone cancers induced by ^{224}Ra (Th X) in children and adults. Health Phys. 19:713, 1970.
242. Bove, K. E., and McAdams, A. J.: The nephroblastomatosis complex and its relationship to Wilms' tumor: a clinicopathologic treatise. Perspect. Pediatr. Pathol. 3:185, 1976.
243. Breslow, N. E., and Bechwith, J. B.: Epidemiological features of Wilms' tumor: results of the national Wilms' tumor study. J. Natl. Cancer Inst. 68:429, 1982.
244. Pilling, G. P.: Wilms' tumor in seven children with congenital aniridia. J. Pediatr. Surg. 10:87, 1975.
245. Fraumeni, J. F., Jr.: The aniridia-Wilms' tumor syndrome. In Birth Defects: Original Article Series, Vol. V. Bergsma, D. (ed.), National Foundation-March of Dimes, 1969, p. 198.
245a. Yunis, J. J., Ramsay, N. K., et al.: Familial occurrence of the aniridia-Wilms tumor syndrome with deletion 11p13-14.1. J. Pediatr. 96:1027, 1980.
246. Barakat, A. Y., Papadopoulou, Z. L., et al.: Pseudohermaphroditism, nephron disorder and Wilms' tumor: a unifying concept. Pediatrics 54:366, 1974.
247. Meadows, A. T., Lichtenfeld, J. L., et al.: Wilms' tumor in three children of a woman with congenital hemihypertrophy. New Engl. J. Med. 291:23, 1974.
247a. Orkin, S. H., Goldman, D. S., et al.: Development of homozygosity for chromosome 11p markers in Wilms' tumor. Nature 309:172, 1984.
248. Newell, G. R., Roberts, J. D., et al.: Retinoblastoma: presentation and survival in Negro children compared with whites. J. Natl. Cancer Inst. 49:989, 1972.
249. Editorial. The changing pattern of retinoblastoma. Lancet 2:1016, 1971.
249a. Motegi, T., Yanagawa, Y., et al.: A recognizable pattern of the midface of retinoblastoma patients with interstitial deletion of 13q. Hum. Genet. 64:160, 1983.
250. Dryja, T. P., Cavenee, W., et al.: Homozygosity of chromosome 13 in retinoblastoma. New Engl. J. Med. 310:550, 1984.
251. Benedict, W. F., Murphree, A. L., et al.: Patient with 13 chromosome deletion. Science 219:973, 1983.
252. Abramson, D. H., Ellsworth, R. M., et al.: Nonocular cancer in retinoblastoma survivors. Trans. Am. Acad. Ophthalmol. Otol. 81:454, 1976.
253. Gordon, H.: Family studies in retinoblastoma. In Birth Defects: Original Article Series, Vol. X, No. 10. Bergsma, D. (ed.), National Foundation-March of Dimes, 1974, p. 185.
254. Chan, H., and Pratt, C. B.: A new familial cancer syndrome? A spectrum of malignant and benign tumors including retinoblastoma, carcinoma of the bladder and other genitourinary tumors, thyroid adenoma, and a probable case of multifocal osteosarcoma. J. Natl. Cancer Inst. 58:205, 1977.
255. Exelby, P. R., Filler, R. M., et al.: Liver tumors in children in the particular reference to hepatoblastoma and hepatocellular carcinoma: American Academy of Pediatrics Surgical Section Survey. J. Pediatr. Surg. 10:329, 1975.
256. Arthur, M. J. P., Hall, A. J., et al.: Hepatitis B, hepatocellular carcinoma, and strategies for prevention. Lancet 1:607, 1984.
257. Farber, E.: On the pathogenesis of experimental hepatocellular carcinoma. In Hepatocellular Carcinoma. Okuda, K., and Peters, R. L. (eds.), New York, John Wiley and Sons, 1976, p. 3.
258. Berk, P. D., Martin, J. F., et al.: Vinyl chloride liver disease. Ann. Intern. Med. 84:717, 1976.
259. Johnson, F. L., Lerner, K. G., et al.: Association of androgenic-anabolic steroid therapy with development of hepatocellular carcinoma. Lancet 2:1273, 1972.
260. Christopherson, W. M., and Mays, E. T.: Liver tumors and contraceptive steroids: experience with the first one hundred registry patients. J. Natl. Cancer Inst. 58:167, 1977.
261. Schottenfeld, D., Warshauer M. E., et al.: The epidemiology of testicular cancer in young adults. Am. J. Epidemiol. 112:232, 1980.
262. Tulinius, H., Day, N., et al.: Rarity of testis cancer in Negroes. Lancet 1:35, 1973.
263. Morrison, A. S.: Cryptorchidism, hernia, and cancer of the testis. J. Natl. Cancer Inst. 56:731, 1976.
264. Dow, J. A., and Mostofi, F. K.: Testicular tumors following orchiopexy. South. Med. J. 60:193, 1967.
264a. Gilbert, J. B., and Hamilton, J. B.: Studies in malignant testis tumors. III—Incidence and nature of tumors in ectopic testes. Surg. Gynecol. Obstet. 71:713, 1940.
264b. Beard, C. M., Benson, R. C., Jr., et al.: The incidence and outcome of mumps orchitis in Rochester, Minnesota, 1935–1974. Mayo Clin. Proc. 52:3, 1977.
265. Anderson, K. C., Li, F. P., et al.: Dizygotic twinning, cryptorchism, and seminoma in a sibship. Cancer 53:374, 1984.
265a. Schimke, R. N., Madigan, C. M., et al.: Choriocarcinoma, thyrotoxicosis, and the Klinefelter syndrome. Cancer Genet. Cytogenet. 9:1, 1983.
266. Li, F. P., Fraumeni, J. F., Jr., et al.: Ovarian cancers in the young: epidemiologic observations. Cancer 32:969, 1973.
267. Lingeman, C.: Etiology of cancer of the human ovary: a review. J. Natl. Cancer Inst. 53:1603, 1974.
268. Joly, D. J., Lilienfeld, A. M., et al.: An epidemiologic study of the relationship of reproductive experience to cancer of the ovary. Am. J. Epidemiol. 99:190, 1974.
269. Li, F. P., Rappaport, A. H., et al.: Familial ovarian carcinoma. J.A.M.A. 214:1559, 1970.
270. Schweisguth, O., Gerard-Marchant, R., et al.: Bilateral non-functioning thecoma of the ovary in epileptic children under anticonvulsant therapy. Acta Paediatr. Scand. 60:6, 1971.
271. Miller, R. W.: Peculiarities in the occurrence of adrenal cortical carcinoma. Am. J. Dis. Child. 132:235, 1978.
272. Feinman, N. L., and Yakovac, W. C.: Neurofibromatosis in childhood. J. Pediatr. 76:339, 1970.
273. Fraumeni, J. F., Jr., Li, F. P., et al.: Teratomas in children: epidemiologic features. J. Natl. Cancer Inst. 51:1425, 1973.
274. Linder, D., McCaw, B., et al.: Pathenogenic origin of benign ovarian teratomas. New Engl. J. Med. 292:63, 1975.
275. Mintz, B., Illmensee, K., et al.: Developmental and experimental potentialities of mouse teratocarcinoma cells from embryoid body cores. In Teratomas and Differentiation. Sherman, M. I., and Solter, D. (eds.), New York, Academic Press, Inc., 1975, p. 59.
276. Meadows, A. T., D'Angio, G. J., et al.: Patterns of second malignant neoplasms in children. Cancer 40:1903, 1977.
277. Li, F. P., Corkery, J., et al.: Breast carcinoma after cancer therapy in childhood. Cancer 51:521, 1983.
278. Jaffe, N.: Late side effects of treatment. Pediatr. Clin. North Am. 23:233, 1976.

279. Pastore, G., Antonelli, R., et al.: Late effects of treatment of cancer in infancy. Med. Pediatr. Oncol. *10*:369, 1982.
280. Riseborough, E. J., Grabias, S. L., et al.: Skeletal alterations following irradiation for Wilms' tumor, with particular reference to scoliosis and kyphosis. J. Bone Joint Surg. *58*:526, 1976.
281. Meadows, A. T., Massari, D. J., et al.: Declines in IQ scores and cognitive dysfunctions in children with acute lymphocytic leukemia treated with cranial radiation. Lancet *2*:1015, 1981.
282. Gangji, D., Reaman, G. H., et al.: Leukoencephalopathy and elevated levels of myelin basic protein in the cerebrospinal fluid of patients with acute lymphoblastic leukemia. New Engl. J. Med. *303*:19, 1980.
283. Editorial: Long-term effects of cancer treatment. Lancet *1*:1108, 1982.
284. Kaplan, M. M., Garnick, M. B., et al.: Risk factors for thyroid abnormalities after neck irradiation for childhood cancer. Am. J. Med. *74*:272, 1983.
285. Stillman, R. J., Schinfeld, J. S., et al.: Ovarian failure in long-term survivors of childhood malignancy. Am. J. Obstet. Gynecol. *139*:62, 1981.
286. Li, F. P., Fine, W., et al.: Offspring of patients treated for cancer in childhood. J. Natl. Cancer Inst. *62*:1193, 1979.
287. Green, D. M., Fine, W. E., et al.: Offspring of patients treated for unilateral Wilms' tumor in childhood. Cancer *49*:2285, 1982.
288. Duffner, P. K., Cohen, M. E., et al.: Late effects of treatment on the intelligence of children with posterior fossa tumors. Cancer *51*:233, 1983.

ONCOLOGY

CHAPTER 31
Oncogenes and the Molecular Biology of Cancer

SHELLY C. BERNSTEIN

INTRODUCTION 942
ONCOGENIC VIRUSES 942
DNA Tumor Viruses
  Papovaviruses
  Human Adenoviruses
  Herpesviruses
  Hepatitis B Virus
RNA Tumor Viruses
  Characteristics and Molecular Biology
  Retroviral Transforming Genes and Their Products
CELLULAR ONCOGENES 957
Detection of Cellular Oncogenes in Tumors of Nonviral Etiology
Characterization and Molecular Biology
  Proteins Encoded by Cellular Oncogenes
Cellular Oncogenes and Cancer
  Mechanisms of Proto-oncogene Activation
  Cooperation of Oncogenes
  Tissue Specificity and Oncogenes
Role of Cellular Oncogenes in the Normal Cell
Clinical Applications

INTRODUCTION

The search for the cause of cancer has stimulated much speculation and investigation. The previous chapter identified various host and environmental factors implicated in the development of human cancers, based on epidemiologic studies, and alluded to certain viruses that appear to play a role. A steadily increasing number of viruses able to induce tumors in a range of animals have been identified. More recently, specific viral genes have been implicated in the transformation of cells by certain oncogenic viruses. While most naturally occurring human malignancies do not appear to be caused by viruses, related cellular genes with potential oncogenic activity have been identified.

Many human malignant tumors and cell lines exhibit activated cellular oncogenes. Some of these activated oncogenes may exert their effects by expressing gene products that are "inappropriate" to the differentiated state of the cell. Whether the expression of a particular oncogene or group of oncogenes is actually inappropriate must first be confirmed by the analysis of normal cells at the same stage of differentiation. This is not a simple task. Assignment of a pathophysiologic role to a particular oncogene is also rendered complex. Different oncogene proteins belonging to different functional groups may act in concert on their appropriate targets in order to achieve full transformation of the cell. The association of several cellular oncogenes with cellular growth factors suggests that at least some of the products of these genes have an important function in normal cellular growth control; abnormal regulation of these genes may stimulate malignant growth. The study of aberrant gene activity in tumor cells in vitro should lead to an understanding of gene regulation in both normal and abnormal cells. But appropriate controls and conservative conclusions must be adopted as these exciting experiments unfold.

This chapter will begin by reviewing the role of viruses and viral oncogenes in neoplasia. The discussion will then turn to cellular oncogenes to give a preliminary picture of some of the molecular lesions involved in neoplasia.

ONCOGENIC VIRUSES

Viruses that cause cancer can be divided into two general categories, the DNA viruses and the RNA viruses (Table 31–1). The oncogenic DNA

Table 31-1. ONCOGENIC VIRUSES*

Type of Virus	Species of Isolation
I. Oncogenic RNA viruses	
A. Acute type[1]	
Rous sarcoma	Chicken
Fujinami sarcoma	Chicken
Reticuloendotheliosis	Chicken/ turkey
Avian erythroblastosis	Chicken
Avian myeloblastosis	Chicken
Avian myelocytomastosis	Chicken
Moloney sarcoma	Mouse
Abelson leukemia	Mouse
FBJ osteosarcoma[2]	Mouse
Harvey/Kirsten sarcoma	Rat
Rat sarcoma	Rat
Feline sarcoma	Cat
Woolly monkey sarcoma	Woolly monkey
B. Subacute type[3]	
Avian leukosis	Chicken
Mouse leukemia[4]	Mouse
Feline leukemia	Cat
Bovine leukemia	Cow
Gibbon ape leukemia[5]	Gibbon ape
Mouse mammary tumor	Mouse
Human T cell lymphotropic	Human
II. Oncogenic DNA viruses	
A. Papovaviruses	
Papilloma	Rabbit, human, dog, cow, and others
Polyoma	Mouse
Simian virus 40	Monkey
JC[2]	Human
BK[2]	Human
B. Adenoviruses	Human[6], monkey, bird, cow
C. Herpesviruses	
Epstein-Barr virus	Human
Lucké carcinoma	Frog
Marek's disease	Chicken

*Modified from Ruddon, R. W.: *Cancer Biology*. New York, Oxford University Press, 1981, p. 239.

[1]Acute type viruses transform cells in vitro, produce rapid disease induction in vivo, and carry a "transforming gene" related to the cell gene. Most are replication defective but can be isolated free of helper virus.

[2]Designated by the initials of investigators or person from whom virus was obtained.

[3]Subacute type viruses do not transform cells in vitro; they have a long latency period in vivo and show no evidence of a transforming gene. These viruses all appear to be horizontally transmitted; in some cases, related sequences are found in cell DNA.

[4]The Friend leukemia virus complex contains a defective genome, codes for a smaller envelope glycoprotein not incorporated into virions, does not transform cells in vitro, and perhaps should be placed in a separate category.

[5]Viruses show distant relationship to mouse DNA, but not to DNA of primates; this indicates "ancient" horizontal transmission.

[6]There are 31 members of the human adenovirus group, and at least 12 of these induce tumors in newborn animals and/or cells in vitro.

productive infection. These host cells are known as permissive cells. By contrast, cells of other species are more or less nonpermissive. They do not support efficient multiplication. Instead, the viral DNA becomes integrated into that of the host, creating genetically altered virus-transformed cells capable of forming tumors in animals. With RNA tumor viruses, DNA transcribed from viral RNA by the enzyme reverse transcriptase is integrated into the cellular genome. An important distinction between the DNA and RNA tumor viruses is that the oncogenes of DNA viruses are contained within their genome as part of their lytic cycle. In contrast, retroviral oncogenes are acquired by recombinational events and are not part of the normal viral life cycle. In both cases the infected cells are altered in several fundamental charactcristics and are said to be transformed. Most work with oncogenic viruses is based on the in vitro model of cellular transformation. Virus-transformed cells develop a number of aberrant properties, as shown in Table 31–2 and Figure 31–1. Tumor cells and virus-transformed cells share many properties, and although the relationship is not precise, the ability of a virus to transform cells, particularly if the transformed cells can be shown to be tumorigenic in vivo, provides at least circumstantial evidence that the virus has the potential to induce tumors under natural conditions.

A detailed review of virology is beyond the scope of this chapter. For further details, the reader is referred to recent textbooks on this subject.*

DNA Tumor Viruses

The DNA tumor viruses serve as important models for understanding the mechanisms of viral oncogenesis. Three types of DNA viruses may be distinguished: the papovaviruses, the adenoviruses, and the herpesviruses. The DNA is double-stranded in all of these. It is circular and superhelical in the papovaviruses and linear in the other types. They all consist of a DNA and protein core surrounded by a protein and membrane coat. The coat of papovaviruses and adenoviruses has only protein, whereas that of herpesviruses also has a lipid component. Infection of cells by these DNA tumor viruses involves uncoating, possibly within the cell nucleus. Since the genome is too small to code for all necessary enzymes, the virus makes use of the host cell enzymes for its synthesis. RNA synthesized in the nucleus using host RNA poly-

viruses include papovaviruses, adenoviruses, and herpesviruses. The only RNA viruses known to cause cancer are retroviruses. When DNA tumor viruses infect cells of their natural hosts, viral DNA replicates, viral proteins are made, progeny virus particles are formed, and the cells lyse, initiating

*Luria, S.E., Darnell, J.E., et al.: *General Virology*, 3rd ed., New York, Wiley, 1978; Tooze, J.: *DNA Tumor Viruses. Molecular Biology of Tumor Viruses*, 2nd ed., Part 2, New York, Cold Spring Harbor Laboratory, 1980; Weiss R., Teich, N., et al.: *RNA Tumor Viruses. Molecular Biology of Tumor Viruses*, 2nd ed., New York, Cold Spring Harbor Laboratory, 1984.

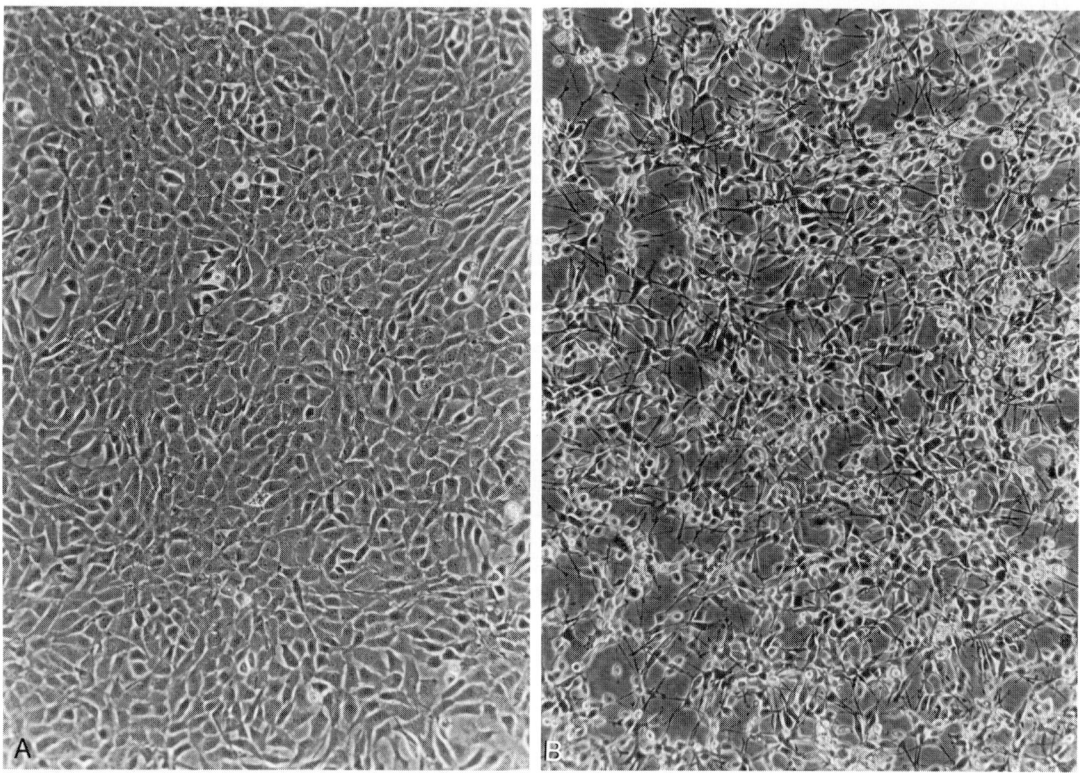

Figure 31–1. Morphologic changes in normal and transformed established cell lines. *A*, NIH 3T3 mouse fibroblasts, nearly confluent. *B*, NIH 3T3 cells transformed by Harvey murine sarcoma virus, nearly confluent. Phase contrast.

merase is of very high molecular weight and is processed into a cytoplasmic messenger RNA. Proteins are formed on polyribosomes in the cytoplasm and are then transported into the nucleus where the virions are assembled. Transformation is manifested by the appearance of changes outlined in Table 31–2.

PAPOVAVIRUSES

Papilloma viruses, polyoma viruses, and simian virus 40 (SV40) are classified as the papovaviruses (1).

Papilloma Virus. Warts (papillomas) are commonly found in many species of mammals. They arise by excessive proliferation of epithelial tissue and are usually benign growths that only rarely give rise to invasive cancers. Papilloma virus was first isolated and characterized from wild cottontail rabbits (2). It was the first tumor virus to be studied at the molecular level (3, 4).

The virus responsible for human contagious warts is very similar in its structure to the Shope papilloma virus (5–7). Formation of a human wart most likely starts by the transformation of a single basal cell into a cell that has lost its normal control over cell division. A wart is probably a clone of descendants from a single transformed cell (8). The benign tumors induced by human papilloma

Table 31–2. CHANGED PROPERTIES IN TRANSFORMED CELLS*

Morphologic and Behavioral Changes
Become more rounded, have looser attachment to substratum
Mutual orientation more random; lose contact inhibition of movement
Grow on top of each other
Grow in suspension; lose anchorage dependence
Grow to high or indefinite saturation density; kill themselves rather than stop growth
Have decreased serum requirement
Become invasive

Surface Alterations
Hyaluronic acid increased
Protein-linked sialic acid decreased
Ganglioside content of lipids decreased
250,000-dalton surface protein disappears
Sugar transport increased
More easily agglutinated by plant lectins
Surface proteins more mobile
Lipid fluidity not changed
Microfilaments (actin) cables disappear, but diffuse actin remains
Myosin-like filaments disappear
Microtubules disaggregate
Fetal antigens become evident
Virus-specific transplantation-rejection antigens appear

Nonsurface Biochemical Changes
Release of proteases
Transcription of fetal genes

*From Luria, S. E., Darnell, J. E., Jr., et al.: *General Virology,* 3rd ed. New York, John Wiley & Sons, 1978, p. 437.

viruses (HPV) rarely convert into malignant tumors, and common skin warts never become malignant (9–11). However, warts carried by people with epidermodysplasia verruciformis progress to invasive squamous cell carcinomas or intraepidermal carcinomas in about 25 per cent of cases (12, 13). There is strong evidence that HPV plays a role in genital neoplasias. DNA hybridization with HPV probes has demonstrated HPV in biopsy specimens of premalignant cervical lesions (14, 15). The genomes of two HPV types, HPV16 and HPV18, have been found to be associated with about 70% of invasive carcinomas of the uterine cervix (16–18, 148).

Polyoma Virus. A virus isolated by Gross (19, 20) was capable of producing parotid adenocarcinomas in mice. A variety of other tumors occasionally develop in newborn animals only, including medullary adrenal tumors, epithelial thymic tumors, mammary gland carcinomas, renal carcinomas, liver hemangiomas, and subcutaneous fibrosarcomas (21); therefore the virus was named polyoma virus. Tumor cells from polyoma virus–infected newborn mice do not contain mature viral particles (22, 23), suggesting that polyoma virus, and the morphologically similar papilloma virus, are present in tumor cells either as proviruses or as defective viruses lacking the late region of their genomes.

A set of antigens called the T (tumor) antigens was recognized in cells transformed by polyoma virus (24). When extracts from cells infected or transformed by polyoma virus are treated with sera from animals bearing tumors induced by polyoma virus, three major proteins with molecular weights of about 22,000, 55,000, and 100,000 daltons are immunoprecipitated. These are referred to as "small" T antigen, "middle" T antigen, and "large" T antigen, respectively (25–29). Middle T antigen is a transforming protein that transforms established cell lines (30–34). Middle T is associated with a tyrosine-specific kinase activity in vitro and is located at the plasma membrane (27, 35–38). A fraction of middle T has been shown to form a stable complex with pp60^{c-src}, the cellular homologue of the transforming protein of Rous sarcoma virus. The middle T–associated kinase may at least in part be a property of pp60^{c-src} rather than middle T itself (39). The biochemical basis of its ability to transform still remains unclear. Whereas middle T is sufficient to transform cells of established lines, the transformants are serum dependent. Middle T alone cannot transform primary rat embryo fibroblasts. Although large T lacks intrinsic oncogenic potential, it can relieve the serum dependence of normal and transformed cells, and leads to establishment/immortalization (40, 41). These two separate functions of establishment/immortalization and transformation will be discussed in greater detail below.

Simian Virus 40. Simian virus 40 (SV40) was discovered as an agent that multiplied silently in rhesus monkey kidney cultures used for propagating poliovirus for the development of a polio vaccine. SV40 was found to induce tumors when injected into newborn hamsters (42, 43) and can transform rodent fibroblasts.

SV40 and polyoma virus have similar structures, chemical compositions, and interactions with host cells. SV40 has not been associated with any disease in adult monkeys; its relationship with its natural hosts closely parallels the relationship between polyoma virus and the mouse. Under normal circumstances, neither polyoma virus nor SV40 behaves as a tumor virus in its natural host species. However, the oncogenic potential of both of these viruses can be revealed by injecting high concentrations of virus into either foreign hosts or natural hosts lacking a functional immune system. The similarities of tumors induced in vivo and those induced from cell lines transformed in vitro suggest the important relationship between viral transformation and tumorigenesis. Different lines of cells transformed by SV40 have different numbers of integrated copies of SV40 DNA at different chromosomal locations (44, 45). The only common feature of viral DNA in transformed cells is the presence of the early region of the SV40 genome, a section of viral DNA encoding early proteins. Cells can be transformed with that portion of the viral DNA molecule that contains the origin of viral DNA replication and the sequences that code for the T antigens (46, 46a).

While the genome of polyoma virus specifies the three early proteins (large, middle, and small T antigens), SV40 has only two early proteins, large and small T antigens. In SV40, the role of small T antigen is unclear. It may affect the cell cycle while large T brings about other changes required for transformation (47). The large T antigen seems to be required for both establishment and maintenance of transformation in SV40 (48–50).

Human Papovaviruses. Viruses related to SV40 and polyoma virus, or to antigens that cross-react with antisera against SV40, or both, have been detected in human tissues (51–54). JC virus was isolated from the brain tissue of a patient with progressive multifocal leukoencephalopathy. Another human papovavirus, BK, has been isolated from the urine of immunosuppressed renal transplant patients (52, 55–57) as well as from the urine of recipients with hemorrhagic cystitis who received bone marrow transplants (149). Both BK virus and JC virus can induce tumors in newborn hamsters (58, 59) and have been shown to transform hamster cells in vitro (60–63). BK and JC induce T antigens that cross-react with each other as well as with SV40 T antigen. There is significant sequence homology among the DNAs of JC, BK, and SV40 (64–68). There is no clear evidence associating human papovaviruses with human cancer.

HUMAN ADENOVIRUSES

Several types of human adenoviruses cause tumors when inoculated into newborn rodents (6, 70). Numerous serotypes of human adenoviruses differ greatly in their oncogenic potential (71). All adenoviruses, including those that do not cause tumors, can transform rodent cells in vitro (72, 73). The viral DNA sequences are integrated into cellular DNA (74, 75), and the early sequences are transcribed in transformed cells (76, 77). The presence of adenoviral DNA and messenger RNA within transformed hamster cells raised the possibility that adenoviral sequences might be found in certain human tumors if these were caused by human adenoviruses. So far, however, hybridization tests using viral DNA probes and DNA or RNA from over 200 different human cancers have given negative results (78).

Only a fraction of the adenovirus genome is required for transformation in vitro. The leftmost 11 per cent of the genome, including the two transcriptional units E1A and E1B, appears to be sufficient for transformation (79–82). The E1A region encodes three highly related viral proteins. All appear to be required for complete transformation by adenovirus 2 (83). The adenovirus E1A proteins have some structural resemblance to the proteins encoded by the *myc* and *myb* oncogenes, described below, suggesting that oncogenes of RNA and DNA tumor viruses may, at least in some instances, share evolutionary origins and functions (84). As with polyoma large T antigens, the adenovirus E1A has an establishment function, allowing primary cells to grow indefinitely in culture (85). As is the case with papovaviruses, transformation by adenovirus does not involve a unique site in the cellular DNA to which viral sequences are joined (86, 87).

Although expression of the left end of the adenoviral genome, consisting of the E1A and E1B regions, is essential for transformation of rodent cells in vitro, the relationship between transformation and the ability of transformed cells to cause tumors when injected into animals is not so clear. Cells transformed by the highly oncogenic adenovirus type 12, compared with the nononcogenic type 5, appear to be oncogenic because they escape from T cell immunity. This may be brought about by a reduction in the expression of Class I transplantation antigens and appears to be a function of the protein encoded by the E1A region (88). This difference in oncogenicity has also been attributed to differential killing of infected cells by natural killer cells and macrophages (89, 150).

HERPESVIRUSES

The herpesviruses are the largest and structurally most complex of the DNA tumor viruses. Some of these viruses can transform cells in vitro, or induce tumors, or both.

Renal adenocarcinomas of the leopard frog (*Rana pipiens*) have a probable viral origin, the Lucké herpesvirus (90). Marek's disease virus (MDV), the causative agent of avian neurolymphomatosis (Marek's disease), has been successfully grown in culture and has the morphology of typical herpesviruses (91–93).

Herpesviruses and Human Cancers

Human Herpes Simplex Virus. Indirect evidence suggests that herpesviruses may also be oncogenic for humans. Transformation of rodent cells is obtained with either herpes simplex virus (HSV) type 1 or HSV type 2 if the ability of the virus to multiply and kill the cells is reduced either by ultraviolet irradiation or by using temperature-sensitive mutants at the nonpermissive temperature (94–97). These transformed cells produce no infectious virus, and they contain one or a few copies of the HSV genomes.

A fragment of HSV-1 DNA has been shown to transform rodent cells (98–99). However, attempts to detect viral sequences in cells transformed by this HSV-1 fragment have been unsuccessful. Two different fragments of HSV-2 DNA, neither homologous to the HSV-1 fragment, have been found to transform rodent cells (99–102). The mechanism of HSV transformation is not clear. Failure to detect a consistent set of viral sequences or a specific protein in transformed cells or human tumors suggests a "hit-and-run" mechanism whereby HSV may act as a mutagen, or may induce cellular oncogenes by the expression or insertion of HSV sequences (101).

HSV-2 has been implicated in the etiology of squamous cell carcinoma of the uterine cervix, initially by seroepidemiologic studies (103–107). Viral antigens are expressed in tumor cells (108–111) and viral RNA and DNA have been detected in some tumors (111–113). Studies in mice show that repeated application of inactivated HSV-2 to the cervix produces premalignant and malignant lesions. Immunization prior to exposure of the cervix to virus confers a protection against the induction of cervical carcinoma, strongly supporting a causative role of HSV-2 in cervical carcinoma in mice (114).

Epstein-Barr Virus. The Epstein-Barr virus (EBV), widespread in humans, is associated with three diseases: infectious mononucleosis, Burkitt's lymphoma, and nasopharyngeal carcinoma. Infectious mononucleosis is an extensive but self-limited lymphoid proliferation (115). Burkitt's lymphoma is a B-cell lymphoma endemic in central Africa and New Guinea and sporadic throughout the world (see Chapter 30). Most endemic lymphomas contain EBV DNA, whereas most of the sporadic ones do not. The host range of EBV in vitro is restricted to B lymphocytes of human origin (116–120) and to lymphocytes of some nonhuman primates (121–123). When normal lymphocytes are exposed to EBV, the cells, previously unable to grow in culture, change into lymphoblast-like cells capable of continuous culture (116, 124, 125). The cells of most EBV-transformed cell lines established from tissue of tumors contain from 20 to 60 EBV genomes per cell. Whether the EBV DNA in transformed cells is integrated into the cellular DNA remains to be established. Cell lines containing EBV DNA also contain the EBV nuclear antigen(s) (EBNAs) in their nuclei. A specific region of the EBV genome was demonstrated to immortalize monkey kidney cells (126). However, following isolation and propagation, these cells had a finite capacity to grow in soft agar and failed to produce tumors in mice. Examination of the cell line for EBNA proved negative. The EBV genome specifying latent infection membrane protein (LMP) appears to be a transforming gene, which may account for many aspects of EBV-induced cell transformation (415).

After EBV infection initiates a block in B lymphocyte differentiation, a genetic rearrangement involving a cellular oncogene may lead directly or indirectly to lymphoma formation. In Burkitt's lymphoma cells, reciprocal translocations are observed between the long arm of chromosome 8 (8q24) and either the long arm of chromosome 14 (14q32), the short arm of chromosome 2 (2p12), or the long arm of chromosome 22 (22q11) (127, 128) (see Chapter 43). Gene mapping studies have shown that c-*myc*, the cellular homologue of the avian myelocytomatosis retrovirus transforming gene, is localized at 8q24 (129–131) and that the three immunoglobulin gene loci map at breakpoints involved in the translocation: immunoglobulin heavy-chain genes are located at 14q32 (132, 133), kappa light chains at 2p12 (134), and lambda light chains at, or close to, 22q11, (135, 136). This correlation suggests an association of immunoglobulin gene rearrangements with the occurrence of these specific translocations. There appear to be substantial differences between translocated c-*myc* genes in Burkitt's lymphoma compared with normal sequences. These differences presumably arise from somatically introduced mutations associated with the DNA joining during chromosomal translocation. In several Burkitt's lymphoma cell lines, the sequence of the first exon differs from the normal exon 1 sequence (137, 138). No coding function can be assigned to exon 1 of c-*myc*, suggesting that this segment has a role in the control of transcription of c-*myc* (139). The rearranged c-*myc* is often placed so that it cannot utilize immunoglobulin regulatory elements (140, 141). Since the level of c-*myc* messenger RNA is often, but not always, elevated in Burkitt cells (137, 142–144), the translocation may lead to a deregulation of the c-*myc* gene (137–145). Even though there may be no unifying hypothesis to account for both the variety of translocation points and the apparent consistent activation of the c-*myc* gene, the common feature is probably deregulation of the translocated gene. Indeed, there may be several ways in which chromosomal translocation can achieve this deregulation (416). While c-*myc* expression is dependent on the normal cellular growth cycle, it may lose its cycle-dependent regulation in transformed cells (146, 147). However, the specific role that the c-*myc* protein plays in normal cells is still obscure (see below).

The human c-*fgr* oncogene, corresponding to the viral v-*fgr* oncogene of Gardner-Rasheed feline sarcoma virus, is expressed in Burkitt's lymphoma cell lines naturally infected with EBV. Moreover, when Burkitt's lymphoma cell lines are deliberately infected with EBV, a 50-fold increase of the steady-state c-*fgr* mRNA concentration is observed (417). This demonstrates the induction of a proto-oncogene in response to infection by a DNA tumor virus and suggests that one step in EBV-induced B-cell immortalization may involve transcriptional activation of the *fgr* oncogene in response to an EBV-encoded function.

EBV and Nasopharyngeal Carcinoma. Nasopharyngeal carcinoma, consisting of anaplastic epithelial cells abundantly infiltrated with lymphocytes, is most frequently seen in Southeast Asia, particularly among Cantonese Chinese. Patients with this tumor have elevated titers of antibodies against EBV antigens (151–158). After successful radiotherapy, the titers usually decline (154–156). Multiple copies of the EBV genome (100 to 150 per cell) are present in the epithelial cells, which have receptors for EBV (159) and contain EBNA (160–162), but are not present in the infiltrating lymphocytes (163–165). These observations suggest a strong causal relationship between EBV and the development of nasopharyngeal carcinoma. As with Burkitt's lymphoma, EBV may represent the "first hit" of a multistep process leading to transformation.

Another undifferentiated tumor with histopathologic characteristics similar to those of undifferentiated nasopharyngeal carcinoma is the lymphoepithelioma-like carcinoma of the thymus. The serologic profile, presence of EBNA in the carcinoma cells, and high level of viral genomes detected in the DNA of a patient suggest a role of the Epstein-Barr virus in the genesis of a thymic carcinoma, similar to its role in undifferentiated nasopharyngeal carcinoma (418).

HEPATITIS B VIRUS

Hepatitis B virus (HBV) exhibits characteristics associated with oncogenic viruses. Chronic infection with this virus incurs a high risk of hepatocellular carcinoma (approximately 40 per cent). The finding of viral integrations in genomic DNA prepared from primary hepatomas of chronically infected patients has suggested a possible role of these integrations in hepatocarcinogenesis (419, 421). While integration can occur at variable sites for both the cellular and viral DNAs (165a, 165b, 419–423), integration may place the viral sequence next to a liver sequence that bears a striking resemblance to both an oncogene (v-erbA) and the supposed DNA-binding domain of the human glucocorticoid receptor and human estrogen receptor genes (165c). This suggests that this gene, which is usually silent or transcribed at a very low level in normal hepatocytes, becomes inappropriately expressed as a consequence of HBV integration, contributing to cell transformation and thus relating hormonal and HBV carcinogenesis. However, no HBV oncogene has yet been identified (421–423).

RNA Tumor Viruses

In 1908, Ellermann and Bang first demonstrated a viral cause for avian myeloblastosis (166). Three years later Rous induced sarcomas in chickens from cell-free extracts (167). In 1936 Bittner demonstrated the transmission of mouse mammary carcinoma through the milk of mothers to offspring (168). Based on the experiments of Bittner, Gross postulated that mouse leukemia was also caused by a virus and that occurrence of the disease in successive generations of mice was due to transmission of virus from parents to offspring (169). Since these initial studies, much has been learned about this group of viruses, subsequently demonstrated to be RNA viruses, and their role in the causation of tumors.

CHARACTERISTICS AND MOLECULAR BIOLOGY

Taxonomy, Structure and Replication. Retroviruses, or RNA tumor viruses, are characterized by the presence of an enzyme, reverse transcriptase, in the virions. Various oncoviruses induce tumors. In addition, this family contains nononcogenic members. The virions are enveloped and are about 100 nm in diameter. The capsid encloses the single-stranded RNA genome. These viruses are classified according to their appearance in thin-section electron microscopy (Table 31–3): Mature virions of B particles have an eccentric core and C particles a central core; D particles have a morphology intermediate between B and C particles; A particles, found only within cells, have a double shell with a clear core.

The viral genome consists of two identical strands of RNA, which are held together by a dimer linkage near the 5' end. Three viral genes participate in the replication of viruses (Fig. 31–2): *gag* (for *g*roup-specific *a*nti*g*ens), which encodes structural proteins located in the interior of the virus particle; *pol*, which encodes a virus-associated polymerase, reverse transcriptase; and *env*, which encodes the glycoprotein constituents of the membranous envelope that encloses the virus particle. Some retrovirus genomes contain these genes alone; others contain an additional transforming gene or oncogene, v-*onc*, that may transform the host cell but is not required for viral replication (see below).

RNA-directed DNA synthesis is a central event in the replication of retroviruses. Reverse transcriptase copies the RNA genome of the virus into DNA. As a consequence, retroviruses are the only viruses whose genomes assume both RNA and DNA forms. Their unique mode of replication consists of an intermediate proviral DNA and integration into the host cell. The ends of retroviral RNA are different from the ends of retroviral DNA. The RNA has a small terminal repeat, while the DNA has a large terminal repeat, or LTR (170, 171) (Fig. 31–2). The LTRs appear to contain regulatory signals for promotion, initiation, and polyadenylation of transcripts (172, 172a). Deletion of specific nucleotides at either end of the LTR results in replication-competent but integration-defective virus, suggesting that the LTRs are required for integration, but that integration of retrovirus DNA is not required for retrovirus gene expression (172a, 173).

The replication of the viral RNA into double-stranded DNA, shown in Figure 31–3, is mediated by the viral polymerase reverse transcriptase (174, 175). The resulting linear or circular DNA is then inserted, at random positions, in the host cell genome (176). The proviral DNA consists of the gene-coding sequences of DNA flanked by the LTR regions, which do not encode for proteins. Progeny RNA is generated by transcription of the integrated provirus.

The virion contains a number of structural proteins, including internal proteins, envelope glycoproteins, and reverse transcriptase. All of the internal proteins are encoded by the *gag* genes, are synthesized as a single high-molecular-weight polyprotein, and are formed by cleavage of this protein. Newly synthesized proteins, along with RNA molecules, organize themselves at the surface of the cell, and this complex buds from the plasma membrane to form an infectious virion. Once established, virus production continues indefinitely and is usually limited by the life span and the growth state of the infected cell.

Pathogenesis. Retroviruses consist of both en-

Table 31–3. RETROVIRIDAE*

Genus	Subgenus	Species
Cisternavirus A Mice, hamsters, guinea pigs		
Oncovirus B Mammary carcinomas in mice		Mouse mammary tumor viruses: MMTV-S (Bittner's virus) MMTV-P (GR virus), MMTV-L
Oncovirus C	Avian	Rous sarcoma virus (RSV)
		Rous-associated virus (RAV)
		Other chicken sarcoma viruses
		Leukosis viruses (ALV)
		Avian erythroblastosis virus (AEV)
		Avian myeloblastosis virus (AMV)
		Avian myelocytomatosis virus
		Reticuloendotheliosis viruses
		Pheasant viruses
	Mammalian	Murine sarcoma viruses (MSV)
		Murine leukosis virus G (Gross or AKR virus)
		Murine leukosis viruses (MLV)—F, M, R (Friend, Moloney, Rauscher viruses)
		Murine radiation leukemia virus
		Murine endogenous viruses
		Rat leukosis virus
		Feline leukosis virus
		Feline sarcoma virus
		Feline endogenous virus (RD114)
		Hamster leukosis virus (HLV)
		Porcine leukosis virus
		Bovine leukosis virus
		Primate sarcoma viruses (woolly monkey, gibbon ape)
		Primate sarcoma-associated virus
		Primate endogenous viruses, baboon endogenous virus (BaEV), stumptail monkey virus (MAC-1), owl monkey virus (OMC-1)
		Human T cell lymphotropic virus (HTLV-I, -II, -III)
	Reptilian	Viper virus
Oncovirus D Primates		Mason-Pfizer monkey virus (MPMV)
		Langur virus
		Squirrel monkey virus
Lentivirus E		Visna virus of sheep
		Maedi virus
Spumavirus F		Foamy viruses of primates, cats, humans, and bovines

*Modified from Davis, B. D., Dulbecco, R., et al.: *Microbiology*, 3rd ed. Hagerstown, MD, Harper & Row, 1980, p. 1244.

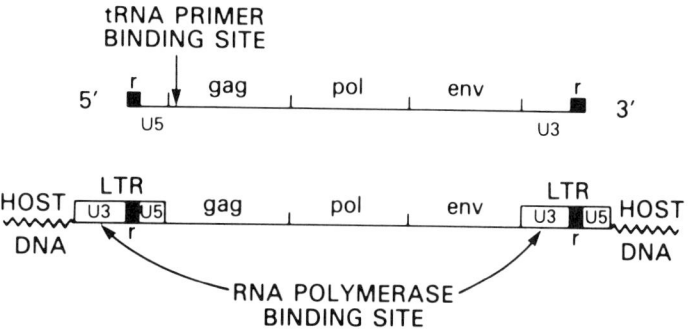

Figure 31–2. Structures of the RNA genome and integrated DNA of retroviruses. LTR, long terminal repeat sequences; U3, unique sequences at 3' end of viral genome; U5, unique sequences at 5' end of viral genome. (From Gallo, R. C., and Wong-Staal, F.: Retroviruses as etiologic agents of some animal and human leukemias and lymphomas and as tools for elucidating the molecular mechanism of leukemogenesis. Blood *60*:547, 1982. Reprinted by permission.)

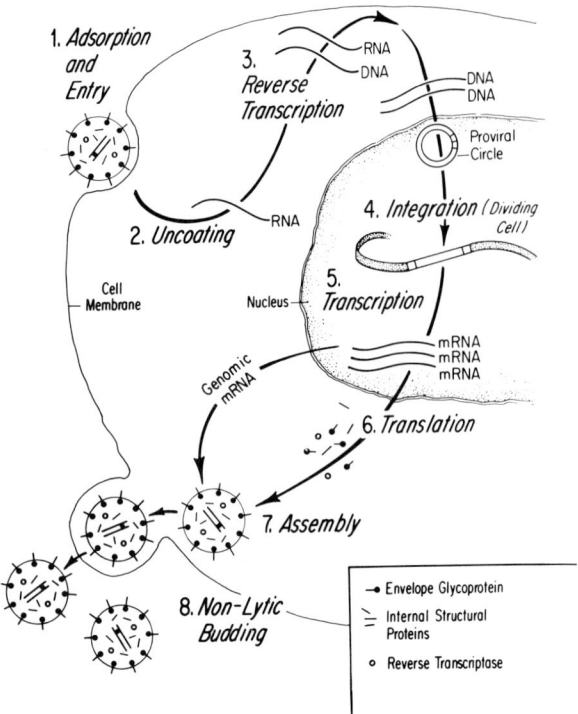

Figure 31–3. An overview of the life cycle of a prototypical wild type retrovirus. A simplified schematic view of the major events in the life cycle of replication-competent retroviruses is shown. Details are described in the text. *1*, Virion particle becomes attached to cell surface via glycoprotein receptor in cell membrane. *2*, Uncoating of particle takes place in cytoplasm of cell, exposing RNA genome. *3*, An exact DNA copy of RNA is produced by viral-encoded reverse transcriptase. *4*, Double-stranded DNA enters nucleus and integrates into infected cell chromosome. *5*, Integrated provirus becomes transcriptionally active, producing genomic RNA and RNA for translation into proteins. *6*, RNA translated into virion proteins and genomic RNA encapsulated into virion particle. *7*, Virion particle shed by non-lytic budding. (Courtesy of Dr. David A. Williams.)

dogenous and exogenous strains. Endogenous viruses are stably integrated proviruses within host cellular DNA in the germ line and are genetically transmitted from one generation to another. On the other hand, exogenous viruses are not incorporated into the cellular genome until after infection of the host cell. Retroviruses may be transmitted horizontally from one host animal to another or vertically by congenital infection of offspring or by genetic transmission through the gametes.

Retroviruses are commonly identified according to the species from which the virus has been isolated. The host range of retroviruses is an important means of classification. The ecotropic viruses are those that will grow in cells of the species from which they are isolated. In contrast, the xenotropic viruses are endogenous to one species but cannot replicate well in that species, generally because of a receptor block. They tend to have a wide range for replication in cells of heterologous species. Rare amphotropic strains multiply in cells of both kinds.

Retroviruses may be replication-defective or nondefective depending on whether or not the viruses possess genomes deficient in the genes that code for structural viral components. Transcription of the integrated viral genome of nondefective viruses leads to the constant production of virus by the transformed cell. When the viral genome is defective, transcription of the integrated viral genome does not result in the production of virus. Virus production may be restored by infection with a second, replication-competent "helper" virus.

Retroviral infections may induce a variety of pathologic syndromes. The diseases most commonly associated with retroviruses are malignant tumors, proliferative diseases, anemias, and slow degenerative diseases. Tumors consist of sarcomas, carcinomas, and leukemias and lymphomas. The majority of retrovirus-induced tumors fall into this third category.

In order to better understand the genetic determinants of retrovirus-induced neoplastic transformation, the role of viral oncogenes, and their relationship to cellular oncogenes, the following is a brief description of some of the more intensively investigated retroviruses.

Some retroviruses cause the appearance of malignant tumors within a few days of infection. These acutely oncogenic viruses induce specific kinds of leukemias or solid tumors in animals. Most of these viruses also transform cells in vitro. The viruses contain a sequence of genetic material (v-*onc* gene) that confers this high oncogenic potential (Fig. 31–4A). In most cases, incorporation of this sequence is accompanied by a loss of other viral genes that are essential for replication; a coinfected nondefective virus is then required as helper. The tumors that appear early after infection are probably not clonal growths but involve transformation of many target cells. Acutely oncogenic retroviruses induce specific kinds of leukemias or solid tumors. They are found only rarely and sporadically in nature, suggesting that each isolate represents a new recombinant virus. They are not naturally transmitted from one host to another. Nevertheless they are powerful tools in studies of experimental and natural oncogenesis (177).

The acute leukemia viruses consist of murine and Avian strains. These viruses have a broader range of target cells than the non-defective viruses, a much higher probability of transformation, and a much shorter latent period before the induction of neoplasia. The Abelson virus, an acute leukemia virus isolated from a steroid-treated, Moloney virus–infected mouse, produces B cell lymphomas,

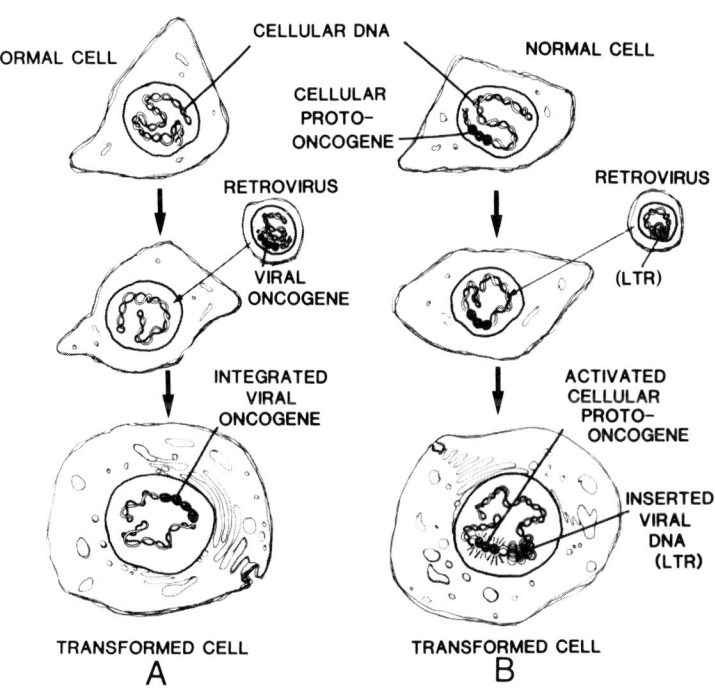

Figure 31-4. Cell transformation by retroviruses. *A*, Mechanism of cell transformation by acutely oncogenic viruses. A retrovirus containing a v-*onc* sequence integrates into cellular DNA and expresses a protein product mimicking the effect of normal cellular genes, leading to cell transformation. *B*, Mechanism of cell transformation by slowly oncogenic viruses. A retrovirus that, in contrast to the acutely oncogenic viruses, does not contain a v-*onc* sequence, integrates into cellular DNA. If a viral LTR is adjacent to the cellular proto-oncogene, excessive quantities of the proto-oncogene product may be synthesized, transforming the cell.

and also transforms fibroblasts in vitro (178, 179). The Abelson virus complex is composed of two viral components, the helper, Moloney murine leukemia virus (Mo-MLV), and a replication-defective virus, Ab-MLV. Ab-MLV contains a gene, v-*abl*, that encodes a phosphorylated protein exhibiting an associated tyrosine-specific protein kinase activity (180–182). Fibroblasts transformed by Ab-MLV lose binding sites for epidermal growth factor (183). Direct transformation of hematopoietic cells in vitro by Ab-MLV has also been demonstrated (184–186). Most Ab-MLV–transformed lymphoid cells resemble an intermediate stage in B lymphocyte development in which both heavy-chain genes, but not light-chain genes, are rearranged (187). It appears that Ab-MLV directly affects a variety of committed progenitor cells from different lineages, rather than the uncommitted stem cell (188, 189). Ab-MLV–induced neoplasms have been shown to contain cellular transforming genes by transfection assay that are distinct from Ab-MLV sequences, suggesting that v-*abl* expression may induce early events in the neoplastic process and that secondary activation of a distinct cellular transforming gene may be involved in progression to neoplasia (190).

The Avian erythroblastosis virus (AEV), the avian myeloblastosis virus (AMV), and the myelocytomatosis virus (MC29) produce leukemias in chickens. Precise identification of the target cells is still somewhat equivocal, but the AEV targets appear to be erythrocyte precursors less mature than the late CFU-E precursors (191). The targets for MC29 are macrophage-like (191), whereas AMV usually transforms an earlier cell of the myeloid lineage (191, 192). Transformation by these different defective leukemia viruses results from blocks at specific points in various hematopoietic lineages (193). These viruses encode putative transforming genes related to genetic material in normal cells (see below); the viral genes appear to mimic the effect of normal cellular genes. The viral genes may be aberrant in function, or, being controlled by viral promoters, they may be inappropriately expressed. They seem to effectively block further maturation of the host cell. Using a temperature-sensitive mutant of AEV, at the nonpermissive temperature, transformed erythroid cells continue along the path of erythrocyte development and synthesize hemoglobin (194).

The sarcoma viruses induce sarcomas in animals with high efficiency and a short latent period, and they transform fibroblasts in vitro. Two groups of avian viruses have been identified: the various strains of Rous sarcoma virus (RSV), most of which are nondefective for growth and have a unique genomic structure, and the defective sarcoma viruses, including Fujinami sarcoma virus (FuSV). RSV has acquired a wide host range accompanied by a broad pathogenic spectrum. The oncogenic range of FuSV is similar to that of RSV. This broad oncogenic potential of RSV is reflected in its ability to transform a wide range of cell types in vitro. The replication-competent RSV strains carry the *src* gene. Other replication-defective avian sarcoma viruses contain distinct oncogenes with tyrosine-specific protein kinase activity: *fps* (found in FuSV), *yes*, and *ros*. These other oncogenes are distantly related to the *src* oncogenes of RSV. Changes in cell phenotype that result from the expression of the RSV *src* gene are discussed below.

The murine sarcoma viruses (MSV), which are all replication-defective, have leukosis virus genomes with large deletions that are partially replaced by the substitution of sequences derived from the cells in which each virus was isolated. Kirsten MSV (Ki-MSV) and Harvey MSV (Ha-MSV) were isolated following passage of MLV in rats. Both isolates contain related oncogene sequences (*ras*; see below), and both produce erythroleukemias as well as sarcomas. Like Ab-MLV–transformed fibroblasts, Ki-MSV–transformed fibroblasts lose epidermal growth factor (EGF) binding sites (195). Cells transformed by Ki-MSV and several other mammalian sarcoma viruses secrete polypeptides capable of inducing morphologic changes and anchorage-independent growth of nontransformed cells (196). These sarcoma growth factors (SGFs) appear to compete with EGF for the same membrane receptors. The role of SGFs in the initiation and maintenance of viral transformation has not yet been defined, but similar factors have been isolated from several human tumors (197). The Moloney strain of MSV (Mo-MSV) was isolated from a mouse infected with Mo-MLV. This replication-defective virus contains *mos* oncogene sequences.

In contrast to the acutely oncogenic viruses, the nonacute or "slow" oncogenic viruses are nondefective leukosis viruses with low oncogenic potential and are often recovered from animals with lymphomas or leukemias. Their genomes carry no identifiable oncogene (Fig. 31–4*B*). They can multiply in cells without causing cell transformation. Because they contain all the genes required for multiplication, they require no helper. These viruses transform only a small proportion of specific target cells (mostly hemopoietic-lymphoid) in certain stages of development. The induced tumors may be fast growing and highly malignant. The "slowness" of these viruses refers to the long latent period between infection and manifestation of disease. Tumors induced by slow retroviruses usually appear in animals that are chronically viremic; yet these tumors appear to be clonal in origin. This means that many more cells become infected with virus than progress to form a malignant tumor.

The nondefective avian lymphoid leukosis viruses (LLVs) produce neoplasms in susceptible flocks. The tumors are typified by an enlarged liver and spleen, infiltrated with B lymphoblasts, and anemia, with a long clinical latency. The LLVs are not known to encode a gene product that mediates this oncogenic change (198–201). Integration of an LLV provirus into the host DNA results in the viral coding sequence being flanked by two LTRs (202, 203). Since the proviral LTRs are identical, it is possible that the downstream (3′) LTR, like its upstream (5′) counterpart, can act as a transcriptional promoter and can stimulate transcription of adjacent cellular genes. The model of insertional mutagenesis ("promoter insertion") predicts that LLV causes neoplasms when this downstream LTR transcribes elevated levels of an adjacent cellular *onc* gene (200) (Fig. 31–5). In support of this, it has been shown that all tumors retain at least one LLV provirus (199–201), and the proviral DNA is found in the same region of the host genome (200, 201), in the vicinity of c-*myc*, the cellular homologue of the transforming gene of the myelocytomatosis virus (204). Most of these tumors contain novel RNAs that appear to have c-*myc* sequences and are more abundant than the usual transcripts of the c-*myc* locus, owing to initiation by the adjacent LTR (204). LLV uses the same mechanism in erythroblastosis induction by activating a different cellular oncogene, c-*erbB* (205). Activated cellular oncogenes, detectable by transfection, have also been reported in B cell lymphomas induced by LLV (206). However, this

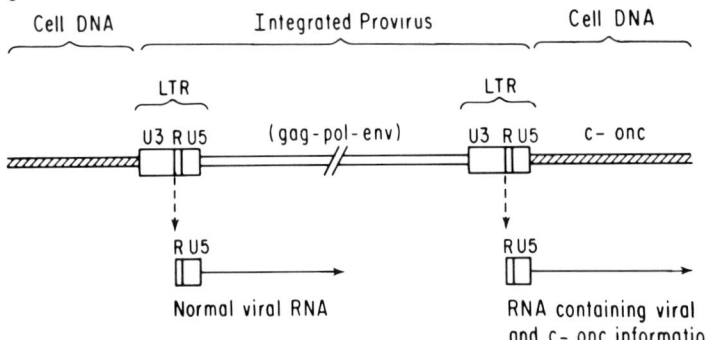

Figure 31–5. Structure and transcriptional products of the integrated avian lymphoid leukosis virus. The LTRs, shown greatly enlarged to emphasize structural details, are approximately 350 base pairs in length, and are composed of sequences derived from the 5′ (U5) and 3′ (U3) ends of genomic RNA, and a short sequence (R) present at both ends of genomic RNA. Synthesis of viral genomic and messenger RNAs initiates within the left LTR. Initiation within the right LTR could result in elevated transcription of adjacent cellular sequences. If, as a rare event, the provirus integrated adjacent to a potentially oncogenic cellular gene (c-*onc*), transcriptional activation of this gene could lead to neoplastic transformation. (From Hayward, W. S., Neel, B. G., et al.: *Advances in Viral Oncology*, Vol. 1, Klein, G. [ed.], New York, Raven Press, 1982, p. 212.)

transforming gene is unrelated to the activated c-*myc* gene (206) and is found at an unlinked chromosomal site.

Moloney (Mo-MLV) and AKR (AKR-MLV) murine leukemia viruses lacking viral transforming genes can also induce lymphomas in a variety of mouse strains after a long latency period. MLV provirus is frequently integrated into a specific chromosomal site (207), and a distinct host gene is activated by the integration of provirus in its vicinity (208). As with LLV, a second cellular transforming gene has been reported to be present, detected by transfection in neoplasms induced by MLV (209).

Feline leukemia virus (FeLV), like LLV and MLV, belongs to the class of slowly oncogenic viruses carrying only replicative genes and no specific transforming gene. The majority of spontaneous lymphoid tumors in the cat are associated with FeLV infection. In contrast to induction of lymphomas by LLV, in which c-*myc* activation occurs by retrovirus promoter insertion near c-*myc*, recombinant FeLV proviruses contain the c-*myc* oncogene in the DNA of naturally occurring feline lymphoid tumors. This suggests that a c-*myc*–containing leukemia virus may be transmitted contagiously between cats (210–212).

Mouse mammary tumor viruses (MMTV) induce mammary adenocarcinomas that derive from the secretory epithelial cells of the mammary gland. This type of virus differs from most other RNA tumor viruses in morphology (B type) and morphogenesis. MMTV can be transmitted by two principal routes: (1) by congenital infection of suckling mice via milk-borne virus, and (2) genetically as an endogenous provirus. Like the avian and murine leukemia viruses that induce tumors after lengthy latency and fail to transform cultured cells, MMTV appears to carry genes required for replication only (213–215). There is no evidence for a viral *onc* gene. Virus-induced tumors almost always carry new proviruses (216, 217). It appears that induction of mammary carcinomas by MMTV involves provirus activation of specific cellular genes. A high percentage of virally induced tumors contain an acquired MMTV provirus inserted in either of two defined integration regions, termed *int-1* and *int-2*, and provirus insertion is accompanied by expression of specific RNA transcripts for these regions (218–220). These regions lack homology with retroviral oncogenes (218–220) and do not appear to be related to a cellular transforming gene detectable by transfection (220, 221). It is suggested that activation of these cellular genes is not sufficient for the development of malignancy and may represent part of a multistage process (222). Glucocorticoid hormones stimulate the production of MMTV in a variety of host cells (223) and boost the concentration of MMTV RNA in these cells (224). This effect on MMTV gene expression appears to be a direct action of the hormone (225), and the MMTV LTR interacts directly with the hormone-receptor complex (226, 227).

Human RNA Tumor Viruses. Numerous claims have been made for evidence of human retrovirus infection. At this time there appear to be several distinct retroviruses occurring as natural infections of human populations. One is a foamy virus with no known associated disease. The others are C type viruses associated with certain forms of adult T cell leukemia and lymphoma, and a related virus associated with the acquired immunodeficiency syndrome (AIDS).

Human T cell lymphotropic virus (HTLV-I) was first isolated in the United States from a patient with an aggressive form of cutaneous T cell lymphoma (228), and was subsequently found to be associated with clusters of adult T cell leukemia-lymphomas (ATL) in various parts of the world, including Japan and the Caribbean (229). While sharing some features with classic chronic lymphocytic leukemia of T cell origin and with typical Sézary syndrome, ATL appears to be a distinct syndrome (230). A subtype of HTLV, termed HTLV-II, has been described from cell lines of two patients with atypical T cell variants of hairy-cell leukemia (231, 231a).

HTLV is not an endogenous virus, but rather is an acquired virus with T cell tropism (228–232). HTLV-related sequences are not present in the DNA of normal uninfected human cells but are readily detected from HTLV-positive tumor cells. Unlike most other nonacute transforming retroviruses, both HTLV-I and HTLV-II are capable of transforming normal human peripheral lymphocytes by co-cultivation with virus-infected cells (233–236). At present, the mechanism of transformation by these retroviruses remains unknown. Neither HTLV-I nor HTLV-II contains a recognized oncogene, nor do these viruses appear to activate cellular oncogenes by *cis*-insertion of retroviral promoter (or enhancer) sequences, since the sites of proviral integration vary from tumor to tumor (236a). An unusual feature of the HTLV-I and HTLV-II viruses is that they encode a gene whose protein product greatly stimulates the expression of other viral genes controlled by the LTRs (236b–236h, 238). The elements of this autostimulatory control mechanism are the *trans*-activator proteins *tat*-I (42 kilodaltons [kD]) and *tat*-II (38 kD), which are encoded by a long open reading frame (LOR) within the pX region (237), at the 3' end of the viral genomes, and the *trans*-acting responsive sequences TAR-I and TAR-II, which are located within the viral LTRs (236i). It has been suggested that the *tat* proteins may also be able to alter the expression of certain cellular genes involved in T cell growth (236j). Introduction of the *tat* gene of HTLV-II into a T lymphoid cell line results in the induction of both interleukin-2 (IL-2) receptor and IL-2 gene expression (236k). Hybridization studies show that the DNA sequences of HTLV-II are distinct from those of HTLV-I (236).

Another related virus, human immunodeficiency virus (HIV, alternatively known as HTLV-III and lymphadenopathy-associated virus [LAV]), has been isolated from patients with AIDS (239–244). The association of HIV and AIDS is discussed in detail in Chapter 28.

RETROVIRAL TRANSFORMING GENES AND THEIR PRODUCTS

As discussed above, the tumor-inducing retroviruses may be divided into two groups: those carrying nucleotide sequences of cellular origin (*onc* genes) that are capable of directing synthesis of all or part of a protein required for oncogenic transformation, and those viruses that do *not* appear to contain coding sequences for proteins other than those normally required for viral replication. This section will focus on the structure of the transforming genes and their protein products.

Viruses possessing *onc* sequences have been isolated from a number of animal species. To distinguish among these *onc* elements, a three-letter designation has been assigned, as listed in Table 31–4 (245). The names for the transforming sequences are derived from the names of the viruses in which the sequences were first encountered. The distinction between viral and cellular versions of related sequences is maintained by using v- and c- as prefixes. Many of the v-*onc* sequences identified are synthesized as part of a fusion protein in which the aminoterminal domain is encoded by viral replicative genes (*gag* or *gag* and *pol*), and the carboxyterminal domain is encoded by the v-*onc* in question. Yet other v-*onc* genes appear to be expressed as proteins encoded entirely by the transforming sequence. Identification of the products of *onc* genes in infected cells has been greatly facilitated by the production of appropriate antisera. In addition, nucleotide sequencing, in vitro translation, and physical characterization of mRNAs have provided further information.

RNA virus oncogenes (v-*onc*) are derived from normal cellular genes, or "proto-oncogenes" (c-*onc*) (246, 247). It appears that in each case, a virus has acquired the cellular gene by transducing the gene as part of its genome during retroviral replication (Fig. 31–6). The exact mechanisms by which v-*onc* proteins transform cells are not known. Several of these proteins display similar functions. In addition, products of some retroviral transforming genes have similar locations within cells. The significance of these homologies among *onc* sequences will now be reviewed.

RSV was the first retrovirus to be isolated and characterized. The product of its oncogene became the first retroviral transforming gene product to be identified. After prolonged efforts, antisera to RSV-induced tumors were obtained that precipitated a 60,000-dalton protein (248). In vitro translation studies showed the immunoprecipitated protein, $pp60^{v-src}$, to be the product of *src* (249). The availability of antisera against the protein product of *src* led to the discovery of an associated protein kinase activity in vitro (250, 251). Modification of proteins by phosphorylation is thought to be a widely used mechanism for regulating the activity of these proteins (252, 253). Studies with temperature-sensitive mutants of *src* indicate that the kinase activity can be attributed to the $pp60^{v-src}$ polypeptide itself, rather than to an associated protein (251, 254, 255). Further evidence was provided by the synthesis of the *src* protein in bacteria and the observation of kinase activity in this protein (256, 257). Unexpectedly, the amino acid acceptor of the phosphate was shown to be tyrosine, rather than the serine or threonine residues that account for over 99 per cent of the phosphoamino acids in avian and mammalian cell proteins (258). The same property was demonstrated for the protein kinase activity encoded by v-*abl*, the oncogene of Ab-MLV (181). The discovery that the polyoma virus middle T protein was phosphorylated in vitro on tyrosine residues (259), and subsequent similar findings with the products of *yes*, *fps*, *ros*, and *fes*, suggest that tyrosine phosphorylation may be an important factor in transformation by many viral proteins. A tenfold rise of total phosphotyrosine occurs upon transformation of RSV-transformed cells (258).

Most evidence indicates that the bulk of $pp60^{v-src}$ in infected cells is bound to the inner surface of the plasma membrane (260, 261). There are probably two major sites of serine phosphorylation and a single phosphotyrosine residue $pp60^{v-src}$. A domain of about 8000 daltons at the amino terminus anchors the protein to the plasma membrane (262, 263). The active site for phosphotransfer resides in the carboxyterminal half of $pp60^{v-src}$ (264, 265). It is possible that the aminoterminal domain regulates both kinetic features and substrate specificity of the kinase activity, perhaps by allosteric effects. It appears that myristylation of $pp60^{v-src}$ at its amino terminus mediates attachment to membranes, and that the latter is in turn required for transformation (265a–d). Transformation by v-*src* can be accounted for by both point mutations and genetic substitution, perhaps by increasing the specific activity of $pp60^{v-src}$, by changing its preference for protein substrates, or by conferring constitutive activity on a protein that

Table 31-4. CELLULAR ONCOGENES*

Acronym	Origin	Species of Isolation	Chromosomal Location		Subcellular Localization of Virally Encoded Protein	Activity of Virally Encoded Protein
			Human	*Mouse*		
src	Rous sarcoma virus	Chicken	20		Plasma membrane	Tyrosine kinase
yes	Y73 sarcoma virus	Chicken	18			Tyrosine kinase
fps = fes	Fujinami (ST feline) sarcoma virus	Chicken (Cat)	15	7	Cytoplasm	Tyrosine kinase
abl	Abelson murine leukemia virus	Mouse	9	2	Plasma membrane	Tyrosine kinase
fgr	Gardner-Rasheed feline sarcoma virus	Cat				Tyrosine kinase
trk	Colon carcinoma	Human			Plasma membrane	Tyrosine kinase
met	Osteosarcoma	Human	7			Tyrosine kinase
kit	H24 feline sarcoma virus	Cat			Cytoplasm	Tyrosine kinase
mos	Moloney murine sarcoma virus	Mouse	8	4	Cytoplasm	Serine/threonine kinase
raf-mil	3611 murine sarcoma virus	Mouse	3	6	Cytoplasm	Serine/threonine kinase
erbB	Avian erythroblastosis virus	Chicken	7		Plasma membrane	Growth-factor receptor
neu	Neuro-, glioblastomas	Rat	17		Plasma membrane	Growth-factor receptor
fms	McDonough feline sarcoma virus	Cat	5		Plasma membrane	Growth-factor receptor
ros	UR II avian sarcoma virus	Chicken			Plasma membrane	Cell surface receptor
sis	Simian sarcoma virus	Woolly monkey	22	15	Cytoplasm	Growth factor
Ha-ras-1	Harvey murine sarcoma virus	Rat	11	7	Plasma membrane	Guanosine triphosphate binding
Ki-ras-2	Kirsten murine sarcoma virus	Rat	12		Plasma membrane	
N-ras	Neuroblastoma, leukemia, sarcoma	Human	1			
myc	Avian MC29 myelocytomatosis virus	Chicken	8	15	Nuclear matrix	DNA binding
N-myc	Neuroblastoma	Human	2		Nuclear matrix	DNA binding
L-myc	Small cell lung cancer	Human	1			
myb	Avian myeloblastosis virus	Chicken	6		Nuclear matrix	
fos	FBJ osteosarcoma virus	Mouse	2		Nucleus	
ski	Avian SKV770 virus	Chicken	1		Nucleus	
ets	Avian myeloblastosis virus	Chicken	11		Nucleus	
p53	—	Mouse	17		Nucleus	
erbA	Avian erythroblastosis virus	Chicken	17		Cytoplasm	
rel	Reticuloendotheliosis	Turkey	2		Cytoplasm	
mam	Mammary carcinoma	Mouse, human				
mas	Epidermoid carcinoma	Human			Plasma membrane	
mel	Melanoma	Human				
dbl	B-cell lymphoma	Human				
mcf-3	Mammary carcinoma	Human				
ref	Lymphoma	Human				

*Modified and expanded from a table originally appearing in Land, H., Parada, L. F., et al.: Science 222:772, 1983. Copyright 1983 by the AAAS.

Note: Other genes that may function as oncogenes have been discovered but are still incompletely characterized: *int-1* and *int-2* are altered by mouse mammary tumor virus provirus insertion; *MLVI-1* and *MLVI-2* are altered by murine leukemia virus provirus insertion. These four genes may therefore be activated in a fashion similar to the avian leukosis virus-mediated activation of *myc*. Two other sequences, human Ha-*ras*-2 and Ki-*ras*-1, are clearly related to two genes listed in this table; it remains unclear whether they are complete genes or pseudogenes.

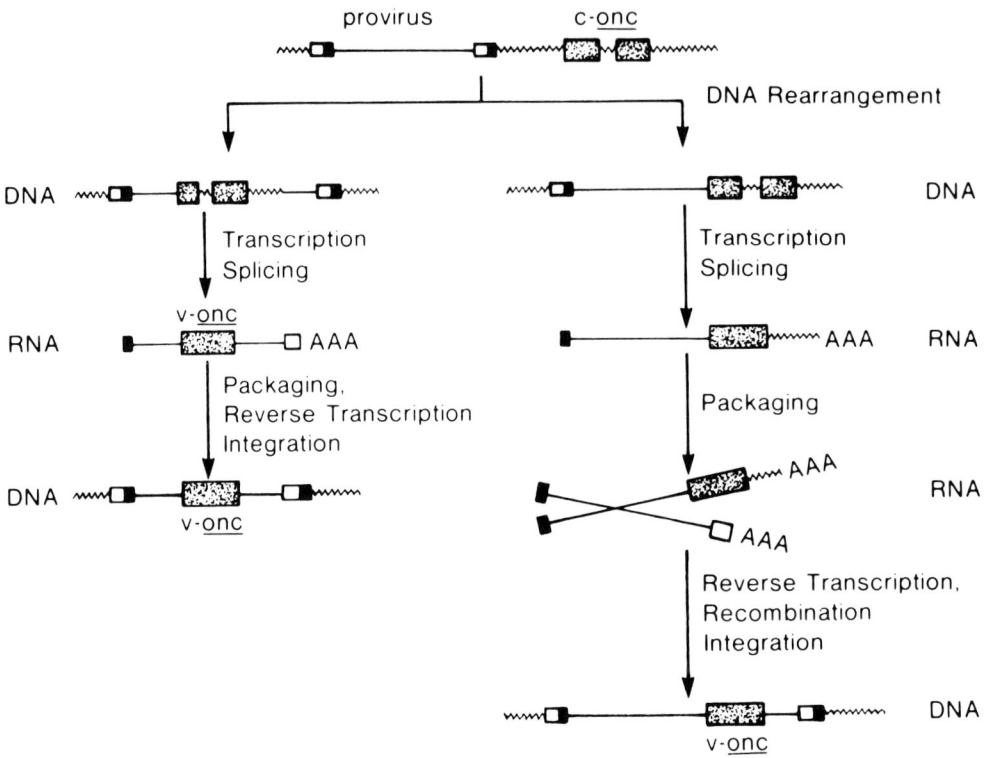

Figure 31–6. Model for transduction by retroviruses. The drawing illustrates how cellular proto-oncogenes might be transduced by pre-existent retroviruses. An intact retroviral provirus fortuitously integrates upstream from a cellular proto-oncogene. The characteristic terminal redundancies of the provirus are illustrated by black and white boxes, exons of the cellular proto-oncogene by stippled boxes, viral nucleic acid by straight lines, and cellular nucleic acid by jagged lines. A postulated rearrangement of DNA begins transduction and could take either of two forms, as illustrated, resulting in the integration of cellular proto-oncogene DNA sequences within the retrovirus genome. (From Bishop, J. M.: Cellular oncogenes and retroviruses. Ann. Rev. Biochem. 52:327, 1983. Reproduced, with permission, from the Annual Review of Biochemistry, Vol. 52. © 1983 by Annual Reviews Inc.)

is normally regulated by allosteric devices (265e, f; 324).

Efforts to identify cellular protein targets of phosphorylation by pp60$^{v\text{-}src}$ yielded a 36,000-dalton phosphoprotein, p36 (266). This protein was later shown to be phosphorylated at tyrosine residues following transformation by several oncogenes or after treatment with epidermal growth factor (267–270). However, the functional role of p36 has yet to be established. Another possible target protein (50,000-dalton) was noted to be associated with pp60$^{v\text{-}src}$ in immunoprecipitates (258). Three proteins phosphorylated at tyrosine in RSV-transformed cells have been shown to be glycolytic enzymes: enolase, phosphoglycerate mutase, and lactate dehydrogenase (271). However, the role of these structural modifications in the regulation of glycolysis is not known. More recently, purified pp60$^{v\text{-}src}$ has been shown to phosphorylate phosphatidylinositol (272). The product of inositol lipid biosynthesis may play an important role in proliferation and other cellular responses and will be discussed in detail below. Several of the identified transforming gene products have proved to be tyrosine-specific protein kinases (Table 31–4). The biochemical functions of the other proteins are currently being investigated.

Studies of simian sarcoma virus (SSV), an acute transforming retrovirus of primate origin, have produced a relationship between oncogenes and growth factors. Biologically active SSV DNA has been isolated by cloning (273), and its nucleotide sequence, including that of its cell-derived transforming sequence, v-*sis*, has been determined (274). Using antisera prepared against synthetic peptides derived from sequence analysis of v-*sis*, the primary v-*sis* gene product in SSV-transformed cells, p28$^{v\text{-}sis}$ was identified (275). Computer comparison of the p28$^{v\text{-}sis}$ amino acid sequence with the partial amino acid sequence determined for purified platelet–derived growth factor (PDGF) (276) revealed extensive homology between these two proteins (277–279). Examination of p28$^{v\text{-}sis}$ in light of this finding has confirmed the close structural and immunologic relationship with PDGF (280). Expression of this PDGF-like molecule appears to be responsible for the abnormal regulation of growth in SSV-transformed cells. This suggests that v-*sis* may induce transformation by causing overproduction of a hormone that stimulates growth of the same cell that has secreted it.

The genome of avian erythroblastosis virus (AEV) contains two putative oncogenes, v-*erbA* and v-*erbB*. The v-*erbA*-oncogene codes for 75,000-

dalton *gag-erbA* fusion protein, p75$^{gag-erbA}$, located predominantly in the cytoplasm (281, 282). There is extensive homology between the thyroid hormone receptor and the v-*erbA* gene (282a, b). The product of the v-*erbB* oncogene is a plasma membrane glycoprotein, gp74^{erbB} (282–284). Studies with viral mutants carrying large deletions in either v-*erbA* or v-*erbB* indicate that v-*erbB* is the principal transforming gene of AEV (285). In the absence of v-*erbA*, v-*erbB* causes fibroblast transformation and induces an aberrant type of leukemic erythroblast, which requires complex growth conditions and which partially differentiates into mature erythrocytes. In contrast, v-*erbA* in combination with v-*erbB* is capable of arresting the leukemic cells in an early stage of differentiation (286). Using temperature-sensitive AEV mutants, it appears that these erythroblasts become insensitive to the transforming functions of gp74^{erbB} after progression to a certain stage of differentiation (287). The amino acid sequence for a portion of the gp74^{erbB} protein suggests that the *erbB* gene is distantly related to the *src* gene family (288). Amino acid sequence analysis demonstrates that peptides for human epidermal growth factor (EGF) receptor very closely match a portion of the v-*erbB* transforming protein (289). The v-*erbB* gene appears to encode only the transmembrane region of the EGF receptor and the internal domain associated with tyrosine kinase activity (288, 289a, 289b). This suggests that the *src* related subset of oncogenes, including v-*erbB*, may be derived from cellular sequences encoding growth factor receptors, inducing transformation through expression of uncontrolled receptor functions. In fact, the kinase activity associated with the v-*erbB* protein is constitutive, and the appearance of this protein on the plasma membrane seems to be a precondition for transformation (289c, d).

In cells transformed by avian myeloblastosis virus MC29, the v-*myc* gene is expressed as a fusion protein containing a transformation-specific region and the aminoterminal region of the *gag* protein (290). The protein, designated p110$^{gag-myc}$, has a molecular weight of 110,000 daltons. It is located in the nucleus and binds to double-stranded DNA (291). The oncogenicity of avian myeloblastosis virus (AMV) has been attributed to the v-*myb* gene, which encodes a 45,000-dalton protein (292). Another avian leukosis virus, E26, also contains the v-*myb* oncogene. While both AMV and E26 induce myeloblastosis in vivo and transform myeloblasts in vitro, E26 has the additional capacity to induce erythroblastosis in vivo and to transform erythroblasts (293, 294). A second putative oncogene, v-*ets*, located adjacent to v-*myb*, has been identified in E26, which may account for the additional transforming properties of E26, or may potentiate the transforming properties of the v-*myb* gene (295). The exact role of v-*myc* and v-*myb* in tumorigenesis is not known, but the function of c-*myc* in malignant neoplasms appears to be an important one and will be discussed below.

The Harvey and Kirsten strains of murine sarcoma virus contain related viral oncogenes, v-Ha-*ras* and v-Ki-*ras*. The only known gene product of the viruses is a 21,000-dalton protein, p21^{ras}, which is required for cellular transformation (296) and is present at relatively high levels in virally transformed cells. A related but distinguishable p21 is constitutively expressed at low levels in normal cells of many vertebrate species (297), as well as in yeast (298–300). The vast majority of p21^{ras} appears to be associated with the inner surface of the plasma membrane and is not exposed on the cell surface (301). Two biochemical properties have been associated with the products of v-*ras*, efficient binding to guanine nucleotides (especially GTP and GDP) (302), and an apparent autophosphorylation at threonine residues (303); however, neither function has been clearly implicated as the mechanism by which p21^{ras} transforms cells. Although the mechanism of cellular transformation remains obscure, strong evidence favors a major role for c-*ras* in a number of human cancers, as discussed below.

CELLULAR ONCOGENES

DNA sequences homologous to v-*onc* genes, termed cellular oncogenes (c-*onc*) or proto-oncogenes, have been identified in normal uninfected cells, including human cells. These cellular oncogenes appear to be the evolutionary progenitors of the v-*onc* genes. Recombinational events between the retroviral genome and these genes lead to their acquisition and activation by retroviruses. These proto-oncogenes are highly conserved in evolution and appear to represent normal cellular genes that are not normally linked to viral DNA. The strong evolutionary conservation as well as the finding that these genes are expressed in many tissues of each species examined suggests an essential function in cellular metabolism for these proto-oncogenes (304, 305). This section will detail what is known about these cellular genes, their relationship with human neoplasms, and their possible role in normal cellular metabolism.

Detection of Cellular Oncogenes in Tumors of Nonviral Etiology

As previously mentioned, nucleic acid hybridization studies revealed that the RSV-associated v-*src* gene is derived by a recombinational event from the normal cellular gene (246). Using the other known retroviral v-*onc* genes as probes, additional cellular oncogenes have been detected by hybridization (245).

Yet another approach to the identification of cellular genes implicated in oncogenesis uses the DNA-mediated gene transfer procedure, DNA transfection (306). High-molecular-weight DNA is prepared from donor cells possessing the transformed phenotype. This DNA is precipitated in calcium phosphate and incubated with untransformed recipient NIH 3T3 mouse fibroblasts. The DNA is introduced into a small proportion of these cells and is stably incorporated into their genomes and expressed. Many of these transfected cells assume the transformed phenotype and can be detected by the formation of foci of refractile cells against a background monolayer of normal fibroblasts. This transfer of phenotype indicates the presence of dominantly acting transforming information in the donor cell DNA. Such transforming genes can then be transmitted at high efficiencies in secondary transfection assays.

Initial attempts using DNA from 3-methylcolanthrene–transformed mouse cells suggested that cellular genes controlling cell proliferation were apparently activated by the process of chemical transformation and could be assayed by DNA transfection (307, 308). These oncogenes were subsequently shown to be versions of the c-Ki-*ras* gene (309, 310). Other tumors induced by chemical carcinogens have also been found to contain *ras* genes (311, 312).

Efforts to demonstrate transforming activity in human tumor DNA resulted in the identification of an activated cellular oncogene from a bladder carcinoma cell line (313, 314). Subsequently, activated oncogenes have been detected by transfection of DNAs from a variety of human malignancies, from both tumor-derived cell lines and freshly obtained specimens, as detailed below. However, only a small proportion of all tumor cell DNAs (10 to 30 per cent) yield transformed foci upon transfection (313–316). Attempts to identify these genes responsible for transformation have in some cases implicated cellular oncogenes, as discussed below (317–319).

Characterization and Molecular Biology

As with other cellular genes, there is great diversity among cellular oncogenes, which range in size from a few kilobase pairs to over 40 kilobase pairs. They contain one or more introns ranging in size from a few base pairs to several thousand base pairs (305). Cellular oncogenes behave as classic Mendelian loci, occupying the same positions within the genome of a given species, and are present in all members of a species (320, 321). Cellular oncogenes are highly conserved over a wide range of species.

Transcription from c-*onc* genes occurs in every vertebrate species examined and in a variety of tissues. The amount of RNA produced is extremely small in many cells (1 to 10 copies per cell), with occasional exceptions in both normal tissues and tumor cells. Each c-*onc* gene gives rise to distinct RNA species whose sizes are generally conserved in various cell types and in different species.

Cellular oncogenes and their viral derivatives are remarkably similar. For example, the nucleotide sequences of v-*mos* and c-*mos* differ at only 25 out of 1157 nucleotides, with the deduced amino acid sequences of the viral and cellular proteins differing by only 11 amino acids (322). Similarly v-*myb* and c-*myb* have 15 differences among 1197 nucleotides, resulting in 11 amino acid substitutions (323). It seems likely that differences between viral and cellular oncogenes have arisen as mutations in the viral genes subsequent to their transduction from cells.

PROTEINS ENCODED BY CELLULAR ONCOGENES

Because of the small quantities available, characterization of oncogene proteins has been difficult. The viral and cellular forms of pp60^{src} have the same molecular weight, display antigenic cross-reactivities, yield closely related peptide maps, are both associated with the plasma membrane, are both phosphorylated with phosphoserine in the aminoterminal and phosphotyrosine in the carboxyterminal domains, and are both protein kinases specific for tyrosine (305). However, the biologic properties of c-*src* and v-*src* may be quite different. A chimeric molecular clone permitting the expression of c-*src* in mammalian cells, under the direction of transcriptional controls derived from SV40, gave rise to substantial quantities of pp60^{c-src} with demonstrable protein kinase activity when introduced into rat cells in culture (324). However, the cells remain phenotypically normal, even though pp60^{c-src} was produced in quantities greater than the amount of pp60^{v-src} required to achieve neoplastic transformation of the same cells, suggesting that the pathogenic properties of v-*src* are attributable to damage inflicted upon the gene during or subsequent to transduction. Further analysis of the differences between v-*src* and c-*src* may help reveal the role of cellular oncogenes in tumorigenesis. The product of *fps* (pp98^{c-fps}) displays tyrosine-specific protein kinase activity (324a). By contrast, the c-*abl* protein has failed in tests for protein kinase (324b), whereas the capability of v-*abl* proteins to phosphorylate tyrosine is well established.

The proteins encoded by the cellular and viral *ras* genes also appear to be similar, with molecular weights of about 21,000 daltons, sharing of some antigenic determinants, related peptide maps and ability to bind guanine nucleotides with high affinity (297, 303, 325, 326). But the proteins encoded by the cellular *ras* do not carry out autophosphorylation described for the viral proteins, apparently because they lack the threonine residue on which the viral proteins are phosphorylated (357). The viral and, presumably, the cellular versions of p21^{ras} are located on the inner plasma membrane (301). Cells of the yeast *Saccharomyces cerivisiae*, which contain disruptions of either of two genes that are members of the *ras* oncogene family, are viable, but haploid yeast spores carrying disruptions of both genes fail to grow (327, 328). This suggests that the gene products may be required early in the cell division cycle. The products of yeast *RAS1* and *RAS2* stimulate the adenylate cyclase of yeast (328a). It has been suggested that *ras* proteins are regulators of adenylate cyclase, with functions similar to those of the G proteins that transmit signals from receptors on the surface of mammalian cells by activating adenylate cyclase (328b). The analogies between the *ras* and G proteins are strong (328c–e); however, there is as yet no direct evidence that *ras* proteins play a role in regulating adenylate cyclase.

While the chicken and human c-*myc* genes share homology with the v-*myc* gene of MC29, they differ in 5' coding regions (329, 330). On this basis it is suggested that their protein products may have different functions. The transforming sequence of the avian acute leukemia virus, E26, contains two distinct oncogenes: v-*myb* and v-*ets*, fused together. The product of the c-*ets* proto-oncogene is a 56-kD polypeptide, p56, which may be involved in regulating the growth of lymphoid cells (330a).

The c-*erbB* gene encodes the cell surface receptor for epidermal growth factor (289, 289a). As described above, v-*sis* has been completely sequenced and shown to code for the protein p28^{v-sis}. This protein is closely related in its amino acid sequence and structural properties to human platelet-derived growth factor (PDGF), implying that the two proteins are derived from the same or closely related cellular genes. The human c-*sis* gene has been molecularly cloned, and it has been demonstrated that this human proto-oncogene is the structural gene encoding one of the two major polypeptides of PDGF (331, 332).

The *mas* oncogene was detected by the tumorigenicity assay, following cotransfection with DNA isolated from a human epidermoid carcinoma. This gene efficiently induces tumorigenicity. The *mas* gene encodes a protein with seven hydrophobic regions that are potential transmembrane domains, suggesting that *mas* is an integral membrane protein. The structure of the *mas* protein is unique among cellular oncoproteins and may represent a new functional class (332a).

A transforming gene present in a human colon carcinoma, *trk*, contains gene sequences of both tropomyosin and a previously unknown protein tyrosine kinase. The predicted protein (641 amino acids) encoded by this oncogene seems to have been formed by a somatic rearrangement that replaced the extracellular domain of a putative transmembrane receptor by the first 221 amino acids of a non-muscle tropomyosin molecule (332b).

The c-*fos* gene, the cellular homolog of the oncogene carried by the FBJ murine osteosarcoma virus, encodes a 55-kD nuclear phosphoprotein, p55$^{c\text{-}fos}$, of unknown function (332c, 332d). A series of observations suggests that c-*fos* gene expression is associated both with specific differentiation pathways and with normal cell growth (332e).

The *neu* oncogene, frequently activated in neuro- and glioblastoma of BDIX rats, is related in DNA sequence to the *erbB* gene (332f). Yet *neu* has only limited homology with *erbB*, the two genes reside on different chromosomes, and the encoded protein, p185, bears only limited homology to the EGF receptor (332g). Rat and human cDNA clones of the *neu* oncogene have been isolated (332h–j). The *neu* product appears to be a transmembrane protein, made up of a cysteine-rich extracellular region, a transmembrane domain, and an intracellular portion consisting in part of a tyrosine kinase domain. p185 has an associated tyrosine-specific kinase activity (332k). It does not, however, bind EGF, and appears to be the receptor for an as yet unidentified growth factor. The activating event is a point mutation converting a valine to a glutamic acid in the transmembrane domain. The same mutation in the *neu* gene occurs in four independent tumor lines (332l). It is assumed that the activated protein has constitutive, rather than ligand-regulated, protein kinase activity. This suggests that the transmembrane domain is much more important in transmembrane signaling than was previously appreciated.

The c-*fms* proto-oncogene product is a 165- to 170-kD glycoprotein with associated tyrosine kinase activity. The murine c-*fms* proto-oncogene product and the cell surface receptor for macrophage colony-stimulating factor (CSF-1) are related and possibly identical molecules (332m). CSF-1 is a lineage-specific macrophage growth factor that stimulates hematopoietic precursor cells to form colonies containing mononuclear phagocytes (332n).

The *met* oncogene activated in vitro by treatment of a human osteogenic sarcoma (HOS) cell line with N-methyl-N'-nitronitrosoguanidine (MNNG) is related to the tyrosine kinase gene family. Treating HOS cells in vitro with MNNG, a known clastogenic carcinogen, resulted in the fusion of two chromosomally disparate loci, *met* and *tpr* (translocated promoter region), generating the active *met* oncogene (332o–q). A tight genetic linkage of the *met* proto-oncogene locus has been established in pedigree analysis to the hereditary genetic disease cystic fibrosis (CF), allowing the assignment of the CF gene to chromosome 7q21-31 (332p).

Little is known of the other cellular oncogene products. One is tempted to deduce their functions from the properties of their viral homologues (305). However, modifications of retroviral transforming proteins and their cellular homologs can also differ. For example, the products of v-*ras*, v-*fps*, and v-*abl* are phosphorylated in vivo, whereas their cellular counterparts are not (324a, b). A number of cellular oncogenes have been located on human chromosomes (see Chapter 43). They appear to be widely dispersed throughout the human genome.

Cellular Oncogenes and Cancer

As mentioned earlier, transfection analysis has allowed the detection of activated oncogenes in a variety of human malignancies, including carcinomas of the lung, breast, bladder, pancreas, and colon, myeloid and lymphoid leukemias, lymphomas, sarcomas, and neuroblastomas, as shown in Table 31–5 (209, 221, 313–316, 318, 333–335, 335a). Examination of homologies by DNA hybridization, schematized in Figure 31–7, between retroviral oncogenes and transforming sequences defined by transfection revealed that the human bladder carcinoma cell line EJ/T24 is homologous to the Harvey murine sarcoma virus oncogene, v-Ha-*ras* (317–319). The oncogene of the EJ/T24

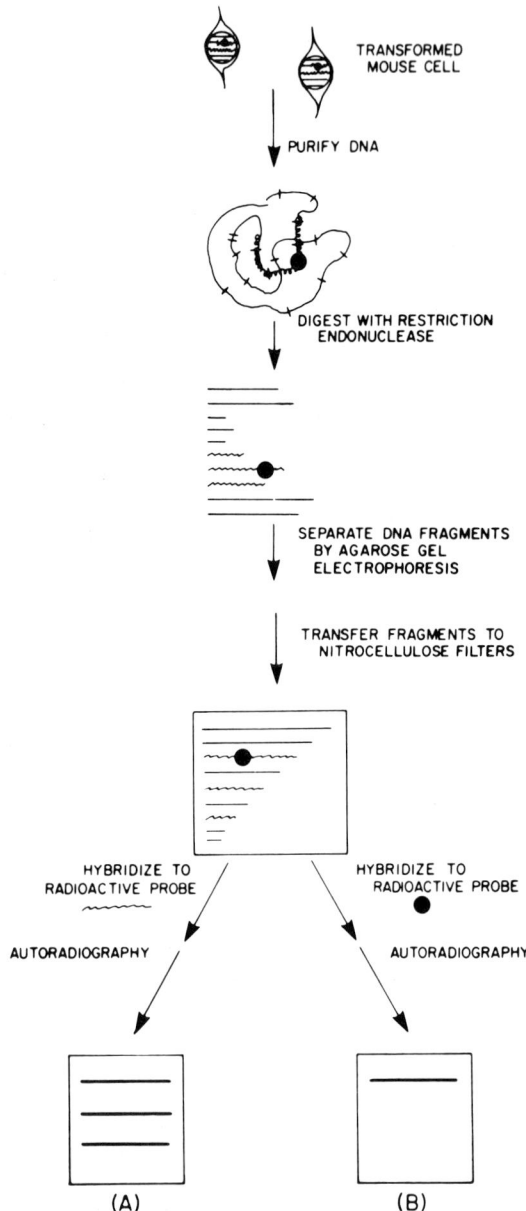

Figure 31–7. Hybridization analysis of human oncogenes. For analysis by nucleic acid hybridization, DNA is purified from mouse cells transformed by human-tumor DNA. Human DNA (represented by the undulating line) containing an oncogene (represented by the circle) has become covalently associated with the mouse genomic DNA. A restriction endonuclease is used to cleave DNA into unique fragments by producing double-stranded breaks at specific recognition sites (hatch marks). The DNA is fractionated by size on an agarose gel and transferred in situ to a nitrocellulose filter. The fragments of human DNA within and near the oncogene will hybridize to a human-DNA probe (Path A). These fragments, which are unique for each oncogene, will be visualized as bands after autoradiography. The DNA may also be hybridized to a probe representing a viral oncogene (Path B). If homology exists, a band will appear. (From Krontiris, T. G.: The emerging genetics of human cancer. New Engl. J. Med. *309*:406, 1983. Reprinted by permission of the New England Journal of Medicine.)

Table 31–5. TRANSFORMING ACTIVITY OF HUMAN-TUMOR DNA*

Source of DNA	No. Positive/No. Tested
Carcinomas	13/49 (27%)
Lung	4/11
Bladder	3/9
Breast	1/6
Colon	4/6
Pancreas	1/2
Other†	0/15
Leukemias and lymphomas	9/18 (50%)
Myeloid	1/3
B cell lineage	6/7
T cell lineage	2/3
Unclassified	0/5
Other‡	4/19 (21%)
Total	26/86 (30%)

*From Krontiris, T. G.: New Engl. J. Med. *309*:405, 1983. Reprinted by permission of the New England Journal of Medicine.

†Cervix, head and neck, kidney, skin, ovary, and esophagus.

‡Glioblastoma, astrocytoma, melanoma, neuroblastoma, rhabdomyosarcoma, osteosarcoma, and fibrosarcoma. One of three neuroblastoma DNAs, two of seven fibrosarcoma DNAs, and a rhabdomyosarcoma DNA were positive.

cell line was isolated by molecular cloning (334, 336, 337) and was shown to consist of a sequence of approximately 6000 nucleotides, which contained the entire transforming activity. When compared with its proto-oncogene, which has no effect on cellular phenotype, the oncogene clone is potently oncogenic. The DNA sequence of the cloned oncogene was compared with the sequence of the normal, nontransforming proto-oncogene, revealing that a single base change in the codon corresponding to amino acid 12 (changing glycine to valine) of the *ras*-associated protein, p21, confers transforming activity on the gene (338–340). This mutation, altering the encoded protein, is sufficient to activate the proto-oncogene. In another experiment, providing the proto-oncogene with new transcriptional controls that elevated the level of p21^{ras} also led to activation of the proto-oncogene and induced tumorigenic transformation (341). Activation of c-Ha-*ras* appears to be the result of a somatic event selected for within the growing tumor. Structural mutations that activate *ras* gene transforming activity do not seem to alter the encoded protein's known biochemical parameters and do not affect its ability to bind guanine nucleotides (342).

Using viral oncogenes to probe the structures of other human oncogenes from transfection assays, the majority of oncogenes detected in solid tumors were identified as human homologues of the *ras* family of retroviral oncogenes (Table 31–6). While the human c-Ha-*ras* gene is responsible for the transforming activity of DNA from three human urinary tract tumors, a single lung carcinoma, and a single melanoma (317–319, 343–345), activation of c-Ki-*ras* seems to be more common, accounting for the transforming activity detected in DNA from human carcinoma cell lines of the colon, lung, gallbladder, and urinary bladder, and from an acute lymphocytic leukemia cell line (316, 318, 346, 347, 357). Activation of the c-Ki-*ras* gene is also present in primary tumor isolates of human lung, colon, pancreatic, and ovarian carcinomas, as well as a rhabdomyosarcoma (316, 349–351). Activation of the third member of the human *ras* gene family, N-*ras*, occurs in many tumor cell types, including neuroblastoma, fibrosarcoma, leukemia, and lymphoma cell lines, as well as primary tumor isolates of colon carcinoma, melanoma, and acute myelogenous leukemia (343, 345, 346, 352, 353, 355, 355a, 355b). The *ras* oncogene protein, p21, has been detected in prostate cancers and correlates strongly with histologic tumor grade (355c). Another study demonstrated that 21 per cent of fresh human tumors expressed elevated levels of *ras* gene proteins (355d). Activation of *ras* genes has been detected in about 20 per cent of all neoplasms. Molecular characterization of the human Ha-*ras*, Ki-*ras*, and N-*ras* loci indicates that these genes acquire malignant properties by single point mutations that affect either the 12th or 61st amino acid residues of their p21 proteins (338–340, 343, 344, 351, 358–360).

The c-*myc* gene is altered (amplified/rearranged) in association with a broad spectrum of human neoplasms, including acute and chronic leukemias, APUDoma, Burkitt's lymphoma, fibrosarcomas, glioblastomas, and lung and ovarian carcinomas (131, 142, 363–367, 367b).

Examination of a variety of freshly obtained human malignancies, including renal, gynecologic, gastrointestinal, lung, breast, sarcomatous, lymphoreticular, and hematologic malignancies, revealed several patterns of expression of c-*onc* genes: c-*fos*, c-Ha-*ras*, and c-Ki-*ras* were expressed in nearly all of the tumors examined; c-*abl*, c-*fes*, c-*fms*, and c-*myb* were expressed infrequently, with c-*fes* and c-*myb* found in 9 out of 10 hematologic malignancies, c-*fes* expressed in all 4 lung malignancies, and c-*abl* found in 2 cases of chronic leukemia and 1 case of acute leukemia; and c-*erbA*, c-*erbB*, c-*mos*, c-*rel*, c-*sis*, and c-*yes* were not detectable in any of the tumors (361). Another study demonstrated alterations of c-*myc*, c-Ha-*ras*, or c-*myb* in more than one third of human solid tumors (362a). The c-*myb* gene is expressed in malignant hematopoietic cell lines and in primary hematopoietic tumors. The c-*myb* gene product has been found within the nucleus of leukemic cells, suggesting that c-*myb* may be involved in human leukemia (362b). Amplification and elevated expression of the c-*erbB*-2 (identical to *neu*) has been observed in the MKN-7 gastric cancer cell line (367c). Similarly, a transforming gene closely related to v-*raf* has been detected and molecularly cloned from a surgically removed stomach cancer (332t). These results suggest that a variety of cellular oncogenes may be important in malignancy. However, until the levels of expression of cellular oncogenes are determined in corresponding normal tissues at the same stage of differentiation, one must be cautious in ascribing oncogene expression as being inappropriate and causal in tumor formation.

MECHANISMS OF PROTO-ONCOGENE ACTIVATION

As previously described, a single point mutation replacing glycine by valine at the 12th amino acid residue converts the Ha-*ras* proto-oncogene into a potent oncogene in the human bladder carcinoma cell line EJ/T24 (338–340). Another activated version of this gene encodes an aspartate residue at this same position (360). Alteration of the 12th residue of the Ki-*ras* gene also leads to oncogenic activation (359, 368). The Ha-*ras* oncogene of a human lung carcinoma has a mutation affecting amino acid 61 (344). These changes appear to affect the structure of the encoded proteins and

Table 31–6. RELATIONSHIPS OF TRANSFECTION EXPERIMENTS WITH RETROVIRUS-ASSOCIATED ONCOGENES

Oncogene	Cell Line	Tumor	Reference
Ha-*ras*	EJ/T24	Bladder carcinoma	317–319, 343
	HS-242	Lung carcinoma	344
	SK-MEL-146	Melanoma	345
Ki-*ras*	CCRF-CEM	ALL cell line	346
	Duke	Colon adenocarcinoma	347
	SW480	Colon carcinoma	343
	SK-CO-1	Colon carcinoma	316
	A2233	Colon carcinoma	
	LX-1	Lung small cell carcinoma	318, 347
	Calu-1	Lung carcinoma	343
	A549	Lung adenocarcinoma	347
	A2182	Lung carcinoma	316
	A427	Lung carcinoma	316
	1615	Lung carcinoma	316
	A1698	Bladder carcinoma	316
	1189	Pancreatic carcinoma	316
	PANC-1	Pancreatic carcinoma	348
	A1604	Gall bladder carcinoma	316
	1085	Rhabdomyosarcoma	316
	OVCA-1	Ovarian carcinoma	349
	LC-10	Lung carcinoma	350
	PR371	Lung adenocarcinoma	351
	PR310	Lung adenocarcinoma	351
N-*ras*	HL-60	Promyelocytic leukemia	352
	AW Ramos	Burkitt's lymphoma	352
	PAC	AML primary tumor	352
	—	AML primary tumor	353
	31-26-146	ALL primary tumor	353
	MOLT-3	ALL cell line	346
	MOLT-4	ALL cell line	346
	IM9	CML cell line	346
	p12	T cell leukemia	354
	8402	T cell leukemia	354
	TALL	T cell leukemia	354
	MALT	Colon adenocarcinoma	352
	1665	Colon carcinoma	316
	PA1	Teratocarcinoma	348
	HT1080	Fibrosarcoma	355
	RD	Rhabdomyosarcoma	355
	SK-N-SH	Neuroblastoma	343
	SK-MEL-119	Melanoma	345
	SK-MEL-147	Melanoma	345
	SK-MEL-93	Melanoma	345
neu	MKN-7	Gastric carcinoma	367c
mas	—	Epidermoid carcinoma	332a
trk	—	Colon carcinoma	332b
mel	NK14	Melanoma	332r
dbl	—	B cell lymphoma	332s
raf-1	—	Stomach carcinoma	332t
met	HOS	Osteosarcoma	332o
mcf-3	MCF-7	Mammary carcinoma	332u

not the levels of expression of these genes, suggesting that amino acids 12 and 61 represent critical sites that may create potent oncogenes when mutated.

A second mechanism of activation involves overexpression of a proto-oncogene following acquisition of a novel transcriptional promoter. Recombinant DNA containing the c-*mos* proto-oncogene of mice is biologically inactive by transfection assay. However, when the cellular oncogene is rearranged by retrovirus-like endogenous genetic elements, the rearranged c-*mos* is active in a transfection assay. The rearranged segment of DNA immediately adjacent to the c-*mos* sequence was shown to be the LTR region from the retrovirus-like endogenous element (369, 370). Similarly, the *mos* proto-oncogene can be converted into a potent oncogene by the experimental addition of a strong transcriptional promoter (371), producing transcripts at much higher levels than normal. The Ha-*ras* proto-oncogene in rats can be activated by a similar mechanism (372). As described above, integration of an avian lymphoid leukosis provirus into host DNA causes neoplasms when the downstream LTR transcribes elevated levels of c-*myc*.

A third mechanism of activation, also described above, consists of chromosomal translocations, as in Burkitt's lymphoma, rearranging the c-*myc* and immunoglobulin genes, resulting in the deregulation of the c-*myc* gene. The c-*abl* gene was mapped in the human genome to a chromosomal site involved in the Philadelphia chromosome (Ph¹) translocation in chronic myelogenous leukemia (CML) (373). In the Ph¹ translocation, the c-*abl* gene is moved from chromosome 9 to chromosome 22. The translocation breakpoints occur in a specific locus, *bcr* (breakpoint cluster region), on chromosome 22 (373a), and near the 5' end of the c-*abl* locus on chromosome 9 (373, 373b). A chimeric *bcr-abl* transcription unit is generated (373c, 373d) whose mature transcript appears as a novel *bcr-abl* m whose product is a 210 kD phosphoprotein (373e). The c-*abl* transcript is found in both the chronic phase and blast crisis, but is absent from Ph¹-negative CML and most other human leukemia cells, as well as from nonhemopoietic cell lines and normal bone marrow samples (374, 375). A patient with Ph¹-negative CML has been described whose leukemic cells exhibit a rearrangement in the *bcr* gene without juxtaposition of c-*abl* sequences (375a).

Other reciprocal chromosomal translocations have been observed in human B cell neoplasms, demonstrating the existence of two commonly translocated loci *bcl*-1 and *bcl*-2 (375b, 375c). Similarly, T cell neoplasms have been associated with the chromosome translocations involving the loci of the α- and β-chains of the T cell receptor (375d–g). Additional translocations involving human oncogenes include: c-*mos* in the 8;21 translocation in acute myeloblastic leukemia (375h); c-*sis* in a 14;22 translocation in a pedigree with familial meningioma (375i); and the p53 gene in the 15;17 translocation in acute promyelocytic leukemia (375j).

Finally, activation may be due to amplification of the proto-oncogene or oncogene, leading to overexpression. The Ki-*ras* gene is amplified 3- to 5-fold in a human colon carcinoma cell line (347) and as much as 60-fold in an adrenocortical tumor of mice (376). The *myc* proto-oncogene is amplified 30 to 50 times in the human promyelocytic leukemia cell line HL-60 (363, 366) in a human colon cancer cell line with neuroendocrine properties (364), and in highly malignant forms of human small cell lung cancers (377). Similarly, c-*myc* was found to be amplified 5- to 10-fold in cells cultured from a patient with acute myelogenous leukemia (378).

Cell lines derived from different human neuroblastomas and fresh tumors contain an altered gene related to the *myc* gene, designated N-*myc*. The N-*myc* gene is often amplified in neuroblastoma, in both cell lines and primary tumors (379–381). In one study, N-*myc* was found to be amplified in neuroblastoma tissue from 24 of 63 untreated patients (382). The extent of amplification appeared bimodal, with amplification of 100- to 300-fold in 12 cases and 3- to 10-fold in 10 others. Amplification was found in 0 of 15 patients with stage 1 or 2 disease, whereas 24 of 48 patients with stage 3 or 4 disease had evidence of N-*myc* amplification, indicating that N-*myc* is highly correlated with advanced stages of disease and the ability to grow in vitro as an established cell line, both of these factors being associated with a poor prognosis (382). A subsequent, larger study continues to demonstrate a significant association between genomic amplification and rapid tumor progression after diagnosis (382a). Additionally, N-*myc* expression, measured by mRNA levels, is elevated in human neuroblastoma (382b–d); elevated levels of N-*myc* RNA are associated with a poor prognosis (382d). The neuroblastoma cell line SK-N-SH does not contain an amplified N-*myc* sequence (379). However, this cell line does contain a transforming gene, N-*ras* (343), suggesting that at least two distinct genetic events involving different oncogenes play a role in the etiology of neuroblastoma. Similarly, c-*myc*, N-*myc*, and L-*myc*, a third *myc*-related gene, have been shown to be amplified and expressed in human small cell lung cancer (SCLC) (377, 382e–g). Bombesin and bombesin-like peptides, such as gastrin-releasing peptide, are produced and secreted by SCLC cell lines, and may function as autocrine growth factors for this tumor (382h).

Retinoblastoma occurs in hereditary, nonhereditary, and chromosomal deletion forms. A retinoblastoma susceptibility gene, *Rb*, recessive-acting, is located at chromosome 13q14 (383–386). Loss of function of this gene ($Rb+/Rb+ \rightarrow rb-/rb-$) is associated with the appearance of malignancy (Table 31-7). Although pedigrees of affected families show typical dominant inheritance of the tumor, the inheritance of one inactive or deleted allele ($Rb+/rb- \rightarrow rb-/rb-$ or $Rb+/- \rightarrow rb-/-$) is not dominant at the cellular level (384, 385). A second event resulting from mitotic nondisjunction or from a mitotic recombination event ($Rb+/rb-$ or $Rb+/- \rightarrow rb-/rb-$ or $rb-/-$) is required for retinoblastoma to develop. The likelihood of this occurring in at least one retinoblast accounts for the observed dominant pattern of inheritance (387). It is suggested that this gene, or anti-oncogene (387a, 387b), possesses a regulatory or suppressor function. When active, it would prevent the expression of a structural transforming gene normally functional only during embryogenesis. Loss or inactivation of both alleles could lead to tumor formation (388). Recombinant DNA probes that recognize individual chromosome-specific markers, termed restriction-fragment-length polymorphisms (RFLPs) (388a), have been used in conjunction with isoenzyme patterns, to compare individual family members and determine which haplotype pattern was associated with the maternally and which with the paternally derived retinoblastoma allele (388b). Based on its chromosomal assignment, a cDNA segment has been isolated that is homologous to the transcript of the retinoblastoma gene (388c), a gene implicated in the etiology of both retinoblastoma and osteosarcoma (388d). This gene is expressed in a wide variety of cell types, but no RNA transcript has been found in retinoblastomas and osteosarcomas. The N-*myc* gene is amplified 10- to 200-fold, and its expression is highly elevated in most retinoblastomas examined (389), suggesting that the N-*myc* gene may have a primary role in the tumorigenesis of retinoblastoma.

Another embryonal tumor, Wilms' tumor, also illustrates how somatic alterations may reveal recessive alleles important in oncogenesis. Wilms' tumor is occasionally associated with aniridia, genitourinary malformations, mental retardation (the WAGR syndrome), and deletion of chromosome 11p13 (390, 391). Although most Wilms' tumors are sporadic and not accompanied by these findings, interstitial deletion of chromosome 11 in tumor cells, but not in normal cells, has been reported (392). Somatic deletions of 11p chromosome markers associated with duplications leading to homozygosity of the nondeleted alleles were found in cells from several Wilms' tumors (393–395, 395a). Close physical linkage has been demonstrated between the gene encoding the β-subunit of follicle stimulating hormone and the WAGR locus (395b). Children with the Beckwith-Wiedemann syndrome have a greatly increased potential for the specific development of the embryonal tumors hepatoblastoma, rhabdomyosarcoma, and Wilms' tumor. The association of these disparate, rare tumor types may reflect a common pathogenetic mechanism that entails the somatic development of homozygosity for a mutant allele at a locus on human chromosome 11 (395c). These studies suggest that abnormal mitotic events that allow expression of recessive mutations predisposing to cancer are involved in at least two types of tumor, retinoblastoma and Wilms' tumor, and may be of more widespread importance in the process of oncogenesis. In a number of cases of Wilms' tumor, insulin-like growth factor–II (IGF-II) transcripts are highly elevated compared with the adjacent normal kidney. The gene for IGF-II maps to chromosome band 11p14-15, suggesting that IGF-II may be involved in the etiology of Wilms' tumor (395d, e). Additionally, the loss of a c-Ha-*ras* allele has been associated with a reciprocal translocation between chromosome 11p13 and chromosome 12 in two cases of Wilms' tumor (396), suggesting that the resulting hemizygosity may have a role in tumor initiation. Whereas the c-Ha-*ras* gene has been excluded from the region deleted in the aniridia-Wilms' tumor complex (397, 398), the exact chromosomal location of the c-Ha-*ras* gene has not been localized with certainty and has been placed at both 11p15.1–11p15.5 (399, 400) and 11p14 (401).

Finally, translocations involving chromosome 22q12 have been found in a majority of cases of Ewing's sarcoma (402–403), suggesting that the c-*sis* gene, located on the long arm of chromosome 22 (404–405) may be implicated in this tumor. However, analysis of tumor biopsy specimens and

Table 31–7. RETINOBLASTOMA GENOTYPES AT THE Rb LOCUS IN 13q14*

Genotype	Sporadic Unilateral	Hereditary Bilateral	13 Deletion
Constitutional	$Rb+/Rb+$	$Rb+/rb-$ †	$Rb+/-$
Tumor	$rb-/rb-$ or $rb-/-$	$rb-/rb-$ or $-/rb-$	$rb-/-$ or $-/-$

*From Murphree, A. L., and Benedict, W. F.: Science 223:1029, 1984. Copyright © 1984 by the AAAS.
†The genotype referred to when a patient is said to carry the retinoblastoma "gene."

tumor cell lines revealed no rearrangement of the c-*sis* gene and no detectable transcript of c-*sis* mRNA (406).

COOPERATION OF ONCOGENES

Numerous examples above indicate that many human malignant cell lines express multiple cellular oncogenes. Additionally, while the Ha-*ras* oncogene causes transformation of NIH 3T3 cells, which are capable of inducing tumors, work with cell lines other than NIH 3T3 suggests that a single oncogene alone may have a limited effect and that cooperative interaction between different oncogenes may be required for transformation and tumorigenesis (407–409). When rat embryo fibroblasts (REFs) were removed from the rat embryo and acquired the Ha-*ras* oncogene by transfection, no foci of transformed cells grew out (407). However, when grown in soft agar, colonies of transformants grew out, indicating that the *ras* oncogene could produce anchorage independence. After several doublings, these cells died. Furthermore, these cells did not cause tumor formation when injected into animals.

As previously described, polyoma virus middle T antigen was found to induce morphologic alteration and anchorage independence, whereas the large T antigen altered serum dependence and life span in culture (40, 41). When the middle T antigen and *ras* oncogene were cotransfected into REFs, no differences were observed beyond those induced by *ras* alone. However, large T antigen and *ras*, cotransfected together, transformed REFs that were capable of forming tumors in animals (407). Adenovirus E1A, acting like polyoma large T antigen (85), produced similar results in cooperation with the *ras* oncogene (407–409). Since the c-*myc* oncogene coexists with other oncogenes in several malignancies (410–352), the *myc* gene was cotransfected with *ras*, again transforming REFs capable of tumorigenesis (407).

Based on their ability to cooperate with *myc* in cotransfection assays, Ha-*ras*, N-*ras*, and polyoma middle T may be placed in one functional class, leading to morphologic transformation (407). These gene products are localized to the plasma membrane. A second group, whose members help *ras* to transform REFs, consists of *myc*, *myb*, p53, polyoma large T, and adenovirus E1A, and has been implicated in establishment/immortalization functions (407–409, 409a). The proteins made by this group are all associated with nuclear structures. These functional groups suggest that one cellular target of oncogene action is in the nucleus and another near the plasma membrane; both targets must be acted on by oncogene proteins in order to achieve full transformation of the cell (411, 411a). In contrast, complete malignant transformation of early passage cells with the mutant c-Ha-*ras*, and induction of properties of transformed cells by either adenovirus E1A, p53, or c-*myc* alone can be accomplished only by linkage of these genes to strong transcriptional promoters/enhancers (411b, c). Comparing the effects of transfected *myc* and *ras* oncogenes on the responsiveness of cells to growth factors suggests that *ras*-like genes induce growth factor production, whereas *myc*-like genes increase the responsiveness of cells to these factors (411d). Similarly, although the v-*mil* oncogene cannot directly transform macrophages, v-*mil* dramatically enhances the capacity of v-*myc* to induce monocytic neoplasms (411e). The introduction of v-*erbA* into erythroblasts transformed with v-*erbB*, v-*src*, v-*sea*, or v-Ha-*ras* induces a fully transformed phenotype (411f).

Chemical carcinogenesis is a multistep process consisting of *initiation,* achieved by a single, subthreshold dose of a carcinogen, and *promotion,* induced by repetitive treatments with a noncarcinogenic tumor promoter. At the cellular level, establishment of the transformed phenotype is also a multistep process, requiring activation of several independent genes (see above). Induction of carcinomas by single exposure to a carcinogen often involves activation of the Ha-*ras* gene. The frequency of the activating mutation was shown to be dependent on the initiating agent used, not on the promoter, suggesting that the mutation occurs at the time of initiation (411g, h, 412). A tumor promoter, TPA (12-*O*-tetradecanoylphorbol-13-acetate), like the *myc* oncogene, is able to collaborate with *ras* to allow focal overgrowth in monolayer culture (411i, j). TPA has been found to induce expression of the normal *myc* gene (146).

TISSUE SPECIFICITY AND ONCOGENES

Initial observations suggested that specific transforming genes are activated in neoplasms of the same differentiated cell type. Several correlations could be made: the Ha-*ras* gene is more commonly associated with urinary tract tumors than is the Ki-*ras* or N-*ras* gene; N-*ras* appears to be the most frequently activated *ras* gene in hematopoietic tumors; and Ki-*ras* predominates in colon and lung carcinomas. However, as the number of human tumors with activated oncogenes expands, these relationships are becoming less precise (Table 31–6). It appears that activated oncogenes are able to affect the behavior of a variety of cell types, very likely through similar mechanisms for a given oncogene.

Role of Cellular Oncogenes in the Normal Cell

Although the functions of proto-oncogenes are unknown, several lines of evidence suggest that the proteins encoded by the corresponding cellular oncogenes participate in normal biochemical pathways essential to the regulation of cell proliferation. Proto-oncogene activation may lead to oncogenesis by altering these pathways.

Proliferation of normal cells in culture is under the control of exogenous growth factors. Transformed cells have a relaxed cell cycle control and may continue through the cell cycle in the absence of these exogenous growth factors. Lack of growth factor requirement seems to be an important feature of transformed cells, contributing to their defective growth control (413).

The cellular events linking growth factors, oncogenes, and the initiation of DNA synthesis have been reviewed in detail (413a) and are schematized in Figure 31–8. What follows is a brief summary. After a growth factor binds to its appropriate receptor, the receptor may undergo an allosteric change, a redistribution to the membrane, or an association with other membrane proteins. In the presence of growth factor, the growth factor receptor complex is internalized (413b), and the activated growth factor receptor activates a number of intracellular substrates. Activation of the receptor may occur in the absence of growth factor. Cells expressing a truncated growth factor receptor might be constitutively activated, even in the absence of the growth factor.

The human c-*sis* gene has been shown to be the structural gene encoding one of the two major polypeptides of platelet-derived growth factor (PDGF) (331, 332). The v-*erbB* gene encodes a protein homologous to the epidermal growth factor (EGF) receptor (289). The *neu* oncogene encodes a growth factor receptor closely related to EGF, although the ligand has yet to be identified (332f, g). The protein product of the c-*fms* oncogene has been identified as the cell surface receptor for the hematopoietic stem cell growth factor (colony-stimulating factor–1 [CSF-1]) (322m). Other oncogenes that have tyrosine-specific protein kinase activity may mimic activities of some activated growth factor receptors (414). However, the significance of tyrosine phosphorylation has not provided the key to growth control as anticipated. Some of these oncogene products, including $pp60^{src}$, may act on a receptor-activated pathway in which the breakdown on an inositol lipid is stimulated, leading to cell proliferation via an increase in cytoplasmic calcium concentration and activation of protein kinase C, and adenyl cyclase (420).

The p21 product of the *ras* gene may be involved in growth factor signal transduction, another step at which a lesion may lead to neoplastic transformation. If a postreceptor mechanism is constitutively activated, the cell may continue to receive a proliferative stimulus without the need for a growth factor or its receptor. This may be the mechanism of transformation by activated *ras*.

One of the most striking consequences of growth factor stimulation is the induction of cellular oncogene transcription. Treatment of fibroblasts with PDGF brings about a 40-fold elevation of c-*myc* mRNA levels within 2 hours (146) and a similar

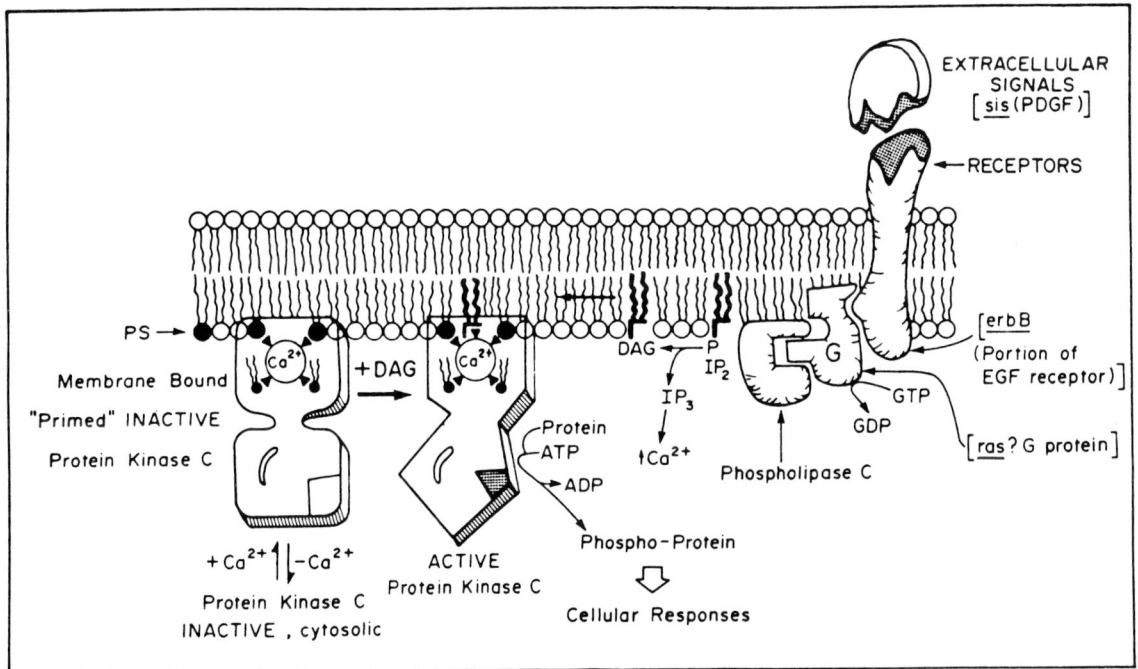

Figure 31–8. Interactions between oncogene products, cell-surface receptors, and inositol lipid metabolism. (From Bell, R. M.: Cell 45:631, 1986.)

increase in c-*fos* mRNA levels within 45 minutes (413c–e). EGF also induces c-*fos* gene transcription (413d). Several growth factor–induced proteins are localized in the nucleus of stimulated cells and may be involved in the activation of growth-regulated genes. The products of the c-*myc* and c-*fos* genes are presumably DNA-binding proteins found in the cell nucleus (413f–h). Constitutive activation of growth factor–regulated genes such as c-*myc* may result in a continuous stimulus to proliferation. In certain B cell tumors, such as Burkitt's lymphoma, the chromosomal rearrangements presumably transcriptionally activate the c-*myc* locus, resulting in a high constitutive level of c-*myc* mRNA, leading to uncontrolled proliferation (142). The constitutive high-level synthesis of *myc* RNA is not sufficient to transform fibroblasts, however, and requires a second cooperating oncogene (407). Introduction of activated c-*myc* genes under the control of the tissue-specific mammary tumor virus (MTV) promoter/enhancer into the genomes of transgenic mice led to the formation of solitary adenocarcinomas of the breast in these animals, suggesting that the deregulated c-*myc* gene was necessary but not sufficient for transforming the mammary epithelium (413i). Similarly, c-*myc* transgenes demonstrated tissue-specific expression in lymphoid cells (413j). These experiments support a multiple hit model for transformation involving c-*myc*. The MTV/c-*myc* fusion gene is expressed in an even wider variety of tissues and has contributed to the development of malignancy in cells of mammary, testicular, mast cell, pre-B cell, B cell, and T cell origin. These results indicate that c-*myc* has the capacity to cause transformation in a wide range of tissues, but transformation is not seen in all tissues in which the fusion gene is expressed. The c-*myc* gene requires additional events to bring about transformation in the ancestral lines of these tumors in vivo (413k).

Growth factors have been divided into two groups (413l, m). Competence factors, such as PDGF, induce a state of "competence" to respond to a second growth factor signal that might come from stimulation by a progression factor, such as EGF or insulin-like growth factors. Similarly, certain oncogene products may be involved in competence (*myc*, *myb*, E1A, *fos*, *sis*) and others in progression (*ras*) (413a). While the biochemical events leading to malignancy remain largely unknown, studies on transforming proteins are beginning to reveal that they have a close relationship with biochemical pathways that are essential to the regulation of normal cell proliferation.

Clinical Applications

As the molecular lesions involved in neoplasia become understood, this information can be transferred to clinical practice in several areas. Patients at risk for certain types of cancer may be screened for the presence of closely linked restriction endonuclease polymorphisms; this screening procedure is currently used to predict the presence of other genetic diseases, including thalassemia, sickle cell anemia, diabetes, and Huntington's disease (424–426). Particular polymorphisms closely linked to oncogenes may be associated with an increased risk of cancer.

Additionally, the association of activated oncogenes with specific tumor types may lead to a more precise classification of tumors and may be useful in determining prognosis as well as choice of therapy. There already appears to be a high correlation between N-*myc* amplification and expression with advanced stages of neuroblastoma (382, 382d). Similarly the *ras* oncogene protein, p21, correlates strongly with histologic tumor grade (355c). The ability of cells to break off from a primary tumor and metastasize may be due to the alteration of specific genes (411, 427). NIH3T3 cells containing the EJ-Ha-*ras* oncogene are metastatic in nude mice (428–428d). Furthermore, transfection of human metastatic tumor DNA into EJ-Ha-*ras*–transformed NIH3T3 cells, which are nonmetastasizing in immunocompetent animals, confers metastatic capability into immunocompetent animals (428). The detection of such genes will undoubtedly have important prognostic and therapeutic implications.

Antigen- or mitogen-induced activation of resting T cells stimulates the synthesis of interleukin-2 (IL-2 or T cell growth factor) (428e). These activation signals also induce the expression of specific membrane receptors for IL-2 on another population of T cells (428f). In the presence of IL-2, the cells with IL-2 receptors proliferate. Adult T cell leukemia (ATL), caused by HTLV-I, constitutively expresses large numbers of IL-2 receptors (428g). Antibodies to IL-2 receptors have been used to treat patients with ATL, leading to reduction in circulating leukemic cells (428h). The systemic administration of autologous lymphokine-activated killer (LAK) cells and recombinant-derived IL-2 can mediate the regression of established pulmonary and hepatic metastases (428i). Expression of mouse major histocompatibility complex Class I antigens (H-2) following transfection in a murine metastatic sarcoma previously lacking H-2 was associated with a profound decrease in metastatic capacity (428j).

Thus, the identification of oncogene products, including growth factors and their mechanisms of action, should direct the development of new therapeutic approaches. These altered proteins may be specific to cancer cells and essential for continued tumor growth. By regulating activated oncogenes or antagonizing their protein products, one may eventually be able to reverse the processes of transformation and tumorigenesis and prevent the progression of benign tumors to malignant forms.

ACKNOWLEDGMENTS

The author is indebted to Dr. Robert A. Weinberg and numerous other colleagues for helpful reviews of the manuscript, and to Ms. Sunny Rose Roberts for secretarial assistance.

References

1. Melnick, J. L.: Papova virus group. Science 135:1128, 1962.
2. Shope, R. E.: Infectious papillomatosis of rabbits. J. Exp. Med. 58:607, 1933.
3. Beard, J. W., Bryan, W. R., et al.: Isolation of the rabbit papilloma virus protein. J. Infect. Dis. 65:43, 1939.
4. Beard, J. W.: Review: Purified animal viruses. J. Immunol. 58:49, 1948.
5. Strauss, M. J., Shaw, E. W., et al.: "Crystalline" virus-like particles from skin papillomas characterized by intramolecular inclusion bodies. Proc. Soc. Exp. Biol. Med. 72:46, 1949.
6. Williams, M. G., Howatson, A. F., et al.: Morphological characterization of the virus of the human common wart. Nature 189:895, 1961.
7. Crawford, L. V.: A study of human papilloma virus DNA. J. Mol. Biol. 13:362, 1965.
8. Murray, R. F., Hubbs, J., et al.: Possible clonal origin of common warts (Verruca vulgaris). Nature 232:50, 1971.
9. Gissman, L., Pfister, H., et al.: Human papilloma viruses (HPV): Characterization of four different isolates. Virology 76:569, 1977.
10. Pass, F., Reissig, M., et al.: Identification of an immunologically distinct papillomavirus from lesions of *epidermodysplasia verruciformis*. Fed. Proc. 36:1084, 1977.
11. Orth, G., Favre, M., et al.: Characterization of a new type of human papillomavirus that causes skin warts. J. Virol. 24:108, 1977.
12. Jablonska, S., Dabrowski, J., et al.: Epidermodysplasia verruciformis as a model in studies of the role of papovaviruses in oncogenesis. Cancer Res. 32:583, 1972.
13. Jablonska, S., Maciejewski, W., et al.: Epidermodysplasia verruciformis. In *Biomedical Aspects of Human Wart Virus Infection*. Prunieras, M. (ed.), Lyon, France, Fondation Merieux, 1976, p. 113.
14. McCance, D. J., Walker, P. G., et al.: Presence of human papillomavirus DNA in cervical intraepithelial neoplasia. Br. Med. J. 287:784, 1983.
15. Gissman, L., Wolnik, L., et al.: Human papillomavirus type 6 and 11 DNA sequences in genital and laryngeal papillomas and in some cervical cancers. Proc. Natl. Acad. Sci. USA 80:560, 1983.
16. Durst, M., Gissman, L., et al.: A papillomavirus DNA from a cervical carcinoma and its prevalence in cancer biopsy samples from different geographic regions. Proc. Natl. Acad. Sci. USA 80:3812, 1983.
17. Crum, C. P., Ikenberg, H., et al.: Human papilloma virus type 16 and early cervical neoplasia. N. Engl. J. Med. 310:880, 1984.
18. Boshart, M., Gissmann, L., et al.: A new type of papillomavirus DNA, its presence in genital cancer biopsies and in cell lines derived from cervical cancer. EMBO J. 3:1151, 1984.
19. Gross, L.: A filterable agent, recovered from AK leukemic extracts, causing salivary gland carcinomas in C3H mice. Proc. Soc. Exp. Biol. Med. 83:414, 1953.
20. Gross, L.: Neck tumors, or leukemia, developing in adult C3H mice following inoculation, in early infancy, with filtered (Berkefeld N), or centrifuged (144,000 × g), AK-leukemic extracts. Cancer 6:948, 1943.
21. Stewart, S. E., Eddy, B. E., et al.: Neoplasms in mice inoculated with a tumor agent carried in tissue culture. J. Natl. Cancer Inst. 20:1223, 1958.
22. Gross, L.: Induction of parotid carcinomas and/or subcutaneous sarcomas in C3H mice with normal C3H organ extracts. Proc. Soc. Exp. Biol. Med. 88:362, 1955.
23. Stewart, S. E., Eddy, B. E., et al.: The induction of neoplasms with a substance released from mouse tumors by tissue culture. Virology 3:380, 1957.
24. Habel, K.: Specific complement-fixing antigens in polyoma tumors and transformed cells. Virology 25:55, 1965.
25. Benjamin, T. L.: Host-range mutants of polyoma virus. Proc. Natl. Acad. Sci. USA 67:394, 1970.
26. Feunteun, J., Sompayrac, L., et al.: Localization of gene functions in polyoma virus DNA. Proc. Natl. Acad. Sci. USA 73:4169, 1976.
27. Ito, Y., Brocklehurst, J. R., et al.: Virus-specific proteins in the plasma membrane of cells lytically infected or transformed by polyoma virus. Proc. Natl. Acad. Sci. USA 74:4666, 1977.
28. Schaffhausen, B. S., Silver, J. E., et al.: T-antigen(s) in cells productively infected by wild-type polyoma virus and mutant NG-18. Proc. Natl. Acad. Sci. USA 75:79, 1978.
29. Hutchinson, M. A., Hunter, T., et al.: Characterization of T antigens in polyoma-infected and transformed cells. Cell 15:65, 1978.
30. Ito, Y.: Organization and expression of the genome of polyoma virus. In *Viral Oncology*. Klein, G. (ed.), New York, Raven Press, 1980, pp. 447–473.
31. Treisman, R., Novak, U., et al.: Transformation of rat cells by an altered polyoma virus genome expressing only the middle-T protein. Nature 292:595, 1981.
32. Eckhart, W.: Polyoma T antigens. Adv. Cancer Res. 35:1, 1981.
33. Griffin, B. E., and Dilworth, S. M.: Polyomavirus: An overview of its unique properties. Adv. Cancer Res. 39:183, 1983.
34. Benjamin, T. L.: The hr-t gene of polyoma virus. Biochem. Biophys. Acta 695:69, 1982.
35. Smith, A. E., Smith, R., et al.: Polyoma virus middle-T has associated protein kinase. Cell 18:915, 1979.
36. Eckhart, W., Hutchinson, M. A., et al.: An actively phosphorylating tryosine in polyoma T antigen immunoprecipitates. Cell 18:925, 1979.
37. Schaffhausen, B. S., Dorai, H., et al.: Studies of polyoma virus middle-T antigen—relationship to cell membranes and apparent lack of ATP binding activity. Mol. Cell. Biol. 2:1187, 1982.
38. Schaffhausen, B. S., and Benjamin, T. L.: Phosphorylation of polyoma T antigens. Cell 18:935, 1979.
39. Courtneidge, S. A., and Smith, A. E.: Polyoma virus transforming protein associates with the product of the c-src cellular gene. Nature 303:435, 1983.
40. Rassoulzadegan, M., Cowie, A., et al.: The roles of individual polyoma virus early proteins in oncogenic transformation. Nature 300:713, 1982.
41. Rassoulzadegan, M., Naghashfar, Z., et al.: Expression of the large T protein of polyoma virus promotes the establishment in culture of "normal" rodent fibroblast cell lines. Proc. Natl. Acad. Sci. USA 80:4354, 1983.
42. Eddy, B. E., Borman, G. S., et al.: Identification of the oncogenic substance in rhesus monkey kidney cell cultures as simian virus 40. Virology 17:65, 1962.
43. Girardi, A. J., Sweet, B. H., et al.: Development of tumors in hamsters inoculated in the neo-natal period with vacuolating virus, SV40. Proc. Soc. Exp. Biol. Med. 109:649, 1962.
44. Ketner, G., and Kelly, T. J., Jr.: Integration of SV40

sequences in transformed cell DNA: Analysis using restriction endonucleases. Proc. Natl. Acad. Sci. USA 73:1102, 1976.
45. Botchan, M., Topp, W., et al.: The arrangement of simian virus 40 sequences in the DNA of transformed cells. Cell 9:269, 1976.
46. Abrahams, P. J., Mulder, C., et al.: Transformation of primary rat kidney cells by fragments of simian virus 40. J. Virol. 16:818, 1975.
46a. Hanahan, D.: Heritable formation of pancreatic β-cell tumours in transgenic mice expressing recombinant insulin/simian virus 40 oncogenes. Nature 315:115, 1985.
47. Seif, R., and Martin, R. G.: Simian virus 40 small T antigen is not required for the maintenance of transformation but may act as a promoter (cocarcinogen) during establishment of transformation in resting rat cells. J. Virol. 32:979, 1979.
48. Lewis, A. M., Jr., and Marting, R. G.: Oncogenicity of simian virus 40 deletion mutants that induce altered 17-kilodalton t-proteins. Proc. Natl. Acad. Sci. USA 76:4299, 1979.
49. Martin, R. G., Setlow, V., et al.: The roles of the simian virus 40 tumor antigens in transformation of Chinese hamster lung cells. Cell 17:635, 1979.
50. Martin, R. G., Setlow, V., et al.: Roles of the simian virus 40 tumor antigens in transformation of chinese hamster lung cells: Studies with simian virus 40 double mutants. J. Virol. 31:596, 1979.
51. Padgett, B. L., Walker, D. L., et al.: Cultivation of papova-like virus from human brain with progressive multifocal leucoencephalopathy. Lancet 1:1257, 1971.
52. Gardner, S. D., Field, A. M., et al.: New human papovavirus (BK) isolated from urine after renal transplantation. Lancet 1:1253, 1971.
53. Weiner, L. P., Herndon, R. M., et al.: Further studies of simian virus 40-like virus isolated from human brain. J. Virol. 10:147, 1972.
54. Weiner, L. P., Herndon, R. M., et al.: Isolation of virus related to SV40 from patients with progressive multifocal leukoencephalopathy. New Engl. J. Med. 286:385, 1972.
55. Takemoto, K. K., and Mullarkey, M. F.: Human papovavirus BK strain: Biological studies including antigenic relationship to simian virus 40. J. Virol. 12:625, 1973.
56. Lecatsas, G., Prozesky, O. W., et al.: Papovavirus in urine after renal transplantation. Nature 241:343, 1973.
57. Jung, M., Krech, U., et al.: Evidence of chronic persistent infections with polyomaviruses (BK type) in renal transplant recipients. Arch. Virol. 47:39, 1975.
58. Shah, K. V., Daniel, R. W., et al.: Sarcoma in a hamster inoculated with BK virus, a human papovavirus. J. Natl. Cancer Inst. 54:945, 1975.
59. Walker, D. L., Padgett, B. L., et al.: Human papovavirus (JC) induction of brain tumors in hamsters. Science 181:674, 1973.
60. Major, E. O. and diMayorca, G.: Malignant transformation of BKH_{21} clone 13 cells by BK virus-A human papovavirus. Proc. Natl. Acad. Sci. USA 70:3210, 1973.
61. Portolani, M., Bardanti-Brodano, G., et al.: Malignant transformation of hamsters kidney cells by BK virus. J. Virol. 15:420, 1975.
62. van der Noorda, J.: Infectivity, oncogenicity and transforming ability of BK virus and BK virus DNA. J. Gen. Virol. 30:371, 1976.
63. Takemoto, K. K., and Martin, M. A.: Transformation of hamster kidney cells by BK papovavirus DNA. J. Virol. 17:247, 1976.
64. Howley, P. M., Mullarkey, M. F., et al.: Characterization of human papovavirus BK DNA. J. Virol. 15:173, 1975.
65. Howley, P. M., Khoury, G., et al.: Polynucleotide sequences common to the genomes of SV40 and the human papovaviruses JC and BK. Virology 73:303, 1976.
66. Khoury, G., Howley, P. M., et al.: An analysis of the homology and relationship between the genomes of papovaviruses BKV and SV40. Proc. Natl. Acad. Sci. USA 72:2563, 1975.
67. Khoury, G., Lai, C.-J., et al.: The human papovaviruses and their potential role in human diseases. Cold Spring Harbor Conf. Cell Proliferation 4:971, 1977.
68. Osborn, J. E., Robertson, S. M., et al.: Comparison of JC and BK human papovaviruses with SV40: DNA homology studies. J. Virol. 19:675, 1976.
69. Trentin, J. J., Yabe, Y., et al.: The quest for human cancer viruses. Science 137:835, 1962.
70. Huebner, R. J., Rowe, W. P., et al.: Oncogenic effects in hamsters of human adenovirus types 12 and 18. Proc. Natl. Acad. Sci. USA 48:2051, 1962.
71. Green, M. L.: Oncogenic viruses. Ann. Rev. Biochem. 39:701, 1970.
72. Freeman, A. E., Black, P. H., et al.: Adenovirus type 12 rat embryo transformation system. J. Virol. 1:362, 1967.
73. McAllister, R. M., Nicholson, M. O., et al.: Transformation of rat embryo cells by adenovirus type 1. J. Gen. Virol. 4:29, 1969.
74. Sambrook, J., Botchan, P., et al.: Viral DNA sequences in cells transformed by simian virus 40, adenovirus type 2 and adenovirus type 5. Cold Spring Harbor Symp. Quant. Biol. 39:615, 1975.
75. Green, M. R., Green, M., et al.: Evidence for post-transcriptional selection of viral mRNA in cells transformed by human adenovirus 12. Nature 261:340, 1976.
76. Green, M., Parsons, J. T., et al.: Transcription of adenovirus genes in productively infected and in transformed cells. Cold Spring Harbor Symp. Quant. Biol. 35:803, 1971.
77. Flint, S. J., Sambrook, J., et al.: Viral nucleic acid sequences in transformed cells. IV. A study of the sequences of adenovirus 5 DNA and RNA in four lines of adenovirus 5–transformed rodent cells using specific fragments of the viral genome. Virology 72:456, 1976.
78. Green, M., and Mackey, J. K.: Are oncogenic human adenoviruses associated with human cancer? Analysis of human tumors for adenoviruses transforming gene sequences. Cold Spring Harbor Conf. Cell Proliferation 4:1027, 1976.
79. Sharp, P. A., Pettersson, V., et al.: Viral DNA in transformed cells. II. A study of the sequences of adenovirus 2 DNA in a line of transformed rat cells using specific fragments of the viral genome. J. Mol. Biol. 86:709, 1974.
80. Gallimore, P. H., Sharp, P. A., et al.: Viral DNA in transformed cells. II. A study of the sequences of adenoviruses 2 DNA in nine lines of transformed rat cells using specific fragments of the viral genome. J. Mol. Biol. 89:49, 1974.
81. Graham, F. L., Abrahams, P. J., et al.: Studies on *in vitro* transformation by DNA and DNA fragments of human adenovirus and SV40. Cold Spring Harbor Symp. Quant. Biol. 39:637, 1974.
82. van der Eb, A. J., van Ormondt, H., et al.: Structure and function of the transforming genes of human adenoviruses and SV40. Cold Spring Harbor Symp. Quant. Biol. 44:383, 1979.
83. Montell, C., Courtois, G., et al.: Complete transformation by adenovirusse 2 requires both E1A proteins. Cell 36:951, 1984.
84. Ralston, R., and Bishop, J. M.: The protein products of the *myc* and *myb* oncogenes and adenoviruses E1a are structurally related. Nature 306:803, 1983.
85. Houweling, A., van den Elsen, P. et al.: Partial transformation of primary rat cells by the leftmost 4.5% fragment of adenovirus 5 DNA. Virology. 105:537, 1980.
86. Sambrook, J., Greene, R., et al.: Analysis of the sites of integration of viral DNA sequences in rat cells transformed by adenovirus 2 or SV40. Cold Spring Harbor Symp. Quant. Biol. 44:569, 1980.

87. Sutter, D., Westphal, M., et al. Patterns of integration of viral DNA sequences in the genomes of adenovirus type 12-transformed hamster cells. Cell 14:569, 1978.
88. Bernards, R., Schrier, P. I., et al.: Tumorigenicity of cells transformed by adenovirus type 12 by evasion of T-cell immunity. Nature 305:776, 1983.
89. Cook, J. L., and Lewis, A. M., Jr: Differential NK cell and macrophage killing of hamster cells infected with nononcogenic or oncogenic adenovirus. Science 224:612, 1984.
90. Lucké, B.: Carcinoma of the kidney in the leopard frog: the occurrence and significance of metastatis. Am. J. Cancer 34:15, 1938.
91. Churchill, A. E., and Biggs, P. M.: Agent of Marek's disease in tissue culture. Nature 215:528, 1967.
92. Epstein, M. A., Achong, B. G., et al.: Structure and development of the herpes-type virus of Marek's disease. J. Natl. Cancer Inst. 41:805, 1968.
93. Nazerian, K., Solomon, J. J., et al.: Studies on the etiology of Marek's disease. II. Finding of a herpesvirus in cell culture. Proc. Soc. Exp. Biol. Med. 127:177, 1968.
94. Munyon, W., Kraiselburd, E., et al.: Transfer of thymidine kinaseless cells by infection with ultraviolet-irradiated herpes simplex virus. J. Virol. 7:813, 1971.
95. Duff, R., and Rapp, F.: Oncogenic transformation of hamster cells after exposure to herpes simplex virus type 2. Nature New Biol. 233:48, 1971.
96. Duff, R., and Rapp, F.: Oncogenic transformation of hamster embryo cells after exposure to inactivated herpes simplex type 1. J. Virol 12:209, 1973.
97. Takahashi, M., and Yamanishi, K.: Transformation of hamster embryo and human embryo cells by temperature-sensitive mutants of herpes simplex virus type 2. Virology 61:306, 1974.
98. Camacho, A., and Spear, P.: Transformation of hamster embryo fibroblasts by a specific fragment of the herpes simplex virus genome. Cell 15:993, 1978.
99. Reyes, G. R., Lafemina, R., et al.: Morphological transformation by DNA fragments of human herpes viruses: Evidence for two distinct transforming regions in HSV-1 and HSV-2 and lack of correlation with biochemical transfer of the thymidine kinase gene. Cold Spring Harbor Symp. Quant. Biol. 44:629, 1979.
100. Galloway, D. A., and McDougall, J. K.: Transformation of rodent cells by a cloned DNA fragment of herpes simplex virus type 2. J. Virol. 38:749, 1981.
101. Galloway, D. A., and McDougall, J. K.: The oncogenic potential for herpes simplex viruses: Evidence for a "hit-and-run" mechanism. Nature 302:21, 1983.
102. Jarriwalla, R. J., Aurelian, L., et al.: Tumorigeneic transformation induced by a specific fragment of DNA from herpes simplex virus type 2. Proc. Natl. Acad. Sci. USA 77:2279, 1980.
103. Rawls, W. E., Laurel, D., et al.: A search for viruses in smegma, premalignant and early malignant cervical tissues. The isolation of herpesviruses with distinct antigenic properties. Am. J. Epidemiol. 87:647, 1968.
104. Rawls, W. E., Gardner, H. L., et al.: Antibodies to genital herpesviruses in patients with carcinoma of the cervix. Am. J. Obstet. Gynecol. 7:710, 1970.
105. Rawls, W. E., Bacchetti, S., et al.: Relation of herpes simplex viruses to human malignancies. Curr. Top. Microbiol. Immunol. 77:71, 1977.
106. Nahmias, A. J., Josey, W. E., et al.: Antibodies to herpesvirus hominis types 1 and 2 in humans. II. Women with cervical cancer. Am. J. Epidemiol. 91:547, 1970.
107. Nahmias, A. J., Shore, S. L., et al.: Immunology of herpes simplex virus infection: Relevance to herpes simplex virus vaccines and cervical cancer. Cancer Res. 36:836, 1976.
108. Aurelian, L.: Virions and antigens of herpes virus type 2 in cervical carcinomas. Cancer Res. 33:1539, 1973.
109. Hollinshead, A. C., and Tarro, G.: Soluble membrane antigens of lip and cervical carcinomas: Reactivity with antibody for herpesvirus nonvirion antigens. Science 179:698, 1973.
110. Dreesman, G. R., Burek, J., et al.: Expression of herpesvirus-induced antigens in human cervical cancer. Nature 283:591, 1980.
111. McDougall, J. K., Galloway, D. A., et al.: Herpes simplex virus expression in latently infected ganglion cells and in cervical neoplasia. In Viruses in Naturally Occurring Cancers. Essex, M., Todaro, G., et al. (eds.), New York, Cold Spring Harbor, 1980, pp. 101–116.
112. Eglin, R. P., Sharp, F., et al.: Detection of RNA complementary to herpes simplex virus DNA in human cervical squamous cell neoplasms. Cancer Res. 41:3597, 1981.
113. Frenkel, N., Roizman, B., et al.: A herpes simplex 2 DNA fragment and its transcription in human cervical cancer tissue. Proc. Natl. Acad. Sci. USA 69:3784, 1972.
114. Wentz, W. B., Heggie, A. D., et al.: Effect of prior immunization on induction of cervical cancer in mice by herpes simplex virus type 2. Science 222:1128, 1983.
115. Niederman, J. C., McCollum, R. W., et al.: Infectious mononucleosis. Clinical manifestations in relation to EB virus antibodies. J.A.M.A. 203:205, 1968.
116. Henle, W., Diehl, V., et al.: Herpes-type virus and chromosome marker in normal leukocytes after growth with irradiated Burkitt cells. Science 157:1064, 1967.
117. Klein, E., Vanfurth, R., et al.: Immunoglobulin synthesis as cellular marker of malignant lymphoid cells. In Oncogenesis and Herpesvirus. Biggs, P. M., et al. (eds.), Lyon, France, International Agency for Research on Cancer, 1972, pp. 253.
118. Jondal, M., and Klein, G.: Surface markers on human B and T lymphocytes. II. Presence of Epstein-Barr virus (EBV) receptors on B lymphocytes. J. Exp. Med. 138:1365, 1973.
119. Moore, G. E., and Minowade, J.: B and T lymphoid cell lines. New Engl. J. Med. 288:106, 1973.
120. Pattengale, P. K., Smith, R. W., et al.: Selective transformation of B lymphocytes by EB virus. Lancet 2:93, 1973.
121. Miller, G., Shope, T., et al.: Epstein-Barr virus: transformation, cytopathic changes and viral antigens in squirrel monkey and marmoset leukocytes. Proc. Natl. Acad. Sci. USA 69:383, 1972.
122. Frank, A., Andiman, W. A., et al.: Epstein-Barr virus and non-human primates: natural and experimental infection. Adv. Cancer Res. 23:171, 1976.
123. Gerber, P., Pritchett, R., et al.: Antigens and DNA of a chimpanzee agent related to Epstein-Barr virus. J. Virol. 19:1090, 1976.
124. Pope, J. H., Horne, M. K., et al.: Transformation of foetal human leukocytes in vitro by filtrates of a human leukaemic cell line containing herpes-like virus. Int. J. Cancer 3:857, 1968.
125. Gerber, P., Whang-Peng, J., et al.: Transformation and chromosome changes induced by Epstein-Barr virus in normal human leukocyte cultures. Proc. Natl. Acad. Sci. USA 63:740, 1969.
126. Griffin, B. E., and Karran, L.: Immortalization of monkey epithelial cells by specific fragments of Epstein-Barr virus DNA. Nature 309:78, 1984.
127. Manolov, G., and Manolova, Y.: Marker bands in one chromosome 14 from Burkitt lymphomas. Nature 237:33, 1974.
128. Bernheim, A., Berger, R., et al.: Cytogenetic studies on African Burkitt's lymphoma cell lines: t(8;14), t(2;8) and t(8;22) translocations. Cancer Genet. Cytogenet. 3:307, 1981.
129. Dalla Favera, R., Bregni, M., et al.: Human c-myc oncogene is located on the region of chromosome 8 that is translocated in Burkitt lymphoma cells. Proc. Natl. Acad. Sci. USA 79:7824, 1982.
130. Neel, B. G., Jhanwar, S. C., et al.: Two human c-onc genes

are located on the long arm of chromosome 8. Proc. Natl. Acad. Sci. USA 79:7842, 1982.
131. Taub, R., Kirsch, I., et al.: Translocation of the c-myc gene into the immunoglobulin heavy chain locus in human Burkitt lymphoma and mouse plasmacytoma cells. Proc. Natl. Acad. Sci. USA 79:7837, 1982.
132. Croce, C. M., Shander, M., et al.: Chromosomal location of the human immunoglobulin heavy chain genes. Proc. Natl. Acad. Sci. USA 76:3416, 1979.
133. Hobart, M. J., Rabbits, T. H., et al.: Immunoglobulin heavy chain genes in humans are located on chromosome 14. Ann. Hum. Genet. 45:331, 1981.
134. Malcolm, S., Barton, P., et al.: Localization of human immunoglobulin light chain variable region genes to the short arm of chromosome 2 by in situ hybridization. Proc. Natl. Acad. Sci. USA 79:4957, 1982.
135. Erikson, J., Martinis, J., et al.: Assignment of the human genes for immunoglobulin chains to chromosome 22. Nature 294:173, 1981.
136. de la Chapelle, A., Lenoir, G., et al.: Lambda Ig constant region genes are translocated to chromosome 8 in Burkitt's lymphoma with t(8;22). Nucleic Acids Res. 11:1133, 1983.
137. Taub, R., Moulding, C., et al.: Activation and somatic mutation of the translocated c-myc gene in Burkitt's lymphoma cells. Cell 36:339, 1984.
138. Rabbits, T. H., Forster, A., et al.: Effect of somatic mutation within translocated c-myc genes in Burkitt's lymphoma. Nature 309:592, 1984.
139. Watt, R., Stanton, L. W., et al.: Nucleotide sequence of cloned cDNA of human c-myc oncogene. Nature 303:725, 1983.
140. Rabbits, T. H., Hamlyn, P. H., et al.: Altered nucleotide sequences of a translocated c-myc gene in Burkitt's lymphoma. Nature 306:760, 1983.
141. Battey, J., Moulding, C., et al.: The human c-myc oncogene: Structural consequences of translocation into the IgH locus in Burkitt's lymphoma. Cell 34:779, 1983.
142. Erikson, J., ar-Rushdi, A., et al.: Transcriptional activation of the translocated c-myc oncogene in Burkitt's lymphoma. Proc. Natl. Acad. Sci. USA 80:820, 1982.
143. Nishikura, K., ar-Rushdi, A., et al.: Differential expression of the normal and of the translocated human c-myc oncogenes in B cells. Proc. Natl. Acad. Sci. USA 80:4822, 1983.
144. ar-Rushdi, A., Nishikura, K., et al.: Differential expression of the translocated and the untranslocated c-myc oncogene in Burkitt's lymphoma. Science 222:390, 1983.
145. Leder, P., Battey, J., et al.: Translocations among antibody genes in human cancer. Science 222:765, 1983.
146. Kelly, K., Cochran, B. H., et al.: Cell-specific regulation of the c-myc gene by lymphocyte mitogens and platelet-derived growth factor. Cell 35:603, 1983.
147. Campisi, J., Gray, H. E., et al.: Cell-cycle control of c-myc but not c-ras expression is lost following chemical transformation. Cell 36:241, 1984.
148. Riou, G., Barrois, M., et al.: Presence of papillomavirus genomes and amplification of the c-myc and c-Ha-ras oncogenes in invasive cancers of the uterine cervix. C. R. Acad. Sci. 229:575, 1984.
149. Arthur, R. R., Shah, K. V., et al.: Association of BK viruria with hemorrhagic cystitis in recipients of bone marrow transplants. New Engl. J. Med. 315:230, 1986.
150. Sawada, Y., Föhring, B., et al.: Tumorigenicity of adenovirus-transformed cells: region E1A of adenovirus 12 confers resistance to natural killer cells. Virology 147:413, 1985.
151. Old, L. J., Boyse, E. A., et al.: Precipitating antibody in human serum to an antigen present in cultured Burkitt's lymphoma cells. Proc. Natl. Acad. Sci. USA 56:1699, 1966.
152. Henle, G., Henle, W., et al.: Relation of Burkitt's tumor associated herpes-type virus to infectious mononucleosis. Proc. Natl. Acad. Sci. USA 59:94, 1968.
153. Henle, W., Henle, G., et al.: Differential reactivity of human sera with EBV-induced "early antigens." Science 169:188, 1970.
154. Henle, W., Henle, G., et al.: Antibodies to Epstein-Barr virus in nasopharyngeal carcinoma, other head and neck neoplasms, and control groups. J. Natl. Cancer Inst. 44:225, 1970.
155. Henle, W., Henle, G., et al.: Antibodies to early antigens induced by Epstein-Barr virus in infectious mononucleosis. J. Infect. Dis. 124:58, 1971.
156. Henle, W., Ho, H. C., et al.: Antibodies to Epstein-Barr virus-related antigens in nasopharyngeal carcinoma. Comparison of active cases with long-term survivors. J. Natl. Cancer Inst. 51:361, 1973.
157. deSchryver, A., Friberg, S., et al.: Epstein-Barr virus-associated antibody patterns in carcinoma of the post-nasal space. Clin. Exp. Immunol. 5:443, 1969.
158. Rocchi, G., Hewetson, J., et al.: Specific neutralizing antibodies in Epstein-Barr virus associated diseases. Int. J. Cancer 11:637, 1973.
159. Glaser, R., de-Thé, G., et al.: Superinfection of epithelial nasopharyngeal carcinoma cells with Epstein-Barr virus. Proc. Natl. Acad. Sci. USA 73:960, 1976.
160. Wolf, H., zur Hausen, H., et al.: EB viral genomes in epithelial nasopharyngeal carcinoma and cells. Nature New Biol. 244:245, 1973.
161. Wolf, H., zur Hausen, H., et al.: Attempts to detect virus-specific DNA sequences in human tumors. III. Epstein-Barr viral DNA in non-lymphoid nasopharyngeal carcinoma cells. Med. Microbiol. Immunol. 161:15, 1975.
162. Huang, D. P., Ho, J. C., et al.: Demonstration of Epstein-Barr virus-associated nuclear antigen in nasopharyngeal carcinoma cells from fresh biopsies. Int. J. Cancer 14:580, 1974.
163. zur Hausen, H., Schulte Holthausen, H., et al.: EBV DNA in biopsies of Burkitt's tumours and anaplastic carcinomas of the nasopharynx. Nature 228:1056, 1970.
164. zur Hausen, H., Schulte Holthausen, H., et al.: Attempts to detect virus specific DNA in human tumors. II. Nucleic acid hybridizations with complementary RNA of human herpes group viruses. Int. J. Cancer 13:657, 1974.
165. Nonoyama, M. and Pagano, J. S.: Homology between Epstein-Barr virus DNA and viral DNA from Burkitt's lymphoma and nasopharyngeal carcinoma determined by DNA-DNA reassociation kinetics. Nature 242:44, 1973.
165a. Shaul, Y., Ziemer, M., et al.: Cloning and analysis of integrated hepatitis virus sequences from a human hepatoma cell line. J. Virol. 51:776, 1984.
165b. Koch, S., Freytag von Loringhoven, A., et al.: The genetic organization of integrated hepatitis B virus DNA in the human hepatoma cell line PLC/PRF/5. Nucleic Acids Res. 12:6871, 1984.
165c. Dejean, A., Bouguerleret, L. et al.: Hepatitis B virus DNA integration in a sequence homologous to v-erb-A and steroid receptor genes in a hepatocellular carcinoma. Nature 322:70, 1986.
166. Ellermann, V., and Bang, O.: Experimentelle Leukämie bei Hühnern. Zentralbl. Bakteriol. 46:595, 1908.
167. Rous, P.: A sarcoma of the fowl transmissible by an agent separable from the tumor cells. J. Exp. Med. 13:397, 1911.
168. Bittner, J. J.: Some possible effects of nursing on the mammary gland tumor incidence in mice. Science 84:162, 1936.
169. Gross, L.: Development and serial cell-free passage of a highly potent strain of mouse leukemia virus. Proc. Soc. Exp. Biol. Med. 94:767, 1957.
170. Hsu, T. W., Sabran, J. L., et al.: Analysis of unintegrated avian RNA tumor virus double-stranded DNA intermediates. J. Virol. 28:810, 1978.

171. Shank, P. R., Hughes, S. H., et al.: Mapping unintegrated avian sarcoma virus DNA: termini of linear DNA bear 300 nucleotides present once or twice in two species of circular DNA. Cell *15*:1383, 1978.
172. Temin, H. M.: Function of the retrovirus long terminal repeat. Cell *28*:3, 1982.
172a. Panganiban, A. T.: Retroviral integration. Cell *42*:5, 1985.
173. Panganiban, A. T., and Temin, H. M.: The terminal nucleotides of retrovirus DNA are required for integration but not virus production. Nature *306*:155, 1983.
174. Baltimore, D.: RNA-dependent DNA polymerase in virions of RNA tumor viruses. Nature *226*:1209, 1970.
175. Temin, H. M., and Mizutani, S.: RNA-directed DNA polymerase in virions of Rous sarcoma virus. Nature *226*:1211, 1970.
176. Varmus, H., and Swanstrom, R.: Replication of retroviruses. In *RNA Tumor Viruses: Molecular Biology of Tumor Viruses,* 2nd ed. Weiss, R., Teich, N., et al. (eds.), New York, Cold Spring Harbor Laboratory, 1982, pp. 423–440.
177. Teich, N., Wyke, J., et al.: Pathogenesis of retrovirus-induced disease. In *RNA Tumor Viruses: Molecular Biology of Tumor Viruses,* 2nd ed. Weiss, R., Teich, N., et al. (eds.), New York, Cold Spring Harbor Laboratory, 1982, pp. 790–792.
178. Abelson, H. T., and Rabstein, L. S.: Influence of prednisolone on Moloney leukemogenic virus in BALB/mice. Cancer Res. *30*:2208, 1970.
179. Abelson, H. T., and Rabstein, L. S.: Lymphosarcoma: virus-induced thymic-independent disease in mice. Cancer Res. *30*:2213, 1970.
180. Witte, O. N., Rosenberg, N., et al.: Identification of an Abelson murine leukemia virus–encoded protein present in transformed fibroblast and lymphoid cells. Proc. Natl. Acad. Sci. USA *75*:2488, 1978.
181. Witte, O. N., Dasgupta, A., et al.: Abelson murine leukemia virus protein is phosphorylated *in vitro* to form phosphotyrosine. Nature *283*:826, 1980.
182. Van de Ven, W. J. M., Reynolds, F. H., Jr., et al.: The nonstructural components of polyproteins encoded by replication defective mammalian transforming retroviruses are phosphorylated and have associated protein kinase activity. Virology *101*:185, 1980.
183. Blomberg, J., Reynolds, F. H., Jr., et al.: Abelson murine leukaemia virus transformation involves loss of epidermal growth factor-binding sites. Nature *286*:504, 1980.
184. Sklar, M. D., White, B. J., et al.: Initiation of oncogenic transformation of mouse lymphocytes *in vitro* by Abelson leukemia virus. Proc. Natl. Acad. Sci. USA *71*:4077, 1974.
185. Rosenberg, N., Baltimore, D., et al.: *In vitro* transformation of lymphoid cells by Abelson leukemia virus. Proc. Natl. Acad. Sci. USA *72*:1932, 1975.
186. Rosenberg, N., and Baltimore, D.: A quantitative assay for transformation of bone marrow cells by Abelson murine leukemia virus. J. Exp. Med. *143*:1453, 1976.
187. Alt, F. W., Rosenberg, N. E., et al.: Organization and reorganization of immunoglobulin genes in Abelson murine leukemia virus-transformed cells: rearrangement of heavy but not light chain genes. Cell *27*:387, 1981.
188. Shinefeld, L. A., Sato, V. L., et al.: Monoclonal rat anti-mouse brain antibody detects Abelson murine leukemia virus target cells in mouse bone marrow. Cell *20*:11, 1980.
189. Paige, C. J., Kincade, P. W., et al.: Precursors of murine B lymphocytes: physical and functional characterization and distinction of myeloid stem cells. J. Exp. Med. *153*:154, 1981.
190. Lane, M.-A., Neary, D., et al.: Activation of a cellular transforming gene in tumours by Abelson murine leukaemia virus. Nature *300*:659, 1982.
191. Graf, T., von Kirchbach, A., et al.: Characterization of the hematopoietic target cells of AEV, MC29, and AMV avian leukemia viruses. Exp. Cell. Res. *131*:331, 1981.
192. Gazzolo, L., Moscovici, C., et al.: Response of hemopoietic cells to avian acute leukemia viruses: effects on the differentiation of the target cells. Cell *16*:627, 1979.
193. Graf, T., and Beug, H.: Avian leukemia viruses. Interaction with their target cells *in vivo* and *in vitro*. Biochem. Biophys. Acta *516*:269, 1978.
194. Savin, K. W., and Beug, H.: Cell-surface glycoprotein synthesis during differentiation of chicken erythroblasts transformed by temperature-sensitive avian erythroblastosis virus. Cell Differ. *10*:163, 1981.
195. Todaro, G. J., DeLarco, J. E., et al.: Transformation by murine and feline sarcoma viruses specifically blocks binding of epidermal growth factor to cells. Nature *264*:26, 1976.
196. DeLarco, J. E., and Todaro, G. J.: Sarcoma growth factor: specific binding to and elution from membrane receptors for epidermal growth factor. Cold Spring Harbor Symp. Quant. Biol. *44*:643, 1980.
197. Todaro, G. J., Fryling, C., et al.: Transforming growth factors produced by certain human tumor cells: polypeptides that interact with epidermal growth factor receptors. Proc. Natl. Acad. Sci. USA *77*:5258, 1980.
198. Neiman, P., Payne, L. N., et al.: Viral DNA in bursal lymphomas induced by avian leukosis viruses. J. Virol. *34*:178, 1980.
199. Neiman, P., Beemon, K., et al.: Independent recombination between avian leukosis virus terminal sequences and host DNA in virus-induced proliferative disease. Proc. Natl. Acad. Sci. USA *78*:1891, 1981.
200. Neel, B. G., Hayward, W. S., et al.: Avian leukosis virus-induced tumors have common proviral integration sites and synthesize discrete new RNAs: oncogenesis by promoter insertion. Cell *23*:323, 1981.
201. Payne, G. S., Courtneidge, S. A., et al.: Analysis of avian leukosis virus DNA and RNA in bursal tumors: viral gene expression is not required for maintenance of the tumor state. Cell *23*:311, 1981.
202. Hughes, S. H., Shank, P. R., et al.: Proviruses of avian sarcoma virus are terminally redundant, co-extensive with unintegrated linear DNA and integrated at many sites. Cell *15*:1397, 1978.
203. Sabran, J. L., Hsu, T. W., et al.: Analysis of integrated avian RNA tumor virus DNA in transformed chick, duck, and quail fibroblasts. J. Virol. *29*:170, 1979.
204. Hayward, W. S., Neel, B. G., et al.: Activation of a cellular *onc* gene by promoter insertion in ALV-induced lymphoid leukosis. Nature *290*:475, 1981.
205. Fung, Y.-K. T., Lewis, W. G., et al.: Activation of the cellular oncogene c-erbB by LTR insertion: molecular basis for induction of erythroblastosis by avian leukosis virus. Cell *33*:357, 1983.
206. Cooper, G. M., and Neiman, P. E.: Transforming genes of neoplasms induced by avian lymphoid leukosis viruses. Nature *287*:656, 1980.
207. Tsichlis, P. N., Strauss, P. G., et al.: A common region for proviral DNA integration in MoMuLV-induced rat thymic lymphomas. Nature *302*:445, 1983.
208. Cuypers, H. T., Selten, G., et al.: Murine leukemia virus-induced T-cell lymphomagenesis: integration of proviruses in a distinct chromosomal region. Cell *37*:141, 1984.
209. Lane, M.-A., Sainten, A., et al.: Stage-specific transforming genes of human and mouse B- and T-lymphocyte neoplasms. Cell *28*:873, 1982.
210. Neil, J. C., and Hughes, D., et al.: Transduction and rearrangement of the *myc* gene by feline leukaemia virus in naturally occurring T-cell leukaemias. Nature *308*:814, 1984.
211. Levy, L. S., Gardner, M. B., et al.: Isolation of a feline leukaemia provirus containing the oncogene *myc* from a feline lymphosarcoma. Nature *308*:853, 1984.
212. Mullins, J. I., Brody, D. S., et al.: Viral transduction of c-*myc* gene in naturally occurring feline leukaemias. Nature *308*:856, 1984.

213. Lasfargues, E. Y., Kramarsky, B., et al.: Detection of mouse mammary tumor virus in cat kidney cells infected with purified B particles from RIII milk. J. Natl. Cancer Inst. 53:1831, 1974.
214. Lasfargues, E. Y., Lasfargues, J. C., et al.: Experimental infection of a cat kidney cell line with the mouse mammary tumor virus. Cancer Res. 36:67, 1976.
215. Vaidya, A. B., Lasfargues, E. Y., et al.: Murine mammary tumor virus: characterization of infection of non-murine cells. J. Virol. 28:911, 1976.
216. Michalides, R., Vlahakis, G., et al.: A biochemical approach to the study of the transmission of mouse mammary tumor viruses in mouse strains RIII and C3H. Int. J. Cancer 18:105, 1976.
217. Morris, V. L., Medeiros, W., et al.: Comparison of mouse mammary tumor virus-specific DNA in inbred, wild and asian mice, and in tumors and normal organs from inbred mice. J. Mol. Biol. 114:73, 1977.
218. Nusse, R., and Varmus, H. E.: Many tumors induced by the mouse mammary tumor virus contain a provirus integrated in the same region of the host genome. Cell 31:99, 1982.
219. Peters, G., Brookes, S., et al.: Tumorigenesis by mouse mammary tumor virus: Evidence for a common region of integration in mammary tumors. Cell 33:369, 1983.
220. Nusse, R., van Ooyen, A., et al.: Mode of proviral activation of a putative mammary oncogene (int-1) on mouse chromosome 15. Nature 307:131, 1984.
221. Lane, M.-A., Sainten, A., et al.: Activation of related cellular transforming genes in mouse and human mammary carcinomas. Proc. Natl. Acad. Sci. USA 78:5185, 1981.
222. Peters, G., Lee, A. E., et al.: Activation of cellular gene by mouse mammary tumour virus may occur early in mammary tumour development. Nature 309:273, 1984.
223. McGrath, C. M.: Replication of mammary tumor virus in tumor cell cultures: dependence of hormone-induced cellular organization. J. Natl. Cancer Inst. 47:455, 1971.
224. Parks, W. P., Scolnick, E. M., et al.: Dexamethasone stimulation of murine mammary tumor virus expression: a tissue culture source of virus. Science 184:158, 1974.
225. Ringold, G. M., Yamamoto, K. R., et al.: Dexamethasone-mediated induction of mouse mammary tumor virus RNA: a system for studying glucocorticoid action. Cell 6:299, 1975.
226. Lee, F., Mulligan, R., et al.: Glucocorticoids regulate expression of dihydrofolate reductase cDNA in mouse mammary tumor chimaeric plasmids. Nature 294:228, 1981.
227. Govindan, M. V., Spiess, E., et al.: Purified glucocorticoid receptor-hormone complex from rat liver cytosol binds specifically to cloned mouse mammary tumor virus long terminal repeats *in vitro*. Proc. Natl. Acad. Sci. USA 79:5157, 1982.
228. Poiesz, B. J., Ruscetti, F. W., et al.: Detection and isolation of type-C retrovirus particles from fresh and cultured lymphocytes of a patient with cutaneous T-cell lymphoma. Proc. Natl. Acad. Sci. USA 77:7415, 1980.
229. Blattner, W. A., Takatsuki, K., et al.: Human T-cell leukemia-lymphoma virus and adult T-cell leukemia. J.A.M.A. 250:1074, 1983.
230. Takatsuki, K., Uchiyama, T., et al.: Adult T-cell leukemia: proposal as a new disease and cytogenetic, phenotypic and functional studies of leukemic cells. Gann. Monograph on Cancer Research 28:13, 1982.
231. Kalyanaraman, V. S., Sarngadharan, M. G., et al.: A new subtype of human T-cell leukemia virus (HTLV-II) associated with a T-cell variant of hairy cell leukemia. Science 218:571, 1982.
231a. Rosenblatt, J. D., Golde, D. W., et al.: A second isolate of HTLV-II associated with atypical hairy cell leukemia. New Engl. J. Med. 315:372, 1986.
232. Gallo, R. C., Mann, D., et al.: Human T-cell leukemia-lymphoma virus (HTLV) is in T- but not B-lymphocytes from a patient with cutaneous T-cell lymphoma. Proc. Natl. Acad. Sci. USA 79:5680, 1982.
233. Miyoshi, I., Kubonishi, I., et al.: Type C virus particles in a cord T-cell line derived by co-cultivating normal human leukocytes and human leukemic T-cells. Nature 294:770, 1981.
234. Yamamoto, N., Okada, M., et al.: Transformation of human leukocytes by cocultivation with an adult T-cell leukemia virus producer cell line. Science 217:737, 1982.
235. Popovic, M., Sarin, P. S., et al.: Isolation and transmission of human retrovirus (human T-cell leukemia virus). Science 219:856, 1983.
236. Chen, I. S. Y., McLaughlin, J., et al.: Molecular characterization of genome of a novel human T-cell leukaemia virus. Nature 305:502, 1983.
236a. Seiki, M., Eddy, R., et al.: Nonspecific integration of the HTLV provirus genome into adult T-cell leukaemia cells. Nature 309:640, 1984.
236b. Sodroski, J., Rosen, C., et al.: A transcriptional activator protein encoded by the *x-lor* region of the human T-cell leukemia virus. Science 288:1430, 1985.
236c. Sodroski, J., Patarca, R., et al.: Location of the *trans*-activating region on the genome of the human T-cell lymphotropic virus type III. Science 229:74, 1985.
236d. Chen, I. S. Y., Slamon, D. J., et al.: The *x* gene is essential for HTLV replication. Science 229:54, 1985.
236e. Seiki, A., Hikikoshi, T., et al.: Expression of the *pX* gene of the HTLV-I: general splicing mechanism in the HTLV family. Science 228:1532, 1985.
236f. Wachsman, W., Golde, D. W., et al.: HTLV *x*-gene product: requirement for the *env* methionine initiation codon. Science 228:1534, 1985.
236g. Fisher, A. G., Collalti, E., et al.: A molecular clone of HTLV-III with biological activity. Nature 316:262, 1985.
236h. Felber, B. K., Paskalis, H., et al.: The pX protein of HTLV-I is a transcriptional activator of its long terminal repeats. Science 229:675, 1985.
236i. Rosen, C., Sodroski, J. G., et al.: Location of *cis*-acting regulatory sequences in human T-cell leukemia virus type I long terminal repeat. Proc. Natl. Acad. Sci. USA 82:6502, 1985.
236j. Wong-Staal, F., and Gallo, R. C.: Human T-lymphotropic retroviruses. Nature 317:395, 1985.
236k. Greene, W. C., Leonard, W. J., et al.: *Trans*-activator gene of HTLV-II induces IL-2 receptor and IL-2 cellular gene expression. Science 232:877, 1986.
237. Seiki, M., Hattori, S., et al.: Human adult T-cell leukemia virus: Molecular cloning of the provirus DNA and the unique terminal structure. Proc. Natl. Acad. Sci. USA 79:6899, 1983.
238. Sodroski, J. G., Rosen, C. A., et al.: *Trans*-acting transcriptional activation of the long terminal repeat of human T lymphotropic viruses in infected cells. Science 225:381, 1984.
239. Schüpbach, J., Popovic, M., et al.: Serological analysis of a subgroup of human T-lymphotropic retroviruses (HTLV-III) associated with AIDS. Science 224:503, 1984.
240. Schüpbach, J., Sarngadharan, M. G., et al.: Antigens on HTLV-infected cells recognized by leukemia and AIDS sera are related to HTLV viral glycoprotein. Science 224:607, 1984.
241. Gallo, R. C., Salahuddin, S. Z., et al.: Frequent detection and isolation of cytopathic retroviruses (HTLV-III) from patients with AIDS and at risk for AIDS. Science 224:500, 1984.
242. Popovic, M., Sarngadharan, M. G., et al.: Detection, isolation, and continuous production of cytopathic retroviruses (HTLV-III) from patients with AIDS and pre-AIDS. Science 224:497, 1984.
243. Barré-Sinoussi, F., Chermann, J. C., et al.: Isolation of a

T-lymphotropic retrovirus from a patient at risk for acquired immune deficiency syndrome (AIDS). Science 220:868, 1983.
244. Vilmer, F., Barré-Sinoussi, F., et al.: Isolation of new lymphotropic retrovirus from two siblings with hemophilia B, one with AIDS. Lancet 1:753, 1984.
245. Coffin, J. M., Varmus, H. E., et al.: A proposal for naming host cell-derived inserts in retrovirus genomes. J. Virol. 40:953, 1981.
246. Stehelin, D., Varmus, H. E., et al.: DNA related to the transforming gene(s) of avian sarcoma viruses is present in normal avian DNA. Nature 260:170, 1976.
247. Bishop, J. M.: Enemies within: the genesis of retrovirus oncogenes. Cell 23:5, 1981.
248. Brugge, J. S. and Erikson, R. L.: Identification of a transformation-specific antigen induced by an avian sarcoma virus. Nature 269:346, 1977.
249. Purchio, A. F., Erikson, E., et al.: Identification of a polypeptide encoded by the avian sarcoma virus *src* gene. Proc. Natl. Acad. Sci. USA 75:1567, 1978.
250. Collett, M. S., and Erikson, R. L.: Protein kinase activity associated with the avian sarcoma virus *src* gene product. Proc. Natl. Acad. Sci. USA 75:2021, 1978.
251. Levinson, A. D., Oppermann, H., et al.: Evidence that the transforming gene of avian sarcoma virus encodes a protein kinase associated with a phosphoprotein. Cell 15:561, 1978.
252. Rubin, C. S., and Rosen, O. M.: Protein phosphorylation. Ann. Rev. Biochem. 44:831, 1975.
253. Weller, M.: *Protein Phosphorylation.* London, Pion, 1979.
254. Rübsamen, H., Friis, R. R., et al.: *src* gene product from different strains of avian sarcoma virus: kinetics and possible mechanism of heat inactivation of protein kinase activity from cells infected by transformation-defective, temperature-sensitive mutant and wild-type virus. Proc. Natl. Acad. Sci. USA 76:967, 1979.
255. Bishop, J. M., Courtneidge, S. A., et al.: Origin and function of avian retrovirus transforming genes. Cold Spring Harbor Symp. Quant. Biol. 44:919, 1980.
256. Gilmer, T. M., and Erikson, R. L.: Rous sarcoma virus transforming protein, pp60^{src}, expressed in *E. coli*, functions as a protein kinase. Nature 294:771, 1981.
257. McGrath, J. P., and Levinson, A. D.: Bacterial expression of an enzymatically active protein encoded by RSV *src* gene. Nature 295:423, 1982.
258. Hunter, T., and Sefton, B. M.: Transforming gene product of Rous sarcoma virus phosphorylates tyrosine. Proc. Natl. Acad. Sci. USA 77:1311, 1980.
259. Smith, A. E., Fried, M., et al.: Is polyoma middle-T antigen a protein kinase? Cold Spring Harbor Symp. Quant. Biol. 44:141, 1980.
260. Beug, H., Peters, J. H., et al.: Expression of virus specific morphological cell transformation induced in enucleated cells. Z. Naturforsch. 31c:766, 1976.
261. Willingham, M. C., Jay, G., et al.: Localization of the ASV *src* gene product to the plasma membrane of transformed cells by electron microscopic immunocytochemistry. Cell 18:125, 1979.
262. Krueger, J. G., Wang, E., et al.: Differences in intracellular location of pp60^{src} in rat and chicken cells transformed by Rous sarcoma virus. Proc. Natl. Acad. Sci. USA 77:4142, 1980.
263. Levinson, A. D., Courtneidge, S. A., et al.: Structural and functional domains of the Rous sarcoma virus transforming protein (pp60^{src}). Proc. Natl. Acad. Sci. USA 78:1624, 1981.
264. Oppermann, H., Levinson, A. D., et al.: The structure and protein kinase activity of proteins encoded by nonconditional mutants and back mutants in the *src* gene of avian sarcoma virus. Virology 108:46, 1981.
265. Garber, E. A., Krueger, J. G., et al.: Only membrane-associated RSV *src* proteins have amino-terminally bound lipid. Nature 302:161, 1983.
265a. Buss, J. E., and Sefton, B. M.: Myristic acid, a rare fatty acid, is the lipid attachment to the transforming protein of Rous sarcoma virus and its cellular homolog. J. Virol. 53:7, 1985.
265b. Pellman, D., Garber, E. A., et al.: An N-terminal peptide from p60^{src} can direct myristylation and plasma membrane localization when fused to heterologous proteins. Nature 314:374, 1985.
265c. Pellman, D., Garber, E. A., et al.: Fine structural mapping of a critical NH$_2$-terminal region of p60^{src}. Proc. Natl. Acad. Sci. USA 82:1623, 1985.
265d. Schultz, A. M., Henderson, L. E., et al.: Amino terminal myristylation of the protein kinase p60^{src}, a retroviral transforming protein. Science 227:427, 1985.
265e. Iba, H., Takeya, T., et al.: Rous sarcoma virus variants that carry the cellular *src* gene instead of the viral *src* gene cannot transform chicken embryo fibroblasts. Proc. Natl. Acad. Sci. USA 81:4424, 1984.
265f. Shalloway, D., Coussens, P. M., et al.: Overexpression of the *c-src* protein does not induce transformation of NIH 3T3 cells. Proc. Natl. Acad. Sci. USA 81:7071, 1984.
266. Radke, K., and Martin, G. S.: Transformation by Rous sarcoma virus: effects of *src* gene expression on the synthesis and phosphorylation of cellular polypeptides. Proc. Natl. Acad. Sci. USA 76:5212, 1979.
267. Radke, K., Gilmore, T., et al.: Transformation by Rous sarcoma virus. A cellular substrate for transformation-specific protein phosphorylation contains phosphotyrosine. Cell 16:821, 1980.
268. Erikson, E., and Erikson, R. L.: Identification of a cellular protein substrate phosphorylated by the avian sarcoma virus–transformating gene product. Cell 21:829, 1980.
269. Erikson, E., Cook, R., et al.: The same normal cell protein is phosphorylated after transformation by avian sarcoma viruses with unrelated transforming genes. Mol. Cell. Biol. 1:43, 1981.
270. Cooper, J. A., and Hunter, T.: Changes in protein phosphorylation in Rous sarcoma virus–transformed chicken embryo cells. Mol. Cell. Biol. 1:165, 1981.
271. Cooper, J. A., Reiss, N. A., et al.: Three glycolytic enzymes are phosphorylated at tyrosine in cells transformed by Rous sarcoma virus. Nature 302:218, 1983.
272. Sugimoto, Y., Whitman, M., et al.: Evidence that the Rous sarcoma virus transforming gene product phosphorylates phosphatidylinositol and diacylglycerol. Proc. Natl. Acad. Sci. USA 81:2117, 1984.
273. Robbins, K. C., Devare, S. G., et al.: Molecular cloning of integrated simian sarcoma virus: genome organization of infectious DNA clones. Proc. Natl. Acad. Sci. USA 78:2918, 1981.
274. Devare, S. G., Reddy, E. P., et al.: Nucleotide sequence of the simian sarcoma virus genome: demonstration that its acquired cellular sequences encode the transforming gene product p28sis. Proc. Natl. Acad. Sci. USA 80:731, 1983.
275. Robbins, K. C., Devare, S. G., et al.: *In vivo* identification of the transforming gene product of simian sarcoma virus. Science 218:1131, 1982.
276. Antoniades, H. N., and Hunkapiller, M. W.: Human platelet-derived growth factor (PDGF): amino terminal amino acid sequence. Science 220:963, 1983.
277. Doolittle, R. F., Hunkapiller, M. W., et al.: Simian sarcoma virus *onc* gene, *v-sis*, is derived from the gene (or genes) encoding a platelet-derived growth factor. Science 221:275, 1983.
278. Waterfield, M. D., Scrace, T., et al.: Platelet-derived growth factor is structurally related to the putative transforming protein p28^{sis} of simian sarcoma virus. Nature 304:35, 1983.
279. Johnsson, A., Heldin, C.-H., et al.: The *c-sis* gene encodes a precursor of the B chain of platelet derived growth factor. EMBO J. 3:921, 1984.
280. Robbins, K. C., Antoniades, H. N., et al.: Structural and

immunological similarities between simian sarcoma virus gene product(s) and human platelet-derived growth factor. Nature 305:605, 1983.
281. Hayman, M. J., Royer-Pokora, B., et al.: Defectiveness of avian erythroblastosis virus: synthesis of a 75K gag-related protein. Virology 92:31, 1979.
282. Hayman, M. J., Ramsay, G., et al.: Identification and characterization of the avian erythroblastosis virus erbB gene product as a membrane glycoprotein. Cell 32:579, 1983.
282a. Green, S., Walter, P., et al.: Human estrogen receptor cDNA: sequence expression and homology to v-erb-A. Nature 320:134, 1986.
283. Hayman, M. J., and Beug, H.: Identification of a form of the avian erythroblastosis virus erb-B gene product at the cell surface. Nature 309:460, 1984.
284. Privalsky, M. L., Sealy, L., et al.: The product of the avian erythroblastosis virus erbB locus is a glycoprotein. Cell 32:1257, 1983.
285. Frykberg, L., Palmieri, S., et al.: Transforming capacities of avian erythroblastosis virus mutants detected in the erbA or erbB oncogenes. Cell 32:227, 1983.
286. Beug, H., Palmieri, S., et al.: Hormone-dependent terminal differentiation in vitro of chicken erythroleukemia cells transformed by ts mutants of avian erythroblastosis virus. Cell 28:907, 1982.
287. Beug, H., and Hayman, M. J.: Temperature-sensitive mutants of avian erythroblastosis virus: surface expression of the erbB product correlates with transformation. Cell 36:963, 1984.
288. Yamamoto, T., Nishida, T., et al.: The erbB gene of avian erythroblastosis virus is a member of the src gene family. Cell 35:71, 1983.
289. Downward, J., Yarden, Y., et al.: Close similarity of epidermal growth factor receptor and v-erb-B oncogene protein sequences. Nature 307:521, 1984.
289a. Ullrich, A., Coussens, L., et al.: Human epidermal growth factor receptor cDNA sequence and aberrant expression of the amplified gene in A431 epidermoid carcinoma cells. Nature 309:418, 1984.
289b. Privalsky, M. L., Ralston, R., et al.: The glycoprotein encoded by the retroviral oncogene v-erb-B is structurally related to tyrosine-protein kinases. Proc. Natl. Acad. Sci. USA 81:704, 1984.
289c. Beug, H., and Hayman, M. J.: Temperature sensitive mutants of avian erythroblastosis virus surface expression of the erbB product correlates with transformation. Cell 36:963, 1984.
289d. Schmidt, J. A., Beug, H., et al.: Effects of inhibitors of glycoproteins processing on the synthesis and biological activity of erb-B oncogene. EMBO J. 4:105, 1985.
290. Bister, K., Hayman, M. J., et al.: Defectiveness of avian myelocytomatosis virus MC29: isolation of long-term nonproducer cultures and analysis of virus-specific polypeptide synthesis. Virology 82:431, 1977.
291. Hann, S. R., Abrams, H. D., et al.: Proteins encoded by v-myc and c-myc oncogenes: identification and localization in acute leukemia virus transformants and bursal lymphoma cell lines. Cell 34:789, 1983.
292. Klempnauer, K.-H., Ramsay, G., et al.: The product of the retroviral transforming gene v-myb is a truncated version of the protein encoded by the cellular oncogene c-myb. Cell 33:345, 1983.
293. Radke, K., Beug, H., et al.: Transformation of both erythroid and myeloid cells by E26, an avian leukemia virus that contains the myb gene. Cell 31:643, 1982.
294. Moscovici, M. G., Jurdic, P., et al.: Organization of the hemopoietic target cells for the avian leukemia virus E26. Virology 129:65, 1983.
295. Leprince, D., Gegonne, A., et al.: A putative second cell-derived oncogene of the avian leukemia retrovirus E26. Nature 306:395, 1983.
296. Shih, T. Y., Weeks, M. O., et al.: Identification of a sarcoma virus–coded phosphoprotein in nonproducer cells transformed by Kirsten on Harvey murine sarcoma virus. Virology 96:64, 1979.
297. Langbeheim, H., Shih, T. Y., et al.: Identification of a normal vertebrate cell protein related to the p21 src of Harvery murine sarcoma virus. Virology 106:292, 1980.
298. DeFeo-Jones, D., Scolnick, E. M., et al.: ras-related gene sequences identified and isolated from Saccharomyces cerevisiae. Nature 306:707, 1983.
299. Gallwitz, D., Donath, C., et al.: A yeast gene encoding a protein homologous to the human c-has/bas proto-oncogene product. Nature 306:704, 1983.
300. Powers, S., Kataoka, T., et al.: Genes in S. cerevisiae encoding proteins with domains homologous to the mammalian ras proteins. Cell 36:607, 1984.
301. Willingham, M. C., Pastan, I., et al.: Localization of the src gene product of the Harvey strain of MSV to the plasma membrane of transformed cells by electron microscopic immunocytochemistry. Cell 18:1005, 1980.
302. Scolnick, E. M., Papageorge, A. G., et al.: Guanine nucleotide-binding activity as an assay for src protein of rat-derived murine sarcoma viruses. Proc. Natl. Acad. Sci. USA 76:5355, 1979.
303. Shih, T. Y., Papageorge, A. G., et al.: Guanine nucleotide binding and autophosphorylating activities associated with the $p21^{src}$ protein of Harvey sarcoma virus. Nature 287:686, 1980.
304. Bishop, J. M.: Retroviruses. Ann. Rev. Biochem. 47:35, 1978.
305. Bishop, J. M.: Cellular oncogenes and retroviruses. Ann. Rev. Biochem. 52:301, 1983.
306. Graham, F. L., and van der Eb, A. J.: A new technique for the assay of infectivity of human adenovirus 5 DNA. Virology 52:456, 1973.
307. Shih, C., Shilo, B.-Z., et al.: Passage of phenotypes of chemically transformed cells via transfection of DNA and chromatin. Proc. Natl. Acad. Sci. USA 76:5714, 1979.
308. Cooper, G. M., Okenquist, S., et al.: Transforming activity of DNA of chemically transformed and normal cells. Nature 284:418, 1980.
309. Eva, A., and Aaronson, S. A.: Frequent activation of c-kis as a transforming gene in fibrosarcomas induced by methylcolanthrene. Science 220:955, 1983.
310. Parada, L. F., and Weinberg, R. A.: Presence of a Kirsten murine sarcoma virus ras oncogene in cells transformed by 3-methylcolanthrene. Mol. Cell. Biol. 3:2298, 1983.
311. Balmain, A., and Pragnell, I. B.: Mouse skin carcinomas induced in vivo by chemical carcinogens have a transforming Harvey-ras oncogene. Nature 303:72, 1983.
312. Sukumar, S., Notario, V., et al.: Induction of mammary carcinomas in rats by nitroso-methylurea involves malignant activation of H-ras-1 locus by single point mutations. Nature 306:658, 1983.
313. Shih, C., Padhy, L. C., et al.: Transforming genes of carcinomas and neuroblastomas introduced into mouse fibroblasts. Nature 290:261, 1981.
314. Krontiris, T. G., and Cooper, G. M.: Transforming activity of human tumor DNAs. Proc. Natl. Acad. Sci. USA 78:1181, 1981.
315. Perucho, M., Goldfarb, M., et al.: Human-tumor-derived cell lines contain common and different transforming genes. Cell 27:467, 1981.
316. Pulciani, S., Santos, E., et al.: Oncogenes in solid human tumors. Nature 300:539, 1982.
317. Parada, L., Tabin, C., et al.: Human EJ bladder carcinoma oncogene is homologue of Harvey sarcoma virus ras gene. Nature 297:474, 1982.
318. Der, C. J., Krontiris, T. G., et al.: Transforming genes of human bladder and lung carcinoma cell lines are homologues to the ras genes of Harvey and Kirsten sarcoma virus. Proc. Natl. Acad. Sci. USA 79:3637, 1982.

319. Santos, E., Tronick, S. R., et al.: T24 human bladder carcinoma oncogene is an activated form of the normal human homologue of BALB- and Harvey-MSV transforming genes. Nature 298:343, 1982.
320. Hughes, S. H., Payvar, F., et al.: Heterogeneity of genetic loci in chickens: Analysis of endogenous viral and nonviral genes by cleavage of DNA with restriction endonucleases. Cell 18:347, 1979.
321. Hughes, S. H., Stubblefield, E., et al.: Gene localization by chromosomal fractionization: Globin genes are on at least two chromosomes and three estrogen-inducible genes are on three chromosomes. Proc. Natl. Acad. Sci. USA 76:1348, 1979.
322. Van Beveren, C., van Straaten, F., et al.: Nucleotide sequence of the genome of a murine sarcoma virus. Cell 27:97, 1981.
323. Klempnauer, K.-H., Gonda, T. J., et al.: Nucleotide sequence of the retroviral leukemia gene v-*myb* and its cellular progenitor c-*myb*: The architecture of a transduced oncogene. Cell 31:453, 1982.
324. Parker, R. C., Varmus, H. E., et al.: Expression of *v-src* and chicken *c-src* in rats demonstrates qualitative differences between pp60$^{v\text{-}src}$ and pp60$^{c\text{-}src}$. Cell 37:131, 1984.
324a. Mathey-Prevot, B., Hanafusa, H., et al.: A cellular protein is immunologically crossreactive with and functionally homologous to the Fujinami sarcoma virus transforming protein. Cell 28:897, 1982.
324b. Ponticelli, A. S., Whitlock, C. A., et al.: In vivo tyrosine phosphorylations of the Abelson virus transforming protein are absent in its normal cellular homolog. Cell 29:953, 1982.
325. Scolnick, E. M., Weeks, M. O., et al.: Markedly elevated levels of an endogenous *sarc* protein in a hematopoietic precursor cell line. Mol. Cell. Biol. 1:66, 1981.
326. Furth, M. E., Davis, L. J., et al.: Monoclonal antibodies to the p21 products of the transforming gene of Harvey murine sarcoma virus and of the cellular *ras* gene family. J. Virol. 43:294, 1982.
327. Tatchell, K., Chaleff, D. T., et al.: Requirement of either of a pair of *ras*-related genes of *Saccharomyces cerevisiae* for spore viability. Nature 309:523, 1984.
328. Kataoka, T., Powers, S., et al.: Genetic analysis of yeast *RAS1* and *RAS2* genes. Cell 37:437, 1984.
328a. Toda, T., Uno, I., et al.: In yeast, *RAS* proteins are controlling elements of adenylate cyclase. Cell 40:27, 1985.
328b. Gilman, A. G.: G proteins and dual control of adenylate cyclase. Cell 36:577, 1984.
328c. Gibbs, J. B., Sigal, I. S., et al.: Intrinsic GTPase activity distinguishes normal and oncogenic *ras* p21 molecules. Proc. Natl. Acad. Sci. USA 81:5704, 1984.
328d. McGrath, J. P., Capon, D. J., et al.: Comparative biochemical properties of normal and activated human *ras* p21. Nature 310:644, 1984.
328e. Sweet, R. W., Yokoyama, S., et al.: The product of *ras* is a GTPase and the T24 oncogenic mutant is deficient in this activity. Nature 311:273, 1984.
329. Watson, D. K., Reddy, E. P., et al.: Nucleotide sequence analysis of the chicken c-*myc* gene reveals homologous and unique coding regions by comparison with the transforming gene of avian myelocytomatosis virus MC29, Δ *gag-myc*. Proc. Natl. Acad. Sci. USA 80:2146, 1983.
330. Watson, D. K., Psallidopoulos, M. C., et al.: Nucleotide sequence analysis of human c-*myc* locus, chicken homologue, and myelocytomatosis virus MC29 transforming gene reveals a highly conserved gene product. Proc. Natl. Acad. Sci. USA 80:3642, 1983.
330a. Chen, J. H.: The proto-oncogene c-*ets* is preferentially expressed in lymphoid cells. Mol. Cell. Biol. 5:2993, 1985.
331. Chiu, I.-M., Reddy, E. P., et al.: Nucleotide sequence analysis identifies the human c-*sis* proto-oncogene as a structural gene for platelet-derived growth factor. Cell 37:123, 1984.

332. Josephs, S. F., Guo, C., et al.: Human proto-oncogene nucleotide seuqences corresponding to the transforming region of simian sarcoma virus. Science 223:487, 1984.
332a. Young, D., Waitches, G., et al.: Isolation and characterization of a new cellular oncogene encoding a protein with multiple potential transmembrane domains. Cell 45:711, 1986.
332b. Martin-Zanca, D., Hughes, S. H., et al.: A human oncogene formed by the fusion of truncated tropomyosin and protein tyrosine kinase sequences. Nature 319:743, 1986.
332c. Curran, T., MacConnell, W. P., et al.: Structure of the FBJ murine osteosarcoma virus genome: molecular cloning of its associated helper virus and the cellular homolog of the c-*fos* gene from mouse and human cells. Mol. Cell. Biol. 3:914, 1983.
332d. Curran, T., Miller, A. D., et al.: Viral expression and cellular *fos* proteins: a comparative analysis. Cell 36:259, 1984.
332e. Verma, I. M.: Proto-oncogene *fos*: a multifaceted gene. Trends Genet. 2:93, 1986.
332f. Schechter, A. L., Stern, D. F., et al.: The *neu* oncogene: an erb-B-related gene encoding a 185,000 M_r tumour antigen. Nature 312:513, 1984.
332g. Schechter, A. L., Hung, M.-C., et al.: The *neu* gene: an *erb*B-homologous gene distinct from and unlinked to the gene encoding the EGF receptor. Science 229:976, 1985.
332h. Bargmann, C. I., Hung, M.-C., et al.: The *neu* oncogene encodes an epidermal growth factor receptor-related protein. Nature 319:226, 1986.
332i. Yamamoto, T., Ikawa, S., et al.: Similarity of protein encoded by the human c-*erb-B-2* gene to epidermal growth factor receptor. Nature 319:230, 1986.
332j. Coussens, L., Yang-Feng, T. L., et al.: Tyrosine kinase receptor with extensive homology to EGF receptor shares chromosomal location with *neu* oncogene. Science 230:1132, 1985.
332k. Stern, D. F., Heffernan, P. A., et al.: p185, a product of the *neu* proto-oncogene, is a receptorlike protein associated with tyrosine kinase activity. Mol. Cell. Biol. 6:1729, 1986.
332l. Bargmann, C. I., Hung, M.-C., et al.: Multiple independent activations of the *neu* oncogene by a point mutation altering the transmembrane domain of p185. Cell 45:1986.
332m. Sherr, C. J., Rettenmier, C. W., et al.: The c-*fms* proto-oncogene product is related to the receptor for the mononuclear phagocyte growth factor, CSF-1. Cell 41:665, 1985.
332n. Stanley, E. R., Guilbert, E. J., et al.: Regulation of macrophage production by a colony-stimulating factor. In *Mononuclear Phagocytes-Functional Aspects, Part 1.* van Furth, R. (ed.), The Hague, Martinus Nijhoff, pp. 417–433.
332o. Cooper, C. S., Park, M., et al.: Molecular cloning of a new transforming gene from a chemically transformed human cell line. Nature 311:29, 1984.
332p. Dean, M., Park, M., et al.: The human *met* oncogene is related to the tyrosine kinase oncogenes. Nature 318:385, 1985.
332q. Park, M., Dean, M., et al.: Mechanism of *met* oncogene activation. Cell 45:895, 19986.
332r. Padua, R. A., Barrass, N., et al.: A novel transforming gene in a human malignant melanoma cell line. Nature 311:671, 1984.
332s. Eva, A., and Aaronson, S. A.: Isolation of a new human oncogene from a diffuse B-cell lymphoma. Nature 316:273, 1985.
332t. Shimizu, K., Nakatsu, Y., et al.: Molecular cloning of an activated human oncogene, homologous to v-*raf*, from primary stomach cancer. Proc. Natl. Acad. Sci. USA 82:5641, 1985.
332u. Fasano, O., Birnbaum, D., et al.: New human transform-

ing genes detected by a tumorigenicity assay. Mol. Cell. Biol. 4:1695, 1984.
333. Murray, M. J., Shilo, B.-Z., et al.: Three different human tumor cell lines contain different oncogenes. Cell 25:355, 1981.
334. Pulciani, S., Santos, E., et al.: Oncogenes in human tumor cell lines: Molecular cloning of a transforming gene from human bladder carcinoma cells. Proc. Natl. Acad. Sci. USA 79:2845, 1982.
335. Marshall, C. J., Hall, A., et al.: A transforming gene present in human sarcoma cell lines. Nature 229:171, 1982.
335a. Trent, J., Meltzer, P., et al.: Evidence for rearrangement, amplification, and expression of c-myc in a human glioblastoma. Proc. Natl. Acad. Sci. USA 83:470, 1986.
336. Shih, C., and Weinberg, R. A.: Isolation of a transforming sequence from a human bladder carcinoma cell line. Cell 29:161, 1982.
337. Goldfarb, M., Shimizu, K., et al.: Isolation and preliminary characterization of a human transforming gene from T24 bladder carcinoma cells. Nature 296:404, 1983.
338. Tabin, C. J., Bradley, S. M., et al.: Mechanism of activation of a human oncogene. Nature 300:143, 1982.
339. Reddy, E. P., Reynolds, R. K., et al.: A point mutation is responsible for the acquisition of transforming properties by the T24 human bladder carcinoma oncogene. Nature 300:149, 1982.
340. Taparowsky, E., Suard, Y., et al.: Activation of the T24 bladder carcinoma transforming gene is linked to a single amino acid change. Nature 300:762, 1982.
341. Chang, E. H., Furth, M. E., et al.: Tumorigenic transformation of mammalian cells induced by a normal human gene homologous to the oncogene of Harvey murine sarcoma virus. Nature 297:479, 1982.
342. Finkel, T., Der, C. J., et al.: Activation of ras genes in human tumors does not affect localization, modification, or nucleotide binding properties of p21. Cell 37:151, 1984.
343. Shimizu, K., Goldfarb, M., et al.: Three human transforming genes are related to the viral ras oncogenes. Proc. Natl. Acad. Sci. USA 80:2112, 1983.
344. Yuasa, Y., Srivastava, S. K., et al.: Acquisition of transforming properties by alternative point mutations within c-bas/has human proto-oncogene. Nature 303:775, 1983.
345. Albino, A. P., LeStrange, R., et al.: Transforming ras genes from human melanoma: a manifestation of tumour heterogeneity? Nature 308:69, 1984.
346. Eva, A., Tronick, S. R., et al.: Transforming genes of human hematopoietic tumors: Frequent detection of ras-related oncogenes whose activation appears to be independent of tumor phenotype. Proc. Natl. Acad. Sci. USA 80:4926, 1983.
347. McCoy, M. S., Toole, J. J., et al.: Characterization of a human colon/lung carcinoma oncogene. Nature 302:79, 1983.
348. Cooper, C. S., Blair, D. G., et al.: The transforming genes of a human pancreatic carcinoma, a teratocarcinoma and a chemically-transformed human cell. Cancer Res. 44:1, 1984.
349. Feig, L. A., Bast, R. C., Jr., et al.: Somatic activation of ras^k gene in a human ovarian carcinoma. Science 223:698, 1984.
350. Santos, E., Martin-Zanca, D., et al.: Malignant activation of a K-ras oncogene in lung carcinoma but not in normal tissue of the same patient. Science 223:661, 1984.
351. Nakano, H., Yamamoto, F., et al.: Isolation of transforming sequences of two human lung carcinomas: Structural and functional analysis of the activated c-K-ras oncogenes. Proc. Natl. Acad. Sci. USA 81:71, 1984.
352. Murray, M. J., Cunningham, J. M., et al.: The HL-60 transforming sequence: A ras oncogene coexisting with altered myc genes in hematopoietic tumors. Cell 33:749, 1983.
353. Gambke, C., Signer, E., et al.: Activation of N-ras gene in bone marrow cells from a patient with acute myeloblastic leukaemia. Nature 307:476, 1984.
354. Souyri, M., and Fleissner, E.: Identification by transfection of transforming sequences in DNA of human T-cell leukemias. Proc. Natl. Acad. Sci. USA 80:6676, 1983.
355. Hall, A., Marshall, C. J., et al.: Identification of transforming gene in two human sarcoma cell lines as a new member of the ras gene family located on chromosome 1. Nature 303:396, 1983.
355a. Bos, J. L., Toksoz, D., et al.: Amino acid substitutions at codon 13 of the N-ras oncogene in human acute myeloid leukaemia. Nature 315:726, 1985.
355b. Hirai, H., Tanaka, S., et al.: Transforming genes in human leukemia cell lines. Blood 66:1371, 1985.
355c. Viola, M. V., Fromowitz, F., et al.: Expression of ras oncogene p21 in prostate cancer. New Engl. J. Med. 314:133, 1986.
355d. Tanaka, T., Slamon, D. J., et al.: Expression of p21 ras oncoproteins in human cancers. Cancer Res. 46:1465, 1986.
356. Fujita, J., Yoshida, O., et al.: Ha-ras oncogenes are activated by somatic alterations in human urinary tract tumours. Nature 309:464, 1984.
357. Der, C. J., and Cooper, G. M.: Altered gene products are associated with activation of cellular ras^k genes in human lung and colon carcinomas. Cell 32:201, 1983.
358. Taparowsky, E., Shimizu, K., et al.: Structure and activation of the human N-ras gene. Cell 34:581, 1983.
359. Capon, D. J., Seeburg, P. H., et al.: Activation of Ki-ras2 gene in human colon and lung carcinomas by two different point mutations. Nature 304:507, 1983.
360. Santos, E., Reddy, E. P., et al.: Spontaneous activation of a human proto-oncogene. Proc. Natl. Acad. Sci. USA 80:4679, 1983.
361. Slamon, D. J., deKernion, J. B., et al.: Expression of cellular oncogenes in human malignancies. Science 224:256, 1984.
362. Dalla Favera, R., Martinotti, S., et al.: Translocation and rearrangements of the c-myc oncogene locus in human undifferentiated B-cell lymphomas. Science 219:963, 1983.
362a. Yokota, J., Tsunetsugu-Yokota, Y., et al.: Alterations of myc, myb, and ras^{Ha} proto-oncogenes in cancers are frequent and show clinical correlation. Science 231:261, 1986.
362b. Slamon, D. J., Boone, T. C., et al.: Studies of the human c-myb gene and its product in human acute leukemia. Science 233:347, 1986.
363. Collins, S., and Groudine, M.: Amplification of endogenous myc-related DNA sequences in a human myeloid leukaemia cell line. Nature 295:679, 1982.
364. Alitalo, K. M., Schwab, M., et al.: Homogeneously staining chromosomal regions contain amplified copies of an abundantly expressed cellular oncogene (c-myc) in malignant neuroendocrine cells from a human colon carcinoma. Proc. Natl. Acad. Sci. USA 80:1707, 1983.
365. Eva, A., Robbins, K. C., et al.: Cellular genes analogous to retroviral onc genes are transcribed in human tumour cells. Nature 295:116, 1982.
366. Dalla Favera, R., Wong-Staal, F., et al.: onc gene amplification in promyelocytic leukaemia cell line HL-60 and primary leukaemic cells of the same patient. Nature 299:61, 1982.
367. Rothberg, P. G., Erisman, M. D., et al.: Structure and expression of the oncogene c-myc in fresh tumor material from patients with hematopoietic malignancies. Mol. Cell. Biol. 4:1096, 1984.
367a. Trent, J., Meltzer, P., et al.: Evidence for rearrangement,

amplification, and expression of c-*myc* in a human glioblastoma. Proc. Natl. Acad. Sci. USA *83*:470, 1986.

367b. Saglio, G., Emanuel, B. S., et al.: 3′ c-*myc* rearrangement in a human leukemic T-cell line. Cancer Res. *46*:1413, 1986.

367c. Fukushige, S.-I., Masubara, K.-I., et al.: Localization of a novel v-*erb*B-related gene, c-*erb*B-2, on human chromosome 17 and its amplification in a gastric cancer cell line. Mol. Cell. Biol. *6*:955, 1986.

368. Shimizu, K., Birnbaum, D., et al.: Structure of the Ki-*ras* gene of the human lung carcinoma cell line Calu-1. Nature *304*:497, 1983.

369. Rechavi, G., Givol, D., et al.: Activation of a cellular oncogene by DNA rearrangement: possible involvement of an IS-like element. Nature *300*:607, 1982.

370. Kuff, E. L., Feenstra, A., et al.: Homology between an endogenous viral LTR and sequences inserted in an activated cellular oncogene. Nature *302*:547, 1983.

371. Blair, D. G., Oskarsson, M., et al.: Activation of the transforming potential of a normal cell sequence: a molecular model for oncogenesis. Science *212*:941, 1981.

372. DeFeo, D., Gonda, M. A., et al.: Analysis of two divergent rat genomic clones homologous to the transforming gene of Harvey murine sarcoma virus. Proc. Natl. Acad. Sci. USA *78*:3328, 1981.

373. deKlein, A., Guerts van Kessel, A., et al.: A cellular oncogene is translocated to the Philadelphia chromosome in chronic myelocytic leukaemia. Nature *300*:765, 1982.

373a. Groffen, J., Stephenson, J. R., et al.: Philadelphia chromosomal breakpoints are clustered within a limited region, bcr, on chromosome 22. Cell *36*:93, 1984.

373b. Heisterkamp, N., Stephenson, J. R., et al.: Localization of the c-*abl* oncogene adjacent to a translocation breakpoint in chronic myelogenous leukaemia. Nature *306*:239, 1983.

373c. Heisterkamp, N., Stam, K., et al.: Structural organization of the *bcr* gene and its role in the Ph′ translocation. Nature *315*:758, 1985.

373d. Shtivelman, E., Lifshitz, D., et al.: Fused transcript of *abl* and *bcr* in chronic myelogenous leukaemia. Nature *315*:550, 1985.

373e. Ben-Neriah, Y., Daley, G. Q., et al.: The chronic myelogenous leukemia-specific P210 protein is the product of the bcr/abl hybrid gene. Science *233*:212, 1986.

374. Bartram, C. R., deKlein, A., et al.: Translocation of c-*abl* oncogene correlates with the presence of a Philadelphia chromosome in chronic myelocytic leukaemia. Nature *306*:277, 1983.

375. Canaani, E., Gale, R. P., et al.: Altered transcription of an oncogene in chronic myeloid leukaemia. Lancet *1*:593, 1984.

375a. Bartram, C. R.: bcr rearrangement without juxtaposition of c-*abl* in chronic myelocytic leukemia. J. Exp. Med. *162*:2175, 1985.

375b. Tsujimoto, Y., Finger, L. R., et al.: Cloning of the chromosome breakpoint of neoplastic B cells with the t(14;18) chromosome translocation. Science *226*:1097, 1984.

375c. Tsujimoto, Y., Jaffe, E., et al.: Clustering of breakpoints on chromosome 11 in human B-cell neoplasms with the t(11;14) chromosome translocation. Nature *315*:340, 1985.

375d. Croce, C. M., Isobe, M., et al.: Gene for α-chain of human T-cell receptor: location on chromosome 14 region involved in T-cell neoplasms. Science *227*:1044, 1985.

375e. Isobe, M., Erikson, J., et al.: Location of gene for β subunit of human T-cell receptor at band 7q35, a region prone to rearrangements in T cells. Science *228*:580, 1985.

375f. Morton, C. C., Duby, A. D., et al.: Genes for β chain of human T-cell antigen receptor maps to regions of chromosomal rearrangements in T cells. Science *228*:582, 1985.

375g. Hecht, F., Morgan, R., et al.: Common region in chromosome 14 in T-cell leukemia and lymphoma. Science *22*:1445, 1984.

375h. Diaz, M. O., LeBeau, M. M., et al.: The role of the c-*mos* gene in the 8;21 translocation in human acute myeloblastic leukemia. Science *229*:767, 1985.

375i. Bolger, G. B., Stamberg, J., et al.: Chromosome translocation t(14;22) and oncogene (c-*sis*) variant in a pedigree with familial meningioma. New Engl. J. Med. *312*:564, 1985.

375j. LeBeau, M. M., Westbrook, C. A., et al.: Translocation of the p53 gene in t(15;17) in acute promyelocytic leukaemia. Nature *316*:826, 1985.

376. Schwab, M., Alitalo, K., et al.: A cellular oncogene (c-Ki-*ras*) is amplified, overexpressed, and located within karyotypic abnormalities in mouse adrenocortical tumour cells. Nature *303*:497, 1983.

377. Little, C. D., Nau, M. M., et al.: Amplification and expression of the c-*myc* oncogene in human lung cancer cell lines. Nature *306*:194, 1983.

378. Pelicci, P.-G., Lanfrancone, L., et al.: Amplification of the c-*myc* oncogene in a case of human acute myelogenous leukemia. Science *224*:1117, 1984.

379. Schwab, M., Alitalo, K., et al.: Amplified DNA with limited homology to *myc* cellular oncogene is shared by human neuroblastoma cell lines and a neuroblastoma tumor. Nature *305*:245, 1983.

380. Montgomery, K. T., Biedler, J. L., et al.: Specific DNA sequence amplification in human neuroblastoma cells. Proc. Natl. Acad. Sci. USA *80*:5724, 1983.

381. Kohl, N. E., Kanda, N., et al.: Transposition and amplification of oncogene-related sequences in human neuroblastomas. Cell *35*:359, 1983.

382. Brodeur, G. M., Seeger, R. C., et al.: Amplification of N-*myc* in untreated human neuroblastomas correlates with advanced disease stage. Science *224*:1121, 1984.

382a. Seeger, R. C., Brodeur, G. M., et al.: Association of multiple copies of the N-*myc* oncogene with rapid progression of neuroblastomas. New Engl. J. Med. *313*:1111, 1985.

382b. Kohl, N. E., Gee, C. E., et al.: Activated expression of the N-*myc* gene in human neuroblastomas and related tumors. Science *226*:1335, 1984.

382c. Schwab, M., Ellison, J., et al.: Enhanced expression of the human gene N-*myc* consequent to amplification of DNA may contribute to malignant progression to neuroblastoma. Proc. Natl. Acad. Sci. USA *81*:4940, 1984.

382d. Grady-Leopardi, E. F., Schwab, M., et al.: Detection of N-*myc* oncogene expression in human neuroblastoma by *in situ* hybridization and blot analysis: relationship to clinical outcome. Cancer Res. *46*:3196, 1986.

382e. Nau, M. M., Brooks, B. J., et al.: Human small-cell lung cancers show amplification and expression of the N-*myc* gene. Proc. Natl. Acad. Sci. USA *83*:1092, 1986.

382f. Wong, A. J., Ruppert, J. M., et al.: Gene amplification of c-*myc* in small cell carcinoma of the lung. Science *233*:461, 1986.

382g. Nau, M. M., Brooks, B. J., et al.: L-*myc*, a new *myc*-related gene amplified and expressed in human small cell lung cancer. Nature *318*:69, 1985.

382h. Cuttitta, F., Carney, D. N., et al.: Bombesin-like peptides can function as autocrine growth factors in human small-cell lung cancer. Nature *316*:823, 1985.

383. Sparkes, R. S., Murphree, A. L., et al.: Gene for hereditary retinoblastoma assigned to chromosome 13 by linkage to esterase D. Science *219*:971, 1983.

384. Benedict, W. F., Murphree, A. L., et al.: Patient with chromosome 13 deletion: evidence that the retinoblastoma gene is a recessive cancer gene. Science *219*:973, 1983.

385. Cavenee, W. K., Dryja, T. P., et al.: Expression of recessive alleles by chromosomal mechanisms in retnoblastoma. Nature 305:779, 1983.
386. Dryja, T. P., Cavenee, W., et al.: Homozygosity of chromosome 13 in retinoblastoma. New Engl. J. Med. 310:550, 1984.
387. Murphree, A. L., and Benedict, W. F.: Retinoblastoma: clues to human oncogenesis. Science 223:1028, 1984.
387a. Knudsen, A. G.: Hereditary cancer, oncogenes, and anti-oncogenes. Cancer Res. 45:1437, 1985.
387b. Green, A. R., and Wyke, J. A.: Anti-oncogenes: a subset of regulatory genes involved in carcinogenesis. Lancet 2:475, 1985.
388. Comings, D. E.: A general theory of carcinogenesis. Proc. Natl. Acad. Sci. USA 70:3324, 1973.
388a. Botstein, D., White, R. L., et al.: Construction of a genetic linkage map in man using restriction fragment length polymorphisms. Am. J. Hum. Genet. 32:314, 1980.
388b. Cavenee, W. K., Murphree, A. L., et al.: Prediction of familial predisposition to retinoblastoma. New Engl. J. Med. 314:1201, 1986.
388c. Friend, S. H., Bernards, R., et al.: A human DNA segment with properties of the gene that predisposes to retinoblastoma and osteosarcoma. Nature 323:643, 1986.
388d. Dryja, T. P., Rapaport, J. M., et al.: Chromosome 13 homozygosity in osteosarcoma without retinoblastoma. Am. J. Hum. Genet. 38:59, 1986.
389. Lee, W.-H., Murphree, A. L., et al.: Expression and amplification of the N-*myc* gene in primary retinoblastoma. Nature 309:458, 1984.
390. Miller, R. W., Fraumeni, J. F., et al.: Association of Wilms' tumor with aniridia, hemihypertrophy and other congenital malformations. New Engl. J. Med. 270:922, 1964.
391. Riccardi, V. M., Sujansky, E., et al.: Chromosomal imbalance in the aniridia-Wilms' tumor association: 11p interstitial deletion. Pediatrics 61:604, 1978.
392. Keneko, Y., Egues, M. C., et al.: Interstitial deletion of short arm of chromosome 11 limited to Wilms' tumor cells in a patient without aniridia. Cancer Res. 41:4577, 1981.
393. Orkin, S. H., Goldman, D. S., et al.: Development of homozygosity for chromosome 11p markers in Wilms' tumour. Nature 309:172, 1984.
394. Fearon, E. R., Vogelstein, B., et al.: Somatic deletion of genes on chromosome 11 in Wilms' tumour. Nature 309:176, 1984.
395. Koufos, A., Hansen, M. F., et al.: Loss of alleles at loci on human chromosome 11 during genesis of Wilms' tumour. Nature 309:170, 1984.
395a. Van Heyningen, V., Boyd, P. A., et al.: Molecular analysis of chromosome 11 deletions in aniridia-Wilms' tumor syndrome. Proc. Natl. Acad. Sci. USA 82:8592, 1985.
395b. Glaser, T., Lewis, W. H., et al.: The β-subunit of follicle-stimulating hormone is deleted in patients with aniridia and Wilms' tumour, allowing a further definition of the WAGR locus. Nature 321:882, 1986.
395c. Koufos, A., Hansen, M. F., et al.: Loss of heterozygosity in three embryonal tumours suggests a common pathogenetic mechanism. Nature 316:330, 1985.
395d. Reeve, A. E., Eccles, M. R., et al.: Expression of insulin-like growth factor–II transcripts in Wilms' tumour. Nature 317:258, 1985.
395e. Scott, J., Cowell, J., et al.: Insulin-like growth factor-II gene expression in Wilms' tumour and embryonic tissues. Nature 317:260, 1985.
396. Reeve, A. E., Housiaux, P. J., et al.: Loss of a Harvey *ras* allele in sporadic Wilms's tumour. Nature 309:174, 84.
397. Huerre, C., Despoisse, S., et al.: c-Ha-*ras*1 is not deleted in aniridia-Wilms' tumour association. Nature 305:638, 1983.
398. deMartinville, B., and Francke, U.: The c-Ha-*ras*1, insulin and β-globin loci map outside the deletion association with aniridia-Wilms' tumour. Nature 305:641, 1983.
399. McBride, O., Swan, D. C., et al.: Localization of the normal allele of T24 human bladder carcinoma oncogene to chromosome 11. Nature 300:773, 1982.
400. deMartinville, B., Giacalone, J., et al.: Oncogene from human EJ bladder carcinoma is located on the short arm of chromosome 11. Science 219:498, 1983.
401. Dean, A., Fordis, C. M., et al.: Localization of genes on human chromosome 11p in normal lymphocytes and K562 human leukemia cells. Clin. Res. 32:492A (abstr.), 1984.
402. Aurias, A., Rimbaut, C., et al.: Chromosomal translocations in Ewing's sarcoma. New Engl. J. Med. 309:496, 1983.
403. Turc-Carel, C., Philip, I., et al.: Chromosomal translocations in Ewing's sarcoma. New Engl. J. Med. 309:497, 1983.
404. Swan, D. C., McBride, O. W., et al.: Chromosomal mapping of the simian sarcoma virus *onc* gene analogue in human cells. Proc. Natl. Acad. Sci. USA 79:4691, 1982.
405. Dalla Favera, R., Gallo, R. C., et al.: Chromosomal localization of the human homolog (c-*sis*) of the simian sarcoma virus *onc* gene. Science 218:686, 1982.
406. Bechet, J.-M., Bornkamm, G., et al.: The c-*sis* oncogene is not activated in Ewing's sarcoma. New Engl. J. Med. 310:393, 1984.
407. Land, H., Parada, L. F., et al.: Tumorigenic conversion of primary embryo fibroblasts requires at least two cooperating oncogenes. Nature 304:596, 1983.
408. Newbold, R. F., and Overell, R. W.: Fibroblast immortality is a prerequisite for transformation by EJ c-Ha-*ras* oncogene. Nature 304:648, 1983.
409. Ruley, H. E.: Adenovirus early region 1A enables viral and cellular transforming genes to transform primary cells in culture. Nature 304:602, 1983.
409a. Parada, L. F., Land, H., et al.: Cooperation between gene encoding p53 tumour antigen and *ras* in cellular transformation. Nature 312:649, 1984.
410. Cooper, G. M., and Neiman, P. E.: Two distinct candidate transforming genes of lymphoid leukosis virus-induced neoplasms. Nature 292:857, 1981.
411. Land, H., Parada, L. F., et al.: Cellular oncogenes and multistep carcinogenesis. Science 222:771, 1983.
411a. Land, H., Chen, A. L., et al.: Behavior of *myc* and *ras* oncogenes in transformation of rat embryo fibroblasts. Mol. Cell. Biol. 6:1917, 1986.
411b. Spandidos, D. A., and Wilkie, N. M.: Malignant transformation of early passage rodent cells by a single mutated human oncogene. Nature 310:469, 1986.
411c. Kelekar, A., and Cole, M. D.: Tumorigenicity of fibroblast lines expressing the adenovirus E1a, cellular p53, or normal c-*myc* genes. Mol. Cell. Biol. 6:7, 1986.
411d. Stern, D. F., Roberts, A. B., et al.: Differential responsiveness of *myc*- and *ras*-transfected cells to growth factors: selective stimulation of *myc*-transfected cells by epidermal growth factor. Mol. Cell. Biol. 6:870, 1986.
411e. Graf, T., Weizsaecker, F. V., et al.: v-*mil* induces autocrine growth and enhanced tumorigenicity in v-*myc*-transformed avian macrophages. Cell 45:357, 1986.
411f. Kahn, P., Frykberg, L., et al.: v-*erbA* cooperates with sarcoma oncogenes in leukemic cell transformation. Cell 45:349, 1986.
411g. Zarbl, H., Sukumar, S., et al.: Direct mutagenesis of Ha-*ras*-1 oncogenes by N-nitroso-N-methylurea during initiation of mammary carcinogenesis in rats. Nature 315:382, 1985.
411h. Quintanilla, M., Brown, K., et al.: Carcinogen-specific mutation and amplification of Ha-*ras* during mouse skin carcinogenesis. Nature 322:78, 1986.
411i. Dotto, G. P., Parada, L. F., et al.: Specific growth response

of *ras*-transformed embryo fibroblasts to tumour promoters. Nature *318*:472, 1985.
411j. Hsiao, W.-L.W., Gattoni-Celli, S., et al.: Oncogene-induced transformation of C3H 10T1/2 cells is enhanced by tumor promoters. Science *226*:552, 1984.
412. Balmain, A., Ramsden, M., et al.: Activation of the mouse cellular Harvey-*ras* gene in chemically induced benign skin papillomas. Nature *307*:658, 1984.
413. Heldin, C.-H., and Westermark, B.: Growth factors: mechanisms of action and relation to oncogenes. Cell *37*:9, 1984.
413a. Goustin, A. S., Leof, E. B., et al.: Growth factors and cancer. Cancer Res. *46*:1015, 1986.
413b. Pastan, I. H., and Willingham, M. C.: Journey to the center of the cell: role of the receptosome. Science *214*:504, 1981.
413c. Greenberg, M. E., and Ziff, E. B.: Stimulation of 3T3 cells induces transcription of the *fos* proto-oncogene. Nature *311*:433, 1984.
413d. Muller, R., Bravo, R., et al.: Induction of c-*fos* gene and protein by growth factors precedes activation of c-*myc*. Nature *312*:716, 1984.
413e. Kruijer, W., Cooper, J. A., et al.: Platelet-derived growth factor induces rapid but transient expression of the c-*fos* gene and protein. Nature *312*:711, 1984.
413f. Persson, H., and Leder, P.: Nuclear localization and DNA binding properties of a protein expressed by human c-*myc* oncogene. Science *225*:718, 1984.
413g. Curran, T., Miller, A. D., et al.: Viral and cellular *fos* proteins: a comparative analysis. Cell *36*:259, 1984.
413h. Abrams, H. D., Rohrschneider, L. R., et al.: Nuclear location of the putative transforming protein of avian myelocytomatosis virus. Cell *29*:417, 1982.
413i. Stewart, T. A., Pattengale, P. K., et al.: Spontaneous mammary adenocarcinomas in transgenic mice that carry and express MTV/*myc* fusion genes. Cell *38*:627, 1984.
413j. Adams, J. M., Harris, A. W., et al.: The c-*myc* oncogene driven by immunoglobulin enhancers induce lymphoid malignancy in transgenic mice. Nature *318*:533, 1985.
413k. Leder, A., Pattengale, P. K., et al.: Consequences of widespread deregulation of the c-*myc* gene in transgenic mice: multiple neoplasms and normal development. Cell *45*:485, 1986.
413l. Pledger, W. J., Stiles, C. D., et al.: An ordered sequence of events is required before BALB/c-3T3 cells become committed to DNA synthesis. Proc. Natl. Acad. Sci. USA *75*:2839, 1978.
413m. Leof, E. B., Wharton, W., et al.: Epidermal growth factor (EGF) and somatomedin-C regulate G_1 progression in competent BALB/c-3T3 cells. Exp. Cell Res. *141*:107, 1982.
414. Rubin, J. A., Shia, M. A., et al.: Stimulation of tyrosine-specific phosphorylation *in vitro* by insulin-like growth factor I. Nature *305*:438, 1983.
415. Wang, D., Liebowitz, D., et al.: An EBV membrane protein expressed in immortalized lymphocytes transforms established rodent cells. Cell *43*:831, 1985.
416. Rabbits, T. H.: The c-*myc* proto-oncogene: involvement in chromosomal abnormalities. Trends Genet. *1*:327, 1985.
417. Cheah, M. S. C., Ley, T. J., et al.: *fgr* proto-oncogene mRNA induced in B lymphocytes by Epstein-Barr virus infection. Nature *319*:238, 1986.
418. Leyvras, S., Henle, W., et al.: Association of Epstein-Barr virus with thymic carcinoma. New Engl. J. Med. *312*:1296, 1985.
419. Ogston, C. W., Jonak, G. J., et al.: Cloning and structural analysis of integrated woodchuck hepatitis virus sequences from hepatocellular carcinomas of woodchucks. Cell *29*:385, 1982.
420. Neidel, J. E., Kuhn, L., et al.: Phorbol diester receptor copurifies with protein kinase C. Proc. Natl. Acad. Sci. USA *80*:36, 1983.
421. Bréchot, C., Hadchovel, M., et al.: State of hepatitis B virus DNA in hepatocytes of patients with hepatitis B surface antigen-positive and -negative liver disease. Proc. Natl. Acad. Sci. USA *78*:3906, 1981.
422. Koch, S., Freytag von Loringhoven, A., et al.: Amplification and rearrangement in hepatoma cell DNA associated with integrated hepatitis B virus DNA. EMBO J. *3*:2185, 1984.
423. Mizusawa, H., Taira, M., et al.: Inversely repeating integrated hepatitis B virus DNA and cellular flanking sequences in the human hepatoma-derived cell line huSP. Proc. Natl. Acad. Sci. USA *82*:208, 1985.
424. Kan, Y. W., Lee, K. Y., et al.: Polymorphism of DNA sequence in the β-globin gene region: application to prenatal diagnosis of $β^0$ thalassemia in Sardinia. New Engl. J. Med. *302*:185, 1980.
425. Rotwein, P. S., Chirgwin, J., et al.: Polymorphism in the 5' flanking region of the human insulin gene: A genetic marker for non-insulin-dependent diabetes. New Engl. J. Med. *308*:65, 1983.
426. Gusella, J. F., Wexler, N. S., et al.: A polymorphic DNA marker genetically linked to Huntington's disease. Nature *306*:234, 1983.
427. Weinberg, R. A.: Alteration of the genomes of tumor cells. Cancer *52*:1971, 1983.
428. Bernstein, S. C., and Weinberg, R. A.: Expression of the metastatic phenotype in cells transfected with human metastatic tumor DNA. Proc. Natl. Acad. Sci. USA *82*:1726, 1985.
428a. Thorgeirsson, U. P., Turpeenniemi-Hujanen, T., et al.: NIH/3T3 cells transfected with human tumor DNA containing activated *ras* oncogenes express the metastatic phenotype in nude mice. Mol. Cell. Biol. *5*:259, 1985.
428b. Greig, R. G., Koestler, T. P., et al.: Tumorigenic and metastatic properties of "normal" and *ras*-transfected NIH/3T3 cells. Proc. Natl. Acad. Sci. USA *82*:3698, 1985.
428c. Bondy, G. P., Wilson, S., et al.: Experimental metastatic ability of Ha-*ras*-transformed NIH3T3 cells. Cancer Res. *45*:6005, 1985.
428d. Bradley, M. O., Kraynak, A. R., et al.: Experimental metastasis in nude mice of NIH 3T3 cells containing various *ras* genes. Proc. Natl. Acad. Sci. USA *83*:5277, 1986.
428e. Morgan, D. A., Ruscetti, F. W., et al.: Selective *in vitro* growth of T lymphocytes from normal human bone marrow. Science *193*:1007, 1976.
428f. Robb, R. J., Munk, A., et al.: T cell growth factor receptors, quantitation, specificity, and biological relevance. J. Exp. Med. *154*:1455, 1981.
428g. Depper, J. M., Leonard, W. J., et al.: Augmented T cell growth factor receptor expression in HTLV-1-infected human leukemia cells. J. Immunol. *133*:1691, 1984.
428h. Waldmann, T. A., Longo, D. L., et al.: Interleukin 2 receptor (Tac antigen) expression in HTLV-1-associated adult T-cell leukemia. Cancer Res. (suppl.) *45*:4559S, 1985.
428i. Rosenberg, S. A., Lotze, M. T., et al.: Observations on the systemic administration of autologous lymphokine-activated killer cells and recombinant interleukin-2 to patients with metastatic cancer. New Engl. J. Med. *313*:1485, 1985.
428j. Wallich, R., Bulbuc, N., et al.: Abrogation of metastatic properties of tumour cells by *de novo* expression of H-2K antigens following *H-2* gene transfection. Nature *315*:301, 1985.

ONCOLOGY

CHAPTER 32
Cancer Chemotherapy and Radiation Therapy

I. Cancer Chemotherapy
HERBERT T. ABELSON

II. Radiation Therapy
NANCY J. TARBELL
J. ROBERT CASSADY

I. CANCER CHEMOTHERAPY
INTRODUCTION 981
HISTORICAL CONSIDERATIONS 982
DEVELOPMENT AND TESTING OF NEW AGENTS 982
Preclinical
Clinical
TREATMENT CONSIDERATIONS 985
Selectivity of Treatment
Control of Toxicity
Nutritional Support
Clinical Pharmacokinetics
Drug Interactions
The Individual Patient
TUMOR GROWTH RATE AND RESPONSE TO CHEMOTHERAPY 988
Volume Doubling Time
Exponential and Gompertzian Growth Patterns
First-Order Kinetics and Protocol Design
Gompertzian Kinetics and Protocol Design
Kinetics of Microscopic Disease and Adjuvant Chemotherapy
The Cell Cycle and Cell Labeling Techniques
Tumor Stem Cells
Chemotherapeutic Agents and the Cell Cycle
Cell Synchronization
Recruitment
Do Cell Kinetics Help?
COMMONLY USED DRUGS IN CHILDHOOD CANCER CHEMOTHERAPY 997
Combination Chemotherapy
Resistance
Therapeutic Strategy
Prospectus

II. RADIATION THERAPY
PHYSICAL PRINCIPLES 1019
Absorption of Radiation by Matter
Particulate Radiation
RADIATION BIOLOGY 1020
Mechanisms and Site of Action of Radiation Damage
Methods of Cell Killing by Irradiation
Cell Survival Curve Characteristics
Repair
Cell Cycle Variations in Radiation Sensitivity
The Oxygen Effect
Radiation Protectors
Radiation Interactions with Chemotherapeutic Agents
Dose-Rate Effect
CLINICAL PRINCIPLES 1024
Complications
TREATMENT PLANNING PRINCIPLES 1025

I. Cancer Chemotherapy
HERBERT T. ABELSON

INTRODUCTION

The vast majority of malignant tumors cannot be cured or adequately controlled by local measures because they have already spread regionally or systemically at the time of diagnosis. Therefore surgery (for biopsy, debulking, or removal of localized tumors), although a cornerstone of sound cancer management, must usually be combined with other treatment modalities to provide effective therapy. Radiation therapy also has its greatest use for treatment of local or circumscribed tumors and therefore, like surgery, is limited by the pernicious biology of most malignant tumors, which renders them systemic rather than local diseases. Chemotherapy is vastly less specific than surgery and is not generally focusable like radiotherapy. However, even with its shortcomings, chemotherapy holds the promise for long-term survival since it is capable of killing tumor cells after they have already been disseminated throughout the body. In fact, the reduction in cancer mortality in the United States since 1970 has been largely attributed to the success of chemotherapy in patients less than 45 years old. For example, the results in treatment of childhood leukemia and lymphoblastic lymphoma (both systemic diseases) have been dramatically improved by chemotherapy (1, 2). Although extremely useful in treating bulk disease in leukemia and lymphoma, chemotherapy may be most effective after tumor burden has been effectively reduced by surgery or radiation therapy, when the drugs are directed against residual micrometastatic disease (adjuvant treatment), as in the treatment of Hodgkin's disease, testicular cancer, osteosarcoma, and premenopausal breast cancer. The indications for and limitations of chemotherapy are given in Table 32–1.

Immunotherapy, like chemotherapy, has the potential to attack tumor cells after they have become widespread; however, most immunotherapy approaches are experimental and have not been

Table 32–1. INDICATIONS FOR AND LIMITATIONS OF CHEMOTHERAPY IN TREATMENT OF CANCER

Indications	Major Limitations
Systemic tumors, e.g., acute leukemia and disseminated solid tumors Adjuvant therapy after definitive surgery, e.g., for osteosarcoma	1. Intrinsic or acquired drug resistance 2. Lack of specificity for tumor cells versus normal cells 3. Inability to reach "sanctuaries" such as the CNS 4. First-order kinetics of cell kill
Reduction in size of solid tumors in order to facilitate surgery or radiology	The above plus: 1. A greater proportion of resting or G_0 cells
Regional perfusion, e.g., of liver or extremities	The above plus: 1. Technical, requiring specialized procedures and personnel 2. Limited to area being perfused
Palliation	1. Temporary 2. Additional side effects

widely tested, and studies have not evaluated dose of agent, immunocompetence of the host, and tumor cell type. Nevertheless, passive approaches utilizing allogeneic or xenogeneic antibodies, which can also be coupled with cytotoxins or chemotherapeutic agents, will be discussed later.

HISTORICAL CONSIDERATIONS

The end of World War II ushered in the era of cancer chemotherapy when the nitrogen mustards were declassified as chemical warfare agents. Shortly thereafter, reviews were published demonstrating that these compounds had activity against lymphomas (3). In 1948, Farber and colleagues demonstrated that the folic acid antagonist aminopterin induced temporary remissions in childhood acute lymphocytic leukemia (4). None of these patients were cured, however, and all eventually relapsed and died. Another crucial milestone was reached in the mid-1950's when it was found that another antifolate, methotrexate, could effect cures in a solid tumor, choriocarcinoma (5). The intervening years to the present time have been punctuated by further advances resulting from the perseverance of individuals who believed that the natural course of other malignant diseases could also be altered by chemotherapy (6, 7). Some highlights of this period were:

1. The early sequence of studies that introduced scientific experimental designs, including criteria for response as well as the development of the principles of sequential and combination chemotherapy during remission and prophylactic treatment of the central nervous system (8, 9, 384, 386–388).

2. The development of combinations of drugs for the curative treatment of acute lymphocytic leukemia (1, 10, 11) and Hodgkin's disease (12, 13).

3. The development of a multidisciplinary approach (surgery, radiation therapy, and chemotherapy) to metastatic Wilms' tumor (14, 15). This concept of multidisciplinary management has now become a fundamental principle of oncology.

4. The development of aggressive adjuvant chemotherapy against micrometastatic disease, which has helped to alter the natural course of some tumors such as osteogenic sarcoma (16, 17).

Thirty years ago, any physician using drugs to treat malignant disease was regarded with suspicion and contempt, not unlike the pessimism that greeted the early attempts for successful chemotherapy of tuberculosis. Even today, reticence is often expressed, e.g., when drugs are referred to as "poisons" and self-fulfilling prophecies of failure are voiced as in years past (18). The issue remains charged. We have learned much about the biochemistry and pharmacology of anticancer drugs; however, many treatment programs have been developed empirically and the data base remains incomplete.

DEVELOPMENT AND TESTING OF NEW AGENTS

Preclinical

The use of massive screening programs to identify substances with anticancer activity has been denigrated by some, but most of the clinically useful agents have been found empirically in this way. Exceptions are L-asparaginase (19) and 5-fluorouracil (20). The evaluation of chemotherapeutic agents in preclinical test systems (i.e., acquisition of agents, choice of screening systems, determination of drug activity and toxicity) (21–23) and their subsequent clinical evaluation (24–26) provide the safeguards as well as the data base for drug use in the clinic. A recent comprehensive review outlines drug development screening procedures, protocols for in vivo and in vitro screening systems, and toxicology, pharmacology, and experimental models, as well as Phase-I to Phase-III clinical trials (26).

The development of antitumor screening systems was detailed in the initial report of Gellhorn and Hirschberg, in which 74 different biologic test systems were presented (27). Additional screening systems were added, but retrospective analysis revealed that the vast majority of clinically active agents would have been identified using only two systems, L1210 leukemia and Walker carcinoma 256, and L1210 is the primary test system in use today. A typical in vivo experiment, utilizing the transplantable murine L1210 leukemia, would be to determine the per cent increase in life span (ILS) of treated mice versus nontreated mice. The size of the L1210 inoculum and the delay in administering therapy are important determinants of response. In general, agents producing a 25 per cent or greater ILS are considered candidates for further study (26). Additional screening systems that identify agents missed by L1210 leukemia and Walker carcinoma 256 are P338 leukemia, L5178Y leukemia, P1798 leukemia, B16 melanoma, Lewis lung tumor, AKR lymphoma, and in vitro KB human epidermal carcinoma (21).

The various in vivo screening systems attempt not only to identify active agents but also to exclude from clinical trials those agents whose toxicity is likely to be excessive. Laboratory animal models often predict toxicity in humans and thereby establish initial drug doses (22, 28). Although the models have some predictive value, the development of better animal models for screening should improve the preclinical accuracy of determining antitumor effects and toxicity of treatment programs. It should be emphasized that fast-growing, transplantable tumor systems (i.e., L1210 leukemia) do not resemble the majority of human tumors, which have low growth fractions (see later section). Experimental tumors with low growth fractions such as the transplanted Lewis lung tumor in mice may be better models of their human counterparts. In addition, human tumor xenographs in nude mice may provide valuable secondary drug screening data (374). It should be emphasized here that an agent could be inactive in a preclinical screening test but effective in human disease; such an agent would not be identified by current procedures. Conversely, some drugs appear extremely promising in the preclinical screening, i.e., N-(phosphonacetyl)-L-aspartate, PALA, but have been relatively disappointing in clinical practice (29).

Clinical

Prompt introduction of new, effective chemotherapeutic agents into clinical use has been facilitated by collaborative studies and rigorous clinical investigative techniques. After an agent has been identified as potentially useful in preclinical screenings and the dose, toxicity, tolerance, tumor spectrum, and delivery route and schedule have been evaluated in animals, it may be subjected to a succession of human clinical trials (30) designated Phase-I, Phase-II, and Phase-III, as outlined in Table 32–2.

Phase-I trials are conducted with patients who have malignant disease resistant to the usual forms of therapy or for whom no known therapy is effective. These studies are primarily pharmacologic and attempt to establish several criteria with respect to the drug being tested: (1) maximum tolerated drug dose for a given route and schedule of administration; (2) drug toxicity, with emphasis on predictability, patterns, and reversibility; and (3) evidence of biologic effect, i.e., myelosuppression, stomatitis, and alopecia (antitumor activity is not usually required). Some European Phase-I trials assess qualitative antitumor effect, and patients must have measurable lesions to be included in the study (31).

There are a number of potentially serious problems with Phase-I trials. First, the patients involved are often dying or have far advanced disease.

Table 32–2. CLINICAL TRIALS IN CANCER CHEMOTHERAPY*

Phase I.	Clinical pharmacology in advanced cancer patients with or without measurable disease:	
	1. Establish maximally tolerated dose	
	2. Establish toxicity	
	3. Establish biologic effect (antitumor activity not necessarily required)	
Phase II.	Survey for clinical activity in patients with measurable or evaluable disease:	
	1. Nonrandomized drug-oriented studies	
	2. Ten to 20 patients with a variety of tumors, e.g., slow-growing and fast-growing:	
	a. Adenocarcinoma of colon	
	b. Bronchogenic carcinoma	
	c. Adenocarcinoma of breast	
	d. Undifferentiated lymphosarcoma	
	e. Acute myelocytic leukemia	
	f. Acute lymphocytic leukemia	
Phase III.	Definitive studies to establish role in cancer therapy:	
	1. Controlled clinical trials	
	2. Combination studies	
	3. Adjuvant applications	

*Modified from Goldin, A., and Carter, S. K.: Screening and evaluation of antitumor agents. In *Cancer Medicine*. Holland, J.F., and Frei, E., III (eds.), Philadelphia, Lea and Febiger, 1982.

Because of their general debility, patients may receive drug doses or courses that are inadequate to evaluate drug activity. In addition, patients may have metabolic derangements (i.e., decreased hepatic or renal function) that alter activation, metabolism, or excretion of the drug being tested. The maximum tolerated drug dose reached in these trials may be influenced to a large degree by prior therapy and patient selection. Unfortunately, in practice, drugs are often administered before assays for the parent compound or its metabolites have been developed. Because of this, data concerning drug levels, metabolism, and excretion are often imprecise at the very time that the study is designed to evaluate dose-related toxicity. In spite of these limitations, it must be emphasized that Phase-I trials have therapeutic intent; they are not exclusively toxicity trials. Patients entered on a trial should have progressive dose escalation to a potentially therapeutic range. Failure to demonstrate antitumor activity, however, does not preclude the passage of a biologically active agent into Phase-II trials.

Phase-II trials attempt to assess the degree of antitumor activity for a new agent by employing a single dose and schedule in a variety of human tumors with different growth rates. These studies may or may not be randomized, and their end point is a measurable, objective response within a specified time period. This type of trial is crucial, as it determines whether or not a drug is evaluated further for a specific tumor. An agent would be considered potentially useful if it appeared to be as good as or better than the best existing treatment or if it showed activity in patients who had already failed on the best available treatment. Criteria for objective responses are:

1. Complete response (CR)—complete disappearance of all evident disease.
2. Partial response (PR)—50 per cent or greater reduction in measurable tumor (product of longest and widest diameters) and no measurable disease progression at other sites.
3. No response (NR)—less than 50 per cent reduction in measurable disease. The minimal duration of partial or complete response is usually taken as 1 month.

Phase-II trials also have a number of inherent problems. Drugs have usually been evaluated in the Phase-I trials on one or few dosage schedules that may not reflect the most effective way to administer the drug. In addition, as noted previously, the maximum tolerated drug dose achieved in Phase-I studies may be a compromise. Since drug dose–response curves are steep (Fig. 32–1) and the schedule of drug administration often crucial (32), it is possible that the chosen drug dose and schedule for the Phase-II trial may be far from optimum.

A second major problem is that of evaluating

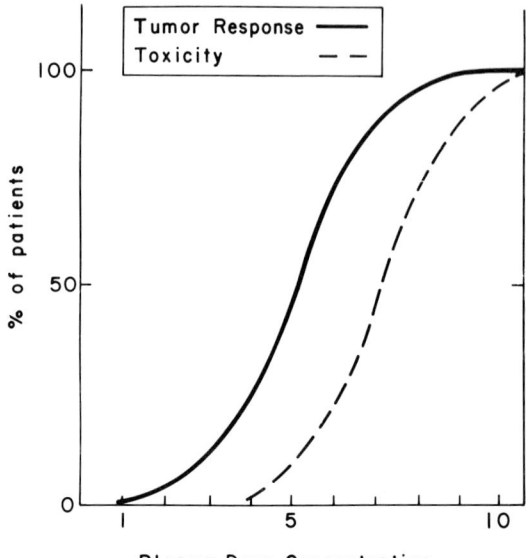

Figure 32–1. Tumor response (solid line) and toxicity (broken line) are related to drug dose. Both curves are steep. The extent to which the toxicity curve is displaced to the right reflects the therapeutic index (median toxic dose/median effective dose), which for most oncolytic drugs is low. An ideal drug would produce 100 per cent tumor response with zero toxicity. Pragmatically, a compromise must be struck as to how much toxicity (and of what type) is acceptable for a given degree of response.

response. Since tumor cross-sectional area and volume are not linearly related (Fig. 32–2), potentially deceptive interpretations about response may be made from measurement of tumor diameter alone. In addition, edges of tumors are often difficult to define, adding further uncertainty to the measurements. The widespread availability of computed tomography scanning should improve the sensitivity and accuracy of these measurements.

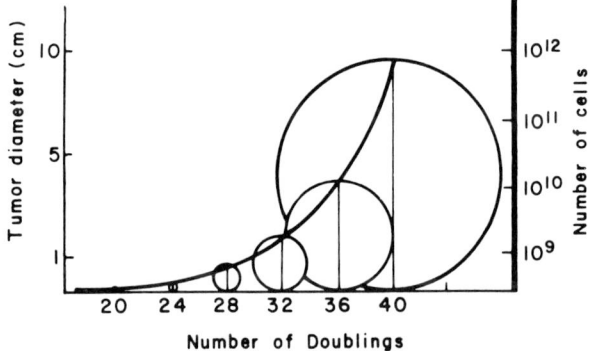

Figure 32–2. Tumor diameter and cell number (volume) are directly but not linearly related. As the diameter doubles, the volume increases eightfold. This may help to explain the so-called rapid tumor growth noted when clinical diagnosis is made. Most of a tumor's history is subclinical (up to about 28 doublings or about 1 cm. in diameter) in a geometrically increasing population of cells. The relationship $N(t) = 2^n$ describes such a population, in which n is the number of divisions in time (t) and N(t) is the total number of cells.

There is another potential problem with Phase-II evaluations. An agent that is not active against *gross* deposits of tumor may be active against *microscopic* deposits of the same disease. In experimental mouse tumors, this scenario has been repeatedly described (33). The probability, therefore, of rejection of an agent that is active or more active only against microscopic deposits of tumor is very great.

Phase-II trials often employ techniques that take into account known prognostic variables for a disease. For example, groups of patients are categorized (stratification), and randomization is used to decrease treatment selection bias (33, 35). Inherent in these trials, whether randomized or not, is a biostatistical design that helps to avoid false-negative results (type 2, β, or rejection error) for an agent. This type of error leads to rejection of an agent for further study when, in fact, additional study is indicated. The number of patients necessary to assess drug activity can be calculated for any predetermined level of drug effectiveness and any percentage of type 2 error (33). For example, a sample of nine patients is required to determine whether a new agent is 25 per cent effective while accepting a 10 per cent chance of having a false-negative result. In a sample of this size, there is a greater than 90 per cent chance that one or more patients will respond if the actual response rate is 25 per cent (34).

Phase-III trials focus on a particular malignancy, utilizing the techniques of stratification and randomization within the setting of a controlled clinical study. The goal of Phase-III trials is to compare a new treatment with other known treatments while confirming and extending the data obtained in Phase-II trials.

A particularly sensitive issue with respect to Phase-II and Phase-III trials is the use of historical controls. Changes in criteria for diagnosis, histopathology, staging, measurement of response, supportive care, physicians involved, referral patterns, a possible change in the natural history of the disease, and the difficulty in matching known prognostic variables between the study group and historical controls contribute in various degrees to the uncertainty of historical control groups for comparison with ongoing studies. Whenever possible, concurrent control or comparison groups should be employed rather than historical controls (364).

TREATMENT CONSIDERATIONS

Selectivity of Treatment

There are now more than 70 drugs shown to be clinically useful in the treatment of human malignancies. The chemotherapeutic approach to an individual patient with cancer requires that a number of priorities be considered when a therapeutic strategy is developed.

The aim of chemotherapy is the cytoreduction of malignant cells with concomitant sparing of normal cells. For the most part, however, this paradigm, which has evolved from the treatment of malaria (36) and bacterial diseases (37, 38), is rarely attainable. Effective chemotherapy almost invariably means that the host will experience side effects (toxicity) to a greater or lesser degree. When differences between normal and tumor cells are identified and exploited, toxicity can be minimized. To be sure, as the mechanism of action of agents becomes better understood and as biologic targets are identified, more rational approaches to chemotherapy will become available, but despite a large body of information concerning the action of chemotherapeutic agents, we are far from this ideal. Therapeutic strategy attempts to balance the probability of tumor response while minimizing complications.

The major enigma of cancer chemotherapy is why it should work at all. In general, normal cells (bone marrow and gastrointestinal tract) divide more rapidly (39–43) than tumor cells. Therefore, agents that are most active against growing cells are apt to be very toxic toward the normal bone marrow and gastrointestinal tract, and, in practice, this is the case.

The number of tumor cells at clinical diagnosis in acute leukemia and multiple myeloma often approximates 5×10^{11} to 10^{12} (44, 45, 388). The total number of normal bone marrow stem cells may be less than 10^9.* Therefore, no bone marrow stem cells could survive an assault that kills all tumor cells (assuming equivalent drug sensitivity and first order kinetics: see later section). However, all tumor cells may not be tumor stem cells. In fact, the proportion may be variable and related to the tumor type; e.g., early L1210 leukemia has a very high percentage of tumor stem cells, whereas the percentage is much lower in plasmacytomas. This may partially account for the success in treating certain malignancies. In addition, differential sensitivity to chemotherapeutic agents has previously been noted for normal versus tumor cell populations (29, 44). Proper scheduling of chemotherapy so that normal cells recover whereas tumor cells do not also contributes to successful treatment. For example, Figure 32–3 shows that a given dose of drug may kill an equivalent fraction of tumor cells and normal cells, but the rate of recovery of normal cells may exceed that of tumor cells. Therefore, the next course of chemotherapy can be delivered when there are fewer tumor cells

---

*This calculation is based on numbers of early erythroid progenitors (BFU-E) and granulocyte progenitors (CFU-C), as there is no appropriate assay for human CFU-S progenitor cells that engraft (see Chapter 6) (365).

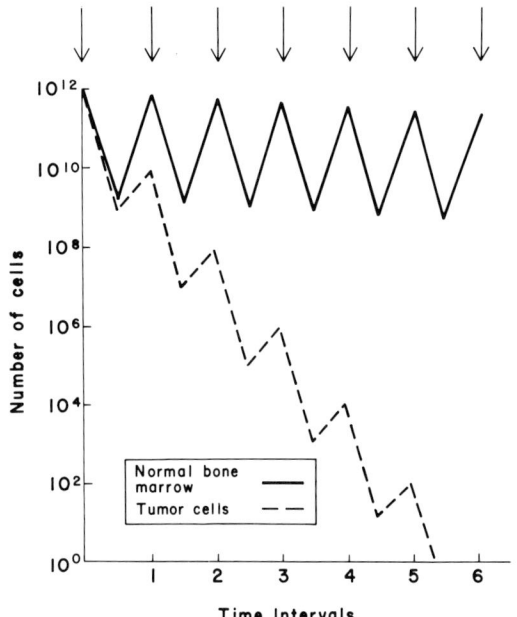

Figure 32–3. Normal bone marrow cell kill and recovery (solid line) are compared with tumor cell kill and recovery (broken line). A course of chemotherapy is given in each time interval, as indicated by the vertical arrows. Each course of chemotherapy produces an equivalent amount of destruction of both normal bone marrow (solid line) and tumor cells (broken line). The rate of recovery of normal bone marrow cells, however, may be greater than that of the tumor cells (39–43) so that with each successive course of chemotherapy, the tumor cell burden is less. It should also be noted that the number of normal bone marrow progenitors does decrease with continued treatment, but at a far slower rate than that of the tumor cells.

present than there were when the previous course was administered. The concepts of first-order kinetics of cell killing and the fact that all tumor cells must be eliminated are discussed in a later section. Despite the fact that the proliferative characteristics of either normal or tumor stem cells are largely unknown (365), chemotherapy can eradicate tumor and allow the host to survive. It has been determined that the four-drug combination of cyclophosphamide, cytosine arabinoside, vincristine, and prednisone (COAP) achieves a 100,000-fold selectivity against tumor cells over normal cells in the treatment of spontaneous AKR leukemia in mice (44).

Control of Toxicity

The relative risks of chemotherapy (e.g., effectiveness, toxicity, availability of supportive measures) must be weighed against the potential benefits in the form of palliation, temporary control, prolonged disease-free survival, or "cure." This relationship is shown in schematic fashion in Figure 32–1. The degree to which the toxicity curve is shifted to the right is a reflection of the therapeutic index, which may be defined as the ratio between the median toxic dose and the median effective dose for a given toxicity. However, drugs usually do not produce single toxic effects, and multiple therapeutic indices must be considered. The lower the therapeutic index, the smaller is the margin of safety for a particular agent in the majority of patients. In general, the therapeutic index of most cytotoxic agents is very low (1.5 to 3); however, in contrast to the generally steep and fixed dose-response curve for tumors, the toxicity curve may be modified by appropriate support measures. These can be pharmacologic (high-dose methotrexate followed by leucovorin rescue [54]) or physiologic (autologous bone marrow stem cell replacement after therapy-induced bone marrow aplasia [55–57]). Blood products (46–49), antibiotics (50, 51), and a sterile environment (52, 53) all help to control morbidity. Some current treatment protocols result in periods of bone marrow hypoplasia or aplasia and necessitate replacement therapy with white blood cells, platelets, and red blood cell transfusions (58). The state of the art is such that patients can now be maintained during these periods of extensive myelosuppression in the same manner that supportive care is available for bone marrow transplant recipients. Very high-dose chemotherapy approaches, however, may be limited by extramedullary toxicities (366).

The major toxicities of selected agents are detailed in a later section. In general, toxicity can be divided into immediate, delayed, and late reactions. Immediate reactions such as nausea and vomiting can produce significant morbidity and reluctance to continue therapy. Antiemetic agents are of considerable importance as adjuncts to therapy. Principles of antiemetic therapy include (1) careful attention to psychologic factors, i.e., the presence of emesis basins, proximity to other patients who are vomiting from their chemotherapy, anticipatory vomiting; (2) prophylactic treatment/continuous treatment/individualized treatment with agents such as antihistamines, barbiturates, phenothiazines, and combinations of metoclopramide with a variety of other agents (59–62); and (3) awareness of other causes of nausea and vomiting. Hyperkalemia, hyperphosphatemia, hyperuricemia, and hypocalcemia, as well as other electrolyte disorders, can be anticipated at the onset of chemotherapy in some patients with acute leukemia, Burkitt's lymphoma, or other tumors in which chemotherapy causes rapid lysis of large numbers of cells (63, 64). Delayed toxicity includes bone marrow suppression; immunosuppression (65); disruption of small intestinal villous structure and function, i.e., interruption of crypt cell replication, decreased mucosal thickness, vacuolated cells, and disaccharide malabsorption (367, 368); stomatitis; hair loss; and cardiac, hepatic, renal, and even brain damage. Adverse interaction of some chemotherapeutic agents (i.e., adriamycin and actinomycin-D) with irradiation can be debilitating (66). Late toxicity may involve major sequelae (67) including disturbances in growth and endocrine function (68, 69), sterility (70), and development of second tumors (71-73). An organ system review of toxic reactions is also available (74).

In addition, some drug toxicities may be related to mechanisms of action that are not obvious at first. Adriamycin, bleomycin, and neocarzinostatin may produce free radicals that result in direct damage to DNA and adjacent macromolecules (75, 76). Methotrexate-related central nervous system toxicity is a complex and controversial issue that may involve drug-irradiation interaction, inhibition of 1-carbon transfer pathways, and biogenic amine and serotonin formation (77). The increased survival of brain tumor patients after treatment with methyl-CCNU has resulted in unexpected late development of bone marrow dyscrasias and renal failure (78, 79).

Nutritional Support

The effect of nutrition and diet on cancer treatment has been treated rather casually. There have been both confusion and controversy about the benefits and potential consequences of aggressive nutritional support for patients during cancer therapy (80). The belief that feeding cancer patients may make their tumor grow more aggressively is prevalent and is partially responsible for some therapeutic conservatism. There is other evidence, however, that patients maintained on optimal diets or by total parenteral nutrition fare much better than their less-well-fed counterparts and, in addition, are able to undergo more intensive chemotherapy (81). Nutritional therapy should be thought of as another support modality during primary treatment. Adequate caloric intake may be impaired by psychologic factors, (including learned food aversions [82]), changes in taste acuity, nausea and vomiting secondary to chemotherapy, and metabolic effects of the disease itself (83, 84). The nutritional consequences of cancer and of cancer therapy are just beginning to be critically explored (84).

Clinical Pharmacokinetics

The optimal therapeutic use of drugs requires knowledge about the following variables: absorption, distribution, metabolism, and elimination (85-87). Absorption, transport, and uptake can be complex processes, since drugs may have to cross several membranes before reaching their targets. Drug uptake is often accomplished by passive diffusion (movement down a concentration or electrochemical gradient without energy expenditure by the cell). Facilitated diffusion (carrier-mediated passive diffusion) and active transport (energy-dependent transport against a concentration gradient) allow for more rapid passage across cell membranes and may also be involved in drug uptake.

A two-compartment open model is used to describe the pharmacokinetics of most drugs (88). It assumes a small central compartment (vascular fluid plus extracellular fluid of highly perfused tissues) and a peripheral compartment of larger apparent volume (less perfused tissues, i.e., skin, fat, and muscle).

Drug distribution is influenced by the binding of the drug to plasma and cellular proteins; the affinity for, as well as the ability of, the drug to cross membranes; the blood flow to component tissues; and the relative partition and apparent volume of the central and peripheral compartments.

First-order kinetic processes describe the exit of most drugs from both compartments as well as the processes of absorption, distribution, metabolism, and elimination. First-order kinetics is defined as follows: the rate of reaction at any time is proportional to the concentration of one reactant, and the half-life (t½) of the process is independent of the concentration. The t½ for elimination is the time required for the quantity of drug in the body to be decreased by half. Thus, after two, three, four, and five half-lives, 75, 87, 94, and 97 per cent of the drug has been eliminated, respectively. The pharmacokinetic concepts of apparent volume of distribution, clearance, extraction ratio, elimination, and t½, as well as modes of drug administration and more complex kinetic models, are covered in detail elsewhere in the literature (85, 86, 88, 89).

Various processes can contribute to the individual variation among patients that makes therapeutic equivalence difficult to achieve with a given drug dose (90). Examples are intrinsic factor deficiency (91); altered receptor levels (92, 93, 415); impaired liver microsomal biotransformation or metabolism (i.e., the mixed function oxidase system involving NADPH, cytochrome P-450, and NADPH cytochrome P-450 reductase) (87, 94, 95); and glucose-6-phosphate dehydrogenase (G6PD) deficiency (97). In addition, the type and stage of disease, concurrent disease or diseases, and presence of hypersensitivity, as well as general nutrition and diet, may be important factors (98).

Drug Interactions

Most drugs probably act independently; however, it is clear that some drugs affect or modify the response to others (99). These drug interactions are infrequently favorable in a therapeutic sense and may be dangerous or life-threatening. Most interactions with anticancer drugs involve

Table 32–3. SELECTED DRUG INTERACTIONS IN CANCER CHEMOTHERAPY

Anticancer Drug	Interacting Drug	Kind of Interaction	Effect	References
Methotrexate	Sulfonamides	Competition for plasma protein binding resulting in larger amount of "free" or active methotrexate	Bone marrow suppression and stomatitis	101
	Aspirin			
	Other salicylate-containing agents			
	Hydralazine			
	Probenecid	Interferes with renal and biliary excretion; prolongs CSF MTX levels	Decreased MTX clearance from CSF	103–106
Cyclophosphamide	Barbiturates	Increased activation	Bone marrow suppression	107
	Corticosteroids			
	Chloramphenicol	Decreased activation	Less antitumor effect	107, 108
	Allopurinol		Bone marrow suppression	109
6-Mercaptopurine	Allopurinol	Blocks detoxification by inhibiting xanthine oxidase	Bone marrow suppression	110, 111

either alterations in protein binding (e.g., displacement reactions) or changes in metabolic activation or detoxification (e.g., enzymatic interactions). Drug interactions may be a factor in the efficacy and toxicity of treatment. Selected examples are listed in Table 32–3 (for an overview see reference 100). The interaction of chemotherapeutic agents will be discussed later under Combination Chemotherapy. The hospitalized patient is particularly prone to exposure to a myriad of potential drug interactions, including combinations of anticancer drugs, analgesics, antipyretics, antimicrobials, sedatives, antiemetics, and tranquilizers.

The Individual Patient

Once a patient is identified as having a malignant disease that might respond to chemotherapy and it is agreed that the patient should be so treated, he or she still remains subject to a rather nascent art. Attempts have been made to develop tests to predict those drugs to which a particular tumor may respond (96, 102, 112–117). Some tests have potential, but there is presently no way to optimize the variables of schedule, dose, and drug combinations for an individual with a particular tumor. The model from microbiology of a rapid, predictive assay for drug sensitivity awaits the development of techniques that allow the reproducible growth of single cells or tumor spheroids from a wide range of cancers.

Many forms of cancer do respond to chemotherapy. Maximizing drug response often depends on understanding both the biochemistry and pharmacology of the chemotherapeutic agents as well as the kinetic behavior of the tumor itself. The factors we understand today that underlie the current success and failure of cancer chemotherapy include (1) the intrinsic drug sensitivity of many childhood cancers; (2) stage of disease (tumor burden) at diagnosis; (3) the availability of multiple agents for combination protocols; (4) the dose and dose rate for each drug; (5) the delay between diagnosis and starting chemotherapy; (6) volume doubling time of the tumor; (7) the emergence and growth of drug-resistant cells; and (8) the heterogeneity of tumor cells (117a). The following sections will focus on an overview of chemotherapy—its promise and its problems. It is not intended to be a comprehensive compendium of drugs used in cancer therapy.

TUMOR GROWTH RATE AND RESPONSE TO CHEMOTHERAPY

Volume Doubling Time

At the time a tumor becomes clinically apparent by either physical examination or conventional radiographic techniques, the tumor mass must be at least 0.5 cm in diameter and would thus be composed of about 1.5×10^8 cells (see Figure 32–2). Assuming that the tumor begins from a single cell; that it obeys ideal growth kinetics, with each cell giving rise to two daughter cells; and that all cells survive: 27 doublings are required to reach this number of cells. The nodule would be palpable after about 30 doublings (10^9 cells) or when it is about 1 cm in diameter. Ten more doublings or only one third again the lifetime of the tumor would result in 1.1×10^{12} cells and a 1-kg mass about 10 cm in diameter. This idealized geometric increase in cell number can be expressed mathematically by the relationship $N(t) = 2^n$, in which n is the number of divisions in time (t) and N(t) is the number of cells present. Thus, when considered in terms of the number of tumor doublings, only a small portion of the life history of a tumor occurs after it becomes clinically evident. In addition, tumor diameter and tumor volume are not linearly related; rather, the tumor volume more than doubles while the tumor diameter increases by only one third (118, 119), as illustrated in Figure 32–2. It must be emphasized, however, that what appears clinically as a rapidly enlarging mass may, in fact, be a tumor whose volume has increased because of hemorrhage, edema, and inflammatory cells. Growth of fibrous tissue and supporting elements also contributes to the increased volume.

Whether the increase in tumor size is due to tumor cell proliferation alone or to a complex admixture of elements, it has become increasingly clear from tumor data from both humans and experimental animals that the response rate to chemotherapy is related to the tumor growth rate (119–121). This relationship can be most easily envisioned cytokinetically by considering the volume doubling time of tumors. Volume measurements can be made of the spherical infiltrates that characterize pulmonary metastases. Utilizing computerized tomographic scanning and ultrasonography, less accessible tumors such as those in the retroperitoneal space and central nervous system can be subjected to the same kind of analysis. Correlation of changes in tumor volume with time has been made for a variety of human tumors (120). For a given tumor histologic type, volume doubling times tend to follow a log-normal distribution. Figure 32–4 shows the distribution and mean volume doubling time for a number of human tumors. These have been arbitrarily divided into three groups: those tumors with doubling times shorter than 30 days (Group I), those with intermediate doubling times (Group II), and those with doubling times exceeding 80 days (Group III).

A correlation of the volume doubling time with response to chemotherapy is shown in Figure 32–5. Metastatic human tumors are ranked in decreasing order with respect to their degree of responsiveness to chemotherapy versus their volume doubling time. Categories are divided into those tumors that can be cured by chemotherapy, those that show substantial tumor regression with chemotherapy, and those that have little response to chemotherapeutic agents. The median doubling times for these three groups are 24, 52, and 93 days, respectively. Therefore, in these groups of metastatic human cancers it seems clear that the response to chemotherapy is related at least in part to the volume doubling time of the tumors. This relationship has also been noted in experimental leukemias as well as in human primary

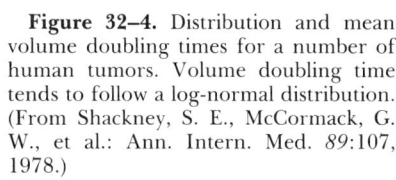

Figure 32–4. Distribution and mean volume doubling times for a number of human tumors. Volume doubling time tends to follow a log-normal distribution. (From Shackney, S. E., McCormack, G. W., et al.: Ann. Intern. Med. 89:107, 1978.)

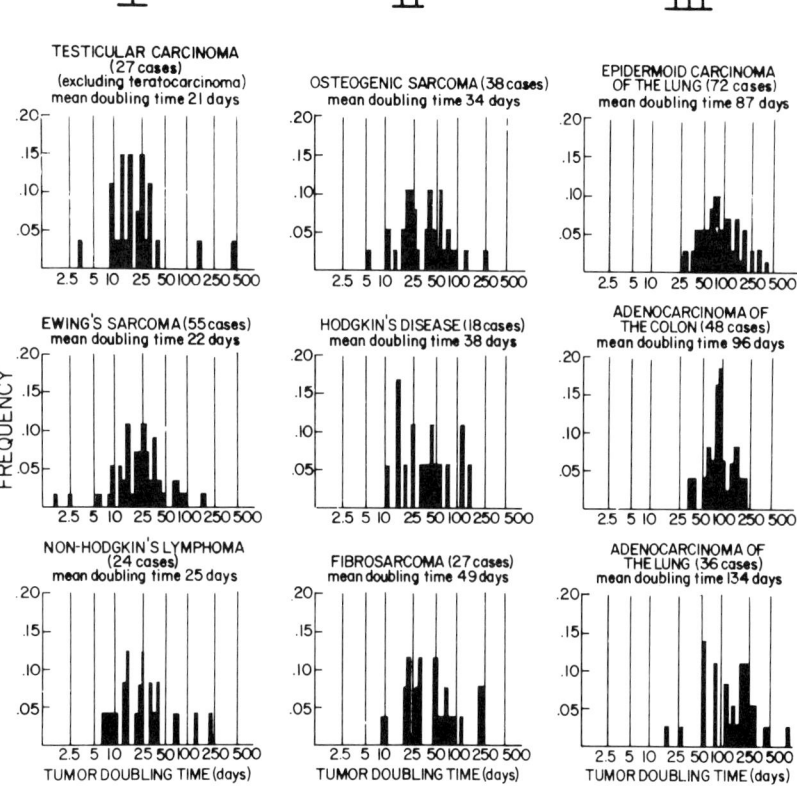

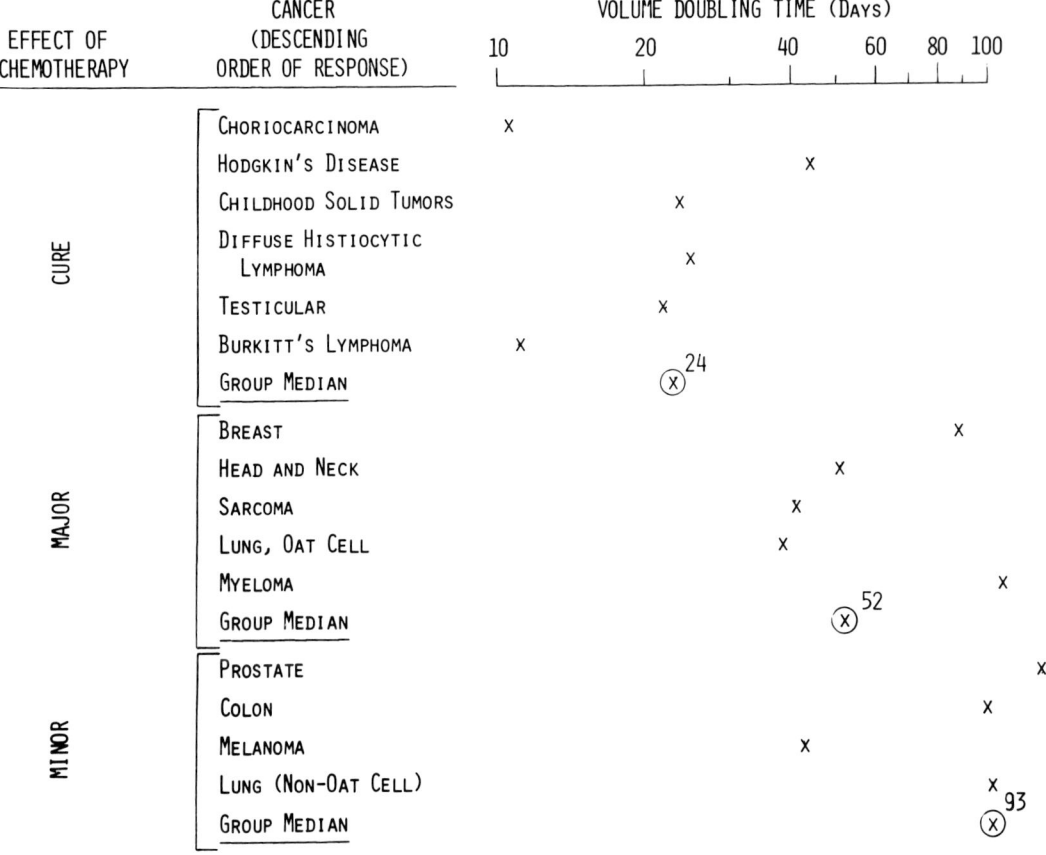

Figure 32–5. Correlation of volume doubling time with response to chemotherapy in metastatic human tumors. The volume doubling time (days) is compared with three groups of human metastatic tumors ranked in decreasing order with respect to curability and major and minor responsiveness to chemotherapy. [E. Frei, from data in Steel (119)].

tumors. The most rapidly growing tumors may be cured by chemotherapy, but more slowly growing tumors tend to be poor responders (see Goldie-Coldman discussion below). Exceptions may be tumors such as childhood B cell lymphomas (short volume doubling time), which are initially very sensitive to chemotherapy but have a high propensity for rapid relapse (376). These concepts may also explain differences between early and late stages of disease. As tumors enlarge, their volume doubling time increases and growth fraction decreases (to be discussed). Both choriocarcinoma (122) and Burkitt's lymphoma (123) are highly curable by single agents when tumors are small and localized; however, large tumor burden (late disease) results in response rates that are more akin to those of slowly growing tumors than to those of rapidly growing ones (120).

Tumor volume doubling time is only one of many variables that help to determine responsiveness to chemotherapy. Other influential factors affect the kinetics of tumor growth by altering either the percentage of cells dividing (growth fraction) or the time between mitosis (cell cycle time). These are listed in Table 32–4.

Exponential and Gompertzian Growth Patterns

There are two principal patterns that must be considered when assessing tumor growth, i.e., exponential and Gompertzian. Exponential growth patterns are usually observed only in transplanted tumors, i.e., early L1210 leukemia. (Exponential growth implies that the tumor doubling time is constant; the rate of cell production increases in direct proportion to the number of cells present).

Most experimental solid tumors, however, have irregular growth patterns and, on the average, seem best to obey Gompertzian kinetics, which dictate a slower rate of growth as the tumor enlarges.

Although little is known about the growth pattern of human tumors, the available data on primary and metastatic lung tumors indicate that growth curves in human tumors are best described by exponential rather than Gompertzian models (119). The lung, however, may not be representative, as it has excellent vascular supply and minimum physical resistance. Indeed, when the rate of myeloma protein synthesis was used as an index

Table 32–4. FACTORS AFFECTING KINETICS OF TUMOR GROWTH*

Perturbing Influence	Primary Kinetic Effect		References
	Growth Fraction	Cell Cycle Time	
Circadian rhythms	+		124, 125
Hormones	+		126
Diet	+	+	127
Vascular supply	+		128, 129
Immunologic	+	+	130, 131
Cytotoxic chemotherapy	+	+	132, 133
Irradiation	+	+	134
Contact inhibition		+	135

*Modified from Silver, R. T., Young, R. C., et al.: Am. J. Med. 63:722, 1977.

of myeloma cell number, the kinetics of tumor growth in untreated patients appeared to be Gompertzian (139).

First-Order Kinetics and Protocol Design

The shape of tumor growth curves has implications with respect to therapeutic approach. If, in fact, tumors follow exponential growth kinetics, the fractional cell kill hypothesis of Skipper, Schabel, and Wilcox assumes paramount importance (140–143). Their concepts predict that a drug's ability to kill tumor cells is dependent on both the dose and schedule of drug administration as well as the number of tumor cells present.

These investigators established that chemotherapeutic agents obey first-order kinetics with respect to cell kill.* Although this was a revelation to cancer chemotherapists, the concept was well known to microbiologists (the effects of disinfectants) and radiation biologists (radiation dose-response) (134). First-order kinetics dictates that increasing the drug dose results in an exponential decrease in the percentage of surviving cells. From this, it is clear that any given dose of drug will result in a constant decrease in the fraction, not the number, of different sized surviving cell populations. For example, a dose of drug that will reduce a population of cells from 1 million to 1000 cells will reduce 1000 cells to only one cell (Fig. 32–6). In order to increase the fractional cell kill with any agent, it is necessary to increase the drug dose, but this is limited by host toxicity (Fig. 32–1). In addition, the number of tumor cells present at the initiation of therapy has a direct bearing on a drug's ability to eradicate tumor. There is, in fact, an inverse relationship between drug effect or curability and the number of viable tumor cells present at the start of therapy (140, 143–146). The potential for destroying all tumor cells at a tolerable drug dose is much greater when the tumor burden is small. First-order kinetics does not imply that it is impossible to kill the last cell (142), but rather that host toxicity may be the limiting factor. The probability of killing the last cell with a given single dose of drug is described by Poisson distributions (140) and by the percentage of surviving

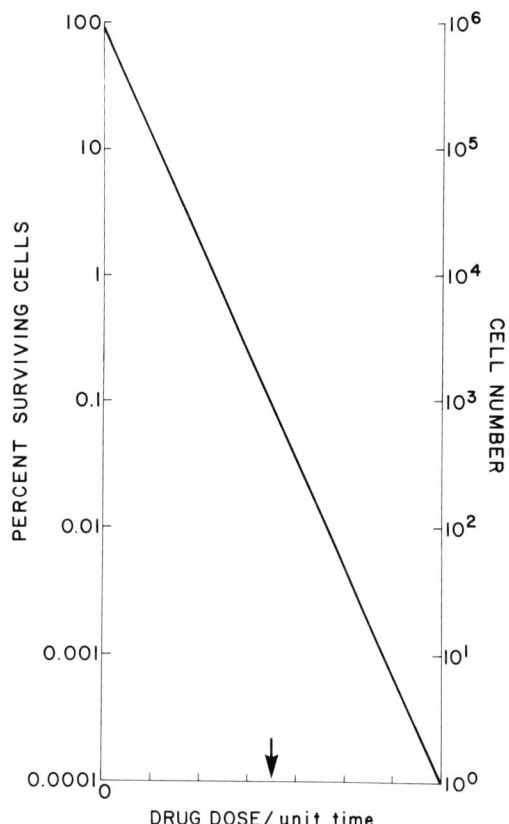

Figure 32–6. First-order decay. A given dose/unit time of chemotherapy will result in a constant percentage cell kill, *not* a constant number of different-sized tumor stem cell populations but only with the proviso that growth fraction and sensitivity to the drug remains the same. For example, a dose/unit time of drug (arrow) that will cause an average decrease of 10^6 to 10^3 cells will also cause an average decrease of 10^3 to 10^0. The actual number of remaining cells, however, is described by a Poisson distribution. This means that a decrease to 10^0 (1 cell), on the average, will result in an actual decrease to less than one cell (cure) in only 30 per cent of cases. Therefore, in reality, treatment must proceed such that cell kill would be 10^{-1} or less to insure a higher percent of cures.

---

*See Skipper (141) for a discussion of pseudo–first-order kinetics, in which two reactants are involved, with one in large excess (drug), and in which the rate of reaction depends on the first power of the second reactant (cell concentration).

cells for a given drug dose (142). For example, if a given drug dose will decrease the percentage of surviving cells by three logs (e.g., 1000 → 1.0), there is a 99.9 per cent chance that one surviving cell would be killed by that same dose of drug. A few (or in some instances, one) viable tumor cells can be lethal; therefore, eradication or cure of tumor requires killing all viable tumor cells (140, 143, 147).

The assumptions of first-order cell kill are valid only for populations of cells in which a constant fraction of cells initiates DNA synthesis per unit time.* Since this applies only to exponentially growing cells, its clinical application to human tumors may be limited. However, the concept of first-order cell kill has helped to form the basis of protocols utilizing combinations of drugs at maximum tolerated doses. This approach overcomes the limiting host toxicity that results from escalating the dose of single agents (to be discussed).

Gompertzian Kinetics and Protocol Design

Solid tumors, however, often undergo progressive growth retardation as they increase in size. This is illustrated in Figure 32–7, which portrays the temporal increase in tumor size. This Gompertzian growth curve indicates that larger tumors have progressively smaller growth fractions and increased doubling times as they approach maximum size, which may be due to increased cell death or movement of cells into G_0. The decrease in growth fraction is not necessarily uniform throughout the tumor, especially as the tumor progressively increases in size. Tumors often retain a highly proliferative rim of cells at their periphery, whereas cells in the interior portions of the tumor are out of cycle or in the process of becoming necrotic.

This discrepancy in growth rates between the interior and exterior portions of the tumor has been clarified to a degree by the demonstration that solid tumors can grow only to a certain defined diameter, after which they are unable to increase further in size without new vascularization (128, 137). Diffusion of nutrients into and removal of waste products from the tumor limit its steady state size. Neovascularization is induced by a tumor angiogenesis factor that is present in both animal and human tumors (137).

As new capillaries approach the tumor, the outer rim of tumor cells grows out around the capillaries, forming a cylindrical shape three to four cells thick. As the tumor expands, its interior may or may not become necrotic, depending on how tightly cells are packed together. This, in turn, depends on a number of factors, including cell-to-cell adhesiveness and mitotic index (376). Tumors with high packing pressures, e.g., Wilms' tumor, are often described as avascular when, in fact, they are actually ischemic, since their capillaries are compressed. Wilms' tumor cells are packed so tightly together that the tumor literally explodes if the surgeon drops it (377). (The inadvertent rupture of a Wilms' tumor during surgical removal has important consequences for both therapy and prognosis [see Chapter 37]).

The growth of experimental tumors in small animals seems to be well described by Gompertzian kinetics (119). These tumors include primary osteosarcomas, mammary carcinomas, and fibroadenomas, as well as numerous transplanted tumors. All show significant departure from exponential growth. Gompertzian growth (Fig. 32–7) has a limiting or plateau size. Norton and Simon (138) have attempted to predict the pattern of Gompertzian growth using the relations in Figure 32–7A to construct Figure 32–7B. It can be seen that growth rate is least for both very small and very large tumors and maximum for tumors of intermediate size (Fig. 32–7A, curve C). Specific growth rate (growth fraction) (Fig. 32–7A, curve C, which is expressed as the increase in tumor volume per unit time) decreases as tumor volume increases, but a large growth fraction does not necessarily imply a large growth rate (Fig. 32–7B, point 1).

If human tumor growth resembles experimental tumors that are described by Gompertzian growth, there may be new therapeutic strategies to consider. Norton and Simon (138) have provided a provocative model for therapeutics based on the relative growth rate of cells at various points on an idealized Gompertzian curve (Fig. 32–7A and B). They point out that large tumors do not usually respond well to chemotherapy, although first-order kinetic theory would predict that such tumors should be most sensitive to therapy in terms of both number of cells killed and rate of regression. In addition, they argue that very small tumors may have a lesser rate of regression (i.e., less sensitivity) than intermediate-sized tumors following a given therapy. Norton and Simon therefore propose that the growth-inhibiting effect of a treatment is proportional to growth rate of the untreated tumor (138). With reference to Figure 32–7A, the volume reduction in a tumor would be proportional to the specific growth rate (curve B) times the total tumor size (curve A). The authors' model dictates that the rate of regression for very large tumors (Fig. 32–7B, points 5 and 6) and very small tumors (Fig. 32–7B, points 1 and 2) will be less than tumors at point 3, Figure 32–7B. The clinical implication of their concepts is that a dose of a chemotherapeutic agent that will cause regression of an intermediate-sized tumor (Fig. 32–7B, point 3) may, when administered to a smaller

---

*This also assumes that no drug-resistant cells have emerged and that there are no pharmacologic sanctuaries (e.g., the central nervous system).

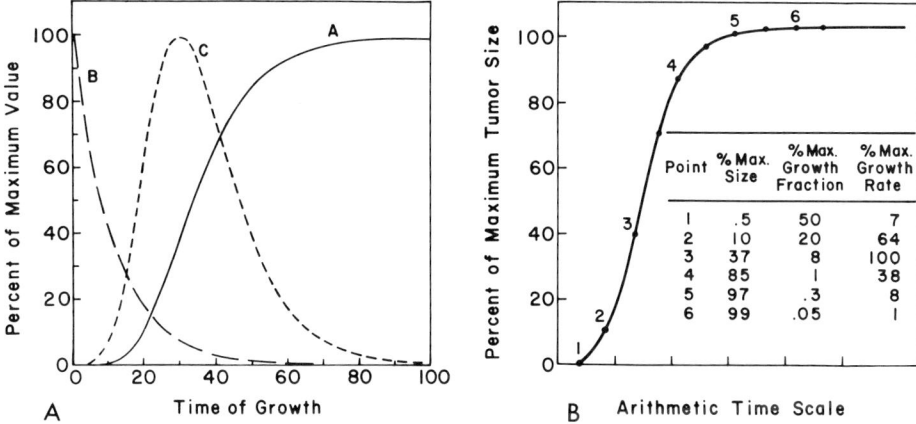

Figure 32–7. A, Relationship between tumor size (curve A), specific growth rate (growth fraction) (curve B), and growth rate (curve C) for unperturbed Gompertzian growth. Although the growth fraction (curve B) is maximal at the time of initiation of growth, the growth rate (curve C) is maximal when the tumor is about 37 per cent of its limiting size. B, Relationship, for Gompertzian growth, between tumor size, growth fraction, and growth rate, presented in tabular form. (From Norton, L., and Simon, R.: Cancer Treat. Rep. 61:1307, 1977.)

tumor volume (Fig. 32–7B, point 1 or 2), produce a more shallow regression rate, resulting in tumor regrowth when therapy is discontinued. In terms of protocol design, Norton and Simon propose pulse high-dose alternating drug therapy during maintenance and a period of late drug intensification. The latter concept is presently incorporated into some protocols for the treatment of acute leukemia (148) and osteosarcoma (17).

It is not possible to generalize as to whether human tumors are best described by exponential or Gompertzian growth. It is clear, however, that a variety of factors are involved in the overall determination of tumor responsiveness (see later section).

Kinetics of Microscopic Disease and Adjuvant Chemotherapy

As emphasized earlier, most of a tumor's history is subclinical and microscopic. The response of macroscopic disease to chemotherapy correlates well with volume doubling time (see Figure 32–5), but the behavior of microscopic disease is not as well defined. The concept of maximum recurrence time or period of risk, introduced by Collins and co-workers (118), is a technique for determining the kinetics of tumors during their early stages of growth. Collins reasoned that the maximum time of recurrence of any tumor would be determined by the growth characteristics of the original tumor. Since the original tumor could have begun no earlier than at the time of conception, the maximum lifetime of the original tumor is the patient's age at the time of clinical diagnosis of the tumor plus 9 months. If, after treatment, a single remaining tumor cell were to give rise to recurrent clinical disease, the maximum time to clinical recurrence should also not exceed the patient's age at diagnosis plus 9 months. This assumes that the growth characteristics of the recurrent tumor are comparable to the original. The corollary of this concept has prognostic significance; if the tumor has not recurred within the maximum time to recurrence or period of risk, it will not recur at all and the patient is cured.

The direct application of Collins' law has limited prognostic value except for several pediatric tumors, e.g., Wilms' tumor (149). However, the concept can be applied to the determination of human tumor subclinical doubling times (120). An example of such an application was developed by Frei and co-workers for osteogenic sarcoma (150). Since osteogenic sarcomas usually occur on an extremity, the primary tumor can be controlled by amputation or wide resection (16, 17), rendering patients totally free of clinical and radiographic evidence of disease. Of these patients, about 20 per cent will remain disease-free indefinitely, i.e., cured by the primary treatment; however, 80 per cent of patients will develop recurrent disease, as evidenced by pulmonary metastases (16, 17). It is assumed that this latter group had clinically undetected microscopic disease in the lungs at the time of primary surgery. The risk of recurrence (pulmonary metastases) is greatest within 9 months of surgery and progressively decreases with time. This pattern of recurrence is similar for other human tumors that also exhibit a reasonably discrete "break point," after which the risk of recurrence is much less. The disease-free survival curve reaches a plateau, and the majority of patients who survive with no evidence of disease after that time are cured of that tumor. The time from initial surgery (control of the primary tumor) to the break point is also a measure of the maximum recurrence time. If the maximum recurrence time represents the interval required for one or a very few tumor stem cells (present in the lungs at the time of primary surgery) to become radiologically detectable, the doubling time of microscopic disease can be calculated from the fact that somewhat less than 1 g of tumor (10^9 cells) is required to permit radiographic visualization (150).

The efficacy of adjuvant treatment for osteosarcoma has been a controversial issue. Recent results from Rosen and Nirenberg (392) have indicated that intensive multiagent chemotherapy given both preoperatively ("neo-adjuvant") and postoperatively (adjuvant) is effective in prolonging the disease-free survival in patients with osteosarcoma. In addition, the preoperative treatment with chemotherapy allows for an in vivo prediction of drug effectiveness. At the time of subsequent removal of the primary tumor, an assessment is made of the degree of tumor destruction secondary to chemotherapy. Those patients who have complete or almost complete destruction of the primary tumor continue their postoperative treatment with the same chemotherapeutic agents used preoperatively. Patients who show a less than optimum response to the preoperative chemotherapy are treated with a different combination of drugs postoperatively. Using this in vivo tumor assay system coupled with individualized therapy, disease-free survival is reported to be better than in any trials utilizing only postsurgical adjuvant chemotherapy.

Preoperative treatment with multiagent chemotherapy is also treatment at the earliest possible time after diagnosis. At this time, there should be the smallest possible tumor burden in the pulmonary metastases and the lowest probability of resistant drug phenotypes (see Goldie-Coldman discussion, below). Using the concepts of Skipper and Schabel that treatment is more efficacious against smaller amounts of disease, that multiple non–cross-resistant agents should be used, and that first-order kinetic kill is operative, together with the hypothesis of Norton and Simon that very intensive treatment needs to be administered to eradicate small amounts of disease, it may be concluded that the preoperative period is the optimum time for administration of chemotherapy to eradicate pulmonary metastatic disease. In patients who are treated with postsurgical adjuvant chemotherapy, the delay from diagnosis until the first administration of chemotherapy is often 3 to 4 weeks. This factor, in conjunction with the volume doubling time for osteosarcoma (Fig. 32–4) and the potential loss of growth control of metastatic disease after removal of the primary tumor, suggests that a significantly increased tumor burden may be present in the micrometastases at the time of initiation of postsurgical adjuvant chemotherapy. This potential increase in tumor burden may allow the spontaneous emergence of drug-resistant cells as predicted by Goldie and Coldman (see below) and may be responsible for the differences in disease-free survival in postoperative adjuvant trials versus Rosen's preoperative chemotherapy studies. It seems clear that a variety of chemotherapeutic agents, administered in different combinations, are active against micrometastatic disease in patients with osteosarcoma and result in prolongation of disease-free and overall survival (393). This conclusion would not be easily anticipated from Phase-II trials of the individual agents against gross deposits of osteosarcoma. This decoupling of the response of micrometastatic disease from gross metastatic disease after chemotherapy should result in a rethinking of our approach to the evaluation of Phase-II trials.

Almost uniformly, the doubling time for microscopic disease is substantially shorter than the doubling time for macroscopic disease. This is consistent with Gompertzian kinetics, as previously discussed in detail (see Figure 32–7A), and suggests that chemotherapy directed at microscopic disease (large growth fraction) following control of the primary tumor (adjuvant chemotherapy) might have a great potential for eradicating the residual tumor. In addition to volume doubling time, there is other substantial evidence to the effect that microscopic disease or minimal disease may be more susceptible to eradication by a given chemotherapeutic program than overt or bulk disease (33, 151). The greater effect of chemotherapeutic agents on microscopic disease is probably related to:

1. Small numbers of cells.
2. High growth fraction, i.e., more cells in cycle versus nonproliferating cells (see later section).
3. More effective delivery of drugs, i.e., better blood supply.
4. Less heterogeneity, i.e., less chance for intrinsically resistant cells to be present (see later section).

The Cell Cycle and Cell Labeling Techniques

The concept of a cell cycle (the interval between the midpoint of mitoses between a cell and its direct descendants) has had considerable impact on the development of chemotherapy (377). As depicted in Figure 32–8, several fundamental issues emerge:

1. There are distinct events that are limited to certain segments of the cell cycle, i.e., nuclear DNA replication during the S phase.
2. Cells may continuously traverse the cycle, may temporarily leave the cycle (G_0) to be recruited by an appropriate stimulus, or may irreversibly differentiate or die.
3. There may be a number of restriction (378) or control points (379) during the G_1 period.
4. Cells may increase in number by increasing

the fraction of cycling cells, shortening the cell cycle length, or decreasing cell loss.

To dissect the cell cycle, tritiated thymidine, an obligate precursor of DNA, can be used to label cells. This procedure provides information about the labeling index, rate of cell production, and intermitotic time. The latter is determined from a per cent labeled mitosis (PLM) curve, which is generated by using tritiated thymidine to follow a cohort of cells through the cell cycle. The PLM technique allows calculation of the average duration of G_2, M, S, and G_1 phases of the cell cycle, and from these the average duration of the cell cycle (T_c) or intermitotic time can be determined (152). It is clear from such labeling studies that there is a wide distribution of intermitotic times within a cohort of cells, which probably best reflects the variable length of G_1. However, within an exponentially growing population of cells in which a reasonably constant fraction of cells enters the S phase per unit time, individual cells show additional variability in their rate of entry into the S phase and the duration of this phase.*

If all the cells are in cycle (as in early L1210 leukemia), the volume doubling time would equal the T_c, but this is approachable only during exponential growth. Growth fraction refers to that fraction of cells within a tumor that is proliferating. The growth fraction, however, gives no clue as to whether the proliferating cells are tumor cells. In addition, if they are tumor cells, it is not known whether they are tumor stem cells capable of unlimited divisions or end-stage cells capable of only a few divisions.

The labeling indices (e.g., the ratios of pulse tritiated thymidine-labeled cells to total cells in tissue autoradiographs) for human leukemias and solid tumors can vary widely but are usually less than those of normal myeloid precursors (164).

---

*The variability associated with the intermitotic times or the duration of the S phase has important implications for the interpretation of tritiated thymidine pulse-labeling studies and is referred to as length-biased sampling (153). Length-biased sampling refers to the fact that when "units" from a population of "units" having length or time as a characteristic are sampled, the probability of a "unit" being sampled is not random but proportional to its length (153). Since the rate of entry of cells into the S phase, the duration of the S phase, and intermitotic times are all variable, pulse-labeling with tritiated thymidine will tend to label those cells whose S phase duration is long relative to their intermitotic time; e.g., the probability of a cell being labeled depends on the ratio (S/T_c). Thus, pulse-labeling is not labeling of a random (or even representative) sample of cells, but is labeling of a selected and biased sample. Therefore, Zelen (153) concludes that the effect of length-biased sampling is to overestimate the mean duration of the S phase or intermitotic times by as much as 100 per cent. Length-biased sampling errors arise also in interpreting the results of early disease detection by screening programs (153, 154). The paradox of "waiting for a bus" (154) (in Zelen's case, the MBTA—means between times of arrival) is another example of length-biased sampling; i.e., the average waiting time for public transportation is twice the MBTA.

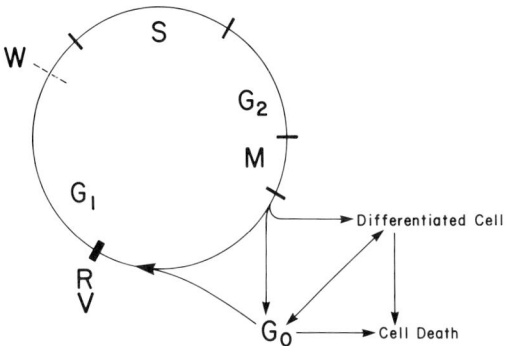

Figure 32–8. Diagram of the mammalian cell cycle. Cells may continuously traverse the cycle (M→G_1→S→G_2→M) or may temporarily or permanently leave the cycle (G_0, cell differentiation, or cell death). R (reference 378), V, and W (reference 379) represent potential growth control points.

Although there is little correlation between the initial labeling index and response to chemotherapy, increases in labeling index after initiation of chemotherapy can be directly correlated with clinical response (155, 156).

Cell loss from tumors can result from actual death of cells (limited blood supply, hypoxia, increased concentration of waste products), from their irreversible movement into G_0, or from differentiation (see Figure 32–8). Cell loss, although difficult to quantitate, helps explain the discrepancy between large growth fraction and long doubling time. In addition, the rate of cell loss may be very important for an accurate assessment of chemotherapy effects; i.e., there would be a more rapid decrease in tumor size after treatment of a tumor with a high rate of cell loss as compared with a tumor with a lower rate of cell loss. Tumors with long doubling times characteristically have small growth fractions, whereas those with short doubling times have a significantly greater growth fraction. However, some tumors have relatively large growth fractions, but their doubling time is also long (375). This is due to a high degree of cell loss.

A rapid and potentially more useful method for determining cytokinetic variables is to use flow microfluorometry (157, 158). The technique measures DNA content per cell and allows many cells to be analyzed at one time. Homogeneous cell populations are, however, required for critical analysis.

Tumor Stem Cells

Tumor stem cells, like normal bone marrow stem cells, are "invisible" using ordinary techniques. Both are capable of producing additional stem cells as well as families of descendants. However, in contrast to normal cell renewal systems, tumor cell renewal systems seem to exhibit a variety of aberrant features, including incomplete and erratic differentiation, aneuploidy, mutation and selection for resistance to therapy, and possibly no true G_0 or resting state (372). All these features suggest escape from normal regulatory mechanisms.

Tumor stem cells or clonogenic cells have been identified from a variety of experimental tumors by techniques such as spleen colony, lung colony, and limiting dilution assays. Recently, human tumor stem cells (clonogenic cells) have come under intensive study because of advances in tissue culture technique (96, 117, 159–161). Using peripheral blood tumor cells or single cell suspensions, antitumor agents can be assayed for their effect on colony formation. In one study, increasing concentrations of several different drugs produced progressive decrease in the number of colonies formed, and there was a strikingly positive correlation between in vitro assays and in vivo response (117). Major criticisms of these clonogenic assay systems as predictors of drug responsiveness include: low plating efficiency; difficulty in preparing single cell suspensions; artifactual cell survival curves with inappropriate inclusion of small colonies or clusters; nonapplicability for drugs that require prior activation; nonphysiologic drug delivery, i.e., lack of influence of vasculature; and wide variation of drug metabolism among patients.

Assay systems need to be improved so that they are more rapid, can accommodate drug combinations and variable drug schedules, and can more selectively grow tumor rather than normal cells (394–396). Although clonogenic cells may represent only a small proportion of the tumor population, they may be largely responsible for the biologic behavior of the tumor, and their drug sensitivity, cytokinetics, and metastatic potential are prime determinants of curability. With respect to metastases:

1. The metastatic process is dependent upon an interplay of properties unique to the tumor cell, as well as upon host factors (369, 370, 397).

2. The metastatic process is not random; i.e., certain cells may have a greater potential to metastasize as well as a specific affinity for one particular organ (369).

3. Establishment of metastases is best correlated with numbers of clumps of tumor cells (six to seven cells or larger), which must contain one or more clonogenic cells (371).

4. Metastases can metastasize (372).

There is evidence from tissue culture systems that transformed cells are unable to leave the replicative cell cycle completely and enter G_0 (373). However, the relationship of tumor stem cells to G_0 cells in vivo is not clear. The small percentage of tumor cells that are stem cells may stoichiometrically differentiate into descendants or may be able to enter a G_0 phase. It is difficult to reconcile the late appearance of breast metastases (15 to 20 years after control of the primary) without the existence of tumor cells in G_0. Regardless, whether tumor stem cells can enter G_0, have very long generation times (with presumably a long G_1 period), or are programmed for differentiation, the problem of therapy for slowly growing tumors remains a central issue (162, 163, 339). Most of our present chemotherapeutic agents are more cytotoxic toward cycling cells than toward cells that are slowly proliferating or are in G_0.

Chemotherapeutic Agents and the Cell Cycle

The classification of drugs by their cell-cycle–dependent cytotoxicity was initiated by Bruce and co-workers (165–167; see also references 168 and 398 for reviews). Using a quantitative spleen colony assay, they compared the lethal effect of a 24-hour exposure of 11 anticancer agents on transplanted lymphoma cells versus normal bone marrow cells. Since the end-point was formation of spleen colonies in lethally irradiated BDF_1 mice, their assay differentiated drug effects on normal stem cells versus tumor stem cells. They proposed three classes of drugs based on differential cell survival and the shape of survival curves (Fig. 32-9):

Class I—*nonspecific*: Members of this class kill proliferating cells and resting cells with equal efficiency and are therefore proliferation-independent.

Class II—*phase-specific*: Agents in this class demonstrated specificity for cells traversing specific parts of the cell cycle, in particular the S phase. The greatest differential effect between normal stem cells and tumor stem cells is exhibited by these agents because experimental tumor cells are actively cycling, whereas only a small percentage of normal stem cells are in cycle. Provided that exposure times are kept short (i.e., 24 hours), a differential cell killing effect of more than 4 logs can be achieved.

Class III—*cycle-specific*: These agents are active against both the tumor cells and normal cells, but there is a sixfold increase in toxicity for the lymphoma cells; therefore, drugs in this class are proliferation-dependent. If exposure times for Class II and Class III agents are prolonged, selectivity for tumor cells versus normal cells is lost. Although many drugs have now been classified by these criteria (151), distinctions between some Class I and Class III agents have become less clear and may be dependent on cell type (329).

Cell Synchronization

Since most agents preferentially kill cells during particular phases of the cell cycle, it would poten-

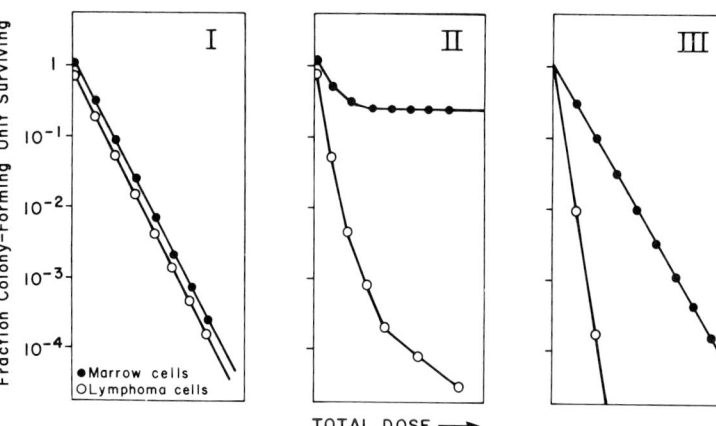

Figure 32–9. Classification of chemotherapeutic agents by their relative effect on normal bone marrow versus lymphoma stem cells. Agents are usually given in fractionated doses over a 24-hour period. Class I agents are proliferation-independent, Class II agents are phase-specific, and Class III agents are proliferation-dependent. (Modified from Bruce, R. W., and Meeker, B. E.: J. Natl. Cancer Inst. 38:401, 1967.)

tially be of great importance to manipulate and temporarily block the progression of cells through the cell cycle. This would alter the proportion of cells within the particular phases (see Figure 32–8), resulting in an accumulation of cells at various points. For example, thymidine causes synchrony by blocking cells in S phase. Cells in other phases of the cell cycle continue cycle traverse and accumulate at G_1/S. Removal of the thymidine blockade results in the semisynchronous progression of cells through S phase and mitosis (325). Selective killing of cells by different phase-specific agents would then be possible as cells enter those sensitive portions of the cell cycle. This concept of cell synchronization has had only limited clinical use, however, since, at best, only limited synchrony occurs, and normal as well as tumor cells are affected. The various agents that have been utilized for synchronization studies are irradiation, cytosine arabinoside, 5-fluorouracil, vincristine, hydroxyurea, and thymidine (326–331).

If better methods (more selective drugs and dose schedules) for producing synchrony are developed, the obvious problems of asynchronous tumor cell growth, wide deviations in single-cell cycle times from mean generation times (see previous discussion of length-biased sampling), and variations in growth fraction can possibly be overcome. Of the currently available agents, thymidine (administered by continuous infusion) may be the most promising (325).

Recruitment

Closely linked to the concept of cell synchrony is cell recruitment. As proliferating cells are destroyed, nonproliferating cells enter the proliferating pool or compartment to replace them (328). In Figure 32–8, this could be envisioned as the reentrance of a G_0 cell (or apparently differentiated cell) into G_1 and therefore into the pool of potentially cycling cells. In a functional sense, this may be related to tumor debulking. As the outer rim of cycling cells is decreased by chemotherapy, nutrient delivery and debris removal by either new or existing vasculature may be improved, resulting in increased cellular activity in deeper areas of the tumor.

In mice, bone marrow is particularly sensitive to destruction of cycling cells and responds within hours of injury by a dramatic increase in CFU-S that are in cycle. Recruitment has also been reported after much longer intervals (4 to 8 days) in experimental tumors and in human leukemia (328). Cell recruitment and synchrony are closely associated responses that unfortunately seem to be most evident in normal bone marrow, as opposed to other normal tissues or tumors.

Do Cell Kinetics Help?

There is far from universal agreement concerning the relevance of of cell kinetics to the design and implementation of our present chemotherapy protocols (398). Two recent critical reviews come to diametrically opposed conclusions (151, 164). Others contend that although much basic tumor biology has been generated by cell kinetic studies, these studies have not "been pursued to the point where serious impact on clinical practice has been achieved" (119).

COMMONLY USED DRUGS IN CHILDHOOD CANCER CHEMOTHERAPY

This section will emphasize principles and problems involved in the use of the most common chemotherapeutic agents for childhood neoplasia. In general, chemotherapeutic agents can be divided into several general categories: (1) alkylating agents, (2) antimetabolites, (3) antibiotics, (4) steroid hormones, (5) plant alkaloids, (6) enzymes, and (7) miscellaneous agents. Mechanisms of action of agents are often ascribed in broad terms with respect to such classifications. However, it is probably more useful to attempt to understand drug effects at a cellular or biochemical level. The important caveat is that most drugs probably have multiple intracellular targets and what has been identified in vitro as a mechanism of action may have little to do with cellular cytotoxicity and antitumor effect.

A statement of general principles for drug use in combinations is given in Table 32–5. A summary of commonly used agents, including their pharmacokinetics, dosages, toxicity, and general modes of action, is given in Table 32–6. Several recent reviews provide detailed information about these and other agents (169, 180, 390, 414).

Combination Chemotherapy

In general, chemotherapeutic agents are not currently used as single agents, although sequential single agent chemotherapy characterized the early development of treatment programs. The use of combinations of drugs to achieve better therapeutic effect is rooted in antiquity, although the present-day rationale for combination cancer chemotherapy derives from combination drug studies for controlling hypertension and delaying or preventing drug resistance in antimicrobial therapy. The delay or prevention of the emergence of drug-resistant cells by combination chemotherapy can perhaps be demonstrated most dramatically by studies of antimetabolite combinations in mice with L1210 leukemia (340).

The use of methotrexate and 6-mercaptopurine for induction of remission in acute lymphocytic leukemia was the first drug combination shown to be conclusively superior to single agents (341). Combining drugs with qualitative as well as quantitative differences in dose-limiting toxicity led to the development of VAMP (vincristine, methotrexate, 6-mercaptopurine, and prednisone) for acute leukemia (10) and MOPP (nitrogen mustard, vincristine, procarbazine, and prednisone) for lymphomas (13).

Although pediatric tumors constitute only a small percentage of overall cancer, the development and implementation of combination chemotherapy and its success in the treatment of acute lymphoblastic leukemia, Wilms' tumor, non-Hodgkin's lymphomas, rhabdomyosarcoma, Ewing's sarcoma, and osteogenic sarcoma have provided the framework for aggressive treatment of other tumors. Several recent reviews describe various aspects of combination chemotherapy for cancer treatment (343–345).

Table 32–5 presents general principles of drug use that are, in effect, the model for drug combinations. General drug interactions were discussed previously, but, specifically, drug effects on both tumor cells and normal cells can be categorized as antagonistic, subadditive, additive, or synergistic (Table 32–7). Ideally, we strive for additive or synergistic effects against tumor cells, with subadditive or antagonistic effects on normal cells. Combinations of cytosine arabinoside and 6-thioguanine and methotrexate with asparaginase for acute leukemia and of MOPP for lymphoma seem to fulfill these criteria (343). Drug combinations have been developed empirically as well as on the basis of cytokinetic, biochemical, pharmacologic, and toxicologic considerations. Contributing factors include:

1. Steep dose-response curves for tumor cells and normal cells (see Figure 32–1).
2. Schedule dependence, which can be a complex multifactorial phenomenon involving host factors and intervals between courses as well as dose and schedule of drugs. Combinations that include antimetabolites are frequently very sensitive to schedule, i.e., methotrexate and cytosine arabinoside, methotrexate and asparaginase, methotrexate and 5-fluorouracil, cytosine arabinoside and daunorubicin, cytosine arabinoside and BCNU, cytosine arabinoside and asparaginase, and cytosine arabinoside and 5-fluorodeoxyuridine (see reference 343 for a review).
3. Biochemical and pharmacologic factors, which take into account transport of agents across cell membranes, biotransformation and excretion, and known major targets of action. An understanding of suspected macromolecular targets of action has led to the formulation of a rationale for drug combinations based on attacking multiple sites within various biochemical pathways and is referred to as sequential, concurrent, and complementary inhibition. Sequential inhibition or blockade (346) refers to the simultaneous action of two inhibitors at different enzymatic steps in a metabolic pathway. Examples of this concept are methotrexate and 5-fluorouracil limiting de novo deoxythymidine monophosphate (dTMP) synthesis, and cytosine arabinoside and hydroxyurea inhibiting DNA polymerase and ribonucleotide reductase, respectively. Concurrent inhibition or blockade (347) refers to end-product inhibition by two alternate pathways, i.e., limitation of dTMP by inhibition of the de novo pathway via thymidylate synthetase and the salvage pathway via thymidine kinase. Although 5-fluorouracil is a potent inhibitor against thymidylate synthetase, no agent is

Table 32–5. GENERAL PRINCIPLES OF DRUG USE

1. Maximum tolerated dosages of known active agents should be administered
2. Combinations of drugs that are known to be individually active should be used
3. If possible, drugs should have different suspected mechanisms of action and cytotoxicity
4. Drug toxicities should overlap as little as possible with respect to either time or organ system involved

Text continued on page 1006

Table 32–6. COMMONLY USED CANCER CHEMOTHERAPEUTIC AGENTS IN PEDIATRIC PATIENTS

Drug[1]	Dosage and Schedule of Administration[2]	Side Effects[3] (*Major)	Indications for Use in Pediatrics	Cell Cycle Effects and Class[1]
Vincristine (VCR) (Oncovin) (1) Plant alkaloid (2) Mitotic arrest; inhibition of tubulin-microtubule polymerization (181, 182); inhibition of macromolecular metabolism (183) (3) Multiphasic with t½'s of 0.85, 7.4, and 164 minutes (184, 185) (4) Liver (5) Biliary, 50–75% within 72 hours (184–186) (6) Decreased hepatic function (193); biliary obstruction; irradiation of liver (7) Not known, but about 30% of dose is excreted as metabolites (184) (8) Peak levels of 3×10^{-7} M (184, 442) (9) Increase cAMP levels (187); affect methotrexate transport (188–190); after levels of hepatic microsomal sulfatase (191); vesicle formation (192)	0.05 mg/kg–0.075 mg/kg (1.0–2.0 mg/m², max. dose 2.0 mg) IV only Continuous infusion may be useful (443, 444)	*Local cellulitis, skin ulceration and necrosis if extravasation present *Neurotoxicity (173, 193) including paresthesias, areflexia, jaw pain, ileus, hoarseness, ptosis, muscle weakness, abdominal pain and muscle cramps, changes in gait, cranial nerve palsy, and depression *Alopecia Seizures Minimal to mild bone marrow suppression SIADH	Acute lymphoblastic leukemia Wilms' tumor Hodgkin's disease (MOPP) Non-Hodgkin's lymphoma Ewing's sarcoma Rhabdomyosarcoma and other soft tissue sarcomas Neuroblastoma	S-phase–dependent, causes metaphase block (132) Class II
Vinblastine (VLB) (Velban) (1) Plant alkaloid (2) Mitotic arrest; inhibition of tubulin-microtubule polymerization (181, 182); inhibition of macromolecular metabolism (183, 197) (3) Multiphasic with t½'s of 3.9, 53, and 1173 minutes (198, 199) (4) Liver (5) Biliary and urine (198) (6) Decreased hepatic function; biliary obstruction; bone marrow depression (7) Deacetylvinblastine (199) (8) $1.0–3.0 \times 10^{-7}$ M (181, 198) (9) Increase cAMP levels (187); vesicle formation (192); inhibition of DNA polymerase (200)	0.1 mg/kg with weekly 0.05 mg/kg increments (4.0–6.0 mg/m²) IV only	*Local cellulitis, skin ulceration and necrosis if extravasation present Anorexia, nausea, and vomiting Less neurotoxicity than VCR (173, 193) Alopecia *Bone marrow suppression, especially leukopenia	Hodgkin's disease Histiocytosis-X Teratocarcinoma Testicular cancer	S-phase–dependent, causes metaphase block Class II
Prednisone (P) (1) Steroid hormone (2) Unknown, but may involve specific cytoplasmic receptors leading to nuclear	40–120 mg/m² PO with variable schedules	Few effects with short-term use (1–2 weeks) but longer exposure results in: fluid	Acute lymphoblastic leukemia Hodgkin's disease	G_1 and S may be most sensitive (212) $G_1 \rightarrow$ S delay

[1]Numbers in parentheses indicate: (1) Class of agent, (2) mechanism of action, (3) plasma clearance, (4) metabolism, (5) excretion, (6) dose alteration, (7) pharmacologically active metabolites, (8) blood levels, and (9) other effects.
[2]For drug infusion technique see reference 381.
[3]See also references 171–173, 176–178, and 180.
[4]See also references 151, 167, 168, 194, and 195.

Table continued on the following page

Table 32–6. COMMONLY USED CANCER CHEMOTHERAPEUTIC AGENTS IN PEDIATRIC PATIENTS *Continued*

Drug[1]	Dosage and Schedule of Administration[2]	Side Effects[3] (*Major)	Indications for Use in Pediatrics	Cell Cycle Effects and Class[1]
Prednisone (P) *(Continued)*				
(3) binding and transcriptional modification (201); free fatty acid accumulation may be important (202)		and electrolyte disturbance including sodium and fluid retention, hypokalemic alkalosis, hyperglycemia, and congestive heart failure in susceptible patients (211)	Non-Hodgkin's lymphoma	
(3) t½ about 132 minutes in children (203), although longer in adults (204, 205) and influenced by dose (205, 206)		Hypertension		
(4) Liver		Proximal myopathy		
(5) Urinary		Peptic ulcer and gastrointestinal bleeding (196)		
(6) Infections, e.g., varicella; hypertension; diabetes		"Cushingoid" appearance		
(7) Prednisolone		Increased susceptibility to infections		
(8) Ten mg. of prednisone results in a plasma cortisol level of $1–4 \times 10^{-6}$ M (207)		CNS disturbance		
(9) Immunosuppression (207, 208); decreased methotrexate transport (209); resistance may be related to numbers of receptors (201, 210) or intracellular free fatty acid levels (202)		Lymphocytopenia		
Methotrexate (MTX) (Amethopterin)				
(1) Antimetabolite (folic acid analog)	*Conventional doses:*	*Bone marrow suppression: WBC nadir 7–10 days; high-dose protocols are not myelosuppressive unless MTX levels persist	Acute lymphoblastic leukemia	S-phase–specific; will not kill resting or G_0 cells (250, 339)
(2) Inhibits dihydrofolate reductase (inhibition constant is about 1×10^{-9} M), thereby limiting the 1-carbon pathways (de novo pyrimidine and purine synthesis), which depend on tetrahydrofolate (190, 213–219, 295)	15–30 mg/m² twice weekly PO, IM, or IV; 60 mg/m² IV or IM weekly; high-dose protocols with leucovorin "rescue" (236–238) begin at MTX doses of 500 mg/m²	*Gastrointestinal effects including stomatitis, diarrhea, and vomiting; most sensitive mucosa is the inner surface of lower lip; also generalized mucositis; in high-dose protocols, *renal toxicity (224, 244, 245) may occur, requiring super rescue techniques (54, 219, 226, 247)	Osteosarcoma Medulloblastoma Burkitt's lymphoma	$G_1 \rightarrow S$ delay Class II
(3) Complex, probably triphasic with t½'s of 0.75, 2–4, and 10.5 hours (220–224); t½ for CSF decay of MTX administered intrathecally is 6–9 hours (264, 265)	and range up to MTX doses greater than 10 g/m² (54, 219, 232, 233, 240); selectivity of high-dose MTX protocols with leucovorin "rescue" may reflect the availability of tetrahydrofolate from 5-methyl tetrahydrofolate via homocysteine-methionine methyl transferase (239, 249); schedules for high-dose MTX range from weekly to every 4 weeks	Early detection of impending MTX toxicity (i.e., serum creatinine level rise of 50% or greater over the baseline value [223] or persistent elevation of serum MTX levels signals the need for additional rescue measures);[5] children clear MTX from their plasma more rapidly than do adults		
(4) Liver and probably gut bacteria				
(5) 50–90% of dose appears unchanged in urine within 24 hours; also enterohepatic circulation (219, 225)				
(6) Impaired renal or hepatic function; drugs that compete for serum protein binding, i.e., sulfonamides and aspirin (101)	*Intrathecal MTX:* 12 mg for patients between 3 and 40 years of age (243); 6 mg for patients age 1 year or younger; 8 mg for patients between ages 1 and 2; and 10 mg for those from 2 to 3 years of age (446); aminopterin may be a pharmacologically superior agent (362)	*Skin rashes ranging from perifolliculitis to exfoliative reactions		
(7) None with greater activity than MTX (227, 228)				
(8) Depends directly on dose, with peak plasma levels ranging from about 10^{-6} M with high-dose protocols to about 10^{-6} M with conventional doses				

| | | Chronic changes may occur in liver and lungs
*Alopecia
*Leukoencephalopathy (77) | | |

(9) May inhibit thymidylate synthetase (229); MTX transport may be altered by many other agents (101, 103–106, 230); potentiate MTX effect with thymidine (231); resistance may be related to decreased drug transport or increased dihydrofolate reductase levels (232, 233); MTX resistance may be related to dihydrofolate reductase gene multiplication (234, 235); schedule-dependent effects of MTX and L-asparaginase (241, 242)

6-Mercaptopurine (6-MP)

(1) Antimetabolite (purine analog)
(2) Activated intracellularly by hypoxanthine guanine phosphoribosyltransferase (HGPRT) to thioinosinic acid; inhibition of de novo purine formation at phosphoribosyl pyrophosphate (PRPP) and other interconversions (251, 252, 254); also incorporated into DNA (253)
(3) $t_{1/2}$ of 90 minutes (110)
(4) Oxidized to 6-thiouric acid by xanthine oxidase; sulfate and other metabolites are also formed (251, 255)
(5) Renal for both 6-MP and its various metabolites; 46% of P.O. dose in urine after 24 hours
(6) Sensitivity to 6-MP (liver abnormalities) may require substitution of 6-thioguanine; concurrent administration of allopurinol, a xanthine oxidase inhibitor, requires up to 75% decrease in dose, although this may not be true when 6-MP is administered IV rather than PO (110, 257)
(7) 6-Thioinosinic acid and others (251, 254)
(8) —
(9) Effect on polymorphonuclear (PMN) function (258); immunosuppression (255); resistance may be associated with the loss of HGPRT activity (251)

2.5 mg/kg/day P.O.
250 mg/m² × 5 days PO or IV
Absorption may be erratic following oral administration

*Bone marrow suppression
Stomatitis (thrushlike)
Hepatic dysfunction

Maintenance in acute lymphoblastic leukemia

S phase
Class II

---

[1] Numbers in parentheses indicate: (1) Class of agent, (2) mechanism of action, (3) plasma clearance, (4) metabolism, (5) excretion, (6) dose alteration, (7) pharmacologically active metabolites, (8) blood levels, and (9) other effects.
[2] For drug infusion technique see reference 381.
[3] See also references 171–173, 176–178, and 180.
[4] See also references 151, 167, 168, 194, and 195.
[5] In our experience (247), MTX-related renal toxicity is nonoliguric and best managed by vigorous hydration (2 × maintenance); alkalization, although this, like hydration (246), does not alter serum MTX pharmacokinetics (248); increasing the leucovorin dose to 150 mg every 3 hours; and the addition of thymidine (8 g/m²/day) by continuous infusion. This regimen is continued until MTX levels have fallen to less than 10^{-7} M. Using this approach, we have been able to prevent patients from developing either stomatitis or myelosuppression despite prolonged elevation of MTX levels.

Table continued on the following page

Table 32-6. COMMONLY USED CANCER CHEMOTHERAPEUTIC AGENTS IN PEDIATRIC PATIENTS *Continued*

Drug[1]	Dosage and Schedule of Administration[2]	Side Effects[3] (*Major)	Indications for Use in Pediatrics	Cell Cycle Effects and Class[4]
Cytosine Arabinoside (Ara-C) (1) Antimetabolite (pyrimidine analog) (2) Activated to the triphosphate (Ara-CTP) (259), which may inhibit DNA polymerase or be incorporated into DNA (169, 260–262); DNA chain initiation may also be a target (263) (3) Biphasic with t½'s of 3–15 minutes and about 2 hours (260, 266); CSF decay of intrathecally administered Ara-C has a t½ of 5.4–11.4 hours (260) (4) Probably hepatic deamination to Ara-U (may be blocked by tetrahydrouridine, Ki of 2×10^{-8} M) (260) (5) About 90% in urine within 24 hours primarily as Ara-U (260) (6) Severe hepatic dysfunction; concomitant administration of tetrahydrouridine (7) Ara-CTP (8) Steady state level at dose of 200 mg/m²/day is between 5×10^{-7} M and 1×10^{-6} M with simultaneous CSF levels 60–70% of plasma (342) (9) Chromatid breakage (267); inhibition of RNA polymerase (268); resistance may be related to decreased levels of deoxycytidine kinase (activation) and/or increased levels of cytidine deaminase (degradation) (169, 260)	Very variable, from 30 mg/m²/day in a 12-hour infusion to 200/mg/m² day for 5–7 days; may be given either IV or subcutaneously; intrathecal dose is 40 mg/m² Low-dose continuous infusion may be efficacious (446)	*Bone marrow suppression Nausea, vomiting, diarrhea, stomatitis Cerebral and cerebellar dysfunction seen with high-dose administration (445)	Acute myelogenous leukemia Acute lymphoblastic leukemia Lymphomas	S and early G_2 $G_1 \rightarrow S$ delay Class II
Adriamycin (ADM) (1) Antibiotic (2) Specifically binds to DNA by intercalation between adjacent base pairs and inhibits DNA, RNA, and protein synthesis (256, 271, 294); free radical formation may be involved (76) (3) Triphasic with t½'s of 12 minutes, 3.3 hours and 29.6 hours (291), although others report biphasic decay with t½'s of 1–1.5 hours and 14–21 hours (269)	45–90 mg/m² IV as single or divided doses, repeated every 3–4 weeks; maximum cumulative dose is 450–550 mg/m²	*Local cellulitis and necrosis if extravasation *Bone marrow suppression *Nausea and vomiting *Stomatitis *Alopecia *Cardiac toxicity ranging from ECG changes and arrhythmias to progressive cardiomyopathy; below 550 mg/m² cumulative dose; congestive heart failure incidence is less than 1% (272, 275); low-dose continuous IV infusion may also reduce cardiac toxicity (447) Pneumonitis, esophagitis, and dermatitis in previously irradiated areas (66)	Acute lymphoblastic leukemia Acute myelogenous leukemia Osteosarcoma Non-Hodgkin's lymphoma Rhabdomyosarcoma Ewing's sarcoma Neuroblastoma	S phase is most sensitive but all phases affected (273) Class III

(4) Hepatic with numerous metabolites formed (i.e., adriamycinol and several aglycones) (270, 274) (5) <10% in urine as parent drug and metabolites at 72 hours (266, 270); biliary is most important, with 35% of the drug excreted intact in the bile at 72 hours (270) (6) Hepatic dysfunction (increased bilirubin); radiation therapy either concomitant or to certain areas, i.e., mediastinum, heart (66) (7) Adriamycinol is the primary metabolite, but it may be less active than adriamycin (269) (8) About $1-2 \times 10^{-6}$ M as a peak level (9) Immunosuppression (271)				
Actinomycin-D (A) (Dactinomycin)				
(1) Antibiotic (2) Binds to G-C rich regions in DNA, inhibiting RNA polymerase and subsequently all macromolecular synthesis (276–278, 294) (3) Niphasic with t½'s of about 1 hour and 36 hours (279) (4) 1–4% metabolism to monolactones (279) (5) 10–30% in urine primarily as actinomycin-D after 72 hours with less recovered in stool (279) (6) Radiation therapy (7) — (8) Peak plasma level of $6-7 \times 10^{-8}$ M after a single dose of 15 μg/kg (279) (9) Selective suppression of erythropoiesis (280)	$0.2–0.3$ μg/m² I.V. daily × 10 days, repeated every 6 weeks; $1.0–1.5$ mg/m² IV as a single dose every 3 weeks	*Local cellulitis and vesicle formation and necrosis if extravasation *Nausea, vomiting, diarrhea, stomatitis, mucositis *Bone marrow suppression, especially thrombocytopenia *Alopecia Skin rash *Radiation recall (66)	Wilms' tumor Rhabdomyosarcoma Ewing's sarcoma Acute lymphoblastic leukemia	G_1/S and early S phase are most sensitive G_1 and $G_2 \rightarrow$ M delay Class III
Cyclophosphamide (CTX) (Cytoxan)				
(1) Alkylating agent (2) Probably substitution of an alkyl group at the N_7 position of guanine (281, 296) (3) t½'s of 4–8.9 hours (282–284); the t½'s may decrease with continued therapy (285) (4) Must be activated in liver microsomal enzymes and subsequent ring modification (4-hydroxylation) (296) (5) About 10% of parent compound and 40% of metabolites are excreted in the urine within 24 hours (286)	Variable from 2.5 mg/kg to 40 mg/kg; may be given by any route since it is inert until activated, although IV is used for high doses; should be accompanied by vigorous hydration	*Nausea and vomiting *Bone marrow suppression *Hemorrhagic cystitis (acrolein) (448) SIADH *Cardiac toxicity (272, 296) *Alopecia *Bladder tumors (292)	Acute lymphoblastic leukemia Burkitt's lymphoma Rhabdomyosarcoma Ewing's sarcoma Hodgkin's disease Non-Hodgkin's lymphoma	All phases are sensitive G_2 block Class III

[1] Numbers in parentheses indicate: (1) Class of agent, (2) mechanism of action, (3) plasma clearance, (4) metabolism, (5) excretion, (6) dose alteration, (7) pharmacologically active metabolites, (8) blood levels, and (9) other effects.
[2] For drug infusion technique see reference 381.
[3] See also references 171–173, 176–178, and 180.
[4] See also references 151, 167, 168, 194, and 195.

Table continued on the following page

Table 32–6. COMMONLY USED CANCER CHEMOTHERAPEUTIC AGENTS IN PEDIATRIC PATIENTS *Continued*

Drug[1]	Dosage and Schedule of Administration[2]	Side Effects[3] (*Major)	Indications for Use in Pediatrics	Cell Cycle Effects and Class[1]
Cyclophosphamide (CTX) (Cytoxan) *(Continued)*				
(6) Impaired hepatic function (must be severe) or renal function; a variety of drugs, i.e., phenobarbital, allopurinol, dilantin, and corticosteroids, have theoretical but few actual interactions, whereas chloramphenicol, nicotine, atropine, ephedrine, and apomorphine may decrease conversion to active metabolites; simultaneous radiation to the pelvic area (293)				
(7) 4-Hydroxycyclophosphamide, aldophosphamide, phosphoramide mustard, and acrolein (282, 287, 288)				
(8) Peak plasma levels of $2-6 \times 10^{-6}$ M				
(9) Circadian dependence of tumor response and host toxicity (289); immunosuppression (288, 290)				
L-Asparaginase (L-ASP)				
(1) Enzyme	Variable from 10 to 1000 IU/kg/day (309) either IV or IM (the latter is associated with fewer side effects)	*Hypersensitivity reactions (312–314) *Antibody formation (315) *Anaphylactic reactions *Pancreatitis *Hyperglycemia and frank diabetes (more common if corticosteroids are given simultaneously) *Liver dysfunction *CNS abnormality (173)	Acute lymphoblastic leukemia	G_1
(2) Inhibits protein synthesis by depleting L-asparagine in extracellular fluids (308–310); normal cells can synthesize L-asparagine, whereas leukemic blasts may be deficient, accounting for selective killing (310)				
(3) $t\frac{1}{2}$'s of 8–30 hours (308)				
(4) —				
(5) Probably cleared by the reticuloendothelial system or immune mechanisms (310)				
(6) —				
(7) —				
(8) Asparagine levels rapidly become undetectable; L-ASP levels range from 1–4 IU/ml serum after 200 IU/kg/day (324)				
(9) The enzyme is usually isolated from either *Escherichia coli* or *Erwinia carotovora*; the former isolate is usually used unless hypersensitivity develops; in general, there is no cross-reactivity; some evidence suggests that the isolates do not have equal anti-tumor activity (311); resistance may be related to induced enzyme synthesis in the leukemic blasts (310); decrease in thyroxine-binding globulin (363); Sequential administration of either MTX or Ara-C followed by L-ASP produces a synergistic therapeutic effect (449)				

BCNU
(1) N-alkyl-N-nitrosourea
(2) Carbamoylation of proteins and alkylation of nucleic acids (305)
(3) t½ approximately 5 minutes (298)
(4) Liver microsomes. Phenobarbital may increase drug metabolism and decrease antitumor activity (450)
(5) Reaction products and degradation products are found primarily in the urine
(6) Myelosuppression
(7) Organic isocyanates; chloroethyl diazohydroxide and carbonium ion (299)
(8) Peak plasma level of 8×10^{-6} M after a 200 mg/m² dose (385)
(9) Cross-linking DNA (300) and production of DNA strand breaks (301); inhibition of DNA repair (302, 303); inhibition of RNA synthesis and processing (304–306)

100–200 mg/m² I.V. every 4–6 weeks; 1.4 g/m² with autologous bone marrow support (297)

*Nausea and vomiting
*Delayed bone marrow suppression (4–6 weeks)
*Possible long-term effects on bone marrow and kidneys (78, 79); possibly mutagenic, teratogenic and carcinogenic (169)

Brain tumors
Lymphomas
Hodgkin's disease

Prolongation of S and G_2 (307)
Class I

CIS-Diamminedichloroplatinum (II)
(1) Metal coordination complex
(2) May react at N_7 and O_6 positions of guanine, producing intrastrand and interstrand crosslinking and DNA synthesis inhibition (316–318, 389)
(3) Biphasic with t½'s of 30–60 minutes and 2–3 days (319, 320, 451); rapidly binds to plasma proteins
(4) —
(5) Urinary excretion is incomplete with 27–45% elimination in 5 days (318)
(6) Renal toxicity
(7) —
(8) Peak plasma level of 1.7–12.0 $\times 10^{-6}$ M after a 100 mg/m² dose (bolus versus 6 hour infusion) (391)
(9) Poor penetration into the CNS

60–120 mg/m² after vigorous hydration and forced mannitol diuresis; drug is also administered in mannitol

*Nausea and vomiting (318, 321)
*Myelosuppression
*Ototoxicity (high frequency range)—dose-related and cumulative
*Renal toxicity—dose related and cumulative
Neurotoxicity
Tetany (322)

Ovarian and testicular tumors (389)
Osteosarcoma
Neuroblastoma
Brain tumors
Wilms' tumor

Nonspecific (323)
Class III

---

[1]Numbers in parentheses indicate: (1) Class of agent, (2) mechanism of action, (3) plasma clearance, (4) metabolism, (5) excretion, (6) dose alteration, (7) pharmacologically active metabolites, (8) blood levels, and (9) other effects.
[2]For drug infusion technique see reference 381.
[3]See also references 171–173, 176–178, and 180.
[4]See also references 151, 167, 168, 194, and 195.

Table 32–7. DRUG INTERACTIONS*

Effect	Cell Kill %	Log
Single Agent:		
A	90	1
B	90	1
Combined:		
A + B – Antagonistic	<90	<1
A + B – Subadditive	<99	<2
A + B – Additive	99	2
A + B – Synergistic	>99	>2

*From Blum R. H., and Frei, E.: Combination therapy. In *Methods in Cancer Research*, Vol. XVII. DeVita, V., and Busch, H. (eds.), New York, Academic Press, 1979.

currently selective against thymidine kinase. Complementary inhibition or blockade (348) refers to different mechanisms of end-product limitation, i.e., intercalating agents (adriamycin) or alkylating agents (nitrogen mustard), which directly interact with DNA and other macromolecules, and antimetabolites (cytosine arabinoside or 5-fluorouracil), which limit biosynthesis.

4. Cytokinetic considerations, which were previously discussed, including cell cycle and phase specificity, kinetics of cell kill, synchronization, and recruitment.

Resistance

The emergence of drug-resistant cells (until mechanisms are known, it may be more accurate to refer to drug-unresponsive cells) is a major limitation of cancer chemotherapy. In every population of tumor cells, the spontaneous occurrence and frequency of drug-resistant cells may be an intrinsic characteristic of the tumor type and is independent of drug treatment (399–401). This type of resistance is a permanent genetic change that has taken place in the tumor cells and was originally described in the fluctuation test of Luria and Delbruck, who were studying the capacity of bacteria to develop resistance to invasion by bacteriophages (402). Goldie and Coldman have used the work of Luria and Delbruck to develop a mathematical model for relating the drug sensitivity of tumors to their spontaneous mutation rate toward pleiotropic drug resistance (403). The latter concept refers to patterns of drug cross-resistance that can include agents from antibiotic, plant alkaloid, and alkylating types. Goldie and Coldman posit that the proportion as well as the absolute numbers of resistant cells will increase with time, and the fraction of resistant cells within tumor colonies of the same size will vary depending on whether mutation to drug resistance occurred as an early or late event. There is the clear implication that a large tumor volume is more apt to contain resistant drug phenotypes than a small tumor volume. The probability of the appearance of resistant drug phenotypes is also dependent on the mutation rate. This concept implies that at certain times in the growth of a tumor population, there is a relatively short period of time in which its susceptibility to chemotherapy changes rapidly. The higher the mutation rate, e.g., one in a thousand cells (10^{-3}) versus one in a million cells (10^{-6}), the earlier this transition will occur in the growth of the tumor. The transition from 5 per cent drug-resistant phenotypes to 95 per cent drug-resistant phenotypes occurs within a period of 5.9 stem cell doublings and is independent of the mutation rate (Fig. 32–10). The implication of this finding is that a delay in the institution of therapy during this critical transition time, i.e., delay of several generation times, may greatly reduce the effectiveness of therapy and therefore the likelihood of cure. This point is clearly emphasized in rodent tumor experimental data that have been plotted using the Goldie-Coldman assumptions for treatment with the drug cyclophosphamide (402). The curability of this rodent tumor diminishes as the tumor cell number increases for any given mutation rate. Using a mutation of 1×10^7 or 1 in 10 million cells, the cure rate drops from 90 per cent to less than 10 per cent as the tumor burden increases from 10^6 to 10^8 cells.

Goldie, Coldman, and Gudauskas have extended these observations and developed the mathematical rationale for use of alternating non–cross-resistant chemotherapy programs (404). This concept is practical only for those neoplastic processes that respond to a large number of different drugs, i.e., acute leukemias, lymphoma, and Hodgkin's disease. For Hodgkin's disease, evidence does exist that alternate cycles of MOPP and ABVD may be superior to either combination used alone (405, 406). This was not true, however, for different combinations in the treatment of ovarian carcinoma (407, 408).

Goldie and Coldman (409) have further refined their mathematical model to include the fact that not all tumor cells are stem cells with unlimited growth potential (see above). Given an equivalent rate of stem cell birth and death processes, the larger the tumor stem cell compartment, the fewer the number of doublings required to achieve any given tumor size. If a tumor of 10^9 cells (1 cm in diameter) is composed of 100 per cent stem cells and there is no cell loss, then about 30 doublings will be required for the tumor to grow to 1 cm (see Figure 32–2). If the same tumor is composed of 51 per cent stem cells, and the death rate of non–stem cells is high (98 per cent), then approximately 1200 doublings are required to reach the 1-cm diameter tumor. The potential for genetic heterogeneity is therefore much greater in the latter case. Assuming there is a fixed mutation rate to drug-resistant phenotypes, the more slowly growing tumor (i.e., more stem cell divisions) has

Figure 32–10. This plot relates the probability of the existence of no resistant phenotypes to various mutation rates and tumor size (N). The almost identical profile of each curve reflects the independence of the time required for a class of tumors to proceed from the state when only 5 per cent have resistant phenotypes to that when 95 per cent have such phenotypes. (Adapted from Goldie and Coldman [403] with the authors' permission.)

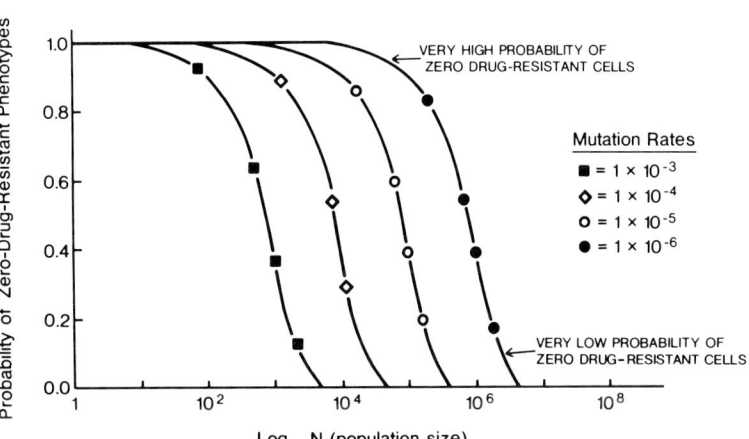

a higher probability of producing these phenotypes. Slowly growing tumors are often well differentiated and only partially responsive to chemotherapy. The Goldie-Coldman model does predict, however, that there should have been a period in the tumor's history when it was sensitive or when the probability of drug-resistant cells was very low (Fig. 32–10). This has very important implications for how we interpret Phase-II drug trials. The latter are conducted in patients with grossly evident, advanced disease—a period of time in the history of the tumor when the probability of drug-resistant phenotypes is high. The criteria for activity, PR and CR (see above), are probably unrealistic in this setting and should be modified to recognize that any antitumor activity is potentially significant.

It is clear from animal tumor models (Lewis lung carcinoma, colon tumor line 26, B16 melanoma, and C3H mammary tumor line 44) that some drugs that are ineffective or only minimally effective against gross tumor deposits can be curative for the same tumor in an adjuvant setting (33). Drugs that have demonstrated this effect include Adriamycin, cyclophosphamide, methyl-CCNU, and BCNU. The obvious concern is that drugs have been labeled as ineffective against a particular tumor because of Phase-II trial results when in fact they are active against microscopic disease (see below). Genes associated with individual drug resistance, e.g., dihydrofolate reductase/methotrexate and Adriamycin pleiotropic drug resistance, are being identified and cloned (410, 411). Probes will thereby become available to test populations of cells for the expression of these genes. Since cells that exhibit pleiotropic drug resistance also have alterations in cell surface glycoproteins, treatment strategies (e.g., monoclonal antibodies) may be specifically designed and directed toward their eradication.

The probability that the same cell is resistant to another agent with an independent mechanism of action is theoretically the product of $10^6 \times 10^6$, or 10^{12} (i.e., one chance in a trillion). Resistance or unresponsiveness can be related to a variety of possible mechanisms (334–337, 399). These include:

1. *Intrinsic factors*, i.e., if 10^6 to 10^7 cells are initially present and if the incidence of drug resistance is 1 in 10^6 cells, the resistant tumor cells will regrow if treatment is continued with the same drug. This commonly occurs in animal leukemias treated with noncurative antimetabolite therapy (338). To overcome this type of resistance, tumors may first be debulked by surgery or radiation (Goldie and Coldman) so that less than 10^6 to 10^7 viable tumor cells remain (the percentage of tumor stem cells is not known). Drug doses must be maximized (first-order kinetics), and combinations of non–cross-resistant drugs should be used.

2. *Resting cells or slowly growing tumors* (162, 163). Most agents, with the possible exception of the nitrosoureas and bleomycin, are more active against cycling than noncycling cells. In fact, many drugs have no activity against resting or G_0 cells (162, 163, 250, 339). The previous section on recruitment indicated that it is difficult to overcome this problem, and clinical experience with such slowly growing tumors is confirmatory. The best approach is probably to begin with an aggressive adjuvant program after all known tumor has been ablated.

3. *Sanctuaries*, i.e., the central nervous system and testes. There may well be many "relative" sanctuaries in which adequate drug concentrations are not always obtained. The best recognized is the central nervous system in acute lymphoblastic leukemia (1, 11; see also Chapter 33). The approach in this case is direct, using either irradiation or intrathecally administered drugs, i.e., methotrexate and cytosine arabinoside.

4. *Acquired resistance* may be due to gene mutations or amplification, chromosomal abnormalities, phenotypic alterations, epigenetic changes, i.e., changes in activation, delivery, half-life, excretion, transport across the cell membrane (methotrex-

ate); binding to specific receptors either on the cell membrane or intracellularly (steroids); conversion to an active metabolite by intracellular enzymes (6-mercaptopurine and cyclophosphamide); decreased activation or increased degradation (cytosine arabinoside); and induced enzyme synthesis (asparaginase and methotrexate). It should be emphasized that normal bone marrow and other normal tissue show no evidence of developing drug resistance. This may be related to normal karyotype, with tumor aneuploidy being a predisposition or facilitating factor in drug resistance.

Therapeutic Strategy

After a definitive diagnosis is made by examination of pathologic material, further characterization of cell surface markers, contents of secretory granules, or other enzymatic markers will help to subtype or classify the precise identity of the neoplasm. It is critical to know the extent of disease (stage) and whether or not there is local, regional, or distant metastatic spread. Tumors that are curable by surgery or radiation therapy alone or in combination are then separated from the subsequent plan. Drug treatment strategies are based on a number of factors, including those given above under the section on the individual patient, and presuppose a thorough understanding of the disease processes themselves as well as the basic and clinical pharmacology of the drugs to be used. There may need to be modifications in treatment because of underlying medical problems or complications from the tumor itself; a need to coordinate therapy with surgeons and radiotherapists, i.e., "sandwiching" of radiation therapy between courses of chemotherapy, and an ability to balance the potential for severe or disabling toxicity with the maximal drug doses usually required to ensure full therapeutic benefit. It would be ideal to be able to design individualized chemotherapy regimens based on biochemical and pharmacologic interactions for the specific tumor in each patient after a pretreatment prediction of tumor response from an in vitro assay followed by the ability to profile drug concentration versus time during therapy. At present, the general approach to chemotherapy should include:

1. Rapid initial cytoreduction by surgery, radiation therapy, or combination chemotherapy, either as single- or multimodality therapy, depending on the disease. The limiting factors may be those imposed by G_0 cells, first-order kinetics, intrinsic resistance, and host toxicity.

2. Treatment of known sanctuaries.

3. Vigorous combination maintenance therapy and possibly late intensification (see earlier section on Gompertzian Kinetics and Protocol Design).

Prospectus

New agents are continually under evaluation in the United States and other countries (349, 350). In addition, new approaches for therapy, such as drugs enclosed in liposomes (351, 352, 412), continuous low-dose drug infusions (380, 413), hyperthermia (353, 430), antitumor antibodies as vehicles for cytotoxic agents or toxins (354), alternative methotrexate (MTX) rescue techniques using carboxypeptidase (355), regional drug administration (416), biologic and immune response modifiers (417–419), radiosensitizers (420), radiolabeled immune molecules (421), and new approaches to radiation therapy (422), are under active consideration. Active immunotherapy has generally been disappointing (423, 424), whether attempted with intralesional BCG (425), regional administration of immunostimulants with or without tumor cell vaccines (427), "immunorestorative agents" such as thymosin and levamisole (428), or interferons (429).

Passive immunotherapy with monoclonal antibodies alone (431–437), or coupled with toxins (438), cytotoxic drugs (439), or isotopes (440, 441), has generated great enthusiasm. Problems include amounts of circulating tumor antigen(s), antigenic modulation (down-regulation), antigen-negative tumor cells, and immune response of host to foreign antibody. Chemotherapy has progressed from infancy to middle age, and the future can only be better.*

---

*Afterthought. As if it weren't enough of a problem to understand the compexities of known active agents, we are at times beset by the specter of trying to explain to patients why unorthodox therapies are of no use. The history of quackery is replete with schemes to take advantage of those who are extraordinarily vulnerable and often gullible. However, none of these (e.g., Harry Hoxie's remedies or Krebiozen) have had the political and social impact of the present-day ruse—Laetrile (356). The following points concerning Laetrile should provide some perspective: Laetrile is a class of cyanogenetic glycosides (these naturally occur in the kernels of apricot pits as well as numerous other sources) of which amygdalin is the principal constituent. Amygdalin is 6 per cent cyanide by weight. Laetrile is also known by a variety of other names such as Aprikern, Bee 17, and Vitamin B_{17}. Laetrile is not a vitamin (357) and the term Vitamin B_{17} is only a trade-name established in an attempt to circumvent FDA constraints on the interstate movement of unproven drugs by claiming that Laetrile is a food. In addition, Laetrile is purported to work by being activated at the tumor site by the enzyme β-glucosidase to yield benzaldehyde and hydrogen cyanide. The hydrogen cyanide then kills the tumor cell. To protect normal tissues from the effects of hydrogen cyanide, the mitochondrial sulfur transferase, rhodanase, is said to detoxify the cyanide to thiocyanate. The theory depends on the differential distribution of β-glucosidase and rhodanase between tumor cells and normal cells, and all available evidence is to the contrary (356, 357). In fact, tumor cells may have very little β-glucosidase, and rhodanase is widely distributed. Also, cyanide is a poor antitumor agent. Laetrile is toxic (358–361) in contrast to the claims of its supporters. This is particularly the case when ingested by mouth so that cyanide can be nonenzymatically released in the gastrointestinal tract.

When administered intravenously, Laetrile is excreted essentially intact in the urine, since β-glucosidase levels in plasma are insignificant. Finally, there is no scientific evidence that Laetrile is useful in the prevention, cure, or palliation of cancer, whether it is used alone or with other "holistic" therapies. Both the American Cancer Society and the American Medical Association maintain files on this and other unproven methods of cancer treatment, and copies of these materials are always available.

References to Part I (Cancer Chemotherapy)

1. Sallan, S., Weinstein, H., et al.: Childhood leukemia. J. Pediatr. *99*:676, 1981.
2. Weinstein, H. J., Vance, Z. B., et al.: Improved prognosis for patients with mediastinal lymphoblastic lymphoma. Blood *53*:687, 1979.
3. Calabresi, P., and Parks, R. E.: Alkylating agents, antimetabolites, hormones, and other antiproliferative agents. In *The Pharmacological Basis of Therapeutics*, 4th Ed. Goodman, L. S., and Gilman, A. (eds.), Toronto, The Macmillan Co., 1970, pp. 1348–1395.
4. Farber, S., Diamond, L. K., et al.: Temporary remissions in acute leukemia in children produced by folic acid antagonist, 4-aminopteroylglutamic acid (Aminopterin). New Engl. J. Med. *238*:787, 1948.
5. Li, M. C., Hertz, R., et al.: Effect of methotrexate upon choriocarcinoma and chorioadenoma. Proc. Soc. Exptl. Bio. Med. *93*:361, 1956.
6. Burchenal, J. H.: The historical development of cancer chemotherapy. Semin. Oncol. *4*:135, 1977.
7. Zubrod, C. G.: Selective toxicity of anticancer drugs: Presidential Address. Cancer Res. *38*:4377, 1978.
8. Brubaker, C. A., Wheeler, H. E., et al.: Cyclic chemotherapy for acute leukemia in children. Blood *22*:820, 1963.
9. Zuelzer, W. W.: Cyclic therapy and long-term survival in childhood leukemia. Blood *22*:840, 1963.
10. Freireich, E. J., Karon, M., et al.: Quadruple combination therapy (VAMP) for acute lymphocytic leukemia of childhood. Proc. Am. Assoc. Cancer Res. *5*:20, 1964.
11. Simone, J.: Acute lymphocytic leukemia in childhood. Semin. Hematol. *11*:25, 1974.
12. Frei, E., III, DeVita, V. T., et al.: Approaches to improving the chemotherapy of Hodgkin's disease. Cancer Res. *26*:1284, 1966.
13. DeVita, V. T., Serpick, A. A., et al.: Combination chemotherapy in the treatment of advanced Hodgkin's disease. Ann. Intern. Med. *73*:881, 1970.
14. Farber, S., D'Angio, G., et al.: Clinical studies of actinomycin D with special reference to Wilms' tumor. Ann. N. Y. Acad. Sci. *89*:421, 1960.
15. Green, D. M., and Jaffe, N.: Wilms' tumor-model of a curable pediatric malignant solid tumor. Cancer Treat. Rev. *5*:143, 1978.
16. Proceedings of the Osteosarcoma Study Group Meeting. Cancer Treat. Rep. *62*:187, 1978.
17. Proceedings of the Osteosarcoma Study Group Meeting. J. Natl. Cancer Inst., 1979.
18. DeVita, V. T.: The evolution of therapeutic research in cancer. New Engl. J. Med. *298*:907, 1978.
19. Broome, J. D.: Evidence that the L-asparaginase activity of guinea pig serum is responsible for its antilymphoma effects. Nature (Lond.) *191*:1114, 1961.
20. Heidelberger, C., Chaudhuri, N. K., et al.: Fluorinated pyrimidines, a new class of tumor-inhibitory compounds. Nature (Lond.) *179*:663, 1957.
21. Goldin, A., Carter, S., et al.: Evaluation of antineoplastic activity: Requirements of test systems. In *Antineoplastic and Immunosuppressive Agents*, Part I. Sartorelli, A. C., and Johns, D. G. (eds.), New York, Springer-Verlag, 1974, pp. 12–32.
22. Homan, E. R.: Quantitative relationship between toxic doses of antitumor chemotherapeutic agents in animals and man. Cancer Chemother. Rep. *3*(3):13, 1972.
23. Driscoll, J. S.: The preclinical new drug research program of the National Cancer Institute. Cancer Treat. Rep. *68*:63, 1984.
24. Marsoni, S., and Wittes, R.: Clinical development of anticancer agents—a National Cancer Institute perspective. Cancer Treat. Rep. *68*:77, 1984.
25. Creaven, P. J., and Mihich, E.: The clinical toxicity of anticancer drugs and its prediction. Semin. Oncol. *4*:147, 1977.
26. U.S.A.–U.S.S.R. Monograph: Methods of development of new anticancer drugs. National Cancer Institute Monograph 45, pp. 5–177, 1977.
27. Gellhorn, A., and Hirschberg, E.: Investigation of diverse systems for cancer chemotherapy screening. Cancer Res. Supp. *3*:1, 1955.
28. Schein, P. S., Davis, R. D., et al.: The evaluation of anticancer drugs in dogs and monkeys for the prediction of qualitative toxicities in man. Clin. Pharmacol. Ther. *11*:3, 1970.
29. Tsuboi, K. K., and Kwong, L. K.: Antiproliferative agents and differential survival between normal and cancer cells. Cancer Res. *38*:3745, 1978.
30. Goldin, A., and Carter, S. K.: Screening and evaluation of antitumor agents. In *Principles of Chemotherapy*, 2nd. Ed. Holland, J. F., and Frei, E., III (eds.), Philadelphia, Lea and Febiger, 1982, pp. 633–663.
31. Mathe, G., and Kenis, Y.: Logistics of clinical trials: The example of cancerology. Biomedicine *18*:181, 1973.
32. Blum, R. H., and Frei, E.: Combination chemotherapy. In *Methods in Cancer Research*, Vol. XVII. DeVita, V., and Busch, H. (eds.), New York, Academic Press, 1979, pp. 215–257.
33. Schabel, F. M., Jr.: Experimental basis for adjuvant chemotherapy. In: *Adjuvant Therapy of Cancer*. Salmon, S. E., and Jones, S. E. (eds.), New York, North-Holland Publishing Co., 1977, pp. 3–14.
34. Gehan, E. A., and Schneiderman, M. A.: Experimental design of clinical trials, 2nd ed. In *Cancer Medicine*. Holland, J. F., and Frei, E. III (eds.), Philadelphia, Lea and Febiger, 1982, pp. 531–553.
35. Zelen, M.: A new design for randomized clinical trials. New Engl. J. Med. *300*:1242, 1979.
36. Shannon, J. A., Earle, D. P., et al.: The pharmacologic basis for the rational use of Atabrine in the treatment of malaria. J. Pharmacol. Exptl. Therap. *81*:307, 1944.
37. Austrian, R., Mirick, A. S., et al.: The efficacy of modified oral penicillin therapy of pneumococcal lobar pneumonia. Bull. Johns Hopkins Hosp. *88*:264, 1951.
38. Park, J. T., and Strominger, J. L.: Mode of action of penicillin. Science. *125*:99, 1957.
39. Gavosto, F., and Pileri, A.: Cell cycle of cancer cells in man. In *The Cell Cycle and Cancer*. Baserga, R. (ed.), New York, Marcel Dekker, 1971, 97–128.
40. Killman, S. A.: Acute leukemia: The kinetics of leukemic blast cells in man. An analytical review. Ser. Haematol. *2*:38, 1968.
41. Saunders, E. F., Lampkin, B. C., et al.: Variation of proliferative activity in leukemic cell populations of patients with acute leukemia. J. Clin. Invest. *46*:1356, 1967.
42. Winawer, S. J., and Liplin, M.: Cell proliferation kinetics in the gastrointestinal tract of man. IV. Cell renewal in the intestinalized gastric mucosa. J. Natl. Cancer Inst. *42*:9, 1969.
43. Clarkson, B., Ohkita, T., et al.: Studies of cellular proliferation in human leukemia. I. Estimation of growth rates of leukemic and normal hematopoietic cells in two adults with acute leukemia given single injections of tritiated thymidine. J. Clin. Invest. *46*:506, 1967.

44. Frei, E., III: Combination cancer therapy: Presidential Address. Cancer Res. *32*:2593, 1972.
45. Salmon, S. E., and Smith, B. A.: Immunoglobulin synthesis and total body tumor cell number in IgG myeloma. J. Clin. Invest. *49*:1114, 1970.
46. Graw, R. G., and Yankee, R. A.: Principles of hematologic supportive care. Symposium on clinical signs of blood disease. Med. Clin. North Am. *57*:441, 1973.
47. Yankee, R. A., Grumet, F. C., et al.: Platelet transfusion therapy: The selection of compatible donors for refractory patients by lymphocyte HL-A typing. New Engl. J. Med. *281*:1208, 1969.
48. Herzig, R. H., Herzig, G. P., et al.: Successful granulocyte transfusion therapy for gram-negative septicemia. A prospectively randomized controlled study. New Engl. J. Med. *296*:701, 1977.
49. Alvai, J. B., Root, R. K., et al.: Randomized clinical trial of granulocyte transfusions for infection in acute leukemia. New Engl. J. Med. *296*:706, 1977.
50. Levine, A. S., Schimpff, S. C., et al.: Hematologic malignancies and other marrow failure states: Progress in the management of complicating infections. Semin. Hematol. *11*:141, 1974.
51. Hughes, W. T., Kuhn, S., et al.: Successful chemoprophylaxis for *Pneumocystis carinii* pneumonitis. New Engl. J. Med. *297*:1419, 1977.
52. Schimpff, S. C., Greene, W. H., et al.: Infection prevention in acute nonlymphocytic leukemia: Laminar air flow room reverse isolation with oral, non-absorbable antibiotic prophylaxis. Ann. Intern. Med. *82*:351, 1975.
53. Pizzo, P. A., and Levine, A. S.: The utility of protected-environment regimens for the compromised host: A critical assessment. Prog. Hematol. *10*:311, 1977.
54. Bertino, J. R.: "Rescue" techniques in cancer chemotherapy: Use of leucovorin and other rescue agents after methotrexate treatment. Semin. Oncol. *4*:203, 1977.
55. Tobias, J. S., Weiner, R. S., et al.: Cryopreserved autologous marrow infusion following high dose cancer chemotherapy. Europ. J. Cancer *13*:269, 1977.
56. Levine, A. S., and Deisseroth, A. B.: Recent developments in the supportive therapy of acute myelogenous leukemia. Cancer *42*:883, 1978.
57. Deisseroth, A., and Abrams, R. A.: The role of autologous stem cell reconstitution in intensive therapy for resistant neoplasms. Cancer Treat. Rep. *63*:461, 1979.
58. Lister, T. A., and Yankee, R. A.: Blood component therapy. Clin. Haematol. *7*:407, 1978.
59. Greenblatt, D., and Miller, R. (eds.): *"Antiemetics," Handbook of Drug Therapy.* New York, Elsevier, 1979, pp. 1060–1074.
60. Seigel, L. J., and Longo, D. L.: The control of chemotherapy-induced emesis. Ann. Intern. Med. *95*:352, 1981.
61. Zeltzer, L., LeBaron, S., et al.: Paradoxical effects of prophylactic phenothiazine antiemetics in children receiving chemotherapy. J. Clin. Oncol. *2*:930, 1984.
62. Gralla, R. J., Tyson, L. B., et al.: Antiemetic therapy: a review of recent studies and a report of a random assignment of trial comparing metoclopramide with delta-9-tetrahydrocannabinol. Cancer Treat. Rep. *68*:163, 1984.
63. Zusman, J., Brown, D. M., et al.: Hyperphosphatemia, hyperphosphaturia and hypocalcemia in acute lymphoblastic leukemia. New Engl. J. Med. *289*:1335, 1973.
64. O'Regan, S., Carson, S., et al.: Electrolyte and acid-base disturbances in the management of leukemia. Blood *49*:345, 1977.
65. Mathe, G.: Chemotherapy, a double agent in respect of immune functions. Cancer Chemother. Pharmacol. *1*:65, 1978.
66. Newburger, P. E., Cassady, J. R., et al.: Esophagitis due to Adriamycin and radiation therapy for childhood malignancy. Cancer *42*:417, 1978.
67. Jaffe, N.: Late side effects of treatment: Skeletal, genetic, central nervous system, and oncogenic. Pediatr. Clin. North Am. *23*:233, 1976.
68. Shalet, S. M., Beardwell, C. G., et al.: Endocrine function following the treatment of acute leukemia in childhood. J. Pediatr. *90*:920, 1977.
69. Dickinson, W. P., Berry, D. H., et al.: Differential effects of cranial radiation on growth hormone response to arginine and insulin infusion. J. Pediatr. *92*:754, 1978.
70. Siris, E. S., Leventhal, B. G., et al.: Effects of childhood leukemia and chemotherapy on puberty and reproductive function in girls. New Engl. J. Med. *294*:1143, 1976.
71. Einhorn, N.: Acute leukemia after chemotherapy (melphalan). Cancer *41*:444, 1978.
72. Toland, D. M., Coltman, C. A., Jr., et al.: Second malignancies complicating Hodgkin's disease: The Southwest Oncology Group Experience. Cancer Clin. Trials *1*:27, 1978.
73. Li, F. P.: Second malignant tumors after cancer in childhood. Cancer *40*:1899, 1977.
74. Perry, M. C.: Toxicity of chemotherapy. In *Seminars in Oncology.* Yarbro, J. W., Bornstein, R. S., et al. (eds.). Philadelphia, W. B. Saunders Co., 1982, pp. 1–154.
75. D'Andrea, A. D., and Haseltine, W. A.: Sequence specific cleavage of DNA by the antitumor antibiotics neocarzinostatin and bleomycin. Proc. Natl. Acad. Sci. USA *75*:3608, 1978.
76. Bachur, N. R., Gordon, S. L., et al.: A general mechanism for microsomal activation of quinone anticancer agents to free radicals. Cancer Res. *38*:1745, 1978.
77. Abelson, H. T.: Methotrexate and central nervous system toxicity. Cancer Treat Rep. *62*:1999, 1978.
78. Osband, M. E., Cohen, H., et al.: Severe and protracted bone marrow dysfunction following long-term therapy with methyl-CCNU. Proc. Am. Assoc. Cancer Res. *18*:303, 1977.
79. Harmon, W. E., Cohen, H. J., et al.: Chronic renal failure in children treated with methyl CCNU. New Engl. J. Med. *300*:1200, 1979.
80. Symposium on nutrition in the causation of cancer. Cancer Res. *35*:231, 1975.
81. Filler, R. M., Jaffe, N., et al.: Parenteral nutritional support in children with cancer. Cancer *39*:2665, 1977.
82. Bernstein, I. L.: Physiological and psychological mechanisms of cancer anorexia. Cancer Res. (Suppl.) *42*:715, 1982.
83. Issell, B. F.: Nutrition in cancer patients. In *Cancer and Chemotherapy,* Vol. II. Crooke, S. T., and Prestayko, A. W. (eds.), New York, Academic Press, 1981, pp. 363–370.
84. Von Eys, J.: Nutrition as part of total care. In *Cancer Therapy in Children.* Pochedly, C. (ed.), Thorofare, NJ, Charles B. Slack, 1983, pp. 210–217.
85. Fingl, E., and Woodbury, D. M.: General principles. In *The Pharmacological Basis of Therapeutics,* 4th ed. Goodman, L. S., and Gilman, A. (eds.), New York, Macmillan, 1970, pp. 1–35.
86. Melmon, K. L., and Morrelli, H. F.: *Clinical Pharmacology,* 2nd Ed. New York, The Macmillan Co., 1978, pp. 3–152.
87. Mihich, E.: Pharmacologic principles and the basis for selectivity of drug action. In *Cancer Medicine.* Holland, J. F., and Frei, E., III (eds.), Philadelphia, Lea and Febiger, 1973, pp. 650–674.
88. Greenblatt, D. J., and Koch-Weser, J.: Clinical pharmacokinetics. New Engl. J. Med. *293*:702, 964, 1975.
89. Carson, E. R., and Jones, E. A.: Use of kinetic analysis and mathematical modeling in the study of metabolic pathways in vivo. New Engl. J. Med. *300*:1016, 1077, 1979.
90. Vesell, E. S.: (1972) Pharmacogenetics: History, definitions, and clinical applications. New Engl. J. Med. *287*:904, 1972.
91. Castle, W. B.: A century of curiosity about pernicious anemia. Trans. Am. Clin. Climatol. Assoc. *73*:54, 1961.
92. Lippman, M. E., Yarbro, G. K., et al.: Clinical implications

of glucocorticoid receptors in human leukemia. Cancer Res. 38:4251, 1978.
93. Crabtree, G. R., Smith, K. A., et al.: Glucocorticoid receptors and sensitivity of isolated human leukemia and lymphoma cells. Cancer Res. 38:4268, 1978.
94. Cohen, J., and Jao, J. Y.: Enzymatic basis of cyclophosphamide activation by hepatic microsomes of the rat. J. Pharmacol. Exp. Ther. 174:206, 1970.
95. Darby, F. J., Newnes, W., et al.: Human liver microsomal drug metabolism. Biochem. Pharmacol. 19:1514, 1970.
96. VonHoff, D. D., and Johnson, G. E.: Secretion of tumor markers in the human tumor stem cell system. Proc. Am. Assoc. Cancer Res. 20:51, 1979.
97. Carson, P. E., Flanagan, C. L., et al.: Enzymatic deficiency in primaquine-sensitive erythrocytes. Science 124:484, 1956.
98. Gillette, J. R.: Individually different responses to drugs according to age, sex and functional or pathologic state. In *Drug Responses in Man*. Ciba Foundation Symposia. Wolstenholme, G. E. W., and Porter, R. (eds.), Boston, Little, Brown & Co., 1967, pp. 24–54.
99. Morrelli, H. F., and Melmon, K. L.: Drug interactions in clinical pharmacology. In *Clinical Pharmacology*, 2nd Ed. Melmon, K. L., and Morrelli, H. F. (eds.), New York, The Macmillan Co., 1978, pp. 982–1007.
100. Hansten, P. D.: *Drug Interactions*. Philadelphia, Lea & Febiger, 1975.
101. Bender, R. A., Zwelling, L. A., et al.: Antineoplastic drugs: Clinical pharmacology and therapeutic use. Drugs. 16:46, 1978.
102. Wheeler, G. P., and Alexander, J.: Rate of DNA synthesis as an indication of drug toxicity and as a guide for scheduling cancer therapy. Cancer Treat. Rep. 62:755, 1978.
103. Leigler, D. G., Henderson, E. S., et al.: The effect of organic acids on renal clearance of methotrexate in man. Clin. Pharmacol. Ther. 10:849, 1969.
104. Bourke, R. S., Chheda, F., et al.: Inhibition of renal transport of methotrexate by probenecid. Cancer Res. 35:110, 1975.
105. Spector, R.: Inhibition of methotrexate transport from cerebrospinal fluid by probenecid. Cancer Treat. Rep. 60:913, 1976.
106. Ramu, A., Fusner, J. E., et al.: Probenecid inhibition of methotrexate-cerebrospinal fluid pharmacokinetics in dogs. Cancer Treat. Rep. 62:1465, 1978.
107. Kaplan, S. R., and Calabresi, P.: Immunosuppressive agents. New Engl. J. Med. 289:952, 1973.
108. Rundles, R. W., Wyngaarden, J. B., et al.: Drugs and uric acid. Ann. Rev. Pharmacol. 9:345, 1969.
109. Boston Collaborative Drug Surveillance Program: Allopurinol and cytotoxic drugs. Interaction in relation to bone marrow depression. J.A.M.A. 227:1036, 1974.
110. Coffey, J. J., White, C. A., et al.: Effect of allopurinol on the pharmacokinetics of 6-mercaptopurine (NSC 755) in cancer patients. Cancer Res. 32:1283, 1972.
111. Calabro, J. J., and Castleman, B.: Case records of the Massachusetts General Hospital (Case 4-1972). New Engl. J. Med. 286:205, 1972.
112. Buskirk, H. H., Crim, J. A., et al.: Rapid in vitro method for determining cytotoxicity of antitumor agents. J. Natl. Cancer Inst. 51:135, 1973.
113. Thirlwell, M. P., Livingston, R. B., et al.: A rapid in vitro labeling index method for predicting response of human solid tumors to chemotherapy. Cancer Res. 36:3279, 1976.
114. Roper, P. A., and Drewinko, B.: Comparison of in vitro methods to determine drug-induced cell lethality. 36:2182, 1976.
115. Ross, D. W.: Cell volume growth after cell cycle block with chemotherapeutic agents. Cell Tissue Kinet. 9:379, 1976.
116. Hall, T. C.: Prediction of responses to therapy and mechanisms of resistance. Semin. Oncol. 4:193, 1977.
117. Salmon, S. E., Hamburger, A. W., et al.: Quantitation of differential sensitivity of human tumor stem cells to anticancer drugs. New Engl. J. Med. 298:1321, 1978.
117a. Schnipper, L. E.: Clinical implications of tumor-cell heterogeneity. New Engl. J. Med. 314:1423, 1986.
118. Collins, V. P., Loeffler, R. K., et al.: Observations on growth rate of human tumors. Am. J. Roentgenol. Radium Ther. Nucl. Med. 76:988, 1956.
119. Steel, G. G.: *Growth Kinetics of Tumors. Cell Population Kinetics in Relation to the Growth and Treatment of Cancer.* Oxford, Clarendon Press, 1977.
120. Shackney, S. E., McCormack, G. W., et al.: Growth rate patterns of solid tumors and their relation to responsiveness to therapy. An analytical review. Ann. Intern. Med. 89:107, 1978.
121. Charbit, A., Malaise, E. P., et al.: Relation between the pathological nature and the growth of human tumors. Eur. J. Cancer 7:307, 1971.
122. Bagshawe, K. D.: Risk and prognostic factors in trophoblastic neoplasia. Cancer 38:1373, 1976.
123. Ziegler, J. L.: Treatment results of 54 American patients with Burkitt's lymphoma are similar to the African experience. New Engl. J. Med. 297:75, 1977.
124. Badran, A. F., and Echave-Llanos, J. M.: Persistence of mitotic circadian rhythm of a transplantable mammary carcinoma after 35 generations: its bearing on the success of treatment with Endoxan. J. Natl. Cancer Inst. 35:285, 1965.
125. Hamilton, E.: Diurnal variation in proliferative compartments and their relation to cryptogenic cells in the mouse colon. Cell Tissue Kinet. 12:91, 1979.
126. Simpson-Herren, L., and Griswold, D. P.: Studies of the cell population kinetics of induced and transplanted mammary adenocarcinomas in rats. Cancer Res. 33:2415, 1973.
127. Stragand, J. J., Braunschweiger, P. G., et al.: Cell kinetic alterations in murine mammary tumors following fasting and refeeding. Eur. J. Cancer 15:281, 1979.
128. Folkman, J., and Cotran, R. S.: Relation of vascular proliferation to tumor growth. In *International Review of Experimental Pathology*. Richter, G. W., and Epstein, M. A. (eds.), New York, Academic Press, 1976, pp. 207–247.
129. Hirst, D. G., and Denekamp, J.: Tumor cell proliferation in relation to the vasculature. Cell Tissue Kinet. 12:31, 1979.
130. Janik, P., and Steel, G. G.: Cell proliferation during immunological perturbation in three transplanted tumours. Br. J. Cancer 26:108, 1972.
131. DeCosse, J. J., and Gelfant, S.: Noncycling tumor cells: mitogenic response to antilymphocyte serum. Science 162:698, 1968.
132. Frei, E., Whang, J., et al.: The stathmokinetic effect of vincristine. Cancer Res. 24:1918, 1964.
133. Young, R. C., and DeVita, V. T.: The effect of chemotherapy on the growth characteristics and cellular kinetics of leukemia L1210. Cancer Res. 30:1789, 1970.
134. Tubiana, M.: The kinetics of tumor cell proliferation and radiotherapy. Br. J. Radiol. 44:325, 1971.
135. Lala, P. K., and Patt, H. M.: Cytokinetic analysis of tumor growth. Proc. Natl. Acad. Sci. USA 56:1735, 1966.
136. Silver, R. T., Young, R. C., et al.: Some new aspects of modern cancer chemotherapy. Am. J. Med. 63:772, 1977.
137. Folkman, J.: Tumor angiogenesis factor. Cancer Res. 34:2109, 1974.
138. Norton, L., and Simon, R.: Tumor size, sensitivity to therapy, and design of treatment schedules. Cancer Treat. Rep. 61:1307, 1977.
139. Sullivan, P. W., and Salmon, S. E.: Kinetics of tumour growth and regression in IgG multiple myeloma. J. Clin. Invest. 51:1697, 1972.

140. Skipper, H. E., Schabel, F. M., Jr., et al.: Experimental evaluation of potential anticancer agents. XIII. On the criteria and kinetics associated with "curability" of experimental leukemia. Cancer Chemother. Rep. 35:1, 1964.
141. Skipper, H. E.: Pharmacological basis of cancer chemotherapy: Closing remarks. Twenty-seventh Annual Symposium on Fundamental Cancer Research, 1974. The University of Texas M. D. Anderson Hospital and Tumor Institute. Baltimore, The Williams and Wilkins Co., 1975, pp. 713–726.
142. Wilcox, W. S.: The last surviving cancer cell: the chances of killing it. Cancer Chemother. Rep. 50:541, 1966.
143. Schabel, F. M., Jr.: Concepts for systemic treatment of micrometastases. Cancer 35:15, 1975.
144. Griswold, D. P., Jr., Schabel, F. M., Jr., et al.: Success and failure in the treatment of solid tumors. I. Effects of cyclophosphamide on primary and metastatic plasmacytoma in the hamster. Cancer Chemother. Rep. 52:345, 1968.
145. Laster, W. R., Jr., Mayo, J. G., et al.: Success and failure in the treatment of solid tumors. II. Kinetic parameters and "cell cure" of moderately advanced carcinoma 755. Cancer Chemother. Rep. 53:169, 1969.
146. Mayo, J. G., Laster, W. R., Jr., et al.: Success and failure in the treatment of solid tumors. III. "Cure" of metastatic Lewis lung carcinoma with methyl CCNU (NSC-95441) and surgery-chemotherapy. Cancer Chemother. Rep. 56:183, 1972.
147. Furth, J., and Kahn, M. C.: The transmission of leukemia of mice with a single cell. Am. J. Cancer 31:276, 1937.
148. Bodey, G. P., Freireich, E. J., et al.: Late intensification therapy for acute leukemia in remission. J.A.M.A. 235:1021, 1976.
149. Collins, V. P.: The treatment of Wilms' tumor. Cancer 11:89, 1958.
150. Frei, E., III, Jaffe, N., et al.: Adjuvant chemotherapy of osteogenic sarcoma. Progress and perspectives. J. Natl. Cancer Inst. 60:3, 1978.
151. Hill, B. T.: Cancer chemotherapy. The relevance of certain concepts of cell cycle kinetics. Biochim. Biophys. Acta 516:389, 1978.
152. Kajewsky, M. F.: Proliferative parameters relevant to cancer therapy. In *The Ambivalence of Cytostatic Therapy*. Grunderman, E. and Gross, R. (eds.), New York, Springer-Verlag, 1975, pp. 156–171.
153. Zelen, M.: *Problems in Cell Kinetics and the Early Detection of Disease. Reliability and Biometry*. Philadelphia, SIAM, 1974, pp. 701–726.
154. Rozencweig, M., Zelen, M., et al.: Waiting for a bus: Does it explain age-dependent differences in response to chemotherapy of early breast cancer. New Engl. J. Med. 229:1363, 1978.
155. Hayes, F. A., Green, A. A., et al.: Correlation of cell kinetic and clinical response to chemotherapy in disseminated neuroblastoma. Cancer Res. 37:3766, 1977.
156. Burke, P. J., Karp, J. E., et al.: Timed sequential therapy of human leukemia based upon the response of leukemic cells to humoral growth factors. Cancer Res. 37:2138, 1977.
157. Krishan, A., Pitman, S. W., et al.: Flow microfluorometric patterns of human bone marrow and tumor cells in response to cancer chemotherapy. Cancer Res. 38:3813, 1976.
158. Horan, P. K., and Wheeless, L. L., Jr.: Quantitative single cell analysis and sorting. Science 198:149, 1977.
159. Jones, S. E., Hamburger, A. W., et al.: Development of a bioassay for putative human lymphoma stem cells. Blood 53:294, 1979.
160. Courtenay, V. D., Selby, P. J., et al.: Growth of human tumour cell colonies from biopsies using two soft-agar techniques. Br. J. Cancer 38:77, 1978.
161. Salmon, S. E.: Human tumor colony assay and chemosensitivity testing. Cancer Treat. Rep. 68:117, 1984.
162. Sarna, G.: The resting cell: A chemotherapeutic problem. Biomedicine 20:322, 1974.
163. van Putten, L. M.: Problems in the treatment of slow-growing tumors. In *The Ambivalence of Cytostatic Therapy*. Grundmann, E., and Gross, R. (eds.), New York, Springer-Verlag 1975, pp. 225–233.
164. Tannock, I.: Cell kinetics and chemotherapy: A critical review. Cancer Treat. Rep. 62:1117, 1978.
165. Bruce, W. R., and Meeker, B. E.: Comparison of the sensitivity of hematopoietic colony-forming cells in different proliferative states to 5-fluorouracil. J. Natl. Cancer Inst. 38:401, 1967.
166. Bruce, W. R., Meeker, B. E., et al.: Comparison of the dose- and time-survival curves for normal hematopoietic and lymphoma colony-forming cells exposed to vinblastine, vincristine, arabinosylcytosine and amethopterin. J. Natl. Cancer Inst. 42:1015, 1969.
167. Bruce, W. R., Meeker, B. E., et al.: Comparison of the sensitivity of normal hematopoietic and transplanted lymphoma colony-forming cells to chemotherapeutic agents administered *in vivo*. J. Natl. Cancer Inst. 37:233, 1966.
168. Valeriote, F., and van Putten, L.: Proliferation-dependent cytotoxicity of anticancer agents: A review. Cancer Res. 35:2619, 1975.
169. Chabner, B. A., Myers, C. E., et al.: Clinical pharmacology of anticancer drugs. Semin. Oncol. 4:165, 1977.
170. Livingston, R. B., and Carter, S. K.: *Single Agents in Cancer Chemotherapy*. New York, Plenum Press, 1970, p. 280.
171. Sieber, S. M., and Adamson, R. H.: Toxicity of antineoplastic agents in man. Chromosomal aberrations, antifertility effects, congenital malformations, and carcinogenic potential. In *Advances in Cancer Research*. Klein, G., Weinhouse, S., et al. (eds.), New York, Academic Press, 1975, pp. 57–155.
172. Sartorelli, A. C., and Johns, D. G. (eds.): *Antineoplastic and Immunosuppressive Agents*. I and II. *Handbook of Experimental Pharmacology*, XXXVIII/2. New York, Springer-Verlag, 1975.
173. Weiss, W. D., Walker, M. E., et al.: Neurotoxicity of commonly used antineoplastic agents. New Engl. J. Med. 291:78, 127, 1974.
174. Cohen, F. B., Lippman, A. J., et al.: New antineoplastic drugs and their proper use. Med. Clin. North Am. 60:959, 1976.
175. DeVita, V. T.: Cell kinetics and the chemotherapy of cancer. Cancer Chemother. Rep. 2:23, 1971.
176. Chabner, B. A., Myers, C. E., et al.: The clinical pharmacology of antineoplastic agents. New Engl. J. Med. 292:1107, 1159, 1975.
177. Bergevin, P. R., Tormey, D. C., et al.: Guide to the use of cancer chemotherapeutic agents. Mod. Treat. 9:185, 1972.
178. Cline, M. J., and Haskell, C. M.: *Cancer Chemotherapy*, 3rd Ed. Philadelphia, W. B. Saunders Co., 1980.
179. Valeriote, F., and Vietti, T. J.: Cellular kinetics and conceptual basis of chemotherapy. In *Clinical Pediatric Oncology*. Sutow, N. W., Vietti, T. J., et al. (eds.), St. Louis, C. V. Mosby Co., 1977, pp. 182–196.
180. Vietti, T. J., Valeriote, F., et al.: General aspects of chemotherapy. In *Clinical Pediatric Oncology*. Sutow, N. W., Vietti, T. J., et al. (eds.), St. Louis, C. V. Mosby Co., 1977, pp. 197–237.
181. Owellen, R. J., Hartke, C. A., et al.: Inhibition of tubulin-microtubule polymerization by drugs of the vinca alkaloid class. Cancer Res. 36:1499, 1976.
182. Himes, R. H., Kersey, R. N., et al.: Action of the vinca alkaloids vincristine, vinblastine, and desacetyl vinblastine amide on microtubules *in vitro*. Cancer Res. 36:3798, 1976.
183. Creasey, W. A.: Vinca alkaloids and colchicine. In *Antineoplastic and Immunosuppressive Agents*. Sartorelli, A., and Johns, D. (eds.), New York, Springer-Verlag, pp. 670–694, 1975.

184. Bender, R. A., Castle, M. C., et al.: The pharmacokinetics of ^{3}H vincristine in man. Clin. Pharmacol. Ther. 22:430, 1977.
185. Owellen, R. J., Root, M. A., et al.: Pharmacokinetics of vindesine and vincristine in humans. Cancer Res. 37:2603, 1977.
186. Jackson, D. V., Jr., Castle, M. C., et al.: Biliary excretion of vincristine. Clin. Pharmacol. Ther. 24:101, 1978.
187. Kotani, M., Koizumi, Y., et al.: Increase of cyclic adenosine 3':5'-monophosphate concentration in transplantable lymphoma cells by vinca alkaloids. Cancer Res. 38:3094, 1978.
188. Warren, R. D., Nichols, A. P., et al.: The effect of vincristine on methotrexate uptake and inhibition of DNA synthesis by human lymphoblastoid cells. Cancer Res. 37:2993, 1977.
189. Bender, R. A., Nichols, A. P., et al.: Lack of therapeutic synergism between vincristine and methotrexate in L1210 murine leukemia in vivo. Cancer Treat. Rep. 62:997, 1978.
190. Goldman, I. D., Gupta, V., et al.: Exchangeable intracellular methotrexate levels in the presence and absence of vincristine at extracellular drug concentrations relevant to those achieved in high-dose methotrexate-folinic acid "rescue" protocols. Cancer Res. 36:276, 1976.
191. Gurtoo, H. L., Gessner, T., et al.: Studies of the effects of cyclophosphamide, vincristine, and prednisone on some hepatic oxidations and conjugations. Cancer Treat. Rep. 60:1285, 1976.
192. Krishan, A., and Frei, E., III: Morphological basis for the cytolytic effect of vinblastine and vincristine on cultured human leukemic lymphoblasts. Cancer Res. 35:497, 1975.
193. Sandler, S. G., Tobin, W., et al.: Vincristine-induced neuropathy: A clinical study of fifty leukemic patients. Neurology 19:367, 1969.
194. Clarysee, A., Kenis, Y., et al.: Classification of chemotherapeutic agents according to their effect on the cell cycle. In *Cancer Chemotherapy*. Clarysee, A., Kenis, Y., et al. (eds.), New York, Springer-Verlag, 1976, pp. 101–111.
195. Madoc-Jones, H., and Mauro, F.: Site of action of cytotoxic agents in the cell life cycle. In *Antineoplastic and Immunosuppressive Agents*. Sartorelli, A., and Johns, D. (eds.), New York, Springer-Verlag., 1975, pp. 205–219.
196. Conn, H. O., and Blitzer, B. L.: Non-association of adrenocorticosteroid therapy and peptic ulcer. New Engl. J. Med. 294:473, 1976.
197. Vassali, J. D., and Silverstein, S. C.: Colcemid and related alkaloids inhibit lectin-mediated stimulation of RNA synthesis in human peripheral blood lymphocytes. Exp. Cell Res. 106:95, 1977.
198. Owellen, R. J., and Hartke, C. A.: The pharmacokinetics of 4-acetyl tritium vinblastine in two patients. Cancer Res. 35:975, 1975.
199. Owellen, R. J., Hartke, C. A., et al.: Pharmacokinetics and metabolism of vinblastine in humans. Cancer Res. 37:2597, 1977.
200. Roodman, G. D., Hutton, J. J., et al.: DNA polymerase activities during erythropoiesis. Effect of erythropoietin, vinblastine, colcemid and daunomycin. Exp. Cell Res. 91:269, 1975.
201. Rosen, F., and Milholland, R. J.: Mechanism of action of glucocorticoids. In *Antineoplastic and Immunosuppressive Agents*. Sartorelli, A., and Johns, D. (eds.), New York, Springer-Verlag, 1975, pp. 85–103.
202. Turnell, R. W., and Burton, A. F.: Studies on the mechanism of resistance to lymphocytolysis induced by corticosteroids. Cancer Res. 34:39, 1974.
203. Green, O. C., Winter, R. J., et al.: Pharmacokinetic studies of prednisolone in children. J. Pediatr. 93:299, 1978.
204. DiSanto, A. R., and DeSante, K. A.: Bioavailability and pharmacokinetics of prednisone in humans. J. Pharm. Sci. 64:109, 1975.
205. Pickup, M. E., Lowe, J. R., et al.: Dose dependent pharmacokinetics of prednisolone. Eur. J. Clin. Pharmacol. 12:213, 1977.
206. Loo, J. C. K., McGilveray, I. J., et al.: Dose dependent pharmacokinetics of prednisone and prednisolone in man. J. Pharm. Pharmacol. 30:736, 1978.
207. Claman, H. M.: Corticosteroids and lymphoid cells. New Engl. J. Med. 287:388, 1972.
208. Tak Yan Yu, D.: Effect of corticosteroids on lymphocyte activation. Blood 49:873, 1977.
209. Bruckner, H. W., Schreiber, C., et al.: Interaction of chemotherapeutic agents with methotrexate and 5-fluorouracil and its effect on *de novo* DNA synthesis. Cancer Res. 35:801, 1975.
210. Kaiser, N., Milholland, R. J., et al.: Glucocorticoid receptors and mechanism of resistance in the cortisol-sensitive and -resistant lines of lymphosarcoma P1798. Cancer Res. 34:621, 1974.
211. Axelrod, L.: Glucocorticoid therapy. Medicine 55:39, 1976.
212. Zaitoun, A. M., Lander, I., et al.: Cell population kinetic profile of the mouse thymus and the changes induced by prednisolone. Cell Tissue Kinet. 12:191, 1979.
213. Bertino, J. R.: The mechanism of action of the folate antagonists in man. Cancer Res. 23:1286, 1963.
214. Tattersall, M. H. N., Jackson, R. C., et al.: Factors determining cell sensitivity to methotrexate: studies of folate and deoxyribonucleoside triphosphate pools in five mammalian cell lines. Eur. J. Cancer 10:819, 1974.
215. White, J. C., Loftfield, S., et al.: The mechanism of action of methotrexate: III. Requirement of free intracellular methotrexate for maximal suppression of ^{14}C formate incorporation into nucleic acids and protein. Mol. Pharmacol. 11:287, 1975.
216. Jackson, R. C., Hart, L. I., et al.: Intrinsic resistance of cultured mammalian cells in relation to the inhibition kinetics of their dihydrofolate reductases. Cancer Res. 36:1991, 1976.
217. Goldman, I. D.: Analysis of the cytotoxic determinants for methotrexate (NSC-740): A role for "free" intracellular drug. Cancer Chemother. Rep. 6:51, 1975.
218. Goldman, I. D.: The mechanism of action of methotrexate. I. Interaction with a low-affinity intracellular site required for maximum inhibition of deoxyribonucleic acid synthesis in L-cell mouse fibroblasts. Mol. Pharmacol. 10:257, 1974.
219. Bleyer, W. A.: The clinical pharmacology of methotrexate: new applications of an old drug. Cancer 41:36, 1978.
220. Huffman, D. H., Wan, S. H., et al.: Pharmacokinetics of methotrexate. Clin. Pharmacol. Ther. 14:572, 1973.
221. Wan, S. H., Huffman, D. H., et al.: Effect of route of administration and effusions on methotrexate pharmacokinetics. Cancer Res. 34:3487, 1974.
222. Stoller, R. G., Jacobs, S. A., et al.: Pharmacokinetics of high-dose methotrexate (NSC-740). Cancer Chemother. Rep. 6:19, 1975.
223. Pitman, S. W., Parker, L. M., et al.: Clinical trial of high-dose methotrexate (NSC-740) with citrovorum factor (NSC-3590)—Toxicologic and therapeutic observations. Cancer Chemother. Rep. 6:43, 1975.
224. Pitman, S. W., and Frei, E., III: Weekly methotrexate-calcium leucovorin rescue: Effect of alkalinization on nephrotoxicity; pharmacokinetics in the CNS; and use in CNS non-Hodgkin's lymphoma. Cancer Treat. Rep. 61:695, 1977.
225. Shen, D. D., and Azarnoff, D. L.: Clinical pharmacokinetics of methotrexate. Clin. Pharmacokinet. 3:1, 1978.
226. Bleyer, W. A.: Methotrexate: Clinical pharmacology, current status and therapeutic guidelines. Cancer Treat. Rep. 4:87, 1977.

227. Jacobs, S. A., Stoller, R. G., et al.: 7-Hydroxymethotrexate as a urinary metabolite in human subjects and rhesus monkeys receiving high dose methotrexate. J. Clin. Invest. 57:534, 1976.
228. Donehower, R. C., Hande, K. R., et al.: Presence of 2,4-diamino-N^{10}-methylpteroic acid in the plasma and urine of patients receiving high dose methotrexate. Proc. Am. Assoc. Cancer Res. 19:687, 1978.
229. McBurney, M. W., and Whitmore, G. F.: Mechanism of growth inhibition by methotrexate. Cancer Res. 35:586, 1975.
230. Bender, R. A., Bleyer, W. A., et al.: Alteration of methotrexate uptake in human leukemia cells by other agents. Cancer Res. 35:1305, 1975.
231. Semon, J. H., and Grindey, G. B.: Potentiation of the antitumor activity of methotrexate by concurrent infusion of thymidine. Cancer Res. 38:2905, 1978.
232. Bender, R. A.: Anti-folate resistance in leukemia: treatment with "high-dose" methotrexate and citrovorum factor. Cancer Treat. Rev. 2:215, 1975.
233. Bertino, J. R.: Toward improved selectivity in cancer chemotherapy: The Richard and Hinda Rosenthal Foundation Award Lecture. Cancer Res. 39:293, 1979.
234. Alt, F. W., Kellems, R. E., et al.: Selective multiplication of dihydrofolate reductase genes in methotrexate-resistant variants of cultured murine cells. J. Biol. Chem. 253:1357, 1978.
235. Kaufman, R. J., Bertino, J. R., et al.: Quantitation of dihydrofolate reductase in individual parental and methotrexate-resistant murine cells. J. Biol. Chem. 253:5852, 1978.
236. Goldin, A.: Studies with high-dose methotrexate—historical background. Cancer Treat. Rep. 62:307, 1978.
237. Capizzi, R. L., DeConti, R. C., et al.: Methotrexate therapy of head and neck cancer: Improvement in therapeutic index by the use of leucovorin "rescue." Cancer Res. 30:1782, 1970.
238. Djerassi, I., and Kim, J. S.: Methotrexate and citrovorum factor rescue in the management of childhood lymphosarcoma and reticulum cell sarcoma (non-Hodgkin's lymphomas). Cancer 38:1043, 1976.
239. Halpern, R. M., Halpern, B. C., et al.: A new approach to antifolate treatment of certain cancers as demonstrated in tissue culture. Proc. Natl. Acad. Sci. USA 72:4018, 1975.
240. Frei, E., III, Jaffe, N., et al.: New approaches to cancer chemotherapy with methotrexate. New Engl. J. Med. 292:846, 1975.
241. Capizzi, R. L.: Schedule-dependent synergism and antagonism between methotrexate and asparaginase. Biochem. Pharmacol. 23(Suppl. 2):151, 1974.
242. Capizzi, R. L., Keiser, L. W., et al.: Combination chemotherapy—Theory and practice. Semin. Oncol. 4:227, 1977.
243. Bleyer, W. A.: Clinical pharmacology of intrathecal methotrexate. II. An improved dosage regimen derived from age-related pharmacokinetics. Cancer Treat. Rep. 61:1419, 1977.
244. Condit, P. T., Chanes, R. E., et al.: Renal toxicity of methotrexate. Cancer 23:126, 1969.
245. Howell, S. B., and Carmody, J.: Changes in glomerular filtration rate associated with high-dose methotrexate therapy in adults. Cancer Treat. Rep. 61:1389, 1977.
246. Romolo, J. L., Goldberg, N. H., et al.: Effect of hydration on plasma-methotrexate levels. Cancer Treat. Rep. 61:1393, 1977.
247. Abelson, H. T., Fosburg, M. T., et al.: Methotrexate-induced renal impairment: clinical studies and rescue from systemic toxicity with high dose leucovorin and thymidine. Oncology 1:208, 1983.
248. Beardsley, G. P., and Abelson, H. T.: Unpublished observations.
249. Groff, J. P., and Blakley, R. L.: Rescue of human lymphoid cells from effects of methotrexase *in vitro*. Cancer Res. 38:3847, 1978.
250. Johnson, L. F., Fuhrman, C. L., et al.: Resistance of resting 3T6 mouse fibroblasts to methotrexate cytotoxicity. Cancer Res. 38:2408, 1978.
251. Paterson, A. R. P., and Tidd, D. M.: 6-Thiopurines. In *Antineoplastic and Immunosuppressive Agents*. Sartorelli, A., and Johns, D. (eds.), New York, Springer-Verlag, 1975, pp. 384–379.
252. Higuchi, T., Nakamura, T., et al.: Metabolism of 6-mercaptopurine in human leukemic cells. Cancer Res. 36:3779, 1976.
253. Nelson, J. A., Carpenter, J. W., et al.: Mechanisms of action of 6-thioguanine, 6-mercaptopurine and 8-azaguanine. Cancer Res. 35:2872, 1975.
254. Roy-Burman, P.: *Analogues of Nucleic Acid Components. Mechanisms of Action*. Berlin, Springer-Verlag, 1970.
255. Elion, G. B.: Biochemistry and pharmacology of purine analogues. Fed. Proc. 26:898, 1967.
256. DiMarco, A.: Daunomycin (Daunorubicin) and Adriamycin. In *Antineoplastic and Immunosuppressive Agents*. Sartorelli, A., and Johns, D. (eds.), New York, Springer-Verlag, 1975, pp. 593–614.
257. Hitchings, G.: Chemotherapy and comparative biochemistry: G. H. A. Clowes Memorial Lecture. Cancer Res. 29:1895, 1969.
258. Losito, A., Williams, D. G., et al.: The effects on polymorphonuclear leukocyte function of prednisolone and azathioprine in vivo and prednisolone, azathioprine and 6-mercaptopurine in vitro. Clin. Exp. Immunol. 32:423, 1978.
259. Chou, T. C., Arlin, Z., et al.: Metabolism of 1-beta-D-arabinofuranosylcytosine in human leukemic cells. Cancer Res. 37:3561, 1977.
260. Creasey, W. A.: Arabinosylcytosine. In *Antineoplastic and Immunosuppressive Agents*. Sartorelli, A., and Johns, D. (eds.), New York, Springer-Verlag, 1975, pp. 232–249.
261. Cohen, S. S.: The mechanisms of lethal action of arabinosyl cytosine (ara-C) and arabinosyl adenine (ara-A). Cancer 40(Suppl. 1):509, 1977.
262. Rashbaum, S. A., and Cozzarelli, N. R.: Mechanism of DNA synthesis inhibition by arabinosyl cytosine and arabinosyl adenine. Nature 264:679, 1976.
263. Fridland, A.: Inhibition of deoxyribonucleic acid chain initiation: a new mode of action for 1-beta-D-arabinofuranosyl-cytosine in human lymphoblasts. Biochemistry 16:5308, 1977.
264. Shapiro, W. R., Young, D. F., et al.: Methotrexate: distribution in cerebrospinal fluid after intravenous, ventricular, and lumbar injections. New Engl. J. Med. 293:161, 1975.
265. Bleyer, W. A., and Dedrick, R. L.: Clinical pharmacology of intrathecal methotrexate. I. Pharmacokinetics of nontoxic patients after lumbar injection. Cancer Treat. Rep. 61:703, 1977.
266. Baguley, B. C., and Falkenhaug, E. M.: Plasma half-life of cytosine arabinoside in patients with leukemia–the effect of uridine. Eur. J. Cancer 11:43, 1975.
267. Benedict, W. F., Harris, N., et al.: Kinetics of 1-β-D-arabino-furanosyl-cytosine-induced chromosome breaks. Cancer Res. 30:2477, 1970.
268. Chuang, R. Y., and Chuang, L. F.: Inhibition of RNA polymerase as a possible anti-leukemic action of cytosine arabinoside. Nature 260:549, 1976.
269. Creasey, W. A., McIntosh, L. S., et al.: Clinical effects and pharmacokinetics of different dosage schedules of Adriamycin. Cancer Res. 36:216, 1976.
270. Glode, L. M., Israel, M., et al.: Hepatobiliary metabolism and excretion of Adriamycin in man. Br. J. Clin. Pharmacol. 4:639, 1977.

271. Carter, S. K.: Adriamycin—a review. J. Natl. Cancer Inst. 55:1265, 1975.
272. Ghione, M.: Cardiotoxic effects of antitumor agents. Cancer Chemother. Pharmacol. 1:25, 1978.
273. Krishan, A., and Frei, E., III.: Effect of Adriamycin on the cell cycle traverse and kinetics of cultured human lymphoblasts. Cancer Res. 36:143, 1976.
274. Riggs, C. E., Jr., Benjamin, R. S., et al.: Biliary disposition of Adriamycin. Clin. Pharmacol. Therap. 22:234, 1977.
275. Bristow, M. R., Mason, J. W., et al.: Doxorubicin cardiomyopathy: Phonocardiography, endomyocardial biopsy, and cardiac catheterization. Ann. Int. Med. 88:168, 1978.
276. Bowen, D., and Goldman, I. D.: The relationship among transport, intracellular binding, and inhibition of RNA synthesis by actinomycin D in Ehrlich ascites tumor cells in vitro. Cancer Res. 35:3054, 1975.
277. Cooper, H. L., and Braverman, R.: The mechanism by which actinomycin D inhibits protein synthesis in animal cells. Nature 269:527, 1977.
278. Goldberg, I. H.: Actinomycin D. In *Antineoplastic and Immunosuppressive Agents*. Sartorelli, A., and Johns, D. (eds.), New York, Springer-Verlag, 1975, pp. 582–589.
279. Tattersall, M. H. N., Sodergren, J. E., et al.: Pharmacokinetics of actinomycin D in patients with malignant melanoma. Clin. Pharmacol. Ther. 17:701, 1975.
280. Zuckerman, K. S., Sullivan, R., et al.: Effects of actinomycin D in vivo on murine erythroid stem cells. Blood 51:957, 1978.
281. Rutman, R. J., and Avadhavi, N. G.: Distinctive effects of mechlorethamine, cyclophosphamide and BCNU on transcription in Ehrlich cells. Cancer Treat. Rep. 60:471, 1976.
282. Cox, P. J., Phillips, B. J., et al.: The enzymatic basis of the selective action of cyclophosphamide. Cancer Res. 35:3755, 1975.
283. Bagley, C. M., Jr., Bostick, F. W., et al.: Clinical pharmacology of cyclophosphamide. Cancer Res. 33:226, 1973.
284. Juma, F. D., Rogers, H. J., et al.: Pharmacokinetics of intravenous cyclophosphamide in man, estimated by gas-liquid chromatography. Cancer Chemother. Pharmacol. 1:229, 1978.
285. D'Incalci, M., Bolis, G., et al.: Decreased half life of cyclophosphamide in patients under continual treatment. Eur. J. Cancer 15:7, 1979.
286. Mouridsen, H. T., Faber, O., et al.: The metabolism of cyclophosphamide dose dependency and the effect of long-term treatment with cyclophosphamide. Cancer 37:665, 1976.
287. Wagner, T., Peter, G., et al.: Characterization and quantitative estimation of activated cyclophosphamide in blood and urine. Cancer Res. 37:2592, 1977.
288. Proceedings of the symposium on the metabolism and mechanism of action of cyclophosphamide. Cancer Treat. Rep. 60:299, 1976.
289. Cardoso, S. S., Avery, T., et al.: Circadian dependence of host and tumor responses to cyclophosphamide in mice. Eur. J. Cancer 14:949, 1978.
290. Gershwin, M. E., Goetzl, E. J., et al.: Cyclophosphamide: Use in practice. Ann. Intern. Med. 80:531, 1974.
291. Benjamin, R. S., Riggs, C. E., Jr., et al.: Plasma pharmacokinetics of Adriamycin and its metabolites in humans with normal hepatic and renal function. Cancer Res. 37:1416, 1977.
292. Wall, R. L., and Clausen, K. P.: Carcinoma of the urinary bladder in patients receiving cyclophosphamide. New Engl. J. Med. 293:271, 1975.
293. Jayalakshmamma, B., and Pinkel, D.: Urinary-bladder toxicity following pelvic irradiation and simultaneous cyclophosphamide therapy. Cancer 38:701, 1976.
294. Schwartz, H. S.: Biochemical action and selectivity of intercalating drugs. In *Advances in Cancer Chemotherapy*. Rosowsky, A. (ed.), Marcel Dekker, Inc., New York and Basel, 1979, pp. 1–60.
295. Ensminger, W. D., Grindey, G. B., et al.: Antifolate therapy: Rescue, selective host protection and drug combinations. In *Advances in Cancer Chemotherapy*. Rosowsky, A. (ed.), Marcel Dekker, Inc., New York and Basel, 1979, pp. 61–109.
296. Friedman, O. M., Myles, A., et al.: Cyclophosphamide and related phosphoramide mustards: Current status and future prospects. In *Advances in Cancer Chemotherapy*. Rosowsky, A. (ed.), Marcel Dekker, Inc., New York and Basel, 1979, pp. 143–204.
297. Canellos, G., and Parker, L.: Personal communications.
298. DeVita, V. T., Denham, C., et al.: The physiological disposition of the carcinostatic 1,3-bis-(2-chloroethyl)-1-nitrosourea (BCNU) in man and animals. Clin. Pharmacol. Ther. 8:566, 1967.
299. Kann, H. E., Jr.: Comparison of biochemical and biological effects of four nitrosoureas with differing carbamoylating activities. Cancer Res. 38:2363, 1978.
300. Kohn, K. W.: Interstrand cross-linking of DNA by 1,3-bis-(2-chloroethyl)-1-nitrosourea and other 1-(2-haloethyl)-1-nitrosoureas. Cancer Res. 37:1450, 1977.
301. Erickson, L. C., Bradley, M. O., et al.: Strand breaks in DNA from normal and transformed human cells treated with 1,3-bis(2-chloroethyl)-1-nitrosourea. Cancer Res. 37:3744, 1977.
302. Kann, H. E., Jr., Kohn, K. W., et al.: Inhibition of DNA repair by the 1,3-bis(2-chloroethyl)-1-nitrosoureas breakdown product, 2-chloroethyl isocyanate. Cancer Res. 34:398, 1974.
303. Erickson, L. C., Bradley, M. O., et al.: Differential inhibition of the rejoining of x-ray-induced DNA strand breaks in normal and transformed human fibroblasts treated with 1,3-bis(2-chloroethyl)-1-nitrosourea in vitro. Cancer Res. 38:672, 1978.
304. Abelson, H. T., Karlan, D., et al.: A comparison of the effects of alkylating agents 1,3-bis(2-chloroethyl)-1-nitrosourea, 1-(2-chloroethyl)-3-cyclohexyl-1-nitrosourea and nitrogen mustard on nuclear RNA synthesis and processing. Biochim. Biophys. Acta 349:389, 1974.
305. Proceedings of the Seventh New Drug Seminar on the Nitrosoureas (Washington D.C., Dec. 15–16, 1975). Cancer Treat Rep. 60:645, 1976.
306. Kann, H. E., Jr., Kohn, K. W., et al.: Effects of 1,3-bis(2-chloroethyl)-1-nitrosourea and related compounds on nuclear RNA metabolism. Cancer Res. 34:1982, 1974.
307. Tobey, R. A., and Crissman, H. A.: Comparative effects of three nitrosourea derivatives on mammalian cell cycle progression. Cancer Res. 35:460, 1975.
308. Capizzi, R. L., Bertino, J. R., et al.: L-Asparaginase. Ann. Rev. Med. 21:433, 1970.
309. Capizzi, R. L., Bertino, J. R., et al.: L-Asparaginase: Clinical, biochemical, pharmacological, and immunological studies. Ann. Intern. Med. 74:893, 1971.
310. Patterson, M. K., Jr.: L-Asparaginase: Basic aspects. In *Antineoplastic and Immunosuppressive Agents*. Sartorelli, A., and Johns, D. (eds.), New York, Springer-Verlag, 1975, pp. 695–722.
311. Roberts, J., Schmid, F. A., et al.: A comparative study of the antitumor effectiveness of *E. coli* and *Erwinia* asparaginases. Cancer Biochem. Biophys. 1:175, 1976.
312. Dellinger, C. T., and Miale, T. D.: Comparison of anaphylactic reactions to asparaginase derived from *E. coli* and from *Erwinia* cultures. Cancer 38:1843, 1976.
313. Land, V. J., Sutow, W. W., et al.: Toxicity of L-Asparaginase in children with advanced leukemia. Cancer 30:339, 1972.
314. Oettgen, H. F.: L-Asparaginase: Current status of clinical evaluation. In *Antineoplastic and Immunosuppressive Agents*. Sartorelli, A., and Johns, D. (eds.), New York, Springer-Verlag, 1975, pp. 723–746.

315. Peterson, R. G., Handschumacher, R. E., et al.: Immunological responses to L-asparaginase. J. Clin. Invest. 50:1080, 1971.
316. Van dan Berg, H. W., and Roberts, J. J.: Investigations into the mechanism of action of anti-tumor platinum compounds: time- and dose-dependent changes in the alkaline sucrose gradient sedimentation profiles of DNA from hamster cells treated with *cis*-platinum diamminechloride. Chem. Biol. Interact. 11:493, 1975.
317. Stone, P. J., Kelman, A. D., et al.: Specific binding of antitumor drug *cis*-pt. $(NH_3)_2 Cl_2$ to DNA rich in guanine and cytosine. Nature 251:736, 1974.
318. Prestayko, A. W., D'Aoust, J. C., et al.: Cis-Platin (*cis*-diamminedichloroplatinum II). Cancer Treat. Rev. 6:17, 1979.
319. Patton, T. F., Himmelstein, K. J., et al.: Plasma levels and urinary excretion of filterable platinum species following bolus injection and I.V. infusion if *cis*-dichlorodiammineplatinum (II) in man. Cancer Treat. Rep. 62:1359, 1978.
320. DeConti, R. C., Toftness, B. R., et al.: Clinical and pharmacological studies with *cis*-diamminedichloroplatinum (II). Cancer Res. 33:1310, 1973.
321. Rozencweig, M., Von Hoff, D. D., et al.: *Cis*-diamminedichloroplatinum (II). A new anticancer drug. Ann. Intern. Med. 86:803, 1977.
322. Hayes, F. A., Green, A. A., et al.: Tetany: A complication of *cis*-dichlorodiammineplatinum (II) therapy. Cancer Treat. Rep. 63:547, 1979.
323. Drewinko, B., and Gottlieb, J. A.: Action of *cis*-dichlorodiammineplatinum (II) at the cellular level. Cancer Chemother. Rep. 59:665, 1975.
324. Miller, H. K., Salser, J. S., et al.: Amino acid levels following L-asparagine amidohydrolase (EC.3.5.1.1) therapy. Cancer Res. 29:183, 1969.
325. Kufe, D. W., Egan, E. M., et al.: Thymidine arrest and synchrony of cellular growth in vivo. Cancer Treat. Rep. (In press).
326. Hall, T.: Limited role of cell kinetics in cancer therapy. In *Prediction of Response in Cancer*. National Cancer Institute Monographs, No. 34., 1971.
327. Klein, H., and Lennartz, K.: Chemotherapy after synchronization of tumor cells. Semin. Hematol. 11:203, 1974.
328. Tubiana, M., Frindel, E., et al.: Critical survey of experimental data on *in vivo* synchronization by hydroxyurea, Rec. Results Cancer Res. 52:187, 1975.
329. Van Putten, L. M.: Are cell kinetic data relevant for the design of tumor chemotherapy schedules? Cell Tissue Kinet. 7:493, 1974.
330. Hopkins, H. A., and Looney, W. B.: Synchronization of host and tumor responses for sequential therapy in experimental solid tumors. Antibiot. Chemother. 23:135, 1978.
331. Wheeler, G. P., and Alexander, J. A.: Rate of DNA synthesis as an indication of drug toxicity and as a guide for scheduling cancer therapy. Cancer Treat. Rep. 62:755, 1978.
332. Hutchison, D. J., and Schmid, F. A.: Cross-resistance and collateral sensitivity. In *Drug-Resistance and Selectivity: Biochemical and Cellular Basis*. Mihich, E. (ed.), New York and London, Academic Press, Inc., 1973, pp. 73–126.
333. Skipper, H. E., Hutchison, D. J., et al.: A quick reference chart on cross resistance between anticancer agents. Cancer Chemother. Rep. 56:493, 1972.
334. Brockman, R. W.: Mechanisms of resistance. In *Handbook of Experimental Pharmacology*. Vol. 38, Part I. Antineoplastic and Immunosuppressive Agents. Berlin, Springer-Verlag, 1974, pp. 352–410.
335. Hall, T. C.: Prediction of responses to therapy and mechanisms of resistance. Semin. Oncol. 4:193, 1977.
336. DeVita, V. T., Jr.: Principles of chemotherapy. In *Cancer: Principles and Practice of Oncology*, 2nd ed. DeVita, V. T., Jr., Hellman, S., et al., (eds.), Philadelphia, J. B. Lippincott, 1985, pp. 257–285.
337. Mihich, E.: *Drug Resistance and Selectivity: Biochemical and Cellular Basis*. New York, Academic Press, 1973.
338. Skipper, H. E., Schabel, F. M., Jr., et al.: Dose-response and tumor cell repopulation rate in chemotherapeutic trials. In *Advances in Cancer Chemotherapy*. Rosowsky, A. (ed.), Marcel Dekker, New York, 1979, pp. 205–253.
339. Schabel, F. M., Jr., Skipper, H. E., et al.: Experimental evaluation of anticancer agents. XIX. Sensitivity of nondividing leukemic cell populations to certain classes of drugs in vitro. Cancer Chemother. Rep. 48:17, 1965.
340. Schmid, F. A., Hutchison, D. J., et al.: Development of resistance to combinations of six antimetabolites in mice with L1210 leukemia. Cancer Treat. Rep. 60:23, 1976.
341. Frei, E., III, Freireich, E. J., et al.: Studies of sequential and combination antimetabolite therapy in acute leukemia: 6-Mercaptopurine and methotrexate. Blood 18:431, 1961.
342. Weinstein, H., Griffin, T., et al.: Pharmacology of cytosine arabinoside (a-C). Proceedings of the Sixty-Ninth Annual Meeting of the American Association for Cancer Research. 19:157, 1978.
343. Capizzi, R. L., Keiser, L. W., et al.: Combination chemotherapy–Theory and Practice. Semin. Oncol. 4:227, 1977.
344. Blum, R. H., and Frei, E., III: Combination chemotherapy. In *Methods in Cancer Research*. Vol. XVII, DeVita, V. T. (ed.), New York, Academic Press, 1978, pp. 215–257.
345. Sartorelli, A. C., and Creasey, W. A.: Combination chemotherapy. In *Cancer Medicine,* 2nd Ed. Holland, J., and Frei, E. (eds.), Philadelphia, Lea and Febiger, 1982, pp. 720–730.
346. Potter, V. R.: Sequential blocking of metabolic pathways in vivo. Proc. Soc. Exp. Biol. Med. 76:41, 1951.
347. Elion, G. B., Singer, S., et al.: Antagonists of nucleic acid derivatives. VIII. Synergism in combinations of biochemically related antimetabolites. J. Biol. Chem. 208:477, 1954.
348. Sartorelli, A. C.: Some approaches to the therapeutic exploitation of metabolic sites of vulnerability of neoplastic cells. Cancer Res. 29:2292, 1969.
349. Carter, S. K.: New drugs under clinical evaluation in the United States. Cancer Chemother. Pharmacol. 1:15, 1978.
350. Mathe, G., and van Putten, L. M.: New cancer chemotherapy drugs in Europe. Cancer Chemother. Pharmacol. 1:5, 1978.
351. Juliano, R. L., and Stamp, D.: Pharmacokinetics of liposome-encapsulated anti-tumor drugs. Studies with vinblastine, actinomycin, cytosine arabinoside, and daunomycin. Biochem. Pharmacol. 27:21, 1978.
352. Papahadjopoulos, D. (ed.): Liposomes and their uses in biology and medicine. Ann N.Y. Acad. Sci. 308:1–441, 1978.
353. Milder, J. W. (ed.): Conference on Hyperthermia in Cancer Treatment. Cancer Res. 39:2235, 1979.
354. Philpott, G., Goldenberg, D., et al.: Anti-CEA antibody enzyme conjugate binding to human tumor cells. Proc. Am. Assoc. Cancer Res. 18:211, 1977.
355. Abelson, H. T., Ensminger, W., et al.: Comparative effects of citrovorum factor and carboxypeptidase G_1 on cerebrospinal fluid-methotrexate pharmacokinetics. Cancer Treat. Rep. 62:1549, 1978.
356. Dorr, R. T., and Paxinos, J.: The current status of Laetrile. Ann. Intern. Med. 89:389, 1978.
357. Greenberg, D. M.: The vitamin fraud in cancer quackery. West J. Med. 122:345, 1975.
358. Smith, F. P., Butler, T. P., et al.: Laetrile toxicity: A report of two patients. Cancer Treat. Rep. 62:169, 1978.
359. Davignon, J. P., Trissel, L. A., et al.: Pharmaceutical assessment of amygdalin (Laetrile) products. Cancer Treat. Rep. 62:99, 1978.
360. Schmidt, E. S., Newton, G. W., et al.: Laetrile toxicity studies in dogs. J.A.M.A. 239:943, 1978.

361. Braico, K. T., Humbert, J. R., et al.: Laetrile intoxication: Report of a fatal case. New Engl. J. Med. *300*:238, 1979.
362. Bleyer, W. A., Savitch, J. L., et al.: Is aminopterin (AMT) a safer drug for intrathecal (IT) injection than methotrexate? Proc. American Association for Cancer Research. *19*:179, 1979.
363. Garnick, M. B., and Larsen, P. R.: Acute deficiency of thyroxine-binding globulin during L-asparaginase therapy. New Engl. J. Med. *301*:252, 1979.
364. Fletcher, R. H., and Fletcher, S. W.: Clinical research in general medical journals: A 30 year perspective. New Engl. J. Med. *301*:180, 1979.
365. Keystone Conference on Autologous Bone Marrow Transplantation. Exp. Hematol. *7*:1, 1979.
366. Glode, L. M.: Dose limiting extramedullary toxicity of high dose chemotherapy. Exp. Hematol. *7*:265, 1979.
367. Slavin, R. E., Dias, M. A., et al.: Cytosine arabinoside-induced gastrointestinal toxic alterations in sequential chemotherapeutic protocols. Cancer *42*:1747, 1978.
368. Trier, J. S.: Morphologic alterations induced by methotrexate in the mucosa of human proximal tubule. Gastroenterology *42*:295, 1962.
369. Fidler, I. J.: Selection of successive tumor lines for metastases. Nature (New Biol.) *242*:148, 1973.
370. Nowel, P. C.: The clonal evolution of tumor cell populations. Science *194*:23, 1976.
371. Fidler, I. J.: Metastases: Quantitative analysis of distribution and fate of tumor emboli labeled with ^{125}I-5-Iodo-2′-deoxuridine. J. Natl. Cancer Inst. *45*:773, 1970.
372. Hoover, H. C., Jr., and Ketchan, A. S.: Metastasis of metastases. Am. J. Surg. *130*:405, 1975.
373. Scher, C. D., Pledger, W. J., et al.: Transforming viruses directly reduce the cellular growth requirement for a platelet-derived growth factor. J. Cell. Physiol. *97*:371, 1978.
374. Ovejera, A. A., Houchens, D. P., et al.: Efficacy of various drugs against xenografts of human tumors in athymic (nude) mice. Proc. Am. Assoc. Cancer Res. *20*:40, 1979.
375. Hoshimo, T.: Therapeutic implications of brain tumor cell kinetics. Natl. Cancer Inst. Monogr. *46*:29, 1977.
376. Murphy, S. B., Melvin, S. L., et al.: Correlation of tumor cell kinetic studies with surface marker results in childhood non-Hodgkin's lymphoma. Cancer Res. *39*:1534, 1979.
377. Baserga, R. (ed.): *The Cell Cycle and Cancer*. New York, M. Dekker, Inc., 1971.
378. Pardee, A. B.: A Restriction point for control of normal animal cell proliferation. Proc. Natl. Acad. Sci. USA *71*:1286, 1974.
379. Pledger, W. J., Stiles, C. D., et al.: An ordered sequence of events is required before Balb/c-3T3 cells become committed to DNA synthesis. Proc. Natl. Acad. Sci. USA *75*:2839, 1978.
380. Buckles, R. G.: A system for the controlled administration of parenteral drugs. J. Pharm. Sci. (In press.)
381. Altman, A. J., and Schwartz, A. D.: *Cancer Chemotherapy in Malignant Diseases of Infancy, Childhood and Adolescence.* Philadelphia, W. B. Saunders Co., 1978, pp. 57–88.
382. Folkman, J.: Tumor invasion and metastases. In *Cancer Medicine*, 2nd Ed. Holland, J., and Frei, E. (eds.), Philadelphia, Lea and Febiger, 1982, pp. 167–177.
383. Folkman, J.: Personal communication.
384. Frei, E. III, Holland, J. F., et al.: A comparative study of two regimens of combination chemotherapy in acute leukemia. Blood *13*:1126, 1958.
385. Ensminger, W. D., Thompson, M., et al.: Hepatic arterial BCNU: A pilot clinical-pharmacologic study in patients with liver tumors. Cancer Treat. Rep. *62*:1509, 1978.
386. Freirich, E. J., et al.: The effect of 6-mercaptopurine on the duration of steroid-induced remission in acute leukemia: A model for evaluation of other potentially useful therapy. Blood *21*:699, 1963.
387. Frei, E., III, et al.: The effectiveness of combinations of antileukemic agents in inducing and maintaining remission in children with acute leukemia. Blood *26*:642, 1965.
388. Frei, E. III., and Freirich, E. J.: Progress and perspectives in the chemotherapy of acute leukemia. Adv. Chemother. *2*:269, 1965.
389. Proceedings of the National Cancer Institute Conference on *cis*-Platinum and Testicular Cancer (Washington, D.C., Sept. 21–22, 1978). Cancer Treat. Rep. *63*:1431, 1979.
390. Pratt, W. B., and Ruddon, R. W. (eds.): *The Anticancer Drugs*. New York, Oxford University Press, 1979.
391. Patton, T. F., Himmelstein, K. J., et al.: Plasma levels and urinary excretion of filterable platinum species following bolus injection and IV infusion of *cis*-Dichlorodiammineplatinum (II) in man. Cancer Treat. Rep. *62*:1359, 1978.
392. Rosen, G., and Nirenberg, A.: Chemotherapy for osteogenic sarcoma: an investigative method, not a recipe. Cancer Treat. Rep. *66*:1687, 1982.
393. Malawer, M. M., Abelson, H. T., et al.: Sarcomas of bone. In *Cancer: Principles and Practice of Oncology*, 2nd ed. DeVita, V. T., Jr., Hellman, S., et al. (eds.), Philadelphia, J. B. Lippincott, 1985, pp. 1293–1342.
394. Selby, P., Buick, R. N., et al.: A critical appraisal of the "human tumor stem-cell assay." New Engl. Med. *308*:129, 1983.
395. Von Hoff, D. D.: Send this patient's tumor for culture and sensitivity. New Engl. J. Med. *308*:154, 1983.
396. Von Hoff, D. D., Clark, G. M., et al.: Prospective clinical trial of a human tumor cloning system. Cancer Res. *43*:1926, 1983.
397. Fidler, I. J.: Recent concepts of cancer metastasis and their implications for therapy. Cancer Treat. Rep. *68*:193, 1984.
398. Shackney, S. E., and Ritch, P. S.: Cell kinetics. In *Pharmacologic Principles of Cancer Treatment*. Chabner, B. (ed.), Philadelphia, W. B. Saunders Co., 1982, pp. 45–76.
399. Ling, V.: Genetic basis of drug resistance in mammalian cells. In *Drug and Hormone Resistance in Neoplasia*, Vol. 1. Bruchousky, V., and Goldie, J. H. (eds.), Florida, CRC Press, 1982, pp. 1–19.
400. Schabel, F. M., Jr., Skipper, H. E., et al.: Establishment of cross-resistance profiles for new agents. Cancer Treat. Rep. *67*:905, 1983.
401. Skipper, H. E., and Schabel, F. M., Jr.: Tumor stem cell heterogeneity: implications with respect to classification of cancers by chemotherapeutic effect. Cancer Treat. Rep. *68*:43, 1984.
402. DeVita, V. T., Jr.: Some new concepts on the development of resistance to chemotherapy. In *Accomplishments in Cancer Research*, 1982. Fortner, J. G., and Rhoads, J. E. (eds.), Philadelphia, J. B. Lippincott, 1983, pp. 99–123.
403. Goldie, J. H., and Coldman, A. J.: A mathematical model for relating the drug sensitivity of tumors to their spontaneous mutation rate. Cancer Treat. Rep. *63*:1727, 1979.
404. Goldie, J. H., Coldman, A. J., et al.: Rationale for the use of alternating non–cross-resistant chemotherapy. Cancer Treat. Rep. *66*:439, 1982.
405. Bonadonna, G., Monfardini, S., et al.: Non–cross-resistant combinations in stage IV non-Hodgkin's lymphomas. Cancer Treat. Rep. *61*:1117, 1977.
406. Santoro, A., Bonadonna, G., et al.: Non–cross-resistant regimens (MOPP and ABVD) vs. MOPP alone in stage IV Hodgkin disease. Proc. Am. Soc. Clin. Oncol. *21*:470, 1980.
407. Young, J. A., Johnson, A., et al.: Alternating combination chemotherapy for stages III and IV ovarian carcinoma. J. Clin. Oncol. *2*:1317, 1984.
408. Dembo, A. J.: Editorial: Spontaneous mutation to chemotherapy resistance. Implications of the Goldie-Coldman model for the management of ovarian cancer. J. Clin. Oncol. *2*:1311, 1984.

409. Goldie, J. H., and Coldman, A. J.: Quantitative model for multiple levels of drug resistance in clinical tumors. Cancer Treat. Rep. 67:923, 1983.
410. Bertino, J. R., Carman, M. D., et al.: Gene amplification and altered enzymes as mechanisms for the development drug resistance. Cancer Treat. Rep. 67:901, 1983.
411. Roninson, I. B., Abelson, H. T., et al.: Amplification of specific DNA sequences correlates with multi-drug resistance in Chinese hamster cells. Nature 390:626, 1984.
412. Weinstein, J. N.: Liposomes as drug carriers in cancer therapy. Cancer Treat. Rep. 68:127, 1984.
413. Samulski, T. V., Lee, E. R., et al.: Hyperthermia as a clinical treatment modality. Cancer Treat. Rep. 68:309, 1984.
414. Bleyer, W. A.: Antineoplastic agents. In *Pediatric Pharmacology, Therapeutic Principles in Practice*. Yaffe, S. J. (ed.), New York, Grune & Stratton, 1980, pp. 349–377.
415. Lippman, M. E., and Kasid, A.: Role of receptors in mediating steroid hormone effects in human breast cancer. Cancer Treat. Rep. 68:265, 1984.
416. Ensminger, W. D., and Gyves, J. W.: Regional cancer chemotherapy. Cancer Treat. Rep. 68:101, 1984.
417. Umezawa, H.: Antitumor antibiotics and low molecular weight immunomodifiers of microbial orgin. Cancer Treat. Rep. 68:137, 1984.
418. Oldham, R. K.: Biologicals and biological response modifiers: fourth Modality of Cancer Treatment. Cancer Treat. Rep. 68:221, 1984.
419. Bloch, A.: Induced cell differentiation in cancer therapy. Cancer Treat. Rep. 68:199, 1984.
420. Phillips, T. L., and Wasserman, T. H.: Promise of radiosensitizers and radioprotectors in the treatment of human cancer. Cancer Treat. Rep. 68:291, 1984.
421. Carrasquillo, J. A., Krohn, K. A., et al.: Diagnosis of and therapy for solid tumors with radiolabeled antibodies and immune fragments. Cancer Treat. Rep. 68:317, 1984.
422. Richter, M. P., and Kligerman, M. M.: Particle-beam radiation therapy 1983: evaluation and recommendations. Cancer Treat. Rep. 68:303, 1984.
423. Terry, W. D., and Hodes, R. J.: Immunotherapy. In *Cancer: Principles and Practice of Oncology*, 2nd ed. DeVita, V. T., Jr., Hellman, S., et al. (eds.), Philadelphia, J. B. Lippincott, 1985, pp. 1788–1810.
424. Oldham, R. K., and Smalley, R. V.: Immunotherapy: the old and the new. J. Biol. Resp. Mod. 2:1, 1983.
425. Herr, H. W., Pinsky, C. M., et al.: Effect of intravesical Bacillus Calmette-Guérin (BCG) on carcinoma in situ of the bladder. Cancer 51:1323, 1983.
426. Bast, R. C., Jr., Berek, J. S., et al.: Intraperitoneal immunotherapy of human ovarian carcinoma with *Corynebacterium parvum*. Cancer Res. 43:1395, 1983.
427. Chirigos, M. A., and Mastrangelo, M. J.: Immunorestoration by chemicals. In *Immunological Approaches to Cancer Therapeutics*. Mihich, E. (ed.), New York, John Wiley & Sons, 1982, pp. 191–240.
428. Zatz, M. M., Low, T. L. K., et al.: Role of thymosin and other thymic hormones in T-cell differentiation. In *Biological Responses in Cancer: Progress Toward Potential Applications*, Vol. I. Mihich, E. (ed.), New York, Plenum Publishing Corp., 1982, pp. 219–248.
429. Kirkwood, J. M., and Ernstoff, M. S.: Interferons in the treatment of human cancer. J. Clin. Oncol. 2:336, 1984.
430. Vogelzang, N. J.: Continuous infusion chemotherapy: a critical review. J. Clin. Oncol. 2:1289, 1984.
431. Bernstein, I. D., Nowinski, R. C., et al.: Monoclonal antibodies: prospects for cancer treatment. In *Immunological Approaches to Cancer Therapeutics*. Mihich, E. (ed.), New York, John Wiley & Sons, 1982, pp. 277–297.
432. Nadler, L. M., Stashenko, P., et al.: Serotherapy of a patient with a monoclonal antibody directed against a human lymphoma associated antigen. Cancer Res. 40:3147, 1980.
433. Ritz, J., Pesando, J. M., et al.: Serotherapy of acute lymphoblastic leukemia with monoclonal antibody. Blood 58:141, 1981.
434. Miller, R. A., Maloney, D. G., et al.: Treatment of B-cell lymphoma with monoclonal anti-idiotype antibody. New Engl. J. Med. 306:517, 1982.
435. Sears, H. F., Mattis, J., et al.: Phase-I clinical trial of monoclonal antibody in treatment of gastrointestinal tumors. Lancet 1:762, 1982.
436. Bast, R. C., Jr., Ritz, J., et al.: Elimination of leukemic cells from human bone marrow using monoclonal antibody and complement. Cancer Res. 43:1389, 1983.
437. Ritz, J., Sallan, S. E., et al.: Autologous bone marrow transplantation in CALLA positive ALL following *in vitro* treatment with J-5 monoclonal antibody and complement. Lancet 2:60, 1982.
438. Vittetta, E. S., Krolick, K. A., et al.: Immunotoxins: a new approach to cancer therapy. Science 219:644, 1983.
439. Bernstein, I., Kersey, J., et al.: Immunodiagnosis and immunotherapy of childhood malignancy. Pediatr. Clin. North Am. 32:575, 1985.
440. Kemshead, J. T., Malpas, J. S., et al.: Targeted radiation therapy to neuroblastoma cells using 131-I conjugated to monoclonal antibody UJ13A. Proc. Am. Soc. Clin. Oncol. 3:79, 1984.
441. Ettinger, D. S., Order, S. E., et al.: Phase I–II study of isotopic immunotherapy for primary liver cancer. Cancer Treat. Rep. 66:289, 1982.
442. Sethi, V. S., Jackson, D. V., et al.: Pharmacokinetics of vincristine sulfate in adult cancer patients. Cancer Res. 41:3551, 1981.
443. Weber W., Nagel, G. A., et al.: Vincristine infusion-A phase I study. Cancer Chemother. Pharmacol. 3:49, 1979.
444. Jackson, D. V., Sethi, V. S., et al.: Intravenous vincristine infusion. Cancer 48:2559, 1981.
445. Lazarus, H. M., Herzig, R. H., et al.: Central nervous system toxicity of high-dose systemic cytosine arabinoside. Cancer 48:2577, 1981.
446. Wisch, J. S., Griffin, J. D., et al.: Response of preleukemic syndromes to continuous infusion of low-dose cytarabine. New Engl. J. Med. 309:1599, 1983.
447. Benjamin, R., Legha, S., et al.: Reduction of Adriamycin cardiac toxicity using a prolonged continuous intravenous infusion. Proc. Am. Assoc. Cancer Res. 22:179, 1981.
448. Cox, P. J.: Cyclophosphamide cystitis—identification of acrolein as the causative agent. Biochem. Pharmacol. 28:2045, 1979.
449. Capizzi, R. L.: Schedule-dependent potentiation of the therapeutic activity of methotrexate and high dose Ara-C by asparaginase in the treatment of the acute leukemias. In *Leukemia Research: Advances in Cell Biology and Treatment*. Murphy, S. B., and Gilbert, J. R. (eds.), New York, Elsevier Science, 1983, pp. 145–155.
450. Levin, V. A., Stearns, J., et al.: The effect of phenobarbital pretreatment on the antitumor activity of 1,3-bis(2-chloroethyl)-1-nitrosourea (BCNU), 1-(2-chloroethyl)-3-cyclohexyl-1-nitrosourea (CCNU) and 1-(2-chloroethyl)-3-(2,6-Dioxo-3-piperidyl)-1-nitrosourea (PCNU), and on the plasma pharmacokinetics and biotransformation of BCNU. J. Pharmacol. Exp. Ther. 208:1, 1979.
451. Pratt, C. B., Hayes, A., et al.: Pharmacokinetic evaluation of cisplatin in children with malignant solid tumors: a phase II study. Cancer Treat. Rep. 65:1021, 1981.

II. Radiation Therapy

NANCY J. TARBELL
J. ROBERT CASSADY

Radiation therapy is a highly effective treatment modality for many pediatric hematologic malignancies. In this section, basic physical and biological aspects of radiation therapy will be considered along with details of patient simulation and treatment.

PHYSICAL PRINCIPLES

Clinically useful radiation produces biological effects through the production of ionization within the exposed tissue. The physical characteristics of ionizing radiation depend on the energy of the machine, and these energy differences have important clinical implications. External radiation is divided into superficial, orthovoltage, and megavoltage radiation. Superficial x-ray beams are in the 50 to 140 kilovolt (kV) range, while beams in the 140 to 500 kV range are referred to as orthovoltage. These low energies are advantageous in the treatment of skin tumors because the dose reaches a maximum at the skin level and falls off rapidly below the surface. Megavoltage radiation refers to radiation energies of greater than 500 kV. The properties of radiation absorption above 500 kV include skin sparing, reduced absorption in bone, and a sharper edge to the radiation field. Skin sparing refers to the fact that the maximum dose occurs below the skin and is delivered with megavoltage energy machines in contrast to the historical use of orthovoltage radiation in which the skin received the maximum dose and frequently was the dose-limiting normal tissue (Fig. 32–11).

The dose of radiation deposited at a specific depth relative to the maximum dose increases as the energy increases. For example, the maximum dose occurs at 0.5 cm below the surface for a ^{60}Co machine, while it occurs at 1 and 2 cm with 4 and 8 MV linear accelerators, respectively. Thus, there is an advantage to having more than one energy available to optimize therapy at different depths (Fig. 32–12).

Linear accelerators (4–20 MV) and ^{60}Co machines currently predominate in radiation therapy practice. In the former, electrons are accelerated to very high energies in an electrical device and then this monoenergetic electron beam strikes a target (usually tungsten), which results in the formation of an x-ray beam. ^{60}Co machines contain a radioactive isotope that emits gamma rays. X-rays and gamma rays differ only in the way in which they are produced: gamma rays are spontaneously emitted by radioactive isotopes and have a defined energy of limited range (e.g., ^{60}Co has 2 photon energies—1.17 and 1.33 MV), while x-ray beams contain photons of varying energies up to the peak energy of that beam.

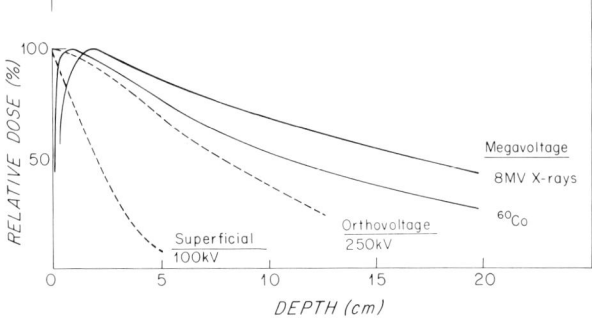

Figure 32–11. Comparison of the relative dose at different depths for different photon energies. Note the skin sparing effect of megavoltage x-rays. The maximum (100 per cent) dose is at 0.5 cm depth for the ^{60}Co and 2 cm for the 8 MV machine; it is at the surface for superficial and orthovoltage x-rays. (Adapted from DeVita, V. T., Jr., and Hellman, S. [eds.]: *Cancer: Principles and Practice of Oncololgy.* Philadelphia, J. B. Lippincott, 1982.)

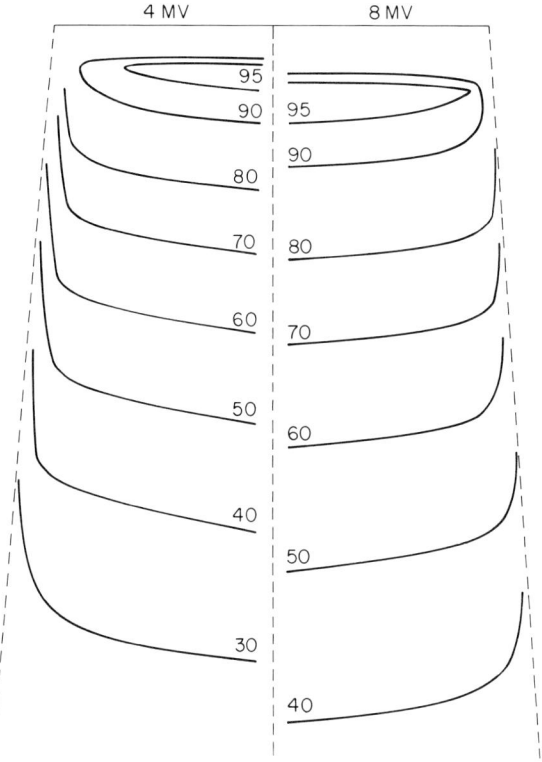

Figure 32–12. Typical single field isodose curves for 4 MV and 8 MV linear accelerators. Numbers represent per cent of maximum dose. Note the greater penetration of the higher energy 8 MV machine as compared to the 4 MV.

Absorption of Radiation by Matter

The amount of energy deposited per unit mass represents the radiation absorbed dose (rad). One rad equals 100 ergs per gm. More recently, the gray has been adopted as the official unit of dose. One joule per kg equals a gray (Gy) and 1 gray equals 100 rads.

Photon (x-ray) and gamma ray beams are absorbed in matter by three distinct means, two of which will be discussed here: the photoelectric process and Compton scattering (1). The relative importance of each process is dependent on the energy of the beam in question. In the photoelectric process, the probability of absorption is proportional to the cube of the atomic number of the absorbing tissue. In Compton scattering; the probability of absorption is independent of the atomic number and proportional to the electron density. Clinically, this difference is of major importance because photons from megavoltage beams are primarily absorbed by the Compton process, while the photoelectric process plays a major role in photons from orthovoltage beams. The dependence of the photoelectric process on the atomic number of the absorber permits the clear delineation of bone in diagnostic x-rays. However, the increased absorption leads to unacceptably high radiation doses in bone when utilized in therapy. Orthovoltage machines, which were used for therapy of deep-seated tumors in the past, did cause a significantly greater dose to bone and a consequent increase in bony complications as compared with today's megavoltage equipment.

Particulate Radiation

A number of charged and uncharged particles have been found to be clinically useful, including neutrons, protons, negative Pi mesons, alpha particles, and electrons. Electrons have the greatest clinical applicability. Unlike high-energy photons, the dose to the skin increases with increasing electron energy and thus electrons have little skin sparing. Electrons also have a relatively sharp fall-off compared with photons and so are useful in treating superficial tumors such as cutaneous lymphomas when a sharp fall-off in dose is desirable. For example, protracted disease-free survival has followed total skin electron therapy in early stage patients with mycosis fungoides (2). Figure 32–13 shows the depth dose characteristics of electrons.

RADIATION BIOLOGY

Mechanisms and Site of Action of Radiation Damage

Experiments using short-range particle beams or the incorporation of radioactive isotopes into DNA have demonstrated that DNA is the critical

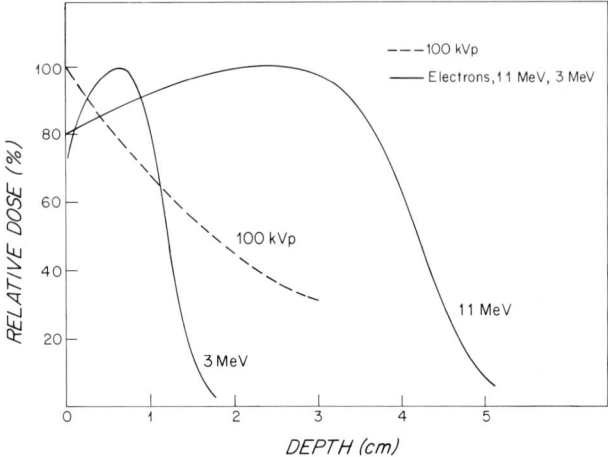

Figure 32–13. Comparison of relative dose at different depths for electrons and orthovoltage x-rays. Note the sharp fall off in dose for the 3 MeV electrons compared to the 11 MeV electrons or the 100 Kv orthovoltage x-rays.

target for radiation inactivation (3). Cellular DNA can be affected in two ways: the DNA molecule may be directly ionized, or it may be altered by ionization of adjacent molecules, which create free radicals. Formation of free radicals constitutes the primary way in which radiation affects the cell, and the most important of these is the hydroxyl radical. The ability of molecular oxygen to increase radiation damage is thought to result from oxygen fixation of the free radicals, which then damage the DNA.

Methods of Cell Killing by Irradiation

Radiation can kill cells by two principal mechanisms: interphase death and mitotic death. With the former, cells fail to divide prior to undergoing lysis. Although this is an uncommon form of cell death, it is the major mechanism for lymphocytes and some spermatocytes. With mitotic death, radiation has damaged the cell's DNA sufficiently to preclude indefinite replication. Although a cell may undergo one or more mitoses, the progeny of division can no longer carry on essential cell functions and ultimately cell death occurs (3). This is the predominant mechanism by which radiation kills cells. Clinically, then, an attempt at cell division must occur in order for cells to manifest the damage imparted by radiation (3,4).

Cell Survival Curve Characteristics

In 1956, Puck and Marcus (3) developed a cell culture technique that has proven invaluable in studying cellular effects of radiation. Clonogenic cells can be grown in vitro and measured by counting colonies. Cells incapable of indefinite replication will fail to form colonies and are thus considered dead. This assay made quantitation of cell killing by a variety of agents possible. A typical radiation cell survival curve is shown in Figure 32–14. The surviving fraction is plotted on a logarithmic scale with the dose of radiation on a linear scale. The resulting cell survival curve has two distinct regions. In the initial "shoulder" portion of the curve, the fraction of cells killed increases slightly with increasing radiation dose. Killing then becomes exponential, which means that a given dose increment kills a constant fraction of cells. The slope of the exponential portion of the survival curve is called the D_0, which indicates the inherent radiosensitivity of the cell. The smaller the D_0, the more sensitive the cells are to radiation. This is in contrast to radioresponsiveness, which refers only to the rate of disappearance of a tumor after irradiation and has no correlation with the innate sensitivity of the cells. The D_0 for mammalian cells in vitro generally falls between 100 and 200 cGy. This relatively narrow range of values for widely varying types of cells is striking.

The fact that the initial portion of the curve is nonexponential is believed to be due to the capacity of most mammalian cells to repair nonlethal radiation injury. Saturation of the repair capability is thought to occur at the point where killing becomes exponential. A quantitative measure of sublethal repair capability is given by the D_9, the quasi-threshold dose (Fig. 32–14).

Repair

A decrease in cell death is noted in most classes of cells when a given dose of irradiation is divided into several fractions rather than given in one large fraction. This decreased lethality appears to be related to the ability of most cells to repair some portion of the radiation damage before it

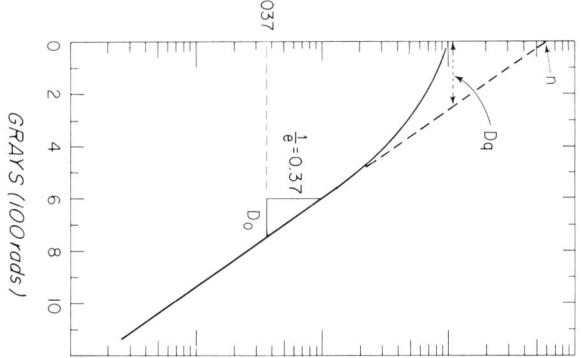

Figure 32–14. Idealized radiation cell survival curve. The fraction of surviving cells is plotted on a logarithmic scale against dose on a linear scale. The D_0 is the dose necessary to reduce the surviving fraction to 0.37 or e^{-1}. The smaller the D_0 the more sensitive the cells are to radiation. The Dq is the quasi-threshold dose and is a quantitative measure of the sublethal repair capability. (Modified from Hall, E. J.: *Radiology for the Radiologist*, 2nd ed. Hagerstown, Md., Harper & Row, 1978.)

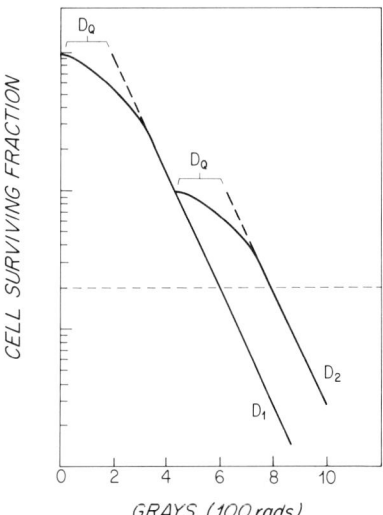

Figure 32–15. Return of the shoulder with two split doses of irradiation. This quantity $D_2-D_1=Dq$ is a reflection of the repair of sublethal damage. (Modified from Hall, E. J.: *Radiology for the Radiotherapist*, 2nd ed. Hagerstown, Md., Harper & Row, 1978.)

proves lethal. Two types of damage repair have been described. The first, reported initially by Elkind and Sutton (5), has been termed sublethal damage repair. If a dose of radiation is administered in a single fraction and compared with two or more equally divided fractions, a significant increase in total dose will be required for equal lethality in the fractionated group. This sublethal damage repair is shown graphically in Figure 32–15. The magnitude of such repair is related to the size of the shoulder of the cell survival curve. Two dose experiments with graded time intervals between the fractions reveal that such repair is relatively rapid and is virtually complete after 3 hours.

Almost all human cells show sublethal repair, with the exceptions of certain germ cells and most lymphocytes. A number of factors can affect the degree of sublethal damage repair, including severe hypoxia or the use of certain chemotherapeutic agents.

The other type of radiation-induced damage repair is potentially lethal damage repair (PLDR). Modification of the postirradiation conditions of cultured cells can allow repair and enhance cell survival. In cultured human tumor cells, PLDR may correlate with the clinical responsiveness of the tumor to radiation. Weichselbaum and colleagues (6, 7) have shown that tumors that appear resistant to radiation have a greater capacity for PLDR than do more radiosensitive tumors.

Cell Cycle Variations in Radiation Sensitivity

Mitotic division has four phases: mitosis (m), gap (G_1), synthesis (S), and gap 2 (G_2). By means

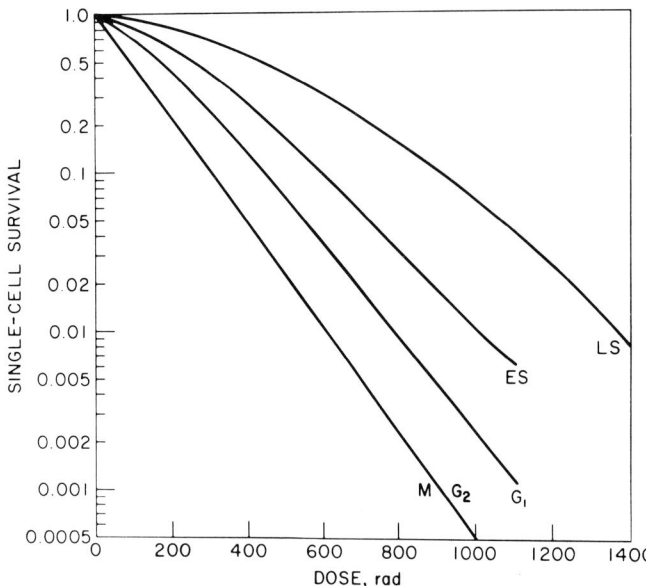

Figure 32–16. Single-cell survival curves of cells irradiated in various stages of the cell cycle. Note maximum sensitivity in G_2 and M (mitosis) and maximum resistance in late S (LS). G_1 and early S (ES) are intermediate in sensitivity. (From Sinclair, W. K., and Morton, R. A.: X-ray sensitivity during the cell generation cycle of cultured Chinese hamster cells. Radiat. Res. 33:620, 1968.)

of synchronization techniques, the radiation sensitivity of cells in each of these phases has been analyzed (8, 9). In general, cells in mitosis are most sensitive, whereas cells in the late synthetic phase are most resistant to irradiation (8) (Fig. 32–16).

The Oxygen Effect

Irradiation is much more lethal in the presence of molecular oxygen and under conditions of severe hypoxia (10–14). The mechanism of the oxygen effect is not definitely established; however, it is generally felt that oxygen interacts with the free radicals formed shortly after irradiation. These important free radicals have a short half-life and they may either return to an innocuous state or remain as highly reactive molecules. Oxygen favors the latter, while sulfhydryl compounds appear to favor the former.

The importance of the oxygen effect was recognized by Thomlinson and Gray when they showed that human tumors frequently had anoxic regions (15). They found that the diffusion capacity of oxygen limits oxygen transfer from vessels to a distance of approximately 100 to 150 μ. Cells closer to the vessel were sufficiently oxygenated, while cells beyond 160 μ were anoxic; cells in the intermediate range showed varying degrees of hypoxia and associated radioresistance (2, 14, 15). After a single dose of radiation, the surviving tumor cells are predominantly the original hypoxic ones. However, after a period of time the proportion of hypoxic cells returns to the preradiation level. This phenomenon of hypoxic cells becoming oxygenated after doses of radiation has been termed reoxygenation (16–18).

Results of several clinical studies support the importance of the oxygen effect. Henk and co-workers (19, 20) conducted a randomized trial in which patients with head and neck cancer were treated with hyperbaric oxygen plus irradiation or with irradiation under normal atmospheric conditions. The hyperbaric oxygen group showed improved local control and survival. Despite these apparent advantages the technique is cumbersome and potentially hazardous. Also, it requires a chamber, which makes precise, multidirectional radiation treatment nearly impossible. Because of these difficulties, a class of agents, best characterized by the nitroimidazole compounds, has been developed. These agents are called hypoxic cell sensitizers because they sensitize hypoxic cells to the effects of radiation but do not affect well-oxygenated cells. Clinical trials of first or second generation compounds have been disappointing; however, dose schedules and drug concentrations were limited by acute gastrointestinal morbidity and neurotoxicity. Pharmacological development of agents with improved activity but less toxicity appears quite possible (21–23).

Radiation Protectors

Sulfhydryl compounds and their thiophosphate derivatives are radioprotectors and are thought to act as free-radical scavengers, thereby minimizing the indirect effects of photon irradiation (24–26). These compounds appear to protect normal tissues to a greater extent than tumors, thereby permitting a differential effect and an improved therapeutic ratio. This preferential protection of normal tissues may occur for several reasons, including (1) deficient vascularity and/or blood flow, which limits the concentration of the drug in the tumor; (2) limited absorption of the drug at the level of the tumor cell membrane; and (3) the existence of hypoxic cells within the tumor (26).

Radiation Interactions with Chemotherapeutic Agents

A number of chemical substances will alter the radiation response of a cell. The effect may be additive, as with most alkylating agents and antimetabolites, or it may be synergistic, as with the antibiotic dactinomycin (27). Doxorubicin and dactinomycin markedly reduce the shoulder region of the radiation cell survival curve (28). Because dactinomycin also steepens the slope of the exponential portion of the cell survival curve and potentiates the radiation effect, it is felt to be a true radiation sensitizer.

An interesting clinical phenomenon known as "recall" has been demonstrated with combinations of radiation and actinomycin-D. Even with wide time intervals between the use of radiation and actinomycin, a brisk reaction can be seen with striking recurrence of the prior radiation reaction (27, 28). Radiation may also alter drug metabolism, thereby increasing the combined toxicity. This has been shown in children with right-sided Wilms' tumor where hepatic irradiation combined with actinomycin and vincristine has resulted in veno-occlusive disease. In addition, the neurotoxicity of vincristine is enhanced, presumably because of delayed metabolism of the drug by the liver (29).

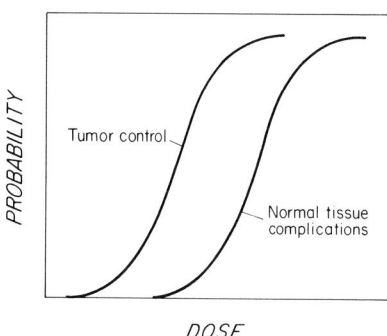

Figure 32–18. Idealized sigmoid curves depicting the probability of tumor control compared to the probability of normal tissue complications. The therapeutic ratio refers to the balance between these curves. Compare with Figure 32–1.

Dose-Rate Effect

The dose rate is a major factor in determining the biological effect of a given absorbed dose of radiation. As the dose rate is reduced, the slope of the survival curve becomes less steep while the extrapolation number tends toward unity. This is illustrated in Figure 32–17. This dose-rate effect is primarily due to repair of sublethal damage and is most dramatic between 1 and 100 cGy per min (4). There is tremendous variation in the magnitude of the dose-rate effect. For example, normal bone marrow stem cells generally demonstrate little dose-rate effect and are characterized by a small shoulder (little repair capacity). This is in contrast to the gastrointestinal (GI) tract, which has a broad shoulder and a correspondingly large dose-rate effect (30, 31). It is this differential sensitivity in repair capacity between GI and bone marrow stem cells that permits a differential effect of total body irradiation for bone marrow transplantation. GI stem cells have been shown to have a striking capacity for sublethal repair (Fig. 32–18) (31–33), whereas normal bone marrow stem cells have minimal sublethal repair capacity (33).

Pulmonary alveolar cells also demonstrate a significant repair capacity, and the incidence of pneumonitis at whole body doses of 900 to 1000 cGy decreases significantly as the dose rate decreases to the 2 to 5 cGy per min level (34). Total body irradiation (TBI) prior to bone marrow transplantation serves two primary purposes: abrogation of host bone marrow stem cells, thereby permitting engraftment and treatment of residual malignant cells residing within the host. The optimum total dose or technique to achieve these two objectives is not known. In his pioneering work, Thomas used cyclophosphamide along with a single fraction of 900 to 1000 cGy delivered at approximately 5 cGy per min using opposing ^{60}Co sources (35). Although this regimen resulted in some cured patients, most died of complications or recurrence

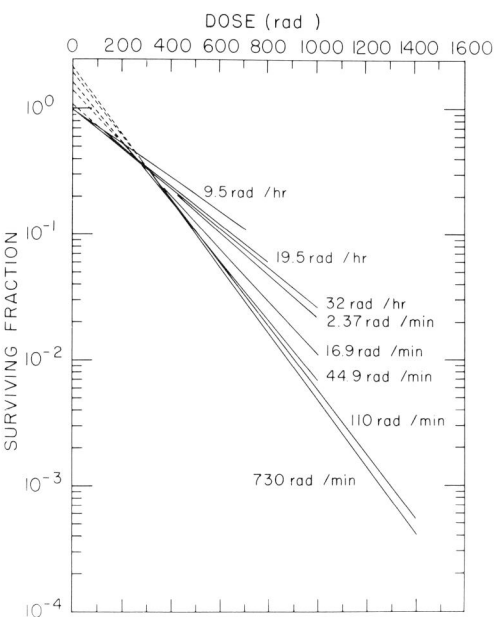

Figure 32–17. Response of irradiated mouse jejunal crypt cells to different dose rates. Note that as the dose rate decreases, the slope becomes less steep. There is a large dose-rate effect. (From Hall, E. J.: *Radiobiology for the Radiologist*, 2nd ed. Hagerstown, Md., Harper & Row, 1978.)

of leukemia. Researchers at the Fred Hutchinson Cancer Research Center in Seattle then designed the only prospective randomized clinical study comparing single-dose TBI with a fractionated schedule (38). Patients with acute nonlymphoblastic leukemia were randomized to receive either 1000 cGy in a single fraction or 1200 cGy given in 200-cGy fractions over 6 days. Survival was significantly better in the fractionated group ($p = 0.05$) with a follow-up of 4 to 27 months. The incidence of leukemic deaths was identical; the improved survival was due to a decrease in deaths from complications. This study suggests that 1200 cGy given over 6 days may be equivalent to 1000 cGy in a single dose for leukemic cell kill but may allow more repair of dose-limiting normal tissues such as the lung. Canadian investigators are using a relatively high dose rate (50 cGy per min) but with a lower total dose, giving a single fraction of 500 cGy (36). Various combinations of fractionated and low dose-rate techniques are currently being used (36–38), and the optimal schedule is still uncertain.

CLINICAL PRINCIPLES

Radiation is a highly active antitumor agent. Virtually all tumors will respond favorably to irradiation and a substantial number will be permanently controlled. For this reason, criteria such as "complete response" or "partial response" have limited value, and permanent or long-term local control is a better gauge of treatment efficacy.

The probability of local tumor control or, conversely, normal tissue complications usually follows a steep sigmoid curve with respect to radiation dose. This relationship is best shown graphically (Fig. 32–18). When the normal tissue complication curve lies far to the right of the tumor control curve, most patients can expect a high probability of uncomplicated control. This balance between tumor control and normal tissue complications is referred to as the therapeutic ratio.

The optimal balance between control and complications varies in different clinical settings, depending on the consequences of local relapse or the complications engendered. When the complication results in severe morbidity (e.g., radiation myelitis), then it must be avoided even at the price of an increased rate of tumor relapse. However, if patients who develop local tumor failure following irradiation can not be salvaged and normal tissue complications can be managed by medical or surgical means (e.g., small bowel obstruction), then a significant rate of complications is a reasonable price for a higher proportion of cured patients. For example, in the treatment of early stage Hodgkin's disease, one can use radiation alone with decreased toxicity. Chemotherapy can then be reserved for salvage. In advanced stage Hodgkin's disease, irradiation of smaller volumes with planned chemotherapy produces an equivalent rate of tumor control with less morbidity than the previously used wide-field irradiation.

Parameters that can be varied during a course of treatment include the volume irradiated, the total dose, the fraction size, and the dose rate to be used at each treatment session. Also, the time interval between each radiation fraction and the overall time between initiation and completion of radiation can vary. Each of these features has a significant bearing on both tumor control probability and normal tissue complications. In general, as treatment volumes increase, the total dose must decrease in order to maintain a given level of complications. Similarly, an increase in radiation fraction size will also result in an increase in late complications if the total dose and/or volume is not reduced. The total dose required for tumor control is largely dependent on the number of tumor cells that are present (i.e., tumor volume).

Generally, these principles of total dose and radiation schedule are not age related. No data are available to justify a variation in radiation dose based on age. The one exception appears to be neuroblastoma in the child less than 12 months old, because the biology of the disease appears to be different than in older children. Modifications of total dose may, however, be justified by age-related toxicity. For example, dose reductions in CNS prophylaxis for acute lymphoblastic leukemia have been made from 2400 cGy to 2000 or 1500 gGy for children less than 24 months of age. This is because myelinization is incomplete and functional impairment in this age group is of great concern. In this case, lower control rates may be justified by the decrease in complications.

Complications

Acute reactions develop as a consequence of radiation damage to proliferating cell renewal systems and are, therefore, most noticeable in tissues with rapid turnover. The skin, bone marrow, and gastrointestinal mucosa are examples of tissues that require continued cellular proliferation for their function and generally show an early acute reaction to irradiation.

In contrast to acute reactions, the late effects of radiation are observed from months to years following irradiation. Although the exact mechanism is unknown, late radiation complications have been thought to be related to either vascular endothelial damage or damage to parenchymal cells of the irradiated organ (39). Each organ appears to have a unique radiation tolerance, and thus vascular injury may not entirely explain the long-term effects of radiation. The late complications of radiation therapy are often the most critical dose- and volume-limiting considerations in clinical practice.

Clinically, late effects appear to be dependent primarily upon the total dose of radiation and the size of the radiation fractions. When the total dose or fraction size is increased but the time protracted to minimize acute effects, unacceptable late complications can ensue. Acute reactions can be misleading and are not a reliable guide to late effects.

In the child, irradiation prior to full development of various tissues can result in failure of normal development. This is most evident in organs such as bone where failure of normal development can be manifested by short stature or, if treatment was unilateral, by varying degrees of asymmetry. The severity of growth retardation is related primarily to the age at treatment, the dose, and the site. Doses of greater than 2000 cGy are felt to have a significant effect on bony growth (40), and the younger the patient, the greater the effect since there is more growth remaining. For example, one epiphysis is often treated in Ewing's sarcoma, and the amount of asymmetry and resulting functional consequences will depend largely on the patient's age. The spine is frequently treated in many pediatric tumors. In patients with Hodgkin's disease a large segment of spine is included in the mantle and para-aortic fields. The whole craniospinal axis is treated in brain tumors with the potential to seed, such as medulloblastoma, or in cases of central nervous system relapse in leukemia. With such treatment the growth retardation is manifested primarily as a reduction in sitting height. A variety of other tissues may not develop fully, such as the brain or, less commonly, the bowel or an artery. Subtle changes include mild learning disabilities and minor growth changes.

In general, tolerance to the acute and subacute effects of irradiation is greater in pediatric patients, but children are susceptible to a wider range and number of late complications. Pediatric patients are at greater risk for treatment-associated malignancies, especially in certain sites such as the thyroid gland.

These late effects have only been appreciated in recent years with the improvement in survival rates in many pediatric malignancies. Late effects may include growth abnormalities, endocrine imbalances, and neuropsychological sequelae. Second malignancies, particularly in the irradiated site, are also being reported with increasing frequency. The actual risk of second malignancies appears to be related to intensity of treatment as well as genetic factors (43–44). However, it now appears that the risk of leukemia is associated primarily with the use of chemotherapy and is rare after radiation therapy alone (41, 42). The actuarial risk of leukemogenesis may approach 4 per cent at 7 years in adult patients treated with intensive chemotherapy with or without radiation.

TREATMENT PLANNING PRINCIPLES

The "patterns of care" study (43) has shown considerable variability in results of treatment, depending on the nature of the institution, the disease being treated, and the experience of the radiation therapists. The excellent treatment results in patients with early stage Hodgkin's disease (with a 10-year relapse-free survival rate of 79 per cent and overall survival rate of 95 per cent in stage IA-IIB disease treated with radiation therapy alone with MOPP reserved for relapse) (46) illustrate the importance of adherence to the general principles of radiation dose and technique discussed in this chapter. Similar variability both in reproducibility of treatment parameters and results has been demonstrated in CNS prophylaxis in children with acute lymphoblastic leukemia. These studies demonstrate that radiation therapy, like surgery, is a technically demanding treatment mode in which precision and accuracy ultimately translate into improved results. Dose-response curves show the potential importance of seemingly small doses of irradiation in markedly affecting tumor control rates. Failure to include a portion of the tumor in the desired high-dose treatment volume even for a small fraction of the total treatments can have major ramifications in ultimate treatment results.

For optimal results, treatment planning is essential. Precise localization of the tumor volume, utilizing both physical examination and diagnostic x-ray procedures, is necessary to insure that the tumor receives the maximum dose relative to the normal tissues. This requires knowledge of the natural history of the tumor plus an understanding of the anatomical considerations and usual routes of local or regional spread. Special attention must be given to symmetry in treatment planning for the pediatric group due to the effects of radiation on growth. In Wilms' tumor, for example, scoliosis can result when only the right or left half of the spine is included in the renal fossa field.

Prior to tumor localization, the patient is placed in a comfortable, reproducible treatment position. Immobilization can be difficult in children, especially those younger than 2½ years of age, and deep sedation or daily anesthesia may be required. Ketamine is generally used because it is short acting, offers optimal immobilization, and causes less respiratory depression than alternative agents. Immobilization devices are very important for daily reproducibility. Head straps and bite blocks are used for cancers in the head and neck region;

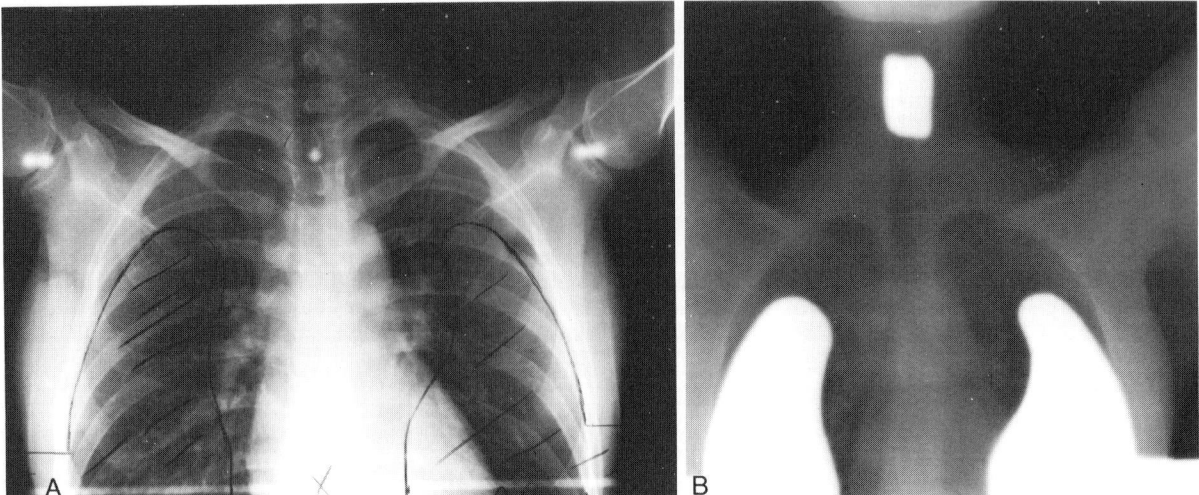

Figure 32–19. *A*, Simulator films for a patient with Hodgkin's disease. Mantle field with outline for shielding blocks. *B*, Portal films to verify field and accurate placement of blocks.

molds and body casts are frequently utilized in the treatment of extremity lesions. Multiple wall- and machine-mounted lasers allow for accurate patient positioning. Critical field margins can be permanently marked with small pin-point "tattoos," which further augment reproducibility of the patient's position.

Following immobilization of the patient, the tumor is localized by a variety of radiographic and physical methods that may include the placement of radiopaque seeds in the tumor or the use of various oral or intravenous contrast media. Computerized tomography (CT) scans are extremely valuable for radiotherapy tumor localization, in part because they provide information in the transverse plane, in which most radiation treatment planning is performed. The use of dedicated CT scanners for radiotherapy treatment planning is an important advance. Radiation therapy planning is usually carried out on a simulator, which allows duplication of the geometry of the treatment but utilizes diagnostic quality radiographs and has fluoroscopic capabilities. Simulation is essential for sophisticated treatment planning.

Once localization is complete, alternative treatment techniques are considered. The selection of the appropriate treatment plan is generally made by the clinician in consultation with the radiologic physicist and dosimetrist. This team decides on the best beam distribution, the homogeneity within the target volume, and methods to minimize the dose distribution in the transit normal tissues.

Various techniques are used to maximize doses in the tumor region, including multiple ports, such as a four-field box technique for the pelvis, the use of fields at right angles to each other, and the use of multiple arcs and 360° rotations of the machine about the target volume. Beam modifiers are selected that help create dose homogeneity, and individual blocks are drawn by the physician on the simulator films to insure protection of normal tissues from unnecessary irradiation. Wedges or tissue compensators can be designed that absorb the beam differentially and lead to a more even dose distribution to compensate for variations in patient contour.

Prior to actual treatment, confirmation of the precise reproducibility of the desired treatment fields is obtained by means of a "port" or verification film, which is a radiograph of the treatment volume obtained using x-rays from the treatment machine. This port film is then compared with the previously obtained diagnostic quality simulator film. These verification films are obtained for each treatment field and are repeated at frequent intervals to insure quality control. Figure 32–19 shows the simulator and port films for a patient who is to receive mantle irradiation for Hodgkin's disease. This illustrates the precision and accuracy necessary for optimal treatment with minimal morbidity.

References to Part II (Radiation Therapy)

1. Johns, H. E., and Cunningham, J. R.: *Physics of Radiology*. Springfield, Ill., Charles C Thomas, 1969.
2. Hoppe, R. T., Cox, R. S., et al.: Electron beam therapy for mycosis fungoides: The Stanford University experience. Cancer Treat. Rep. *63*(4):691, 1979.
3. Puck, T. T., and Marcus, P. I.: Action of x-rays on mammalian cells. J. Exp. Med. *103*:653, 1956.
4. Hall, E. J.: *Radiobiology for the Radiologist*, 2nd ed. Hagerstown, Md., Harper and Row, 1978.
5. Elkind, M. M., and Sutton, H.: Radiation response of mammalian cells grown in culture. 1. Repair of x-ray damage in surviving Chinese hamster cells. Radiat. Res. *13*:556, 1960.
6. Weichselbaum, R. R., Nove, J., et al.: X-ray sensitivity of human tumor cells *in vitro*. Int. J. Radiat. Oncol. Biol. Phys. *6*:437, 1980.

7. Weichselbaum, R. R., Little, J. B., et al.: Response of human osteosarcoma *in vitro* to x-irradiation: Evidence for unusual cellular repair activity. Int. J. Radiat. Biol. *31*:295, 1977.
8. Sinclair, W. K.: Cyclic x-ray responses in mammalian cells *in vitro*. Radiat. Res. *33*:620, 1968.
9. Terishima, R., and Tolmach, L. J.: X-ray sensitivity and DNA synthesis in synchronous population of HeLa cells. Science *140*:490, 1963.
10. Mottram, J. C.: Factors of importance in radiosensitivity of tumors. Br. J. Radiol. *9*:606, 1936.
11. Read, J.: The effect of ionizing radiation on the broad beam root: The dependence of the x-ray sensitivity on dissolved oxygen. Br. J. Radiol. *25*:89, 1952.
12. Gray L. H., Conger A. D., et al.: The concentration of oxygen dissolved in tissues at the time of irradiation as a factor in radiotherapy. Br. J. Radiol. *26*:638, 1953.
13. Crabtree, H. G., and Kramer, W.: Action of radium on cancer cells. Some factors affecting susceptibility of cancer cells to radium. Proc. R. Soc. Lond. (Biol.) *113*:238, 1933.
14. Wright, E. A., and Howard-Flanders, P.: The influence of oxygen on the radiosensitivity of mammalian tissues. Acta Radiol. *48*:26, 1957.
15. Thomlinson, R. H., and Gray, L. H.: The histologic structure of some human lung cancer and possible implications for radiotherapy. Br. J. Cancer *9*:539, 1955.
16. Van Putten, L. M.: Tumor reoxygenation during fractionated radiotherapy. Studies with a transplantable osteosarcoma. Euro. J. Cancer *4*:173, 1968.
17. Kallman, R. F.: The phenomenon of reoxygenation and its implications for fractionated radiotherapy. Radiol. *105*:135, 1972.
18. Thomlinson, R. H.: Reoxygenation as a function of tumor size and histopathological type. In *Proceedings of the Carmel Conference on Time/Dose Relationships and Radiation Biology as Applied to Radiotherapy*. BNL Report 50203 C-57, 1969.
19. Henk, J. M., and Kindler, P. B.: Radiotherapy and head and neck cancer: Final report of the first clinical trial. Lancet *2*:101, 1977.
20. Henk, J., and Smith, C. W.: Radiotherapy and head and neck cancer: Interim report of second clinical trial. Lancet *2*:104, 1977.
21. Brown, J. M., and Yu, N. Y.: Radiosensitization of hypoxic cells in vivo by SR-2508 at low radiation doses: a preliminary report. Int. J. Radiat. Oncol. Biol. Phys. *10*:1207, 1984.
22. Coleman, N. C.: Hypoxic cell radiosensitizers: expectations and progress in drug development. Int. J. Radiat. Oncol. Biol. Phys. *11*:223, 1985.
23. Brown, J. M., Yu, N. Y., et al.: SR-2508: 4-nitroimidazole amide which should be superior to a misonidazole as a radiosensitizer for clinical use. Int. J. Radiat. Oncol. Biol. Phys. *7*:695, 1981.
24. Yuhas, J. M.: Protective drugs in cancer therapy: Optimal clinical testing and future directions. Int. J. Radiat. Oncol. Biol. Phys. *8*:513, 1982.
25. Yuhas, J. M., Davis, M. E., et al.: Circumvention of the tumor membrane barrier to WR-2721 absorption by reduction of drug hydrophilicity. Int. J. Radiat. Oncol. Biol. Phys. *8*:519, 1982.
26. Harris, J. W., and Phillips, T. L.: Radiobiological and chemical studies of thiophosphate compounds related to cysteamine. Radiat. Res. *46*:362, 1971.
27. D'Angio, G. J.: Clinical and biologic studies of actinomycin D and roentgen irradiation. Am. J. Roent. *87*:106, 1962.
28. Elkind, M. M., Whitmore, G. F., et al.: Actinomycin-D: Suppression of recovery in x-irradiated mammalian cells. Science *143*:1454, 1964.
29. Cassady, J. R., Carabell, S., et al.: Chemotherapy irradiation related hepatic dysfunction in patients with Wilms' tumor. Front. Rad. Ther. Onc. *13*:147, Basel, Kargen 1979.
30. Cassady, J. R., Order, S., et al.: Modification of gastrointestinal symptoms following irradiation by low dose rate technique. Int. J. Radiat. Oncol. Biol. Phys. *1*:15, 1976.
31. Withers, H. R., Mason, K., et al.: Response of mouse intestine to neutrons and gamma rays in relation to dose fractionation and division cycle. Cancer *34*:39, 1974.
32. Fu, K., and Phillips, T. L.: Tumor and normal tissue response to irradiation *in vivo*: Variation with decreasing dose rates. Radiol. *114*:709, 1975.
33. McCulloch, E. A., and Till, J. E.: The sensitivity of cells from mouse bone marrow to gamma radiation *in vitro* and *in vivo*. Radiat. Res. *16*:822, 1962.
34. Depledge, M. H., and Barrett, A.: Dose rate dependence of lung damage after TBI in mice. Int. J. Radiat. Biol. *41*:325, 1982.
35. Thomas, E. D., Storb, R., et al.: Total body irradiation in preparation for marrow engraftment. Transplant. Proc. *8*:591, 1976.
36. Rider, W., and Van Dyk, J.: In *Total and Partial Body Irradiation in Radiation Therapy Planning*. Bleehen, N. M., Glatstein, E., et al. (eds.), New York, Marcel Dekker, pp. 559–594.
37. Shank, B., Chu, F. C. H., et al.: Hyperfractionated total body irradiation for bone marrow transplantation: Results in seventy leukemia patients with allogeneic transplants. Int. J. Radiat. Oncol. Biol. Phys. *9(11)*:1607, 1983.
38. Thomas, E. D., Clift, R. A., et al.: Marrow transplantation for acute non-lymphoblastic leukemia in first remission using fractionated or single dose irradiation. Int. J. Radiat. Oncol. Biol. Phys. *8*:817, 1982.
39. Withers, H. R., Peters, L. J., et al.: The pathobiology of late effects of radiation. In *Radiation Biology in Cancer Research*. Meyn, R. E., and Withers, H. E. (eds.), New York, Raven Press, 1980, pp. 439–448.
40. Neuhauser, E. B. D., Wittenborg, M. H., et al.: Irradiation effects of roentgen therapy on the growing spine. Radiol. *59*:637, 1952.
41. Loeffler, J. S., Tarbell, N. J., et al.: Primary lymphoma of bone in children: analysis of treatment results with APO and local radiation therapy. J. Clin. Oncol. *4*:496, 1986.
42. Coltman, C. A., and Dixon, D. O.: Second malignancies complicating Hodgkin's disease: A Southwest Oncology Group 10-year following. Cancer Treat. Rep. *66*:1023, 1982.
43. Meadows, A., Strong, L., et al.: Bone sacromas as a second malignant neoplasm in children: influence of radiation and genetic predisposition. Cancer *46*:2603, 1980.
44. Meadows, A. T., Baum, E., et al.: Second malignant neoplasms in children: an update from the late effects study group. J. Clin. Oncol. *3*:532, 1985.
45. Kinzie, J. J., Hanks, G. E., et al.: Patterns of care study: Hodgkin's disease relapse rates and adequacy of portals. Cancer *52(12)*:2223, 1983.
46. Leslie, N. T., Mauch, P., et al.: Stage IA-IIB supradiaphragmatic Hodgkin's disease: Long term survival and recurrence relapse frequency. Cancer *55*:2072, 1985.

ONCOLOGY

CHAPTER 33
Childhood Acute Leukemia

STEPHEN E. SALLAN
HOWARD J. WEINSTEIN

INTRODUCTION 1028
CLASSIFICATION 1028
  Morphologic and Cytochemical Classification
PATHOPHYSIOLOGY 1030
  Hematopoietic and Lymphoid Progenitors and Precursors
  The Clonal Expansion Theory
  Cellular Heterogeneity
    Surface Markers
    Cytoplasmic Markers
  Chromosomes and Leukemia
CLINICAL MANIFESTATIONS 1035
  Characteristic Findings at Diagnosis
  The Protean Nature of Leukemia
  Extramedullary Leukemia
    Central Nervous System Manifestations
    Genitourinary Tract Manifestations
    Bone and Joint Manifestations
    Gastrointestinal Manifestations
    Oral Manifestations
    Ocular Manifestations
    Cardiac Manifestations
    Pulmonary Manifestations
    Miscellaneous Manifestations
LABORATORY FINDINGS 1040
DIAGNOSIS AND DIFFERENTIAL DIAGNOSIS 1040
TREATMENT 1041
  General Treatment
    The First Day
    The First Month
  Acute Lymphoblastic Leukemia (ALL)
    Remission Induction
    CNS Prophylaxis
    Other Extramedullary "Prophylaxis"
    Treatment in Remission
    Cessation of Therapy
    Relapsed ALL
    Prognosis
  Acute Myelogenous Leukemia (AML)
    Remission Induction
    CNS Prophylaxis
    Continuation Therapy
    Bone Marrow Transplantation
    Prognosis
  Interpretation of Results of Clinical Trials
  Supportive Care
    Hemorrhage
    Infection
  Consequences of Survival

CONGENITAL LEUKEMIA 1052
MANAGEMENT OF THE EMOTIONAL ASPECTS OF
  LEUKEMIA 1053
  The Disease
  The Child
  The Family
  The Staff
  Death, Grief, and Bereavement

INTRODUCTION

The childhood acute leukemias are rare diseases that collectively represent about 35 per cent of all childhood malignancies. Approximately 2500 new cases occur annually in the United States. Since the 1960's, the prognosis for children with acute leukemia has improved dramatically. Diseases that were uniformly fatal are now nearly universally treatable, and many patients have prolonged disease-free survival.

In this chapter, we will review the childhood acute leukemias with respect to classification, pathophysiology, clinical presentation, laboratory findings, differential diagnosis, treatment strategies, and prognosis. Etiology and epidemiologic considerations, including the incidence, prevalence, and life span of afflicted individuals, have been discussed in Chapter 30. Discussion of the cytogenetic aspects of the leukemias appears in Chapter 43, and molecular genetics and oncogenes are considered in Chapter 31. Details concerning the various chemotherapeutic agents are provided in Chapter 32, and the chronic leukemias and myeloproliferative disorders are discussed in Chapter 34.

CLASSIFICATION

The childhood leukemias can be classified as acute, chronic, and congenital. The terms "acute" and "chronic" originally referred to the relative duration of the natural course of the different types of leukemias prior to the advent of successful treatment modalities. However, "acute leukemia" now refers to those diseases characterized by a predominance of immature hematopoietic or lymphoid precursors, whereas "chronic leukemia" refers to those conditions characterized by expansion of mature marrow elements. "Congenital leukemia" describes those diseases diagnosed within the first 4 weeks of life. "Preleukemia" refers to the "smoldering" conditions characterized by unexplained anemia, neutropenia, and/or thrombocytopenia with dysmorphic maturation of hematopoietic elements that may evolve into frank acute leukemia.

The leukemias are also classified morphologically according to the predominant cell lines involved. This classification broadly divides the acute leukemias into lymphoblastic and myelogenous (nonlymphoblastic) forms and the chronic leukemias into lymphocytic and myelogenous forms. Approximately 80 per cent of the acute leukemias in children are lymphoblastic (ALL), 15 per cent are myelogenous (AML), and the remainder are difficult to characterize as either ALL or AML and are therefore classified as undifferentiated (AUL). Advances in identifying lineage-related cell surface antigens and the application of molecular genetics have resulted in a gradual diminution of the number of leukemias that now are classified as AUL. Further subclassification of ALL and AML will be discussed in later sections of this chapter.

The morphologic hallmark of acute leukemia is the blast form, a relatively undifferentiated cell with diffusely distributed nuclear chromatin, one or more nucleoli, and basophilic cytoplasm. Multiple methods exist for characterizing blast cells, including studies of morphology, cytochemistry, immunologic surface markers, biochemical cytoplasmic markers, chromosomes, and immunoglobulin gene rearrangements.

Morphologic and Cytochemical Classification

The blood-forming organs are responsible for the production of several types of cells, with each undergoing various stages of maturation and degrees of differentiation. Defects induced by the malignant transformation in leukemia may result in a variety of clinically and morphologically distinguishable types of leukemia, depending on the cell line involved and the severity of the maturation defect.

Production of blast forms is part of the normal maturational sequence of hematopoietic and lymphoid elements. However, under normal conditions such forms constitute fewer than 5 per cent of the nucleated cells of the bone marrow and are never seen in the peripheral blood except during periods of profound overproduction of blood cells in response to infection or bleeding and to bone marrow invasion by granulomas, fibrosis, or tumor cells (leukoerythroblastic anemia). Blast cells are primitive precursors, lacking many of the features of differentiation. Therefore, it is sometimes difficult to differentiate a lymphoid from a myeloid blast. Because the capacity to distinguish these blasts is of marked therapeutic and prognostic importance, various cytologic criteria have been established to differentiate them, and newer approaches involving enzymatic, surface marker, and scanning electron microscopic (1, 2) techniques also have been employed.

Color plate I (parts *1* to *4*) summarizes standard morphologic and cytochemical differences between lymphoblasts and myeloblasts. Wright-Giemsa–stained lymphoblasts have smooth, homogeneous nuclear material with indistinct nucleoli and only a small rim of light blue–staining cytoplasm without granules. In approximately 80 per cent of cases, lymphoblasts are reactive with periodic acid–Schiff (PAS), and they are usually—but not always (3)—nonreactive with myeloperoxidase and Sudan black. For further discussion, the reader is referred to the excellent monograph by Hayhoe and co-workers on the use of cytochemical techniques (4).

Myeloblasts differ from lymphoblasts in that the former have a lower nuclear:cytoplasmic ratio, more finely developed nuclear chromatin, and more distinct "punched-out" nucleoli. Cytoplasmic granules are often present, and detection of eosinophilic Auer rods is pathognomonic. Myeloblasts may react with PAS, but the staining is fine, as opposed to the clumps of glycogen found in lymphoblasts. Myeloblasts are myeloperoxidase-positive in approximately 75 per cent of patients. Small myeloblasts, so-called micromyeloblasts, may be confused with lymphoblasts morphologically and may be distinguished only by cytochemical studies. Whereas cytochemical stains for granule enzymes (e.g., myeloperoxidase) are usually helpful, other stains for cytoplasmic lipids (e.g., Sudan black stain) and specific and nonspecific esterases also may serve to accentuate the granules or Auer rods of myeloblasts. When immature cells are nonreactive with PAS, myeloperoxidase, nonspecific esterase, and Sudan black stains and the morphologic classification is neither obviously lymphoid nor obviously myeloid, the leukemic blast is considered morphologically and cytochemically undifferentiated.

Attempts have been made to correlate newer cytochemical reactions with both morphology and immunologic cell surface markers. For example, 90 per cent of T cell lymphoblasts may show a positive acid-phosphatase reaction, compared with less than 10 per cent of non T cell lymphoblasts (5).

International collaborative efforts have been undertaken to standardize morphologic classification (color plate I, parts *L1* to *M6*) (6, 7). According to the French-American-British (FAB) classification, ALL has been subdivided into three types, (L1, L2, and L3) and AML has been divided into six subgroups (M1 to M6).

L1 is the most common type of childhood ALL. L1 lymphoblasts are small cells characterized by a high nuclear:cytoplasmic ratio. The pale blue cytoplasm is scanty and limited to a small portion of the perimeter of the cell. The cells have indistinct nucleoli and nuclear membranes that vary from round to clefted. L2 lymphoblasts are larger, often in a more heterogeneous population, with a lower nuclear:cytoplasm ratio (cytoplasm occupies 20 per cent or more of the surface area of the cell), prominent nucleoli (often with perinuclear chromatin condensation), and irregular nuclear membranes that may be reniform or irregular. L3 is a homogeneous group of cells indistinguishable from Burkitt-like leukemia. The L3 lymphoblasts are characterized by deeply basophilic cytoplasm, prominent cytoplasmic vacuolation, the presence of immunoglobulin on the cell surface, and a distinct karyotypic abnormality, a translocation between chromosomes 8 and 14 (8, 9). Morphologic variants, such as "hand mirror" cells, have been reported in ALL (10) and AML (11). Such cells have been correlated with both T and B lymphoblastic surface markers and are of uncertain prognostic significance.

The M1 variant of myeloid leukemia may be indistinguishable from the L2 group morphologically. The differentiation must be made primarily by myeloperoxidase staining. M1 blasts are poorly differentiated, lack maturation, and may have occasional Auer rods. M2 blasts show differentiation beyond the promyelocyte stage (greater than 30 per cent blasts and promyelocytes), and Auer rods are frequently evident. M3 is acute promyelocytic leukemia, and in the most common form the blasts (the hypergranular variant) are packed with azurophilic granules and bundles of Auer rods. The latter finding is often associated with disseminated intravascular coagulation at the time of presentation (12). M4, acute myelomonocytic leukemia, shows myeloblastic and monoblastic differentiation in varying proportions in the bone marrow and peripheral blood. The monocytic component may be more predominant in the peripheral blood than in the bone marrow. The M5 type, monocytic leukemia, consists of poorly differentiated and differentiated subgroups. The poorly differentiated group, the more common variant in childhood, is characterized by large monoblasts with delicate chromatin, folded nucleus, and basophilic, vacuolated cytoplasm with pseudopods. In the differentiated type, 20 per cent or more of the abnormal cells are recognizable "promonocytes" with a folded nucleus, grayish-blue cytoplasm, and scattered azurophilic granules. The M5 form of AML is associated with gingival hypertrophy and leukemic skin infiltrations, the latter especially in neonatal leukemia. The monoblasts of the M4 and M5 types can be differentiated cytochemically from granulocytic cells by the presence of nonspecific esterase activity in the cytoplasm. The diagnosis of the M6 type (erythroleukemia, or Di-Guglielmo's syndrome) is made when a high proportion of the cells in the bone marrow are erythroid. There is bizarre dyserythropoiesis with megaloblastic features, and erythroblasts are often present in the peripheral blood. The granulocytic series shows an increased percentage of myeloblasts and promyelocytes, and Auer rods may be seen.

Acute megakaryoblastic leukemia is a rare subtype of AML. Blood and bone marrow smears may show megakaryoblasts that are undifferentiated or lymphoid in appearance. Bone marrow biopsies show megakaryocytic differentiation and reticulin fibrosis. Cytochemical staining is not specific, and the diagnosis is often made by electron microscopy and ultracytochemistry. Acute megakaryoblastic leukemia is also referred to as acute myelofibrosis (13).

PATHOPHYSIOLOGY

A review of factors that may incite leukemia is presented in Chapter 30, in which epidemiologic considerations are stressed. The molecular basis of leukemic transformation in humans is unknown. In general, the disease results from unbridled proliferation of immature hematopoietic precursors derived in some, if not all, cases from damaged hematopoietic progenitors that lack the capacity to transfer differentiation programs to the precursors to which they give rise. The progenitor/precursor basis of hematopoiesis (14) is examined in some detail in Chapter 6. One concept of the array of hematopoietic and lymphoid progenitors is shown in Figure 6–7 and discussed in detail in the legend to that figure.

Hematopoietic and Lymphoid Progenitors and Precursors

Progenitors are undifferentiated cells that are initially capable of self-renewal. These cells undergo a maturation process in which they become increasingly committed to specific differentiation into recognizable hematopoietic or lymphoid precursors. There are relatively few progenitors, and they are not themselves recognizable morphologically at any stage of their commitment. The pluripotent progenitor is capable of maturation to a multipotent committed myeloid progenitor (CFU-S) (15) of erythroid cells, megakaryocytes, eosinophils, and phagocytes and, in animals, to a bipotent lymphoid progenitor (CFU-L) that gives rise to the committed progenitors of the T and B lymphocytes that populate the marrow, lymph nodes, Peyer's patches, and spleen. The term "precursor," as used here, defines the numerous immature but recognizable nucleated hematopoietic and lymphoid blast cells that also divide in the process of their differentiation into mature circulating blood cells. A leukemia may

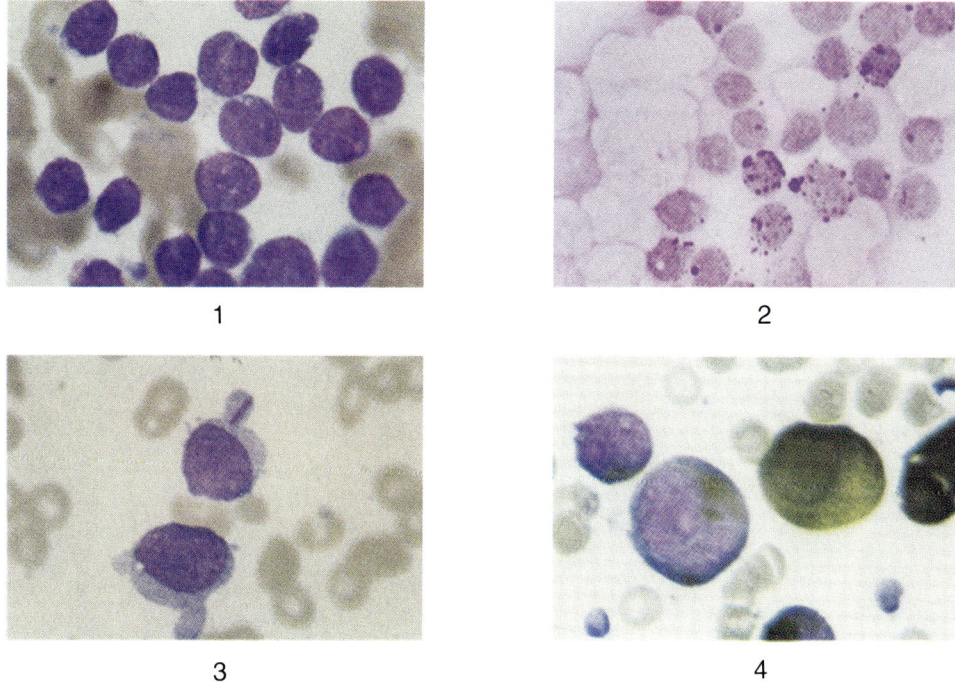

Color Plate I. Blood micrographs 1, 2, 3, and 4 show standard morphologic and cytochemical differences between Wright-Giemsa–stained lymphoblasts and myeloblasts.
1. Lymphoblasts. Note smooth, homogeneous nuclear chromatin with indistinct nucleoli and sparse rim of cytoplasm without granules.
2. Periodic acid-Schiff (PAS)–positive lymphoblasts. Note lumpy character of PAS staining glycogen in cytoplasm.
3. Myeloblasts. Note the greater cytoplasmic to nuclear ratio, the more finely developed nuclear chromatin and distinct nucleoli, and the presence of cytoplasmic granules. An Auer rod can be seen in the cytoplasm.
4. Myeloperoxidase-positive myeloblasts. The granules and Auer rods stain to a golden-yellow color.
Blood micrographs L1 to M6 (see text) illustrate the morphologic classification of leukemia according to the French-American-British (FAB) classification. Types L1, L2, and L3 are subgroups of acute lymphoblastic leukemia (ALL), and types M1 to M6 are subcategories of acute myelogenous leukemia (AML). (See text for additional information.)
L1, Common childhood ALL.
L2, Adult lymphoid leukemia.
L3, Homogeneous group of leukemic cells indistinguishable from Burkitt-type leukemia.
M1, Variant of myeloid leukemia that may be indistinguishable from *L2* on morphologic classification.
M2, Variant showing evidence of maturation and differentiation.
M3, Hypergranular promyelocytic leukemia.
M4, Myelomonocytic leukemia.
M5, Acute monocytic leukemia.
M6, Erythroleukemia, or the Di Guglielmo syndrome.

Color Plate I continued on following page

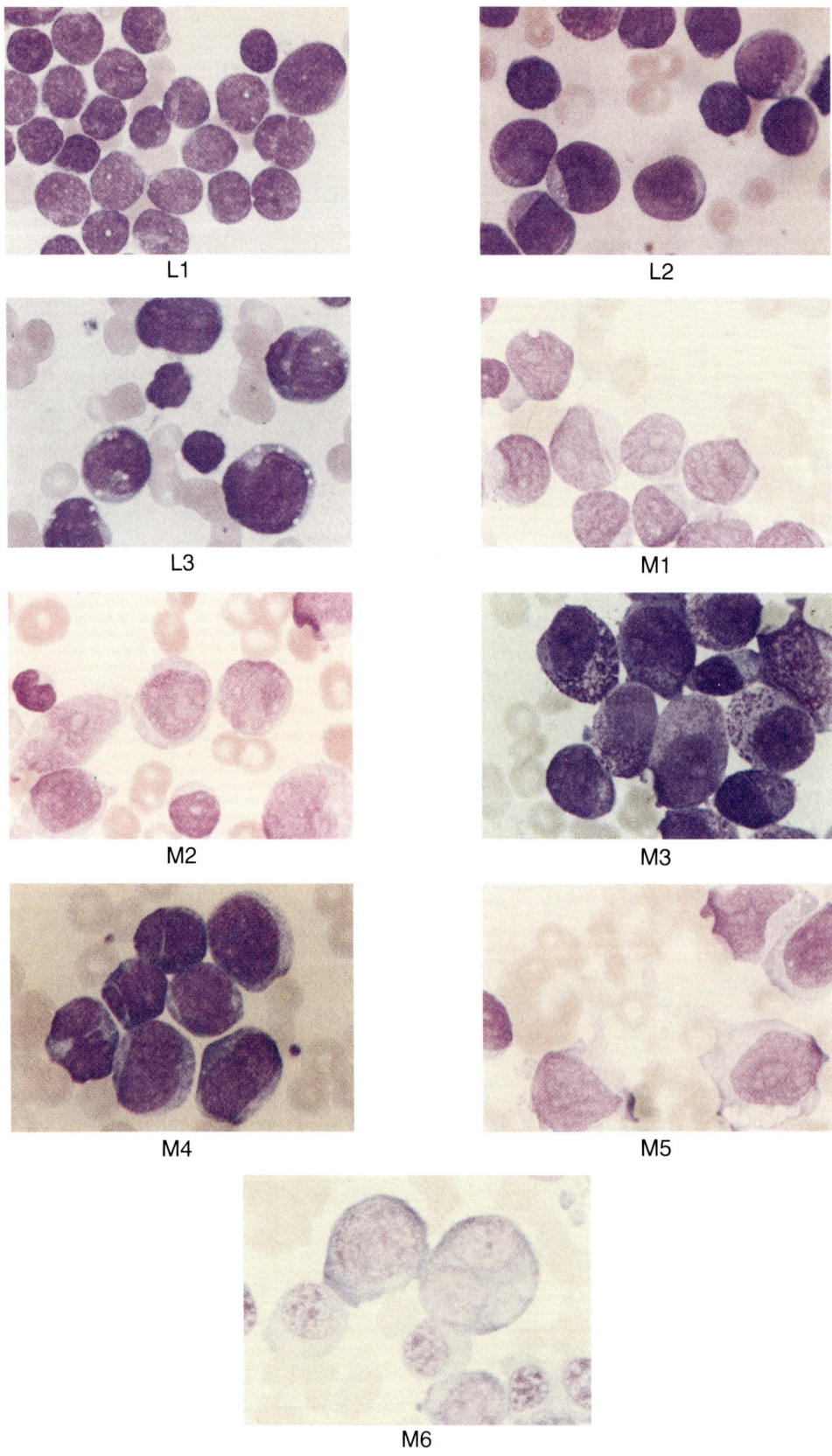

Color Plate I *Continued.*

arise during the maturation of the progenitors from their most primitive to most mature states and at the level of the immature precursor as well.

Numerous studies of human leukemic progenitors have been performed in vitro. Bone marrow cultures from patients with AML have shown abnormal growth patterns in progenitor-derived colonies (16). In semisolid medium, the majority of leukemic cells either fail to proliferate or form small clusters (3 to 40 cells) of poorly differentiated cells. A small number of leukemic cells, however, form colonies (>40 cells) and have several properties that are not shared by the majority of leukemic cells. Many are in S-phase. The cells are able to divide five or more times in vitro, and some have self-renewal capability. These have been termed "clonogenic leukemic cells" and may act in vivo as the leukemic stem cells. It is sometimes possible to distinguish these clonogenic cells from their progeny by their surface antigen phenotype (17).

The leukemic blasts, both in vivo and in vitro, generally demonstrate little maturation to functional end cells. Human myeloid leukemic cell lines have provided unique models for study of whether these blasts are capable of maturation under certain environmental circumstances. HL-60 cells are a line of human acute promyelocytic leukemic cells that can be induced to differentiate into mature neutrophils or macrophages by agents such as dimethylsulfoxide (DMSO), retinoic acid, phorbol esters, and cytosine arabinoside (18, 19). The induction of leukemic cell differentiation has not as yet been clearly demonstrated in the clinical setting.

Suppression of the growth of normal bone marrow progenitor cells has been observed in cocultures of normal bone marrow cells and human myeloid leukemic cells (20). At least one rare form of "leukemia-associated inhibitory activity" has been characterized as acidic isoferritins (21). Decreased normal hematopoiesis in leukemia may in part be explained by these observations. Successful remission induction in AML is usually accompanied by normalization of in vitro bone growth abnormalities (22).

Application of long-term bone marrow culture techniques (23, 24) to the study of normal and leukemic hematopoiesis should provide greater insights into why leukemic cells have a proliferative advantage over normal cells.

The Clonal Expansion Theory

We believe that in most cases of leukemia a single damaged progenitor, capable of expansion by indefinite self-renewal, gives rise to malignant, poorly differentiated precursors. These precursors divide at the same rate or even more slowly than their normal counterparts (25). The body burden of leukemic blasts, therefore, increases at a rate that is a function of their production from the progenitor pool, plus their doubling time, minus their rate of removal.

The clonal origin of leukemia is best demonstrated by glucose-6-phosphate dehydrogenase (G6PD) isoenzyme and cytogenetic studies of leukemic progenitors and precursors (26, 27, 27a, and Chapter 43). In females who are heterozygous for the G6PD gene, the leukemic cells produce only one of the two enzyme types, whereas normal tissues show both enzyme types. Over 75 per cent of children with ALL and AML have clonal chromosomal abnormalities in their bone marrow cells and not in other tissues. The disappearance of these chromosomal abnormalities or the return of two G6PD enzyme types during remission suggests that the clone of leukemic cells is superimposed on a residual normal population (28). One report, however, indicates that restoration of a normal karyotype in marrow cells after chemotherapy need not mean that normal progenitors have repopulated the marrow (29). At relapse, the original clone reappears with or without karyotypic evolution (30, 31).

Cytogenetic and G6PD isoenzyme studies have established that chronic myelogenous leukemia is a clonal proliferative disorder arising from a stem cell with pluripotential capacity (32, 33). Similar studies have shown that AML is heterogeneous with respect to the cell of origin (34, 35). In some patients, the clonal marker is found in erythroid and granulocytic cells, suggesting involvement of a multipotent myeloid stem cell (CFU-S). In other patients, the clonal marker is restricted to the granulocytic/monocytic lineage, suggesting involvement of a more committed progenitor (CFU-GM).

In those cases of acute leukemia that are the result of the expansion of a damaged hematopoietic or lymphoid progenitor, the vast numbers of recognizable "blasts" visible in the marrow, lymph nodes, and blood are not the primary leukemic cells but are instead the poorly differentiated derivatives of the damaged progenitors. The blast cells are obviously clinically important because they divide, migrate, invade, and eventually kill the patient. However, total eradication of the recognizable blasts would not be curative unless the treatment also led to eradication of the invisible clonogenic leukemic cells, the cellular level at which the disease begins (17).

Rare but important cases in which leukemia has appeared in the engrafted donor cells of a leukemic patient who received a marrow transplant from a histocompatible sibling suggest that leukemogenesis may result from unidentified factors that persist in certain susceptible hosts (36–39).

Cellular Heterogeneity

SURFACE MARKERS

Studies of G6PD isoenzymes in informative ALL cases show that the disease arises from a single cell (40), but the complexities of lymphoid ontogeny (as discussed in Chapter 26, Figure 26–7) suggest that a leukemic insult may occur at different stages of B cell differentiation and that the disease must be immunophenotypically heterogeneous. This heterogeneity has been illuminated by study of leukemic cell surface antigens.

Acute Lymphoblastic Leukemia. Immunologic surface marker studies are of biologic and therapeutic significance in the lymphatic leukemias, in which three broad subclasses are defined by cell surface antigens (Table 33–1) (41).

T cell ALL accounts for 15 to 20 per cent of the cases. T lymphoblasts have characteristic antigenic sites that can be recognized by monoclonal antibodies (42–44) and other distinguishing clinical and laboratory characteristics (Table 33–2). The subclassification of T cell leukemia is more complex than that suggested by the data in Table 33–2. By the use of monoclonal antibodies that react with subsets of normal peripheral blood T cells or thymocytes or with leukemic T lymphoblasts, one can demonstrate the broad heterogeneity within the T cell subpopulation (45).

T cell leukemia is characterized by a 4:1 male:female ratio, median age of diagnosis of 12 years, median white blood count >100,000 cells/mm^3, normal hematocrit and hemoglobin level, and a high incidence of anterior mediastinal masses at presentation (see Table 33–2). The normal hemoglobin concentration is probably related to the role of helper T cells in the production of certain molecules that enhance the influence of erythropoietin on erythrocyte production (46, 47). Additional functional and migratory characteristics of T lymphoblasts, such as suppression of antibody production (48) and invasion into the skin, testes, and central nervous system (45, 49, 50), may be intimately related to prognosis.

With the exception of 5 to 10 per cent of the cases that currently defy classification, the remainder of the childhood lymphoblastic leukemias are of B cell lineage (51). They express the Ia antigen (52–54) and other immature B cell surface antigens (51), and they are also characterized by rearrangements of the light chains of the immunoglobulin genes (55) (see Chapter 27). Approximately 15 to 20 per cent of cases contain intracytoplasmic immunoglobulin and are sometimes referred to as "pre B cell" leukemia (56–58). On rare occasions, pre-B cell leukemias with rearranged immunoglobulin genes may exhibit the morphology and gene expression of monocytes (58a).

Most of the immature B cell leukemias express an antigen known as the common ALL antigen (CALLA) (59, 60). This antigen, which has been defined by monoclonal antibodies (59), is also expressed on a small population of mononuclear cells in normal bone marrow (61), as well as on some nonhematopoietic cells (62). The CALLA antigen is also expressed on other malignant cells, including the terminal deoxynucleotidyl transferase–positive lymphoblastic cells of chronic myelogenous leukemia in blast crisis and Burkitt's lymphoma cells and cell lines (59, 63).

Mature B cell leukemias, characterized by monoclonal surface immunoglobulin, are rare in childhood (only 1 to 2 per cent of all cases) and are

Table 33–1. CLASSIFICATION OF CHILDHOOD ACUTE LEUKEMIAS

Diagnosis	% of Patients	FAB Group	Monoclonal Antibody Reactivity						
			Leu 9	Ia	Ig	B4	J5	MY9	TdT
ALL									
T cell	15–20	L1,2	+	−	−	−	±	−	+
B cell	75–80								
mature	1–2	L3	−	+	SIg	+	±	−	+
common	65	L1,2	−	+	−	+	+	−	+
pre B	20	L1,2	−	+	CIg	+	−	−	+
Unclassifiable	<10	L1,2	−	+	−	−	−	−	+
AML									
	45	M1/M2	−	+	−	−	−	+	−
	5	M3	−	−	−	−	−	+	−
	45	M4/M5	−	+	−	−	−	+	−
	<5	M6	−	−	−	−	−	+	−

Notes: ALL is acute lymphoblastic leukemia; AML is acute myelogenous leukemia; FAB is the French-American-British classification (6, 7); Leu 9 is the monoclonal antibody that recognizes T cells and is also known as WT1, Leu, and as 3A1 (42–44); anti-Ia is also known as anti–HLA-DR, BA-3, and as DA-2 (52–54); the anti-immunoglobulin antibody (Ig) reacts with surface immunoglobulin (SIg) or intracytoplasic immunoglobulin (CIg) (56–58); anti-B4 is a marker of B cell lineage (51) and is also known as BA-1; anti-J5 is the anti–common ALL antigen and is also known as anti-CALLA and AL-2 (59, 60); anti-MY9 is a monoclonal antibody that recognizes myeloid cells; and anti-TdT reacts with terminal deoxynucleotidyl transferase (71, 72).

clinically characterized by a distinctive morphology (FAB-L3) (8, 9) and a high incidence of associated central nervous system leukemia. Very rare cases of leukemia that express both T cell and B cell markers on the same cell have been described (64). These may arise from the CFU-L itself.

Acute Myeloblastic Leukemia. The monoclonal antibodies that have identified immunologic subtypes of ALL have in general not reacted with AML blasts. With rare exceptions, T cell antigens, monoclonal immunoglobulin, early B cell differentiation antigens, and CALLA are not found on the surface of myeloid blast cells (65, 66), which do express Ia antigen, with the exception of the malignant promyelocytes in acute promyelocytic leukemia and the erythroblasts of M6 AML.

It has been shown that monoclonal antibodies that recognize surface antigens on normal myeloid cells can be used to identify stages of normal myeloid differentiation (67). Furthermore, AML cells tend to express these antigens in patterns that are characteristic of immature normal myeloid cells. These data suggest that AML may originate at multiple levels in the differentiation pathway from the multipotent myeloid stem cell (CFU-GEMM) to the immature precursor (blast).

Rare cases of leukemia have been reported in which the blast population was found either to be composed of distinct, antigenically distinct subtypes of leukemic cells or to contain a varying portion of cell hybrids expressing both myeloid and lymphoid characteristics (68, 69). An example would be typical AML with increased terminal deoxynucleotidyl transferase activity. These have been referred to as biphenotypic leukemias, or blasts showing lineage infidelity. It is not clear whether these represent progeny of a pluripotent malignant cell or aberrant gene expression in a committed progenitor.

CYTOPLASMIC MARKERS

Acute Lymphoblastic Leukemia. Certain intracellular and ectoenzymes further define the heterogeneity of childhood ALL and aid in the understanding of its pathophysiology (70). At least six such marker enzymes have been described: terminal deoxynucleotidyl transferase, the first enzyme to provide a diagnostic differentiation between ALL and AML (71, 72); hexosaminidase (73); *N*-alkaline phosphatase (74); and three enzymes of the purine pathway: purine nucleoside phosphorylase (75), 5′-nucleotidase (76), and adenosine deaminase (77, 78). The interrelationship between immunologic and biochemical markers has been demonstrated by studies showing that T lymphoblasts have diminished 5′-nucleotidase (76) and increased adenosine deaminase (77). These distinguishing characteristics can be useful clinically. For example, inhibitors of adenosine deaminase, such as deoxycoformycin, have some

Table 33–2. CLINICAL AND LABORATORY DIFFERENCES BETWEEN T CELL AND NON T CELL ACUTE LYMPHOBLASTIC LEUKEMIA (ALL)

Patient Factors*	T Cell	Non T Cell
% of ALL	15	85
Median age (years)	12	4
Presenting WBC/mm^3	>100,000	10,000±
Presenting Hgb	Normal	Low
Presenting thymic mass	+ + +	±
Presenting hepatomegaly and/or splenomegaly	+ + + +	+ +
Male:female	4:1	1.4:1
Complete remissions	<90%	>90%
Extramedullary relapses	+ + +	+

*These data represent the findings in 93 children with ALL followed at the Dana-Farber Cancer Institute and the Children's Hospital, Boston, MA.

efficacy in the treatment of T cell ALL (79). Terminal deoxynucleotidyl transferase activity, however, has been of little value in separating subclasses of ALL because it is positive in over 90 per cent of cases (80). It has been useful, though, in predicting relapse early (81), in correctly defining the lymphoblastic crisis of chronic myelogenous leukemia, and in predicting the efficacy of vincristine and prednisone administration in the management of ALL (82). Purine pathway enzymes also have been studied in AML, but the results are inconsistent and based on a relatively small data base (83, 84).

The leukemic cells of the majority of children with untreated ALL have cytoplasmic glucocorticoid receptor activity (85, 86). Non-T lymphoblasts are likely to have greater numbers of these receptors than T lymphoblasts have. This differential capacity of lymphoblasts to incorporate steroids into receptors may help investigators design therapeutic programs for the subcategories of ALL, although cells with adequate amounts of cytoplasmic receptor activity may still fail to respond to glucocorticoids. Glucocorticoid receptor levels are of limited prognostic importance (87). In AML, the correlation between receptor assays and clinical responsiveness has not been fully elucidated.

Chromosomes and Leukemia

This topic is discussed in detail in Chapter 43 and will not be further elaborated upon here.

CLINICAL MANIFESTATIONS

Characteristic Findings at Diagnosis

Acute leukemia may present insidiously or acutely, as an incidental finding on a routine blood count of an asymptomatic child, or as a life-threatening hemorrhage, infection, or episode of respiratory distress. The presenting signs, symptoms, and physical and hematologic findings of 137 consecutive children with ALL in a 3½-year period are shown in Table 33–3. Similar findings have been reported in childhood AML (88).

The Protean Nature of Leukemia

Although leukemia is primarily a disease of the bone marrow and peripheral blood, any organ or tissue may be infiltrated by the abnormal cells. Such infiltration may be clinically apparent by physical examination or may be occult and detectable only by histologic sampling. Autopsy studies of patients who died without having had antemortem clinical evidence of leukemia (89, 90), as well as reports of extensive tissue biopsies in leukemic patients who were alive and presumably in complete remission (91–93), demonstrate evidence of residual leukemic foci in extramedullary sites. This involvement during bone marrow remission is of great importance therapeutically and prognostically. Such occult disease means that leukemic cells from extramedullary sites may seed other sites, including the bone marrow, and result in hematologic relapse or that any other involved site may become clinically apparent and result in extramedullary relapse.

Extramedullary Leukemia

CENTRAL NERVOUS SYSTEM MANIFESTATIONS

In the era preceding effective systemic control of leukemia, CNS disease was a rare and usually preterminal event. However, with progressively longer periods of hematologic remission, the incidence of CNS leukemia increased, so that by the late 1960's the incidence of CNS relapse approximated 4 per cent each month in remission (94). Although fewer than 10 per cent of children with acute leukemia have clinical CNS involvement at the time of diagnosis, it remains the most common site of clinically apparent extramedullary leukemia.

Some children, such as those under age 2 years and those with T cell ALL and M4 or M5 AML, may have a higher incidence of CNS leukemia at the time of either diagnosis or relapse. The propensity of T cells (49) and monoblasts (95) to migrate to extramedullary sites may explain the increased incidence of CNS disease in the latter groups. The relationship of the initial leukocyte count to the frequency of CNS relapse was statistically significant in the era prior to CNS prophylaxis (96). Although children with markedly elevated initial leukocyte counts who are treated with preventive CNS therapy continue to be at an increased risk for CNS leukemia, the overall frequency has been markedly diminished.

The pathophysiology of CNS leukemia has been elegantly delineated by Price and Johnson (97). The disease process originates in the cranial arachnoid and is first seen in the walls of superficial arachnoid veins. It then progresses, with extension into the surrounding deep arachnoid blood vessels as they course through the brain. The blasts then invade the cerebrospinal fluid. Increasing numbers of cells eventually penetrate vessel walls in the deep arachnoid and, after disrupting the pia-glia, invade brain parenchyma.

There are two major models for the pathogenesis of meningeal leukemia: (1) Leukemic cells are already present within the leptomeninges at the time of diagnosis, as a result of direct perivascular invasion or deposition from hemorrhage secondary to thrombocytopenia; or (2) leukemic cells invade the leptomeninges from the periphery as part of the process of relapse. The second alternative has been suggested because (a) most patients show no signs of meningeal leukemia at the time of initial diagnosis, and (b) there is a relatively long interval between initial diagnosis and the development of meningeal leukemia in most patients who have not received CNS prophylaxis—an interval longer than that anticipated if leukemic cells, initially present as a focus in the CNS, were

Table 33–3. CHARACTERISTICS AT THE TIME OF DIAGNOSIS OF 137 CONSECUTIVE CHILDREN WITH ACUTE LYMPHOBLASTIC LEUKEMIA (ALL)

Characteristics	Patients
Signs and Symptoms	
Lethargy/malaise	50
Fever/infection	43
Extremity/joint pain	31
Bleeding manifestations	24
Anorexia	17
Abdominal pain	9
CNS manifestations	3
Physical Findings	
Pallor	39
Hepatosplenomegaly	36
Ecchymoses/petechiae	24
Lymphadenopathy	12
Hematologic Findings	
Hematocrit (%)	
>35	9
30–34	7
21–29	41
<20	43
White Blood Count (mm^3)	
<1000	3
1000–500	25
5100–25,000	45
25,000–100,000	19
>100,000	8
Platelet Count (mm^3)	
>100,000	26
50,000–100,000	25
10,000–49,000	34
<10,000	15

to continue their proliferation uninhibited by systemic medication. The marked clinical success of CNS prophylaxis suggests that the first alternative is more probable and that, in patients who do not receive CNS prophylaxis, the leukemic cell proliferation within the CNS is not a linear process.

Leukemic cells persist in the CNS throughout induction of hematologic remission because most drugs used in the treatment of acute leukemia inadequately penetrate the CNS. This allows progressive growth of cells or emergence of resistant clones. Karyotypic studies (98) and patterns of systemic relapse following the appearance of CNS disease strongly suggest that the hematologic recurrence is due to reseeding of leukemic cells from the CNS to the marrow (99).

Children with CNS leukemia present with diffuse or focal neurologic signs and symptoms. Approximately 90 per cent of patients will have manifestations of increased intracranial pressure (vomiting, headache, papilledema, and lethargy) (96, 100), whereas convulsions and nuchal rigidity are infrequent. Cranial nerve palsies are rare, with the facial nerve being most frequently involved. When it is affected, unilateral facial nerve paralysis may precede the symptoms and signs of increased intracranial pressure.

Localizing signs from parenchymal involvement include hemiparesis, hemisensory losses, and convulsions. CNS leukemia may rarely present with hypothalamic involvement, resulting in excessive weight gain, behavior disturbances, and hirsutism (101). Other uncommon manifestations of CNS leukemia include central pontine myelinosis (102), cerebellar involvement, multifocal leukoencephalopathy (103), and diabetes insipidus (104). Eighty-five per cent of patients with CNS leukemia have cerebrospinal fluid pleocytosis as a result of the presence of leukemic blast cells (96, 100). These cells can usually be identified with certainty by the use of cytocentrifugation (105) and Wright-Giemsa staining. Such morphologic evaluation is used to distinguish the pleocytosis of leukemic meningitis from that induced as a reaction to intrathecal chemotherapeutic agents or from other CNS infections. At times when the diagnosis of CNS relapse may be difficult, specific tests for the identification of individual cells in the cerebrospinal fluid may be enhanced by immunofluorescent staining for terminal transferase (106) or the detection of increased levels of beta$_2$-microglobulin in the cerebrospinal fluid (107, 108). Neither spinal fluid protein nor glucose concentration alone is useful in the diagnosis of meningeal leukemia (100).

Clinically significant spinal cord involvement is very unusual in leukemia (109, 110). Localized epidural leukemic infiltrates (tumors) compressing the cord are the most common finding and most often involve the thoracic segments. Symptoms include back and radicular pain, weakness, paralysis, and bladder and bowel incontinence. Myelography is helpful in localizing the lesion. Epidural cord compression is more common in AML than in ALL.

The epidural tumors in AML are composed of immature myeloid cells and have been called "chloromas," or "granulocytic sarcomas." They were originally described and so named because of their green color secondary to the presence of myeloperoxidase (111). However, many granulocytic sarcomas are colorless. These tumors frequently are located in the head and neck (in the retro-orbital area or sinuses) and in extradural structures, but they may occur anywhere in the body (112). Chloromas may precede systemic manifestations of AML by months or years or occur as extramedullary relapses early in the course of the disease.

The differential diagnosis includes epidural hematoma, especially in thrombocytopenic patients following lumbar puncture (113), as well as vincristine neurotoxicity and vertebral body collapse.

GENITOURINARY TRACT MANIFESTATIONS

Testicle. The clinical presentation of testicular leukemia is a painless enlargement of one or both testes. Although rare, testicular enlargement has been reported as an initial manifestation of both ALL and AML (114, 115). Testicular relapse may be the first identifiable site of recurrent leukemia. Although more commonly reported in patients with ALL, leukemic involvement of the testes in males with AML during bone marrow remission also has been reported (116, 117). Testicular involvement in AML may become more frequent as the number of patients with long-term remissions increases. Because the clinical incidence of testicular leukemia in ALL ranges from 5 to 40 per cent and because microscopic infiltrates seen at autopsy have been reported in 64 to 92 per cent of male patients (118, 119), it is thought that testicular infiltrates often escape clinical detection until the organ size is several times normal. Autopsy findings in patients who died while presumably in complete remission (89, 90) as well as multiple organ biopsies in patients who were in hematologic remission (91) have demonstrated that occult testicular leukemic infiltration may occur but that it is usually accompanied by microscopic involvement of other organs as well, most often the kidney. Exploratory laparotomies performed on children with "isolated" testicular relapse showed that most patients had other organ involvement as well (93). The existence of isolated testicular leukemia is extremely rare, if it exists at all.

Several histopathologic studies have examined the microscopic findings of testicular leukemia (120–122). The leukemic infiltration is mainly in the interstitial spaces, but it has also been observed to invade and accumulate beneath the Sertoli cell layer. Destruction of the tubules by the infiltrate occurs in advanced cases, and postirradiation biopsies are characterized by fibrosis (120). Of 49 boys who had bilateral wedge testicular biopsies at the time of diagnosis and again 3 to 3½ years later while in continuous complete remission, occult testicular leukemia was found in 10 per cent of the patients, all of whom were on maintenance therapy at the time of biopsy (122). In another 44 patients, among whom half were receiving chemotherapy and half had electively stopped their drugs, leukemic infiltrations of the testes were seen in 11 per cent, interstitial fibrosis in 55 per cent, and basement-membrane thickening in 14 per cent (121). Bilateral microscopic testicular involvement is common despite unilateral clinical testicular enlargement.

Other Genitourinary Tract Sites of Involvement. Renal infiltrates are generally asymptomatic and discovered at the time of diagnosis as enlarged kidneys by ultrasonography. Renal enlargement in acute leukemia is not due to infiltration by tumor cells only; noninfiltrative causes related to hyperuricemia, hemorrhage, and pyelonephritis also must be considered. Renal involvement has been found in asymptomatic patients who are presumably in complete remission (84, 87), as well as in findings at autopsy series. Hypertension is more commonly associated with the treatment of leukemia, especially with prolonged use of corticosteroids, than with renal involvement. Although bladder infiltration may rarely result in hematuria (123), the latter is most often associated with either thrombocytopenia or hemorrhagic cystitis induced by cyclophosphamide.

Priapism is seen in ALL (124), AML (125), and chronic myelogenous leukemia (126, 127), usually in association with an elevated white blood count. The pathogenesis may be due to involvement of sacral nerve roots, or it may be related to mechanical obstruction of the corpora cavernosa and dorsal veins by leukemic infiltration or leukostasis.

Ovarian involvement has been found at the time of autopsy in 30 per cent of girls with leukemia (99). Reports of "isolated" ovarian involvement are rare, and most of the girls have had other extramedullary sites involved as well (128). Leukemic involvement of the fallopian tubes, uterus, broad ligaments, and pelvic lymph nodes also has been described (99, 128).

BONE AND JOINT MANIFESTATIONS

As many as 30 per cent of patients with childhood leukemia initially present with a limp or painful bones or joints (129, 130). Some patients may have characteristic radiologic changes in the absence of bone pain, whereas others may have bone pain unaccompanied by radiologic changes. These changes are most easily seen in the long bones, especially around the areas of rapid growth (e.g., the knees, wrists, and ankles) and include (1) subperiosteal new bone formation, (2) transverse metaphyseal radiolucent bands, (3) osteolytic lesions involving the medullary cavity and cortex, (4) diffuse demineralization, and (5) transverse metaphyseal lines of increased density ("growth arrest lines") (131–133). These bands probably represent regions of growth arrest during active phases of the disease rather than direct infiltration by leukemic cells. Bone necrosis also may produce bone pain, which is more frequently associated with ALL (134), usually occurs at a time of leukopenia, does not respond to radiation therapy by relief of pain, and tends to be related to a poor response to chemotherapy. With the possible exceptions of necrosis and widespread bony lesions (135, 136), there is no correlation between initial radiologically evident bone disease and prognosis (133). Pathologic fractures occur secondary to severe osteoporosis and are frequently the end result of long-term methotrexate therapy (137). Marked point tenderness frequently occurs and may be due to local periosteal elevation caused by stripping of the periosteum by infiltrates of leukemic cells or by hemorrhage. Such painful lesions readily respond to palliative radiation therapy. Pain and swelling of the joint are less frequent but may be presenting manifestations of disease and can initially cause confusion in the diagnosis (138). Migratory joint pain accompanied by swelling and tenderness can be misdiagnosed as juvenile rheumatoid arthritis or as rheumatic fever. These symptoms may be the result of direct leukemic infiltration of the periosteum, periosteal elevation of underlying cortical disease, bone infarction, or expansion of the marrow cavity by the leukemic cells.

GASTROINTESTINAL MANIFESTATIONS

Leukemic infiltrates in the lower gastrointestinal tract are commonly observed at autopsy but rarely cause clinical problems except in the terminally ill, relapsed patient. Such individuals may develop symptoms of an acute abdomen secondary to perforation of the small bowel or infarction or infection from infiltrated bowel wall.

The most common gastrointestinal manifestation of leukemia is bleeding as reflected by gross or occult blood in the stool. This is usually secondary to thrombocytopenia, disseminated intravascular coagulopathy, or the toxic effects of chemotherapy on the gastrointestinal mucosa. A specific syndrome of right lower quadrant pain with rebound tenderness, abdominal distention, vomiting, and sepsis is seen and often referred to as "typhlitis," or "necrotizing enterocolitis" (139). Plain abdominal x-ray films may show a paucity of air in the right lower quadrant (140). The pathogenesis of typhlitis is most likely related to mucosal and bowel wall damage secondary to chemotherapy. It can also occur in the setting of prolonged neutropenia. Typhlitis has been associated with several antileukemic drugs, including doxorubicin, daunorubicin, and cytosine arabinoside. Management includes bowel rest, intravenous fluids, and broad-spectrum antibiotics. Surgery is usually not indicated except in the rare case of perforation, uncontrolled bleeding, or abdominal wall cellulitis (141). In the differential diagnosis of typhlitis one must also consider common surgical conditions of childhood, including appendicitis and intussusception, as well as rare problems related to leukemia or antileukemic therapy, such as pancreatitis (142) and acute cholangitis (143).

Other gastrointestinal lesions that are generally associated with neutropenia or chemotherapy or both are mouth ulcers or esophagitis (usually as a result of methotrexate, doxorubicin, and/or radiation) (144, 145), oral and esophageal moniliasis (usually as a result of prednisone and/or antibiotic therapy), and perirectal inflammation or abscess (146–148). Antileukemic chemotherapy can also lead to lactose malabsorption, characterized by cramps and diarrhea (149).

Hepatic fibrosis is a common autopsy finding and, except in occasional patients (150, 151), is of no clinical significance. Chemotherapy with methotrexate and 6-mercaptopurine has been implicated as a cause of this complication (137).

ORAL MANIFESTATIONS

With the exception of gingival hypertrophy seen in monocytic and myelomonocytic leukemia, infection is probably the single most important oral problem in leukemia (152–154). The use of broad-spectrum antiseptic agents can markedly improve the management of patients with oral infections (155). Other oral lesions are generally nonspecific and include mucosal petechiae as a manifestation of thrombocytopenia, buccal ulcerations associated with antileukemic drug toxicity, oral moniliasis related to relapse and/or treatment, and Mikulicz's syndrome (bilateral salivary and lacrimal gland enlargement due to leukemic invasion) (156).

OCULAR MANIFESTATIONS

Hemorrhage and papilledema are the most common ocular findings. Retinal hemorrhages, the most frequent ocular abnormality, are presumably due to thrombocytopenia or anemia. However, local infiltration of the capillary vessel walls with subsequent rupture and hemorrhage also may occur, especially in patients with very high numbers of circulating blasts. Retinal leukemic infiltrates are uncommon and, when they do occur, are usually associated with systemic relapse or uncontrolled primary disease (157, 158). Ocular motor palsies and papilledema are frequently indicative of meningeal leukemia. On occasion, the optic disc or anterior chamber may be directly involved by leukemic infiltration, usually accompanied by signs of meningeal involvement (157, 159). In such situations, visual acuity may be markedly affected, whereas the cerebrospinal fluid pressure and protein content remain normal. Prompt radiation therapy may be necessary to salvage useful vision. Histologic examination reveals infiltration of the optic nerve by leukemic cells (160, 161). The ophthalmoscopic appearances are presumably caused by obstruction of exoplasmic flow. Loss of vision may rarely be related to retinal pigment epitheliopathy (162). Leukemic iritis has been described (99, 100, 163), at times associated with the development of glaucoma (164). Clinically inapparent choroid involvement also has been found in 43 per cent of patients at autopsy (165). This was invariably associated with systemic involvement but was unrelated to preterminal leukocyte counts.

Orbital chloromas are generally associated with AML and chronic myelogenous leukemia and may precede the peripheral blood and bone marrow manifestations of leukemia by as much as 2 years (166, 167). The most common presenting feature of ocular chloroma is proptosis (168). Occasionally, AML relapse may be heralded by an isolated chloroma.

CARDIAC MANIFESTATIONS

One half to two thirds of patients with leukemia have demonstrable cardiac involvement at autopsy (169, 170), although symptomatic heart disease occurs in fewer than 5 per cent. Pathologic findings include leukemic infiltration and hemorrhage. Pericardial infiltration may be a presenting feature of disease (167, 171) or occur during remission (172), and pericardial effusion may occasionally lead to cardiac tamponade. The pathophysiology of cardiac involvement is thought to begin with an obstruction to normal lymphatic flow between the endocardium and epicardium (173). Cardiomyopathy in leukemia is most commonly induced by therapy, especially with the anthracyclines doxorubicin and daunorubicin (174).

PULMONARY MANIFESTATIONS

Pulmonary complications in leukemia are most often of infectious origin (175, 176), but pulmonary leukemic infiltration may occur even during hematologic remission (177, 178). Pulmonary hemorrhage, usually as a consequence of thrombocytopenia, is found in 50 per cent of patients at autopsy (176). Roentgenographic distinction among infection, leukemic infiltration, and hemorrhage may be impossible.

MISCELLANEOUS MANIFESTATIONS

Skin infiltration is uncommon in childhood leukemia with the exception of congenital leukemia, in which it has been reported in approximately half the cases, including both AML and ALL (see later section on congenital leukemia). Pleural effusion may be associated with thymic enlargement in some patients (179). Involvement of the inner ear may result in vertigo or hearing loss (180). Infiltration of the breasts has occurred in girls with ALL (181) and AML (182). Chloromas also have been described in the breasts and ovaries during apparent clinical remission (183). Rib involvement with a clinical picture resembling florid rickets has been described (184). The evolution of a monoclonal gammopathy has been described in ALL (185, 186). Neither the mechanism nor the significance is known.

LABORATORY FINDINGS

Clinical laboratory data often provide a broad spectrum of abnormal findings at the time of diagnosis of leukemia (see Table 33–3). Anemia, abnormal white cell and differential blood counts, and thrombocytopenia are common. However, as many as 10 per cent of children with ALL may have normal routine blood counts at the time of diagnosis, even when the bone marrow is replaced by leukemic cells.

The red blood cells are usually normochromic and normocytic. Failure of erythroid production is manifested by a low reticulocyte count, and "tear-drop" and nucleated red cells may provide the tell-tale traces of marrow invasion.

Leukocyte counts at the time of diagnosis can vary from 100 to 1,000,000 cells per mm^3, often with absolute granulocytopenia. Approximately 20 per cent of children with ALL present with white blood counts greater than 50,000 cells per mm^3. This is an important group because of the known adverse effect of an elevated white blood count on long-term prognosis in ALL.

Blast forms may not be present on routine smears of peripheral blood of leukopenic patients; however, buffy coat smears may be more rewarding. In any case, the peripheral blasts may not accurately reflect the status of the bone marrow because the morphologic appearance of the peripheral blast forms sometimes differs from that seen on marrow smears. For example, normal myeloblasts may be detected in the circulation when lymphoblasts invade the marrow as part of the so-called leukoerythroblastic response to marrow invasion. The same response occurs in other infiltrative diseases of the marrow, including osteopetrosis, myelofibrosis, granulomatous infections, sarcoidosis, and metastatic tumor. Thus, the definitive diagnosis of leukemia should not be made from the peripheral smear.

Platelet counts also vary from normal to extremely low, the majority of children have fewer than 100,000 cells per mm^3 at presentation, and the platelets are usually of normal size.

Inspection of smears of bone marrow aspirates is essential to establishment of the diagnosis of leukemia. Whereas normal bone marrow has fewer than 5 per cent blast forms, leukemic marrow generally has 30 to 50 per cent or more blasts. The marrow specimen is usually hypercellular and characterized by a homogeneous population of cells. Leukemia must be suspected in patients whose marrows contain greater than 5 per cent blasts, but the diagnosis should not be made on the basis of a single marrow smear with fewer than 30 per cent blasts.

A bone marrow aspirate may be difficult to obtain at the time of diagnosis. This is commonly thought to be due to the density of blast forms in the marrow, but it may be caused by bone infarction or fibrosis (187). In such cases, a bone marrow biopsy should be performed with a Jamshidi or other type of needle. "Touch preps" of the biopsy specimen can be stained for morphologic diagnosis.

Differences in the leukemic involvement of the marrow aspirates from widely separated sites may occur. Site-to-site morphologic discordance may be seen at presentation (188, 189), after radiation therapy (190), or during presumed complete remission (191, 192). If clinical findings suggest relapse but the bone marrow is normal, the marrow should be sampled at additional sites.

Hypereosinophilia has been described in association with ALL, AML, and chronic myelogenous leukemia (193–197). In ALL, the hypereosinophilia is thought to be "reactive" because the eosinophils have a normal karyotype, whereas the lymphoblasts may be aneuploid (194). The eosinophilia may appear at presentation and disappear with successful remission induction (197). The stimulus for such eosinophilia is unknown. In AML, true eosinophilic leukemia has been reported (198) as well as dysplastic marrow eosinophils in patients with the M4 subtype and an inversion in chromosome 16 (199).

DIAGNOSIS AND DIFFERENTIAL DIAGNOSIS

A careful history and physical examination, as well as an examination of the peripheral blood and bone marrow, result in a straightforward diagnosis of leukemia in approximately 90 per cent of cases. However, for the 10 per cent of difficult cases, other diagnoses must be entertained and systematically excluded. These include idiopathic thrombocytopenic purpura, neuroblastoma, juvenile rheumatoid arthritis, aplastic anemia, infectious mononucleosis, and various infections that result in leukemoid reactions or neutropenia.

Idiopathic Thrombocytopenic Purpura (ITP). ITP is the most common cause of the acute onset of petechiae and purpura in children. There is often a history of a recent viral infection. Ordinarily, children with ITP have no evidence of anemia. Bone marrow smears reveal normal hematopoiesis and a normal to increased number of megakaryocytes. Peripheral blood smears of these patients may reveal large "young" platelets.

Neuroblastoma. Because ALL and neuroblastoma may have similar modes of presentation, differentiation between lymphoblasts and neuroblasts occasionally results in perplexing problems. Bone marrow neuroblasts usually form discrete clumps or rosettes, whereas lymphoblasts diffusely infiltrate the bone marrow. Circulating neuroblasts are rare, but, when present, they also can be confusing. The differential diagnosis can be facilitated by the determination of urinary catecholamines, by radiologic findings of a posterior mediastinal or suprarenal mass with calcifications, and by the use of antisera that distinguish neuroblasts from lymphoblasts (200).

Juvenile Rheumatoid Arthritis. Because many patients with ALL present with joint or extremity complaints (especially limp, arthritis, or arthralgia) and often manifest fever, pallor, splenomegaly, and leukocytosis, the disease may be confused with juvenile rheumatoid arthritis. Until a reliable, positive test for juvenile rheumatoid arthritis becomes available, that diagnosis should not be made unless a bone marrow aspirate has been done to exclude leukemia. Similarly, some children presenting with painful and swollen joints who had positive tests for antinuclear antibody and were presumed to have systemic lupus erythematosus have subsequently been shown to have ALL (201).

Aplastic Anemia and Myeloproliferative Disorders. Both patients with leukemia and those with aplastic anemia may present with pancytopenia and have fevers or infections associated with granulocytopenia. Both lymphadenopathy and hepatosplenomegaly are unusual in aplastic anemia. The roentgenographic skeletal changes usually seen in leukemia do not occur in aplastic anemia (202). Bone marrow smears may be confusing because the only cells remaining in the marrow of some children with aplastic anemia are lymphocytes, and the unwary may make the diagnosis of leukemia in such circumstances. Biopsy of the marrow may be rewarding when the aspirate is hypocellular. Infrequently, the two diseases cannot be differentiated initially because a small number of children with acute leukemia present with a hypocellular bone marrow that eventually becomes hypercellular with blasts. Indeed, children with "aplastic anemia" who respond very rapidly to steroid therapy should be suspected of having ALL.

Myeloproliferative and "preleukemic" syndromes are rare in childhood but are part of the differential diagnosis and are discussed in detail in Chapter 34.

Infectious Mononucleosis and Other Viral Infections. Childhood infectious mononucleosis and other viral illnesses can masquerade as leukemia. Patients may have generalized lymphadenopathy, splenomegaly, skin rash, fevers, and peripheral blood lymphocytosis. This differential diagnosis is particularly difficult in the rare patient with a viral illness whose disease is complicated by thrombocytopenic purpura or immunohemolytic anemia. The presence of a positive mononucleosis spot test or the detection of antibodies to Epstein-Barr virus is helpful in establishing the correct diagnosis. In addition, the morphology of the young lymphocytes seen in infectious mononucleosis and other viral diseases is usually distinguishable from that of lymphoblasts. The viral lymphocytes are larger than normal lymphocytes, are pleomorphic in size and shape, and have pale blue and often vacuolated cytoplasm; these atypical cells are admixed with normal lymphocytes. Usually, these diseases can be differentiated without a bone marrow aspiration, but the procedure is sometimes necessary for accurate diagnosis.

Leukemoid Reactions and Sepsis-Induced Neutropenia. Some diseases unrelated to a malignant blood dyscrasia may occasionally be associated with a peripheral white blood count of greater than 50,000 cells per mm^3 and/or immature granulocytic precursors in the peripheral blood (leukemoid reaction) (203, 204). Bacterial infections, acute hemolysis, granulomatous disease (tuberculosis, sarcoidosis, and histoplasmosis), vasculitis, and metastatic tumor to the marrow all have been associated with leukemoid reactions. Bone marrow aspirates show myeloid hyperplasia with normal maturation. Bacterial sepsis, in addition to causing a leukemoid reaction, may cause profound neutropenia. In this circumstance, the bone marrow picture may be confusing. There may be a transient "maturation arrest" of the granulocyte precursors at the promyelocyte stage associated with toxic granulation. This morphologic picture has been confused with that of acute promyelocytic leukemia. With treatment of the sepsis, normal granulocyte maturation returns. In general, the diagnosis of leukemia is strongly suggested when a so-called leukemic hiatus exists in the peripheral smear. This hiatus is characterized by the presence of blasts and mature forms in the blood with few, if any, intermediate forms present.

TREATMENT

The symptoms of acute leukemia are due to accumulation of poorly differentiated hematopoietic or lymphoid blast cells that arise from leukemic progenitors and invade organs, particularly marrow, blood, liver, spleen, and the central nervous system. Fatal pancytopenia results from marrow replacement and probably from suppression of the development of normal hematopoietic progenitors (20). The purpose of therapy is to eradicate the invading leukemic cells and their progenitors while preserving the expression of normal progenitors.

General Treatment

THE FIRST DAY

From the time of diagnosis, the most critical issues of management pertain to complications of the leukemic cell burden. The major clinical problems are metabolic and those complications resulting from leukemic infiltration of nonhematopoietic organs. Issues pertaining to hemorrhagic and infectious complications are discussed further on under Supportive Care.

Metabolic Complications. Life-threatening and other serious metabolic complications of acute leukemia result from both spontaneous and chemotherapeutically induced leukemic cell lysis. The latter may result in hyperuricemia, hyperkalemia, hyperphosphatemia with concomitant hypocalcemia, and hyperphosphaturia (205).

Elevated serum levels and increased urinary excretion of uric acid result from increased cell lysis, release of deoxyribonucleic acid (DNA), and accelerated intrahepatic purine catabolism. Massive release of intracellular nucleic acids and their conversion to uric acid may result in precipitation of uric acid in the renal collecting system and the ureters. This occurs most frequently when the urine is concentrated and acidic. Careful hydration and alkalinization of the urine with bicarbonate, together with administration of allopurinol prior to chemotherapy, help avert this complication. Allopurinol treatment should be discontinued after the leukemic cell burden is decreased because it perturbs the pharmacology of some chemotherapeutic agents.

Abnormalities of potassium and calcium metabolism have been reported during remission induction (205, 206). Potassium is released from lysed cells, but the resultant hyperkalemia is usually not a threat unless there is concomitant decreased renal function. However, cardiac arrest due to hyperkalemia has been reported following the institution of chemotherapy for childhood ALL (206). Hypokalemia also may occur, especially in patients in relapse (207). The rapid breakdown of leukemic cells also causes hyperphosphatemia with secondary hypocalcemia (205). In addition, drugs such as cyclophosphamide or vincristine (208, 209) induce inappropriate secretion of antidiuretic hormone, and certain antibiotics sometimes result in hypokalemia (210).

Hyperleukocytosis. In patients with markedly elevated peripheral white blood counts, usually greater than $100,000/mm^3$, blood flow in the microcirculation can be impeded by intravascular clumping or plugging by the poorly deformable blasts (211, 212). This may result in local hypoxemia, endothelial damage, hemorrhage, and infarction. Any organ can show pathologic evidence of leukostasis, but clinical symptomatology is usually related to the CNS and lung. Leukostasis is most common in patients with AML, but has been reported in ALL (213). Treatment consists of the immediate institution of therapy that will result in rapid cytoreduction. This can be accomplished with standard remission induction agents or with hydroxyurea (214). In some patients, the response to chemotherapy may be delayed, whereas in others it is difficult to begin chemotherapy because of severe metabolic problems or renal insufficiency. In the latter, emergency leukapheresis has been utilized to stabilize or lower the white blood cell count (see Chapter 51). One should administer red blood cell transfusions cautiously to avoid increasing whole blood viscosity and worsening symptoms.

Leukemic Infiltration of Organs. Extensive leukemic infiltrates in the bowel, liver, spleen, and lymph nodes usually cause little morbidity at the time of presentation. Skeletal infiltration may cause bone pain, and kidney infiltration can lead to renal failure. In addition, infiltration of the mediastinal structures may cause life-threatening tracheobronchial or cardiovascular compression. Prompt application of systemic chemotherapy or local irradiation is necessary to deal with such emergencies. A second cause of respiratory distress at presentation is pulmonary leukostasis, which has been reported in patients with hyperleukocytic granulocytic leukemias (215).

Leukemic Infiltration of the Central Nervous System. Clinical symptoms of CNS leukemia (leptomeningeal involvement) are rare at the time of diagnosis. When they do occur, signs and symptoms may include headache, vomiting, meningismus, and cranial nerve palsies. Lumbar puncture is indicated for diagnostic and therapeutic purposes when CNS symptoms are present. At the time of the procedure, intrathecal methotrexate or cytosine arabinoside should be administered (216, 217). Cranial irradiation should be added in the event of a cranial nerve palsy.

Leukemic invasion of the optic nerve or retina or both at the time of presentation is rare, but when either exists, immediate radiation therapy and intrathecal chemotherapy are indicated to prevent blindness (157, 158). Compression of the spinal cord by masses of leukemic cells, especially in AML, may cause paraplegia—again demanding immediate radiotherapeutic intervention.

THE FIRST MONTH

Generally, no more than 24 hours are necessary to control the urgent problems associated with hemorrhage, metabolic imbalances, and complications of extensive leukemic infiltration of organs. Antileukemic chemotherapy should be begun without delay.

The introduction of combination chemotherapy has been one of the most important contributions to the improved prognosis of childhood leukemia (Fig. 33–1). The rationale for chemotherapy and the mode of action of individual chemotherapeutic agents are discussed in detail in Chapter 32 and will be treated very briefly here, with emphasis on clinical applications. Three pharmacologic principles that underlie the choice and scheduling of *combinations* of agents must be emphasized. First, particular combinations of active drugs are chosen because each of the drugs in the combination attacks leukemic cells by different mechanisms, including cell cycle–specific agents that kill cells in the process of DNA synthesis and cell cycle–independent agents that kill resting cells (129, 218–220). In ideal combinations, the drugs should not exhibit additive toxicity. This permits administration of each drug at *full dose* without intolerable side effects. Reduction of a particular drug dose to avoid toxicity may destroy the therapeutic value of the combination. Finally, the *schedule* is as important as the choice of drugs. Chemotherapeutic drugs are cytotoxic agents. They kill or inhibit the growth of both leukemic and normal progenitors and precursors. The relative sensitivities and the recovery rates of leukemic and normal cells may differ, and the extent of these differences establishes the therapeutic:toxic ratio. Failure to maintain a schedule permits resurgence of leukemic cells and development of resistant clones.

Acute Lymphoblastic Leukemia (ALL)

Therapy is divided into three phases: remission induction, central nervous system prophylaxis, and treatment in remission.

REMISSION INDUCTION

The initial phase of treatment, remission induction, is designed to reduce the leukemic cell burden to a clinically and hematologically undetectable level. Complete remission is the absence of clinical signs and symptoms of disease and the presence of normal blood counts and a normocellular bone marrow with 5 per cent or fewer blasts. There is no evidence, however, that clinical disappearance of leukemic cells is indicative of their total eradication or, more particularly, of the eradication of their progenitors. Indeed, the latter cell population is quite likely to be much more resistant to the agents used in remission induction than are the actively metabolizing precursors themselves. The rapid return of hematopoiesis following remission induction could indicate excellent preservation of progenitor pools (both normal and leukemic) during this early stage of treatment.

Clinical trials have demonstrated that combinations of two agents have been consistently superior to single agents for inducing complete remission in children with ALL. The most effective combination has been vincristine and prednisone because (1) individually these drugs are active as single agents; (2) their toxicity is not additive, so that they can be given at full dose; and (3) they are not myelosuppressive. Thus, vincristine and prednisone can produce complete remission in more than 90 per cent of pediatric patients with ALL (221). Older patients, individuals with morphologically undifferentiated leukemia, and those with T cell disease remain relatively resistant to this induction therapy. For these populations, the addition of a third drug may be indicated. In various clinical trials, three or more agents have been used during initial treatment (222, 223). The improved outcome for children treated with these combinations suggests a therapeutic advantage for early intensive therapy for all patients with ALL.

Attempts have been made to correlate pretreatment cytokinetic measurements with the ultimate outcome of therapy. However, such measurements are of uncertain value (224, 225), and it is unclear whether the fraction of cells in DNA synthesis (probably a function of the leukemic cell renewal rate) correlates either with susceptibility of these cells to cytolysis or with prognosis. Because progenitor kinetics are not measured in such studies,

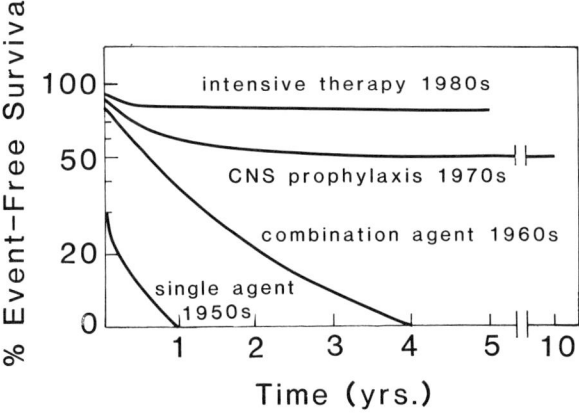

Figure 33–1. Historical perspective of the treatment of childhood acute lymphoblastic leukemia. The single-agent era resulted in few complete remissions and no cures. The combination-agent era resulted in high complete remission rates but nearly uniform mortality. Between the mid 1960's and mid 1970's, combination chemotherapy and CNS prophylaxis resulted in prolonged, disease-free survival for approximately 50 per cent of children.

their prognostic value must be fairly limited. However, in one treatment program, prolonged disease-free survival occurred more frequently in children who had very rapid initial cytoreduction and who entered complete remission within 1 month (129).

If strict attention to detail is maintained, the initial course of patients with ALL is usually relatively uncomplicated from the time of diagnosis until the time of complete remission 3 to 4 weeks thereafter. Exceptions are patients who develop infections during periods of granulocytopenia and those who develop metabolic complications during induction.

CNS PROPHYLAXIS

This phase of antileukemic treatment became an integral component of ALL therapy when CNS sequestration of leukemic cells became evident (226) and the pattern of systemic relapse following the appearance of CNS disease strongly suggested that recurrence was due to reseeding of leukemia cells from the CNS to the bone marrow (99). Therefore, it was postulated that early eradication of these cells (CNS "prophylaxis") might result in prolonged disease-free survival.

Several CNS prophylaxis treatment regimens have been employed, including the use of intrathecal drugs (220), moderate and high doses of systemically administered drugs (227–229), craniospinal irradiation (230), and combinations of intrathecal drugs and cranial irradiation (230, 231).

Since the institution of routine CNS prophylaxis, the incidence of CNS leukemia as a primary site of relapse has been reduced from more than 50 per cent (230) to 5 to 10 per cent (220, 227, 229, 231, 232). The introduction of this phase of therapy has unequivocally increased the numbers of long-term disease-free survivors of childhood ALL and constituted a major therapeutic advance (232a). The promising results of prophylaxis without cranial irradiation (220) and the late effects of combined modality treatment may necessitate a reappraisal of the "optimal" method of CNS prophylaxis. Specifically, patients at low risk of CNS relapse may require less intensive prophylactic therapy (232). It should be emphasized that CNS prophylaxis results must be interpreted in the context of the overall treatment results.

The failure of previous efforts to control CNS leukemic relapse completely has led to new approaches, particularly in patients at increased risk for CNS leukemia. For example, it has been demonstrated that the use of intrathecal drugs administered into the lumbar subarachnoid space results in lower and less predictable concentrations of drug in the ventricular fluid (233). These findings furnished a rationale for the use of drugs administered via intraventricular reservoirs (220). However, long-term evaluation of patients treated in this manner failed to show a clinical advantage over those treated with lumbar subarachnoid-administered drugs. Further exploration of modes of CNS therapy has included the investigation of high doses of systemically administered drugs, such as methotrexate (227–229) and cytosine arabinoside (234, 235), as well as pharmacokinetically derived drug dosage regimens (236). At the same time that these chemotherapeutic approaches have met with success, the morbidity of craniospinal irradiation became apparent. Patients undergoing craniospinal irradiation experienced increased immunosuppression and infections (237), and significant amounts of vertebral body bone marrow had been irradiated, resulting in increased myelosuppression and subsequent inability to deliver full therapeutic doses of systemic drugs.

The presence of symptoms or signs referable to the CNS warrants an immediate lumbar puncture. Although some neurologists are reluctant to carry out lumbar puncture in individuals with classic signs of increased intracranial pressure because of fear of uncal herniation, experience indicates that this procedure is quite safe in the leukemic patient because the increased pressure is evenly distributed throughout the cerebrospinal fluid rather than caused by a mass exerting pressure above the tentorium. If deemed necessary, computed tomography can be performed prior to the lumbar puncture and a determination of pressure on the cerebral ventricles can be made prior to the procedure.

OTHER EXTRAMEDULLARY "PROPHYLAXIS"

Because of the variable incidence of occult testicular involvement in patients still receiving chemotherapy, some investigators have advocated the use of prophylactic gonadal irradiation. Presymptomatic testicular irradiation therapy significantly decreases the incidence of testicular relapse (238), but because testicular involvement is rarely an isolated event, such prophylaxis may not influence life span and the irradiation causes permanent sterility. The development of male secondary sexual characteristics is thought to be unimpaired because the testosterone-secreting Leydig cells are considered to be relatively radioresistant (118). It must be noted that the low incidence of testicular relapse in some studies that do not include testicular irradiation (223, 239) suggests that routine gonadal irradiation is not necessarily justified. The conflicting findings among various groups are probably due to differences in treatment programs. This emphasizes that the course of leukemia must be reviewed in the context of particular treatment regimens.

Testicular biopsies performed at the time of cessation of antileukemic chemotherapy for ALL demonstrated histologic damage mainly to germinal cells, although thickening of the tunica propria of the seminiferous tubules also was commonly found. These findings occurred independent of the patient's age at diagnosis and in the absence of endocrinologic abnormalities (240).

TREATMENT IN REMISSION

General Considerations. Following remission induction and CNS prophylaxis, treatment in remission is begun. In many trials, this consists of intensive, multidrug therapy of variable duration (222, 223, 241), followed by "continuation," or "maintenance," therapy. The rationale for treatment in remission is based on historical studies in which therapy was discontinued immediately (242) or 6 months (243) after induction of remission. In both studies, relapse rapidly followed discontinuation. Presumably, the failure was due to the growth of residual leukemic cells not destroyed during the remission induction phase or the resurgence of progenitors that were only partially affected. Therapeutic research now focuses on optimal combinations and doses of chemotherapeutic agents that will most effectively kill leukemic blasts and their progenitors, spare normal marrow, and preserve the patient's immune response.

Clinical Application. The use of two or more drugs, either continuously or intermittently, produces prolonged disease-free survival for at least 40 to 50 per cent of those who enter complete remission (129, 220, 222, 223, 244) (Fig. 33–2), but several uncertainties have arisen, including the choice of appropriate drugs and schedules for administration. Continuation therapy usually consists of daily administration of 6-mercaptopurine and weekly methotrexate (223, 244). An early, randomized study that compared a two-drug maintenance regimen (methotrexate and 6-mercaptopurine) to a three- or four-drug combination (the aforementioned drugs plus cyclophosphamide and cytosine arabinoside) failed to confirm the value of the addition of the third and fourth drugs (244). However, trials that include three-drug induction, early intensification with multiple agents, and four-drug continuation therapy appear to result in improved disease-free survival (222, 223, 241). A comparison of clinical trials for childhood ALL conducted during the 1970's has been reported (245), but results of subsequent trials are too immature for meaningful interpretation.

Immunotherapy. Some clinics have investigated nonspecific immunotherapy as part of remission maintenance programs (246). The various approaches have been designed to enhance the antileukemic cytotoxic capacity of the host cellular immune system and to lend support to chemotherapeutically compromised immune function. With a single exception in a childhood ALL treatment program (247), the results of multiple trials

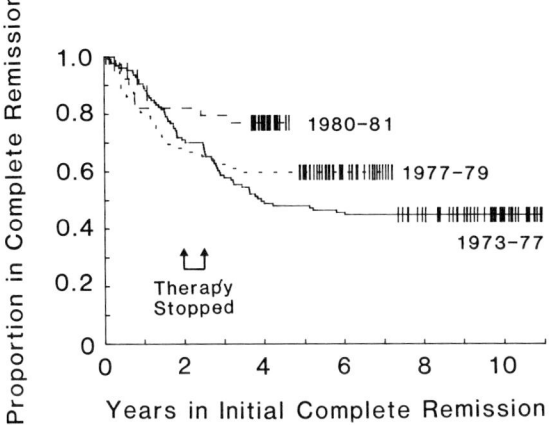

Figure 33–2. The impact of therapy in childhood ALL. The curves demonstrate the proportion of children with acute lymphoblastic leukemia that remain in initial complete remission in three separate programs at The Children's Hospital and The Dana-Farber Cancer Institute, Boston, as of October, 1984. Tick marks represent individual patients. The curve drops with any relapse or death in remission. The regimens have been reported in references 129, 222, and 245, and have been updated in reference 241.

utilizing various forms of nonspecific immunotherapy, such as bacille Calmette-Guerin (BCG) vaccine and allogeneic tumor cells, have produced no obvious therapeutic benefits in the treatment of childhood leukemia.

The development of monoclonal antibodies to leukemia-associated antigenic sites (59) led to therapeutic trials of serotherapy. Patients in relapse were treated by the intravenous injection of monoclonal antibodies, but the clinical outcome was disappointing (248). Problems encountered included the modulation of the antigens from the cell surface and ineffective cytolysis. More promising use of antileukemic antibodies has emerged from their in vitro application to autologous bone marrow in the course of transplantation (249, 249a). Finally, such antibodies may be used as leukemia cell–specific therapy-delivery vehicles (250).

CESSATION OF THERAPY

An important observation has been that chemotherapy need not be continued indefinitely. In deciding to prolong treatment, one must consider both the acute and the cumulative effects of antileukemic drugs—infection, carcinogenicity, brain and other organ toxicity, and psychosocial debilitation—versus the risk of reemergence of leukemia after drugs are stopped. At present, the optimal duration of therapy remains unknown, in part because of inability to assess minimal residual disease, including both leukemic blasts and their progenitors. A major contribution of the discovery of the monoclonal antibody against CALLA may be its use in determining residual leukemic cells in the marrow by means of a radioimmunoassay.

The ability to assay very small numbers of monoclonal cells, otherwise undetectable morphologically, in patients with lymphoma has already been demonstrated (251). It is possible that therapy might be stopped in CALLA-positive patients when CALLA-positive cells are no longer detectable in the marrow. Such a decision would, of course, rest on the assumption that the CALLA-positive cells are not sequestered elsewhere and on the further assumption that the progenitors of CALLA-positive leukemic blasts are detectable with the antibody. An additional approach to the evaluation of minimal residual disease involves the serial assessment of biochemical markers, such as terminal deoxynucleotidyl transferase, in patients who are in remission (81, 252).

Logic dictates that the optimal duration of treatment must depend on the nature of the therapeutic program at its inception. If a particular program kills leukemic blasts and progenitors so completely that resistant populations of cells cannot emerge, the duration of treatment can be much shorter and achieve the same, if not better, results than a considerably less aggressive program that suppresses, but does not eradicate, the disease. In treatment programs at the Dana-Farber Cancer Institute and The Children's Hospital in Boston, treatment for ALL is stopped after 2 years. In earlier studies of ALL, 25 per cent of patients relapsed following cessation of therapy, resulting in apparent cure in over 40 per cent of patients (231). More recent and intensive therapy programs result in fewer relapses during and after discontinuation of treatment (241).

Clinical trials that randomized treatment durations and evaluated outcome for children with ALL have led to equivocal results. One such study found that disease-free survival was improved, especially for boys, if treatment was for 5 rather than 3 years (253). However, as previously noted, changes in therapy, such as early intensive chemotherapy, may confound such observations. Investigators at St. Jude Children's Research Hospital found that 20 per cent of children with ALL relapsed after therapy was stopped following 2½ to 3 years of continuous complete remission (254). The majority of relapses occurred within 1 year after cessation of chemotherapy, and no relapses occurred in patients followed for more than 4 years after cessation (255). All such findings must be tempered by anecdotal reports of relapses occurring from 10 to 15 years after cessation of therapy (256, 256a).

RELAPSED ALL

Most patients who relapse have a grave prognosis. However, factors such as the duration of first remission, whether relapse occurred during or after cessation of therapy, and the site of relapse may have some predictive value in determining the outcome of subsequent therapy.

Relapse After Cessation of Therapy. Children who relapse more than 6 to 12 months after cessation of therapy have a somewhat better prognosis than those who relapse while receiving drugs (255). Of the former group, almost all reenter complete remission, and a few have actually stopped treatment for a second time (257).

The majority of relapses first appear in the bone marrow, although an increasing percentage of them have been found in the testes (238, 254, 258, 259). Relapse at any site must be presumed to be associated with systemic reseeding of leukemic cells. Therefore, patients with clinically localized relapses must be treated both locally and systemically.

It is unusual for children who have received adequate CNS prophylaxis to have a primary CNS relapse after cessation of therapy. However, if a bone marrow relapse occurs after cessation of therapy, the patient is again as susceptible to CNS relapse as he was at the time of diagnosis. Therefore, CNS reprophylaxis is recommended (257). However, this should not include reirradiation because of the risk of CNS damage. It is particularly important to avoid irradiation for reprophylaxis in patients for whom bone marrow transplantation is contemplated.

Relapse During Therapy. Relapses that occur during maintenance combination chemotherapy are presumed to be due to the emergence of a resistant clone of leukemic cells. The mechanisms of clinical resistance to most of the antileukemic drugs are poorly understood. Exceptions include methotrexate resistance, which may occur because of an increase in dihydrofolate reductase activity (260) or a decrease in drug transport (261), and cytosine arabinoside resistance, which results from induction of drug-inactivating cytidine deaminase (262) or deletion of the activating enzyme deoxycytidine kinase (263, 264).

Patients who experience bone marrow relapse while on chemotherapy have a particularly grave prognosis (265, 266). Most patients who have ALL can readily be induced into a second remission; however, the duration of these remissions is generally less than 1 year, and long-term remissions are infrequent.

Extramedullary Relapse. Although signs and symptoms of extramedullary leukemia may occur at any site, the CNS and testes are the most common sites. The so-called isolated extramedullary relapse should be considered as a localized manifestation of systemic leukemia, and treatment of extramedullary relapse should always include systemic therapy as well as local therapy.

As shown in Figure 33–3, CNS relapse has a major adverse impact on survival in ALL (267,

267a), especially when relapses occur following CNS prophylaxis (268). Treatments for CNS relapse, including the use of intrathecal (269), intraventricular (270), or high-dose systemic (235, 270a) drugs or craniospinal irradiation (271), not only have been relatively ineffective but also often result in severe and chronic CNS morbidity among the survivors (272).

Like CNS leukemia, testicular involvement probably arises as a metastatic phenomenon in a "sanctuary" area, and its frequency is directly proportional to the duration of survival (99, 120). The incidence of testicular relapse varies from as low as 5 to 9 per cent to as high as 13 to 40 per cent (238, 258, 259, 273).

Although "late" testicular relapses, especially those that occur after the elective cessation of therapy (258, 273), have a relatively favorable prognosis compared with late hematologic relapses (259), testicular relapses can be of ominous prognostic importance when they occur while the patients are receiving chemotherapy (258, 259). The median time to testicular relapse is 36 months, with a range of 3 to 66 months, and is on the shorter end of the spectrum in patients with initially elevated white blood counts (99). Testicular relapse may also be more likely to occur if the initial platelet count was less than 100,000 cells per mm^3 (273, 274). Unless systemic therapy is reinstituted, bone marrow relapse follows testicular relapse with a median interval of 1 to 6 months (122, 275).

The occurrence of testicular relapse appears to be temporally bimodal (238, 239). Early testicular relapse occurs in T cell disease and may be explained by the propensity of T lymphoblasts to migrate to extramedullary sites (49). The generally less successful treatment of T cell leukemia and its pattern of early relapse suggest that late testicular relapse occurs mainly in patients with non T cell leukemia, but it can also occur in patients with B cell ALL (276). Testicular relapse in AML may be more common in patients with monocytic or myelomonocytic disease. This pattern of failure, analogous to that seen in T cell ALL, suggests that the leukemic monocyte also may have a propensity for extramedullary migration.

The pathophysiology of testicular relapse is unknown. It has been postulated that chemotherapeutic agents may not reach maximum concentration in the testes because of a "blood-gonad barrier." However, the fact that testicular relapse responds to systemic chemotherapy tends to refute this theory. The influence of body temperature on chemotherapeutic efficacy remains questionable: Testicular leukemia has occurred in a descended testis with sparing of a cryptorchid testis (277), as well as in the cryptorchid testis with sparing of the descended testis (278).

Bone Marrow Transplantation for Relapsed ALL. Bone marrow transplantation is the preferred alternative to chemotherapy for patients with ALL and AML who have had a bone marrow relapse while receiving chemotherapy. Except for anecdotal reports (266, 266a, 279), transplantation has been the only modality that has resulted in long-term disease-free survival for such patients. Controversy exists whether transplantation is indicated for patients whose initial relapse during therapy occurs at an extramedullary site. However, long-term follow-up data suggest that although prolonged survival can occur after a CNS relapse, "cure" is elusive when conventional treatment modalities are employed (267, 268). Whether bone marrow transplantation will result in a better prognosis remains uncertain.

Approximately 25 per cent of patients with ALL transplanted either in second or subsequent remission have prolonged, leukemia-free survival, compared with 10 to 15 per cent of those transplanted in relapse (280). An advantage of transplantation in second remission, as opposed to third or subsequent remission, also has been suggested (281). The reasons for this improvement include a healthier host, a lower number of leukemia cells, and transplantation at a time in the course of disease when drug resistance is less likely. Eighty per cent of failures in ALL are due to leukemic relapse. This finding suggests that a single exposure to high-dose cyclophosphamide and total body irradiation, the "standard" pretransplantation treatment regimen, is insufficient to eradicate the aberrant progenitors and precursors in most children with relapsed ALL.

The progressively diminishing likelihood of reinducing complete remissions after repeated re-

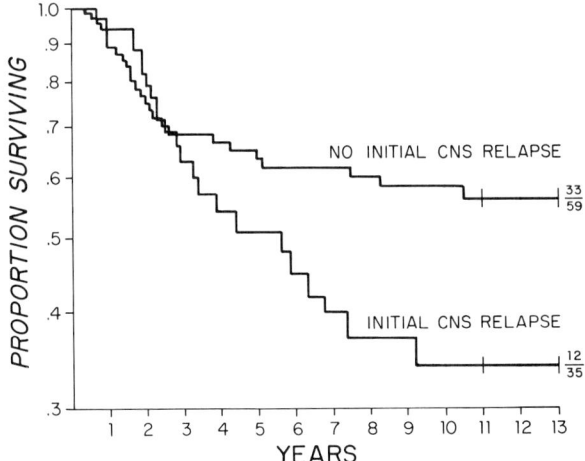

Figure 33–3. The impact of central nervous system relapse in childhood ALL. (Data shown are from St. Jude Children's Research Hospital, Memphis, TN, and used with the permission of Dr. Joseph Simone.)

lapses mitigates in favor of transplantation in second remission. The possible exceptions to this recommendation are patients whose initial relapse occurred after a prolonged initial remission and late after the cessation of therapy. Patients who relapse after transplantation can be retreated with chemotherapy, but their prognosis is extremely grave.

Patients with relapsed CALLA-positive ALL, as well as those with AML or T cell ALL who do not have allogeneic donors may undergo autologous transplantation. By the use of immunologic (249, 249a) and pharmacologic (282, 282a) purging of autologous marrow in vitro, the option of the transplantation modality of treatment has vastly expanded the potential recipient population. Interestingly, long-term disease-free survival following autologous transplantation appears to be about 30 per cent, the same as that achieved in allogeneic transplantation in second remission.

PROGNOSIS

The likelihood of long-term survival for a child with ALL in 1970 was less than 10 per cent and by 1986 approached 70 per cent. This major but incomplete improvement resulted from an unraveling of the clinical and cellular heterogeneity of leukemia, which suggested that, within the generic category of ALL, there are multiple subpopulations of patients with different prognoses and different treatment requirements.

Various clinical and laboratory findings at the time of diagnosis—such as white blood count (283), organ infiltration (especially spleen, liver, thymus, and lymph nodes) (283), lymphoblast morphology and cytochemistry (284, 285), sex (286, 287), age (288), race (283, 289), and immunoglobulin levels (290)—have been correlated with prognosis. Although the relative importance, if any, of a given factor varies among treatment programs (223, 239, 291, 292), certain features appear to be consistently valuable. The latter are measures of total leukemic cell burden, especially white blood count. Certain groups of patients, such as those less than 1 year old at diagnosis, have poor outcomes irrespective of treatment regimens (241, 293, 293a). For the latter group, differences in the biology of the leukemic cells and/or the host have been postulated.

The addition of more sophisticated laboratory measures such as cell surface antigens (see Table 33–1) and cytogenetics (see Chapter 43) have further elucidated the heterogeneity of the childhood acute leukemias and emphasized the relative long-term responses in various subsets of patients. The concomitant appreciation of biologic markers of disease and improved treatment programs has resulted in a continual reappraisal of all prognostic factors. Modern chemotherapy programs that treat such subgroups with different drug programs based on the clinical and laboratory characteristics at the time of diagnosis have made comparisons of treatment programs quite difficult.

Table 33–4. PROGNOSTIC FACTORS IN CHILDHOOD ACUTE LYMPHOBLASTIC LEUKEMIA (ALL)

Factors	Standard Risk	High Risk
WBC	$<50,000/mm^3$	$>50,000/mm^3$
Age	2–9 years	<2 or >9 years
Organ involvement (liver/spleen)	0 to +	++ to +++
Thymic mass	Absent	Present
CNS involvement	Absent	Present
Chromosomal translocation	Absent	Present (?)
Surface markers		
T cell	−	+
Mature B cell	−	+
Pre B cell	−	?
CALLA	+	−
Undifferentiated	−	+

Although much overlap exists among the individual prognostic factors, a summary is shown in Table 33–4.

Early programs of less intensive chemotherapy demonstrated that patients with T cell ALL responded poorly to a therapeutic program that was quite effective for non T cell patients (239). Subsequently, more intensive regimens have obviated such findings (241). Thus, treatment, per se, may be an important prognostic factor, and all prognostic factors should be considered protocol-specific. Clinical trials to establish the most effective and least morbid therapies must be designed with great caution to ensure that in the course of protecting patients from treatment toxicity one does not jeopardize the likelihood for cure.

One perplexing clinical presentation is that of "lymphoma-leukemia." The distinction between leukemia and lymphoma is often made on a rather arbitrary basis. The diagnostic criteria usually pertain to the extent of bone marrow involvement and the degree of organ infiltration. Because children with lymphoma-like presentation of leukemia often respond poorly to treatment (129), interpretations of results of different leukemia and lymphoma treatment programs must be influenced by the entry criteria used in individual institutions.

Acute Myelogenous Leukemia (AML)

Since the 1960s, progress in the treatment of children with AML has not equalled the advances discussed in the management of childhood ALL. However, new chemotherapeutic strategies, better supportive care, and bone marrow transplantation have resulted in an increase in the overall survival for children with AML. As in ALL, therapy is divided into remission induction, CNS prophylaxis, and continuation therapy.

REMISSION INDUCTION

The effective chemotherapeutic agents in AML have a narrow therapeutic index. Therefore, the drug doses that are necessary to kill myeloid leukemic blasts cause marked bone marrow hypoplasia. The normal multipotent myeloid progenitors in the marrow must have the ability to recover more rapidly than their leukemic counterparts in order to attain a complete remission. With rare exceptions, complete remission in AML involves repopulation of the marrow by normal stem cells. This is supported by the restoration of a normal karyotype in marrow cells and normal in vitro growth or cultured myeloid colonies after chemotherapy (294).

Approximately 70 to 80 per cent of children with AML achieve complete remission with protocols that include daunomycin or doxorubicin combined with cytosine arabinoside (295). The duration of peripheral pancytopenia during AML induction ranges from 21 to 35 days. Of the 20 to 30 per cent of children who fail to achieve remission, approximately 50 per cent have leukemic blasts refractory to the specific drug regimen, and the others succumb to either leukostasis, bleeding, or infection. The aggressive use of broad-spectrum antibiotics; red blood cell, platelet, and granulocyte transfusions; and cardiorespiratory support by highly experienced clinicians is essential to a successful outcome.

CNS PROPHYLAXIS

Approximately 10 to 30 per cent of children with AML will have their initial relapse detected in the CNS if they do not receive some form of CNS prophylaxis (295–297). In several studies, effective CNS prophylaxis regimens consisted of (1) intrathecal methotrexate or cytosine arabinoside or (2) cranial irradiation and intrathecal methotrexate (297–300). It has not been demonstrated, however, in a prospective clinical trial that children who are treated with CNS prophylaxis have improved leukemia-free survival compared with children who do not receive CNS prophylaxis. The value of CNS prophylaxis may not become apparent until duration of hematologic remission becomes significantly longer. Both children and adults with myelomonocytic or monocytic leukemia are at increased risk for CNS leukemia.

CONTINUATION THERAPY

The principles of treatment in remission in AML are similar to those in ALL, but the strategy differs. Much more intensive treatment appears necessary to achieve prolonged remission durations in AML. Chemotherapy programs that did not induce severe myelosuppression resulted in fewer than 30 per cent of children remaining in remission for 2 or more years. The addition of nonspecific immunotherapeutic agents, such as BCG, have failed to increase remission durations (301).

Clinical studies employing 1 year of intensive sequential combination chemotherapy show an actuarial leukemia-free survival of 40 to 50 per cent for children with AML who achieve complete remission (300). As in ALL, the optimal duration of treatment is unknown but must depend on the nature of the therapeutic program at its inception.

BONE MARROW TRANSPLANTATION

An alternative therapeutic approach after remission is achieved is bone marrow transplantation from an HLA-identical donor. Reports suggest that 50 to 60 per cent of children with AML who were treated by bone marrow grafting soon after the chemotherapeutic induction of complete remission are surviving free of leukemia for 5 or more years (302–304). Although this yield seems slightly higher than that achieved with chemotherapy, the transplanted patient pool does not include infants with monocytic leukemia. The chemotherapy pool does include these patients, and they do poorly. Graft-versus-host disease and interstitial pneumonia account for the majority of deaths in the transplanted group. This is in contrast to the transplantation experience for second-remission ALL, in which recurrent leukemia is the major cause of failure following marrow grafting.

Whether children with AML who do have donors should be transplanted as soon as they enter remission or whether they should first receive a trial of intensive chemotherapy and be transplanted only if they relapse remains uncertain. Bone marrow transplantation does offer the chance of long-term leukemia-free survival for as many as 30 per cent of children grafted in early second remission (305). We therefore recommend the procedure as a second approach for patients who fail chemotherapy.

There are some groups of children, such as those with therapy-linked preleukemia or leukemia with monosomy 7, who are very unlikely to achieve a complete remission with chemotherapy (306). For these children, perhaps bone marrow transplantation should be the initial therapeutic approach.

Additional trials of marrow grafting, intensive chemotherapy, and longer follow-up evaluation will be needed before the most advantageous treatment modality becomes certain. Appropriate determination of histocompatibility should be performed in all family members of children with AML so that options can be established and potentially hazardous transfusions from donors or family members excluded.

PROGNOSIS

There have been no consistently observed clinical or laboratory features that predict for duration of remission in children with AML. A preleukemic syndrome or monosomy 7 or both predict for a low likelihood of remission. In one study, a large spleen size (>5 cm) and a high myeloblast-labeling index (>10 per cent at diagnosis) were significantly related to shorter durations of remission (298). In other studies, children with M5 leukemia and those less than 2 years of age had statistically significant shorter durations of remission than patients with other FAB subtypes and those from 2 to 17 years of age (307).

Interpretation of Results of Clinical Trials

The relative efficacy of one treatment program compared with another is determined by analysis of life tables (308), success ratios, and median event-free intervals. These techniques permit the determination of the probability of event-free survival within confidence limits established by the number of patients entered in the analysis and the length of follow-up. All such analyses presume uniform patient entry criteria. However, even within clinically homogeneous subsets of patients, one must assume that there is variability among individuals. Thus, reported successes and failures should include a description of the uncertainty of the results.

The duration of survival after relapse is, in part, a measure of the intensity of chemotherapy and supportive care. Therefore, assessment of the efficacy of a treatment program is more meaningful when event-free (or relapse-free) survival is determined. Because relapse-free survival curves begin at the time of complete remission (and not at diagnosis), it is necessary to know the proportion of patients who enter complete remission. This is of particular importance to the evaluation of AML treatment programs because of the previously noted relatively lower proportion of AML patients who enter complete remission (296, 299, 300). For example, a given maintenance therapy might appear to be much better than it really is if the patients admitted to that maintenance program are selected from low-yield remission induction programs, because such referrals would represent a set of patients whose disease responds relatively easily to therapy.

Supportive Care

HEMORRHAGE

Hemorrhagic manifestations in the child with leukemia are usually due to thrombocytopenia, the differential diagnosis of which includes decreased production (secondary to leukemia or chemotherapy-induced bone marrow hypoplasia, or both), disseminated intravascular coagulation, and septicemia.

Significant visceral bleeding is unusual, and generally the hemorrhagic manifestations are limited to the skin and mucous membranes, in which ecchymoses and petechiae are common. Of grave concern are intracranial hemorrhages secondary to thrombocytopenia or to leukostasis—intravascular clumping of blasts, especially within small vessels of the brain, leading to infarction and hemorrhage (211, 212). The latter appears more commonly in AML than in ALL.

Patients with acute promyelocytic leukemia characteristically present with hemorrhagic manifestations secondary to disseminated intravascular coagulation. The abnormal granules of the promyelocyte contain and release tissue thromboplastins that initiate intravascular clotting (12). For these exceptional patients, prophylactic heparin has been advocated (309), in addition to more conventional supportive care with fresh frozen plasma or procoagulant concentrates and platelets. There is no convincing evidence, however, that heparin improves survival, increases remission rates, or decreases the incidence of CNS bleeding in childhood AML. Ultimately, correction of the disseminated intravascular coagulopathy depends on appropriate treatment of the underlying leukemia.

There is an inverse correlation between the platelet count and the likelihood of hemorrhage in patients with leukemia (310). Control of bleeding due to thrombocytopenia has been achieved by the administration of platelet concentrates donated by ABO-compatible donors (311).

The use of "prophylactic" platelet transfusions in the absence of overt bleeding remains controversial. The theoretical advantage of the use of prophylactic transfusions is avoidance of the morbidity associated with spontaneous bleeding. Randomized studies comparing the use of prophylactic transfusions with therapeutic platelet transfusions have demonstrated that the former either decrease the incidence of bleeding and morbidity (312, 313) or show no effect on morbidity (314). Arguments against prophylactic platelet transfusions are based on the risk of alloimmunization (315) and transmission of hepatitis.

Patients receiving frequent transfusions may become sensitized to HLA or other antigens on platelet surfaces (316). Attempts to reduce alloimmunization by transfusing leukocyte-poor or single-donor platelets have generally been unsuccessful. In most cases of platelet refractoriness, one can accomplish successful platelet transfusions with platelets matched at the HLA-A and HLA-B loci, using family and nonrelated donors (317). Autologous frozen platelets also may be of value in the management of alloimmunized patients (318).

In general, the condition of the patient and the anticipated clinical course should be used as guidelines for platelet transfusions rather than the absolute platelet count. Indications for platelets in the thrombocytopenic patient include fresh bleeding, fever, infection, and anticipated protracted thrombocytopenia as a result of therapy. Platelet transfusions have markedly decreased the incidence of major hemorrhage in patients with acute leukemia. However, the use of these transfusions has resulted in a relative increase in infection as a cause of morbidity and mortality.

INFECTION

Infection due to granulocytopenia is an important early complication of leukemia. Most early infections are presumably bacterial (319), but specific etiologic agents are usually not found. Therefore, any febrile patient with an absolute granulocyte count of less than 500 cells per mm^3 must be considered septic. Cultures should be obtained promptly, and the patient should be begun immediately on broad-spectrum antibiotics with activity against bowel and respiratory organisms. The specific choice of drugs varies among institutions, based in part on local patterns of antibiotic resistance (320).

In addition to bacterial infections, a variety of nonbacterial opportunistic organisms invade the immunosuppressed host (321). Chickenpox complicated by pneumonitis, hepatitis, or cerebritis may be particularly devastating. Treatment has been effective with either vidarabine or acyclovir (322, 323). The latter may also be effective in the treatment of herpes zoster and herpes simplex (324).

Pneumocystis carinii is another organism found to cause severe, often fatal interstitial pneumonitis in children receiving multiagent chemotherapy (325), and rarely this infection may occur at the onset of leukemia. The incidence of *P. carinii* pneumonia may increase in proportion to the number of immunosuppressive antileukemic drugs used (326). Controlled studies of prophylaxis involving trimethoprim-sulfamethoxazole have clearly demonstrated that infection with *P. carinii* can be markedly reduced. The only complications of prophylaxis appear to be increased myelosuppression and a minor increase in oral moniliasis (327). This drug combination is also effective in the prevention and treatment of certain bacterial infections and should be used promptly in children with leukemia who present with interstitial pneumonia and reduced arterial oxygen saturation. With the exception of this drug combination, routine antibiotic prophylaxis during drug-induced granulocytopenia is not recommended.

In the past, invasive fungal infections were an important cause of mortality in children with relapsed leukemia. However, fungal disease has been increasingly observed during the initial treatment of leukemia for several reasons: the use of intensive chemotherapy leading to prolonged periods of neutropenia and immunosuppression; the use of broad-spectrum antibiotics; and the frequent use of central venous catheters. The major fungal pathogens in these patients include *Candida* and *Aspergillus* species. Administration of amphotericin B is the treatment of choice for invasive fungal disease. Its empirical use may also be indicated for patients who are granulocytopenic and remain febrile after 1 week of broad-spectrum antibiotics.

Consequences of Survival

With prolonged survival have come reports of late effects of antileukemic therapy (328). These are related to drugs, radiation therapy, and possible genetic or induced immunologic abnormalities in the host.

Although a list of late effects might include involvement of any organ, the number of patients with organ dysfunction after completing antileukemic therapy is very small. Reports suggest that some patients may be at increased risk of a second malignancy (329). This may be treatment-related or represent a manifestation of impaired host surveillance mechanisms that permit the occurrence of multiple malignancies or autoimmune diseases.

There are several long-term problems associated with CNS prophylaxis. Computed tomographic scans have shown that 50 per cent of tested asymptomatic patients treated with cranial irradiation and intrathecal drugs for ALL have abnormalities, including brain atrophy, ventricular dilatation, and cerebral calcifications (330); however, another study failed to confirm these findings (331). In addition, leukoencephalopathy (332), mineralizing microangiopathy (333), postirradiation somnolence syndrome (334), seizures, and neuropsychiatric problems (335) have been reported. The neuropsychiatric problems are characterized by easy distractibility and minor impairment of memory, which can result in school problems (336). These consequences may be remediable and are not reasons to alter successful programs. Although such findings are often attributed to cranial irradiation, one report showed no difference in neuropsychologic sequelae between patients who did receive such treatment and those who did not (337). Major intellectual deficits are rare in our experience, and their relationship to radiotherapy is yet to be established. It is possible that the use of high doses of systemic chemotherapy and intrathecal drugs in lieu of irradiation may obviate some of these effects, but the costs in terms of CNS relapse and other toxic effects will have to be evaluated. One study that used computerized tomography to evaluate patients who received either systemic and intrathecal methotrexate for CNS prophylaxis or cranial irradiation demonstrated no major differences between the two groups (338). Another trial showed no difference in the incidence of computerized tomography abnormalities between patients who had received cranial irradiation and those who had not (339).

Endocrine function usually has remained normal in children who have completed therapy for ALL (340). Exceptions include the findings of abnormal growth hormone responses, but the effect on linear growth has varied markedly, especially in children treated after the age of 5 years (341–343). Normal sexual development can be expected in girls diagnosed after menarche (344). Sexual maturation in boys is normal, although those who received cyclophosphamide are at risk for spermatogenic dysfunction (345). Successful fatherhood during and following chemotherapy for ALL has been reported (346, 347). The progeny of survivors of childhood leukemia are few, but there has been no excess of offspring with congenital anomalies (348). In young girls, obesity and early onset of menstruation seem to occur with increased frequency.

Late psychiatric effects of surviving life-threatening disease, without the certainty of cure, are being investigated at this time. For the vast majority of patients, regardless of whether or not they do well, leukemia is a long-term problem that requires prolonged follow-up and careful observation. Patients and their families must be counseled in these terms, and the psychologic effects of leukemia on parents and siblings of the affected child suggest that the impact is shared by the entire family (349).

CONGENITAL LEUKEMIA

Incidence. Congenital leukemia (diagnosed from birth to 4 weeks of age) is rare, with just over 100 cases reported to date (350). The majority of patients described had AML, but newborns with ALL have been observed. Leukemia in the newborn period has been associated with Down's syndrome (351–353), Turner's syndrome (354), mosaic monosomy 7 (355), and trisomy 9 (356).

Etiology. The etiology of congenital leukemia, like that of other leukemias, is unknown. No reported cases of congenital leukemia have occurred in infants whose mothers had leukemia before or during pregnancy. Fetal x-ray exposure has not consistently been associated with an increased incidence of leukemia.

Clinical Manifestations. Most neonates with leukemia die within a few days to months after diagnosis. The clinical manifestations are somewhat different from those seen in older infants and children. Approximately 50 per cent of newborns with leukemia have nodular skin infiltrates. These are blue to slate-gray in color and are palpated as fibroma-like tumors of the deep skin (357). Other signs and symptoms in the newborn period include petechiae, purpura, hepatosplenomegaly, lethargy, pallor, and poor feeding. In the past, many infants with leukemia died of respiratory distress, which was thought to be secondary to pulmonary leukostasis.

Laboratory Findings. The laboratory findings are similar to those seen in older children with leukemia. Morphologic, cytochemical, and immunologic data are not available for most of the reported cases of congenital leukemia. The majority of recently reported cases of congenital AML were of the monocytic (FAB-M5) subtype, and all showed leukemia cutis (358). There is frequently complete or partial spontaneous regression of leukemia cutis in newborns with this disease, but this is usually followed in a few weeks by reappearance of skin nodules and bone marrow involvement. Two neonates with ALL were reported in whom the blasts in each case had immunologic markers consistent with the pre B phenotype (359).

Differential Diagnosis. A variety of disorders in the newborn can mimic leukemia. A leukoerythroblastic peripheral blood smear is commonly seen in response to bacterial infection, hypoxemia, or severe hemolysis in the neonate. Other differential diagnoses include congenital syphilis, intrauterine viral diseases, neuroblastoma, and the transient myeloproliferative syndrome associated with Down's syndrome (351). Congenital syphilis is associated with a positive VDRL and abnormal bone marrow. Intrauterine infections may present with chorioretinitis, intracerebral calcifications, congenital defects, positive serologic tests for cytomegalic inclusion disease, rubella, or toxoplasmosis and with normal bone marrow. Neuroblastoma is diagnosed by the findings of elevated urinary catecholamine metabolites, biopsy of the primary tumor, and/or the presence of neuroblastoma cells in the marrow.

Myeloproliferative disorders, described as transient acute leukemia or ineffective regulation of granulopoiesis masquerading as congenital leukemia (360), have been reported in newborns with Down's syndrome and also in several phenotypically normal babies with trisomy 21 mosaicism in either blood cells or skin fibroblasts (361). Myeloproliferative disorders are often clinically and hematologically indistinguishable from congenital AML. In contrast to congenital AML, these disorders are characterized by complete clinical and hematologic recovery within weeks or months of diagnosis without specific antileukemia treatment. The white blood count in infants with these disorders can be markedly elevated, and the peripheral blood may contain up to 95 per cent myeloblasts. The bone marrow may manifest erythroid or myeloid hyperplasia without an increase in blasts or may contain 10 to 60 per cent myeloblasts with a decrease in other hematopoietic precursors.

In one review of neonates with Down's syndrome, half the patients died within 2 weeks to 6 years following diagnosis, but none had evidence of leukemia at autopsy (351). The causes of death were secondary to infectious diseases or congenital cardiac anomalies. On the basis of our current understanding of the clinical course of leukemia, it is doubtful that these infants with Down's syndrome had true congenital leukemia.

The neonate with Down's syndrome and the hematologic and clinical picture of congenital AML presents a major diagnostic and therapeutic dilemma. Because one cannot clinically or biologically identify the group of these infants with true congenital leukemia from those who will have spontaneous regression of their "myeloproliferative disorder," judicious supportive care and clinical monitoring for 3 to 6 weeks constitute the preferred treatment. If clinical or hematologic deterioration ensues, appropriate chemotherapy can be instituted.

Treatment. The treatment of congenital leukemia in the newborn should be identical with that of leukemia occurring in the older child, with the exception of cranial irradiation (which is contraindicated in the newborn because it would limit subsequent brain and skull growth). Because congenital leukemia is rare, treatment reviews are limited to case reports. Thus, the prognosis for the newborn with leukemia remains unknown (362–364). Several newborns with monocytic leukemia have been successfully treated with an epipodophyllotoxin: VP-16 or VM-26 (358).

MANAGEMENT OF THE EMOTIONAL ASPECTS OF LEUKEMIA

Those responsible for the care of the child with leukemia must understand the emotional connotations of the disease and its treatment, be comfortable and skilled with children and their families, and above all know themselves.

The Disease

Substantive therapeutic advances in the past decade have caused "acute" leukemia to become a chronic disease of childhood. The initial treatment of all children with leukemia is given with curative intent. Because such treatment often necessitates discomfort, disfigurement (especially alopecia), and a change in life pattern, it is incumbent upon the physician to convey to the child and family both the intent and the complications of this intensive therapy (365). For the majority of patients, early therapy will result in prolonged complete remission. Often the leukemia itself is perceived as being less problematic than its treatment. This perception may cause patients and their families to seek alternative, unconventional antileukemic therapies from charlatans to obviate the unpleasantness of chemotherapy or transplantation.

The Child

The age of the child is of great importance in the assessment of psychologic issues (366). Children under 5 years old may be particularly concerned about the separation from parents and the painful aspects of treatment. Even older children may be more concerned about being physically assaulted with chemotherapy than about issues of life or death. Regardless of age, most children will express two universal feelings—anger and guilt. "Why did you let this happen to me?" "What did I do wrong to deserve this awful illness?" It is important to learn to listen to what the child means rather than to the content of what is said.

Adolescents with leukemia are a particularly challenging group (367). At their developmental stage they want autonomy and control, yet they are forced into a dependent position because of their illness. Any means of including them in the treatment decision-making process is helpful. They, even more than young children, need complete explanations about the effects of the disease or chemotherapy on their bodies.

Communication with the child and the family should be honest and gentle. Studies of children who survive malignancy underscore the importance of openness, honesty, consistent support, and the maintenance of hope by a primary physician or nurse (368). As soon as the child has begun chemotherapy, every effort should be made to encourage him to return to normal social and physical activities (369, 370). Failure to do so may result in pathologic behavior patterns, such as withdrawal from peers, regression, and school phobia (371). The majority of children with leukemia adjust well to their disease and function like their peers.

The Family

At the time of diagnosis, the clinician and members of the team who will care for the patient, including nurses and social workers, should confer with parents to explain the diagnosis and its significance. Prognosis should be discussed in general terms, and the family should be prepared for the likelihood of coping with a chronic illness as well as the possibility of the child's facing an early death. The initial response of most parents to the diagnosis of leukemia in their child is one of shock. They, like their child, experience strong feelings of anger and guilt: How can this disease strike their child? Are they in some way responsible for the leukemia? After much reassurance, most parents accept and deal with the circumstances quite well. Soon after the diagnosis, the parents have the disagreeable task of telling the child's other relatives, including grandparents, and his or her friends. This task can be eased if the parents are alerted to anticipate the concentric circles of disbelief that grow as more and more people beyond the child's group of close family and friends learn of the illness.

A period of severe psychologic stress has been newly recognized—that immediately preceding the time of elective cessation of therapy. This event usually occurs 1 or more years after diagnosis, at a time when the child and family have adapted to the chemotherapy regimen and life style. Several weeks or months prior to the anticipated time of stopping treatment, parents feel a heightened level of anxiety. In a sense they have developed a "love/hate" relationship with the drugs: They are reassured by their success yet fearful of failure after they are stopped. For many families, this is the second most stressful period, with the first being the time of initial diagnosis. Although the familial stresses caused by leukemia are obviously greater than those for most other families, measures of stability, such as divorce rates, appear to be similar to those of the general population (372).

The Staff

Physicians, nurses, psychologists, social workers, play therapists, dietitians, and other hospital and clinic personnel all have a role in the care of the child with leukemia. All these professionals should be cognizant of classic defense mechanisms such as denial and intellectualization and how they are used in caretaking situations and should be honestly aware of their own feelings. The complete integration of all these individuals into the caretaking team, as well as aids such as teaching seminars for oncology fellows (373, 374), results in more effective care of the patient.

A distressing new phenomenon has appeared in some oncology units. Occasionally, young, inexperienced personnel partially trained in "thanatology" emerge on the ward having learned by rote the "stages of dying" (375) and other systematic approaches to the evaluation of the ill child. Although such education can be advantageous, it is no substitute for sensitivity, understanding, and, above all, experience in direct patient contact.

Also relatively new are feelings of profound shock and disturbance on the part of staff members on leukemia services with respect to unexpected relapses in some children. In an era of high expectations for "cure" in certain favorable-risk groups, long-term event-free survival that is eventually interrupted by relapse in some ways seems more devastating to the staff than the expected failures of patients whose diseases are known from the beginning to be relatively resistant to therapy and for whom expectations are appropriately guarded.

Death, Grief, and Bereavement

Death from leukemia occurs in approximately 50 per cent of the affected children. Several studies have concluded that even very young children have a substantial awareness of the seriousness of their illness and may anticipate their own premature death (376–379). The child becomes more anxious as clinic visits increase in frequency (379), and with each successive hospitalization he or she experiences increasing isolation from both family and staff members (380).

As one relapse follows another, it is incumbent upon the physician to focus on palliation, respect individual wishes, and assure that the child and family will not be abandoned. The last responsibility is of the utmost importance.

The chronicity of leukemia results in the development of close relationships among families, clinicians, and supporting personnel. After the child dies, many families feel lonely, yet they may feel that there is no longer a medical indication to return to the treatment center. The center should "give permission" to families to maintain contact with one another after the child's death. This provides time for people to come to terms with painful feelings. The close attachments between caretakers and families necessitate maintenance of contact following the child's death. Above all, families want to be certain that investigators are making progress in treating leukemia and improving survival rates. Contact with a treatment center over the years gives them some assurance that other children may live because of their child's participation in therapy and that their loss was not entirely in vain.

References

1. Glick, A. D.: Acute leukemia: electron microscopic diagnosis. Semin. Oncol. 3:229, 1976.
2. Polliack, A., Formimovici, M., et al.: Acute lymphoblastic leukemia: a study of 25 cases by scanning electron microscopy. Blut 33:359, 1976.
3. Stass, S. A., Pui, C. H., et al.: Sudan black B positive acute lymphoblastic leukaemia. Br. J. Hematol. 57:413, 1984.
4. Hayhoe, F. G. J., Wintrobe, M. F., et al.: The cytology and cytochemistry of acute leukaemias: a study of 140 cases. London, Her Majesty's Stationery Office, 1964.
5. Catovsky, D., Greaves, M. F., et al.: Acid-phosphatase reaction in acute lymphoblastic leukaemia. Lancet 1:749, 1978.
6. Bennett, J. M., Catovsky, D., et al.: The morphological classification of acute lymphoblastic leukaemia: concordance among observers and clinical correlations. Br. J. Hematol. 47:553, 1981.
7. Gralnick, H. R., Galton, D. A. G., et al.: Classification of acute leukemia. Ann. Int. Med. 87:740, 1977.
8. Preud'homme, J. L., Brouet, J. C., et al.: Acute lympho-

blastic leukemia with Burkitt's lymphoma cells: membrane markers and serum immunoglobulin. J. Natl. Cancer Inst. 66:261, 1981.
9. Berger, R., Bernheim, A., et al.: t(8;14) translocation in a Burkitt's type of lymphoblastic leukaemia (L3). Br. J. Haematol. 43:87, 1979.
10. Stass, S. A., Perlin, E., et al.: Acute lymphoblastic leukemia—hand mirror cell variant: a detailed cytological and ultrastructural study with an analysis of the immunologic surface markers. Am. J. Hematol. 4:67, 1978.
11. Norberg, R., Brand, L., et al.: Hand-mirror blast cells in acute leukemia. Lancet 1:957, 1977.
12. Gralnick, H. R., and Abrell, E.: Studies of the procoagulant and fibrinolytic activity of promyelocytes in acute promyelocytic leukaemia. Br. J. Haematol. 24:89, 1973.
13. den Ottolander, G., TeVelde, J., et al.: Megakaryoblastic leukaemia (acute myelofibrosis): a report of 3 cases. Br. J. Haematol. 42:9, 1979.
14. Quesenberry, P., and Levitt, L.: Hematopoietic stem cells. New Engl. J. Med. 301:755, 1979.
15. Fauser, A. A., and Messner, H. A.: Identification of megakaryocytes, macrophages, and eosinophils in colonies of human bone marrow containing neutrophilic granulocytes and erythroblasts. Blood 53:1023, 1979.
16. Moore, M. A. S., Spitzer, G., et al.: Agar culture studies of 127 cases of untreated acute leukemia: the prognostic value of reclassification of leukemia according to in vitro growth characteristics. Blood 44:1, 1974.
17. Sabbath, K., Ball, E., et al.: Heterogeneity of clonogenic cells in acute myeloblastic leukemia. J. Clin. Invest. 75:746, 1985.
18. Collins, S. J., Ruscetti, F. W., et al.: Terminal differentiation of human promyelocytic leukemia cells induced by dimethyl sulfoxide and other polar compounds. Proc. Natl. Acad. Sci. U.S.A. 75:2458, 1978.
19. Griffin, J., Monroe, D., et al.: Induction of differentiation of human myeloid leukemia cells by inhibitors of DNA synthesis. Exp. Hematol. 10:744, 1982.
20. Morris, T. C. M., McNeill, T. A., et al.: Inhibition of normal in vitro–colony forming cells by cells from leukaemic patients. Br. J. Cancer 31:641, 1975.
21. Broxmeyer, J., Bognacki, J., et al.: Identification of leukemia-associated inhibitory activity as acidic isoferritins. A regulatory role of acidic isoferritins in the production of granulocytes and macrophages. J. Exp. Med. 153:1426, 1981.
22. Metcalf, D.: The clonal cultures in vitro of human leukaemic cells. In Methods in Hematology, vol. 2. Catovsky, E. (ed.), Edinburgh, Churchill-Livingstone, 1981.
23. Dexter, T. M., Allen, T. D., et al.: Conditions controlling the proliferation of haemopoietic stem cells in vitro. J. Cell Physiol. 91:335, 1977.
24. Coulombel, L., Kalousek, D., et al.: Long-term marrow culture reveals chromosomally normal hemopoietic progenitor cells in patients with Ph¹–positive chronic myelogenous leukemia. New Engl. J. Med. 308:1493, 1983.
25. Saunders, E. F., Lampkin, B. C., et al.: Variation of proliferative activity in leukemic cell populations of patients with acute leukemia. J. Clin. Invest. 46:1356, 1967.
26. Fialkow, P. J.: Cell lineages in hematopoietic neoplasia studied with glucose-6-phosphate dehydrogenase cell markers. J. Cell Physiol. 1(suppl):37, 1982.
27. Rowley, J. D.: The cytogenetics of acute leukemia. Clin. Haematol. 7:385, 1978.
27a. Reid, M. M., Tantravahi, R., et al.: Detection of leukemia-related karyotypes in granulocyte/macrophage colonies of a patient with acute myelogenous leukemia. New Engl. J. Med. 308:1324, 1983.
28. Fialkow, P. J., Singer, J. W., et al.: Acute nonlymphocytic leukemia. Expression in cells restricted to granulocytic and monocytic differentiation. New Engl. J. Med. 301:1, 1979.
29. Jacobson, R., Temple, M., et al.: A clonal complete remission in a patient with acute nonlymphocytic leukemia originating in a multipotent stem cell. New Engl. J. Med. 310:1513, 1984.
30. Zuelzer, W. W., Inoue, S., et al.: Long-term cytogenetic studies in acute leukemia of children: the nature of relapse. Am. J. Hematol. 1:143, 1976.
31. Cimino, M. C., Rowley, J. D., et al.: Banding studies of chromosomal abnormalities in patients with acute lymphocytic leukemia. Cancer Res. 39:227, 1979.
32. Fialkow, P., Jacobson, R., et al.: Chronic myelocytic leukemia: clonal origin in a stem cell common to the granulocyte, erythrocyte, platelet, and monocyte/macrophage. Am. J. Med. 63:125, 1977.
33. Fialkow, P. J., Denman, A. M., et al.: Chronic myelocytic leukemia. Origin of some lymphocytes from leukemic stem cells. J. Clin. Invest. 62:815, 1978.
34. Blackstock, A. M., and Garson, O. M.: Direct evidence for involvement of erythroid cells in acute myeloblastic leukaemia. Lancet 2:1178, 1974.
35. Fialkow, P., Singer, J., et al.: Acute nonlymphocytic leukemia: Heterogeneity of stem cell origin. Blood 57:1068, 1981.
36. Fialkow, P. J., Thomas, E. D., et al.: Leukaemic transformation of engrafted human marrow cells in vivo. Lancet 1:251, 1971.
37. Thomas, E. D., Bryant, J. I., et al.: Leukaemic transformation of engrafted human marrow cells in vivo. Lancet 1:1310, 1972.
38. Newburger, P. E., Latt, S., et al.: Leukemic relapse in donor cells after allogeneic bone marrow transplantation. New Engl. J. Med. 304:712, 1981.
39. Marmont, A., Frassoni, F., et al.: Recurrence of a Ph¹-positive leukemia in donor cells after marrow transplantation for chronic granulocytic leukemia. New Engl. J. Med. 310:903, 1984.
40. Dow, L. W., Martin, P., et al.: Evidence for clonal development of childhood acute lymphoblastic leukemia. Blood 66:902, 1985.
41. Chan, L. C., Pegram, S. M., et al.: Contribution of immunophenotype to the classification and differential diagnosis of acute leukaemia. Lancet 1:475, 1985.
42. Link, M., Warnke, R., et al.: A single monoclonal antibody identifies T-cell lineage of childhood lymphoid malignancies. Blood 62:722, 1983.
43. Vodinelich, L., Tax, W., et al.: A monoclonal antibody (WT1) for detecting leukemias of T-cell precursors (T-ALL). Blood 62:1108, 1983.
44. Meuer, S. C., Hussey, R. E., et al.: An alternative pathway of T-cell activation: a functional role for the 50 KD T11 sheep erythrocyte receptor protein. Cell 36:897, 1984.
45. Reinherz, E. L., Kung, P. S., et al.: Discrete stages of human intrathymic differentiation: analysis of normal thymocytes and leukemic lymphoblasts of T lineage. Proc. Natl. Acad. Sci. U.S.A. 77:1588, 1980.
46. Nathan, D. G., Chess, L., et al.: Human erythroid burst-forming unit: T-cell requirement for proliferation in vitro. J. Exp. Med. 147:324, 1978.
47. Golde, D. W., Quan, S. G., et al.: Human T lymphocyte cell line producing colony-stimulating activity. Blood 52:1068, 1978.
48. Broder, S., Poplack, D., et al.: Characterization of a suppressor-cell leukemia: evidence for the requirement of an interaction of two T-cells in the development of human suppressor cells. New Engl. J. Med. 298:66, 1978.
49. Bhan, A. K., Reinisch, C. L., et al.: T-cell migration into allografts. J. Exp. Med. 141:1210, 1975.
50. Lilleyman, J. S., and Sugden, P. J.: T lymphoblastic leukaemia and the central nervous system. Br. J. Cancer 43:320, 1981.
51. Nadler, L. M., Korsmeyer, S. J., et al.: B cell origin of non-T-cell acute lymphoblastic leukemia. A model for discrete stages of neoplastic and normal pre-B cell differentiation. J. Clin. Invest. 74:332, 1984.

52. Schlossman, S. F., Chess, L., et al.: Distribution of Ia-like molecules on the surface of normal and leukemic human cells. Proc. Natl. Acad. Sci. U.S.A. 73:1288, 1976.
53. Janossy, G., Goldstone, A. H., et al.: Differentiation-linked expression of p28,33 (Ia-like) structures on human leukaemic cells. Br. J. Haematol. 37:391, 1977.
54. Newman, R. A., Greaves, M. F.: Characterization of HLA-DR antigens on leukaemic cells. Clin. Exp. Immunol. 50:41, 1982.
55. Korsmeyer, S. J., Arnold, A., et al.: Immunoglobulin gene rearrangement and cell surface antigen expression in acute lymphocytic leukemia of T-cell and B-cell precursor origins. J. Clin. Invest. 71:301, 1983.
56. Vogler, L. B., Crist, W. M., et al.: Pre-B-cell leukemia. A new phenotype of childhood lymphoblastic leukemia. New Engl. J. Med. 298:872, 1978.
57. Greaves, M., Verbi, W., et al.: Antigenic and enzymatic phenotypes of the pre-B subclass of acute lymphoblastic leukaemia. Leuk. Res. 3:353, 1979.
58. Brouet, J. C., Preud'homme, J. L., et al.: Acute lymphoblastic leukemia with pre-B-cell characteristics. Blood 54:269, 1979.
58a. Srivastava, B. I. S., Wright, J. J., et al.: Immunoglobulin chain gene rearrangements in a t(4;11) acute leukaemia with monocytoid blasts. Br. J. Haematol. 63:321, 1986.
59. Ritz, J., Pesando, J. M., et al.: A monoclonal antibody to human acute lymphoblastic leukaemia antigen. Nature 283:583, 1980.
60. Greaves, M. F., Hariri, G., et al.: Selective expression of the common acute lymphoblastic leukemia (gp 100) antigen on immature lymphoid cells and their malignant counterparts. Blood 61:628, 1983.
61. Hokland, P., Nadler, L., et al.: Purification of common acute lymphoblastic leukemia antigen positive cells from normal human bone marrow. Blood 64:662, 1984.
62. Metzgar, R. S., Borowitz, M., et al.: Distribution of the common acute lymphoblastic leukemia antigen in non-hematopoietic tissues. J. Exp. Med. 154:1249, 1981.
63. Ritz, J., Nadler, L. M., et al.: Expression of common acute lymphoblastic leukemia antigen (CALLA) by lymphomas of B-cell and T-cell lineage. Blood 58:648, 1981.
64. Shevach, E. M., Edelson, E., et al.: A human leukemia cell with both B and T cell surface receptors (lymphocytic leukemia: Sézary's syndrome). Proc. Natl. Acad. Sci. U.S.A. 71:863, 1974.
65. Griffin, J., Mayer, R., et al.: Surface marker analysis of acute myeloblastic leukemia: identification of differentiation-associated phenotypes. Blood 62:557, 1983.
66. Foon, K., Schroff, R., and Gale, R.: Surface markers on leukemia and lymphoma cells: recent advances. Blood 60:1, 1982.
67. Griffin, J., Ritz, J., et al.: Expression of myeloid differentiation antigens on normal and malignant myeloid cells. J. Clin. Invest. 68:932, 1981.
68. Pui, C., Dahl, G., et al.: Acute leukaemia with mixed lymphoid and myeloid phenotype. Br. J. Haematol. 56:121, 1984.
69. Lanham, G., Bollom, F., et al.: Simultaneous occurrence of terminal deoxynucleotidyl transferase and myeloperoxidase in individual leukemic blasts. Blood 64:318, 1984.
70. Blatt, J., Reaman, G., et al.: Biochemical markers in lymphoid malignancy. New Engl. J. Med. 303:918, 1980.
71. McCaffrey, R., Harrison, R. A., et al.: Terminal deoxynucleotidyl transferase activity in human leukemic cells and in normal human thymocytes. New Engl. J. Med. 292:775, 1975.
72. Bollum, F. G.: Terminal deoxynucleotidyl transferase as a hematopoietic cell marker. Blood 54:1203, 1979.
73. Ellis, R. B., Rapson, H. T., et al.: Expression of hexosaminidase isoenzymes in childhood leukemia. New Engl. J. Med. 298:476, 1978.
74. Neumann, H., Klein, E., et al.: N-alkaline phosphatase: a potential marker for lymphoproliferative disorders. Br. J. Haematol. 41:519, 1979.
75. Blatt, J., Reaman, G., et al.: Purine nucleoside phosphorylase activity in T cell acute lymphoblastic leukemia. Blood 56:380, 1980.
76. Reaman, G. H., Levin, N., et al.: Diminished lymphoblast 5'-nucleotidase in acute lymphoblastic leukemia with T-cell characteristics. New Engl. J. Med. 300:1374, 1979.
77. Smyth, J. F., Poplack, D. G., et al.: Correlation of adenosine deaminase activity with cell surface markers in acute lymphoblastic leukemia. J. Clin. Invest. 62:710, 1978.
78. Coleman, M. S., Greenwood, M. F., et al.: Adenosine deaminase, terminal deoxynucleotidyl transferase (TdT), and cell surface markers in childhood acute leukemia. Blood 52:1125, 1978.
79. Poplack, D. G., Sallan, S. E., et al.: Phase I study of 2'deoxycoformycin in acute lymphoblastic leukemia. Cancer Res. 42:3343, 1981.
80. Kalwinsky, D. K., Weatherred, W. H., et al.: Clinical utility of initial terminal deoxynucleotidyl transferase determinations in childhood acute leukemias. Cancer Res. 41:2877, 1981.
81. Froehlich, T. W., Buchanan, G. R., et al.: Terminal deoxynucleotidyl transferase–containing cells in peripheral blood: implications for the surveillance of patients with lymphoblastic leukemia or lymphoma in remission. Blood 58:214, 1981.
82. Marks, S. M., Baltimore, D., et al.: Terminal transferase as a predictor of initial responsiveness to vincristine and prednisone in blastic chronic myelogenous leukemia. New Engl. J. Med. 298:812, 1978.
83. Sylwestrowicz, T. A., Ma, D. D. F., et al.: 5' Nucleotidase, adenosine deaminase and purine nucleoside phosphorylase activities in acute leukemia. Leuk. Res. 6:475, 1982.
84. Mejer, J., and Nygaard, P.: Adenosine deaminase and purine nucleoside phosphorylase levels in acute myeloblastic leukemia cells. Relationship to diagnosis and clinical course. Leuk. Res. 4:211, 1979.
85. Bloomfield, C. D.: Glucocorticoid receptors in leukemia and lymphoma. J. Clin. Oncol. 2:323, 1984.
86. Homo-Delarche, G.: Glucocorticoid receptors and steroid sensitivity in normal and neoplastic human lymphoid tissues: a review. Cancer Res. 44:431, 1984.
87. Pui, C. H., Ochs, J. J., et al.: Impact of treatment efficacy on the prognostic value of glucocorticoid receptors levels in childhood acute lymphoblastic leukemia. Leuk. Res. 8:345, 1984.
88. Choi, S., and Simone, J.: Acute non-lymphocytic leukemia in 171 children. Med. Pediatr. Oncol. 2:119, 1976.
89. Nies, B. A., Bodey, G. P., et al.: The persistence of extramedullary leukemic infiltrates during bone marrow remission of acute leukemia. Blood 26:133, 1965.
90. Simone, J. V., Holland, E., et al.: Fatalities during remission of childhood leukemia. Blood 39:759, 1972.
91. Mathe, G., Schwarzenberg, L., et al.: Extensive histological and cytological survey of patients with acute leukaemia in "complete remission." Br. Med. J. 1:640, 1966.
92. Sharp, H. L., Nesbit, M. E., et al.: Renal and hepatic pathology following initial remission of acute leukemia induced by prednisone. Cancer 20:1395, 1967.
93. Baum, E., Nesbit, M., et al.: Extent of disease in pediatric patients with acute lymphocytic leukemia experiencing an isolated testicular relapse. Am. Soc. Clin. Oncol. 20:435, 1979.
94. Evans, A. E., Gilbert, E. S., et al.: The increasing incidence of central nervous system leukemia in children. Cancer 26:404, 1970.
95. Schiffer, C. A., Sanel, F. T., et al.: Functional and morphologic characteristics of the leukemia cells of a patient with acute monocytic leukemia. Blood 46:17, 1975.
96. Hardisty, R. M., and Norman, P. M.: Meningeal leukaemia. Arch. Dis. Child. 42:441, 1967.

97. Price, R. A., and Johnson, W. W.: The central nervous system in childhood leukemia: I. The arachnoid. Cancer 31:520, 1973.
98. Mastrangelo, R., Zuelzer, W. W., et al.: Chromosomes in the spinal fluid: evidence for metastatic origin of meningeal leukemia. Blood 35:227, 1970.
99. Hustu, H. O., and Aur, R. J. A.: Extramedullary leukemia. Clin. Haematol. 7:313, 1978.
100. Hyman, C. B., Bogle, J. M., et al.: Central nervous system involvement by leukemia in children. Blood 25:1, 1965.
101. Greydanus, D. E., et al.: Hypothalamic syndrome in children with acute lymphocytic leukemia. Mayo Clin. Proc. 53:217, 1978.
102. Rosman, N. P., Kakulas, B. A., et al.: Central pontine myelinolysis in a child with leukemia. Arch. Neurol. 14:273, 1966.
103. Kanner, S. P., Wiernick, P. H., et al.: CNS leukemia mimicking multifocal leukoencephalopathy. Am. J. Dis. Child. 119:264, 1970.
104. Miller, V. I., and Campbell, W. G., Jr.: Diabetes insipidus as a complication of leukemia. A case report with a literature review. Cancer 28:666, 1971.
105. Komp, D. M.: Cytocentrifugation in the management of central nervous system leukemia. J. Pediatr. 91:992, 1972.
106. Bradstock, K. F., Papageorgiou, E. S., et al.: Diagnosis of meningeal involvement in patients with acute lymphoblastic leukemia: immunofluorescence for terminal transferase. Cancer 47:2478, 1981.
107. Mavligit, G. M., Stuckey, S. E., et al.: Diagnosis of leukemia or lymphoma in the central nervous system by beta$_2$-microglobulin determination. New Engl. J. Med. 303:718, 1980.
108. Koch, T. R., Lichtenfeld, K. M., et al.: Detection of central nervous system metastasis with cerebrospinal fluid beta-2-microglobulin. Cancer 52:101, 1983.
109. Wilhyde, D. E., Jane, J. A., et al.: Spinal epidural leukemia. Am. J. Med. 34:281, 1963.
110. Petursson, S. R., and Boggs, D. R.: Spinal cord involvement in leukemia: a review of the literature and a case of Ph^1+ acute myeloid leukemia presenting with a conus medullaris syndrome. Cancer 47:346, 1981.
111. Ioachim, H. L., Keller, S., et al.: Myeloperoxidase and crystalline bodies in the granules of DMBA-induced rate chloroma cells. Am. J. Pathol. 66:147, 1972.
112. Muss, H., and Moloney, W.: Chloroma and other myeloblastic tumors. Blood 42:721, 1973.
113. Pochedly, C.: Neurotoxicity due to CNS therapy for leukemia. Med. Pediatr. Oncol. 3:101, 1977.
114. Jampol, M. L., and Ohnysty, J.: Acute leukemia seen as testicular tumor. N.Y. State J. Med. 67:1903, 1967.
115. DeVillez, R., Lufkin, E., et al.: Symmetrical enlargement of breasts and testes due to leukemic infiltrations. South. Med. J. 65:341, 1972.
116. Dublin, T., Movassaghini, N., et al.: Leukemic infiltration of the testis in acute myelocytic leukemia during bone marrow remission. J. Pediatr. 83:886, 1973.
117. Wagner, V. M., and Baehner, R. L.: Leukemic infiltration of the testes in acute nonlymphocytic leukemia. Med. Pediatr. Oncol. 12:166, 1984.
118. Finkelstein, J. Z., Dyment, P. G., et al.: Leukemic infiltration of the testes during bone marrow remission. Pediatrics 43:1042, 1969.
119. Givler, R. L.: Testicular involvement in leukemia and lymphoma. Cancer 23:1290, 1969.
120. Kuo, T., Tschang, T. P., et al.: Testicular relapse in childhood acute lymphocytic leukemia during bone marrow remission. Cancer 38:2604, 1976.
121. Lendon, M., Palmer, M. K., et al.: Testicular histology after combination chemotherapy in childhood for acute lymphoblastic leukaemia. Lancet 2:439, 1978.
122. Kim, T. H., Lui, B. K. S., et al.: Testicular biopsy prior to termination of leukemic therapy. J. Pediatr. 94:95, 1979.
123. Troup, C. W., Thatcher, G., et al.: Infiltrative lesion of the bladder presenting as gross hematuria in a child with leukemia: case report. J. Urol. 107:314, 1972.
124. Vadakan, V. V., and Ortega, J.: Priapism in acute lymphoblastic leukemia. Cancer 30:373, 1972.
125. Jaffe, N., and Kim, B. S.: Priapism in acute granulocytic leukemia. Am. J. Dis. Child. 118:619, 1969.
126. Graw, R. G., Jr., Skeel, R. T., et al.: Priapism in a child with chronic granulocytic leukemia. J. Pediatr. 74:788, 1969.
127. Ritz, N. D., and Purfar, M.: Chronic myeloid leukemia with priapism in an eight year old child. N.Y. State J. Med. 64:553, 1964.
128. Cepalupo, A. J., Frankel, L. S., et al.: Pelvic and ovarian extramedullary leukemic relapse in young girls. A report of four cases and review of the literature. Cancer 50:587, 1982.
129. Sallan, S. E., Camitta, B. M., et al.: Intermittent combination chemotherapy with adriamycin for childhood acute lymphoblastic leukemia: clinical results. Blood 51:425, 1978.
130. Thomas, L. B., Forkner, C. E., Jr., et al.: The skeletal lesions of acute leukemia. Cancer 14:608, 1961.
131. Wilson, J. V. K.: The bone lesions of childhood leukemia. A survey of 140 cases. Radiology 72:672, 1959.
132. Kushner, D. C., Weinstein, H. J., et al.: The radiologic diagnosis of leukemia and lymphoma in children. Semin. Oncol. 15:316, 1980.
133. Aur, R. J. A., Westbrook, H. W., et al.: Childhood acute lymphocytic leukemia. Am. J. Dis. Child. 124:653, 1972.
134. Nies, B. A., Kundel, D. W., et al.: Leukopenia, bone pain, and bone necrosis in patients with acute leukemia. A clinicopathologic complex. Ann. Intern. Med. 62:698, 1965.
135. Masera, G., Carnelli, V., et al.: Prognostic significance of radiologic bone involvement in childhood acute lymphoblastic leukemia. Arch. Dis. Child. 52:530, 1977.
136. Hann, I. M., Gupta, S., et al.: The prognostic significance of radiological and symptomatic bone involvement in childhood acute lymphoblastic leukaemia. Med. Pediatr. Oncol. 6:51, 1979.
137. Nesbit, M., Krivit, W., et al.: Acute and chronic effect of methotrexate on hepatic, pulmonary, and skeletal systems. Cancer 37:1048, 1976.
138. Schaller, J.: Arthritis as a presenting manifestation of malignancy in children. J. Pediatr. 81:793, 1972.
139. Lea, J. W., Jr., Masys, D. R., et al.: Typhlitis: a treatable complication of acute leukemia therapy. Cancer Clin. Trials 2:355, 1980.
140. Wagner, J. L., Rosenberg, H. S., et al.: Typhlitis: a complication of leukemia in childhood. Am. J. Roentgenol. Rad. Therm. Nucl. Med. 109:341, 1970.
141. Shamberger, R. C., Weinstein, H. J., et al.: The medical and surgical management of typhlitis in children with acute nonlymphocytic (myelogenous) leukemia. Cancer 57:603, 1986.
142. Weetman, R. M., and Baehner, R. L.: Latent onset of clinical pancreatitis in children receiving L-asparaginase therapy. Cancer 34:780, 1974.
143. Kosloske, A. M., and Zwartjes, W. J.: Acute abdomen due to acute cholangitis in a leukemic child. Pediatrics 56:469, 1975.
144. Al-Rasgud, R. A., and Harned, R. K.: Dysphagia due to leukemic involvement of the esophagus. Am. J. Dis. Child. 121:75, 1971.
145. Newburger, P. E., Cassady, J., et al.: Esophagitis due to adriamycin and radiation therapy for childhood malignancy. Cancer 42:417, 1978.
146. Sehdev, M. K., Dowling, M. D., Jr., et al.: Perianal and anorectal complications in leukemia. Cancer 31:149, 1973.
147. Schimpff, S. C., Wiernik, P., et al.: Rectal abscesses in cancer patients. Lancet 2:844, 1972.

148. Merrill, J. M., Brereton, H. D., et al.: Anorectal disease in patients with non-haematologic malignancy. Lancet *1*:1105, 1976.
149. Hyams, J. S., Batrus, C. L., et al.: Cancer chemotherapy-induced lactose malabsorption in children. Cancer *49*:646, 1982.
150. Wetherley-Mein, G., and Cottom, D. G.: Portal fibrosis in acute leukaemia. Br. J. Haematol. *2*:345, 1956.
151. Hutter, R. V. P., Shipkey, F. H., et al.: Hepatic fibrosis in children with acute leukemia. A complication of therapy. Cancer *13*:288, 1960.
152. Curtis, A. B.: Childhood leukemias: initial oral manifestations. J. Am. Dent. Assoc. *83*:159, 1971.
153. Segelman, A. E., and Doku, H. C.: Treatment of the oral complications of leukemia. J. Oral Surg. *35*:469, 1977.
154. Dreizen, S., Bodey, G. P., et al.: Oral complications of cancer chemotherapy. Postgrad. Med. *58*:75, 1975.
155. Shepard, J. P.: The management of oral complications in leukemia. Oral Surg. *45*:543, 1978.
156. Cocchi, R., and Borgueresi, S.: The Mikulicz syndrome in the course of leukemia. Minerva Pediatr. *18*:997, 1966.
157. Ridgeway, E. W., Jaffe, N., et al.: Leukemia ophthalmopathy in children. Cancer *38*:1744, 1976.
158. Murray, K. M., Goldman, J. M., et al.: Ocular involvement in leukaemia. Report of three cases. Lancet *1*:829, 1977.
159. Ninane, J., Taylor, D., et al.: The eye as a sanctuary in acute lymphoblastic leukaemia. Lancet *1*:452, 1980.
160. Chalfin, A. I., Nash, B. M., et al.: Optic nerve head involvement in lymphocytic leukemia. J. Pediatr. Ophthalmol. *10*:39, 1973.
161. Rosenthal, A. R., Egbert, P. R., et al.: Leukemic involvement of the optic nerve. Trans. Pac. Coast Otoophthalmol. Soc. *55*:137, 1974.
162. Clayman, H. M., Flynn, Y. T., et al.: Retinal pigment epithelial abnormalities in leukemic disease. Am. J. Ophthalmol. *74*:416, 1972.
163. Gruenwald, R. L., Perry, M. C., et al.: Leukemic iritis with hypopyon. Cancer *44*:1511, 1979.
164. Fonken, H. A., and Ellis, P. P.: Leukemic infiltrates in the iris. Successful treatment of secondary glaucoma with x-irradiation. Arch. Ophthalmol. *76*:32, 1966.
165. Robb, R. M., Ervin, L. D., et al.: A pathological study of eye involvement in acute leukemia of childhood. Med. Pediatr. Oncol. *6*:171, 1979.
166. Mason, T. E., Demaree, R. S., Jr., et al.: Granulocytic sarcoma (chloroma) two years preceding myelogeneous leukemia. Cancer *31*:423, 1973.
167. Krause, J. R.: Granulocytic sarcoma preceding acute leukemia: a report of six cases. Cancer *44*:1017, 1979.
168. Lusher, J. M.: Chloroma as a presenting feature of acute leukemia. A report of two cases in children. Am. J. Dis. Child. *108*:62, 1964.
169. Summers, J. E., Johnson, W. W., et al.: Childhood leukemic heart disease. A study of 116 hearts of children dying of leukemia. Circulation *40*:575, 1969.
170. Roberts, W. C., Bodey, G. P., et al.: The heart in acute leukemia. A study of 250 autopsy cases. Am. J. Cardiol. *21*:388, 1968.
171. Jaffe, N., Traggis, D. G., et al.: Acute leukemia presenting with pericardial tamponade. Pediatrics *45*:461, 1970.
172. Armata, J., Zajaczkowski, J., et al.: Pericardial involvement during remission in acute leukemia. Haematologia *5*:425, 1971.
173. Miller, A. J.: Some observations concerning pericardial effusions and their relationship to the nervous and lymphatic circulation of the heart. Lymphology *3*:76, 1970.
174. Goorin, A. M., Borow, K. M., et al.: Congestive heart failure due to adriamycin cardiotoxicity: its natural history in children. Cancer *47*:2810, 1981.
175. Klatte, E. C., Yardley, J., et al.: The pulmonary manifestations and complications of leukemia. Am. J. Roentgenol. *89*:598, 1963.
176. Bodey, G. P., Powell, R. D., Jr. et al.: Pulmonary complications of acute leukemia. Cancer *19*:781, 1966.
177. Georgitis, J., Eigen, H., et al.: Isolated pulmonary leukemic relapse following successful bone marrow transplant in a child with acute lymphoblastic leukemia. Pediatrics *64*:913, 1979.
178. Wells, R. J., Weetman, R. M., et al.: Pulmonary leukemia in children presenting as diffuse interstitial pneumonia. J. Pediatr. *96*:262, 1980.
179. Mainzer, R., and Taybi, H.: Thymic enlargement and pleural effusion: an unusual roentgenographic complex in childhood leukemia. Am. J. Roentgenol. *112*:35, 1971.
180. LaVenuta, F., and Moore, J. A.: Involvement of the inner ear in acute stem cell leukemia. Report of two cases. Ann. Otol. *81*:132, 1972.
181. Kennedy, B. J., Borenstein, R., et al.: Breast involvement in acute lymphatic leukemia. Daunorubicin-induced remission: *Pneumocystis carinii* pneumonia. Cancer *25*:693, 1970.
182. Larson, S. M., Graff, K. S., et al.: Positive gallium-67 photoscan in myeloblastoma. J. A. M. A. *222*:321, 1972.
183. Gralnick, H. R., and Dittmar, K.: Development of myeloblastoma and massive breast and ovarian involvement during remission in acute leukemia. Cancer *24*:746, 1969.
184. Austin, J. H. M.: Chloroma. Report of a patient with unusual rib lesions. Radiology *93*:671, 1969.
185. Stoop, J. W., Zegers, B. J. M., et al.: Monoclonal gammopathy in a child with leukemia. Blood *32*:774, 1968.
186. Lindquist, K. J., Ragab, A. H., et al.: Paraproteinemia in a child with leukemia. Blood *35*:213, 1970.
187. Hann, I. M., Evans, D. I. K., et al.: Bone marrow fibrosis in acute lymphoblastic leukaemia of childhood. J. Clin. Pathol. *31*:313, 1978.
188. Raney, R. B., and McMillan, C. W.: Simultaneous disparity of bone marrow specimens in acute leukemia. Am. J. Dis. Child. *117*:548, 1969.
189. Ragab, A. H., and Crist, W. M.: Morphologic discordance in acute leukemia. New Engl. J. Med. *287*:1134, 1972.
190. Ellman, L., and Carey, R. W.: Morphological discordance in acute leukemia. Blood *48*:621, 1976.
191. Hann, I. M., Morris-Jones, P. H., et al.: Discrepancy of bone marrow aspirations in acute lymphoblastic leukaemia in relapse. Lancet *1*:1215, 1977.
192. Golombe, B., Ramsay, N. K. C., et al.: Localized bone marrow relapse in acute lymphoblastic leukemia. Med. Pediatr. Oncol. *6*:229, 1979.
193. Rickles, F. R., and Miller, D. R.: Eosinophilic leukemoid reaction. J. Pediatr. *80*:418, 1972.
194. Spitzer, G., and Garson, D. M.: Lymphoblastic leukemia with marked eosinophilia: a report of two cases. Blood *42*:377, 1973.
195. Nelken, R. P., and Stockman, J. A.: The hypereosinophilic syndrome in association with acute lymphoblastic leukemia. J. Pediatr. *89*:771, 1976.
196. Pereira, F., Moreno, H., et al.: Loffler's endomyocardial fibrosis, eosinophilia, and acute lymphoblastic leukemia. Pediatrics *59*:950, 1977.
197. Wimmer, W. S., Raney, R. B., Jr., et al.: Hypereosinophilia with acute lymphocytic and acute myelocytic leukemia in childhood. J. Pediatr. *92*:244, 1978.
198. Weinger, R. S., Andre-Schwartz, J., et al.: Acute leukaemia with eosinophilic leukaemia: a dilemma. Br. J. Haematol. *30*:65, 1975.
199. LeBeau, M. M., Larson, R. A., et al.: Association of an inversion of chromosome 16 with abnormal marrow eosinophils in acute myelomonocytic leukemia. A unique cytogenetic clinicopathological association. New Engl. J. Med. *309*:630, 1983.
200. Kemshead, J. T., Goldman, A., et al.: Use of panels of monoclonal antibodies in the differential diagnosis of neuroblastoma and lymphoblastic disorders. Lancet *1*:12, 1983.

201. Saulsbury, F. T., Sabio, H., et al.: Acute leukemia with features of systemic lupus erythematosus. J. Pediatr. *105*:57, 1984.
202. Shackelford, G. D., Bloomberg, G., et al.: The value of roentgenography in differentiating aplastic anemia from leukemia masquerading as aplastic anemia. Am. J. Roentgenol. *116*:651, 1972.
203. Holland, P., and Mauer, A. M.: Myeloid leukemoid reactions in children. Am. J. Dis. Child. *105*:568, 1963.
204. Hilts, S. V., and Shaw, C. C.: Leukemoid blood reactions. New Engl. J. Med. *249*:434, 1953.
205. Zusman, J., Brown, D. M., et al.: Hyperphosphatemia, hyperphosphaturia and hypocalcemia in acute lymphoblastic leukemia. New Engl. J. Med. *289*:1335, 1973.
206. Wilson, D., Stewart, A., et al.: Cardiac arrest due to hyperkalemia following therapy for acute lymphoblastic leukemia. Cancer *39*:2290, 1977.
207. O'Regan, S., Kaplan, B. S., et al.: Hypokalemia in children with leukemia in relapse. Am. J. Dis. Child. *130*:937, 1976.
208. DeFronzo, R. A., Braine, H., et al.: Water intoxication in man after the cyclophosphamide therapy: time course and relation to drug activation. Ann. Intern. Med. *78*:861, 1973.
209. Stuart, M., Cuaso, C., et al.: Syndrome of recurrent increased secretion of antidiuretic hormone following multiple doses of vincristine. Blood *45*:315, 1975.
210. Stapleton, F. B., Nelson, B., et al.: Hypokalemia associated with antibiotic treatment: evidence in children with malignant neoplasms. Am. J. Dis. Child. *130*:1104, 1976.
211. McKee, L. C. Jr., and Collins, R. D.: Intravascular leukocyte thrombi and aggregates as a cause of morbidity and mortality in leukemia. Medicine *53*:463, 1974.
212. Lichtman, M., and Rowe, J.: Hyperleukocytic leukemias: rheological, clinical and therapeutic considerations. Blood *60*:279, 1982.
213. Dearth, J. C., Fountain, K. S., et al.: Extreme leukemic leukocytosis (blast crisis) in childhood. Mayo Clin. Proc. *53*:207, 1978.
214. Gruno, F. M., Armitage, J. O., et al.: Hydroxyurea in the prevention of the effects of leukostasis in acute leukemia. Arch. Intern. Med. *137*:1246, 1977.
215. Vernant, J. P., Brun, B., et al.: Respiratory distress of hyperleukocytic granulocytic leukemias. Cancer *44*:264, 1979.
216. Hyman, C. B., Boule, J. M., et al.: Central nervous system involvement in children. II. Therapy with intrathecal methotrexate. Blood *24*:13, 1965.
217. Wang, J. J., and Pratt, C. B.: Intrathecal arabinosyl cytosine in meningeal leukemia. Cancer *25*:531, 1970.
218. Mauer, A.: Cell kinetics and practical consequences for therapy of acute leukemia. New Engl. J. Med. *293*:389, 1975.
219. Saunders, E. F., and Mauer, A. M.: Re-entry of nondividing leukemic cells into a proliferative phase in acute childhood leukemia. J. Clin. Invest. *48*:1299, 1969.
220. Haghbin, M., Murphy, M. L., et al.: A long-term clinical follow-up of children with acute lymphoblastic leukemia treated with intensive chemotherapy regimens. Cancer *46*:241, 1980.
221. Selawry, O. S., Hananian, J., et al.: New treatment schedule with improved survival in childhood leukemia. J. A. M. A. *194*:75, 1965.
222. Sallan, S. E., Hitchcock-Bryan, S., et al.: Influence of intensive asparaginase in the treatment of childhood non-T-cell acute lymphoblastic leukemia. Cancer Res. *43*:5601, 1983.
223. Riehm, H., Feikert, H.-J., et al.: Acute lymphoblastic leukaemia. In *Cancer in Children: Clinical Management*. Voute, P. A., Barrett, A., et al. (eds.), Heidelberg, Springer-Verlag, 1986, pp. 101–108.
224. Hart, J. S., Livingston, R. B., et al.: Neoplasia kinetics and chemotherapy. Semin. Oncol. *3*:259, 1976.
225. Murphy, S. B., Aur, R. J. A., et al.: Pre-treatment cytokinetic studies in 94 children with acute leukemia: Relationship to other variables at diagnosis and outcome of standard treatment. Blood *49*:683, 1977.
226. Frei, E., III, Karon, M., et al.: The effectiveness of combinations of antileukemia agents in inducing and maintaining remission in children with acute leukemia. Blood *26*:642, 1965.
227. Moe, P. J., Seip, M., et al.: Intermediate dose methotrexate in childhood acute lymphocytic leukemia. Eur. Paediatr. Haematol. Oncol. *1*:113, 1984.
228. Freeman, A. I., Weinberg, V., et al.: Comparison of intermediate-dose methotrexate with cranial irradiation for the post-induction treatment of acute lymphocytic leukemia in children. New Engl. J. Med. *308*:477, 1983.
229. Poplack, D. G., Reaman, G. H., et al.: Central nervous system (CNS) preventive therapy with high dose methotrexate (HDMTX) in acute lymphoblastic leukemia (ALL): a preliminary report (abstr.). Proc. Am. Soc. Clin. Oncol. *3*:204, 1984.
230. Aur, R. J. A., Simone, J. V., et al.: A comparative study of central nervous system irradiation and intensive chemotherapy early in remission of childhood acute lymphocytic leukemia. Cancer *29*:381, 1972.
231. Inati, A., Sallan, S. E., et al.: Efficacy and morbidity of central nervous system "prophylaxis" in childhood acute lymphoblastic leukemia: eight years' experience with cranial irradiation and intrathecal methotrexate. Blood *61*:297, 1983.
232. Sullivan, M. P., Chen, T., et al.: Equivalence of intrathecal chemotherapy and radiotherapy as central nervous system prophylaxis in children with acute lymphocytic leukemia: a Pediatric Oncology Group Study. Blood *60*:948, 1982.
232a. Editorial: Leukaemia and the central nervous system. Lancet *i*:1196, 1985.
233. Shapiro, W. R., Young, D. R., et al.: Methotrexate: distribution in cerebrospinal fluid after intravenous ventricular and lumbar injections. New Engl. J. Med. *293*:161, 1975.
234. Weinstein, H. J., Griffin, T. W., et al.: Pharmacokinetics of continuous intravenous and subcutaneous infusions of cytosine arabinoside. Blood *59*:1351, 1982.
235. Frick, J., Ritch, P. S., et al.: Successful treatment of meningeal leukemia using systemic high dose cytosine arabinoside. J. Clin. Oncol. *2*:365, 1984.
236. Bleyer, W. A., Coccia, P. F., et al.: Reduction in central nervous system leukemia with a pharmacokinetically derived intrathecal methotrexate dosage regimen. J. Clin. Oncol. *1*:317, 1983.
237. Baehner, R. L., Neiburger, R. G., et al.: Transient bacterial defect of peripheral blood phagocytes from children with acute lymphoblastic leukemia receiving craniospinal irradiation. New Engl. J. Med. *289*:1209, 1973.
238. Nesbit, M. E., Robinson, L. L., et al.: Testicular relapse in childhood acute lymphoblastic leukemia: association with pretreatment patient characteristics and treatment. Cancer *45*:2009, 1980.
239. Sallan, S. E., Ritz, J., et al.: Cell surface antigens: implications in childhood acute lymphoblastic leukemia. Blood *55*:395, 1980.
240. Uderzo, C., Lasciulli, A., et al.: Correlation of gonadal function with histology of testicular biopsies at treatment discontinuation in childhood acute leukemia. Med. Pediatr. Oncol. *12*:97, 1984.
241. Clavell, L. A., Gelber, R. D., et al.: Four-agent induction and intensive asparaginase therapy for treatment of childhood acute lymphoblastic leukemia. New Engl. J. Med. *315*:657, 1986.

242. Freireich, E. J., Gehan, E., et al.: The effect of 6-mercaptopurine on the duration of steroid-induced remission in acute leukemia. A model for evaluation of other potentially useful therapy. Blood 21:699, 1963.
243. Lonsdale, D., Gehan, E. A., et al.: Interrupted vs. continued maintenance therapy in childhood acute leukemia. Cancer 36:341, 1975.
244. Aur, R. J. A., Simone, J. V., et al.: Childhood acute lymphocytic leukemia. Cancer 42:2123, 1978.
245. Niemeyer, C. M., Hitchcock-Bryan, S., et al.: Comparative analysis of treatment programs for childhood acute lymphoblastic leukemia. Semin. Oncol. 12:122, 1985.
246. Alexander, P., and Powles, R.: Immunotherapy of human acute leukaemia. Clin. Haematol. 17:275, 1978.
247. Mathe, G., deVassal, F., et al.: 1975 current results of the first 100 cytologically typed acute lymphoid leukemias submitted to BCG active immunotherapy. Cancer Immunol. Immunother. 1:77, 1976.
248. Ritz, J., Pesando, J. M., et al.: Serotherapy of acute lymphoblastic leukemia with monoclonal antibody. Blood 58:141, 1981.
249. Ritz, J., Sallan, S. E., et al.: Autologous bone marrow transplantation in CALLA-positive acute lymphoblastic leukaemia after in vitro treatment with J5 monoclonal antibody and complement. Lancet 2:60, 1982.
249a. Ramsay, N., LeBien, T., et al.: Autologous bone marrow transplantation for patients with acute lymphoblastic leukemia in second or subsequent remission: results of bone marrow treated with monoclonal antibodies BA-1, BA-2, and BA-3, plus complement. Blood 66:508, 1985.
250. Muirhead, M., Martin, P. J., et al.: Use of an antibody-ricin A-chain conjugate to delete neoplastic B cells from human bone marrow. Blood 62:327, 1983.
251. Ault, K. A.: Detection of small numbers of monoclonal B-lymphocytes in the blood of patients with lymphoma. New Engl. J. Med. 300:1401, 1979.
252. Barr, R. D., and Koekebakker, M.: Detection of circulating "terminal transferase–positive" cells does not predict relapse in acute lymphoblastic leukemia. Leuk. Res. 8:1051, 1984.
253. Nesbit, M. E., Jr., Sather, H. N., et al.: Randomized study of 3 years versus 5 years of chemotherapy in childhood acute lymphoblastic leukemia. J. Clin. Oncol. 1:308, 1983.
254. Simone, J. V., Aur, R. J. A., et al.: Three to ten years after cessation of therapy in children with leukemia. Cancer 42:839, 1978.
255. George, S. L., Aur, R. J. A., et al.: A reappraisal of the results of stopping therapy in childhood leukemia. New Engl. J. Med. 330:269, 1979.
256. Carcassonne, Y.: Relapse after presumed cure of lymphoblastic leukaemia. Lancet 2:473, 1981.
256a. Burton, G. V., Weinberg, J. B., et al.: Extramedullary recurrence of acute lymphoblastic leukemia 15 years after initial diagnosis. Med. Pediatr. Oncol. 12:255, 1984.
257. Rivera, G., Aur, R. J. A., et al.: Second cessation of therapy in childhood lymphocytic leukemia. Blood 53:1114, 1979.
258. Land, V. J., Berry, D. H., et al.: Long-term survival in childhood acute leukemia: "late relapses." Med. Pediatr. Oncol. 7:19, 1979.
259. Bowman, W. P., Aur, R. J. A., et al.: Isolated testicular relapse in acute lymphocytic leukemia of childhood: categories and influence on survival. J. Clin. Oncol. 2:924, 1984.
260. Bertino, J. R.: Toward improved selectivity in cancer chemotherapy: The Richard and Linda Rosenthal Foundation Award Lecture. Cancer Res. 39:293, 1979.
261. Bender, R. A.: Anti-folate resistance in leukemia: treatment with "high dose" methotrexate and citrovorum factor. Cancer Treat. Rev. 2:215, 1975.
262. Stewart, C. D., and Burke, P. J.: Cytidine deaminase and the development of resistance to arabinosyl cytosine. Nature 233:109, 1971.
263. Chabner, B. A., Myers, C. E., et al.: Clinical pharmacology of anticancer drugs. Semin. Oncol. 4:165, 1977.
264. Tattersall, M. N. H., Ganeshaguru, K., et al.: Mechanism of resistance of human acute leukemia cells to cytosine arabinoside. Br. J. Haematol. 27:39, 1974.
265. Sallan, S. E., Camitta, B. M., et al.: Chemotherapy with cyclophosphamide, vincristine, cytosine arabinoside and prednisone (COAP) in childhood acute lymphoblastic leukemia (ALL). Med. Pediatr. Oncol. 3:359, 1977.
266. Rivera, G., Murphy, S. B., et al.: Recurrent childhood lymphocytic leukemia. Cancer 42:252, 1978.
266a. Rivera, G. K., Buchanan, G., et al.: Intensive retreatment of childhood acute lymphoblastic leukemia in first bone marrow relapse. A Pediatric Oncology Group Study. New Engl. J. Med. 315:274, 1986.
267. Simone, J. V.: Leukaemia remission and survival. Lancet 2:531, 1981.
267a. George, S. L., Ochs, J. J., et al.: The importance of an isolated central nervous system relapse in children with acute lymphoblastic leukemia. J. Clin. Oncol. 3:776, 1985.
268. Nesbit, M. E., D'Angio, G. J., et al.: Effect of isolated central nervous system leukaemia on bone marrow remission and survival in childhood acute lymphoblastic leukaemia. Lancet 1:1386, 1981.
269. Sullivan, M. P., Vietti, T. J., et al.: Clinical investigations in the treatment of meningeal leukemia: radiation therapy regimen vs. conventional intrathecal methotrexate. Blood 34:301, 1969.
270. Green, D. M., West, C. R., et al.: The use of subcutaneous cerebrospinal fluid reservoirs for the prevention and treatment of meningeal relapse of acute lymphoblastic leukemia. Am. J. Pediatr. Hematol. Oncol. 4:147, 1982.
270a. Balis, F. M., Savitch, J. L., et al.: Remission induction of meningeal leukemia with high-dose intravenous methotrexate. J. Clin. Oncol. 3:485, 1985.
271. Kun, L. E., Camitta, B. M., et al.: Treatment of meningeal relapse in childhood acute lymphoblastic leukemia. I. Results of craniospinal irradiation. J. Clin. Oncol. 2:359, 1984.
272. Pizzo, P. A., Poplack, D. G., et al.: Neurotoxicities of current leukemia therapy. Am. J. Pediatr. Hematol. Oncol. 1:127, 1979.
273. Medical Research Council's Working Party on Leukaemia in Childhood: Testicular disease in acute lymphoblastic leukaemia in childhood. Br. Med. J. 1:334, 1978.
274. Steinfeld, A. D.: Radiation therapy in the treatment of leukemic infiltrates of the testes. Radiology 120:681, 1976.
275. Stoffel, T. J., Nesbit, M. E., et al.: Extramedullary involvement of the testes in childhood leukemia. Cancer 35:1203, 1975.
276. Shaw, M. T., Dwyer, J. M., et al.: Terminal deoxyribonucleotidyl transferase activity in B-cell acute lymphocytic leukemia. Blood 51:181, 1978.
277. vanEys, J., and Sullivan, M.: Testicular leukaemia and temperature. Lancet 2:256, 1976.
278. Garwicz, S., and Hedling, L.: Testicular leukaemia and temperature. Lancet 2:630, 1976.
279. Reaman, G. H., Ladisch, S., et al.: Improved treatment results in the management of single and multiple relapses of acute lymphoblastic leukemia. Cancer 45:3090, 1980.
280. Thomas, E. D., Sanders, J. E., et al.: Marrow transplantation for patients with acute lymphoblastic leukemia: a long-term follow-up. Blood 62:1139, 1983.
281. Dinsmore, R., Kirkpatrick, D., et al.: Allogeneic bone marrow transplantation for patients with acute lymphoblastic leukemia. Blood 62:381, 1983.
282. Yeager, A. M., Kaizer, H., et al.: Autologous bone marrow transplantation in patients with acute nonlymphocytic leukemia, using ex vivo marrow treatment with 4-hydro-

peroxycyclophosphamide. New Engl. J. Med. *315*:141, 1986.
283. Simone, J. V., Verzosa, M. S., et al.: Initial features and prognosis of 363 children with acute lymphocytic leukemia. Cancer *36*:2099, 1975.
284. Lee, S. L., Kopel, S., et al.: Cytomorphological determinants of prognosis in acute lymphoblastic leukemia of children. Semin. Oncol. *3*:209, 1976.
285. Shaw, M. T.: The cytochemistry of acute leukemia: a diagnostic and prognostic evaluation. Semin. Oncol. *3*:219, 1976.
286. Baumer, J. H., and Mott, M. G.: Sex and prognosis in childhood acute lymphoblastic leukaemia. Lancet *2*:128, 1978.
287. Baum, E., Sather, H., et al.: Relapse rates following cessation of chemotherapy during complete remission of acute lymphocytic leukemia. Med. Pediatr. Oncol. *7*:25:1979.
288. George, S. L., Fernbach, D. J., et al.: Factors influencing survival in pediatric acute leukemia: the SWCCSG experience 1958–1970. Cancer *32*:1542, 1973.
289. Walters, T., Bushore, M., et al.: Poor prognosis in Negro children with acute lymphocytic leukemia. Cancer *29*:210, 1972.
290. Hann, I. M., Morris-Jones, P. H., et al.: Low IgE or IgA. A further indicator of a poor prognosis in childhood acute lymphoblastic leukaemia. Br. J. Cancer *41*:317, 1980.
291. Heideman, R. L., Falletta, J. M., et al.: Lymphocytic leukemia in children: prognostic significance of clinical and laboratory findings at the time of diagnosis. J. Pediatr. *92*:540, 1978.
292. Miller, D. R., Leikin, S., et al.: Prognostic factors and therapy in acute lymphoblastic leukemia of childhood: CCG-141. Cancer *51*:1041, 1983.
293. Reaman, G., Zeltzer, P., et al.: Acute lymphoblastic leukemia in infants less than one year of age: a cumulative experience of the Children's Cancer Study Group. J. Clin. Oncol. *3*:1513, 1985.
293a. Crist, W., Pullen, J., et al.: Clinical and biologic features predict a poor prognosis in acute lymphoid leukemias in infants: A Pediatric Oncology Group Study. Blood *67*:135, 1986.
294. Testa, J. R., Mintz, U., et al.: Evolution of karyotypes in acute nonlymphocytic leukemia. Cancer Res. *39*:3619, 1979.
295. Lampkin, B. C., Woods, W., et al.: Current status of the biology and treatment of acute nonlymphocytic leukemia in children (report from the ANLL Strategy Group of the Children's Cancer Study Group). Blood *61*:215, 1983.
296. Weinstein, H. J., Mayer, R. J., et al.: Chemotherapy for acute myelogenous leukemia in children and adults: VAPA update. Blood *62*:315, 1983.
297. Dahl, G. V., Simone, J. V., et al.: Preventive central nervous system irradiation in children with acute nonlymphocytic leukemia. Cancer *42*:2187, 1978.
298. Dahl, G. V., Kalwinsky, D. K., et al.: Cytokinetically based induction chemotherapy and splenectomy for childhood acute nonlymphocytic leukemia. Blood *60*:856, 1982.
299. Creutzig, U., Ritter, J., et al.: Improved treatment results in childhood acute myelogenous leukemia: a report of the German Cooperative Study AML BFM 78. Blood *65*:298, 1985.
300. Grier, H., Camitta, B., et al.: A seven year experience with intensive post-remission chemotherapy for childhood acute myelogenous leukemia (abstr.). Proceedings at the American Society of Hematology. Blood *62*:203a, 1984.
301. Baehner, R. L., Bernstein, I. D., et al.: Improved remission induction rate with D-ZAPO but unimproved remission duration with addition of immunotherapy to chemotherapy in previously untreated children with ANLL. Med. Pediatr. Oncol. *7*:127, 1979.
302. Thomas, E. D., Buckner, C. D., et al.: Marrow transplantation for acute nonlymphoblastic leukemia in first remission. New Engl. J. Med. *301*:597, 1979.
303. Thomas, E. D.: Marrow transplantation for acute nonlymphoblastic leukemia in first remission: a follow-up. New Engl. J. Med. *308*:1539, 1983.
304. Dinsmore, R., Kirkpatrick, D., et al.: Allogeneic bone marrow transplantation for patients with acute nonlymphocytic leukemia. Blood *63*:649, 1984.
305. Appelbaum, F. R., Clift, R. A., et al.: Allogeneic marrow transplantation for acute nonlymphoblastic leukemia after first relapse. Blood *61*:949, 1983.
306. Woods, W., Nesbit, M., et al.: Correlation of chromosome abnormalities with patient characteristics, histological subtype, and induction success in children with acute nonlymphocytic leukemia (ANLL). J. Clin. Oncol. *3*:3, 1985.
307. Gelber, R., Grier, H., et al.: Prognostic factors for childhood acute myelogenous leukemia (abstr.). Proc. Am. Soc. Clin. Oncol. *3*:186, 1984.
308. Peto, R., Pike, M. C., et al.: Design and analysis of randomized clinical trials requiring prolonged observation of each patient. II. Analysis and Examples. Br. J. Cancer *35*:1, 1977.
309. Drapkin, R. L., Gee, T. S., et al.: Prophylactic heparin therapy in acute promyelocytic leukemia. Cancer *41*:2484, 1978.
310. Gaydos, L., Freireich, E. J., et al.: Quantitative relation between platelet count and hemorrhage in patients with acute leukemia. New Engl. J. Med. *266*:905, 1962.
311. Lohrman, H. P., Decter, M. I., et al.: Platelet transfusion from HLA compatible unrelated donors to alloimmunized patients. Ann. Intern. Med. *80*:9, 1974.
312. Higby, D. J., Cohen, E., et al.: The prophylactic treatment of thrombocytopenic leukemic patients with platelets: a double blind study. Transfusion *14*:440, 1974.
313. Murphy, S., Koch, P. A., et al.: Randomized trial of prophylactic vs. therapeutic platelet transfusion in childhood acute leukemia (abstr.). Clin. Res. *24*:379, 1976.
314. Solomon, J., Bentler, E., et al.: Indications for the administration of platelet transfusions during remission induction therapy of acute leukemia (abstr.). Blood *50*:210, 1977.
315. Dutcher, J.: Platelet transfusion therapy. In *Neoplastic Diseases of the Blood*, Vol. 2. Wiernik, P., Canellos G. (eds.), Edinburgh, Churchill-Livingstone, 1985, p. 1039.
316. Yankee, R. A., Grumet, F. C., et al.: Platelet transfusion therapy—the selection of compatible platelet donors for refractory patients by lymphocyte HLA typing. New Engl. J. Med. *281*:1208, 1969.
317. Yankee, R. A., Graff, K. S., et al.: Selection of unrelated compatible platelet donors by lymphocyte HLA matching. New Engl. J. Med. *288*:760, 1973.
318. Daly, P. A., Schiffer, C. A., et al.: Successful transfusion of platelets cryopreserved for more than 3 years. Blood *54*:1023, 1979.
319. Hughes, W., and Smith, D.: Infection during induction of remission in acute lymphocytic leukemia. Cancer *31*:1008, 1973.
320. Pizzo, P. A., Robichaud, K. J., et al.: Duration of empiric antibiotic therapy in granulocytopenic patients with cancer. Am. J. Med. *67*:194, 1979.
321. Bodey, G. P., Rodriguez, V., et al.: Fever and infection in leukemic patients: a study of 494 consecutive patients. Cancer *41*:1610, 1978.
322. Whitley, R., Hilty, M., et al.: Vidarabine therapy of varicella in immunosuppressed patients. J. Pediatr. *101*:125, 1982.
323. Prober, C. G., Kirk, L. E., et al.: Acyclovir therapy of chickenpox in immunosuppressed children—a collaborative study. J. Pediatr. *101*:622, 1982.

324. Balfour, H. H., Jr., Bean, B., et al.: Acyclovir halts progression of herpes zoster in immunocompromised patients. New Engl. J. Med. *308*:1448, 1983.
325. Pifer, L. L., Hughes, W. T., et al.: *Pneumocystis carinii* infection: evidence for high prevalence in normal and immunosuppressed children. Pediatrics *61*:35, 1978.
326. Simone, J. V., Aur, R. J. A., et al.: Acute lymphocytic leukemia in children. Cancer *36*:770, 1975.
327. Hughes, W. T., Kuhn, S., et al.: Successful chemoprophylaxis for *Pneumocystis carinii* pneumonitis. New Engl. J. Med. *297*:1419, 1977.
328. Chessells, J. M.: Childhood acute lymphoblastic leukaemia: the late effects of treatment. Br. J. Haematol. *53*:369, 1983.
329. Mosijczuk, A. D., and Ruymann, F. B.: Second malignancy in acute lymphocytic leukemia: A review of 33 cases. Am. J. Dis. Child. *135*:313, 1981.
330. Riccardi, R., Brouwers, P., et al.: Abnormal computed tomography brain scans in children with acute lymphoblastic leukemia: serial long-term follow-up. J. Clin. Oncol. *3*:12, 1985.
331. Day, R. E., Kingston, J., et al.: CAT brain scans after central nervous system prophylaxis for acute lymphoblastic leukaemia. Br. Med. J. *2*:1752, 1978.
332. Price, R. A., and Jamieson, P. A.: The central nervous system in childhood leukemia. II. Subacute leukoencephalopathy. Cancer *35*:306, 1975.
333. Price, R. A., and Birdwell, D. A.: The central nervous system in childhood leukemia. III. Mineralizing microangiopathy and dystrophic calcification. Cancer *42*:717, 1978.
334. Freeman, J. E., Johnston, P. G. B., et al.: Somnolence after prophylactic cranial irradiation in children with acute lymphoblastic leukemia. Br. Med. J. *1*:523, 1973.
335. McIntosh, S., Klatskin, E. H., et al.: Chronic neurologic disturbance in childhood leukemia. Cancer *37*:853, 1976.
336. Eiser, C., Lansdown, R. G., et al.: Retrospective study of intellectual development of children treated for acute lymphoblastic leukaemia. Arch. Dis. Child. *52*:525, 1977.
337. Whitt, J. K., Wells, R. J., et al.: Cranial irradiation in childhood acute lymphocytic leukemia. Neuropsychologic sequelae. Am. J. Dis. Child. *138*:730, 1984.
338. Ochs, J. J., Parvey, L. S., et al.: Serial cranial computed tomography scans in children with leukemia given two different forms of central nervous system therapy. J. Clin. Oncol. *1*:793, 1983.
339. Esseltine, D. W., Freeman, C. R., et al.: Computerized tomography brain scans in long-term survivors of childhood acute lymphoblastic leukemia. Med. Pediatr. Oncol. *9*:429, 1981.
340. Muhlendahl, K. E., Gadner, H., et al.: Endocrine function after antineoplastic therapy in 22 children with acute lymphoblastic leukaemia. Helv. Paediatr. Acta *31*:463, 1976.
341. Shalet, S. M., Price, D. A., et al.: Normal growth despite abnormalities of growth hormone secretion in children treated for acute leukemia. J. Pediatr. *94*:719, 1979.
342. Dickinson, W. P., Berry, D. H., et al.: Differential effects of cranial irradiation on growth hormone response to arginine and insulin infusion. J. Pediatr. *92*:754, 1978.
343. Wells, R. J., Foster, M. B., et al.: The impact of cranial irradiation on the growth of children with acute lymphocytic leukemia. Am. J. Dis. Child. *137*:37, 1983.
344. Siris, E. S., Leventhal, B. G., et al.: Effects of childhood leukemia and chemotherapy on puberty and reproductive function in girls. New Engl. J. Med. *294*:1143, 1976.
345. Lentz, R. D., Bergstein, J., et al.: Postpubertal evaluation of gonadal function following cyclophosphamide therapy before and during puberty. J. Pediatr. *91*:385, 1977.
346. Lilleyman, J. S.: Male fertility after successful chemotherapy for lymphoblastic leukaemia. Lancet *2*:1125, 1979.
347. Matthews, J. H., and Wood, J. K.: Male fertility during chemotherapy for acute leukemia. New Engl. J. Med. *303*:1235, 1980.
348. Li, F. P., Fine, W., et al.: Offspring of patients treated for cancer in childhood. J. Natl. Cancer Inst. *62*:1193, 1979.
349. Sourkes, B.: Siblings of the pediatric cancer patient. In *Psychological Aspects of Childhood Cancer*. Kellerman, J. (ed.), Springfield, IL, Charles C Thomas, 1980.
350. Weinstein, H. J.: Congenital leukaemia and the neonatal myeloproliferative disorders associated with Down's syndrome. Clin. Haematol. *7*:147, 1978.
351. Rosner, F., Lee, S. L., et al.: Down's syndrome and acute leukemia: myeloblastic or lymphoblastic. Am. J. Med. *53*:203, 1972.
352. Conen, P. E., and Erkman, B.: Combined mongolism and leukemia. Am. J. Dis. Child. *112*:429, 1966.
353. Holland, W., Doll, R., et al.: The mortality from leukaemia and other cancers among patients with Down's syndrome and among their parents. Br. J. Cancer *16*:178, 1962.
354. van den Berghe, H., Fryns, J., et al.: Congenital leukaemia with 46,XX,t (Bq+ Cq−) cells. J. Med. Genet. *9*:468, 1978.
355. MacDougall, L., Brown, J., et al.: C-monosomy myeloproliferative syndrome: a case of 7-monosomy. J. Pediatr. *84*:256, 1974.
356. Djernes, B. W., Soukup, S. W., et al.: Congenital leukemia associated with mosaic trisomy 9. J. Pediatr. *88*:596, 1972.
357. Reimann, D. L., Clemmens, R. L., et al.: Congenital acute leukemia. Skin nodules, a first sign. J. Pediatr. *46*:415, 1959.
358. Odom, L., and Gordon, E.: Acute monoblastic leukemia in infancy and early childhood: successful treatment with an epipodophyllotoxin. Blood *64*:875, 1984.
359. Spier, C. M., Kjeldsberg, C. R., et al.: Pre-B-cell acute lymphoblastic leukemia in the newborn. Blood *64*:1064, 1984.
360. Ross, J. D., Moloney, W. C., et al.: Ineffective regulation of granulopoiesis masquerading as congenital leukemia in a mongoloid child. J. Pediatr. *63*:1, 1963.
361. Brodeur, G. M., Dahl, D., et al.: Transient leukemoid reaction and trisomy 21 mosaicism in a phenotypically normal newborn. Blood *55*:691, 1980.
362. Honda, F., Punnett, H. H., et al.: Serial cytogenetic and hematologic studies on a mongol with trisomy-21 and acute congenital leukemia. J. Pediatr. *65*:880, 1964.
363. Wolk, R., Stuart, M., et al.: Congenital and neonatal leukemia—lymphocytic or myelocytic? Am. J. Dis. Child. *128*:864, 1974.
364. Toch, R.: Case records of the Massachusetts General Hospital (Case 37-1976). New Engl. J. Med. *295*:608, 1976.
365. Holland, J.: Psychological aspects of oncology. Med. Clin. North Am. *61*:737, 1977.
366. Spinetta, J.: Adjustment in children with cancer. J. Pediatr. Psychol. *2*:49, 1977.
367. Karon, J.: The physician and the adolescent with cancer. Pediatr. Clin. North Am. *20*:965, 1973.
368. O'Malley, J. E., Koocher, G., et al.: Psychiatric sequelae of surviving childhood cancer. Am. J. Orthopsychiatry *49*:608, 1979.
369. Kagan-Goodheart, L.: Reentry: living with childhood cancer. Am. J. Orthopsychiatry *47*:651, 1977.
370. Katz, E., Kellerman, J., et al.: School intervention with pediatric cancer patients. J. Pediatr. Psychol. *2*:72, 1977.
371. Lansky, S. B., Lowman, J. T., et al.: School phobia in children with malignant neoplasms. Am. J. Dis. Child. *129*:42, 1975.
372. Lansky, S. B., Cairns, J. U., et al.: Childhood cancer: parental discord and divorce. Pediatrics *62*:184, 1978.

373. Wise, T. N.: Training oncology fellows in psychological aspects of their specialty. Cancer *39*:2584, 1977.
374. Artiss, K. L., and Levine, A. S.: Doctor–patient relation in severe illness. New Engl. J. Med. *288*:1210, 1973.
375. Kübler-Ross, E.: On Death and Dying. New York, Macmillan Publishing Co., 1969.
376. Binger, C. M., Ablin, A. R., et al.: Childhood leukemia: emotional impact on patient and family. New Engl. J. Med. *280*:414, 1969.
377. Koocher, G. P.: Childhood, death, and cognitive development. Dev. Psychol. *9*:369, 1973.
378. Spinetta, J. J.: The dying child's awareness of death: a review. Psychol. Bull. *81*:256, 1973.
379. Spinetta, J. J., and Maloney, L. J.: Death anxiety in the outpatient leukemic child. Pediatrics *65*:1034, 1975.
380. Spinetta, J. J., Rigler, D., et al.: Anxiety in the dying child. Pediatrics *52*:841, 1973.

ONCOLOGY

CHAPTER 34
Chronic Myeloproliferative Disorders and Myelodysplasia

HOLCOMBE E. GRIER

INTRODUCTION 1064
CHRONIC MYELOPROLIFERATIVE DISORDERS 1064
Adult Type Chronic Myelogenous Leukemia (CML)
   Clinical Presentation
   Pathophysiology
   Differential Diagnosis
   Clinical Course
   Treatment
Juvenile Chronic Myelogenous Leukemia
   Clinical Presentation
   Treatment
Polycythemia Vera
   Clinical Presentation
   Etiology
   Clinical Course
   Treatment
Essential Thrombocythemia
   Clinical Presentation
   Course and Treatment
Agnogenic Myeloid Metaplasia/Myelofibrosis
   Clinical Presentation
   Etiology
   Course and Treatment
THE MYELODYSPLASTIC SYNDROMES 1075
Clinical Presentation
Pathophysiology
   Bone Marrow Culture Systems
   Cytogenetics and Preleukemia
   Clonal Nature of Myelodysplasia
Differential Diagnosis
Clinical Course
Treatment
Monosomy 7

INTRODUCTION

The chronic myeloproliferative disorders (chronic myelogenous leukemia, polycythemia vera, essential thrombocythemia, and agnogenic myeloid metaplasia/myelofibrosis) and the myelodysplastic syndromes are diseases observed mainly in adults and characterized by (1) a clonal proliferation of an abnormal multipotent stem cell (Table 34–1) and (2) a propensity to develop syndromes similar to acute leukemia. Although these disorders are rare in childhood, they provide important insights into the biology of the hematopoietic system.

CHRONIC MYELOPROLIFERATIVE DISORDERS

In 1951, Dameshek introduced the idea that chronic myelogenous leukemia (CML), polycythemia vera (PV), essential thrombocythemia (ET), and agnogenic myeloid metaplasia (AMM), are related "myeloproliferative syndromes" (1). Although each has distinct clinical, laboratory, and biological features, much information gathered since the 1950's provides further evidence for their linkage (2). Each is manifested by clonal proliferation of an abnormal cell, a panmyelopathy (albeit with unique peripheral blood manifestations), and a variable tendency to develop acute leukemia. In addition, patients may rarely present with mixed manifestations of the various disorders, or patients with one disorder may develop symptoms more typical of a different myeloproliferative disease during the course of their illness (3). Basic biological abnormalities may be strikingly similar as in the example of decreased platelet lipoxygenase deficiency (4). The factors that create and select for the increased expansion of abnormal stem cells and the pressures that force the specific peripheral manifestations of the particular syndromes (CML—increased granulocytes; ET—increased platelets; PV—increased red cells) are completely unknown.

Adult Type Chronic Myelogenous Leukemia

Chronic myelogenous leukemia (CML) constitutes 2 to 5 per cent of all childhood leukemia. In childhood the disorder may present as two distinct clinical syndromes: adult type CML (ACML), a disease virtually indistinguishable from that seen in older patients, and juvenile CML (JCML), a disease relatively restricted to children and with

Table 34–1. CLONAL DISEASES INVOLVING A MULTIPOTENT STEM CELL PROGENITOR

Disease	Reference
Chronic myelogenous leukemia (adult type)	64
Polycythemia vera	172
Essential thrombocythemia	217
Myelofibrosis/myeloid metaplasia	235
Myelodysplastic syndromes	301–303
Paroxysmal natural hemoglobinuria	320
Acute myelogenous leukemia (variable involvement)	321

distinct clinical, laboratory, and cytogenetic characteristics. The two diseases are compared in Table 34–2. The incidence of ACML is 1 to 2 cases per 100,000 between ages 20 to 50 years with a slow rise thereafter. The incidence among those younger than 20 is <1 per 100,000. The male to female ratio in adult studies is 1.8:1 (5).

CLINICAL PRESENTATION

The presenting signs and symptoms of ACML are attributable to the excessive accumulation of both mature and immature granulocytic cells. Anemia, pain, dysphagia, or increased abdominal girth from splenomegaly, or hypermetabolic symptoms such as fever, night sweats, and weight loss may bring the patient to medical attention. In adults, approximately 20 per cent of diagnoses are made when an elevated white blood count is found on routine examination (6). Malaise, abdominal discomfort, bleeding diathesis, and bone and joint pains were the most common symptoms at diagnosis in a series of 39 children with ACML (7). Splenomegaly is present in most patients at diagnosis and may be more frequent in children. Hepatomegaly and lymphadenopathy occur less commonly (6, 7).

The majority of patients have white blood cell counts greater than 100,000 cells per mm^3 at diagnosis (6), and children tend to present with even higher counts (7, 8). Thrombocytosis is common with average platelet counts above 400,000 cells per mm^3 in most pediatric and adult series. Occasionally white counts of ACML patients may fluctuate spontaneously on a regular cycle. The platelet count may also fluctuate but with a periodicity different from that of the white count. Such fluctuations may make therapy difficult (9). The presence of anemia is quite variable; hematocrits tend to average 35 per cent in adult series and are frequently lower in children (7, 8, 10, 11).

Leukostasis, a syndrome commonly seen in acute myelogenous leukemia with high blast counts, is rarely found in adults presenting with CML (12). The syndrome is more common in childhood, and papilledema, strokes, cerebellar signs, decreased cerebral function, ischemic digits, and priapism have all been noted (7, 8, 13). Rarely skin nodules, representing extramedullary hematopoiesis, may be seen (14).

The most prominent feature of the bone marrow at diagnosis is granulocytic hyperplasia; megakaryocytic hyperplasia may also be seen occasionally (6). About one of six patients with ACML has lipid-laden macrophages similar to Gaucher cells or sea-blue histiocytes (15). Marrow basophils and eosinophils may be increased (8). Myelofibrosis is unusual at diagnosis, although a mild increase in reticulum may be seen; the development of myelofibrosis during the course of CML frequently heralds a blast crisis (16, 17). Although the peripheral blood differential contains the entire spectrum of the granulocytic series, blasts are usually less than 5 per cent (8). Dysplastic eosinophils and basophilia are common. Rare patients may present in blast crisis (see below).

Approximately 85 per cent of ACML patients demonstrate the Philadelphia chromosome (Ph^1) on cytogenetic analysis of their bone marrow or peripheral blood (18, 19) (see Chapter 41). Ph^1 refers to the shortened chromosome 22 formed by a reciprocal translocation of genetic material between chromosomes 9 and 22 [t(9q+;22q−)] (20). The cytogenetic abnormality is limited to hematopoietic cells; lymphocytes, marrow fibroblasts, and other somatic cells are diploid (21, 22). The Ph^1 chromosome usually does not disappear during hematologic "remission" although it may decrease in frequency. In 8 per cent of cases the Ph^1 chromosome is formed from variant translocations involving other chromosomes in addition to or instead of 9 (19). Recent evidence shows that chromosomes 9 and 22 may both always be involved in the variant translocation even when not

Table 34–2. CLINICAL CHARACTERISTICS OF ADULT TYPE CHRONIC MYELOGENOUS LEUKEMIA (ACML) AND JUVENILE CHRONIC MYELOGENOUS LEUKEMIA (JCML) IN CHILDHOOD

Characteristics at Diagnosis	JCML	ACML
Age	Usually <4	Usually >4
Lymphadenopathy	Common	Unusual
Skin lesions	Common	Unusual
Bleeding	Common	Unusual
Bacterial infection	Common	Unusual
WBC >100 K	Unusual	Common
Hg <12	Common	Variable
Platelets	Usually Decreased	Usually Increased
Monocytosis	Common	Unusual
Circulating pronormoblasts	Common	Unusual
Hg F% increased	Common	Unusual
Philadelphia chromosome	Absent	>90%
Leukocyte alkaline phoshatase Decreased	Variable	Common
Clinical Course		
Median Survival	1–2 years	4–5 years
Blastic phase	Unusual	Common

apparent by usual techniques (23). In general Ph^1-negative patients are older, more anemic, have lower white blood cell counts at presentation, and have a shorter survival than Ph^1-positive cases (24). Indeed, Ph^1-negative ACML is likely a different syndrome entirely.

Leukocyte alkaline phosphatase activity (LAP) is reduced at diagnosis in most patients with ACML. When the white count is lowered with therapy, the LAP returns to normal levels in 30 per cent of cases (25, 26). LAP levels also may increase during accelerated and blast phases (25) or during any inflammatory response (27, 28). LAP activity may rise when leukocytes of CML patients are transfused into neutropenic hosts, suggesting the existence of an "extrinsic" cause for the low LAP levels (29, 30) or selection for survival of LAP-positive cells.

Neutrophils from patients with ACML display many other functional and biochemical abnormalities in addition to decreased LAP activity (31). The exact etiology of these defects remains unclear but may be related to an increase in circulating early myeloid forms (31). The clinical consequence of the abnormalities is not severe, since neither chronic nor acute infections pose particular problems to the non-neutropenic ACML patient in chronic phase (6) and transfused CML cells are useful in the treatment of septic neutropenic patients.

The expanded granulocytic mass results in an increase in white cell–derived B_{12} binding protein (32). Increased transcobalamin I is responsible for most of the increased binding. B_{12} binding falls as the white count decreases with therapy (33). Hemoglobin F may be slightly increased in ACML, but generally to a much lower level than that commonly seen in JCML (34, 35).

PATHOPHYSIOLOGY

Etiology. The etiology of ACML is unknown in the majority of patients. Ionizing radiation can increase its incidence; a seven-fold increase in incidence was seen in the survivors of the nuclear blasts at both Nagasaki and Hiroshima (36). The incidence was highest in young people, especially children less than 5 years old (37). There was no increase of ACML in children exposed in utero (38). The increase of CML peaked at 5 to 10 years postexposure and then returned to expected levels; this is in marked contrast to the incidence of acute myelogenous leukemia, which continues to be abnormal 40 years later (37).

The role of genetic influences in ACML is unclear. There is one reported instance of two identical twins and another sibling developing ACML (39), although other families have been reported in which the second twin did not develop the disease (39, 40).

The high correlation between ACML and the Philadelphia chromosome [t(9;22)] implies but does not prove an etiologic link. Two cellular oncogenes, c-*abl* and c-*sis* are located on chromosomes 9 and 22 respectively (41, 42). Although both have been found translocated to the opposite chromosome in some cases of CML, the movement of c-abl to chromosome 9 appears to be the more constant change, occurring even in variant translocations not including chromosome 9 by standard cytogenetic techniques (43). C-abl, in fact, always moves to a very limited area on chromosome 22, termed the breakpoint cluster region or bar (43a). This translocation results in the transcription of an abnormal chimeric bcr/c-abl messenger RNA (43b). The link between translocation of oncogenes and oncogenesis is discussed in Chapter 31.

Progenitor Culture System. The exact mechanism for expansion of the granulocytic series and preferential growth of leukemic cells in ACML is unknown. CML precursors do not divide more rapidly than normal precursors (44). Studies using blood and bone marrow in vitro culture systems (reviewed in Chapter 6) revealed an increased frequency of granulocyte-macrophage progenitors (CFU-GM) (44) as well as erythroid progenitors (45). These derived colonies display normal maturation in vitro, and there is a direct correlation between CFU-GM numbers and peripheral white cell count (46). Studies in children with ACML show similar results (47, 48).

The interrelationship between the findings of increased numbers of precursors, increased positive regulators of granulopoiesis such as colony-stimulating activity (49, 50), and decreased inhibitors of granulopoiesis such as lactoferrin (51, 52) is unclear (53). In addition ACML cells may produce an inhibitor that suppresses the growth of normal progenitors (54, 55, 56). Nevertheless, normal progenitors that give rise to Ph^1 negative precursors are present at diagnosis and persist throughout the chronic phase in most patients as demonstrated by emergence of Ph^1 negative cells in long-term marrow culture and the return of Ph^1 negative cells in heavily treated patients (57, 58).

Clonal Nature of CML. The clonal origin of ACML has been well demonstrated. Philadelphia chromosomes have been found in granulocytic and erythoid colonies (57, 59–63). Fibroblast colonies do not contain the Ph^1, indicating they are not part of the neoplastic clone (21).

Further work on clonality has focused on female CML patients whose X chromosome inactivation mosaicism is delineated by a glucose-6-phosphatase dehydrogenase (G6PD) marker. Early in embryogenesis each cell undergoes a random inactivation of one X chromosome. Any single cell and all of its progeny continue to express only one specific X chromosome. G6PD is encoded on the X chromosome and women with electrophoretically distinct G6PD types thus have a marker for their two populations of cells. A tumor arising from a single cell should therefore have only one G6PD type, while a tumor arising from multiple cells would display both types. In CML, granulocytes, platelets, red blood cells, and in vitro erythroid and granulocyte-macrophage colonies all display only one G6PD type in patients heterozygous for the enzyme (64, 65). Marrow fibroblasts, however, display both G6PD types (65). Nonclonal hematopoiesis can be restored transiently by intensive chemotherapy (66). A patient with Ph¹-negative CML has been studied and this disease was also found to be clonal at the level of a multipotent stem cell (67).

Involvement of lymphoid cells in the malignant CML clone has been more difficult to prove. Indirect evidence is provided by the fact that blastic transformation in CML is lymphoid in one third of cases as analyzed by surface markers, including the common acute lymphoblastic leukemia antigen (CALLA), and by increased terminal deoxytransforase enzyme levels (see below) (68). Furthermore, lymphocytes staining for surface IgM may contain the Ph¹ chromosome (69). Similarly lymphocytes from an ACML patient that were enriched for B cells were monoclonal for G6PD; T lymphocytes from the same patient were polyclonal (70). B lymphocyte cell lines derived from a patient with Ph¹-positive CML had a preponderance of the malignant G6PD type (71). So far, evidence for lymphoid involvement in Ph¹-negative ACML is limited to the existence of lymphoblastic crisis (72).

The B lymphocyte cell lines derived from the patient with Ph¹-positive CML mentioned above did not contain the Ph¹ chromosome, although they did show a propensity for chromosomal aberration (71). This finding, along with the existence of patients with CML in whom the Ph¹ appears late in the disease (73) and patients with mixed Ph¹+ and Ph¹– blast crisis, argues strongly for a multistep pathogenesis. In this model, clonal expansion as exemplified by the development of only one G6PD type is the first step. The second step is the subsequent development of the Ph¹ chromosome.

Peripheral blood T lymphocytes studied by G6PD are not clonal in CML (70). A recent report has confirmed T cell involvement in CML, however (74). The T cells studied were cultured from the cells of multilineage hematopoietic colonies (CFU-GEMMT) grown from a patient with Ph¹-positive CML. All of the T cells in these colonies contained only Ph¹ positive karyotypes. A possible explanation for these discrepant findings rests on the long life of T cells. Most of the T cells in CML patients may have derived from normal stem cells long before leukemic transformation. Rare cases of T cell lymphoblastic crises in Ph¹-positive CML confirm involvement of the T cell in the neoplastic process (75, 76, 77).

DIFFERENTIAL DIAGNOSIS

A diagnosis of ACML is self evident in the patient with the typical picture of a white blood count over 100,000 cells per mm³, a differential spanning the myeloid series, a low leukocyte alkaline phosphatase, a large spleen, and the Ph¹ chromosome. Even in a young child, attention to the distinct differences between ACML and JCML usually makes the correct diagnosis clear (see Table 34–2). Occasionally patients with severe infections, congenital heart disease, or metastatic cancer will present with a "leukemoid" reaction (78). In these disorders, the peripheral blood differential rarely contain blasts and promyelocytes, the white cell count is usually somewhat lower, a source of infection is frequently found, and LAP scores and cytogenetics are normal. Since ACML may present in blast crisis, the patient with Philadelphia chromosome–positive acute lymphoblastic leukemia presents a particular problem in differential diagnosis (79, 80). Since in ACML the Ph¹ chromosome rarely disappears for more than a few months even with very aggressive therapy (58), we believe a lengthy conversion to a Ph¹-negative state after remission induction excludes ACML as the diagnosis.

CLINICAL COURSE

The course in ACML is quite variable. The time span from malignant transformation of a single cell to the development of clinically detectable disease has been estimated at 6 years (81). After clinical detection, patients still enjoy control of their disease with unimpaired lifestyles for periods of many months to years. Inevitably, however, patients develop a more malignant form of their disease, a phase difficult to control with therapy and leading to death within a short period (6). Children with ACML are not protected from this unfortunate outcome (7). This blastic phase occurs at a median of about 3 years and may be heralded by a 3 to 6 month transitional phase (6). Findings during the transitional period may include basophilia, new-onset thrombocytosis, thrombocytopenia, leukocytosis refractory to previous therapy, anemia, and splenomegaly (6, 82). Biopsy of the marrow may show myelofibrosis (16, 17), and cytogenetic analyses may reveal new abnormalities. No therapy short of bone marrow transplantation has been shown to prevent the inevitable development of a blastic phase and death in ACML (83).

Chronic Phase. Several studies have attempted to identify factors at diagnosis that will predict which patients' chronic phase will be longer than average (84–88). It is well established that ACML patients without the Ph¹ chromosome have a significantly shorter course (85). Other negative factors include tumor burden (white blood cell count, spleen size, liver size) and a high myeloblast count (84–87). A multivariant analysis of several clinical studies found spleen size and circulating blasts the most important negative prognostic indicators (88). Reports of particularly long survival in patients with a mixture of Ph^1-positive and Ph^1-negative marrow cells at diagnosis are not substantiated in a larger series (89, 90).

Blast Phase. The terminal phase may occur abruptly or have a slow onset over months. Common clinical and laboratory findings of the accelerated phase are reviewed above. The blasts in ACML may be hard to characterize, but they are usually morphologically similar to those of acute myeloblastic leukemia (91). In about a third of cases the blasts resemble lymphoblasts (92); this ratio has been further confirmed by terminal transference levels and surface marker analysis (see Chapter 33) (93–96). The mean age of patients with a lymphoblastic crisis is younger than that of patients with myeloblastic crisis (95). The lymphoblasts are primarily of the pre-B cell type, but three cases with T cell markers have been noted (75–77, 97).

Tumors composed of primitive blast cells may occur simultaneously with or even precede the blast phase in over a tenth of ACML patients. Common extramedullary sites include lymph nodes, bone, soft tissue, skin, and the paravertebral area (91, 98). These chloromas or myeloblastomas may be more common in blast phase CML than in acute myelogenous leukemia (99). Meningeal leukemia occurs most frequently after lymphoid blast crisis, usually as a primary relapse site (100, 101).

Further chromosomal abnormalities frequently accompany the accelerated or blastic phase of ACML. The most common new findings are a second Ph^1 chromosome, isochromosome 17, and trisomy 8 (19, 102–104). Leukocyte alkaline phosphatase frequently rises during blast crisis, and in vitro growth patterns begin to resemble those seen in acute myelogenous leukemia (6, 54). The mix of lymphoid to myeloid blast crisis in childhood ACML appears to be the same as in adult series (7).

TREATMENT

Chronic Phase. The majority of patients with chronic phase ACML do not need immediate treatment, since symptoms are mild and complications rare at diagnosis. Occasionally signs of leukostasis are present at diagnosis and more rapid institution of therapy is indicated. This may be especially true in children (8). If the white count must be lowered quickly leukophoresis and/or immediate chemotherapy with high doses of hydroxyurea may be used (105, 106). Proper hydration and the use of allopurinol to avoid hyperuricemia are imperative before rapid lysis of cells with chemotherapy. For years splenic radiation was the mainstay of therapy for chronic ACML (83), but it has been supplanted by chemotherapy. Many chemotherapeutic agents are effective in chronic phase CML (107). Busulfan and hydroxyurea are the most frequently used drugs (107); median survival of patients treated with either drug is similar (108). The busulfan side effects of skin hyperpigmentation and, rarely, interstitial pneumonitis have led many clinicians to favor hydroxyrea as the treatment of choice (68).

Patients in chronic phase are best managed by periods of chemotherapy followed by rest periods. Excessive therapy with marked leukopenia or thrombocytopenia is more dangerous than mild elevation of counts, and care must be exercised (68). Remission is usually not associated with disappearance of the Ph^1 chromosome; in fact most patients continue to have 100 per cent Ph^1 metaphases in bone marrow. Splenectomy may be very effective for complications of the disease, but it has not in general had a marked influence on median survival (109–112).

Several groups have used aggressive therapy in chronic phase ACML in an attempt to forestall the development of blastic transformation (58, 113, 114). A transient (several months) decrease or disappearance of the Philadelphia chromosome is seen in many patients, but median survival as compared with historical controls is only slightly altered, and cure does not appear likely (115). This loss of the Ph^1 chromosome has also been noted during treatment of the chronic phase with human recombinant alpha-interferon (115a). In general aggressive therapy is indicated only in the research setting. Bone marrow transplantation for ACML will be discussed later.

Blast Phase. The blastic phase of ACML is quite refractory to chemotherapy. Leukostasis is more common in the blastic phase, and very high blast counts must be treated aggressively with hydration, allopurinol, and leukophoresis and/or high dose chemotherapy (105, 106). Lymphoid blast morphology, pre–B cell surface antigens, and high terminal deoxynucleotydal transferase all predict for good response to drugs effective in lymphoblastic leukemia, such as vincristine and prednisone (92, 95, 96). Patients with myeloblastic crisis respond poorly to any form of therapy. Median survival after blastic transformation is only 8 months for patients with myeloblastic morphology and 6 months for patients with lymphoblastic morphology (92). In vitro growth studies show that peripheral blood collected during the chronic phase of ACML has many colony-forming cell (45). Theoretically, aggressive chemotherapy fo blastic phase with reinfusion of chronic phase cel might re-establish chronic phase and prolong su vival. But cure obviously cannot be effected with this technique, and although median survival may be slightly improved, the results have in general been disappointing (68). Curative autologous transplant for CML awaits an ability to select nonleukemic (Ph¹-negative) progenitors with high accuracy and in large numbers (57, 116).

Bone Marrow Transplantation. The first ACML patients to receive allogeneic bone marrow transplants (see Chapter 8) were in accelerated or blastic phase. Results were initially disappointing, but some long-term remissions were obtained (117, 118). Fefer and colleagues reported excellent success with syngeneic transplants of patients in chronic phase who had identical twin donors (119). Many groups have since used allogeneic transplants for ACML patients in chronic phase (120–124), and early results show excellent survival with most patients free of Philadelphia chromosomes. We currently recommend bone marrow transplantation in chronic phase for any child with ACML who has an HLA matched donor.

Juvenile Chronic Myelogenous Leukemia

Juvenile chronic myelogenous leukemia (JCML) is a myeloproliferative disorder that presents in the first few years of life. Alternate terms used to describe JCML include infantile chronic myelogenous leukemia and subacute and chronic myelomonocytic leukemia in children (4, 125, 127); the latter is a much more accurate term, as the disease is quite distinct from the adult form of CML. A high male-to-female ratio is seen in most series. The characteristics of JCML and adult chronic myelogenous leukemia are contrasted in Table 34–2.

CLINICAL PRESENTATION

Common presenting complaints in JCML include fever, persistent infections, organomegaly, skin rash, bleeding, and failure to thrive (4, 125–127). The hematologic profile usually reveals a white blood count of 15,000 to 85,000 cells per mm³, a platelet count of 25,000 to 100,000 cells per mm³, and a hemoglobin of 8 to 10 g per dl. The bone marrow is hypercellular with myeloid hyperplasia and decreased megakaryocytes (11). The peripheral blood differential reveals immature myeloid cells, many immature monocytes, nucleated red blood cells, and occasionally pronormoblasts (4, 125–127) (Fig. 34–1). Presentation of JCML may occur at birth (128), and teenagers with JCML have been described (129). Xanthomata and eczematoid rashes are common findings (126), and multiple cafe-au-lait spots characteristic of neurofibromatosis may also be seen (130–132).

Median fetal hemoglobin is 38 per cent and may be as high as 70 per cent; distribution of fetal hemoglobin is uniform throughout the red cells

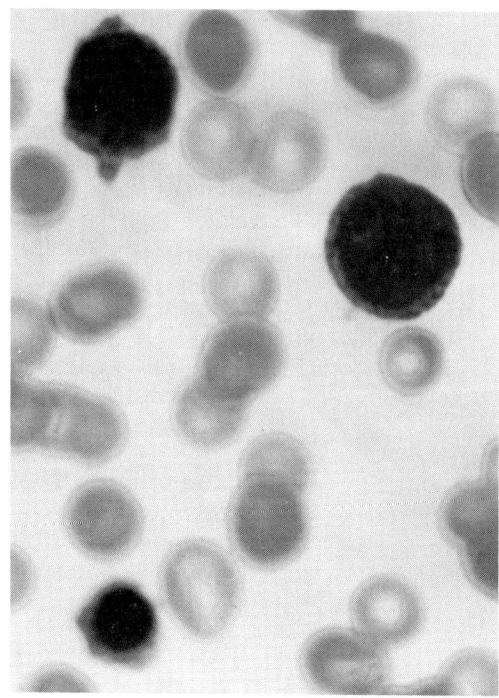

Figure 34–1. Pronormoblasts and nucleated red blood cells in the peripheral blood of a patient with juvenile chronic myelogenous leukemia.

(34, 35). Although some authors consider the elevation of fetal hemoglobin a sine qua non for the diagnosis of JCML, others disagree and consider patients with normal fetal hemoglobin levels to have the disease. Fetal hematopoiesis may be mirrored in other metabolic and antigenetic abnormalities of the red cell (133–135). Colonies of progenitor-derived erythroblasts occur in cultures independent of added erythopoietin as is observed in polycythemia vera and in cultures of fetal marrow (136). The Philadelphia chromosome is not present. A number of different cytogenetic abnormalities may occur in JCML, although the incidence appears low (127, 137, 138). The multiple red cell anomalies argue for erythroid involvement in the malignant clone with transformation to a fetal phenotype; however, neither G6PD studies nor cytogenetic studies of the type described for ACML have been performed in JCML.

Monocytic colonies predominate over granulocyte colonies when peripheral blood and bone marrow from JCML patients are grown in vitro, reflecting the peripheral monocytosis frequently seen (139, 140). Large numbers of granulocytic colonies may be seen in some JCML patients, however (141). Cytogenetic changes seen in the whole bone marrow may also be noted in the granulocyte/macrophage colonies, indicating their derivation from the malignant clone. Co-culture of JCML marrow with normal marrow leads to suppression of normal colony growth, implying an inhibitory effect by abnormal cells (141a).

The clinical picture of JCML is quite characteristic. Combined immune deficiency or congenital viral infections may present a picture quite similar to JCML in the very young child. Similarly, persistent Epstein-Barr virus infections may provoke clinical and laboratory findings very like those in JCML (142). However, in none of these conditions does fetal hemoglobin reach the levels seen in JCML. These disorders should be ruled out before the diagnosis of JCML is made. A disease similar to JCML has been seen in two pairs of siblings (11). This familial chronic myeloid leukemic syndrome differs from JCML mainly by virtue of the very long survival of two of the sibs (> 9 years).

TREATMENT

Unlike ACML patients, those with JCML usually do not respond to busulfan or hydroxyurea with reversion to a normal hematopoietic and clinical profile. Although response to a combination of cytarabine and mercaptopurine has been noted, the median survival for most treated or untreated patients is between 1 and 2 years (143). Most series report almost universal fatality, although in a more recent study Castro-Malaspina and colleagues note a subset of patients whose course may not be so virulent (127). Death is usually due to infection or progression of disease; a distinct blast phase as in ACML is uncommon, however. The exact etiology of the frequent infections in JCML is not clear. Bone marrow transplantation has been successful in patients with JCML (144), and we would suggest transplantation for any patient who has a histocompatible donor (see Chapter 8).

Polycythemia Vera

Polycythemia has been variously defined as an increase in erythrocyte mass, hemoglobin, or hematocrit. Normal values for hemoglobin and hematocrit vary with the altitude at which a person lives and, in pediatrics, with age. The normal values for hemoglobin and hematocrit by age are listed in the Appendix. For adults at sea level hematocrit values above 52 per cent in men and 47 per cent in women require attention since they lie outside the 95 per cent confidence levels of the population (145).

There are three types of polycythemia: (1) polycythemia vera (PV), or primary polycythemia; (2) secondary polycythemia; and (3) relative polycythemia (146) (Table 34–3). The first two types are associated with an increase in red cell mass, while in the third the red cell mass is normal and the plasma volume reduced. Secondary polycythemia is due to an excess of erythropoietin that may be either a manifestation of decreased tissue oxygenation (physiologically appropriate) or inappropriate erythropoietin secretion from a tumor. Hemoglobins with abnormal oxygen affinity are

Table 34–3. CLASSIFICATION OF THE POLYCYTHEMIAS*

I. Primary Polycythemia
   A. Polycythemia vera
   B. Familial polycythemia
II. Secondary Polycythemia
   A. Physiologically appropriate (decreased tissue oxygenation)
      1. Hypoxemia
         a. Cardiac disease with left to right shunting
         b. Pulmonary disease
         c. High altitude
         d. Alveolar hypoventilation (Pickwickian syndrome)
      2. Normal arterial oxygenation
         a. High oxygen affinity hemoglobinopathy
         b. Carboxyhemoglobin, methemoglobin
         c. Low cardiac output
         d. Decreased red cell 2, 3 DPG
         e. Decreased tissue oxygen utilization, such as seen in cobalt therapy
   B. Physiologically inappropriate (normal tissue oxygenization)
      1. Tumors producing excess erythropoietic substances
         a. Wilms' tumor
         b. Cerebellar hemangioblastoma
         c. Hepatoma
         d. Tumors rarely seen in children: renal cell carcinoma, uterine leiomyomas, ovarian carcinoma
      2. Renal disease with increased erythropoietic synthesis
         a. Cysts
         b. Hydronephrosis
         c. Bartter's syndrome
      3. Endocrine disorders
         a. Adrenocorticoid excess
         b. Testosterone administration
         c. Growth hormone administration
         d. Pheochromocytoma
III. Relative Polycythemia
   A. Loss of water and/or electrolytes (GI loss, renal loss diuretics, poor intake)
   B. Loss of plasma (burns, GI loss)
   C. Spurious or stress erythrocytosis (Gaisbocks's syndrome)

*Adapted from References 145, 146, and 159.

discussed in Chapter 20. Relative, or spurious, polycythemia occurs almost exclusively in middle-aged men (147). Confirmation of increased erythrocyte mass usually requires formal measurement with radioactively labeled red cells. An exception is the hematocrit value of greater than 60 per cent, which is pathognomonic for increased red cell mass unless the patient is severely dehydrated (146).

Many patients previously classified as having "familial polycythemia" instead had abnormal hemoglobins, decreased erythrocyte diphosphoglycerate (DPG), increased erythropoietin production, or polycythemia vera in multiple family members. Even when these causes are excluded, however, there are still some families with polycythemia of unknown etiology (148). In most patients with polycythemia, a careful history, physical examination, and measurements of (1) total red cell volume with labeled red cells, (2) arterial blood oxygen saturation, and (3) the oxygen pressure at which hemoglobin is 50 per cent saturated (P50) will lead to appropriate classification (146).

CLINICAL PRESENTATION

Polycythemia vera (PV) is a myeloproliferative disease caused by clonal expansion of an abnormal multipotent stem cell. The main manifestation of disease is a primary increase in erythrocyte mass. Strict criteria for the diagnosis of PV have been developed by the Polycythemia Vera Study Group and are presented in Table 34–4 (146). In addition to the criteria listed, all pediatric patients should have either a normal P50 measurement or, preferably, a normal hemoglobin dissociation curve. Hemoglobin electrophoresis alone is inadequate to rule out a hemoglobin with abnormal oxygen affinity since many abnormal hemoglobins migrate with hemoglobin A (145).

The incidence of PV is approximately 1 per 100,000 people. PV is uncommon in children; less than 1 per cent of all PV patients are less than 25 years old and the median age at presentation in most series is around 60 (146, 149). Nevertheless several childhood cases have been reported (150–158). The male-to-female ratio in PV is elevated in most adult series (146).

Clinical findings in PV are due to increased red cell mass and blood volume, increased blood viscosity, and hypermetabolism (159). The most common symptoms in PV include headache, weakness, pruritus, and dizziness; all occur in greater than 40 per cent of cases. Night sweats and weight loss are also frequent (160). On physical examination, most patients are plethoric, 70 per cent have large spleens, 40 per cent large livers, and a third will have diastolic blood pressures above 90 mm of mercury (146, 160).

By definition all patients have an increased red cell volume unless previously treated. At diagnosis the white cell count is greater than 12,000 in nearly half and the platelet count over 400,000 in almost two thirds of the patients (146, 160, 161). Similarly, leukocyte alkaline phosphatase score is increased in 70 per cent of the patients; the increase is not necessarily correlated with the white blood cell count (146, 160). Serum B_{12} values are elevated in approximately one third of the patients (160). Hypercellularity, an increase in megakaryocyte number and size, and an absence of iron stores are the usual bone marrow findings. Bone marrow reticulum may be slightly increased at diagnosis, but a marked increase is uncommon (162). Serum uric acid is elevated in over half the patients with PV, and gout may be a presenting symptom (146).

Clonal chromosomal abnormalities are seen in 10 to 25 per cent of patients at diagnosis (163–165); the incidence is higher in previously treated patients (25–40 per cent) (164, 165). The changes are nonrandom and include trisomy 8 (a finding common in acute leukemia), trisomy 9, and loss of part of chromosomes 5 or 22 (5q− and 22q−) (164–167). Cytogenetic abnormalities do not predict for leukemic transformation (164). When acute myelogenous leukemia intervenes in PV, cytogenetic abnormalities are almost universal and may be quite complex (167). Findings seen in therapy-related acute myelogenous leukemia such as a loss of part or all of chromosomes 5 and 7 are common (−5, −7, 5q−, 7q−) (164, 167). Although fetal hemoglobin levels may be somewhat elevated in PV at presentation, they do not reach the levels seen in juvenile CML.

ETIOLOGY

As with all the myeloproliferative diseases, the exact cause of PV is unknown. Several reports of PV in monozygotic twins as well as an increased rate in family members hint at some genetic influence on etiology (168–171). Using G6PD heterozygosity as a marker (see discussion of CML), PV has clearly been shown to be due to the clonal expansion of a single abnormal multipotent stem cell capable of differentiation into red cells, platelets, and white cells (172).

Expansion of the red cell mass in secondary polycythemia is due to increased erythropoietin. In contrast, erythropoietin is usually normal or decreased in PV (173). Both red cell precursors and multipotent precursors of PV patients are hypersensitive to erythropoietin in vitro; erythroid colonies will grow at concentrations of erythropoietin undetectable except by depletion with antibodies (174–180). Colonies grown at low erythropoietin concentration derive exclusively from the abnormal clone (181). Studies to determine the contribution of increased cycling of erythroid and multipotent progenitors to the increased erythroid pool have yielded conflicting results (177, 182). The cycling index of abnormal granulocytic colony-forming cells appears to exceed that of their normal counterparts, and unlike the erythroid

---

Table 34–4. POLYCYTHEMIA VERA: CRITERIA FOR DIAGNOSIS*

Category A
1. Increased red cell volume (males ≥36 ml/kg; females ≥32 ml/kg)
2. Arterial oxygen saturation ≥92%
3. Splenomegaly

Category B
1. Thrombocytosis (>400,000 cells mm³)
2. Leukocytosis (>12,000 cells mm³)
3. Increased leukocyte alkaline phosphatase
4. Increased vitamin B_{12} (>900 pg/ml) or unsaturated B_{12} binding capacity (>2200 pg/ml)

For diagnosis patient must have: A1+, A2+, A3+ or A1+, A2+, and any two from Category B

*Adapted from Reference 146.

progenitors, these cells can be separated from normal progenitors by physical properties (183, 184). Normal progenitors of all types seem to decrease over time when the same patient is tested (185). An increased proportion of erythrocyte and megakaryocyte cells in multipotent colonies reflects the situation in the whole bone marrow (179). Finally, the increased sensitivity to erythropoietin is not lost during the "spent" phase of PV (see next section) (186).

CLINICAL COURSE

Long survival after the diagnosis of PV is quite common (148). Vascular occlusive episodes are an important cause of morbidity and mortality. Occlusive episodes are related to hematocrit, and efforts should be made to keep the hematocrit of PV patients less than 45 per cent (187). The proper management of the hematocrit in patients with secondary polycythemia is more controversial, since the increased erythrocyte mass is due to a physiologic attempt to provide increased tissue oxygenation. Blood viscosity may become so high that tissue oxygen delivery is paradoxically decreased due to impaired cardiac output and altered regional blood flow (145).

Hematocrit values greater than 60 per cent may be deleterious, and patients often benefit from phlebotomy (188, 189). Phlebotomy in young children, especially those with compromised cardiac function or threatened infarction, should be performed with isovolemic replacement by colloid or crystalloid solutions in order to maintain the flow of oxyhemoglobin. In any patient undergoing chronic phlebotomy, the resultant iron deficiency must be corrected, since it can lead not only to disturbing nonhematopoietic symptoms but also to increased blood viscosity (190). The replacement of iron stores increases the required incidence of phlebotomy.

Fatal complications of PV include bleeding, thrombosis, myelofibrosis with count depression, and acute leukemia (149, 191, 192). The "spent" phase of PV is poorly defined, but usually refers to a decrease in hematocrit (often secondary to an increase in plasma volume rather than a decrease in red cell volume), variable depression in other blood cell counts, and enlargement of the spleen (193, 194). Myelofibrosis may not be present initially in "spent" PV, but usually an increase in bone marrow fibrosis or transition to acute leukemia eventually occurs (193, 194). Acute leukemia may occur in PV patients without a history of exposure to chemotherapy or radioisotopes, but an increased incidence is apparently seen in patients receiving alkylating agents (191).

TREATMENT

Effective treatment of PV can be accomplished by phlebotomy alone (see previous section), radioactive phosphorous, or chemotherapy (148, 191, 192). The Polycythemia Vera Study Group randomized patients into three treatment categories: phlebotomy alone, radiophosphorus therapy, or chlorambucil therapy. There was no significant difference in survival among the groups despite an increase in leukogenesis with chlorambucil. The equalization of survival is due in part to an increase in thrombotic complications in the phlebotomy-only group (160). In contrast, a European group randomized patients to receive busulfan or radioactive phosphorus; busulfan treatment was associated with a statistically significant improved survival rate (149). Other alkylating agents, 6 thioguinine, and hydroxyurea have all been used for PV (194–196), and optimal therapy is far from established (197). We would advise phlebotomy alone as initial therapy in young patients. If complications such as symptomatic splenomegaly or extreme thrombosis (platelet counts >1,000,000 cells per mm^3) occur, we would advise addition of hydroxyurea, an agent not yet associated with leukemogenesis.

Essential Thrombocythemia

Essential thrombocythemia (ET) is a myeloproliferative disorder characterized by a rise in platelet count unattributable to any other cause (198–201). Since high platelet counts are associated with other myeloproliferative diseases, polycythemia vera, chronic myelogenous leukemia, and myeloid metaplasia must be excluded before the diagnosis of ET can be made. The requirements for the diagnosis of ET should thus include (1) a platelet count of more than 1,000,000 cells per mm^3; (2) normal red cell mass; (3) no Philadelphia chromosome or extensive marrow fibrosis; (4) normal iron stores; and (5) no other identifiable cause of thrombocytosis (199–201). Although ET may occur in childhood, it is very rare (202–206). The common causes of increased platelet counts in children are listed in Table 34–5 (207).

CLINICAL PRESENTATION

The most common presenting symptoms in ET are bleeding, arterial or venous thrombosis, paresthesias, and general malaise (199–201). Diagnosis may be made incidentally in asymptomatic patients following routine complete blood count for unrelated problems. Thrombotic events may include venous thrombosis, transient ischemic attacks, stroke, and gangrene of the fingers (200, 201, 208). Bleeding occurs in about one fourth of the patients and is frequently mild. The gastrointestinal tract is the site of most severe bleeds (200, 201). The exact cause of excess bleeding is unclear, although multiple abnormalities in platelet function have been noted (209–212). More recent studies have found that bleeding and thrombosis are less common in these disorders than previously suspected (199, 213). Splenomegaly is noted in 50 to 75 per cent of patients, and hepatomegaly is seen in approximately 10 per cent. Although platelet counts may go very high, most patients present with counts less than 1,750,000 cells per mm^3 (199–201). A mild leukocytosis is common (median:12,000 cells per mm^3) and anemia may occur (199–201). The bone marrow is hypercellular, has increased numbers of dysplastic megakaryocytes, and may show a mild increase in reticular staining (200).

Chromosomes from the bone marrow of more than two thirds of ET patients are normal (201, 214). Extra C group chromosomes have been seen, including trisomy 9 (215). Zaccaria and Tura found a loss of part of chromosome 21 (21q−) in five patients with ET (216). As is the case in CML, chromosomal abnormalities in ET do not disappear when chemotherapeutic treatments lower the platelet count (216). G6PD studies have clearly demonstrated that ET is a clonal hematopoietic disease with involvement of granulocytes, red cells, and platelets (217–219). Why the megakaryocytes preferentially proliferate in ET is not at all clear.

COURSE AND TREATMENT

The clinical course of ET is highly variable. Some patients have been followed for more than 10 years without therapy and without problems, and in fact, a benign course may be more common in young patients (204). However morbidity and mortality secondary to thrombosis or hemorrhage occasionally occur, and acute leukemia can follow ET even in untreated patients (220–222). The incidence of leukemic transformation is unknown, but is probably very low. Treatment with chemotherapeutic agents or radioactive phosphorus will transiently reduce the platelet count in nearly every patient, but most patients require frequent retreatment. The influence of such treatments (most of the drugs used are alkylating agents) on eventual leukogenesis is unknown (199–201). Prostaglandin inhibitors are sometimes used to treat or prevent thrombosis but may increase the hemorrhagic problems inherent in the disease (213).

Agnogenic Myeloid Metaplasia/Myelofibrosis

CLINICAL PRESENTATION

Agnogenic myeloid metaplasia (AMM) is a myeloproliferative disease characterized by (1) leukoerythroblastosis, (2) tear drop erythrocytes, (3) extramedullary hematopoiesis, and (4) varying degrees of myelofibrosis (160, 223–226). Median age at presentation is approximately 60 years in all series; pediatric AMM is rare but reports of typical cases in children exist (227). Twenty per cent or more of patients at presentation may be asymptomatic. When they do occur, symptoms include malaise, weight loss, night sweats, and upper abdominal discomfort from splenomegaly, which is nearly universal and may be massive (223, 226). Spleen size is believed to correlate with duration of disease (223). Hepatomegaly occurs in over half the patients (223, 225, 226).

The peripheral blood in AMM is characterized by Pelger-Huet cells, leukoerythroblastosis, and prominent tear drop formation (Fig. 34–2). Immature granulocytes, nucleated red blood cells, and large platelets are prominent and megakaryocytes may circulate (228). Blood counts vary more in AMM than in any other myeloproliferative disease; normal counts, anemia (most common), polycythemia, leukocytosis (usually mild), leukopenia, thrombocytosis, and thrombocytopenia may all occur (226). The bone marrow is hard to aspirate in most patients, but biopsies will provide accurate diagnosis. Although some series include

Table 34–5. CAUSES OF THROMBOCYTOSIS IN CHILDHOOD*

Nutritional	*Neoplastic*
Iron deficiency	Myeloproliferative diseases
Megaloblastic anemia	Hepatoblastoma
Vitamin E deficiency	Neuroblastoma
Metabolic	Histiocytosis
Hyperadrenalism	Lymphoma
Infectious	Carcinoma
Viral	*Drugs*
Bacterial	Corticosteroids
Mycobacterial	Vinca alkaloids
Traumatic	Citrovorum factor
Surgery	*Miscellaneous*
Fractures	Splenectomy/congenital asplenia
Hemorrhage	Infantile cortical hyperostosis (Caffey's disease)
Inflammatory	Pulmonary embolism/thrombophlebitis
Collagen vascular disease	Cerebral vascular accident
Inflammatory bowel disease	Hemolytic anemias
Sarcoidosis	
Any inflammatory condition	

*Adapted from Reference 207.

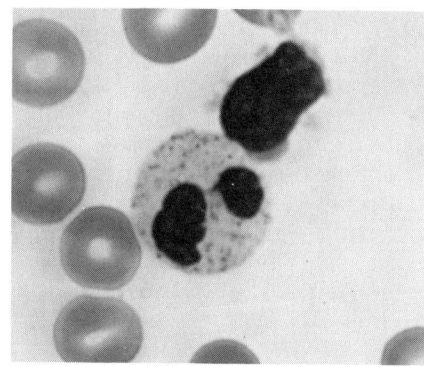

Figure 34–2. Typical Pelger-Hüet neutrophil demonstrating bilobate nucleus. (Smear kindly provided by Pearl R. Leavitt.)

marrow fibrosis as a requirement for diagnosis, up to one third of patients with AMM may have hyperplastic marrows with minimal to no fibrosis (228, 229). The marrow fibrosis may vary from this minimal amount to the extreme of myelosclerosis with almost no normal marrow elements present except scattered islands of megakaryocytes (229). As in polycythemia vera, osteosclerosis may be detectable on chest radiographs in about one third of patients. It is most noticeable in the vertebrae, pelvis, ribs, and metaphases of the femur and humerus. Uric acid is frequently increased in AMM (228). Ham's test for paroxysmal nocturnal hemoglobinuria may be positive in some patients with AMM; the exact link between these disorders is unknown (230). Leukocyte alkaline phosphatase scores are usually high, but vary with white blood cell count (228). Because of the likelihood of dry taps in AMM, cytogenetic data from analysis of bone marrow is scant. Although abnormalities are frequent no characteristic changes have been noted (231). Patients with AMM may have multiple immunologic abnormalities, including polyclonal increases in immunoglobulin, autoantibodies, circulating immune complexes, and complement consumption (232–234).

AMM has been shown to be a clonal disease involving red cells, platelets, and white cells in a patient studied by G6PD heterozygosity (see previous section on CML) (235). Marrow fibroblasts in this patient were not clonal by G6PD or cytogenetic marker, highlighting the secondary nature of the fibrosis. In fact, bone marrow fibroblasts are not primary hematopoietic cells as evidenced by continued recipient karyotype after bone marrow transplantation, and there are no physical in vitro growth differences between fibroblasts in AMM patients and normals (236–238). Increased numbers of granulocyte-macrophage progenitors circulate in AMM (239, 240). Erythroid progenitors do not show erythropoietin hypersensitivity as they do in polycythemia vera (239, 241).

ETIOLOGY

The causes of myelofibrosis in childhood are outlined in Table 34–6. Acute myelofibrosis is a condition characterized by pancytopenia and myelofibrosis without marked splenomegaly or leukoerythroblastosis. Proliferation of an immature myeloid cell occurs and the situation rapidly evolves into acute leukemia. Histochemical stains and electron microscopy of bone marrow cells have shown that most cases of acute myelofibrosis are associated with megakaryoblasts, and acute myelofibrosis and acute megakaryocytic leukemia may be the same disease (242, 243). The incidence of acute myelofibrosis may be increased in Down's syndrome (244).

The cause of the secondary myelofibrosis in AMM remains a mystery (3, 245, 246). The etiology of fibrosis in metastatic disease and AMM may be very different (247). One theory for the production of fibrosis in AMM postulates that platelet-derived growth factor (a product of megakaryocytes as well as platelets) may stimulate proliferation of fibroblasts. This theory suggests that the increased megakaryocytes frequently seen in AMM cause the fibrosis (248, 249). In addition megakaryocytes may release platelet factor 4, an inhibitor of collagenase; this could inhibit collagen breakdown and increase the fibrosis (245). These mechanisms do not explain the relative lack of fibrosis in essential thrombocytosis, a myeloproliferative disease with a marked increase in megakaryocytes. The fact that myelofibrosis associated with metastases can disappear with chemotherapy just as the myelofibrosis associated with CML regresses after bone marrow transplantation (250–253) argues that the fibrosis in both situations is a secondary phenomenon (246).

Table 34–6. CAUSES OF MYELOFIBROSIS*

Metabolic	Hematologic Disorders
Hypoparathyroidism	Agnogenic myeloid metaplasia
Chronic renal failure	Other myeloproliferative diseases
Vitamin deficiency	Acute myelofibrosis (megakaryoblastic leukemia)
Bone Diseases	Acute leukemia (rarely)
Osteopetrosis	Myelodysplasia
Paget's disease	**Other**
Osteomalacia	Connective tissue disorders (e.g., lupus erythematosis)
Metastatic Tumor	Granulomatous diseases
Neuroblastoma	
Lymphoma	
Breast, prostate	

*Adapted from References 3, 245, 246.

COURSE AND TREATMENT

The natural history of AMM can be quite variable. Median survivals from clinical series vary from less than 1½ years to over 5 years (226), and very long survival is possible. Complications include bleeding, intercurrent infection, acute leukemic transformation, and portal hypertension (224, 226). The etiology of portal hypertension in ET is unclear but may be linked to increased portal blood flow from the enlarged spleen (254). Anemia or thrombocytopenia at diagnosis reliably predicts for a poorer outcome (225, 226). The influence of age, spleen size, and systemic symptoms on survival is less clear. The incidence of leukemic transformation varies from less than 5 per cent to 12 per cent and so far has been independent of cytotoxic therapy (160). Androgen therapy has been used extensively, and although it may produce an increase in hematocrit, it has little effect on platelet count or spleen size (228, 255). Splenectomy will not cause further depression in blood counts and should be considered for treatment of (1) mechanical symptoms, (2) portal hypertension, (3) refractory thrombocytopenia, and (4) hemolytic anemia (254). However, a risk of mortality from splenectomy is seen even in modern series (226). The role of chemotherapy in this disorder is ill defined, but judicious use of rapidly reversible agents such as hydroxyurea may be effective.

THE MYELODYSPLASTIC SYNDROMES

The myelodysplastic syndromes (MDS) are a variety of hematologic entities characterized by abnormal bone marrow and peripheral blood morphology, various and frequently progressive cytopenias, and a propensity in some cases for transformation into acute myelogenous leukemia (256). They are frequently classified as preleukemias, although leukemic transformation is by no means universal (257). The syndromes are most common in patients over 50, and are quite unusual in childhood (256, 258). Patients previously treated with alkylating agents have an increased incidence of myelodysplastic syndromes (259).

There have been many attempts to classify the myelodysplastic syndromes by various clinical, biological, and morphological criteria. In 1982, the French-American-British (FAB) cooperative group defined five categories for the myelodysplastic syndromes: refractory anemia, refractory anemia with ringed sideroblasts, refractory anemia with excess blasts, refractory anemia with excess blasts in transformation, and chronic myelomonocytic leukemia (260). The salient features of each category are outlined in Table 34–7. Bone marrow cellularity in all five categories is usually normal to increased except in patients previously treated with radiotherapy or chemotherapy (260).

Clinical Presentation

Most patients with MDS present with the signs and symptoms of bone marrow failure (i.e., malaise and weakness, recurrent infections, and signs and symptoms of bleeding) (256). Symptoms may be so insidious that the diagnosis is made incidentally following blood tests for unrelated problems. Physical examination frequently reveals pallor and/or increased bruising. Splenomegaly may be present but is uncommon, usually seen in less than 20 per cent of patients (256, 261, 262). Hepatomegaly is even less frequent (263). The male-to-female ratio is increased in nearly every series (261–264, 275).

Peripheral blood testing reveals anemia, neutropenia and/or thrombocytopenia. Macrocytosis, tear drop formations, and moderate poikilocytosis are common. Reticulocyte counts usually are low. "Megaloblastoid" nucleated red blood cells are frequently detected (256, 265). The mean corpuscular volume is usually normal or slightly increased. Neutrophils may display decreased lobulation (the Pelger-Huet abnormality) and the neutrophil granules are frequently either absent or very large (260, 265). "Giant" platelets may also be seen (265).

Bone marrow cellularity is usually normal to increased, and excessive reticulin is present in most cases (266). Dysmorphology may be present in one, two, or (most frequently) all three cell lines. Erythroid abnormalities are the most common, and include (1) "megaloblastoid" to frankly megaloblastic changes; (2) increased iron stores frequently distributed in a ringlike manner around the nuclei (ringed sideroblasts); (3) multinucleation; (4) nuclear fragments; and (5) an overabundance of premature forms (256, 260, 265) (Figure 34–3). The anemia in MDS is due to ineffective erythropoiesis as demonstrated by low reticulocyte counts despite normal numbers of erythroid progenitors. This is an example of relative bone marrow failure. Megakaryocytic dysplasia is common

Table 34–7. PERIPHERAL BLOOD AND BONE MARROW FINDINGS IN THE MYELODYSPLASTIC SYNDROMES*

	RA[1]	RARS[2]	RAEB[3]	RAEBIT[4]	CMML[5]
Anemia	+	+	+	+	+/−
Granulocytopenia	+/−	+/−	usually +	usually +	+/−
Thrombocytopenia	+/−	+/−	usually +	usually +	+/−
Marrow dysplasia					
erythroid	+	+	usually +	usually +	+/−
myeloid	+/−	+/−	usually +	usually +	+/−
megakaryocytic	+/−	+/−	usually +	usually +	+/−
Auer rods	−	−	−	+/−	−
Ringed sideroblasts >15%	−	+	+/−	+/−	+/−
Peripheral blood blasts	≤1%	≤1%	<5%	may be >5%	<5%
Abnormal marrow blasts	<5%	<5%	5–20%	5–30%	<5 to 20%
Peripheral blood monocytosis (>1 × 10⁹/l)	—	—	—	—	+

*Adapted from Reference 260.
[1] RA = refractory anemia.
[2] RARS = refractory anemia with ringed sideroblasts.
[3] RAEB = refractory anemia with excess blasts.
[4] RAEBIT = refractory anemia with excess blasts in transformation. RAEBIT is distinguished from RAEB by either (1) presence of Auer rods; (2) >5% blasts in the peripheral blood; or (3) 20–30% abnormal blasts in the bone marrow.
[5] CMML = chronic myelomonocytic leukemia.

and may be more easily appreciated on biopsy specimens than on aspirates (266). Small forms, increased nuclear-to-cytoplasmic ratios, marked variation in size, and hypo- or hyperlobulated nuclei are seen (256, 266). Bone marrow abnormalities of the granulocyte series can be more subtle (256). Increased numbers of immature cells may be present, granules are frequently absent or abnormally large, and cell numbers are often increased (267)

Transmission electron microscopy of the bone marrow may reveal abnormalities in all three cell lines (268, 269, 270). Table 34–7 outlines the distribution of peripheral blood and bone marrow abnormalities within the FAB subclassifications of myelodysplasia (260). The presenting signs and symptoms and hematologic findings in patients previously treated with chemotherapy are not markedly different from the de novo group (259).

Myelodysplastic syndromes in childhood present with clinical peripheral blood and bone marrow findings similar to those in adult patients (271, 272). Cases of refractory anemia with excess blasts alone or in transformation seem to predominate (271, 272). Blank and Lange argue that preleukemia may be more common in childhood than previously noted. In their retrospective review of all patients diagnosed with acute nonlymphocytic leukemia (ANLL) at Children's Hospital of Philadelphia, six patients (17 per cent of ANLL cases) had clear evidence of preleukemic states (272). This incidence is quite similar to that in adult series of ANLL cases (273).

Kobrinsky and co-workers have described seven children with a unique presentation of myelodysplasia. Six of the seven had major constitutional abnormalities including unusual facies, short stature, and mental retardation. In contrast to most cases of MDS, the bone marrow cellularity in these patients was decreased. Although some hematologic responses were seen to folic acid, androgens, or steroids, most patients developed leukemic transformation or died from problems secondary to pancytopenia (274).

HgF is increased in as many as 80 per cent of cases, although the elevation is mild compared to that seen in juvenile CML (35). The reason for this increase is unclear, but it is likely due to the "stress" of chronic anemia (see Chapters 7 and 8). Other red cell defects occasionally seen include (1) alterations in certain enzyme activity (276); (2) changes in erythrocyte antigens such as an increase in "i" antigen (276, 277); and (3) increased susceptibility to sugar water hemolysis (Ham's test) (265). Most studies have recorded decreased myeloperoxidase content in neutrophils (270, 278). An extensive study of neutrophil function in 20 patients with myelodysplasia revealed multiple defects: decreased adhesion, deficient chemotaxis, decreased enzyme content, slower chemiluminescence, decreased phagocytosis, and impaired microbicidal capacity (279). Whether any of these are primary defects is uncertain. Others have found that the neutrophil defects are linked to a specific chromosomal defect, monosomy 7 (see concluding section) (278, 280). Muramidase is increased in about 20 per cent of patients (281). Decreased natural killer cell activity has been noted (282, 283). Abnormalities in chromosomes and cell culture systems are discussed in the next section.

Pathophysiology

Just as the molecular basis of leukemia is unknown, the exact cause of MDS is unclear. The syndromes are clearly linked with acute nonlymphocytic leukemia, not only by their propensity to evolve into that clinical condition but also by similar inciting conditions (such as previous treatment with chemotherapeutic agents) and common cytogenetic changes. In fact it has been argued that the myelodysplastic syndromes are not a distinct entity but merely an early form of acute leukemia (284).

BONE MARROW CULTURE SYSTEMS

In vitro culture systems have provided certain insights into the pathophysiology of the myelodysplastic syndromes. The techniques and theories

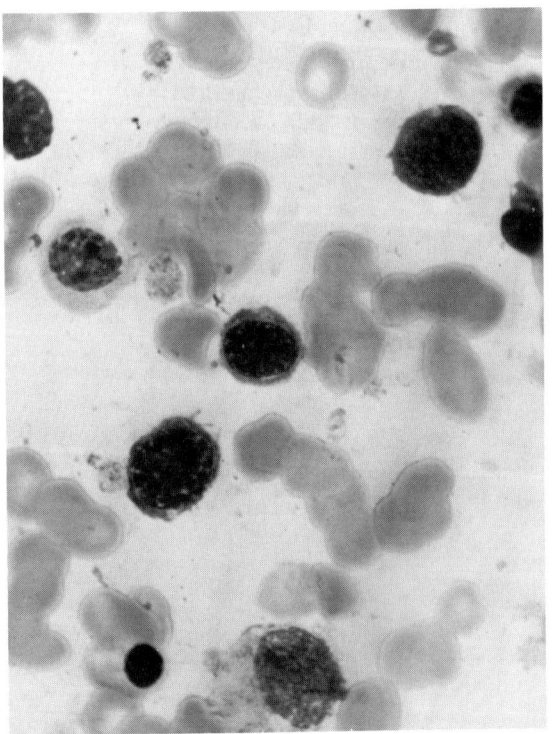

Figure 34–3. "Megaloblastoid" changes in the erythroid series from a bone marrow sample of a patient with myelodysplasia. (Bone marrow smear kindly provided by Pearl R. Leavitt.)

of bone marrow culture systems have been reviewed in Chapter 7. In general, CFU-G/M colonies in myelodysplasia are reduced in number, with cluster formation disproportionately prominent (285–288). This growth pattern is similar to that seen in acute nonlymphocytic leukemia and is more common in refractory anemias with excess blasts than in refractory sideroblastic anemia (288). An increase in cluster to colony ratio may predict transformation into acute leukemia (290). In addition, elevated urinary colony-stimulating factor output (286) or an increased endogenous colony-stimulating activity (289) may also predict the onset of leukemic transformation. Studies of erythroid colony growth reveal normal CFU-E formation but a profound depression of BFU-E–derived colonies (291, 292). Thus hematopoietic studies reveal a selected loss or dysfunction of immature committed progenitors strongly suggesting that the defect begins in a progenitor cell common to at least two cell lines (granulocyte-erythroid). This increased production and excretion of hematopoietic growth factor is probably secondary to relative bone marrow failure (286).

CYTOGENETICS AND PRELEUKEMIA

The chromosomal abnormalities observed in MDS are reviewed in Chapter 43. Clonal cytogenetic abnormalities in the marrow cells (but not the PHA-stimulated T cells) are found in about half the patients with myelodysplasia (293–295). The most frequent abnormalities found involve chromosome 5 (5q− or monosomy 5), chromosomy 7 (7q− or monosomy 7), and chromosome 8 (trisomy 8). Trisomy 8 is also a frequent finding when ANLL presents de nova, and the abnormalities of chromosomes 5 and 7 are particularly common in ANLL occurring after exposure to previous chemotherapy or other known leukemogenic toxins (296). Less common findings such as t(1;3) or the development of new abnormalities in addition to established ones (such as the appearance of trisomy 1 and 11 in the setting of 5q−) have been reported (297, 298). It is quite curious that other nonrandom chromosomal abnormalities found commonly in ANLL such as t(8;21) and t(15;17) have not been frequently reported in MDS (293).

Unlike the situation in CML, progression to ANLL is not commonly heralded by additional cytogenetic changes (294). An exception is the report by Rowley of six patients with preleukemia. Five developed additional karyotypic abnormalities when transformation to ANLL occurred (296). Patients developing myelodysplasia after previous chemotherapy or radiation therapy have cytogenetic changes similar to those of patients presenting without such exposures with the exception of a higher frequency of loss of all or part of chromosomes 5 or 7 (293). There appears to be an increased incidence of progression to ANLL in myelodysplastic patients with a detectable cytogenetic abnormality compared to those without (257, 293, 294, 299).

A study of 10 children with preleukemia, all meeting the FAB criteria of refractory anemia with excess blasts (RAEB) or refractory anemia with excess blasts in transformation (RAEBIT), found karyotypic changes similar to those in adult patients, including three with monosomy 7. Four patients did not display any obvious karyotypic abnormality (300).

CLONAL NATURE OF MYELODYSPLASIA

The above-mentioned cytogenetic changes support a clonal derivation of the myelodysplastic disorders (see previous section on CML and Chapter 43). Furthermore, the myriad abnormalities in the erythroid, megakaryocytic, and granulocytic-monocytic cell lines already described argue for involvement of a progenitor common to all three lines. These changes could be a secondary phenomenon, however, and direct evidence for involvement is needed. Two case reports speak to this point (301–303). The granulocytes from a black female heterozygous for G6PD (see section on CML) with refractory anemia were monoclonal (type B). During 5 years of follow-up, a progressive predominance of type B G6PD in the granulocytic colonies in culture occurred and eventually peripheral blood, platelets, red cells, and granulocytes exhibited only type B G6PD (301, 302). A second patient previously treated with alkylating agents developed refractory anemia with excess blasts. All of the karyotypes examined from the whole bone marrow revealed monosomy 7. The cells from individually analyzed erythroid and myeloid colonies also had monosomy 7 karyotypes exclusively, confirming that the abnormal progenitor in this case could give rise to at least two different blood lines (303).

Differential Diagnosis

A careful history and physical examination along with evaluation of the peripheral blood smear, bone marrow aspirate, and bone marrow biopsy will yield a clear diagnosis of myelodysplasia in the majority of cases. The possibility of folate or vitamin B_{12} deficiency should be eliminated, since the "megaloblastoid" appearance of the erythroid series in these syndromes could easily be confused with myelodysplasia. Pyridoxine-dependent anemia and riboflavin deficiency should also be ruled out. Exact differentiation between myelodysplasia and acute leukemia is occasionally difficult. Evidence of extramedullary invasion strongly suggests that leukemic transformation has occurred.

Clinical Course

The clinical course in the myelodysplastic syndromes is very varied. Patients may experience a rapid fatal progression to ANLL, death from complications of cytopenias, or a slow drawn-out course requiring multiple transfusions but terminating in death from a totally unrelated problem. Although rare patients with MDS are alive and well 10 to 15 years after initial diagnosis (262), median survival in most series varies from 20 to 36 months (257, 304, 305).

Determining prognosis has proven difficult. When bone marrow morphologic findings are classified as primary "erythroid" abnormalities versus "myeloid" abnormalities, transformation to acute leukemia is more prominent in the myeloid group (261). Similarly, as mentioned above, leukemic patterns of in vitro growth, increased CSA (colony-stimulating activity) production, or cytogenetic abnormalities also predict for both acute leukemic transformation and poor outcome (289, 290, 300). Surprisingly the presence of Auer rods in the myeloblasts may not impart a poorer prognosis (see Chapter 33) (271). Pediatric patients apparently have no special protection from poor outcome and develop acute leukemia at a rate similar to that of adult patients with MDS (258, 300). Loss of chromosome material as measured by flow cytometry portends a poor course. This DNA loss correlates with chromosomal abnormalities, especially loss of chromosome 7 (305a) (see Cytogenetics, above).

Treatment

The mainstay of therapy for all patients with myelodysplasia is supportive care, including blood product transfusions and antibiotics. Androgenic steroids have not been proven beneficial (306). Likewise aggressive chemotherapy, usually reserved for patients with leukemic evolution, has with few exceptions been ineffective (307, 308). More recently enthusiasm has been generated for the use of drugs that enhance differentiation of hematopoietic cells in vitro. Low-dose cytosine arabinoside has produced an improvement of peripheral counts and a decrease of marrow blast percentage in several patients with preleukemia (309, 310). Whether low-dose cytosine arabinoside works by forcing differentiation of abnormal cells or by direct cytotoxic effects is unclear (311, 312). The effect may be far from universal and is frequently short lived (313, 314). Stereoisomers of retinoic acid, another inducer of hematopoietic differentiation in vitro, are also being used in early clinical trials (315).

Despite the varied course of myelodysplasia, the nearly inexorable deterioration makes a search for a curative therapy very important. Bone marrow transplantation is currently not a viable option for the elderly majority of patients with MDS, but may be used in younger patients with success (316, 317).

Monosomy 7

In 1981, Sieff and colleagues described six patients with monosomy 7 and presented a review of several similar previously reported patients (318). A fairly specific clinical presentation was found. The patients were mainly young (5 of 6 were 1 year or less), suffered from recurrent infections, and had hepatosplenomegaly, increased white blood cell count, anemia, thrombocytopenia, and hypercellular marrow with either myeloid or erythroid predominance. Dyspoiesis was not prominent. Three of the six patients developed acute nonlymphocytic leukemia. The syndrome resembles juvenile CML but differs in that fetal hemoglobin is normal or only slightly elevated. Furthermore, juvenile CML does not typically transform into ANLL as does the monosomy 7 syndrome. Although monosomy 7 is a frequent finding in more typical myelodysplastic syndromes even in childhood (306), the increased WBC and hepatosplenomegaly seen in these cases are unusual in MDS. Sieff also found a decrease in neutrophil mobility similar to that in adults with monosomy 7 (278).

Linch and co-workers reported a similar case in 1982 (319). An unusual finding in their case was a reversion to a diploid karyotype at the time of acute transformation. This development argues for the existence in this patient of a leukemic stem cell clone with a diploid karyotype that sequentially gave rise initially to a clone of monosomy 7 cells and later to a diploid acute leukemic clone.

References

1. Dameshek, W.: Some speculations on the myeloproliferative syndromes. Blood 6:372, 1951.
2. Adamson, J. W., and Fialkow, P. J.: The pathogenesis of myeloproliferative syndromes. Br. J. Haematol. 38:299, 1978.
3. Editorial: Myelofibrosis. Lancet 1:127, 1980.
4. Schaeffer, A. I.: Deficiency of platelet lipoxygenase activity in myeloproliferative disorders. New Engl. J. Med. 306:381, 1982.
5. Li, F. P.: The chronic leukemias: etiology and epidemiology. In Neoplastic Diseases of the Blood. Wiernik, P. H., Canellos, G. P., et al. (eds.), New York, Churchill Livingstone, 1985, p. 7.
6. Canellos, G. P.: Chronic granulocytic leukemia. Med. Clin. North Am. 60:1001, 1976.
7. Castro-Malaspina, H., Schaison, G., et al.: Philadelphia chromosome positive chronic myelocytic leukemia in children. Survival and prognostic factors. Cancer 52:721, 1983.
8. Rowe, J. M., and Lichtman, M. A.: Hyperleukocytosis and leukostasis: common features of childhood chronic myelogenous leukemia. Blood 63:1230, 1984.

9. Vodopick, H., Rupp, E. M., et al.: Spontaneous cyclic leukocytosis and thrombocytosis in chronic granulocytic leukemia. New Engl. J. Med. 286:284, 1972.
10. Sokal, J. E., Cox, E. B., et al.: Prognostic discrimination in "good-risk" chronic granulocytic leukemia. Blood 63:789, 1984.
11. Smith, K. L., and Johnson, W.: Classification of chronic myelocytic leukemia in children. Cancer 34:670, 1974.
12. Hild, D. H., and Myers, T. J.: Hyperviscosity in chronic granulocytic leukemia. Cancer 46:1418, 1980.
13. Suri, R., Goldman, J. M., et al.: Priapism complicating chronic granulocytic leukemia. Am. J. Hematol. 9:295, 1980.
14. Barton, J. C., Conrad, M. E., et al.: Pseudochloroma: extramedullary hematopoietic nodules in chronic myelogenous leukemia. Ann. Intern. Med. 91:735, 1979.
15. Dosik, H., Rosner, F., et al.: Acquired lipidosis: Gaucher-like cells and "blue cells" in chronic granulocytic leukemia. Semin. Hematol. 9:309, 1972.
16. Gralnick, H. R., Harbor, J., et al.: Myelofibrosis in chronic granulocytic leukemia. Blood 37:1039, 1971.
17. Clough, V., Geary, C. G., et al.: Myelofibrosis in chronic granulocytic leukaemia. Br. J. Haematol. 42:515, 1979.
18. Nowell, P. C., and Hungerford, D. A.: A minute chromosome in human chronic granulocytic leukemia. Science 132:1497, 1960.
19. First International Workshop on Chromosomes in Leukaemia: Chromosomes in Ph¹-positive chronic granulocytic leukaemia. Br. J. Haematol. 39:305, 1978.
20. Rowley, J. D.: A new consistent chromosomal abnormality in chronic myelogenous leukaemia identified by quinacrine fluorescence and Giemsa staining. Nature 243:290, 1973.
21. Greenberg, B. R., Wilson, F. D., et al.: Cytogenetics of fibroblastic colonies in Ph¹ positive chronic myelogenous leukemia. Blood 51:1039, 1978.
22. Maniatis, A. K., Amsel, S., et al.: Chromosome pattern of bone marrow fibroblasts in patients with chronic granulocytic leukemia. Nature 222:1278, 1969.
23. Hagemeijer, A., Bartram, C. R., et al.: Is the chromosome region 9q34 always involved in variants of the Ph¹ translocation? Cancer Genet. Cytogenet. 13:1, 1984.
24. Canellos, G. P., Whang-Peng, J., et al.: Chronic granulocytic leukemia without the Philadelphia chromosome. Am. J. Clin. Pathol. 65:467, 1976.
25. Rosner, F., Schreiber, Z. R., et al.: Leukocyte alkaline phosphatase. Arch. Intern. Med. 130:892, 1972.
26. Xefteris, E., Mitus, W. J., et al.: Leukocytic alkaline phosphatase in busulfan induced remissions of chronic granulocytic leukemia. Blood 18:202, 1961.
27. Kenny, J. J., and Maloney, W. C.: Leukocytic alkaline phosphatase. Behavior during prolonged incubation and infection in normal and leukemic leukocytes. Blood 12:295, 1957.
28. Dosik, H., Hurewitz, D. J., et al.: Bullous eruption and elevated leukocyte alkaline phosphatase in the course of bulsulfan-treated chronic granulocytic leukemia. Blood 35:543, 1970.
29. Schiffer, C. A., Aisner, J., et al.: Increased leukocyte alkaline phosphatase activity following transfusion of leukocytes from a patient with chronic myelogenous leukemia. Am. J. Med. 66:519, 1979.
30. Rustin, G. J. S., Goldman, J. M., et al.: An extrinsic factor controls neutrophil alkaline phosphatase synthesis in chronic granulocytic leukaemia. Br. J. Haematol. 45:381, 1980.
31. Pedersen, B.: Functional and biochemical phenotype in relation to cellular age of differentiated neutrophils in chronic myeloid leukaemia. Br. J. Haematol. 51:339, 1982.
32. Corcino, J., Krauss, S., et al.: Release of vitamin B12-binding protein by human leukocytes in vitro. J. Clin. Invest. 49:2250, 1970.
33. Chikkappa, G., Corcino, J., et al.: Correlation between various blood white cell pools and the serum B12-binding capacity. Blood 37:142, 1971.
34. Sheridan, B. L., Weatherall, D. J., et al.: The patterns of fetal haemoglobin production in leukaemia. Br. J. Haematol. 32:487, 1976.
35. Newman, D. R., Pierre, R. V., et al.: Studies on the diagnostic significance of hemoglobin F levels. Mayo Clin. Proc. 48:199, 1973.
36. Bizzozero, O. J., Jr., Johnson, K. G., et al.: Radiation-related leukemias in Hiroshima and Nagasaki, 1946–1964. II. Observations on type-specific leukemia, survivorship, and clinical behavior. Ann. Intern. Med. 66:522, 1967.
37. Kamada, N., and Kimio, T.: Cytogenetic studies of hematological disorders in atomic bomb survivors. In Radiation-Induced Chromosome Damage in Man. Ishihara, T., and Sasaki, M. S. (eds.), New York, A. R. Liss, 1983, p. 455.
38. Jablon, S., and Kato, H.: Childhood cancer in relationship to prenatal exposure to atomic-bomb radiation. Lancet 2:1000, 1970.
39. Tokuhata, G. K., Neely, C. L., et al.: Chronic myelocytic leukemia in identical twins and a sibling. Blood 31:216, 1968.
40. Goh, K., Swisher, S. N., et al.: Chronic myelocytic leukemia and identical twins: additional evidence of the Philadelphia chromosome as postzygotic abnormality. Arch. Intern. Med. 120:214, 1967.
41. Heisterkamp, N., Groffen, J., et al.: Chromosome localization of human cellular homologues of two viral oncogenes. Nature 299:747, 1982.
42. Swan, D. C., McBride, O. W., et al.: Chromosome mapping of the simian sarcoma oncogene analogue in human cells. Proc. Natl. Acad. Sci. USA 79:4691, 1982.
43. Bartram, C. R., de Klein, A., et al.: Localization of the human c-sis oncogene in Ph¹-positive and Ph¹-negative chronic myelocytic leukemia by in situ hybridization. Blood 63:223, 1984.
43a. Groffen, J., Stephenson, J. R., et al.: Philadelphia chromosomal breakpoints are clustered within a limited region, bcr, on chromosome 22. Cell 36:93, 1984.
43b. Stam, K., Heisterkamp, N., et al.: Evidence of a new chimeric bcr/c-abl mRNA in patients with chronic myelocytic leukemia and the Philadelphia chromosome. New Engl. J. Med. 313:1429, 1985.
44. Chervenick, P. A., and Boggs, D. R.: Granulocyte kinetics in chronic myelocytic leukemia. Ser. Haematol. 1:24, 1968.
45. Eaves, A. C., and Eaves, C. J.: Abnormalities in the erythroid progenitor compartments in patients with chronic myelogenous leukemia (CML). Exp. Hematol. 7(Suppl. 5):65, 1979.
46. Olofsson, T., and Olsson, I.: Granulopoiesis in chronic myeloid leukemia. II. Serial cloning of blood and bone marrow cells in agar culture. Blood 48:351, 1976.
47. Christ, W. M., Ragab, A., et al.: Granulopoiesis in chronic myeloproliferative disorders in children. Pediatrics 61:889, 1978.
48. Altman, A. J., and Baehner, R. L.: In vitro colony forming characteristics of chronic granulocytic leukemia in childhood. J. Pediatr. 86:221, 1975.
49. Robinson, W. A., and Pike, B. L.: Leucopoietic activity in human urine: the granulocytic leukemias. New Engl. J. Med. 282:1291, 1970.
50. Metcalf, D., Moore, M. A. S., et al.: Responsiveness of human granulocytic leukemic cells to colony-stimulating factor. Blood 43:847, 1974.
51. Broxmeyer, H. E., Grossbard, E., et al.: Evidence for a proliferative advantage of human leukemia colony-forming cells in vitro. J.N.C.L. 60:513, 1978.
52. Broxmeyer, H. E., and Smithyman, A.: Identification of lactoferrin as the granulocyte-derived inhibitor of colony-stimulating activity product. J. Exp. Med. 148:1052, 1978.

53. Koeffler, H. P., Golde, D. W.: Chronic myelogenous leukemia—new concepts. New Engl. J. Med. *304*:1201, 1981.
54. Broxmeyer, H. E., Mendelsohn, N., et al.: Abnormal granulocyte feedback regulation of colony forming and colony stimulating activity–producing cells from patients with chronic myelogenous leukemia. Leukemia Res. *1*:3, 1977.
55. Quesenberry, P. J., Rappeport, J. M., et al.: Inhibition of normal murine hematopoesis by leukemic cells. New Engl. J. Med. *299*:71, 1978.
56. Olofsson, T., and Olsson, I.: Suppression of normal granulopoiesis *in vitro* by a leukemia-associated inhibitor (LAI) of acute and chronic leukemia. Blood *55*:975, 1980.
57. Dube, I. D., Kalousek, D. K., et al.: Cytogenetic studies of early myeloid progenitor compartments in Ph^1-positive chronic myeloid leukemia. II. Long term culture reveals the persistence of Ph^1-negative progenitors in treated as well as newly diagnosed patients. Blood *63*:1172, 1984.
58. Goto, T., Nishikori, M., et al.: Growth characteristics of leukemic and normal hematopoietic cells in Ph^1-positive chronic myelogenous leukemia and effects of intensive treatment. Blood *59*:793, 1982.
59. Whang-Peng, J., Frei, E., III, et al.: The distribution of the Philadelphia chromosome in patients with chronic myelogenous leukemia. Blood *22*:664, 1963.
60. Chervenick, P. A., Ellis, L. D., et al.: Human leukemic cells: *In vitro* growth of colonies containing the Philadelphia (Ph^1) chromosome. Science *174*:1134, 1971.
61. Grilli, G., Carbonell, F., et al.: Studi citogenetici sui progenitori eritropoietici e mielopoietici *in vitro* nella leucemia mieloide cronica. Haematologica *66*:733, 1981.
62. Dube, I. D., Eaves, C. J., et al.: A method for obtaining high quality chromosome preparations from single hemopoietic colonies on a routine basis. Cancer Genet. Cytogenet. *4*:157, 1981.
63. Dube, I. D., Gupta, C. M., et al.: Cytogenetic studies of early myeloid progenitor compartments in Ph^1 positive chronic myeloid leukaemia. Br. J. Haematol. *56*:633, 1984.
64. Fialkow, P. J., Jacobson, R. J., et al.: Chronic myelocytic leukemia: clonal origin in a stem cell common to the granulocyte, erythrocyte, platelet, and monocyte/macrophage. Am. J. Med. *63*:125, 1977.
65. Douer, D., Levin, A. M., et al.: Chronic myelocytic leukaemia: a pluripotent haemapoietic cell is involved in the malignant clone. Br. J. Haematol. *49*:615, 1981.
66. Singer, J. W., Adamson, J. W., et al.: Chronic myelogenous leukemia. In vitro studies of hematopoietic regulation in a patient undergoing intensive chemotherapy. J. Clin. Invest. *67*:1593, 1981.
67. Fialkow, P. J., Jacobson, R. J., et al.: Philadelphia chromosome (Ph^1)-negative chronic myelogenous leukemia (CML): a clonal disease with origin in a multipotent stem cell. Blood *56*:70, 1980.
68. Canellos, G. P.: Diagnosis and treatment of chronic granulocytic leukemia. In *Neoplastic Diseases of the Blood*. Wiernik, P. H., Canellos, G. P., et al., (eds.), New York, Churchill Livingstone, 1985, p. 81.
69. Bernhein, A., Berger, R., et al.: Philadelphia chromosome positive blood B lymphocytes in chronic myelocytic leukemia. Leukemia Res. *5*:331, 1981.
70. Fialkow, P. J., Denman, A. M., et al.: Chronic myelocytic leukemia. Origin of some lymphocytes from leukemic stem cells. J. Clin. Invest. *62*:815, 1978.
71. Fialkow, P. J., Martin, P. J., et al.: Evidence for a multistep pathogenesis of chronic myelogenous leukemia. Blood *58*:158, 1981.
72. Hughes, A., McVerry, B. A., et al.: Heterogeneous blast cell crises in Philadelphia negative chronic granulocytic leukaemia. Br. J. Haematol. *47*:563, 1981.
73. Lisker, R., Casas, L., et al.: Late appearing Philadelphia chromosome in two patients with chronic myelogenous leukemia. Blood *56*:812, 1980.
74. Fauser, A. A., Kanz, L., et al.: T cells and probably B cells arise from the malignant clone in chronic myelogenous leukemia. J. Clin. Invest. *75*:1080, 1985.
75. Hernandez, P., Carnot, J., et al.: Chronic myeloid leukaemia blast crisis with T-cell features. Br. J. Haematol. *51*:175, 1982.
76. Griffin, J. D., Tantravahi, R., et al.: T-cell surface antigens in a patient with blast crisis of chronic myeloid leukemia. Blood *61*:640, 1983.
77. Herrmann, F., Komischke, B., et al.: Ph^1 positive blast crisis of chronic myeloid leukaemia exhibiting features characteristic of early T blasts. Scand. J. Haematol. *32*:411, 1984.
78. Weick, J. K., Hagedorn, A. B., et al.: Leukoerythroblastosis. Diagnostic and prognostic significance. Mayo Clin. Proc. *49*:110, 1974.
79. Bloomfield, C. D., Peterson, L. C., et al.: The Philadelphia chromosome (Ph^1) in adults presenting with acute leukaemia: a comparison of Ph^1+ and Ph^1- patients. Br. J. Haematol. *36*:347, 1977.
80. Priest, J. R., Robinson, L. L., et al.: Philadelphia chromosome positive childhood acute lymphoblastic leukemia. Blood *56*:15, 1980.
81. Kamada, N., and Uchino, H.: Chronologic sequence in appearance of clinical and laboratory findings characteristic of chronic myelocytic leukemia. Blood *51*:843, 1978.
82. Marks, S. M., McCaffrey, R., et al.: Blastic transformation in chronic myelogenous leukemia: experience with 50 patients. Med. Pediatr. Oncol. *4*:159, 1978.
83. Galton, D. A. G.: Chemotherapy of chronic myelocytic leukemia. Semin. Hematol. *6*:323, 1969.
84. Tura, S., Baccarani, M., et al.: Staging of chronic myeloid leukaemia. Br. J. Haematol. *47*:105, 1981.
85. Gomez, G. A., Sokal, J. E., et al.: Prognostic features at diagnosis of chronic myelocytic leukemia. Cancer *47*:2470, 1981.
86. Oguma, S., Takatsuki, K., et al.: Factors influencing survival in Philadelphia chromosome positive chronic myelocytic leukemia. Cancer *50*:2928, 1982.
87. Cervantes, F., Rozman, C.: A multivariate analysis of prognostic factors in chronic myeloid leukemia. Blood *60*:1298, 1982.
88. Theoligides, A.: Unfavorable signs in patients with chronic myelocytic leukemia. Ann. Intern. Med. *76*:95, 1972.
89. Appelbaum, F. R., Najfeld, V., et al.: Chronic myelogenous leukemia. Prolonged survival with spontaneous decline in the frequency of Ph^1-positive cells and subsequent development of mixed Ph^1-positive and Ph^1-negative blast crisis. Cancer *51*:149, 1983.
90. Sokal, J. E.: Significance of Ph^1-negative marrow cells in Ph^1-positive chronic granulocytic leukemia. Blood *56*:1072, 1980.
91. Rosenthal, S., Canellos, G. P., et al.: Characteristics of blast crisis in chronic granulocytic leukemia. Blood *49*:705, 1977.
92. Rosenthal, S., and Canellos, G. P.: Blast crisis of chronic granulocytic leukemia. Morphologic variants and therapeutic implications. Am. J. Med. *63*:542, 1977.
93. Marks, S. M., Baltimore, D., et al.: Terminal transferase as a predictor of initial responsiveness to vincristine and prednisone in blastic chronic myelogenous leukemia. New Engl. J. Med. *298*:812, 1978.
94. Janossy, G., Greaves, M. F., et al.: Blast crisis of chronic myeloid leukaemia. II. Cell surface marker analysis of "lymphoid" and myeloid cases. Br. J. Haematol. *34*:179, 1976.
95. Janossy, G., Woodruff, R. K., et al.: Relation of "lymphoid" phenotype and response to chemotherapy incorporating vincristine-prednisone in the acute phase of Ph^1 positive leukemia. Cancer *43*:426, 1979.

96. Griffin, J. D., Todd, R. F., III, et al.: Differentiation patterns in the blastic phase of chronic myeloid leukemia. Blood 61:85, 1983.
97. Bakhshi, A., Minowada, J., et al.: Lymphoid blast crises of chronic myelogenous leukemia represent stages in the development of B-cell precursors. New Engl. J. Med. 309:826, 1983.
98. Neiman, R. S., Barcos, M., et al.: Granulocytic sarcoma: a clinicopathologic study of 61 biopsied cases. Cancer 48:1426, 1981.
99. Muss, H. B., and Maloney, W. C.: Chloroma and other myeloblastic tumors. Blood 42:721, 1973.
100. Schwartz, J. H., Canellos, G. P., et al.: Meningeal leukemia in the blastic phase of chronic granulocytic leukemia. Am. J. Med. 59:819, 1975.
101. Smith, A. G., Prentice, A. G., et al.: Meningeal relapse in Ph[1] positive acute lymphoblastic and lymphoid blast crisis of chronic granulocytic leukemia. Cancer 51:2031, 1983.
102. Olah, E., and Rak, K.: Prognostic value of chromosome findings in the blast phase of Ph[1] positive chronic myeloid leukaemia (CML). Int. J. Cancer. 27:287, 1981.
103. Alimena, G., Dallapiccola, B., et al.: Chromosomal, morphological and clinical correlations in blastic crisis of chronic myeloid leukaemia. A study of 69 cases. Scand. J. Haematol. 28:103, 1982.
104. Sadamori, N., Gomez, G. A., et al.: Chromosomes and causation of human cancer and leukemia. II. Therapeutic and prognostic value of chromosome findings during acute phase in Ph[1]-positive chronic myeloid leukemia. Hematol. Oncol. 1:77, 1983.
105. Lowenthal, R. M., Buskard, N. A., et al.: Intensive leukophoresis as initial therapy for chronic granulocytic leukemia. Blood 46:835, 1975.
106. Grund, F. M., Armitage, J. O., et al.: Hydroxyurea in the prevention of the effects of leukostasis in acute leukemia. Arch. Intern. Med. 137:1246, 1977.
107. Stryckmans, P. A.: Treatment of chronic myeloid leukemia. Ann. Rev. Med. 31:159, 1980.
108. Rushing, D., Goldman, A., et al.: Hydroxyurea versus busulfan in the treatment of chronic myelogenous leukemia. Am. J. Clin. Oncol. 5:307, 1982.
109. Spiers, A. S. D., Baikie, A. G., et al.: Splenectomy for complications of chronic granulocytic leukaemia. Lancet 2:627, 1975.
110. Gomez, G. A., Sokal, J. E., et al.: Splenectomy for palliation of chronic myelocytic leukemia. Am. J. Med. 61:14, 1976.
111. Ihde, D. C., Canellos, G. P., et al.: Splenectomy in the chronic phase of chronic granulocytic leukemia. Ann. Intern. Med. 84:17, 1976.
112. Italian Cooperative Study Group on Myeloid Leukemia: Results of a prospective randomized trial of early splenectomy in chronic myeloid leukemia. Cancer 54:333, 1984.
113. Cunningham, I., Gee, T., et al.: Results of treatment of Ph[1]+ chronic myelogenous leukemia with an intensive treatment regimen (L-5 protocol). Blood 53:375, 1979.
114. Kantarjian, H. M., Vellekoop, L., et al.: Intensive combination chemotherapy (ROAP 10) and splenectomy in the management of chronic myelogenous leukemia. J. Clin. Oncol. 3:192, 1985.
115. Clarkson, B.: Chronic myelogenous leukemia: is aggressive treatment indicated? J. Clin. Oncol. 3:135, 1985.
115a. Talpaz, M., Kantarjian, H. M., et al.: Hematologic remission and cytogenetic improvement induced by recombinant human interferon alpha$_A$ in chronic myelogenous leukemia. New Engl. J. Med. 314:1065, 1986.
116. Degliantoni, G., Mangoni, L., et al.: In vitro restoration of polyclonal hematopoiesis in a chronic myelogenous leukemia after in vitro treatment with 4-hydroperoxycyclophosphamide. Blood 65:753, 1985.
117. Doney, K., Buckner, C. D., et al.: Treatment of chronic granulocytic leukemia by chemotherapy, total body irradiation and allogeneic bone marrow transplantation. Exp. Hematol. 6:738, 1978.
118. Doney, K. C., Buckner, C. D., et al.: Allogeneic bone marrow transplantation for chronic granulocytic leukemia. Exp. Hematol. 9:966, 1981.
119. Fefer, A., Cheever, M. A., et al.: Treatment of chronic granulocytic leukemia with chemoradiotherapy and transplantation of marrow from identical twins. New Engl. J. Med. 306:63, 1982.
120. Clift, A., Buckner, C. D., et al.: Treatment of chronic granulocytic leukaemia in chronic phase by allogeneic marrow transplantation. Lancet 2:622, 1982.
121. Goldman, J. M., Baughan, A. S. J., et al.: Marrow transplantation for patients in the chronic phase of chronic granulocytic leukaemia. Lancet 2:623, 1982.
122. McGlave, P. B., Arthur, D. C., et al.: Successful allogeneic bone marrow transplantation for patients in the accelerated phase of chronic granulocytic leukaemia. Lancet 2:625, 1982.
123. Champlin, R., Ho, W., et al.: Allogeneic bone marrow transplantation for chronic myelogenous leukemia in chronic or accelerated phase. Blood 60:1038, 1982.
124. Speck, B., Bortin, M. M., et al.: Allogeneic bone marrow transplantation for chronic myelogenous leukaemia. Lancet 1:665, 1984.
125. Reisman, L. E., and Trujillo, J. M.: Chronic granulocytic leukemia in childhood. Clinical and cytogenetic studies. J. Pediatr. 62:710, 1963.
126. Hardisty, R. M., Speed, D. E., et al.: Granulocytic leukemia in childhood. Br. J. Haematol. 10:551, 1964.
127. Castro-Malaspina, H., Schaison, G., et al.: Subacute and chronic myelomonocytic leukemia in children (juvenile CML). Cancer 54:675, 1984.
128. Clark, R. H., Taylor, L. L., et al.: Congenital juvenile chronic myelogenous leukemia: case report and review. Pediatrics 73:324, 1984.
129. Bennett, A. J., Jason, M., et al.: Infantile type of chronic myelogenous leukemia in a 16-year-old boy. Am. J. Pediatr. Hematol. Oncol. 1:369, 1979.
130. Mays, J. A., Neerhout, R. C., et al.: Juvenile chronic granulocytic leukemia. Emphasis on cutaneous manifestations and underlying neurofibromatosis. Am. J. Dis. Child. 134:654, 1980.
131. Bestak, M., Miller, D. R., et al.: Juvenile chronic myelogenous leukemia and dermal histiocytosis in von Recklinghousen's disease. Am. J. Dis. Child. 133:831, 1979.
132. Clark, R. D., Hutter, J. J., Jr.: Familial neurofibromatosis and juvenile chronic myelogenous leukemia. Hum. Genet. 60:230, 1982.
133. Dover, G. J., Boyer, S. H., et al.: Changing erythrocyte populations in juvenile chronic myelocytic leukemia: evidence for disordered regulation. Blood 49:355, 1977.
134. Terasawa, T., Ito, T., et al.: Characterization of the erythropoietic precursors (BFU-E) in a patient with juvenile chronic myelogenous leukemia by the analysis of Gy and Ay globin chains. Br. J. Haematol. 54:269, 1983.
135. Travis, S. F.: Fetal erythropoiesis in juvenile chronic myelocytic leukemia. Blood 62:602, 1983.
136. Symann, M., de Montpellier, C., et al.: "Spontaneous" erythroid progenitor cells in the circulation and monosomy 7 in juvenile chronic myelogenous leukemia. Cancer Genet. Cytogenet. 6:183, 1982.
137. Brodeur, G. M., Dow, L. W., et al.: Cytogenetic features of juvenile chronic myelogenous leukemia. Blood 53:812, 1979.
138. Inoue, S., Ravindranath, Y., et al.: Cytogenetics of juvenile type chronic granulocyte leukemia. Cancer 39:2017, 1977.
139. Altman, A. J., Palmer, C. G., et al.: Juvenile "chronic granulocytic" leukemia: a panmyelopathy with prominent monocytic involvement and circulating monocyte colony forming cells. Blood 43:341, 1974.

140. Suda, T., Miura, Y., et al.: Characterization of hemopoietic precursor cells in juvenile type chronic myelocytic leukemia. Leuk. Res. *6*:43, 1982.
141. Barak, Y., Levin, S., et al.: Juvenile and adult types of chronic granulocytic leukemia of childhood: growth patterns and characteristics of granulocyte-macrophage colony forming cells. Am. J. Hematol. *10*:269, 1981.
141a. Estrou, Z., Grunberger, T., et al.: Juvenile chronic myelogenous leukemia: characterization of the disease using cell cultures. Blood *67*:1382, 1986.
142. Herrod, H. G., Dow, L. W., et al.: Persistent Epstein-Barr virus infection mimicking juvenile chronic myelogenous leukemia: immunologic and hematologic studies. Blood *61*:1098, 1983.
143. Lilleyman, J. S., Harrison, J. F., et al.: Treatment of juvenile chronic myeloid leukemia with sequential subcutaneous cytarabine and oral mercaptopurine. Blood *49*:559, 1977.
144. Sanders, J. E., Buckner, C. D., et al.: Successful treatment of juvenile chronic granulocytic leukemia with marrow transplantation. Pediatrics *63*:44, 1979.
145. Golde, D. W., Hocking, W. G., et al.: Polycythemia: mechanisms and management. Ann. Intern. Med. *95*:71, 1981.
146. Berlin, N. I.: Diagnosis and classification of the polycythemias. Semin. Hematol. *12*:339, 1975.
147. Weinrib, N. J., and Shih, C.-F.: Spurious polycythemia. Semin. Hematol. *12*:397, 1975.
148. Adamson, J. W.: Familial polycythemia. Semin. Hematol. *12*:383, 1975.
149. Leukemia and Hematosarcoma Cooperative Group, EORTC: Treatment of polycythaemia vera by radiophosphorus or busulfan: a randomized trial. Br. J. Cancer *44*:75, 1981.
150. Modan, B.: The Polycythemia Disorders. Springfield, Il, Charles C Thomas, 1971.
151. Dykstra, O. H., and Halbertsma, T.: Polycythemia vera in childhood. Report of a case with changes in the skull. Am. J. Dis. Child. *60*:907, 1940.
152. Marlow, A. A., and Fairbanks, V. F.: Polycythemia vera in an eleven year old girl. New Engl. J. Med. *263*:950, 1960.
153. Marlow, A. A.: Letter. Blood *45*:463, 1975.
154. Aggeler, P. M., Pollycove, M., et al.: Polycythemia vera in childhood. Studies of iron kinetics with Fe-59 and blood clotting factors. Blood *17*:345, 1961.
155. Natelson, E. A., Lynch, E. C., et al.: Polycythemia vera in childhood. Am. J. Dis. Child. *122*:241, 1971.
156. Hann, H. L., Festa, R. S., et al.: Polycythemia vera in a child with acute lymphocytic leukemia. Cancer *43*:1862, 1979.
157. Danish, E. H., Rasch, C. A., et al.: Polycythemia vera in childhood: case report and review of the literature. Am. J. Hematol. *9*:421, 1980.
158. Heilmann, E., Klein, C. E., et al.: Primary polycythemia in childhood and adolescence. Folia Haematol. (Leipzig) *110*:935, 1983.
159. Castle, W. B.: The polycythemias. In *Hematology*, 2nd ed. Beck, W. S. (ed.), Cambridge, MA, MIT Press, 1977, pp. 393–411.
160. Silverstein, M. N.: Diagnosis and treatment of polycythemia vera, agnogenic myeloid metaplasia and primary thrombocythemia. In *Neoplastic Diseases of the Blood*. Wiernik, P. H., Canellos, G. P., et al. (eds.), New York, Churchill Livingstone, 1985, p. 135.
161. Leblond, P. F., and Weed, R. I.: The peripheral blood in polycythemia vera and myelofibrosis. Clin. Hematol. *4*:353, 1975.
162. Ellis, J. T., Silver, R. T., et al.: The bone marrow in polycythemia vera. Semin. Hematol. *12*:433, 1975.
163. Wurgter-Hill, D., Whang-Peng, J., et al.: Cytogenetic studies in polycythemia vera. Semin. Hematol. *13*:13, 1976.
164. Testa, J. R., Kanofsky, J. R., et al.: Karyotypic patterns and their clinical significance in polycythemia vera. Am. J. Hematol. *11*:29, 1981.
165. Berger, R., Bernheim, A., et al.: Chromosome studies in polycythemia vera patients. Cancer Genet. Cytogenet. *12*:217, 1984.
166. Shiraishi, Y., Hayata, I., et al.: Chromosomes and causation of human cancer and leukemia. XII. Banding analysis of abnormal chromosomes in polycythemia vera. Cancer *36*:199, 1975.
167. Berger, R., Bernheim, A., et al.: Cytogenetic studies on acute nonlymphocytic leukemias following polycythemia vera. Cancer Genet. Cytogenet. *11*:441, 1984.
168. Fairre, G., Black, A. J., et al.: Polycythaemia rubra vera and congenital deafness in monozygotic twins. Br. Med. J. *283*:192, 1981.
169. Burnside, P., Salmon, D. C., et al.: Polycythaemia rubra vera in monozygotic twins. Br. Med. J. *283*:560, 1981.
170. Friedland, M. L., Wittels, E. G., et al.: Polycythemia vera in identical twins. Am. J. Hematol. *10*:101, 1981.
171. Brubaker, L. H., Wasserman, L. R., et al.: Increased prevalence of polycythemia vera in parents of patients on polycythemia vera study group protocols. Am. J. Hematol. *16*:367, 1984.
172. Adamson, J. W., Fialkow, P. J., et al.: Polycythemia vera: stem-cell and probable clonal origin of the disease. New Engl. J. Med. *295*:913, 1976.
173. de Klerk, G., Rosengarten, P. C. J., et al.: Serum erythropoietin (ESF) titers in polycythemia. Blood *58*:1171, 1981.
174. Golde, D. W., and Cline, M. J.: Erythropoietin responsiveness in polycythemia vera. Br. J. Hematol. *29*:567, 1975.
175. Golde, D. W., Bersch, N., et al.: Polycythemia vera: hormonal modulation of erythropoiesis in vitro. Blood *49*:399, 1977.
176. Zanjani, E. D., Lutton, J. D., et al.: Erythroid colony formation by polycythemia vera in bone marrow *in vitro*. Dependence on erythropoietin. J. Clin. Invest. *59*:841, 1977.
177. Fauser, A. A., and Messner, H. A.: Pluripotent hemopoietic progenitors (CFU-GEMM) in polycythemia vera: analysis of erythropoietin requirement and proliferative activity. Blood *58*:1224, 1981.
178. Casadevall, N., Vainchenker, W., et al.: Erythroid progenitors in polycythemia vera: demonstration of their hypersensitivity to erythropoietin using serum free cultures. Blood *59*:447, 1982.
179. Ash, R. C., Detrick, R. A., et al.: *In vitro* studies of human pluripotential hematopoietic progenitors in polycythemia vera. J. Clin. Invest. *69*:1112, 1982.
180. Beckman, B., Anderson, W. F., et al.: Mixed myeloid-lymphoid colonies in a patient with polycythemia vera. Am. J. Hematol. *12*:419, 1982.
181. Prchal, J. F., Murphy, S., et al.: Polycythemia vera. The *in vitro* response of normal and abnormal stem cell lines to erythropoietin. J. Clin. Invest. *61*:1044, 1978.
182. Singer, J. W., Fialkow, P. J., et al.: Polycythemia vera. Increased expression of normal committed granulocytic stem cells in vitro after exposure of marrow to tritiated thymidine. J. Clin. Invest. *64*:1320, 1979.
183. Singer, J. W., Adamson, J. W., et al.: Polycythemia vera. Physical separation of normal and neoplastic committed granulocyte-macrophage progenitors. J. Clin. Invest. *66*:730, 1980.
184. Mladenovic, J., and Adamson, J. W.: Characteristics of circulating erythroid colony forming cells in normal and polycythaemic man. Br. J. Haematol. *51*:377, 1982.
185. Adamson, J. W., Singer, J. W., et al.: Polycythemia vera. Further in vitro studies of hematopoietic regulation. J. Clin. Invest. *66*:1363, 1980.
186. Kornberg, A., Fibach, E., et al.: Circulating erythroid progenitors in patients with "spent" polycythaemia vera

and myelofibrosis with myeloid metaplasia. Br. J. Haematol. 52:573, 1982.
187. Pearson, T. C., and Wetherley-Mein, G.: Vascular occlusive episodes and venous haematocrit in primary proliferative polycythaemia. Lancet 2:1219, 1978.
188. Rosenthal, A., Nathan, D. G., et al.: Acute hemodynamic effects of red cell volume reduction in polycythemia of cyanotic congenital heart disease. Circulation 42:297, 1970.
189. Kontras, S. B., Bodenbender, J. G., et al.: Hyperviscosity in congenital heart disease. J. Pediatr. 76:214, 1970.
190. Hutton, R. D.: The effect of iron deficiency on whole blood viscosity in polycythemic patients. Br. J. Haematol. 43:191, 1979.
191. Beck, R. D., Goldberg, J. D., et al.: Increased incidence of acute leukemia in polycythemia vera associated with chlorambucil therapy. New Engl. J. Med. 304:441, 1981.
192. Wasserman, L. R.: The treatment of polycythemia vera. Semin. Hematol. 13:57, 1976.
193. Silverstein, M. N.: The evolution into and the treatment of late stage polycythemia vera. Semin. Hematol. 13:79, 1976.
194. Najean, Y., Arrago, J. P., et al.: The "spent' phase of polycythaemia vera: hypersplenism in the absence of myelofibrosis. Br. J. Haematol. 56:163, 1984.
195. Najman, A., Stachowiak, J., et al.: Pipobroman therapy of polycythemia vera. Blood 59:890, 1982.
196. Mulligan, D. W., Thein, S. L., et al.: Secondary treatment of polycythemia rubra vera with 6-thioguinine. Cancer 50:836, 1982.
197. Brodsky, I.: Busulfan treatment of polycythaemia vera. Br. J. Haematol. 52:1, 1982.
198. Silverstein, M. N.: Primary or hemorrhagic thrombocythemia. Arch. Intern. Med. 122:18, 1968.
199. Murphy, S., Rosenthal, D. S., et al.: Essential thrombocythemia: response during first year of therapy with melphalan and radioactive phosphorus. A Polycythemia Vera Study Group report. Cancer Treat. Rep. 66:1495, 1982.
200. Case, D. C.: Therapy of essential thrombocythemia with thiotepa and chlorambucil. Blood 63:51, 1984.
201. Brusamolina, E., Canevari, A., et al.: Efficacy trial of pipobroman in essential thrombocythemia: a study of 24 patients. Cancer Treat. Rep. 68:1339, 1984.
202. Ozner, F. L., Truax, W. E., et al.: Primary hemorrhagic thrombocythemia. Am. J. Med. 28:807, 1960.
203. Freedman, M. H., Olivares, R. S., et al.: Primary thrombocytosis in a child. J. Pediatr. 83:163, 1973.
204. Hoagland, H. C., and Silverstein, M. N.: Primary thrombocythemia in the young patient. Mayo Clin. Proc. 53:578, 1978.
205. Sceats, D. J., and Baitlon, D.: Primary thrombocythemia in a child. Clin. Pediatr. 19:298, 1980.
206. Linch, D. L., Hutton, R., et al.: Primary thrombocythemia in childhood. Scand. J. Haematol. 28:72, 1982.
207. Addiego, J. E., Mentzer, W. C., et al.: Thrombocytosis in infants and children. J. Pediatr. 85:805, 1974.
208. Preston, F. E., Emmanuel, I. G., et al.: Essential thrombocythemia and peripheral gangrene. Br. Med. J. 3:548, 1974.
209. Speat, T. H., Lejnieks, I., et al.: Defective platelets in essential thrombocythemia. Arch. Intern. Med. 124:135, 1969.
210. Weinfeld, A., Branehog, I., et al.: Platelets in the myeloproliferative syndrome. Clin. Haematol. 4:373, 1975.
211. Kaywin, P., McDonough, M., et al.: Platelet function in essential thrombocythemia. Decreased epinephrine responsiveness associated with a deficiency of platelet alpha-adrenergic receptors. New Engl. J. Med. 299:505, 1978.
212. Wu, K. K.: Platelet hyperaggregability and thrombosis in patients with thrombocythemia. Ann. Intern. Med. 88:7, 1978.
213. Kessler, C. M., Klein, H. G., et al.: Uncontrolled thrombocytosis in chronic myeloproliferative disorders. Br. J. Haematol. 50:157, 1982.
214. Mark, J.: Chromosomal abnormalities and their specificity in human neoplasms: an assessment of recent observations by banding techniques. Adv. Cancer Res. 24:165, 1977.
215. Rowley, J. D.: Acquired trisomy 9. Lancet 2:390, 1973.
216. Zaccaria, A., and Tura, S.: A chromosome abnormality in primary thrombocythemia. New Engl. J. Med. 298:1422, 1978.
217. Fialkow, P. J., Faguet, G. B., et al.: Evidence that essential thrombocythemia is a clonal disorder with origin in a multipotent stem cell. Blood 58:916, 1981.
218. Gaetani, G. F., Ferraris, A. M., et al.: Primary thrombocythemia: clonal origin of platelets, erythrocytes, and granulocytes in a Gd^B/Gd Mediterranean subject. Blood 59:76, 1982.
219. Singal, U., Prasad, A. S., et al.: Essential thrombocythemia: a clonal disorder of hematopoietic stem cell. Am. J. Hematol. 14:193, 1983.
220. McCabe, W. R., and McLaughlin, R. A.: Is primary hemorrhagic thrombocythemia a clinical myth? Ann. Intern. Med. 43:182, 1955.
221. Geller, S. A., and Shapiro, E.: Acute leukemia as a natural sequel to primary thrombocythemia. Am. J. Clin. Pathol. 77:353, 1982.
222. Frei-Lahr, D., Barton, J. C., et al.: Blastic transformation of essential thrombocythemia: dual expression of myelomonoblastic/megakaryoblastic phenotypes. Blood 63:866, 1984.
223. Ward, H. P., and Block, M. H.: The natural history of agnogenic myeloid metaplasia (AMM) and a critical evaluation of its relationship with myeloproliferative syndrome. Medicine 50:357, 1971.
224. Takacsi-Nagy, L., and Graf, F.: Definition, clinical features and diagnosis of myelofibrosis. Clin. Hematol. 4:291, 1975.
225. Njoku, O. S., Lewis, S. M., et al.: Anaemia in myelofibrosis: its value in prognosis. Br. J. Haematol. 54:79, 1983.
226. Varki, A., Lottenberg, R., et al.: The syndrome of idiopathic myelofibrosis. A cliniopathologic review with emphasis on the prognostic variables predicting survival. Medicine 62:353, 1983.
227. Boxer, L. A., Camitta, B. M., et al.: Myelofibrosis-myeloid metaplasia in childhood. Pediatrics 55:861, 1975.
228. Lazlo, J.: Myeloproliferative disorders (MDP): myelofibrosis, myelosclerosis, extramedullary hematopoiesis, undifferentiated MDP and hemorrhagic thrombocythemia. Semin. Hematol. 12:409, 1975.
229. Skarin, A. T.: Pathology and morphology of chronic leukemias and related disorders. In *Neoplastic Diseases of the Blood*. Wiernik, P. H., Canellos, G. P., et al. (eds.), New York, Churchill Livingstone, 1985, p. 19.
230. Van Voolen, G. A., Hellstrom, H. R., et al.: Paroxysmal nocturnal hemoglobinuria and the myeloproliferative syndrome. Ann. Intern. Med. 96:792, 1982.
231. Whang-Peng, J., Lee, E., et al.: Cytogenetic studies in patients with myelofibrosis and myeloid metaplasia. Leukemia Res. 2:41, 1977.
232. Gordon, B. R., Coleman, M., et al.: Immunological abnormalities in myelofibrosis with activation of the complement system. Blood 58:904, 1981.
233. Cappio, F. C., Vigliani, R., et al.: Idiopathic myelofibrosis: a possible role for immune-complexes in the pathogenesis of bone marrow fibrosis. Br. J. Haematol. 49:17, 1981.
234. Rondeau, E., Solal-Celigny, P., et al.: Immune disorders in agnogenic myeloid metaplasia: relations to myelofibrosis. Br. J. Haematol. 53:467, 1983.
235. Jacobson, R. J., Salo, A., et al.: Agnogenic myeloid metaplasia: a clonal proliferation of hematopoietic stem cells with secondary myelofibrosis. Blood 51:189, 1978.

236. Friedenstein, A. J., Ivanov-Smolenski, A. A., et al.: Origin of marrow stromal mechanocytes in radiochimeras and heterotopic transplants. Exp. Hematol. 6:440, 1978.
237. Golde, D. W., Hocking, W. G., et al.: Origin of human bone marrow fibroblasts. Br. J. Haematol. 44:183, 1980.
238. Castro-Malaspina, H., Gay, R. E., et al.: Characteristics of bone marrow fibroblast colony-forming cells (CFU-F) and their progeny in patients with myeloproliferative disorders. Blood 59:1046, 1982.
239. Croizat, H., Amato, D., et al.: Differences among myeloproliferative disorders in the behavior of their restricted progenitor cells in culture. Blood 62:578, 1983.
240. Wang, J. C., Cheung, C. P., et al.: Circulating granulocyte and macrophage progenitor cells in primary and secondary myelofibrosis. Br. J. Haematol. 54:301, 1983.
241. Kornberg, A., Fibach, E., et al.: Circulating erythroid progenitors in patients with "spent' polycythemia vera and myelofibrosis with myeloid metaplasia. Br. J. Haematol. 152:573, 1982.
242. Bain, B. J., Catovksy, D., et al.: Megakaryoblastic leukemia presenting as acute myelofibrosis—a study of four cases with the platelet peroxidase reaction. Blood 58:206, 1981.
243. Mirchandani, I., Palutke, M., et al.: Acute megakaryoblastic leukemia. Cancer 50:2866, 1983.
244. Evans, D. I. K.: Acute myelofibrosis in children with Down's syndrome. Arch. Dis. Child. 50:458, 1975.
245. McCarthy, D. M.: Fibrosis of the bone marrow: content and causes. Br. J. Haematol. 59:1, 1985.
246. Editorial: Reversible myelofibrosis? Lancet 1:497, 1985.
247. Wang, J. C., Aung, M. K., et al.: Urinary hydroxyproline excretion in myelofibrosis. Blood 55:383, 1980.
248. Castro-Malaspina, H., Rabellino, E. M., et al.: Human megakaryocyte stimulation of proliferation of bone marrow fibroblasts. Blood 57:781, 1981.
249. Groopman, J. E.: The pathogenesis of myelofibrosis in myeloproliferative disorders. Ann. Intern. Med. 92:857, 1980.
250. Kiang, D. T., McKenna, R. W., et al.: Reversal of myelofibrosis in advanced breast cancer. Am. J. Med. 64:173, 1978.
251. Rappeport, J., Parkman, R., et al.: Reversibility of myelofibrosis (MF) after bone marrow transplantation. Blood 52(Suppl. 1):271(Abstr. 589), 1978.
252. McGlave, P. B., Brunning, R. D., et al.: Reversibility of severe bone marrow fibrosis and osteosclerosis following allogeneic bone marrow transplantation for chronic granulocytic leukemia. Br. J. Haematol. 52:189, 1982.
253. Oblon, D. J., Elfenbein, G. J., et al.: The reversal of myelofibrosis associated with chronic myelogenous leukemia after allogeneic bone marrow transplantation. Exp. Hematol. 11:681, 1983.
254. Silverstein, M. N., Wollaeger, E. E., et al.: Gastrointestinal and abdominal manifestations of agnogenic myeloid metaplasia. Arch. Intern. Med. 131:532, 1973.
255. Brubaker, L. H., Briere, J., et al.: Treatment of anemia in myeloproliferative disorders. A randomized study of fluoxymesterone versus transfusions only. Arch. Intern. Med. 142:1533, 1982.
256. Linman, J. W., Bagby, G. C., Jr.: The preleukemic syndrome: clinical and laboratory features, natural course, and management. Blood Cells 2:11, 1976.
257. Pierre, R. V.: Preleukemic syndrome. Virchows Arch. (Cell Pathol.) 29:29, 1978.
258. Cantu-Rajnoldi, A., Porcelli, P., et al.: Myelodysplastic syndromes in children: observations on five cases. Eur. Paediatr. Haematol. Oncol. 1:71, 1984.
259. Pedersen-Bjergaard, J., Olesen-Larsen, S.: Incidence of acute nonlymphocytic leukemia, preleukemia and acute myeloproliferative syndrome up to 10 years after treatment of Hodgkin's disease. New Engl. J. Med. 307:965, 1982.
260. Bennett, J. M., Catovsky, D., et al.: Proposal for the classification of the myelodysplastic syndromes. Br. J. Haematol. 51:189, 1982.
261. Rosenthal, D. S., and Moloney, M. C.: Refractory dysmyelopoietic anemia and acute leukemia. Blood 63:314, 1984.
262. Linman, J. W., and Bagby, G. C., Jr.: The preleukemic syndrome (hemopoietic dysplasia). Cancer 42:854, 1978.
263. Barlogie, B., Johnston, D. A., et al.: Evolution of oligoleukemia. Cancer 53:2115, 1984.
264. Coiffier, B., Adeleine, P., et al.: Dysmyelopoietic syndromes: a search for prognostic factors in 193 patients. Cancer 52:83, 1983.
265. Koeffler, H. P., and Golde, D. W.: Human preleukemia. Ann. Intern. Med. 93:347, 1980.
266. Tricot, G., De Wolfe-Peters, C., et al.: Bone marrow histology in myelodysplastic syndromes. I. Histological findings in myelodysplastic syndromes and comparison with bone marrow smears. Br. J. Haematol. 57:423, 1984.
267. Yoo, D., and Lessin, L. S.: Bone marrow mast cell content in preleukemic syndrome. Am. J. Med. 73:539, 1982.
268. Maldonado, J. E.: Platelet granulopathy: a new morphologic feature in preleukemia and myelomonocytic leukemia; light microscopy and ultrastructural morphology and cytochemistry. Mayo Clin. Proc. 51:452, 1976.
269. Maldonado, J. E., Maigne, J., et al.: Comparative electron-microscopic study of the erythrocytic line in refractory anemia (preleukemia) and myelomonocytic leukemia. Blood Cells 2:167, 1976.
270. Breton-Gorius, J., Houssay, D., et al.: Partial myeloperoxidase deficiency in a case of preleukemia. I. Studies of fine structure and peroxidase synthesis of promyelocytes. Br. J. Haematol. 30:273, 1975.
271. Weisdorf, D. J., Oken, M. M., et al.: Auer rod positive dysmyelopoietic syndrome. Am. J. Hematol. 11:397, 1981.
272. Blank, J., and Lange, B.: Preleukemia in children. J. Pediatr. 98:565, 1981.
273. Schmalzl, F., and Hellriegel, K.-P. (eds.): *Preleukemia*. New York, Springer-Verlag, 1978, p. 1979.
274. Kobrinsky, N. L., Nesbit, M. E., et al.: Hematopoietic dysplasia and marrow hypocellularity in children: a preleukemic condition. J. Pediatr. 100:907, 1982.
275. Geary, C. G.: The diagnosis of preleukaemia. Br. J. Haematol. 55:1, 1983.
276. Dreyfus, B., Sultan, C., et al.: Abnormalities of blood group antigens and erythrocyte enzymes in two types of chronic refractory anaemia. Br. J. Haematol. 16:303, 1969.
277. Salmon, C.: Blood group changes in preleukemic states. Blood Cells 2:211, 1976.
278. Ruutu, P., Ruutu, T., et al.: Function of neutrophils in preleukemia. Scand. Haematol. 18:317, 1977.
279. Boogaerts, M. A., Nelissen, V., et al.: Blood neutrophil function in primary myelodysplastic syndromes. Br. J. Haematol. 55:217, 1983.
280. Ruutu, P., Ruutu, T., et al.: Defective neutrophil migration in monosomy-7. Blood 58:739, 1981.
281. Youman, J. D., III, Saarni, M. I., et al.: Diagnostic value of muramidase (lysozyme) in acute leukemia and preleukemia. Mayo Clin. Proc. 45:219, 1970.
282. Anderson, R. W., Volsky, D. J., et al.: Lymphocyte abnormalities in preleukemia. I. Decreased NK activity, anomalous immunoregulatory cell subsets and deficient EBV receptors. Leukemia Res. 7:389, 1983.
283. Kerndrup, G., Meyer, K., et al.: Natural killer (NK)–cell activity and antibody-dependent cellular cytotoxicity (ADCC) in primary preleukemic syndrome. Leukemia Res. 8:239, 1984.
284. Killman, S. A.: Preleukemia: does it exist? Blood Cells 2:81, 1976.
285. Greenberg, P. L., Nichols, W. C., et al.: Granulopoiesis in acute myeloid leukemia and preleukemia. New Engl. J. Med. 284:1225, 1971.

286. Greenberg, P., Mara, B., et al.: The myeloproliferative disorders. Correlation between clinical evolution and alterations of granulopoiesis. Am. J. Med. 61:878, 1976.
287. Spitzer, G., Verma, D. S., et al.: Culture studies in vitro in human leukemia. Semin. Hematol. 15:352, 1978.
288. Senn, J. S., Curtis, J. E., et al.: The distribution of marrow granulopoietic progenitors among patients with preleukemia. Leukemia Res. 4:409, 1980.
289. Francis, G. E., Wing, M. A., et al.: Use of bone marrow culture in prediction of acute leukaemia transformation in preleukemia. Lancet 1:1409, 1983.
290. Greenberg, P. L.: The smoldering myeloid leukemic states: clinical and biologic features. Blood 61:1035, 1983.
291. Koeffler, H. P., Cline, M. J., et al.: Erythropoiesis in preleukemia. Blood 51:1013, 1978.
292. Chui, D. H. K., and Clark, B. J.: Abnormal erythroid progenitor cells in human preleukemia. Blood 60:362, 1982.
293. Nowell, P. C.: Cytogenetics of preleukemia. Cancer Genet. Cytogenet. 5:295, 1982.
294. Second International Workshop on Chromosomes in Leukemia, 1979: Chromosomes in preleukemia. Cancer Genet. Cytogenet. 2:108, 1980.
295. Sokal, G., Michaux, J. L., et al.: The karyotype in refractory anemia in preleukemia. Clin. Haematol. 9:129, 1980.
296. Rowley, J. D., Golomb, H. M., et al.: Nonrandom chromosome abnormalities in acute leukemia and dysmyelopoietic syndromes in patients with previously treated malignant disease. Blood 58:759, 1981.
297. Moir, D. J., Jones, P. A. E., et al.: A new translocation, t(1;3) (p36:q21) in myelodysplastic disorders. Blood 64:553, 1984.
298. Bernard, P., Reiffers, J., et al.: Associated abnormalities of chromosomes 1, 5, and 11 in dysmyelopoietic syndromes. Cancer Genet. Cytogenet. 12:31, 1984.
299. Anderson, R. L., and Bagby, G. C., Jr.: The prognostic value of chromosome studies in patients with the preleukemia syndrome (hematopoietic dysplasia). Leukemia Res. 6:175, 1982.
300. Nowell, P., Wilmoth, D., et al.: Cytogenetics of childhood preleukemia. Cancer Genet. Cytogenet. 10:261, 1983.
301. Jacobson, R., Raskind, W. H., et al.: Refractory anemia (RA), a myelodysplastic syndrome: clinical development with progressive loss of normal committed progenitors. Blood 60(Suppl. 1):129a(Abstr.), 1982.
302. Raskind, W. H., Tirumali, N., et al.: Evidence for a multistep pathogenesis of a myelodysplasia syndrome. Blood 63:1318, 1984.
303. Grier, H. E., Weinstein, H. J., et al.: Cytogenetic evidence for involvement of erythroid progenitors in a child with therapy linked myelodysplasia. Br. J. Haematol. 64:513, 1986.
304. Weber, R. F. A., Geraedts, J. P. M., et al.: The preleukemia syndrome. I. Clinical and hematological findings. Acta Med. Scand. 207:391, 1980.
305. Joseph, A. S., and Cinkotai, K. L.: Natural history of smouldering leukaemia. Br. J. Cancer 46:160, 1982.
305a. Clark, R., Peters, S., et al.: Prognostic importance of hypodiploid hemopoietic precursors in myelodysplastic syndromes. New Engl. J. Med. 314:1472, 1986.
306. Cooperative Group for the Study of Aplastic and Refractory Anemia. Najean, Y., and Pecking, A. (eds.): Refractory anemia with excess of blast cells: prognostic factors and effect of treatment with androgens or cytosine arabinoside. Cancer 44, 1976.
307. Cohen, J. R., Creger, W. P., et al.: Subacute myeloid leukemia. A clinical review. Am. J. Med. 66:959, 1979.
308. Murray, C., Cooper, B., et al.: Remission of acute myelogenous leukemia in elderly patients with prior refractory dysmyelopoietic anemia. Cancer 52:967, 1983.
309. Wisch, J. S., Griffin, J. D., et al.: Response of preleukemia syndromes to continuous infusion of low-dose cytarabine. New Engl. J. Med. 309:1599, 1983.
310. Castaigne, S., Daniel, M. T., et al.: Does treatment with ARA-C in low dosage cause differentiation of leukemic cells? Blood 62:85, 1983.
311. Editorial: Treatment for preleukemia? Lancet 1:943, 1984.
312. Desforges, J. F.: Cytarabine: Low-dose, no dose. New Engl. J. Med. 309:1637, 1983.
313. Baccarani, M., Zaccaria, A., et al.: Low dose arabinosyl cytosine for treatment of myelodysplastic syndromes and subacute leukemia. Leukemia Res. 7:539, 1983.
314. Jehn, U., De Bock, R., et al.: Clinical trials of low-dose ARA-C in the treatment of acute leukemia and myelodysplasia. Blut 48:255, 1984.
315. Gold, E. J., Mertelsmann, R. H., et al.: Phase I clinical trial of 13-cis-retinoic acid in myelodysplastic syndromes. Cancer Treat. Rep. 67:981, 1983.
316. Gyger, M., Perreault, C., et al.: Restoration of normal hematopoiesis by bone marrow ablation and allogeneic marrow transplantation in a case of Hodgkin's disease therapy related preleukemia. Blood 61:1279, 1983.
317. Appelbaum, F. R., Storb, R., et al.: Allogeneic marrow transplantation in the treatment of preleukemia. Ann. Intern. Med. 100:689, 1984.
318. Sieff, C. A., Chessells, J. M., et al.: Monosomy 7 in childhood: a myeloproliferative disorder. Br. J. Haematol. 49:235, 1981.
319. Linch, D. C., Walker, H., et al.: A chronic myeloproliferative disorder associated with monosomy 7 in the bone marrow cells; normal karyotype in acute transformation. Br. J. Haematol. 51:439, 1982.
320. Dessypris, E. N., Clark, D. A., et al.: Increased sensitivity to complement of erythroid and myeloid progenitors in paroxysmal nocturnal hemoglobinuria. New Engl. J. Med. 309:690, 1983.
321. Fialkow, P. J.: Clonal evolution of myeloid leukemias. In *Genes and Cancer,* Vol. 17. Bishop, J. M., Rowley, J. D., et al. (eds.), New York, A. R. Liss, 1984, p. 215.

ONCOLOGY

CHAPTER 35
The Lymphomas and Lymphadenopathy

SHARON B. MURPHY

INTRODUCTION 1086
LYMPHADENOPATHY 1087
  Anatomy and Physiology of the Lymphoid System
  Non-neoplastic Lymph Node Enlargement
    Approach to the Patient
    Differential Diagnosis
  Mediastinal Masses
NON-HODGKIN'S LYMPHOMA 1091
  Definition
  Immunohistopathology and Classification
    Cellular Lymphoid Origins
    Lymphoblastic Lymphomas
    Undifferentiated Lymphoma, Burkitt's Type
    Large Cell or "Histiocytic" Lymphomas
  Clinical Presentations
  Laboratory Findings
  Staging
  Treatment and Results of Modern Therapy
  Complications
HODGKIN'S DISEASE 1101
  Definition
  Evidence for Altered Immunity in HD
  Cellular Origins and Histopathology
  Clinical Presentations
  Laboratory Findings
  Staging
  Treatment and Results of Modern Therapy
  Complications
UNRESOLVED CONTROVERSIES IN THE
  MANAGEMENT OF LYMPHOMAS 1111

INTRODUCTION

The malignant lymphomas are a diverse group of disorders affecting the lymphoid system. The nonmalignant forms of lymphadenopathy are much more common in childhood and are discussed in this chapter because of the frequent overlap of many of their clinical and pathologic features with the malignant disorders. In the early stages of malignant lymphomas, few, if any, clinical features are present that permit differentiation from non-neoplastic lymph node enlargement. Partial or complete obliteration of normal lymph node architecture is common to all types of malignant lymphoma but is not pathognomonic, as chronic lymphadenitis and infectious mononucleosis may also obscure or obliterate lymph node architecture. The classic Reed-Sternberg cells of Hodgkin's disease (Fig. 35–1) may even be observed in lymph node biopsy specimens from those patients with infectious mononucleosis (1). The difficulties of distinguishing lymph node neoplasms from non-neoplastic reactive states, particularly infections, are underscored by the later recognition (2) of syphilis in one and tuberculosis in another of the original six cases described by Thomas Hodgkin (3).

The unique anatomic arrangement and physiologic function of the components of the lymphoid system are responsible for many of the clinicopathologic features of the group of disorders discussed in this chapter. These include the frequent systemic involvement of lymph nodes, spleen, and bone marrow, as well as the possibility of extranodal disease produced by lymphoid tissue aggregates in the sinusoidal system of the liver, respiratory and digestive tracts, and thymus. Common to all these disorders is the oftentimes difficult task of distinguishing an apparently localized and isolated lymph node enlargement or tumor from a systemic, usually neoplastic, proliferation of lymphoreticular cells. The distinction has important diagnostic, therapeutic, and prognostic implications. As a result of recent major advances, the majority of children with lymphomas are curable with modern multidisciplinary treatment. Consequently, precision in assessment of the immunohistopathologic subtype and extent of disease is of the utmost importance.

In this chapter, the normal anatomy and physiologic functioning of the immune system will first be discussed as a basis for understanding lymphadenopathy. An understanding of normal lymphocyte differentiation is also an essential basis for comprehension of lymphoid neoplasia, since lym-

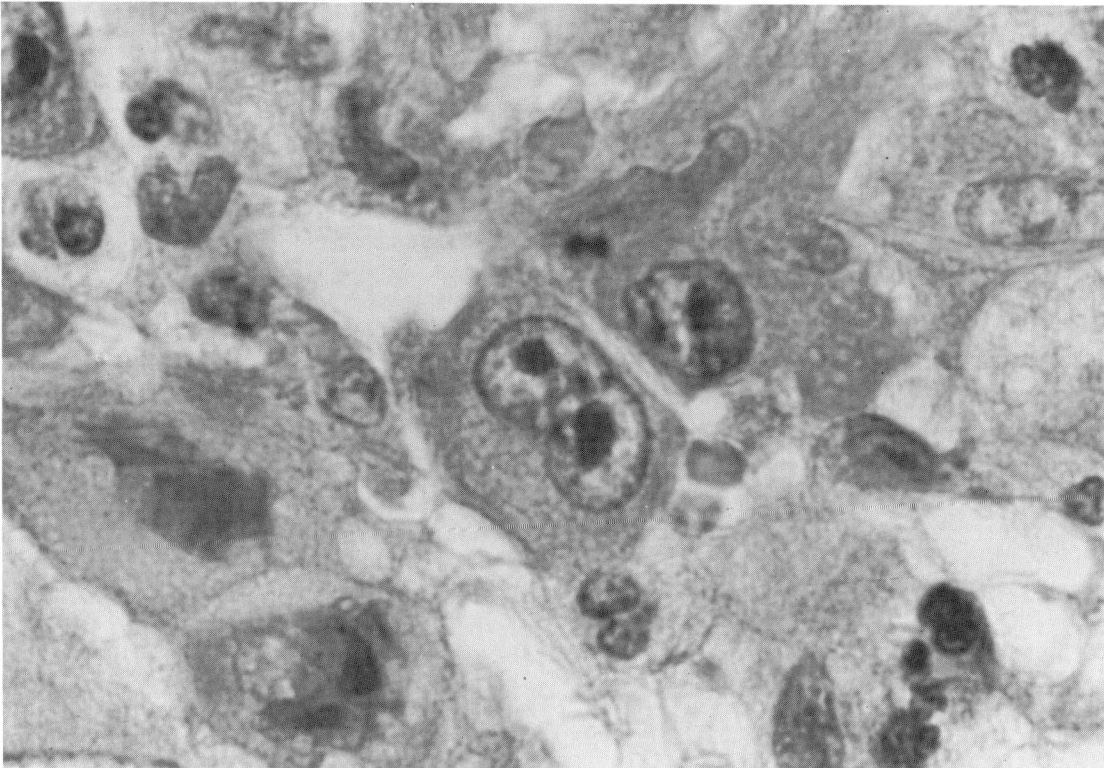

Figure 35–1. A Reed-Sternberg cell. These cells are characterized by large size (15 to 45 μ), amphophilic cytoplasm, binucleate or multinucleate appearance, vesicular nuclei, and prominent nucleoli (hematoxylin-eosin, ×400).

phomas are tumors of the immune system (4, 5). There has been remarkable progress in our understanding of the origins of malignant lymphomas as either thymic-dependent (T cell) or bursal equivalent (B cell), or, far more rarely, of monocyte-macrophage origin. To a remarkable degree, lymphomas behave as expanded clones that mirror their normal counterpart lymphoid cell in the expression of morphologic diversity, phenotypic characteristics, proliferative capacity, anatomic localization, and functional capabilities.

Hodgkin's disease (HD) will be discussed separately from other non-Hodgkin's lymphomas (NHL) because of important biologic and clinical differences governing a separate approach. The reader is referred to references 6 to 10 for complete reviews of the lymphomas.

LYMPHADENOPATHY

Anatomy and Physiology of the Lymphoid System

The lymphoid system may be divided anatomically and functionally into three compartments (11):

1. The *stem cells*, progenitors of all classes of lymphocytes.
2. The *central lymphoid organs*, which are responsible for fostering the development of immature lymphocytes into either T or B cells. In birds and mammals, the thymus is the central lymphoid organ responsible for the maturation of T cells, which are subsequently seeded to the T-dependent areas of peripheral lymphoid tissues and to the recirculating lymphocyte pool. For B cells, the central lymphoid organ is considered to be a "bursal equivalent," an anatomically vague counterpart of the bursa of Fabricius in birds.
3. The *peripheral lymphoid system*, consisting of lymphocyte populations already processed by the central lymphoid organs and capable of generating the immune response following antigenic challenge. The peripheral lymphoid system consists of lymph nodes; the spleen; pulmonary lymphoid tissue; gut-associated lymphoid tissues along the entire alimentary tract, including most notably the lingual, palatine, and pharyngeal tonsils, intestinal Peyer's patches, and appendix; and less well defined collections of lymphocytes in numerous other organs, including the skin. All of the lymphoid organs have a blood and lymphatic circulation and drainage system that assists internal cellular migration and movement, accounting for extensive lymphocyte trafficking and characteristic homing patterns.

Lymph nodes are individual encapsulated anatomic units distributed along lymphatic vessels. The structure of a lymph node consists of highly organized collections of cells supported by a network of interdigitating reticulum cells (Fig. 35–2). The composition and size of different components of a lymph node vary in relation to age, site in the body, and antecedent infections, inflammations, or immunologic events. The processes of specific antigen processing and T and B cell activation leading to cell proliferation and differentiation of effector functions, such as immunoglobulin synthesis, are more completely detailed in Chapters 26 and 27.

Lymph node enlargement thus results either from (a) proliferation of cells *intrinsic* to the node, either normally in response to antigenic stimulation, or apparently autonomously in lymphomas, or (b) from invasion of the node by *extrinsic* cells, e.g., neutrophils, histiocytes, metastatic tumor cells, etc.

Non-neoplastic Lymph Node Enlargement

APPROACH TO THE PATIENT

It is characteristic of infancy and childhood that lymph glands are prone to swelling and hyperplasia. In fact, cervical lymph nodes are nearly universally palpable in children. In 1899, Holt used the term "lymphatism" to refer to this "exaggerated susceptibility of lymphoid tissue in childhood to respond to any inflammation by hyperplasia, which may be out of proportion to the exciting cause and which continues after the cause has ceased to operate" (12). Now, more than 80 years later, the practicing pediatrician is less commonly faced with massive cervical lymph node enlargement from diphtheria or acute bacterial adenitis, as a result of widespread immunization and common use of antibiotics for upper respiratory tract infections and pharyngitis. Nevertheless, the problem of lymphadenopathy, or the lump in the neck, in particular, continues to pose diagnostic dilemmas.

Although the majority of instances of lymph node enlargement in children are transient, benign, and self-limited, a minority are serious, even life-threatening. A systematic history and careful, complete physical examination may provide the diagnosis in many cases. The history should emphasize particularly any preceding acute infection, such as otitis or pharyngitis, associated with tenderness, warmth, or redness of the nodes. Associated constitutional complaints, such as persistent fevers, weight loss, leg pains, or weakness suggest a more serious underlying disorder. The distribution of the adenopathy and whether it is regional or generalized may also be helpful diagnostically. For example, enlarged upper cervical nodes usually are caused by upper respiratory tract infections, whereas supraclavicular adenopathy suggests mediastinal pathology and the prompt necessity of x-ray examination of the chest. A hard neck mass associated with epistaxis, middle ear disease, sinusitis, or trismus suggests a nonlymphomatous head and neck malignancy of childhood, such as rhabdomyosarcoma or an undifferentiated nasopharyngeal carcinoma, so-called lymphoepithelioma. In cases in which clinical fea-

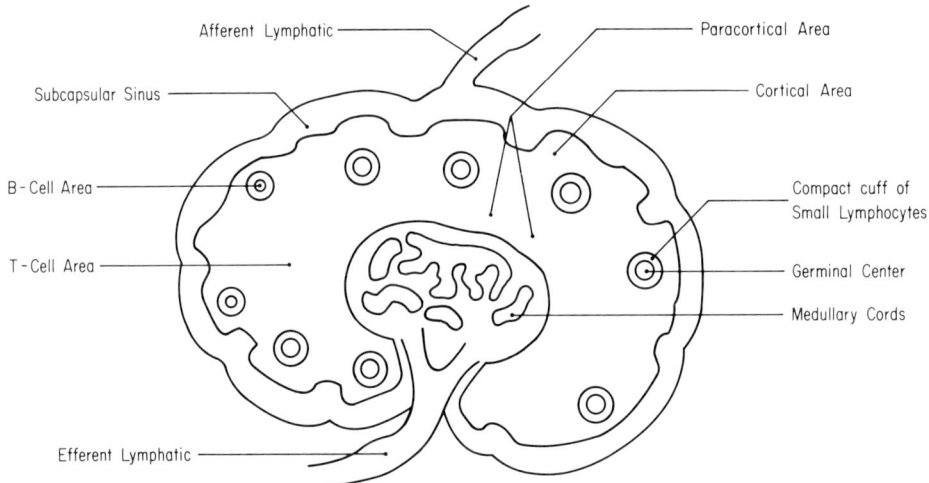

Figure 35–2. A schematic outline of discrete anatomic and functional areas of a lymph node is shown. An outer cortical layer lying beneath the subcapsular sinus contains a dense population of predominantly small lymphocytes and an array of lymphocytic follicles and germinal centers, an area that is functionally a B-cell domain. Germinal centers are spherical or oval structures surrounded by a dense cuff of mainly small lymphocytes and containing densely packed large lymphoid cells, many of which are in mitosis. Germinal centers enlarge in size and increase in number following intense and persistent antigenic stimulation. The paracortical area is an inner cortex that lies beneath and interdigitates with the cortical area and is the main site of proliferation of lymphocytes in cell-mediated immune responses, an area considered to be a T-dependent zone. Under the paracortex lie the medullary cords, stringlike arrays of lymphocytes, plasma cells, and macrophages that converge on the hilus. Medullary cords are the main site of plasma cell proliferation. Afferent lymphatic vessels enter the node and empty into the subcapsular sinus. Lymph flows radially along reticular channels that exit at the node at the hilus via a single efferent lymphatic.

tures provide no clues, a simple work-up should be performed, including complete blood count, inspection of the blood smear, tuberculin skin testing, throat culture, and heterophile antibody studies. Observation with careful measurement of lymph node size in two dimensions, and possibly involving an empiric trial of antibiotic therapy, should persist no longer than 1 to 2 weeks, and a definite follow-up visit to the office or clinic should be scheduled. If nonerythematous, nonfluctuant lymph node enlargement persists or increases, excisional biopsy should be undertaken, selecting a node of the largest size and obtaining material for appropriate culture as well as for pathologic examination.

DIFFERENTIAL DIAGNOSIS

Table 35–1 lists causes of lymphadenopathy in children, practically all of which may be confused with malignant lymphoma, either clinically or pathologically, or in both respects. Excluded from the list is acute lymphadenitis, usually secondary to infection with *Staphylococcus aureus* or *Streptococcus*. This is a straightforward diagnosis, the management of which has been reviewed elsewhere (13, 14). Also excluded are congenital causes for neck masses, such as thyroglossal duct cysts, epidermoid cysts, branchial cleft cysts, or cystic hygromas. Recognition of these entities is based upon their characteristic anatomic features, and management consists of complete surgical excision (15, 16). Other conditions listed in Table 35–1 are discussed in more detail in the following sections and have been reviewed elsewhere (1, 17, 18).

Reactive hyperplasia of lymph nodes is exceedingly common in children. In two large retrospective series of children undergoing excisional biopsy of enlarged peripheral lymph nodes (19, 20), the single most frequent pathologic diagnosis recorded was nonspecific hyperplasia, accounting for approximately one half of all cases. Very likely, this high proportion of cases lacking a specific diagnosis could be reduced with improved serologic and microbiologic techniques. Careful follow-up of children with nondiagnostic reactive lymph node hyperplasia is necessary, since in two series significant and severe disease was ultimately provided in 17 and 25 per cent of the cases, respectively (19, 20).

Infectious mononucleosis may simulate lymphoma rather closely, producing generalized proliferation of lymphoid tissue throughout the entire body, especially the spleen and lymph nodes, along with an absolute lymphocytosis of many immature and highly abnormal-appearing lymphocytes. In the usual case, the clinical picture of lymphadenopathy, fever, pharyngitis, and malaise; the presence of atypical lymphocytosis; and the determination of a positive differential heterophile titer or positive Epstein-Barr virus titer provides an unequivocal diagnosis of infectious mononucleosis. Rarely, it may be more difficult to distinguish the lymphadenopathy of mononucleosis from that of lymphoma. In their review of 11 patients with mononucleosis subjected to lymph node biopsy because of persistence of adenopathy, weight loss, or increased fatigue, Salvador and co-workers stressed the importance of histologic recognition of the mixed cell proliferation seen in mononucleosis, with a prominent component of immunoblasts (21). These large cells (15 to 20 μ in diameter), with vesicular nuclei and one or two prominent nucleoli, may particularly be confused with mononuclear Hodgkin's cells or even classic Reed-Sternberg cells. Such cells may also occur in other viral-induced lymphdenopathies, such as postvaccinial lymphadenitis or herpes zoster adenitis. (See Chapter 52 for a more complete discussion of infectious mononucleosis.)

Sarcoidosis is quite rare in children and is diagnosed infrequently. Its presence is suggested by findings of a multisystem disease manifested primarily by bilateral cervical and hilar adenopathy, pulmonary parenchymal infiltrate, hepatosplenomegaly, and uveitis. Most childhood cases occur in blacks. Organ or node biopsy demonstrates characteristic noncaseating granuloma (22). Tuberculosis adenitis is becoming increasingly frequent among immigrant populations.

Exposure to hydantoin drugs, such as phenytoin, rarely may produce a benign pseudolymphoma, a hypersensitivity reaction characterized by lymphadenopathy, fever, skin rash, eosinophilia, and hepatosplenomegaly, which generally regresses upon drug withdrawal (23). There is also apparently a small excess risk of genuine malignant lymphoma as well (24, 25).

Castleman's disease (giant lymph node hyperplasia or angiomatous lymphoid hamartoma) is a

Table 35–1. CAUSES OF LYMPHADENOPATHY (1, 17, 18)

Nonspecific reactive hyperplasia
Infectious mononucleosis
Cat scratch disease
Secondary syphilis
Mycobacterial infection
Toxoplasmosis
Brucellosis
Histoplasmosis
Postvaccinial lymphadenitis
Rheumatoid arthritis, systemic lupus erythematosus
Autoimmune hemolytic anemia
Sarcoidosis (22)
Hyperthyroidism
Hydantoin hypersensitivity (23)
Sinus histiocytosis with massive lymphadenopathy (31)
Giant lymph node hyperplasia (Castleman's disease) (26)
Metastatic malignancy
Histiocytosis X
Storage diseases

poorly understood condition that has been inadequately studied. The nature of the lesion remains an enigma. It most resembles an enlarged, hyperplastic, somewhat altered lymph node, the median size of excised specimens being 6 cm, although specimens reaching 10 to 16 cm have been observed. Pathologically, two variants exist, either the hyaline-vascular or plasma-cell type (26). The most common anatomic location is the mediastinum, but such lesions may occur in other areas of the body where lymph nodes are found. Frequently systemic manifestations are present, and case reports in the pediatric literature have described the occurrence of fever, anemia, hyperglobulinemia, and altered hemostasis (27–30). Treatment consists of surgical excision.

Sinus histiocytosis with massive lymphadenopathy is a benign condition, the true frequency of which is unknown. Reported cases have commonly been in black children and have been characterized by painless cervical lymphadenopathy of massive proportions, fever, leukocytosis, and hypergammaglobulinemia (31). The disease regresses spontaneously after a protracted course. The histologic picture of excised nodes is distinctive, revealing dilated lymph node sinuses filled with histiocytes; the cytoplasm of many of the histiocytes is distended by lymphocytes exhibiting apparent emperipolesis. The etiology of sinus histiocytosis is obscure.

Histiocytosis X will be dealt with in greater detail in Chapter 36 but is mentioned in this context because it must be included in the differential diagnosis of lymphadenopathy in the child. Williams and Dorfman have recently reviewed the features of lymph nodes biopsied in histiocytosis X (32).

Mediastinal Masses

The differential diagnosis of mediastinal masses in children is enhanced by consideration of the age of the child, presenting symptoms, and the site of the mass on lateral chest roentgenography, i.e., whether located anteriorly, posteriorly, or in the middle. Performance of a barium swallow to outline the esophagus in relation to the mass may also facilitate diagnosis. Table 35–2 lists the differential diagnosis of mediastinal masses according to location within the mediastinum (33). Note that for practical purposes the posterior paravertebral sulci are included as part of the posterior mediastinum, since neurogenic tumors arising from the paravertebral sympathetic nerve trunks typically grow forward. Occasionally they may grow backward as well, in dumbbell fashion, extending through an intervertebral foramen.

The thymus may be the site of a variety of tumors, both benign and malignant, including thymic cysts, lymphomas, germinomas, and carcinoid tumors, as well as true thymomas, i.e., neoplasms of thymic epithelial cells. Thymomas are exceedingly rare in childhood (34, 35) and often present clinicopathologic difficulties in diagnosis. Histologically, thymomas are composed of malignant epithelial cells, admixed in varying proportions with T lymphocytes. The morphology of the epithelial cell component may vary from round cells to ovoid or spindle-shaped cells. Ultrastructural examination of the tumor and demonstration of tonofilaments inserting into desmosomes of the neoplastic epithelial cells may be extremely helpful in confirming the diagnosis. Thymomas may be either grossly encapsulated or invasive, involving the pleura, mediastinal nodes, lungs, trachea, or esophagus and commonly producing the superior vena cava syndrome. Distant metastases are rare. A systemic illness may precede the appearance of or coexist with thymoma, the three most commonly associated conditions being myasthenia gravis, red cell hypoplasia and hypogammaglobulinemia. The treatment of choice of thymomas is total surgical excision, followed postoperatively by radiotherapy (4000 cGy) if the tumor is infiltrative.

The finding of a mediastinal mass in a child is a matter of grave concern, which may require different forms of surgical and nonsurgical intervention. A systematic approach is necessary, with close cooperation between oncologist, surgeon, radiologist, and anesthesiologist, as these children may present special problems related to compression of the trachea, induction of anesthesia, and other potential pitfalls associated with the institution of empiric therapy (36). In two reports of large series of mediastinal masses in infants and children, roughly half of the cases were malignant (37, 38).

Table 35–2. DIFFERENTIAL DIAGNOSIS OF MEDIASTINAL MASSES*

Anterior	Middle	Posterior
Thymic enlargement	Lymphoma	Neurogenic tumors
Thymoma	Lymphadenitis (Tbc, sarcoid, histoplasmosis)	Duplications of the foregut
Lymphoma		Bronchogenic cysts
Lymphangioma		Anterior meningoceles
Teratoma		Diaphragmatic hernia (foramen of Bochdalek)
Diaphragmatic hernia (foramen of Morgagni)		

*Modified from Hope, J. W., and Koop, C. E.: Pediatr. Clin. North Am. 6:379, 1959.

NON-HODGKIN'S LYMPHOMA

Definition

Non-Hodgkin's lymphoma (NHL) is the term used to refer to all malignant lymphomas other than those definable as Hodgkin's disease. The rubric thus covers an array of heterogeneous neoplasms arising from a great many different primary sites and displaying a variable immunohistopathologic picture and clinical course in children. Included in this category are such diverse diagnostic terms as lymphoblastic lymphosarcoma, reticulum cell sarcoma, histiocytic lymphoma, and undifferentiated lymphomas, both the Burkitt and non-Burkitt type.

Immunohistopathology and Classification

CELLULAR LYMPHOID ORIGINS

Prior to the advent of modern immunologic methods for identification of lymphoid cells, Rappaport proposed a comprehensive classification system based entirely on morphology (39). Although many clinical studies have since confirmed the clinical relevance of the Rappaport classification in adult NHL, the same has not been found in series of childhood cases (40, 41). Furthermore, acquisition of modern data permitted development of functional immunologic classification schemes for lymphoma, based on T and B cell lineages and morphologic alterations associated with lymphocyte transformation and activation (4, 5, 42). Indeed, during the decade of the 1970's, a glut of lymphoma classification schemes appeared in the literature, several of which have been conceptually analyzed by Nathwani (43). The diversity of classification schemes and crises in nosology led to the international, multi-institutional clinicopathologic study of 1175 cases of NHL, each case classified by a panel of experts according to six different schemes, with clinical correlates (44). The resulting Working Formulation recognizes 10 major categories of NHL and a number of minor miscellaneous types. The clinical usefulness of the Working Formulation, other than as a means of classifying equivalent or related terms of histologic types of NHL, has not been evaluated in childhood NHL.

Fortunately for the pediatrician, the array of lymphomas commonly seen in children is more limited than that in adults, because more than 95 per cent of cases are diffuse, histologically high-grade tumors. Nodular or follicular lymphomas derived from germinal center cell origin are rare in children, accounting for only 2.5 per cent of cases (45). The major recognizable immunopathologic subtypes of non-Hodgkin's lymphoma observed in childhood are listed in Table 35-3 and are illustrated in Figures 35-3, 35-4, and 35-5. Most cases of childhood NHL are clearly of either T or B cell origin (41, 49, 50). Furthermore, although there may be considerable heterogeneity in expression of immune markers and certain exceptions, broad correlations exist between histologic class and phenotype, the cytology often being predictive of the cellular origin of the lymphoma (41, 51). Considering further information regarding the primary anatomic site of tumor in relation to the anatomy of the immune system, the correlations become even more evident. Bernard and co-workers (50), in their survey of the pattern of reactivity of lymphoma cells from 116 children with a battery of immunologic markers, observed that all children with primary mediastinal (thymic) tumors had T cell (lymphoblastic) lymphomas. By contrast, 44 of the 45 children with abdominal tumors (of gut-associated lymphoid tissues) had B cell (SIg+) lymphomas. The level of differentiation achieved by the T or B tumor cells of childhood NHLs in general is not far removed from that seen with lymphocytic progenitor cells (5), in contrast to most of the lymphomas seen in adult years, which are the neoplastic counterparts of more mature, immunocompetent lymphoid cells.

NHL is clonal in origin, a conclusion based on a variety of lines of evidence, including the display of the exclusive presence of only one immunoglobulin light chain type (κ or λ) and a unique idiotype of the surface immunoglobulin of B cell tumors, by demonstration of clonal karyotypic markers, and by study of tumors from G6PD heterozygotes (5). Recently, the study of DNA rearrangements of immunoglobulin genes within lymphomas has provided an additional sensitive marker for both clonality and B cell lineage (52). Demonstration of clonality in T cell lymphomas

Table 35-3. CLASSIFICATION OF CHILDHOOD NHL (46, 47, 48)

Histologic Type	Immunophenotype	Approximate Frequency of Cases
Lymphoblastic	Usually T, rarely pre-B or non-T, non-B	30–35%
Undifferentiated* (small non-cleaved cell) Burkitt and non-Burkitt pleomorphic	B	40–50%
Large cell* Immunoblastic	Usually B, rarely non-T, non-B or post-thymic T, or more rarely of phagocytic origin	20–25%

Editor's Note: The undifferentiated and large cell types are often referred to as "nonlymphoblastic lymphomas." This leads to the use of the term "nonlymphoblastic non-Hodgkin's lymphoma." Since some of these tumors are of phagocytic origin, they are also "non-lymphomas," a triple negative that could only be invented by groups of oncologists in full cry.

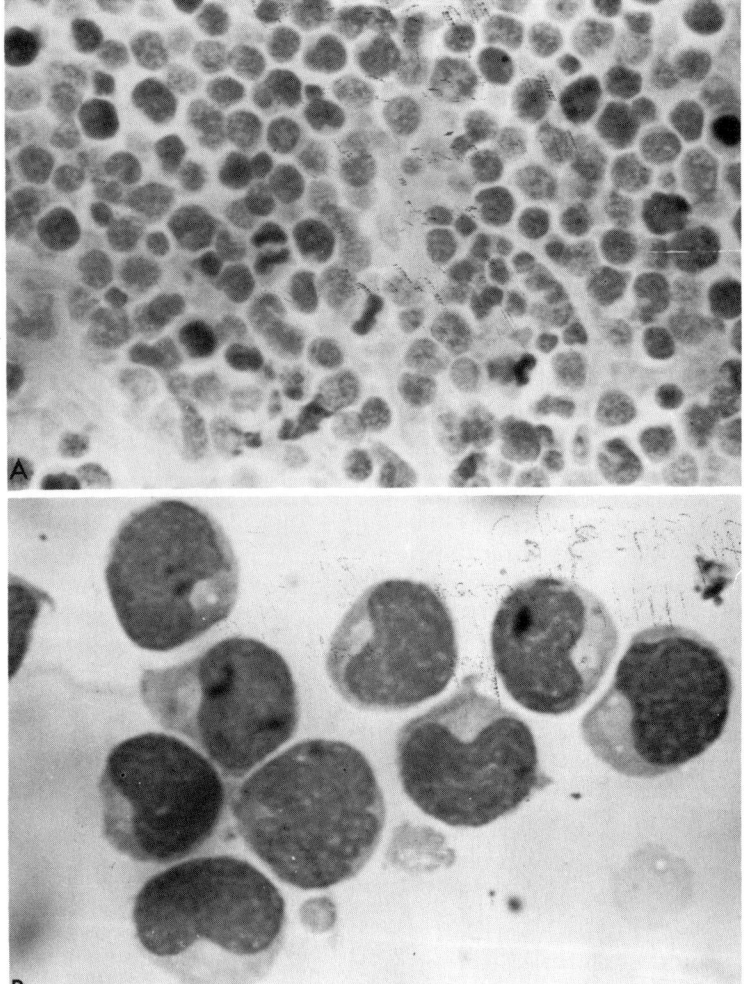

Figure 35–3. Non-Hodgkin's lymphoma, lymphoblastic type. *A*, Cervical lymph node biopsy specimen from a 3-year-old white boy with a mediastinal mass, showing replacement by lymphoid cells exhibiting fine chromatin, scanty cytoplasm, and a high mitotic index (hematoxylin-eosin, ×400). *B*, Cytocentrifuged specimen of lymphoblasts from the cerebrospinal fluid of the same patient, exhibiting nuclear infolding (Wright's stain, ×1000). Thirty per cent of these lymphoblasts formed spontaneous rosettes with sheep red cells at 37°C, a characteristic of normal thymocytes and T lymphoblasts.

rests mainly on demonstration of a predominant cell type that phenotypically closely resembles a normal cell in the T cell differentiation sequence (53, 54), although the availability of molecular probes hybridizing to specific T cell genes (e.g., to the T antigen receptor) would establish conclusively the unique monoclonal nature of individual tumors.

Prior to a further discussion of the common pathologic types of childhood NHL, it is necessary to make some general comments about proper techniques for conclusively establishing the diagnosis and further subclassification of lymphoma. The importance of proper specimen handling and good communication between the pediatrician, oncologist, surgeon, and pathologist can scarcely be overemphasized. The lymph node or tumor specimen should be delivered to the pathologist intact and freshly after removal, and, *Prior to fixation*, it should be divided into multiple samples for cytochemical, immunologic, and additional other studies to complement and correlate with the histopathologic interpretation of the case. If the special expertise in performance and interpretation of these studies is not available locally, there should be consideration of immediate referral of the child *prior to biopsy* or dispatch of the fresh (or freshly frozen) specimen to a reference laboratory.

The identification of cell markers in lymphoma and proper subclassification is more than an academic exercise, as the information obtained has significant implications for the accuracy of diagnosis, for predicting clinical characteristics, and for proper selection of therapy (48). Detection of immunologic markers of T or B cell origin on tumor cells from a child with a small round cell tumor can furthermore also be extraordinarily helpful in conclusively establishing the diagnosis of lymphoma and excluding neuroblastoma, rhabdomyosarcoma, or Ewing's sarcoma (55).

LYMPHOBLASTIC LYMPHOMAS

Lymphoblastic lymphomas of childhood are cytologically indistinguishable from acute lymphoblastic leukemia (ALL) (156) (see Figure 35–3). These lymphomas have previously been classified as poorly differentiated lymphocytic tumors but are now recognized as constituting a distinct clinicopathologic entity (40, 56, 57). The presence of nuclear convolutions is a characteristic, but not invariable, feature of the tumor cells, which are recognizable by their fine nuclear chromatin, inconspicuous nucleoli, and minimal cytoplasm. Mitoses are usually frequent, and a "starry-sky" appearance of sectioned tissue may be present but is generally not striking. The immunophenotype of the majority of cases of lymphoblastic lymphoma in children corresponds to that of cortical thymocytes, predominantly at mid- or later stages of thymic differentiation, i.e., the tumor cells form rosettes with sheep erythrocytes and express a variety of either pan-T or thymocyte surface antigens (OKT3+, T6+, T4+, T8+) (49, 54, 58, 59, 59a). The tumor cells are further distinguished by strong, focally positive acid phosphatase reactivity. It has also been recognized recently that elevated levels of the enzyme terminal deoxynucleotidyl transferase are also characteristic of lymphoblastic lymphomas and thus may provide a useful biochemical marker (61, 62).

Lymphoblastic lymphomas are associated with the presence of an anterior mediastinal mass in the majority of cases, frequent cervical and supraclavicular adenopathy, and notable absence of primary involvement of the gastrointestinal tract or abdominal lymph nodes (56, 57). A high frequency of leukemic evolution and central nervous system involvement has likewise been noted. The overlap in many of the clinical and biologic characteristics of lymphoblastic lymphomas of T cell origin in children with cases of T cell acute lymphoblastic leukemia (58, 59) naturally leads to the not illogical supposition that the leukemic cases merely represent the natural evolution of lymphoma and that the differences between T-NHL and T-ALL are merely related to the degree of disease dissemination present at diagnosis. Although this certainly must be true in some cases of T-ALL, it may not

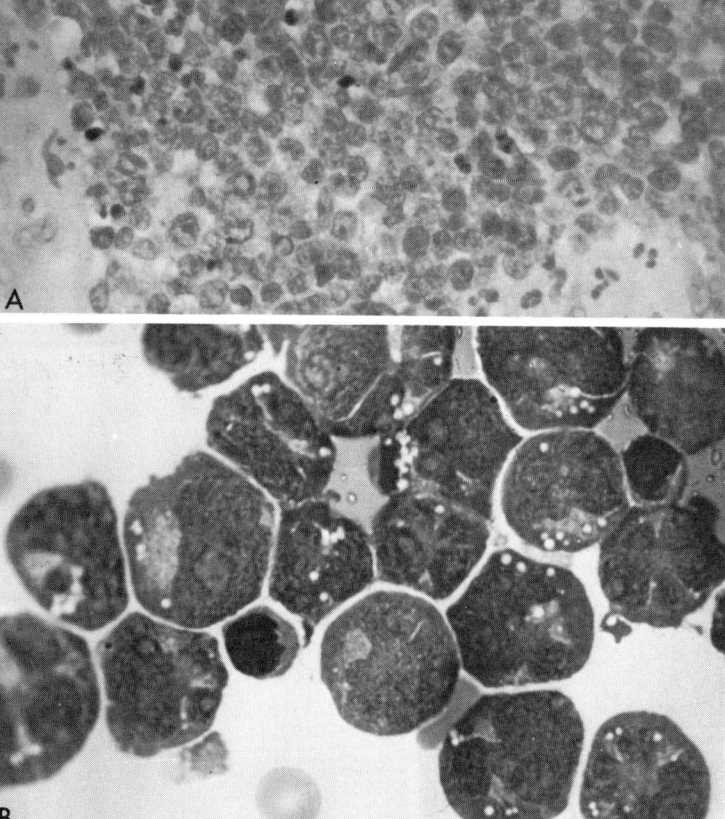

Figure 35–4. Non-Hodgkin's lymphoma, Burkitt's type. *A*, Gingival biopsy specimen from a 10-year-old white boy, showing a uniform tumor cell population with normal phagocytic histiocytes interspersed (hematoxylin-eosin, ×400). *B*, A cytocentrifuged specimen of pleural fluid blast cells from the same patient, which exhibits vacuolated blasts with basophilic systems (Wright's stain, ×1000). Seventy-three per cent of these pleural fluid blasts were positive for surface immunoglobulins by direct immunofluorescence.

be universally true, as there are many cases of T-ALL, for instance, lacking mediastinal masses.

A minority of the lymphoblastic lymphomas that have been studied are non-T, and instead express the common acute lymphoblastic leukemia antigen (cALLa) and are Ia-positive (63). In two reports, these cases have been associated with cutaneous lymphomas in young children (50, 64).

UNDIFFERENTIATED LYMPHOMA, BURKITT'S TYPE

Burkitt's lymphoma (BL) is named for Denis Burkitt, a British surgeon working in Uganda, who first described the tumor more than two decades ago (65). While particularly common in certain endemic areas such as tropical Africa and New Guinea, where it is seen in association with holoendemic malaria, it is now recognized that BL has a worldwide distribution. The chief difference between endemic and nonendemic forms of BL rests in the association with the Epstein-Barr virus (EBV). The vast majority of African cases studied have arisen from a neoplastic clone of EBV-carrying B cells, whereas the tumor cells from nonendemic cases are EBV-negative. Comparisons of established BL cell lines show a much lower level of expression of surface receptors for EBV by EBV-negative lines than by EBV-positive lines, perhaps accounting for the infrequent association of the virus with American cases (66). The epidemiologic, immunologic, etiologic, and clinical features of BL have recently been extensively reviewed (67).

The gross anatomic pathology and histologic, histochemical, and cytologic criteria for the diagnosis of BL have been defined in detail in a memorandum from the World Health Organization (68). Anatomically, there is prominent extranodal involvement, particularly of the gastrointestinal tract and other abdominal, retroperitoneal, and pelvic viscera, kidneys, gonads, jaws, thyroid gland, and central nervous system. The tumor is composed of primitive, so-called "undifferentiated," small, round, noncleaved lymphoid cells (Fig. 35–4A). A "starry-sky" appearance is invariably and characteristically found in tumor sec-

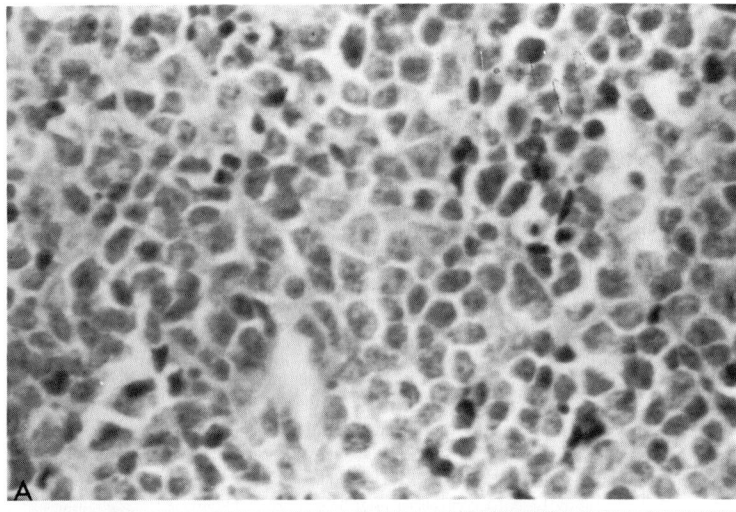
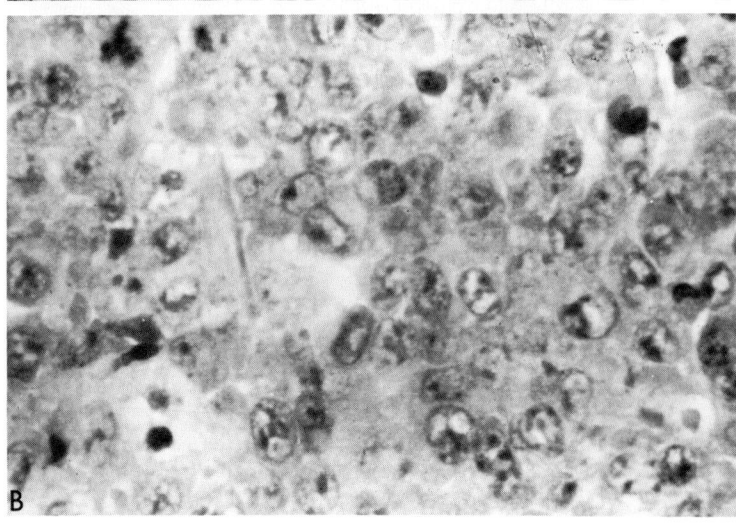

Figure 35–5. Non-Hodgkin's lymphoma, histiocytic or large lymphoid cell type. *A*, Biopsy specimen of a retroperitoneal presacral mass from a 4-year-old boy. The tumor cells are nonuniform and possess moderately abundant methyl-green-pyronine-positive cytoplasm (hematoxylin-eosin, ×400). Sixty per cent of blast cells from pleural fluid from this patient were positive for surface immunoglobulins by direct immunofluorescence, indicating that these large tumor cells are of lymphoid origin. *B*, Axillary lymph node biopsy specimen from an 11-year-old boy with isolated adenopathy. Specimen classified as histiocytic, diffuse, according to Rappaport's scheme, by light microscopic appearance (hematoxylin-eosin, ×400).

tions, owing to the presence of uniformly scattered macrophages laden with cellular debris. A histopathologic distinction between undifferentiated lymphomas of Burkitt's type and those of non-Burkitt's type has been made based on the degree of variation in the size and shape of the nuclei of the malignant cells, the non-Burkitt's type of diffuse undifferentiated tumor exhibiting a greater degree of pleomorphism (47). From a practical standpoint, however, the further subclassification of childhood diffuse undifferentiated lymphomas into Burkitt's and non-Burkitt's pleomorphic types is often subtle, largely subjective, and poorly reproducible (48), and furthermore appears intuitively illogical and artificial, in view of the considerable overlap in morphologic, immunologic, and clinical features (69).

Immunologic studies of BL reveal a B cell origin, the tumor cells typically displaying high-density surface IgM, corresponding either to an immature B lymphocyte precursor or a transformed B lymphocyte (70, 71). Monoclonal immunoglobulin bands are detectable in the serum of some patients, particularly those with extensive tumor (72). There is a direct relationship between the expression of immunoglobulin-chains in Burkitt lymphoma cells and the type of specific chromosomal translocation present (73). Burkitt tumor cells characteristically have one of three specific reciprocal chromosomal translocations, t(8;14), t(2;8) or t(8;22), involving the chromosomes known to carry the genes for immunoglobulin heavy chains, κ and λ light chains, respectively. Whereas tumor cells with the t(8;14) bear surface μ with either κ or λ light chains, BL cells bearing the t(8;22) exclusively express surface λ chains, and those with t(2;8) express κ.

A frankly leukemic blood picture is rare in BL, although bone marrow involvement by tumor cells occurs not infrequently, particularly with extensive or progressive disease. In biopsy material treated with Wright's stain, the cytomorphology of the tumor cells closely conforms to the L3-(FAB) type of acute lymphoblastic leukemia (74–76), the cells exhibiting a moderate amount of deeply basophilic cytoplasm typically containing a number of clear vacuoles (Fig. 35–4B). The relationship of Burkitt's lymphoma with marrow involvement to acute B cell leukemia with bulky extramedullary disease has been extensively reviewed (75, 76). It seems clear that in children the two conditions are generally indistinguishable.

LARGE CELL OR "HISTIOCYTIC" LYMPHOMAS

The pathologic subgroup of NHL that was termed histiocytic according to Rappaport's original classification and termed reticulum cell sarcoma, large cleaved or noncleaved follicular center cell lymphomas, and centroblastic or immunoblastic lymphoma in other classification schemes is now known to be derived from large lymphoid cells. Histologically, the tumors are composed of large cells with vesicular nuclei, prominent nucleoli, and moderately abundant cytoplasm (see Figure 33–5). A battery of cytochemistry tests and immunologic investigations appear necessary in order to achieve distinctions between the various large cell lymphomas. Such studies have shown that few of the tumors are indeed "histiocytic," i.e., few are composed of mononuclear phagocytic cells of the monocyte-macrophage series. A better term for them might be phagocytic rather than histiocytic. The majority are B cell–derived, as evidenced by surface immunoglobulins, but a minority bear T cell markers, and some are devoid of surface markers (4, 77–79). In their review of a series of 31 cases of childhood lymphomas, Murphy and co-workers reclassified 9 of 12 histiocytic lymphomas as "large basophilic cell" on the basis of well-delimited, strongly basophilic and pyroninophilic cytoplasm; large nucleoli; and clumped chromatin. Almost without exception, such lymphomas arose in gut-associated lymphoid tissue, namely tonsils, adenoids, or Peyer's patches (40). A minority of large-cell lymphomas in children involve the skin, mediastinum, bone, and other sites.

Clinical Presentations

The clinical presentation of childhood NHL may be extremely varied, depending upon the dominant anatomic site or sites involved and the extent of disease. Virtually any lymphatic tissue of the body may be involved, including lymph nodes, spleen, Peyer's patches, tonsils, and thymus. Disseminated NHL that is noncontiguous, particularly disease involving the central nervous system and bone marrow, is extremely common. In some cases it is impossible to specify exactly the primary site of the tumor, owing to its extensive, apparently multifocal distribution from the onset. In a large series of 102 children, Jenkin reported a typical distribution of anatomic sites involved at diagnosis: 23 per cent of cases presented with massive anterior mediastinal disease; 20 per cent with nodal involvement in one or more regions, with or without liver and spleen involvement; 22 per cent with primary involvement of the gastrointestinal tract; 18 per cent with extensive intra-abdominal disease of uncertain origin; 11 per cent with the apparent primary site in Waldeyer's ring or the jaw; and 6 per cent with other primary sites, such as bone, breast, skin, or gonads, or with mixed presentations (80).

Painless peripheral lymph node enlargement, usually cervical, is the most common clinical presentation. Cervical lymphadenopathy may be solitary or a reflection of regional disease, in association with a tumor of either the head or neck or the mediastinum. NHL of the head and neck may primarily involve the sinuses, jaws, orbit, nasopharynx, tonsils, or adenoids and is often initially misdiagnosed as a comparatively trivial pediatric complaint, such as tonsillitis with peritonsillar abscess, serous otitis, or a dental problem. Mediastinal tumors are usually associated with upper torso adenopathy. When massive mediastinal tumors are present, stridor, dyspnea, a brassy cough, and venous engorgement and edema of the upper half of the body constitute a medical emergency and are an indication for immediate therapy to relieve the respiratory embarrassment (36).

Abdominal NHL in children typically is associated with abdominal pain and a palpable mass. Vomiting, weight loss, and ascites may also be present. Tumors localized to the gastrointestinal tract generally involve the distal ileum, cecum, and mesenteric nodes and often produce intussusception. Retroperitoneal and renal involvement is commonly greater than appreciated clinically.

The usual interval of symptoms prior to the diagnosis of childhood NHL is brief, less than 4 to 6 weeks. Some children are desperately ill, having rapidly progressive widespread disease within 1 to 2 weeks of their first symptoms.

Laboratory Findings

In the usual case of childhood NHL, the laboratory findings are entirely normal, with the possible exception of an elevation in the serum levels of lactic dehydrogenase and uric acid. Both are elevated because of the often high rate of cell proliferation and the spontaneous tumor cell lysis and necrosis present. The level of the lactic dehydrogenase, in fact, is correlated roughly with the bulk of the tumor burden, and levels exceeding 1000 IU per ml are not uncommonly observed in patients with massive abdominal disease (81).

Peripheral blood findings are unremarkable in the absence of bone marrow involvement by tumor. A typical leukemic blood and bone marrow picture is found when tumor cells disseminate to widely replace normal marrow elements.

Staging

An expeditious investigation should be carried out in the child newly diagnosed as having NHL in order to determine the anatomic extent of disease and the degree of organ impairment or biochemical disturbance present. Every child should have, as a minimum, a complete blood count, including platelet enumeration; tests of renal and liver function; a chest roentgenogram, skeletal survey, or radionuclide bone scan; a bone marrow aspiration; and a lumbar puncture with examination of a cytocentrifuged specimen of spinal fluid. In the author's experience, performance of a bone marrow biopsy practically never reveals marrow involvement by tumor that is not already apparent from an inspection of the smeared aspirate (82).

A variety of other roentgenographic and imaging techniques are useful to demonstrate areas of tumor involvement. These studies include excretory urography, barium studies of the gastrointestinal tract, lateral soft tissue views of the nasopharynx, Panorex views of the mandible and maxilla, lymphangiography, myelography, bone scanning, whole-body gallium scanning, and whole body computed tomography. Typical results of such studies in children with NHL have been reported (83, 84). Disease is seldom demonstrated on such investigations that was not already suspected clinically, except for the occasional otherwise occult finding of nephromegaly or hydronephrosis and hydroureter from retroperitoneal or pelvic disease. Lymphangiography is of considerably more limited usefulness in childhood NHL than in HD, and the procedure should not be done routinely in staging children with NHL. Certainly its performance contributes nothing other than increased hazard to the management of children with primary mediastinal NHL. In other circumstances, the yield of lymphangiography in children with NHL appears low. In the author's experience, no positive lymphangiograms have been found in 10 children with clinically localized supradiaphragmatic disease outside the mediastinum. Jaffe and coworkers also reported negative lymphangiographic studies in seven children with NHL, three with apparent localized tonsillar disease, three with disseminated disease, and one with positive inguinal nodal disease (85). The effectiveness of computed tomography for the accurate delineation of tumor extent, for treatment planning, and for monitoring response in lymphoma patients has been established (86–88). The technique is particularly useful for imaging tumor in the head and neck, mediastinum, and/or abdominal and pelvic viscera.

Laparotomy and splenectomy for staging childhood NHL are not indicated, although many children with abdominal lymphomas undergo exploratory laparotomy for diagnosis, biopsy, relief of intestinal obstruction, and partial or complete excision of abdominal tumor. For children with tumor localized to the gastrointestinal tract, complete excision of the tumor, along with the distal ileum, cecum, appendix, and a portion of the ascending colon and associated mesentery, and performance of an ileocolonic reanastomosis are the generally preferred procedure, when surgically feasible. When only biopsy or incomplete surgical excision of abdominal lymphoma is possible in a child, the prognosis is not as favorable (89–92). Failure to achieve complete excision of abdominal tumor in unfavorable cases is due to the extension of tumor to para-aortic and retroperitoneal tissues, mesentery, and omentum and to the associated malignant ascites.

The Ann Arbor system for staging HD (see Table 35–9) is not well suited for use in NHL, even though it has been used widely for that purpose. Reasons for the lack of suitability of the Ann Arbor system for NHL have been discussed in detail elsewhere (93) and include the diversity of NHL, the frequency of advanced disease in lymphocytic pathologic subgroups, and the great rarity of genuine Stage III disease in childhood. Furthermore, mediastinal NHL would be classified as Stage I or II in the Ann Arbor system; it is, in fact, a form of disease known to confer a poor prognosis and to be associated with a great tendency for leukemic evolution and involvement of the central nervous system.

An alternative clinical staging system for childhood NHL is shown in Table 35–4. The system is based upon a recognition of the typical patterns of disease presentation and extent and an appreciation of the relapse hazard (93). When combined with information regarding the primary site of tumor and immunohistopathologic subtype of disease, the system has great utility in enhancing the clear communication of end results of clinical trials and in developing strategies for planning therapy. When compared with other alternative staging classifications for children with NHL (92, 94, 95), similarities emerge in the common recognition of the good prognosis conferred by grossly complete excision of all abdominal tumor and the determination of Stage IV disease on the basis of involvement of the central nervous system or marrow, or both, at the time of diagnosis. The system shown in Table 35–4 and others like it have powerful prognostic utility, the end results of treatment of children with localized Stage I and II disease being statistically significantly far superior to results in children with more advanced Stage III and Stage IV disease, as outlined in Table 35–5 (91–105).

The clinical importance of distinguishing between partial (< 25 per cent) or complete marrow replacement by blasts, i.e., between Stage IV lymphoma or "leukemia," is debatable (5, 75, 95). Admittedly the distinction is often merely semantic or taxonomic, not resting on a biologic basis. Depending on the treatment, the distinction between Stage IV lymphoma and a frankly leukemic picture (termed IVB, by Wollner) may have no clinical prognostic significance either (95, 106). There is little doubt, however, that bone marrow involvement per se confers a worse prognosis, compared with cases in which there is no marrow involvement (92, 94, 98). The presence of initial CNS disease is particularly ominous.

Table 35–4. A STAGING SYSTEM FOR CHILDHOOD NHL

Stage I
A single tumor (extranodal) or single anatomic area (nodal), with the exclusion of mediastinum or abdomen.

Stage II
A single tumor (extranodal) with regional node involvement.
Two or more nodal areas on the same side of the diaphragm.
Two single (extranodal) tumors with or without regional node involvement on the same side of the diaphragm.
A primary gastrointestinal tract tumor, usually in the ileocecal area, with or without involvement of associated mesenteric nodes only, grossly completely excised.*

Stage III
Two single tumors (extranodal) on opposite sides of the diaphragm.
Two or more nodal areas above and below the diaphragm.
All the primary intrathoracic tumors (mediastinal, pleural, thymic).
All extensive primary intra-abdominal disease.*
All paraspinal or epidural tumors, regardless of other tumor site(s).

Stage IV
Any of the above with initial CNS and/or bone marrow involvement.†

*A distinction is made between apparently localized GI tract lymphoma versus more extensive intra-abdominal disease, because of their quite different pattern of survival after appropriate therapy. Stage II disease typically is limited to a segment of the gut plus or minus the associated mesenteric nodes only, and the primary tumor must be completely removed grossly by segmental excision. Stage III disease typically exhibits spread to para-aortic and retroperitoneal areas by implants and plaques in mesentery or peritoneum, or by direct infiltration of structures adjacent to the primary tumor. Ascites may be present, and complete resection of all gross tumor is not possible.
†If marrow involvement is present initially, the number of abnormal cells must be 25% or less in an *otherwise* normal marrow aspirate with a normal peripheral blood picture.

Treatment and Results of Modern Therapy

The majority of children with NHL are curable with modern treatment (Table 35–5). Hence, the goal of therapy must be prompt attainment and maintenance of a complete remission, the aim being cure, not palliation. Since appropriate treatment planning properly requires precise determination of the immunohistopathologic type, and extent of disease and management entails the use of multiple modalities requiring considerable expertise, the chance for cure of a child with NHL is likely to be significantly enhanced by initial referral to a comprehensive tertiary care center.

All children with NHL should be treated systemically with multiple-drug combination chemotherapy because of the high likelihood of disseminated disease, even with clinically localized presentations. Current regimens use high-dose cyclophosphamide, adriamycin, moderate-to-high dose methotrexate, vincristine, and prednisone, as well as other agents, in continuous or cyclic fashion for periods from 2 to 3 years from the time of diagnosis. Regimens of chemotherapy in current use (Table 35–5) vary extensively in drug dose and scheduling, in toxicity, and in efficacy.

Radiotherapy has occupied a traditional role in management of childhood NHL, since it has demonstrated that radiation is capable of curing a fraction of patients with clinically localized, favorable presentations of disease (107). However, no child, no matter how favorable the presentation, should be managed with radiation therapy alone because of the notorious tendency for recurrence of disease outside the irradiated fields, leading to death. Combined-modality approaches to management of childhood NHL, which include the majority of those outlined in Table 35–5, have led to significant improvements in survival (94–105). In such regimens, radiation is delivered to clinically localized bulky tumor masses, with curative intent in the early stages of disease, and to areas of bulky tumor involvement in the more advanced stages. The volume, dose, and timing of the radiotherapy are adjusted, depending on the intensity of the chemotherapeutic regimen employed. Elective irradiation of areas uninvolved by tumor is not carried out, although the whole abdomen is treated in children with abdominal disease.

The actual contribution that radiation therapy makes to the success of intensive combined-modality regimens is controversial, and current trends are in the direction of reduced doses or deletion of involved field radiotherapy altogether. Treatment failure is seldom due to lack of local control of tumor, but more typically is the result of generalized relapse of disease. Results of irradiation of mediastinal NHL, in particular, fail to support the continued role for involved-field radiation therapy in a combined-modality approach. Rather, such results suggest that treatment should be with multiple drugs alone, much as treatment for "high-risk" acute lymphoblastic leukemia (108–110). Ziegler employed whole-abdomen radiation (2100 cGy) as a form of consolidation following initial intensive chemotherapy of intra-abdominal American Burkitt's lymphoma, but was unable to conclude that such treatment was actually indicated, particularly in view of the acute toxicity produced (91). In a randomized trial in children, Murphy and Hustu observed no significant improvement in complete remission frequency or survival when involved-field radiotherapy (3000 to 3500 cGy) was combined with four-drug induction therapy for advanced stages, compared with the same multiple drug treatment alone (99). Similarly, Sullivan and co-workers from the Pediatric Oncology Group could demonstrate no therapeutic role for radiation in a group of 107 children with non-Burkitt's NHL, roughly half of whom received involved field radiation in a nonrandomized fashion, while all received 10-drug LSA_2-L_2 therapy (98). Mott and colleagues in the United Kingdom tested the role of radiation (1500 cGy as consolidation to areas of bulky disease) in children with Stages II to IV NHL in a randomized trial and found no benefit whatsoever (104). When used in combined modality approaches with multiple drugs, concomitant radiation treatment unquestionably increases the frequency and severity of toxic side effects like mucositis, pneumonitis, cardiomyopathy, neutropenia, and weight loss, particularly when combined with certain drugs such as Adriamycin or Bleomycin.

A rational strategy for treatment of the child newly diagnosed with NHL can be based upon a consideration of the site of the primary tumor, the extent of disease (or stage), and the immunohistopathologic classification (111). After expeditious staging (see above), the child with a good prognosis with localized disease (Stages I and II) can readily be recognized. Jenkin and co-workers have recently reported only one treatment failure out of 32 children with nonlymphoblastic lymphomas who were treated with a 4-drug regimen (cyclophosphamide, vincristine, methotrexate, prednisone [COMP]) (97). Similarly, Hvizdala recently reported a 98 per cent disease-free survival rate (46/47) for children with Stage I and II lymphomas who were treated with an alternative 4-drug (ACOP+) regimen of Adriamycin, cyclophosphamide, vincristine and prednisone (98a). Since 9 out of 10 such children can be cured with modern treatment (Table 35–5) (96, 97, 98a), there is consequently a greater degree of concern regarding the acute and long-term adverse consequences of intensive combined modality therapy. Present approaches to management include consideration of a lowered dose or elimination of involved field radiation therapy, reduction of the number of agents and drug dosages, and shortening of the overall duration of treatment. Recently Link and co-workers have shown the feasibility of treating children with Stage I and II disease with a chemotherapy regimen of 6 months duration (112). Prophylactic treatment of the central nervous system does not appear indicated for children whose localized tumors are outside the region of the head and neck or for those with Stage II localized and completely resected gastrointestinal tract tumors, as the risk of primary relapse within the central nervous system is remote for these children.

Optimal therapy for children with Stage III–IV disease requires further subclassification according to the primary site of tumor and histopathologic subtype of disease, as it has commonly been observed that the response of patients with lymphoblastic tumors differs significantly from that of children with nonlymphoblastic lymphomas when treated with the same treatment regimen. This has

Table 35-5. RESULTS OF MODERN TREATMENT OF CHILDHOOD NHL*

Source	Number of Patients	Complete Remission Rate	Percentage of Patients with 2-Year Disease-Free Survival				Therapy	Reference(s)
			Overall	Localized I–II	Nonlocalized III–IV			
Children's Cancer Study Group	234	Not stated	60%	84%		47%	Two-arm, randomized, LSA_2-L_2 vs. COMP, plus IF RT (2000–3000 cGy)[a]	94
Pediatric Oncology Group	107[b]	85%	66%	100%	67%	57%	39%	LSA_2-L_2 ± IF RT (3000 cGy)	98
Memorial Sloan-Kettering Cancer Center	135	95%	75%	90%		75%	65%	LSA_2-L_2, plus IF RT (2000 cGy)	95, 106
St. Jude Children's Research Hospital	69	88%	55%	90%		40%		Cyclophosphamide, vincristine, prednisone ± Adriamycin, mercaptopurine & methotrexate, ± IF RT (3000–3500 cGy) ± CrRT + IT MTX	99
National Cancer Institute, Pediatric Branch	65[c]	89%	60%	86%		64%	20%	Cyclophosphamide, Adriamycin, vincristine & prednisone cycles, alternating with HDMTX plus IT MTX & ara-C	92
Dana-Farber Cancer Center	32	90%	67%	Not stated		Not stated		APO, plus L-asparaginase and IF RT (3500–4000 cGy) and CrRT	102, 103
Multi-Institutional West German (BFM) Group	116	Not stated	61%	Not stated		Not stated		Prednisone, vincristine, daunomycin, L-asparaginase, cytarabine, methotrexate, mercaptopurine, CrRT	100
Institut Gustave-Roussy, Villejuif, France	204	91%	44%	Not stated		Not stated		COPAD	101
United Kingdom Children's Cancer Study Group	104	Not stated	59%	100%	81%	51%	54%	Cyclophosphamide, Adriamycin, vincristine, prednisone, cytarabine, thioguanine, L-asparaginase, CCNU, VM-26, methotrexate, plus IT MTX ± IF RT (1500 cGy)	104
Istituto Nazionale Tumori, Milan	79	97%	61%	87%[d] 100%[e]	73.9%[e]	38%[d] 48%[e]	16%[d] 0%[e]	Cyclophosphamide, Adriamycin, Vincristine, prednisone, methotrexate, thioguanine, bleomycin, cytarabine, IT MTX, plus IF RT (3000–3500 cGy)	105

[a] Results of treatment were significantly influenced by histologic subtype of disease and therapeutic regimen followed (see text).
[b] Excluded patients with Burkitt's lymphomas.
[c] Included predominantly patients with diffuse undifferentiated Burkitt's lymphomas.
[d] Results by Ziegler staging system for Burkitt's lymphomas: 87% for Stages A, B, and AR combined; 38% for Stage C; 16% for Stage D.
[e] Results by staging classification of Table 35–4 for non-Burkitt's lymphomas.

Key to Abbreviations: IF RT = involved field radiotherapy; CrRT = cranial radiotherapy; IT MTX = intrathecal methotrexate; ara-C = cytarabine; HDMTX = high-dose methotrexate; LSA_2-L_2 = a 10-drug regimen containing: cyclophosphamide, vincristine, methotrexate, daunomycin, prednisone, cytarabine, thioguanine, asparaginase, carmustine, and hydroxyurea with IT MTX; COMP = cyclophosphamide, vincristine, methotrexate, prednisone; COPAD = cyclophosphamide, vincristine, Adriamycin, prednisone, cytarabine, asparaginase, IT methotrexate; APO = Adriamycin, prednisone, vincristine.

been most convincingly demonstrated by members of the Children's Cancer Study Group in relation to the 10-drug LSA_2-L_2 regimen (94), a finding confirmed by the Pediatric Oncology Group in another large series (98, 98a). Anderson and colleagues reported a 2-year disease-free survival rate of 76 per cent for children with disseminated lymphoblastic disease who were treated with the 10-drug LSA_2-L_2 regimen, compared with only a 26 per cent disease-free survival rate for such patients who were treated with a 4-drug COMP program, a statistically highly significant difference. Just the reverse relationship held true for advanced stages of nonlymphoblastic lymphomas (diffuse undifferentiated, Burkitt's, and large cell), in which cases the 4-drug regimen was superior to LSA_2-L_2: 57 versus 28 per cent respectively (94). The same finding, i.e., that Burkitt's lymphomas respond differently, has also been observed with other multiple-drug regimens (100, 101, 105).

Based on this evidence and other similar findings, it follows that children with lymphoblastic, primarily mediastinal and nodal primaries should not receive the same treatment as those with nonlymphoblastic, primarily intra-abdominal tumors of the Burkitt or large cell type. Treatment for advanced stage lymphoblastic disease should be as for high-risk acute lymphoblastic leukemia, consisting of multiple drugs in high dose and combinations for from 2 to 3 years, with prophylactic treatment of the central nervous system. Using such an approach, the 2-year disease-free survival for children with disseminated lymphoblastic disease, predominantly with mediastinal primaries, is in the range of 60 to 75 per cent (94, 100, 108, 109, 110). Management of advanced Stage III–IV nonlymphoblastic tumors should be based upon intensive combination chemotherapy relying on high doses of cyclophosphamide and methotrexate, and intensive intrathecal chemoprophylaxis (92, 113–115). The overall duration of treatment may be shorter, in the range of 6 to 15 months, in view of the well-known earlier relapse hazard of Burkitt's lymphoma and the lack of proven benefit of maintenance chemotherapy.

Central nervous system involvement is observed in approximately 30 to 45 per cent of children with NHL without prophylactic treatment (99, 103, 116, 117), and is correlated with the histopathology, site of primary tumor, and concomitant presence of bone marrow involvement or progressive disease (116, 117, 118). Symptoms of central nervous system involvement by lymphoma include headache, evidence of increased intracranial pressure, seizures, and focal neurologic deficits, particulary of the VIIth cranial nerve (119). Patients at high risk of CNS disease, such as those with advanced stages of lymphoblastic or Burkitt-type tumors, should definitely receive prophylactic treatment with either cranial irradiation and/or intrathecal medication. Management of central nervous system relapse involves the use of these same measures. In addition, high-dose dexamethasone treatment may be particularly useful for relief of acute symptoms, when used in conjunction with either external beam or intrathecal therapy (117–119).

Ablative treatments, incorporating massive doses of chemotherapy and total body irradiation, followed by either autologous or allogeneic marrow rescue, have been used with some success in patients with refractory or recurrent disease and in those considered at extremely high risk for treatment failure (120, 121). This type of approach should be reserved for extreme circumstances, as it is not without hazards, such as early death from infection and other treatment-related complications. Further refinements in techniques are particularly needed, such as the use of monoclonal antitumor antibodies to purge autologous bone marrow prior to reinfusion.

Complications

The management of the child with non-Hodgkin's lymphoma may be beset by a variety of acute and long-term complications, related either to the underlying disease or to the applied treatment modalities.

Children with generalized, massive, or bulky disease are prone to develop a variety of serious, even fatal, acute metabolic and renal problems (81, 122). Such complications may be present prior to treatment but occur more commonly when therapy is initiated, owing to massive tumor cell lysis. Hyperuricemia and urate nephropathy are the most frequent complications, although hyperkalemia, hyperphosphatemia, hypocalcemia, fluid overload, uremia, and lactic acidosis may also be observed. Treatment should be aimed at prevention, with hydration, urinary alkalinization, and administration of allopurinol. If urinary output decreases, a mannitol-induced osmotic diuresis should be forced. If acute renal failure supervenes, vigorous management with peritoneal or hemodialysis should be instituted, since specific therapy for the tumor may produce gratifyingly long remissions in the majority of patients, and all the renal and metabolic complications are reversible with proper management.

The use of combination drugs in high dosages, particularly when combined with radiotherapy, is naturally associated with myelosuppression and the associated risk of infectious complications with neutropenia. The occurrence of mucositis, esophagitis, and weight loss may necessitate nutritional supplementation or intravenous total parenteral nutrition.

A variety of long-term adverse late consequences of treatment may be observed in children cured of lymphoma, necessitating the need for long-term surveillance and appropriate intervention as needed. These effects include growth retardation, infertility, second malignancies, and neuropsychologic or psychosocial dysfunction (123, 124).

HODGKIN'S DISEASE

Definition

Hodgkin's Disease (HD) is a malignant lymphoma with distinctive clinical and pathologic characteristics, possessing features of a neoplasm, an infectious granulomatous disease, and an immunologic disorder. There is now general agreement that HD is a malignancy, since the giant cells (see Figure 35–1) have aneuploid karyotypes and produce tumors when heterotransplanted into nude mice (125). The heterogeneous cellular infiltrates represent nonmalignant reactions to the tumor cells.

An infectious etiology for HD has been proposed in view of the commonly associated pyrexia, the occasional granuloma formation, and the histologic evidence of variable admixtures of presumably reactive normal cells (lymphocytes, eosinophils, plasma cells, neutrophils, and fibroblasts). Initially, the tubercle bacillus was considered the causative organism of HD, although it is now appreciated that the two conditions may coexist.

Evidence for Altered Immunity in HD

The association of an altered immune status with HD has been appreciated since the observation of absent cutaneous delayed hypersensitivity to the tubercle bacillus, even in HD patients with active tuberculosis. Table 35–6 summarizes the evidence for altered immunity in HD. In general, humoral immunity is intact, and T cell–mediated immune function is impaired. It is an unproven but likely speculation that the alteration in immunity is related to the genesis of HD. The nature of the defect is unclear. The severity of the impairment increases with the increasing stage of the disease; with unfavorable histologic subtypes of HD, such as mixed and lymphocyte-depleted patterns; and with disease progression or recurrence. In treated patients, the immunosuppressive effects of radiotherapy and chemotherapy worsen the impairment, which is demonstrable even in successfully treated patients who are in long-lasting unmaintained remissions following intensive therapy (126, 127). However, defects are demonstrable even in untreated patients with active HD (128–133). The estimate of cutaneous anergy in untreated HD patients is influenced by the number and type of skin tests used. Using a battery of six

Table 35–6. EVIDENCE FOR ALTERED IMMUNITY IN HD

Finding	Reference(s)
Lymphopenia	6, 134
Anergy	6, 128, 130
Delayed homograft rejection	6, 134
Impaired in vitro lymphocyte response to phytohemagglutinin	129, 130
Defective binding of sheep erythrocytes to peripheral T lymphocytes, mediated by serum factors	131, 133
Increased in vitro total splenic IgG synthesis	132
Increased infectious complications	135
Elevation of EBV-related antibody titers	136a

recall antigens plus contact sensitization to dinitrochlorobenzene, Young and associates in fact found that absolute anergy was relatively uncommon, i.e., only 13.5 per cent of 103 untreated patients having no skin test reactivity whatsoever (128). The observation of increased splenic production of immunoglobulin with specificity for homologous lymphocytes (132), coupled with the demonstration of a reduction in sheep red cell rosette formation by T lymphocytes, which is mediated by serum factors (133), lends support to the hypothesis that the pathogenesis of HD is related to some aberrant host response to an autologous lymphoreticular cell (of lymphatic system origin) that has undergone malignant transformation.

Cellular Origins and Histopathology

The diagnosis of HD rests upon demonstration of the characteristic pathology in involved tissues, preferably an excisional lymph node biopsy specimen of an enlarged node (136). The pathology of HD is unique and notable for the diversity of morphologic findings, consisting of a complex association of abnormal cells of the Reed-Sternberg type and a mixed inflammatory cell infiltrate. The presence of Reed-Sternberg cells (Fig. 35–1) is necessary for the diagnosis of HD. Atypical mononuclear variants, with identical nuclear and nucleolar characteristics, may also be observed, but such cells are not as diagnostically reliable. A characteristic variant, the lacunar cell, is encountered in the nodular sclerosing type of HD. These lacunar cells have abundant clear cytoplasm, a lobulated nucleus, and small nucleoli (137).

It has recently been proposed that HD is a lymphoma composed of cells of the afferent limb of the immune system and, specifically, that Reed-Sternberg or Hodgkin's cells are the neoplastic counterparts of interdigitating reticulum cells or so-called dendritic cells, the antigen-trapping and presenting cells normally found in the paracortical T-dependent zones of lymph nodes and spleen

(138). Studies of cultured Hodgkin's cell lines have suggested that the cell of origin of HD may be related to a mononuclear phagocyte or macrophage (125) or to a unique cell type of unknown origin and function present around cortical follicles (139). The defects in T cell–mediated immunity so commonly observed in HD may be the result of any malignant transformation of a cell that results in diminished antigen-presenting capacity.

The histologic classification recommended for HD is that of Lukes and Butler (140, 141), which was adopted at the Rye Conference in 1965 and has achieved universal usage. The classification, which originally recognized six histologic expressions of HD, was consolidated into four groups: (a) lymphocytic predominance, (b) nodular sclerosis, (c) mixed cellularity, and (d) lymphocytic depletion (Fig. 35–6). The histologic subtypes, except nodular sclerosis, represent expressions of

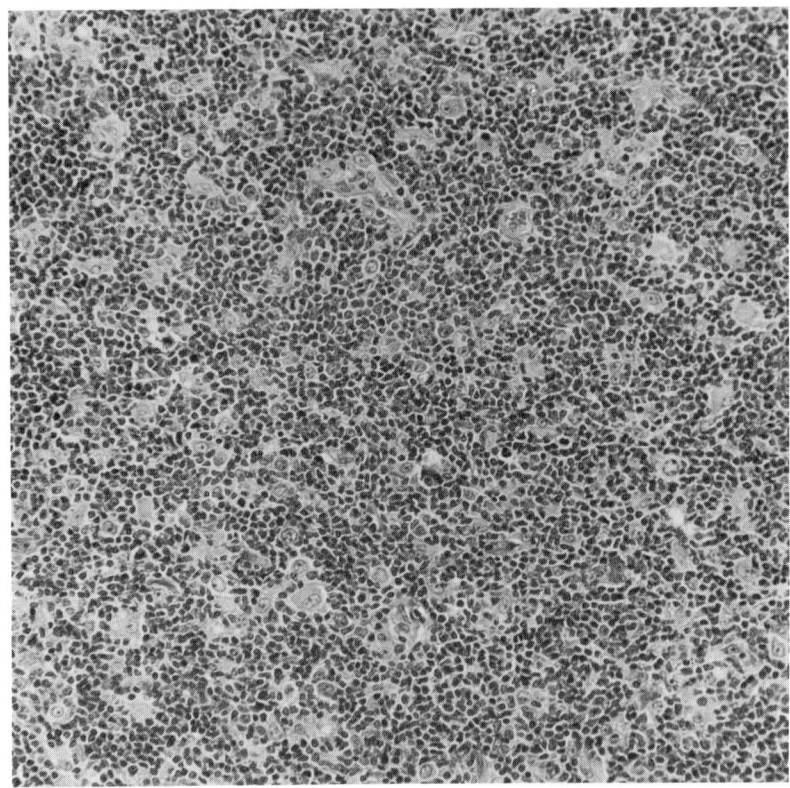

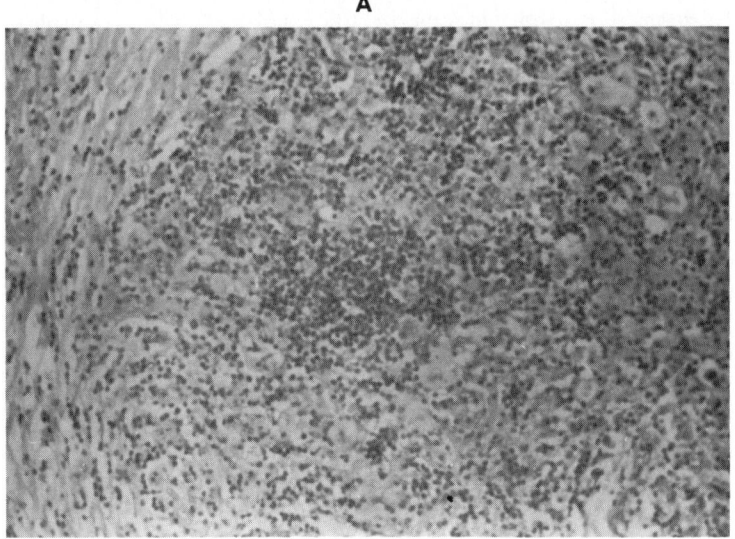

Figure 35–6. The four histologic subtypes of Hodgkin's disease recognized in the classification of Lukes and Butler (41) are shown for comparison: *A*, lymphocytic predominance, showing many diverse lymphocytes and only occasional Reed-Sternberg cells (hematoxylin-eosin, ×50), *B*, nodular sclerosis, showing collagen bands surrounding a lymphoid nodule (hematoxylin-eosin, ×100), *C*, mixed cellularity with lymphocytes and histiocytes in almost equal numbers and readily identifiable Reed-Sternberg cells (hematoxylin-eosin, ×100), and *D*, lymphocyte depletion, in which Reed-Sternberg cells predominate and few lymphocytes occur (hematoxylin-eosin, ×100).

Illustration continued on opposite page

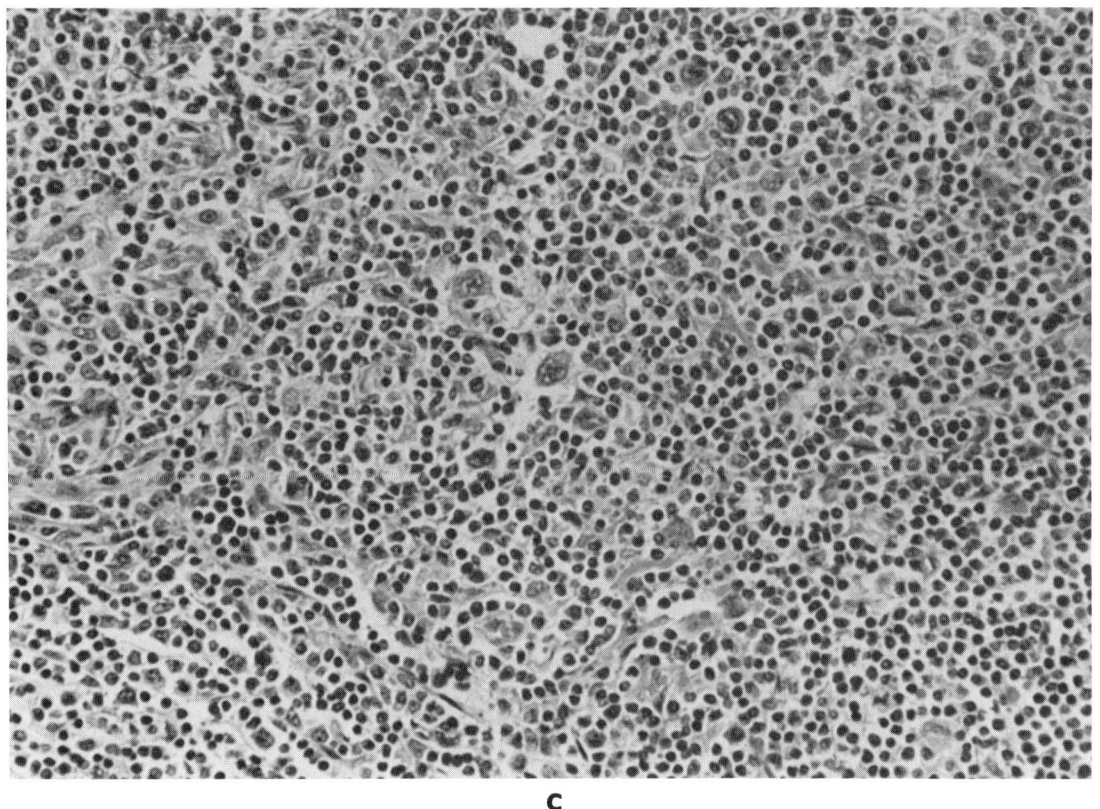

C

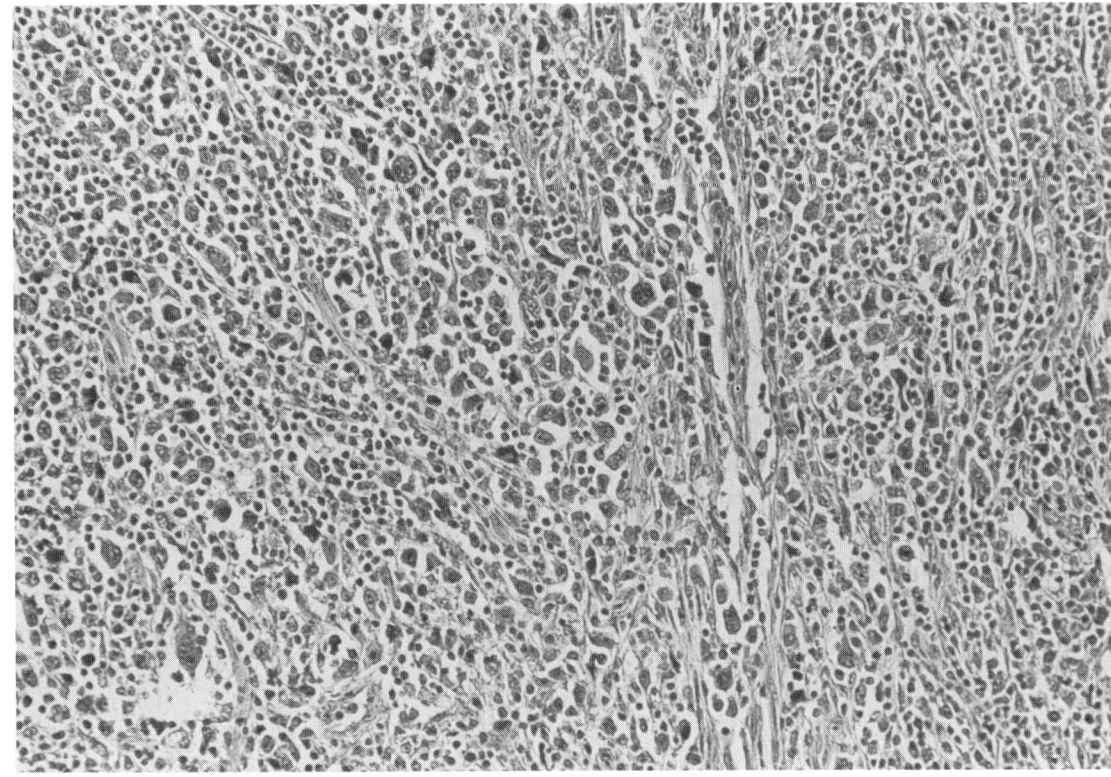

D

Figure 35–6 *Continued*

the inverse relationship that exists between the frequency of lymphocytes and of Reed-Sternberg cells. The lymphocytic-predominant form of HD is characterized mainly by a proliferation of mature-appearing lymphocytes associated with varying numbers of reactive histiocytes, only rare Reed-Sternberg cells, uncommon eosinophils, and essentially no fibrosis. The mixed cellularity type exhibits an intermediate picture of histiocytes, mature neutrophils, eosinophils, plasma cells, and lymphocytes in varying proportions, often associated with rather numerous and prominent Reed-Sternberg cells. Fibrosis in HD occurs in two distinct patterns, either nodular or diffuse. Diffuse and disorderly fibrosis is associated with the lymphocytic depletion subtype. Nodular sclerosis is recognized by orderly, dense, collagenous bands of connective tissue that subdivide abnormal lymphoid tissue into cellular nodules varying widely in their composition but typically manifesting the distinctive lacunar cell.

The Lukes-Butler classification has been related to clinical stage and to prognosis, even within staging groups (140–143). The lymphocytic-predominant form of HD has the best prognosis and is most commonly observed with clinical Stage I disease. At the opposite extreme, lymphocytic depletion has the poorest prognosis and is associated with rapid progression and wide dissemination (144). Mixed cellularity is a reflection of intermediate disease evolution, with an approximately equal distribution between stages of disease. Nodular sclerosis has the second most favorable prognosis and exhibits a typical regional expression, most frequently involving the anterosuperior mediastinum and scalene, supraclavicular, and lower cervical regions.

The distribution of histologic subtypes of HD, classified according to the Lukes-Butler scheme and collected from 10 childhood series, is shown in Table 35–7 (145–154). In comparison with older age groups, lymphocytic predominance is more commonly observed in children (143, 146), although it remains comparatively rare, accounting for 16.4 per cent of a total of 717 cases classified. Nodular sclerosis is the most common histologic subtype of HD observed in children in the collected series, although the mixed cellularity subtype was numerically most frequent in the two European series (153, 154). Lymphocytic depletion is the least prevalent subtype of HD, both in children and adults, and must be carefully distinguished from non-Hodgkin's lymphomas composed of pleomorphic large lymphoid cells.

Clinical Presentations

Painless progressive lymph node enlargement, usually cervical, is the most common presenting symptom of HD in children. The order of frequency of involvement of superficial lymph node groups is cervical (60 to 80 per cent), axillary (6 to 20 per cent), and inguinal (6 to 12 per cent) (155). A mediastinal mass or evidence of widening on chest roentgenogram is found in 20 to 50 per cent of children at the time of diagnosis (152–154) and may produce symptoms such as dyspnea, cough, dysphagia, and the superior vena cava syndrome. Retroperitoneal lymph nodes, spleen, and liver are less commonly involved clinically in the early phases of the disorder. The adenopathy may or may not be accompanied by systemic symptoms such as weight loss, night sweats, fever, and pruritus. The duration of symptoms and physical findings prior to diagnosis is variable, ranging from a few weeks to several months and, occasionally, more than a year. The apparent growth rate of the lymph nodes is also variable. Nodes may even wax and wane.

Fever occurs in 30 to 50 per cent of cases (6, 155). It may be cyclic, continuous, or intermittent. More rarely, Pel-Ebstein fever, a classic characteristic of HD, occurs. These cyclic bouts of high fever last 1 to 2 weeks and are separated by afebrile intervals of similar duration. Fever in HD is usually low grade. However, high, fluctuating fevers with extreme diurnal swings ranging to 40 to 41°C may occur, often accompanied by drenching night sweats.

Laboratory Findings

Routine laboratory findings at the initial presentation of the child with early HD are relatively unrevealing, although scrutiny of the complete blood count, erythrocyte sedimentation rate, and other acute-phase reactants may provide clues to the disease activity. Anemia is an uncommon, but serious, finding and may be attributable to either excessive destruction or inadequate production of red cells. Hemolytic anemia, with normochromic, normocytic erythrocytes; reticulocytosis; and increased unconjugated bilirubin, is rare in those with localized disease but may be present in 80 per cent of patients in later stages of disease (155).

Table 35–7. FREQUENCY OF HISTOLOGIC SUBTYPES OF HD OBSERVED IN CHILDHOOD, CLASSIFIED ACCORDING TO LUKES AND BUTLER*

Subtype	Number	Per Cent
Lymphocytic predominant	118	16.4
Nodular sclerosis	329	46.0
Mixed cellularity	220	30.7
Lymphocytic depletion	43	6.0
Unclassifiable	7	0.9
Total	717	100.0

*A compilation of 10 series (references 145–154), composed of children generally aged 15 years or less at diagnosis.

The Coombs' test is usually not positive. Inadequate production of red cells is due to infiltration of the marrow by Hodgkin's tissue and accompanying myelofibrosis. Pretreatment examination of the bone marrow, by both aspirate and biopsy, is mandatory in all children, and it may provide the only evidence of disseminated extranodal disease. Marrow specimens not demonstrably involved by HD may nevertheless show eosinophilia, plasmacytosis, granulomas, and/or benign lymphocytic aggregates (156, 157).

The total and differential leukocyte counts in HD are variable and nondiagnostic. Leukocytosis with neutrophilia may be observed in more than 50 per cent of patients. Leukopenia and absolute lymphocytopenia (below 1000 lymphocytes per mm^3) generally indicate advanced disease and a poor prognosis (6, 115)

The erythrocyte sedimentation rate is a nonspecific indicator of disease activity and is elevated in the presence of active disease, falling slowly to normal in patients exhibiting a complete response to specific therapy. It has also been noted that a variety of other serum values are elevated with active HD, including serum copper; α_1-, α_2-, and β_2-globulins; haptoglobin; fibrinogen; and C-reactive protein. None of these indicators appears to be a more sensitive or specific indicator of disease activity than the sedimentation rate. However, a multitude of other infections and nonspecific conditions may elevate the sedimentation rate and serum copper level, so that isolated fluctuations must not be given undue weight.

Staging

Once the diagnosis of HD is established, an evaluation is undertaken, referred to as staging, to determine the extent of disease. Staging allows for rational determination of the treatment in individual patients, provides prognostic information, and permits comparative clinical investigations and reporting of end results. Therapy is ordinarily not started until staging procedures are completed. Staging involves a sequential combination of clinical, radiographic, and surgical techniques and pathologic interpretation, as outlined in Table 35–8 (6, 88, 158–161).

Routine radiologic investigation of the child newly diagnosed as having HD is commonly rewarding and plays a major role in staging. Parker and co-workers have reported the pretreatment roentgenographic findings of a series of 105 children with HD who were evaluated at Stanford University from 1962 to 1974 (162). Demonstrable mediastinal and/or hilar adenopathy was found in 36 per cent of children aged less than 10 years at diagnosis and in 76 per cent of the children aged 11 to 15 years. Ten patients had pulmonary parenchymal disease. Pleural effusions were noted in four children (3.8 per cent), always in association with mediastinal disease. Routine skeletal surveys were normal in 104 of the 105 children at diagnosis. Inferior venacavography, excretory urography, and barium studies on the gastrointestinal tract were not useful in demonstrating disease.

Table 35–8. PROCEDURES IN STAGING CHILDREN WITH HODGKIN'S DISEASE

A. Recommended for all patients
  1. History and physical examination
  2. Lymph node biopsy establishing diagnosis
  3. Laboratory studies
    a. Complete blood count, including platelets
    b. Erythrocyte sedimentation rate
    c. Renal and liver function studies
  4. Radiologic studies
    a. Chest roentgenogram (posteroanterior and lateral views) and chest computed tomography
    b. Bilateral lower extremity lymphogram and/or whole-body computed tomography (see text for indication)
  5. Bone marrow aspirate and biopsy
B. Necessary, under certain conditions
  1. Exploratory laparotomy with splenectomy, multiple lymph node biopsies, wedge and needle liver biopsy and, in girls, oophoropexy
C. Occasionally useful ancillary studies
  1. Skeletal, hepatic, and splenic scintigrams
  2. Whole-body^{67} gallium scanning

Lymphography is technically feasible in most children, although the technique is invasive and requires a small cutdown and young patients may require general anesthesia. In two series of children with HD evaluated at diagnosis, 32 of a total of 136 patients studied (23.5 per cent) had abnormal lymphograms (162, 163). Parker and associates reported a lymphographic-histologic correlation of 98 per cent in childhood HD (162), illustrating the high degree of accuracy possible with lymphography performed by experienced radiologists. The lymphogram is also of importance in the planning of radiotherapy portals and the follow-up of the patient. Lymphography, however, cannot be totally relied upon to provide information regarding involvement of the abdomen by HD, as numerous nodal groups are not reliably opacified, including the mesenteric nodes, splenic hilar nodes, celiac axis nodes, and nodes in the region of the porta hepatis.

Computed tomographic (CT) scanning has an established role in staging HD (86–88) and is particularly helpful, for instance, in radiotherapy treatment planning for the mediastinum, by virtue of its cross-sectional display, which provides greater appreciation of the local extent of disease in mediastinal lymph nodes and adjacent pulmonary parenchyma (160). The relative merit of CT scanning versus lymphography for imaging the abdomen in children with HD is rather more controversial (88, 164). Lymphography possesses the advantage of displaying disease within lymph nodes of normal size, but the disadvantages of lymphography are not trivial. CT scanning of the abdomen in HD has the ability to detect enlarged lymph nodes, thereby providing important information for staging, treatment planning, and surveillance, but CT scanning is marginally less sensitive, less specific, and less accurate in detecting disease in retroperitoneal lymph nodes than is lymphography. The CT scan is also insensitive for detection of disease in the spleen or liver (88, 164).

Whole-body scanning with ^{67}gallium citrate is sometimes useful as a tumor-localizing procedure and for monitoring the effectiveness of therapy in individual patients, but low true-positive and high false-negative rates associated with its use suggest that it is not sufficiently reliable to replace other established staging methods (165). Liver and spleen scanning in HD is of quite limited usefulness, since only pathologic examination of adequate liver biopsy specimens and of spleens removed at surgery can be considered definitive evaluation for the presence or absence of HD (166).

Unquestionably, the accuracy of staging HD is improved by staging laparotomy and splenectomy (167–170). The procedure itself involves abdominal exploration; splenectomy with removal of splenic hilar nodes; sampling of multiple intra-abdominal lymph nodes from the para-aortic, iliac, porta hepatis, and celiac regions; wedge and needle biopsies from both hepatic lobes; and surgical bone marrow biopsy. In girls the ovaries may also be repositioned outside of expected radiation portals. Approximately 35 to 50 per cent of patients may have assessment of the stage of their disease altered by the findings from laparotomy and splenectomy. The most significant information gained from exploratory laparotomy and splenectomy concerns involvement of the spleen. Approximately 50 per cent of patients suspected of splenic involvement preoperatively on the basis of enlargement are found to have a spleen uninvolved by HD. Conversely, approximately one patient in four will be found to have splenic involvement by HD when none was suspected; often such patients have a spleen of normal size (167). In addition, splenic involvement may be the only evidence of HD below the diaphragm. Liver involvement is seldom found in untreated patients.

The decision to perform a staging laparotomy and splenectomy in an untreated child with HD should be individualized, in the context of local and current therapeutic philosophy. Justification for the procedure depends on likely alteration of the treatment, not just the stage, of the disease. If the therapeutic plan is to use radiotherapy only to known sites of HD, laparotomy and splenectomy are indispensable to accurately determine the extent of disease. If, however, the therapeutic plan calls for prophylactic irradiation of abdominal lymph node groups, or so-called total lymphoid irradiation, and/or the concomitant use of combination chemotherapy, then the surgical procedure has only limited value. It is possible to estimate the likelihood of a positive abdominal exploration based upon the clinical presentation. For example, Gamble and co-workers observed no evidence of abdominal disease in 16 lymphogram-negative Stage I patients with upper cervical or inguinal presentations, compared with 43 per cent for Stage I patients with supraclavicular or lower cervical adenopathy (169). In general, however, patients with clinical Stage I or Stage II HD must either be explored or be treated for abdominal involvement (170).

The risks and benefits involved in performance of laparotomy and splenectomy in children with HD need careful consideration. Although ordinarily unassociated with operative morbidity and mortality (171), a variety of surgical complications may ensue (172), and postoperative intestinal obstruction occurs not infrequently, particularly if abdominal radiation portals are employed. It should be appreciated that splenectomy per se is not a therapeutic procedure in HD, since follow-up studies of splenectomized HD patients and HD control patients who were similarly treated but who had not had splenectomies show no important differences in long-term remission status or survival (173). Nor does splenectomy improve tolerance to subsequent combination chemotherapy, as originally supposed (174). A minor benefit accruing from the removal of an enlarged spleen is the elimination of a splenic portal of irradiation, thereby sparing the radiation effect on normal gastrointestinal, left renal, and lower lung tissue. The hazard of serious or fatal postsplenectomy infection is not trivial, however, particularly in children receiving intensive myelosuppressive therapy. Of 200 children with HD subjected to splenectomy, Chilcote and associates reported 20 episodes of septicemia or meningitis in 18 patients, with 10 fatalities (175).

Thus, the specified sequence of staging procedures and the indications for laparotomy and splenectomy should be critically examined in each individual case, weighing the risks, costs, and benefits of invasive staging procedures against the likelihood that the resulting pathologic staging will significantly influence the treatment plan and the chance for cure (159, 160, 176). Children with supradiaphragmatic clinical Stages IA and IIA disease (Table 35–9) may be considered candidates for laparotomy and splenectomy to detect occult upper abdominal disease, since there is no other reliable means to detect involvement of high para-aortic, porta hepatis, and splenic pedicle lymph nodes or spleen. Provided mediastinal involvement is not bulky (i.e., does not exceed one third of the diameter of the thoracic cavity) and there is no extension to lung parenchyma, such children and

Table 35–9. STAGING CLASSIFICATION OF HODGKIN'S DISEASE AS RECOMMENDED BY THE ANN ARBOR SYMPOSIUM*

Stage I	Involvement of a single lymph node region (I) or of a single lymphatic organ or site (I_E)
Stage II	Involvement of two or more lymph node regions on the same side of the diaphragm (II) or localized involvement (by direct extension) of an extralymphatic organ or site and one or more lymph node regions on the same side of the diaphragm (II_E).
Stage III	Involvement of lymph node regions on both sides of the diaphragm (III), which may also be accompanied by localized involvement (by direct extension) of an extralymphatic organ or site (III_E) or by the involvement of the spleen or both.
Stage IV	Diffuse or disseminated involvement of one or more extralymphatic organs or tissues with or without associated lymph node enlargement

All stages are subclassified as "A" or "B" to indicate the absence or presence, respectively, of these systemic symptoms: (1) unexplained fever, (2) night sweats, and/or (3) weight loss greater than 10 per cent of normal body weight.

*From Carbone, P. P., Kaplan, H. S., et al.: Cancer Res. 31:1860, 1971.

adolescents with asymptomatic early stage HD may be cured with radiation alone. Thus, the surgical staging potentially spares these patients the major long-term morbidities of combined modality treatments. Laparotomy also allows for segregation of pathologic substage $IIIA_1$ (disease limited to the spleen, splenic, celiac, and/or portal nodes) from $IIIA_2$ (disease also involving lower abdominal nodes, i.e., para-aortic, iliac, and inguinal), a distinction that has prognostic and therapeutic significance (177). Patients with clinical Stage IIIB or unequivocal evidence of $IIIA_2$ disease or Stage IVA or B disease do not require surgical staging, since they need combined modality treatment with chemotherapy—their disease not being readily curable with radiotherapy alone.

The assignment of the stage of HD is based upon the Ann Arbor Staging Classification (178) shown in Table 35–9. Assignment of a clinical stage (CS) in every patient is based upon history, physical examination, radiologic studies, laboratory tests, and initial biopsy results. Patients who undergo further surgical staging procedures also have assigned a more precise pathologic stage (PS), classified by subscript symbols indicating the tissue sample and the results of histopathologic examination. Each stage is further subdivided into A and B categories, based upon absence or presence, respectively, of systemic symptoms of unexplained fevers above 38° C, night sweats, or unexplained weight loss of more than 10 per cent of body weight. For example, the staging designation CSIIIB PSIV H+M−S+ refers to a symptomatic patient with clinically evident lymphatic disease on both sides of the diaphragm who was found to have a spleen and liver positive for HD at laparotomy but an uninvolved marrow. Localized extralymphatic involvement caused by direct invasion of neighboring organs and tissues from affected lymph nodes is classified in accordance with the extent of the associated lymphatic involvement and is separately denoted by the suffix "E" (for Extralymphatic). Involvement of the liver and involvement of marrow are always considered disseminated, however, implying Stage IV disease. According to Kaplan (6) the decision to classify extralymphatic disease as Stage II_E or III_E instead of IV sometimes requires careful judgment and usually depends upon the extralymphatic disease being of limited enough extent to still be treated definitively with radiotherapy. For example, direct invasion of the lung associated with mediastinal and/or ipsilateral hilar adenopathy may be designated "E."

The results of complete clinical and pathologic staging of a total of 163 children collected from four published series are shown in Table 35–10 (150, 151, 168, 179). All children underwent laparotomy and splenectomy. More than half (60 per cent) of the children had localized or regional HD at diagnosis, either Stage I or II, A or B. Only 8.5 per cent of children who underwent laparotomy and splenectomy were found to have Stage IV disease.

Table 35–10. RESULTS OF STAGING OF CHILDHOOD HD, EMPLOYING STAGING LAPAROTOMY AND SPLENECTOMY*

	Number of Patients							
	Stage I		Stage II		Stage III		Stage IV	
Series	A	B	A	B	A	B		Totals
Tan, D'Angio, et al. (151)	9	3	11	4	7	3	8	45
Donaldson, Glatstein, et al. (150)	5	0	11	7	9	5	4	41
Lanzkowsky, Shende, et al. (168)	3	1	5	4	6	6	0	25
Botnick, Goodman, et al. (179)	5	0	26	5	4	10	2	52
Totals	22	4	53	20	26	24	14	163

*According to Ann Arbor Staging Classification (73).

Treatment and Results of Modern Therapy

All children with HD deserve adequate primary therapy with curative intent, based upon consideration of the primary site, extent of disease, symptomatology, and histopathology. Such treatment involves the use of megavoltage extended-field radiotherapy or multiple-drug combination chemotherapy, or both. The best results (Table 35–11) have been achieved by centers employing a multidisciplinary approach to care, involving the cooperation of expert oncologists, diagnostic and therapeutic radiologists, pathologists, and surgeons. Each newly diagnosed child with HD should be considered for prompt referral to such a comprehensive childhood cancer center. Initial palliative approaches employing local radiotherapy to conspicuously enlarged nodes or single-drug chemotherapy are strictly to be deplored. The policy of treating a newly diagnosed child with lymphoma in the local community by whatever methods are readily available and deferring referral to a major medical center until relapse supervenes leads almost inevitably to disaster. Treatment of HD has traditionally rested upon high-dose extended field radiotherapy for Stages I to III, generally with combination chemotherapy reserved for Stages IIIB and IV. The best results reported, however, have resulted from combined modality approaches, incorporating both chemotherapy and comparatively lower dose radiotherapy, while omitting laparotomy and splenectomy, for nearly all stages of disease except localized favorable presentations of Stages IA or IIA disease (180–185). (See Table 35–11.)

Radiation therapy alone can cure localized HD, when coupled with scrupulous pathologic staging. Treatment should be delivered by 4 to 8 MeV linear accelerator, using an opposed field (usually anterior and posterior) technique, with routine field simulation and frequent film verification. Technical details, such as dosimetry, fraction size, volume to be irradiated, beam alignment, shielding, and so on (6, 186, 187) are beyond the scope of this discussion but are crucial to achievement of a successful end result with minimal complications. Based on Kaplan's analysis, a radiation dose of 4000 to 4400 cGy, delivered in 4 to 4½ weeks, provides a reasonable estimate of the optimal tumoricidal dose and ensures 98 per cent freedom from true recurrence of HD in the irradiated field (6). Although there is thus little debate regarding the dose of radiation necessary, the exact technique to be applied in determining the extent of radiation for early-stage HD is still somewhat controversial. Numerous studies have shown that treatment of the so-called extended-field type, as opposed to the involved field, results in superior disease-free survival rates. In a national collaborative trial of Stage I and II HD, 224 eligible patients were randomized to receive involved-field radiotherapy, while 243 received extended-field therapy, either mantle for upper torso HD or inverted-Y for lower torso disease (188). Complications of therapy are significantly more frequent with extended fields of treatment, whereas extensions of HD are more frequent with limited fields. Results from Stanford University of a comparison of involved versus extended fields for Stage I and Stage II HD indicate a significant difference in freedom from progression (82 vs. 32 per cent) in favor of extended fields and subtotal lymphoid or total nodal approaches (6, 189). Other experiences with Stage I and II patients with supradiaphragmatic HD confirm the excellent results obtained with extended prophylactic irradiation, reporting 90 to 98 per cent survival using upper mantle plus para-aortic fields (186, 190).

Sullivan and co-workers have advocated selective modification of treatment plans for children based on prognostic factors in order to ensure maximum freedom from adverse long-term consequences of therapy (191). According to their recommended guidelines, children with "favorable" Stage I or II presentations, e.g., unilateral upper neck lymphocyte predominance, receive involved-field radiotherapy only. In this author's opinion, however, published results of treatment of localized childhood HD with involved-field radiotherapy alone have not appeared promising. In a series of 47 children with clinical Stage I and II HD, who were treated from 1949 to 1969 (prior to the use of staging laparotomy and splenectomy), Fuller and co-workers reported uniform local control, but 22 of 47 children developed extensions of HD and 10 died (192). In a more recently published series of children with Stage I and II HD who underwent staging laparotomy and were treated with involved-field irradiation only, 8 of 20 relapsed—i.e., there was only a 57 per cent actuarial relapse-free survival estimate with only a 3-year follow-up (193).

Combination chemotherapy is highly effective in HD (194–196) and is indicated for the primary control of advanced, symptomatic stages. Furthermore, it is of demonstrated benefit in ensuring freedom from progression when combined with radiotherapy for Stages I to III (186, 189, 197) and is thus beneficial in combined-modality regimens for patient subgroups unlikely to be cured by radiotherapy alone (such as IIB, IIIA$_2$, and IIIB). Chemotherapy is, of course, also a cornerstone of management for patients with HD exhibiting progression following radiation (see below, Salvage Therapies).

Introduction of the four-drug MOPP regimen (acronym for *M*ustargen, *O*ncovin, *p*rocarbazine, and *p*rednisone) (Table 35–12), devised by DeVita and co-workers of the National Cancer Institute, signaled a breakthrough in the management of

Table 35–11. RESULTS OF MODERN TREATMENT OF CHILDHOOD HODGKIN'S DISEASE*

Source	Number of Patients	Stages	Overall 5-Year Survival/DFS	Therapy	Reference
Roswell Park Memorial Institute, 1965–1973	37	I–IV	86%/86%	IA, IIA: RT alone IIB, III: RT + MOPP IV: MOPP (+ Vbl, CCNU)	147
Memorial Sloan-Kettering Cancer Center, 1970–1975	45	I–IV	80%/not stated	I, II: IF or EF RT III: TNI IIIB–IV: ACOPP	151
Toronto 1969–1973	52	PS I–IV	89%/54%	PS I–IIIA: EF RT (3500 cGy) PS IIIB, IV: EF RT + MOPP	180
1973–1977	41	I–IV	89%/85%	CS I IV (except favorable CS IA): MOPP × 3, then EF RT (2000–2500 cGy), then MOPP × 3	180
Stanford University 1962–1972	79	PS I–IV	89%/66%	PS I–III: EF RT or TNI (3500–4400 cGy) PS IV: MOPP	150
1972–1982	48	PS I–IV	96%/93%	EF RT (1500–2500 cGy) + MOPP × 6	181
Children's Hospital of Philadelphia, 1977–1983	16	IA–IIA	100%/86%	PS IA–IIA, pubertal and postpubertal: EF RT (3600–4400 cGy)	206
	32	IIB–IVB	86%/60%	CS IA–IVB, prepubertal, and CS IIA (large MM)–IVB, postpubertal: COPP × 3, then IF RT (2000 cGy), then COPP × 3	
National Cancer Institute, 1964–1973	38	I–IV	63%/not stated	CS I–II: EF RT or TNI (3500–4000 cGy) CS IIIA: TNI CS IIIB–IVB: MOPP	145
Joint Center for Radiation Therapy, 1968–1977	83	IA–IIIB	95%/77%	IA–IIA: EF RT (3600–4000 cGy) IIB, IIIA, IIIB: TNI or EF RT + MOPP	204
St. Jude Children's Research Hospital, 1967–1972	54	I–IV	80%/75%	I–II: EF RT (3500–4000 cGy) + CO III–IV: TNI (3500–4000 cGy) + COP	205
German Cooperative Group, 1978–1981	170	I–IV	92%/96%†	I–IV: 2 cycles of OPPA + IF RT (3600–4000 cGy), then either 3600–4000 cGy to EF or 1800–2000 cGy to EF, then: IA, IB, IIA: No further therapy IIB, III, IV: 4 additional cycles COPP	182
Istituto Nazionale Tumori, Milan, 1979–1982	34	I–III	100%/97%†	I–IIA: ABVD × 3 + EF RT (2500–3500 cGy) IIIA and/or IIIB symptoms: ABVD × 3, then EF RT, then ABVD × 3	183
Institut Gustave-Roussy, Villejuif, and Hôpital Saint-Louis, Paris, 1969–1978	72	CS IA–IIB	92%/85%	MOPP + EF or IF RT (3000–4000 cGy)	184
Children's Solid Tumor Group, Great Britain, 1974–1982	80	I–IV	94%/82%	ChlVPP + IF RT (3000 cGy)	185

*Key to Abbreviations: DFS = disease-free survival; CS = clinical stage; PS = pathologic stage; RT = radiotherapy; IF = involved field; EF = extended field; TNI = total nodal irradiation; MM = mediastinal mass; Vbl = vinblastine; MOPP = nitrogen mustard, vincristine, procarbazine, prednisone; CO = cyclophosphamide, vincristine; COP = cyclophosphamide, vincristine, procarbazine; COPP = COP + prednisone; A = Adriamycin; ABVD = Adriamycin, bleomycin, vinblastine, DTIC; ChlVPP = chlorambucil, vinblastine, procarbazine, prednisone; OPPA = vincristine, procarbazine, prednisone, Adriamycin.
†Reported results from 3 to 4 years follow-up (not 5).

HD. In their original report of 43 patients treated with six cycles of MOPP, 35 or 43 (81 per cent) achieved a complete remission, and the median length of survival for responding patients was 42 months (198). In a follow-up report of a total of 198 patients treated with MOPP, complete responses persisted in 68 per cent of patients at 5 years. This work has been amply confirmed by numerous groups in large numbers of patients. Attempts to improve upon these results have been made by altering the MOPP combination; using three-, four-, and five-drug regimens; and deleting, substituting, or adding other agents active in HD, such as vinblastine, bleomycin, Adriamycin, nitrosoureas, cyclophosphamide, and dimethyl-triazeno-imidazole-carboxamide (DTIC) (196). An alternative, non–cross-resistant four-drug combination, ABVD (Adriamycin, bleomycin, vinblastine, and dacarbazine [imidazole carboxamide or DTIC]; see Table 35–12), is equivalent to MOPP in effectiveness in a head-on comparison in previously untreated patients with advanced HD. Furthermore, ABVD produces a 75 per cent complete response rate in MOPP-failures (195). For stages IIB, IIIA, and IIIB, the combination of ABVD plus radiotherapy is significantly better than MOPP plus radiotherapy, the former producing 91 per cent relapse-free survival at 5 years, versus 82 per cent survival with the latter mode of treatment (195). In the treatment group of 34 children with HD Stages I to III, Fossati-Bellani and coworkers (183) recently reported outstanding success with ABVD plus low-dose radiotherapy (97 per cent disease-free survival for 3 to 4 years following diagnosis).

In patients with Stage IV disease, alternating the two non–cross-resistant drug combinations, MOPP and ABVD, has produced results significantly superior to those seen with MOPP alone (195, 200). In a recent 7-year follow-up report of 88 patients with PS (pathologic stage) IV HD who were randomized to receive either MOPP or alternating MOPP and ABVD for 12 cycles, 72 per cent of the MOPP-ABVD treated patients remained free of evidence of progressive HD, compared with only 35 per cent of the MOPP group (201).

The known radiocurability of HD, coupled with the success of multiple-agent chemotherapy, naturally has led to combined modality approaches aimed at increasing long-term disease-free survival and achieving cure of HD. Such combined regimens of radiation and chemotherapy are particularly useful in the treatment of patients with unfavorable presentations of HD, such as disease above and below the diaphragm or that associated with systemic symptoms, and a number of reports confirm the superior disease-free survival achieved (177, 180–186, 189, 197, 202, 203). Regimens have been variable, employing either radiation first, followed by chemotherapy or vice versa or sandwiching radiation between cycles of drugs. From these studies, we can safely conclude that the addition of effective combination chemotherapy can replace extended field irradiation to clinically uninvolved sites. In Stage IV patients, the complete response rate achievable with drugs alone can be significantly improved by subsequent administration of low-dose radiotherapy to all pretreatment nodal and extranodal sites involved except marrow. Such an approach also obviates the tendency for recurrence in sites of initial bulky tumor, so characteristic of HD patients treated with chemotherapy alone. The success of such combined modality approaches, even with unfavorable presentations of HD, has led to their use in early-stage HD, with concomitant de-emphasis on scrupulous surgical staging to delineate areas of known disease.

Delivery of intensive combined modality therapy is difficult and must be carried out with considerable caution to avoid undue toxicity. Full doses of chemotherapy and conventional doses of radiation are generally not well tolerated and may be associated with severe and prolonged hematologic depression; unacceptable enhancement of normal tissue reactions, such as pneumonitis, enteritis, pericarditis, and cardiomyopathy; and treatment-related deaths (203). It is now increasingly appreciated that a variety of antineoplastic drugs enhance radiation effects, whether given before, concurrently, or after radiation therapy. Consequently, some reduction in radiation dose is prudent and is commonly practiced (180–183, 207), along with interruptions of therapy as necessary to permit recovery from hematologic toxicity.

The results of modern multidisciplinary treatment of HD from 12 major centers or cooperative groups treating children and adolescents are summarized in Table 35–11. Details of reported treatment policies and regimens differ, but the overall results indicate that 9 out of every 10 children who are carefully staged and treated for HD are curable with modern management.

Table 35–12. CHEMOTHERAPY OF HODGKIN'S DISEASE

MOPP (198)
  Vincristine, 1.4 mg/m^2, intravenously on days 1 and 8
  Nitrogen mustard, 6 mg/m^2, intravenously on days 1 and 8
  Procarbazine, 100 mg/m^2, orally, days 1 through 14
  Prednisone, 40 mg/m^2, orally, days 1 through 14, during cycles one and four
  Each cycle is repeated monthly for a total of 6 cycles

ABVD (195)
  Adriamycin, 25 mg/m^2, days 1 and 14
  Bleomycin, 10 mg/m^2, days 1 and 14
  Vinblastine, 6 mg/m^2, days 1 and 14
  DTIC, 150 mg/m^2, days 1 through 5
  All drugs are given intravenously in monthly cycles

The success of a second course of treatment for patients with HD who have suffered a relapse depends upon the pathologic stage and the extent and nature of the initial treatment, as well as the site or sites of failure (208–210). In a series of 179 children treated for HD at Stanford University from 1961 to 1980, children who underwent only clinical staging and were managed with primary radiation therapy alone had the highest risk for relapse (210). The best disease-free survival rate at 10 years (89 per cent) was seen in the group of laparotomy-staged patients receiving combined modality treatment, as compared with 69 per cent for the surgically staged radiation patients, and only 42 per cent for the clinically staged radiation patients. Weller and co-workers have reported the results of second treatment of 243 HD patients treated initially with radiation therapy who relapsed out of a total of 701 HD patients treated at Stanford University from 1961 to 1973 (211). Most relapses occurred within 3 years of initial therapy. The best results of retreatment resulted from use of MOPP, either alone or in conjunction with radiotherapy, which provided a 5-year relapse-free survival rate of 40 to 50 per cent, measured from the time of second treatment. The freedom from further progressive disease is superior for relapsing patients with HD initially treated with radiotherapy alone, compared with patients relapsing and requiring retreatment after an initial combined modality approach (212). Also, not unexpectedly, the outcome of retreatment of recurrent HD still limited to nodes is superior to that with recurrent HD involving the marrow (73 versus 27 per cent at 2 years) (212). Patients in relapse following chemotherapy may often be successfully retreated with MOPP or with one of the alternative non–cross-resistant combination drug regimens (196). Therapeutic recommendations for previously treated patients in relapse have been well outlined by Kaplan and Rosenberg (213). Skillful use of available options for retreatment can provide months or even years of high-quality survival, even in patients destined ultimately to die of HD.

Complications

The underlying immune defects in HD, aggravated by the immunosuppressive effects of therapy, predispose the child with HD to a variety of infectious complications. The infections are frequently opportunistic and include viral diseases (notably herpes zoster and cytomegalic inclusion disease) and protozoal (*Pneumocystis carinii* pneumonitis and toxoplasmosis), mycobacterial, and fungal (candidiasis and cryptococcosis) infections (135). Herpes-zoster–varicella infections, in particular, are distressing frequent; Donaldson and associates observed an incidence of 35 per cent in a total of 179 children treated for HD (214). It must also constantly be borne in mind that in children who have been splenectomized, fever may be the only sign of overwhelming pneumococcal sepsis. Prompt cultures and initiation of penicillin therapy are mandatory until the origin of the fever is established.

Long-term sequelae of treatment for HD have been recognized with increasing frequency, particularly with the use of extended radiation fields and multiagent chemotherapy. Adverse effects include acute pneumonitis and subsequent pulmonary fibrosis (215); pericarditis (216); and thyroid dysfunction, as evidenced by depressed concentrations of serum thyroxine and/or elevated levels of thyroid-stimulating hormone (214, 215). Oophoropexy prior to pelvic node and para-aortic irradiation may successfully prevent ovarian failure, and successful pregnancy has ensued (217, 218). Combination drug therapy, however, may result in ovarian or testicular failure (214, 219, 220). The adverse long-term consequences on axial skeletal growth for the preadolescent child with HD who receives high-dose (3000–4000 cGy) extended field radiotherapy are particularly pronounced, resulting in diminished sitting and standing height, shortening of the clavicles, small thorax, and fibrosis and atrophy of neck muscles (221). Reluctance to accept this severe consequence of large-volume, high-dose radiotherapy has led many centers to adopt a policy of low-dose (<2500 cGy) limited radiotherapy combined with chemotherapy (180, 181, 206) for management of the preadolescent with HD.

The occurrence of secondary malignant neoplasms can be expected with increased frequency following treatment for HD. The increased risk is related to the intensity of therapy administered and is due primarily to the increased late occurrence of acute nonlymphocytic leukemia (124, 214, 222). Coleman and co-workers have estimated the actuarial probability of development of acute leukemia at 5 and 7 years post-treatment to be 2.9 and 3.9 per cent, respectively, for patients treated with combined radiation and chemotherapy (222). The increased occurrence of other tumors, including bone and soft tissue sarcomas within or near fields of previous irradiation, thyroid carcinomas, and non-Hodgkin's lymphoma, has also been reported (124, 214, 223).

UNRESOLVED CONTROVERSIES IN THE MANAGEMENT OF LYMPHOMAS

Despite unqualified successes achieved in the past 10 to 15 years in the management of lymphomas in children, considerable controversy still surrounds certain issues. The unquestioned goal of management is to achieve cure. Questions surround the methods that will achieve this goal with the lowest risk, least acute morbidity, and with minimal long-term complications. The issues of cost and complexity of current approaches are also nontrivial.

The decision to rely on combined modality therapy, radiation alone, or chemotherapy alone is a crucial one, since the frequency and severity of complications is greater with combined modality approaches than with either radiation therapy or chemotherapy alone. For NHL, the issue is not as agonizing, because it is evident that all children should be treated with combination chemotherapy and that involved field radiotherapy contributes little to the overall success of reported regimens. Furthermore, the child with NHL must receive initial treatment that is likely to be successful, since salvage is practically nonexistent. For HD, the issues are more controversial, since patients with HD who relapse after primary irradiation programs may be salvaged by subsequent therapy. Issues surrounding the choice of single- or combined modality therapy for HD have been extensively reviewed (209, 224–226), and the perplexity of the trade-offs involved has even driven some investigators to adopt a formal decision analysis technique (227).

The decision to rely on radiation therapy alone for children with HD depends on the child's age and stage of disease, the estimate of the risk for relapse, and assessment of the feasibility of surveillance and likelihood of success of subsequent salvage therapies. In order to attempt to minimize therapy, one must maximize the pathologic staging of HD. To rely on clinical staging alone and to use combined modality approaches with low-dose, involved-field radiotherapy for all children with HD (except those with asymptomatic Stage IA or IIA disease, without bulky mediastinal masses) will likely cure 90 to 95 per cent, but will assuredly "overtreat" some fraction who would have been cured by radiotherapy alone. The price of such overtreatment may include sterility, increased infectious complications, increased organ toxicity, enhanced risk of second malignancies, and increased expense and duration of primary treatment. Balanced against this must be the certain realization that relapse of HD constitutes a serious and possibly life-threatening event. For this not to be true would require 100 per cent success of salvage therapies, an intrinsically unlikely event considering what is currently known regarding the development of somatic mutations in cancer cells and the development of drug resistance. Furthermore, reported results of salvage approaches used in retreating relapsed HD patients do not come near to 100 per cent success. In 22 children with recurrent HD, Jenkin and Barry, for instance, have reported a median duration of second complete remissions of only 3 years, and more than half of the children with a first relapse experienced multiple relapses (180). In a series of 178 children with HD treated in Paris, the overall 5-year survival for 47 patients following relapse is 69 per cent, without evidence of a plateau (184).

In the absence of well-controlled, long-term, large-scale randomized studies, stratified for staging and directly comparing one approach with another, it is impossible to define with certainty the precise risk-to-benefit ratio of current mangement approaches for childhood lymphoma. Further trials are needed that explore reductions in the dose and volume of radiation therapy, and alternative non–cross-resistant drug combinations of equal efficacy but less toxicity require investigation. Some reduction in the length of planned therapies, e.g., from six cycles to three, for children with localized lymphomas should be tested by controlled trials.

In the meantime, the excellent expectation for cure of childhood lymphomas of all histologic types and all stages provides grounds for optimism in the approach to the newly diagnosed cases.

References

1. Dorfman, R. F., and Warnke, R.: Lymphadenopathy simulating the malignant lymphomas. Hum. Pathol. 5:519, 1974.
2. Fox, H.: Presentation of microscopical preparations made from some of the original tissue described by Thomas Hodgkin, 1832. Ann. Med. Hist. 8:370, 1926.
3. Hodgkin, T.: On some morbid appearances of the absorbant glands and spleen. Trans. Med. Chir. Soc. Edinb. 17:68, 1832.
4. Mann, R. B., Jaffe, E. F., et al.: Malignant lymphomas—a conceptual understanding of morphologic diversity. Am. J. Pathol. 94:105, 1979.
5. Magrath, I. T.: Lymphocyte differentiation: an essential basis for the comprehension of lymphoid neoplasia. J. Natl. Cancer Inst. 67:501, 1981.
6. Kaplan, H. S.: *Hodgkin's Disease*, 2nd ed. Cambridge, Harvard University Press, 1980.
7. Rosenberg, S. A., and Kaplan, H. S. (eds.): *Malignant Lymphomas: Etiology, Pathology, Treatment.* New York, Academic Press, 1982.
8. Coltman, C. A., and Golomb, H. M. (eds.): *Hodgkin's and Non-Hodgkin's Lymphomas.* Seminars in Oncology, VII (2&3), New York, Grune & Stratton, 1980.
9. Conference on Non-Hodgkin's Lymphomas. Proceedings. Cancer Treat. Rep. 61:935, 1977.
10. Symposium on Contemporary Issues in Hodgkin's Disease: Biology, Staging and Treatment. Cancer Treat. Rep. 66:601, 1982.
11. Kay, N. E., Ackerman, S. K., et al.: Anatomy of the immune system. Semin. Hematol. 16:252, 1979.
12. Holt, L. E.: *The Diseases of Infancy and Childhood.* New York, D. Appleton and Co., 1899, pp. 816–818.
13. Barton, L. L., and Feigin, R. D.: Childhood cervical lymphadenitis: A reappraisal. J. Pediatr. 84:846, 1974.
14. Schmitt, B. D.: Cervical adenopathy in children. Postgrad. Med. 60:251, 1976.
15. Moussatos, G. H., and Baffes, T. G.: Cervical masses in infants and children. Pediatrics 33:251, 1963.
16. Knight, P. J., Hamoudi, A. B., et al.: The diagnosis and treatment of mid-line neck masses in children. Surgery 93:603, 1983.
17. Zuelzer, W. W., and Kaplan, J.: The child with lymphadenopathy. Semin. Hematol. 12:323, 1975.
18. Butler, J. J.: Non-neoplastic lesions of lymph nodes of

man to be differentiated from lymphomas. Natl. Cancer Inst. Monogr. 32:233, 1969.
19. Lake, A. M., and Oski, F. A.: Peripheral lymphadenopathy in childhood: Ten year experience with excisional biopsy. Am. J. Dis. Child. 132:357, 1978.
20. Knight, P. J., Mulne, A. F., et al: When is lymph node biopsy indicated in children with enlarged peripheral nodes? Pediatrics 69:391, 1984.
21. Salvador, A., Harrison, E., et al.: Lymphadenopathy due to infectious mononucleosis: Its confusion with malignant lymphoma. Cancer 27:1029, 1971.
22. Kendig, E. L.: The clinical picture of sarcoidosis in children. Pediatrics 54:289, 1974.
23. Choovivathanavanich, P., Wallace, E. M., et al.: Pseudolymphoma induced by the diphenylhydantoin. J. Pediatr. 72:621, 1970.
24. Li, F. P., Willard, D. R., et al.: Malignant lymphoma after diphenylhydantoin (Dilantin) therapy. Cancer 36:1359, 1975.
25. Hyman, G. A., and Sommers S. C.: The development of Hodgkin's disease and lymphoma during anticonvulsant therapy. Blood 28:416, 1960.
26. Keller, A. R., Hochholzer, L., et al.: Hyaline-vascular and plasma-cell types of giant lymph node hyperplasia. Cancer 29:670, 1972.
27. Ballow, M. Parks, B. H., et al.: Benign giant lymphoid hyperplasia of the mediastinum with associated abnormalities of the immune system. J. Pediatr. 84:418, 1974.
28. Burgert, E. O., Gilchrist, G. S., et al.: Intraabdominal angiofollicular lymph node hyperplasia (plasma-cell variant) with an antierythropoietic factor. Mayo Clin. Proc. 50:542, 1975.
29. Miller, J. S., and Miller, J. J.: Benign giant lymph node hyperplasia presenting as fever of unnoticed origin. J. Pediatr. 87:237, 1975.
30. Buchanan, G. R., Tipman, T. T., et al.: Angiomatous lymphoid hamartoma: inhibitory effects on erythropoiesis, growth and primary hemostasis. J. Pediatr. 99:382, 1981.
31. Rosai, J., and Dorfman, R. F.: Sinus histiocytosis with massive lymphadenopathy. A pseudolymphomatous benign disorder. Analysis of 34 cases. Cancer 30:1174, 1972.
32. Williams, J. W., and Dorfman, R. F.: Lymph node involvement by histiocytosis X. Lab. Invest. 36:352, 1977.
33. Hope, J. W., and Koop, C. E.: Differential diagnosis of mediastinal masses. Pediatr. Clin. North Am. 6:379, 1959.
34. Rosai, J., and Levine, R.: Tumors of the thymus. In: *Atlas of Tumor Pathology*, Section 2, Fascicle 13. Washington, D.C., Armed Forces Institute of Pathology, 1975.
35. Dehner, L. P., Martin, S. A., et al.: Thymus related tumors and tumor-like lesions in childhood with rapid clinical progression and death. Hum. Pathol. 8:53, 1977.
36. Halpern, S., Chatten, J., et al.: Anterior mediastinal masses: anesthesia hazards and other problems. J. Pediatr. 102:407, 1983.
37. Haller, J. A., Mazur, D. O., et al.: Diagnosis and management of mediastinal masses in children. J. Thorac. Cardiovasc. Surg. 58:385, 1969.
38. Pokorney, W. J., and Sherman, J. O.: Mediastinal masses in infants and children. J. Thorac. Cardiovasc. Surg. 68:869, 1974.
39. Rappaport, H.: Tumors of the hematopoietic system. In *Atlas of Tumor Pathology*, Section 3, Fascicle 8. Washington, D.C., U.S. Armed Forces Institute of Pathology, 1966.
40. Murphy, S. B., Frizzera, G., et al.: A study of childhood non-Hodgkin's lymphoma. Cancer 36:2121, 1975.
41. Dura, W. T., Gladkowska-Dura, M. J., et al.: Non-Hodgkin's lymphoma in the first two decades. Morphologic and immunocytochemical studies. Virchows Arch. (Pathol. Anat.) 390:23, 1981.
42. Lukes, R. J., and Collins, R. D.: Immunologic characterization of human malignant lymphomas. Cancer 34:1488, 1974.
43. Nathwani, B. N.: A critical analysis of the classifications of non-Hodgkin's lymphomas. Cancer 44:347, 1979.
44. Non-Hodgkin's Lymphoma Pathologic Classification Project. National Cancer Institute sponsored study of classifications of non-Hodgkin's lymphomas. Summary and description of the working formulation for clinical usage. Cancer 49:2112, 1982.
45. Frizzera, G., and Murphy, S. B.: Follicular (nodular) lymphoma in childhood: a rare clinical-pathological entity. Cancer 44:2218, 1979.
46. Callihan, T. R., and Berard, C. W.: Childhood non-Hodgkin's lymphomas in current histological perspective. In *Perspectives in Pediatric Pathology*, Vol. 7. Rosenberg, H. S., and Bernstein, J. (eds.), New York, Masson Publishing, 1982, pp. 259–277.
47. Kjeldsberg, C. R., Wilson, J. S., et al.: Non-Hodgkin's lymphoma in children. Hum. Pathol. 14:612, 1983.
48. Wilson, J. F., Jenkin, R. D. T., et al.: Studies on the pathology of non-Hodgkin's lymphoma of childhood. I. The role of routine histopathology as a prognostic factor. A report from the Children's Cancer Study Group. Cancer 53:1695, 1984.
49. Bernard, A., Boumsell, L., et al.: Subsets of malignant lymphomas in children related to the cell phenotype. Blood 54:1058, 1979.
50. Bernard, A., Murphy, S. B., et al.: Non-T, non-B lymphomas are rare in childhood and associated with cutaneous tumor. Blood 59:549, 1982.
51. Lukes, R. J., Taylor, C. R., et al.: A morphologic and immunologic surface marker study of 299 cases of non-Hodgkin's lymphoma and related leukemias. Am. J. Pathol. 90:461, 1978.
52. Arnold, A., Cossman, J., et al.: Immunoglobulin gene rearrangements as unique clonal markers in human lymphoid neoplasm. New Engl. J. Med. 309:1593, 1983.
53. Nadler, L. M., Reinherz, E. L., et al.: Heterogeneity of T-cell lymphoblastic malignancies. Blood 55:806, 1980.
54. Greaves, M. F., Rao, J., et al.: Phenotypic heterogeneity in cellular origins of T-cell malignancies. Leuk. Res. 5:281, 1981.
55. Andres, T. L., and Kadin, M. E.: Immunological markers in the differential diagnosis of small round cell tumors from lymphocytic lymphoma and leukemia. Am. J. Clin. Pathol. 79:546, 1983.
56. Nathwani, B. N., Kim, H., et al.: Malignant lymphoma, lymphoblastic. Cancer 38:964, 1976.
57. Nathwani, B. N., Diamond, L. W., et al.: Lymphoblastic lymphoma: a clinical pathological study of 95 patients. Cancer 48:2347, 1981.
58. Bernard, A., Boumsell, L., et al.: Cell surface characterization of malignant T-cells from lymphoblastic lymphoma using monoclonal antibodies: evidence for phenotypic differences between malignant T-cells from patients with acute lymphoblastic leukemia and lymphoblastic lymphoma. Blood 57:1105, 1981.
59. Roper, M., Crist, W. M., et al.: Monoclonal antibody characterization of surface antigens in childhood T-cell lymphoid malignancies. Blood 61:830, 1983.
59a. Foon, K. A., Todd, R. F., III: Immunologic classification of leukemia and lymphoma. Blood 68:1, 1986.
60. Stein, H., Petersen, N., et al.: Lymphoblastic lymphoma of convoluted or acid phosphatase type-A tumor of T precursor cells. Int. J. Cancer 17:292, 1976.
61. Murphy, S. B., and Mauer, A. M.: Terminal transferase and lymphoblastic neoplasms. New Engl. J. Med. 297:502, 1977.
62. Braziel, R. M., Keneklis, T., et al.: Terminal deoxynucleotidyl transferase in non-Hodgkin's lymphoma. Am. J. Clin. Pathol. 80:655, 1983.
63. Cossman, J., Chused, T. M., et al.: Diversity of immunological phenotypes of lymphoblastic lymphoma. Cancer Res. 43:4486, 1983.

64. Link, M. P., Roper, M., et al.: Cutaneous lymphoblastic lymphoma with pre-B markers. Blood 61:838, 1983.
65. Burkitt, D.: A sarcoma involving the jaws in the African children. Br. J. Surg. 46:218, 1958.
66. Magrath, I. T., Freeman, C. B., et al.: Characterization of lymphoma-derived cell lines: comparison of cell lines positive and negative for Epstein-Barr virus nuclear antigen. II. Surface markers. J. Natl. Cancer Inst. 64:477, 1980.
67. Lenoir, G., and O'Conor, G. (eds.): *Burkitt's Lymphoma: A Human Cancer Model.* Oxford, IARC Scientific Publications, Oxford University Press, 1985.
68. Memoranda: Histopathologic definition of Burkitt's tumour. Bull. WHO 40:601, 1969.
69. Grogan, T. M., Warnke, R. N., et al.: A comparative study of Burkitt's and non-Burkitt's "undifferentiated" malignant lymphoma: immunologic, cytochemical, ultrastructural, cytologic, histopathologic, clinical and cell culture features. Cancer 49:1817, 1982.
70. Mann, R. B., Jaffe, E. S., et al.: Non-endemic Burkitt's lymphoma. A B-cell tumor related to germinal centers. New Engl. J. Med. 295:685, 1976.
71. Preud'homme, J. L., Dellagi, K., et al.: Immunological markers of Burkitt's lymphoma cells. In *Burkitt's Lymphoma: A Human Cancer Model.* Lenoir, G. M., O'Conor, G. T., et al. (eds.). Oxford, IARC Scientific Publications, Oxford University Press, 1985, pp. 47–64.
72. Magrath, I., Benjamin, B., et al.: Serum monoclonal immunoglobulin bands in undifferentiated lymphomas of Burkitt's and non-Burkitt's types. Blood 61:726, 1983.
73. Lenoir, G. M., Preud'homme, J. L., et al.: Correlation between immunoglobulin light-chain expression and variant translocations in Burkitt's lymphoma. Nature 298: 474, 1982.
74. Bennett, J. M., Catovsky, D., et al.: Proposals for the classification of acute leukemias. French-American-British (FAB) cooperative group. Br. J. Haematol. 33:451, 1976.
75. Magrath, I., and Ziegler, J. L.: Bone marrow involvement in Burkitt's lymphoma and its relationship to acute B-cell leukemia. Leuk. Res. 4:33, 1979.
76. Preud'homme, J., Brouet, J., et al.: Acute lymphoblastic leukemia with Burkitt's lymphoma cells: membrane markers and serum immunoglobulin. J. Natl. Cancer Inst. 66:261, 1981.
77. Habeshaw, J. A., and Stuart, A. E.: Cell receptor studies on 7 cases of diffuse histiocytic malignant lymphoma (reticulum cell sarcoma). J. Clin. Pathol. 28:289, 1975.
78. Morris, M. W., and Davey, F. R.: Immunologic and cytochemical properties of histiocytic and mixed histiocytic-lymphocytic lymphomas. Am. J. Clin. Pathol. 63:403, 1975.
79. Warnke, R., Miller, R., et al.: Immunologic phenotype in 30 patients with diffuse large cell lymphoma. New Engl. J. Med. 393:293, 1980.
80. Jenkin, R. D. T.: The management of malignant lymphoma in childhood. In *Modern Radiotherapy—Malignant Disease in Children.* Deeley, T. J. (ed.), London, Butterworths and Co., 1974. pp. 341–359.
81. Arseneau, T. C., Canellos, G. P., et al.: American Burkitt's lymphoma: A clinicopathologic study of 30 cases. I. Clinical factors relating to prolonged survival. Am. J. Med. 58:314, 1975.
82. Murphy, S. B., and Caces, J.: Limited utility of bone marrow biopsy in staging children with non-Hodgkin's lymphoma. Blood 52:573, 1978.
83. Castellino, R. A., Bellani, F. F., et al.: Radiographic findings in previously untreated children with non-Hodgkin's lymphoma. Radiology 117:657, 1975.
84. Martin, D. J., and Ash, J. M.: Diagnostic radiology in non-Hodgkin's lymphoma. Semin. Oncol. 4:297, 1977.
85. Jaffe, N., Buell, D., et al.: Role of staging in childhood non-Hodgkin's lymphoma. Cancer Treat. Rep. 61:1001, 1977.
86. Pilepich, M. V., Rene, J. B., et al.: Contribution of computed tomography to the treatment of lymphomas. Am. J. Roentenol. 131:69, 1978.
87. Ellert, J., and Kreel, L.: The role of computed tomography in the initial staging and subsequent management of the lymphomas. J. Comput. Assist. Tomogr. 4:368, 1980.
88. Castellino, R. A.: Imaging techniques for extent determination of Hodgkin's disease and non-Hodgkin's lymphomas. Prog. Clin. Biol. Res., 13th International Cancer Congress, Part D, Research and Treatment. New York, A. R. Liss, 1983, pp. 365–372.
89. Zea, J. M., Exelby, P. R., et al.: Abdominal non-Hodgkin's lymphoma in childhood. J. Pediatr. Surg. 11:363, 1976.
90. Jenkin, R. D. T., Sonley, M. J., et al.: Primary gastrointestinal tract lymphoma in childhood. Radiology 92:763, 1969.
91. Ziegler, J. L.: Treatment results of 54 American patients with Burkitt's lymphoma are similar to the African experience. New Engl. J. Med. 297:75, 1977.
92. Magrath, I. T., Janus, C., et al.: An effective therapy for both undifferentiated (including Burkitt's) lymphomas and lymphoblastic lymphomas in children and young adults. Blood 63:1102, 1984.
93. Murphy, S. B.: Prognostic features and obstacles to cure of childhood non-Hodgkin's lymphoma. Semin. Oncol. 4:265, 1977.
94. Anderson, J. R., Wilson, J. F., et al.: Childhood non-Hodgkin's lymphoma. The results of a randomized therapeutic trial comparing a four-drug regimen (COMP) with a 10-drug regimen (LSA$_2$-L$_2$). New Engl. J. Med. 308:559, 1983.
95. Wollner, N.: LSA$_2$-L$_2$ in childhood non-Hodgkin's lymphoma. In: *Malignant Lymphomas.* Rosenberg, S. A., and Kaplan, H. S. (eds.), New York, Academic Press, 1982, pp. 603–626.
96. Murphy. S. B., Hustu, H. O., et al.: End results of treating children with localized non-Hodgkin's lymphoma with a combined modality approach of lessened intensity. J. Clin. Oncol. 1:326, 1983.
97. Jenkin, R. D. T., Anderson, J. R., et al.: The treatment of localized non-Hodgkin's lymphoma in children: a report from the Children's Cancer Study Group. J. Clin. Oncol. 2:88, 1984.
98. Sullivan, M. P., Boyett, J., et al.: Pediatric Oncology group experience with modified LSA$_2$-L$_2$ therapy in 107 children with non-Hodgkin's lymphoma (Burkitt's lymphoma excluded). Cancer, 55:323, 1985.
98a. Hvizdala, E., Berard, C., et al.: Histology and stage related response to therapy in children with non-Hodgkin's lymphoma. Blood 62:213a, 1983.
99. Murphy, S. B., and Hustu, H. O.: A randomized trial of combined modality therapy of childhood non-Hodgkin's lymphoma. Cancer 45:630, 1980.
100. Muller-Weihrich, S., Henze, G., et al.: The BFM studies 1975–1981 on the treatment of high grade non-Hodgkin's lymphomas of children and young adults. Klin. Paediatr. 194:219, 1982 (in German).
101. Patte, C., Rodary, C., et al.: Résultats du traitement de 178 lymphomes malins non-Hodgkiniens de l'enfant de 1973 à 1978. Arch. Fr. Pediatr. 38:321, 1981.
102. Carabell, S. C., Cassady, J. R., et al.: The role of radiation therapy in the treatment of pediatric non-Hodgkin's lymphomas. Cancer 42:2193, 1978.
103. Weinstein, A. J., and Link, M. P.: Non-Hodgkin's lymphoma in childhood. Clin. Haematol. 8:699, 1979.
104. Mott, M., Eden, O. B., et al.: Adjuvant low dose radiation in childhood non-Hodgkin's lymphoma. Br. J. Cancer 50:463, 1984.
105. Gasparini, M., Lombardi, F., et al.: Childhood non-Hodgkin's lymphoma: prognostic relevance of clinical stages and histologic subgroups. Am. J. Pediatr. Hematol. Oncol. 5:161, 1983.
106. Duque-Hammershaimb, L., Wollner, N., et al.: LSA$_2$-L$_2$

protocol treatment of Stage IV non-Hodgkin's lymphoma in children with partial and extensive bone marrow involvement. Cancer 52:39, 1983.
107. Jenkin, R. D. T.: Radiation in the treatment of non-Hodgkin's lymphoma in children. Semin. Oncol. 4:311, 1977.
108. Weinstein, H. J., Vance, Z. B., et al.: Improved prognosis for patients with mediastinal lymphoblastic lymphoma. Blood 53:687, 1979.
109. Weinstein, H. J., Cassady, J. R., et al.: Long-term results of the APO protocol (vincristine, doxorubicin [Adriamycin], and prednisone) for treatment of mediastinal lymphoma. J. Clin. Oncol. 1:537, 1983.
110. Dahl, G. V., Rivera, G., et al.: A novel treatment of childhood lymphoblastic non-Hodgkin's lymphoma: early and intermittent use of Temposide plus Cytarabine. Blood 66:1110, 1985.
111. Murphy, S. B.: Strategies for management of childhood non-Hodgkin's lymphomas based upon stage and immunopathologic subtype: rationale and current results. In *Malignant Lymphomas and Hodgkin's Disease: Experimental and Therapeutic Advances.* Cavalli, F. (ed.), Boston, Martinus Nijhoff Publ., 1985, pp. 627–632.
112. Link, M., Donaldson, S., et al.: Effective therapy with reduced toxicity for children with localized non-Hodgkin's lymphoma. Proc. Am. Soc. Clin. Oncol., 3:251, 1984.
113. Murphy, S. B., Bowman, W. P., et al.: Results of advanced stage Burkitt's lymphoma and B-cell (SIq+) acute lymphoblastic leukemia with high-dose fractionated cyclophosphamide and coordinated high-dose methotrexate and cytarabine. J. Clin. Oncol., in press, 1986.
114. Ramirez, I., Sullivan, M. P., et al.: Effective therapy for Burkitt's lymphoma: high-dose cyclophosphamide plus high-dose methotrexate with coordinated intrathecal therapy. Cancer Chemother. Pharmacol. 3:103, 1979.
115. Lemerle, J.: The treatment of B-cell non-Hodgkin's malignant lymphomas of childhood in Europe—recent and ongoing studies. In *Burkitt's Lymphoma: A Human Cancer Model.* Lenoir, G. M., O'Conor, G. T., et al. (eds.), Oxford, IARC Scientific Publications, Oxford University Press, 1985, pp. 47–64.
116. Hutter, J. J., Favara, B. E., et al.: Non-Hodgkin's lymphoma in children. Correlation of CNS disease with initial presentation. Cancer 36:2132, 1975.
117. Willoughby, M.: Bone marrow and CNS involvement in non-Hodgkin's lymphoma. In *Non-Hodgkin's Lymphomas in Children.* Graham-Pole, J. (ed.), New York, Masson Publishing, 1980, pp. 147–163.
118. Ziegler, J. L., Bluming, A. Z., et al.: Central nervous involvement in Burkitt's lymphoma. Blood 36:718, 1970.
119. Paryani, S. B., Donaldson, S. S., et al.: Cranial nerve involvement in children with leukemia and lymphoma. J. Clin. Oncol. 1:542, 1983.
120. O'Leary, M., Ramsey, N. K. C., et al.: Bone marrow transplantation for non-Hodgkin's lymphoma in children and young adults. A pilot study. Am. J. Med. 74:497, 1983.
121. Philip, T., Pinkerton, R., et al.: The role of massive therapy with autologous bone marrow transplantation. Clin. Haematol. 15:205, 1986.
122. Lynch, R. E., Kjellstrand, C. M., et al.: Renal and metabolic complications of childhood non-Hodgkin's lymphoma. Semin. Oncol. 4:325, 1977.
123. D'Angio, G. J.: Complications of treatment encountered in lymphoma-leukemia long term survivors. Cancer 42:1015, 1978.
124. Simone, J. V.: Late complications of treatment of children with leukemia and lymphoma. In *Malignant Lymphomas.* Rosenberg, S. A., and Kaplan, H. S. (eds.), New York, Academic Press, 1982, pp. 663–673.
125. Kaplan, H. S.,: Hodgkin's disease: biology, treatment, prognosis. Blood 57:813, 1981.
126. Fuks, Z., Strober, S., et al.: Long-term effects of radiation on T and B lymphocytes in peripheral blood of patients with Hodgkin's disease. J. Clin. Invest. 58:803, 1976.
127. King, G. W., Yanes, B., et al.: Immune function of successfully treated lymphoma patients. J. Clin. Invest. 57:1451, 1976.
128. Young, R. C., Corder, M. P., et al.: Immune alterations in Hodgkin's disease. Arch. Intern. Med. 131:446, 1973.
129. Levy, R., and Kaplan, H. S.: Impaired lymphocyte function in untreated Hodgkin's disease. New Engl. J. Med. 290:81, 1974.
130. Holm, G., Mellstedt, H., et al.: Lymphocyte abnormalities in untreated patients with Hodgkin's disease. Cancer 37:751, 1976.
131. Bobrove, A. M., Fuks, Z., et al.: Quantitation of T and B lymphocytes and cellular immune function in Hodgkin's disease. Cancer 36:169, 1975.
132. Longmire, R. L., McMillan, R., et al.: *In vitro* splenic IgG synthesis in Hodgkin's disease. New Engl. J. Med. 289:763, 1973.
133. Fuks, Z., Strober, S., et al.: Interaction between serum factors and T lymphocytes in Hodgkin's disease. New Engl. J. Med. 295:1273, 1976.
134. Aisenberg, A. C.: Immunologic status of Hodgkin's disease. Cancer 19:385, 1966.
135. Casazza, A., Duvall, C. P., et al.: Summary of infectious complications occurring in patients with Hodgkin's disease. Cancer Res. 26:1290, 1966.
136. Lukes, R. S.: Criteria for involvement of lymph node, bone marrow, spleen and liver in Hodgkin's disease. Cancer Res. 31:1755, 1971.
136a. Henle, W., and Henle, G.: Epstein-Barr virus–related serology in Hodgkin's disease. In *International Symposium on Hodgkin's Disease.* Natl. Cancer Inst. Monogr. 36, U.S. Dept. of Health, Education and Welfare, 1973, pp. 79–84.
137. Anagnostou, D., Parker, J., et al.: Lacunar cells of nodular sclerosing Hodgkin's disease. Cancer 39:1032, 1977.
138. Kadin, M.: Possible origin of the Reed-Sternberg cell from an interdigitating reticulum cell. Cancer Treat. Rep. 66:601, 1982.
139. Stein, H., Gerdes, J., et al.: Identification of Hodgkin's and Sternberg-Reed cells as a unique cell type derived from a newly detected small cell population. Int. J. Cancer 30:445, 1982.
140. Lukes, R. J., and Butler, J. J.: The pathology and nomenclature of Hodgkin's disease. Cancer Res. 26:1063, 1966.
141. Lukes, R. J., Butler, J. J., et al.: Natural history of Hodgkin's disease as related to its histologic picture. Cancer 19:317, 1966.
142. Butler, J. J.: Relationship of histologic findings to survival in Hodgkin's disease. Cancer Res. 31:1770, 1971.
143. Keller, A. R., Kaplan, H. S., et al.: Correlation of histopathology with other prognostic indicators in Hodgkin's disease. Cancer 22:487, 1968.
144. Nieman, R. S., Rosen, P. J., et al.: Lymphocyte-depletion Hodgkin's disease. A clinicopathological entity. New Engl. J. Med. 288:751, 1973.
145. Young, R. C., DeVita, V. T., et al.: Hodgkin's disease in childhood. Blood 42:163, 1973.
146. Strum, S., and Rappaport, H.: Hodgkin's disease in the first decade of life. Pediatrics 46:748, 1970.
147. Shah, N. K., Freeman, A. I., et al.: Hodgkin's disease in children. Med. Pediatr. Oncol. 2:87, 1976.
148. Smith, K. C., and Rivera, G.: Comparison of the clinical course of Hodgkin's disease in children and adolescents. Med. Pediatr. Oncol. 2:361, 1976.
149. Norris, D. G., Burgert, E. O., et al.: Hodgkin's disease in childhood. Cancer 36:2109, 1975.
150. Donaldson, S. S., Glatstein, E., et al.: Pediatric Hodgkin's disease. II. Results of therapy. Cancer 37:2436, 1976.
151. Tan, C., D'Angio, G. J., et al.: The changing management of childhood Hodgkin's disease. Cancer 35:808, 1975.

152. Schnitzer, B., Nishizama, R. H., et al.: Hodgkin's disease in children. Cancer *34*:560, 1973.
153. Teillet, F., and Schweisguth, O.: Hodgkin's disease in children. Clin. Pediatr. *8*:698, 1969.
154. Garwicz, S., Lanberg, T., et al.: Malignant lymphomas in children. A clinico-pathologic retrospective study. I. Hodgkin's disease. Acta Paediatr. Scand. *63*:673, 1974.
155. Ultmann, J. E., Cunningham, J. K., et al.: The clinical picture of Hodgkin's disease. Cancer Res. *26*:1047, 1966.
156. O'Carroll, D. I., McKenna, R. W., et al.: Bone marrow manifestations of Hodgkin's disease. Cancer *38*:1717, 1976.
157. Kass, L., and Votaw, M. L.: Eosinophilia and plasmacytosis of the bone marrow in Hodgkin's disease. Am. J. Clin. Pathol. *64*:248, 1975.
158. Rosenberg, S. A., Boiron, M., et al.: Report of the committee on Hodgkin's disease staging procedures. Cancer Res. *31*:1862, 1971.
159. Desforges, J. S., Rutherford, C. J., et al.: Hodgkin's disease. New Engl. J. Med. *301*:1212, 1979.
160. Rostock, R. A.: New aspects of Hodgkin's disease: staging for conservative management. Crit. Rev. Oncol. Hematol. *1*:295, 1984.
161. Green, D. M., Ghoorah, J., et al.: Staging laparotomy with splenectomy in children and adolescents with Hodgkin's disease. Cancer Treat. Rev. *10*:23, 1983.
162. Parker, B. R., Castellino, R. A., et al.: Pediatric Hodgkin's disease. I. Radiographic evaluation. Cancer *37*:2430, 1976.
163. Musumeci, R., Fossati-Bellani, F., et al.: Usefulness of lymphography in childhood neoplasia. Cancer *29*:51, 1972.
164. Castellino, R. A., and Marglin, S. I.: Imaging of abdominal and pelvic lymph nodes: lymphography or computed tomography? Invest.Radiol. *17*:433, 1982.
165. Horn, N. L., Ray, G. R., et al.: Gallium-67 citrate scanning in Hodgkin's disease and non-Hodgkin's lymphoma. Cancer *37*:250, 1976.
166. Milder, M. S., Larson, S. M., et al.: Liver-spleen scan in Hodgkin's disease. Cancer *31*:826, 1973.
167. Rosenberg, S. A.: Splenectomy in the management of Hodgkin's disease. Br. J. Haematol. *23*:271, 1972.
168. Lanzkowsky, P., Shende, A., et al.: Staging laparotomy and splenectomy: Treatment and complications of Hodgkin's disease in children. Am. J. Hematol. *1*:393, 1976.
169. Gamble, J. F., Fuller, L. M., et al.: Influence of staging celiotomy in localized presentations of Hodgkin's disease. Cancer *35*:817, 1975.
170. Aisenberg, A. C., and Qazi, R.: Abdominal involvement at the onset of Hodgkin's disease. Am. J. Med. *57*:870, 1974.
171. Hayes, D. M., Karon, M., et al.: Hodgkin's disease. Technique and results of staging laparotomy in childhood. Arch. Surg. *106*:507, 1973.
172. Dent, D. M., King, H. S., et al.: The value of laparotomy in staging lymphoma. Surg. Gynecol. Obstet. *145*:179, 1977.
173. Panettiere, F., Coltman, C. A., et al.: Splenectomy, chemotherapy, and survival in Hodgkin's disease. Arch. Intern. Med. *137*:341, 1977.
174. Ihde, D. C., DeVita, V. T., et al.: Effect of splenectomy on tolerance to combination chemotherapy in patients with lymphoma. Blood *47*:211, 1976.
175. Chilcote, R. R., Baehner, R. L., et al.: Septicemia and meningitis in children splenectomized for Hodgkin's disease. New Engl. J. Med. *295*:798, 1976.
176. Larson, R. A., and Ultmann, J. E.: The strategic role of laparotomy in staging Hodgkin's disease. Cancer Treat. Rep. *66*:767, 1982.
177. Stein, R. S., Golomb, H. M., et al.: Anatomic substages of Stage IIIA Hodgkin's disease: follow-up of a collaborative study. Cancer Treat. Rep. *66*:733, 1982.
178. Carbone, P. P., Kaplan, H. S., et al.: Report of the committee on Hodgkin's disease staging classification. Cancer Res. *31*:1860, 1971.
179. Botnick, L. E., Goodman, R., et al.: Stages I-III Hodgkin's disease in children. Results of staging and treatment. Cancer *39*:599, 1977.
180. Jenkin, R. D. T., and Barry, M. T.: Hodgkin's disease in children. Semin. Oncol. *7*:202, 1980.
181. Donaldson, S. S.: Hodgkin's disease. Treatment with low-dose radiation and chemotherapy. Front. Radiat. Ther. Oncol. *16*:122, Basel, Karger, 1982.
182. Breu, H., Schellong, G., et al.: Graduated chemotherapy and reduced radiation dose in Hodgkin's disease in children: report on 170 patients in a cooperative study HD-78. Klin. Paediatr. *194*:233, 1982.
183. Fossati-Bellani, F., Kenda, R., et al.: ABVD combined with low-dose limited field radiotherapy for Stage I, II, III childhood Hodgkin's disease. Proc. Am. Assoc. Cancer Res. *25*:195, 1984.
184. Bayle-Weisgerber, C., Lemercier, N., et al.: Hodgkin's disease in children. Results of therapy in a mixed group of 178 clinical and pathologically staged patients over 13 years. Cancer *54*:215, 1984.
185. Robinson, B., Kingston, J., et al.: Chemotherapy and irradiation in childhood Hodgkin's disease. Arch. Dis. Child. *59*:1162, 1984.
186. Hellman, S., and Mauch, P.: Role of radiation therapy in the treatment of Hodgkin's disease. Cancer Treat. Rep. *66*:915, 1982.
187. Hoppe, R. T.: Radiation therapy in the treatment of Hodgkin's disease. Semin. Oncol. *7*.144, 1980.
188. A collaborative study. Survival and complications of radiotherapy following involved and extended field therapy of Hodgkin's disease. Stages I and II. Cancer *38*:288, 1976.
189. Rosenberg, F. A., Kaplan, H. S., et al.: The Stanford randomized trials of the treatment of Hodgkin's disease: 1967–1980. In *Malignant Lymphomas*. Rosenberg, S. A., and Kaplan, H. S. (eds.) New York, Academic Press, 1982, pp. 513–522.
190. Hoppe, R. T.: Stage I–II Hodgkin's disease: current therapeutic options and recommendations. Blood *62*:32, 1983.
191. Sullivan, M. P., Fuller, L. M., et al.: Prognostic factors and late effects: Innovative guidelines for selective, age-conditioned therapy for Hodgkin's disease in children. In *Conflicts in Childhood Cancer*, Vol. 4, Sinks, L. F., and Godden, J. O. (eds.), Progress in Clinical and Biological Research. New York, Alan R. Liss, Inc., 1975, pp. 103–115.
192. Fuller, L. M., Sullivan, M. P., et al.: Results of regional radiotherapy in localized Hodgkin's disease in children. Cancer *32*:640, 1973.
193. Cham, W. C., Tan, C. T. C., et al.: Involved field radiation therapy for early stage Hodgkin's disease in children. Cancer *37*:1625, 1976.
194. DeVita, V. T., Hubbard, S. M., et al.: The cure of Hodgkin's disease with drugs. Adv. Intern. Med. *28*:277, 1983.
195. Bonadonna, G.: Chemotherapy strategies to improve the control of Hodgkin's disease. Cancer Res. *42*:4309, 1982.
196. Coltman, C. A.: Chemotherapy of advanced Hodgkin's disease. Semin. Oncol. *7*:155, 1980.
197. Canellos, G. P., Come, S. E., et al.: Chemotherapy in the treatment of Hodgkin's disease. Semin. Hematol. *20*:1, 1983.
198. DeVita, V. T., Serpick, A. A., et al.: Combination chemotherapy in the treatment of advanced Hodgkin's disease. Ann. Intern. Med. *73*:881, 1970.
199. DeVita, V. T., Simon, R., et al.: Curability of advanced Hodgkin's disease with chemotherapy: long-term follow-up of MOPP-treated patients at the National Cancer Institute. Ann. Intern. Med. *92*:587, 1980.
200. Santoro, A., Bonadonna, G., et al.: Alternating drug

200. combinations in the treatment of advanced Hodgkin's disease. New Engl. J. Med. *306*:770, 1982.
201. Bonadonna, G., Viviani, S., et al.: Alternating chemotherapy with MOPP/ABVD in Hodgkin's disease. Proc. Am. Soc. Clin. Oncol. *3*:254, 1984.
202. Tubiana, M., and Mathe, G.: Combined radiotherapy and chemotherapy in the treatment of Hodgkin's disease. Ser. Haematol. *VI*:202, 1973.
203. Kun, L. E., DeVita, V. T., et al.: Treatment of Hodgkin's disease using intensive chemotherapy followed by irradiation. Int. J. Radiat. Oncol. Biol. Phys. *1*:619, 1976.
204. Mauch, P. M., Weinstein, H., et al.: An evaluation of long-term survival and treatment complications in children with Hodgkin's disease. Cancer *51*:925, 1983.
205. Wilimas, J., Thompson, E., et al.: Long-term results of treatment of children and adolescents with Hodgkin's disease. Cancer *46*:2123, 1980.
206. Lange, B., and Littman, P.: Management of Hodgkin's disease in children and adolescents. Cancer *51*:1371, 1983.
207. Prosnitz, L. R.: Radiation doses following intensive chemotherapy in the treatment of Hodgkin's disease. Int. J. Radiat. Oncol. Biol. Phys. *1*:803, 1976.
208. Mauch, P., Ryback, M. E., et al.: The influence of initial pathologic stage on the survival of patients who relapse from Hodgkin's disease. Blood *56*:892, 1980.
209. Levi, J. A., Wiernik, P. H., et al.: Patterns of relapse in Stages I, II, and IIIA Hodgkin's disease: influence of initial therapy and implications for the future. Int. J. Radiat. Oncol. Biol. Phys. *2*:853, 1977.
210. Russell, K. J., Donaldson, S. S., et al.: Childhood Hodgkin's disease: patterns of relapse. J. Clin. Oncol. *2*:80, 1984.
211. Weller, S. A., Glatstein, E., et al.: Initial relapses in previously treated Hodgkin's disease. I. Results of second treatment. Cancer *37*:2840, 1976.
212. Portlock, C. S., Rosenberg, S. A., et al.: Impact of salvage treatment on initial relapses in patients with Hodgkin's disease, Stages I–III. Blood *51*:825, 1978.
213. Kaplan, H. S., and Rosenberg, S. A.: The management of Hodgkin's disease. Cancer *36*:796, 1975.
214. Donaldson, S. S., and Kaplan, H. S.: Complications of treatment of Hodgkin's disease in children. Cancer Treat. Rep. *66*:977, 1982.
215. Carmel, R. J., and Kaplan, H. S.: Mantle irradiation in Hodgkin's disease. An analysis of technique, tumor eradication, and complications. Cancer *37*:2813, 1976.
216. Byhardt, R., Brace, K., et al.: Dose and treatment factors in radiation-related pericardial effusion associated with mantle technique for Hodgkin's disease. Cancer *35*:795, 1975.
217. Thomas, P. R. M., Winstanly, D., et al.: Reproduction and endocrine function in patients with Hodgkin's disease: Effects of oophoropexy and irradiation. Br. J. Cancer *33*:226, 1976.
218. LeFloch, O., Donaldson, S. S., et al.: Pregnancy following oophoropexy and total nodal irradiation in women with Hodgkin's disease. Cancer *38*:2263, 1976.
219. Schein, P. S., and Winokur, S. H.: Immunosuppressive and cytotoxic chemotherapy: Long-term complications. Ann. Intern. Med. *82*:84, 1975.
220. Sherins, R. J., and DeVita, V. T.: Effect of drug treatment for lymphoma on male reproductive capacity: Studies of men in remission after therapy. Ann. Intern. Med. *79*:216, 1973.
221. Probert, J. C., and Parker, B. R.: The effect of radiation therapy on bone growth. Radiology *114*:155, 1975.
222. Coleman, C. N., Williams, C. J., et al.: Hematologic neoplasia in patients treated for Hodgkin's disease. New Engl. J. Med. *297*:1249, 1977.
223. Arseneau, J. C., Sponzo, R. W., et al.: Non-lymphomatous malignant tumors complicating Hodgkin's disease. Possible association with intensive therapy. New Engl. J. Med. *287*:1119, 1972.
224. Greenberger, J. S., Come, S. E., et al.: Issues of controversy in radiation therapy and combined modality approaches to Hodgkin's disease. Clin. Haematol. *8*:611, 1979.
225. Mauch, P., Goodman, R., et al.: The significance of mediastinal involvement in early stage Hodgkin's disease. Cancer *42*:1039, 1978.
226. Glick, J. H.: The treatment of Stage IIIA Hodgkin's disease: What is the role of combined modality therapy? Int. J. Rad. Oncol. Biol. Phys. *4*:909, 1978.
227. Rutherford, C. J., Desforges, J. F., et al.: The decision between single- and combined modality therapy in Hodgkin's disease. Am. J. Med. *72*:63, 1982.

ONCOLOGY

CHAPTER 36
Lymphohistiocytic Disorders

JOHN L. SULLIVAN
BRUCE A. WODA

INTRODUCTION 1118
THE MONONUCLEAR PHAGOCYTIC SYSTEM 1118
Cellular Components
  Monocytes and Macrophages
  Dendritic Cells
Lymphoreticular Responses to Viral Infections
REACTIVE LYMPHOHISTIOCYTOSES 1121
Familial Erythrophagocytic Lymphohistiocytosis
X-linked Lymphoproliferative Syndrome
Virus-Associated Hemophagocytic Syndrome
Sinus Histiocytosis with Massive Lymphadenopathy
Lymphomatoid Granulomatosis
Differential Diagnosis of Reactive Lymphohistiocytoses
LANGERHANS HISTIOCYTOSES (HISTIOCYTOSES X) 1129
Eosinophilic Granuloma
Hand-Schüller-Christian Disease
Letterer-Siwe Disease
MALIGNANT HISTIOCYTOSES (HISTIOCYTIC MEDULLARY RETICULOSIS) 1131

INTRODUCTION

Immunologic and virologic studies performed in patients suffering from lymphohistiocytic disorders have provided new information regarding their pathogenesis. This chapter will focus on the clinical and immunopathologic features of the reactive and neoplastic lymphohistiocytic syndromes. Included in these syndromes are disorders of the lymphocytic and mononuclear phagocyte–dendritic cell systems.

THE MONONUCLEAR PHAGOCYTIC SYSTEM

Cellular Components

Macrophages, the cells of the phagocytic system, are bone marrow–derived cells that share a common progenitor with granulocytes; together these cells make up the colony-forming unit–granulocyte-macrophge (CFU-GM) (1). Promonocytes leave the marrow and enter the blood as monocytes. They remain in the blood pool for a relatively short period of time (2) and then enter the tissues, where they reside as macrophages. The macrophages that populate the liver are known as Kupffer's cells; those in the lung are termed alveolar macrophages. The microglial cells of the brain may be derived from marrow progenitors, but this is not yet firmly established. In the spleen, macrophages reside in the red pulp and line the sinusoids. In lymph nodes, macrophages reside predominantly in the sinusoids (3, 4, 5).

MONOCYTES AND MACROPHAGES

Monocytes and macrophages can be identified by morphologic, histochemical, or immunologic methods. Monocytes, which are circulating cells, measure 12 to 15 μ. They have kidney-shaped nuclei and abundant cytoplasm that appears blue-gray when stained with hematoxylin-eosin. They may have cytoplasmic vacuoles and small azurophilic granules. Ultrastructural studies have identified numerous lysosomes and a well-developed Golgi apparatus within these cells. They have a well-developed cytoskeletal system (6). Monocytes contain many enzymes that are useful for their characterization, such as nonspecific esterase activity, which is sodium-fluoride sensitive. They also contain peroxidase, lysozyme, β-glucuronidase, aryl sulfatase, acid phosphatase, and α-1-antitrypsin. They may stain weakly for 5′-nucleotidase and adenosine triphosphatase (ATPase). Monocytes are adherent cells and have phagocytic activity.

They may be identified by their surface receptors (e.g., Fc and C3 receptors) and by monocyte-specific proteins identifiable with monoclonal antibodies (7, 8, 9).

Macrophages, which are fixed in tissues, represent a further maturational stage of monocytes. They vary in size from 20 to 80 μ. As seen by light microscopy they have a homogeneously staining, vesicular nucleus, often with a small nucleolus. They have pale pink cytoplasm that may contain phagocytosed debris. Ultrastructural studies demonstrate that, compared with their monocytic precursors, these cells have an increased amount of rough endoplasmic reticulum and more ribosomes. They contain many lysosomes, phagocytic vacuoles, endosomes, and mitochondria. Mature macrophages have little peroxidase. The plasma membrane has numerous microvilli (6). These cells are adherent and more motile than monocytes, and they have increased numbers of Fc and C3 receptors. They possess receptors for IgG_{1-2b}, IgG_{2a}, IgG_3, and IgE (10, 11, 12). A subset of macrophages express surface HLA-DR antigen. The expression of HLA-DR is dependent on the release of interferon by immune T lymphocytes. It is the HLA-DR–bearing subset of macrophages that is active in antigen presentation (13). Recent data demonstrate that the DR^+DQ^+ macrophage is also active in antigen presentation (14). Macrophages secrete many biologically active substances and have important immunoregulatory, phagocytic, and microbicidal functions. Histiocytes, which are fixed in tissues, represent a further maturational stage of macrophages. They are larger, have abundant eosinophilic cytoplasm, are avidly phagocytic, and have increased numbers of lysosomes. In certain locations, such as lymph node sinuses, cells of this series are always referred to as histiocytes.

DENDRITIC CELLS

Dendritic cells have not been studied as extensively as macrophages, because purification techniques for these cells have only recently been devised. Hence, less is known about dendritic cell function. They are bone marrow–derived cells (15) that are found in blood, lymph, skin, and peripheral lymphoid organs (16). The cells of the dendritic cell series are antigen-presenting cells and do not function as phagocytic elements. This series has been subdivided into Langerhans cells, interdigitating reticulum cells, and follicular dendritic cells, based predominantly on their location and minor structural and enzymatic differences. The most extensively studied dendritic cell is the Langerhans cell of the skin (17). In lymph, dendritic cells are referred to as veiled cells. In the lymph node paracortex, dendritic cells are called interdigitating reticulum cells, and the dendritic cells surrounding lymphoid follicles are referred to as follicular dendritic cells. It is thought that Langerhans cells and interdigitating reticulum cells present antigen to T cells, whereas the dendritic reticulum cells present antigen to B cells. Morphologically dendritic cells are aptly named, as they have a dendritic structure that is shown to best advantage with immunologic stains. Under light microscopy with hematoxylin-eosin stain, these cells are seen to have pink cytoplasm and a folded nucleus with granular chromatin. Electron microscopic study has shown that they have an irregular plasma membrane and variable amounts of lysosomes, lipids, and glycogen. They do not have the microvilli of macrophages. The dendritic cells of the skin contain Birbeck granules, which are pentalaminar membranous rod-shaped structures, 180 to 360 nm in length, with a central striated line (Fig. 36–1). A vesicular expansion of the membrane at one end results in a typical racquet shape. The dendritic reticulum cell has an elongated nucleus with scant cytoplasm and long cell processes (18, 19).

Dendritic cells have characteristic physical and immunologic properties (20). They are low-density cells that are adherent for short periods of time; however, they become nonadherent after prolonged incubation. Dendritic cells are nonphagocytic and show little pinocytotic activity. They have ATPase activity. They have weak acid phosphatase and nonspecific esterase activity. They do not contain peroxidase. These cells have C3 receptors and variable Fc receptor activity. They have a high density of HLA-DR (16, 18, 19). Interdigitating reticulum cells have identifiable ATPase and S-100 protein. Langerhans cells, like interdigitating reticulum cells, have ATPase activity and express

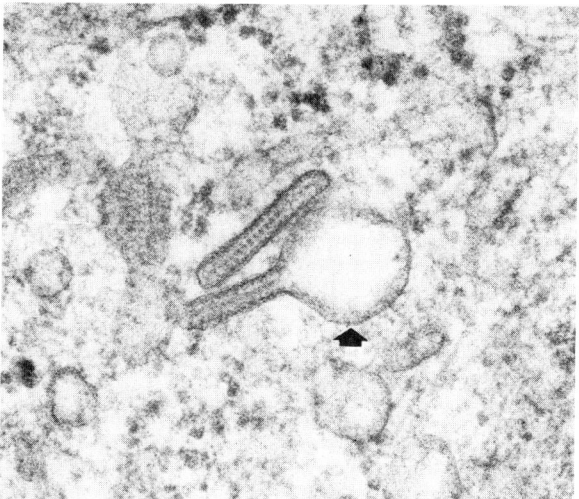

Figure 36–1. Electron micrograph showing Birbeck granules in a dendritic cell. These granules are membranous rod-shaped structures 180–360 nm in length with a central striated line. A vesicular expansion of the membrane at one end results in a typical racket shape (arrow) (×125,000.)

T-6 (21), a protein also found on immature thymocytes, and the S-100 protein (22, 23), a protein found on glial cells of the central nervous system. Dendritic reticulum cells are identifiable by monoclonal antibodies (24, 25) and by their 5'-nucleotidase activity. They secrete both interleukin I and prostaglandin E_2 (25a).

Profound reactive proliferative disorders are seen in cells of the macrophage-dendritic series, with some of these disorders resulting in appreciable morbidity and mortality. As of yet we know little about the pathogenesis or regulation of these reactive processes.

Lymphoreticular Responses to Viral Infections

Murine macrophages can be transformed into malignant histiocytes by a particular murine spleen focus forming RNA tumor virus (25b). Herpesvirus infections of man are among the most studied of human virus infections, and as such serve as prototypes for the study of lymphoreticular responses to viral infections (26–29). Of particular importance to the lymphoreticular system are the herpesviruses Epstein-Barr virus (EBV) and cytomegalovirus (CMV). Both of these viruses replicate in the lymphoreticular system and provoke intense immunologic responses that are responsible for the immunopathology and clinical symptomatology of herpes infections. These viruses remain latent in the lymphoreticular system following host recovery and can be reactivated during periods of immunosuppression, leading to further disease manifestations.

EBV and CMV are both acquired by oropharyngeal contact of a susceptible individual with a virus-containing secretion from a previously infected individual (26, 29). In the case of EBV, saliva appears to be the most common vehicle of viral spread, whereas for CMV, breast milk and saliva are the important infectious secretions. EBV and CMV infection of the host oropharyngeal tissue begins with the initial infection of the nasopharyngeal epithelial cells (30). Through this epithelial cell intermediate, the viruses gain access to the lymphoreticular system. In the case of EBV, infection of the B lymphocyte–rich tonsillopharyngeal tissue occurs, and viral replication is initiated. EBV-infected B lymphocytes are disseminated throughout the lymphoid system, with large numbers of EBV-infected B cells appearing in the circulation. The specific cell in which CMV replicates is not known. Virus has been recovered from polymorphonuclear leukocyte–rich fractions and mononuclear leukocyte–rich fractions (31, 32). Infection of peripheral blood monocytes has been demonstrated. Persistence of EBV infection in B lymphocytes has been demonstrated for the lifetime of an infected individual, while persistence of CMV infection in the peripheral blood has been documented up to 3 months following the onset of acute infection. The incubation period from initial contact with a virus excretor to the appearance of large numbers of EBV-infected B cells in the circulation is approximately 30 to 50 days.

In both acute EBV and CMV mononucleosis, the onset of clinical symptoms (fever, sore throat, lymphadenopathy, splenomegaly, and malaise) is associated with the presence of atypical lymphocytes in the peripheral blood. Epstein-Barr virus infects and replicates only in B lymphocytes. CMV infects and replicates in monocytes. Whether infection and replication in lymphocytes occur remains unanswered. EBV-infected B lymphocytes account for only a minority of the atypical lymphocytes found in the peripheral blood during acute EBV-induced infectious mononucleosis, yet nearly 20 per cent of all B cells in the circulation may be infected with the virus. The majority of the atypical lymphocytes appearing in both EBV and CMV infection are T lymphocytes. During the acute phase of both EBV- and CMV-induced infectious mononucleosis, there is a marked depression of cell-mediated immunity that can be clinically demonstrated by anergy to delayed cutaneous hypersensitivity skin tests. In vitro lymphocyte responses to plant mitogens, the mixed leukocyte reaction, and responses to soluble antigens are markedly depressed. During CMV-induced infectious mononucleosis it appears that infected monocyte-macrophages play a role in the suppression of T lymphocyte responses to the lectin concanavalin A (33). In both infections the majority of atypical lymphocytes belong to the T cytotoxic/suppressor cell population. There is an increase in the absolute numbers of T cytotoxic/suppressor cells, resulting in altered T helper/suppressor ratios, usually below 1.0, which may persist for weeks. Functional studies carried out in individuals with acute EBV-induced infectious mononucleosis have demonstrated that these cytotoxic/suppressor T cells can lyse EBV-infected B lymphocytes and suppress the polyclonal immunoglobulin secretion of EBV-infected B lymphocytes (26, 27). Cytotoxic T cells appearing during acute EBV infection behave differently from classic cytotoxic T cells in that they are not histocompatibility restricted. Classic cytotoxic T cells lyse virus-infected target cells only when the target cells bear one or more identical histocompatibility antigens. The function of cytotoxic/suppressor T cells induced during acute CMV monocleosis is less well characterized. It is known that HLA-restricted cytotoxic T lymphocytes are induced early during the course of cytomegalovirus infection in bone marrow transplant recipients (28). In addition to cytotoxic T lymphocytes, both CMV and EBV appear to induce natural killer cells, which lyse permissively infected target cells. There is strong evidence that natural killer cells play an important role in limiting virus spread early in the course of murine cytomegalovirus infection, and a similar role has also been suggested in the bone marrow transplant recipient experiencing cytomegalovirus infection (34, 35). Both CMV and EBV stimulate the production of interferons, which are important immunoregulatory molecules interacting with virtually every cell of the lymphoreticular system. Of particular interest are the recent observations demonstrating that gamma interferon produced by activated T lymphocytes is a potent activator of the monocyte-macrophage system. Gamma-interferon has been shown to be a necessary factor in inducing intracellular monocyte killing of certain microbial pathogens (36).

The cellular immune responses that occur following EBV and CMV are complex, and it is likely that these cellular events result in the immunopathologic process that accompanies acute infection. Although humoral immune responses appear to be important in preventing recurrent infections, current evidence suggests that cellular mechanisms are responsible for the control of acute and reactivation infections with these herpesviruses. Perturbations of these cellular immune responses may result in poorly controlled infections or in immunologic disease clinically manifested as one of the lymphohistiocytic disorders, discussed in the following section.

REACTIVE LYMPHOHISTIOCYTOSES

Familial Erythrophagocytic Lymphohistiocytosis

The name "familial erythrophagocytic lymphohistiocytosis" (FEL) was coined in 1963 by Mac-Mahon and colleagues (37), who noted that this disease entity was a "narrow but distinct category of uncommon familial diseases of infants and childhood involving primarily the lympho-reticuloendothelial system." While a similar group of diseases have been described under various other names (familial hemophagocytic reticulosis [23], generalized lymphohistiocytosis of infancy, familial lymphohistiocytosis), the term familial erythrophagocytic lymphohistiocytosis is most widely used because it describes the pathology characteristic of this syndrome.

This syndrome, like many other of the lymphohistiocytosis disorders, is characterized by fever, failure to thrive, hepatosplenomegaly, and anemia (37, 38, 39). Clinical discrimination from malignant histiocytosis is frequently difficult. Patients with FEL may have lymphoid, pulmonary, central nervous system, pericardial, bone and soft tissue, and gastrointestinal involvement. Leukopenia and a coagulopathy may be present. Circulating atypical or bizarre-appearing mononuclear cells are frequently present. Liver dysfunction is common with jaundice and elevated transaminases. A common laboratory finding in clinically severe FEL is elevation of plasma triglycerides and cholesterol with a Type IV lipoprotein electrophoresis pattern indicating an elevated pre-beta fraction (40). The distinguishing features of this syndrome, which may be helpful in the differential diagnosis, are the early age at onset, with the majority of patients presenting in the first 3 months of life, and the familial pattern of disease, indicating an autosomal recessive mode of inheritance. The onset of illness in patients suffering FEL may be abrupt or insidious. The duration of disease is extremely variable; however, survival for several months to years has been reported in a number of cases. The major clinical feature distinguishing this entity from malignant histiocytosis is the age of onset. Malignant histiocytosis is extremely rare in patients less than 1 year of age.

Pathologically the most consistent finding is widespread evidence of histiocytic proliferation with erythro- and leukophagocytosis. Virtually all reticuloendothelial organs are involved, and central nervous system infiltration is extremely common (41). In the cases of FEL that we have studied there is a profound generalized lymphoid depletion of the lymphoreticular organs, with infiltration of these organs by well-differentiated histiocytes (Fig. 36–2). These histiocytes have bland nuclei with abundant eosinophilic cytoplasm. The tissue infiltration by these cells varies from moderate to massive organ involvement. Lymph nodes from these cases showed a prominent sinusoidal infiltration by histiocytes. In some lymph nodes massive infiltration with marked replacement of the entire lymph node by bland histiocytes is apparent. The infiltration of spleen, liver, and bone marrow also may vary from mild to massive involvement. Examination of the thymus demonstrates severe lymphoid depletion. Infiltration of visceral organs by histiocytes is commonly seen. The histiocytes in this disease have not been studied using modern immunologic methods.

Immunologic studies have demonstrated a variety of cellular immune defects, which include depressed lymphocyte proliferation, mitogenic and antigenic anergy, and loss of delayed cutaneous hypersensitivity (39, 40, 42). Ladisch and co-workers have demonstrated that plasma from cases of clinically severe FEL inhibit in vitro antigen-induced proliferation of normal lymphocytes and that this inhibitory factor can be reduced following exchange transfusion (40). Cell-mediated cytotoxicity, including monocyte and natural killer cell activity, is severely depressed in the majority of patients with FEL (42). Humoral immune defects have been reported but are difficult to interpret because of the normal age dependence of humoral immune responses to certain antigens (39).

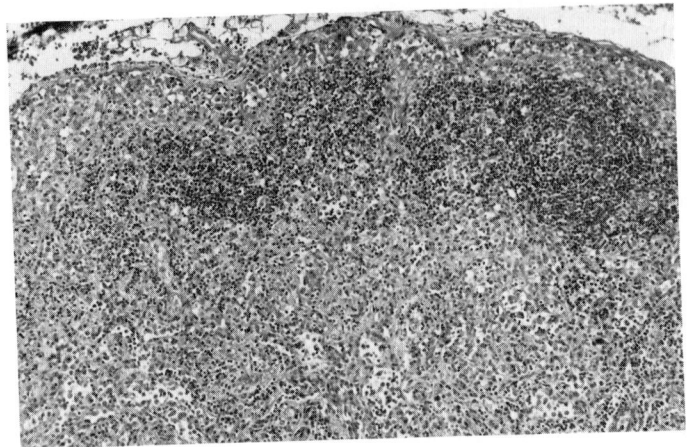

Figure 36–2. This lymph node section from a patient with familial erythrophagocytic leukohistiocytosis exhibits massive infiltration by mature histiocytes ($\times 100$).

Presently there is no proven effective therapy for FEL. Initial clinical responses reported with epipodophyllotoxin (VP16) have not been uniformly observed (43). Temporary improvement in clinically severe cases have been observed with repeated exchange transfusions; however, subsequent worsening and ultimately fatal outcomes persist in spite of repeated exchange transfusion therapy. It is not likely that effective therapy will become available until further understanding of the pathogenesis of this genetic disorder is available.

X-Linked Lymphoproliferative Syndrome

In 1974 and 1975 three families were described as having an X-linked immunodeficiency to Epstein-Barr virus that resulted in fatal infectious mononucleosis in young male children (44, 45, 46). These descriptions occurred 10 years after the discovery of Epstein-Barr virus by Epstein (1964) and represent the initial description of a new X-linked primary immunodeficiency syndrome. Since these first families were described there are now over 25 kindreds that have been reported, with more than 100 affected males. The most recent report of the X-linked lymphoproliferative (XLP) syndrome registry, established by Purtilo and colleagues, gives details on approximately 100 cases of XLP (47). Table 36–1 summarizes the phenotypes and approximate mortalities seen in families with XLP.

Table 36–1. PHENOTYPES EXPRESSED IN X-LINKED LYMPHOPROLIFERATIVE SYNDROME*

Phenotype	Cases	Mortality
Infectious mononucleosis	75%	90%
—with bone marrow aplasia	25%	100%
—with lymphoma	15%	—
—with hypogammaglobulinemia	10%	—
Lymphoma alone	15%	65%
Hypogammaglobulinemia alone	10%	—

*Adapted from reference 46.

The most common presentation of XLP is severe fatal infectious mononucleosis, which occurs in 75 per cent of patients. The mean age of presentation is 6.5 years, which suggests in itself an aberrant immune response to Epstein-Barr virus, since the infectious mononucleosis syndrome as the manifestation of primary Epstein-Barr virus infection is less common in children than in young adults. Massive hepatic necrosis is frequently observed at autopsy. Many patients experiencing fatal infectious mononucleosis will also demonstrate additional phenotypic manifestations such as bone marrow aplasia (25 per cent), lymphoma (15 per cent), or hypogammaglobulinemia. Retrospective studies have suggested that 15 per cent of XLP patients develop lymphoma alone or become hypogammaglobulinemic following EBV infection. The clinical presentation of most patients with the X-linked lymphoproliferative syndrome is one of a severe acute Epstein-Barr virus infection. Patients frequently have high fevers with elevated white counts with marked atypical lymphocytosis. Abnormal liver function tests are present, and a faint maculopapular rash is frequently observed. The clinical course is one of toxicity, with progressive liver damage resulting in jaundice and ultimately liver failure. The typical course in a child suffering fatal EBV infection usually lasts 2 to 3 weeks. The diagnosis of Epstein-Barr virus infection is not usually difficult, with readily detectable heterophil antibody, IgM antibody against viral capsid antigen, and antibodies against early antigens being present. In addition to fulminant liver failure, other causes of death include bleeding secondary to a coagulopathy, secondary bacterial sepsis, and a fulminant lymphoma-like disease.

Patients with fatal X-linked lymphoproliferative syndrome may have widespread infiltration of lymphoreticular organs with immunoblasts. There is evidence for proliferation of both T and B immunoblasts. In most cases the liver shows widespread hepatocyte necrosis (Fig. 36–3) with periportal infiltration by small lymphocytes and

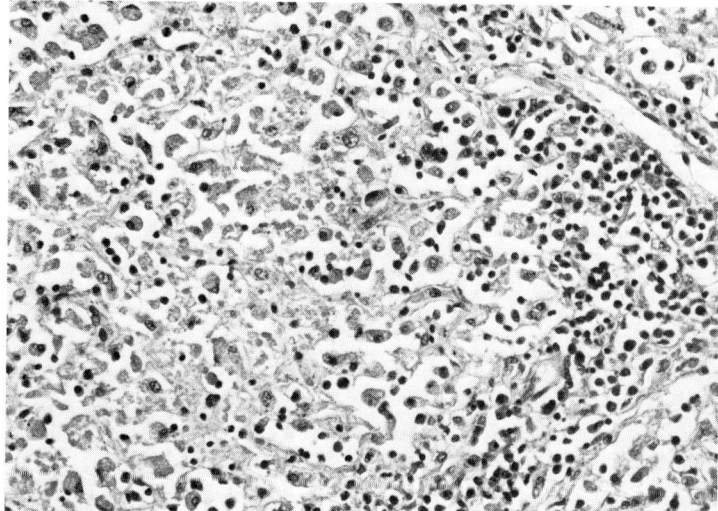

Figure 36–3. This liver section from a patient with X-linked lymphoproliferative syndrome shows massive hepatic necrosis with a focal lymphocytic infiltrate (×252).

immunoblasts. EBV-infected B lymphocytes have been demonstrated in liver specimens obtained at autopsy. In addition to infiltration of lymphoreticular organs, patients suffering fatal XLP may also show lymphoid infiltration of the central nervous system, lungs, and heart. Lymph node pathology during acute infection may reveal total effacement of the lymph node architecture with evidence of necrosis and proliferation of immunoblasts (Fig. 36–4). In other patients profound lymphoid depletion is found at autopsy. In addition to lymphoid depletion, necrosis of splenic white pulp and lymph node follicles may be seen (Fig. 36–5). In patients with lymphoid depletion, lymph node sinus histiocytosis and histiocytic infiltration of the splenic red pulp are usually seen (Fig. 36–6). In some patients, some lymph node groups may show lymphoproliferative changes while others show lymphoid depletion, suggesting that these are evolutionary changes in patients who succumb to this devastating disease. Several studies describing the immunology of patients with XLP have emanated from our laboratory and Purtilo's laboratory (48). We have studied six members of a large family in which 20 males have been affected with XLP (49). An updated pedigree is shown in Figure 36–7. Two members of this family were studied before their encounter with Epstein-Barr virus and during the acute phase of fatal EBV-induced infectious mononucleosis. In both patients, normal numbers of T and B lymphocytes were present before Epstein-Barr virus infection and functional studies demonstrated normal lymphocyte proliferative responses to the mitogens phytohemagglutinin, concanavalin A, and pokeweed. Responses to soluble antigen and alloantigens were also nor-

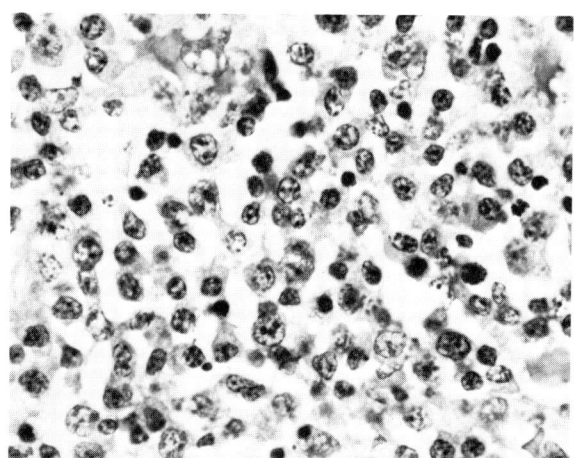

Figure 36–4. This lymph node section exhibits the immunoblastic and plasma cell proliferation seen in patients with the immunoproliferative phenotype of X-linked lymphoproliferative syndrome and shows massive hepatic necrosis with a focal lymphocytic infiltrate (×252).

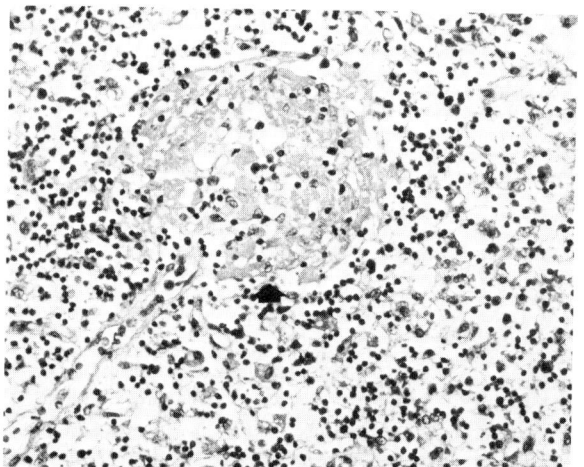

Figure 36–5. This lymph node section exhibits the lymphoid depletion seen in patients with X-linked lymphoproliferative syndrome who die of fatal infectious mononucleosis. Necrosis of lymphoid follicles (arrow) is commonly seen (×252).

mal. Humoral immune function was intact, as demonstrated by normal quantitative immunoglobulins, normal B cell numbers, and normal proliferative responses to anti-immunoglobulin. Further evidence of intact cellular and humoral immune responses included the clinical history of uncomplicated varicella infection at age 6½ years in one patient. In addition, in the single patient studied, natural killer cell activity was intact. During acute Epstein-Barr virus infection, both patients demonstrated suppressed responses to mitogens and antigens. These responses were typical of those observed in normal individuals with acute infectious mononucleosis. In addition, both patients demonstrated normal or exaggerated cell-mediated cytotoxic reactions to EBV-infected target cells and natural killer–sensitive target cells. Cell surface marker studies carried out in a single patient demonstrated a marked increase in the cytotoxic/suppressor cells during acute EBV infection. These cytotoxic T cells were capable of killing an autologous EBV-infected B cell line as well as a primary hepatocyte culture obtained from autopsy tissue. Normal interferon production was also observed in these patients.

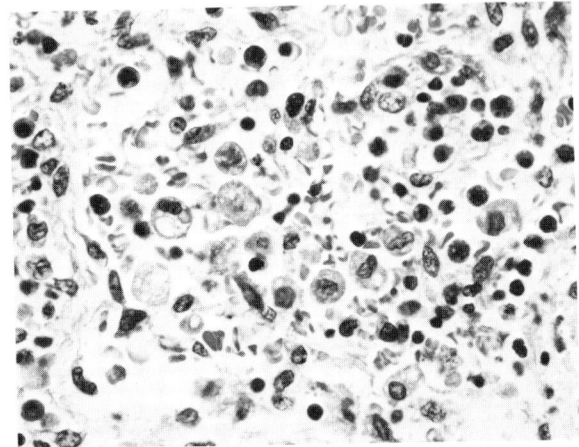

Figure 36–6. This lymph node section shows the lymphoid depletion and histiocytic proliferation characteristic of the fatal infectious mononucleosis phenotype of X-linked lymphoproliferative syndrome (×400).

Comprehensive immunologic studies on 14 affected males with XLP who survived their initial encounter with Epstein-Barr virus have also been reported (48). Lymphocyte surface marker analysis revealed normal percentages of T and B lym-

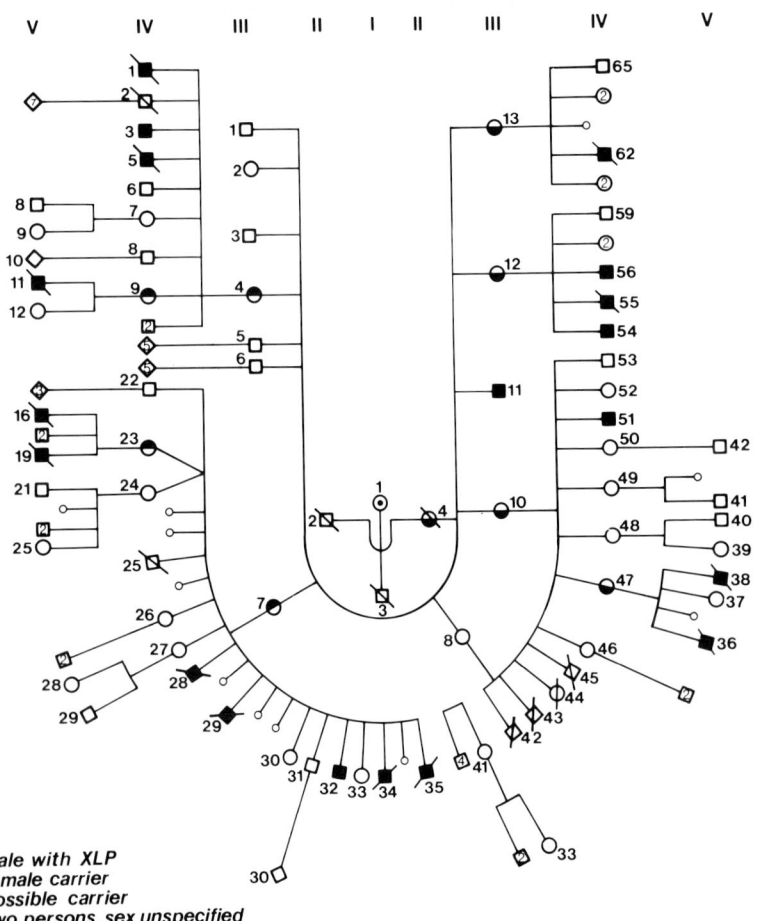

Figure 36–7. Pedigree of a large family in which 20 males are affected with X-linked lymphoproliferative syndrome.

phocytes. Enumeration of lymphocyte subsets has demonstrated increased numbers of cytotoxic/suppressor T cells and reduced helper/suppressor cell ratios. Assessment of quantitative immunoglobulins and polyclonal B cell activation has demonstrated abnormalities of one or more isotypes. Thus many patients with XLP meet the criteria for common variable immunodeficiency with normal numbers of B lymphocytes and decreased IgG levels. Lymphocyte proliferative responses to graded amounts of mitogens and antigens have been shown to be significantly depressed in males with XLP. In addition to these T cell defects, Sullivan and co-workers have shown 5 out of 8 surviving XLP males to have deficient EBV-specific T memory cells (48). Natural killer cell activity has been reported to be markedly deficient in 10 of 12 patients studied. Evaluation of a primary humoral immune response with immunization with bacteriophage OX174 has demonstrated deficient primary immune responses with normal anamnestic responses after secondary immunization. However, severely deficient IgG production following secondary immunization has been observed. Table 36–2 summarizes the immunologic defects observed in patients with the X-linked lymphoproliferative syndrome prior to infection with Epstein-Barr virus and following infection with Epstein-Barr virus. It appears that individuals affected with XLP have normal humoral and cell-mediated immune functions prior to EBV infection, but those patients with XLP who survive their initial infection with Epstein-Barr virus become globally immunodeficient, with defects in both cellular and humoral immunity.

Initial hypotheses concerning the pathogenesis of XLP envisaged a generalized X-linked immune defect that resulted in a predisposition to B cell lymphoproliferative disorders triggered by EBV infections or B cell aplasia when T cell immunoregulation was disturbed by measles virus or other infectious agents (46, 48). These hypotheses were based on immunologic studies reported in patients who had survived their initial encounter with Epstein-Barr virus. It is clear from the reported prospective studies that XLP patients studied in early and late childhood prior to infection with Epstein-Barr virus have intact cellular and humoral immune systems. Normal in vivo responses to polio virus, measles virus, rubella virus, mumps virus, and varicella virus, as well as to bacterial polysaccharide antigens, have been documented. We currently favor the hypothesis that Epstein-Barr virus infection triggers an aberrant T cell–mediated immune response (controlled by an X-linked gene) that mediates lysis of autologous lymphoid and nonlymphoid targets (hepatocytes) (49). This uncontrolled anomalous killer cell activity results in fatal infectious mononucleosis or immune deficiency in those males surviving EBV infections. This mechanism would explain the variation and the severity of the immune deficiency observed within affected kindreds. Secondary immune defects may predispose surviving males with XLP to opportunistic infections and perhaps to lymphoreticular malignancies.

A variety of therapeutic agents have been tried unsuccessfully in XLP patients experiencing acute EBV infection. It is clear that high-dose immunosuppressive therapy predisposes these individuals to fatal B cell lymphoproliferative disorders (49). This effect has been observed with the use of high-dose corticosteroids and antithymocyte globulin. The development of acyclovir, a potent anti-herpesvirus chemotherapeutic agent with activity against Epstein-Barr virus in vitro, has stimulated clinical trials in patients suffering severe life-threatening EBV infections. Acyclovir treatment of two such patients, including one patient with the XLP syndrome, has been reported (50). In each case, objective evidence of clinical improvement was not apparent. More recently, we have treated a third XLP patient who was suffering from fatal infectious mononucleosis (51). This patient died with disseminated Epstein-Barr virus–infected B lymphocytes throughout the lymphoreticular organs in spite of a 2-week course of acyclovir (1500 mg per m^2 per day). Virologic studies in this patient revealed that the virus in infected B lymphocytes was in a nonproductive state and mature virus particles were not being produced. In view of these results, it is likely that acyclovir will prove to be efficacious only in those patients suffering unusually productive EBV infections. Plasma and gammaglobulin preparation containing high-titered antibodies to EBV capsid antigen and early antigen have been tried unsuccessfully (48, 50). There is at present no evidence to suggest that patients with XLP experience un-

Table 36–2. IMMUNOLOGIC DEFECTS IN X-LINKED LYMPHOPROLIFERATIVE SYNDROME

	Before EBV Infection	After EBV Infection
T Cell		
Numbers	Normal	Normal
Function		
Mitogen	Normal	Abnormal
Antigen	Normal	Abnormal
T memory (EBV)	—	Abnormal
B Cell		
Numbers	Normal	Normal
Function		
Primary response	Normal	Abnormal
Secondary response	Normal	Abnormal
NK Cell		
Numbers	—	Normal
Function	Normal	Abnormal

usually productive Epstein-Barr virus infections. Interferon is another candidate for the treatment of life-threatening EBV infections. In addition to its general effects on the prevention of cellular infection, recent studies have shown that interferons can inhibit EBV-induced transformation of B lymphocytes and are strong stimulators of natural killer cell activity (27). In a double-blind placebo-controlled prophylactic trial of human leukocyte interferon in renal transplant recipients, EBV excretion diminished during interferon treatment (52). The efficacy of interferons in the treatment of patients with XLP experiencing EBV infections has not been reported.

Currently efforts are under way using molecular biologic techniques to identify a marker on the X chromosome for the XLP gene. It is likely that such a marker will become available in the near future. The identification of affected males early in infancy, prior to infection with Epstein-Barr virus, will permit immunoprophylaxis with immunoglobulin containing EBV antibodies or immunization with a subunit DNA-free EBV vaccine currently under development (53).

Virus-Associated Hemophagocytic Syndrome

The term "virus-associated hemophagocytic syndrome" (VAHS) was introduced by Risdall and coworkers (54) in 1979 to describe a disorder characterized by a benign generalized histiocytic proliferation with marked hemophagocytosis associated with a systemic virus infection. Since this first description, several case reports have appeared describing the syndrome in immunosuppressed as well as normal individuals (55–57). Thus far, Epstein-Barr virus, cytomegalovirus, herpes simplex virus, and adenovirus have been the most commonly implicated infectious agents (54, 55, 57, 58). The syndrome is characterized by fever and by generalized constitutional symptoms with myalgias and malaise. Physical examination reveals an enlarged liver and spleen with generalized lymphadenopathy. Laboratory studies commonly demonstrate abnormal liver function tests with a coagulopathy that is more severe than that expected on the basis of the abnormal liver function. The patient is usually pancytopenic and may appear very toxic. This syndrome has been most frequently observed in individuals with underlying immunosuppression, including allograft recipients, leukemics, and patients with severe collagen vascular disease receiving high-dose corticosteroids. The mortality in patients experiencing VAHS has been high; however, it is likely that the use of immunosuppressive agents in patients experiencing VAHS has contributed to the high mortality.

There has been some controversy regarding the pathologic differentiation between virus-associated hemophagocytic syndrome and malignant histiocytosis. The pathologic features of VAHS vary with the time that biopsies are performed (58). Early in the disease the bone marrow may be hypercellular with few infiltrating histiocytes. Erythrophagocytosis is usually best demonstrated in aspirate smears. Later in the disease the bone marrow is hypocellular and shows varying numbers of infiltrating histiocytes (Fig. 36–8). Lymph nodes early in the disease may exhibit an intense immunoblastic proliferative response with partial effacement of the lymph node architecture (Fig. 36–9). The numbers of histiocytes early in the disease may be low. Later in the disease, lymphoid depletion supervenes, and there may be a massive sinusoidal infiltration by benign-appearing histiocytes, many of them exhibiting erythrophagocy-

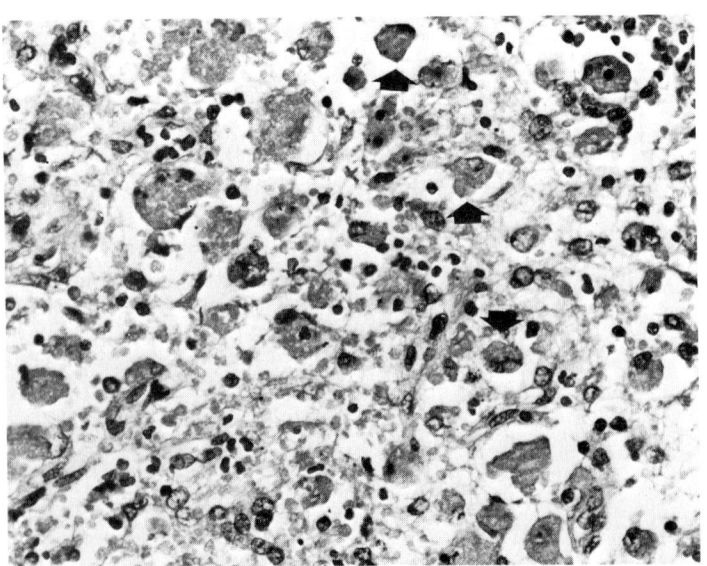

Figure 36–8. Bone marrow section of a patient with virus-associated hemophagocytic syndrome, showing the typical hypocellularity and massive infiltration by mature histiocytes (arrow) (×400).

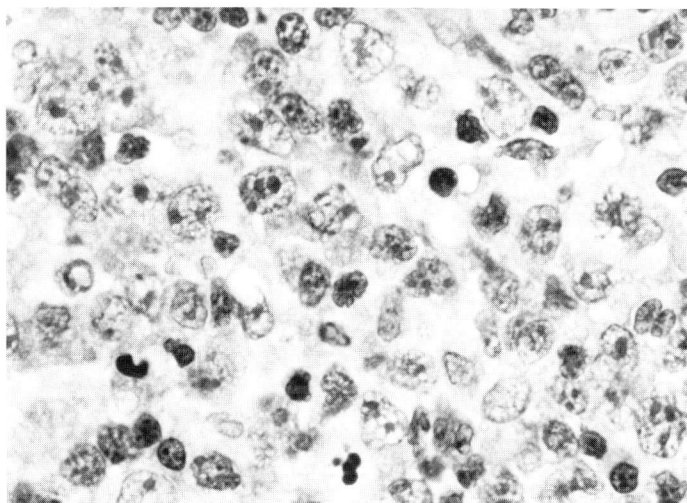

Figure 36–9. Lymph node section from a patient with virus-associated hemophagocytic syndrome shows a florid immunoblastic proliferation (×670).

tosis (Fig. 36–10). Liver biopsy reveals large portal infiltrates of lymphocytes, immunoblasts, and histiocytes. Histiocytes, many of which exhibit erythrophagocytosis, are seen in liver sinusoids. Mild fatty metamorphosis may also be present.

Immunologic studies have been reported only in the two patients studied in our institution (58). In each of these cases, Epstein-Barr virus was the associated infectious agent. Atypical lymphocytes characteristic of acute Epstein-Barr virus infection were notably absent in the peripheral blood of both patients, and cytotoxic T cells, which normally lyse Epstein-Barr virus–infected B cells, were also absent from the peripheral circulation. We have speculated that immunodeficiency or underlying immunosuppression may play a role in the pathogenesis of VAHS. Both Epstein-Barr virus and cytomegalovirus are potent stimulators of the immune system and require complex interactions of immunoregulatory cells for host recovery. Underlying immunoregulatory disturbances may allow an inappropriate antiviral response. As this response progresses, cytokines secreted by activated T lymphocytes may elicit the proliferation and activation of histiocytes.

There is at present no specific treatment for VAHS; however, it appears that the use of immunosuppressive therapy may be deleterious. Immunosuppressive therapy has been used when the diagnosis of VAHS has been confused with malignant histiocytosis. Patients presenting with symptoms compatible with VAHS should be thoroughly studied for evidence of acute EBV, CMV, adenovirus, or other viral infections before immunosuppressive therapy is initiated. Individuals with evidence of acute virus infection should not receive immunosuppressive therapy. There is some suggestion that in VAHS associated with Epstein-Barr virus infection, permissive infection may take place in the lymphoreticular tissues (58). In such cases a trial of the antiviral agent acyclovir may be beneficial. Those individuals who survive their acute infection without any underlying immunodeficiency have an excellent prognosis.

Sinus Histiocytosis with Massive Lymphadenopathy (SHML)

This syndrome was first described by Rosai and Dorfman (59) and consists of a usually benign chronic massive enlargement of cervical lymph nodes frequently accompanied by fever, leukocytosis, elevated sedimentation rate, and hyperglobulinemia (60, 61). This disorder has been found worldwide and is most commonly seen in the first decade of life. More than 90 per cent of patients present with cervical lymph node enlargement, which is usually bilateral and painless. Rarely is a single node involved. Low-grade fever (less than

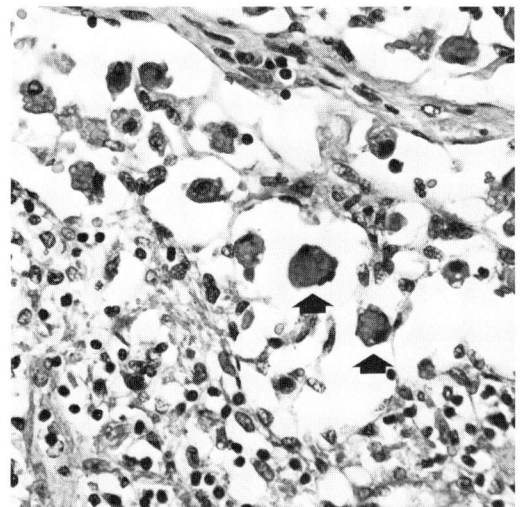

Figure 36–10. Lymph node section from a patient with virus-associated hemophagocytic syndrome, showing sinusoidal histiocytic proliferation with erythrophagocytosis. Note accompanying lymphoid depletion (arrow) (×400).

38°C) is frequently present, and the patient may be found to have a mild normochromic anemia with a leukocytosis and relative lymphopenia. The erythrocyte sedimentation rate is elevated, usually greater than 50 mm per hr. A polyclonal hyperglobulinemia is observed in most patients. The prognosis in most patients is excellent; however, the course is usually protracted, lasting 3 to 9 months. A few individuals with lymphadenopathy persisting greater than 5 years have been described. One case of progression to a malignant lymphoma and one case of amyloidosis have been described in patients with SHML.

The immunopathology of SHML consists of progressive dilatation of lymph node sinuses with histiocytes and lymphocytes until there is almost total effacement of the lymph node architecture (Fig. 36–11). The histiocytes have a benign appearance, with abundant cytoplasm and normal bland nuclei. Leukocytophagocytosis is the hallmark of this disease. Erythrophagocytosis may be observed. Increased numbers of plasma cells and diffuse fibrosis are occasionally seen within the lymph node parenchyma. No etiologic agent has been identified in cases of SHML. Elevated antibody titers to Epstein-Barr virus and measles virus have been observed repeatedly, but evidence to incriminate these as etiologic agents is lacking (62). A defect in immunoregulation is suggested by the exaggerated antibody response to rubella virus in a child with SHML following immunization with an attenuated rubella vaccine (63). Autoimmune phenomena, including hemolytic anemia and glomerulonephritis, are seen in 10 per cent of patients (64).

A variety of treatments have been tried in patients with SHML, without proven benefit. Corticosteroids have not been beneficial, and the usually benign course militates against the use of immunosuppressive agents.

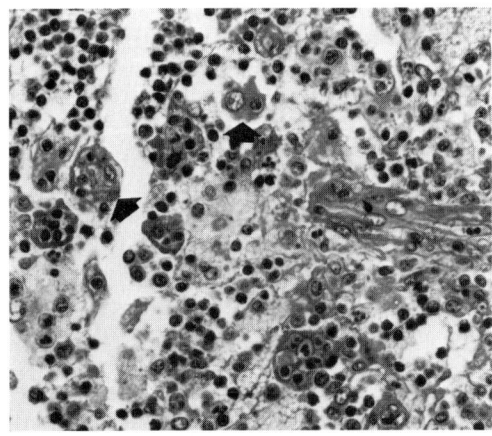

Figure 36–11. Sinus histiocytosis with massive lymphadenopathy: Note sinusoidal histiocytic proliferation with leukophagocytosis (arrow) (×400).

Lymphomatoid Granulomatosis

Lymphomatoid granulomatosis is a disorder characterized by infiltration of the tissues, with atypical lymphocytes and plasmacytoid cells accompanied by granulomatous inflammation in an angiocentric and angiodestructive pattern. First described in 1972 by Liebow and co-workers (64), this entity affects predominantly middle-aged adults, but rare cases in childhood have been described (66, 67, 68). The major organ system involved is the pulmonary system, with virtually all patients demonstrating pulmonary nodules. Constitutional symptoms, including fever, cough, malaise, and weight loss, are common. Lesions in the skin and central nervous system may also develop. Lymphomatoid granulomatosis may be seen in individuals with an underlying malignant or chronic inflammatory process. The chest x-ray most frequently demonstrates multiple bilateral nodular lesions in the lower and peripheral lung fields. Pathologic studies commonly reveal infiltration of the lungs and skin. These infiltrates consist of atypical lymphocytes, most with features of immunoblasts and plasmacytoid cells. Mitoses are frequent, and a vasculitis with infiltration of small and medium-sized arteries and veins may lead to extensive necrosis and vessel obliteration. Other laboratory findings are usually not helpful. A few immunologic studies have appeared (69). Hyperglobulinemias have been reported with rare monoclonal gammopathies. Hypogammaglobulinemia has also been rarely reported. Delayed cutaneous hypersensitivity skin tests are frequently negative. In the few patients studied, no consistent abnormalities in T helper/T suppressor cell ratios have been observed; however, most patients have abnormalities in T cell subsets.

Reactivation of Epstein-Barr virus has been reported in association with lymphomatoid granulomatosis, and we have observed a case of lymphomatoid granulomatosis in association with acute Epstein-Barr virus infection in an immunodeficient host. The prognosis in patients with lymphomatoid granulomatosis is poor, with a mortality rate approaching 60 per cent. A variety of immunosuppressive agents have been tried, and a recent prospective study has demonstrated that cyclophosphamide in combination with corticosteroids can induce long-term remissions in some patients (67). Lymphoma has developed in 15 to 50 per cent of patients, suggesting that this disorder might represent a prelymphomatous process that later eventuates in lymphoma.

Differential Diagnosis of Reactive Lymphohistiocytosis

Each of the lymphohistiocytic disorders may present with overlapping clinical symptoms, making diagnosis difficult. The characteristics of each of the major reactive lymphohistiocytic disorders that may be helpful in diagnosis are shown in Table 36–3. It is possible that certain of these syndromes may be linked to one another. For example, it is possible that sinus histiocytosis with massive lymphadenopathy may be a localized response to an infectious agent, while the virus-associated hemophagocytic syndrome represents a systemic response to the same infectious agent.

At the time of presentation it is essential that a good genetic history and thorough investigation for a viral infection be performed. Definitive diagnosis of familial erythrophagocytic lymphohistiocytosis and X-linked lymphoproliferative syndrome can be accomplished only with a family history of such disorders. Laboratory studies that may be helpful include serum lipoprotein profiles, which show high levels of tryglycerides in cases of familial erythrophagocytic lymphohistiocytosis. There is a great deal of overlap in the pathology of FEL, VAHS, and XLP. VAHS and XLP, being responses to systemic viral infections early in their course, show a florid immunoblastic response that may eventuate in lymphoid depletion with histiocytic proliferation. The degree of histiocytic proliferation may vary from case to case; however, in some cases the degree of histiocytic proliferation in VAHS may be similar to that seen in FEL. The histiocytic proliferation in XLP does not reach that shown in the most florid cases of FEL and VAHS. Necrosis of the splenic white pulp and lymph node follicles, although most often seen in XLP and VAHS, may also be seen in FEL. Thymic atrophy is found in all three of these diseases. Because of the great degree of overlap in the pathology of these diseases, the correct diagnosis depends upon careful study of the pathologic and immunologic processes involved, as well as family history and virologic investigations. The overlap between these diseases suggests that they may have a common pathogenesis. Immunologic studies may be helpful in differentiating familial erythrophagocytic lymphohistiocytosis, X-linked lymphoproliferative syndrome, and virus-associated hemophagocytic syndrome. In FEL, generalized defects in mitogen responses and deficiencies in natural killer and monocyte killing activities are usually present. In X-linked lymphoproliferative syndrome, natural killer cell activity is normal or increased, and high levels of EBV-related anomalous killer cell activity is present. Severe progressive hepatitis is commonly seen in patients with the X-linked lymphoproliferative syndrome. In the virus-associated hemophagocytic syndrome, evidence for acute infection with Epstein-Barr virus, cytomegalovirus, herpes simplex virus, or adenovirus should be sought. Immunologic studies show normal natural killing in EBV-induced virus-associated hemophagocytic syndrome, whereas anomalous EBV-related killing is abnormally low. Clinically, the coagulopathy observed early in the course of VAHS may be helpful in differentiating this disorder from X-linked lymphoproliferative syndrome.

LANGERHANS CELL HISTIOCYTOSIS (HISTIOCYTOSIS X)

Langerhans cell histiocytosis or histiocytosis X is a disease complex comprising eosinophilic granuloma, Hand-Schüller-Christian disease, and Letterer-Siwe disease (71, 72). Most authors believe that the benign forms of these diseases, eosinophilic granuloma and Hand-Schüller-Christian disease, should be separated from the frequently fatal systemic disorder, Letterer-Siwe disease. It is likely that these entities are as different from one another as the reactive lymphohistiocytoses, since

Table 36–3. DISTINGUISHING CHARACTERISTICS OF THE REACTIVE LYMPHOHISTIOCYTOSES*

	Genetic History	Virus Infection	Cellular Immune Function	Miscellaneous
FEL	Autosomal recessive	None	↓ CMI ↓ NK activity ↓ Monocyte killing	Triglycerides
XLP	X-linked recessive	EBV	↓ CMI NL or ↑ NK NL or ↑ anomalous EBV-related killing	Severe, often fatal hepatitis
VAHS	Sporadic	EBV CMV HSV Adenovirus	↓ CMI NL or ↑ NK In cases associated with EBV ↓ Anomalous EBV-related killing	Coagulopathy early in the course of the disease
SHML	Sporadic	?EBV	Not reported	Autoimmune phenomena
LG	Sporadic	EBV	↓ CMI	Lymphoma development

*Key: FEL—familial erythrophagocytic lymphohistiocytosis; CMI—cell-mediated immunity; NK—natural killer; XLP—x-linked lymphoproliferative syndrome; EBV—Epstein-Barr virus; NL—normal; VAHS—virus-associated hemophagocytic syndrome; CMV—cytomegalovirus; HSV—herpes simplex virus; SHML—sinus histiocytosis with massive lymphadenopathy; LG—lymphomatoid granulomatosis.

it is a true rarity to see cases of transition from eosinophilic granuloma to Letterer-Siwe disease. In spite of these criticisms, most workers in the field have accepted Lichtenstein's nosology (72), and several excellent reviews have recently appeared (73, 74, 75).

Eosinophilic Granuloma

Lichtenstein and Jaffe described eosinophilic granuloma of bone in 1940 (76). This is the most common and most benign form of the Langerhans cell histiocytoses (73, 74, 75). This disorder is seen most frequently in children and adolescents. It is characterized by a lytic lesion of bone that is usually discovered because of pain and swelling in the affected area. There is a predilection for lesions to occur in the skull, femur, rib, pelvis, vertebrae, and mandible. Systemic symptoms are unusual. The lesions of eosinophilic granuloma consist of varying proportions of blood histiocytes and eosinophils that destroy the tissues involved (Fig. 36–12). The major cell type involved is the large mononuclear cell, the Langerhans cell. These cells appear benign, with an irregular folded or grooved nucleus and finely dispersed chromatin. The nucleolus is usually single. The cytoplasm is abundant and acidophilic. The cells are grouped in foci or in clusters. Electron microscopy and immunohistochemical techniques are most useful in demonstrating the presence of Langerhans cells in lesions. Electron microscopic studies can be used to demonstrate the pentalaminar marker organelle referred to variously as the Birbeck granule, Langerhans cell granule, X body, and X granule (74, 75) (see Figure 36–1). The function of this organelle remains obscure, but it may represent a plasma membrane invagination. Immunohistochemical analyses may be useful to demonstrate Langerhans cells in lesions. They express HLA-DR antigens, T-6 (thymocyte antigen), and S-100 antigen (77, 78). In addition to Langerhans cells, the cellular infiltrate contains numerous eosinophils and other inflammatory cells. The lytic lesions of bone may be due to Il-1 and PGE_2 secreted by the infiltrating Langerhans cells (25a).

The treatment of eosinophilic granuloma is usually complete curettage of the lesion. In cases in which the lesion is inoperable, irradiation has also been successful.

More recently, a localized extraosseous form of eosinophilic granuloma has been described involving only the lung and has been termed pulmonary histiocytosis X (75). Predominantly a disease of adolescents and young adults, histiocytosis X may present on a routine chest x-ray, appearing as bilateral reticular and micronodular infiltrates. Spontaneous pneumothorax and occasionally cough, fatigue, and weight loss may be the presenting symptoms. The prognosis in pulmonary histiocytosis X is varied, with one fourth of the patients showing spontaneous healing without sequelae, one half showing stable disease with restrictive and/or obstructive lung disease, and one fourth showing progressive, usually fatal, disease.

Hand-Schüller-Christian Disease

This is a chronic, multifocal, eosinophilic granulomatous disease that affects predominantly older children and young adults (71–75). The classically described triad of lytic skull lesions, exophthalmos, and diabetes insipidus is very rare, and one or more of these lesions are usually seen in association with extracranial bone, cutaneous, or pulmonary lesions. The cutaneous lesions may resemble those of Letterer-Siwe disease and are of the seborrheic or eczematoid type. There is a propensity for bone lesions to involve the head, possibly suggestive of a local reaction to an agent

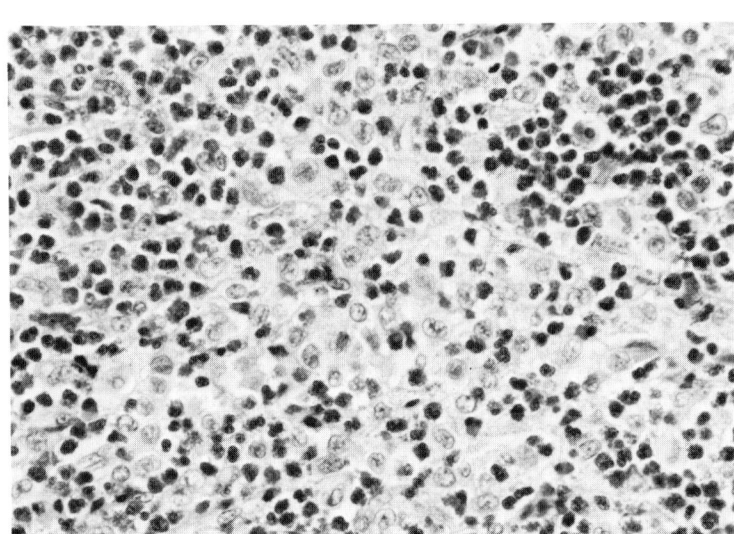

Figure 36–12. Eosinophilic granuloma: Note mixture of histiocytes and eosinophils ($\times 252$).

entering the nasopharynx or oropharynx. Involvement of the central nervous system may result in complex endocrine dysfunction as well as cerebral and cerebellar complications.

Hepatosplenomegaly and lymphadenopathy occur infrequently. Laboratory studies are normal or mildly abnormal, with slightly increased erythrocyte sedimentation rates and mild leukocytosis. There are no abnormalities in lipid metabolism. The course of chronic disseminated histiocytosis X is related to the number, localization, and severity of the lesions. The prognosis is usually good, with diabetes insipidus and growth retardation being the most commonly seen sequelae. Bony lesions and diabetes insipidus (if treated early) may respond to irradiation. Cytotoxic therapy should be reserved for those cases in which the disease is highly aggressive and progressive.

Letterer-Siwe Disease

Between 1924 and 1933, Letterer and Siwe independently described seven infants with a symptom complex that included fever, diffuse purpura, purulent otitis media, lymphadenopathy, and hepatosplenomegaly (79, 80). Each patient demonstrated diffuse tissue infiltration by histiocytes. This disorder is most commonly seen in young infants. The clinical presentation is one of an acute febrile disorder with hepatosplenomegaly, pulmonary bullous lesions, adenopathy, osteolytic lesions, otomastoiditis, and stomatitis. There is frequently a diffuse eruption over the front and back of the trunk, and scalp lesions resembling a purpuric seborrheic rash. Laboratory evaluation may reveal leukocytosis or a pancytopenia. Hepatomegaly may occur in the absence of abnormal liver function tests.

The histopathology of the disseminated form of histiocytosis X mirrors that described for the localized form in each of the involved tissues (74, 75). However, hemophagocytosis may be prominent, and few eosinophils may be present in tissue lesions. Immunologic studies in individuals with histiocytosis X have demonstrated relatively normal numbers of T lymphocytes, with intact in vitro responses to plant mitogens, antigens, and allogeneic cells (81). Several more subtle abnormalities of T lymphocytes have been demonstrated, including elevation of the T helper/T suppressor cell ratio above 3.0, and decreased numbers of histamine H2 receptors on circulating T lymphocytes (81). In addition, increased levels of spontaneous cytotoxicity to cultured fibroblasts and of circulating antibodies to autologous erythrocytes have been reported. Further evidence for thymic dysfunction has come from examination of thymic biopsies and autopsy materials from patients with histiocytosis X (74, 82). Such studies have reported loss of thymic architecture and an absence of Hassall's corpuscles. Histiocytic infiltration with clefts and pseudocysts in thymic lobules has been observed. Thymocyte depletion and destruction of epithelium have been reported.

The differential diagnosis of Letterer-Siwe disease may at times be difficult, and confusion with the reactive lymphohistiocytic syndromes and malignant histiocytosis may occur. The course is commonly fulminant and fatal. Several cases have demonstrated long-lasting spontaneous regressions of disease (83). Treatment of Letterer-Siwe disease has been disappointing; however, the use of chemotherapeutic agents (vinca alkaloids, cyclophosphamide, and chlorambucil singly or in combination with corticosteroids) have been considered to be of benefit, with a remission rate approximating 50 per cent (73–75).

MALIGNANT HISTIOCYTOSIS (HISTIOCYTIC MEDULLARY RETICULOSIS)

Malignant histiocytosis (MH), an uncommon form of lymphoma, is an aggressive disease that is usually rapidly fatal. This disease was first described by Robb-Smith in 1939 as histiocytic medullary reticulosis (84). In 1966, Byrne and Rappaport (85) introduced the term malignant histiocytosis and characterized the disease as a malignant proliferation of cytologically neoplastic histiocytes within lymphoid organs.

The disease has been reported in all decades. The clinical features of MH are protean. In most patients the disease presents as the classically described fulminant systemic disease, although in some the disease is localized as a "true" histiocytic lymphoma. Most patients present with fever, malaise, wasting, hepatosplenomegaly, and lymphadenopathy (85–91). Abdominal pain is a common symptom in the pediatric age group (89). The lymphadenopathy is occasionally tender. Extranodal disease is common. Pulmonary (88–92) and skin (88–90, 93) manifestations are frequent. Central nervous system, pericardial, bone, soft tissue, and gastrointestinal involvement have also been reported. Anemia and thrombocytopenia are common. Patients may have leukopenia or leukocytosis. Circulating atypical mononuclear cells are demonstrable in some patients. Patients may have liver dysfunction manifested by increased alkaline phosphatase, increased transaminases, and hyperbilirubinemia.

The diagnosis of MH depends upon the examination of an appropriate biopsy. The diagnosis is most easily made by the examination of a lymph node biopsy. The pathology of MH is that of a systemic neoplastic proliferation of histiocytes and their precursors (85–88, 90, 94). Early in the disease the neoplastic histiocytes occur as noncohesive cell clusters in the subcapsular and medul-

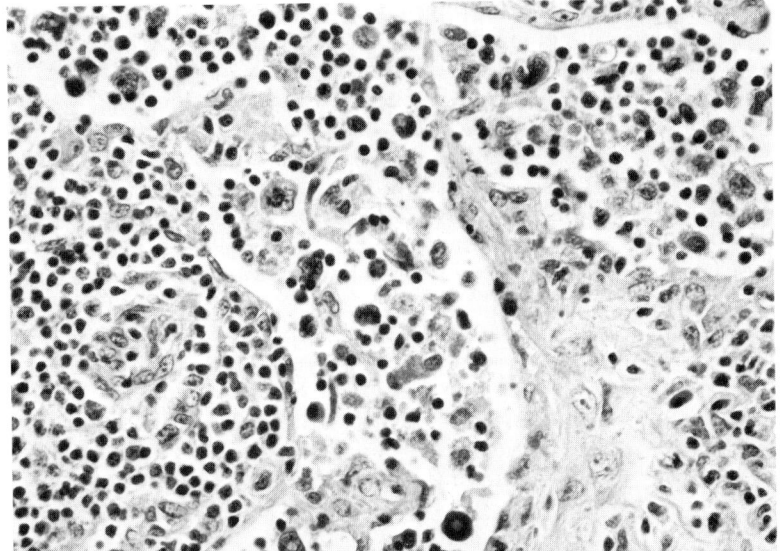

Figure 36-13. Malignant histiocytosis: Note sinusoidal proliferation of malignant histiocytes (×400).

lary sinuses (Fig. 36-13). The lymph node capsule is usually intact. Later in the disease there is extension into the lymph node parenchyma, eventuating in complete effacement of the lymph node architecture. In many patients the initial biopsy shows a diffuse lymphoid neoplasm (Fig. 36-14), and recognition of these cases as MH requires careful cytologic, histochemical and immunologic evaluation. The neoplastic histiocytes exhibit cytologic atypia in all cases; however, there may be great variability in the number of atypical histiocytes and in the degree of cytologic atypia. The cells in MH may be bland, with cleaved nuclei and abundant cytoplasm. It is these better differentiated cells that contain ingested erythrocytes, leukocytes, lipids, and other debris. The most anaplastic forms have a higher nuclear to cytoplasmic ratio, may have prominent nucleoli, and have a high mitotic rate. Anaplastic multinucleated horseshoe forms are commonly seen. It is difficult to identify phagocytosis in these less well differentiated forms. In the pathologic definition of MH by Byrne and Rappaport (85), phagocytosis was an essential criterion in establishing a diagnosis. In subsequent studies it has become evident that a diagnosis of MH may be established without erythrophagocytosis in cases in which the neoplastic cells have the appropriate cytologic features and tissue distribution. Care must be taken to show that it is the neoplastic cells and not the benign reactive histiocytes that are phagocytic. Phagocytosis may be more easily identified in touch preparations or cytocentrifuge preparations than in tissue sections. Variable numbers of plasma cells are seen in most cases. Eosinophils, fibroblasts, and areas of fibrosis are occasionally evident. Focal necrosis may be seen.

The diagnosis of MH can be confirmed by

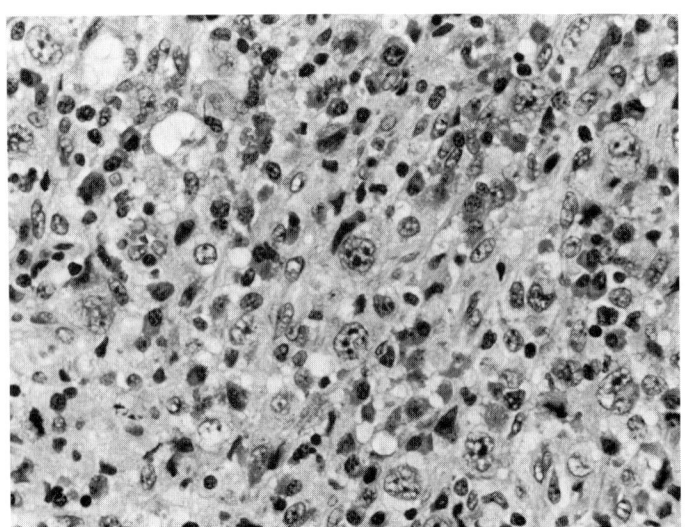

Figure 36-14. Malignant histiocytosis: Note effacement of the lymph node architecture by neoplastic histiocytes (×400).

determining the cell phenotype with immunologic and histochemical studies (87, 90, 91, 94–97). Unfortunately, spotty results have been obtained with immunologic and histochemical studies. Variable numbers of cells in up to 50 per cent of cases express macrophage markers such as lysozyme, alpha$_1$-antitrypsin, and those identifiable with monoclonal antibodies (94).

In a study by Turner and co-workers (94), 14 cases of lymphoma with morphologic features of MH were studied by histochemical, immunologic, and ultrastructural methods. In 5 cases the cells had a mature monocyte/macrophage phenotype; 2 cases had the phenotype of interdigitating reticulum cells; 3 cases were probable T cell lymphomas; and in 4 cases differentiation could not be detected. These cases were classified as lymphomas arising from primitive hemopoietic cells. The clinical and prognostic significance of the phenotypic diversity apparent in MH remains to be determined.

In the differential diagnosis of MH, several other diseases must be considered. The disease that may cause the greatest problem in the differential diagnosis is the virus-associated hemophagocytic syndrome (VAHS) (54, 57). VAHS may have clinical features similar to those of MH, i.e., fever, cytopenias, lymphadenopathy, hepatosplenomegaly, liver dysfunction, and a coagulopathy. The distinction between MH and VAHS is important, as VAHS is an acute life-threatening but potentially reversible disease. Chemotherapy may be contraindicated in VAHS. There are several differences between VAHS and MH. VAHS is associated with a documentable viral infection, severe cytopenias, and a coagulopathy. Skin involvement has not been seen in VAHS. The lymph node involvement in VAHS shows sinusoidal infiltration, but not the destructive infiltration seen in MH. Total effacement of lymph node architecture is usually not seen in VAHS. An early lymph node biopsy is recommended, as VAHS may evolve from an immunoblastic reaction early in the disease to a sinusoidal histiocytic proliferation with lymphoid depletion later in the course. The previously reported cases of MH associated with viral infections may actually have been cases of VAHS.

The histologic overlap between T cell lymphomas (94, 98, 99) and some cases of MH may require specialized histochemical and immunochemical studies for their separation.

MH should be differentiated from reactive disorders such as sinus histiocytosis with massive lymphadenopthy (SHML) (59). The histiocytes in SHML are cytologically benign and show prominent leukophagocytosis. In the majority of cases of SHML there is limited disease distribution, and there is usually no involvement of the liver, spleen, or bone marrow.

MH can be differentiated from histiocytosis X by its cytologic atypia, by the presence of phagocytic cells, and by phenotypic studies. Cells in histiocytosis X have the characteristics of dendritic cells, whereas cells in only some cases of MH have the characteristics of mononuclear phagocytes. The absence of markers for the detection of a clonal expansion of cells in the monocyte/macrophage system contributes to the difficulty in differential diagnosis. Immunoglobulin gene (100) and antigen receptor rearrangement are clonal markers present in the B and T cell system that allow for the detection of clonal malignancy.

It is difficult to make any definitive statements about therapy for MH, as most of the reported series of cases are small and retrospective. The patients are a heterogeneous group, have been treated at different times, and have received different therapies. Unless well-documented, the diagnosis in these cases may be open to some question. MH is an aggressive disease, with death occurring within 6 months. It is resistant to single agent chemotherapy (86). Complete responses have been seen with regimens containing Adriamycin (88, 89). CHOP-based therapy has been used with some success (87, 89, 101). In a recent series consisting of 24 patients receiving CHOP therapy, a median survival of 2 years and a 5-year actuarial survival of 40 per cent have been achieved (91).

References

1. Quesenbery, P., and Levitt, L.: Hematopoietic stem cells. New Engl. J. Med. *301*:755, 819, 868, 1979.
2. Nichols, B. A., and Bainton, D. F.: Differentiation of human monocytes in bone marrow and blood. Lab. Invest. *29*:27, 1973.
3. Strand, F. L., and Bell, E. B.: Studies on the distribution of macrophages derived from rat bone marrow cells in xenogeneic radiation chimaeras. Immunology *22*:549, 1972.
4. Hocking, W. G., and Golde, D. W.: The pulmonary alveolar macrophage. New Engl. J. Med. *301*:580, 639, 1979.
5. Diesselhoff-den Dulk, M. M., Crofton, R. W., et al.: Origin and kinetics of Kupffer cells during an acute inflammatory response. Immunology *37*:7, 1979.
6. Nichols, B. A., and Bainton, D. F.: Ultrastructure and cytochemistry of mononuclear phagocytes. In *Mononuclear Phagocytes in Immunity, Infection and Pathology*. Van Furth, R. (ed.), Oxford, Blackwell Scientific Publications, 1975, p. 17.
7. Huber, H., Polley, M., et al.: Human monocytes: distinct receptor sites for the third component of complement and for immunoglobulin G. Science *162*:1281, 1968.
8. Phillips-Quagliata, J. M., Levine, B. B., et al.: Mechanisms underlying binding of immune complexes to macrophages. J. Exp. Med. *133*:589, 1971.
9. Todd, R. F., Schlossman, S. F.: Analysis of antigenic determinants on human monocytes and macrophages. Blood *59*:775, 1982.
10. Unkeless, J. C.: The presence of two Fc receptors on mouse macrophages: evidence from a variant cell line and different trypsin activity. J. Exp. Med. *142*:931, 1977.
11. Diamond, B., and Yelton, D. E.: A new Fc receptor on mouse macrophages. J. Exp. Med. *153*:514, 1981.

12. Melewicz, F., and Spiegelberg, H. L.: Fc receptors specific for IgE on a subpopulation of human peripheral blood monocytes. J. Immunol. *125*:1026, 1980.
13. Unanue, E. R.: Symbiotic relationships between macrophages and lymphocytes. In *Macrophages and Natural Killer Cells*. Norman, S. J., and Serkin, E. (eds.), New York, Plenum Publishing Corp., 1982, p. 49.
14. Gonwa, T. A., Picker, L. J., et al.: Antigen-presenting capabilities of human monocytes correlates with their expression of HLA-DS, an Ia determinant distinct from HLA-DR. J. Immunol. *130*:706, 1983.
15. Katz, S. I., Tamaki, K., et al.: Epidermal Langerhans cells are derived from cells originating in bone marrow. Nature *282*:324, 1979.
16. Van Voorhis, W. C., Witmer, M. D., et al.: The phenotype of dendritic cells and macrophages. Fed. Proc. *42*:3114, 1983.
17. Rowden, J.: The Langerhans cell. CRC Crit. Rev. Immunol. *3*:95, 1981.
18. Silberberg-Sinakin, I., Gigli, I., et al.: Langerhans cells: role in contact hypersensitivity and relationship to lymphoid dendritic cells and to macrophages. Immunol. Rev. *53*:203, 1980.
19. Steinman, R. M., and Nussenzweig, M. C.: Dendritic cells: features and functions. Immunol. Rev. *53*:205, 1980.
20. Van Voorhis, W. V., Hair, L. S., et al.: Human dendritic cells. Enrichment and characterization from peripheral blood. J. Exp. Med. *155*:1172, 1982.
21. Murphy, G. F., Bhan, A. K., et al.: Characterization of Langerhans cells by the use of monoclonal antibodies. Lab. Invest. *45*:465, 1981.
22. Nakajima, T., Watanabe, S., et al.: S-100 protein in Langerhans cells, interdigitating reticulum cells and histiocytosis X cells. Gann Monograph Cancer Res. *73*:429, 1982.
23. Takahashi, K., Yamaguchi, H., et al.: Immunohistochemical and immunoelectron microscopic localization of S-100 protein in the interdigitating reticulum cells of the human lymph node. Virchows Arch. B (Cell Pathol.) *37*:125, 1981.
24. Flotte, T. J., Springer, T. A., et al.: Dendritic cell and macrophage staining by monoclonal antibodies in tissue sections and epidermal sheets. Am. J. Pathol. *111*:112, 1983.
25. Van Voorhis, W. C., Steinman, R. M., et al.: Specific antimononuclear phagocyte monoclonal antibodies. Application to the purification of dendritic cells and the tissue localization of macrophages. J. Exp. Med. *158*:126, 1983.
25a. Arenzana-Seisdedos, F., Barbey, S., et al.: Histiocytosis X. J. Clin. Invest. *77*:326, 1986.
25b. Franz, T., Löhler, J., et al.: Transformation of mononuclear phagocytes in vivo and malignant histiocytosis caused by a novel murine spleen focus-forming virus. Nature *315*:149, 1985.
26. Sullivan, J. L.: Epstein-Barr virus and the X-linked lymphoproliferative syndrome. In *Advances in Pediatrics*. Barness, L. A. (ed.), Chicago, Year Book Medical Publishers, 1984, p. 365.
27. Sullivan, J. L.: Cellular immune responses and Epstein-Barr virus. In *Human Immunity to Viruses*. Ennis, F. A. (ed.), New York, Academic Press, 1983, p. 279.
28. Rook, A. H., and Quinnan, G. V.: Cell mediated immunity to human cytomegalovirus. In *Human Immunity to Viruses*. Ennis, F. A. (ed.), New York, Academic Press, 1983, p. 241.
29. Sullivan, J. L., and Hanshaw, J. B.: Human cytomegalovirus infections. In *Human Herpesvirus Infections: Clinical Aspects*. Glaser, R., and Gotleib-Stematsky, T. (eds.), New York, Marcel Dekker, 1982, p. 57.
30. Sixbey, J. W., Nedrud, J. G., et al.: Epstein-Barr virus replication in oropharyngeal epithelial cells. New Engl. J. Med. *310*:1225, 1984.
31. Rinaldo, C. R., Carney, W. B., et al.: Mechanisms of immunosuppression in cytomegaloviral mononucleosis. J. Infect. Dis. *141*:488, 1980.
32. Carney, W. P., and Hirsch, M. S.: Mechanisms of immunosuppression in cytomegalovirus mononucleosis. II. Virus-monocyte interactions. J. Infect. Dis. *144*:47, 1981.
33. Rinaldo, C. R., and DeBiasio, R. L.: Alteration of immunoregulatory mechanisms during cytomegalovirus mononucleosis: effect of in vitro culture on lymphocyte blastogenesis to viral antigens. Clin. Immunol. Immunopathol. *28*:46, 1983.
34. Bukowski, J. F., Woda, B. A., et al.: Pathogenesis of murine cytomegalovirus infection in natural killer cell–depleted mice. J. Virol. *52*:119, 1984.
35. Quinnan, G. V., Kirmani, N., et al.: Cytotoxic T cells in cytomegalovirus infection. HLA-restricted T-lymphocyte and non–T-lymphocyte cytotoxic responses correlate with recovery from cytomegalovirus infection in bone-marrow–transplant recipients. New Engl. J. Med. *307*:7, 1982.
36. Nathan, C. F., Murray, H. W., et al.: Identification of interferon-gamma as the lymphokine that activates human macrophage oxidative metabolism and antimicrobial activity. J. Exp. Med. *158*:670, 1983.
37. MacMahon, H. E., Bedizel, M., et al.: Familial erythrophagocytic lymphohistiocytosis. Pediatrics *32*:868, 1963.
38. Farquhar, J. W., MacGregor, A. R., et al.: Familial haemophagocytic reticulosis. Br. J. Med. *2*:1561, 1958.
39. Ladisch, S., Holiman, B., et al.: Immunodeficiency in familial erythrophagocytic lymphohistiocytosis. Lancet *1*:581, 1978.
40. Ladisch, S., Ho, W., et al.: Immunologic and clinical effects of repeated blood exchange in familial erythrophagocytic lymphohistiocytosis. Blood *60*:814, 1982.
41. Akima, M., and Sumi, S. M.: Neuropathology of familial erythrophagocytic lymphohistiocytosis. Six cases and review of the literature. Hum. Pathol. *15*:162, 1984.
42. Perez, N., Virelizier, J. L., et al.: Impaired natural killer activity in lymphohistiocytosis syndrome. J. Pediatr. *104*:569, 1984.
43. Ambruso, D. R., Hays, T., et al.: Successful treatment of lymphohistiocytic reticulosis with phagocytosis with epipodophylotoxin V6 16-213. Cancer *45*:2516, 1980.
44. Bar, R. S., Delor, R. S., et al.: Fatal infectious mononucleosis in a family. New Engl. J. Med. *290*:363, 1974.
45. Provisor, A. J., Iacuone, J. J., et al.: Acquired agammaglobulinemia after a life-threatening illness with clinical and laboratory features of infectious mononucleosis in three related male children. New Engl. J. Med. *293*:62, 1975.
46. Purtilo, D. T., Yang, J. P., et al.: X-linked recessive progressive combined variable immunodeficiency. Lancet *1*:935, 1975.
47. Purtilo, D. T., Sakamoto, K., et al.: Epstein-Barr virus–induced diseases in boys with the X-linked lymphoproliferative syndrome XLP. Am. J. Med. *73*:49, 1982.
48. Sullivan, J. L., Byron, K. S., et al.: X-linked lymphoproliferative syndrome. J. Clin. Invest. *83*:1765, 1983.
49. Sullivan, J. L.: Epstein-Barr virus and the X-linked lymphoproliferative syndrome, Vol. 4. In *The Herpesviruses*. Roizman, B. (ed.), New York, Plenum Press, 1985, p. 229.
50. Sullivan, J. L., Byron, K. S., et al.: Treatment of life-threatening Epstein-Barr virus infections with acyclovir. Am. J. Med. *73*:262, 1982.
51. Sullivan J. L., Medveczky, P., et al.: Epstein-Barr virus induced lymphoproliferation: implications for anti-viral chemotherapy. N. Engl. J. Med. *311*:1163, 1984.
52. Cheeseman, S. H., Rubin, R. H., et al.: Controlled trial of human-leukocyte interferon in renal transplantation. New Engl. J. Med. *300*:1345, 1979.
53. Thorley-Lawson, D. A.: A virus-free immunogen effective against Epstein-Barr virus. Nature *281*:486, 1979.
54. Risdall, R. J., McKenna, R. W., et al.: Virus associated

hemophagocytic syndrome. A benign histiocytic proliferation distinct from malignant histiocytosis. Cancer 44:993, 1979.
55. McKenna, R. W., Risdall, R. J., et al.: Virus associated hemophagocytic syndrome. Hum. Pathol. 12:395, 1981.
56. Liu Yin, J. A., Kumaran, T. O., et al.: Complete recovery of histiocytic medullary reticulosis-like syndrome in a child with acute lymphoblastic leukemia. Cancer 51:200, 1983.
57. Reisman, R. P., and Greco, M. A.: Virus associated hemophagocytic syndrome due to Epstein-Barr virus. Hum. Pathol. 15:290, 1984.
58. Sullivan, J. L., Woda, B. A., et al.: Epstein-Barr virus associated hemophagocytic syndrome: virological and immunopathological studies. Blood 65:1097, 1985.
59. Rosai, J., and Dorfman, R. F.: Sinus histiocytosis with massive lymphadenopathy: a pseudolymphomatous benign disorder. Cancer 30:1176, 1972.
60. Sanchez, R., Rosai, J., et al.: Sinus histiocytosis with massive lymphadenopathy: an analysis of 113 cases with special emphasis on its extranodal manifestations. Lab. Invest. 36:349, 1969.
61. Karpas, A., Worman, C., et al.: Sinus histiocytosis with massive lymphadenopathy: virological, immunological and morphological studies. Br. J. Haematol. 45:195, 1980.
62. Foucer, E., Rosai, J., et al.: Sinus histiocytosis with massive lymphadenopathy. An analysis of 14 deaths occurring in a patient registry. Cancer 54:1834, 1984.
63. Sumaya, C. V., Cherry, J. D., et al.: Exaggerated antibody response following rubella vaccination in a child with sinus histiocytosis with massive lymphadenopathy. J. Pediatr. 89:81, 1976.
64. Liebow, A. A., Carrington, C. R. B., et al.: Lymphomatoid granulomatosis. Hum. Pathol. 3:457, 1972.
65. Lee, S. C., Roth, L. M., et al.: Lymphomatoid granulomatosis: a clinicopathologic study of four cases. Cancer 38:846, 1976.
66. Foucer, E., Rosai, J., et al.: Immunologic abnormalities and their significance in sinus histiocytosis with massive lymphadenopathy. Am. J. Clin. Pathol. 82:515, 1984.
67. Fauci, A. S., Haynes, B. F., et al.: Lymphomatoid granulomatosis. Prospective clinical and therapeutic experience over 10 years. New Engl. J. Med. 306:68, 1982.
68. Patton, W. F., and Lynch J. P.: Lymphomatoid granulomatosis. Clinicopathologic study of four cases and literature review. Medicine 61:1, 1982.
69. Sordillo P. P., Epremian, B., et al.: Lymphomatoid granulomatosis: an analysis of clinical and immunologic characteristics. Cancer 49:2070, 1982.
70. Veltri, R. W., Raich, P. C., et al.: Lymphomatoid granulomatosis and Epstein-Barr virus. Cancer 50:1513, 1982.
71. Lichtenstein, L.: Histiocytosis X. Integration of eosinophilic granuloma of bone, "Letterer-Siwe disease," and "Schüller-Christian disease" as related manifestations of a single nosologic entity. Arch. Pathol. 56:84, 1953.
72. Lichtenstein, L.: Histiocytosis X eosinophilic granuloma of bone, Letterer-Siwe disease, and Schüller-Christian disease. J. Bone Joint Surg. 46:76, 1964.
73. Groopman, J. E., and Golde, D. W.: The histiocytic disorders: a pathophysiologic analysis. Ann. Intern. Med. 94:95, 1981.
74. Favara, B. E., McCarthy R. C., et al.: Histiocytosis X. Hum. Pathol. 14:663, 1983.
75. Basset, F., Nezelof, C., et al.: The histiocytoses. In Pathology Annual. Sommers, S. L., and Rosen, P. P. (eds.), Norwalk, Appleton-Century-Crofts, 1983, p. 27.
76. Lichtenstein, L., and Jaffe, H. L.: Eosinophilic granuloma of bone, with report of a case. Am. J. Pathol. 16:595, 1940.
77. Rowden, G., Connelly, E. M., et al.: Cutaneous histiocytosis X. The presence of S-100 protein and its use in diagnosis. Arch Dermatol. 199:553, 1983.
78. Ide, F., Iwase, T., et al.: Immunohistochemical and ultrastructural analysis of the proliferating cells in histiocytosis X. Cancer 53:917, 1984.
79. Letterer, E.: Aleukämische Retikulose ein Beitrag zu den proliferatioven Erkrakugen des Retikuloendothelialapparates. Frankfurt Z. Pathol. 30:377, 1924.
80. Siwe, S. A.: Die Reticuloendotheliose—ein neues Kranksheitsbild unter den Hepatosplenomegalien. Z. Kinderheilkd. 55:212, 1933.
81. Osband, M. E., Lipton, J. M., et al.: Histiocytosis-X. Demonstration of abnormal immunity, T-cell histamine H2-Receptor deficiency, and successful treatment with thymic extract. New Engl. J. Med. 304:146, 1981.
82. Hamoudi, A. B., Newton, W. A., et al.: Thymic changes in histiocytosis. Am. J. Clin. Pathol. 77:169, 1982.
83. Broadbent, V., Pritchard, J., et al.: Spontaneous remission of multi-system histiocytosis X. Lancet 1:253, 1984.
84. Scott, R. B., and Robb-Smith, A. H. T.: Histiocytic medullary reticulosis. Lancet 2:194, 1939.
85. Byrne, G. E., and Rappaport, H.: Malignant histiocytosis. Gann Monograph Cancer Res. 15:145, 1973.
86. Warnke, R. A., Kim, H., et al.: Malignant histiocytosis histiocytic medullary reticulosis. Cancer 35:215, 1975.
87. Lampert, I. A., Catovsky, D., et al.: Malignant histiocytosis: a clinico-pathological study of 12 cases. Br. J. Hematol. 40:65, 1978.
88. Rilke, F., Carbone, A., et al.: Malignant histiocytosis: a clinicopathologic study of 18 consecutive cases. Tumori 64:211, 1978.
89. Zucker, J. M., Caillaux, J. M., et al.: Malignant histiocytosis in childhood. Clinical study and therapeutic results in 22 cases. Cancer 45:2821, 1980.
90. Ducatman, B. S., Wich, M., et al.: Malignant histiocytosis: a clinical, histologic, and immunohistochemical study of 20 cases. Hum. Pathol. 15:368, 1984.
91. Tseng, A., Coleman, C. N., et al.: The treatment of malignant histiocytosis. Blood 64:48, 1984.
92. Colby, T. V., and Carrington, C. B.: Pulmonary involvement in malignant histiocytosis: a clinicopathologic spectrum. Am. J. Surg. Pathol. 5:61, 1981.
93. Wick, M. R., Sanchez, N. P., et al.: Cutaneous malignant histiocytosis: a clinical and histopathologic study of 8 cases, with immunohistochemical analysis. J. Am. Acad. Dermatol. 8:50, 1983.
94. Turner, R. R., Wood, G. S., et al.: Histiocytic malignancies: morphologic, immunologic, and enzymatic heterogeneity. Am. J. Surg. Pathol. 8:485, 1984.
95. Carbone, A., Micheau, C., et al.: A cytochemical and immunohistochemical approach to malignant histiocytosis. Cancer 47:2862, 1981.
96. Huhn, D., and Meister, P.: Malignant histiocytosis: morphologic and cytochemical findings. Cancer 42:1341, 1978.
97. Risdall, R. J., Sibley, R. K., et al.: Malignant histiocytosis: a light- and electron-microscopic and histochemical study. Am. J. Surg. Pathol. 4:439, 1980.
98. Costa, J., Jaffe, E., et al.: Peripheral T-cell lymphoma with pulmonary involvement and erythrophagocytosis mimicking malignant histiocytosis. (Abstract.) Lab Invest. 42:12, 1980.
99. Kadin, M. E., Kamoun, M., et al.: Erythrophagocytic T gamma lymphoma, a clinicopathologic entity resembling malignant histiocytosis. New Engl. J. Med. 304:648, 1981.
100. Cleary, M. L., Warnke, R., et al.: Monoclonality of lymphoproliferative lesions in cardiac-transplant recipients: clonal analysis based on immunoglobulin-gene rearrangements. New Engl. J. Med. 310:477, 1984.
101. Alexander, M., and Daniels, J. R.: Chemotherapy of malignant histiocytosis in adults. Cancer 39:1011, 1977.

ONCOLOGY

CHAPTER 37
Management of Malignant Solid Tumors

ARNOLD J. ALTMAN

INTRODUCTION 1136
Presentation
Treatment
NEUROBLASTOMA 1138
Cytogenetics
Pathology
Clinical Features
Routes of Metastasis
Biochemical Features
Biologic Behavior
Role of the Immune System
Clinical Staging
Prognosis
Management
Special Locations
New Therapeutic Strategies
WILMS' TUMOR 1145
Genetics
Pathology
Clinical Features
Management
Renal Cell Carcinoma (Hypernephroma)
SOFT TISSUE SARCOMAS 1152
Rhabdomyosarcoma
Fibrosarcoma
Synovial Sarcoma
Soft Tissue Tumors of Neural Origin
Ewing's Sarcoma of Soft Tissue (Extraskeletal Ewing's Sarcoma)
BONE TUMORS 1161
Osteosarcoma
Ewing's Sarcoma
TUMORS OF GERM CELL ORIGIN 1169
Histologic Variants
Tumor Markers
Anatomic Distribution
LIVER TUMORS 1179
Pathology
Clinical Features
Therapy
RETINOBLASTOMA 1181
Genetics
Clinical Features
Staging
Routes of Metastasis
Prognosis
Treatment
CENTRAL NERVOUS SYSTEM TUMORS 1186
Clinical Manifestations
Prognosis
Treatment
Treatment of Specific CNS Tumors

INTRODUCTION

Cancer kills more children between the ages of 1 and 15 years than any other disease. The annual incidence of malignant tumors in the United States for children younger than 15 years is 12.1 per 100,000 white children and 9.3 per 100,000 black children (1); this results in approximately 6000 to 7000 newly diagnosed cases of childhood cancer annually in the United States.

The types of cancers seen in children (Fig. 37-1) are quite different from those seen in adults, possibly reflecting differences in etiology and pathogenesis. The common childhood tumors have many of the features associated with experimentally induced tumors produced by infection of laboratory animals with viruses (2), whereas the "adult-type" tumors (e.g., lung cancer, breast cancer, colon cancer) are more frequently associated with prolonged exposure to environmental chemical carcinogens.

Pediatric cancer is most prevalent in patients up to 4 years of age; approximately 40 per cent of all malignancies occur during this period. Tumors such as neuroblastoma, Wilms' tumor, testicular germ cell tumors, acute lymphocytic leukemia, retinoblastoma, sacrococcygeal teratoma, medulloblastoma, CNS gliomas, rhabdomyosarcomas, and hepatoblastoma have their peak frequency in the child under 5 years of age; prenatal factors affecting embryogenesis may be implicated in their pathogenesis. Other tumors, such as ovarian germ-cell tumors, lymphomas, bone sarcomas, thyroid cancer, acute myelogenous leukemia, and most brain tumors, do not exhibit frequency peaks in younger children, possibly reflecting the role of postnatal (environmental) factors.

A comparison of the incidence rates of the various childhood malignancies in the United States (Table 37-1) shows that many tumors have almost identical frequency in white and black children. However, there are some interesting variations between the races—for instance, the incidence of leukemia in whites is almost twice as high as it is in blacks, and certain other tumors (melanoma, Ewing's sarcoma, and testicular cancers) are absent or very rare in blacks.

Presentation

Cancer may be considered to present in one of three ways in childhood: (1) as a mass lesion; (2) with symptoms directly related to the tumor; or (3) with nonspecific symptoms (paraneoplastic syndromes).

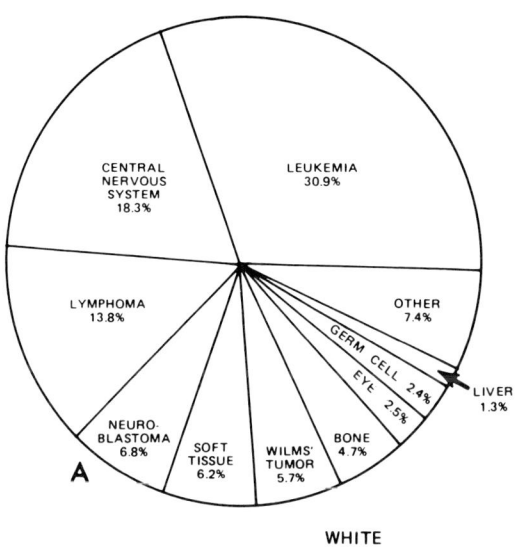 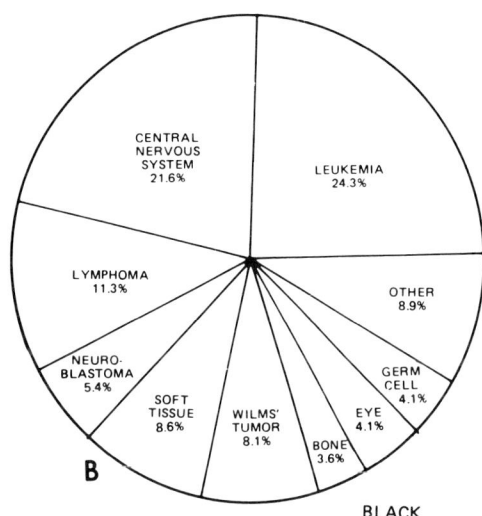

Figure 37–1. Relative frequency of major forms of cancer in the United States: *A*, in white children; *B*, in black children. (From Altman, A. J., and Schwartz, A. D.: Malignant Diseases of Infancy, Childhood and Adolescence. Philadelphia, W. B. Saunders Co., 1983.)

In general, the presence of a mass lesion should alert the physician quickly to the possibility of malignancy, since there are only a few mass lesions that can be considered benign on the basis of location or physical appearance alone. When pondering the possible histology of a mass lesion, it is useful to recognize that most childhood malignancies are essentially single-site tumors and therefore enter consideration for only specific locations or organs. However, there are a few that must be considered in the differential diagnosis of a mass in almost any location. Among these ubiquitous tumors are neuroblastoma, soft tissue sarcomas, germ-cell tumors, and lymphomas.

Symptoms directly referrable to the tumor may include gastrointestinal bleeding, neurologic signs resulting from brain or spinal cord lesions, hematuria from a Wilms' tumor or bladder rhabdomyosarcoma, obstructive symptoms, or endocrinologic symptoms resulting from hormone production by the tumor.

Unfortunately, some cancers may present with very nonspecific symptoms that give no clue as to their nature or location. Such paraneoplastic symptoms include weight loss, diarrhea, low-grade fever, failure to thrive, rheumatoid-like symptoms, and opsomyoclonus. The use of careful physical examination and appropriate radiologic studies, as well as screening laboratory tests, may permit earlier diagnosis of these occult neoplasms.

Treatment

Optimal treatment involves a rapid definitive attack upon the primary lesion and measures to prevent or eradicate metastases. Surgery and radiotherapy are the major weapons of primary treatment. However, their utility is limited because they are effective only against localized disease. To eradicate occult disease, adjuvant chemotherapy is administered simultaneously with, or following treatment of, the primary tumor.

Table 37–1. INCIDENCE OF MALIGNANT TUMORS IN U.S. CHILDREN: RATE PER 100,000 PER YEAR*

Category	Whites	Blacks
Leukemia	3.74	2.27
ALL	2.47	1.05
ANLL	0.55	0.46
CML	0.09	0.08
Unclassified	0.63	0.68
CNS	2.22	2.02
Lymphoma	1.68	1.05
Non-Hodgkin's	0.93	0.58
Hodgkin's	0.75	0.46
Neuroblastoma	0.95	0.67
Soft Tissue	0.75	0.80
Rhabdomyosarcoma	0.37	0.38
Fibrosarcoma	0.05	0.08
Other	0.33	0.34
Wilms' tumor	0.69	0.76
Bone tumors	0.57	0.34
Osteosarcoma	0.31	0.25
Ewing's sarcoma	0.21	—
Other	0.05	0.09
Retinoblastoma	0.30	0.38
Gonadal and germ cell	0.28	0.39
Liver	0.16	—
Melanoma	0.12	0.04
Miscellaneous	0.66	0.63
Thyroid	0.19	0.08
Nasopharynx	0.02	—
Other	0.45	0.55
Total	12.12	9.33

*Based on data from reference 1.

The biologic behavior of most childhood tumors suggests that disseminated microscopic foci of disease are present in the majority of patients at diagnosis. Thus, adjuvant chemotherapy should be initiated early, as it is more effective when the tumor burden is small. The general principles of chemotherapy and specific pharmacology or antineoplastic agents are discussed in Chapter 32.

NEUROBLASTOMA

Neuroblastoma is a malignant tumor of sympathetic neuroblasts. The majority of neuroblastomas are encountered in children under 5 years of age, and at least half are manifested clinically in children under 2 years of age; congenital and even fetal neuroblastomas have been described. Jaffe (3), pooling data from several studies, found that 60 per cent of neuroblastoma cases occurred in children under 1 year of age, 27 per cent in children between 1 and 2 years of age, and 13 per cent in those older than 2 years.

Cytogenetics

The most consistent chromosomal abnormalities associated with neuroblastoma appear to involve loss of genetic material in the short arm of chromosome 1 distal to band 1p31; abnormalities of other chromosome segments, notably 1q, 17q, and 22q, have also been reported (4, 5, 6). In addition, many neuroblastomas and neuroblastoma cell lines contain long nonbanding homogeneously staining chromosome regions and double minute chromosomes that represent amplified genetic material, including many copies of the N-*myc* oncogene (5, 6, 7).

It has been proposed that structural rearrangements of chromosome 1p may play a primary role in the development of neuroblastoma, possibly through loss or inactivation of suppressor genes located in the chromosomal region 1p32 → ter and that the gene changes produced by abnormalities in chromosomes 1q and 17q and by the amplified N-*myc* oncogenes may contribute to tumor progression (6). Indeed, there is a striking correlation between the number of copies of the N-*myc* oncogene and the extent of disease at diagnosis as well as the risk of subsequent tumor progression (6a).

Pathology

Neuroblastomas are small primitive round cell tumors. As such, they must be distinguished from the other small round cell malignancies of childhood (lymphoma, Ewing's sarcoma, embryonal rhabdomyosarcoma). The presence of rosette formation or neurofibrils is a useful diagnostic feature; however, often the cells are too undifferentiated for conventional light microscopic examination to provide a definitive diagnosis. Histochemical stains demonstrating the presence or absence of glycogen may be helpful, since Ewing's sarcoma and rhabdomyosarcoma contain glycogen and are therefore periodic acid–Schiff (PAS)–positive, whereas neuroblastomas are generally PAS-negative (rare cases of glycogen-containing neuroblastomas have been reported (8). The electron microscopic picture of neuroblastoma is distinctive, the tumor cells showing cytoplasmic extensions resembling neural processes with neurofilaments, neurotubules, mitochondria, and occasionally neurosecretory granules. A particularly useful feature is the presence of small, spherical, membrane-bound granules with electron-dense cores, representing cytoplasmic accumulations of catecholamines (9).

Shimada and colleagues (9a) have recently described a histopathologic classification for neuroblastoma that appears to correlate well with prognosis. This system is based on degree of differentiation and nuclear morphology of neuroblastic cells and organization pattern of the "stromal" tissue. Some tumors of sympathetic nervous tissue show differentiation beyond the neuroblast stage and are classified as ganglioneuroblastoma or ganglioneuroma. Ganglioneuroma is the most benign form, being composed of large, mature ganglion cells with abundant cytoplasm. Ganglioneuroblastoma is a transitional tumor that contains both malignant neuroblastomatous and benign ganglioneuromatous elements. Two subtypes with very different biologic behaviors have been described (10, 11): (1) *composite*—this is identical with classic ganglioneuroma, but contains one or more discrete nodules of pure neuroblastoma; (2) *diffuse* ("imperfect")—consisting of a diffuse mixture of primitive and differentiating neuroblasts with bizarre, immature, and mature ganglion cells. The composite form is considered to have a worse prognosis than the diffuse form; overall, 65 to 75 per cent of composite ganglioneuroblastomas exhibit metastatic behavior compared with only 4 to 18 per cent of diffuse ganglioneuroblastomas (10, 11).

Clinical Features

As a consequence of the embryonic migration of neural crest derivatives, sympathetic nervous tissue is distributed within the adrenal medulla as well as throughout the paraspinal sympathetic ganglia extending from the superior cervical ganglion in the neck to the organ of Zuckerkandl in the pelvis. The relative frequency with which neuroblastoma arises in these various anatomic sites is as follows (12):

Adrenal medulla—40%
Paraspinal sympathetic ganglia—25%
Mediastinal ganglia—15%

Pelvic ganglia—5%
Cervical ganglia—3%
Other—12%

The signs and symptoms of neuroblastoma vary with these anatomic locations. Tumors arising in the abdomen tend to be silent until the mass is quite large, unless a sudden hemorrhage into the tumor causes the child to develop acute abdominal pain. When the tumor is intrathoracic the patient is frequently asymptomatic, and the posterior mediastinal mass may be discovered only serendipitously following a chest x-ray for some other indication; very large mediastinal tumors may cause respiratory symptoms. Tumors occurring high in the thorax or in the neck can cause a Horner's syndrome, and the child may present with ptosis. Paravertebral tumors may present with neurologic signs suggestive of spinal cord compression. In some situations, a site of metastatic disease brings the child to the attention of a physician with complaints of bone pain, periorbital ecchymosis, or limp. Nonspecific presenting features of neuroblastoma include fever, weight loss, and irritability. A small number of patients will present with paraneoplastic features such as opsomyoclonus (13), intractable diarrhea, or hematologic abnormalities (14).

Routes of Metastasis

Neuroblastoma may spread by contiguous extension or via hematogenous or lymphatic routes. In contrast to Wilms' tumor, which usually grows as a single encapsulated expansile mass, neuroblastoma usually has no capsule and infiltrates along tissue planes to encase major blood vessels. The sites of distant metastasis vary with the age of the patient. Under 1 year of age, the common metastatic foci are liver, skin, and bone marrow. Above the age of 1 year, regional lymph nodes and bone cortex (axial skeleton, ribs, skull, proximal long bones) are the common metastatic sites.

Biochemical Features

Catecholamines such as dopamine and the epinephrines play an important role in the functioning of the sympathetic nervous system. Many neuroblastomas are characterized by excessive production and excretion of these molecules and their metabolites—vanillylmandelic acid (VMA), metanephrine, and homovanillic acid (HVA). Analysis of urinary excretion of catecholamines is a useful diagnostic procedure, as up to 90 per cent of neuroblastoma patients will have elevation of either VMA and HVA at the time of initial presentation. Attention should also be paid to the ratio between the derivatives of the epinephrines (e.g., VMA) and of dopamine (e.g., HVA); a high VMA/HVA ratio (>1.5) suggests a better prognosis (15, 16). Urinary excretion of the amino acid cystathionine has also been reported in neuroblastoma patients; a low level is correlated with a more favorable prognosis (16).

Elevations of blood levels of various molecules have also been noted in neuroblastoma patients; among those noted to have prognostic import are lactic dehydrogenase (17), ferritin (18, 19), and neuron-specific enolase (NSE) (20). Of these, NSE appears to be a particularly useful disease marker and prognostic indicator in infants with Stage IV disease; in one study, all 7 of such individuals with serum NSE levels of less than 100 ng per ml were alive up to 36 months after diagnosis, whereas 7 of the 8 with serum NSE greater than 100 ng per ml dies within 12 months of diagnosis (20).

Biologic Behavior

One of the most intriguing aspects of neuroblastoma is the remarkable age-related variability of its biologic behavior. This tumor, which is ordinarily highly malignant, often pursues a paradoxically benign course in young infants. Several manifestations of this phenomenon, which may or may not be interrelated, are: (1) the discrepancy between the relatively high incidence of "neuroblastoma in situ" found in infants under the age of 3 months and the subsequent incidence of clinically apparent neuroblastoma; (2) the relatively favorable prognosis at all clinical stages for infants less than 1 year of age; and (3) spontaneous regression of apparently widely disseminated tumor (Stage IVS) in a high proportion of infants less than 6 months of age.

"Neuroblastoma in Situ." When careful autopsies are performed on neonates (below 3 months of age) succumbing to a variety of causes, approximately 0.5 per cent of cases are found to have clusters of primitive neuroblasts ("neuroblastoma in situ") in the adrenal glands (21). However, the actual incidence of clinically apparent neuroblastoma is approximately 40-fold less than that anticipated based on these figures. Furthermore, autopsies performed on older children fail to demonstrate either "neuroblastoma in situ" or expansile neuroblastoma in numbers anywhere approaching the neonatal incidence. Therefore, it has been suggested that the vast majority of these neonatal neuroblastomas disappear without clinical expression (21).

The spontaneous resolution of so many apparent cases of neonatal neuroblastoma may be a reflection of immunologic host defense or cellular maturation, but a more likely explanation is that it is a continuation of a normal embryologic process. During early embryonic life, adrenomedullary tissue is composed of large, tightly packed clusters of neuroblasts. The number and size of these neuroblastic nodules increases until the 15th to 17th week of gestation and thereafter decreases as the nodules break up into smaller nests of cells. Neuroblast clusters closely resembling "neuroblastoma in situ" have been found in all fetuses examined at 14 to 18 weeks of gestation (22); therefore, it is very likely that so-called "neuroblastoma in situ" represents persistence into the neonatal period of these hyperplastic nodules before they break up into individual cells (23).

Spontaneous Regression of Disseminated (IVS) Neuroblastoma. Infants less than 1 year of age fare substantially better than do older children with comparable disease dissemination for all clinical stages. Of particular interest are those infants with apparently widely disseminated disease (Stage IVS) whose tumors completely regress even in the absence of systemic therapy; this phenomenon may occur in association with tumor necrosis, hyalinization, cyst formation, or maturation to ganglioneuroma. As originally defined by Evans and co-workers (24), Stage IVS neuroblastoma consisted of a small primary tumor associated with remote disease involving liver, bone marrow, or skin. Subsequent reports, however, have shown that other sites, such as the pancreas, pleura, or bowel serosa, can be involved without worsening the prognosis (25, 26). Most of these patients are infants in the first few months of life.

In addition to its relatively benign behavior, Stage IVS neuroblastoma also exhibits measurable biochemical differences from true Stage IV neuroblastoma, including reduced production of ferritin and E-rosette inhibitory factor (18). This biologic variability has led Knudson and Meadows (27) to propose that IVS neuroblastoma represents a benign polyclonal proliferative disorder, derived from cells bearing only a single gene mutation, whereas other forms of neuroblastoma are true monoclonal malignancies induced by a critical second mutation ("second-hit"). In support of this hypothesis are the data of Balaban and Gilbert (4, 5), who have demonstrated normal karyotypes in cases of regressing IVS neuroblastoma but consistent chromosomal abnormalities in other forms of neuroblastoma. Lack of amplification of the N-*myc* oncogene in IVS neuroblastoma is also consistent with a more benign phenotype (6a). On the other hand, Look and associates (28) have demonstrated hyperdiploid cells of clonal origin (a universally accepted marker of malignancy) in four infants with IVS neuroblastoma.

Cassady (29) has proposed a cellular kinetic basis for the phenomena of spontaneous regression and maturation of neuroblastoma in the young infant. In this hypothesis, malignant potential is a reflection of the relative proportion of clonogenically viable tumor stem cells (i.e., cells with a capacity for infinite replication). It is postulated that the neuroblastomas of early infancy have a relative paucity of these tumor stem cells. As a consequence, most of the neoplastic proliferation results from cellular elements with a limited capacity for cell division; the progeny of these cells are ultimately destined to differentiate or disappear. By contrast, the more aggressive neuroblastomas seen in older children may have many tumor stem cells and therefore behave like true malignant tumors.

Role of the Immune System

Numerous observations suggest that the host's immune system may play a major role in control of neuroblastoma. Neuroblastoma may elicit both cell-mediated and humoral immune responses. Some of these responses, such as generation of lymphocytes that are cytotoxic to neuroblastoma cells (30), may help the host to control the tumor. Indeed, the presence of a high total peripheral lymphocyte count (>3000 per mm^3) (31), or a high percentage of lymphoblasts in the bone marrow aspirate (32) or in the tumor itself (33), has been correlated with a more favorable prognosis. In addition, some patients respond to the presence of neuroblastoma by producing antibodies directed against tumor-associated antigens on neuroblastoma cells (30). Some immune responses may interfere with tumor control; for example, neuroblastoma patients with advanced disease appear to have a "blocking" factor in their sera (possibly an antigen-antibody complex) that binds to the neuroblasts and inhibits the cytotoxic effect of host lymphocytes (30).

These studies suggest that manipulation of the immune system may offer hope as a form of treatment for neuroblastoma; to date, however, no clinically useful application of immunotherapy in neuroblastoma has been demonstrated.

Clinical Staging

The staging system used most frequently is that of Evans and co-workers (24) (Table 37–2), which is based on the size and extent of the tumor; it does not include lymph node status, operability criteria, or completeness of removal as a determining factor. By contrast, the St. Jude Children's Research Hospital staging system subdivides Stage II patients according to histologic or gross evidence of residual disease and upgrades any patient with lymph node involvement to Stage III (34).

One of the major problems in treating neuroblastoma is the fact that most children have ad-

Table 37–2. STAGING OF NEUROBLASTOMA

	Evans Stage*		St. Jude Stage†
I	Tumor confined to the organ or structure of origin	I	Localized tumor completely resected without local invasion
II	Tumor extending in continuity beyond the organ or structure of origin but not crossing the midline; regional lymph nodes on the ipsilateral side may be involved	IIA	Localized tumor resected with residual microscopic tumor
III	Tumor extending in continuity beyond the midline; regional lymph nodes may be involved bilaterally	IIB	Localized tumor partially or not resected
IV	Remote disease involving skeleton, organs, soft tissues, or distant lymph node groups	IIIA‡	Regional or systemic spread of disease, e.g., metastasis to liver, lymph nodes, or skin without bone or bone marrow involvement
IVS	Same as I or II, but with remote disease confined to one or more of the following sites: liver, skin, or bone marrow	IIIB	Same as IIIA, but with evidence of a single localized destructive lesion of bone, no bone marrow involvement
		IIIC	Generalized tumor in bone and marrow or in marrow only

*Reference 24.
†Reference 34.
‡Stage IIIA (N) = dissemination to regional lymph nodes only.

vanced disease at the time of diagnosis. Using the Evans criteria, the distribution is as follows (35):

Clinical Stage	Relative Frequency (%)
I	9
II	14
III	11
IV	55
IVS	11

Prognosis

The two most important independent variables in predicting the outcome of neuroblastoma are stage and age. Other factors that influence prognosis, albeit to a lesser degree, are histology, primary site, biochemical characteristics, and immunologic status. As seen in Figure 37–2, patients with localized disease (Evans Stages I and II) have an excellent prognosis, whereas those with advanced local disease (Evans Stage III) or metastatic disease (Evans Stage IV) have a more guarded prognosis. Stage IVS patients have an excellent survival (approximately 90 per cent) (24, 25, 26).

When patients are staged according to the St. Jude system, the prognosis for long-term survival is again excellent for patients with truly localized disease (87 per cent for Stages I and IIA). In the St. Jude experience, patients with lymph node involvement (Stage III) have a poor prognosis (33 per cent), even in the absence of more widely disseminated disease to bone or bone marrow (34). On the other hand, Rosen and colleagues (36) have not found regional node involvement to significantly affect prognosis; they have reported an 84 per cent 2-year disease-free survival for such patients. These more favorable results may be attributable to their use of an intensive treatment protocol that included surgical resection of the primary tumor, wide-field radiotherapy, and chemotherapy.

Age of the patient at diagnosis is inversely correlated with survival (Fig. 37–2). Children under 1 year of age have a particularly good prognosis even in the presence of advanced disease, whereas

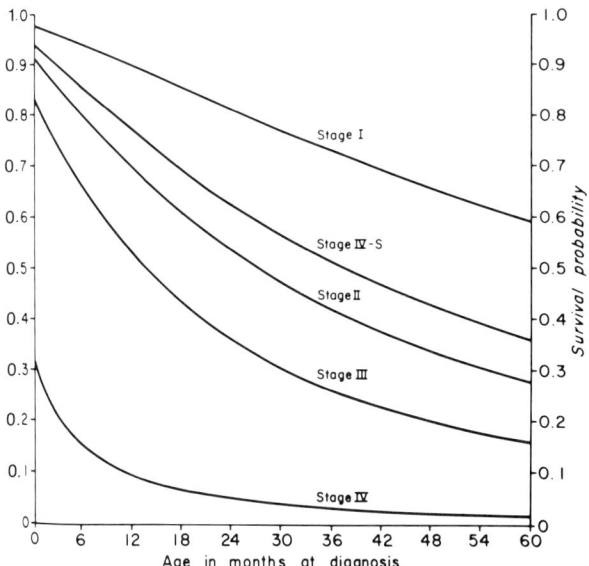

Figure 37–2. Effect of age and stage on prognosis of neuroblastoma. (From Breslow, N., and McCann, B.: Statistical estimation of prognosis for children with neuroblastoma. Cancer Res. 31:2098, 1972.)

children above the age of 1½ to 2 years have a much poorer prognosis.

As mentioned, certain biochemical features, including VMA/HVA ratio (16) and serum levels of lactic dehydrogenase (17), ferritin (19), and neuron-specific enolase (20), have been correlated with prognosis in neuroblastoma. More recently, the presence of hyperdiploid DNA content in the malignant tumor cells has been found to predict a relatively favorable response to chemotherapy (28). There is also a strong correlation between the number of N-*myc* gene copies and prognosis (6a).

Prognosis of neuroblastoma is also influenced by site of the primary disease. Patients with primary neoplasms arising in the cervical region or thorax have a more favorable outlook than those with tumors located within the abdomen. The management of neuroblastoma at these specific locations will be discussed later in this chapter.

Management

Dramatic regression of neuroblastoma can be achieved with radiotherapy as well as with a variety of chemotherapeutic agents. Nonetheless, the long-term outlook for most patients with advanced stages of this disease has not substantially improved over the past several decades. Consequently, the roles of radiotherapy and chemotherapy in the management of neuroblastoma remain poorly defined. Since major toxicities are encountered with each of these modalities, it is incumbent upon the physician caring for the child with neuroblastoma to recognize that a significant subpopulation of patients (approximately 25 per cent) will not require any therapy beyond surgery to achieve long-term control of disease; among this group are the majority of patients with completely resected Stage I–II disease, many patients with Stage IVS disease, and some patients with Stage III disease (particularly those under 1 year of age) (37).

STAGES I–III

Surgical excision is indicated as initial therapy for all children with Stage I–II neuroblastoma. Surgery alone has produced 2-year disease-free survival in the range of 95 to 100 per cent for patients with Stage I and Stage II disease whose tumors were completely excised. As this excellent cure rate is not improved by the addition of adjuvant chemotherapy or radiotherapy, these modalities are not recommended in this situation (38–44).

Excision of the primary tumor (when feasible) also plays an important role in management of the Stage III patient. While this is achievable in less than 25 per cent of patients at the time of diagnosis, subsequent chemo/radiotherapy may eventually render another 25 per cent of tumors resectable at second- or third-look surgery (45). For Stage III patients whose tumors can be resected, the survival rate approaches 80 per cent, versus 31 per cent for those with unresectable tumors (39, 43, 45).

Many centers still advocate radiotherapy to the tumor bed for patients with residual Stage II–III disease, particularly for those above 1½ to 2 years of age. The dose of radiation required to achieve local control appears to be age-related. For children under 1 year, 1200 to 1500 cGy appears to be adequate, while children 1 to 2 years old need slightly higher doses (1500 to 2500 cGy); for older children, doses as high as 4000 cGy (2 to 5 years) to 5000 cGy (>5 years) may be required (45a). At St. Jude Children's Cancer Research Hospital, Stage II–III patients are treated initially with chemotherapy (Cytoxan/Adriamycin) followed by second-look surgery 4 months later. Of 16 patients treated in this fashion, 86.5 per cent survive free of disease; the majority of these were spared radiotherapy (41).

STAGE IV

The primary mode of therapy for the patient with Stage IV neuroblastoma is chemotherapy. Although many chemotherapeutic agents have been tested against neuroblastoma, only 6 have shown significant effectiveness (complete or partial remission rate of >20 per cent) when used as single agents; these are Cytoxan, Adriamycin, cis-platinum, VM26, vincristine, and peptichemio (46–53). Slightly higher response rates have been reported with combination chemotherapy protocols such as Cytoxan/DTIC/ vincristine (48, 55), VAM-DTIC (vincristine/Adriamycin/nitrogen mustard/DTIC) (3, 56), MADDOC (nitrogen mustard/Adriamycin/DTIC/cis-platinum/vincristine/Cytoxan) (54), and Cytoxan/Adriamycin (41). Overall, these combinations produce complete remission in 30 to 40 per cent of patients and partial remission in another 30 per cent; however, recurrences commonly occur within the first year of treatment.

The use of second-look surgery with total resection of residual tumor does not appear to confer significant advantage in terms of long-term survival. In a series of patients reported by the Children's Cancer Study Group, total resection of residual tumor at second-look surgery was achieved in 55 per cent of Stage IV patients, but only 17.6 per cent of these patients had remained disease-free at the time of their report (56).

Overall, about 20 per cent of Stage IV patients are surviving free of disease for 2 or more years (54, 55); however, the prognosis may be more favorable (>40 per cent long-term survival) for

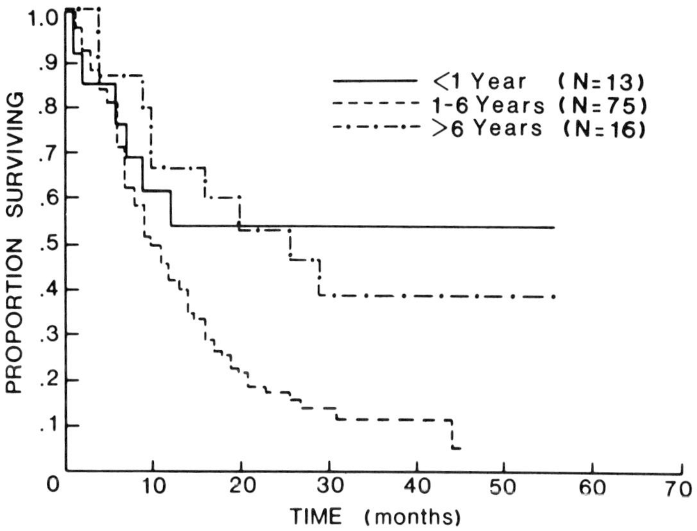

Figure 37–3. Effect of age on prognosis of Stage IV neuroblastoma. (From Finklestein, J. Z., Klemperer, M. R., et al.: Multiagent chemotherapy for children with metastatic neuroblastoma: a report from Children's Cancer Study Group. Med. Ped. Oncol. 6:179, 1979.)

those under 1 year of age or over 6 years of age (54, 55, 56) (Fig. 37–3). Recently, Kretschmar and colleagues (57) have reported a 90 per cent long-term disease-free survival rate for 11 infants with Stage IV neuroblastoma treated with intensive multiagent chemotherapy plus radiotherapy to symptomatic foci of tumor.

Radiotherapy has a clear-cut role for palliation of bone pain and other distressing symptoms such as spinal compression. Single treatments of 300 to 500 cGy are sufficient to palliate bone pain, but doses up to 2000 to 3000 cGy may be required to treat some specific metastatic deposits, particularly when involvement on long bones has the potential to produce pathologic fracture.

STAGE IVS

Management of Stage IVS neuroblastoma remains controversial. Most of these patients will do well, even with minimal treatment. In 1981, Evans and colleagues (25) reviewed a series of 31 patients under the age of 12 months, and found an 87 per cent projected 2-year survival. Treatment varied among the patients in this series. Nine had resection of the primary tumor as their only form of treatment, and all of these patients survived. Among the other patients, 19 had resection of the primary tumor, 21 had liver irradiation (median dose, 450 cGy), and 15 received chemotherapy. Nine patients had progression of tumor, and 4 died. Stokes and colleagues reported a comparable survival rate in a series of 14 patients receiving chemotherapy, radiotherapy, or a combination of the two (57a). The recommendation from these series is that infants with IVS neuroblastoma be managed by close observation only, unless life-threatening complications occur.

The major life-threatening events in IVS neuroblastoma relate to mechanical complications caused by the massive hepatomegaly; these include cardiorespiratory embarrassment by diaphragmatic elevation, hepatic dysfunction, and compression of the inferior vena cava, renal vasculature, and/or stomach. One approach towards shrinkage of the hepatomegaly is the use of low-dose (450 cGy over 3 days) irradiation to a portion of the liver through tangential ports; this approach is designed to minimize spine, gastrointestinal, and renal exposure to radiation. It is particularly important to avoid irradiating the kidney since it has a low threshold for radiation damage in infants under 6 months of age (58). Another approach is to insert a large Silastic patch in the abdominal wall to provide decompression while waiting for liver regression to occur (58a). Chemotherapy with low dose oral Cytoxan (5 mg per kg per day for 5 days, repeated every 2 to 3 weeks if necessary), or vincristine/Cytoxan may be utilized as well.

Factors that may augur a poor prognosis include age less than 6 weeks or over 1 year, presence of bone marrow metastases, or absence of skin metastases (59, 59a). Stephenson and colleagues (59a), after a review of the literature, divided Stage IVS patients into high-risk and low-risk groups. High-risk patients (less than 6 weeks of age and lacking skin metastases) had a 32 per cent survival rate, whereas low-risk patients (7 weeks to 12 months of age regardless of metastases, or less than 6 weeks of age with skin metastases) had an 86 per cent survival rate. Patients in the high-risk group or those with bone marrow metastases may benefit from chemotherapy.

Special Locations

CERVICAL NEUROBLASTOMA

Cervical neuroblastoma is generally diagnosed in the first 3 years of life (usually within the first

6 months of life) and is the most common primary malignancy of the neck in children under 5 years of age. It may present either as an indolent lateral neck mass or with acute airway obstruction or feeding difficulties.

The prognosis for patients with cervical neuroblastoma is relatively good. Review of the literature on this tumor (60) shows that 68 per cent of patients presenting with involvement of only the cervical region survived for more than 2 years. Surgery alone may be curative in patients with localized disease; this is an important consideration, as at least two patients treated with irradiation for cervical neuroblastoma subsequently have developed papillary carcinoma of the thyroid (60).

THORACIC NEUROBLASTOMA

Approximately 14 to 20 per cent of neuroblastomas are found in the thoracic area (3, 61–63). The prognosis for these patients is generally good. Age appears to be a major prognostic feature for patients with thoracic neuroblastoma. In Catalono's series (62), there was an 87 per cent 2-year survival rate in patients under 2 years of age versus a 37 per cent rate in patients above 2 years of age; in Filler's study (63), there were no deaths in patients under 2 years of age, whereas 50 per cent of patients over 2 years of age died. The histologic pattern may also be important in prognosis, the diffuse ganglioneuroblastoma pattern being particularly favorable (10).

When thoracic neuroblastoma patients are divided by clinical stage, the overall survival rates are as follows: Stage I—93.4 per cent; Stages II and III—92.8 per cent; Stage IV—25 per cent (10, 62–64). Although the majority of these patients have been treated with surgical debulking and postoperative radiotherapy (sometimes with chemotherapy as well), there are no available data to suggest significant improvement in relapse-free survival rates by the addition of radiotherapy or chemotherapy. However, postoperative radiotherapy is probably indicated when the patient is above the age of 2 years, when the tumor has a composite pattern, or when there has been significant bulk of tumor left behind (10).

INTRASPINAL (DUMBBELL) EXTENSION

Extradural neuroblastoma is one of the most common causes of spinal cord compression in the pediatric years; however, as a presenting feature of neuroblastoma, it involves only 1 to 4 per cent of cases (65). Prognosis, as in many other forms of neuroblastoma, is largely dependent upon age, with the survival rate of 85 per cent for children under 12 months of age, dropping to 37.5 per cent for children above the age of 2 years (65, 66).

Total removal of tumor is rarely possible, and residual tumor is usually left around nerve roots, ventral to the spinal cord, and in the foramina. Although spontaneous maturation of the unresected paraspinal portion of the tumor to benign ganglioneuroma has been reported (60), postoperative radiotherapy is usually administered to reduce the risk of local recurrence. Low-dose radiotherapy (2000 cGy) appears to be as effective as higher dosages (66), with a much reduced potential for producing gross deformities when delivered to the growing spine. Chemotherapy is not recommended for Stage I and Stage II tumors (65, 66), as no demonstration of improved survival is evident when it is used in these cases, but it is used for unresectable Stage III and Stage IV disease.

New Therapeutic Strategies

Large-Field Irradiation. Several investigators have used large-field radiation therapy techniques, including segmental, hemi-, and total body irradiation to deliver low to moderately high doses of total body irradiation (TBI) at a single defined time during the course of chemotherapy (67–70). To date, these approaches have not only failed to improve survival rates but have also compromised additional chemotherapy administration. A more recent approach has been to deliver fractionated low doses of TBI in 3-week cycles, much as a fourth drug might be added to the three "standard" chemotherapy agents (Cytoxan/DTIC/vincristine). This technique seeks to exploit a potential, albeit small, difference in the sensitivity to radiotherapy of neuroblastoma cells when compared with the response of bone marrow stem cells in tissue culture (71, 72). The projected survival at 2 years is 33 per cent with this approach (67), which is not significantly better than the 25 per cent reported for chemotherapy alone (55).

Bone Marrow Transplantation. The development of bone marrow transplantation techniques has allowed for an escalation of chemotherapy dosage beyond the limits of bone marrow stem-cell tolerance. Therapeutic regimens have utilized supralethal doses of chemotherapy with or without total body irradiation, followed by "rescue" with allogeneic or autologous bone marrow. Preliminary results are encouraging when this approach is employed as early consolidation therapy for patients in complete remission or with minimal residual disease, but are generally poor for patients with persistent bulk disease (73–75a). An obvious concern with the use of autologous bone marrow is contamination with tumor cells; various purging techniques, including the use of immunomagnetic beads, monoclonal antibody and complement, lectin separation, or specific neural toxins, are being employed to deal with this problem (73b).

Maturational Agents. Several physiologic agents influence the proliferation and phenotype of human neuroblastoma cells in tissue culture; in vitro treatment of neuroblastoma cells with agents such as papavarine, prostaglandin E, butyric acid, nerve growth factors, and vitamins C and E can reduce proliferation rates and cause structural alterations such as neurite extension, which are generally associated with differentiation (76, 77). Clinical trials with some of these agents are in progress.

WILMS' TUMOR

Wilms' tumor is an embryonal neoplasm of the kidney. It occurs at an annual rate of 6.9 cases per million white children and 7.6 cases per million black children in the United States, with very little variation in other parts of the world (1). The majority of cases are diagnosed in children between 1 and 5 years of age, with the peak incidence occurring at 3 to 4 years.

Genetics

There are three recognized genetic patterns for Wilms' tumor: *hereditary*, *sporadic*, and *aniridia–Wilms' tumor syndrome*. While the majority of Wilms' tumors arise in a sporadic fashion, approximately 38 per cent of cases are associated with a hereditary propensity; patients with the hereditary form of the disease are more likely to develop multifocal tumors and to develop their tumors at a relatively early age (78).

Individuals with the syndrome of sporadic congenital aniridia, hemihypertrophy, microcephaly, mental retardation, and genitourinary tract anomalies have an extremely high incidence (approximately 33 per cent) of Wilms' tumor (78a). This *aniridia–Wilms' tumor syndrome* is often associated with various interstitial deletions in the short arm of chromosome 11, all of which appear to involve band 11p13 (79); this relationship suggests that the putative Wilms' tumor locus resides in the 11p13 band and that it is a recessive cancer gene whose normal function involves suppression of an oncogene. This hypothesis has been supported by the demonstration of loss of genetic material and resultant homozygosity for the 11p region in Wilms' tumor cells derived from individuals of normal constitutional phenotype and genotype (79a, 79b, 80). The chromosomal events leading to homozygosity for 11p may constitute the "second hit" in the Knudson model of tumorigenesis (80a). (See also Chapter 31.)

Pathology

Wilms' tumor is thought to derive from metanephric blastema, i.e., the precursor tissue for both the stromal and epithelial (renal tubular) elements of the developing metanephron. As a consequence, the tumor usually is composed of a mixture of blastemal, stromal, and epithelial cell types. The histologic appearance consists of an embryonic type of malignant stroma containing undifferentiated spindle-shaped cells surrounding epithelial cells arranged as tubules of various shapes or sizes; abortive glomeruli may be found among these epithelial cells. There may also be smooth and striated muscle, myxomatous tissue, fat, bone, and/or cartilage.

The First National Wilms' Tumor Study (NWTS-1) (81, 82) has reported that certain histologic features of Wilms' tumor, especially the degree of cellular anaplasia and presence of sarcomatous features in the stroma, are of prognostic importance (Table 37–3). The major unfavorable histology variants are classified as *focal anaplasia*, *diffuse anaplasia*, *"rhabdoid" sarcoma*, and *clear-cell sarcoma* (81, 82, 82a). Approximately 12 per cent of Wilms' tumor cases are of unfavorable histology; anaplastic histology comprises about 4 per cent of all cases, clear-cell sarcoma approximately 6 per cent, and rhabdoid tumor about 2 per cent (82a).

Anaplastic Wilms' Tumor. The diagnosis of anaplasia is based on cytologic criteria, including cellular pleomorphism, nuclear enlargement, hyperchromatism, and the presence of bizarre mitotic figures (81). The presence of focal anaplasia has prognostic significance similar to that for diffuse anaplasia (82a). Compared with their counterparts, children with anaplastic Wilms' tumor are generally 1 to 2 years older at diagnosis, are more likely to be non-white, and have a higher frequency of lymph node metastases at diagnosis (82b).

The poor prognosis for anaplastic Wilms' tumor appears to relate more to resistance of the tumor to chemotherapy than to early dissemination of micrometastases. Thus, patients with Stage I anaplastic tumors have a prognosis similar to that for favorable histology tumors of the same stage, and do not appear to require treatment beyond conventional favorable histology chemotherapy (82a). On the other hand, anaplastic tumors of more advanced stage have a very poor prognosis, even when treated extremely intensively (82a). Some of

Table 37–3. EFFECT OF TUMOR HISTOLOGY AND LYMPH NODE STATUS ON PROGNOSIS OF PATIENTS WITH NONMETASTATIC WILMS' TUMOR

Variable	Number of Patients	Relapses (%)	Deaths (%)
Histology			
Sarcomatous	30	63.3	50.0
Anaplastic	40	42.5	37.5
Unknown	46	17.4	15.2
Favorable	516	11.4	8.9
Lymph Nodes			
Positive	90	40.0	32.2
Unknown	7	14.3	14.3
Negative	535	12.3	9.9

these patients may be salvaged with ifosfamide or a combination of cis-platinum/VP-16 (82b).

Flow cytometric studies show a striking association between DNA content, histologic subtype, and prognosis. Hyperdiploidy (>70 chromosomes) appears to be a characteristic feature of anaplastic Wilms' tumor; anaplastic tumors that, in addition, have complex chromosomal rearrangements are the most likely to recur (82c).

Rhabdoid Tumor (Rhabdoid Sarcoma). This highly malignant tumor was originally considered to be a monophasic sarcomatous variant of Wilms' tumor. This histogenesis is unlikely, however, as morphologically similar neoplasms have been found to arise in nonrenal tissues (thymus, soft tissues, central nervous system) (82, 82a).

The distinctive cells of rhabdoid sarcoma are characterized by a single prominent nucleolus and large globular cytoplasmic inclusions composed of whorls of intermediate filaments (83); although the cells resemble rhabdomyoblasts histologically, no evidence of muscle differentiation is present.

Rhabdoid sarcoma has a propensity to afflict the young child; the mean age of patients in NWTS-1 was 18 months (16 out of 21 patients were younger than 2 years at diagnosis) (84). It carries an extremely unfavorable prognosis—the appearance of metastatic disease, often to multiple sites, is very rapid (mean, 4 months), and subsequent survival is short (84). The most common sites of metastasis are liver and lungs (84a). The mortality rate approximates 90 per cent (82a, 84a).

A unique feature of this tumor is its high frequency of central nervous system involvement; in some cases this is a consequence of metastatic disease from the renal primary tumor, but in others it may occur as an independently arising primitive neuroectodermal tumor (82, 82a).

Clear-Cell Sarcoma. Unlike rhabdoid tumor, clear-cell sarcoma occurs solely in the kidneys; it has a predilection for male patients, and the mean age of presentation is 3 to 4 years (82, 85, 85a, 85b). In contrast to the abundant eosinophilic cytoplasm of the malignant rhabdoid tumor, the smaller cells of clear-cell sarcoma have relatively inconspicuous cytoplasm, which may appear to be optically clear.

This tumor has a propensity for bone and possibly lymph node metastasis. In NWTS-1 and NWTS-2, the actuarial 2-year survival rates were 39 and 49 per cent respectively (85b). Preliminary data from NWTS-3 indicate that the prognosis has been distinctly improved by the intensification of chemotherapy through the use of Adriamycin as a third agent (82a).

RENAL TUMORS RELATED TO WILMS' TUMOR

In addition to the spectrum of tumors classified as part of the Wilms' tumor complex, there is a group of renal tumors, also of blastemal origin, whose histology superficially resembles Wilms' tumor but whose natural history is much more benign. Such tumors are classified as *persistent renal blastema/nephroblastomatosis complex* and *mesoblastic nephroma*.

Nodular Renal Blastema/Nephroblastomatosis. In this condition, foci of persistent blastemal cells appear as subcapsular nodules or as sheets of primitive metanephric epithelium. When the nodules are small and localized, the condition is called *nodular renal blastema*; the diffuse form is called *nephroblastomatosis* (86–88). The typical patient is less than 2 years of age and presents with bilateral palpable renal masses and enlarged polycystic-like kidneys on IVP. Actinomycin D and vincristine have been very effective, either alone or in conjunction with radiotherapy, in producing resolution of the process (86, 89).

Nodular renal blastema and nephroblastomatosis are apparently the result of a developmental disturbance occurring relatively late in embryogenesis. They may be precursor lesions of Wilms' tumor, possibly representing the first "hit" in the sequence that leads to true malignancy. Nodular blastema and nephroblastomatosis have been found in kidneys containing a Wilms' tumor (86, 87) and in "uninvolved" contralateral kidneys as well (88); the latter association may account for the phenomenon of bilateral Wilms' tumor. Progression of nodular blastema and nephroblastomatosis to Wilms' tumor has been documented (90, 91).

Mesoblastic Nephroma. Mesoblastic nephroma is usually diagnosed during the first few weeks of life, and it can usually be distinguished from Wilms' tumor by both gross and microscopic appearance. It is composed of interlacing fibrous or mesenchymal stroma; spindle cells are invariably the dominant feature and may represent fibroblasts, smooth muscle cells, or both. These renal mesenchymal tumors span the entire gamut from benign, morphologically quiescent lesions to outright malignant sarcomatous disease with a high risk of distant spread; between these extremes are so-called "gray zone lesions" of indeterminant biologic significance (92). Histologic features that suggest a more malignant variant include irregularly massed cells with high nuclear/cytoplasmic ratio, focal and confluent foci of ischemic necrosis, and mitotic counts of >10 mitoses per 10 high-power fields (93).

Mesoblastic nephroma is usually not encapsulated, and therefore complete surgical removal generally necessitates total nephrectomy. This lesion is a neoplasm of limited capacity for metastasis; consequently, if it is well circumscribed, morphologically well differentiated, and completely removed in an infant less than 3 months of age, it may be safely assumed that no further therapy is necessary (94).

Beckwith (82a) has identified several situations in which the risk of recurrence or metastasis might warrant adjuvant chemotherapy. These include (1) incomplete resection of tumor, (2) intraoperative rupture of tumor, and (3) tumor of dense cellularity and high mitotic index occurring in a patient above the age of 3 months. Vincristine/actinomycin D (in half dosage for infants under 1 year) may be a useful adjuvant regimen, as this combination has been successful in salvaging patients with recurrences. In view of the major sequelae that may complicate irradiation of the infant abdomen, this modality is perhaps best reserved for chemotherapy failures.

NWTS-1 reviewed 51 patients with mesoblastic nephroma. The mean patient age at operation was approximately 3 months, as compared with 3½ years for patients with Wilms' tumor (95). Local extension was noted in 8 patients, and rupture of the tumor at surgery occurred in 10 (20 per cent). No bilateral tumors were found, and no positive lymph nodes were identified; however, few of the specimens were limited by the renal capsule, and in many there were strands of neoplastic tissue extending into the renal sinus or perineal fat. No child suffered metastatic spread of tumor, and there was only one case of local recurrence (a small peritoneal spill occurred at the primary operation). Ninety-eight per cent of patients survive, the only death having occurred secondary to sepsis in association with severe neutropenia following chemotherapy.

Malignant Mesenchymal Nephroma. It is sometimes difficult to distinguish this tumor from "cellular variants" of congenital mesoblastic nephroma; however, the distinction is important, as recurrences and metastases seen in association with malignant mesenchymal nephroma constitute indisputable proof of its aggressive nature (92, 93).

Clinical Features

Wilms' tumor most commonly presents as an asymptomatic abdominal mass; occasionally, patients will present with pain, hematuria, fever, anorexia, or weight loss. Gross hematuria is rare in Wilms' tumor, but about one third of children will have microscopic hematuria. Hypertension, often mild but occasionally severe, is found in as many as 75 to 90 per cent of Wilms' tumor patients (96). This symptom is often associated with elevated plasma renin levels and may reflect renin production either by neoplastic cells or by normal renal parenchyma whose blood supply has been compressed by the surrounding tumor. Less common symptoms include malaise, anemia, erythrocytosis, dysuria, and polyuria.

Wilms' tumor is associated with certain congenital anomalies with unusually high frequency; among these are hemihypertrophy, aniridia, genitourinary anomalies, and Beckwith's syndrome.

METASTATIC SPREAD

Wilms' tumor may metastasize by a variety of routes. Local extension may occur by direct infiltration into the renal pelvis and ureter or through the renal capsule into the perinephric tissues. Preoperative rupture or intraoperative spillage of tumor cells may result in extensive involvement of the ipsilateral flank area. Regional lymph node involvement has been documented in approximately 15 per cent of patients at diagnosis (97, 98); this is an especially poor prognostic feature in patients with otherwise localized tumor (Table 37–3).

Hematogenous metastases result from invasion of the renal veins and inferior vena cava. The lungs and liver are the most common sites of distant spread, pulmonary metastases being demonstrable in approximately 10 per cent of patients at diagnosis and in another 20 per cent within the subsequent 18 months (98–100). In rare instances, Wilms' tumor metastases can be found in bone marrow, salivary glands, tonsils, and other sites (100a). Metastases to cortical bone are generally found only in patients with the clear-cell sarcoma variant (82, 85) and central nervous system involvement in patients with the rhabdoid sarcoma variant (84).

Table 37–4 lists the criteria used by the National Wilms' Tumor Study Group for assessing tumor progression. The staging system has been modified in NWTS-3 to recognize the ominous implications of regional lymph node involvement (upgraded to Stage III) and the less serious implications of localized tumor spillage (downgraded to Stage II).

Management

When children with Wilms' tumor are managed according to modern treatment schedules, the cure rate approaches 90 per cent. The major adverse prognostic features are unfavorable histology and the presence of tumor in regional lymph nodes. In NWTS-2, the mortality rate for favorable histology Wilms' tumor was 8.9 per cent, as compared with 45.6 per cent for unfavorable histology Wilms' tumor (100b).

PREOPERATIVE TREATMENT

Tumor rupture, either preoperatively or during surgery, has been reported to complicate from 16 to 32 per cent of Wilms' tumor cases (101, 103–105). The International Society of Pediatric Oncology (SIOP) has demonstrated that a marked reduction in the frequency of this adverse event can be achieved by shrinking the tumor with either radiotherapy or chemotherapy prior to surgery (103, 105). However, to date, there are no data to suggest that such preoperative therapy will effect an ultimate survival advantage. Furthermore, in the absence of a tissue confirmation, this approach

Table 37–4. NWTS-1 AND -2 GROUPING METHOD AND NWTS-3 STAGING SYSTEM

Group	(NWTS-1 and -2)	Stage*	(NWTS-3)
I	Tumor limited to kidney and completely resected. The surface of the renal capsule is intact. The tumor was not ruptured before or during removal. There is no residual tumor apparent beyond the margins of resection.	I	Tumor limited to kidney and completely excised. The surface of the renal capsule is intact. Tumor was not ruptured before or during removal. There is no residual tumor apparent beyond the margins of resection.
II	Tumor extends beyond the kidney but is completely resected. There is local extension of the tumor, i.e., penetration beyond the pseudocapsule into the perirenal soft tissues, or periaortic lymph node involvement. The renal vessel outside the kidney substance is infiltrated or contains tumor thrombus. There is no residual tumor apparent beyond the margins of resection.	II	Tumor extends beyond the kidney but is completely excised. There is regional extension of the tumor, i.e., penetration through the outer surface of the renal capsule into perirenal soft tissues. Vessels outside the kidney substances are infiltrated or contain tumor thrombus. The tumor may have been biopsied or there has been local spillage of tumor confined to the flank. There is no residual tumor apparent at or beyond the margins of excision.
III	Residual nonhematogenous tumor confined to abdomen. Any one or more of the following occur: (a) The tumor has ruptured before or during surgery, or a biopsy has been performed. (b) Implants are found on peritoneal surfaces. (c) Lymph nodes are involved beyond the abdominal periaortic chains. (d) The tumor is not completely resectable because of local infiltration into vital structures.	III	Residual nonhematogenous tumor confined to abdomen. Any one or more of the following occur: (a) Lymph nodes on biopsy are found to be involved in the hilus, the periaortic chains, or beyond. (b) There has been diffuse peritoneal contamination by tumor, e.g., by spillage of tumor beyond the flank before or during surgery, or by tumor growth that has penetrated through the peritoneal surface. (c) Implants are found on the peritoneal surfaces. (d) The tumor extends beyond the surgical margins either microscopically or grossly. (e) The tumor is not completely excisable because of local infiltration into vital structures.
IV	Hematogenous metastases. Deposits beyond Group III, e.g., in lung, liver, bone, and brain.	IV	Hematogenous metastases. Deposits beyond Stage III, e.g., lung, liver, bone, and brain.
V	Bilateral renal involvement either initially or subsequently on study.	V	Bilateral renal involvement at diagnosis. An attempt should be made to stage each side according to the above criteria on the basis of extent of disease prior to biopsy.

*Staging, which is on the basis of gross and microscopic tumor distribution, is the same for tumors with favorable and with unfavorable histologic features. The patient should be characterized, however, by a statement of both criteria; e.g. Stage II, favorable histology, or Stage III, favorable histology. Tumors of unfavorable type are those with focal or diffuse anaplasia, or those of sarcomatous histology.

incurs an approximately 6 to 10 per cent risk of inappropriately treating benign disease or a malignant tumor other than Wilms' tumor (105, 106). Therefore, preoperative therapy is probably indicated only to facilitate removal of the rare tumor that is too large for safe primary surgical resection (106a).

SURGICAL APPROACH

The initial goal of therapy is to remove the primary tumor, even if distant metastases are present. Surgery should be performed as soon as the patient's condition has been stabilized and the initial evaluation has been completed.

The current recommended approach is via a transabdominal incision. This has the advantage of providing adequate exposure, permitting a thorough exploration of the abdominal contents and opposite kidney as well as a sweeping dissection of the affected renal fossa for removal of the involved kidney and any associated lymph nodes. Careful attention to the renal vein and inferior vena cava is recommended in order to avoid dislodging any tumor that is propagating intraluminally. Tumor that extends into the inferior vena cava is not usually adherent to the vascular endothelium; consequently, it can be removed relatively easily by gentle traction with a forceps after venotomy and control of the vena cava above and below.

The contralateral kidney should be carefully examined. If a small, easily resectable tumor is found in it, then the nodule and a small margin of normal kidney should be excised. Otherwise, the tumor should be biopsied and marked with radio-opaque clips for subsequent radiotherapy.

RADIOTHERAPY

Radiotherapy is not currently recommended for Stage I favorable histology patients of any age, provided 2-drug (vincristine/actinomycin D) adjuvant chemotherapy is given postoperatively. Preliminary data from NWTS-3 suggest that appropriate chemotherapy may obviate the need for radiotherapy for favorable histology Stage II patients as well (107). However, radiotherapy is still recommended for more advanced (Stage III–IV) disease.

It is important to avoid excessive delay (i.e., more than 10 days) in instituting radiotherapy. The radiotherapy field should be large enough to encompass all potential tumor volume, while sparing as much normal tissue as possible, particularly the contralateral kidney and the femoral heads. For localized tumors, the field should include the tumor bed and adjacent para-aortic lymph nodes (107a). The field should be extended to include the entire ipsilateral flank area when localized (confined to the flank) spillage has occurred. With more extensive spread, total abdominal irradiation may be required (108).

When treating favorable histology tumors, there does not appear to be any advantage to using dosages in excess of 2400 cGy, provided adjuvant chemotherapy is also administered; indeed, 1000 to 2000 cGy may be sufficient when no gross residual disease is present (107, 107a, 109, 110). The NWTS modifies dosage according to age in order to minimize disturbance of local bone growth and development, but some authorities (111) do not follow this practice.

Higher doses of radiotherapy are indicated when tumor histology is unfavorable or there is residual bulk tumor. For favorable histology patients, NWTS-3 uses up to 3000 cGy when bulky tumor growth (>3 cm in diameter) is left behind; for unfavorable histology patients, a dosage as high as 4000 cGy is used in children above 3½ years of age.

CHEMOTHERAPY

The chemotherapeutic agents that have achieved response rates in excess of 20 per cent in children with Wilms' tumor are vincristine (71 per cent), Adriamycin (61 per cent), actinomycin D (40 per cent), Cytoxan (33 per cent), and VP-16 (28 per cent) (112, 113).

The use of adjuvant chemotherapy for Wilms' tumor was pioneered by Farber and colleagues in 1966 (113a). This study reported a 70 per cent 2-year relapse-free survival rate for children treated with radiotherapy and a single postoperative course of actinomycin D. However, there were no concurrent controls, and disease stage was not clear. Green and Jaffe's subsequent analysis of these results indicates that the improved prognosis was not attributable to prevention of tumor recurrence, but to other factors, including aggressive treatment of pulmonary metastases by surgical excision and whole lung irradiation (112).

Subsequent to Farber's study, Wolff and colleagues (113b) reported that multiple courses of actinomycin D produced greater relapse-free survival rates than a single course; however, their report did not take into consideration variables that are important in predicting tumor recurrence. Furthermore, subsequent studies (112, 113c) have failed to confirm these results. On balance, actinomycin D appears to increase relapse-free survival by only 10 per cent when used in conjunction with surgery and radiotherapy for Stage I to Stage III Wilms' tumor (112). However, multiple courses of actinomycin D can eliminate the need for radiotherapy in Group I favorable-histology Wilms' tumor patients under 2 years of age (114).

Vincristine has also been used as a single agent for adjuvant therapy of Wilms' tumor. In NWTS-1 (114, 115), patients with Group II and Group III disease treated with radiotherapy and multiple courses of vincristine achieved a 4-year relapse-free survival (57 per cent) that was equal to that achieved with radiotherapy and multiple courses of actinomycin D (56 per cent).

NWTS-2 (114, 115) has shown that double-agent (vincristine/actinomycin D) chemotherapy is superior to the use of single-agent therapy with either of these agents for adjuvant treatment of Wilms' tumor (Table 37–5). In Group I favorable-histology patients, double-agent chemotherapy obviates the need for postoperative radiotherapy in patients of all ages and achieves 90 per cent 4-year survival. In Group II and Group III patients, double-agent chemotherapy in conjunction with radiotherapy achieves 79 per cent 4-year relapse-free survival. Preliminary results from NWTS-3 (107) suggest that double-agent chemotherapy may eliminate the need for radiotherapy in Group II patients.

The role of Adriamycin in the primary treatment of Wilms' tumor has been the focus of several recent studies. Camitta and colleagues (116) have reported encouraging results using a double-agent (vincristine/doxorubicin [Adriamycin]) regimen in a series of 31 patients with disease ranging from Stage I to Stage IV. Adriamycin has also been incorporated with vincristine and actinomycin D into a triple-agent adjuvant regimen. In NWTS-2 (114, 115), patients with Group II and Group III disease who were treated with the triple-agent regimen achieved a higher rate of relapse-free survival than did those treated with the double-agent regimen (Table 37–5). However, this apparent advantage may have derived from the relatively poor performance of the 2-drug regimen in NWTS-2 (which gave actinomycin D in a less intensive schedule than in NWTS-1). In NWTS-3 (107), the schedules for both vincristine and actinomycin D have been intensified, and there is no statistical difference at 2 years in the relapse-free survival rates between the 2- and 3-drug regimens. Likewise, the addition of Adriamycin as a third agent (114) or Cytoxan as a fourth agent (107) has

Table 37–5. RESULTS OF NWTS-1 AND NWTS-2*

Group	Regimen†	Percent Relapse-Free Survival	Percent Survival‡
NWTS-1			
I (<2 years)	RT + Act D (×15 months)	89	94
	Act D (×15 months)	88	90
I (>2 years)	RT + Act D (×15 months)	76	98
	Act D (×15 months)	57	81
II, III	RT + Act D (×15 months)	56	71
	RT + Vcr (×15 months)	57	71
	RT + Act D/Vcr (×15 months)	79	84
NWTS-2			
I	Act D/Vcr (×6 months)	96	97
	Act D/Vcr (×15 months)	90	91
II, III, IV	RT + Act D/Vcr (×15 months)	65	74
	RT + Act D/Vcr/Adria (×15 months)	79	84

*Based on data from reference 114.
†Key: RT = radiotherapy; Act D = actinomycin D; Vcr = vincristine; Adria = Adriamycin.
‡4 years for NWTS-1; 3 years for NWTS-2.

not improved relapse-free survival rates for patients with Stage IV disease or unfavorable histology tumors (with the exception of clear cell sarcoma) (82a).

CURRENT THERAPEUTIC APPROACH — NWTS-3

The goal of treatment of Wilms' tumor is to achieve maximum tumor-free survival with a minimum of iatrogenic complications. NWTS-3, currently in progress, has integrated the results of previous studies to produce the following strategy based on clinical stage and histology:

Favorable Histology Stage I. No postoperative radiotherapy is given; the patients are treated with double-agent chemotherapy (vincristine/actinomycin D) for either 10 weeks or 6 months on a randomized basis. Preliminary results (107) show a 2-year relapse-free survival rate of approximately 90 per cent for these patients, with no significant difference based on length of treatment.

Favorable Histology Stage II. Patients are randomized to receive either no postoperative radiotherapy or 2000 cGy to the tumor bed (or a larger field as dictated by gross and microscopic findings). Chemotherapy is randomized between a triple-agent (vincristine/actinomycin D/Adriamycin) regimen or a double-agent (vincristine/actinomycin D) regimen for 15 months. Preliminary results (107) show 2-year relapse-free survival to be approximately 90 per cent, with no apparent benefit from the addition of radiotherapy or Adriamycin.

Favorable Histology Stage III. All patients receive postoperative radiotherapy, either 1000 cGy or 2000 cGy, to the tumor bed (or larger field) as dictated by gross and microscopic findings. Chemotherapy is randomized as for Stage II. Preliminary results (107) show a 2-year relapse-free survival rate of approximately 76 per cent, with no apparent benefit from addition of Adriamycin or use of the higher dose of radiotherapy.

Favorable Histology Stage IV. Radiotherapy is given to the tumor bed (or appropriate field) using age-adjusted doses (ranging from 1200 cGy in the newborn to 4000 cGy in children above the age of 3½ years). Both lung fields are irradiated with 1200 cGy given in 8 fractions. Chemotherapy is randomized between triple-agent (vincristine/actinomycin D/Adriamycin) or quadruple-agent (vincristine/actinomycin D/Adriamycin/Cytoxan) regimens for 15 months. Preliminary results (107) show 2-year relapse-free survival of approximately 70 per cent with no apparent benefit from the addition of Cytoxan.

Unfavorable Histology Patients. The tumor bed is irradiated in all patients, using age-adjusted doses as discussed for Stage IV. Patients also receive triple-agent therapy with vincristine/actinomycin D/Adriamycin for 15 months.

BILATERAL WILMS' TUMOR

In approximately 5 per cent of cases, nodules of Wilms' tumor of varying sizes may be found in the contralateral kidney. Since this finding is rarely associated with metastatic disease in other areas (even when there is delayed discovery of the contralateral tumor), the most likely interpretation of bilateral Wilms' tumor is that it is consistent with multifocal development of these lesions from embryonic rests (nephroblastomatosis) (90, 91).

Detection of the second tumor may be difficult. Only 9 of 30 patients in NWTS-1 had the second tumor palpable transabdominally, and 10 of 30 did not have obvious roentgenographic signs of disease in the less involved kidney (117). For this reason, it is essential that the contralateral kidney be subjected to direct inspection and palpation during surgery.

In NWTS-1 (117), the prognosis for patients with bilateral Wilms' tumor was excellent, 87 per cent of patients surviving for 2 years or more. Asch and colleagues (117a), in a review of their own patients and of 61 other cases in the literature, came to a less optimistic conclusion (60 per cent 2-year survival). Prognosis is influenced by the patient's age at diagnosis and the stage of the more advanced tumor.

The goal of treatment in all patients is preservation of as much normal renal tissue as possible; however, the therapeutic approach must be individualized, using a judicious combination of chemotherapy, radiotherapy, and surgery. Chemotherapy and radiotherapy recommendations should follow the NWTS guidelines (discussed above). The usual surgical approach is removal of the more involved kidney with heminephrectomy or biopsy of the opposite kidney. In some patients, less extensive surgical procedures, such as bilateral partial nephrectomy and bilateral biopsy, have been employed; these approaches must be followed by intensive chemotherapy and close monitoring of the residual lesions (CT scan every 6 to 8 weeks). If follow-up studies show the tumors to be decreasing in size, chemotherapy should be continued until partial nephrectomy is feasible; if regression is not satisfactory, consideration should be given to radiotherapy followed by partial or complete nephrectomy of the more involved kidney and rebiopsy of the other kidney (117a). Bilateral nephrectomy followed by chemotherapy and renal allotransplantation may be considered for the patient in whom therapy has failed to control local disease or in whom irreversible renal failure has developed; however, the prognosis is poor for such patients (118, 118a).

METASTATIC DISEASE

Even with modern aggressive therapy, approximately 20 per cent of patients with Stages II–III Wilms' tumor, and 50 per cent or more of those with Stage IV disease or unfavorable histology are destined to relapse (119, 119a).

A pulmonary nodule is often the first sign of metastatic or recurrent Wilms' tumor. Whenever possible, this complication should be approached in an aggressive manner with curative intent. The patient with pulmonary metastasis at diagnosis is treated with bilateral whole lung irradiation regardless of the number and the distribution of the metastatic foci. The portal should extend from the apices to the inferior costophrenic recess, and the total dose should not exceed 1200 cGy (higher dosage has been associated with a 10 per cent incidence of clinically overt radiation pneumonitis) (100). However, supplementary dosage can be delivered to residual nodules. Persistent nodules, if few in number, may be removed surgically.

The patient in whom pulmonary metastasis develops as a sign of recurrence during or following chemotherapy should also receive bilateral pulmonary irradiation. Solitary nodules may be removed surgically prior to radiotherapy; however, because of the likelihood that multiple occult foci of disease are present in such patients, pulmonary radiation and possible chemotherapy are still indicated (120). When pulmonary metastases develop in patients who have already received maximal whole lung irradiation, they may be treated with localized radiotherapy, chemotherapy, or surgical resection. Numerous patients have benefited from surgical excision of focal metastases even when they have appeared as sequential solitary metastases.

The choice of chemotherapy for the patient with relapsed Wilms' tumor will be influenced to a certain extent by prior chemotherapy and the timing of the relapse. Combinations that have been used successfully include: vincristine/actinomycin/Adriamycin; vincristine/actinomycin/Cytoxan; vincristine/Cytoxan/DTIC; and cisplatin/VP-16 (100, 101, 119, 121, 122, 122a).

The presence of metastatic disease does not necessarily preclude the possibility of cure. Some reports have indicated a long-term survival rate of 38 to 50 per cent for patients treated for a first episode of pulmonary metastasis with surgery, pulmonary radiotherapy, and chemotherapy (100, 112, 119). However, in a more recent report (119a), the long-term survival rate was only 25 per cent, possibly reflecting the increasing difficulty of salvaging patients who have relapsed despite treatment with the newer, more aggressive chemotherapy regimens. Factors that appear to correlate with survival following relapse include: *duration of initial remission, site of relapse, initial stage of disease,* and *tumor histology* (Fig. 37–4).

Cure of patients with metastasis to nonpulmonary sites is considerably more difficult to achieve, but reports indicate that use of aggressive surgical techniques has resulted in salvage of patients with extensive intra-abdominal spread or extension of metastases to the heart (100, 123).

It is generally accepted that 2 years of survival without recurrence after treatment for Wilms' tumor is a measure of successful therapy. However, 1.4 to 5.0 per cent of patients suffer a recurrence after more than 24 months following treatment (119, 124).

Renal Cell Carcinoma (Hypernephroma)

Since this tumor is presumably derived from renal blastema, it may be regarded as a more differentiated epithelial form of Wilms' tumor in which the cells have acquired a more abundant vesicular or granular cytoplasm (82). It is a rare tumor of childhood, accounting for less than 7 per cent of all primary kidney tumors (125).

The presentation and radiologic appearance may be very similar to that of Wilms' tumor. Although the average age at presentation (11 years) (125, 125a) is considerably higher than that

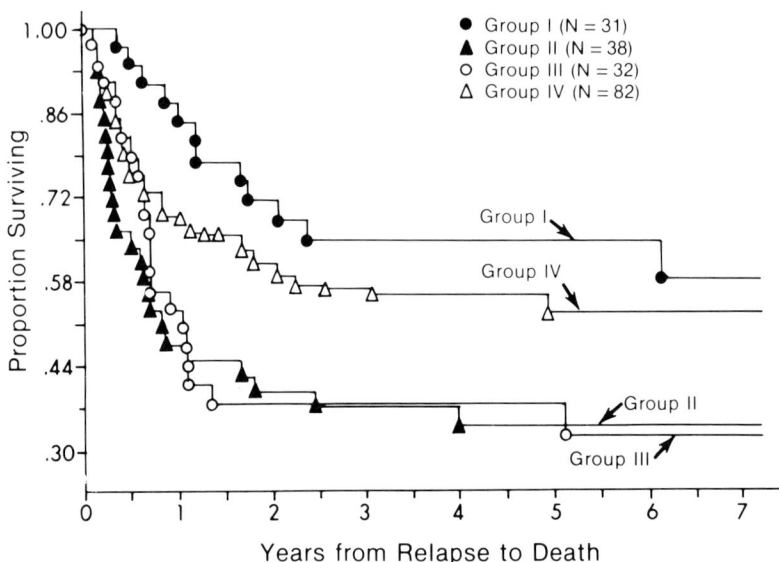

Figure 37-4. Effect of initial stage on subsequent survival of patients with metastatic Wilms' tumor. (Modified from Sutow, W. W., Breslow, N. E., et al.: Prognosis in children with Wilms' tumor metastases prior to or following primary treatment. Am. J. Clin. Oncol. 5:339, 1982.)

for Wilms' tumor, patients as young as 14 months have been reported (125). An abdominal mass is the most common presenting feature, and the classic triad of gross hematuria, pain, and abdominal mass is seldom seen. The tumor spreads by direct extension or by invasion of the renal veins to lungs, liver, bone, and the abdominal cavity, as well as by lymphatic extension to the periaortic lymph nodes (125, 126).

The treatment of choice for patients with localized disease is radical nephrectomy (125a); regional lymphadenectomy would also seem advisable, both to ablate a possible focus of metastatic disease and to identify patients with occult metastatic disease. Adjuvant radiotherapy has been used both pre- and postoperatively, but has not been proved to affect survival (125, 125a, 127). The role of chemotherapy is also yet to be established; however, in one series (128), an 80 per cent survival was reported with the use of surgery, radiotherapy, and actinomycin D.

Survival figures of childhood renal cell carcinoma, although based on relatively few cases, seem to correlate with those seen in adult patients with this tumor. Approximately 50 to 65 per cent of pediatric patients achieve a 2-year disease-free survival (125, 125a); prolonged survival after a recurrence is rarely seen. Prognosis is influenced primarily by clinical and pathologic stage at diagnosis. In regard to histopathologic features, Dehner and colleagues (129) found that the single most important anatomic feature relating to survival was the presence or absence of vascular invasion; however, Lack and co-workers (125a) did not find renal vascular invasion to be an adverse prognostic finding. Another prognostic feature may be the age of the patient, with a young age more consistent with a good prognosis; in the NWTS series (125), all 6 patients under 11 years of age achieved a 2-year relapse-free survival.

Renal cell carcinoma is the second most common tumor (after neuroblastoma) to undergo spontaneous regression, with approximately 70 cases of spontaneous regression having been reported in the literature. Most were adult male patients, and almost all involved regression of pulmonary metastases. However, regression is a rare occurrence when the total number of patients is considered, involving less than 1 per cent of all patients (127).

SOFT TISSUE SARCOMAS

Soft tissue sarcomas account for approximately 6.5 per cent of all malignant neoplasms in children in the United States, with an annual incidence of 0.84 per 100,000 whites and 0.39 per 100,000 blacks (1). Despite the diversity of their apparent tissue of origin (fat, muscle, blood vessels, connective tissue, etc.), the soft tissue sarcomas (Fig. 37-5) share many morphologic and behavioral characteristics as a reflection of their common descent from primitive mesenchyme.

Rhabdomyosarcoma

Rhabdomyosarcoma is, by far, the most common soft tissue malignancy seen in childhood. Although it is frequently described as a tumor of striated muscle origin, there is little evidence in support of this concept. It appears more likely that this tumor arises from primitive or undifferentiated mesenchyme with the capacity for differentiation into muscle; this would explain why rhabdomyosarcoma may originate in areas lacking striated muscle tissue (e.g., common bile duct, urinary bladder, and vagina).

PATHOLOGY

The characteristic cellular element of rhabdomyosarcoma is the rhabdomyoblast, a primitive skeletal muscle cell with eosinophilic cytoplasm and (depending upon the degree of differentiation) cross-striations or longitudinal myofibrils, or some suggestion of their formation. Glycogen granules may be present in the cytoplasm. Within individual tumors, these cells may vary in morphologic appearance. They have been described as round cells, spindle cells, tadpole or racquet cells, spider-web cells, and multinucleated giant cells. The electron microscopic appearance of these cells is more highly characteristic. They have eccentric nuclei, abundant mitochondria, and large numbers of thick and thin cytoplasmic filaments that tend to form so-called Z-bands.

The traditional histologic classification of rhabdomyosarcoma is based upon tissue patterns; the major variants have been called *embryonal, alveolar, pleomorphic*, and *mixed*. The first Intergroup Rhabdomyosarcoma Study (IRS-I) identified three additional types: *sarcoma of undetermined histogenesis*, and *special undifferentiated Types I and II* (extraskeletal Ewing's sarcoma) (130, 131). Nearly two thirds of all childhood rhabdomyosarcoma cases are of embryonal histology; however, the relative proportion of each subtype varies at different primary sites (130, 131). Thus, the embryonal subtype accounts for the vast majority of head and neck, orbital, and genitourinary tumors, whereas the alveolar subtype is found more frequently in the trunk, extremities, and perianal area.

A more recent classification of rhabdomyosarcoma has focused on cytologic features (131a). Three different patterns have been defined: *anaplastic, monomorphous round cell*, and *mixed*. The anaplastic and monomorphous round cell variants make up about 20 per cent of all rhabdomyosarcoma cases and are considered to represent unfavorable histology, whereas the mixed variant is associated with a more favorable prognosis.

CLINICAL MANIFESTATIONS

Although rhabdomyosarcomas may arise anywhere in the body, they occur predominantly in three regions: (1) the head and neck; (2) the retroperitoneum and genitourinary tract; and (3) the upper and lower extremities. In children younger than 10 years of age, rhabdomyosarcoma presents most frequently in the head and neck or genitourinary tract, whereas adolescents more commonly develop truncal, extremity, or paratesticular primaries. The presenting signs and symptoms are variable and reflect the location of the tumor rather than its histology.

ROUTES OF METASTASIS

Rhabdomyosarcoma may spread either by local extension or by metastasis via the venous and lymphatic systems. When metastases develop, 74 per cent will appear within 6 months of diagnosis, and 83 per cent by 1 year (132).

Local extension may follow fascial or muscle planes or may directly infiltrate regional structures. The most frequent sites involved by distant metastases are the regional lymph nodes, lungs, liver, bone marrow, bones, and brain. The incidence of lymphatic spread correlates strongly with the anatomic site of origin of the primary tumor (133). The highest incidence of regional lymph node involvement (40 per cent) has been reported for paratesticular rhabdomyosarcoma; this is undoubtedly a consequence of the rich lymphatic supply of the testis. There is a 15 to 20 per cent incidence of regional lymph node involvement in children with head and neck, extremity, truncal, and genitourinary primary tumors. By contrast, orbital rhabdomyosarcoma, reflecting the paucity of lymphatic vessels in the orbit, is rarely associated with regional lymphatic involvement.

Rhabdomyosarcomas arising in head and neck structures that are adjacent to meningeal surfaces (i.e., the nasopharynx, paranasal sinuses, and middle ear) may extend directly into the central ner-

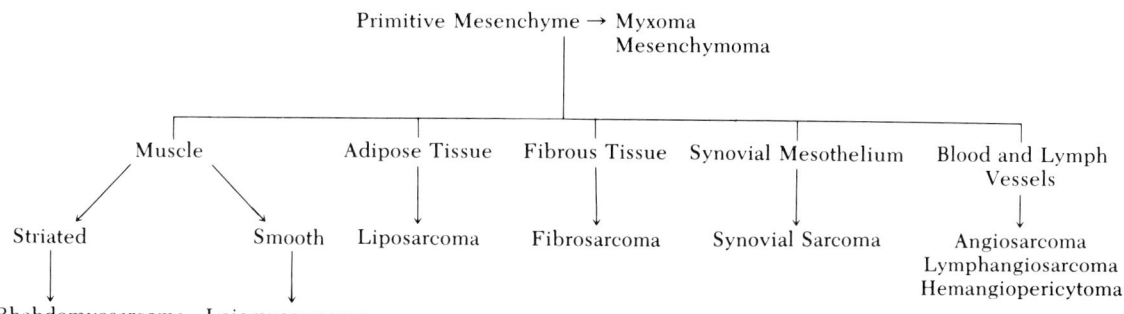

Figure 37–5. Histogenetic classification of soft tissue sarcomas. (From Altman, A. J., and Schwartz, A. D.: Malignant Diseases of Infancy, Childhood and Adolescence. Philadelphia, W. B. Saunders Co., 1983.)

vous system; in the Intergroup Rhabdomyosarcoma Study (134), this complication developed in 35 per cent of such cases.

Because bone does not constitute an effective barrier to the growth of rhabdomyosarcoma, bone invasion is a frequent finding, particularly with lesions of the head and neck region and of the hands and feet. Bone marrow metastases are detectable by routine marrow aspiration in approximately 30 per cent of patients; they may appear individually or in clumps as tadpole-shaped or racquet-shaped cells, primitive monoblast-like cells, or multinucleated cells (136). Cardiac metastases may also develop, and these can result in congestive heart failure (136).

PROGNOSTIC FACTORS

The major factors related to prognosis appear to be (1) age; (2) primary site; (3) histologic type; (4) stage of disease at the time of diagnosis; and (5) treatment.

Age. In early reports, children between the ages of 1 and 7 years had a better prognosis than those above or below these ages (137, 138). This was attributed to less extensive disease at the time of diagnosis and lower rates of tumor recurrence and metastasis, as well as to a higher frequency of the more favorable tumor types in this age group. As treatment has become more intensive, age has become a less important prognostic factor, with the possible exception of a relatively poor outlook for infants with clinical Group III disease (138a).

Primary Site. The anatomy of the primary site appears to influence both the timing of the onset of symptoms and the opportunities for metastasis. As a general rule, sarcomas arising in locations that produce symptoms early and that offer relatively limited opportunities for spread (e.g., orbit) are associated with a better prognosis than are those that arise in deep, poorly confined areas (e.g., retroperitoneum).

Histologic Type. When histologic classification is based on tissue pattern, the best survival rate is associated with the sarcoma botryoides variant of embryonal rhabdomyosarcoma, and the poorest is associated with alveolar rhabdomyosarcoma (139). The new cytologic classification recognizes two unfavorable histology variants: *anaplastic* and *monomorphous round cell.* Combining patients in Groups I to III, the survival rate at 3 years in IRS-I was 47 to 49 per cent for these unfavorable histology variants, compared with 78 per cent for patients with mixed histology (131a, 139a).

Stage of Disease. Accurate staging at the time of diagnosis (see Table 37–6) is critically important, both as a guide to therapy and as probably the most significant determinant of prognosis (140–142). Localized (Group I) and regionally resectable (Group II) tumors are frequently curable with methods presently available. Aggressive multidisciplinary treatment has recently produced some long-term survivors, even among patients with more extensive disease, but the prognosis for these groups still remains guarded.

TREATMENT

In recent years, it has become common practice to employ concurrent prophylactic irradiation and combination chemotherapy in the initial management of all stages of rhabdomyosarcoma rather than reserve them for delayed palliative management of recurrence and metastasis. The goal of these multidisciplinary programs is cure of the patient by the complete eradication of all tumor; indeed, more than half of all children with rhabdomyosarcoma can now be expected to be alive without disease 5 years after initiation of such therapy. Some groups have even reported long-term disease-free survival in over 70 per cent of their patients (132, 141, 142).

Surgery. The efficacy of radiotherapy and chemotherapy has had a major impact on the surgical approach to rhabdomyosarcoma. Formerly, radical operations were the only means to achieve

Table 37–6. INFLUENCE OF CLINICAL GROUP ON PROGNOSIS OF RHABDOMYOSARCOMA (IRS-I)*

Clinical Group	Staging Criteria	3-Year Relapse-Free Survival (%)
I	Localized disease, completely resected (regional nodes not involved) (a) Confined to muscle or organ of origin (b) Contiguous involvement—infiltration outside the muscle or organ of origin	83
II	Localized disease, microscopic residual, or regional disease (a) Grossly resected tumor with microscopic residual disease (nodes negative) (b) Regional disease completely resected (nodes positive or negative) (c) Regional disease with involved nodes, grossly resected, but with evidence of microscopic residual disease	68
III	Incomplete resection or biopsy with gross residual disease	37
IV	Metastatic disease present at onset	19

*Based on data from references 140 and 140a.

cure, often through extensive and disfiguring or disabling procedures. Even then, the results were poor, with high rates of local recurrence and distant metastasis. At present, more conservative surgery is possible in the context of a "total" treatment plan that incorporates multiagent chemotherapy and sometimes radiotherapy.

The role of surgery varies with the anatomic location, size, and extent of the primary tumor. When excision is feasible without producing cosmetic deformity or derangement of function, it remains the most effective mode of therapy for localized rhabdomyosarcoma. For paratesticular and limited truncal or extremity lesions, surgical excision of all gross disease is the primary therapeutic modality, while for certain sites such as the orbit, nasopharynx, prostate, bladder, or female genitourinary tract, the role of surgery is generally confined to biopsy confirmation or limited resection.

With a primary surgical approach, as with other malignancies, the basic principle is wide resection of the primary tumor with an adequate margin of normal tissue; because rhabdomyosarcoma infiltrates diffusely into surrounding tissue, evidence of encapsulation must be regarded as misleading, and the adequacy of resection cannot be fully gauged until it is determined by histologic examination whether any of the margins of the specimen are involved by tumor.

Lymph node evaluation is gaining in importance for staging of rhabdomyosarcoma. Although elective en bloc lymph node dissection is not generally a routine procedure, regional node dissection is appropriate if there are enlarged nodes, if nodes are shown to be positive on biopsy, if the primary tumor is in an area with high propensity to lymph node involvement (133) (e.g., extremity, paratesticular region, spermatic cord, genitourinary system), or if the primary site is in immediate proximity to regional nodes (e.g., axilla, mid-neck, pelvis, para-aortic area).

Radiation Therapy. Early radiotherapists pronounced rhabdomyosarcoma a radioresponsive, but not a radiocurable, lesion, However, in 1968, Cassady and co-workers (143) demonstrated that localized orbital rhabdomyosarcoma could be controlled with adequate radiation therapy doses and field in 90 per cent of cases. Subsequently, Donaldson and co-workers (142) reported a similar local control rate in pediatric head and neck rhabdomyosarcomas treated with surgery, aggressive chemotherapy, and large volume irradiation.

Previously, it had been felt necessary to deliver radiotherapy doses in the range of 5000 to 6000 cGy (over a period of 5 to 6 weeks) in order to effect complete tumor destruction; however, the enhancing effects of concomitant chemotherapy allow for modifications in the radiotherapy approach. Experience in IRS-I and IRS-II has shown that the use of adjuvant chemotherapy can eliminate the need for radiotherapy in "favorable histology" patients who have achieved complete resection of their primary lesion (Group I) (130, 131, 140, 144, 144a) and can allow for reduction in radiotherapy dosage (to 4000 to 5000 cGy) for patients with Group II to Group IV disease (144, 145). The radiotherapy port should include the tissue at risk with a margin of no more than 2 to 5 cm.

Modifications of radiotherapy technique are required when the location or extent of the tumor precludes full dosage. In some instances, variations in the time-dose relationship are necessary to minimize injury to normal tissue (therapy should not exceed 1800 cGy to both lungs, 1500 to 2000 cGy to the kidneys, or 3000 cGy to the liver). In other instances (e.g., irradiation of large areas of mucosa), suitable modifications of the chemotherapy schedule are required to prevent disabling mucositis.

Chemotherapy. The four most effective drugs against rhabdomyosarcoma (and other soft tissue sarcomas as well) are cyclophosphamide, vincristine, actinomycin D, and Adriamycin; imidazole carboxamide (DTIC), cis-platinum, and VP-16 have also shown some activity against soft tissue sarcomas (146, 146a, b).

The chemotherapy regimens that have been used most commonly involve combinations of vincristine, actinomycin D, and cyclophosphamide (VAC). The Standard VAC protocol (Fig. 37–6, Regimen A) has proved very successful for Group I and Group II disease, but a 2-drug vincristine/actinomycin (VA) regimen (Fig. 37–6, Regimen C) appears to be as effective for patients with limited residual disease (140). Patients with Group III and Group IV disease have been treated with the more intensive Pulse VAC regimen (Fig. 37–6, Regimen E) (130, 131); the addition of Adriamycin to this combination (Fig. 37–6, Regimen F) does not appear to confer any added benefit (140, 144a).

Therapeutic Strategy:IRS-II. After analysis of the results of the first Intergroup Rhabdomyosarcoma Study (IRS-I), a second Intergroup Rhabdomyosarcoma Study (IRS-II) was initiated in November, 1978. This study refined the therapeutic approach by (1) eliminating radiotherapy for all Stage I patients, (2) eliminating cyclophosphamide from the chemotherapy regimen of half of the Group I and Group II patients, (3) intensifying the chemotherapy regimen for Group III and Group IV patients, (4) using lower doses of radiotherapy for Group II to Group IV patients (144a, 147).

Group I. Once the primary tumor has been resected, treatment is directed toward eradication of occult metastatic disease with adjuvant chemotherapy (144a). Using the 2-drug VA regimen, the 2-year relapse-free survival rate was 83 per cent,

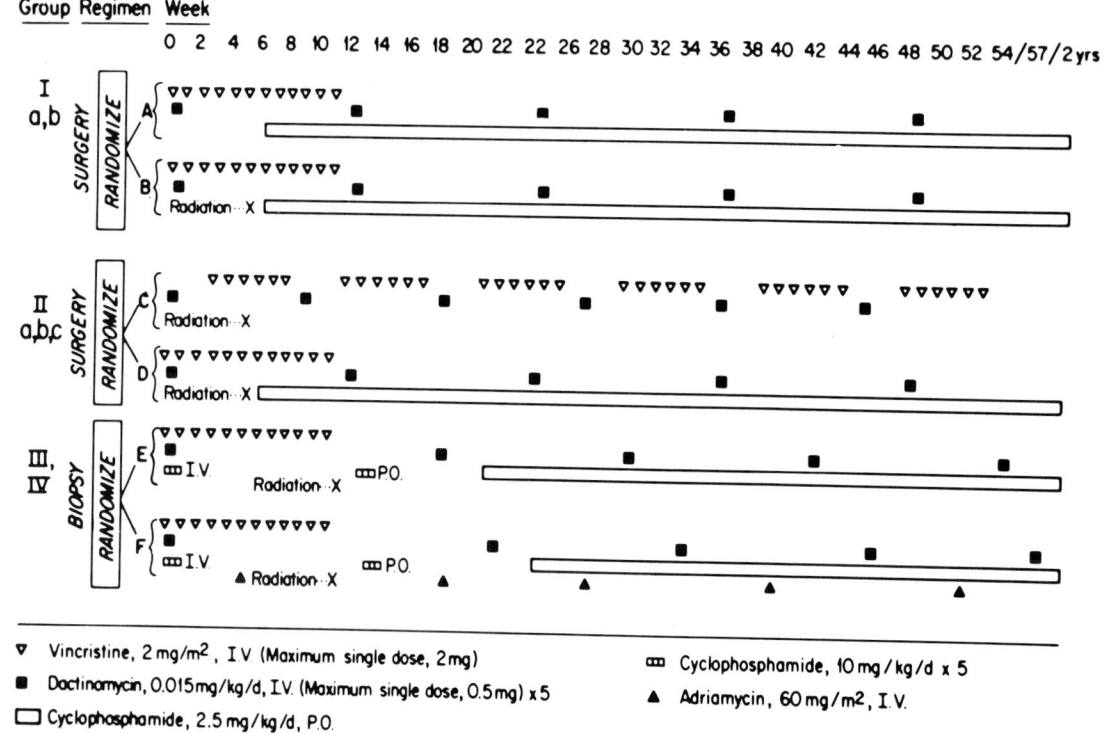

Figure 37–6. Treatment schedules for Intergroup Rhabdomyosarcoma Study. (From Tefft, M. D., Hays, D., et al.: Radiation to regional nodes for rhabdomyosarcoma of the genitourinary tract in children: is it necessary? Cancer 45:3065, 1980.)

versus 87 per cent for patients receiving Standard VAC; this difference is not statistically significant. Group I patients with alveolar, anaplastic, or monomorphous histology represent a subgroup with a high recurrence rate of 43 per cent (147); this has caused the IRS to consider use of more intensive chemotherapy as well as radiotherapy for this subgroup of unfavorable histology patients.

Group II. Since microscopic residual disease is present, radiotherapy (4000 to 4500 cGy) is administered to the tumor bed in all patients. Chemotherapy (either repetitive Pulse VAC or intensive VA) is given to all patients for 1 year. To date, the intensive VA regimen appears to achieve results that are as good as, and possibly better than, those obtained with VAC (144a).

Group III. Intensive chemotherapy (repetitive Pulse VAC with or without Adriamycin) is used to shrink gross residual tumor and to treat occult metastatic foci. After 6 weeks of chemotherapy, the primary tumor is irradiated. Radiation dosage varies from 4000 to 5500 cGy, based on the age of the child and the amount of residual tumor (145). Approximately 75 per cent of patients remain alive after 2 years of follow-up (144a).

Group IV. Intensive chemotherapy, as for Group III disease, is given. The primary site as well as bulk metastatic disease receives radiotherapy as well. With this approach, 61 to 72 per cent of patients show an initial response to chemotherapy. but the relapse rate is high and less than 40 per cent will be alive 2 years following diagnosis (144a).

Relapses. In the IRS-I study, the site of first clinical recurrence was local in 24 per cent of patients, regional in 12.5 per cent, regional and distant in 12.5 per cent, and distant alone in 50 per cent (140). Any recurrence, whether it was local, regional, or distant, augured a poor prognosis, with a median survival of approximately 20 weeks (140). Nonetheless, local and regional recurrences should be approached as potentially curable and treated aggressively with surgery, radiotherapy, and adjuvant chemotherapy.

Ninety per cent of deaths from rhabdomyosarcoma occur within the 2-year period following diagnosis (148, 149), and, for this reason, patients surviving free of disease beyond this point are considered to be long-term survivors with a high probability of cure. However, late relapses (as long as 5 and 6 years after diagnosis) have been reported; patients with parameningeal primary tumors appear to be particularly prone to late relapses (150).

Special Sites

Orbit. The orbit (which has bony confines and a paucity of lymphatics) limits both local extension and lymphatic metastasis of a tumor. The relatively small area resulting from these bony confines also results in early recognition due to exophthalmos. Consequently, orbital tumors have a very good prognosis (137, 142).

At one time, exenteration of the orbital contents was regarded as the primary procedure in the management of orbital rhabdomyosarcoma; however, the recognition that radiotherapy and chemotherapy can achieve excellent disease control has resulted in a more conservative surgical approach. Surgery should generally be limited to obtaining a tissue diagnosis and removing as much tissue as possible without affecting visual function. This is followed by external beam radiotherapy and combination chemotherapy (usually VA or VAC). With this type of therapy, the survival rates are in excess of 80 per cent (151).

Head and Neck (Nonorbital and Nonparameningeal). Children with nonorbital, nonparameningeal head and neck soft tissue sarcomas have an excellent rate of local control and survival when treated with judicious surgery and combination chemotherapy/radiotherapy. Patients with primary tumor arising in the oral cavity, oropharynx, larynx, parotid region, cheek, and scalp have an actuarial 5-year complete remission rate exceeding 90 per cent (152); the results are less good in patients with cervical primaries, for whom the 5-year complete remission rate is 54 per cent (152).

Cosmetic and functional considerations make it difficult to achieve surgical excision with sufficiently wide margins to permit elimination of irradiation. The use of conservative radiotherapy portals and dosage allows minimization of the late effects of combined therapy on facial bones, salivary glands, dentition, and cartilaginous structures. The IRS has found that radiation ports need only subtend the primary tumor with a moderate margin, and the dose to control the primary tumor can be as low as 4100 cGy in patients with only microscopic residual tumor (Group II), provided adjuvant chemotherapy is used (152).

Head and Neck (Parameningeal). Parameningeal sites include the middle ear, auditory canal, mastoid, nasal cavity, paranasal sinuses, nasopharynx, and infratemporal fossa. The nasal cavity, nasopharynx, and maxillary antrum have abundant lymphatics and a lack of anatomic confines; consequently, tumors arising in these locations can easily extend to neighboring structures and lymphatic channels. Moveover, they usually do not produce symptoms until they are fairly far advanced, and thus they have a very poor prognosis. Rhabdomyosarcoma of the ear also is associated with anatomic features that augur a poor prognosis; these lesions exhibit aggressive destructive local growth and metastasis through lymphatic and hematogenous routes.

Patients who have no clinical or radiologic evidence of intracranial extension have an excellent prognosis (153), provided the radiotherapy field extends beyond the primary site and to a margin of meninges limited to 2 cm above the skull base. Approximately 35 per cent of patients with lesions in parameningeal locations will show signs of meningeal extension (cranial nerve palsy, bone erosion at base of skull, intracranial tumor extension, increased intracranial pressure), and the prognosis is extremely poor for such patients (134).

In an effort to improve the prognosis of patients with documented parameningeal extension, some groups have adopted CNS prophylaxis regimens incorporating both radiotherapy and intrathecal chemotherapy. The IRS (154) has treated a series of 61 children with craniospinal radiotherapy and triple-agent (methotrexate, cytosine arabinoside, hydrocortisone) intrathecal chemotherapy; initial results are encouraging, with a relapse-free survival rate of 67 per cent at a median follow-up interval of 96 weeks. Similar results in a small series have been achieved by Gasparini and colleagues (155) using radiotherapy to the brain and single-agent (methotrexate) intrathecal chemotherapy.

Trunk and Thorax. The trunk is an uncommon location for childhood rhabdomyosarcoma; when such involvement does occur, it tends to be located in the chest wall or paraspinal region. The histologic subtype is often alveolar or pleomorphic rhabdomyosarcoma.

Because of a relatively high rate of local recurrence, all visible tumor should be completely excised whenever possible. This is often more easily accomplished after chemotherapy or radiation therapy has caused shrinkage of the tumor (154); however, aggressive surgical procedures such as full-thickness resection of the chest wall and pleura with reconstruction of the chest wall may sometimes be required. If tissue margins are widely adequate, no postoperative irradiation appears necessary so long as aggressive systemic chemotherapy is administered (156). If margins are inadequate, irradiation is necessary; 5000 cGy will generally suffice if only microscopic residual is present.

Patients with tumors arising in the trunk have an overall 50 per cent long-term tumor-free survival (157, 158). However, there is considerable anatomic variation, with prognosis being most favorable when the tumor arises in the paraspinal region, intermediate when it arises on the abdominal wall, and poor when it arises on the chest wall or in the retroperitoneal region (158, 159). These prognostic differences appear to be influenced by extent of disease at diagnosis, histologic subtype, and frequency of life-threatening complications of treatment, such as cardiomyopathy and radiation enteritis.

Tumors arising within the thorax (mediastinum, lung, pleura) are frequently associated with advanced disease at presentation and have a very high mortality rate. If it is at all feasible, surgical removal of all or most of the tumor bulk offers the best hope of cure; residual tumor should then be treated by radiotherapy (with generous margins) and combination chemotherapy (157).

Extremity. Extremity rhabdomyosarcoma is seen mainly in adolescents and is associated with a relatively high incidence of alveolar histology (44 per cent versus 16 per cent for all other sites) (160), a relatively high incidence of dissemination at diagnosis, and a generally poor prognosis (160, 161). Histology is of particular importance for prognosis of extremity rhabdomyosarcoma, as alveolar histology tumors have a relapse rate (65 per cent) that is twice that of tumors with embryonal histology (35 per cent) (160).

These tumors should be treated by wide surgical excision if this can be achieved without producing major functional defect. Amputation is rarely appropriate, but may be considered if irradiation will lead to functionally unacceptable growth discrepancies. In general, however, extensive surgical resection (including amputation) has not improved the prognosis for this group; indeed, patients requiring primary amputation have had lower survival rates than those undergoing primary local excisions. This is because the major problem in management of extremity rhabdomyosarcoma has been failure to control systemic disease, especially in patients with alveolar histology. In IRS-II, extremity rhabdomyosarcomas that exhibit alveolar histology or require primary amputation are being treated with very intensive chemotherapy (160).

Bladder and Prostate. Bladder lesions tend to remain superficial, so that regional or distant metastases do not develop until the primary tumor is far advanced. By contrast, prostatic rhabdomyosarcoma disseminates rapidly through tissue planes into the bladder neck and urethra; lymphatic involvement occurs in about 20 per cent of patients, and distant metastases in 40 per cent (162).

Prior to the development of effective chemotherapy regimens, limited forms of surgery for bladder rhabdomyosarcoma were uniformly followed by local recurrence and death (162, 163), while more radical exenterative procedures achieved only modest success (10 to 40 per cent survival) (163, 164). Likewise, treatment of prostatic rhabdomyosarcoma by surgery alone or by surgery and local radiotherapy resulted in few long-term survivors (163, 165). However, when combination chemotherapy such as VAC is employed in conjunction with exenterative procedures and radiotherapy, survival rates for bladder and prostatic rhabdomyosarcoma are improved to the extent that they are comparable, or superior, to those attained for rhabdomyosarcoma of other sites (149, 166).

Following up on the encouraging results achieved with combined modality treatment, various groups (140, 166–170) have attempted to use a primary chemotherapy approach to obviate the need for radical exenterative surgery and high-dose radiotherapy. To date, these studies indicate that primary chemotherapy, as a single modality, is inadequate to achieve durable local tumor control; for example, only 18 per cent of patients in the IRS-II study achieved pathologically documented complete remission after chemotherapy (Pulse VAC) alone (169, 171). Thus, the overwhelming majority of patients with bladder or prostatic rhabdomyosarcoma will still require radiotherapy or surgery following chemotherapy. However, with a coordinated plan of management, it may be possible to minimize the detrimental effects of surgery and radiotherapy on the pelvic organs.

Perineal-Anal. Sarcomas arising in this region have a poor prognosis (31 per cent relapse-free survival); this probably reflects the relatively high frequency of alveolar histology (171a).

Female Genital Tract. Rhabdomyosarcoma may arise in the wall of the vagina, bladder, uterus, or cervix. Abnormal vaginal bleeding is the most common presenting complaint, although sometimes a polypoid mass lesion may actually protrude through the vaginal opening. Spread occurs by direct infiltration of the vaginal wall and pelvic structures, by lymphatic spread to regional nodes, and by vascular routes to the lungs, bone marrow, and other distant sites.

The "gold standard" for treatment of female genital tract sarcomas has been radical surgery (anterior exenteration) followed by combination chemotherapy and radiotherapy; with this approach, the long-term survival rate approximates 90 per cent. Attempts to modulate the mutilative sequelae of surgery by using chemotherapy or radiotherapy, or both, as the primary modalities of treatment led to encouraging early results; however, longer follow-up has indicated that not all female genital tumors are susceptible to this approach (172, 173, 173a). Indeed, vaginal and uterine sarcomas appear to be clinically distinct in both their epidemiology and response to therapy.

Vaginal sarcomas appear early in life (mean age 1.8 years) and respond well to combination chemotherapy. In IRS-1, excellent results were obtained with primary Pulse VAC or VADRC followed by limited surgery (hystero/vaginectomy for proximal lesions and vaginectomy for distal lesions), local radiotherapy, or both. Among 24 evaluable patients, there were 6 relapses and 2 deaths (173a). A French group (174) has been able to avoid surgery entirely by using systemic chemotherapy and local irradiation (^{192}Iridium wire implants); however, the long-term consequences of this mode of irradiation are unknown at present.

Primary *uterine* sarcomas generally occur in adolescence (mean age >14 years) and have a relatively poor response to chemotherapy. Over 60 per cent of patients treated with primary chemotherapy had progression of tumor and died within 1 year of diagnosis (173a); extensive surgical resection may remain the primary mode of therapy for these patients.

Paratesticular. Most of these tumors occur as painless unilateral masses, arising above the testis and below the superficial inguinal ring. The major pathway of metastasis for paratesticular rhabdomyosarcoma is via the lymphatics; 40 to 45 per cent of patients have demonstrable retroperitoneal node involvement, as compared with only a 15 per cent incidence of histologically demonstrable venous invasion (175, 176). Distant metastasis to bone and lung occurs frequently in the late stages of the disease, after local recurrence cannot be controlled or when retroperitoneal disease becomes extensive.

Adequate surgical removal of this lesion requires radical orchiectomy with early clamping and high ligation of the spermatic cord. Unless there is evidence of systemic metastases, retroperitoneal lymph node dissection is done for both staging and therapeutic purposes. Opinion differs as to whether a unilateral or bilateral dissection should be performed (175, 176).

The role and appropriate dosage of radiotherapy have yet to be defined adequately. Delivery of the standard rhabdomyosarcoma dose (5000 cGy over 5 weeks) to the retroperitoneal area along with chemotherapy can result in considerable morbidity, involving such complications as enteritis, bowel obstruction, fistula formation, and myelosuppression. It has been suggested that radiotherapy can be eliminated from the treatment regimen after a negative node dissection for Group I disease, and the dose reduced for the remaining groups (176).

Combination chemotherapy should be part of the treatment plan of all patients with paratesticular rhabdomyosarcoma; all patients should receive at least vincristine and actinomycin D for 1 to 2 years, with Cytoxan added for patients with advanced disease.

By judicious combination of surgery, chemotherapy, and sometimes radiotherapy, the IRS has achieved 87 per cent disease-free survival at a median of 3½ years for patients with paratesticular rhabdomyosarcoma (176). Relapse rates vary from 3 per cent for patients with Group I tumors to 40 per cent for those with Group III and Group IV tumors (177).

Fibrosarcoma

Fibrous tissue tumors of childhood range from the relatively benign fibromas and fibromatoses to the more aggressive fibrosarcomas. *Fibrosarcomas* are cellular fibroblastic tumors that manifest significant anaplasia, marked variation of cytologic size and shape, and frequent mitotic figures; the histologic features of these lesions do not always correlate well with their clinical behavior, especially in infancy and early childhood (178, 178a–c).

Although common in adults, this tumor is rare in the pediatric age group. A retrospective epidemiologic study conducted by the National Cancer Institute (NCI) found only 182 patients below the age of 19 years reported over a 20-year period (178).

TREATMENT

The initial approach to this tumor should be total surgical excision, if this can be achieved without jeopardizing significant function of the affected part. Radical excision of the local area should be carried out with removal of all possible areas of direct spread, without regard to nodal drainage (179–181). For superficial lesions, wide excision should include the underlying fascia and frequently requires a split-thickness skin graft for closure, with proper precautions to avoid seeding of tumor in the donor site; for deeper lesions, involved muscle bundles should be removed at their origins and insertions.

Extremities should not be amputated without first exhausting the possibilities of less drastic measures (182, 183). If recurrence follows radical local excision of fibrosarcoma in an extremity, some authors (180) would then recommend amputation; others (182) feel it is justifiable to continue repeated local excisions as long as the extremity is functional. Unfortunately, even with this latter approach, with which every attempt is made to salvage the extremity, a number of children with fibrosarcoma in an extremity will ultimately require amputation (180).

There is a relative paucity of published data concerning the use of chemotherapy in infantile fibrosarcoma. However, individual reports document temporary remissions, reduction of tumor bulk sufficiently to permit total surgical excision, and induction of complete long-lasting clinical responses without resort to surgical excision (180, 183a, 183b). While surgical excision (when feasible) remains the treatment of choice for infantile fibrosarcoma, a primary chemotherapeutic approach may allow for less radical surgery in selected patients (183a,b). Radiation therapy may be of benefit in patients with recurrent disease (180, 182, 184) or with unresectable tumors (181).

PROGNOSIS OF FIBROSARCOMA IN CHILDREN

In contrast to the highly anaplastic fibrosarcoma found in adults, the pediatric variant tends to behave in a relatively indolent fashion. In the NCI review, 80 per cent of patients had localized disease, 8 per cent had regional spread, and only 12 per cent had disseminated disease at the time of diagnosis (178). Likewise, in Stout's series of 54 cases, only 18 per cent had demonstrable metastases (183).

Prognosis is dependent mainly upon site of origin and extent of disease at diagnosis. In the NCI series (178), 80 per cent of patients were alive 5 years after diagnosis, but survival was much better for patients with truncal, lower extremity, and head and neck tumors than for those with retroperitoneal disease; the poor prognosis for the retroperitoneal lesions appears to relate mainly to late diagnosis after there has been tumor invasion of adjacent vital structures. Despite the favorable prognosis for survival, local recurrences may present problems, and these have been known to develop as late as 31 years after resection of the primary tumor (185).

Synovial Sarcoma

Synovial sarcoma is an uncommon mesenchymal malignancy that occurs in the vicinity of joints, bursae, and tendon sheaths. Despite its name, it does not arise from synovial membrane but from primitive mesenchymal cells that have partially differentiated into a tissue resembling synovium (186). The histology is characteristically biphasic, with both epithelial and spindle cell components.

CLINICAL FEATURES

Clinical symptomatology includes a painless mass, a tender mass, or pain preceding the development of a mass. The common sites of involvement are the knee, thigh, foot, and hand (synovial sarcoma is the most common soft tissue sarcoma of the hands and feet). Approximately 15 per cent of synovial sarcomas arise in unexpected sites, such as the back, chest, abdominal wall, and head and neck region, that are distant from synovium-lined spaces (187, 188); presumably such tumors originate from undifferentiated mesenchyme that has retained the potential for synovioblastic differentiation.

Metastasis occurs chiefly via the blood stream. In almost every case in which distant metastases have been reported, the lungs have been involved. Metastasis to regional nodes occurs in 20 to 23 per cent of cases (186, 189), and bone metastases appear in 20 per cent (186). The tumor also spreads locally along fascial and muscle planes for extraordinary distances and is notorious for its high frequency of local recurrence (66 to 77 per cent) (186, 189).

THERAPY

The optimal management of synovial sarcoma remains a matter of debate. Some authors advocate radical surgical excision (including amputation if necessary) as the primary therapeutic modality (189, 190), while others advise wide local "en bloc" excision in combination with radiotherapy and possibly chemotherapy (186, 190a,b). In recent years the tendency has been to reserve amputation for recurrences. Regional lymph node dissection may also be indicated (189).

Patients whose tumors have not invaded bone, major blood vessels, or nerve have generally done well with the limited surgical approach, especially if the tumors are <5 cm in size, are well to moderately differentiated, and are at the elbow or knee and below (190a). On the other hand, those whose tumors are more extensive, less differentiated, or located on the thigh, upper arm, or buttock have fared poorly, even when subjected to amputation (190a,c).

Since distant metastasis is common, it is reasonable to begin adjuvant chemotherapy at the time of diagnosis. Pending definitive controlled studies, combination chemotherapy regimens similar to those used for rhabdomyosarcoma may be considered.

Several reviews have emphasized the long natural history of this tumor and its propensity to recur after a long latent period (186, 190, 191). Consequently, 5-year or even 10-year disease-free survival may not necessarily represent "cure." In the series of Cameron and Kostuik (190), for instance, the average survival rate at 5 years was 45 per cent, but this fell to 30 per cent at 10 years and to 10 per cent after 10 years.

Soft Tissue Tumors of Neural Origin

Askin and colleagues (192) have described a unique malignant small cell tumor of the thoracopulmonary region in 20 children and adolescents. This tumor appeared to originate in the soft tissues of the chest wall or the peripheral lung and tended to recur locally. Although systemic dissemination was unusual, median survival was only 8 months. The histogenesis of this neoplasm is uncertain; some evidence suggests a neuroepithelial derivation.

Other authors (193, 194, 195) have also described primitive neuroectodermal tumors arising in soft tissues; these may originate in peripheral nerves and typically present in adolescents and young adults as a large tumor mass, usually in an extremity. They bear a strong histopathologic resemblance to neuroblastoma.

Recent cytogenetic evidence indicates that the Askin tumor and the primitive neuroectodermal tumors known as neuroepithelioma, adult neuroblastoma, or medulloepithelioma may all be identical tumors. In each case studied, a reciprocal (11;22) (q24;q12) translocation has been identified (195a,b). Interestingly, this same translocation is also characteristic of Ewing's sarcoma.

The prognosis for these tumors, now classified as peripheral neuroectodermal tumors (PNETs), has been poor. They tend to metastasize to bone (195c,d) and do not respond to neuroblastoma-type chemotherapy (195c). Recently, however, regimens including those used for Ewing's sarcoma have been reported (193, 195b,d).

Ewing's Sarcoma of Soft Tissue (Extraskeletal Ewing's Sarcoma)

This tumor is composed of primitive small round cells identical to those of Ewing's sarcoma of bone. It is classified by the IRS as an undifferentiated variant of rhabdomyosarcoma; however, it exhibits no evidence of skeletal muscle organelles and, unlike other soft tissue sarcomas, has no discernible cytoskeleton, intracellular collagen, or collagenous intracellular matrix at the ultrastructural level (196, 197).

The IRS approach to this tumor is to attempt a wide local excision followed by chemotherapy. Local radiotherapy is used only if gross or microscopic residual tumor is left behind or if there is regional lymph node involvement. With this approach, a local control rate of 76 per cent and a disease-free survival of 71 per cent was achieved (3 to 7 year follow-up) for truncal and extremity extraskeletal Ewing's sarcoma (158).

At the National Cancer Institute (198), wide local excision is not routinely performed. Instead, patients are treated with high-dose local radiotherapy and VAC chemotherapy. The results achieved are comparable to the IRS results, with 82 per cent local control and 64 per cent disease-free survival after 3 to 7 years of follow-up.

BONE TUMORS

Primary cancers of bone are uncommon malignancies in children; they are, however, the second most common group of solid malignant neoplasms to occur in adolescents and young adults. In the United States, the annual incidence is 5.7 cases per million white children and 3.4 cases per million black children under 15 years of age (1).

The two most common bone tumors are osteosarcoma, a tumor composed of large spindle cells that produce osteoid, and Ewing's sarcoma, a small round cell tumor. Ewing's sarcoma is the more common of the two in patients under 10 years of age, while osteosarcoma is the more common in teenagers. Ewing's sarcoma tends to involve flat bones (vertebrae, ribs, pelvis) or the midshaft (diaphysis) of long bones, whereas osteosarcoma primarily involves the distal portion (metaphysis) of long bones.

Osteosarcoma

EPIDEMIOLOGY

Development of osteosarcoma is closely correlated with linear bone growth. It is rarely seen in the prepubertal child, but after puberty the incidence rises with age to peak at 15 to 19 years, after which a sharp decline occurs (199). Up to the age of 13, both sexes have similar growth rates and a similar incidence of osteosarcoma. After this age, however, the figure for females plateaus while it continues to increase for males, reflecting their more rapid growth rate during this period. The result is an overall preponderance of males afflicted with osteosarcoma, with a male:female ratio of 1.5:1 (200).

The correlation between bone growth and osteosarcoma incidence suggests that a locally high growth rate may predispose a bony site to neoplasia, possibly by affording increased opportunities for mutation to occur. Consistent with this is the fact that the most common sites of osteosarcoma are the rapidly growing ends of the most rapidly growing bones (distal femur, proximal humerus, proximal tibia).

Genetic factors are clearly involved in the pathogenesis of osteosarcoma. At least 16 sets of siblings with this malignancy have been reported (200a). In addition, patients with the hereditary form of retinoblastoma manifest a predisposition to development of osteosarcoma that is roughly 500 times that seen in the general population (201); loss of genetic material in the q14 region of chromosome 13 has been described in retinoblastoma, osteosarcoma associated with retinoblastoma, and sporadic osteosarcoma and may be the pathogenetic mechanism these tumors have in common (201a).

The only environmental factor to have been definitely implicated in the pathogenesis of osteosarcoma is irradiation. Approximately 4 per cent of all osteosarcomas arise in previously irradiated bone (200). In approximately half of these cases, the radiation had been administered for treatment of another primary tumor such as retinoblastoma or Wilms' tumor. The latent period between radiotherapy and diagnosis of osteosarcoma averages 14.2 years (202) but is significantly shortened for children with a genetic predisposition and in preadolescent and adolescent children (who are closer to the age-appropriate occurrence of the tumor) (203). Development of osteosarcoma has also been associated with the therapeutic use of radium in patients with ankylosing spondylitis (204).

PATHOLOGY

Osteosarcoma is a malignant spindle-cell neoplasm that arises from bone-producing mesenchymal cells. It is characterized by the production of osteoid substance in at least some portion of the tumor; this is identifiable on hematoxylin and eosin stained sections as extracellular pink hyaline matrix that may or may not calcify.

Osteosarcoma is not a single disease entity; the basic histologic classification includes at least 9 variants. Approximately 75 per cent of the cases form a relatively homogeneous group considered to represent "classic" osteosarcoma; these may be subdivided according to the appearance of the predominant matrix into three types: *osteoblastic, chondroblastic,* and *fibroblastic.* The remaining 25 per cent form a heterogeneous group of variants, each of which has a unique malignant potential; included in this group are *telangiectatic, low-grade intraosseous, periosteal, parosteal, small cell,* and *malignant fibrous histiocytoma.*

Telangiectatic osteosarcoma is a predominantly lytic tumor with large areas of dilated vascular channels; it has a very poor prognosis. *Low-grade intraosseous osteosarcoma* is a rare variant characteristically confined to the marrow cavity. It has a limited propensity for metastasis, but tends to recur following limited resection. Early definitive surgery will usually result in cure (205).

Periosteal osteosarcoma arises from the periosteum of the bone and extends away from it without invasion of the cortex. It usually occurs in the proximal metaphysis of the tibia and is seen most commonly in adolescents (205). It is a less aggressive tumor than conventional osteosarcoma and may require no treatment beyond wide resection (205a). *Parosteal osteosarcoma* originates on the external surface of the bone in close association to the periosteum, but it is not directly connected to it. It is characterized radiologically by a zone of lucency between the dense tumor mass and the bone of origin. It is found primarily in the metaphyseal region of the femur in older patients (median age, 30 years) (206). This tumor grows relatively slowly but recurs frequently after limited resection and, in cases of delayed or inappropriate therapy, may be followed eventually by pulmonary metastasis. Early definitive surgical therapy is virtually always curative (80 to 90 per cent) (207). Determination of cellular DNA content may serve an adjunctive role to conventional histologic evaluation for differentiating between classic and parosteal osteosarcomas (208).

Small cell osteosarcoma resembles Ewing's sarcoma in cell composition but produces osteoid matrix. It may be less responsive to chemotherapy (especially high-dose methotrexate/citrovorum factor rescue) than are other forms of osteosarcoma (209); however, at least some patients who receive adjuvant chemotherapy with vincristine/Cytoxan/Adriamycin have achieved long-term relapse-free survival (210).

CLINICAL FEATURES

Osteosarcoma often presents with slow, progressively increasing, aching discomfort in an extremity; occasionally, erythema, tenderness, warmth, or limitation of movement is also encountered. Less commonly, the patient may present with a pathologic fracture.

Approximately 50 to 80 per cent of osteosarcomas present in the area around the knee (distal femur or proximal tibia or fibula) and 9 to 15 per cent in the proximal humerus; central axis lesions account for less than 10 per cent of the primary sites in patients under 20 years of age (211–213).

Although no laboratory finding is a specific marker for osteosarcoma, approximately 50 to 60 per cent of patients have an elevated serum alkaline phosphatase level at the time of diagnosis; in general, the degree of elevation correlates roughly with the amount of osteoblastic activity and the size of the tumor mass. Extreme elevations in the serum alkaline phosphatase level in a patient who has osteogenic sarcoma in one symptomatic site should suggest a very rare variant called *multifocal sclerosing osteogenic sarcoma* (201). This type of osteogenic sarcoma usually occurs in very young patients and has a rapidly lethal outcome. Simultaneous or synchronous metastases in the metaphyses of multiple long bones, pulmonary metastases, and resistance to chemotherapy are characteristic features (201, 213a).

On radiologic examination, osteosarcoma typically appears as an eccentric metaphyseal lesion, apparently well localized, consisting of radiodense bony material interspersed with radiolucent regions. The eroded cortex may be traversed by horizontal bone spicules that extend into the surrounding soft tissue and present the so-called "sunburst" appearance. At the tumor margins, there is often a triangular region of periosteal new bone (Codman's triangle).

The most commonly used bone scanning agents in current use are complexes of technetium-99m with polyphosphate, diphosphonate, or pyrophosphate. These agents are deposited in proximity to sites of osteoblastic activity, and any abnormal increase of osteoblastic activity is reflected in increased uptake of the scanning material; this is a nonspecific finding and must be differentiated from arthritis, fracture, osteomyelitis, and metastatic tumor. Bone scanning is useful in detecting bone metastases, since scanning is more sensitive than the conventional x-ray, which requires approximately 30 per cent decalcification of bone before changes can be detected (214).

ROUTES OF METASTASIS

Osteosarcoma may spread through the marrow cavity of the bone of origin by invasion of marrow sinusoids and intraosseous embolization. On rare occasions, this can result in clinically undetectable intraosseous "skip lesions" (i.e., secondary, smaller foci of osteosarcoma that are anatomically separate from the primary lesion and are separated by grossly normal medullary tissue [215]).

Distant metastasis occurs most often via the hematogenous route; either through caval vessels or through the wide network of the vertebral venous system (Batson's veins). In the prechemotherapy era, metastatic disease virtually always initially became manifest in the lungs; approximately 50 per cent of patients developed evidence of pulmonary involvement within 6 to 9 months of diagnosis, and 80 per cent developed pulmonary disease and died within 2 years of diagnosis. Although extrapulmonary metastases (mainly osseous) did occur, these were usually found in patients with preterminal disease or at autopsy. Subsequent to the introduction of adjuvant chemotherapy, there has been an alteration in the pattern of metastatic disease, with a relative increase in the proportion of patients who present with extrapulmonary metastasis alone or with simultaneous extrapulmonary and pulmonary metastasis as the initial site of recurrence (216, 216a); bone, brain, liver, mesenteric lymph nodes, kidney, heart, pericardium, and pleura are among the areas that have been involved by metastatic disease. It is likely that this alteration in metastatic pattern reflects the effect of adjuvant chemotherapy in suppressing pulmonary metastatic disease and prolonging survival.

Lymphatic spread is relatively uncommon, particularly early in the course. Only about 3 per cent of patients show clinically apparent lymph node metastases at the time of presentation (216), whereas lymph node involvement is found in 6 per cent of amputation specimens (217) and in 26 per cent of cases at autopsy (216).

PROGNOSTIC FACTORS

The major factors recognized to adversely affect the prognosis of osteosarcoma are: age less than 10 years, male sex, proximal location of tumor, large tumor size (>15 cm in diameter), duration of symptoms 2 months or less, and unfavorable histologic subtype (201, 217a, 218, 219, 220, 221, 222).

In many series, the most significant prognostic variable for osteosarcoma is the location of the primary lesion; in general, the further the primary site is from the axial skeleton, the better the prognosis (218, 219). Thus, the largest proportion of cures have been reported for tumors below the knee and elbow. Tumors arising in the distal femur also have done reasonably well, whereas the prognosis of shoulder, hip, scapular, clavicular, pelvic, and vertebral primaries has been poor (less than 10 per cent 5-year survival [218]).

Tumor size also appears to be an important variable. Patients with smaller tumors generally do better following surgery than do those with large tumors (220). The most striking example of this is classic osteosarcoma, for which the 5-year relapse-free survival rate has been 44 to 50 per cent for tumors whose greatest diameter is less than 5 cm, but 0 per cent when the greatest tumor diameter is greater than 15 cm.

Tumor histology also appears to influence prognosis. A relatively good prognosis is reported for periosteal, parosteal, and low-grade intraosseous osteosarcoma, whereas a relatively poor prognosis is seen for telangiectatic, extraosseous, small cell, osteoblastic, chondroblastic, and irradiation-induced osteosarcoma (201, 217a, 221, 222).

TREATMENT

Surgery. Historically, amputation has been the procedure of choice for achieving surgical ablation of primary osteosarcoma of an extremity. This can be accomplished through removal of the entire bone by disarticulation at the proximal joint or by transmedullary (cross-bone) amputation 7 to 10 cm above the proximal extension of tumor. While the transmedullary approach preserves the integrity of the proximal joint and thereby permits better functional restoration of the limb, the specter of intramedullary extension or "skip" metastases has led some authors (215) to favor disarticulation amputation. However, as "skip" metastases are relatively uncommon and can usually be ruled out by careful radiologic evaluation with CT scan and bone scan, the necessity for disarticulation may be questioned. Instead, many centers are now advocating transmedullary amputation for distal lesions of the long bones (201, 207, 223–225). This approach has achieved local control of tumor in over 90 per cent of patients.

Limb Salvage. With modern approaches, including adjuvant chemotherapy, it may be possible to avoid amputation entirely for selected patients. In these limited surgical procedures, the tumor-bearing bone is resected en bloc and replaced with a cadaver allograft (226) or a custom-made prosthesis (227). Such limb-sparing surgery is performed only if careful evaluation with bone scans, arteriograms, and CT scanning has demonstrated a strong likelihood that there is no metastatic disease present and that the primary tumor can be resected with tumor-free margins. In addition, the patient should have completed, or nearly completed, linear growth. Recent advances, including the use of intra-arterial cisplatin (227a), may facilitate resection of primary tumors and thereby make more patients eligible for limb-sparing operations.

Limb-salvage procedures may not be appropriate for all primary sites. For example, lesions of the proximal tibia may be handled with an above-the-knee amputation and a good prosthesis with achievement of a very functional lower extremity; likewise, certain expendable bones such as the fibula, ulna, or clavicle may be treated adequately with en bloc resection alone (228).

Although there has been a remarkably low incidence of tumor recurrence and an overall disease-free rate equal to that seen in studies employing amputation, the long-term function of cadaver allografts has been disappointing. In Eilber's series (229), at least 80 per cent of allografts loosened or fractured within 3 years of insertion. The metallic prostheses have functioned relatively well to date, but structural fractures have occurred in approximately 5 per cent, and rotation secondary to loosening at the methacrylate/bony interface has occurred in 30 per cent of the weight-bearing bones over 3 years (230).

Radiotherapy. Osteosarcoma is a relatively radioresistant tumor, with tumoricidal dose in the range of 6000 to 12,000 cGy; viable tumor cells have been found in some cases after doses as high as 10,000 cGy (231).

There are few evaluable series in which radiotherapy has been used as a single modality for local control. Sweetnam and colleagues (232) reported a 12 per cent 5-year survival rate for patients treated with radiotherapy alone; there were considerable variations in the dosage of radiotherapy in this series. Breuer (233) treated patients with 8000 to 9000 cGy and found that 23 per cent achieved 2-year relapse-free survival; however, 43 per cent of the patients eventually required amputation because of radiation-related complications. As the overall success of radiotherapy alone is significantly less than with surgical therapy (at least with respect to ultimate limb function), currently radiotherapy is used only when a surgical procedure cannot create a disease-free state—e.g., for pelvic, skull, or some rib primaries. In these situations, at least 7000 cGy should be used for local control (234).

Breuer and colleagues (235) studied the efficacy of radiotherapy as an adjuvant modality for occult pulmonary metastasis. In their study, patients were randomized following radical treatment of the primary site by either amputation or radiotherapy to receive either no additional treatment or radiotherapy to the lungs (an effective dose of 2000 cGy over 12 days). After a follow-up period of greater than 3 years, 43 per cent of patients receiving pulmonary radiation remained metastasis-free, as compared with only 28 per cent of patients who did *not* receive pulmonary irradiation. However, this study was inconsistent in that at least one major participant did not notice a beneficial effect of radiotherapy. Furthermore, other groups (236, 237) have not found significant benefit from prophylactic pulmonary radiation.

Chemotherapy. The role of adjuvant chemotherapy in the treatment of osteosarcoma has been the topic of much discussion during the past decade. Historically, only 20 per cent of osteosarcoma patients with tumor apparently limited to the primary site at diagnosis and treated with amputation alone achieved long-term relapse-free survival. The implication of these poor results is that 80 per cent of these patients had occult metastatic disease. Efforts to eradicate these micrometastatic foci with adjuvant therapy produced 5-year relapse-free survival rates in the range of 40 per cent with single-agent chemotherapy (high-dose methotrexate with citrovorum factor rescue or Adriamycin) (240a,b) and 60 per cent with combination chemotherapy (240a, 241–245).

In the mid-1970s, Rosen and colleagues (246) introduced the T-7 regimen, which was used in a *neoadjuvant* (preoperative) fashion. The rationale for this approach was that it might allow for more effective and less mutilative surgery, permit earlier treatment of systemic micrometastases, and provide an opportunity to gauge the effectiveness of the chemotherapy regimen against the tumor in vivo. Thus, definitive surgery was delayed while the patient received four weekly cycles of very high dose methotrexate (12 g per M^2 for young children or 8 g per M^2 for fully grown adolescents and adults) with citrovorum rescue. Following surgery, the resected bone was subjected to extensive histopathologic review to determine its response to chemotherapy; responses were graded from I (little or no effect) to IV (no viable-appearing tumor cells noted in any histologic section). Regardless of histologic response, all patients were continued on chemotherapy with high-dose methotrexate, Adriamycin, and BCD (bleomycin, Cytoxan, actinomycin D) postoperatively. The result was an overall 84 per cent disease-free survival over a median period of 36 months. Results were poor for poor histologic responders (Grades I and II), with only a 26 per cent relapse-free survival, but excellent for good responders (Grades III and IV), with 95 per cent relapse-free survival.

In a subsequent protocol (T-10), the postoperative chemotherapy regimen was modified according to the histologic response to the primary chemotherapy regimen (Fig. 37–7). Histologic responders were treated with high-dose methotrexate/citrovorum factor rescue, Adriamycin, and BCD, achieving a 98 per cent relapse-free survival. Patients with a poor histologic response to the primary chemotherapy regimen received a maintenance regimen that substituted cis-platinum for methotrexate; this group also has had an excellent

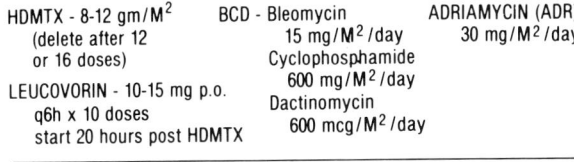
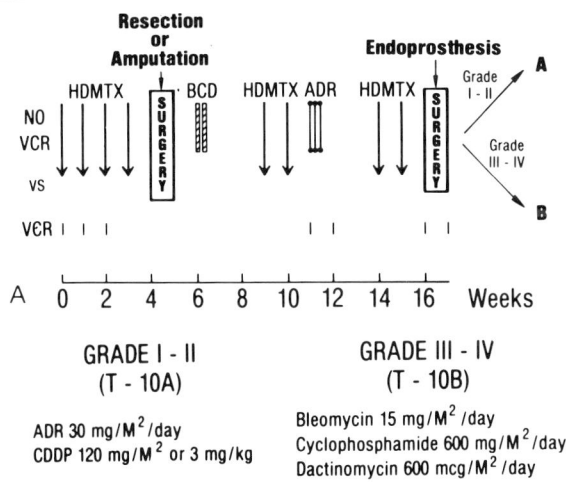
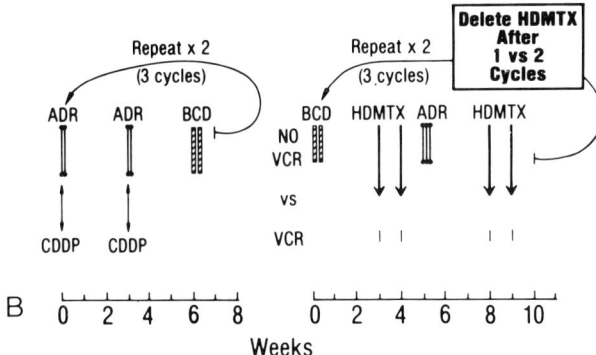

Figure 37–7. The T-10 protocol for treatment of osteosarcoma. *A*, Induction regimen. *B*, Maintenance regimen based on histologic response of primary tumor. (From Rosen, G., Caparros, B., et al.: Preoperative chemotherapy for osteogenic sarcoma. Cancer 49:1221, 1982.)

result, with 93 per cent relapse-free survival at a median follow-up time of 18 months (209). These data seem to indicate the importance of an appropriate postoperative adjuvant chemotherapy regimen individualized on the basis of the response to preoperative chemotherapy.

Since historically the results with surgical therapy alone have been very poor, none of the studies alluded to above used a concurrent control arm. However, a report from the Mayo Clinic (247) has brought into question the validity of historical controls. In this study, Taylor and colleagues reviewed all cases of primary osteosarcoma treated at the Mayo Clinic since 1962 and found evidence of improvements in both overall survival and postoperative disease-free interval over time, unrelated to adjuvant treatment. In their retrospective analysis, disease-free survival at 2 years increased progressively from 13 per cent for 1963–1968 to 43 per cent for 1972–1974. The latter figure was statistically not significantly different from the results achieved by many adjuvant regimens.

It has been hypothesized that the apparent improvement in survival seen during the era of adjuvant chemotherapy may be due to the fortuitous selection of a group of patients with a better prognosis; that is, the use of more sensitive diagnostic tests (e.g., bone scan, CT scan) may have eliminated patients with metastatic disease at presentation. However, this is unlikely to be an adequate explanation, as the sensitivity of pulmonary tomography and CT scan for detecting occult metastases probably does not exceed that of the standard chest x-ray by more than 5 to 10 per cent (248–250). Other possibilities, such as earlier referral to major therapy centers, more rapid and extensive patient evaluation and therapy, and different surgical approaches to the primary tumor, may also have contributed to the apparent improvement in survival.

A controlled study by the Mayo Clinic comparing adjuvant chemotherapy (high-dose methotrexate) versus observation alone has shown no difference in 5-year relapse-free survival (42 per cent) between the two approaches (251). However, it should be noted that this pilot study included only 38 patients, and that the "high-dose" methotrexate dosage ranged between 3 and 7.5 g per M^2, which is significantly below the 8 to 12 g per M^2 recommended by Rosen. Because of the relatively small number of patients included in this study and the relatively less intense chemotherapy used in the treatment wing, it is difficult to compare these results with those of the best chemotherapy results (209). Thus, while it is possible to say that chemotherapy as administered at the Mayo Clinic did not show any advantage over observation alone, the higher doses of methotrexate used by Rosen and colleagues, as well as the inclusion of other chemotherapeutic agents in their T-10 protocol, make direct comparisons difficult.

Two recent clinical trials appear to have confirmed the importance of adjuvant chemotherapy in the treatment of osteosarcoma. Both of these studies randomized patients to either a control or an adjuvant chemotherapy arm. In a multi-institutional study (252), patients were treated with primary amputation and then randomized either to receive a six-drug chemotherapy regimen or to receive no further therapy. At 2 years, the relapse-free survival was 66 per cent for the group receiving adjuvant chemotherapy versus 17 per cent for the control group. The second study was performed at a single institution (252a). Patients were treated initially with intra-arterial Adriamycin, radiotherapy to the primary tumor, and surgery. The control group received no further chemotherapy and had a 39 per cent relapse-free survival at 16 months versus 59 per cent for the group receiving adjuvant chemotherapy.

Immunotherapy. Immunotherapy is based on the concept that osteosarcoma cells contain antigens that are relatively unique to the tumor cells and are sufficiently different from normal cells to elicit cytotoxic immune responses to the tumor cells. The immunologic approach has included attempts to stimulate the immune system with nonspecific agents such as BCG, C. parvum, interferon (253), and transfer factor, as well as specific agents such as tumor cell vaccine (254). Survival rates in the range of 40 per cent with most of these approaches appear favorable in comparison with historical controls, but as yet no randomized prospective trials have been performed, and long-term follow-up has not conclusively demonstrated that this therapy significantly influenced the outcome for these patients.

A monoclonal antibody has been prepared to a tumor-specific antigen on the osteosarcoma cell line 719T (255, 256). This antibody is cytotoxic to osteosarcoma cells in the presence of complement and can also be chemically linked to chemotherapeutic agents (e.g., methotrexate [257, 258]). This technology may open the way for a new immunotherapeutic approach to osteosarcoma by which treatment may be specifically directed against tumor cells while toxicity to normal tissues is minimized.

Treatment of Patients with Frank Pulmonary Metastasis. Aggressive use of multiple or bilateral thoracotomies has resulted in prolonged survival and potential cure in 25 to 50 per cent of those patients who have resectable pulmonary metastases (259, 260, 261). Schaller (260) has suggested that if the disease is bilateral and rapidly growing, a period of intensive chemotherapy should precede thoracotomy to see if the disease is responsive. Although patients with metastatic disease can be kept alive for as long as 8 or 9 years with such aggressive surgical therapy, the majority will eventually succumb to recurrent disease (262). Therefore, survival data must be interpreted with caution unless very long follow-up periods are used.

Regression of metastatic osteosarcoma has been demonstrated following the use of single agents such as high-dose methotrexate with citrovorum factor rescue (263), Adriamycin (239), or cis-platinum (264), as well as following the use of combination regimens such as bleomycin/Cytoxan/actinomycin D (BCD) (265). Although early studies documented response rates of 40 to 80 per cent, recent, more conservative estimates suggest that objective tumor regression occurs in only about 10 to 20 per cent of patients treated with single agents and in 37 per cent of patients treated with the multi-agent BCD regimen (265, 266). Rosen (267) advocates chemotherapy for all patients who develop pulmonary metastases, including those with single pulmonary nodules; it is likely that deposits of metastatic tumor in the lung may range from those visible on x-ray (1 cm in diameter or larger) to subclinical nodules of only a few cells, and that chemotherapy might eradicate these smaller microfoci of metastatic disease.

Ewing's Sarcoma

Ewing's sarcoma, a highly malignant small round cell tumor of bone, is thought to arise from the primitive mesenchyme of the medullary cavity. It has been reported in almost every bone, but it is found most frequently in the midshaft (diaphysis) of long bones, especially the femur. Unlike osteosarcoma, Ewing's sarcoma not uncommonly effects flat bones such as vertebrae, ribs, and the pelvis. A tumor of similar morphology that arises in soft tissue sites, initially called *extraosseous Ewing's sarcoma*, is now considered to be an undifferentiated form of rhabdomyosarcoma; its histologic similarity to Ewing's sarcoma of bone is probably a reflection of the fact that these tumors are both derived from primitive mesenchymal elements (268, 269).

CYTOGENETICS

Cytogenetic analysis of fresh Ewing's sarcoma tissue (270), as well as continuous cell lines of Ewing's sarcoma (271), has demonstrated consistent rearrangements of chromosome 22, most commonly reciprocal translocations between it and chromosome 11. Although the c-*sis* oncogene (whose normal locus is at 22q13) is involved in this t[11;22] translocation, it is not rearranged at the molecular level or activated (271a).

NATURAL HISTORY

Ewing's sarcoma occurs most frequently in the second decade of life; 75 per cent of cases are diagnosed before the age of 20 years, and 90 per cent before the age of 30 years. The most common presenting symptoms are pain and swelling of relatively short duration; patients may also present with associated systemic symptoms such as fever, weight loss, and general fatigue.

Ewing's sarcoma is fundamentally a systemic disease. Up to one third of patients will have evidence of metastatic disease in the lungs or other bones at presentation (273–277). The incidence of overt metastases at presentation is much greater among patients with a primary tumor of the proximal extremity or central axis (up to 50 per cent) than among those whose tumor arises in a distal extremity (approximately 10 per cent) (276). Historically, patients with metastatic disease at diagnosis have had a very poor prognosis, with about 35 per cent survival at 3 years and 0 to 5 per cent survival at 5 years (273–278).

Even patients with apparently localized tumors

at diagnosis are at high risk of eventually developing metastatic disease. Prior to the introduction of adjuvant chemotherapy in 1973, the 5-year survival rate in patients with apparently localized Ewing's sarcoma was in the range of 10 to 25 per cent, with the majority of patients ultimately expiring from pulmonary metastases (274, 279). Although there appeared to be a plateau in survival at 5 years, 21 per cent of patients alive at this point subsequently succumbed to tumor, suggesting that even 5-year disease-free survival was not synonymous with cure (274).

ROUTES OF METASTASIS

Ewing's sarcoma is characterized by intraosseous medullary cavity spread, extraosseous soft tissue spread, and distant metastasis via the blood stream. The soft tissue component, representing tumor infiltration of adjacent muscles and spread along fascial planes, may be quite extensive, often crossing the joint space proximally. The most common sites of distant metastasis are the lungs and bones; involvement of other visceral organs also occurs, but generally late in the course of disease. A very small proportion of patients (approximately 2 per cent) will develop central nervous system involvement (272); in most instances, this is a consequence of soft tissue extension of vertebral disease that produces extradural spinal cord compression.

TREATMENT

Surgery. The surgical approach to Ewing's sarcoma is largely dependent upon the location of the primary tumor. Lesions that are amenable to surgical removal without producing severe functional disability should be treated by amputation or wide excision; examples of these are tumors of rib, clavicle, fibula, ulna, or small bones of the hand or foot (280, 281). For bulky lesions at these sites, preoperative chemotherapy or radiotherapy may be used to reduce tumor mass prior to definitive surgery. Surgery is not the primary modality of treatment for lesions of the tibia or radius unless the lesion is large and destructive, is associated with a pathologic fracture, or occurs in a very young patient (<6 to 8 years), for whom primary radiotherapy would likely result in substantial growth discrepancy (282).

Approximately two thirds of Ewing's sarcomas involve bones such as the humerus, femur, vertebrae, and pelvis, where primary extirpative surgery either is not possible or produces severe functional disability. Since soft tissue spread from such lesions may be massive, with extension proximal to the joint space, definitive surgical excision may require hemipelvectomy, high above-knee amputation, or forequarter amputation (278, 283). Unfortunately, sometimes even the most radical surgical procedure may not be locally curative. An alternative treatment plan would use radiotherapy and chemotherapy, but this may produce substantial functional disability as well as risk development of a second malignancy. In some cases, deferral of definitive local therapy pending assessment of response of the primary tumor to 3 to 5 cycles of combination chemotherapy may allow for subsequent successful surgical excision (284, 285).

Radiotherapy. Despite decades of experience in the use of radiotherapy for treatment of Ewing's sarcoma, there is still no general agreement on either treatment field or dosage. Traditionally, the entire length of the involved bone was encompassed in the treatment portal, with doses in the range of 6000 to 7000 cGy delivered to the primary lesion. Unfortunately, this approach often resulted in severe functional disability as well as failure to control the primary tumor. With the advent of adjuvant chemotherapy, the radiotherapeutic management of Ewing's sarcoma is being re-evaluated with regard to both field and dosage.

With combined multi-agent chemotherapy/radiotherapy protocols, delivery of 4000 to 5000 cGy to the entire affected bone followed by an additional 1000 to 1500 cGy to successively small "conedown" fields has resulted in local control rates in the range of 86 to 91 per cent and good-to-excellent functional results in most patients (275, 286–288); sparing of an adequate strip of skin and subcutaneous tissue is an important precaution if late constrictive fibrosis and lymphedema are to be avoided. However, growth disparities may be anticipated when an entire bone is irradiated.

The necessity for irradiation of the entire involved bone has been based on the presumption that Ewing's sarcoma, which arises in the bone marrow, has the potential to spread throughout the entire medullary cavity. However, the general experience has been that local recurrences are consistently observed at the center of the lesion and not in areas of apparently uninvolved bone. Therefore, whole bone irradiation may offer no advantage over treatment of a more restricted field with very high dose radiation delivered to the center of the lesion (286, 289, 290), particularly when the patient is also receiving adjuvant chemotherapy. This approach has some preliminary support from data of the Intergroup Ewing's Sarcoma Study (IESS) showing that 11 of 12 patients treated with limited field radiotherapy and concurrent adjuvant chemotherapy have remained free of local recurrence (286). Therefore, it may be possible to spare at least the epiphyseal center at the furthermost point from the primary lesion and allow more normal bone growth. However, further studies and longer follow-up will be necessary before this can be accepted as a standard approach.

Chemotherapy. Response rates of 40 to 60 per cent have been reported for single-agent therapy of Ewing's sarcoma with vincristine, actinomycin D, Cytoxan, Adriamycin, BCNU, and mithramycin (291–297). Vincristine (V), actinomycin-D (A), Cytoxan (C), and Adriamycin are currently the most active and effective agents; the VAC and VAC + Adriamycin regimens represent two of the most commonly used combinations (286, 291, 298).

The largest report of combined modality therapy is that of the IESS (298). In this study, 264 patients with previously untreated localized Ewing's sarcoma were randomized to one of three regimens: (1) VAC; (2) VAC + Adriamycin; or (3) VAC + bilateral pulmonary radiation. All groups were treated with radiotherapy to the primary lesion, given concurrently with the beginning of chemotherapy. Local control was good for all groups, but was particularly good for the VAC + Adriamycin group (96 per cent versus 86 per cent in the other two groups) (286). The VAC + Adriamycin regimen was also most effective in achieving long-term survival, with 74 per cent of patients surviving free of disease at 2 years versus 58 per cent for VAC + pulmonary irradiation and 35 per cent for VAC alone.

Comparable results have been reported by other groups using a variety of combined modality protocols (275, 280, 281, 299). The 5-year tumor-free survival in many series is now in the range of 50 to 70 per cent for patients with localized disease at diagnosis (273, 275, 284, 286, 298, 299). However, prognosis remains strongly correlated with the site of the primary tumor. The best results are achieved with lesions of the skull or distal extremities, where the local recurrence rate is 0 to 11 per cent and the incidence of hematogenous metastasis is less than 40 per cent (280, 299a). By contrast, proximal extremity, axial skeleton, and pelvic primary tumors have both a high local recurrence rate (16 to 27 per cent) and a high incidence of distant metastasis (55 to 65 per cent) (276, 280, 299a, 300–303).

The poor prognosis of pelvic and axial skeleton primaries may be a reflection of the relatively greater tumor bulk and degree of extraosseous extension often associated with tumors in these locations; both of these factors are correlated with a higher frequency of local recurrence and distant metastasis (299a, 304). Difficulty in delivery of high-dose radiotherapy to pelvic and vertebral primaries, as well as the impaired capacity of the bone marrow to subsequently tolerate aggressive chemotherapy, might also contribute to the poor outcome for these patients.

With these considerations in mind, some groups (284, 285) have adopted a primary (preoperative, pre-radiotherapy) chemotherapy approach, delaying definitive local therapy of the primary site until the patient has received several cycles of chemotherapy. This approach has the following theoretical advantages: (1) a decrease in the size of the primary tumor often makes surgical excision possible; (2) the delay allows pathologically eroded bone to heal prior to the initiation of radiotherapy; (3) the high-risk patient with an axial spine or pelvic primary tumor might better tolerate aggressive chemotherapy; (4) the radiotherapy port to areas of residual disease might be decreased; and (5) improved oxygenation of residual tumor cells might make them more sensitive to lower doses of radiotherapy.

Using a primary chemotherapy approach with the T-9 protocol (vincristine/bleomycin/Cytoxan/methotrexate/actinomycin D/Adriamycin), Rosen and colleagues (284) achieved an overall 2-year disease-free survival of 79 per cent in 67 consecutive patients presenting with nonmetastatic Ewing's sarcoma. However, prognosis continued to be affected by the site of the primary lesion, as reflected in the 2-year disease-free survival rates of 95 per cent for distal extremity lesions, 79 per cent for proximal extremity lesions, and 65 per cent for axial primaries.

Hayes and colleagues (285) have also employed a primary chemotherapeutic approach. In their series of 24 patients, radiotherapy and definitive surgery were delayed until after the patient had received a trial of induction chemotherapy (Cytoxan/Adriamycin). Nineteen of 23 evaluable patients had no gross residual tumor following this therapy, and 2 of the remaining 4 had complete surgical excision of residual gross disease.

Treatment of Metastatic Disease. Metastatic disease is often responsive to aggressive combination chemotherapy. In an early study, Rosen (305), using combination chemotherapy, achieved complete remission in 8 patients with metastatic Ewing's sarcoma; however, 7 of these patients relapsed within 4 to 5 months of achieving complete remission, with tumors recurring mainly at the sites of initial metastatic involvement.

The IESS has used combination chemotherapy/radiotherapy to treat patients with metastatic disease (306). Thirty-six patients with metastatic disease and 8 patients with advanced regional disease were treated with intensive chemotherapy (VAC + Adriamycin) and radiotherapy (3500 cGy) to all sites of overt disease. Seventy per cent of these patients achieved complete remission, and 18 have remained disease-free after a median follow-up of 34 months.

New Approaches to Treatment of Ewing's Sarcoma

Total Body Irradiation. Attempts to integrate total body irradiation (TBI) with systemic chemotherapy for treatment of Ewing's sarcoma began with the reports of Jenkin and colleagues (307, 308), who achieved long-term survival in 2 of 3 patients with metastatic disease treated with local irradiation to the primary lesion, supplemented with single-fraction TBI (350 cGy).

Lombardi and co-workers (309) used sequential hemi-body irradiation to treat 18 patients with metastatic Ewing's sarcoma who relapsed following radiotherapy and multidrug chemotherapy; an overall response rate of 50 per cent with 25 per cent complete responses was achieved. Preliminary data from a subsequent pilot study have indicated that *adjuvant* chemotherapy and sequential hemi-body irradiation might improve the survival rate for patients with poor-prognosis tumors (309a).

Autologous Bone Marrow Transplantation. Cornbleet and colleagues (310) treated 5 patients with advanced Ewing's sarcoma refractory to conventional chemotherapy with high-dose melphalan followed by autologous bone marrow transplantation; 4 of these patients achieved complete remission, and 1 received partial remission. However, at the time of publication only 1 of these patients had remained in complete remission, and for a follow-up period of only 3 months.

Investigators at the National Cancer Institute have treated 24 high-risk Ewing's sarcoma patients with low-dose fractionated TBI (30 cGy per week; 150 cGy total) and autologous bone marrow infusion (310a). Although 83 per cent of these patients achieved a complete clinical response in the primary and/or metastatic sites following induction therapy, approximately 70 per cent of the patients subsequently have relapsed and died of disease. Thus, despite good control of local disease, this treatment failed to control microscopic systemic disease. The NCI group is now trying a new combined modality protocol with high-dose "therapeutic" TBI (800 cGy/2 fractions).

QUALITY OF SURVIVAL

Quality of survival of patients with Ewing's sarcoma is compromised by the long-term complications following radiotherapy of the growing bones of a child. Among these are contracture, multiple fractures, limb length discrepancy, soft tissue atrophy, chronic pain and edema, neurologic lesions, and radiation-induced secondary tumor.

The volume of bone treated may be even more critical than the dose. While a small volume of bone can tolerate doses in the range of 5000 to 6000 cGy, more than 3000 cGy to a growing epiphyseal plate produces serious growth disturbance. At a dose of 5000 cGy, approximately 3 per cent of patients will develop severe functional disability, and this figure increases with increasing dose (311); Rosen (305) found that 26 per cent of patients develop severe functional disability following irradiation to 7000 cGy in conjunction with combination chemotherapy.

The risk of secondary bone tumors (particularly osteogenic sarcoma) appears to be dose-related. Greene (311) found a 3 per cent risk of secondary bone cancer with doses of 5000 cGy, while Strong (312) found that 13 per cent of patients who had received a median dose of 6000 cGy to the primary tumor developed bone cancer with a median follow-up time of 5.3 years. In the IESS, in which only 27 per cent of patients received doses in excess of 6000 cGy, only 1.2 per cent of patients have developed second malignancies (282). There is hope that, as radiotherapy dosage is reduced in conjunction with combination chemotherapy regimens, the carcinogenic risk will decline.

TUMORS OF GERM CELL ORIGIN

Tumors of germ cell origin account for approximately 3 per cent of childhood malignancies (1). These fascinating neoplasms are characterized by a marked diversity in histologic pattern, anatomic distribution, and clinical behavior (313–315). Therefore, it is inappropriate to make general statements regarding their management. A thorough understanding of the natural history and therapeutic responsiveness of each histologic subtype in relation to its primary site and age at presentation is necessary to plan treatment for an individual patient.

Histologic Variants

The germ cells, as the precursors of the sperm and ova, retain the potential to produce all of the somatic (embryonic) and supporting (extraembryonic) structures of a developing embryo; as shown in Figure 37–8, this totipotentiality allows for expression of a bewildering array of neoplastic histologic patterns. The major morphologic categories are *embryonal carcinoma*, *germinoma*, *teratoma*, *endodermal sinus (yolk sac) tumor*, *choriocarcinoma*, and *gonadoblastoma*; mixtures and transitions between the various types (*mixed germ cell tumors*) are also observed.

Embryonal carcinoma is composed of highly anaplastic primordial germ cells that retain the potential to develop along either embryonal (somatic) or extraembryonal lines. One of the most common variants of nonseminomatous testicular tumors in young adults, it is rarely found in pure form in patients under the age of 15 years (316).

Germinoma is a general designation for a monomorphous primitive germ cell tumor that is generally known as seminoma in the testis, dysgerminoma in the ovary, and germinoma when it occurs in extragonadal sites. In childhood, germinoma occurs most commonly in the ovary of an early pubertal or adolescent girl (317) or in the pineal region of an adolescent boy (318); less common sites in the first two decades of life are the anterior mediastinum and the testis.

Teratomas contain derivatives of at least two of the three primary germ layers (ectoderm, mesoderm, endoderm), often arranged in a haphazard manner. The biologic behavior of these tumors

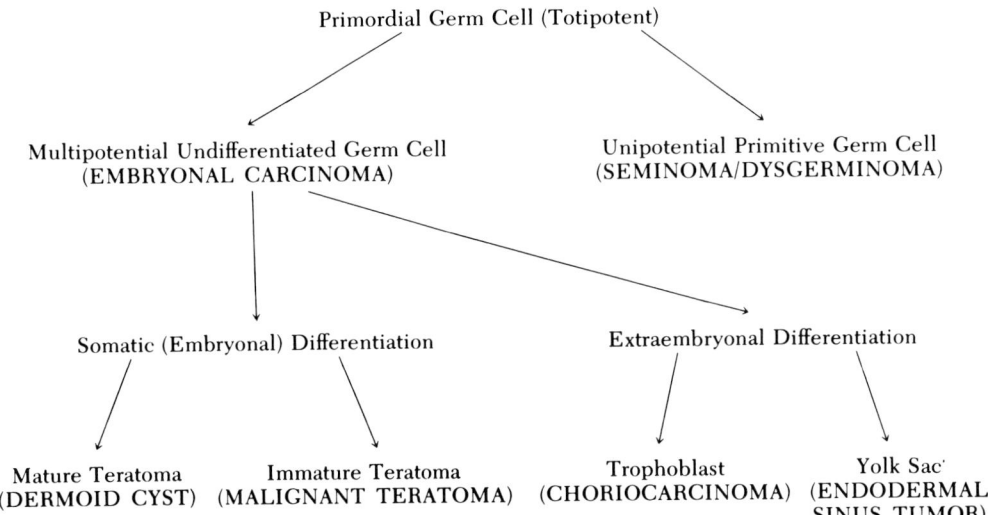

Figure 37-8. Histogenetic classification of germ cell tumors. (From Altman, A. J., and Schwartz, A. D.: Malignant Diseases of Infancy, Childhood and Adolescence. Philadelphia, W. B. Saunders Co., 1983.)

generally reflects the makeup of the component tissues. Teratomas composed entirely of mature, fully differentiated tissues behave in a benign fashion. It is more difficult to generalize on the prognostic implications of teratomas that contain immature (fetal) somatic tissue components (immature neuroectoderm, metanephric areas, embryonic mesenchyme), as the natural history of such tumors varies according to anatomic site and patient age (314, 314a). In general, the presence of fetal tissues does not indicate malignancy in infants and young children, but it does have ominous implications in older children and adults. On the other hand, nonsomatic patterns (germinoma, embryonal carcinoma, endodermal sinus tumor, choriocarcinoma), by their very presence in a teratoma, indicate malignancy.

Endodermal sinus (yolk sac) tumor partially or completely recapitulates the structure of yolk sac; the histologic pattern is characterized by a labyrinthine pattern containing tubular structures, papillary processes, and Schiller-Duval bodies (small cavities lined by a layer of endothelium-like cells), supported by a loose myxoid or vascular stroma (319). Alpha-fetoprotein (AFP) has been demonstrated in the cytoplasm of individual cells, and in PAS-positive, diastase-resistant eosinophilic globules associated with Schiller-Duval bodies (320, 321); it has also been found in the serum of patients with endodermal sinus tumors. Endodermal sinus tumor in childhood is most commonly found in the ovary, testis, and sacrococcygeal areas; less common sites are the pineal region, the anterior mediastinum, the vagina, and the liver (314). The clinical behavior of these tumors is generally highly aggressive, with the exception of pure endodermal sinus tumor of the infantile testis.

Choriocarcinoma, like endodermal sinus tumor, is a manifestation of extraembryonal differentiation of a malignant germ cell tumor. In this case, the tissue recapitulated is the chorion layer of the placenta. Like normal chorionic tissue, choriocarcinoma is capable of producing human chorionic gonadotropin (hCG). Choriocarcinoma may arise (1) within the placenta of a pregnant female (gestational), or (2) within a primary germ cell tumor in a nonpregnant individual (nongestational). In rare instances, an infant may present with widespread visceral metastases from a metastatic maternal gestational choriocarcinoma (322). In the early pediatric years, choriocarcinoma usually occurs as a nongestational tumor of the pineal region, the anterior mediastinum, or the ovary. Gestational choriocarcinoma occurs most commonly in girls from 15 to 19 years of age (323).

Gonadoblastoma is an intratubular neoplasm that occurs most frequently in dysgenetic gonads (324, 325). Primordial germ cells and stromal cells resembling Sertoli cells are the two basic components of the neoplasm; when the germ cells predominate in one or more nests, the lesion is classified as intratubular germ cell neoplasm or germinoma in situ and is considered to be the preinvasive stage of germinoma (seminoma) (314). Approximately 100 cases of gonadoblastoma have been reported, most of which have been found in patients under 20 years of age; in 75 per cent of these cases, the karyotype of the patient has been 46,XY (male pseudohermaphroditism) or 46,XY/45,XO mosaicism (314, 324, 326).

Non–germ cell malignancies may develop within germ cell tumors; these include embryonal rhabdomyosarcoma, Wilms' tumor, chondrosarcoma, adenocarcinoma, and hematologic malignancies (326a, 326b). This may be the result of malignant transformation of mature teratoma or partial dif-

Table 37-7. IMMUNOHISTOLOGIC CLASSIFICATION OF GERM CELL TUMORS*

Tumor	AFP	hCG
Embryonal carcinoma	+	+
Endodermal sinus tumor	+ + + +	−
Choriocarcinoma	−	+ + + +
Teratoma	−	−
Seminoma	−	−

*Based on data from reference 321.

ferentiation of a malignant totipotent germ cell. Of particular interest is the association of hematologic malignancy (especially megakaryocyte leukemia) with primary mediastinal germ cell tumors (326b).

Tumor Markers

It has been proposed (321) that the current classification criteria for germ cell tumors be revised to recognize the diagnostic value of the tumor markers AFP and hCG (Table 37-7). Production of AFP and hCG may be assessed with immunohistologic staining of tissue sections or measurement of blood levels. Using these criteria, endodermal sinus tumor elements would be recognized by the production of AFP, choriocarcinoma elements by the production of hCG, and embryonal carcinoma by the production of small amounts of both these markers. Pure germinomas and teratomas are not associated with production of either AFP or hCG; consequently, elevation of serologic levels or demonstration in histologic sections of either of these markers should prompt a careful reassessment of the histologic material for the presence of one of the more malignant germ cell elements.

AFP and hCG levels may also be used to assess tumor bulk, persistence of residual tumor following surgery, response to chemotherapy and radiotherapy, and recurrence of tumor. To be of maximal utility, serum AFP and hCG should be obtained prior to surgery and then followed serially every 1 to 2 months. When elevated levels persist beyond their expected decay period* after surgical resection of the primary tumor, it is likely that occult metastatic disease is present. If the level has been normal and subsequently rises, then tumor recurrence is likely.

Anatomic Distribution

Germ cell tumors arise not only in the gonads but also in extragonadal locations. Most primary extragonadal germ cell tumors are found in midline structures (sacrococcyx, neck, mediastinum, retroperitoneum, pineal gland), but occasionally they appear in other sites, such as the lung, liver, or stomach. In adults, 90 per cent of germ cell tumors arise in the gonads, but in the pediatric years there is a predilection for extragonadal sites (Table 37-8) (314, 327). An early peak incidence between birth and 3 years of age reflects neoplasms mainly in the sacrococcygeal and head and neck regions; a second peak occurs during puberty, with a predominance of ovarian and testicular tumors.

Explanations for the appearance of primary germ cell tumors in extragonadal locations include (1) origin from ectopic totipotent cells left behind during the embryonic migration of the primordial germ cells from the hindgut yolk sac region to the genital ridge (313), (2) origin from totipotent cells of the early embryo that escaped the regulatory influence of the "primary organizer" in Hensen's node (313), and (3) incomplete twinning.

SACROCOCCYGEAL GERM CELL TUMORS.

Sacrococcygeal germ cell tumors are relatively rare lesions, with an estimated incidence of 1:40,000 live births (328). Nonetheless, they are the most common germ cell tumors of childhood and the most common solid tumor in the newborn infant (329). Females are affected four times as frequently as males (329).

The treatment of these tumors is primarily surgical; the techniques for removal have been discussed in detail by Gross and colleagues (330) and by Donnellan and Swenson (331). Sacrococcygeal neoplasms should be excised as soon as possible, since small, undifferentiated foci in them may proliferate and become more aggressive. It is important to emphasize the attachment of sacrococcygeal germ cell tumors to the coccyx, which necessitates the removal of the entire coccyx as an essential part of any surgical procedure; failure to do so will result in a high rate of local tumor recurrence (31 to 38 per cent) (330, 331).

Prognosis. Prognosis of sacrococcygeal germ cell tumors is dependent upon histologic appearance, the patient's age, and location of the lesion. In general, older age at diagnosis and internal location are associated with a higher incidence of malignancy and a poorer survival.

Table 37-8. ANATOMIC DISTRIBUTION OF PEDIATRIC GERM CELL TUMORS*

Site	Percentage of Total
Sacrococcygeum	42
Ovary	24
Testis	9
Mediastinum	7
CNS	6
Retroperitoneum	4
Other	8

*Based on data from reference 314.

*Half-life for AFP = 5 days; half-life for hCG = 30 hours.

Approximately 60 to 70 per cent of sacrococcygeal teratomas are benign as determined by the presence of mature tissues, and these tumors can be cured by surgical excision alone. Another 10 to 15 per cent are unequivocally malignant by virtue of the presence of endodermal sinus tumor, embryonal carcinoma, or very primitive neuroectodermal tissue (318). The course for these patients is often rapidly fatal, as surgery alone is inadequate for successful management (322, 333); even when the tumor appears localized and is susceptible to apparently complete excision, the recurrence rate is high. The remaining 10 to 15 per cent of cases contain embryonic or immature somatic tissues whose prognostic significance may be difficult to assess. A method of histologic grading has been proposed by Gonzalez-Crussi and colleagues (334) based on a semi-quantitative assessment of the amount of immature tissues, principally neuroectoderm. For many of these patients, the prognosis remains favorable if the tumor is totally excised in early infancy, even when immature tissues resembling neuroblastoma, Wilms' tumor, or embryonal rhabdomyosarcoma are present.

The incidence of malignancy is strongly correlated with the patient's age at diagnosis. Whereas only 10 per cent of sacrococcygeal teratomas treated prior to 2 months of age are malignant (331, 335), after this age the incidence of malignancy rises to 67 per cent for males and 48 per cent for females (335). In Altman's series (335) of 398 cases of sacrococcygeal germ cell tumor, patients with the benign lesions had a mortality rate of only 5 per cent, the deaths in this group resulting from surgical complications and infections. By contrast, 60 per cent of the patients with malignant tumors had died within 10 months of operation, and only 11 per cent were surviving without residual disease.

Combination chemotherapy regimens that have demonstrated activity against malignant sacrococcygeal germ cell tumors include: VAC (vincristine/actinomycin/Cytoxan), VAC + Adriamycin, and various combinations of cisplatin, bleomycin, vinblastine, and VP-16 (336, 337, 337a). These are sometimes used in association with radiotherapy. However, great care must be exercised when using these modalities, as young infants are especially susceptible to hemorrhagic, pulmonary, renal, and cardiac toxicity.

OVARIAN GERM CELL TUMORS

Ovarian tumors account for 1 per cent of all childhood tumors. Although these neoplasms may occur at any time in the pediatric years, they tend to present most frequently at puberty (between the ages of 10 and 14 years). Approximately 10 to 30 per cent of childhood ovarian tumors are malignant.

Diagnosis. Because of their anatomic position, ovarian neoplasms are less easily detected than are testicular ones. Consequently, they are usually discovered at a later age and in a more advanced state than are the corresponding testicular neoplasms.

Since the ovaries have their embryologic origin at the level of the tenth thoracic vertebra and are located within the abdomen during childhood, the most common presenting features are abdominal pain or mass. In about half the patients, the pain is of acute onset, is associated with nausea and vomiting, and may be related to ovarian torsion. Ovarian tumors that contain stromal elements may be endocrinologically functional and may produce precocious puberty, vaginal bleeding, or masculinization. Precocious puberty due to ovarian cyst or tumor may be differentiated from that due to pituitary axis dysfunction by the fact that in the former, only estrogen levels are elevated, while in the latter both pituitary hormones and estrogens are elevated (338).

Preoperative evaluation of a girl with a suspected ovarian tumor should include a thorough physical examination, with special attention paid to signs of precocious puberty or virilism. A careful search of the abdominal radiograph for calcifications or teeth within the mass should also be performed, as these suggest the likelihood of a teratoma. Measurement of alpha-fetoprotein (AFP) and human chorionic gonadotropin (hCG) levels in the blood preoperatively is useful for predicting tumor histology as well as establishing baseline values of these biochemical markers so that they can be used to follow the patient's response to therapy and detect early recurrences.

Diagnostic ultrasound scanning may provide additional useful information, including the outline, size, location, and nature of the mass (cystic or solid), the presence of ascites, and the presence of metastatic disease within the pelvis or abdomen.

Classification. Ovarian tumors arise from (1) the germ cells (oocytes), (2) the coelomic epithelium of the ovarian surface, (3) the mesenchymal ovarian stroma, (4) mesonephric rests, or (5) accessory tissues. In adult females, 90 per cent of ovarian tumors are of epithelial origin; in contrast, the majority of ovarian tumors of childhood are of germ cell origin. While 95 per cent of all ovarian germ cell tumors are benign cystic teratomas, the younger the patient, the more likely the tumor is to be malignant. Kurman and Norris (339) found 84 per cent of ovarian germ cell tumors in girls under 10 years of age to be malignant.

Routes of Metastasis. Extraovarian spread of malignant germ cell tumors usually involves the adnexal surfaces by direct extension, the retroperitoneal lymph nodes by lymphatic spread, and the peritoneal surfaces of the abdomen and pelvis by either lymphatic or transperitoneal seeding. The peritoneal surfaces of the bladder, uterus, and sigmoid colon are probably the most frequent metastatic sites, but the peritoneal surfaces of the diaphragm, liver, and small intestine are also commonly involved. Distant sites of metastasis include lung, liver, bone, and mediastinum.

Neoplasms that contain mixtures of different germ cell elements can metastasize as any of the malignant components; the metastases may contain complex aggregates of tissues derived from several germ layers, or pure carcinoma, sarcoma, or neuroepithelioma. Frequently, only the most malignant element of the original neoplasm is evident in the metastases. When metastasis is limited to peritoneal implants composed exclusively or predominantly of mature neuroglial tissue, the implications are not nearly so grave as they are with other types of metastases, and most such patients do well (340). The reason for this may be that these implants represent extrusion of mature glia through a defect in the primary tumor rather than true metastatic seeding.

Dysgerminoma. Dysgerminoma corresponds histogenetically and morphologically to seminoma of the testis. However, unlike seminoma, which occurs almost exclusively in postpubertal males, dysgerminoma not uncommonly develops prior to puberty. This may reflect the fact that meiotic events occur in the ovary during intrauterine life, whereas meiotic events in the testis begin at puberty (341).

Dysgerminoma is the only malignant germ cell tumor of the ovary that has a significant incidence of bilaterality. Kurman and Norris (339) found 14 per cent of Stage I dysgerminomas to be bilateral, and in one third of these the involvement was evident only microscopically. It is not uncommon for dysgerminoma to appear within 2 years in the clinically uninvolved ovary when pathologic examination is not thorough (342). Bilateral involvement is particularly common in young women with dysgenetic streak gonads and a Y chromosome (343).

Conservative surgery, that is, unilateral salpingo-oophorectomy with bisection and biopsy of the opposite ovary, is reasonable treatment for the patient with a small (<10 cm) encapsulated unilateral tumor, a normal female 46XX karyotype, and no evidence of spread in the abdominal cavity or to draining lymph nodes (344–348). At the time of exploration, the parametrium, retroperitoneum, and para-aortic lymph nodes should be carefully palpated in view of the propensity of dysgerminoma to disseminate via retroperitoneal lymphatics (339). Because of the high incidence of bilateral involvement in patients with dysgenetic streak gonads and a Y chromosome, such patients should be managed by bilateral salpingo-oophorectomy; as the gonads are functionally and hormonally inactive, no advantage would be gained by preserving them (343).

If the tumor is bilateral, larger than 10 cm, has metastasized locally or to regional nodes, or has caused bloody ascites, then total abdominal hysterectomy and bilateral salpingo-oophorectomy with postoperative radiotherapy have generally been recommended (344, 346). However, this approach has been recently challenged by Weinblatt and Ortega (349), who were able to produce regression of widespread dysgerminoma with chemotherapy. This was then followed by limited surgery and/or radiotherapy for residual disease, thereby preserving as much reproductive endocrine function as possible.

Dysgerminoma is the most radiosensitive of the ovarian germ cell tumors. Although postoperative radiotherapy is not considered necessary if the tumor is unilateral and localized inside the ovarian capsule, more advanced cases are usually treated with radiotherapy to the abdomen, pelvis, and para-aortic nodes, depending upon the histology of the tumor and the presence and location of metastases (346). Generally, the entire abdomen is treated with 2500 to 3000 cGy, with a boost of 1500 cGy to the para-aortic region and an additional 1500 to 2000 cGy to the pelvis (345). When para-aortic nodes are involved, strong consideration should be given to treating the mediastinal and supraclavicular lymph nodes prophylactically with 2500 cGy (345).

Prognosis is excellent (over 96 per cent survival) for patients with tumor confined to one ovary (342, 346). However, if the tumor is bilateral or shows local extension, the chance of a 5-year cure drops to 64 per cent (342). Careful follow-up of these patients is imperative, as they are potentially salvageable if recurrences are detected early. The most frequent sites of recurrence are the abdomen and pelvis, followed by the para-aortic and supraclavicular nodes (347); metastases to bone, liver, lung, and brain are late manifestations of disease. Recurrent disease should be treated with curative intent with surgical resection when possible, followed by further irradiation or chemotherapy (345, 347).

Teratoma. Teratomas account for 40 to 50 per cent of reported ovarian masses in children. Of these, the majority (approximately 80 per cent) are mature cystic lesions (dermoid cysts) with a very low incidence of malignancy; however, solid teratomas, which have a much higher incidence of malignancy, are not uncommon in childhood.

Optimal treatment of *mature teratoma* depends upon the age of the patient and the desire to conserve reproductive function. In young girls and women of childbearing age, cystectomy (enucleation) or oophorocystectomy can be done, with care to preserve as much functional ovarian tissue as possible. If the contralateral ovary appears normal, a wedge biopsy is not considered necessary in most cases (350).

Table 37–9. HISTOLOGIC GRADING OF IMMATURE TERATOMAS*

Grade 0: All tissues mature; no mitotic activity
Grade 1: Minor foci of abnormally cellular or embryonal tissue mixed with mature elements; rare mitoses
Grade 2: Moderate quantities of embryonal tissue mixed with mature elements; moderate mitotic activity
Grade 3: Large quantities of embryonal tissue present

*Based on data from reference 340.

In an *immature teratoma*, at least one of the germ cell layers lacks full differentiation; most often, the immature component is neuroepithelial, and it often forms neuroblastic rosettes. It is important to recognize that immaturity of tissues within an ovarian teratoma reflects metastatic capability, and therefore the immature elements should be considered evidence of malignancy. The grading system proposed by Robboy and Scully (340) (Table 37–9), which quantitates the degree of immaturity and the presence of neuroepithelial components, appears to correlate well with the clinical behavior of these tumors (Fig. 37–9). The prognosis also depends upon the types of immature cells that are present; elements of endodermal sinus tumor, embryonal carcinoma, or choriocarcinoma imply a much poorer prognosis than do immature neural or thyroid elements.

Unilateral salpingo-oophorectomy appears to be adequate surgical treatment for an immature teratoma that is confined within a single ovary (Stage Ia) (345, 350); although the opposite ovary is rarely involved by occult disease, biopsy may be useful in documenting this (346, 351). Adjuvant chemotherapy using combinations of VAC (vincristine/actinomycin D/Cytoxan) or VBP (vinblastine/bleomycin/cis-platinum) may be indicated for patients with Stage I tumors of a high histologic grade, as these are more likely to manifest extra-ovarian spread (350). Adjuvant chemotherapy (350, 352–356) is definitely indicated for patients with advanced stage disease and for patients with ruptured tumors. Preliminary results suggest that VBP may be superior to VAC for patients with Stage III–IV disease (356).

Endodermal Sinus Tumor. Endodermal sinus (yolk sac) tumor is characterized by rapid growth; there is often extensive intra-abdominal and intra-pelvic spread, with widespread involvement of peritoneal surfaces. Because these tumors are rarely bilateral, unilateral salpingo-oophorectomy may be chosen as initial treatment for unilateral encapsulated tumors (348). All patients should receive adjuvant chemotherapy as well.

A decade ago, Kurman and Norris (357) reported that overall survival for patients with this tumor was 13 per cent, with only 16 per cent survival for patients with Stage I disease. Recent reports (345, 358–360b) indicate that the use of adjuvant chemotherapy (VAC or VBP) following surgery has improved the disease-free survival rate. To date, VBP appears to be superior to VAC both for Stage I–II tumors (100 per cent survival rate versus 73.5 per cent for VAC) and for Stage III–IV tumors (78 per cent survival versus 40 per cent for VAC) (356). Patients whose tumors are resistant to these protocols may sometimes be salvaged with regimens containing VP-16 (360c).

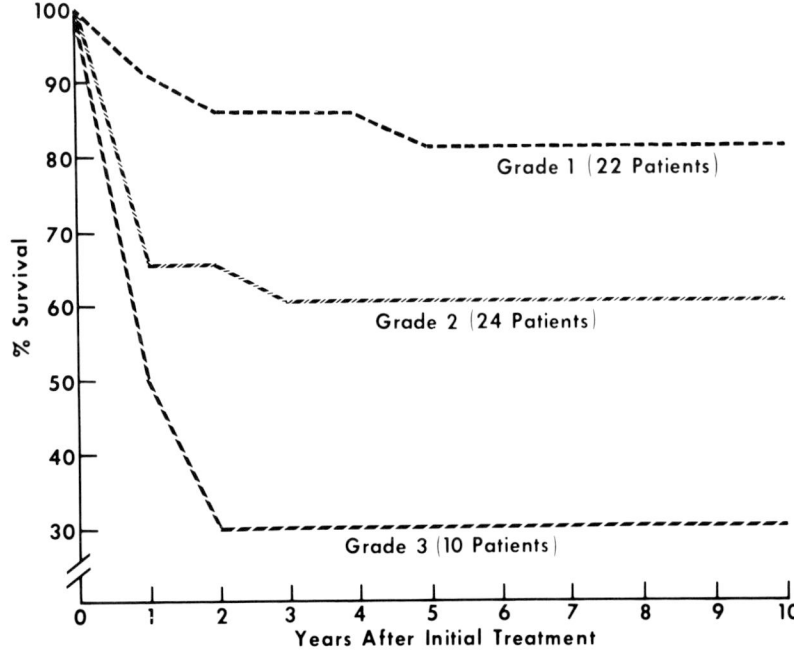

Figure 37–9. Effect of histologic grade on prognosis of ovarian teratomas. (From Norris, H. J., Zirkin, H. J., et al.: Immature (malignant) teratoma of the ovary: a clinical and pathologic study of 58 cases. Cancer 37:2359, 1976; Armed Forces Institute of Pathology Neg. No. 3653.)

TESTICULAR GERM CELL TUMORS

Testicular tumors are relatively uncommon in infants and children, accounting for only 1 to 2 per cent of all pediatric solid tumors. Of those that do occur in the pediatric years, over half are detected before the age of 5 years. After puberty, the incidence of testicular malignancy increases significantly.

In most patients, testicular tumors present as a painless scrotal swelling, and in over half of the cases this symptom has been present at least 3 months before the patient seeks treatment. Rarely, a testicular tumor may be endocrinologically active and produce precocious puberty or feminizing effects. A tumor may also arise in an undescended testis and present as an abdominal mass.

Classification. The normal testis is composed primarily of (1) germ cells (spermatozoa), (2) sex cord (Sertoli) cells, and (3) stromal interstitial testosterone-secreting (Leydig) cells. Neoplasms may arise from any of these elements. In the adult, 98 per cent of testicular tumors are of germ cell origin, whereas in children germ cell tumors account for approximately 60 to 80 per cent of testicular neoplasms, with non–germ cell tumors making up the other 20 to 40 per cent (361–364).

There are three main histologic variants of testicular germ cell malignancy in childhood and adolescence: (1) endodermal sinus (yolk sac) tumor, (2) embryonal carcinoma, and (3) teratoma. Endodermal sinus tumor is by far the most common testicular malignancy seen in the first 4 years of life, whereas embryonal carcinoma and malignant teratoma are the predominant malignancies seen in older children, adolescents, and young adults. Mature testicular teratomas are virtually always benign in infancy but are potentially malignant when they occur in adolescents or young adults. Seminoma is rarely seen in childhood; approximately 25 cases have been reported in patients ranging in age from 2½ to 25 years (365). It appears to be more common in boys in whom puberty and spermatogenesis occurred early.

Routes of Metastasis. Testicular tumors rarely spread by direct extension to the scrotal sac, because the tunica albuginea and tunica vaginalis act as barriers: the primary routes of metastasis are hematogenous and lymphatic. Endodermal sinus tumor usually spreads along vascular channels and metastasizes to the lungs or liver in about 14 per cent of cases (366). In contrast, embryonal carcinoma, malignant teratoma, and seminoma spread primarily via the long efferent lymphatic channels paralleling the testicular vessels, up to the para-aortic nodes at the level of the renal hilum. Spread to inguinal nodes is unusual, unless the scrotal sac has been invaded by tumor or the lymphatic drainage of the testis has been altered by prior surgery (e.g., herniorrhaphy or orchidopexy).

Staging. There have been many staging systems proposed for testicular cancer. The one used most commonly is a composite of those proposed by Boden (367) and Maier (368), which stratifies patients as follows:

Stage I_A —tumor confined to the testis
Stage I_B —microscopic involvement of retroperitoneal nodes
Stage II —bulky involvement of retroperitoneal nodes
Stage III—extension beyond retroperitoneal nodes

Preoperative evaluation of a child with a suspected malignant testicular germ cell tumor would include measurement of serum AFP and hCG levels, chest x-ray, and ultrasound of the abdomen with particular attention to the retroperitoneal nodes; computed tomography of the chest and abdomen should also be strongly considered if there is a high likelihood of malignancy.

The initial surgical approach to a potentially malignant testicular tumor is radical orchiectomy with high ligation of the spermatic cord at the internal inguinal ring. Orchiectomy through the scrotal sac or trans-scrotal biopsy is contraindicated because of the danger of local tumor spill or dissemination to regional lymphatics.

Since the lymphatic channels of the testis drain via the para-aortic nodes, evaluation of the retroperitoneal lymph nodes has become a particularly important part of both the staging and therapy of testicular tumors. Retroperitoneal nodes can be evaluated by ultrasound, computed tomography, or lymphangiography. As these nonoperative approaches yield a 10 to 20 per cent rate of error (368a), surgical staging (retroperitoneal lymphadenectomy) has traditionally been incorporated into the management plan. However, this procedure may have unpleasant sequelae, including ejaculatory dysfunction and subsequent infertility. There is currently much discussion about the indications and proper technique for retroperitoneal lymphadenectomy.

Several reports (363, 366, 369) indicate that less than 6 per cent of young children with endodermal sinus tumor clinically limited to the testis are found to have positive retroperitoneal nodes at surgery; thus, such patients should be spared this procedure. As will be discussed below, selected older patients with testicular tumors may also be managed without operative staging.

The debate regarding the proper technique for retroperitoneal sampling concerns the relative merits of bilateral versus unilateral lymphadenectomy. Ever since the work of Jamieson and Dobson (370) in 1910, it has been recognized that there is a cross-communication between the lymphatic channels of the testes, and it has also been demonstrated that when the *ipsilateral* nodes are positive, 15 to 30 per cent of *contralateral* nodes also will be positive (371, 372). These considerations have led to the recommendation for *bilateral* retroperitoneal dissection. In actuality, however, the incidence of lymphatic crossover when the *ipsilateral* nodes are negative appears to be extremely small. Ray and colleagues (372) in a review of 283 postlymphadenectomy specimens, found only 1 patient to have positive *contralateral* nodes when the *ipsilateral* nodes were negative, and Maier and associates (373) were unable to demonstrate that the bilateral approach improved survival when the results of unilateral and bilateral lymphadenectomies were compared in 213 patients with testicular germ cell neoplasms. Consequently, a modified unilateral lymphadenectomy, which avoids some of the complications of the bilateral procedure and appears to provide equally accurate staging and therapeutic efficacy (when ipsilateral nodes are negative) may be the preferable procedure for those patients who require surgical evaluation of the retroperitoneal nodes (369, 374).

Management

In order to properly manage a pediatric testicular germ cell tumor, it is necessary to consider the age of the patient, the histology of the tumor, and the extent of progression. Unfortunately, many of the reported studies (361, 363, 364, 369, 374–377a) are standardized for neither age groups nor histology; therefore it is difficult to make comparisons between them and to derive clear-cut conclusions from them. However, certain general impressions appear to be valid: (1) boys under 2 years of age with endodermal sinus tumors represent a special subgroup with a very good prognosis; (2) radiotherapy does not appear to be indicated in the initial management of the young infant with localized endodermal sinus tumor (359) and may not have a role in the treatment of the adolescent or adult with a nonseminomatous germ cell tumor either (374); and (3) combination chemotherapy has had a major impact on the prognosis of testicular germ cell tumors. The regimens that have proved to be successful include T-2 (vincristine/Adriamycin/actinomycin D/Cytoxan) (361), VBP (vinblastine/bleomycin/cis-platinum) (359, 374), and VAB-6 (vinblastine/actinomycin/bleomycin/cis-platinum/Cytoxan) (375).

Two major concerns with the use of VBP and VAB regimens in the young child are the nephrotoxicity of cis-platinum and the pulmonary toxicity of bleomycin. The former may be ameliorated by dose modification, careful monitoring of renal function prior to each treatment, and vigorous hydration and diuresis when cis-platinum is being administered. The pulmonary toxicity of bleomycin is accentuated by irradiation of the lungs or mediastinum; the use of these modalities concurrently or sequentially should be avoided if possible.

It has also been suggested that exposure to high oxygen concentrations and the injudicious use of fluids during prolonged surgical procedures predispose to a pulmonary capillary leak syndrome in patients previously treated with bleomycin; this synergistic toxicity may be diminished by limiting the FIO_2 to no greater than 24 per cent intraoperatively and avoiding overhydration (378).

Endodermal Sinus Tumor. Eighty-five per cent or more of infants with localized endodermal sinus tumor of the testis may be cured by radical orchiectomy alone (359, 376, 377a). Retroperitoneal lymph node dissection or chemotherapy or both are rarely indicated if chest x-ray and whole lung tomography are negative, the hCG level is normal, the alpha-fetoprotein (AFP) level returns to normal following surgery, and there is no evidence of retroperitoneal adenopathy on abdominal CT scan and ultrasound. The small proportion of patients that do relapse appear to be salvageable with combination chemotherapy (359, 377a).

For the child above 2 years of age with negative chest x-ray, extended unilateral retroperitoneal lymphadenectomy should be considered if the AFP level is elevated. Such patients should also be considered for adjuvant chemotherapy with T-2 (361), VBP (359, 374), or VAB-6 (375). For any patient with evidence of retroperitoneal lymph node involvement or positive chest x-ray, surgical debulking of gross disease should be followed by combination chemotherapy.

Embryonal Carcinoma and Teratoma. The most common histologies seen in the testicular tumors of adolescent and adult males are embryonal carcinoma and teratoma. These may occur in pure form or in combination in a mixed germ cell tumor (teratocarcinoma). It is unusual to find pure testicular choriocarcinoma or endodermal sinus tumor in this age group, but these elements are not infrequently found as components of mixed germ cell tumors.

Overall, 95 per cent or more of patients with malignant testicular germ cell tumors are curable with current therapeutic modalities. The standard approach to the patient whose physical examination and radiologic assessment have shown disease limited to the testis (Clinical Stage I) or to the testis and retroperitoneal nodes (Clinical Stage II) has been to proceed with radical orchiectomy followed by retroperitoneal lymphadenectomy. The need for, and duration of, adjuvant chemotherapy is then determined by the results of the pathologic staging. Patients with Clinical Stage III disease have been managed with a primary chemotherapy approach followed by selective debulking procedures. As will be discussed below, management of testicular tumors has been evolving and has become more complex as investigators have attempted to minimize iatrogenic complications while maintaining maximal survival rates.

Clinical Stage I patients can be stratified into high-and low-risk groups for relapse, based on histologic and serologic factors. Unfavorable histologic features include evidence of vascular or lymphatic invasion, extension of tumor along the spermatic cord, and presence of pure embryonal carcinoma or embryonal carcinoma with choriocarcinoma (368a, 383a–d). Unfavorable serologic features include extremely high AFP (>2000 mg/ml) or hCG (>10,000 U/ml) level at diagnosis or failure of marker levels to return to normal following orchiectomy (383e). Although the standard approach to Clinical Stage I disease has employed retroperitoneal lymphadenectomy, selected patients (i.e., those who lack unfavorable prognostic features and can be relied upon to comply with a careful monitoring regimen) may require no therapy beyond orchiectomy, as few of these will relapse and most relapsed patients are salvaged by chemotherapy (368a, 379–383a–e). Although the avoidance of lymphadenectomy is an appealing concept, it must be emphasized that the above approaches are still experimental and require careful monitoring of the patient by an experienced oncologist.

When retroperitoneal lymphadenectomy is performed and shows no evidence of nodal involvement (Surgical Stage Ia), the cure rate is 80 to 100 per cent, even without the use of adjuvant chemotherapy. Therefore, Stage Ia patients may be managed by close clinical, radiologic, and serologic monitoring (368a, 383a–c); VBP-based chemotherapy regimens will salvage most of the patients who relapse (379–383a).

Patients with microscopically positive retroperitoneal nodes (Stage Ib) have a 60 to 80 per cent cure rate with surgery alone, but this increases to virtually 100 per cent when two courses of adjuvant VBP chemotherapy are given. Patients not given adjuvant chemotherapy initially and who subsequently relapse have been salvaged (with few exceptions) with four courses of VBP (384). Stage Ib patients with high-risk factors for recurrence (see above) are candidates for adjuvant chemotherapy (2 courses); the rest could conceivably be managed by careful monitoring with chemotherapy (4 courses) reserved for those patients who relapse. VP-16–based salvage chemotherapy in which this agent is combined with cis-platinum and bleomycin, with or without Adriamycin, has been found to be effective in patients with persistent tumor following VBP therapy (381, 385).

The management approach to the patient with Clinical Stage II disease is also evolving as high-risk factors predicting relapse are identified; in addition to those discussed above, these include large nodal size (>2 cm in diameter) or involvement of more than 5 nodes (368a, 385a,b). Current therapeutic options include: (1) the standard approach—retroperitoneal lymphadenectomy followed by adjuvant chemotherapy (2 to 3 cycles); (2) a potential modification for patients who lack high-risk factors—lymphadenectomy followed by careful monitoring only, with chemotherapy (4 cycles) reserved for patients with recurrent disease; (3) an experimental approach—primary chemotherapy followed by selective lymphadenectomy (385a,b).

Patients with Stage III disease should receive chemotherapy. Regimens utilizing high doses of vinblastine, bleomycin, and cis-platinum alone (VBP) or in combination with actinomycin D and Cytoxan (VAB-6) have induced complete remissions in 60 to 70 per cent of patients, and another 10 to 15 per cent have subsequently been rendered disease-free by surgical removal of residual tumor (375, 386). Generally, 3 to 4 cycles of chemotherapy are sufficient to achieve maximal benefits, and maintenance chemotherapy is not required for patients who achieve complete remission (375, 387, 387a).

Despite the advances in treatment of testicular germ cell tumors, there remains a clinically definable subset of patients for whom current combination chemotherapy regimens have been relatively unsuccessful. These patients are characterized by the presence of bulky disease (palpable abdominal mass or intrathoracic metastases greater than 2 cm in diameter), visceral metastases, and/or marked elevation in serum levels of hCG and AFP (388). For such patients, new combination chemotherapy regimens such as (PVeBV) (388), which incorporates very high doses of cis-platinum with vinblastine, bleomycin, and VP-16, and the cyclical $CISCA_{II}/VB_{IV}$ regimen (388a), which alternates Cytoxan/Adriamycin/cis-platinum with vinblastine/bleomycin, have produced promising initial results.

Seminoma. Current therapeutic strategy for seminoma is influenced by two of its prominent features: (1) a marked proclivity for lymphatic spread, and (2) extreme radiosensitivity. In view of the radiosensitivity of this tumor, patients with Stages Ia and Ib pure seminoma (based on radiologic evaluation) can be spared retroperitoneal lymphadenectomy. Instead, they are treated with radiotherapy following radical orchiectomy (365, 379, 389, 390). A relatively modest dose (2500 to 3500 cGy) of megavoltage radiation at the midplane level is usually tumoricidal. When treated in this manner, patients with localized (Stage I) testicular seminoma have a 5-year survival rate approaching 100 per cent. For patients with positive lymphangiograms, the results are almost as good, with approximately 80 to 90 per cent alive and tumor-free after 5 years.

The radiotherapy field for localized testicular seminoma (negative lymphangiogram and CT scan) encompasses the periaortic and ipsilateral iliac nodes. If the lymphangiogram shows lymphatic spread to the periaortic region, then the practice has been to administer "prophylactic" treatment to the mediastinal and lower neck nodes (389, 390). However, this approach has the disadvantage of increasing the risk of bleomycin pulmonary fibrosis should the patient subsequently relapse and require chemotherapy with bleomycin. Because the VBP regimen has been effective in salvaging relapsed seminoma patients as well as in shrinking bulky tumor masses (391–393), it may be reasonable to avoid supradiaphragmatic irradiation for minimal Stage II seminoma, provided the patient is followed carefully (378).

MEDIASTINAL GERM CELL TUMORS

The mediastinum is the third most common location for germ cell tumors in children (after the sacrococcygeal area and the gonads). As this area affords an ample space for expansion before a mass causes symptoms, mediastinal germ cell tumors may achieve enormous dimensions prior to detection. These tumors are usually found in the anterior mediastinum and manifest the same histologic spectrum as do germ cell tumors found in other locations. Most are benign dermoid cysts, but approximately 20 per cent are malignant. Overall, mediastinal germ cell tumors are slightly more common in females, but malignant lesions are much more common in males (a situation analogous to that of sacrococcygeal tumors in young infants and gonadal tumors in adolescents). Treatment and prognosis depend upon the histology and extent of the tumor.

Mediastinal germinomas generally expand within the confines of the thorax; they may invade adjoining structures, but more often they encroach upon them. Hematogenous metastasis may occur but is relatively uncommon with germinomas in comparison with other mediastinal germ cell malignancies. Surgical excision, when it can be accomplished, may be curative in 66 to 81 per cent of cases (394). However, the enormous bulk of many of these tumors, as well as their proximity to great vessels and other vital structures, generally renders complete surgical excision impossible. Such cases are often managed by radiotherapy, sometimes preceded by surgical debulking. Mediastinal germinoma appears to be as radioresponsive as testicular seminoma; however, very bulky tumors may require higher dosages than are used for testicular tumors. Doses should be individualized and tailored to tumor volume, ranging from 3000 cGy for minimal disease to 4500 to 5000 cGy (with reduced portals) for larger tumors (395, 396). Overall, 5- to 10-year survival rates for patients treated with surgery and radiotherapy are in the range of 52 to 58 per cent (395, 396). Combination chemotherapy using high doses of cis-platinum seems to be effective in shrinking large primary mediastinal germinoma as well as eradicating distant metastases (397). It is thus possible that chemotherapy alone may be sufficient in the management of at least some of these patients, and that initial chemotherapy followed by local regional surgery or radiotherapy (if necessary) may improve the survival rate of the others.

Mediastinal germ cell tumors other than germinoma are not very radiosensitive and tend to recur both locally and at distant sites if treated only with surgery and irradiation; consequently, combination chemotherapy should be part of the initial treatment plan. The response rate of mediastinal germ cell tumors to conventional VBP regimens is inferior to that reported for germ cell tumors of comparable histology arising in other sites (397); endodermal sinus tumor and choriocarcinoma of the mediastinum have particularly poor prognoses. Some reports (394, 398) suggest that modified VBP-type regimens that utilize very intensive cis-platinum schedules may improve the treatment results for mediastinal germ cell tumors (excluding endodermal sinus tumor and choriocarcinoma). The very intensive cyclic $CISCA_{II}/VB_{IV}$ regimen (399) has been reported to be effective in the treatment of mediastinal germ cell tumors (including endodermal sinus tumor). Nonetheless, the single most important prognostic determinant for mediastinal endodermal sinus tumor remains the potential for complete excision, either before or after chemotherapy (399a,b).

The patient's age at diagnosis appears to be a critical prognostic factor for *immature teratoma* of the mediastinum. As reviewed by Carter and colleagues (400), all 13 reported cases of immature mediastinal teratoma in patients 15 years or older had a fatal outcome within 1 year of diagnosis. On the other hand, only 2 of 53 patients under the age of 15 had a fatal outcome, and both of these individuals succumbed to surgical complications. Thus, immature mediastinal teratomas of infancy and early adolescence appear to behave as space-occupying, but not malignant, neoplasms. For patients above the age of 15 years, such tumors behave as true malignancies and must be treated as such.

GERM CELL TUMORS OF THE HEAD AND NECK

Although germ cell tumors are a rare cause of head and neck masses, they frequently enter into the differential diagnosis of lesions in this area because of their occurrence in a variety of sites (cranial cavity, orbit, nasopharynx, face, oral cavity, thyroid gland, soft tissues of the neck). Nearly 10 per cent of all childhood teratomas occur above the level of the clavicles (327), and the majority of these are recognized in the newborn or very young infant. Neck teratomas may cause life-threatening airway obstruction in the neonate.

Quick recognition of a cervical germ cell tumor is essential, since early operation can be life-saving.

Delay of surgery in the presence of respiratory obstruction is virtually always fatal (401, 402). In the preoperative phase, tracheal aspiration and oxygen administration are advisable; laying the infant on the side with the tumor may help to relieve the tracheal compression. Surgery consists of "shelling out" the tumor and is accompanied by a mortality rate of 17 per cent (402).

In the infant, the presence of immature components in a head or neck teratoma does not necessarily portend malignant behavior. However, there may be a greater potential for malignancy if the tumor is not removed in the neonatal period or if endodermal sinus tumor elements are present (403, 403a).

Intracranial germ cell tumors usually arise in the pineal region or in other midline locations. These tumors will be discussed with the other CNS tumors in a subsequent section of this chapter.

RETROPERITONEAL AND INTRA-ABDOMINAL GERM CELL TUMORS

Abdominal germ cell tumors are usually located posterolaterally in the retroperitoneal tissues; about 10 per cent show malignant changes (404). Although they are quite rare in this location, germ cell tumors are nonetheless the third most common malignancy of the retroperitoneal space (after neuroblastoma and Wilms' tumor) (329). Presenting symptoms are usually vague and frequently secondary to the pressure effects of the tumor on neighboring structures. Patients may thus complain of abdominal or back pain, nausea, vomiting, constipation, and urinary tract symptoms (404).

Intra-abdominal germ cell tumors are quite unusual. Fifty-one cases of gastric teratoma have been described to date. Teratomas of the liver and kidney have also been reported (405).

LIVER TUMORS

Primary tumors of the liver are rare in childhood, accounting for less than 5 per cent of cancer in the young. The majority of primary liver tumors are of hepatocyte origin (hepatomas). Hepatomas are divided into two major histologic types: *hepatoblastoma* and *hepatocellular carcinoma*. Hepatoblastoma appears largely in the infant population and is seldom seen after 3 years of age; it generally occurs in otherwise normal livers. Hepatocellular carcinoma is seen most often in children above the age of 5 years and is often superimposed upon cirrhotic changes in the liver.

Pathology

Hepatoblastoma consists of tumor cells that are smaller than normal liver cells. It may be purely epithelial in nature or it may contain an admixture of mesenchymal (bone, cartilage, muscle) elements. The malignant hepatocytes that make up the epithelial component may be *fetal* or *embryonal* in pattern. Tumor histology is considered to be of prognostic importance. Hepatoblastomas with a purely fetal pattern have a better prognosis than do those with embryonal, mesenchymal, or anaplastic elements. Complete surgical resection is tantamount to cure for the vast majority of purely fetal hepatoblastomas, whereas less than 10 per cent of patients with embryonal or other undifferentiated patterns survive 5 years when treated with surgical resection alone (406–408).

Hepatocellular carcinoma in the pediatric age group generally is histologically similar to hepatocellular carcinoma in adults. However, a significant proportion of childhood cases are associated with the histologic variant known as *fibrolamellar carcinoma* or *polygonal cell tumor with fibrous stroma* (409, 410), which is associated with a relatively favorable prognosis. In Berman's series (409), 82 per cent of these patients exhibited 2-year survival and 63 per cent 5-year survival.

A less common form of malignant liver tumor is called *undifferentiated sarcoma* or *malignant mesenchymoma* (411). This tumor is composed primarily of immature mesenchyme and may represent a malignant variant of the more common benign mesenchymal hamartoma of childhood. The majority of cases of this tumor occur between 6 and 10 years of age and are associated with a particularly poor prognosis (median survival less than 1 year).

Clinical Features

EPIDEMIOLOGY

Hepatoblastoma is a tumor of early infancy; 60 per cent of cases are found in patients under 1 year of age, and 90 per cent in those under 3 years. It is sometimes seen in association with congenital anomalies such as hemihypertrophy and Beckwith's syndrome (412).

Hepatocellular carcinoma is seen most often in children older than 5 years. It is found more commonly in conditions associated with childhood cirrhosis, such as chronic active hepatitis (413), biliary atresia (414), alpha$_1$ antitrypsin deficiency (415), and Byler's disease (progressive familial cholestatic cirrhosis) (416). Hereditary tyrosinemia has a particular predisposition for development of malignancy; nearly one third of children surviving longer than 2 years with the chronic form of this disease develop hepatocellular carcinoma (417). However, cirrhosis per se may not be the predisposing factor to malignancy, for the risk is dissimilar for different causes of cirrhosis, and some conditions associated with childhood cirrhosis, such as Wilson's disease, cystinosis, galactosemia, cystic fibrosis, and Hurler's disease, are rarely associated with hepatic tumors (414).

In many areas of the world, particularly Africa and Asia, hepatocellular carcinoma is associated with infection by the hepatitis B virus (HBV). Chronic carriers of HBV have a risk approximately 22.6 times that of the uninfected population for developing this tumor (413). Integration of the DNA of the hepatitis B virus with the nuclear DNA of human hepatocellular carcinoma cells further strengthens the association between these two entities (418). HBV infection acquired by the fetus through maternal vertical transmission may be particularly carcinogenic, possibly because of an impaired immune response (419); however, because of the long latent period between HBV infection and the development of malignancy, most cases occur beyond the pediatric years (usually in the fourth decade of life).

The role of chemical carcinogens in producing liver tumors may be superimposed upon the damage produced by HBV. In many areas of the world, the incidence of primary hepatic tumors is correlated with exposure to aflatoxin, a substance produced by the mold *Aspergillus flavus*, which grows in any warm, moist area where grain is stored. It is common in parts of Africa, where hepatocellular carcinoma is also common (420) and may act as a co-carcinogen with HBV in producing liver tumors in these areas.

Pharmacologic agents such as androgens and estrogenic steroids have also been associated with the induction of liver tumors (406, 414).

PRESENTATION

The most common presentation for hepatic malignancies is abdominal distention with a palpable right upper quadrant mass. Other findings directly related to the presence of the tumor are anorexia, weight loss, pain, and vomiting; jaundice and ascites are seen less frequently. Extrahepatic manifestations include paraneoplastic endocrinopathies (hypoglycemia, hypercalcemia, precocious puberty in males) and hematologic abnormalities (erythrocytosis, thrombocytosis).

METASTATIC SPREAD

Hepatoblastoma and hepatocellular carcinoma may spread by direct extension into contiguous areas of the liver or by intrahepatic vascular or lymphatic channels into other parts of the liver. Extrahepatic spread is usually to regional lymph nodes in the porta hepatis or by vascular routes to the lung. Since liver tumors are well vascularized, distant metastasis may already be present at diagnosis; spread may also occur at the time of surgery, as it is impossible to ligate all veins draining the liver. Intra-abdominal spread to either lymph nodes or viscera may also occur. Less common is involvement of the central nervous system, bone, and bone marrow.

EVALUATION

On plain x-rays of the abdomen, the liver shadow is often enlarged, with displacement of the stomach or colon, and calcifications in the liver are occasionally seen. Radionuclide imaging of the liver with ^{99m}Tc sulfur colloid shows a "cold" space-occupying lesion, but there is increased uptake in the mass when ^{67}Ga is used as the scanning agent. Probably the most important preoperative diagnostic procedure is hepatic angiography, which not only can be useful in establishing the diagnosis but also can aid in determining the feasibility of complete surgical excision. Abdominal CT scan is also useful in assessing extent of the tumor.

Elevated alpha-fetoprotein (AFP) levels have been observed in 84 to 91 per cent of patients with hepatoblastoma (421) and in 80 to 90 per cent of patients with hepatocellular carcinoma (422, 423). The short half-life of AFP (4 to 6 days) makes it a valuable marker for monitoring residual or metastatic disease following resection of the primary tumor, as well as for following the response of an unresectable primary tumor to chemotherapy.* However, it is also important to realize that AFP-negative metastases may be seen following the resection of an AFP-producing tumor (425).

PROGNOSTIC FEATURES

The most favorable prognostic feature is confinement of the tumor to one lobe of the liver, with the potential for total excision. Cure can be achieved in 30 to 50 per cent of hepatoblastoma patients on whom successful surgery is performed (406, 426–428) and in 33 per cent of patients with hepatocellular carcinoma (426, 427). Prolonged survival for patients with unresectable or incompletely excised tumors is unusual. Prognosis is not influenced by tumor size so long as the tumor is resectable. On the other hand, the presence of multiple tumors, nodal metastases, or pulmonary metastases augurs a particularly poor prognosis.

Therapy

Surgery. Complete surgical resection is the mainstay of therapy for liver tumors. Unfortunately, at the time of presentation only about 54 per cent of children have operable tumors and only 49 per cent are susceptible to total excision (427, 428). Surgical risks are considerable, with operative and postoperative mortality rates in the range of 15 to

---

*The production of AFP by hepatoblastoma (and certain germ cell tumors) may offer possibilities for a combined chemotherapy-immunotherapy attack on the neoplasm, while minimizing toxicity to normal cells. In this approach, a chemotherapeutic agent is bound to a carrier (e.g., an antibody to AFP) that has a specific affinity for the tumor cells (424).

33 per cent (427, 429, 430). Massive hemorrhage is a particular problem, with some patients requiring replacement of more than their total blood volume during the procedure. On the other hand, infants and children who survive the surgery tolerate removal of large volumes of liver better than adults, and the liver will often regenerate to its original volume within a few months, even when as much as 85 per cent of it has been removed.

Radiotherapy. Radiotherapy alone is generally ineffective in the treatment of malignant liver tumors of childhood, primarily because the effective tumor dose exceeds hepatic tolerance. However, it may be of palliative value; on occasion, inoperable tumors have responded for up to 2 years following radiotherapy (426). Radiotherapy has also been used in association with chemotherapy to shrink an initially inoperable tumor in order to allow total resection at a second surgical procedure (426, 431–433).

Several novel forms of internal radiation are currently under investigation. Nolan and colleagues (434) have injected microspheres coated with radioactive yttrium into the hepatic artery for local deposition of radiation. Order and colleagues (435) are administering radiolabeled immunoglobulin (^{131}I anti-ferritin) in conjunction with external irradiation (2100 cGy) and chemotherapy (Adriamycin/5-FU).

Chemotherapy. Although not considered a primary mode of therapy in liver cancer, chemotherapy has been used with some success in converting inoperable tumors into surgically resectable ones (436–438).

The most active agent to date in the treatment of liver tumors is Adriamycin. When used as a single agent, it produced complete remission or good partial remission in 5 of 11 children with hepatomas (437) and in 11 of 14 children with hepatocellular carcinoma (438). It has also been found to be active against metastatic disease and, in at least one case, has produced disease-free survival in excess of 3 years in a patient with pulmonary metastasis (439, 440). Adriamycin in combination with Cytoxan, vincristine, and 5-FU produced a clinical response in 7 of 8 patients with primary unresectable hepatic malignancies, 4 of whom were able to subsequently undergo complete excision of residual disease (430). In another study (441), 44 per cent of patients with residual disease after surgery responded to this regimen. Adriamycin in combination with cis-platinum has also achieved long-term disease-free survival in 3 patients with unresectable primary tumors, one of whom had pulmonary metastases at diagnosis (442). These results suggest that chemotherapy used for initial cytoreduction may reduce the operative and postoperative mortality in paients with extensive primary tumors as well as permit curative surgery in some patients.

Investigators have also employed chemotherapy in an adjuvant fashion after complete tumor excision. The Children's Cancer Study Group employed the combination of vincristine/Adriamycin/Cytoxan/5-FU (441) in 24 patients who had no measurable disease after surgical excision; at the time of the report, 83 per cent had remained free of disease, with a median follow-up period of 30 months. Holton and colleagues (443) also employed an adjuvant chemotherapy regimen using vincristine/Cytoxan/5-FU in a series of 7 patients and were encouraged to find 3 long-term survivors among 7 patients, in comparison with no survivors among 20 children treated prior to the use of adjuvant therapy. The Adriamycin/cis-platinum combination also shows promise as an adjuvant regimen for hepatoblastoma (442).

RETINOBLASTOMA

Retinoblastoma is a malignant neoplasm arising from primitive neuroectodermal tissue within the nuclear layer of the retina (444). In its histology it is quite similar to neuroblastoma, medulloblastoma, and pineoblastoma, three other highly malignant and relatively radioresponsive neoplasms of neural origin (445, 446). Ultrastructural studies have demonstrated the presence of cells with features of photoreceptor cells as well as primitive neuroblasts within retinoblastoma tissue (447).

Genetics

There are three recognized genetic patterns of retinoblastoma: sporadic, autosomal dominant, and 13q− syndrome (448–450). The majority of cases (approximately 60 per cent) arise sporadically, presumably as new somatic mutations, and are virtually always associated with unilateral disease. Approximately 40 per cent of patients are felt to have a hereditary form of the disease—this includes the 10 per cent of patients with a positive family history as well as the 30 per cent who have multifocal tumors with a negative family history. The attack rate of the hereditary form is found to be 40 per cent, consistent with an autosomal dominant pattern with 80 per cent penetrance (450). Tumor development in these individuals follows a Poisson distribution, with lesions randomly distributed between the two eyes; the mean number of tumors that develop is five (451). Approximately 15 per cent of patients with unilateral tumors may also transmit the disease to their offspring (448).

Although most retinoblastoma patients have a normal constitutional karyotype, a small proportion manifest the 13q− syndrome; these individuals have multiple malformations, including mental and physical retardation, microcephaly, cardiac and eye defects, and various skeletal deformities. The deletion of the long arm of chromosome 13 is congenital and occurs in all cells of the body. As techniques of increased sensitivity have been applied, progressively smaller deletions have been identified (452), all of which include band 14. These data would suggest that at least one of the genes responsible for retinoblastoma is located in chromosome band 13q14.

The enzyme esterase D, whose genetic locus has also been assigned to band 13q14, has proved to be a useful marker for study of this particular chromosomal region (453, 454). The linkage between the putative retinoblastoma gene and the esterase D gene has enabled investigators to demonstrate 13q14 deletions beyond the resolution of chromosome banding in some retinoblastoma patients (455) and may permit identification of carriers of the retinoblastoma gene. Esterase D isoenzyme studies have also demonstrated homozygosity or hemizygosity for the malignant allele in approximately one half to two thirds of retinoblastomas (455–458). These findings suggest that retinoblastoma may develop as a result of loss or inactivation of suppressor genes that are normally present in band 13q14; this may allow subsequent overexpression of a putative oncogene (457, 459, 459a).

Other nonrandom chromosomal abnormalities that have been demonstrated in retinoblastoma cells include *additional copies of 1q, isochromosome 6p(iso6p), monosomy 16, marker 1p+, homogeneously staining regions,* and *double minutes* (457, 460, 460a). The *iso6p* mutation, which appears to be fairly specific for retinoblastoma, provides two extra copies of the 6p region; it has been proposed (459a) that retinoblastoma development may reflect an imbalance between an "expressor" gene (i.e., oncogene) on region 6p and the suppressor genes on 13q14. Some of the other genetic changes described above could also result in increased proliferative potential and tumor progression. The putative suppressed gene of retinoblastoma (and osteosarcoma) that is present in chromosome 13 has recently been cloned, and RNA transcript was found to be absent in the cases of retinoblastoma and osteosarcoma tested to date. This finding has obvious broad implications for our understanding of many childhood tumors. The protein produced by this gene may be a vital regulator of cell growth. Individuals who are heterozygous deficient may be predisposed to the second "hit," a cross-over in a single cell that renders it homozygous deficient and therefore the stem cell of a tumor clone (461a,b).

The cytogenetic data reviewed above are consistent with Knudson's "two-hit" model of carcinogenesis, which proposes that two distinct mutational events are required for malignant transformation (461). In the case of retinoblastoma, the "hits" would represent loss or inactivation of regulator genes at the 13q14 locus. In the hereditary form of the disease, one of these defective alleles would be inherited via the germ cells. Since one "hit" would then already be present in all somatic cells, only a single postzygotic "hit," i.e., inactivation of the homologous normal allele, would be required to transform a normal retinal cell into a retinoblastoma cell. The development of sporadic retinoblastoma, on the other hand, would require that both "hits" occur in a single retinal cell.

The mutation responsible for producing hereditary retinoblastoma is also associated with induction of malignancy in other tissues. The most frequent second malignancy is osteosarcoma, the incidence of which in these patients is about 500 times that seen in the general population (462). A review of survivors of hereditary retinoblastoma (462a) reported the incidence of second tumors to be 20 per cent at 10 years, 50 per cent at 20 years, and 90 per cent at 30 years. Radiotherapy clearly plays a role in tumorigenesis, as two thirds of these tumors develop in the radiotherapy field; however, it is significant to note that the other one third occur outside the radiotherapy field or in patients who have never received radiotherapy.

Clinical Features

In the majority of children with retinoblastoma, the condition is diagnosed within the first 2 years of life, and over 80 per cent are diagnosed before age 3 years. The major presenting features are leukocoria (white pupil), strabismus, a red painful eye, or poor vision. Strabismus is more commonly a presenting feature in patients with early-stage disease, whereas leukocoria is almost always associated with advanced disease.

As Ellsworth (463–465) has stressed, the most important tool in the diagnostic evaluation of suspected retinoblastoma is indirect ophthalmoscopy with 360-degree scleral depression; as this is best performed while the patient is under anesthesia, a bone marrow aspirate and lumbar puncture (with cytocentrifuge preparation) may be performed at the same time for staging purposes.

It is no longer necesary to enucleate the eye in order to establish a diagnosis, since with ultrasonography, the electroimmunofluorescent test for *Toxocara* (466), and LDH isoenzyme studies (467), it is possible in most cases to confirm a diagnosis without histologic sampling.

X-rays of the orbit will often demonstrate calcification in retinoblastoma; computed tomography (CT) is even more sensitive to the presence of calcification and may detect extrascleral extension of tumor as well (468). An unusual, but significant, radiologic finding is erosion of the bony wall of the orbit or of the optic foramen on plain x-ray or CT scan; this virtually always indicates extraorbital spread of tumor and little hope of cure.

Additional studies, such as bone scan and skeletal series, may be performed if there is suspicion that disease has extended beyond the globe.

Staging

The staging system most commonly used for retinoblastoma is that proposed by Reese and Ellsworth (469) (Table 37–10). This system recognizes five groups based on the size, location, and number of tumors in each eye. Bedford and associates (470) have added a sixth group to this staging system to include patients with residual and metastatic disease. It is extremely rare to find unilateral disease of limited extent (Groups I to III) unless the patient presents with strabismus or is being examined because of a positive family history. Diagnosis of retinoblastoma at an early age does not preclude the discovery of advanced disease on initial examination, as 68 per cent of infants diagnosed under 6 months of age have been found to have Group V disease (451).

Routes of Metastasis

Retinoblastoma grows in a roughly spherical manner and may demonstrate either an *endophytic* or *exophytic* growth pattern. *Endophytic* tumors grow from the retina inward to the vitreous cavity; as they become larger, they may seed tumor cells into the vitreous cavity. These vitreous seeds are associated with large tumors (usually >5 disc diameters) and are a bad prognostic sign; they may survive as floating spheroidal tumor clumps until they nest into the surface of the retina or move into the anterior or posterior chambers of the eye and form sheets or nodules of tumor cells on the endothelial surface of the cornea or the iris. *Exophytic* retinoblastomas grow from the retina outward into the subretinal space; such tumors produce a progressive retinal detachment and occasionally seed into the anterior chamber, where they may produce nodules at the pupillary margin. Progressive growth of tumor is associated with extension into the choroid or sclera.

Spread of retinoblastoma beyond the globe follows an orderly path through the lamina cribrosa sclerae along the optic nerve to the base of the brain, and from there to the subarachnoid space and then to systemic sites. Distant metastases from hematogenous spread may develop in the bone marrow, long bones, and liver, but usually spare the lungs (a pattern similar to that seen in neuroblastoma). Lymphatic spread follows invasion of the orbit and face.

Approximately 4 per cent of children with bilateral retinoblastoma develop lesions in the pineal region (471a). These do not usually represent metastatic spread, but are the consequence of retinoblastoma arising independently within the vestigial photoreceptor tissue of the pineal region (the "third eye"). This is known as the *trilateral retinoblastoma syndrome* and has a poor prognosis because of dissemination of tumor along the neuraxis (446, 471a,b).

Prognosis

Successful treatment of retinoblastoma is gauged by two criteria: (1) patient survival—the primary concern; and (2) preservation of useful vision—usually defined as visual acuity of at least 20/200.

The prognosis for 5-year survival (Table 37–11) in patients with Group I to Group IV retinoblastoma is virtually 100 per cent. Survival drops to 83 to 87 per cent for patients with Group V disease (464); this relatively high mortality is particularly significant because the majority of patients with retinoblastoma fall into this group.

Prognosis for survival can also be correlated with the extent of tumor spread evident in the enucleated specimen. Approximately two thirds of

Table 37–10. STAGING SYSTEM FOR RETINOBLASTOMA*

Group I	(A)	Solitary tumor, <5 disc diameters in size, at or behind the equator†
	(B)	Multiple tumors, none >4 disc diameters in size, all at or behind the equator
Group II	(A)	Solitary tumor, 4 to 10 disc diameters in size, at or behind the equator
	(B)	Multiple tumors, 4 to 10 disc diameters in size, behind the equator
Group III	(A)	Any lesion anterior to the equator
	(B)	Solitary tumors >10 disc diameters behind the equator
Group IV	(A)	Multiple tumors, some >10 disc diameters
	(B)	Any lesion extending anteriorly to the ora serrata‡
Group V	(A)	Massive tumors invading over half the retina
	(B)	Vitreous seeding
Group VI	(A)	Residual orbital disease
	(B)	Optic nerve involvement and extrascleral extension

*Based on data from references 463 and 470.
†Equator: the midplane of the eye.
‡Ora serrata: junction of the retina and ciliary body.

Table 37–11. RESULTS OF TREATMENT OF RETINOBLASTOMA*

Group	Preservation of Normal Vision (%)	5-Year Survival (%)	
		Unilateral	Bilateral
I	95–100	100	100
II	87–100	100	100
III	67–86	100	100
IV	69–75	100	(33)†
V	34–75	83	87

*Based on data from references 463, 464, and 470.
†Only 3 cases.

all enucleated eyes show evidence of involvement of the choroid (471); however, choroidal involvement does not suggest a poor prognosis unless there is involvement of the sclera, iris, ciliary body, or the cut end of the optic nerve. The mortality rate is about 15 per cent for tumors involving the sclera if they do not extend beyond the lamina cribrosa, but rises to 40 per cent for tumors that extend beyond this point, and to about 60 per cent for tumors that extend to the cut end of the optic nerve (464, 472–474). Once the disease has invaded the orbit, mortality exceeds 90 per cent and reaches virtually 100 per cent for patients with distant metastases (464).

In assessing the ultimate prognosis in retinoblastoma patients, it is necessary to recognize the impact of second malignancies on long-term survival. Although the likelihood of survival of retinoblastoma is not influenced by whether the tumor was unilateral or bilateral, the patient with bilateral (i.e., hereditary) disease is clearly at a disadvantage in terms of ultimate survival. Indeed, in one long-term follow-up study of patients with bilateral retinoblastoma, the mortality rate from second malignancies exceeded that due to the retinoblastoma itself within 5 years of diagnosis, and by 35 years from diagnosis, 59 per cent of the patients had died (474a).

The prognosis for preserving useful vision is excellent for Group I and Group II patients but is progressively less favorable for patients in Groups III, IV, and V (Table 37–11). This reflects the larger areas of the retina involved by the more advanced tumors, difficulties in designing radiotherapy fields that avoid the lens, and higher recurrence rates that necessitate enucleation to control tumor progression.

Treatment

The primary treatment modalities for retinoblastoma are enucleation and irradiation; other modes of treatment, such as chemotherapy, photocoagulation, cryotherapy, and cobalt-60 plaques, may be used in special situations, but almost always in conjunction with one of the primary treatment approaches.

In the past, all unilateral retinoblastomas were managed by enucleation. However, radiotherapy has proved successful in salvaging useful vision without compromising survival in unilateral cases of Stage I to Stage III disease (463, 470, 475). Unfortunately, it is uncommon for unilateral tumors to present when still this small. Close follow-up of radiotherapy-treated retinoblastoma is mandatory; if the tumor has not shown signs of response 6 to 8 weeks after the start of radiotherapy, alternative forms of treatment and possibly enucleation should be considered (473). In addition to the requirement for frequent follow-up examinations under anesthesia, radiotherapy also is associated with long-term consequences affecting the development of facial bones and the risk of radiation-induced second neoplasms. This has led some authorities (476) to reconsider enucleation as the primary mode of treatment, even for early stage unilateral tumors, provided there is no family history of retinoblastoma and, hence, a low risk of involvement of the remaining eye.

Radiotherapy is relatively unsuccessful in salvaging useful vision in Group IV and Group V disease, so that enucleation is the more common approach to these tumors (463, 464, 477). However, some authors (470) advocate avoiding enucleation unless there is evidence of optic nerve involvement.

The traditional approach to bilateral retinoblastoma has been to enucleate the eye with the more advanced disease and to irradiate the remaining eye. More recently, there has been a tendency to manage each eye independently according to its potential for preserving vision and to reserve enucleation for those eyes in which there is no hope of preserving vision. Overall, the use of bilateral irradiation may salvage sufficient visual acuity in at least one eye for more than 50 per cent of patients to lead a normal life (478). Enucleation may be avoided in as many as 85 to 93 per cent of eyes in which the disease does not exceed Group IV. Careful follow-up of such patients is indicated, however, as over half will require further treatment (479, 480). Group V tumors may also be treated by irradiation if there is potentially good retina remaining in each eye; however, only about 10 per cent of such eyes can be salvaged in this fashion (480). For the rare unfortunate case in which disease in both eyes is so extensive that no vision is likely to be saved in either, bilateral enucleation may be necessary.

Surgery. When enucleation is performed, removal of as long a segment of optic nerve as possible (at least 10 mm) is essential. As it is not uncommon to find tumor extending for only a few millimeters beyond the lamina cribrosa, this approach often totally removes a tumor that might otherwise eventually have spread to the subarachnoid space. The presence of tumor cells at the cut end of the optic nerve has generally been considered to be an indication of extraocular spread, requiring postoperative radiotherapy.

Radiotherapy. Since the disease can be multifocal, the field of radiotherapy should encompass all of the retina. Conventional dosage ranges from 3500 cGy in 3 weeks, for Group I to Group III disease, to 4500 cGy in 4 weeks for Group IV and Group V disease. Higher doses have been used with more prolonged fractionation (e.g., 5000 to 6000 cGy in 5 to 6 weeks using 200 to 250 cGy fractions) in an attempt to minimize the complications of large fraction treatment while providing good local control of tumor (448).

An alternative to external beam irradiation is the use of radioactive applicators of cobalt 60, which are sutured to the sclera and removed 7 days later. They are able to deliver an extremely high dose to the immediate area where the applicator is sutured (25,000 to 30,000 cGy to the tumor base and 4000 cGy to the tumor apex), but distribution is nonhomogeneous, with rapid dose fall-off within a millimeter's distance. Thus a large tumor, or multiple tumors, cannot be adequately treated by this technique. These applicators may cause nerve fiber damage at the site of treatment and hemorrhage from large retinal vessels if placed near the optic disc, and therefore they are not recommended for tumors near the macula or optic disc.

Intraocular Recurrences Following Radiotherapy. Intraocular recurrences may result from failure to completely kill all the tumor in the treated field or from unrecognized tumor outside the field of treatment. Even when disease is detected and treated at an early stage (Groups I to III), more than 50 per cent of eyes will require further treatment (470, 479). Approximately two thirds of these failures result from residual tumor and one third from new tumors outside the treatment field (479, 481). The majority of recurrences develop within 6 months after treatment, and few are seen beyond 24 months after treatment.

Radiotherapy failures can sometimes be managed with phototherapy, cryotherapy, or local ^{60}Co implants; however, in some instances enucleation is eventually required. Only as a last resort should a second course of radiotherapy be undertaken (464).

Phototherapy. Photocoagulation is a method of destroying small retinal tumors by obliterating their nutrient vessels with the use of a powerful xenon arc light beam (482, 483). Tumors are considered suitable for control by this method if they (a) are greater than 4 disc diameters in size, (b) are distinct from the optic nerve head and macula, (c) do not contain large nutrient vessels, and (d) do not involve the choroid. The major use of this method has been to treat small recurrences after external beam or cobalt applicator therapy has failed (470, 475) and to treat the less involved eye in patients with bilateral retinoblastoma (484).

Cryotherapy. Cryotherapy is believed to destroy tumor cells by interrupting their microcirculation and causing mechanical cellular damage from the thaw of intracellular ice crystals. It has been reported to be of value in the treatment of small, anteriorly located tumors (485).

Chemotherapy. The role of chemotherapy in the treatment of retinoblastoma remains undefined. Its use can be considered to serve at least three functions: (1) to enhance the effect of radiotherapy on advanced intraocular disease; (2) to treat clinically evident orbital disease or metastatic disease; and (3) to reduce mortality due to unrecognized micrometastatic disease.

Intra-arterial triethylenemelamine (TEM) is the agent that has been used most widely for treatment of local disease, particularly in patients with Group IV or Group V disease and in those with residual or recurrent orbital disease (463, 464, 475). However, TEM administered by intracarotid injection in conjunction with radiation therapy has shown no clear-cut advantage over radiation alone (464).

Usually the presence of meningeal involvement or systemic metastases is fatal. In one report (486), a child with meningeal involvement by retinoblastoma responded to a treatment program of intrathecal methotrexate, intravenous Cytoxan, oral CCNU, and cranial/orbital radiation, with a remission persisting in excess of 20 months; however, 5 other patients treated in this fashion failed to survive. Two other patients with metastatic disease treated with Adriamycin, vincristine, and Cytoxan were reported to be disease-free after 2 years (464), and one child with skeletal metastases responded to radiation therapy and chemotherapy (487). Other agents that have been used in the treatment of metastatic retinoblastoma include Cytoxan alone or in combination with vincristine (474, 475, 488) and methotrexate alone (489) or in combination with actinomycin D and chlorambucil (490); these have been reported to result in transient responses in a number of patients with widespread metastatic disease.

Since long-term survival for less advanced stages of retinoblastoma using either enucleation or radiotherapy techniques is so good, it has been difficult to define a role for adjuvant chemotherapy. To date, there has been no prospectively randomized trial that has proved the value of adjuvant chemotherapy in reducing the mortality of localized retinoblastoma.

Wolff and colleagues (474) were unable to demonstrate that addition of adjuvant chemotherapy (vincristine/Cytoxan) to standard surgical enucleation significantly improved the survival rate for patients with Group V retinoblastoma. All relapses in this study occurred in patients who had involvement of the retinal pigment epithelium, choroid, or optic nerve distal to the lamina cribrosa in the enucleated specimen; the authors felt that chemotherapy should be recommended only for this group. Howarth and colleagues (491), in a nonrandomized study of adjuvant chemotherapy (vincristine/Cytoxan) in 32 retinoblastoma patients of all stages, reported an overall survival of 92 per cent; of particular significance in this study was the survival rate of 94 per cent for patients with extraretinal extension of tumor and with extensive choroidal involvement in comparison with the 78 per cent survival reported for historical controls (492). As a result of their study, these investigators recommended that adjuvant chemotherapy be considered for patients with: (1) multiple tumors involving more than 25 per cent of the retina (when radiotherapy is not being used); (2) Group IV and Group V non-enucleated tumors; (3) extensive tumor involvement of the choroid; or (4) extraocular disease.

CENTRAL NERVOUS SYSTEM TUMORS

Primary malignancies of the central nervous system (CNS) compose the largest group of solid tumors occurring in children, with an annual incidence of 22.2 per million white children and 20.2 per million black children in the United States (1). These tumors may be categorized by histologic features (Table 37–12) or by anatomic location (Fig. 37–10).

In one representative series (493), five major histologic types accounted for about 80 per cent of all pediatric brain tumors: astrocytoma (28 per cent), medulloblastoma (25 per cent), ependymal neoplasm (9 per cent), craniopharyngioma (9 per cent), and glioblastoma multiforme (9 per cent). Overall, the majority of pediatric brain tumors originate in the posterior fossa; however, the reverse is true for the first year of life (493, 494, 495). From 2 to 12 years of age, infratentorial tumors (mainly cerebellar astrocytomas, medulloblastomas, and brainstem gliomas) account for approximately 85 per cent of CNS tumors. After puberty, there is a sharp decline in the incidence of infratentorial tumors; the most common CNS malignancies seen during this period are cerebral astrocytoma and craniopharyngioma.

Clinical Manifestations

SIGNS AND SYMPTOMS

Because of the relative flexibility of the cranium and nonunion of the sutures, infants and young children are able to adapt their intracranial contents to large space-occupying lesions. The early signs and symptoms in these patients are generally nonspecific in nature and include malaise, failure to thrive, irritability, vomiting, ataxia, or clumsiness. Signs of increased pressure, including marked increase in head size and focal symptoms, are not noted until there is obstruction of the flow of cerebrospinal fluid (CSF).

In older children, whose sutures have fused, increased intracranial pressure is usually manifested by headache and vomiting; these symptoms may awaken the child at night or appear early in the moning and are not usually accompanied by nausea. The headache of increased intracranial pressure is commonly accentuated by stooping or straining. When symptoms or signs suggestive of a brain tumor are noted, a thorough neurologic examination will often elicit evidence of localizing neurologic signs.

Table 37–12. HISTOLOGIC CLASSIFICATION OF BRAIN TUMORS

Tissue of Origin	Tumor
Neuroglia	Astrocytoma
	Glioblastoma multiforme
	Oligodendroglioma
	Ependymoma
Neuronal	Medulloblastoma
	Primitive neuroectodermal tumor (neuroblastoma)
Mesodermal	Meningioma
	Sarcoma
Cranial nerves and nerve roots	Schwannoma
	Neurofibroma/Neurofibrosarcoma
Choroid plexus	Choroid plexus papilloma
Pineal region	Germ cell tumors
	Pineocytoma/Pineoblastoma
	Glial tumors
Blood vessel	Hemangioblastoma
Microglia	Microgliomatosis (reticulum cell sarcoma)
Miscellaneous	Craniopharyngioma
	Lipoma

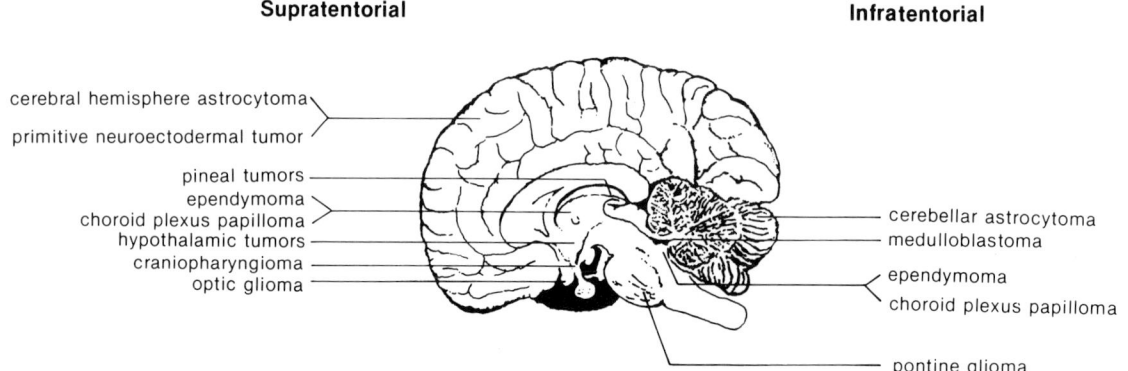

Figure 37–10. Anatomic distribution of brain tumors in children.

EVALUATION

Accurate localization of the site and extent of an intracranial lesion is best accomplished through the use of computed tomography (CT). Procedures that may supplement the CT scan are angiography, radionuclide scanning, and nuclear magnetic resonance (NMR). NMR, which uses high frequency radiowaves rather than ionizing radiation, may soon replace CT scan as the diagnostic procedure of choice in evaluation of brain tumors. Its major advantages over CT include (1) greater sensitivity to blood flow, edema, hemorrhage and myelination; (2) more thorough depiction of tumor extent; (3) better depiction of brainstem and posterior fossa anatomy; and (4) superior delineation of associated abnormalities such as hydrocephalus. Disadvantages of NMR include longer data acquisition times as well as failure to detect foci of tumor calcification and to demonstrate the severity of bone destruction (496, 497, 497a).

Tumor markers that have proved to be of value in evaluating CNS tumors include alpha-fetoprotein (AFP), human chorionic gonadotropin (hCG), and certain polyamines (spermine, spermidine, putrescine) (497b,c). Although these markers are most often measured in the CSF, in some instances they are in the serum in high concentrations. AFP and hCG are most useful in assessment and follow-up of germ cell tumors, whereas the polyamines find their greatest application in medulloblastoma and other primitive neuroectodermal tumors.

As will be discussed below, certain brain tumors have a propensity to seed early and diffusely via CSF pathways. Myelography and cytologic examination of CSF may be helpful in staging and follow-up of such patients (497b,d).

ROUTES OF METASTASIS

The major mode of spread of brain tumors is via infiltration into adjacent brain parenchyma, which lacks limiting membranes and therefore offers little impedance to cellular migration from an adjoining malignancy. Infiltrative cells generally appear in advance of histologically apparent neovascularization and have a high growth fraction in comparison with cells more centrally located in the main tumor mass (495).

Brain tumors may also shed cells into the cerebrospinal fluid (CSF), and these may implant anywhere within the subarachnoid space. Such behavior is most common with medulloblastomas, ependymal tumors, and pineal tumors. The risk of dissemination is particularly high for undifferentiated variants (desmoplastic medulloblastoma, ependymoblastoma, pineoblastoma) and for tumors growing near the meningeal space (498).

Compared with spread by direct infiltration and CSF seeding, systemic metastasis of brain tumors via vascular or lymphatic channels is a relatively uncommon event; the overall incidence of extracranial metastasis associated with childhood brain tumors is only 2.3 per cent (499). There are no lymphatic vessels in the CNS, and the thin-walled blood vessels are easily compressed by enlarging brain tumors, which flatten and effectively obliterate their lumens instead of invading them. Thus, tumor cells escape into the systemic circulation most commonly when vessels are transected in the course of surgery or when a shunt permits direct access of CSF into vascular channels or the peritoneal cavity.

Prognosis

Published reports vary considerably with regard to survival data for childhood brain tumors. These discrepancies no doubt relate to differences in the abilities of neurosurgeons and radiotherapists, as well as differences in the impact of various treatment modalities. Furthermore, the biasing effects of referral patterns, small sample size, and the tendency of some authors to report only those patients who survived surgery and radiotherapy compound the difficulty of obtaining a true picture of the current state of the art. The survival data of the Surveillance, Epidemiology, End Result (SEER) registries (495), shown in Fig. 37–11, probably represent the most comprehensive picture of the current treatment results for childhood brain tumors in the United States.

Treatment

GENERAL PRINCIPLES

Surgery. The invasive nature of many CNS malignancies, and the fact that the surrounding normal brain cannot be resected without producing significant deficit, clearly limit the effectiveness of surgery. In general, the role of surgery is threefold: (1) relief of pressure; (2) establishment of diagnosis; and (3) debulking.

Radiotherapy. Decisions regarding dosimetry and field of radiation are based upon the location, histology, and volume of the tumor as well as the tolerance of the various regions of the CNS for radiotherapy. The treatment port may be limited to the tumor bed for lesions that do not widely infiltrate surrounding parenchyma (e.g., craniopharyngioma), but much larger volumes of the brain must be irradiated when a highly infiltrative malignancy (e.g., glioblastoma multiforme) is to be treated. When the tumor is known to spread via the CSF, the entire neuraxis must be included in the treatment plan.

Short-term effects of cranial radiotherapy are seen 4 to 6 weeks following treatment; these include fever, somnolence, and anorexia, which usu-

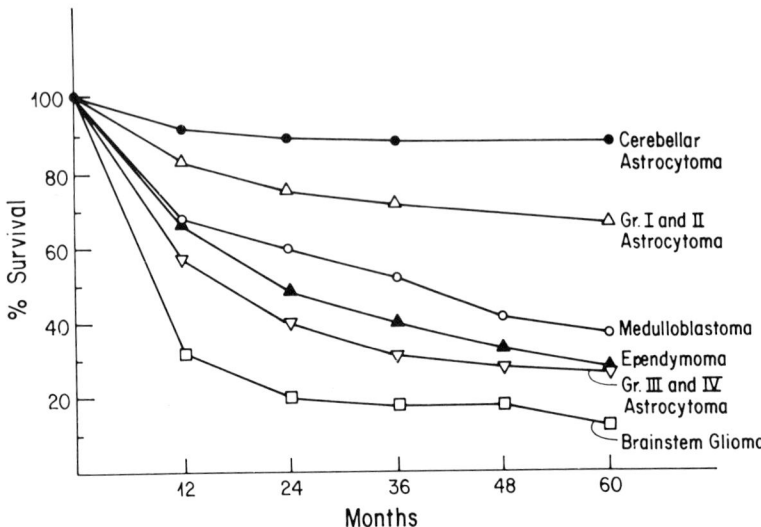

Figure 37–11. Survival data for brain tumors based on life tables from the SEER registries. (From Cohen, M. E., and Duffner, P. K.: Brain Tumors in Children: Principles of Diagnosis and Treatment. New York, Raven Press, 1984.)

ally last from 1 to 2 weeks. When total neuraxis radiotherapy is employed, effects on hematopoietic elements, bone growth, and soft tissues may further complicate the patient's course. However, it is the long-term cumulative effect on the cerebral vasculature that is the major dose-limiting factor. Small vessel adventitial fibrosis, arteriosclerotic changes, and occlusive disease begin to appear 1 to 3 years following radiotherapy and may lead to necrosis of brain, transverse myelopathy, impaired spinal cord growth, endocrine hypofunction (most commonly, growth hormone hyposecretion), and defects in cognitive and neuropsychological development. Recent reviews (500–503) report that at least 70 to 80 per cent of long-term survivors of childhood brain tumors have normal or near-normal global function; however, many of these individuals also can be shown to have deficits in intellectual or emotional capabilities when carefully tested for these parameters. Such deficits are more common and more severe in children who were below the age of 5 years at the time of treatment. For the child less than 2 years of age, the consequences of radiotherapy are so severe that serious consideration should be given to primary chemotherapy (503a).

Chemotherapy. As yet, chemotherapy has not established an impact on the treatment of CNS tumors that is comparable to its role in the management of other childhood malignancies. There are several reasons for this. In the first place, chemotherapy has traditionally been reserved as a modality of last resort for patients whose tumors have become refractory to surgery and radiotherapy; this psychologic barrier has impeded the integration of chemotherapy into the primary therapeutic strategy. More formidable obstacles to the development of successful chemotherapeutic regimens have been the blood-brain barrier (504–508), which interferes with delivery of drugs into CNS tumors, and the variable kinetics (509, 510) and heterogeneous sensitivities of brain tumor cells (511–513), which prevent maximal cytoreduction.

The blood-brain barrier, which excludes from the CNS all water-soluble (polar) molecules with a molecular weight of over 200, is a consequence of the unique structure of the cerebral vasculature. Unlike the endothelial cells of systemic capillaries, those of the CNS are characterized by tight intercellular junctions and a relative paucity of membrane fenestrations and cytoplasmic vesicles, resulting in a continuous cellular layer between blood and brain. The glial sheath that surrounds cerebral capillaries forms a further obstacle to molecular transport. Thus, under normal conditions, the drugs most likely to penetrate the CNS are those that have one or more of the following features: lipid solubility, low molecular weight, weak ionization in plasma, and poor binding to plasma proteins (507, 508).

The integrity of the blood-brain barrier is often compromised within the parenchyma of a brain tumor. As a result, substances such as contrast-enhancing agents, scanning radionuclides, and large water-soluble molecules may diffuse into portions of the neoplasm (504–508). However, the permeability of the *blood-tumor barrier* is highly variable for different brain tumors as well as within different regions of a given tumor. Permeability does not necessarily correlate with tumor histology or size, but does reflect regional variations in vascularity (507a,b; 508). Thus, the neovascularized central zone of a tumor may develop capillaries with open intercellular junctions, increased numbers of pinocytic vesicles, and fenestrated endothelium whose permeability characteristics are similar to those of systemic capillaries. In contrast, the rapidly proliferating peripheral margin of the tumor, which is capable of considerable infiltration into normal brain prior to the development of new vessels, receives its blood supply from the adjacent parenchyma with an intact blood-brain barrier; drug delivery to this critical brain adjacent tumor (BAT) is therefore poor and is further impeded by extracellular edema, which increases the distance between the cerebral capillaries and the tumor cells.

Clinically, the most effective agents for treatment of brain tumors have been the lipid-soluble nitrosoureas (BCNU, CCNU). Unfortunately, these agents are cell-cycle–nonspecific, and therefore they are more likely to be effective against the resting (G_0) cells in the relatively avascular center of the tumor than against the actively proliferating infiltrating cells of the BAT. None of the cell-cycle–specific drugs (except for vincristine and possibly epipodophyllotoxin) are lipophilic; the antimetabolites are water-soluble and vary in molecular weight from approximately 76 (hydroxyurea) to 454 (methotrexate). In order to achieve maximal effectiveness, many current chemotherapeutic regimens combine lipid-soluble drugs with various cell-cycle–specific agents.

New strategies for treatment of brain tumors are directed toward increasing the intracerebral concentration of drug sufficiently to kill all malignant cells prior to the development of resistance. Techniques to accomplish this objective include use of very high-dose BCNU followed by autologous bone marrow transplantation (513a,b); intra-arterial infusion of chemotherapy (514, 515); and osmotic disruption of the blood-brain barrier by infusion of hypertonic solutions (e.g., mannitol) (516–518). Direct instillation of drugs into the CSF by lumbar puncture or via an Ommaya reservoir is effective for treatment of cells circulating in the CSF or lodged within the meninges, but has proved less effective in controlling mass lesions within the CNS. This is probably because intrathecal medications can penetrate only the first few millimeters of brain parenchyma deep to the CSF pathway (518a).

Treatment of Specific CNS Tumors

CEREBRAL ASTROCYTOMA

Astrocytomas may arise anywhere in the neuraxis; in childhood they are found most commonly in the brainstem and cerebellum, but they may arise in the cerebral hemispheres, optic chiasma, or hypothalamus as well. They vary in degree of anaplasia from the benign low-grade (Grade I) astrocytoma to the highly malignant glioblastoma multiforme (Grade IV astrocytoma). Prognosis is clearly correlated with degree of anaplasia (Fig. 37–11).

In childhood, cerebral hemisphere astrocytomas tend to have a poorer prognosis than do the more benign lesions arising in the cerebellum. The signs and symptoms accompanying hemispheric supratentorial astrocytomas relate to the area of cortical involvement. Headache, vomiting, and seizures are the most common presenting symptoms, while focal motor deficits, visual field abnormalities, and papilledema are the most common physical signs (495).

Surgery. Surgery is the initial mode of therapy for cerebral astrocytoma, not only to provide tissue or histologic grading but also to debulk as much of the tumor as possible. Since astrocytomas in children frequently have a large cystic component, surgical drainage often provides relief of increased intracranial pressure. Complete removal is rarely accomplished with high-grade gliomas, because of their infiltrative nature; complicating the problem is the fact that 20 to 25 per cent of these tumors may spread to the contralateral hemisphere via the corpus callosum (519).

Radiotherapy—Grade I and Grade II Astrocytomas. Radiotherapy does not improve the already excellent survival rate achieved with *completely resected* low-grade astrocytomas (520, 521). Although to date there is no properly conrolled study documenting the benefit of postoperative radiotherapy for patients with *partially resected* low-grade cerebral astrocytoma, several studies suggest that it can improve 5-year survival from 25 to 50 per cent, and 10-year survival from 10 to 25 per cent (520, 522, 523). The radiotherapy plan usually followed is to deliver 4000 to 4500 cGy to the involved hemisphere in children less than 3 years of age, and 4500 to 5000 cGy for children over 3 years of age; treatment is given over a 6- to 7-week period. When the radiotherapy field is plotted with the use of CT, a more limited radiation port confined to the primary tumor, with a margin of several centimeters of normal tissue, may be equally effective (524).

Radiotherapy—Grade III and Grade IV Astrocytomas. Because of the infiltrative nature of high-grade astrocytoma, all cases of this type should receive postoperative radiotherapy, even when the surgeon has apparently achieved complete removal. The radiotherapy field should include a large volume (the tumor plus a generous margin of at least 4 cm of normal surounding tissue). If contralateral involvement is present, whole brain irradiation is given in older children and adults; however, more limited ports may be appropriate in young children in whom rapid brain growth and myelination are still in progress. The dose for adults and older children is 5000 to 6000 cGy over 6 to 7 weeks; for children under 5 years of age, the dose is limited to 4500 cGy. Although this approach may produce remissions, the ultimate prognosis for these patients remains poor (524–526); half of these children die within 15 months of diagnosis and almost all within 5 years.

Chemotherapy. Chemotherapy of supratentorial astrocytomas has been carried out in only a limited number of cases, usually at the time of recurrence, after both surgery and radiotherapy have failed. Beneficial responses (usually temporary) have been reported in 13 to 60 per cent of patients following administration of nitrosoureas, nitrogen mustard, vincristine, procarbazine, methotrexate (intrathecally or systemically), and VM-26 when given alone or in various combinations including MOPP (527–531). High-dose methotrexate with citrovorum rescue has also produced clinical responses in patients with astrocytoma (531a).

Studies of the use of adjuvant chemotherapy in high-grade astrocytomas have generally failed to demonstrate significant improvement in survival (532–536). In these studies, radiotherapy alone was more effective than chemotherapy alone, and the addition of adjuvant chemotherapy to radiotherapy produced only a modest prolongation of median survival. Chemotherapy was most effective in prolonging survival time when used after relapse had occurred following radiotherapy. In a recent study (537), however, patients who received adjuvant chemotherapy with vincristine/prednisone/CCNU had a significantly prolonged disease-free survival in comparison with those treated with radiotherapy alone. At 30 months, the disease-free survival was 43.8 per cent for the chemotherapy arm and 21.3 per cent for the radiation therapy arm.

OPTIC GLIOMA

Gliomas of the anterior visual pathway are usually low-grade astrocytomas; these may arise from the optic nerve, the optic chiasm, or the optic tract. Approximately 30 to 55 per cent are associated with neurofibromatosis.

The most common symptom is decreased visual acuity. A presumptive diagnosis is based on finding enlargement of an optic foramen, evidence of a suprasellar space-occupying lesion, and/or enlargement of the optic nerve on CT scan. Lesions of the posterior chiasm may involve the hypothalamus and produce signs of hypothalamic dysfunction, including diabetes insipidus or "diencephalic syndrome." These lesions appear to have a different histopathology from those of the anterior chiasm or those restricted to the optic nerve (538).

Surgery. When the tumor is localized to an optic nerve and there is a clear margin between tumor and the optic chiasm, surgical resection should achieve excellent control, but at the cost of unilateral blindness. No further therapy is required when complete resection has been achieved (529, 539). Radiotherapy may be an effective alternate therapy for such patients in an effort to preserve vision; however, the patient must be monitored closely.

For lesions involving the chiasm, excision is usually not feasible. Consequently, surgery is limited to biopsy or partial resection. A shunt may be required for posterior chiasmal lesions that produce ventricular obstruction.

Radiotherapy. The role of radiotherapy for optic gliomas is incompletely defined, since the majority are slow growing and prolonged survival is achieved even following incomplete removal. However, in the situation of an incompletely resected lesion of the optic nerve or of a chiasmal lesion in which resection is not possible, high-dose radiation therapy may achieve arrest of visual loss, restoration of vision, decrease in proptosis, and reduction in tumor mass (529, 538, 540).

HYPOTHALAMIC ASTROCYTOMA

Hypothalamic tumors of early infancy often present with the "diencephalic syndrome," which is characterized clinically by marked emaciation, euphoria, general hyperactivity, and alert appearance; approximately 50 per cent of patients also exhibit nystagmus. Most cases of diencephalic syndrome have been due to low-grade astrocytomas arising from the anterior hypothalamus or involvement of this region by optic nerve tumors. In late childhood, tumors in the hypothalamic region present with hyperphagia and obesity, often associated with short stature, hypogonadism, and diabetes insipidus.

Because of the tumor locations, surgery has been of little value in treatment, and the prognosis has generally been considered to be poor. However, radiotherapy has proved to be effective for some of these tumors (529, 541), with 5-year survival rates of 83 per cent being reported for intrinsic hypothalamic tumors when "radical" radiotherapy is used (529).

CEREBELLAR ASTROCYTOMA

This tumor may arise in the midline (vermis) or within the cerebellar hemispheres. The gross appearance may be either solid or cystic in nature; the cystic variant often harbors a solid mural nodule. Cerebellar astrocytoma is the intracranial tumor with the most favorable outlook in childhood (Fig. 37–11), mainly because of the high proportion of cases with slow-growing, well-circumscribed cystic lesions.

Surgery. Complete resection of cystic cerebellar astrocytoma is possible in 50 to 75 per cent of cases. There is a 10- to 20-year survival rate of greater than 90 per cent in this group (542, 543), and therefore further therapy does not appear to be indicated. However, when the cerebellar astrocytoma is a diffuse low-grade lesion, it may be infiltrative and can rarely be resected, resulting in a much higher recurrence rate (542, 543).

Radiotherapy. Radiotherapy is not necessary for completely resected cystic cerebellar astrocytomas (495, 542, 543). However, for partially resected cystic, and for diffuse, astrocytomas, radiotherapy appears to improve the prognosis (495, 523). The entire posterior fossa should be included in the port, and radiotherapy doses similar to those used for cerebral astrocytoma are used. The 5-year survival rate for patients treated with surgery alone is 30 to 50 per cent; with postoperative radiotherapy this rate improves to greater than 80 per cent.

Like other childhood posterior fossa tumors, the rare malignant cerebellar astrocytoma can involve supratentorial areas of the brain as well as cervical subarachnoid spaces by direct extension; seeding via CSF spread may then occur. Such tumors should be treated by total neuraxis radiotherapy (544).

BRAINSTEM GLIOMA

Brainstem gliomas typically present with the clinical triad of *long-tract signs, multiple cranial nerve palsies,* and *cerebellar ataxia.* Approximately two thirds of these lesions are low-grade astrocytomas, and one third are high-grade astrocytomas and glioblastomas. Different grades of malignancy are sometimes present within a single tumor. Although CT scan accurately indicates the presence of a brainstem tumor, it cannot be relied upon to characterize tumor histology or to reliably differentiate a brainstem glioma from brainstem encephalitis or hemorrhage (545).

Brain-stem tumors may occur anywhere in the region extending from the aqueduct of Sylvius to the fourth ventricle. Epstein and McCleary (545a) have subclassified them into three groups: *focal* (circumscribed mass <2 cm in diameter and without associated edema), *diffuse* (>2 cm and associated with a large area of apparent edema on CT scan), and *cervicomedullary* (located at the junction of the medulla and the spinal cord). In their report, virtually all focal and cervicomedullary tumors were of Grade II histology, whereas all of the diffuse tumors were of a higher degree of malignancy (Grade III–IV).

Although brainstem glioma is not generally recognized as a tumor that manifests clinical signs of widespread CNS dissemination, tumors with very anaplastic histology may exhibit a propensity for diffuse spread via the CSF. Packer and colleagues (546) found 5 of 15 brainstem glioma patients to have developed symptoms of meningeal spread. These authors advocate that the CSF be examined for cells, sugar, and protein prior to therapy and, if abnormalities are encountered, that a myelogram be performed.

Surgery. Because of the difficulties in taking biopsies of lesions in the brainstem, many patients have been treated on the basis of physical and neuroradiologic findings without confirmation of diagnosis by tissue examination. However, with the use of corticosteroids and the operating microscope, some authors (545) now feel that a biopsy can be performed with acceptable morbidity and essentially no operative mortality. Biopsy of the brainstem is useful for ruling out brainstem encephalitis or demyelinating disease, as well as for clarifying tumor histology.

Surgery does not usually play a major therapeutic role in brain-stem glioma. However, surgical shunting is necessary when significant obstruction to CSF flow has produced hydrocephalus. Some patients with relatively benign (Grade I–II) cervicomedullary or focal tumors may benefit from surgical excision (545a); decompression of an exophytic lesion or drainage of a surgically significant cyst can also produce neurologic improvement and contribute to prolongation of survival (545, 547).

Radiotherapy. Radiotherapy is the main modality of treatment for brainstem glioma. The maximum dose using conventional daily fractionation is 5000 to 6000 cGy over 6 to 7 weeks (548, 549). CT scanning is useful in accurate treatment planning, as it may show extension into the cerebellar peduncles and hypothalamus (550); for most patients, limited radiation fields designed to cover the CT scan definition of tumor with an appropriate margin are adequate (550a). Craniospinal irradiation and possibly adjuvant chemotherapy should be administered to patients with abnormal CSF cytologic or myelographic findings (546). Care must be taken to avoid brainstem edema during radiotherapy, particularly in patients who do not have shunts in place. High-dose steroids may be useful in this regard.

Overall 5-year survival rates generally range from 5 to 20 per cent but are as high as 30 to 45 per cent in some centers (545, 549, 550) for patients who have survived long enough to complete radiotherapy. Tumor location has an influence on survival; patients with tumors of the midbrain, thalamus, and third ventricle area have a significantly better 5-year survival than do those whose tumors are in the pons or medulla (550a).

Chemotherapy. Chemotherapy trials have mainly consisted of preliminary reports with small numbers of patients and little long-term follow-up information. Shapiro (511) obtained a 30 per cent response rate with BCNU or CCNU and also found that 5 of 6 patients responded to intrathecal methotrexate. Djerassi obtained an occasional favorable response with high-dose methotrexate followed by citrovorum rescue (551).

While the above studies have shown some benefits for chemotherapy in producing objective responses in patients whose disease recurred after radiotherapy, to date no study has demonstrated that adjuvant chemotherapy can improve the long-term survival rate.

MEDULLOBLASTOMA

Medulloblastoma accounts for 40 per cent of posterior fossa tumors and 53 per cent of all tumors in the cerebellum. The tumor arises from the neuroepithelial roof of the fourth ventricle and can extend into the fourth ventricle, cerebellar vermis, and cerebellar hemispheres. It may also spread into the subarachnoid space, from which it may disseminate widely via the CSF to the cerebral hemispheres and spinal cord. Systemic metastases to lymph nodes, bone, and bone marrow may also develop.

The extent of disease should be evaluated with pre- and postoperative CT scan, CSF cytology, bone marrow aspiration, and possibly myelography. Measurement of CSF polyamines (spermine, spermidine, putrescine) has proved to be a sensitive marker of tumor activity and of response to therapy (497b,c). Harisiadis and Chang (552) have defined a "T" and "M" staging system for medulloblastoma based on the extent of the primary tumor and the degree of spread within the CSF (Table 37-13). The 5-year survival rate for their patients progressively declined from 75 per cent for T_1 to 0 per cent for T_4 disease; there was also a dramatic decline in prognosis when gross nodular seeding of the CSF was present (M_2–M_3).

Prognosis varies also with the age of the patient. Children under 5 years of age tend to have relatively advanced disease and a poor prognosis, whereas children over 11 years of age tend to have more limited disease and a relatively good prognosis (553).

Surgery. Surgical cure by complete resection is often precluded by the location and infiltrative nature of medulloblastoma; the primary role of the surgeon in such cases is to relieve increased intracranial pressure and to debulk the tumor within the limits of acceptable neurologic dysfunction. However, complete macroscopic excision is possible in 38 to 47 per cent of patients (554, 555). Several recent studies (556, 557) have shown improved survival in patients who had radical excision of tumor.

Radiotherapy. Because of the propensity of this tumor to spread along CSF pathways, complete neuraxis radiotherapy is mandatory. At present, there is no agreement on the optimal dose. The usual dose given to older children is 4000 cGy to the cranium, with a boost of 1000 to 1500 cGy to the posterior fossa over 6 to 7 weeks, and 3500 cGy to the spinal cord over 5 to 6 weeks. For children under 3 years of age, the total dose to the posterior fossa is usually limited to 4000 to 4500 cGy, with 3000 cGy to the cord. Survival statistics for patients treated in this fashion show a 5-year survival rate of 30 to 40 per cent and a 10-year survival rate of 20 to 25 per cent (495, 522, 558–561).

The major cause of treatment failure is inability to control tumor in the posterior fossa; 70 to 80 per cent of first recurrences are in this region (495, 529, 562). The cribriform plate and adjoining frontal lobes may be the site of recurrence in as many as 15 per cent of patients (562), possibly reflecting inadequate radiotherapy dosage to this area. In addition, approximately 5 to 12 per cent of patients develop recurrences outside the CNS (562, 563).

Recent therapeutic approaches designed to improve tumor control by use of radical surgery, megavoltage radiotherapy, and modification of the radiotherapy field have reported 5-year survival rates in the range of 50 to 60 per cent (529, 556, 562, 563). It must be recognized that these studies reflect patients who survived long enough to complete surgery and radiotherapy. Even higher survival rates (77 to 84 per cent) have been reported for small subsets of patients treated with complete surgical resection and/or posterior fossa doses in excess of 5200 rad (529, 549, 556, 563). Careful design of the cribriform plate area field may also augment survival (562). The cost of these aggressive measures in terms of serious late sequelae, particularly in young children, is unknown at present.

Chemotherapy. Initial efforts at chemotherapy were instituted in patients with recurrent disease; in this setting, a number of drugs have proved capable of producing significant regression of recurrent or metastatic medulloblastoma. Among

Table 37-13. OPERATIVE STAGING SYSTEM FOR CEREBELLAR MEDULLOBLASTOMA*

T_1	Tumor less than 3 cm in diameter, and limited to the classic midline position in the vermis, the roof of the fourth ventricle, and less frequently to the cerebellar hemispheres.
T_2	Tumor 3 cm or greater in diameter, further invading one adjacent structure or partially filling the fourth ventricle.
T_3	(a) Tumor further invading two adjacent structures or completely filling the fourth ventricle, with extension into the aqueduct of Sylvius, foramen of Magendie, or foramen of Luschka, thus producing marked internal hydrocephalus.
	(b) Tumor arising from the floor of the fourth ventricle or brainstem and filling the fourth ventricle.
T_4	Tumor further spreading through the aqueduct of Sylvius to involve the third ventricle or midbrain, or tumor extending to the upper cervical cord.
M_0	No evidence of gross subarachnoid or hematogenous metastasis.
M_1	Microscopic tumor cells found in cerebrospinal fluid.
M_2	Gross nodular seeding demonstrated in the cerebellar, cerebral subarachnoid space, or in the third or lateral ventricles.
M_3	Gross nodular seeding in spinal subarachnoid space.
M_4	Metastasis outside the cerebrospinal axis.

*Based on data from reference 552.

these agents are vincristine, VM-26, procarbazine, methotrexate, cis-platinum, and cyclophosphamide. These agents have been shown to reduce bulky disease in the posterior fossa and spinal subarachnoid space, but they rarely produce permanent disease control. They do appear to be more effective in permanently eradicating systemic metastases. Thus, their main use has been to prolong life and improve the neurologic dysfunction associated with recurrence.

In planning chemotherapy, it is important to bear in mind that patients who have received spinal cord irradiation have a decreased bone marrow reserve and, therefore, an increased risk of myelosuppression. The use of chemotherapy in patients who have received cranial irradiation may also lead to dementia or leukoencephalopathy, particularly when methotrexate is one of the agents used (548).

In the past decade, several large multicenter trials have been in progress to evaluate the use of adjuvant chemotherapy in patients with primary medulloblastoma. Among these are studies by the Children's Cancer Study Group (CCSG), using vincristine/CCNU/prednisone (554), and the International Society of Pediatric Oncology (SIOP) (529, 555, 564), using vincristine/CCNU. In neither of these studies was there a demonstrable benefit of chemotherapy when the overall patient group was analyzed; however, patients with advanced (T_3–T_4) tumors or otherwise poor prognostic indicators (incomplete resection, brainstem involvement, age <2 years) had a significant benefit from chemotherapy in terms of event-free survival.

Currently, CCSG and the Pediatric Oncology Group (POG) are separating medulloblastoma patients into good- and poor-risk groups based on "T" and "M" staging. Good-risk patients (T_1–T_2, M_0) are considered to have at least a 75 per cent 5-year disease-free survival. These patients will be treated with radiotherapy alone. All will receive 5000 cGy to the posterior fossa, but the group will be randomized between conventional dosage (3600 cGy) and lower dosage (2400 cGy) to the craniospinal axis. For poor-risk patients (T_3–T_4, M_1–M_3), the large collaborative groups are using combinations of chemotherapy and radiotherapy. CCSG is currently planning a two-arm randomized study comparing vincristine/prednisone/CCNU with a new multiple-drug regimen combining 8 drugs in 1 day ("8 in 1"), to be administered both prior and subsequent to radiotherapy (565). POG is comparing radiotherapy alone versus radiotherapy plus the MOPP (nitrogen mustard, vincristine, prednisone, procarbazine) regimen (527). SIOP is exploring a sandwich chemotherapy protocol that combines preradiation high-dose intravenous methotrexate, procarbazine, and vincristine with postradiation CCNU and vincristine (566).

PRIMITIVE NEUROECTODERMAL TUMORS (PNET)

PNET were first described by Hart and Earle (567) in 1973 as a group of tumors found in the cerebrum and characterized histologically by a high proportion of undifferentiated small dark cells with a high mitotic index. It is often difficult to distinguish PNET histologically from other primitive CNS tumors such as cerebellar medulloblastoma, cerebral neuroblastoma, ependymoblastoma, and pineal parenchymal tumors. While some authors (568) feel that cerebral neuroblastoma and PNET are essentially the same tumor, others (495) differentiate between them on the basis of the presence of mesenchymal elements in PNET and the more benign biologic behavior of cerebral neuroblastoma.

PNET usually occur in children and young adults ranging from birth to 24 years of age; their location is usually supratentorial, with the frontoparietal region being the most common location (569). The tumors have a tendency to spread along CSF pathways; distant metastases to lungs, lymph nodes, pericardium, diaphragm, and liver have also been reported (569).

Therapy. Gross total surgical excision is desirable for these tumors. Because of their tendency to spread along CSF pathways, craniospinal irradiation has been advocated by most authors (569, 570); however, others recommend only local irradiation unless CSF cytology or myelogram is abnormal (571).

Reports on the use of chemotherapy in this tumor have been sporadic, and results have been generally unsuccessful (569). The histologic and biologic similarities between supratentorial neuroectodermal tumors and medulloblastoma suggest that similar treatment protocols may be pursued for both these tumor types.

EPENDYMOMA

Ependymomas arise from cells lining the ventricular system and central spinal cord. They can occur in supratentorial or infratentorial locations; the most common location in children is in the floor of the fourth ventricle. The median age at diagnosis is 5 years, with a peak incidence during the first year.

Signs and symptoms are dependent upon location. Tumors arising in the posterior fossa will mimic the symptoms of medulloblastoma and present with ataxia, meningism, headache, and nausea and vomiting; those arising supratentorially will more frequently produce lethargy or focal signs.

The risk of CSF seeding depends upon the location and histologic grading of the primary tumor: (1) low-grade supratentorial ependymomas rarely seed; (2) malignant supratentorial ependymomas (ependymoblastomas) seed more commonly (approximately 12 per cent), but usually to supratentorial locations; (3) infratentorial ependymomas quite commonly seed to intraspinal locations—this may occur in 50 per cent or more of the high-grade ependymoblastomas, but also in 15 per cent of low-grade infratentorial ependymomas (572, 573, 574).

Surgery. The primary treatment of ependymoma is a judicious resection of as much tumor as possible. However, total removal is rarely accomplished, especially with tumors that lie in close continuity with vital structures of the fourth ventricle; attempted total resection can have a morbidity and mortality rate as high as 20 to 30 per cent.

Radiotherapy. Postoperative radiotherapy appears to improve the chances for survival. However, the nature of the radiotherapy field is still a matter of conjecture. Based on the relative propensity of neuraxis seeding of various sites and histologic classifications (discussed above), it would appear that local large-volume radiotherapy is sufficient for low-grade supratentorial ependymomas. On the other hand, the field should encompass the whole brain (with a boost to the tumor site) or the entire neuraxis for high-grade supratentorial ependymomas, and the posterior fossa and spine or entire neuraxis for all infratentorial ependymomas (572, 573–575).

Overall prognosis for low-grade ependymoma is 70 per cent survival at 5 years and 50 to 70 per cent survival at 10 years. The 5-year survival falls to 10 to 20 per cent for high-grade ependymoblastomas (572–575).

Chemotherapy. Single agents that have produced tumor regression in recurrent ependymomas include BCNU, CCNU, and VM-26, and there have also been responses to a combination chemotherapy protocol using vincristine, CCNU, and intrathecal methotrexate and also to methotrexate given via Ommaya reservoir (576). Intrathecal methotrexate may also be useful in patients with extensive meningeal disease. Studies are currently in progress to test the adjuvant use of vincristine, CCNU, and prednisone in combination for preventing recurrence.

OLIGODENDROGLIOMA

In adults, the vast majority of oligodendrogliomas arise in the cerebral hemispheres; however, posterior fossa origin is relatively more common in childhood (576a). Posterior fossa lesions and high-grade tumors may spread along CSF pathways in a fulminant manner similar to that of medulloblastoma or may leave implants that lie dormant within the meninges for years (576b).

Surgery. The therapy of choice for this tumor is total resection. Radical tumor removal has been shown to prolong survival in several series and is advocated when tumor location permits (577, 578). If total resection is not possible, subtotal removal with decompression can produce prolonged survival.

Radiotherapy. Radiotherapy does not appear to be necessary for cerebral hemisphere lesions if complete removal has been achieved. For patients who have undergone incomplete resection, local postoperative radiotherapy (5000 to 5500 cGy over 6 to 7 weeks) may prolong survival, but this has not been demonstrated as yet in a prospective randomized study. Both local and presymptomatic craniospinal irradiation may be indicated for children with high-grade lesions or with posterior fossa tumors (576a).

Oligodendroglioma is generally a slow-growing lesion, and consequently long-term survival with or without radiotherapy occurs in a large percentage of cases—70 per cent survival at 5 years and 58 per cent at 10 years in children (579).

Chemotherapy. Responses to the combination of CCNU, vincristine, and procarbazine have been reported (580).

CHOROID PLEXUS PAPILLOMA

This tumor occurs wherever choroid plexus is located. Approximately 80 per cent of childhood cases occur in the lateral ventricles, with 16 per cent in the fourth ventricle and 4 per cent in the third ventricle (581). The most striking clinical manifestation is a progressive hydrocephalus; the diagnosis may be made by CT scan, which shows an intraventricular mass of high density that markedly enhances with contrast (495).

The majority of these tumors (approximately 83 per cent) are benign and can be treated successfully with surgical excision. However, because of the tumor's vascularity, operative mortality remains high. If total removal is accomplished, late recurrences are unusual. Unfortunately, many patients suffer significant sequelae, including mental retardation, epilepsy, pyramidal tract dysfunction, and sensory disturbances following surgery. Radiotherapy is reserved for cases that develop evidence of recurrence or in the rare malignant form of choroid plexus papilloma.

PINEAL TUMORS

Four major tumor types occur in the pineal region: (1) pineoblastoma/pineocytoma; (2) germ cell tumors; (3) benign cysts; and (4) glial tumors. Pineoblastoma and pineocytoma are of neural origin, deriving from parenchymal pineal cells. Germ cell tumors are presumably derived from germ cell rests that become sequestered in midline intracranial structures during embryonic life; the histologic spectrum encountered here is identical to that seen in germ cell tumors arising in other sites. Miscellaneous tumors, usually arising from glial elements in the pineal region or in the posterior third ventricle, are also encountered. Pineal tumors arising in young males are likely to be of germ cell origin, whereas those arising in females more often derive from pineal parenchyma (582).

Pineal tumors can give rise to the symptoms of increased intracranial pressure as well as produce precocious puberty, hypogonadism, diabetes insipidus, and anterior pituitary insufficiency. Parinaud's syndrome (paralysis of conjugate upward gaze, absent pupillary reaction to light, and retraction nystagmus) is also characteristic of tumors in this location, particularly germinomas and teratomas (582). Ectopic pinealomas may be located in the area of the hypothalamus; these tumors often produce a characteristic triad of diabetes insipidus, bitemporal hemianopsia, and hypopituitarism (583).

In common with germ cell tumors at other locations, germ cell tumors of the pineal region produce biochemical markers (e.g., alpha fetoprotein and human chorionic gonadotropin) that are of diagnostic, prognostic, and therapeutic utility, particularly when simultaneous CSF and blood levels are compared (584). Neuroradiologic studies, when evaluated in conjunction with clinical features and biochemical markers, permit categorization of some pineal tumors without the need for invasive procedures; however, a firm diagnosis is not always possible in individual cases.

Although the incidence of clinical spinal cord metastasis is generally about 12 per cent (586), the overall frequency of tumor spread in the ventricles and in the cerebral and spinal subarachnoid space is much higher; it may reach 50 to 60 per cent for germinomas and 30 to 50 per cent for pineal parenchymal tumors (586).

Management. Over the past several decades, the approach to pineal area tumors has been to employ a therapeutic trial of low-dose (2000 to 3000 cGy) radiotherapy as the primary mode of treatment (usually without prior biopsy), reserving surgery for relief of hydrocephalus and for management of tumors unresponsive to radiotherapy. The rationale for this approach has been (1) the high mortality (30 to 70 per cent) associated with conventional pineal area surgery (584–586); (2) the concern that surgical manipulation may contribute to neuraxial dissemination of tumor cells (586a, 586b); and (3) the relatively high proportion (50 to 60 per cent) of pineal tumors that are radiosensitive germinomas.

When empiric radiotherapy is employed, the overall 5-year survival for pineal tumors has been 50 to 75 per cent (586). However, determination of tumor histology, when feasible (see below), clearly has a considerable influence on prognosis. For example, verified germinomas have a 5-year survival rate approaching 80 per cent, whereas only 25 to 30 per cent of patients with anaplastic germ cell tumors treated with radiotherapy will survive for 5 years (586). Prognosis for some pineal tumors (e.g., germinomas, pineal parenchymal tumors, and teratomas with malignant elements) may be improved by administering total neuraxis radiotherapy.

In recent years, there has been a renewed interest in histologic diagnosis of pineal tumors, so that appropriate therapy can be planned from the start. This is entirely reasonable, as 20 to 25 per cent of pineal tumors are benign, encapsulated, or relatively radioresistant (582, 586). Advances in microsurgical techniques have reduced the operative mortality to less than 5 per cent (582, 587, 588). Thus, in selected cases in which the diagnosis is uncertain, the risks of surgery are acceptable. Likewise, it would also be appropriate to use a surgical approach with tumors that appear benign and well-demarcated based on their clinical presentation, neuroradiologic features, and biochemical markers. Mature teratomas, meningiomas, and epidermoid cysts, for example, may be cured by surgical excision alone. Germinomas, on the other hand, often completely resolve with low doses of radiation, and the prognosis is not improved by surgical resection (585, 586, 588a, 590). Consequently, a therapeutic trial of radiotherapy (2000 to 3000 cGy) followed by reassessment with CT scan may be the best approach for pineal tumors that have the neuroradiologic features of germinoma and do not express tumor markers (586, 586c). If the tumor does not respond, then relative radioresistance is implied and operative intervention is indicated.

In patients with gliomas, embryonal carcinomas, and pineal parenchymal tumors, attempts at excision often amount to only a debulking procedure that may be of therapeutic value as a preliminary step to radiotherapy and in planning chemotherapy (588a, 589). Choriocarcinoma can usually be diagnosed based on elevated hCG levels in blood and CSF; the surgical approach to these tumors is hazardous, as they are highly vascular and prone to uncontrollable bleeding following manipulation (584). Optimal therapy of choriocarcinoma, embryonal cell carcinoma, and endodermal sinus tumors remains uncertain; some reports (586c, 589) suggest that a combination of radiotherapy, chemotherapy, and surgical excision may offer the best chance of success.

Chemotherapy. Experience with chemotherapy for these tumors has been limited. It is conceivable that intracranial germ cell tumors may show a sensitivity to chemotherapy comparable to that seen in germ cell tumors arising outside the central nervous system. Excellent responses have been obtained in a small group of patients with pineal germ cell tumors treated with the combination of cis-platinum, bleomycin, and vinblastine (591, 592). However, particular care must be taken with the use of bleomycin, as these patients seem to be unduly susceptible to fatal pulmonary toxicity.

CRANIOPHARYNGIOMA

Craniopharyngioma is a benign congenital tumor that develops from the squamous cell remnants of Rathke's pouch. The tumor arises in the pituitary fossa and suprasellar area; by virtue of its relation to the optic chiasm, pituitary, and hypothalamic areas, it may produce visual, endocrine, or hypothalamic symptoms, as well as increased intracranial pressure. Skull films will often show calcification in the suprasellar region and/or erosion of the sella turcica; the demonstration on CT scan of a contrast-enhancing centrally located suprasellar mass containing calcification and cystic areas is virtually diagnostic.

Management. The surgical approach to craniopharyngioma is complicated by the hazardous location of the tumor as well as its tendency to adhere firmly to adjacent structures, including the hypothalamus and carotid artery. With meticulous preparation of the patient, including hormonal support and control of cerebral edema, as well as use of the operating microscopic, surgical mortality has been reduced to approximately 10 per cent (529, 593); however, many patients will suffer serious neurologic, visual, and endocrine complications. In general, only 35 to 45 per cent of children with craniopharyngioma are candidates for total excision (594), and only 75 per cent of those in whom apparent "total" excision has been achieved will actually experience long-term tumor-free recurrence (595).

Many reports have documented the radioresponsiveness of craniopharyngioma (529, 558, 595–598); indeed, the results of conservative surgery plus radiotherapy compare favorably with those achieved by radical "total" excision, with 60 to 94 per cent long-term survival and less disability. Furthermore, this approach is applicable to virtually all patients rather than to only a selected few. Particularly noteworthy are the results of the Royal Marsden Series (329) (85 per cent 5-year survival and 72 per cent 10-year survival) and of the Joint Center for Radiation Therapy (598) (all of 25 patients alive without documented recurrence up to 10 years) for patients treated primarily with conservative surgery and radiotherapy.

In summary, craniopharyngioma is a most unusual tumor. Although histologically benign, its management by surgical excision alone has often been unsatisfactory, but it has proved surprisingly responsive to radiotherapy. The goal of treatment should be complete surgical excision if this can be accomplished without producing serious sequelae; otherwise, the surgeon should withdraw at the stage of subtotal resection and refer the patient for radiotherapy.

SPINAL CORD TUMORS

Spinal cord tumors present with signs of progressive loss of cord function. Motor weakness, pain, and loss of sphincter control are among the symptoms that may be present, depending upon the site of the tumor and rapidity of tumor growth.

Intramedullary tumors arise within the cord itself. The same histologic spectrum is encounterd here as is seen in brain tumors, the common tumors being low-grade astrocytoma (which usually is located in the cervical or upper thoracic region) and ependymoma (which more commonly involves the lumbar region around the roots of the cauda equina). The goal of surgical treatment for these tumors is to decompress the cord, obtain a tissue diagnosis, and remove as much tumor as the tumor site and extent permit; this is usually more complete for ependymoma of the cauda equina than it is for other intramedullary tumors. The dose of radiation therapy should never exceed 4500 cGy over 4½ weeks, in order to avoid radiation myelitis. Ependymomas, which are generally histologically more malignant than astrocytomas, are usually more responsive to radiation therapy.

Extramedullary (but intradural) tumors include benign meningiomas and neuromas. "Drop" metastases from intracranial medulloblastomas, ependymomas, choroid plexus papillomas, and pineal tumors may implant with the subarachnoid space.

Extradural tumors of the vertebral bodies (Ewing's sarcoma and osteogenic sarcoma), bone cysts, and vertebral eosinophilic granuloma, as well as dumbbell neuroblastoma and metastatic rhabdomyosarcoma and non-Hodgkin's lymphoma, may also cause extradural compression of the cord.

Clearly, the development of effective treatment and better understanding of the principles of neuro-oncology represent the next important challenge of pediatric oncology. It is reasonable to hope that important clues will be derived from family studies such as recent analyses of the frequency of brain tumors in individuals with neurofibromatosis (599).

References

1. Young, J. L., Heise, H. W., et al.: Incidence, survival and mortality for children under 15 years of age. Am. Cancer Soc. Prof. Ed. Publ., 1978.
2. Doll, R.: An epidemiological perspective of the biology of cancer. Cancer Res. *38*:3573, 1978.
3. Jaffe, N.: Neuroblastoma: review of the literature and an examination of factors contributing to its enigmatic character. Cancer Treat. Rev. *3*:61, 1976.
4. Balaban, P., and Gilbert, F.: Chromosomes, genes, and cancer: anomaly of stage IVS neuroblastoma. Am. J. Hum. Genet. *34*:66a, 1982.
5. Balaban, P., and Gilbert, F.: Neuroblastoma IV-S: chromosome analysis. New Engl. J. Med. *309*:989, 1983.
6. Gilbert, F., Feder, M., et al.: Human neuroblastomas and abnormalities of chromosomes 1 and 17. Cancer Res. *44*:5444, 1984.
6a. Seeger, R. C., Brodeur, G. M., et al.: Association of multiple copies of the N-myc oncogene with rapid progression of neuroblastomas. New Engl. J. Med. *313*:1111, 1985.

7. Schwab, M., Alitalo, K., et al.: Amplified DNA with limited homology to myc cellular oncogene is shared by human neuroblastoma cell lines and a neuroblastoma tumor. Nature 305:245, 1983.
8. Triche, T. J., and Ross, W. E.: Glycogen-containing neuroblastoma with clinical and histopathologic features of Ewing's sarcoma. Cancer 41:1425, 1978.
9. Misugi, K., Misugi, M., et al.: Fine structural study of neuroblastoma, ganglioneuroblastoma, and pheochromocytoma. Arch Pathol. 86:160, 1968.
9a. Schimada, H., Chatten, J., et al.: Histopathologic prognostic factors in neuroblastic tumors: definition of subtypes of ganglioneuroblastoma and an age-linked classification of neuroblastomas. JNCI 73:405, 1984.
10. Adam, A., and Hochholzer, L.: Ganglioneuroblastoma of the posterior mediastinum: a clinicopathologic review of 80 cases. Cancer 47:373, 1981.
11. Stout, A. P.: Ganglioneuroma of the sympathetic system. Surg. Gynecol. Obstet. 84:101, 1947.
12. Seeger, R. C. (moderator): Neuroblastoma: clinical perspectives, monoclonal antibodies, and retinoic acid. Ann. Intern. Med. 97:873, 1982.
13. Altman, A. J., and Baehner, R. L.: Favorable prognosis for survival in children with coincident opso-myoclonus and neuroblastoma. Cancer 37:846, 1976.
14. Quinn, J. J., and Altman, A. J.: The multiple hematologic manifestations of neuroblastoma. Am. J. Pediatr. Hematol. Oncol. 1:201, 1979.
15. LaBrosse, E. H., Com-Nougué, C., et al.: Urinary excretion of 3-methoxy-4-hydroxy mandelic acid and 3-methoxy-4-hydroxy phenylacetic acid by 288 patients with neuroblastoma and related neural crest tumors. Cancer Res. 40:1995, 1980.
16. Laug, W. E., Wiegel, S. E., et al.: Initial urinary catecholamine metabolite concentrations and prognosis in neuroblastoma. Pediatrics 62:77, 1978.
17. Quinn, J. J., Altman, A. J., et al.: Serum lactic dehydrogenase: an indicator of tumor activity in neuroblastoma. J. Pediatr. 97:89, 1980.
18. Hann, H. L., Evans, A. E., et al.: Biologic difference between neuroblastoma Stages IV-S and IV. New Engl. J. Med. 305:425, 1981.
19. Hann, H. L., Levy, H. M., et al.: Serum ferritin as a guide to therapy in neuroblastoma. Cancer Res. 40:1411, 1980.
20. Zeltzer, P. M., Marangos, P. J., et al.: Serum neuron-specific enolase in children with neuroblastoma. Relationship to stage and disease control. Cancer 57:1230, 1986.
21. Beckwith, J. B., and Perrin, E. V.: In situ neuroblastoma: A contribution to the natural history of neural crest tumors. Am. J. Pathol. 43:1089, 1963.
22. Ikeda, Y., Lister, J., et al.: Congenital neuroblastoma, neuroblastoma in situ, and the normal fetal development of the adrenal. J. Pediatr. Surg. 16:636. 1981.
23. Turkel, S. B., and Itabashi, H. H.: The natural history of neuroblastic cells in the fetal adrenal gland. Am. J. Pathol. 76:225, 1974.
24. Evans, A. E., D'Angio, G. J., et al.: A proposed staging for children with neuroblastoma. Cancer 27:324, 1971.
25. Evans, A. E., Baum, E., et al.: Do infants with Stage IV-S neuroblastoma need treatment? Arch. Dis. Child. 56:271, 1981.
26. Evans, A. E., Chatten, J., et al.: A review of 17 IV-S neuroblastoma patients at the Children's Hospital of Philadelphia. Cancer 45:833, 1980.
27. Knudson, A. G., Jr., and Meadows, A. T.: Regression of neuroblastoma IV-S: a genetic hypothesis. New Engl. J. Med. 302:1254, 1980.
28. Look, A. T., Hayes, F. A., et al.: Cellular DNA content as a predictor of response to chemotherapy in infants with unresectable neuroblastoma. New Engl. J. Med. 311:231, 1984.
29. Cassady, J. R.: A hypothesis to explain the enigmatic natural history of neuroblastoma. Med. Pediatr. Oncol. 12:64, 1984.
30. Hellström, I., Hellström, K. E., et al.: Studies on cellular immunity to human neuroblastoma cells. Int. J. Cancer 6:172, 1970.
31. Koop, C. E., Kiesewetter, W. B., et al.: Neuroblastoma in childhood: survival after major surgical insult to tumor. Surgery 38:171, 1955.
32. Evans, A. E., and Hummeler, K.: The significance of primitive cells in marrow aspirates of children with neuroblastoma. Cancer 32:906, 1973.
33. Martin, R. F., and Beckwith, J. B. Lymphoid infiltrates in neuroblastomas: their occurrence and prognostic significance. J. Pediatr. Surg. 3:161, 1968.
34. Hayes, F. A., Green, A., et al.: Surgicopathologic staging of neuroblastoma: prognostic significance of regional lymph node metastases. J. Pediatr. 102:59, 1983.
35. Breslow, N., and McCann, B.: Statistical estimation of prognosis for children with neuroblastoma. Cancer Res. 31:2098, 1971.
36. Rosen, E. M., Cassady, J. R., et al.: Influence of local-regional lymph node metastases on prognosis in neuroblastoma. Med. Pediatr. Oncol. 12:260, 1984.
37. Nitschke, R., Humphrey, G. B., et al.: Neuroblastoma: therapy for infants with good prognosis. Med. Pediatr. Oncol. 11:154, 1983.
38. D'Angio, G. J.: The role of radiation therapy in neuroblastoma. In *Pediatric Oncology: Proceedings of the XIIIth Meeting of the International Society of Pediatric Oncology, Marseilles, September 15–19, 1981*. Raybaud, C., Clement, R., et al. (eds.), Amsterdam, Excerpta Medica, 1982.
39. Evans, A. E., D'Angio, G. J., et al.: The role of multimodal therapy in patients with local and regional neuroblastoma. J. Pediatr. Surg. 19:77, 1984.
40. Koop, C. E., and Johnson, D. G.: Neuroblastoma: an assessment of therapy in reference to staging. J. Pediatr. Surg. 6:595, 1971.
41. Hayes, R. A., and Green, A. A.: Neuroblastoma. Pediatr. Ann. 12:366, 1983.
42. Zucker, J. M., and Margolis, E.: Radiochemotherapy of postoperative minimal residual disease in neuroblastoma. Recent Results Cancer Res. 68:423, 1979.
43. Zucker, J. M. Retrospective study of 462 neuroblastomas treated between 1950 and 1970. Maandschr. Kindergeneesk. 42:369, 1974.
44. Rosen, E. M., Cassady, J. R., et al.: Improved survival in neuroblastoma using multimodality therapy. Radiother. Oncol. 2:189, 1984.
45. Haase, G., Wong, K., et al.: Improvement in survival after excision of primary tumor in stage III neuroblastoma. Proc. ASCO 5:831a, 1986.
45a. Jacobson, G. M., Sause, W. T., et al.: Dose response analysis of pediatric neuroblastoma to megavoltage radiation. Am. J. Clin. Oncol. 7:693, 1984.
46. Carli, M., Pastore, G., et al.: The role of chemotherapy in neuroblastoma. In *Pediatric Oncology: Proceedings of the XIIIth Meeting of the International Society of Pediatric Oncology, Marseilles, September 15–19, 1981*. Raybaud, C., Clement, R., et al. (eds.), Amsterdam: Excerpta Medica, 1982.
47. Bernardi, B., Pastore, G., et al.: Effect of peptichemio in nonlocalized neuroblastoma. Cancer 50:10, 1982.
48. Evans, A. E., Brand, W., et al.: Results in children with local and regional neuroblastoma managed with and without vincristine, cyclophosphamide, and imidazolecarboxamide. A report from the Children's Cancer Study Group. Am. J. Clin. Oncol. 6:3, 1984.
49. Evans, A. E., Heyn, R. M., et al.: Vincristine sulfate and cyclophosphamide for children with metastatic neuroblastoma. J. A. M. A. 207:1325, 1969.
50. Green, A. A., Hayes, F. A., et al.: Sequential cyclophosphamide and doxorubicin for induction of complete remission in children with disseminated neuroblastoma. Cancer 48:2310, 1981.

51. Hayes, F. A., Green, A. A., et al.: Clinical evaluation of sequentially scheduled cisplatin and VM 26 in neuroblastoma: response and toxicity. Cancer 48:1715, 1981.
52. Sawitsky, A.: Vincristine and cyclophosphamide therapy in generalized neuroblastoma. A collaborative study. Am. J. Dis. Child. 119:308, 1970.
53. Sullivan, M. P., Nora, A. M., et al.: Evaluation of vincristine sulfate and cyclophosphamide chemotherapy for metastatic neuroblastoma. Pediatrics 44:685, 1969.
54. Frantz, C. N., Gelber, J. A., et al.: Aggressive treatment of neuroblastoma. In *Pediatric Oncology: Proceedings of the XIIIth Meeting of the International Society of Pediatric Oncology, Marseilles, September 15–19, 1981.* Raybaud, C., Clement, R., et al. (eds.), Amsterdam, Excerpta Medica, 1982.
55. Finkelstein, J. Z., Klemperer, M. R., et al.: Multiagent chemotherapy for children with metastatic neuroblastoma: a report from the Children's Cancer Study Group. Med. Pediatr. Oncol. 6:179, 1979.
56. Sitarz, A., Finklestein, J., et al.: An evaluation of the role of surgery in disseminated neuroblastoma: a report from the children's cancer study group. J. Pediatr. Surg. 18:147, 1983.
57. Kretschmar, C. S., Frantz, C. N., et al.: Improved prognosis for infants with stage IV neuroblastoma. J. Clin. Oncol. 2:799, 1984.
57a. Stokes, S. H., Thomas, P. R., et al.: Stage IV-S neuroblastoma. Results with definitive therapy. Cancer 53:2083, 1984.
58. Peschel, R. E., Chen, M., et al.: The treatment of massive hepatomegaly in Stage IV-S neuroblastoma. Int. J. Radiat. Oncol. Biol. Phys. 7:549, 1981.
58a. Schnaufer, L., and Koop, C. E.: Silastic abdominal patch for temporary hepatomegaly in Stage IV-S neuroblastoma. J. Pediatr. Surg. 10:73, 1975.
59. Grosfeld, J. L., Schatzlein, N., et al.: Metastatic neuroblastoma: factors influencing survival. J. Pediatr. Surg. 13:59, 1978.
59a. Stephenson, S. R., Cook, B. A., et al.: The prognostic significance of age and pattern of metastases in Stage IV-S neuroblastoma. Cancer 58:372, 1986.
60. Cushing, B. A., Slovis, T. L., et al.: A rational approach to cervical neuroblastoma. Cancer 50:785, 1982.
61. Castleberry, R. P., Crist, W. M., et al.: Management of localized thoracic neuroblastoma. Med. Pediatr. Oncol. 7:153, 1979.
62. Catalano, P. W., Newton, W. A. Jr., et al.: Reasonable surgery for thoracic neuroblastoma in infants and children. J. Thorac. Cardiovasc. Surg. 76:459, 1978.
63. Filler, R. M., Traggis, D. G., et al.: Favorable outlook for children with mediastinal neuroblastoma. J. Pediatr. Surg. 7:136, 1972.
64. Carachi, R., Campbell, P. E., et al.: Thoracic neural crest tumors. A clinical review. Cancer 51:949, 1983.
65. Punt, J., Pritchard, J., et al.: Neuroblastoma. A review of 21 cases presenting with spinal cord compression. Cancer 45:3095, 1980.
66. Holgersen, L. O., Santulli, T. V., et al.: Neuroblastoma with intraspinal (dumbbell) extension. J. Pediatr. Surg. 18:406, 1983.
67. D'Angio, G. J., and Evans, A. E.: Cyclic, low-dose total body irradiation for metastatic neuroblastoma. Int. J. Radiat. Oncol. Biol. Phys. 9:1961, 1983.
68. Helson, L., Jereb, B., et al.: Sequential hemi-body irradiation (HBI) in treatment of advanced neuroblastoma: a pilot study. Int. J. Radiat. Oncol. Biol. Phys. 7:531, 1981.
69. Green, A. A., Hustu, H. G., et al.: Total body sequential segmental irradiation and combination chemotherapy for children with disseminated neuroblastoma. Cancer 38:2250, 1976.
70. Wharam, M. D., Kaizer, H., et al.: Systemic irradiation for selected Stage IV and recurrent pediatric solid tumors: method, toxicity, and preliminary result. Int. J. Radiat. Oncol. Biol. Phys. 6:217, 1980.
71. Ohnuma, N., Tsutoma, K., et al.: Radiosensitivity of human neuroblastoma cell line (NB-1). Gan 68:711, 1977.
72. McColloch, A. E., and Till, J. E.: The sensitivity of cells from normal mouse bone marrow to gamma radiation in vitro and in vivo. Radiat. Res. 16:822, 1962.
73. Spruce, W. E., Blume, K. G., et al. Syngeneic bone marrow transplantation in a patient with metastatic neuroblastoma refractory to conventional therapy. Pediatrics 65:573, 1980.
74. August, C. S., Serota, F. T., et al.: Treatment of advanced neuroblastoma with supralethal chemotherapy, radiation, and allogeneic or autologous marrow reconstitution. J. Clin. Oncol. 2:609, 1984.
75. Pritchard, J., McElwain, T. J., et al.: High-dose melphalan with autologous marrow for treatment of advanced neuroblastoma. Br. J. Cancer 45:86, 1982.
75a. Hartmann, O., Kalifa, C., et al.: Treatment of advanced neuroblastoma with high-dose melphalan and autologous bone marrow transplantation. Cancer Chemother. Pharmacol. 16:165, 1986.
75b. Helson, L.: Autologous bone marrow transplantation. A maximal therapy design for disseminated neuroblastoma. Am. J. Ped. Hem. Oncol. 7:49, 1985.
76. Prasad, K. N.: Control mechanisms of malignancy and differentiation in cultures of nerve cells. In *Advances in Neuroblastoma Research.* Evans, A. E. (ed.), New York, Raven Press, 1980.
77. Botterstein, J. E.: Differentiated properties of neuronal cell lines. In *Functionally Differentiated Cell Lines.* Sate, G. H. (ed.), New York, A. R. Liss, 1981.
78. Knudson, A. G., Jr., and Strong L. C.: Mutation and cancer: a model for Wilms' tumor of the kidney. J. Natl. Cancer Inst. 48:313, 1972.
78a. Pilling, G. P.: Wilms' tumor in seven children with congenital aniridia. J. Pediatr. Surg. 10:87, 1975.
79. Yunis, J. J., and Ramsay, N. K.: Familial occurrence of the aniridia–Wilms' tumor syndrome with deletion 11p13 –14.1. J. Pediatr. 96:1027, 1980.
79a. Koufos, A., Hansen, M. F., et al.: Loss of alleles at loci on human chromosome 11 during genesis of Wilms' tumour. Nature 309:170, 1984.
79b. Orkin, S. H., Goldman, D. S., et al.: Development of homozygosity for chromosome 11p markers in Wilms' tumor. Nature 309:172, 1984.
80. Kaneko, Y., Egues, M. C., et al.: Interstitial deletion of short arm of chromosome 11 limited to Wilms' tumor cells of a patient without aniridia. Cancer Res. 41:4577, 1981.
80a. Knudson, A. G., Jr.: Mutagenesis and embryonal carcinogenesis. Natl. Cancer Inst. Monograph 15:19, 1979.
81. Beckwith, J. B., and Palmer, N. F.: Histopathology and prognosis of Wilms' tumor. Results from the First National Wilms' Tumor Study. Cancer 41:1937, 1978.
82. Beckwith, J. B.: Wilms' tumor and other renal tumors of childhood: a selective review from the National Wilms' Tumor Study Pathology Center. Hum. Pathol. 14:481, 1983.
82a. Beckwith, J. B.: Wilms' tumor and other renal tumors of childhood: an update. J. Urol. 136:320, 1986.
82b. Bonadio, J. F., Storer, B., et al.: Anaplastic Wilms' tumor. Clinical and pathological studies. J. Clin. Oncol. 3:513, 1985.
82c. Douglass, E. C., Look, A. T., et al.: Hyperdiploidy and chromosomal rearrangements define the anaplastic variant of Wilms' tumor. J. Clin. Oncol. 4:975, 1986.
83. Haas, J. E., Palmer, N. F., et al.: Ultrastructure of malignant rhabdoid tumor of the kidney: a distinctive renal tumor of childhood. Hum. Pathol. 12:646, 1981.
84. Palmer, N. F., and Sutow, W.: Clinical aspects of the rhabdoid tumor of the kidney: a report of the National

Wilms' Tumor Study Group. Med. Pediatr. Oncol. 11:242, 1983.
84a. Sotelo-Avila, A., Gonzalez-Crussi, F., et al.: Renal and extra-renal rhabdoid tumors in children: a clinicopathologic study of 14 patients. Semin. Diagnostic. Pathol. 3:151, 1986.
85. Carcassonne, N., Raybaud, C., et al.: Clear cell sarcoma of the kidney in children: a distinct entity. J. Pediatr. Surg. 16:645, 1981.
85a. Schmidt, D., Harms, D., et al.: Bone metastasizing renal tumor (clear cell sarcoma) of childhood with epithelioid elements. Cancer 56:609, 1985.
85b. Haas, J., Bonadio, J. F., et al.: Clear cell sarcoma of the kidney with emphasis on ultrastructural studies. Cancer 54:2978, 1984.
86. Kumar, A. P. M., Pratt, C. B., et al.: Treatment strategy for nodular renal blastema and nephroblastomatosis associated with Wilms' tumor. J. Pediatr. Surg. 13:281, 1978.
87. Bolande, R. P.: Neoplasia of early life and its relationships to teratogenesis. In *Perspectives in Pediatric Pathology*. Rosenberg, R. S., and Bolande, R. P. (eds.), Chicago, Year Book Medical Publishers, 1976.
88. Bove, K. E., and McAdams, A. J.: Multifocal nephroblastic neoplasia. J. Natl. Cancer. Inst. 61:285, 1978.
89. DeChadarévian, J. P., Fletcher, B., et al.: Massive infantile nephroblastomatosis: a clinical, radiological, and pathological analysis of four cases. Cancer 39:2294, 1977.
90. Rosenfield, N. S., Shimkin, P., et al.: Wilms tumor arising from spontaneously regressing nephroblastomatosis. AJR 135:381, 1980.
91. Kulkarni, R., Bailie, M. D., et al.: Progression of nephroblastomatosis to Wilms' tumor. J. Pediatr. 96:178, 1980.
92. Beckwith, J. B.: Mesenchymal renal neoplasms of infancy revisited. J. Pediatr. Surg. 9:803, 1974.
93. Gonzalez-Crussi, F., Sotelo-Avila, C., et al.: Malignant mesenchymal nephroma of infancy: report of a case with pulmonary metastases. Am. J. Surg. Pathol. 4:185, 1980.
94. Gonzalez-Crussi, F., Sotelo-Avila, C., et al.: Mesenchymal renal tumors in infancy: a reappraisal. Hum. Pathol. 12:78, 1981.
95. Howell, C. G., Othersen, H. B., et al.: Therapy and outcome in 51 children with mesoblastic nephroma: a report of the National Wilms' Tumor Study. J. Pediatr. Surg. 17:826, 1982.
96. Dibbins, A. W., and Wiener, E. S.: Retroperitoneal tumors in children. In *Current Problems in Surgery*. Ravitch, M. M. (ed.), Chicago, Year Book Medical Publishers, 1973, pp. 1–70.
97. Jereb, B., Tournade, M. F., et al.: Lymph node invasion and prognosis in nephroblastoma. Cancer 45:1632, 1980.
98. Breslow, N., Churchill, G., et al.: Prognosis for Wilms' tumor patients with nonmetastatic disease at diagnosis — results of The Second National Wilms' Tumor Study. J. Clin. Oncol. 3:521, 1985.
99. Bond, J. V., and Martin, E. C.: Pulmonary metastases in Wilms' tumor. Clin. Radiol. 27:191, 1976.
100. D'Angio G. J., Evans, A., et al.: The treatment of Wilms' tumor: Results of the Second National Wilms' Tumor Study. Cancer 47:2302, 1981.
100a. Movassaghi, N., Leikin, S., et al.: Wilms' tumor metastasis to uncommon sites. J. Pediatr. 84:416, 1974.
100b. Breslow, N., Churchill, G., et al.: Prognosis for Wilms' tumor patients with nonmetastatic disease at diagnosis—results of the second National Wilms' Tumor Study. J. Clin. Oncol. 3:521, 1985.
101. D'Angio, G. J., Evans, A., et al: Biology and management of Wilms' tumor. In *Cancer in the Young*. Levin, A. S. (ed.), New York, Masson Publishing, 1982.
102. Breslow, N. E., Palmer, N. F., et al.: Wilms' tumor: prognostic factors for patients without metastases at diagnosis. Results of the National Wilms' Tumor Study. Cancer 41:1577, 1978.
103. Voûte, P. A., Lemerle, J. et al.: Preoperative chemotherapy in Wilms' tumour. In *Pediatric Oncology: Proceedings of the XIIIth Meeting of the International Society of Pediatric Oncology, Marseilles, September 15–19, 1981*. Raybaud, C., Clement, R., et al. (eds.), Amsterdam, Excerpta Medica, 1982.
104. Lemerle, J., Voûte, P., et al.: Preoperative versus postoperative radiotherapy, single versus multiple courses of Actinomycin-D in the treatment of Wilms' tumor. Preliminary results of a controlled trial conducted by the International Society of Pediatric Oncology (SIOP). Cancer 38:647, 1976.
105. Lemerle, J., Voûte, P. A., et al.: Effectiveness of preoperative chemotherapy in Wilms' tumor: results of an International Society of Pediatric Oncology (SIOP) clinical trial. J. Clin. Oncol. 1:604, 1983.
106. D'Angio, G. J.: Wilms' tumor—a review. The Cancer Bulletin of the M.D. Anderson Hospital and Tumor Institute 34:104, 1982.
106a. Bracken, R. B., Sutow, W. W., et al.: Preoperative therapy for Wilms' tumor. Urology 19:55, 1982.
107. D'Angio, G. J., Evans, A. E., et al.: Results of the Third National Wilms' Tumor Study (NWTS-3): A preliminary report. Proc. AACR 25:183, 1984.
107a. D'Angio, G. J., Tefft, M., et al.: Radiation therapy of Wilms' tumor: results according to dose, field, postoperative timing, and histology. Int. J. Radiat. Oncol. Biol. Phys. 4:769, 1978.
108. Tefft, M.: Postoperative radiation therapy for residual Wilms' tumor. Review of Group III patients in the National Wilms' Tumor Study. Cancer 37:2768, 1976.
109. Hussey, D. H., Castro, J. R., et al.: Radiation therapy in management of Wilms' tumor. Radiology 101:663, 1971.
110. Jeal, P. N., and Jenkins, R. D. T.: Abdominal radiation in the treatment of Wilms' tumor. Int. J. Radiat. Oncol. Biol. Phys. 6:655, 1980.
111. Cassady, J. R., and Belli, J. A.: Radiation in the management of children with Wilms' tumor. Int. J. Radiat. Oncol. Biol. Phys. 4:907, 1978.
112. Green, D. M., and Jaffe, N.: The role of chemotherapy in the treatment of Wilms' tumor. Cancer 44:52, 1979.
113. Chard, R. L., Krivit, W., et al.: Phase II study of VP-16-213 in childhood malignant disease. Cancer Treat. Rep. 63:1755, 1979.
113a. Farber, S.: Chemotherapy in the treatment of leukemia and Wilms' tumor. JAMA 198:826, 1966.
113b. Wolff, J. A., D'Angio, G. J., et al.: Long-term evaluation of single versus multiple courses of actinomycin D therapy of Wilms' tumor. New Engl. J. Med. 290:84, 1976.
113c. Lemerle, J., Voûte, P. A., et al.: Preoperative versus postoperative radiotherapy, single versus multiple courses of actinomycin D in the treatment of Wilms' tumor. Cancer 38:647, 1976.
114. Belasco, J., and D'Angio, G. J.: Wilms' tumor. CA 31:258, 1981.
115. D'Angio, G. J., Evans, A., et al.: The treatment of Wilms' tumor. Cancer 47:2302, 1981.
116. Camitta, B., Kun, L., et al.: Doxorubicin-vincristine therapy for Wilms' tumor: a pilot study. Cancer Treat. Rep. 66:1791, 1982.
117. Bishop, H. C., Tefft, M., et al.: Survival in bilateral Wilms' tumor—review of 30 National Wilms' Tumor Study cases. J. Pediatr. Surg. 12:631, 1977.
117a. Asch, M. J., Siegel, S., et al.: Prognostic factors and outcome in bilateral Wilms' tumor. Cancer 56:2526, 1985.
118. Penn, I.: Renal transplantation for Wilms' tumor: report of 20 cases. J. Urol. 122:793, 1979.
118a. DeMaria, J. E., Brezinski, H. A., et al.: Renal transplantation in patients with bilateral Wilms' tumor. J. Pediatr. Surg. 14:577, 1979.

119. Sutow, W. W., Breslow, N. E., et al.: Prognosis in children with Wilms' tumor metastases prior to or following primary treatment. Results from the First National Wilms' Tumor Study (NWTS-1). Am. J. Clin. Oncol. 5:339, 1982.

119a. Wilimas, J. A., Douglass, E. C., et al.: Relapsed Wilms' tumor. Factors affecting survival and cure. Am. J. Clin. Oncol. 8:324, 1985.

120. Monson, K. J., Brand, W. N., et al.: Results of small-field irradiation of apparent solitary metastasis from Wilms' tumor. Radiology 104:157, 1972.

121. Ortega, J., Higgins, G. R., et al.: Vincristine, dactinomycin, and cyclophosphamide (VAC) chemotherapy for recurrent metastatic Wilms' tumor in previously treated children. J. Pediatr. 96:502, 1980.

122. Cangir, A., Morgan, S. K., et al.: Combination chemotherapy with adriamycin (NSC-123127) and dimethyl triazeno imidazole carboxamide (DTIC) (NSC-45388) in children with metastatic solid tumors. Med. Pediatr. Oncol. 2:183, 1976.

122a. Douglass, E. C., Wilimas, J. A., et al.: Efficacy of combination cisplatin (DDP) and VP-16 in the treatment of recurrent and advanced Wilms' tumor. Proc. ASCO 5:789, 1986.

123. Schullinger, J. N., Santulli, T. V., et al.: Wilms' tumor: the role of right heart angiography in the management of selected cases. Ann. Surg. 18:451, 1977.

124. Clausen, N.: Late recurrence of Wilms' tumor. Med. Pediatr. Oncol. 10:557, 1982.

125. Raney, R. B., Jr. Palmer, N., et al.: Renal cell carcinoma in children. Med. Pediatr. Oncol. 11:91, 1983.

125a. Lack, E. E., Cassady, J. R., et al.: Renal cell carcinoma in childhood and adolescence; a clinical and pathological study of 17 cases. J. Urol. 133:822, 1985.

126. Lang, E. K.: Renal cell carcinoma presenting with metastases to pulmonary hilar nodes. J. Urol. 118:543, 1977.

127. DeKernion, J. B., and Berry, D.: The diagnosis and treatment of renal cell carcinoma. Cancer 45:1947, 1980.

128. Cassady, J. R., Filler, R., et al.: Carcinoma of the kidney in children. Results of an interdisciplinary approach to management. Radiology 112:691, 1974.

129. Dehner, L. P., Leestma, J. E., et al.: Renal cell carcinoma in children: a clinicopathologic study of 15 cases and review of the literature. J. Pediatr. 75:358, 1970.

130. Maurer, H. M., Donaldson, M., et al.: Rhabdomyosarcoma in childhood and adolescence. In *Current Problems in Cancer*. Hickey, R. C. (ed.), Chicago, Year Book Medical Publishers, 1978.

131. Maurer, H. M., Moon, T., et al.: The Intergroup Rhabdomyosarcoma Study. A preliminary report. Cancer 40:2015, 1977.

131a. Palmer, N. F., and Foulkes, M.: Histopathology and prognosis in the Second Intergroup Rhabdomyosarcoma Study (IRS-II). Proc. ASCO 2:C-897, 1983 (Abstr.).

132. Heyn, R. M., Holland, R. et al.: The role of combined chemotherapy in the treatment of rhabdomyosarcoma in children. Cancer 34:2128, 1974.

133. Lawrence, W., Jr., Hays, D. M., et al.: Lymphatic metastasis with childhood rhabdomyosarcoma. Cancer 39:556, 1977.

134. Tefft, M., Fernandez, C., et al.: Incidence of meningeal involvement by rhabdomyosarcoma of the head and neck in children. A report of the Intergroup Rhabdomyosarcoma Study (IRS). Cancer 42:253, 1978.

135. Ruymann, F. B., Newton, W. A., Jr., et al.: Bone marrow metastases at diagnosis in children and adolescents with rhabdomyosarcoma. A report from the Intergroup Myosarcoma Study. Cancer 53:368, 1984.

136. Pratt, C. B., Dugger, D. L., et al.: Metastatic involvement of the heart in childhood rhabdomyosarcoma. Cancer 31:1492, 1973.

137. Ehrlich, F. E., Haas, J. E., et al.: Rhabdomyosarcoma in infants and children: factors affecting long-term survival. J. Pediatr. Surg. 6:571, 1971.

138. Grosfeld, J. L., Clatworthy, H. W., Jr., et al.: Combined therapy in childhood rhabdomyosarcomas: an analysis of 42 cases. J. Pediatr. Surg. 4:637, 1969.

138a. Regab, A., Heyn, R., et al.: Infants under one year of age with soft tissue sarcomas: a report from the Intergroup Rhabdomyosarcoma Study (IRS) Committee. Proc. ASCO 5:807a, 1986.

139. Enzinger, F. M., and Shiraki, M.: Alveolar rhabdomyosarcoma: an analysis of 110 cases. Cancer 24:18, 1969.

139a. Maurer, H. M.: Personal communication.

140. Maurer, M. H.: The Intergroup Rhabdomyosarcoma Study. The Cancer Bulletin of the University of Texas M.D. Anderson Hospital and Tumor Institute at Houston 34:108, 1982.

140a. Gehan, E. A., Glover, F. N., et al.: Prognostic factors in children with rhabdomyosarcoma. Natl. Cancer Inst. Monogr. 56:83, 1981.

141. Clatworthy, H. W., Jr., Braren, V., et al.: Surgery of bladder and prostatic neoplasms in children. Cancer 32:1157, 1973.

142. Donaldson, S., Castro, J. R., et al.: Rhabdomyosarcoma of head and neck in children. Combination treatment by surgery, irradiation, and chemotherapy. Cancer 31:26, 1973.

143. Cassady, J. R., Sagerman, R. H., et al.: Radiation therapy for rhabdomyosarcoma. Radiology 91:116, 1968.

144. Tefft, M., Lingberg, R. D., et al.: Radiation therapy combined with systemic chemotherapy of rhabdomyosarcoma in children: local control in patients enrolled in the Intergroup Rhabdomyosarcoma Study. Natl. Cancer Inst. Monogr. 56:75, 1981.

144a. Maurer, H., Foulkes, M., et al.: Intergroup Rhabdomyosarcoma Study (IRS)-II: Preliminary Report. Proc. ASCO 2:C-274, 1983 (Abstr.).

145. Tefft, M., Lindberg, R. D., et al.: Radiation therapy combined with systemic chemotherapy of rhabdomyosarcoma in children: local control in patients enrolled in the Intergroup Rhabdomyosarcoma Study. Natl. Cancer Inst. Monogr. 56:75, 1981.

146. Gottlieb, J., Baker, L., et al.: Chemotherapy of sarcomas with a combination of adriamycin and dimethyltriazeno imidazole carboxamide. Cancer 30:1632, 1972.

146a. Baum, E. S., Gaynon, P., et al.: Phase II trial of cis-dichlorodiammine-platinum II in refractory childhood cancer. Children: Cancer Study Group report. Cancer 65:815, 1981.

146b. Chard, R. L., Krivit, W., et al.: Phase II study of VP-16-213 in childhood malignant disease: a CCSG report. Cancer Treat. Rep. 63:1755, 1979.

147. Ruymann, F., Heyn, R., et al.: Completely resected rhabdomyosarcoma: the effect of unfavorable histology on recurrence. A report from the Intergroup Rhabdomyosarcoma Study. Proc. ASCO 3:C-334, 1984 (Abstr.).

148. Hornback, N. B., and Shidnia, H.: Rhabdomyosarcoma in the pediatric age group. AJR 126:542, 1976.

149. Jaffe, N. J., Filler, R. M., et al.: Rhabdomyosarcoma in children. Improved outlook with a multidisciplinary approach. Am. J. Surg. 125:482, 1973.

150. Sutow, W. W., Lindberg, R. D., et al.: Three-year relapse-free survival rates in childhood rhabdomyosarcoma of the head and neck. Report from the Intergroup Rhabdomyosarcoma Study. Cancer 49:2217, 1982.

151. Hays, D. M.: The management of rhabdomyosarcoma in children and young adults. World J. Surg. 4:15, 1980.

152. Wharam, M. D., Jr., Foulkes, M. A., et al.: Soft tissue sarcoma of the head and neck in childhood: nonorbital and nonparameningeal sites. A report of the Intergroup Rhabdomyosarcoma Study (IRS-1). Cancer 53:1016, 1984.

153. Littman, P., Raney, B., et al.: Soft-tissue sarcomas of the head and neck in children. Int. J. Radiat. Oncol. Biol. Phys. 9:1367, 1983.

154. Raney, R. B., Tefft, M., et al.: Results of intensive treat-

ment of children with cranial parameningeal sarcoma: a report from the Intergroup Rhabdomyosarcoma Study (IRS) (Abstr). Proc. AACR 471:120, 1982.
155. Gasparini, M., Lombardi, F., et al.: Childhood rhabdomyosarcoma with meningeal extension: results of combined therapy including central nervous system prophylaxis. Am. J. Clin. Oncol. 6:393, 1983.
156. Masson, J. K., and Soule, E. H.: Embryonal rhabdomyosarcoma of the head and neck: report on 88 cases. Am. J. Surg. 110:585, 1965.
157. Crist, W. M., Raney, R. B., Jr., et al.: Intrathoracic soft tissue sarcomas in children. Cancer 50:598, 1982.
158. Raney, R. B., Jr., Ragab, A. H., et al.: Soft-tissue sarcoma of the trunk in childhood. Results of the Intergroup Rhabdomyosarcoma Study. Cancer 49:2612, 1982.
159. Ransom, J. L., and Pratt, C. B., et al.: Retroperitoneal rhabdomyosarcoma in children. Results of multimodality therapy. Cancer 45:845, 1980.
160. Hays, D. M., Soule, E. H., et al.: Extremity lesions in the Intergroup Rhabdomyosarcoma Study (IRS-1): a preliminary report. Cancer 48:1, 1982.
161. Ransom, J. L., Pratt, C. B., et al.: Childhood rhabdomyosarcoma of the extremity: results of combined modality therapy. Cancer 40:2810, 1977.
162. Tefft, M., and Jaffe, N.: Sarcoma of the bladder and prostate in children. Rationale for the role of radiation therapy based on a review of the literature and a report of 14 additional patients. Cancer 32:1161, 1973.
163. Mackenzie, A. R., Whitmore, W. F., Jr., et al.: Myosarcomas of the bladder and prostate. Cancer 22:833, 1968.
164. Ghazali, S.: Embryonic rhabdomyosarcoma of the urogenital tract. Br. J. Surg. 60:124, 1973.
165. Lemmon, W. T., Jr., Holland, J. M., et al.: Rhabdomyosarcoma of the prostate. Surgery 59:736, 1966.
166. Hays, D. M., Raney, R. B., Jr., et al.: Bladder and prostatic tumors in the Intergroup Rhabdomyosarcoma Study (IRS-1). Results of therapy. Cancer 50:1472, 1982.
167. Ortega, J. A.: A therapeutic approach to childhood pelvic rhabdomyosarcoma without pelvic exenteration. J. Pediatr. 94:205, 1979.
168. Hays, D. M., and Ortega, J.: Primary chemotherapy in the management of pelvic rhabdomyosarcoma in infancy and early childhood. In *Adjuvant Therapy of Cancer*. Salmon, S. E., and Jones, S. E. (eds.), Amsterdam, Elsevier-North Holland Biomedical Press, 1977.
169. Raney, R. B., and Duckett, J. W.: Editorial comment. J. Urol. 132:319, 1984.
170. Ghavimi, F., Herr, H., et al.: Treatment of genitourinary rhabdomyosarcoma in children. J. Urol. 132:313, 1984.
171. Hays, D., Raney, R. B., Jr., et al.: Primary chemotherapy in the treatment of children with bladder-prostate tumors in the Intergroup Rhabdomyosarcoma Study (IRS II). J. Pediatr. Surg. 17:812, 1982.
171a. Raney, B., Crist, W., et al.: Soft tissue sarcoma of the perineal-anal region in childhood: a report from the Intergroup Rhabdomyosarcoma Study (IRS) Committee. Proc. ASCO 5:822a, 1986.
172. Hays, D. M., Raney, R. B., Jr., et al.: Rhabdomyosarcoma of the female urogenital tract. J. Pediatr. Surg. 16:828, 1981.
173. Kumar, A. P. M., Wrenn, E. L., Jr., et al.: Combined therapy to prevent complete pelvic exenteration for rhabdomyosarcoma of the vagina or uterus. Cancer 37:118, 1976.
173a. Hays, D. M., Shimada, H., et al.: Sarcomas of the vagina and uterus: the Intergroup Rhabdomyosarcoma Study. J. Pediatr. Surg. 20:718, 1985.
174. Flamant, F., Chassagne, D., et al.: Embryonal rhabdomyosarcoma of the vagina in children. Conservative treatment with curietherapy and chemotherapy. Eur. J. Cancer 15:527, 1979.
175. Cromie, W. J., Raney, R. B., Jr., et al.: Paratesticular rhabdomyosarcoma in children. J. Urol. 122:80, 1979.
176. Raney, R. B., Hays, D. M., et al.: Paratesticular rhabdomyosarcoma in childhood. Cancer 42:729, 1978.
177. Raney, R. B., Jr., Tefft, M., et al.: Therapy results in paratesticular sarcoma of children and adolescents: a report of the IRS-I and -II. Proc. AACR 25:724, 1984 (Abstr.).
178. Niefeld, J. P., Berg, J. W., et al.: A retrospective epidemiologic study of pediatric fibrosarcomas. J. Pediatr. Surg. 13:735, 1978.
178a. Chung, E. B., and Enzinger, F. M.: Infantile fibrosarcoma. Cancer 38:728, 1976.
178b. Soule, E. H., and Pritchard, D. J.: Fibrosarcoma in infants and children: A review of 110 cases. Cancer 40:1711, 1977.
178c. Dehner, L. P., and Askin, F. B.: Tumors of fibrous tissue origin in children. A clinicopathologic study of cutaneous and soft tissue neoplasms in 66 children. Cancer 38:888, 1976.
179. Fu, Y. S., and Perzin, K. H.: Nonepithelial tumors of the nasal cavity, paranasal sinuses, and nasopharynx. A clinico-pathologic study. VI. Fibrous tissue tumors (fibroma, fibromatosis, fibrosarcoma). Cancer 37:2912, 1976.
180. Hays, D. M., Mirabel, V. O., et al.: Fibrosarcoma in infants and children. J. Pediatr. Surg. 5:176, 1970.
181. Swain, R. E., Sessions, D. G., et al.: Fibrosarcoma of the head and neck in children. Laryngoscope 86:113, 1976.
182. Exelby, P. R., Knapper, W. H., et al.: Soft tissue fibrosarcoma in children. J. Pediatr. Surg. 8:415, 1973.
183. Stout, A. P.: Fibrosarcoma in infants and children. Cancer 15:1028, 1962.
183a. Grier, H. C., Perez-Atayde, A. R., et al.: Chemotherapy for inoperable infantile fibrosarcoma. Cancer 56:1507, 1985.
183b. Ninane, J., Gosseye, S., et al.: Congenital fibrosarcoma. Preoperative chemotherapy and conservative surgery. Cancer 58:1400, 1986.
184. Senyszyn, J. J., and O'Conor, G.: Fibrosarcoma of the brain. A case report describing response of the primary and metastatic tumors to radiotherapy. Oncology 24:431, 1970.
185. Renaud, J., Van Slooten, E. A., et al.: The treatment of fibrosarcoma of soft tissues: a survey of 39 patients. Arch. Chir. Neerl. 15:187, 1963.
186. Cadman, S. L., Soule, E. H., et al.: Synovial sarcoma. An analysis of 134 tumors. Cancer 18:613, 1965.
187. Roth, J. A., Enzinger, F. M., et al.: Synovial sarcoma of the neck: follow-up study of 24 cases. Cancer 35:1243, 1975.
188. Shmookler, B. M., Enzinger, F. M., et al.: Orofacial synovial sarcoma. A clinicopathologic study of 11 new cases and review of the literature. Cancer 50:269, 1982.
189. Morton, D. L.: Soft tissue sarcomas. In *Cancer Medicine*. Holland, J. F., and Frei, E., III (eds.), Philadelphia, Lea & Febiger, 1973.
190. Cameron, H. U., and Kostuik, J. P.: A long-term follow-up of synovial sarcoma. J. Bone Joint Surg. 56B:613, 1974.
190a. Carson, J. H., Harwood, A. R., et al.: The place of radiotherapy in the treatment of synovial sarcoma. Int. J. Radiat. Oncol. Biol. Phys. 7:49, 1981.
190b. Raney, R. B., Jr.: Synovial sarcoma. Med. Pediatr. Oncol. 9:41, 1981.
190c. Shui, M. H., McCormack, P. M., et al.: Surgical treatment of tendosynovial sarcoma. Cancer 43:889, 1979.
191. Gerner, R. E., and Moore, G. E.: Synovial sarcoma. Ann. Surg. 181:22, 1975.
192. Askin, F. B., Rosai, J., et al.: Malignant small cell tumor of the thoracopulmonary region in childhood. A distinctive clinicopathologic entity of uncertain histogenesis. Cancer 43:2438, 1979.
193. Womer, R. B.: Extracranial primitive neuroectodermal tumor. Med. Pediatr. Oncol. 12:119, 1984.

194. Seemayer, T. A., Thelmo, W. L., et al.: Peripheral neuroectodermal tumors. Perspect. Pediatr. Pathol. 2:151, 1975.
195. Nesbitt, K. A., and Vidone, R. A.: Primitive ectodermal tumor (neuroblastoma) arising in the sciatic nerve of a child. Cancer 37:1562, 1976.
195a. Israel, M. A.: The evaluation of clinical molecular genetics. Am. J. Pediatr. Hem. Oncol. 8:163, 1986.
195b. Israel, M. A., Triche, T. J., et al.: Treatment of peripheral neuroepithelioma in children and young adults: a genetically determined approach. Proc. ASCO 5:71a, 1986.
195c. Kretschmar, C., Perez-Atayde, A., et al.: Extracranial primitive neuroectodermal tumors (PNET) in childhood. Proc. ASCO 5:815a, 1986.
195d. Göbel, V., Jürgens, H., et al.: Malignant peripheral neuroectodermal tumors (MPNT) of childhood and adolescence: retrospective analysis of treatment results in 30 patients. Proc. ASCO 5:810a, 1986.
196. Triche, T. J.: Round cell tumors in childhood: the application of newer techniques to the differential diagnosis. Perspect. Pediatr. Pathol. 7:279, 1980.
197. Dickman, P.S., and Triche, T. J.: Ultrastructural comparison of Ewing's sarcoma of bone with diverse pediatric soft tissue sarcoma resembling Ewing's sarcoma. Lab. Invest. 44:15A, 1981 (Abstr.).
198. Kinsella, T. J., Triche, T. J., et al.: Extraskeletal Ewing's sarcoma: results of combined modality treatment. J. Clin. Oncol. 1:489, 1983.
199. Dahlin, D. C.: Bone Tumors. General Aspects and Data on 3987 Cases, 2nd ed. Springfield, IL, Charles C Thomas, 1967.
200. Dahlin, D. C., and Coventry, M. B.: Osteosarcoma. A study of 600 cases. J. Bone Joint Surg. 49A:101, 1967.
200a. Colyer, R. A.: Osteogenic sarcoma in siblings. Johns Hopkins Med. J. 145:131, 1979.
201. Rosen, G.: Spindle cell sarcoma—osteogenic sarcoma. In Clinical Pediatric Oncology. Sutow, W. W., Fernbach, D. J., et al. (eds.), St. Louis, C. V. Mosby Co., 1984.
201a. Hansen, M. F., Koufos, A., et al.: Osteosarcoma and retinoblastoma: a shared chromosomal mechanism revealing recessive predisposition. Proc. Natl. Acad. Sci. USA 82:6216, 1985.
202. Weatherby, R. P., Dahlin, D. C., et al.: Postradiation sarcoma of bone: review of 78 Mayo Clinic cases. Mayo Clin. Proc. 56:294, 1981.
203. Meadows, A. T., Strong, L. C., et al.: Bone sarcoma as a second malignant neoplasm in children: influence of radiation and genetic predisposition. Cancer 46:2603, 1980.
204. Mueller, W. A.: Epidemiologische erhebungen ueber spaetschaeden bei mit radium 224 behandelten personen. Z. Orthop. 116:619, 1978.
205. Unni, K., Dahlin, D. C., et al.: Periosteal osteogenic sarcoma. Cancer 37:2466, 1976.
205a. Hall, R. B., Robinson, L. H., et al. Peritoneal osteosarcoma. Cancer 55:165, 1985.
206. Ahuja, S. C., Villacin, A. B., et al. Juxtacortical (parosteal) osteogenic sarcoma. J. Bone Joint Surg. 59A:632, 1977.
207. Dahlin, D. C. Osteosarcoma of bone and a consideration of prognostic variables. Cancer Treat. Rep. 62:189, 1978.
208. Kreicbergs, A., Broström, L. A., et al.: Cellular DNA content in human osteosarcoma. Aspects on diagnosis and prognosis. Cancer 50:2476, 1982.
209. Rosen, G., Caparros, B., et al.: Preoperative chemotherapy for osteogenic sarcoma: selection of postoperative adjuvant chemotherapy based on the response of the primary tumor to preoperative chemotherapy. Cancer 49:1221, 1982.
210. Martin, S. E., Dwyer, A., et al.: Small-cell osteosarcoma. Cancer 50:990, 1982.
211. Bode, U., and Levine, A. S.: The biology and management of osteosarcoma. In Cancer in the Young. Levine, A. S. (ed.), New York, Masson Publishing, 1982.
212. Goorin, A. M., Frei, E., III, et al.: Adjuvant chemotherapy for osteosarcoma: a decade of experience. Surg. Clin. North Am. 61:1379, 1981.
213. Huvos, A. G.: Bone Tumors: Diagnosis, Treatment and Prognosis. Philadelphia, W. B. Saunders Co., 1979.
213a. Parham, D. M., Pratt, C. B., et al.: Childhood multifocal osteosarcoma. Clinicopathologic and radiologic correlates. Cancer 55:2653, 1985.
214. Heyman, S., and Treves, S.: Scintigraphy in pediatric bone tumors. In Pediatric Hematology/Oncology. Jaffe, N. (ed.), Littleton, MA, PSG Publishing Co., 1979.
215. Enneking, W. F., and Kagan, A.: "Skip" metastases in osteosarcoma. Cancer 36:2192, 1975.
216. Jeffree, G. M., Price, C. H. G., et al.: The metastatic patterns of osteosarcoma. Br. J. Cancer 32:87, 1975.
216a. Giuliano, A. E., Feig, S., et al.: Changing metastatic patterns of osteosarcoma. Cancer 54:2160, 1984.
217. Schwinn, G. P., and McKenna, R. J.: The biologic behavior of osteosarcoma. In Seventh National Cancer Conference Proceedings. Clark, R. L., Stanley, W. M., et al. (eds.), Philadelphia, J. B. Lippincott, 1973.
217a. Taylor, W. F., Ivins, et al.: Trends and variability in survival among patients with osteosarcoma: a 7-year update. Mayo Clin. Proc. 60:91, 1985.
218. Lockshin, M. D., and Higgins, I. T. T.: Prognosis in osteogenic sarcoma. Clin. Orthop. Rel. Res. 58:85, 1968.
219. Simon, R.: Clinical prognostic factors in osteosarcoma. Cancer Treat. Rep. 62:193, 1978.
220. McKenna, R. J., Schwinn, C. P., et al.: Sarcomata of the osteogenic series (osteosarcoma, fibrosarcoma, chondrosarcoma, parosteal osteogenic sarcoma, and sarcoma arising in abnormal bone): an analysis of 552 cases. J. Bone Joint Surg. 48A:1, 1966.
221. Cortes, E. P., and Holland, J. F.: Adjuvant chemotherapy for primary osteogenic sarcoma. Surg. Clin. North Am. 61:1391, 1981.
222. Dahlin, D. C., and Unni, K. K.: Osteosarcoma of bone and its important recognizable varieties. Am. J. Surg. Pathol. 1:61, 1977.
223. Eilber, F. R., and Morton, D. L.: Osteosarcoma: results of treatment employing adjuvant immunotherapy. Clin. Orthop. 111:94, 1975.
224. Watts, H. G.: Surgical management of malignant bone tumors in children. In Bone Tumors in Children. Jaffe, N. (ed.), Littleton, MA, PSG Publishing Co., 1979.
225. Pratt, C., Shanks, E., et al.: Adjuvant multiple drug chemotherapy for osteosarcoma of the extremity. Cancer 39:51, 1977.
226. Morton, D. L., Eilber, F. R., et al.: Limb salvage from a multidisciplinary treatment approach for skeletal and soft tissue sarcomas of the extremity. Ann. Surg. 184:268, 1976.
227. Marcove, R. C., and Rosen, G.: En bloc resections for osteogenic sarcoma. Cancer 45:3040, 1980.
227a. Jaffe, N., Murray, J., et al.: Limb salvage utilizing preoperative intra-arterial cis-diamminedichloroplatinum-II, local en bloc resection and endoprosthetic replacement in pediatric osteosarcoma. Proc. ASCO 5:802a, 1986.
228. Ettinger, L. J.: Osteosarcoma. Pediatr. Ann. 12:374, 1983.
229. Eilber, F. R.: Is amputation necessary for extremity sarcomas? A seven-year experience with limb salvage. Ann. Surg. 192:431, 1980.
230. Eilber, F. R., and Weisenburger, T.: Osteosarcoma. In Cancer Treatment, 2nd ed. Haskell, C. M. (ed.), Philadelphia, W. B. Saunders Co., 1985.
231. Suit, H. D.: Radiation therapy given under conditions of local tissue hypoxia for bone and soft tissue sarcoma. In Tumors of Bone and Soft Tissue (papers presented at Eighth Clinical Conference on Cancer, 1963, at the University

of Texas, M. D. Anderson Hospital and Tumor Institute). Chicago, Year Book Medical Publishers, 1965.
232. Sweetnam, R., Knowelden, J., et al.: Bone sarcoma: treatment by irradiation, amputation, or a combination of the two. Br. Med. J. 2:363, 1971.
233. Breuer, K., and Van der Schueren, E.: Adjuvant therapy in the management of osteosarcoma: need for critical reassessment. Rec. Results Cancer Res. 68:5, 1979.
234. Tefft, M., Chabora, B. M., et al.: Radiation in bone sarcomas. A reevaluation in the era of intensive systemic chemotherapy. Cancer 39:806, 1977.
235. Breuer, K., Cohen, P., et al.: Irradiation of the lungs as an adjuvant therapy in the treatment of osteosarcoma of the limbs. An EORTC randomized study. Eur. J. Cancer. 14:461, 1978.
236. Caceras, E., Zaharia, M., et al.: Adjuvant whole lung radiation with or without adriamycin treatment in osteogenic sarcoma. Cancer Treat. Rep. 62:297, 1978.
237. Rab, G. T., Ivins, J. C., et al.: Elective whole lung irradiation in the treatment of osteogenic sarcoma. Cancer 38:939, 1976.
238. Jaffe, N., Frei, E., III, et al.: High-dose methotrexate in osteogenic sarcoma: a 5-year experience. Cancer Treat. Rep. 62:259, 1978.
239. Cortes, E. P., Holland, J. F., et al.: Adriamycin (NSC-123127) in 87 patients with osteosarcoma. Cancer Chemother. Rep. 6:305, 1975.
240. Cortes, E. P., Holland, J. F., et al.: Amputation and adriamycin in primary osteosarcoma: a 5-year report. Cancer Treat. Rep. 62:271, 1978.
240a. Goorin, A. M., Abelson, H. T., et al.: Osteosarcoma: fifteen years later. New Engl. J. Med. 313:1637, 1985.
240b. Cortes, E. P., Holland, J. F., Glidewell, O.: Adjuvant therapy of operable primary osteosarcoma—cancer and Leukemia Group B experience. Recent Results Cancer Res. 68:16, 1978.
241. Herson, J., Sutow, W. W., et al.: Adjuvant chemotherapy in nonmetastatic osteosarcoma: a Southwest Oncology Group study. Med. Pediatr. Oncol. 8:343, 1980.
242. Benjamin, R. S., Baker, L. H., et al.: Chemotherapy for metastatic osteosarcoma—studies of the M. D. Anderson Hospital and the Southwest Oncology Group. Cancer Treat. Rep. 62:237, 1978.
243. Murphy, W. K., Benjamin, R. S., et al.: Adjuvant chemotherapy in osteosarcoma of adults. In *Adjuvant Chemotherapy of Cancer*. Salmon, S. E., and Jones, S. E. (eds.), Amsterdam, Elsevier/North Holland Biomedical Press, 1977.
244. Ettinger, L. J., Douglass, H. O. et al.: Adjuvant adriamycin and cisplatin in newly diagnosed, nonmetastatic osteosarcoma of an extremity. J. Clin. Oncol. 4:353, 1986.
245. Cortes, E. P., and Holland, J. F.: Adjuvant chemotherapy for primary osteogenic sarcoma. Surg. Clin. North Am. 61:1391, 1981.
246. Rosen, G., Marcove, R. C., et al.: Primary osteogenic sarcoma; the rationale for preoperative chemotherapy and delayed surgery. Cancer 43:2163, 1979.
247. Taylor, W. F., Ivins, J. C., et al.: Trends and variability in survival from osteosarcoma. Mayo Clin. Proc. 53:695, 1978.
248. Jaffe, N., van Eys, J., et al.: Response to: "Is it ethical not to conduct a prospectively controlled trial of adjuvant chemotherapy in osteosarcoma?" Cancer Treat. Rep. 67:743, 1983.
249. Cohen, M., Provisor, A., et al.: Efficacy of whole lung tomography in diagnosing metastases from solid tumors in children. Radiology 141:375, 1981.
250. Cohen, M., Grosfeld, J., et al.: Lung CT for detection of metastases: solid tissue neoplasms in children. AJR 139:895, 1982.
251. Edmonson, J. H., Green, S. J., et al.: A controlled pilot study of high-dose methotrexate as postsurgical adjuvant treatment for primary osteosarcoma. J. Clin. Oncol. 2:152, 1984.
252. Eilber, F. R., and Eckardt, J.: Adjuvant therapy for osteosarcoma: a randomized prospective trial. Proc. ASCO 4:C-561, 1985 (Abstr.).
252a. Link, M., Goorin, A., et al.: The effect of adjuvant chemotherapy on relapse-free survival in patients with osteosarcoma of an extremity. New Engl. J. Med. 314:1600, 1986.
253. Strander, H., Adamson, U., et al.: Adjuvant interferon treatment of human osteosarcoma. Rec. Results Cancer Res. 68:40, 1979.
254. Marcove, R. C., Mike, V., et al.: Vaccine trials for osteogenic sarcoma—a preliminary report. Cancer 23:74, 1973.
255. Price, M. R., Campbell, D. G., et al.: Characteristics of a cell surface antigen defined by an anti-human osteogenic sarcoma monoclonal antibody. Eur. J. Cancer Clin. Oncol. 19:81, 1983.
256. Rosenberg, S. A., Brown, J., et al.: Serologic studies of the antigens on human osteosarcoma cells. In *Serologic Analysis of Human Cancer Antigens*. Rosenberg, S. A. (ed.), New York, Academic Press, 1980.
257. Price, M. R., Pinum, M. V., et al.: Complement-dependent cytotoxicity of anti-human osteogenic sarcoma monoclonal antibodies. Br. J. Cancer 44:601, 1982.
258. Garnett, M. C., Embleton, M. J., et al.: Preparation and properties of a drug-carrier-antibody conjugate showing selective antibody-directed cytotoxicity in vitro. Int. J. Cancer 31:661, 1983.
259. Han, M., Telander, R. L., et al.: Aggressive thoracotomy for pulmonary metastatic osteogenic sarcoma in children and young adolescents. J. Pediatr. Surg. 16:928, 1981.
260. Schaller, R. T., Jr., Haas, J., et al.: Improved survival in children with osteosarcoma following resection of pulmonary metastases. J. Pediatr. Surg. 17:546, 1982.
261. Putnam, J. B., Jr., Roth, J. A., et al.: Survival following aggressive resection of pulmonary metastases from osteogenic sarcoma: analysis of prognostic factors. Ann. Thorac. Surg. 36:516, 1983.
262. Rosen, G., Marcove, R. C., et al.: Primary osteogenic sarcoma: eight-year experience with adjuvant chemotherapy. J. Cancer Res. Clin. Oncol. 106 (Suppl.):55, 1983.
263. Jaffe, N., Traggis, D., et al.: Favorable response of metastatic osteogenic sarcoma to pulse high-dose methotrexate with citrovorum rescue and radiation therapy. Cancer 31:1367, 1973.
264. Ochs, J. J., Freeman, A., et al.: Cis-dichlorodiammineplatinum (II) in advanced osteogenic sarcoma. Cancer Treat. Rep. 62:239, 1978.
265. Mosende, C., Gutierrez, M., et al.: Combination chemotherapy with bleomycin, cyclophosphamide, and dactinomycin for the treatment of osteogenic sarcoma. Cancer 40:2779, 1977.
266. Cortes, F. P., Holland, J. F., et al.: Doxorubicin in disseminated osteosarcoma J.A.M.A. 221:1132, 1972.
267. Rosen, G., Huvos, A. G., et al.: Chemotherapy and thoracotomy for metastatic osteogenic sarcoma. A model for adjuvant chemotherapy and the rationale for the timing of thoracic surgery. Cancer 41:841, 1978.
268. Soule, E. H., Newton, W., Jr., et al.: Extraskeletal Ewing's sarcoma. A preliminary review of 26 cases encountered in the Intergroup Rhabdomyosarcoma Study. Cancer 42:259, 1978.
269. Navas-Palacios, J. J., Aparicio-Duque, R., et al.: On the histogenesis of Ewing's sarcoma. An ultrastructural, immunohistochemical, and cytochemical study. Cancer 53:1882, 1984.
270. Aurias, A., Rimbaut, G., et al.: Translocation involving chromosome 22 in Ewing's sarcoma. A cytogenetic study of four fresh tumors. Cancer Genet, Cytogenet. 12:21, 1984.
271. Turc-Carel, C., Philip, I., et al.: Chromosome study of

Ewing's sarcoma (ES) cell lines. Consistency of a reciprocal translocation t(11;22)(q24; q12). Cancer Genet. Cytogenet. 12:1, 1984.
271a. Bechet, J. M., Bornkamm, G., et al.: The c-sis oncogene is not activated in Ewing's sarcoma. New Engl. J. Med. 310:393, 1984.
272. Trigg, M. E., Glaubiger, D., et al.: The frequency of isolated CNS involvement in Ewing's sarcoma. Cancer 49:2404, 1982.
273. Pomeroy, T. C., and Johnson, R. E.: Combined modality therapy of Ewing's sarcoma. Cancer 35:36, 1975.
274. Pritchard, D. J., Dahlin, D. C., et al.: Ewing's sarcoma. A clinocopathological and statistical analysis of patients surviving five years or longer. J. Bone Joint Surg. 57(A):10, 1975.
275. Glaubiger, D. L., Tepper, J., et al.: Ewing's sarcoma. In Cancer in the Young. Levine, A. S. (ed.), New York, Masson Publishing, 1982.
276. Glaubiger, D. L., Makuch, R. W., et al.: Influence of prognostic factors on survival in Ewing's sarcoma. Natl. Cancer Inst. Monogr. 56:285, 1981.
277. Gehan, E. A., Nesbit, M. E., et al.: Prognostic factors in children with Ewing's sarcoma. Natl. Cancer Inst. Monogr. 56:273, 1981.
278. Pritchard, D. J.: Indications for surgical treatment of localized Ewing's sarcoma of bone. Clin. Orthop. 153:39, 1980.
279. Phillips, R. E., and Higginbotham, N. L.: The curability of Ewing's endothelioma of bone in children. J. Pediatr. 70:391, 1967.
280. Graham-Pole, J.: Ewing sarcoma: treatment with high dose radiation and adjuvant chemotherapy. Med. Pediatr. Oncol. 7:1, 1979.
281. Zucker, J. M., Henry-Amar, M., et al.: Intensive systemic chemotherapy in localized Ewing's sarcoma in childhood. A historical trial. Cancer 52:415, 1983.
282. Thomas, P. R., Perez, C. A., et al.: The management of Ewing's sarcoma: role of radiotherapy in local tumor control. Cancer Treat. Rep. 68:703, 1984.
283. Marcove, R. S., and Rosen, G.: Radical en bloc excision of Ewing's sarcoma. Clin. Orthop. 153:86, 1980.
284. Rosen, G., Caparros, B., et al.: Ewing's sarcoma: ten-year experience with adjuvant chemotherapy. Cancer 47:2204, 1981.
285. Hayes, F. A., Thompson, E. I., et al.: The response of Ewing's sarcoma to sequential cyclophosphamide and Adriamycin induction therapy. J. Clin. Oncol. 1:45, 1983.
286. Razek, A., Perez, C. A., et al.: Intergroup Ewing's Sarcoma Study: local control related to radiation dose, volume, and site of primary lesion in Ewing's sarcoma. Cancer 46:516, 1980.
287. Perez, C. A., Tefft, M., et al.: The role of radiation therapy in the management of non-metastatic Ewing's sarcoma of bone. Report of the Intergroup Ewing's Sarcoma Study. Int. J. Radiat. Oncol. Biol. Phys. 7:141, 1981.
288. Cassady, J. R.: Ewing's sarcoma—the place of radiation therapy. In Bone Tumors in Children. Jaffe, N. (ed.), Littleton, MA, PSG Publishers, 1979.
289. Suit, H. D.: Role of therapeutic radiology in cancer of bone. Cancer 35:930, 1975.
290. Tefft, M., Chabora, B. M., et al.: Radiation in bone sarcomas—a reevaluation in the era of intensive systemic chemotherapy. Cancer 39:424, 1977.
291. Rosen, G., Wollner, N., et al.: Combination chemotherapy and radiation therapy in the treatment of metastatic osteogenic sarcoma treated with radiation therapy and adjuvant four-drug sequential chemotherapy. Cancer 33:384, 1974.
292. Jenkin, R. D. T.: Ewing's sarcoma. A study of treatment methods. Clin. Radiol. 17:97, 1966.
293. Haggard, M. E.: Cyclophosphamide (NSC 26271) in the treatment of children with malignant neoplasms. Cancer Chemother. Rep. 51:403, 1967.
294. Kofman, S., Perlia, C. P., et al.: Mithramycin in the treatment of metastatic Ewing's sarcoma. Cancer 31:889, 1973.
295. Sutow, W. W.: Vincristine therapy for malignant solid tumors in children (except Wilms' tumor). Cancer Chemother. Rep. 52:485, 1968.
296. Oldham, R. K., and Pomeroy, T. C.: Treatment of Ewing's sarcoma with Adriamycin (NSC-123127). Cancer Chemother. Rep. 56:635, 1972.
297. Palma, J., and Gailani, S.: Treatment of metastatic Ewing's sarcoma with BCNU. Cancer 30:909, 1972.
298. Nesbit, M. E., Jr., Perez, C. A., et al.: Multimodal therapy for the management of primary, nonmetastatic Ewing's sarcoma of bone: an Intergroup Study. Natl. Cancer Inst. Monogr. 56:255, 1981.
299. LeMevel, B. P., Hoerni, B., et al.: EORTC/GTO adjuvant chemotherapy program for primary Ewing's sarcoma: results at 5 years. Rec. Results Cancer Res. 68:52, 1979.
299a. Evans, R., Nesbit, M., et al.: Local recurrence, rate and sites of metastases, and time to relapse as a function of treatment regimen, size of primary and surgical history in 62 patients presenting with non-metastatic Ewing's sarcoma of the pelvic bones. Int. J. Radiat. Oncol. Biol. Phys. 11:129, 1985.
300. Kinsella, T. J., Lichter, A. S., et al.: Local treatment of Ewing's sarcoma: radiation therapy versus surgery. Cancer Treat. Rep. 68:695, 1984.
301. Tefft, M., Razek, A., et al.: Local control and survival related to radiation dose and volume and to chemotherapy in non-metastatic Ewing's sarcoma of pelvic bones. Int. J. Radiat. Oncol. Biol. Phys. 4:367, 1978.
302. Thomas, P. R. M., Foulkes, M. A., et al.: Primary Ewing's sarcoma of the ribs. A report from the Intergroup Rhabdomyosarcoma Study. Cancer 51:1021, 1983.
303. Pilepich, M. V., Vietti, T. S., et al.: Ewing's sarcoma of the vertebral column. Int. J. Radiat. Oncol. Biol. Phys. 7:27, 1981.
304. Mendenhall, C. N., Marcus, R. B., Jr., et al.: The prognostic significance of soft tissue extension in Ewing's sarcoma. Cancer 51:913, 1983.
305. Rosen, G., Caparros, B., et al.: Curability of Ewing's sarcoma and considerations for further therapeutic trials. Cancer 41:888, 1978.
306. Pilepich, M. V., Vietti, T. J., et al.: Radiotherapy and combination chemotherapy in advanced Ewing's sarcoma—Intergroup Study. Cancer 47:1930, 1981.
307. Jenkin, R. D. T., Rider, W. D., et al.: Ewing's sarcoma. A trial of adjuvant total body irradiation. Radiology 96:151, 1970.
308. Jenkin, R. D. T., Rider, W. D., et al.: Ewing's sarcoma. Adjuvant total body irradiation, cyclophosphamide, and vincristine. Int. J. Radiat. Oncol. Biol. Phys. 1:407, 1976.
309. Lombardi, F., Lattuada, A., et al.: Sequential half-body irradiation as systemic treatment of progressive Ewing's sarcoma. Int. J. Radiat. Oncol. Bio. Phys. 8:1679, 1982.
309a. Berry, M. P., Jenkin, R. D. T., et al.: Ewing's sarcoma: A trial of adjuvant chemotherapy and sequential half-body irradiation. Int. J. Radiat. Oncol. Biol. Phys. 12:19, 1986.
310. Cornbleet, M. A., Corringham, R. E. T., et al.: Treatment of Ewing's sarcoma with high-dose melphalan and autologous bone marrow transplantation. Cancer Treat. Rep. 65:241, 1981.
310a. Kinsella, T. J., Glaubiger, D., et al.: Intensive combined modality therapy including low-dose TBI in high-risk Ewing's sarcoma patients. Int. J. Radiat. Oncol. Biol. Phys. 9:1955, 1983.
311. Greene, M. H., Glaubiger, D. L., et al.: Subsequent cancer in patients with Ewing's sarcoma. Cancer Treat. Rep. 63:2043, 1979.
312. Strong, L. C., Herson, J., et al.: Risk of radiation-related subsequent malignant tumors in survivors of Ewing's sarcoma. J. Natl. Cancer Inst. 62:1401, 1979.

313. Brown, N. J.: Teratomas and germ cell tumors. J. Clin. Pathol. *29*:1021, 1976.
314. Dehner, L.: Gonadal and extragonadal germ cell neoplasia of childhood. Hum. Pathol. *14*:493, 1983.
314a. Bale, P. M.: Sacrococcygeal developmental abnormalities and tumors in children. Perspect. Pediatr. Pathol. *1*:9, 1984.
315. Berry, C. L., Keeling, J., et al.: Teratomata in infancy and childhood: a review of 91 cases. J. Pathol. *98*:241, 1969.
316. Kurman, R. J., and Norris, H. J.: Embryonal carcinoma of the ovary. A clinicopathologic entity distinct from endodermal sinus tumor resembling embryonal carcinoma of the adult testis. Cancer *38*:2420, 1976.
317. Kurman, R. J., and Norris, H. J.: Germ cell tumors of the ovary. Pathol. Annu. *13* (Part 1):291, 1978.
318. Wara, W. M., Jenkins, R. D. T., et al.: Tumors of the pineal and suprasellar region: Children's Cancer Study Group treatment result, 1960–1975. Cancer *43*:698, 1979.
319. Roth, L. M., and Panganiban, W. G.: Gonadal and extragonadal yolk sac carcinomas. A clinicopathologic study of 14 cases. Cancer *37*:812, 1976.
320. Kurman, R. J., Scardino, P. T., et al.: Malignant germ cell tumors of the ovary and testis: an immunohistologic study of 69 cases. Ann. Clin. Lab. Sci. *9*:462, 1979.
321. Kurman, R. J., Scardino, P. T., et al.: Cellular localization of alpha-fetoprotein and human chorionic gonadotropin in germ cell tumors of the testis using an indirect immunoperoxidase technique. A new approach to classification utilizing tumor markers. Cancer *40*:2136, 1977.
322. Witzleben, C. L., and Bruninga, G.: Infantile choriocarcinoma: a characteristic syndrome. J. Pediatr. *73*:374, 1968.
323. Hayashi, F., Bracken, M. B., et al.: Hydatidiform mole in the United States (1970–1977): a statistical and theoretical analysis. Am. J. Epidemiol. *115*:67, 1982.
324. Scully, R. E.: Gonadoblastoma: a review of 74 cases. Cancer *25*:1340, 1970.
325. Mandell, J., Stevens, P. S., et al.: Childhood gonadoblastoma and seminoma in a dysgenetic cryptorchid gonad. J. Urol. *117*:674, 1977.
326. Robboy, S. J., Miller, T., et al.: Dysgenesis of testicular and streak gonads in the syndrome of mixed gonadal dysgenesis: perspective derived from a clinicopathologic analysis of twenty-one cases. Hum. Pathol. *13*:700, 1982.
326a. Ulbright, T. M., Loehrer, P. J., et al.: The development of non-germ cell malignancies within germ cell tumors. A clinicopathologic study of 11 cases. Cancer *54*:1824, 1984.
326b. Nichols, C. R., Hoffman, R., et al.: Hematologic malignancies associated with primary mediastinal germ-cell tumors. Ann. Intern. Med. *102*:603, 1985.
327. Ashley, D. J. B.: Origin of teratomas. Cancer *32*:390, 1973.
328. Gelb, A., Rosenblum, H., et al.: Sacrococcygeal teratoma. Del. Med. J. *36*:119, 1964.
329. Allen, J. E.: Teratomas in infants and children. In *Cancer Medicine*. Holland, J. F., and Frei, E., III (eds.), Philadelphia, Lea & Febiger, 1973.
330. Gross, R. E., Clatworthy, H. W., Jr. et al.: Sacrococcygeal teratomas in infants and children. A report of 40 cases. Surg. Gynecol. Obstet. *92*:341, 1951.
331. Donnellan, W. A., and Swenson, O.: Benign and malignant sacrococcygeal teratomas. Surgery *64*:834, 1968.
332. Noseworthy, J., Lack, E. E., et al.: Sacrococcygeal germ cell tumors in childhood: an updated experience with 118 patients. J. Pediatr. Surg. *16*:358, 1981.
333. Valdiserri, R. O., and Yunis, E. J.: Sacrococcygeal teratomas: a review of 68 cases. Cancer *48*:217, 1981.
334. Gonzalez-Crussi, F., Winkler, R. F., et al.: Sacrococcygeal teratomas in infants and children; relationship of histology and prognosis in 40 cases. Arch. Pathol. Lab. Med. *102*:420, 1978.
335. Altman, R. P., Randolph, J. G., et al.: Sacrococcygeal teratomas: American Academy of Pediatrics Surgical Section Survey, 1973. J. Pediatr. Surg. *9*:389, 1974.
336. Raney, R. B. Jr., Chatten, J., et al.: Treatment strategies for infants with malignant sacrococcygeal teratoma. J. Pediatr. Surg. *16*:573, 1981.
337. Beddis, I. R., Noblett, H., et al.: Effective chemotherapy for metastatic malignant sacrococcygeal tumor. Med. Pediatr. Oncol. *12*:231, 1984.
337a. Pinkerton, C. R., Pritchard, J., et al.: High complete response rate in children with advanced germ cell tumors using cisplatin-containing combination chemotherapy. J. Clin. Oncol. *4*:194, 1986.
338. Towne, B. H., Mahour, G. H., et al.: Ovarian cysts and tumors in infancy and childhood. J. Pediatr. Surg. *10*:311, 1975.
339. Kurman, R. J., and Norris, H. J.: Malignant germ cell tumors of the ovary. Hum. Pathol. *8*:551, 1977.
340. Robboy, S. J., and Scully, R. E.: Ovarian teratoma with glial implants on the peritoneum. Hum. Pathol. *1*:643, 1970.
341. Erickson, R. P., and Gondos, B.: Alternative explanations of the differing behavior of ovarian and testicular teratomas. Lancet *1*:407, 1976.
342. Asadourian, L. A., and Taylor, H. B.: Dysgerminoma: an analysis of 105 cases. Obstet. Gynecol. *33*:370, 1969.
343. Talerman, A.: Germ cell tumors of the ovary. In *Pathology of the Female Genital Tract*, 2nd ed. Blaustein, A. (ed.), New York, Springer-Verlag, 1982.
344. Barber, H. R. K., and Kwon, R. H.: Current status of the treatment of gynecologic cancer by site: ovary. Cancer *38*:610, 1976.
345. Slayton, R. E.: Management of germ cell and stromal tumors of the ovary. Semin. Oncol. *11*:299, 1984.
346. Smith, J. P., Rutledge, F., et al.: Malignant gynecologic tumors in children: current approaches to treatment. Am. J. Obstet. Gynecol. *116*:261, 1973.
347. Krepart, G., Smith, J. P., et al.: The treatment for dysgerminoma of the ovary. Cancer *41*:986, 1928.
348. Barber, H. R. K.: Ovarian cancer: diagnosis and management. Am. J. Obstet. Gynecol. *150*:910, 1984.
349. Weinblatt, M. E., and Ortega, J. A.: Treatment of children with dysgerminoma of the ovary. Cancer *49*:2608, 1982.
350. Lack, E. M., and Goldstein, D. P.: Primary ovarian tumors in childhood and adolescence. Curr. Prob. Obstet. Gynecol. *7*:10, 1984.
351. Norris, H. J., Zirkin, H. J., et al.: Immature (malignant) teratoma of the ovary. A clinical and pathologic study of 58 cases. Cancer *37*:2359, 1976.
352. Cangir, A., Smith, J., et al.: Improved prognosis in children with ovarian cancer following modified VAC (vincristine sulfate, dactinomycin, and cyclophosphamide) chemotherapy. Cancer *42*:1234, 1978.
353. Jereb, B., Wollner, N., et al.: Radiation in multidisciplinary treatment of children with malignant ovarian tumors. Cancer *43*:1037, 1979.
354. Slayton, R. E., Hreshchyshyn, M. M., et al.: Treatment of malignant ovarian germ cell tumors. Response to vincristine, dactinomycin, and cyclophosphamide (preliminary report). Cancer *42*:390, 1978.
355. Vriesendorp, R., Aalders, J. G., et al.: Treatment of malignant germ cell tumors of the ovary with cisplatin, vinblastine, and bleomycin (PVB). Cancer Treat. Rep. *68*:775, 1984.
356. Taylor, M. H., Depetrillo, A. D., et al.: Vinblastine, bleomycin, and cisplatin in malignant germ cell tumors of the ovary. Cancer *56*:1341, 1985.
357. Kurman, R. J., and Norris, H. J.: Endodermal sinus tumor of the ovary. A clinical and pathologic analysis of 71 cases. Cancer *38*:2404, 1976.

358. Lakey, J. L., Baker, J. J., et al.: Cisplatin, vinblastine, and bleomycin for endodermal sinus tumor of the ovary. Ann. Intern. Med. 94:56, 1981.
359. Green, D. M.: The diagnosis and treatment of yolk sac tumors in infants and children. Cancer Treat. Rev. 10:265, 1983.
360. Ungerleider, R. S., Donaldson, S. S., et al.: Endodermal sinus tumor. The Stanford experience and the first reported case arising in the vulva. Cancer 41:1627, 1978.
360a. Gallion, H., VanNagell, J. R., Jr., et al.: Therapy of endodermal sinus tumor of the ovary. Am. J. Obstet. Gynecol. 135:447, 1979.
360b. Karlen, J. R., and Kastelic, J. E.: Endodermal sinus tumor of the ovary. An improving prognosis. Gynecol. Oncol. 10:206, 1980.
360c. Smith, E. B., Clarke-Pearson, D. L., et al.: A VP-16-213-cisplatin-containing regimen for treatment of refractory ovarian germ cell malignancies. Am. J. Obstet. Gynecol. 150:927, 1984.
361. Exelby, P. R.: Testis cancer in children. Semin. Oncol. 6:116, 1979.
362. Johnson, D. E. (ed.): *Testicular Tumors*, 2nd ed. Flushing, NY, Medical Examination Publishing Co., 1976.
363. Brosman, S. A.: Testicular tumors in prepubertal children. Urology 13:581, 1979.
364. Colodny, A., and Hopkins, T. B.: Testicular tumors in infants and children. Urol. Clin. North Am. 4:347, 1977.
365. Viprakasit, D., Navarro, C., et al.: Seminoma in children. Urology 9:568, 1977.
366. Bracken, R. B., and Johnson, D. E., et al.: Regional lymph nodes in infants with embryonal carcinoma of testis. Urology 11:376, 1978.
367. Boden, G., and Gibb, R.: Radiotherapy and testicular neoplasms. Lancet 2:1195, 1951.
368. Maier, J. G., and Sulak, M. H.: Radiation therapy in malignant testis tumors. Cancer 32:1212, 1973.
368a. Javadpour, N., and Young, J.: Prognostic factors in nonseminomatous testicular cancer. J. Urol. 135:497, 1986.
369. Filler, R. M., and Hardy, B. E.: Testicular tumors in children. World J. Surg. 4:63, 1980.
370. Jamieson, J. K., and Dobson, J. F.: The lymphatics of the testicle. Lancet 1:493, 1910.
371. Staubitz, W. J., Early, K. S., et al.: Surgical management of testis tumors. J. Urol. 111:205, 1974.
372. Ray, B., Hajdu, S. I., et al.: Distribution of retroperitoneal lymph node metastases in testicular germinal tumors. Cancer 33:340, 1974.
373. Maier, J. G., van Buskirk, K. E., et al.: An evaluation of lymphadenectomy in the treatment of malignant testicular germ cell neoplasms. Trans. Am. Assoc. Genitourin. Surg. 60:71, 1968.
374. Richie, J. P., and Garnick, M. B.: Changing concepts in the treatment of nonseminomatous germ cell tumors of the testis. J. Urol. 131:1089, 1984.
375. Vugrin, D., Whitmore, W. F., Jr., et al.: VAB-6 combination chemotherapy without maintenance in treatment of disseminated cancer of the testis. Cancer 51:211, 1983.
376. Jeffs, R. D.: Management of embryonal adenocarcinoma of the testis in childhood: an analysis of 164 cases. In *Cancer in Childhood*. Gooden, J. A., (ed.), Toronto, The Ontario Cancer Treatment and Research Foundation, 1972.
377. Drago, J. R., Nelson, R. P., et al.: Childhood embryonal carcinoma of testes. Urology 12:499, 1978.
377a. Flamant, F., and Diez, B.: Cure of testicular stage I yolk sac tumor (endodermal sinus tumor) in children by conservative treatment. Proc. ASCO 4:Abstr. C:916, 1985.
378. Garnick, M.: Personal communication.
379. Hainsworth, J. D., and Greco, F. A.: Testicular germ-cell neoplasms. Am. J. Med. 75:817, 1983.
380. Einhorn, L.: Testicular cancer as a model for a curable neoplasm: the Richard and Hinda Rosenthal Foundation Award Lecture. Cancer Res. 41:3275, 1981.
381. Donohue, J. P.: Editorial comment. J. Urol. 131:1092, 1984.
382. Sogani, P. C., Whitmore, W. F., Jr., et al.: Orchiectomy alone in the treatment of clinical stage I nonseminomatous germ cell tumor of the testis. J. Clin. Oncol. 2:267, 1984.
383. Peckham, M. J., Barret, A., et al.: Orchiectomy alone in testicular stage I nonseminomatous germ cell tumors. Lancet 2:678, 1982.
383a. Pizzocaro, G., Zanomi, F., et al.: Orchiectomy alone in clinical Stage I nonseminomatous testis cancer: a critical appraisal. J. Clin. Oncol. 4:35, 1986.
383b. Hoskin, P., Dilly, S., et al.: Prognostic factors in Stage I non-seminomatous germ-cell testicular tumors managed by orchiectomy and surveillance: implications for adjuvant chemotherapy. J. Clin. Oncol. 4:1031, 1986.
383c. Garnick, M., Richie, J. P.: Toward more rational management for Stage I testis cancer: watch out for "watch and wait"! J. Clin. Oncol. 4:1021, 1986.
383d. Medical Research Council Working Party on Testicular Tumours: Prognostic factors in advanced non-seminomatous germ-cell testicular tumours: Results of a multicentre study. Lancet 1:8, 1985.
383e. Ozols, R. F., Ihde, D., et al.: Randomized trial of PVe BV [high dose (HD) cisplatin (P), vinblastine (Ve), bleomycin (B), VP-16 (V)] versus testicular cancer (NSTC). Proc. Soc. Clin. Oncol. 3:155, 1984.
384. DeWys, W. D., Green, S. B., et al.: Prediction of nodal involvement and of relapse after lymphadenectomy in early stage testicular cancer. Proc. ASCO 2:Abstr. C-525, 1983.
385. Varini, M., and Cavelli, F.: Etoposide for therapy-resistant testicular tumors. Cancer Treat. Rev. 9:1, 1982.
385a. Logothetis, C. J., Samuels, M. L., et al.: Primary chemotherapy followed by selective retroperitoneal lymphadenectomy in the management of clinical stage II testicular carcinoma: a preliminary report. J. Urol. 134:1127, 1985.
385b. Javadpour, N.: Predictors of recurrence in Stage II nonseminomatous testicular cancer after lymphadenectomy: implications for adjuvant chemotherapy. J. Urol. 134:629, 1985.
386. Einhorn, L. H., and Donohue, J.: Cis-diamminedichloroplatinum, vinblastine, bleomycin combination chemotherapy in disseminated testicular cancer. Ann. Intern. Med. 87:293, 1977.
387. Einhorn, L., Williams, S. D., et al.: The role of maintenance therapy in disseminated testicular cancer. New Engl. J. Med. 305:727, 1981.
387a. Bosl, G. J., Gluckman, R., et al.: VAB-6: an effective chemotherapy regimen for patients with germ cell tumors. J. Clin. Oncol. 4:1493, 1986.
388. Ozols, R. F., Deisseroth, A. B., et al.: Treatment of poor prognosis nonseminomatous testicular cancer with a "high dose" platinum combination chemotherapy regimen. Cancer 51:1803, 1983.
388a. Logothetis, C. J., Samuels, M. L., et al.: Improved survival with cyclic chemotherapy for nonseminomatous germ cell tumors of the testis. J. Clin. Oncol. 3:326, 1985.
389. Anderson, T. (moderator): Testicular germ-cell neoplasms: recent advances in diagnosis and therapy. Ann. Intern. Med. 90:373, 1979.
390. Fraley, E. E., Lange, P. H., et al.: Germ cell testicular cancer in adults. New Engl. J. Med. 301:1370, 1420, 1979.
391. Einhorn, L.: Management of difficult and unusual problems in testicular cancer. Paper Presented at the Nineteenth Annual ASCO Meeting, May, 1983.
392. Ball, D., Barrett, A., et al.: The management of metastatic seminoma testis. Cancer 50:2289, 1982.

393. Stanton, G. F., Bosl, G. J., et al.: Treatment of patients (pts) with advanced seminoma with cyclophosphamide, bleomycin, actinomycin D, vinblastine, and cisplatin (VAB-6). Proc. Am. Soc. Clin. Oncol. 2:141, 1983. (Abstr.).
394. Daugaard, G., Rorth, M., et al.: Therapy of extragonadal germ-cell tumors. Eur. J. Cancer Clin. Oncol. 19:859, 1983.
395. Aygun, C., Slawson, R. O., et al.: Primary mediastinal seminoma. Urology 23:109, 1984.
396. Bush, S. E., Martinez, A., et al.: Primary mediastinal seminoma. Cancer 48:1877, 1981.
397. Feun, L. G., Samson, M. K., et al.: Vinblastine (VLB) Bleomycin (BLEO), cis-diamminedichloro-platinum (DDP) in disseminated extragonadal germ cell tumors. A Southwest Oncology Group Study. Cancer 45:2543, 1980.
398. Hainsworth, J. D., Einhorn, L. H., et al.: Advanced extragonadal germ cell tumors. Successful treatment with combination chemotherapy. Ann. Intern. Med. 97:7, 1982.
399. Logothetis, C. J., Samuels, M. L., et al.: Chemotherapy of extragonadal germ cell tumors. J. Clin. Oncol. 3:316, 1985.
399a. Noronha, P. A., Noronha, R., et al.: Primary anterior mediastinal endodermal sinus tumors in childhood. Am. J. Pediatr. Hematol. Oncol. 7:312, 1985.
399b. Truong, L. D., Harris, L., et al.: Endodermal sinus tumor of the mediastinum. A report of seven cases and review of the literature. Cancer 58:730, 1986.
400. Carter, D., Bibro, M. C., et al.: Benign clinical behavior of immature mediastinal teratoma in infancy and childhood: report of two cases and review of the literature. Cancer 49:398, 1982.
401. Hajdu, S. I., Farugue, A. A., et al.: Teratoma of the neck in infants. Am. J. Dis. Child. 111:412, 1966.
402. Hurlbut, J. H., Webb, H. W., et al.: Cervical teratoma in infant siblings. J. Pediatr. Surg. 5:460, 1970.
403. Gundry, S. R., Wesley, J. R., et al.: Cervical teratomas in the newborn. J. Pediatr. Surg. 18:382, 1983.
403a. Lack, E. E.: Extragonadal germ cell tumors of the head and neck region: review of 16 cases. Hum. Pathol. 16:56, 1985.
404. Polsky, M. S., Shackelford, G. D., et al.: Retroperitoneal teratoma. Urology 8:618, 1976.
405. Dehner, L. P.: Intrarenal teratoma occurring in infancy: report of a case with discussion of extragonadal germ cell tumors in infancy. J. Pediatr. Surg. 8:369, 1973.
406. Weinberg, A. G., and Finegold, M. J.: Primary hepatic tumors of childhood. Hum. Pathol. 14:512, 1983.
407. Lack, E. E., Neave, C., et al.: Hepatoblastoma: a clinical and pathological study of 54 cases. Am. J. Surg. Pathol. 6:693, 1982.
408. Watanabe, I.: Histopathologic features of liver cell carcinoma in infancy and childhood and their relations to surgical prognosis. Jpn. J. Cancer Clin. 23:691, 1977.
409. Berman, M. M., Libbey, N. P., et al.: Hepatocellular carcinoma: polygonal cell type with fibrous stroma—an atypical variant with a favorable prognosis. Cancer 46:1448, 1980.
410. Farhi, D. C., Shikes, R. H., et al.: Hepatocellular carcinoma in young people. Cancer 52:1516, 1983.
411. Stocker, J. T., and Ishak, K. G.: Undifferentiated (embryonal) sarcoma of the liver. Report of 31 cases. Cancer 42:336, 1978.
412. Fraumeni, C. F., Jr., Miller, R. W., et al.: Primary carcinoma of the liver in childhood: an epidemiologic study. J. Natl. Cancer Inst. 40:1087, 1968.
413. Szmuness, W.: Hepatocellular carcinoma and the hepatitis B virus—evidence for a causal association. Prog. Med. Virol. 24:40, 1978.
414. Landing, B. H.: Tumors of the liver in childhood. In Hepatocellular Carcinoma. Okuda, K., and Peters, R. (eds.), New York, John Wiley & Sons, 1976.
415. Rubel, L. R., Ishak, K. G., et al.: α_1-antitrypsin deficiency and hepatocellular carcinoma. Arch. Pathol. Lab. Med. 106:678, 1982.
416. Ugarte, N., and Gonzalez-Crussi, F.: Hepatoma in siblings with progressive familial cholestatic cirrhosis of childhood. Am. J. Clin. Pathol. 76:172, 1981.
417. Weinberg, A. G., Mize, C. E., et al.: The occurrence of hepatoma in the chronic form of hereditary tyrosinemia. J. Pediatr. 88:434, 1976.
418. Edman, J. C., Gray, P., et al.: Integration of hepatitis B virus sequences and their expression in a human hepatoma cell. Nature 286:535, 1980.
419. Larouze, B., Saimot, G., et al.: Host responses to hepatitis-B infection in patients with primary hepatic carcinoma and their families. Lancet 2:534, 1976.
420. Linsell, A.: The mycotoxins as a human health hazard. In Human Cancer. Its Characterization and Treatment. Vol. 5 of Advances in Tumour Prevention, Detection, and Characterization. Davis, W., Harrap, K. R., et al. (eds.), Amsterdam, Excerpta Medica, 1980, pp. 114–120.
421. Ishak, K. G.: Primary hepatic tumors in childhood. In Progress in Liver Disease, Vol. 5. Popper, H., and Schaffner, F. (eds.), New York, Grune & Stratton, 1976.
422. Ruoslahti, E., and Hirai, H.: Alpha-fetoprotein. Scand. J. Immunol. 8(Suppl. 8):3, 1978.
423. Altman, D.: Hepatoma—Medical Staff Conference, University of California, San Francisco. West. J. Med. 132:514, 1980.
424. Tsukada, Y., Bischof, W. K. D., et al.: Effect of a conjugate of daunomycin and antibodies to rat-α-fetoprotein on the growth of α-fetoprotein–producing tumor cells. Proc. Natl. Acad. Sci. USA 79:621, 1982.
425. Murthy, A. S., Vawter, G. F., et al.: Biochemical studies on liver tumors in children. Arch. Pathol. 96:48, 1973.
426. Exelby, P. R., el-Domeri, A., et al.: Primary malignant tumors of the liver in children. J. Pediatr. Surg. 6:272, 1971.
427. Exelby, P. R., Filler, R. M., et al.: Liver tumors in children with particular reference to hepatoblastoma and hepatocellular carcinoma: American Academy of Pediatrics Surgical Section Survey, 1974. J. Pediatr. Surg. 10:329, 1975.
428. Randolph, J., Chandra, R., et al.: Malignant liver tumors in infants and children. World J. Surg. 4:71, 1980.
429. Lin, T., Chen, C., et al.: Primary carcinoma of the liver in infancy and childhood. Surgery 60:1275, 1966.
430. Weinblatt, M. E., Siegel, S. E., et al.: Preoperative chemotherapy for unresectable primary hepatic malignancies in children. Cancer 50:1061, 1982.
431. Hermann, R. E., and Lonsdale, D.: Chemotherapy, radiotherapy, and hepatic lobectomy for hepatoblastoma in an infant: report of a survival. Surgery 68:383, 1970.
432. Ikeda, K., Suita, S., et al.: Preoperative chemotherapy for initially unresectable hepatoblastoma in children. Arch. Surg. 114:203, 1979.
433. Shafer, A. D., and Selinkoff, P. M.: Preoperative irradiation and chemotherapy for initially unresectable hepatoblastoma. J. Pediatr. Surg. 12:1001, 1977.
434. Nolan, T. R., Grady, E. D., et al.: Internal hepatic radiotherapy. Am. J. Roentgenol. 124:590, 1975.
435. Order, S. E., Ettinger, D., et al.: Radiolabeled antibodies in the treatment of hepatic malignancies. Radiat. Oncol. Biol. Phys. 8:121, 1982.
436. Lascari, A. D.: Vincristine therapy in a child with probable hepatoblastoma. Pediatrics 45:109, 1970.
437. Tan, C., Rosen, G., et al.: Adriamycin (NSC-123127) in pediatric malignancies. Cancer Chemother. Rep. 6:259, 1975.
438. Olweny, C. L., Toya, T., et al.: Treatment of hepatocellular carcinoma with Adriamycin. Cancer 36:1250, 1975.
439. Pritchard, J., da Cunha, A., et al.: Alpha Feto (α FP) monitoring of response to Adriamycin in hepatoblastoma. J. Pediatr. Surg. 17:429, 1982.
440. Siegel, M. M., Siegel, S. E., et al.: Primary chemothera-

peutic management of unresectable and metastatic hepatoblastoma in children: report of four cases. Med. Pediatr. Oncol. *4*:297, 1978.
441. Evans, A. E., Land, V. J., et al.: Combination chemotherapy (vincristine, adriamycin, cyclophosphamide and 5-fluorouracil) in the treatment of children with malignant hepatoma. Cancer *50*:821, 1982.
442. Quinn, J. J., Altman, A. J., et al.: Adriamycin and cisplatin for hepatoblastoma. Cancer *56*:1926, 1985.
443. Holton, C. P., Burrington, J. D., et al.: A Multiple chemotherapeutic approach to the management of hepatoblastoma—a preliminary report. Cancer *35*:1083, 1975.
444. Kyritsis, A. P., Tsokos, M., et al.: Retinoblastoma—origin from a primitive neuroectodermal cell? Nature *307*:471, 1984.
445. Molnar, M. L., Stefansson, K., et al.: Immunohistochemistry of retinoblastomas in humans. Am. J. Ophthalmol. *97*:301, 1984.
446. Bader, J. L., Miller, R. W., et al.: Trilateral retinoblastoma. Lancet *1*:582, 1980.
447. Ts'o, M. O. M., Zimmerman, L. E., et al.: The nature of retinoblastoma. II. Photoreceptor differentiation. An electron microscopic study. Am. J. Ophthalmol. *69*:350, 1970.
448. Donaldson, S. S.: Retinoblastoma. In *Cancer in the Young*. Levine, A. S. (ed)., New York, Masson Publishing, 1982.
449. Kitchin, F. D.: Genetics of retinoblastoma. In *Tumors of the Eye*, 3rd ed. Reese, A. B. (ed), New York, Harper & Row, 1976.
450. Nussbaum, R., and Puck, J.: Recurrence risks for retinoblastoma: a model for autosomal dominant disorders with complex inheritance. J. Pediatr. Ophthalmol. *13*:89, 1976.
451. Abramson, D. H., Notterman, R. B., et al.: Retinoblastoma treated in infants in the first six months of life. Arch. Ophthalmol. *101*:1362, 1983.
452. Yunis, J. J., and Ramsay, N. K.: Retinoblastoma and subband deletion of chromosome 13. Am. J. Dis. Child. *132*:161, 1978.
453. Sparkes, R. S., Sparkes, M. C., et al.: Regional assignment of genes for human esterase D and retinoblastoma to chromosome band 13q14. Science *208*:1042, 1980.
454. Sparkes, R. S., Murphree, A. L., et al.: Gene for hereditary retinoblastoma assigned to human chromosome 13 by linkage to esterase D. Science *219*:971, 1983.
455. Benedict, W. F., Murphree, A. L., et al.: Patient with 13 chromosome deletion: evidence that the retinoblastoma gene is a recessive cancer gene. Science *219*:973, 1983.
456. Cavenee, W. K., Dryja, T. P., et al.: Expression of recessive alleles by chromosomal mechanisms in retinoblastoma. Nature *305*:779, 1983.
457. Murphree, A. L., and Benedict, W. F.: Retinoblastoma: clues to human oncogenesis. Science *223*:1028, 1984.
458. Dryja, T. P., Cavenee, W., et al.: Homozygosity of chromosome 13 in retinoblastoma. New Engl. J. Med. *310*:550, 1984.
459. Godbout, R., Dryja, T. P., et al.: Somatic inactivation of genes on chromosome 13 is a common event in retinoblastoma. Nature *304*:451, 1983.
459a. Murphree, A. L., and Benedict, W. F.: Retinoblastoma: clues to human oncogenesis. Science *223*:1028, 1984.
460. Squire, J., Phillips, R. A., et al.: Isochromosome 6p, a unique chromosomal abnormality in retinoblastoma: verification by standard staining techniques, new densitometric methods, and somatic cell hybridization. Hum. Genet. *66*:46, 1984.
460a. Potluri, V. R., Helson, L., et al.: Chromosomal abnormalities in retinoblastoma. A review. Cancer *58*:663, 1986.
461. Knudson, D.: Genetics and the etiology of childhood cancer. Pediatr. Res. *10*:513, 1976.
461a. Friend, S. H., and Bernards, R.: A human DNA segment with properties of the gene that predisposes to retinoblastoma and osteosarcoma. Nature *323*:643, 1986.
461b. Cavenee, W. K., Murphree, A. L., et al.: Prediction of familial predisposition to retinoblastoma. New Engl. J. Med. *314*:1201, 1986.
462. Abramson, D. H., Ellsworth, R. M., et al.: Nonocular cancer in retinoblastoma survivors. Trans. Am. Acad. Ophthalmol. Otolaryngol. *81*:454, 1976.
462a. Abramson, D. H., Eilsworth, R. M., et al.: Second nonocular tumors in retinoblastoma survivors: are they radiation induced? Ophthalmology *91*:1351, 1984.
463. Ellsworth, R. M: The practical management of retinoblastoma. Trans. Am. Ophthalmol. Soc. *67*:462, 1969.
464. Ellsworth, R. M.: Retinoblastoma. Mod. Probl. Ophthalmol. *18*:94, 1977.
465. Ellsworth, R. M.: Staging and treatment of retinoblastoma. Paper Presented at the Ninth Annual Meeting of International Society of Pediatric Oncology, Philadelphia, 1977.
466. Schantz, P. M., Meyer, D., et al.: Clinical serologic and epidemiologic characteristics of ocular toxocariasis. Am. J. Trop. Med. Hyg. *28*:24, 1979.
467. Dias, P. L. R.: Prognostic significance of aqueous humour lactic dehydrogenase activity. Br. J. Ophthalmol. *63*:571, 1979.
468. Goldberg, L., and Danziger, A.: Computed tomographic scanning in the management of retinoblastoma. Am. J. Ophthalmol. *84*:380, 1977.
469. Reese, A. B., and Ellsworth, R. M.: The evaluation and current concept of retinoblastoma therapy. Trans. Am. Acad. Ophthalmol. Otolaryngol. *67*:164, 1963.
470. Bedford, M. A., Bedotto, C., et al.: Retinoblastoma: a study of 139 cases. Br. J. Ophthalmol. *55*:19, 1971.
471. Redler, L. D., and Ellsworth, R. M.: Prognostic importance of choroidal invasion in retinoblastoma. Arch. Ophthalmol. *90*:294, 1973.
471a. Kingston, J. E., Plowman, P. N., et al.: Ectopic intracranial retinoblastoma in children. Br. J. Ophthalmol. *69*:10, 1985.
471b. Johnson, D. L., Chandra, R., et al.: Trilateral retinoblastoma: ocular pineal retinoblastomas. J. Neurosurg. *63*:367, 1985.
472. Stannard, C., Lipper, S., et al.: Retinoblastoma: correlation of invasion of the optic nerve and choroid with prognosis and metastases. Br. J. Ophthalmol. *63*:560, 1979.
473. Rosenbaum, A. L., Arenson, E. B., et al.: Retinoblastoma. In *Cancer Treatment*, 2nd ed. Haskell, C. M. (ed.), Philadelphia, W. B. Saunders Co., 1985.
474. Wolff, J. A., Boesel, C. P., et al.: Treatment of retinoblastoma. A preliminary report. In *Pediatric Oncology: Proceedings of the XIIIth Meeting of the International Society of Pediatric Oncology, Marseilles, September 15–19, 1981*. Raybaud, C., Clement, R., et al. (eds.) Amsterdam, Excerpta Medica, 1982.
474a. Abramson, D. H., Ellsworth, R. M., et al.: Retinoblastoma: survival, age at detection and comparison 1914–1958, 1958–1983. J. Pediatr. Ophthalmol. Strabismus *22*:246, 1985.
475. Tapley, N. du V and Tretter, P.: Retinoblastoma. In *Clinical Pediatric Oncology*. Sutow, W. W., Vietti, T. J., et al. (eds.), St. Louis, C. V. Mosby, 1973.
476. Cassady, J. R.: Personal communication.
477. Cassady, J. R., Sagerman, R. H., et al.: Radiation therapy in retinoblastoma. *93*:405, 1969.
478. Migdal, C.: Bilateral retinoblastoma: the prognosis for vision. Br. J. Ophthalmol. *67*:592, 1983.
479. Abramson, D. H., Ellsworth, R. M., et al.: Treatment of bilateral groups I through III retinoblastoma with bilateral radiation. Arch. Ophthalmol. *99*:1761, 1981.
480. Abramson, D. H., Ellsworth, R. M., et al.: Simultaneous bilateral radiation for advanced bilateral retinoblastoma. Arch. Ophthalmol. *99*:1763, 1981.

481. Salmonsen, P. C., Ellsworth, R. M., et al.: The occurrence of new retinoblastoma after treatment. Ophthalmology (Rochester) *86*:837, 1979.
482. Höpping, W., and Meyer-Schwickerath, G.: Light coagulation treatment in retinoblastoma. In: *Ocular and Adrenal Tumors*. Boniuk, M. (ed.), St. Louis, C.V. Mosby, 1964.
483. Margo, C., Hidayat, A. A., et al.: Cryotherapy and photocoagulation in the management of retinoblastoma: treatment failure and unusual complication. Ophthalmic Surg. *14*:336, 1983.
484. Char, D.: Current concepts in retinoblastoma. Ann. Ophthalmol. *12*:792, 1980.
485. Tolentino, F. L., Jr., and Tablante, R. T.: Cryotherapy of retinoblastoma. Arch. Ophthalmol. *87*:52, 1972.
486. Stannard, C. E., Sealy, R., et al.: Treatment of malignant meningitis in retinoblastoma. Br. J. Ophthalmol. *59*:362, 1975.
487. Freeman, C. R., Esseltine, D. L., et al.: Retinoblastoma: the case for radiotherapy and adjuvant chemotherapy. Cancer *46*:1913, 1980.
488. Lonsdale, D., Berry, D. H., et al.: Chemotherapeutic trials in patients with metastatic retinoblastoma. Cancer Chemother. Rep. *52*:631, 1968.
489. Wolff, J. A., Pratt, C. B., et al.: Chemotherapy of metastatic retinoblastoma. Cancer Chemother. Rep. *16*:435, 1962.
490. Sitarz, A. L., Heyn, R., et al.: Triple drug therapy with actinomycin D (NSC-3053), chlorambucil (NSC-3088), and methotrexate (NSC-740) in metastatic solid tumors in children. Cancer Chemother. Rep. *45*:45, 1965.
491. Howarth, C., Meyer, D., et al.: Stage-related combined modality treatment of retinoblastoma. Results of a prospective study. Cancer *45*:851, 1980.
492. Hopping, W., and Schmitt, G.: The treatment of retinoblastoma. Mod. Probl. Ophthalmol. *18*:106, 1977.
493. Farwell, J. R., Dohrmann, G. J., et al.: Central nervous system tumors in children. Cancer *40*:3123, 1977.
494. Hooper, R.: Intracranial tumours in childhood. Child's Brain *1*:136, 1975.
495. Cohen, M. E., and Duffner, P. K.: Brain tumors in children. Principles of diagnosis and treatment. New York, Raven Press, 1984.
496. Gooding, C. A., Brasch, R. C., et al.: Nuclear magnetic resonance imaging of the brain in children. J. Pediatr. *104*:589, 1984.
497. Brant-Zawadzki, M., Badami, J. P., et al.: Primary intracranial tumor imaging: a comparison of magnetic resonance and CT. Radiology *150*:435, 1984.
497a. Holland, B. A., Brandt-Zawadzki, M., et al.: Magnetic resonance imaging of primary intracranial tumors: a review. Int. J. Radiat. Oncol. Biol. Phys. *11*:315, 1985.
497b. Edwards, M. S. B., Davis, R. L., et al.: Tumor markers and cytologic features of cerebrospinal fluid. Cancer *56*:1773, 1985.
497c. Phillips, P. C., Kremzner, L. T., et al.: Cerebrospinal fluid polyamines: biochemical markers of malignant childhood brain tumors. Ann. Neurol. *19*:360, 1986.
497d. Deutsch, M., Laurent, J. P., et al.: Myelography for staging medulloblastoma. Cancer *56*:1763, 1985.
498. Calvo, F. A., Hornedo, J., et al.: Intracranial tumors with risk of dissemination in neuroaxis. Int. J. Radiat. Oncol. Biol. Phys. *9*:1297, 1983.
499. Campbell, A. N., Chan, H. S. L., et al.: Extracranial metastases in childhood primary intracranial tumors. A report of 21 cases and review of the literature. Cancer *53*:974, 1984.
500. Deutsch, M.: Radiotherapy for primary brain tumors in very young children. Cancer *50*:2785, 1982.
501. Danoff, B. E., Cowchock, F. S., et al.: Assessment of the long-term effects of primary radiation therapy for brain tumors in children. Cancer *49*:1580, 1982.
502. Duffner, P. K., Cohen, M. E., et al.: Late effects of treatment on the intelligence of children with posterior fossa tumors. Cancer *51*:233, 1983.
503. Kun, L. E., Mulhern, R. K., et al.: Quality of life in children treated for brain tumors. Intellectual, emotional and academic function. J. Neurosurg. *58*:1, 1983.
503a. Van Eys, J., Cangir, A., et al.: MOPP regimen as primary chemotherapy for brain tumors in infants. J. Neuro-Oncol. *3*:237, 1985.
504. Long, J. M.: Capillary ultrastructure and blood-brain barrier in human brain tumours. J. Neurosurg. *32*:127, 1970.
505. Milhorat, T., Davis, D., et al.: Experimental intracerebral movement of electron microscopic tracers of various molecular sizes. J. Neurosurg. *42*:315, 1975.
506. Schut, L., and Rosenstock, J. G.: Treatment of intracranial neoplasms in children. Semin. Oncol. *1*:9, 1974.
507. Crane, C.: The permeability of brain capillaries to non-electrolytes. Acta Physiol. Scand. *64*:407, 1956.
507a. Levin, V. A., Landahl, H. D., et al.: Drug delivery to CNS tumors. Cancer Treat. Rep. *65*:19, 1981.
507b. Levin, V., Freeman-Dove, M., et al.: Permeability characteristics of brain adjacent to tumors in rats. Arch. Neurol. *32*:785, 1975.
508. Rall, D. P., and Zubrod, C. G.: Mechanism of drug absorption and excretion, passage of drugs in and out of the central nervous system. Ann. Rev. Pharmacol. *2*:109, 1962.
509. Hoshino, T., Barker, M., et al.: The kinetics of cultured human glioma cells. Acta Neuropathol. *32*:235, 1975.
510. Hildebrand, J., and deBeyl, D. Z.: Rationale of combined chemotherapy of brain tumours. In: *Tumours of the Central Nervous System in Infancy and Childhood*. Voth, D., Gutjahr, P., et al. (eds.), Berlin, Springer-Verlag, 1982, p.376.
511. Shapiro, W. R.: Chemotherapy of primary malignant brain tumors in children. Cancer *36*:965, 1975.
512. Shapiro, J. R., Yung, A., et al.: Isolation, karyotype and clonal growth of heterogeneous subpopulations of human malignant gliomas. Cancer Res. *41*:2349, 1981.
513. Yung, W.-K., Shapiro, J. R., et al.: Heterogeneous chemosensitivities of subpopulations of human glioma cells in culture. Cancer Res. *42*:992, 1982.
513a. Hochberg, F. H., Parker, L. M., et al.: High dose BCNU with autologous bone marrow rescue for recurrent glioblastoma multiforme. J. Neurosurg. *54*:455, 1981.
513b. Phillips, G. L., Wolff, S. N., et al.: Intensive 1,3-bis (2-chloroethyl)-1-nitrosorea (BCNU) monochemotherapy and autologous bone marrow transplantation for malignant glioma. J. Clin. Oncol. *4*:639, 1986.
514. Levin, V. A., Kabra, P. M., et al.: Pharmacokinetics of intracarotid artery ^{14}C-BCNU in the squirrel monkey. Neurosurgery *48*:587, 1978.
515. Feun, L. G.: Intra-arterial chemotherapy for primary and metastatic brain cancer. The Cancer Bulletin *36*:57, 1984.
516. Fenstermacher, J., and Gazendam, J.: Intra-arterial infusions of drugs and hypertonic solutions as ways of enhancing CNS chemotherapy. Cancer Treat. Rep. *65* (Suppl. 2):27, 1981.
517. Neuwelt, E. A., Hill, S. A., et al.: Osmotic blood-brain barrier disruption: pharmacodynamic studies in dogs and a clinical phase I trial in patients with malignant brain tumors. Cancer Treat. Rep. *65*(Suppl.2):39, 1981.
518. Neuwelt, E. A., Howieson, J., et al.: Therapeutic efficacy of multiagent chemotherapy with drug delivery enhancement by blood-brain barrier modification in glioblastoma. Neurosurgery *19*:573, 1986.
518a. Bleyer, W. A.: Current status of intrathecal chemotherapy for human meningeal neoplasms. In *Modern Concepts in Brain Tumor Therapy: Laboratory and Clinical Investigations*. Natl. Cancer Inst. Monogr. *46*:171, 1977.
519. Klein, M., and Festa, R.: Central nervous system malignancies. In *Pediatric Oncology*. Lanzkowsky, P. (ed.), New York, McGraw-Hill, 1983.

520. Fazekas, J. T.: Treatment of grades I and II astrocytomas. Role of radiotherapy. Radiat. Oncol. Biol. Phys. 2:661, 1972.
521. Shin, K. H., and Webster, J. H.: Astrocytoma in children. J. Can. Assoc. Radiol. 30:167, 1979.
522. Sheline, G. E.: Radiation therapy of brain tumors. Cancer 39:873, 1977.
523. Leibel, S. A., Sheline, G. E., et al.: The role of radiation therapy in the treatment of astrocytomas. Cancer 35:1551, 1975.
524. Phupanich, S., Edwards, M., et al.: Supratentorial malignant gliomas of childhood: results of treatment with radiation therapy and chemotherapy. J. Neurosurg. 60:495, 1984.
525. Scanlon, P. W., and Taylor, W. F.: Radiotherapy of intracranial astrocytomas: analysis of 417 cases treated from 1960–69. Neurosurgery 5:301, 1979.
526. Uihlein, A., Colby, M. Y., Jr., et al.: Comparison of surgery and surgery plus irradiation in the treatment of supratentorial gliomas. Acta Radiol. Therapy Phys. Biol. 5:67, 1966.
527. Cangir, A., Ragab, A. H., et al.: Combination chemotherapy with vincristine (NSC-67574), procarbazine (NSC-77213), prednisone (NSC-10023) with or without nitrogen mustard (NSC-762) (MOPP vs OPP) in children with recurrent brain tumors. Med. Pediatr. Oncol. 12:1, 1984.
528. Sumer, T., Freeman, A. I., et al.: Chemotherapy in recurrent noncystic low-grade astrocytomas of the cerebrum in children. J. Surg. Oncol. 10:45, 1978.
529. Bloom, H. J. G.: Intracranial tumors: response and resistance to therapeutic endeavors 1970–1980. Int. J. Radiat. Oncol. Biol. Phys. 8:1083, 1982.
530. Bloom, H. J. G.: Management of some intracranial tumors in children and adults. In *Recent Advances in Clinical Oncology.* Hazra, T. A., Beachley, M. C. (eds.), New York: A. R. Liss, 1978, p. 55.
531. Bloom, H. J. G.: SIOP brain tumour trial. In *Abstracts of the 10th Meeting of the International Society of Pediatric Oncology.* Bruxelles, 1978.
531a. Djerassi, I., Kim, J. S., et al.: Response of astrocytoma to high-dose methotrexate with citrovorum factor rescue. Cancer 55:2741, 1985.
532. Levin, V. A., Wilson, C. B., et al.: A phase III comparison of BCNU, hydrosyurea, and radiation therapy for treatment of primary malignant gliomas. J. Neurosurg. 51:526, 1979.
533. EORTC Brain Tumor Group. Effect of CCNU on survival rate of objective remission and duration of free interval in patients with malignant brain glioma — spinal evaluation. Eur. J. Cancer 44:851, 1978.
534. Reagan, T. J., Bisel, H. F., et al.: Controlled study of CCNU and radiation therapy in malignant astrocytoma. J. Neurosurg. 44:186, 1976.
535. Seiler, R. W., Greiner, R. H., et al.: Radiotherapy combined with procarbazine, bleomycin, and CCNU in the treatment of high-grade supratentorial astrocytomas. J. Neurosurg. 48:861, 1978.
536. Walker, M. D., Alexander, E., Jr., et al.: Evaluation of BCNU and/or radiotherapy in the treatment of anaplastic gliomas. J. Neurosurg. 49:333, 1978.
537. Ertel, I., Boesel, C., et al.: Adjuvant chemotherapy of high grade astrocytomas in children: radiation therapy with or without CCNU, vincristine, and prednisone. Proc. ASCO 3:Abstr. C-309, 1984.
538. Sung, D. I.: Suprasellar tumors in children. A review of clinical manifestations and management. Cancer 50:1420, 1982.
539. Keiskaren, O., Raitta, C., et al.: The management and prognosis of gliomas of the optic pathways in children. Acta Neurochir. (Wien) 43:193, 1978.
540. Montgomery, A. B., Griffin, T., et al.: Optic nerve glioma: the role of radiation therapy. Cancer 40:2079, 1977.
541. Markesberry, W. R., and MacDonald, V.: Diencephalic syndrome. Long-term survival. Am. J. Dis. Child. 125:123, 1973.
542. Fjerris, F., and Klinker, L.: Long-term prognosis in children with benign cerebellar astrocytoma. J. Neurosurg. 49:179, 1978.
543. Griffin, W. T., Beaufait, D., et al.: Cystic cerebellar astrocytomas in childhood. Cancer 44:276, 1979.
544. Salazar, O. M.: Primary malignant cerebellar astrocytomas in children: a signal for postoperative craniospinal irradiation. J. Radiat. Oncol. Biol. Phys. 7:1661, 1981.
545. Albright, A. L., Price, R. A., et al.: Brain stem gliomas of children. A clinicopathological study. Cancer 52:2313, 1983.
545a. Epstein, F., and McCleary, E. L.: Intrinsic brain-stem tumors of childhood: surgical indications. J. Neurosurg. 64:11, 1986.
546. Packer, R. J., Allen, J., et al.: Brainstem glioma: clinical manifestations of meningeal gliomatosis. Ann. Neurol. 14:177, 1983.
547. Lassiter, K. R. L., Alexander, E., Jr., et al.: Surgical treatment of brain stem gliomas. J. Neurosurg. 34:719, 1971.
548. Gumbinas, M.: Tumors of the central and peripheral nervous system. In *Malignant Diseases of Infancy, Childhood and Adolescence.* Altman, A. J., and Schwartz, A. D. (eds.), Philadelphia, W. B. Saunders Co., 1983.
549. Sheline, G. E.: Radiation therapy of tumors of the central nervous system in childhood. Cancer 35:957, 1975.
550. Littman, P., Jarrett, P., et al.: Pediatric brain stem gliomas. Cancer 45:2787, 1980.
550a. Halperin, E. C.: Pediatric brain stem tumors: patterns of treatment failure and their implications for radiotherapy. Radiat. Oncol. Biol. Phys. 11:1293, 1985.
551. Djerassi, I., Kim, J. S., et al.: High dose methotrexate-citrovorum factor rescue in the management of brain tumors. Cancer Treat. Rep. 61:691, 1977.
552. Harisiadis, L., and Chang, C. H.: Medulloblastoma in children: a correlation between staging and results of treatment. Radiat. Oncol. Biol. Physiol. 2:833, 1977.
553. Allen, J. C., and Epstein, F.: Medulloblastoma and other primary malignant neuroectodermal tumors of the CNS. The effect of patients' age and extent of disease on prognosis. J. Neurosurg. 57:446, 1982.
554. Allen, J. C.: Current status of clinical trials in newly diagnosed and recurrent brain tumors. In *Symposium on Pediatric Oncology.* Altman, A. J. (ed.), Pediatr. Clin. North Am. 32:633, 1986.
555. Bloom, H. J. G., Thornton, H., et al.: SIOP medulloblastoma and high grade ependymoma therapeutic trial: preliminary results (1975–1981). In *Pediatric Oncology: Proceedings of the XIIIth Meeting of the International Society of Pediatric Oncology, Marseilles, September 15–19, 1981.* Raybaud, C., Clement, R., et al. (eds.), Amsterdam, Excerpta Medica, 1982.
556. Berry, M. P., Jenkin, D. T., et al.: Radiation treatment for medulloblastoma. J. Neurosurg. 55:43, 1981.
557. Park, T. S., Hoffman, H. J., et al.: Medulloblastoma: clinical presentation and management. Experience at the Hospital for Sick Children, Toronto, 1950–1980. J. Neurosurg. 58:543, 1983.
558. Bloom, H. J. G.: Combined modality therapy for intracranial tumors. Cancer 35:111, 1975.
559. McIntosh, N.: Medulloblastoma — a changing prognosis? Arch. Dis. Child. 54:200, 1979.
560. Raimondi, A. J., and Tomita, T.: Medulloblastoma in childhood. Acta Neurochir. (Wien) 50:127, 1979.
561. Cohen, M., Duffner, P., et al.: SEER Registry results in children with brain tumors, 1973–1981. Proc. Am. Soc. Clin. Oncol. 3:79, 1984.
562. Jereb, B., Reid, A., et al.: Patterns of failure in patients with medulloblastoma. Cancer 50:2941, 1982.

563. Silverman, C. L., and Simpson, J. R.: Cerebeller medulloblastoma: the importance of posterior fossa dose to survival and patterns of failure. Int. J. Radiat. Oncol. Biol. Phys. 8:1869, 1982.
564. Bloom, H. J. G.: Medulloblastoma in children: increasing survival rates and further prospects. Int. J. Radiat. Oncol. Biol. Phys. 8:2023, 1982.
565. Bleyer, W., Millstein, J., et al.: 8 drugs in 1 day chemotherapy for brain tumors: a new approach and rationale for pre-radiation chemotherapy. Med. Pediatr. Oncol. 11:213, 1983.
566. Neidhart, M., Hanefeld, F., et al.: Treatment of medulloblastoma with postoperative combination chemotherapy before neuroaxis irradiation: an interim progress report on the Berlin pilot study and the West German cooperative trial. In *Pediatric Oncology: Proceedings of the XIIIth Meeting of the International Society of Pediatric Oncology, Marseilles, September 15–19, 1981.* Raybaud, C., Clement, R., et al. (eds.), Amsterdam, Excerpta Medica, 1982.
567. Hart, M. N., and Earle, K. M.: Primitive neuroectodermal tumors of the brain in children. Cancer 32:890, 1973.
568. Becker, L. E., and Hinton, D.: Primitive neuroectodermal tumors of the central nervous system. Hum. Pathol. 14:538,1983.
569. Duffner, P. K., Cohen, M. E., et al.: Primitive neuroectodermal tumors of childhood. An approach to therapy. J. Neurosurg. 55:376, 1981.
570. Parker, J. C., Jr.: Mortara, R. H., et al.: Biological behavior of the primitive neuroectodermal tumors: significant supratentorial childhood gliomas. Surg. Neurol. 4:387, 1975.
571. Wara, W. M., Edwards, M. S., et al.: Treatment of cerebral neuroblastomas. In *Pediatric Oncology. Proceedings of the XIIIth Meeting of the International Society of Pediatric Oncology, Marseilles, September 15–19, 1981.* Raybaud, C., Clement, R., et al. (eds.), Amsterdam, Excerpta Medica, 1982.
572. Pierre-Kahn, A., Hirsch, J. F., et al.: Intracranial ependymomas in childhood. Survival and functional results of 47 cases. Child's Brain 10:145, 1983.
573. Salazar, O. M., Rubin, P., et al.: Improved survival of patients with intracranial ependymomas by irradiation: dose selection and field extension. Cancer 35:1563, 1975.
574. Schuman, R. M., Ellsworth, C. A., et al.: The biology of childhood ependymomas. Arch. Neurol. 32:731, 1975.
575. Sagerman, R. H., Bagshaw, M. A., et al.: Considerations in the treatment of ependymomas. Radiology 84:401, 1965.
576. Van Eys, J.: Chemotherapy for gliomas in children. Cancer Bull. 27:16, 1975.
576a. Packer, R. J., Sutton, L. N., et al.: Oligodendroglioma of the posterior fossa in childhood. Cancer 56:195, 1985.
576b. Ludwig, C. L., Smith, M. T., et al.: A clinicopathological study of 323 patients with oligodendrogliomas. Ann. Neurol. 19:15, 1986.
577. Reedy, D. P., Bay, J. W., et al.: Role of radiation therapy in the treatment of cerebral oligodendroglioma: an analysis of 57 cases and a literature review. Neurosurgery 13:499, 1983.
578. Horrax, G., and Wu, W. G.: Postoperative survival of patients with intracranial oligodendroglioma with special reference to radical tumor removal: a study of 26 patients. J. Neurosurg. 8:473, 1951.
579. Dohrmann, G. J., Farwell, J. R., et al.: Oligodendrogliomas in children. Surg. Neurol. 10:21, 1978.
580. Gutin, P. H., Wilson, C. B., et al.: Phase II study of procarbazine, CCNU, and vincristine combination chemotherapy in the treatment of malignant brain tumors. Cancer 35:1398, 1975.
581. Pascual-Castroviejo, I., Villarejo, F., et al.: Childhood choroid plexus neoplasms. A study of 14 cases less than 2 years old. Eur. J. Pediatr. 140:51, 1983.
582. Jooma, R., and Kendall, B. E.: Diagnosis and management of pineal tumors. J. Neurosurg. 58:654, 1983.
583. Rubin, P., and Kramer, S.: Ectopic pinealoma: a radiocurable neuroendocrinologic entity. Radiology 85:512, 1965.
584. Allen, J. C., Nisselbaum, J., et al.: Alphafetoprotein and human chorionic gonadotropin determination in cerebrospinal fluid. An aid to the diagnosis and management of intracranial germ-cell tumors. J. Neurosurg. 51:368, 1979.
585. Rao, Y. T. R., Medini, E., et al.: Pineal and ectopic pineal tumors: the role of radiation therapy. Cancer 48:708, 1981.
586. Bloom, H. J. G.: Primary intracranial germ cell tumours. Clin. Oncol. 2:233, 1983.
586a. Wara, W. M., Jenkin, R. D., et al.: Tumors in the pineal and suprasellar region: Children's Cancer Study Group treatment results, 1960–1975. Cancer 43:698, 1979.
586b. Hitchon, P. W., Abu-Yousef, M. M., et al.: Management and outcome of pineal region tumors. Neurosurgery 13:248, 1983.
586c. Rich, T. A., Cassady, J. R., et al.: Radiation therapy for pineal and suprasellar germ cell tumors. Cancer 55:932, 1985.
587. Stein, B. M.: Supracerebellar-infratentorial approach to pineal tumors. Surg. Neurol. 11:331, 1979.
588. Stein, B. M.: Pineal region tumors. In *Pediatric Neurosurgery: Surgery of the Developing Nervous System.* American Association of Neurological Surgeons, Section of Pediatric Neurosurgery (eds.), New York, Grune & Stratton, 1982.
588a. Packer, R. J., Sutton, L. N., et al.: Pineal region tumors of childhood. Pediatrics 74:97, 1984.
589. Murovic, J. A., Ongley, J. P., et al.: Manifestations and therapeutic considerations in pineal yolk-sac tumors. Case report. J. Neurosurg. 1981; 55:303, 1981.
590. Jenkin, R. D. T., Simpson, W. J. K., et al.: Pineal and suprasellar germinomas: results of radiation treatment. J. Neurosurg. 48:99, 1978.
591. Neuwelt, W. A., Frenkel, E. P., et al.: Suprasellar germinomas: aspects of immunological characterization and successful chemotherapeutic responses in recurrent disease. Neurosurgery 7:352, 1980.
592. Kasper, C. S., Schneider, N. R., et al.: Suprasellar germinoma. Unresolved problems in diagnosis, pathogenesis, and management. Am. J. Med. 75:705, 1983.
593. Thomsett, M. J., Conte, F. A., et al.: Endocrine and neurologic outcome in childhood craniopharyngioma: review of effect of treatment in 42 patients. J. Pediatr. 97:728, 1980.
594. Sung, D. I.: Suprasellar tumors in children. A review of clinical manifestations and managements. Cancer 50:1420, 1982.
595. Amacher, A. L.: Craniopharyngioma: the controversy regarding radiotherapy. Child's Brain 6:57, 1980.
596. Shapiro, K., Till, K., et al.: Craniopharyngiomas in childhood: a rational approach to treatment. J. Neurosurg. 50:617, 1979.
597. Thompson, I. L., Griffin, T. W., et al.: Craniopharyngiomas: the role of radiation therapy. Int. J. Radiat. Oncol. Biol. Phys. 4:1059, 1978.
598. Cassady, J. R., Eifel, P., et al.: Progress and problems of the treatment of brain stem glioma, medulloblastoma, and craniopharyngioma in childhood. In *Recent Trends in Radiation Oncology.* Amendola, B. E., and Amendola, M. A. (eds.), New York, Elsevier Scientific, 1983.
599. Sørensen, S. A., Mulvihill, J. J., et al.: Long-term follow-up of von Recklinghausen neurofibromatosis. Survival and malignant neoplasms. New Engl. J. Med. 314:1010, 1986.

STORAGE DISEASE

CHAPTER 38
Storage Diseases of the Reticuloendothelial System*

EDWIN H. KOLODNY
ROSE-MARY BOUSTANY

INTRODUCTION 1212
GENERAL CONCEPTS OF STORAGE DISEASES 1213
Lysosomes
Pathogenesis
Genetics
Clinical Diagnosis
Laboratory Diagnosis
Treatment
Prevention
SPHINGOLIPIDOSES 1224
Gaucher's Disease (Glucosylceramide Lipidosis)
Niemann-Pick Disease (Sphingomyelin Lipidosis)
Farber's Disease (Lipogranulomatosis)
G_{M1}-Gangliosidosis
G_{M2}-Gangliosidosis, Sandhoff Variant
MUCOPOLYSACCHARIDOSES 1230
Hurler's Disease, Scheie's Disease, and Hurler-Scheie Compound
Hunter's Disease
Sanfilippo's Disease
Morquio's Syndrome
Maroteaux-Lamy Syndrome
β-Glucuronidase Deficiency
Mucosulfatidosis
MUCOLIPIDOSES AND OTHER DISEASES OF COMPLEX CARBOHYDRATE METABOLISM 1235
Sialidoses
Mucolipidosis II (I-Cell Disease)
Mucolipidosis III (Pseudo-Hurler Polydystrophy)
Mucolipidosis IV
Fucosidosis
Mannosidosis
Aspartylglucosaminuria
ACID LIPASE DEFICIENCY 1240
Wolman's Disease
Cholesterol Ester Storage Disease
NEURONAL CEROID-LIPOFUSCINOSES 1241
Infantile Type (Haltia-Santavuori Syndrome)
Late Infantile Type (Jansky-Bielschowsky Syndrome)
Juvenile Type (Spielmeyer-Sjögren Syndrome)
Adult Type (Kufs' Disease)

---

*During the preparation of this manuscript, the authors received support from the Department of Mental Health, Commonwealth of Massachusetts, and from U.S.P.H.S. grants HD 05515 and HD 04147.

INTRODUCTION

Storage diseases of children may produce dramatic changes in circulating blood and in the organs of the reticuloendothelial system. These include pancytopenia, vacuolization of mononuclear cells, storage of foam cells, and enlargement of the liver, spleen, and lymph nodes. Storage diseases may also affect other organ systems, particularly the central nervous system.

The pathogenesis of each condition is similar. A specific hydrolytic enzyme that is normally present in lysosomal particles of the cell cytoplasm is inactive. Consequently, products of cellular metabolism that are ordinarily degraded by this enzyme remain undigested and overload the lysosomes, causing severe disruption of the cellular architecture. These diseases are therefore referred to as the lysosomal storage diseases.

In recent years, the lysosomal storage diseases have been the object of intensive study by morphologists, biochemists, cell biologists, and geneticists. Their investigations have established the following for each disease: the mode of inheritance, histologic and ultrastructural features, chemical structure of the stored materials, and properties of the missing enzyme and its molecular genetics. Simple definitive laboratory methods have been developed that permit accurate diagnosis of these conditions, in some cases prenatally. As a result, these diseases are now being diagnosed in many more patients, including individuals with perplexing clinical manifestations representing variant forms of lysosomal storage diseases.

A hematologic perspective is particularly pertinent to the diagnosis of inherited storage diseases. The natural products that accumulate in these diseases are normally present in cell membranes; however, their reduced metabolic turnover in lysosomal enzyme deficiency states causes them to pile up. Circulating leukocytes have not only a rapid metabolic rate but also the capacity to phagocytize nondegradable materials. Therefore, these cells are doubly vulnerable, and so it is not surprising that various morphologic changes are observed in leukocytes from patients with storage diseases. Bone marrow–derived macrophages are the sites of the quietus of blood cells that deposit their effete membranes in these littoral scavengers. Consequently, the bone marrow and other tissues of the hematopoietic system reflect the storage phenomenon, and their examination further aids in the workup of a patient with storage disease.

Biochemical studies are usually required to

reach a definitive diagnosis, and here too the circulating blood may serve an important function. Serum, plasma, and mixed leukocyte fractions provide a rich and readily available source of material for substrate analyses and enzymatic assays. Blood enzyme testing is also helpful in identifying relatives who are heterozygous for the storage disease gene. The incidence of one disease, the Tay-Sachs variant of G_{M2}-gangliosidosis, has actually been reduced by large-scale public screening of serum and, in some situations, leukocytes of at-risk populations. Couples discovered to be doubly heterozygous for the Tay-Sachs gene and therefore at risk for bearing affected children can elect to have an amniocentesis performed for prenatal diagnosis and, if the fetus is affected, accept pregnancy termination. Through the use of more efficient and economical testing methods, this prototype program of genetic disease prevention may become applicable to other storage diseases that are fatal in early childhood. However, for the present, we can still reduce the burden of these diseases by properly testing and counseling family members of individuals known to have these disorders. This should include a full disclosure concerning the prenatal diagnosis option as soon as possible after a diagnosis has been made.

Bone marrow transplantation represents a promising new approach for treatment of storage diseases. In disorders primarily affecting the reticuloendothelial system, the new cell line could colonize the liver, spleen, and bone marrow with cells competent to degrade the natural products being stored and to reduce through a concentration gradient their accumulation in these and other tissues. Indeed, preliminary results in Gaucher's disease (1) and Maroteaux-Lamy syndrome (2) appear to substantiate this theory. As techniques for marrow transplantation improve and we learn better how to handle graft-versus-host reactions, this mode of therapy may become increasingly attractive. It is therefore important to know as much as possible about the pathophysiology and biochemistry of these diseases so appropriate patient selection and therapeutic monitoring can be done.

Considerable phenotypic heterogeneity characterizes each of the storage diseases. The case descriptions presented in this chapter are derived from the authors' own clinical experiences and in some instances may deviate from classic textbook descriptions. As specific molecular probes become available, it is likely that a variety of different genetic lesions will be found to produce superficially similar diseases. However, close clinical scrutiny will almost invariably reveal differences from case to case. Therefore, the physician faced with a perplexing case of suspected storage disease should not exclude otherwise similar conditions because of a few phenotypic dissimilarities. Consequently, blood enzyme assays will remain a cornerstone in the classification of these diseases.

To properly understand the pathophysiology of reticuloendothelial storage diseases, the reader must grapple with some rather unfamiliar biochemistry. One of the purposes of this chapter is to guide the reader through some of the complex chemical pathways involved in these diseases. The references provided at the end of the chapter reflect the most recent findings in this rapidly developing field of medicine, and these should be consulted for further clinical and biochemical details of the storage diseases.

GENERAL CONCEPTS OF STORAGE DISEASES

Lysosomes

Morphology and Physiology. Lysosomes are found in all cells, including leukocytes, erythrocytes, and platelets. They account for the characteristic azurophilic-staining granules in polymorphonuclear leukocytes and eosinophils and are much more numerous in reticulocytes, especially after splenectomy, than in mature red blood cells (3).

The formation of primary lysosomes begins in ribosomes attached to the limiting membrane of the rough endoplasmic reticulum (RER). The proteins synthesized in the RER proceed to the smooth endoplasmic reticulum where the signal sequence for peptides destined to form lysosomal enzymes is removed and oligosaccharide chains high in mannose are added. The nascent enzyme is further modified in the Golgi apparatus with the addition of mannose-6-phosphate residues. Additional processing occurs after the proenzyme is released from the Golgi apparatus and is packaged into the lysosomal vesicle (4). Electron microscope studies reveal that these vesicles are delineated by a single membrane that may condense with pinocytotic vesicles containing ingested foreign material (heterophagy) or with vacuoles containing cellular metabolites destined for further catabolism (autophagy). The secondary lysosomes formed during the processes of heterophagy and autophagy are polymorphic in size. The undigested material that remains in the secondary lysosomes after their hydrolytic enzymes have acted then coalesces into a residual body. This residue can be regurgitated from the cell if an excretory pathway exists; for example, in bile from the liver and urine from the kidney.

Enzymes. The complement of hydrolytic enzymes within lysosomes functions as a digestive system for the cell, but normal cell constituents are protected from their destructive action by the lysosomal membrane. At least 50 enzymes acting on lipids, carbohydrates, proteins, and nucleotides are present in lysosomes. In vitro, their activity is optimal in an acid pH environment. Each enzyme functions as a hydrolase with a high degree of specificity for one particular linkage. However, the structural requirements for the remainder of the molecule are less and less stringent the greater the distance from the point of hydrolysis. Therefore, small synthetic substrates can frequently substitute for more complex natural products in assays of lysosomal enzyme activity. However, complex isozyme systems exist in which two or more enzymes act on a single substrate. The β-N-acetylhexosaminidases, arylsulfatases, α-galactosidases, α-mannosidases, and neuraminidases are examples. By altering reaction conditions to take advantage of subtle differences in their properties, or by choosing as an enzyme source a tissue or fluid that contains only the enzyme component of interest, it is generally possible to quantitate the activity of individual enzyme components that have similar substrate specificities.

An active two-way exchange of lysosomal enzyme apparently occurs within cells (4a) and between cells and the extracellular environment. This exchange is readily demonstrable in skin fibroblast cultures. Release of enzyme from the cell can be demonstrated in culture media that do not initially contain any activity of the relevant enzyme. Cell uptake of enzyme from the nutrient media has been shown with cells that are genetically deficient in a single enzyme activity. Entry of lysosomal enzymes into cells is believed to be a specific process. Receptors exist on the cell surface that recognize a particular type of carbohydrate moiety on the enzyme; for example, mannosyl phosphate residues in the case of human fibroblasts (5). Release of lysosomal enzyme activity occurs during phagocytosis, on exposure to membrane-disruptive agents or immune complexes (6), or during treatment with acetylcholine and cyclic guanosine monophosphate (cyclic GMP) in the presence of calcium (7). Epinephrine, isoproterenol, cyclic adenosine monophosphate (cyclic AMP) (7), and anti-inflammatory drugs (8) inhibit lysosomal enzyme release. Some of these factors could be involved in regulating the levels of lysosomal enzyme activity present in body fluids such as plasma, urine, and tears.

Pathogenesis

Based upon his studies of Type II (Pompe) glycogen storage disease, Hers proposed in 1965 the concept of inborn lysosomal disease (9). He concluded that the deficiency of a single lysosomal enzyme (α-glucosidase) resulted in the accumulation of its substrate (glycogen) within membrane-bound vesicles of lysosomal origin. According to this concept, continued lysosomal uptake of the nonmetabolizable material leads to lysosomal hypertrophy, which produces mechanical crowding within the cell, disrupting its normal functions and possibly also destroying it.

The signs and symptoms produced by each of the storage diseases primarily reflect the pattern of distribution of the non-degradable natural products. In Gaucher's disease and Niemann-Pick disease, the turnover of erythrocyte and leukocyte membranes leads to the formation of lipids that become trapped within the visceral organs principally involved in their metabolism. However, in disorders of ganglioside metabolism, the principal pathologic changes occur in the central nervous system, because the ganglioside concentrations in this tissue under normal circumstances are much greater than in extraneural tissues. Glycoproteins are abundant in nearly all tissues, both inside and outside the nervous system. Hence, diseases caused by the storage of mucopolysaccharides and other complex carbohydrates derived from glycoproteins affect a variety of different organ systems.

Natural materials with apparently intact pathways for their metabolism sometimes accumulate as secondary products in certain of the lysosomal storage diseases. Cholesterol is closely associated with sphingomyelin in membranes and apparently for this reason also accumulates in Niemann-Pick disease (sphingomyelin lipidosis). High concentrations of mucopolysaccharide can inhibit G_{M1}-ganglioside β-galactosidase so that the brain tissue of patients with mucopolysaccharidoses accumulates not only mucopolysaccharide but also G_{M1}-ganglioside.

Genetics

Interspecies somatic cell hybrids have been employed in gene mapping experiments to make specific chromosome assignments for genes that code for several of the lysosomal hydrolases (Table 38–1). Nearly all the lysosomal storage diseases are transmitted as autosomal recessive traits. Two

Table 38–1. CHROMOSOME ASSIGNMENT OF GENES CODING FOR CERTAIN LYSOSOMAL ENZYME ACTIVITIES

Enzyme	Chromosome Number
α-L-Fucosidase	1
Acid β-Glucosidase	1
β-Galactosidase	3
Aspartylglucosaminidase	4
Arylsulfatase B	5
Hexosaminidase B	5
β-Glucuronidase	7
Acid lipase A	10
Hexosaminidase A (α-chain only)	15
α-Glucosidase	17
α-Mannosidase	19
α-Galactosidase A	X
Iduronate sulfatase	X

exceptions, Fabry's disease (α-galactosidase deficiency) and Hunter's disease (iduronate sulfatase deficiency), follow an X-linked pattern of inheritance.

Two or more enzyme activities can be affected by a single mutation in a particular gene locus. One explanation is that under ordinary circumstances the gene involved in such situations regulates the synthesis of a subunit that is shared by more than one enzyme. For example, in Sandhoff's disease, failure to properly code for the β-subunit of hexosaminidases A and B accounts for deficiencies of both these enzymes. Alternatively, the mutation could affect a post-translational event such as the attachment or removal of carbohydrate residues in conversion of the enzyme to its final glycoprotein form. This could result in an enzyme molecule that is catalytically active but can be neither retained nor selectively taken up by the cell. This type of defect occurs in mucolipidoses II and III and probably accounts for the altered electrophoretic properties of lysosomal enzymes in these diseases.

In several of the lysosomal storage diseases, catalytically inactive enzyme protein can be detected by using antibodies to normal purified enzyme. Although the substrate binding and/or catalytic sites of this cross-reacting material may be altered, its antigenic sites are intact. Immunoassays for cross-reacting material are therefore an additional means for classifying variants of individual lysosomal storage diseases.

Several heat-stable protein factors have been shown to stimulate the enzymatic hydrolysis of individual sphingoglycolipids. A deficiency in one of these factors had been implicated in the pathogenesis of the AB variant of G_{M2}-gangliosidosis (10). In another form of lysosomal storage disease, Morquio disease type B, the mutant protein is activated sufficiently by the G_{M1}-activator to protect patients with this form of β-galactosidase deficiency from G_{M1}-ganglioside storage (11).

These various mechanisms allow for enormous genetic heterogeneity and are, in fact, reflected in the marked phenotypic variations that distinguish many of the storage diseases. With recombinant DNA techniques it has become possible to clone genes for lysosomal enzymes (12–14) and to use the molecular information from these clones to classify the defects occurring in the various mutant forms of lysosomal storage disease. This technology has opened up a new era of discovery for these and other inherited metabolic diseases and has provided tools for more precise diagnosis as well as the potential for definitive therapy through gene transfer.

Clinical Diagnosis

The various macromolecules that accumulate in the storage diseases are not uniformly distributed in all tissues. Instead, they are deposited in certain preferred anatomic sites that in normal persons actively metabolize these substances or utilize them as structural components. The involvement of specific tissues and organs thus determines the manner of clinical presentation in each of the storage diseases (Table 38–2).

Dysmorphic facial features and hepatomegaly are two common features. The former occurs in type 1 G_{M1}-gangliosidosis, the mucopolysaccharidoses, mucolipidoses II and III, mannosidosis, and fucosidosis. Many of these diseases also display other evidence of connective tissue infiltration, such as joint contractures, skeletal dysplasia, and corneal clouding. Some degree of liver enlargement also occurs in most of these disorders, including Gaucher's disease, Niemann-Pick disease, sialidosis type 2, and Wolman's disease. Splenomegaly is also a common presenting sign in Gaucher's disease, Niemann-Pick disease, and Wolman's disease. Lymphadenopathy and granulomatous joint deposits are characteristic in Farber's disease.

Signs of central nervous system dysfunction occur in many patients, particularly the very young. Slowed development, hypotonia, and an excessive startle response in an infant may suggest gangliosidosis. Actual regression in neurologic functioning with loss of previously acquired developmental milestones eventually occurs in these gangliosidoses as well as in type A Niemann-Pick disease and several of the mucopolysaccharidoses. Seizures, megacephaly, and blindness result later in the course of the ganglioside storage diseases. Vomiting may be a presenting sign in type A Niemann-Pick disease and Wolman's disease.

Generally, the later clinical signs appear, the slower the progression and the less severe the disease process. In contrast to the severely retarded epileptic infant with a gangliosidosis and life expectancy measured in months, the patient who presents in late childhood or early adolescence with seizures because of juvenile Gaucher's disease (type 3) or the cherry-red macula–myoclonus forms of sialidosis may survive 10 or more years without loss of intellect. Although mental retardation does occur in aspartylglucosaminuria, fucosidosis, mannosidosis, and the less severe form of Hunter's disease, these diseases evolve slowly and affected patients survive into adulthood. In the adult form of Gaucher's disease (type 1) and Niemann-Pick disease (type B), splenic lipid storage may evolve very slowly, no mental deficiency occurs, and a normal life span is possible.

Knowledge of the patient's family history is often helpful in arriving at a diagnosis. The majority of patients with adult Gaucher's disease and type A Niemann-Pick disease are of northeastern European Jewish ancestry. A Scandinavian background is common among patients with aspartylglucosaminuria, and many patients with fucosi-

Table 38–2. STORAGE DISEASES OF THE RETICULOENDOTHELIAL SYSTEM

Age of Onset	Presenting Signs
FIRST YEAR	
Niemann-Pick disease, type A	Slow development, hepatosplenomegaly
Gaucher's disease, type 2	Failure to thrive, hepatosplenomegaly, brain stem signs
Farber's disease	Hoarseness, vomiting, swollen joints, lymphadenopathy
G_{M1}-gangliosidosis, type 1	Coarse facies, increased startle, hepatosplenomegaly
G_{M2}-gangliosidosis, Sandhoff variant	Slow development, increased startle, cherry-red macula
Hurler's disease	Coarse facies, stiff joints
Hunter's disease	Coarse facies, stiff joints
Sanfilippo's disease	Coarse facies, stiff joints, severe mental retardation
Mucosulfatidosis	Slow development, coarse facies
Sialidosis II, late-infantile type	Slow development, coarse facies, hepatomegaly
Mucolipidosis II	Wizened face at birth, gingival hyperplasia, stiff joints
Mucolipidosis IV	Slow development, corneal clouding
Fucosidosis, type 1	Slow development, coarse facies
Mannosidosis	Slow development, coarse facies, hepatosplenomegaly
Wolman's disease	Vomiting, diarrhea, hepatosplenomegaly, calcified adrenals
Neuronal ceroid-lipofuscinosis, infantile type	Slow development, poor vision
SECOND YEAR	
Niemann-Pick disease, type B	Hepatosplenomegaly
C_{M1}-gangliosidosis, type 2	Slow development, increased startle
Morquio's syndrome	Dwarfism, skeletal abnormalities, loose joints
Maroteaux-Lamy syndrome	Coarse facies, stiff joints, corneal clouding
Mucolipidosis III	Stiff hands and shoulders
Fucosidosis, type 2	Slow neurologic deterioration
Aspartylglucosaminuria	Slow development, coarse facies, aggressive behavior
Neuronal ceroid-lipofuscinosis, late infantile type	Seizures, myoclonus, decreased vision, decreased intellect
CHILDHOOD	
Niemann-Pick disease, chronic neuronopathic form	Tetraparesis, decreased intellect, hepatomegaly
Gaucher's disease, type 1	Splenomegaly, anemia, thrombocytopenia
Scheie's disease	Claw hands
Cholesterol ester storage disease	Hepatomegaly, increased plasma cholesterol and triglycerides
Neuronal ceroid-lipofuscinosis, juvenile type	Blindness, seizures, decreased intellect
ADOLESCENCE	
Gaucher's disease, type 3	Splenomegaly, seizures, myoclonus
Cherry-red spot myoclonus syndrome	Unexplained falls, seizures, cherry-red macula
Galactosialidosis	Corneal clouding, coarse facies, seizures, cherry-red macula

dosis are of Italian extraction. If the patient is a male with Hurler-like physical features and a similarly affected maternal uncle, Hunter's disease with X-linked inheritance should be suspected.

Therefore, in the clinical evaluation of patients with possible storage disease particular attention should be devoted to a review of the chronology of the disease and the family background and a careful assessment made of the neurologic, visceral, and skeletal manifestations. However, because of considerable genetic heterogeneity, the physical signs and severity of the lysosomal storage diseases vary considerably, thus confounding the clinician attempting to arrive at a specific diagnosis. For this reason, laboratory studies play an important role in the diagnosis of these conditions.

Laboratory Diagnosis

MORPHOLOGIC FINDINGS

The histologic changes observed in the storage diseases are especially pronounced in those organs with a significant reticuloendothelial component, such as the liver, spleen, lymph nodes, and bone marrow. The accumulating natural products form inclusions that display specific staining characteristics and a defined ultrastructure. These may be readily observed using easily accessible tissues such as peripheral blood, bone marrow, liver, and skin (Table 38–3).

Peripheral Blood. Vacuolated lymphocytes are a common finding in the storage diseases (15–25). Those present in Sandhoff's disease and the sialidoses contain periodic acid-Schiff (PAS)–positive granules. Electron microscopic examination of the lymphocytic vacuoles generally reveals dense cytoplasmic bodies or lamellar arrays surrounded by a single limiting membrane. In Wolman's disease, both intracytoplasmic and intranuclear lymphocytic vacuoles may occur. Other types of circulating monocytes, in addition to lymphocytes, may also form vacuoles. This change occurs, for example, in the sialidoses and mucolipidosis II.

Excessive granulation of circulating neutrophils helps to distinguish several of the storage diseases. In the mucopolysaccharidoses and in mucosulfatidosis, metachromatic granules known as Alder-Reilly bodies are present (26, 27). Azurophilic hypergranulation of neutrophils is a characteristic feature in many patients with the neuronal ceroid-lipofuscinoses. Ultrastructural studies of buffy coat preparations from peripheral blood are also utilized in the study of certain storage diseases, such as the neuronal ceroid-lipofuscinoses (28), to detect the abnormal intracytoplasmic inclusions typical of these diseases.

Bone Marrow. The foam cell, a lipid-laden macrophage often called a histiocyte, provides perhaps the most dramatic and convincing histologic evidence of a storage disease. It may be easily recognized in unstained preparations of bone marrow aspirate as a round or oval cell measuring 20 to 90 μ in diameter. It generally has a single eccentric nucleus with a prominent nucleolus, but foam cells with two or more nuclei are not uncommon. Under darkfield microscopy, these cells appear as large white spheres on a dark background (Color Plate II, 1). They may be distinguished on phase contrast microscopy as large, glittering cells with numerous cytoplasmic droplets or particles. These droplets are fairly uniform in size and when viewed under polarization microscopy are often birefringent (Color Plate II, 2). They impart a mulberry- or honeycomb-like appearance to the cell, having a finely reticulated cytoplasmic web that is better seen in stained preparations (Color Plate II, 3). Under the electron microscope, the droplets appear as polymorphic lipid cytosomes ranging from less than 1 μ to more than 5 μ in diameter and consisting of both concentrically laminated myelin-like membranous arrays and dense homogeneous residual bodies.

The staining properties of the foam cells in each of the storage diseases may differ. They frequently stain red with oil-red-O and black with Sudan black B, indicating that sudanophilic material is

Table 38–3. LABORATORY FINDINGS IN THE STORAGE DISEASES.
I. PRESENCE OF INCLUSIONS IN READILY ACCESSIBLE TISSUES

Disease	Peripheral Blood		Bone Marrow	Liver		Skin	
	Vacuolated Lymphocytes	Granulated* Neutrophils	Foam Cells	Kupffer Cells	Hepatocytes	Biopsy	Culture
Gaucher's disease			Gaucher cell	Gaucher cell	Gaucher cell		+
Niemann-Pick disease	Nova Scotia variant		+	+	+		+
Farber's disease			+	+	+	+	+
G_{M1}-gangliosidosis	+		+	+	+	+	+
Sandhoff variant G_{M2}-gangliosidosis,	+		+	+	+	+	+
Hurler's disease		+		+	+	+	+
Hunter's disease				+	+	+	+
Sanfilippo's disease, type A	+			+		+	+
Sanfilippo's disease, type B						+	+
Morquio's syndrome				+	+	+	+
Maroteaux-Lamy syndrome		+		+	+		+
β-Glucuronidase deficiency		+					+
Mucosulfatidosis	+	+	Granulated myeloid cells	+	+		+
Sialidosis I	+		+	+			+
Sialidosis II, late infantile type	+	+	+	+	+		+
Mucolipidosis II	+		+				+
Mucolipidosis III			Vacuolated plasma cells				+
Mucolipidosis IV			+; vacuolated plasma cells	+	+		+
Fucosidosis	+		+	+	+	+	+
Mannosidosis	+	+	+				+
Aspartylglucosaminuria	+				+		
Wolman's disease	+		+	+			
Neuronal ceroid-lipofuscinosis	+	+	+			+	+

*Coarse granulations characteristic of Alder-Reilly bodies are seen in granulocytes of patients with a mucopolysaccharidosis. In Sialidosis II fine granulations are present in granulocytes, lymphocytes, and monocytes. The leukocytes in the neuronal ceroid-lipofuscinoses show azurophilic granulation.

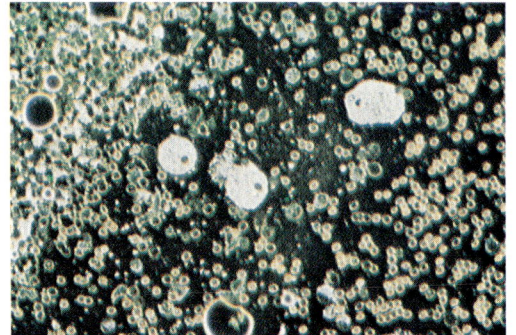
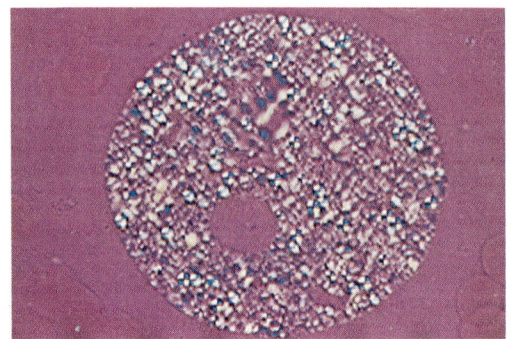
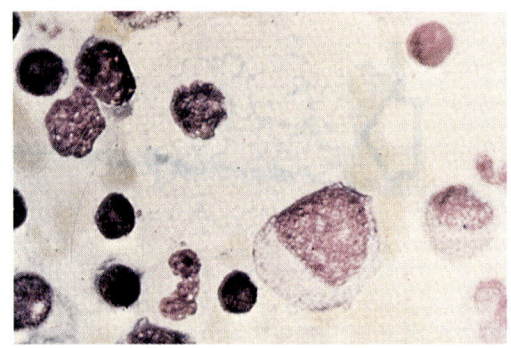
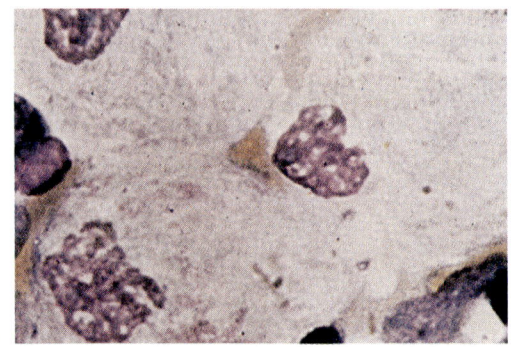

Color Plate II. Photomicrographs of storage cells.
1. Foam cells—Niemann-Pick disease, type B—darkfield (photomicrograph).
2. Foam cell—Niemann-Pick disease, type A—polarization (photomicrograph).
3. Foam cell—Giemsa-stained—Niemann-Pick disease, type B (photomicrograph).
4. Gaucher cell—Giemsa-stained—Gaucher's disease, type 1 (photomicrograph).

present. The PAS reaction may be weakly positive. The presence of lipofuscin is indicated by the appearance of autofluorescence under ultraviolet light. These histochemical reactions may be lost if alcohol or other lipid solvents are used to fix the bone marrow smears or tissue sections prior to staining. Therefore, for examining the staining properties of biopsy specimens from patients with storage diseases, formalin-fixed frozen-section slices are preferable to alcohol-treated paraffin-embedded material.

Occasionally, sea-blue histiocytes (29, 30) are noted in bone marrow preparations of patients with Niemann-Pick disease (31, 32) and other systemic lipidoses (33–37). These are large cells, measuring up to 60 μ in diameter, that contain several to many large, homogeneous granules that have a blue or blue-green color with Giemsa or Wright stains. Ultrastructural investigations indicate that these granules consist of lamellar as well as amorphous and granular cytosomes. Their major chemical constituent is believed to be ceroid, but increased tissue stores of phospholipids and glycolipids in diseases associated with this abnormal cell also implicate these substances in their pathogenesis.

The Gaucher cell is sometimes mistakenly identified as a foam cell. It is also a large histiocyte, measuring 20 to 100 μ in diameter, but instead of lipid droplets its cytoplasm contains striated rod-shaped inclusion bodies that give it a wrinkled tissue paper or crumpled silk appearance (Color Plate II, 4). The Gaucher cell stains pale pink with hematoxylin and eosin and stains only slightly with oil-red-O and Sudan black B. The inclusions are autofluorescent and PAS positive.

Electron microscopic studies indicate that these deposits are composed of hollow tubules contained within a limiting membrane. Analysis of purified preparations of these deposits by freeze-fracture and x-ray diffraction techniques suggests that they exist as a series of gradually twisting membranous bilayers 60 Å thick (38). They are composed of glucocerebroside (66 per cent), phospholipid (17 per cent), cholesterol (6 per cent), and protein and glycoprotein (11 per cent) (39). Strong acid phosphatase activity (40) and iron deposition (41, 42) have also been demonstrated in the Gaucher cell by use of histochemical staining methods.

Unlike the foam cell, which is found in many lipid storage diseases, the Gaucher cell is unique to the Gaucher form of inherited lipidosis. However, it cannot be regarded as entirely specific for Gaucher's disease for it has also been observed in the bone marrow of some patients with certain blood disorders, including chronic myelogenous leukemia (43, 44) and thalassemia (45), and in one patient who had both Gaucher's disease and coexistent Philadelphia positive chronic granulocytic leukemia (46). Presumably Gaucher cells can form when the breakdown of blood cells exceeds the capacity of macrophages to metabolize the effete lipids. Since Gaucher cells are detected in marrow preparations of only a few of the patients just described, it remains possible that these patients are actually heterozygotes for glucocerebrosidase deficiency.

A careful examination of the bone marrow smear is therefore an essential part of a storage disease workup. In addition to the foam cell, sea-blue histiocyte, and Gaucher cell, other abnormal structures can be detected in the bone marrow, such as the Alder-Reilly bodies characteristic of Hurler's disease and mucosulfatidosis and the vacuolated plasma cells associated with mucolipidoses III and IV.

Liver. In many storage diseases, an enlarged liver provides a tempting target for a diagnostic biopsy in spite of the fact that many of the cellular changes occurring in the liver are similar to those present in the bone marrow. This is because a liver biopsy has the additional advantage of allowing access to a solid tissue for biochemical analysis. A needle biopsy can yield 10 to 25 mg of fresh tissue that could be divided equally between the biochemistry and pathology laboratories. The specimen for biochemical studies must be preserved frozen in a sealed container, preferably one flushed with nitrogen gas prior to sealing to displace oxygen and prevent oxidation and dehydration during storage. One segment of the tissue destined for the pathology laboratory is immediately immersed in buffered glutaraldehyde for electron microscopy. The remainder is fixed in formalin and further subdivided into two specimens. Half the specimen is routinely processed and embedded in paraffin. The other half of the formalin-fixed material is used to prepare frozen sections, with care taken to avoid exposure to alcohol or other lipid solvents.

Liver involvement may be reflected in changes in the Kupffer cells, hepatocytes, and endothelial cells. The Kupffer cells are enlarged, containing membrane-limited vacuoles of various sizes. Electron microscopic studies of their ultrastructure demonstrate cytoplasmic bodies ranging from membranous and granuloreticular lamellar structures to more polymorphous and homogeneous dense bodies. Vacuolated histiocytes may infiltrate the sinuses, appearing as discrete islands of light-staining cells in routinely stained sections. Hepatic parenchymal cell involvement is variable. A mild vacuolar change may be noticed, or more extensive infiltration can occur in these cells, indicated by obvious enlargement and foamy metamorphosis.

On electron microscopy, dense bodies and osmophilic bodies are present. Vascular endothelial cells in the liver may also contain inclusions, and in some cases the lobular architecture of the liver itself is disturbed. The typical appearance of the Gaucher cell in liver specimens from patients with Gaucher's disease distinguishes this condition from other forms of storage disease, but in all other instances the histologic changes in the liver are not distinctive enough to permit the diagnosis of a specific storage disease.

Skin. Many different cell types are present in skin, including epithelial cells, hair follicles, fibroblasts, eccrine sweat glands, smooth muscle cells, sebaceous glands, vascular cells, and nerve bundles, making skin biopsy an extremely useful technique for histologic diagnosis of storage diseases (21, 47–49). Vacuoles may be found in the secretory coils of eccrine sweat glands, bulbs of hair follicles, fibroblasts, and Schwann cells in a number of diseases. Biopsy specimens from patients with the ganglioside storage diseases contain complex osmiophilic lipid deposits in axons, Schwann cells, and nerve fascicles. Study of skin ultrastructure is particularly helpful in the diagnosis of the neuronal ceroid-lipofuscinoses because the same distinctive pattern of inclusions present in the nervous system may be evident in skin (21, 49–52), and the enzymatic diagnosis of these diseases is not yet possible.

Cultured skin fibroblasts are less informative, but ultrastructural changes have been noted in these cells also. The membrane-bound, electron-dense inclusions of mucolipidoses II (53) and IV (54) and the curvilinear profiles of neuronal ceroid-lipofuscinoses (52) are examples of this phenomenon. However, not all storage diseases produce histologic changes in the skin; for example, none have been found in Gaucher's disease (21). Nevertheless, as electron microscopists have become more proficient in examining this tissue and cell culture specialists and biochemists have come to appreciate the usefulness of cultured skin fibroblasts for metabolic studies, diagnostic skin biopsy has increased in popularity.

BIOCHEMICAL STUDIES

Storage Substances. Morphologic studies will suggest the presumptive diagnosis of a storage disease, but biochemical studies are required for a specific diagnosis. For the majority of the storage diseases, structural identification of the major accumulating substances preceded elucidation of the enzyme defects. Characterization of these compounds is generally more difficult than assaying the relevant enzyme, so that for diagnostic purposes determination of enzyme activity is preferred. However, a number of laboratory techniques have been developed that facilitate screening for storage substances in readily available tissue and fluid specimens.

The urine of patients with sphingolipidoses, mucopolysaccharidoses, mucolipidoses, and other oligosaccharidoses is a rich source of storage material. The sphingolipids present in a filtered 24-hour urine specimen can be extracted from the filter paper, separated from other lipids on a silicic acid column, and quantitated by a combination of thin-layer and gas-liquid chromatography (55). An excess of mucopolysaccharides is recognized in the urine by a positive Berry spot test (56), and these substances can be isolated by precipitation with quaternary ammonium salts and fractionated into separated species by gel chromatography (57) and partitioning in a butanol-aqueous salt phase system (58). Simple thin-layer chromatography methods employing microliter quantities of whole desalted urine have been described for separating the oligosaccharides excreted in fucosidosis (59), mannosidosis, G_{M1}-gangliosidosis (59, 60), and the sialidoses (61) into patterns distinctive for each disease. The presence of aspartylglucosamine on a urinary amino acid chromatogram aids in the diagnosis of aspartylglucosaminuria.

Sphingoglycolipids present in plasma can be quantitated by high performance liquid chromatography (HPLC) (62, 63). The procedure requires less than 1 ml of plasma and permits the detection of elevated ceramide, cerebroside, and globoside levels in Farber's disease (62), Gaucher's disease (63), and the Sandhoff variant of G_{M2}-gangliosidosis, respectively. The HPLC technique has also been used to demonstrate elevated sphingomyelin levels in cultured skin fibroblasts from patients with type A Niemann-Pick disease (64).

In other storage diseases as well, cultured skin fibroblasts provide an opportunity for biochemical documentation of the storage phenomenon and for turnover studies of the accumulating material. The kinetics of $^{35}SO_4$ accumulation has been used as an indicator of defective degradation of polysaccharides in the mucopolysaccharidoses (65) and mucolipidoses (66, 67). In Gaucher's disease cells, the metabolic utilization of radioactively labeled glucocerebroside is reduced (68) and in vivo studies of Farber's disease cells reveal a defect in their ability to metabolize the ceramide portion of a fatty acid labeled precursor (69). Fucosidosis fibroblasts store abnormal quantities of tritiated fucose (70), and Wolman's disease cell lines incorporate increased amounts of ^{14}C-mevalonate into cholesterol (71).

In certain instances, solid tissues may need to be analyzed. This step is required when a strong clinical presumption of storage disease exists but studies of body fluids and more readily accessible tissues, such as leukocytes and cultured fibroblasts, disclose neither the nature of the stored substance nor the presence of a deficient enzyme. This situation occurs, for example, in the chronic neuronopathic form of Niemann-Pick disease (type C). A liver biopsy is most commonly done in such circumstances. Biopsy of cerebral tissue is no longer warranted except in very rare instances of neurodegenerative disease without extraneural morphologic or biochemical stigmata.

Deficient Enzyme Activity. Specific enzyme defects have been clearly established for all the lysosomal storage diseases except Niemann-Pick disease types C and D and the neuronal ceroid-lipofuscinoses. Even in this latter group, in spite of the fact that the basic molecular defects are not fully understood, the types of storage bodies formed suggest that the primary defect is a lysosomal enzyme deficiency. Therefore, enzymatic assays are an especially convincing means for confirming the diagnosis of a storage disease. These can be performed in vitro using readily accessible sources of patient enzyme such as serum, plasma, leukocytes, lymphocytes, cultured skin fibroblasts, and tears.

The chemical linkage that each lysosomal enzyme attacks is quite specific for that particular enzyme. However, the structural requirements for the remainder of the molecule are less rigorous, so that in many instances artificial substrates can substitute for natural substrates of the enzyme. The chromogenic p-nitrophenyl and fluorogenic 4-methylumbelliferyl derivatives are commonly employed for this purpose because they are more easily cleaved in vitro than are the natural substrates and the aglycone product of their hydrolysis can readily be quantitated by colorimetry or fluorometry. When natural substrates are used, they generally carry a radioactive label. Assays with these compounds are processed by separating the reaction products and quantitating the labeled component in a liquid scintillation spectrometer.

Reviews are available that describe the methodology employed in assaying most of the enzymes shown in Table 38-4 (72, 73). These techniques are usually beyond the scope of a routine clinical chemistry laboratory and are most competently performed in a research laboratory setting, preferably one devoted to lysosomal enzymology. Fortunately, most lysosomal enzymes are quite stable upon freezing (α-neuraminidase is an exception) so that, if necessary, enzyme preparations can be shipped to distant localities for assay.

A leukocyte pellet sufficient for several different assays can be isolated from 10 ml of fresh whole heparinized blood by the dextran sedimentation procedure (74). A repeat sedimentation step can double the yield of leukocytes, an especially valuable consideration when the amount of blood obtainable is limited because of the size, age, or medical condition of the patient (usually a child). Specimens of blood should also be obtained from

Table 38–4. LABORATORY FINDINGS IN THE STORAGE DISEASES. II. BIOCHEMISTRY

Disease	Stored Material	Enzyme Deficiency	Substrates Used in Enzyme Assays	
			Natural	Artificial*
Sphingolipidoses				
Gaucher's disease	Glucocerebroside	Glucocerebrosidase	Glucocerebroside	4-MU-β-glucoside
Niemann-Pick disease	Sphingomyelin	Sphingomyelinase	Sphingomyelin	2-N-hexadecanoyl-amino-4-nitrophenyl-phosphorylcholine monohydrate
Farber's disease	Ceramide	Ceramidase	Ceramide	
G_{M1}-gangliosidosis	G_{M1}-ganglioside, glycoprotein	G_{M1}-ganglioside–β-galactosidase	G_{M1}-ganglioside	pNP-β-galactoside, 4-MU-β-galactoside
G_{M2}-gangliosidosis, Sandhoff variant	G_{M2}-ganglioside, globoside	Hexosaminidases A + B	Asialo-G_{M2}-ganglioside, globoside	pNP-β-N-acetylglucosamine, 4-MU-β-N-acetylglucosamine
Mucopolysaccharidoses				
Hurler's and Scheie's diseases	Dermatan sulfate, heparan sulfate	α-Iduronidase		4-MU-α-L-iduronide
Hunter's disease	Dermatan sulfate, heparan sulfate	Iduronosulfate sulfatase	^{35}S-Heparin	
Sanfilippo's disease				
Type A	Heparan sulfate	Sulfamidase	Unacetylated trisaccharide isolated from heparin	
Type B	Heparan sulfate	N-acetyl-α-glucosaminidase	6-Sulfo-acetylgalactosamine-glucuronic-acid-β-sulfa-N-acetylgalactosaminatol	pNP-α-N-acetylglucosaminide
Type C	Heparan sulfate	Heparan N-acetyl transferase		
Type D	Heparan sulfate	Heparan-6-sulfate sulfatase	Heparan-6-sulfate	
Morquio's syndrome				
Type A	Keratan sulfate	N-acetylgalactosamine-6-SO$_4$ sulfatase	Chondroitin-6-SO$_4$	
Type B	Keratan sulfate	β-galactosidase		4-MU-β-galactoside
Maroteaux-Lamy syndrome	Dermatan sulfate	Arylsulfatase B	Chondroitin-4-SO$_4$	p-Nitrocatechol sulfate, 4-MU-sulfate
β-Glucuronidase deficiency disease	Dermatan sulfate, heparan sulfate	β-Glucuronidase		pNP-glucuronide, 4-MU-glucuronide
Mucosulfatidosis	Sulfatides, mucopolysaccharides	Arylsulfatase A, B, and C, other sulfatases	Disulfated disaccharide, heparan, sulfatide	p-Nitrocatechol sulfate, 4-MU-sulfate
Mucolipidoses				
Sialidoses	Sialyloligosaccharides, glycoproteins,	α-Neuraminidase		
Mucolipidosis II	Sialyloligosaccharides, glycoproteins, glycolipids	High serum, low fibroblast enzymes; N-acetylglucosamine-1-phosphate transferase		4-MU-glycosides
Mucolipidosis III	Glycoproteins, glycolipids	Same as above		
Mucolipidosis IV	Glycolipids, glycoproteins	Ganglioside neuraminidase	G_{M3}-ganglioside	
Other Diseases of Complex Carbohydrate Metabolism				
Fucosidosis	Fucoglycolipids, fucosyloligosaccharides	α-Fucosidase		pNP-α-L-fucoside, 4-MU-α-fucoside
Mannosidosis	Mannosyloligosaccharides	α-Mannosidase		pNP-α-mannoside, 4-MU-α-mannoside
Aspartylglucosaminuria	Aspartylglucosamine	Aspartylglucosamine amidase		1-Aspartamido-β-N-acetyl-glucosamine
Wolman's disease	Cholesterol esters, triglycerides	Acid lipase	Glyceryl tripalmitate	pNP-palmitate, 4-MU-oleate
Neuronal ceroid-lipofuscinoses	Ceroid-lipofuscin pigments	Unknown		

*pNP = nitrophenyl; 4-MU = 4-methylumbelliferyl.

the child's parents to be used in confirming any enzyme defect discovered in the child's blood. When tested for activity of the relevant enzyme, the parents' specimens should demonstrate intermediate levels of enzyme activity, indicative of their heterozygote status. However, detection of heterozygotes in X-linked conditions such as Hunter's disease is more difficult because of the overlap with normal values that can occur as a result of mosaicism in the expression of the X-chromosome in females (75).

Treatment

SYMPTOMATIC TREATMENT

After the diagnosis of a storage disease is made, the physician often feels that the family must be given a prognosis. Since none of the storage diseases can be cured and their progressive course cannot be halted, a bleak outlook is presented, and the distraught family trudges off without a clear understanding of how to manage their child's illness. Actually, the clinical state is quite stable in a number of the storage diseases: e.g., adult Gaucher's disease, type B Niemann-Pick disease, mannosidosis, and the cherry-red spot myoclonus–epilepsy variant of sialidosis. Moreover, no two patients with the same storage disease follow the same timetable of clinical signs. Instead of prognostication, attention should be focused on alleviating or ameliorating existing signs and symptoms.

Feeding problems may arise because of bulbar paralysis, necessitating changes in the consistency of the child's food and in feeding techniques. Consultation with a nutritionist may be needed to insure that the child continues to receive an adequate fluid and caloric intake. Chronic constipation must be managed, the skin surface protected from ulcerations, and dental hygiene maintained to prevent caries. Seizures occurring in the course of gray matter storage disease of the brain generally respond to combinations of certain drugs, including diazepam (Valium), mephobarbital (Mebaral), and clonazepam (Clonopin). To prevent joint contractures, a regular program of physical therapy should be established. Orthopedic corrective procedures, otorhinolaryngologic surgery, and other types of operative intervention should not be withheld if they will make nursing care easier or bring relief to the child who has a clinically vexing problem.

The child's education is also important. Infant stimulation programs in day care centers, as well as special nursery school and kindergarten programs, are available for handicapped children through the Easter Seal Society, Cerebral Palsy Association, and similar organizations. By taking advantage of these resources the family and child can feel that they are not missing out on opportunities for self expression and achievement available to other children.

ENZYME REPLACEMENT THERAPY

There is strong theoretical justification for the use of enzyme replacement therapy in the lysosomal storage diseases. By means of a secretory process, hydrolytic enzymes may leave one cell only to be taken up by the same or another cell. Transport of enzyme molecules into the cell occurs via pinocytotic vacuoles formed from the cell membrane. Intracellular vacuoles containing macromolecular products of cell metabolism may fuse with these vacuoles, or they may enter from the cell exterior within the pinocytotic vacuole. This mechanism thus brings together hydrolytic enzymes and their natural substrates in the same subcellular compartment. Presumably, exogenously administered enzyme could take the same route to reach and remove intracellular accumulations in each of the storage diseases.

Deposits of mucopolysaccharides that build up in fibroblasts cultured from the skin of patients with various mucopolysaccharidoses can be removed by exposure of these cells to corrective factors secreted by normal or other mutant cell lines. These corrective factors are identical to the enzymes missing in each of the diseases (76). Cell surface recognition of lysosomal enzymes is a specific process that involves a carbohydrate moiety on the enzyme. Removal of the carbohydrate recognition marker from the enzyme converts it from a high uptake to a low uptake form. The fibroblast cell receptor shows a preference for phosphomannosyl residues, whereas in mammalian liver, galactosyl terminals are preferred by the hepatocyte receptor, and mannosyl and N-acetylglucosaminyl residues bind to the Kupffer cell receptor (5).

The promise of enzyme replacement therapy engendered by the in vitro fibroblast model has not come close to expectations. Infusions of fresh plasma into patients with mucopolysaccharidosis, for example, have produced only transient clinical improvement or no improvement at all (77–79). One reason for the failure of enzyme therapy has been the very short half-life of the infused enzyme activity. The half-life of purified hexosaminidase A given to a child with the Sandhoff variant of G_{M2}-gangliosidosis was only 7.5 minutes (80). Similarly, human placental glucocerebrosidase administered intravenously to two children with Gaucher's disease had a half-life of only 20 minutes in the circulation (81). Most of the infused enzyme concentrated in the liver. Furthermore, a check of the spinal fluid in the patient with Sandhoff disease indicated that the enzyme had not crossed the blood-brain barrier.

Leukocyte infusions have been tried in patients with mucopolysaccharidoses in an attempt to provide a more continuous, longer-lived source of enzyme activity (82). The unsuccessful outcome of such infusions is not surprising, however, in view of the finding of Jolly and co-workers that a twin male calf had all the manifestations of mannosidosis even though it had circulating lymphocytes acquired as a fetal transplant from its normal female co-twin (83).

Liposomes (84) and erythrocyte ghosts (85) have been suggested as biodegradable vehicles for enzyme loading in the storage diseases. This approach also suffers from the difficulty of targeting a limited amount of enzyme to the proper cells.

Initial successes in kidney transplantation for Fabry's disease encouraged the trial of organ transplantation for Gaucher's disease (86, 87) and Niemann-Pick disease (88). However, neither a kidney transplant in an infant with Gaucher's disease (87) nor a spleen transplant in a patient with the juvenile form of Gaucher's disease (86) produced any long-term benefit. In a 2-year-old child with Niemann-Pick disease, type A, liver transplantation restored sphingomyelinase activity to normal in serum and cerebrospinal fluid but not in leukocytes and tears. During the first 6 months after transplantation some improvement was noticed, but the child subsequently died (88).

Histocompatible skin fibroblasts have been transplanted into three patients with Hunter's syndrome (89) and three with Sanfilippo A disease (90). In each case, increases in enzyme activity and catabolism of mucopolysaccharide were observed but clearance of stored material and actual clinical improvement could not be demonstrated.

BONE MARROW TRANSPLANTATION

In properly selected cases, bone marrow transplantation may be an effective means of metabolic correction. In diseases of the reticuloendothelial system (RES), donor macrophages could wander throughout the viscera to repopulate the Kupffer cells of the liver and other RES-derived elements, exocytose and degrade the stored metabolite, and secrete enzyme to be taken up by deficient lysosomes in distant cells. Promising results have been obtained in Hurler's disease (91) and Maroteaux-Lamy syndrome (2), but this form of treatment has not been successful in many other cases, either because the lysosomal storage disease affected the central nervous system (1) or because of the increased mortality associated with the graft-versus-host reaction (> 40 per cent) (92).

There is no evidence that enzymes in blood can reach the brain, nor do marrow-derived elements appear to cross the blood-brain barrier. Therefore, bone marrow transplantation is most likely to succeed where there is an HLA-identical (MLC) negative donor (93), the disease to be treated does not affect the nervous system, and the treatment is performed before severe structural damage has occurred (1). The popularity of this procedure will undoubtedly increase as the present high rate of complications declines and methods are worked out in conjunction with molecular biologists for the use of marrow replacement for specific gene therapy (94).

Prevention

An autosomal recessive mechanism of inheritance characterizes each of the storage diseases of the RES with the exception of Hunter's disease, a mucopolysaccharidosis that is transmitted through the X chromosome. In most instances, the amount of lysosomal enzyme activity correlates with the dosage of the wild-type gene present. For example, enzyme levels in carriers of the abnormal gene (heterozygotes) are approximately half those in normal individuals. Thus, heterozygotes for specific recessive disease traits can be diagnosed by enzyme assay. This requires that there be no overlap between the enzyme levels in heterozygotes and those in normal or diseased individuals.

Heterozygote detection by enzyme assay serves several functions. The finding of heterozygosity in the parents of an individual with a storage disease helps to confirm the diagnosis in that individual. This method of testing is particularly valuable when the propositus has died without enzymatic confirmation of a diagnosis. Siblings, cousins, and other close relatives of a patient with a storage disease can be told specifically whether or not there is a chance that they can pass the abnormal gene on to their offspring. Carrier relatives who are married will probably also want their spouses to be tested.

In those rare instances in which both spouses are heterozygotes, each pregnancy carries a 25 per cent risk of producing an affected offspring. In such circumstances, chorionic biopsy performed about the eighth week or amniocentesis done at the fifteenth to sixteenth week of gestation permits biochemical determinations to be made on cells of fetal origin. In this way, a prenatal diagnosis can be made in sufficient time to terminate a pregnancy if the fetus is affected. Families previously struck by the tragedy of an infant with a fatal form of storage disease may thus be spared the burden of additional progeny having the same disease and can anticipate having healthy children without fear. Happily, the outcome in the majority (75 per cent) of prenatal diagnostic investigations for these high-risk situations is a clinically unaffected child. This reduces the incidence of abortion in families who are determined to avoid such disasters, because without this assurance such families often terminate all pregnancies.

Prenatal diagnosis has been accomplished, or is theoretically possible, for each of the storage diseases. It is important that the parents of a child with a sphingolipidosis, mucopolysaccharidosis, or oligosaccharidosis be carefully counseled and informed of the availability of prenatal diagnosis for future pregnancies as soon as possible after the diagnosis is made in their child. Otherwise, it often happens that one or both parents will elect to undergo a sterilization procedure in the mistaken belief that all their subsequent offspring will be similarly affected. In addition, the mother might already be pregnant or might become pregnant and be unaware of the prenatal diagnostic option until after the optimal time for conducting such studies has passed. Often, one of the factors motivating parents to obtain a specific diagnosis in their young child with a storage disease is a current pregnancy. This circumstance may place a severe time constraint on the laboratory by requiring diagnosis of the affected child before the pregnancy passes the mid-trimester point, after which prenatal diagnostic amniocentesis is no longer practical.

Thus far, it has been possible to screen large populations for heterozygotes only in Tay-Sachs disease. The circumstances that have made this practicable are a high gene frequency in a small subgroup of the population (Ashkenazi Jews) and the availability of a simple, dependable, and economical test for heterozygotes. Testing for other storage diseases cannot meet these prerequisites either because the disease trait is very rare and distributed equally throughout the general population or because the enzyme assay for heterozygotes is complicated and cannot be automated or in some other way performed inexpensively. Also, without the advantage of an index case in the family, interpretation of enzyme tests for heterozygotes may be difficult. This is because carriers of two diseases with very different clinical consequences, such as Hurler's disease and Scheie's disease or the infantile and adult forms of Gaucher's disease, may be indistinguishable. Therefore, at present, prevention of the storage diseases relies upon the concepts of early case identification, screening of close relatives for heterozygotes, and prenatal diagnosis during pregnancies in which both spouses carry the same recessive trait.

SPHINGOLIPIDOSES

The sphingolipidoses account for 10 categories of storage disease, each characterized by the accumulation of a particular sphingolipid in neural and/or extraneural tissues. The basic unit of the stored material, ceramide, is composed of the long-chain amino alcohol sphingosine joined to a fatty acid of 16 to 26 carbon atoms by an amide linkage at the nitrogen atom on carbon 2 of sphingosine (Fig. 38–1).

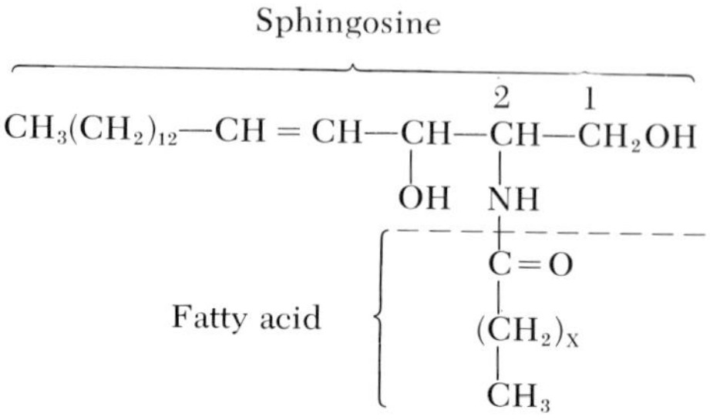

Individual sphingolipids belong to one of four subgroups, depending upon the types of substi-

$$CH_3(CH_2)_{12}-CH=CH-\overset{\text{Sphingosine}}{\overset{2}{C}H}-\overset{1}{C}H-CH_2OH$$

Figure 38–1. Chemical structure of ceramide.

tuents joined to the primary alcohol on carbon 1 of sphingosine, i.e., sphingomyelin, neutral glycosphingolipids, sulfatoglycosphingolipids, and gangliosides. Sphingomyelin is a phospholipid component of cell membranes. The neutral glycosphingolipids are found in many body tissues, with normally high concentrations of globoside in red blood cell membranes and of ceramide trihexoside in kidney. The sulfolipids and galactolipids are important in the formation of myelin. Gangliosides are located in nervous system tissues.

Catabolism of the sphingolipids occurs by the stepwise hydrolysis of linkages joining the various components of the molecule. The sequence of cleavage is from the terminal nonreducing hydrophilic end of the molecule toward the hydrophobic sphingosine portion. The structure of the individual sphingolipids, their degradative pathway, and the reactions blocked in each of the sphingolipidoses are shown in Figure 38–2.

Not all the sphingolipidoses cause lipid storage in RES cells. The pathologic findings in metachromatic leukodystrophy and Krabbe's disease are confined to the nervous system, with the occurrence of severe myelin destruction and a segmental peripheral neuropathy. Clinically, blindness, long tract signs, and loss of reflexes occur. Elevation in spinal fluid protein concentration and delayed nerve conduction velocities are early diagnostic findings.

Tay-Sachs disease, the most common form of G_{M2}-gangliosidosis, results in ballooning of nerve cells throughout the neuraxis. Psychomotor retardation and a cherry-red spot in the macula are early signs. Eventually, seizures, megacephaly, blindness, and flaccid quadriparesis develop before the affected child dies, usually between the ages of 3 and 5 years. Before heterozygote testing for the Tay-Sachs trait become widely available, the majority of cases occurred among the offspring of Ashkenazi Jews. As a result of carrier testing and prenatal diagnosis among this population, the number of Tay-Sachs cases has declined, with a much greater proportion now observed in children of non-Jewish parentage.

The lesions in Fabry's disease are predominantly extraneural, primarily in the vascular endothelium

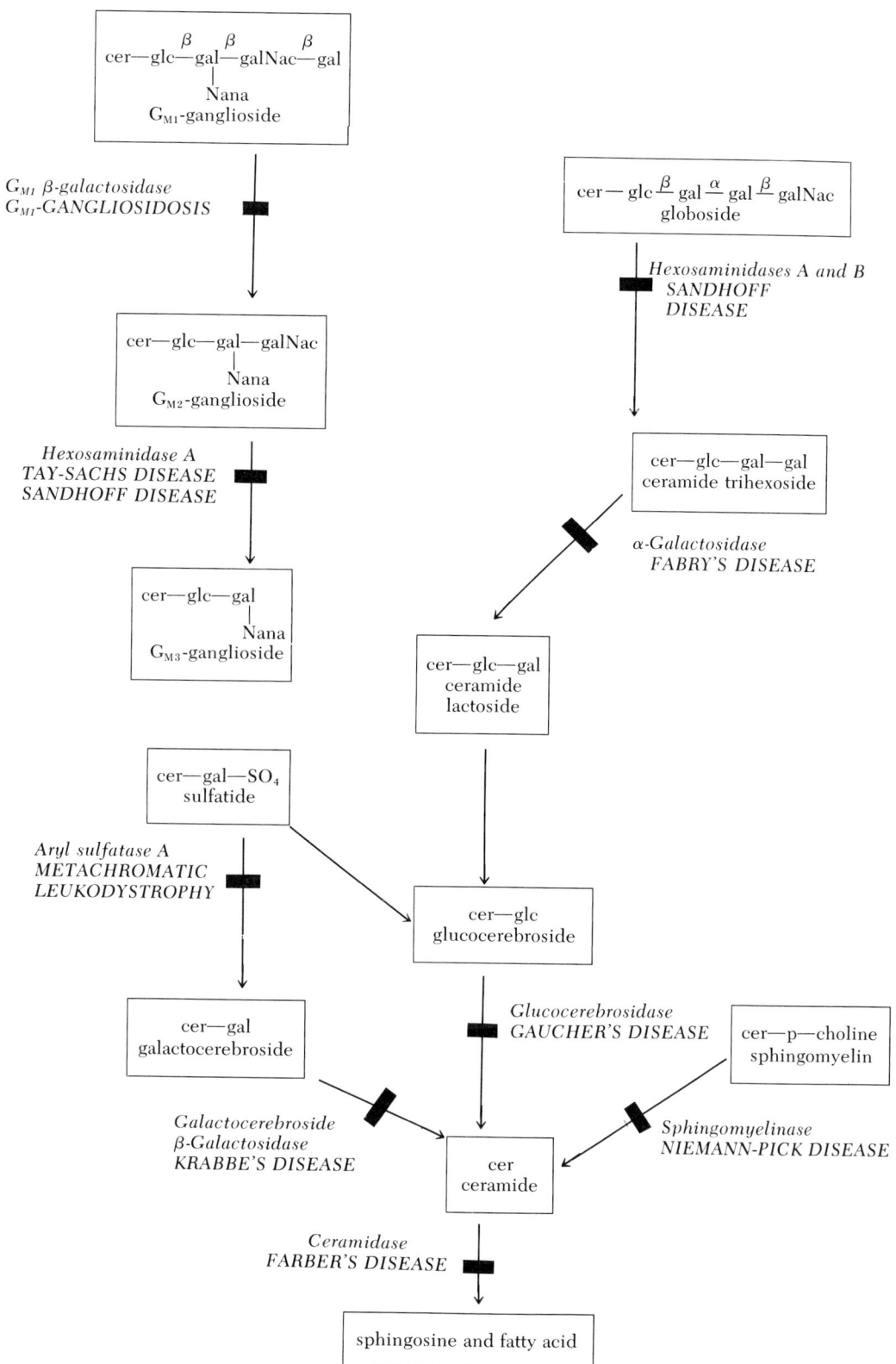

Figure 38–2. Pathways and diseases of sphingolipid metabolism. The enzymes involved are shown in italics. Listed below each enzyme is the disease that results from deficiency of that enzyme. KEY: *cer* = ceramide; *glc* = glucose; *gal* = galactose; *galNac* = N-acetylgalactosamine; *Nana* = N-acetylneuraminic acid.

and kidneys. It is an X-linked disease that is usually recognized in early-adolescent boys by the onset of intermittent pains in the hands and feet and the appearance of clusters of purple punctate angiokeratomas. The presence of feathery corneal opacities on slit-lamp examination helps to establish the diagnosis in hemizygotes and to confirm heterozygosity in their mothers and sisters.

Another of the sphingolipidoses, fucosidosis, will be discussed with the oligosaccharidoses.

Gaucher's Disease (Glucosylceramide Lipidosis)

Gaucher's disease is the oldest known and most frequently encountered type of inherited lipidosis. Phillipe C. E. Gaucher, who first described the disease in 1882 as an epithelioma of the spleen without leukemia, did not recognize its systemic nature or its predilection for the RES (95). Individual patients differ greatly in their degree of clinical involvement but nearly all have hepatosplenomegaly, Gaucher cells in their bone marrow, and accumulation of glucocerebroside due to a deficiency of the enzyme glucocerebroside β-glucosidase. The glucocerebroside is derived from (1) lactosylceramide, the major glycolipid of leukocytes; (2) globoside, the principal red blood cell glycolipid; and (3) the blood-group glycosphingolipids.

TYPE 1: CHRONIC NON-NEURONOPATHIC (ADULT) GAUCHER'S DISEASE

Three separate and distinct clinical varieties of Gaucher's disease have been recognized. The great majority of cases belong to type 1, the chronic non-neuronopathic form of the disease. Hematologic findings dominate the clinical picture of patients in this category. The spleen may be enlarged from an early age and in some patients can become so huge that it causes abdominal distension and pain. An anemia is usually present because of decreased red cell survival. The anemia may be either normocytic or microcytic and hypochromic and is probably due to hypersplenism rather than to the crowding out of erythropoiesis in the bone marrow by Gaucher cells. Although iron therapy may temporarily help the anemia, it is not recommended because Gaucher cells avidly take up iron, reducing its availability for erythropoiesis and leading to hemachromatosis.

A bleeding tendency resulting from thrombocytopenia is a more serious consequence of the hypersplenism that occurs in Gaucher's disease. Easy bruisability and epistaxis are also common complaints in childhood. Trauma to the enlarged spleen is a special danger because of the possibility of rupture and hemorrhage. This hazard also exists when a Gaucher's disease patient with hypersplenism develops acute infectious mononucleosis. Bleeding into other organs and metrorrhagia may also occur. In one patient with portal hypertension, hematemesis occurred from rupture of esophageal varices (96). Possibly contributing to the bleeding tendency in Gaucher's disease is a deficiency of Factor IX (plasma thromboplastin component). This abnormality was found in vitro in the plasma of 8 of 11 Gaucher's disease patients studied (97). Splenectomy is often performed because of thrombocytopenia with recurrent bleeding or because of marked abdominal pain and discomfort produced by the large spleen. Platelet counts rise after splenectomy, and episodes of bleeding no longer occur.

Bone complications are common. As Gaucher cells infiltrate the medullary cavity, there is loss of bone density, thinning of the cortex, loss of the normal trabeculations, patchy myelosclerosis, bone infarcts, and osteonecrosis. At least half of all patients show an Erlenmeyer flask deformity. The midshaft of the femur has a tapered appearance and the distal end is widened due to failure of trabeculation. This same change may also be seen in the proximal ends of the tibia and fibula. Aseptic necrosis of the head and neck of the femur can occur, causing such disability and pain as to require surgical arthroplasty. Other forms of pathological fracture are also seen as well as bone infarcts that cause episodes of severe incapacitating bone and joint pain (98).

In some patients, the basic disease clearly worsens following splenectomy, and the liver increases in size more rapidly. This has fueled arguments pro and con regarding the efficacy of splenectomy for Gaucher's disease. Conventional wisdom suggests that the loss of the spleen diverts the accumulating lipid to the liver and bone marrow, further compromising these tissues. However, not all splenectomized patients develop serious problems with their liver or bones. Nevertheless, treatment strategies designed to allow some of the benefits of splenectomy without total loss of spleen tissue might conceivably protect patients against bone disease. If an accessory spleen is present, it might be left in situ during surgical removal of the main splenic mass. Alternatively, a small part of the spleen might be detached at the time of splenectomy and reimplanted into the omentum so that a nidus of spleen tissue remains behind to proliferate as a new storage depot for the glucocerebroside excess. The usefulness of these approaches needs to be tested.

Most patients have some degree of hepatosplenomegaly, and portal hypertension sometimes occurs, but liver failure with abnormal liver function tests is rare. A few patients develop diffuse pulmonary infiltration. Renal disease and central nervous system involvement are unusual. Older patients may develop hypergammaglobulinemia and a few individuals with coexistent multiple myeloma have been reported (99, 100). There is also an increase in other malignancies such as leukemia (101) and Hodgkin's disease (102).

Approximately 60 per cent of patients with type 1 Gaucher's disease are of Ashkenazi Jewish ancestry. Among this population the gene frequency may be as high as 8 per cent (98), but the actual disease incidence is much less than expected because the clinical spectrum includes many mildly affected individuals who may remain undiagnosed until late in life or may never become symptomatic. The variability in clinical expression is evident in families in which several members are affected; one may have severe incapacitating bone disease while another has only mild hypersplenism and occasional joint pains. A particularly malignant form of the disease is seen in non-Jewish children who develop considerable splenomegaly by age 3 years and portal hypertension by age 10. These patients have massive abdominal swelling and stunted linear growth and are good candidates for bone marrow transplantation.

Laboratory diagnosis depends upon the presence of Gaucher cells in the bone marrow and the demonstration of a deficiency in lysosomal β-glucosidase activity measured in leukocytes or cultured skin fibroblasts. Other helpful procedures include a liver and spleen scan for organ size and zones of hemorrhage, a bone scan for microinfarctions, and analysis of plasma glycolipids by HPLC to demonstrate the increase in glucocerebroside (usually two- to three-fold). Ancillary findings in the serum include elevations in activities of nontartrate-inhibitable acid phosphatase, angiotensin-converting enzyme (103), and transcobalamin II (104).

TYPE 2: ACUTE NEURONOPATHIC (INFANTILE) GAUCHER'S DISEASE

The child with the acute neuronopathic variety of Gaucher's disease (type 2) presents between birth and 6 months of age with failure to thrive, hepatosplenomegaly, muscular hypertonicity, and signs of brain stem dysfunction, including strabismus and retroflexion of the head. Other nervous system signs include dysphagia, laryngospasm, dyspnea, vomiting, and generalized spasticity. In addition, there are feeding difficulties, inanition, and weight loss. Death is inevitable before 2 years of age. A later-onset form has also been recognized in which strabismus develops during the first year but the children are otherwise normal until the second or third year.

Nerve cells in the brains of these children are swollen by a PAS-positive, weakly sudanophilic material. Brain concentrations of glucocerebroside and psychosine (sphingosine-glucose) are increased in all types of Gaucher's disease, but the highest levels are found in the cerebral and cerebellar cortex of patients with the acute neuronopathic variety (105). As in type 1 Gaucher's disease, the activities of serum acid phosphate and angiotensin-converting enzyme are markedly elevated (106). Because of its early onset and fatal outcome, prenatal diagnosis of type 2 Gaucher's disease provides a feasible alternative to families at risk for additional children with this disorder.

TYPE 3: SUBACUTE NEURONOPATHIC (JUVENILE) GAUCHER'S DISEASE

In rare cases, nervous system involvement has occurred in older children and adults with Gaucher's disease. Neurologic findings have included decreased mental abilities, seizures, poor coordination, and an increase in muscle tone. Certain cases most closely resemble the acute neuronopathic variety of Gaucher's disease (107), whereas in others the clinical course is similar in many respects to the more common adult non-neuronopathic variety of the disease (108).

However, one subgroup of patients with neurologic signs does differ significantly enough from those with types 1 and 2 Gaucher's disease to justify classifying them separately. These patients develop a mixed seizure disorder in late childhood or early adolescence that includes frequent staring spells as well as grand mal convulsions. Mentation and voluntary motor movements are slowed. Myoclonus develops, producing rapid asynchronous jerks of the extremities, trunk, and face that interfere with all activities including walking, speaking, feeding, and dressing. The majority of these patients have a history of splenectomy at some time prior to the onset of their neurologic symptoms.

Genetically, this particular syndrome is probably distinct from type 1 adult Gaucher's disease. It has been identified in several related patients from Northern Sweden but has not been reported in Ashkenazi Jews. This form of Gaucher's disease is also distinguished from types 1 and 2 by the response of monoclonal antibodies to the residual β-glucosidase present. After separation by polyacrylamide gel electrophoresis, the three molecular forms of the enzyme form different patterns of banding in the three diseases (109). Because of the relentlessly progressive neurologic deterioration that occurs in type 3 patients, they have been prime candidates for therapeutic experimentation such as enzyme replacement (81), organ transplantation (86), and bone marrow transplantation (1). Whether marrow transplantation would improve neurologic function in storage disease is currently unknown and under limited study in metachromatic leukodystrophy (109a).

Niemann-Pick Disease (Sphingomyelin Lipidosis)

Niemann-Pick disease comprises a group of disorders that have in common infiltration of the RES by foam cells containing sphingomyelin and to a lesser extent cholesterol and other cell membrane lipids. The eponym refers to Albert Niemann, the German pediatrician who published the first clinical description in 1914 (110), and Ludwig Pick, whose histologic studies published in 1922 (111) and 1927 (112) differentiated this disease from Gaucher's disease.

Sphingomyelin is both a phospholipid and a sphingolipid. Its two major components are ceramide and phosphorylcholine, which are linked by a phosphodiester bond to the first carbon atom of sphingosine. Any interference in the normal process of cell membrane turnover may cause sphingomyelin, cholesterol, and other membrane constituents to accumulate. The enzyme sphingomyelinase is deficient in some forms of Niemann-Pick disease, but no abnormality in sphingomyelin catabolism can be demonstrated in other variants associated with sphingomyelin accumulation. Therefore, the different forms of Niemann-Pick disease are grouped together because of similarities in clinical features, including hepatosplenomegaly and foam cell infiltration of the bone marrow, not because each variant shares the same enzyme deficiency.

In 1961, Crocker proposed a division of Niemann-Pick disease into four clinical subtypes (113); a fifth (adult non-neuronopathic) form was later added. Clinical and biochemical studies carried out since then suggest that this classification should be modified to include: (1) two forms with severe sphingomyelinase deficiency, i.e., classic Niemann-Pick disease (type A) and a chronic form in infancy without nervous system involvement (type B); (2) a third form with partial sphingomyelinase deficiency manifested by moderate visceral involvement and variable central nervous system degeneration in early childhood; and (3) a category for other forms with sphingomyelin storage, few (if any) neurologic findings, and normal sphingomyelinase activity.

ACUTE NEURONOPATHIC FORM (TYPE A)

Patients with the classic infantile form of Niemann-Pick disease present at 3 to 6 months of age with feeding difficulties, liver and spleen enlargement, and developmental delay. Lymphadenopathy may be found, and in half the cases a cherry-red macula is noted. During the succeeding months, the abdomen becomes protuberant, and there is general inanition with wasting of the extremities and frequent infections. Death occurs by age 2 to 3 years. At postmortem examination, there is ascites fluid in the abdomen; the liver, spleen, and lymph nodes are enlarged, yellow, and fatty; and foam cells are present in many different tissues. The vast majority of these patients are of Ashkenazic Jewish parentage, but this disease is considerably less common than Tay-Sachs or adult (type 1) Gaucher's disease, two other sphingolipidoses with a higher frequency among Ashkenazim.

CHRONIC FORM WITHOUT CENTRAL NERVOUS SYSTEM INVOLVEMENT (TYPE B)

Patients with this variant usually present in early childhood with abdominal distention due to liver and spleen enlargement. Foam cell infiltration of the lungs may occur, but survival with preservation of intellect for many years is common. Massive enlargement of the spleen in these patients may necessitate splenectomy, but curiously, plasma sphingomyelin levels are not elevated. Bone pathology of the type seen in Gaucher's disease does not occur but osteoporosis, widening of the medullary cavities and modelling defects can be demonstrated radiologically. Occasionally, a macular halo may be found in the fundus but vision is not disturbed. Sea-blue histiocytes are present in the bone marrow of some patients. The bluish cast revealed by the Giemsa stain results from the accumulation of ceroid within these cells.

CHRONIC NEURONOPATHIC FORM

The largest group of sphingomyelin lipidosis patients probably belongs in this category. After a variable period of normal development usually lasting 1 to 3 years, the affected child develops ataxia, progressive tetraparesis, loss of speech, and deterioration of mental functions. Older children may present with a vertical gaze paresis, dysarthria, dysphagia, incoordination, seizures, and involuntary movements (114). There may be a history of jaundice during the neonatal period, and a liver biopsy may show chronic hepatitis with giant cells (115). Hepatomegaly is usually present. Sphingomyelinase activity is normal or partially deficient, depending upon the tissue examined. Crocker's type C and D patients and some patients with the sea-blue histiocyte syndrome are in this category.

ADULT NON-NEURONOPATHIC FORM

These patients have normal sphingomyelinase activity but store sphingomyelin in organs of the RES. They usually have no neurologic involvement and several have survived to old age.

Niemann-Pick disease must be suspected in infants and children with hepatosplenomegaly and bone marrow findings of enlarged foamy or sea-blue histiocytes. The diagnosis may be confirmed by use of leukocytes or cultured skin fibroblasts to assay sphingomyelinase activity. If no deficiency is found and other causes of hepatomegaly and foam cell infiltration can be ruled out, evidence of sphingomyelin storage can be obtained by analyzing a liver biopsy specimen. Ancillary findings that are helpful in some cases include lymphocytic vacuolization in peripheral blood smears and an increase in the sphingomyelin content of the urinary sediment.

Heterozygotes for the A and B types can be identified by the reduced levels of sphingomyelinase activity present in their leukocytes or cultured skin fibroblasts, using ^{14}C-sphingomyelin as substrate. Prenatal diagnosis of type A Niemann-Pick disease is also possible (116).

Farber's Disease (Lipogranulomatosis)

Painful swollen joints in the hands and feet, hoarseness, and vomiting are early presenting signs of Farber's disease. These difficulties may be present as early as a few weeks after birth. As the disease progresses, subcutaneous and periarticular nodules develop, especially near the interphalangeal, ankle, wrist, and elbow joints, leading to flexion contractures. Swelling and granuloma formation in the epiglottis and larynx cause swallowing and respiratory disturbances. Foam cell infiltration and granulomatous deposits in the lungs further complicate the pulmonary problem. The tongue, heart, and liver may become enlarged, and granulomatous lesions of the heart valves also develop.

There are few central nervous system signs in Farber's disease. Joint pain limits movement, but psychomotor development in most patients is normal. In some patients a peripheral neuropathy occurs, with a decrease in response of the deep tendon reflexes and electromyographic signs of denervation. The electroencephalogram is normal, and seizures have not been reported.

The principal finding in pathologic studies is the presence of granulomatous infiltrates composed of foam cells containing a PAS-positive material that is extractable with lipid solvents. Analysis of this material by electron microscopy suggests a heterogeneous ultrastructure composed principally of membrane-bound inclusions. Neuronal cytoplasm is also filled with PAS-positive storage material.

Chemical studies of the subcutaneous nodules indicate that ceramides account for 10 to 20 per cent of the total lipids present. Increased ceramide concentrations in the urine, brain, and organs of Farber's disease patients have also been demonstrated. Two enzymes, with pH optima of 4 and 9, have been described that are capable of catalyzing ceramide hydrolysis. Leukocytes, cultured skin fibroblasts, and solid tissue specimens from patients with Farber's disease are deficient in the acid ceramidase.

To date, 29 cases of this disease have been reported since Farber's original report in 1957 (117–119). Death generally occurs before age 2 years. Tracheostomy may be useful in managing upper airway obstruction, and some relief of joint pains may be obtained with prednisone.

G_{M1}-Gangliosidosis

Central nervous system signs dominate the clinical picture in both the infantile type 1 and late infantile–juvenile type 2 forms of G_{M1}-gangliosidosis. The gray matter of the brain in both disorders contains approximately 10 times the normal amount of G_{M1}-ganglioside, owing to deficiency of G_{M1}-ganglioside β-galactosidase. However, there are major differences in these two diseases that relate primarily to the age of onset and degree of visceral involvement.

INFANTILE G_{M1}-GANGLIOSIDOSIS, TYPE 1

A child with this form of G_{M1}-gangliosidosis may appear edematous at birth and have a weak suck, poor feeding, and slow weight gain. Hypotonia, increased startle response, and hepatosplenomegaly may be noticed within the first 2 months. Development will be delayed because of inability to crawl or sit unsupported. The child's facial features are coarse and distinguished by frontal bossing and a depressed nasal bridge. Bony deformities include stubby hands, broad wrists, anterior beaking of the lumbar vertebrae, thickening of the midshaft of the humerus, and spatulate ribs. A cherry-red macula occurs in half the type 1 cases; nystagmus and an esotropia may also be present. Clonic-tonic convulsions develop, and if the child survives beyond age 1 year, decerebrate rigidity, deafness, blindness, and spastic quadriplegia occur. Death usually results from bronchopneumonia between 1 and 2 years of age.

LATE INFANTILE-JUVENILE G_{M1}-GANGLIOSIDOSIS, TYPE 2

The early development of a patient with type 2 G_{M1}-gangliosidosis may be normal, but careful review of the history usually discloses an exaggerated startle response and hypotonia from an early age. Toward the end of the first year, the child may lose the ability to crawl, sit, and stand, and language development ceases. The plantar responses become extensor, and seizures develop later. Some pallor of the optic discs may be noted, but a cherry-red spot is absent. Corneal clouding and rotatory nystagmus may occur. In most cases the liver is not enlarged, and there are no skeletal abnormalities. Survival for 3 to 10 years is possible.

A third group of older patients with G_{M1}-gangliosidosis has also been described. These patients have progressive pyramidal and extrapyramidal disease beginning late in childhood or in adolescence. Skeletal changes and visceromegaly do not occur in this group.

The RES in both childhood types of G_{M1}-gangliosidosis contains foamy histiocytes filled with strongly PAS-positive granular material. In addition, the hepatocytes, renal tubule and skin epithelial cells, and other cells contain PAS-positive intracellular vacuoles. The liver of patients with type 1 (but not type 2) G_{M1}-gangliosidosis contains an excess of G_{M1}-ganglioside. Accumulations of other galactose-containing oligosaccharides have been found in the viscera and urine of individuals with both types of G_{M1}-gangliosidosis. Several of these oligosaccharides appear to be derived from the incomplete degradation of certain erythrocyte glycoproteins and plasma immunoglobulins (120).

The diagnosis of the G_{M1}-gangliosidoses may be confirmed by assay of plasma, leukocyte, or fibroblast β-galactosidase activity (121).

G_{M2}-Gangliosidosis, Sandhoff Variant

The G_{M2}-gangliosidoses include five diseases resulting from impaired degradation of G_{M2}-ganglioside, a minor brain glycolipid containing both sialic acid and N-acetylgalactosamine in the terminal portion of its oligosaccharide side chain. In the classic and most common form, Tay-Sachs disease, hexosaminidase A is deficient. Hexosaminidase A activity is also reduced or absent in cases of the juvenile and adult variants of G_{M2}-gangliosides. Patients with the much rarer AB variant lack a factor that stimulates the hexosaminidase-A–catalyzed hydrolysis of G_{M2}-ganglioside and of its asialo derivative G_{A2} (10). In each of these four forms of G_{M2}-gangliosidosis, G_{M2}-ganglioside and smaller amounts of G_{A2} accumulate in brain and, to a considerably lesser extent, in visceral organs. Consequently, the clinical signs in these diseases are confined to the central nervous system, and obvious infiltration of the RES has not been noted.

However, considerable involvement of extraneural tissues does occur in the Sandhoff variant of G_{M2}-gangliosidosis. This disorder is associated with more marked accumulation of G_{A2} in both the brain and viscera than occurs in any of the other variants. In addition, levels of globoside, the major red blood cell glycolipid, are markedly elevated, particularly in the liver, spleen, and kidney. These lipid abnormalities result from the absence of hexosaminidases A and B and produce signs of RES involvement, including foam cells in the bone marrow and other organs. In all other respects, the infant with Sandhoff's disease is clinically indistinguishable from the child with Tay-Sachs disease.

The Tay-Sachs or Sandhoff's disease infant may appear normal at birth, but an alert parent or an experienced professional can detect hypotonia and an exaggerated startle response within the first 2 months. Between 3 and 6 months of age, motor weakness and then listlessness become evident. The child may roll from side to side but cannot turn over completely. He or she slumps forward when placed in a sitting position and cannot crawl or stand. There is poor visual fixation with roving eye movements. Quite early in the course of the disease and definitely by 4 months a cherry-red spot with a white perimacular halo can be observed in both fundi. Weakness, spasticity, and increased deep tendon reflexes develop, and feeding difficulties with associated gagging become a concern.

At approximately 1 year of age seizures are first noted, excessive drooling begins, and bouts of unmotivated laughter occur. During the second year the head begins enlarging disproportionately. The optic discs become pale and atrophic, and cortical blindness ensues. After age 2 years there are episodes of autonomic dysfunction with unexplained temperature elevations; spells of rubor, pallor, or cyanosis; and irregular breathing. Although visceral lipid storage occurs in Sandhoff's disease, the liver and spleen are not clinically enlarged, and there are no obvious skeletal changes. Great efforts must be expended to maintain hydration and nutrition, control constipation and seizures, and prevent infection. These children rarely survive beyond age 3 or 4 years.

Sandhoff's disease can be distinguished from other forms of G_{M2}-gangliosidosis by the presence of foam cells in the bone marrow and the total absence of β-N-acetylhexosaminidase from serum, leukocytes, cultured fibroblasts, tears, and urine. HPLC analysis of plasma glycolipids will demonstrate an increased globoside content in Sandhoff's disease but not in Tay-Sachs disease.

Persons heterozygous for the gene for Sandhoff's disease can usually be identified by a reduced level of total serum hexosaminidase (A and B forms) and a higher than normal percentage (greater than 70 per cent) of hexosaminidase in the A form. The same test used to screen for carriers of Tay-Sachs can be used to detect Sandhoff carriers. No cases of Sandhoff's disease have been recorded in children of Jewish parents. This contrasts with Tay-Sachs disease, which until recently was much more frequent among Ashkenazic Jewish offspring.

MUCOPOLYSACCHARIDOSES

The coarse facial features, skeletal dysplasia, and limitation of joint motion that dominate the clinical picture of the mucopolysaccharidoses clearly distinguish this group of lysosomal storage diseases from the sphingolipidoses. The urine of these patients contains excessive amounts of mucopolysaccharides, which are complex carbohydrates found in various types of connective tissue, including cartilage and bone.

The typical mucopolysaccharide contains a core polypeptide to which a number of polysaccharide chains are attached by a xylose link. Each polysac-

DERMATAN SULFATE

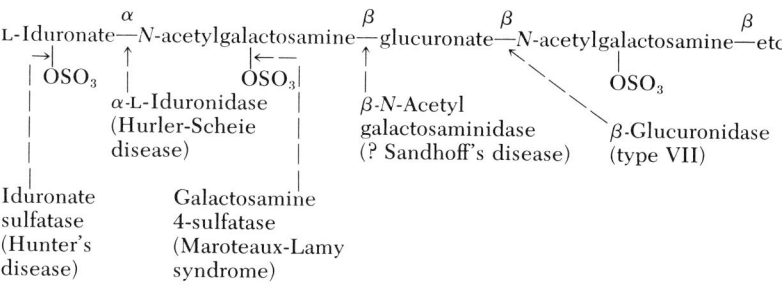

HEPARAN SULFATE

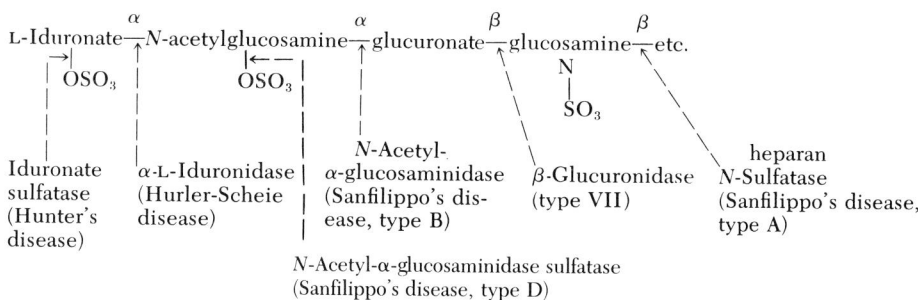

Figure 38–3. Pathways for the enzymatic degradation of dermatan sulfate and heparan sulfate. Deficiencies of each of the enzyme activities shown are correlated with specific mucopolysaccharidoses.

charide chain may contain 100 or more sugar residues joined together in repeating disaccharide units consisting of a uronic acid (glucuronic or L-iduronic acid) alternating with a sulfated hexosamine (glucosamine or galactosamine) (Fig. 38–3). The hexosamine in dermatan sulfate is N-acetyl-β-D-galactosamine; in heparan sulfate, it is N-acetyl-α-D-glucosamine. Iduronic acid is occasionally sulfated, but glucuronic acid is not. In heparan sulfate, sulfate may be present on the amino nitrogen in place of an acetyl group. Fragments from one or both of these mucopolysaccharides accumulate in each of the mucopolysaccharidoses (Table 38–5) because of a block in their sequential hydrolysis due to a lysosomal enzyme deficiency (Fig. 38–3). An exception is Morquio's syndrome, which is characterized by the accumulation of two other mucopolysaccharides, keratan sulfate and chondroitin-6-sulfate. In keratan sulfate, galactose substitutes for the uronic acid moiety (Fig. 38–4).

Mucopolysaccharide storage leads to several alterations of cell morphology in the blood and bone marrow. Azurophilic granulations are present in polymorphonuclear leukocytes and lymphocytes (Alder-Reilly bodies) (26, 27). Vacuoles with basophilic granulations are also found in circulating lymphocytes, bone marrow reticulocytes (Gasser cells), and bone marrow plasma cells (Buhot cells). Circulating lymphocytes may also contain metachromatic vacuoles without granulation (Mittwoch cells).

Other cells also manifest changes associated with excessive tissue mucopolysaccharide. Clouding of the cornea, thickening of the leptomeninges with hydrocephalus, alterations in bone architecture, thickening of heart valves, ballooning of neurons, and RES foam cell infiltration are some of the changes observed. The salient clinical and biochemical features of each mucopolysaccharidosis are presented in Table 38–5.

Hurler's Disease (1H), Scheie's Disease (1S) and Hurler-Scheie Compound (1H/S)

Three diseases of α-L-iduronidase deficiency are recognized: Hurler's disease, Scheie's disease, and the Hurler-Scheie compound. Both dermatan and heparan sulfate are increased in the urine of these patients, but the heparan sulfaturia is much greater in Hurler's patients than in patients with Scheie's disease and Hurler-Scheie compound (122). Corresponding enzyme deficiencies can also be demonstrated. The α-iduronidase activity in fibroblasts of patients with Scheie and Hurler-Scheie diseases effectively hydrolyzes desulfated heparin but this same activity is deficient in Hurler's disease fibroblasts. Other substrates for α-iduronidase, such as dermatan sulfate and 4-MU-α-L-iduronide, an artificial fluorogenic compound, do not distinguish between the three diseases; with these substrates, the α-iduronidase deficiency in each variant is equally profound. Complementa-

Table 38–5. THE MUCOPOLYSACCHARIDOSES

Class	Eponym	Enzyme Defect	Urinary Mucopolysaccharides*	Mental Retardation	Corneal Clouding	Skeletal Dysplasia	Life Expectancy (Years)
I-H	Hurler's disease	α-L-iduronidase	DS, HS	+ +	+	+ + +	<10
I-S	Scheie's disease	α-L-iduronidase	DS, HS	−	+	+	normal
I-H/S	Hurler-Scheie compound	α-L-iduronidase	DS, HS	+	+	+ +	20's
II-Severe	Hunter's disease	iduronate sulfatase	DS, HS	+ +	−	+ +	<15
II-Mild	Hunter's disease	iduronate sulfatase	DS, HS	+	−	+	adulthood
III-A	Sanfilippo's disease	heparan N-sulfamidase	HS	+ + +	−	+	<20
III-B	Sanfilippo's disease	N-acetyl-α-D-glucosaminidase	HS	+ + +	−	+	<20
III-C	Sanfilippo's disease	heparin N-acetyl transferase	HS	+ +	−	+	adulthood
III-D	Sanfilippo's disease	N-acetyl-α-D-glucosamine sulfatase	HS	+ +	−	+	<20
IV	Morquio's syndrome	hexosamine-6-sulfatase	KS, CS	−	−	+ + +	20–40
VI	Maroteaux-Lamy syndrome	galactosamine-4-sulfatase	DS	−	+	+ +	20's
VII	Sly's disease	β-glucuronidase	DS	+	+/−	+	?
Mucosulfatidosis		multiple sulfatases	DS, HS Cholesterol S, sulfatide	+ +	−	+	3–12

*DS = dermatan sulfate; HS = heparan sulfate; KS = keratan sulfate; CS = chondroitin-6-sulfate; cholesterol S = cholesterol sulfate.

tion studies performed by fusing fibroblasts from patients with each of the three clinical types support the idea that they are allelic mutants (123). However, the Hurler-Scheie phenotype is probably not a genetic compound since it has been observed in children of a consanguineous marriage (124, 125) and the heparan α-iduronidase activity in this variant is not diminished (122).

Infants with Hurler's disease appear normal during the first few months of life, but they may be brought to medical attention because of persistent rhinorrhea, frequent middle ear infections, or stertorous breathing. Later during the first year, coarsening of the facial features, stiffening of the joints, and a thoracolumbar kyphosis become evident. Examination during the second year of life will reveal a large head with flat nasal bridge, broad nose and upturned nares, ocular hypertelorism, corneal clouding, hepatosplenomegaly, a gibbus deformity, and dwarfism. X-ray studies show that the skull sutures close early and the sinuses are poorly developed. Other radiologic signs include a J-shaped sella turcica, oar-shaped ribs, rounding and anterior beaking of the vertebrae, and shortening of the metacarpals and phalanges. These patients develop heart valve involve-

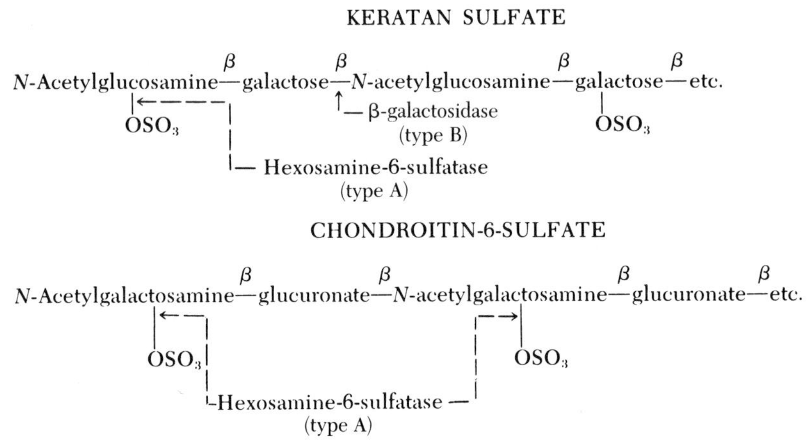

KERATAN SULFATE

N-Acetylglucosamine—β—galactose—β—N-acetylglucosamine—β—galactose—β—etc.
  | |
  OSO$_3$ OSO$_3$
                    └— β-galactosidase
                        (type B)
           └— Hexosamine-6-sulfatase
                    (type A)

CHONDROITIN-6-SULFATE

N-Acetylgalactosamine—β—glucuronate—β—N-acetylgalactosamine—β—glucuronate—β—etc.
  | |
  OSO$_3$ OSO$_3$
           └—Hexosamine-6-sulfatase—┘
                    (type A)

Figure 38–4. Glycosaminoglycans stored in Morquio's disease, and sites for the probable action of the enzyme deficiencies in this disease.

ment with murmurs and cardiac enlargement, which contributes to death before age 10 years.

Scheie's disease is less common than Hurler's disease. It usually presents in the school-aged child as difficulty in fine motor dexterity in the hands and fingers because of a claw hand deformity and carpal tunnel syndrome. The child's height is usually normal or only slightly below the norm, and the intellect is preserved. The neck may be very short. Corneal clouding is present, and some hearing loss may be noted. Aortic regurgitation may develop, and facial features eventually become coarse. Patients usually survive into adult life.

As in Hurler's disease, patients with the Hurler-Scheie phenotype have corneal clouding, hepatosplenomegaly, and dysostosis multiplex, but they are less retarded, not as dwarfed, have no gibbus deformity, and may live into their twenties. A receding chin and arachnoid cyst formation in the region of the sella turcica have been reported in several of these patients. There are also some forms of α-L-iduronidase deficiency of intermediate clinical severity that do not fit into the 1H, 1S, or 1H/S syndromes.

Diagnosis of patients and detection of carriers for each of the recognized clinical forms may be performed by assay of leukocyte or fiboblast α-L-iduronidase activity. Prenatal diagnosis has also been successfully performed (126). Bone marrow transplantation, though still controversial as a form of therapy (see section on treatment), has been successfully carried out in Hurler's disease (125, 127), but further followup is required before the therapy can be evaluated.

Hunter's Disease

Hunter's disease is an X-linked disorder of males that may take a severe or mild form. In the severe type, coarse facial features, stiff joints, and hepatosplenomegaly occur, but the changes are less severe than in Hurler's disease. Patients with Hunter's disease are hirsute and have nodular white skin lesions on the posterior thorax and upper arms. Atypical retinitis pigmentosa and progressive deafness occur; however, the corneas remain clear. Mental retardation is progressive, and survival beyond adolescence is rare.

The mild form of Hunter's disease is compatible with low-normal intelligence and survival into adult life. Limitation of joint mobility and hepatosplenomegaly occur. The older adult patient has rosy cheeks and a hoarse voice. Degenerative arthritis in the hips and heart disease may also occur.

In keeping with the X-chromosome locus for the Hunter gene and the Lyon hypothesis, the Hunter heterozygote has two populations of cells, one containing iduronate sulfatase and the other deficient in this enzyme. Therefore, heterozygosity for the Hunter gene is valid only when enzyme activity is reduced to levels below 50 per cent of normal. Normal levels of iduronate sulfatase activity in a female relative of a Hunter's disease patient do not rule out heterozygosity. A new, though tedious, method using ^{35}S-sulfate incorporation into fibroblasts in the presence of fructose-1-phosphate seems suitable for carrier diagnosis. Uptake of the iduronate sulfatase produced by the normal cells in the culture is prevented and ^{35}S-labelled acid mucopolysaccharide therefore accumulates in the Hunter population of cells (128).

Sanfilippo's Disease (Types A, B, C, and D)

The physical stigmata of Sanfilippo's disease are milder than those observed in either Hurler's or Hunter's disease, but the degree of mental retardation is usually more extreme and survival to adulthood is possible. Delay in development occurs early in childhood. Joint stiffness and, in some cases, hepatosplenomegaly are present. Radiologic signs include thickening of the calvarium and biconvex configuration of the dorsolumbar vertebral bodies.

All cases of Sanfilippo's disease seem to conform to a single phenotype, yet four forms can be distinguished enzymatically. In the type A variant, an N-sulfatase is deficient; in the type B variant, an α-N-acetylglucosaminidase is absent; in the type C variant, heparan N-acetyl transferase is missing; and in the type D variant the deficient enzyme is N-acetyl-α-D-glucosaminide-6-sulfatase (129). Carriers of these diseases can be diagnosed by enzyme assay, and prevention of each type is possible by prenatal detection.

Morquio's Syndrome (Types A and B)

The child with Morquio's syndrome may be differentiated easily from children with other forms of mucopolysaccharidoses. Intelligence is usually normal. In type A, skeletal deformities begin to appear between 1 and 2 years of age, and skeletal growth generally ceases by age 7 to 8 years. The neck and trunk are short, the sternum is prominent, and the knees bowed. Absence or severe hypoplasia of the odontoid process of the second cervical vertebra results in atlantoaxial subluxation, leading to cervical myelopathy. The maxilla is broad, and the dental enamel is abnormally thin. Joints are loose and hypermobile. The facial features become coarse, and deafness and mild corneal clouding develop. The major medical problem in adult life is cardiorespiratory insufficiency due to valvular heart disease and restrictions in the size and motion of the thoracic cage. The deficient enzyme in this form of Morquio's syndrome (Type A) is galactosamine-6-sulfatase.

A clinically milder form (type B) due to a β-galactosidase deficiency is also encountered. The G_{M1}-ganglioside β-galactosidase activity of these patients is preserved and therefore they are not neurologically impaired (11).

Maroteaux-Lamy Syndrome

Many of the physical signs of Hurler's disease are also present in patients with Maroteaux-Lamy syndrome, who have short stature, coarse facies, joint stiffness, marked corneal clouding, and deafness. Contractions of the knees and hips and a claw hand deformity result. However, the preservation of intellect in this disease clearly differentiates it from Hurler's disease. As in Morquio's syndrome, there is hypoplasia of the odontoid process with subluxation of the C_1 vertebra onto C_2. Involvement of the heart valves with associated murmurs and heart disease is common. There are severe, mild and intermediate forms.

Leukocytes from patients with Maroteaux-Lamy syndrome present a more striking picture of metachromatic inclusions than do the leukocytes in most other mucopolysaccharidoses. Both arylsulfatase B and galactosamine-4-sulfatase are deficient in this disease. Since the activity of arylsulfatase B is measured with an artificial substrate, its assay simplifies the diagnosis of this disease. Bone marrow transplantation in a 13-year-old girl with the severe form of the disease resulted in restitution of arylsulfatase B levels in both circulating leukocytes and liver. Clinical improvement occurred with regression of hepatosplenomegaly and improved joint mobility, and in ultrastructural studies evidence was obtained for disappearance of storage material from bone marrow cells and lymphocytes (2). Long-term follow-up will be of great interest.

β-Glucuronidase Deficiency

At least 18 cases of a mucopolysaccharidosis with β-glucuronidase deficiency have been observed since publication of Sly's original case in 1973 (130). The clinical presentation of each has differed. The original patient had slowing of development at age 2 to 3 years, coarse facial features, anterior chest deformity, hepatosplenomegaly, bilateral inguinal hernias, and clear corneas. Other patients have had infantile onset, clouding of the corneas, and dysostosis multiplex. Hydrops fetalis has been described in two infants, one whose death occurred less than one hour after delivery, the other at 6 months (131). Two teen-aged patients with normal intelligence have also been described. One had hypertension and an aortic graft because of fibromuscular dysplasia; the other was well except for bilateral clubfoot and genu valgum. All had had repeated bouts of pneumonia in infancy and manifested abundant coarse granulations characteristic of Alder-Reilly bodies in their granulocytes. Prenatal diagnosis for β-glucuronidase deficiency is possible (132).

Mucosulfatidosis

The clinical phenotype of patients with mucosulfatidosis, also known as multiple sulfatase deficiency, combines the features of late infantile metachromatic leukodystrophy with those of mucopolysaccharidosis. Metachromatic leukodystrophy, by itself, does not affect the RES. This disease results from a failure to degrade cerebroside sulfate due to a deficiency of arylsulfatase A. There is widespread degeneration of both central and peripheral myelin, causing spastic tetraparesis, blindness, peripheral neuropathy, and an elevation of the cerebrospinal fluid protein. Development is delayed from early infancy. The child may learn to sit and stand but does not develop speech and regresses after the second year, losing previously acquired skills. The forehead is prominent and the nasal bridge flattened. There may be an excessive startle reaction, spasticity, and extensor plantar responses. Seizures eventually appear. Hepatosplenomegaly has been found in some but not all patients. Many have had ichthyosis. The corneas are clear and the maculae abnormally gray. The skeletal changes are similar to those found in the mucopolysaccharides and include lumbar kyphosis, prominent sternum, broad phalanges, and a J-shaped sella turcica. Clinical involvement is therefore more severe than in either late infantile metachromatic leukodystrophy or the mucopolysaccharidoses.

The child with mucosulfatidosis accumulates not only cerebroside sulfate but also cholesterol sulfate and sulfated mucopolysaccharides because of deficiencies of at least seven different sulfatases, including arylsulfatases A, B, and C, steroid sulfatase, heparan N-sulfamidase, and iduronate sulfatase. In tissue culture, these deficiencies can be partially corrected by maintaining the cells in a high pH medium (7.4) or by the addition of sodium thiosulfate. These observations suggest that a factor that is necessary for the expression of the various sulfatases may be deficient. Complementation studies indicate that the genetic defect is different from that responsible for metachromatic leukodystrophy, Hunter's disease and type A Sanfilippo disease.

The laboratory work-up for this disease should include a search for Alder-Reilly bodies in the circulating granulocytes and the bone marrow, a Berry spot test for mucopolysacchariduria, and determinations of aryl sulfatases A and B activity in leukocytes or cultured skin fibroblasts.

MUCOLIPIDOSES AND OTHER DISEASES OF COMPLEX CARBOHYDRATE METABOLISM

In 1970, Spranger and Wiedemann established a new category of storage disease for patients who exhibit the clinical features of Hurler's disease without an excess of urinary mucopolysaccharides (133). The term "mucolipidosis" was selected to indicate the coexistence in these patients of signs and symptoms typical of both the mucopolysaccharidoses and sphingolipidoses. The urine of these patients contains large quantities of oligosaccharides identical in structure to the carbohydrate side chains in glycoproteins. The oligosaccharides are of two types, sialyloligosaccharides and neutral oligosaccharides.

High sialyloligosaccharide concentrations correlate with deficiencies in acid neuraminidase activity, a finding that is characteristic of the sialidoses and mucolipidosis IV and also occurs secondarily in mucolipidoses II and III. The enzyme deficiency in the sialidoses is in the lysosomal neuraminidase specific for glycoproteins and oligosaccharides with a terminal sialic acid. A second neuraminidase specific for gangliosides is deficient in mucolipidosis IV. In mucolipidoses II and III, the primary defect is in the post-translational modification of the carbohydrate unit that is common to most lysosomal enzymes. The mannose-6-phosphate recognition marker required for uptake of these enzymes from the cell surface is not formed, and consequently the intracellular content of neuraminidase as well as other lysosomal enzymes is reduced.

The accumulation of neutral oligosaccharides occurs in G_{M1}-gangliosidosis, the Sandhoff variant of G_{M2}-gangliosidosis, fucosidosis, mannosidosis, aspartylglucosaminuria, and Pompe's disease. The tissue of patients with each of these diseases is deficient in one or more of the glycosidases that act on the oligosaccharide unit of glycoproteins (Fig. 38–5 and Table 38–4) or glycogen side chains (Pompe's disease). Although these diseases (with the exception of Pompe's) also fulfill the criteria established by Spranger and Wiedemann for a mucolipidosis (133) they are commonly designated by the principal substance stored in the disease. Clinical descriptions of the gangliosidoses may be found earlier in this chapter in the section on the sphingolipidoses.

Sialidoses

TYPE I (NORMOMORPHIC SIALIDOSIS, CHERRY-RED-SPOT MYOCLONUS SYNDROME)

Patients with this disease have few if any bony changes and their intelligence is normal or only slightly impaired. It presents in later childhood or adolescence with unexpected falls and decreased visual acuity (134–137). The visual loss is progressive and is associated with bilateral macular cherry-red spots that may fade later in the course of the disease. In some patients small punctate opacities occur in the lens.

The most striking clinical feature is myoclonus, which may be precipitated by voluntary movements, the thought of movement, passive joint movements, or light touch or sound stimuli. Initially there are intention tremors and difficulty with fine motor movements, but eventually the myoclonus becomes so disabling that in spite of continued normal muscle strength patients cannot speak, feed themselves, walk, or even roll over in bed. The deep tendon reflexes are increased. Leg tremors and generalized seizures may occur in the early morning prior to awakening. Myoclonic jerking is more severe in the premenstrual phase of the monthly cycle. As the disease progresses, the

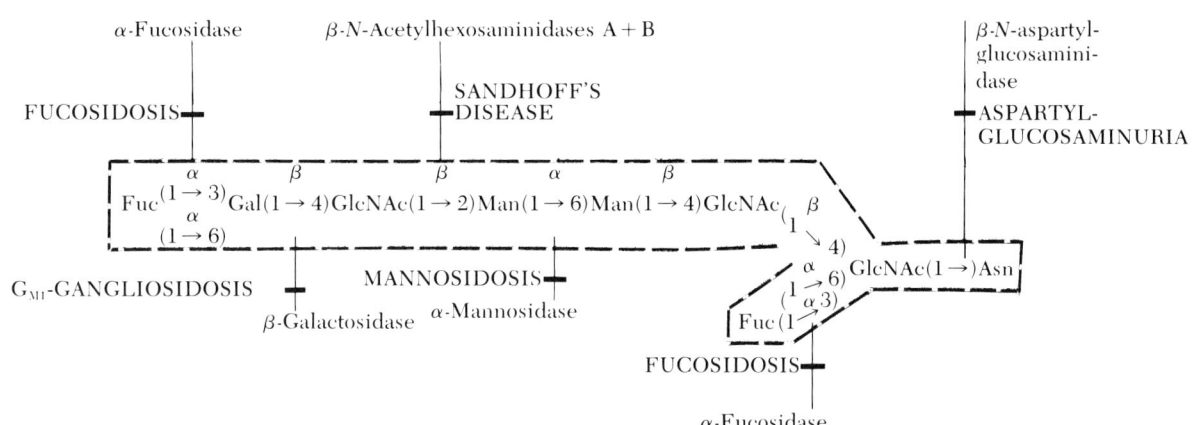

Figure 38–5. Fucosyloligosaccharide unit (125) of a hypothetical glycoprotein indicating the sites of catabolic block in fucosidosis, G_{M1}-gangliosidosis, Sandhoff's disease, mannosidosis, and aspartylglucosaminuria. Abbreviations: Fuc = fucose, Gal = galactose, GlcNAc = N-acetylglucosamine, Man = mannose, and Asn = asparagine.

patient is confined to a wheelchair and is helped by passive restraints on the limbs. Anticonvulsants and tranquilizers, including valproic acid, clonazepam, and diazepam, do not improve the myoclonus dramatically, although generalized seizure activity can be controlled by phenytoin.

Although disabled, patients have continued with their schoolwork. Two men with this disease were still employed in their late twenties, some time after signs of the disease first appeared, one as a mechanical surveyor (135), the other as a machinist (137). Sensation is normal and there are no Hurler-like features such as corneal cloudiness, hepatomegaly, or bone or joint abnormalities. A few patients have developed scoliosis late in the course of the disease. Some patients have complained of severe pains in the hands and feet during hot weather of the type observed in Fabry's disease. In seven of ten reported cases the patients were of Italian extraction.

A few vacuolated lymphocytes may be seen in the peripheral blood smear, and foamy histiocytes have been described in the bone marrow. Nerve cells contain PAS-positive material that is removed with alcohol fixation. Electron microscopy discloses vacuoles in the abnormal bone marrow cells and in Kupffer cells. Most of these vacuoles are empty, but some contain fine fibrillar material or electron-dense bodies. The sialic acid content of cultured fibroblasts may be normal (137) or elevated (141), but there is an increase in sialic-acid–containing compounds in urine. A convenient technique to screen for these compounds involves the use of silica gel thin layer plates (20 × 20 cm). Urine (20 microliters) is spotted on the plate, dried, and then run in butanol:acetic acid:water 3:3:2 for 2 hours. The plate is air dried and stained with resorcinol. A blue color indicates the presence of sialylated oligosaccharides (59).

The α-neuraminidase deficient in this disease normally acts on terminal α-(2- →3) and α-(2- →6) sialyl linkages present in glycoproteins and oligosaccharides. Assays for the disease and for carriers can be reliably performed using homogenates of freshly harvested cultured skin fibroblasts and the artificial substrate 4-methylumbelliferyl-α-N-acetylneuraminic acid.

TYPE II (DYSMORPHIC SIALIDOSIS, GALACTOSIALIDOSIS)

Sialidosis II (formerly termed mucolipidosis I) can be subdivided into congenital, infantile, and juvenile types, all of which feature dysmorphic facies and α-neuraminidase deficiency. Two cases of congenital sialidosis type II have been reported; both infants were stillborn, with hydrops fetalis, ascites, hepatosplenomegaly, stippling of the epiphyses and periosteal cloaking of the long bones (138). In cultured skin fibroblasts from these patients, there is a complete deficiency of α-neuraminidase activity and their β-galactosidase activity is reduced to 5 to 10 per cent of normal. Prenatal diagnosis of this disorder has been accomplished.

At birth, the infants with the late infantile type already have coarse puffy facies, depressed nasal bridge, and broad maxilla. Development is slow, but by age 2 years the child can walk and speak single words. Many skeletal abnormalities are found, and the radiologic examination reveals findings typical of dysostosis multiplex. The trunk is short and the extremities relatively long. There may be a thoracic deformity of either the pectus excavatum or carinatum type, and a thoracic kyphosis is present. Joint mobility is mildly restricted. X-ray signs include stippled epiphyses, ovoid vertebral bodies, and a thickened calvarium. The eye examination discloses punctate lens opacities and a macular cherry-red spot. Other signs include an inner ear hearing loss, mild gingival hyperplasia, widely spaced teeth, and hepatomegaly.

Mental retardation is evident from an early age, and progressive neurologic deterioration occurs during childhood. Initially the gait is broad based and waddling, but as muscle wasting and weakness develop, there is further unsteadiness and then inability to walk. Slowing in nerve conduction velocity suggests that these neurologic difficulties may be due to a degenerative neuropathy. Gross myoclonus and a tonic clonic seizure disorder may develop and death comes later in childhood or in adolescence.

In peripheral blood smears, a small number of lymphocytes and monocytes may contain large cytoplasmic vacuoles. Fine abnormal granulations may also be present in these cell types and granulocytes. Foam cells are found in the bone marrow, which contain vacuoles of different sizes that appear under the electron microscope as single membrane-bound clear inclusions. Similar cytoplasmic inclusions have also been found in liver, cartilage, and cultured fibroblasts. Neuronal storage has been demonstrated, and a sural nerve biopsy has revealed myelin and axonal degeneration.

The quantity of bound sialic acid in the leukocytes and fibroblasts of these patients is increased several fold (139–141), whereas the sialyloligosaccharide content of their urine is several hundred fold greater than normal (142). Thin-layer chromatography of urine (cf., sialidosis type I) is therefore a very useful diagnostic test. There is a marked deficiency of α-neuraminidase activity in fibroblasts and a partial deficiency of this enzyme in obligate heterozygotes. Thus, in the late infantile form of sialidosis type II, the primary defect is in α-neuraminidase. Except for a single case, β-galactosidase activity has been normal (143).

In the juvenile form of sialidosis type II, onset is between the ages of 8 and 15, although it can also be present in adult life. Patients typically exhibit mildly coarse facies. Bony changes are usually limited to the lumbar vertebra and scoliosis. Macular cherry-red spots, corneal clouding, cerebellar ataxia, myoclonus, and convulsions are usually present. The progression of the disease is slow and mentation is mildly impaired if at all. Ten out of fourteen reported patients have been Japanese (144), and there is a high incidence of consanguinity among the parents, making an autosomal recessive pattern of inheritance likely.

Vacuolation of peripheral lymphocytes and foamy cells in the bone marrow are consistently present. Autopsy studies have shown the presence of fibroblasts and macrophages in lymph nodes, liver, and spleen containing cytoplasmic vacuoles limited by a unit membrane. The brain stem nuclei and anterior horn cells are swollen with Sudan black B stain–positive granular material. Ultrastructurally, these inclusions consist of membranous lamellar structures and multilamellar arrangements mixed with vacuole-like granules of low electron density (145).

Enzyme determinations have shown deficiencies of both β-galactosidase and α-neuraminidase in most cases. The primary defect could be a deficiency of a glycoprotein that normally prevents degradation of β-galactosidase and neuraminidase (146). In cultured fibroblasts from these patients β-galactosidase activity can be restored to normal by protease inhibitors (147) or by complementation through fusion with fibroblasts from patients with sialidosis type I or G_{M1}-gangliosidosis (148). An alternative explanation is that the basic defect is in a post-translational step in the processing of neuraminidase (152).

Mucolipidosis II (I-Cell Disease)

The appearance of peculiar cytoplasmic granular inclusions in phase micrographs of cultured skin fibroblasts from a child first believed to have Hurler's disease prompted Leroy and Demars to reclassify this patient's disorder into a new nosologic entity that they designated I-cell disease (inclusion cell disease) (149, 150). This child and others with I-cell disease have many of the clinical features of Hurler's disease but do not have mucopolysacchariduria. Other features that set this disorder apart from Hurler's disease are its clinical appearance at a younger age, striking gingival hyperplasia, less apparent corneal clouding, faster progression, and earlier death, usually by age 8 years (150).

From birth, dysmorphic facial features, tight hip muscles with hip dislocation, joint stiffness, hernias, downy hirsutism, and tight, thickened skin may already be present. Two neonates have been described, who had erythroblastosis with persistence beyond age 1 year of a normochromic, normocytic anemia and reticulocytosis (151). Mental and physical development are delayed, and there are dwarfism, mental retardation, and a failure to progress neurologically beyond age 1 year. The child with I-cell disease is recognized after age 6 months by an abnormal low-pitched cry, a small triangular shaped head, mild corneal clouding, constantly present nasal discharge, hypertrophied maxillary alveolar ridge, enlarged tongue, kyphoscoliosis, a protuberent abdomen, hepatomegaly, and hypotonicity. Head control is poor. By age 2 to 3 years, the child is able to sit but walking is not achieved. There are systolic murmurs and frequent respiratory tract infections. Death usually results from cardiopulmonary complications.

Among the many roentgenographic signs of skeletal dysplasia in this disease are a thickening of the calvarium, cone-shaped phalanges, proximal pointing of metacarpals, V-shaped deformity of the wrist joints; short rounded vertebral bodies with anterior-inferior beaking of T_{12} or L_1; flaring of the iliac wing; dysplasia of the acetabulum; wide ribs; and cortical thickening in the diaphyses of the long bones. Computer-assisted tomography of the brain demonstrates cerebral atrophy and mild ventricular dilatation.

Vacuolated lymphocytes are abundant in the circulating blood (20), but there are no foam cells in the bone marrow. The dense cytoplasmic inclusions in cultured fibroblasts stain positively with PAS and Sudan black but are negative with alcian blue, indicating that glycolipids but not mucopolysaccharides are stored in these cells. Foam cells staining positively with PAS are found in various tissues including the spleen and portal spaces of the liver, but Kupffer cell and neuronal storage is variable.

Many acid hydrolases are deficient in the fibroblasts of these patients including α-neuraminidase. Two exceptions are β-glucosidase and acid phosphatase. In contrast, acid hydrolase activity in their serum is increased many times normal levels. Leukocyte enzyme activity is generally normal. The laboratory diagnosis of I-cell disease is usually made by demonstrating a marked discrepancy between serum and fibroblast levels of several lysosomal enzyme activities. The defect is in the post-translational modification of acid hydrolases interfering with cell surface recognition and uptake of these enzymes. The enzyme UDP-N-acetylglucosamine (lysosomal enzyme N-acetylglucosamine 1-phosphate transferase, which phosphorylates the oligosaccharide portion of lysosomal enzymes to produce mannose-6-phosphate termini) is deficient in I-cell disease so that these enzymes cannot be transferred into lysosomes (152). Carrier detection is not reliable, but prenatal diagnosis has been done successfully by assaying amniotic fluid cells for multiple deficiencies of lysosomal enzymes.

Mucolipidosis III (Pseudo-Hurler Polydystrophy)

This disorder was first described in 1966 by Maroteaux and Lamy as "la pseudopolydystrophie de Hurler." It is now recognized as an attenuated form of mucolipidosis II (153). The first clinical signs are stiffness of the hands and shoulders appearing between ages 2 and 4 years. Coarsening of facial features becomes noticeable by age 6 years. There is progressive joint stiffness, and consequently, restriction in joint mobility. A claw hand deformity and a carpal tunnel syndrome usually appear before 12 years of age. Other clinical features include mild mental retardation, mild corneal clouding, retinal degeneration detectable by an electroretinogram, cardiac murmurs of aortic or mitral valvular disease, short stature, and progressive skeletal dysplasia, particularly of the spine and pelvis. Survival into the thirties and as late as the sixties has been described.

Peripheral leukocytes in this disease are normal, but vacuolated plasma cells are found in bone marrow specimens. Cultured skin fibroblasts manifest the same phase-dense inclusions seen in I-cell disease, although the findings are not always as prominent.

As in I-cell disease, there are also multiple acid hydrolase deficiencies in cultured fibroblasts and a marked elevation in lysosomal enzyme activity in serum. The defect is also thought to be in the phosphorylation of acid hydrolases, although there is some residual phosphorylation detected in fibroblasts from patients with mucolipidosis III (154). Like mucolipidosis II, mucolipidosis III is an autosomally inherited disorder. The two diseases could be produced by different mutations at the same locus. Carrier detection is unavailable for this rare disease.

Mucolipidosis IV

This disorder was first described in four children of Ashkenazi Jewish parentage whose ancestry was traced to southern Poland (155). Since then additional cases have been described in both Jews and non-Jews (156). Physical signs include corneal clouding from birth or early infancy and psychomotor retardation noted at the end of the first year. An alternating esotropia or convergent squint and signs of retinal degeneration may also develop. Mental retardation is profound. The child may acquire a few words, learn to sit, crawl, or walk with support but does not achieve further developmental milestones. Muscle tone is normal or decreased, and the deep tendon reflexes are increased. The face is full, but there is no organomegaly and no skeletal deformities of the type seen in the mucopolysaccharidoses or other mucolipidoses.

The original report of this disease described numerous large histiocyte-like cells in the bone marrow containing small sudanophilic, weakly PAS-positive vacuoles. These cells also showed weak metachromasia after staining with toluidine blue (157). However, bone marrow studies in another patient did not reveal storage cells. Blood smears from this patient were also normal when examined by light microscopy, but under the electron microscope dense lamellar inclusion bodies were observed in lymphocytes of the buffy coat (158). Ultrastructural changes have also been observed in various other tissues, including brain, conjunctiva, and cultured fibroblasts (155, 157–159). These consist of concentric laminated lipid-like bodies and vacuoles containing amorphous sparse fibrillo-granular material. In the liver, the multilamellar cytosomes are present in the hepatocytes, whereas the clear vacuoles are seen in the Kupffer cells. Both types of inclusions appear in the epithelial and stromal cells of the conjunctiva, which may be biopsied as an aid to diagnosis (155).

Gangliosides, mainly G_{M3} and G_{D3}, accumulate in brain and cultured fibroblasts. Mucopolysaccharides, particularly hyaluronic acid, also accumulate in cultured fibroblasts, probably as a secondary phenomenon (67). The defect is in ganglioside-specific sialidase. Mucolipidosis IV heterozygotes show a partial deficiency of the ganglioside sialidase. Glycoprotein sialidase, deficient in the sialidoses, is normal (160). Prenatal diagnosis has been accomplished by demonstration of abnormal storage bodies in cultured amniotic fluid cells of two fetuses at risk for this disease (161).

Fucosidosis

Fucosidosis is commonly identified as both a sphingolipidosis and an oligosaccharidosis (162). One form of this disease (type 1) is recognized by a delay in psychomotor development toward the end of the child's first year. Hypotonia progresses to hypertonia, then to severe spasticity, and finally to decerebrate rigidity. Thick skin, coarse facial features, skeletal abnormalities, and growth retardation occur. Other signs are a nonfunctioning gallbladder and hyperhidrosis. One or more patients have also had seizures, cardiomegaly, hepatomegaly, and corneal opacities. Respiratory tract infections are frequent, with survival in most cases being limited to 4 or 5 years.

A second clinically milder variant (type 2) has also been described (163). The onset is later in the second year, neurologic deterioration is slower, and patients may survive beyond adolescence. A distinguishing feature is the presence of angiokeratomas in the gums and conjunctiva and on the external genitalia, abdomen, buttocks and thighs. A significant number of patients with both clinical types have been of Italian ancestry.

Sweat electrolytes are increased early in the course of type 1 disease, but with progressive damage to the sweat glands by storage material, the sweat test may become normal, and in the terminal stage anhidrosis may even develop. Many lymphocytes contain cytoplasmic vacuoles, and foam cells may be present in the bone marrow. Biopsy studies of liver indicate the presence of foamy cytoplasm in some hepatocytes and Kupffer cells. Ultrastructural studies demonstrate the presence of vacuoles with heterogeneous content, some appearing empty and some containing reticular or lamellar structures. Postmortem examination of type 1 patients has revealed enlargement of the brain, heart, liver, spleen, and pancreas. The gallbladder appears strawberry-like. Heterogeneity in the appearance of storage vacuoles has also been observed in ultrastructural studies of brain tissues (164). Vacuolization of the epithelial cells of sweat glands and of the conjunctiva is also quite prominent (165).

Excess amounts of two fucose-containing glycosphingolipids have been isolated from various tissues (166). One of these glycosphingolipids, a pentahexosylceramide, is the H-antigen glycolipid. Also, Lewis blood group activity is increased in fucosidosis tissues, and elevated levels of Le^a and Le^b activity have been found in the sera, erythrocytes, and saliva of fucosidosis patients (162). However, the major products stored in tissues are the fucosyl disaccharide, Fuc-GlcNac, and the fucodecasaccharide (Fuc-Gal-GlcNAc-Man)$_2$Man-GlcNAc (166). Large concentrations of nine different fucose-containing oligosaccharides and glycopeptides have been found in urine from two patients (167).

The inheritance pattern is autosomal recessive, and both forms of the disease, which may exist in the same pedigree but not the same sibship, are characterized by total deficiency of α-L-fucosidase activity. The structural gene for the enzyme has been mapped to human chromosome 1 (168). Isoelectric focusing of leukocyte extracts reveals three common α-fucosidase phenotypes best explained by the existence of three alleles Fu^1, Fu^2, and Fu^0, the last being a silent allele associated with fucosidosis (169, 170). There is, in addition, evidence for a polymorphism affecting the level of α-fucosidase in plasma (171). Individuals with the low activity variant are healthy. Carrier testing is possible using leukocytes and fibroblasts. Prenatal diagnosis performed on amniotic fluid cells has been successful (172).

Mannosidosis

Clinically and biochemically, mannosidosis conforms to the stereotype of an oligosaccharide storage disease. As in fucosidosis and aspartylglucosaminuria, there are skeletal changes, a dysmorphic facial appearance, moderate to severe mental retardation, vacuoles in the lymphocytes, foam cell infiltration of the bone marrow, and normal mucopolysacchariduria (173–175).

Mannosidosis is recognizable in the first year of life by progressive coarsening of the facial features, slow mental and motor development, and mild hepatosplenomegaly that tends to disappear after age 2 or 3 years. In some patients, early growth is accelerated and bilateral spoke-shaped lens opacities are found. These children have recurrent infections but enjoy an otherwise benign medical course. They usually learn to speak in single words or short sentences, although this simple speech is garbled, possibly because of concomitant sensorineural hearing loss. They walk with an awkward wide-based gait and use their upper extremities clumsily. Older children and adults with this disease have a high prominent forehead, forward protruding jaw, and prominent alveolar ridge. In adulthood massive gum hyperplasia may occur (175). Skeletal abnormalities include a lumbar kyphosis, abnormally thickened calvarium especially at the base, coarsened trabeculation of the long bones with thinning of the cortical margins, and beaking of the vertebrae. Once the disease is fully expressed, the progression is slow and survival into adulthood is the rule. One 29-year-old man with this disease developed a communicating hydrocephalus and progressive gait ataxia that improved following a ventriculoperitoneal shunt (177).

Vacuoles are found in 80 per cent of circulating lymphocytes and in mononuclear cells of the bone marrow. These vacuoles remain PAS-positive after fixation with alcohol. They have also been found in hepatocytes and Kupffer cells, and in the nervous system they are associated with widespread ballooning of nerve cell cytoplasm in cerebral cortex, brain stem, spinal medulla, and pituitary (173, 177). Abnormalities in chemotactic function of neutrophils may account for the increased susceptibility to infection of these patients. Hypogammaglobulinemia has been described as well.

Excessive amounts of mannose-containing oligosaccharides have been found in various tissues and urine of patients with mannosidosis. Thinlayer chromatography of a few drops of urine will easily disclose a pattern of glycoconjugates, which is distinctive for this particular type of oligosacchariduria (60). The major oligosaccharide excreted is a trisaccharide. A defect in the hydrolysis of this compound has been demonstrated using an enzyme preparation from the liver of a patient with mannosidosis.

The deficient enzyme, lysosomal acidic α-mannosidase, may be assayed using leukocytes or cultured fibroblasts as the enzyme source. However, if serum or plasma is used as the enzyme source, the diagnosis may be missed since the lysosomal enzyme is not the major α-mannosidase in these fluids. Heterozygote detection is available and prenatal diagnosis has been performed successfully (178, 179). The acid mannosidase gene has been mapped to human chromosome 19 by somatic cell hybridization (180). Animal models of mannosidosis have been described in Angus cattle (181), in the goat (182), and in cattle who have grazed on a legume of the genus *Swainsona,* which is a potent inhibitor of lysosomal α-mannosidase (183). The residual α-mannosidase activity in mannosidosis can be stimulated and stabilized by zinc ions (175, 184) but long-term therapy in two patients using oral zinc sulfate failed and caused no change in clinical status or biochemical findings (185).

Aspartylglucosaminuria

About 130 patients, nearly all from Finland, have been identified as having the disease aspartylglucosaminuria (186, 187). Two patients from England, two from Italy, and one from the United States have been reported (188). The disease begins between ages 2 and 6 years with slow progressive psychomotor retardation, resulting in severe mental retardation before puberty. The clinical features include episodic aggressive behavior, coarse facies with sagging cheeks, short neck, and scoliosis. Some patients exhibit cutaneous manifestations, including large nevi, acne, and photosensitive pigmentation. Recurrent diarrhea and respiratory tract infections occur. The circulating lymphocytes are vacuolated. Patients with this disease may live for many years.

The principal storage product is aspartylglucosylamine, which may be detected on urine chromatograms for amino acids (189). The storage material has been found in kidney, liver, spleen, peripheral nerves, spinal cord, and brain (190). This compound serves as the link between the carbohydrate group and the peptide chain in glycoproteins and keratan sulfate. Lesser amounts of other glycoasparagines containing galactose, N-acetylneuraminic acid, and additional N-acetylglucosamine residues have also been isolated from the urine of patients with aspartylglucosaminuria (191).

The enzyme deficient in this autosomal recessive disease is the amidase N-aspartyl-β-glucosaminidase, which hydrolyzes aspartylglucosamine to aspartate, ammonia, and aspartylglucosamine. Serum, fibroblasts, and leukocytes of affected patients show less than 10 per cent enzyme activity. Heterozygotes are best diagnosed using fibroblasts or lymphocytes (192).

ACID LIPASE DEFICIENCY

Allelic genes probably account for the occurrence of Wolman's disease and cholesterol ester storage disease. These diseases share a deficiency of lysosomal acid esterase and massive accumulation of cholesterol esters and triglycerides in tissues but differ considerably in their clinical expression.

Wolman's Disease

Signs of Wolman's disease appear as early as the second month of life (193). The disease begins with severe vomiting and frequent, foul-smelling stools, and the liver and spleen rapidly assume massive proportions. X-ray examination shows the adrenal glands to be grossly enlarged and seeded with finely stippled or punctate calcific deposits. The vomiting and diarrhea continue and the infant fails to gain weight. Progression of the disease is marked by abdominal distention, recurrent anemia, persistent low-grade fever, and wasting, culminating in death before the age of 1 year.

Lymphocytes contain both intranuclear and intracytoplasmic lipid vacuoles. Lipid droplets are also present in neutrophils and monocytes. Enlarged vacuolated histiocytes appear in the bone marrow and in all organs. In contrast to other diseases characterized by vacuolated cells, the vacuoles in Wolman's disease are strongly sudanophilic. They stain positively with oil-red-O and with stains for cholesterol, and their lysosomal origin is indicated by a strong reaction to staining for acid phosphatase activity. In some patients, plasma high-density and low-density lipoproteins are reduced.

Extracts of cultured fibroblasts contain at least three electrophoretically dissimilar acid lipase components: A, B and C. Only one of these, the least anodal band A, is totally deficient in Wolman's disease. The other two components are retained, although their activity is reduced. These findings have important implications for prenatal diagnosis because amniotic fluid cells from a Wolman's disease pregnancy may contain activity that is 30 to 40 per cent that found in controls, especially if the artificial substrate is used. This finding alone, without electrophoresis of the acid lipase activity, could result in an erroneous diagnosis of a clinically unaffected fetus. Prenatal diagnosis combining both methods has been successfully performed in four cases (194, 195).

Additional confirmation of a prenatal diagnosis may be obtained by staining the cultured amniotic fluid cells with oil-red-O to demonstrate intracellular neutral lipid accumulation. Subnormal levels of acid lipase activity have been found in obligate heterozygotes for Wolman's disease in cultured skin fibroblasts and leukocytes (196, 197).

Cholesterol Ester Storage Disease

The major finding in patients with cholesterol ester storage disease is hepatomegaly, which is first noticeable early in childhood and increases with time (198). Splenomegaly and esophageal varices may also occur. In some patients, hepatic fibrosis results, but liver function is normal. Plasma levels of cholesterol, triglyceride, and low density lipoproteins are elevated, and foam cells may be found in the bone marrow. In some patients bone marrow aspirates contain numerous large macrophages filled with birefringent droplets. Hepatic acid esterase activity is reduced but clearly detectable and is substantially greater than in Wolman's disease liver (199). Most patients with this variant live beyond childhood.

NEURONAL CEROID-LIPOFUSCINOSIS

Lysosomal accumulation of lipopigments is characteristic of the neuronal ceroid-lipofuscinoses, a group of neurodegenerative conditions whose biochemical basis is not yet well understood. The stored material resembles both ceroid and lipofuscin. Upon extraction with chloroform:methanol, these deposits yield insoluble, autofluorescent, retinoid-like complexes and soluble polyisoprenols known as dolichols (200). The latter are lipid intermediates in the biosynthesis of glycoproteins and are a helpful biochemical marker for the disease (201). The residual bodies formed have a heterogenous ultrastructural appearance. They are present in all tissues but are particularly abundant in the neuronal perikaryon, where they continue to accumulate until the nerve cell degenerates. Types of deposits found include curvilinear bodies, zebra bodies, fingerprint profiles, homogenous osmiophilic bodies, and osmiophilic granular deposits.

Clinically, the neuronal ceroid-lipofuscinoses represent a broad spectrum of diseases varying in age of onset; visual, mental, and motor signs; and types of inclusions present. With some exceptions (202), patients who become symptomatic before adulthood develop blindness, and for this reason older texts frequently grouped these diseases with the familial amaurotic idiocies. Eponyms used have included the names of Batten, Spielmeyer, Vogt, and Mayou, but the term neuronal ceroid-lipofuscinosis is now preferred for it emphasizes the nature of the stored material. The absence of ganglioside storage and the marked brain atrophy that occur in the neuronal ceroid-lipofuscinoses clearly set the syndrome apart from the classic forms of gangliosidoses. A deficiency of leukocyte peroxidase activity has been reported in certain cases (203), but other studies have not been able to confirm this finding (204, 205), which probably represents a secondary manifestation rather than a primary defect.

Each of the clinical variants of neuronal ceroid-lipofuscinoses—infantile, late infantile, juvenile, or adult—is probably the result of a different mutated gene, but the accumulation of autofluorescent storage material is common to all. The diagnosis of these relatively common disorders depends primarily upon the clinical features, but the examination of a skin biopsy by electron-microscopy (206) and measurement of urinary dolichols are also of great help (200). Brain dolichol levels are also increased but since dolichols increase with age (207) and are also elevated out of proportion to age in Alzheimer's disease (208), they cannot be relied upon for the diagnosis of the adult variant. Lymphocyte vacuolization and azurophilic hypergranulation of neutrophils are frequent findings in the peripheral blood smear except in the infantile form (209, 210). Electron microscopic studies of these blood elements (23–25) and of urinary sediment (211), liver, skeletal muscle (212), and sural nerve (213) have also aided in the diagnosis. Retinal degeneration can be followed with the electroretinogram (ERG). With complete degeneration of the outer retinal layer, the ERG response is totally abolished. Another useful test is the electroencephalogram, which may be abnormal even before the development of dementia.

Infantile Type (Haltia-Santavuori Syndrome)

This is the most common progressive encephalopathy in Finnish children under 2 years of age (209). Developmental delay, impaired vision, and a squint may suggest the diagnosis at or before age 1 year. Thereafter, there is rapid psychomotor deterioration with hypotonia and ataxia of the trunk and limbs. By 18 months to 2 years of age, myoclonic jerks are evident. Within a few more months, rigidity, spastic tetraparesis, and blindness are noted. The optic discs are pale, the retinal vessels are narrowed, and the retina itself is hypopigmented. Severe neuronal destruction occurs with almost total loss of cortical neurons and cerebellar Purkinje cells, resulting in brain atrophy, subsequent microcephaly (214), and EEG findings of diminution in amplitude and rhythmic activity approaching isoelectricity. The urine content of dolichols is increased. A prolonged stationary burnt-out phase precedes death, which may not come until age 9 or 10 years.

Neuropathologic studies show great numbers of phagocytes between the remaining cortical neurons. Their cytoplasm is is distended by a granular material that under the electron microscope resembles conglomerations of small spherical membrane-bound globules. Hypertrophic fibrillary astrocytes are abundant and these also contain granular storage material. Ultrastructural study of skin biopsies demonstrates membrane-bound, irregular granular bodies.

Late Infantile Type (Jansky-Bielschowsky Syndrome)

The patient with this syndrome presents with seizures at age 3 to 4 years. Manifestations include episodes of staring, absence attacks with frequent falls, and myoclonic jerking. There is increasing clumsiness, tremulousness, and dysarthria. Thereafter, the child is hyperactive, sleeps little, and fails to gain weight. He or she becomes ataxic and then loses the ability to walk and speak. By age 5 years there is loss of intellect, visual failure, and incontinence. The eye examination at this stage reveals optic atrophy and a granular or pigmentary degeneration of the macula.

Ultrastructural studies demonstrate the presence of curvilinear bodies in a variety of cell types including skin, which is often biopsied for diagnostic purposes. High levels of urinary dolichols are also characteristic. Autopsy studies have disclosed storage material in the bone marrow parenchyma and Kupffer cells of the liver, and in the spleen, lymph nodes, and the renal parenchyma.

Juvenile Type (Spielmeyer-Sjögren Syndrome)

The juvenile type of neuronal ceroid-lipofuscinosis is first suspected in the child between ages 3 and 8 years who presents with declining central visual acuity. Initially, a granular macular degeneration may be observed. During the next several years the optic discs atrophy and pigmentary changes occur in the peripheral part of the retina. By age 10 to 12 years, only light perception remains and a low frequency nystagmus is present. At about this same age, convulsions first appear and mental capacity declines. Thereafter, memory, school performance, and behavior steadily deteriorate. By their midteens these patients are moderately mentally retarded. Their speech is slurred and monotonous with stammering, perseveration, and echolalia, and their thoughts become incoherent. An extrapyramidal syndrome develops that is characterized by a dull facial expression, peculiar postures, paratonic rigidity, and a Parkinsonian-like gait. Cerebellar disturbances are also noticed, including clumsiness in all movements, progressive ataxia, and compulsive, dysarthric speech. Approximately 10 years after the onset of symptoms the patient becomes bedridden in a semiflexed posture with frequent seizures. These seizures are difficult to control and may be accompanied by opisthotonic posturing and prolonged spells of apnea.

Laboratory findings include vacuolization in approximately 20 per cent of circulating lymphocytes, increased thickness of the skull, an absent ERG, abnormal EEG, and often, decreased motor nerve conduction velocities (215). The predominant type of ultrastructural inclusion in biopsy specimens such as skin and sural nerve are fingerprint profiles (213). Dolichols are elevated in the brain and urinary sediment. Treatment with antioxidants (216), and in later stages, L-dopa may slow the progress of this disease in some patients.

Adult Type (Kufs' Disease)

Rarely, neuronal ceroid-lipofuscinosis may present in adulthood as a psychologic or motor disturbance. There are no visual complaints or retinal changes. The disease becomes manifest at about age 30 years. Symptoms develop insidiously and are highly variable. Initially, the patient's strange affect may be interpreted as depression or paranoid psychosis, but eventually a mild progressive dementia is recognized. The intracellular inclusions are of several types, including dense amorphous membrane-vesicular and curvilinear cytosomes. In one family with an unusual dominantly inherited form of Kufs' disease, leukocytic azurophilic hypergranulation was present in all 11 affected members (217). Recent evidence in a small number of cases suggests that the dolichol content of urine in this form may also be elevated. The earlier onset, milder course, relatively preserved mentation, and hematologic findings differentiate this form of neuronal ceroid-lipofuscinosis from Alzheimer's disease.

References

1. Rappeport, J. M., and Ginns, E. I.: Bone-marrow transplantation in severe Gaucher's disease. New Engl. J. Med. *311*:84, 1984.
2. Krivit, W., Pierpont, M. E., et al.: Bone-marrow transplantation in the Maroteaux-Lamy syndrome (mucopolysaccharidosis type VI): Biochemical and clinical status 24 months after transplantation. New Engl. J. Med. *311*:1606, 1984.
3. Kornfeld, S., and Gregory, W.: The identification and partial characterization of lysosomes in human reticulocytes. Biochim. Biophys. Acta *177*:615, 1969.
4. Goldberg, D. E., and Kornfeld, S.: Evidence for extensive subcellular organization of asparagine-linked oligosaccharide processing and lysosomal enzyme phosphorylation. J. Biol. Chem. *258*:3159, 1983.
4a. Kornfeld, S.: Trafficking of lysosomal enzymes in normal and disease states. J. Clin. Invest. *77*:1, 1986.
5. Sly, W. S., and Fischer, H. D.: The phosphomannosyl recognition system for intracellular and intercellular transport of lysosomal enzymes. J. Biochem. *18*:67, 1982.
6. Weissmann, G., Zurier, R. B., et al.: Mechanisms of lysosomal enzyme release from leukocytes exposed to immune complexes and other particles. J. Exper. Med. *134*:149, 1971.
7. Smith, R. J., and Ignarro, L. J.: Bioregulation of lysosomal enzyme secretion from human neutrophils: roles of guanine 3′:5′-monophosphate and calcium in stimulus-secretion coupling. Proc. Natl. Acad. Sci. USA *72*:108, 1975.
8. Smith, R. J., Sabin, C., et al.: Effect of antiinflammatory drugs on lysosomes and lysosomal enzymes from rat liver. Biochem. Pharmacol. *25*:2171, 1976.
9. Hers, H. G.: Inborn lysosomal diseases. Gastroenterology *48*:625, 1965.

10. Conzelman, E., and Sandhoff, K.: AB variant of infantile G_{M2} gangliosidosis: deficiency of a factor necessary for stimulation of hexosaminidase A-catalyzed degradation of ganglioside G_{M2} and glycolipid G_{A2}. Proc. Natl. Acad. Sci. USA 75:3979, 1978.

11. Paschke, E., and Kresse, H.: Morquio disease, type B: activation of G_{M1}-β-galactosidase by G_{M1}-activator protein. Biochem. Biophys. Res. Commun. 109:568, 1982.

12. Ginns, E. I., Choudary, P. V., et. al.: Isolation of cDNA clones for human β-glucocerebrosidase using the λgt 11 expression system. Biochem. Biophys. Res. Commun. 123:574, 1984.

13. Konings, A., Hypkes, P., et. al.: Cloning a cDNA for the lysosomal α-glucosidase. Biochem. Biophys. Res. Commun. 119:252, 1984.

14. Fukushima, H., deWet, J., et. al.: Molecular cloning of a human α-fucosidase cDNA. Am. J. Hum. Genet. 36:137s, 1984.

15. Lazarus, S. S., Vethamany, V. G., et al.: Fine structure and histochemistry of peripheral blood cells in Niemann-Pick disease. Lab. Invest. 17:155, 1967.

16. Witzleben, C. L., Smith, K., et al.: Ultrastructural studies in late-onset amaurotic idiocy. Lymphocyte inclusions as a diagnostic marker. J. Pediatr. 79:285, 1971.

17. Vethamany, V. G., Welch, J. P., et al.: Type D Niemann-Pick disease (Nova Scotia variant). Ultrastructure of blood, skin fibroblasts, and bone marrow. Arch. Pathol. 93:537, 1972.

18. Belcher, R. W.: Ultrastructure and cytochemistry of lymphocytes in the genetic mucopolysaccharidoses. Arch. Pathol. 93:1, 1972.

19. Heyne, K., Kemmer, C., et al.: Generalisierte G_{M1}-Gangliosidose. Feinstruktur und differential diagnostische Bedeutung speichernder Lymphozyten und Knochenmarkszellen. Pädiatr. Pädol. 8:272, 1973.

20. Rapola, J., Autio, S., et al.: Lymphocytic inclusions in I-cell disease. J. Pediatr. 85:88, 1974.

21. Dolman, C. L., MacLeod, P. M., et al.: Skin punch biopsies and lymphocytes in the diagnosis of lipidoses. J. Can. Sci. Neurol. Feb., 1975, pp. 67–73.

22. Noonan, S. M., Weiss, L., et al.: Ultrastructural observations of cytoplasmic inclusions in Tay-Sachs lymphocytes. Arch. Pathol. Lab. Med. 100:595, 1976.

23. Schwendemann, G.: Lymphocyte inclusions in the juvenile type of generalized ceroid-lipofuscinosis. An electron microscopic study. Acta Neuropathol. 36:327, 1976.

24. Stekhoven, J. H. S., van Haelst, U. J. G. M., et al.: Ultrastructural study of so-called curvilinear bodies and fingerprint structures in lymphocytes in late-infantile amaurotic idiocy. Acta Neuropathol. 35:295, 1976.

25. Stekhoven, J. H. S., van Haelst, U. J. G. M., et al.: Ultrastructural study of the vacuoles in the peripheral lymphocytes in juvenile amaurotic idiocy. Juvenile form of generalized ceroid lipofuscinosis. Acta Neuropathol. 38:137, 1977.

26. Alder, A.: Konstitutinell bedingte Granulationsveränderungen der Leukocyten und Knochenveränderungen. Schweiz. Med. Wochenschr. 80:1095, 1950.

27. Reilly, W. A.: The granules in the leukocytes in gargoylism. Am. J. Dis. Child. 62:489, 1941.

28. Curless, R. G., Parker, J. C., Jr., and Flynn, J. T.: Neuronal ceroid lipofuscinosis. Diagnosis by semi-thin plastic-embedded sections of peripheral blood lymphocytes from a patient with a normal blood smear. Arch. Neurol. 39:308, 1982.

29. Sawitsky, A., Hymen, G. A., et al.: An unidentified reticuloendothelial cell in bone marrow and spleen: report of two cases with histochemical studies. Blood 9:977, 1954.

30. Silverstein, M. N., Ellefson, R. D., et al.: The syndrome of the sea-blue histiocyte. New Engl. J. Med. 282:1, 1970.

31. Golde, D. W., Schneider, E. L., et al.: Pathogenesis of one variant of sea-blue histiocytosis. Lab. Invest. 33:371, 1975.

32. Ellender, M., Hrodek, J., and Cihula, J.: Niemann-Pick disease: lipid storage in bone marrow macrophages. Histochem. J. 15:1065, 1983.

33. Neville, B. G. R., Lake, B. D., et al.: A neurovisceral storage disease with vertical supranuclear ophthalmoplegia, and its relationship to Niemann-Pick disease—a report of nine patients. Brain 96:97, 1973.

34. Smith, H.: Sea-blue histiocytes in marrow in Batten-Spielmeyer-Vogt disease. Pathology 6:323, 1974.

35. Kornfeld, M., Appenzeller, O., et al.: Sea-blue histiocytes and sural nerve in neurovisceral storage disorder with vertical ophthalmoplegia. J. Neurol. Sci. 25:291, 1975.

36. Swaiman, K. F., Garg, B. P., et al.: Sea-blue histiocyte and posterior column dysfunction: A familial disorder. Neurology 25:1084, 1975.

37. Miley, C. E., Gilbert, E. F., et al.: Clinical and extraneural histologic diagnosis of neuronal ceroid-lipofuscinosis. Neurology 28:1008, 1978.

38. Lee, R. E., Worthington, C. R., et al.: The bilayer nature of deposits occurring in Gaucher's disease. Arch. Biochem. Biophys. 159:259, 1973.

39. Glew, R. H., and Lee, R. E.: Composition of the membranous deposits occurring in Gaucher's disease. Arch. Biochem. Biophys. 156:626, 1973.

40. Hibbs, R. G., Ferrans, V. J., et al.: A histochemical and electron microscopic study of Gaucher cells. Arch. Pathol. 89:137, 1970.

41. Lorber, M., and Neimes, J. L.: Identification of ferritin within Gaucher cells: An electron microscopic and immunofluorescent study. Acta Haematol. 37:189, 1967.

42. Lorber, M.: Iron distribution in adult-type Gaucher's disease. New Engl. J. Med. 292:110, 1975.

43. Albrecht, M.: Gaucher-Zellen bei chronisch myeloischer Leukämie. Blut 13:169, 1966.

44. Lee, R. E., and Ellis, L. D.: The storage cells of chronic myelogenous leukemia. Lab. Invest. 24:261, 1971.

45. Zaino, E. C., Rossi, M. B., et al.: Gaucher's cells in thalassemia. Blood 38:457, 1971.

46. Shinar, E., Leibovitz-Ben Gershon, Z., et al.: Coexistence of Gaucher disease and Philadelphia positive chronic granulocytic leukemia. Am. J. Hematol. 12:199, 1982.

47. O'Brien, J. S., Bernett, J., et al.: Lysosomal storage disorders: diagnosis by ultrastructural examination of skin biopsy specimens. Arch. Neurol. 32:592, 1975.

48. Lasser, A., Carter, D. M., et al.: Ultrastructure of the skin in mucopolysaccharidoses. Arch. Pathol. 99:173, 1975.

49. Martin, J. J., and Ceuterick, C.: Morphological study of skin biopsy specimens: A contribution to the diagnosis of metabolic disorders with involvement of the nervous system. J. Neurol. Neurosurg. Psychiat. 41:232, 1978.

50. Martin, J. J., and deGroote, Ch.: Involvement of the skin in late infantile and juvenile amaurotic idiocies (neuronal ceroid-lipofuscinoses). Pathol. Europ. 9:263, 1974.

51. Arsénio-Nunes, M. L., and Goutières, F.: An ultramicroscopic study of the skin in the diagnosis of the infantile and late infantile types of ceroid-lipofuscinosis. J. Neurol. Neurosurg. Psychiat. 38:994, 1975.

52. Miley, C. E., Gilbert, E. F., et al.: Clinical and extraneural histologic diagnosis of neuronal ceroid-lipofuscinosis. Neurology 28:1008, 1978.

53. Nanai, J., Leroy, J., et al.: Ultrastructure of cultured fibroblasts in I-cell disease. Am. J. Dis. Child. 122:34, 1971.

54. Berman, E. R., Livni, N., et al.: Congenital corneal clouding with abnormal systemic storage bodies: A new variant of mucolipidosis. J. Pediatr. 84:519, 1974.

55. Desnick, R. J., Dawson, G., et al.: Diagnosis of glycosphingolipidoses by urinary-sediment analysis. New Engl. J. Med. 284:739, 1971.

56. Berry, H. K., and Spinayer, J. J.: A paper spot test useful

in study of Hurler's syndrome. J. Lab. Clin. Med. 55:136, 1960.
57. Hurst, R. E., Settine, J. M., et al.: A method for the quantitative determination of urinary glycosaminoglycans. Clin. Chim. Acta 70:427, 1976.
58. Hurst, R. E., Jennings, G. C., et al.: Partition techniques for isolation and fractionation of urinary glycosaminoglycans analysis. Anal. Biochem. 79:502, 1977.
59. Humbel, R., and Collart, M.: Oligosaccharides in urine of patients with glycoprotein storage diseases. I. Rapid detection by thin-layer chromatography. Clin Chim. Acta 60:143, 1975.
60. Friedman, R. B., Williams, M. A., et al.: Improved thin-layer chromatographic method in the diagnosis of mannosidosis. Clin. Chem. 24:1576, 1978.
61. O'Brien, J. S.: The cherry red spot–myoclonus syndrome: a newly recognized inherited lysosomal storage disease due to acid neuraminidase deficiency. Clin. Genet. 14:55, 1978.
62. Sugita, M., Iwamori, M., et al.: High performance liquid chromatography of ceramides: Application to analysis in human tissues and demonstration of ceramide excess in Farber's disease. J. Lipid Res. 15:223, 1974.
63. Ullman, M. D., and McCluer, R. H.: Quantitative analysis of plasma neutral glycosphingolipids by high performance liquid chromatography of their perbenzoyl derivatives. J. Lipid Res. 18:371, 1977.
64. Jungalwala, F. B., and Milunsky, A.: High performance liquid chromatography for the detection of homozygotes and heterozygotes of Niemann-Pick disease. Pediatr. Res. 12:655, 1978.
65. Fratantoni, J. C., Hall, C. W., et al.: The defect in Hurler's and Hunter's syndromes: Faulty degradation of mucopolysaccharides. Proc. Natl. Acad. Sci. USA 60:699, 1968.
66. Schmickel, R. D., Distler, J. J., et al.: Accumulation of sulfate containing acid mucopolysaccharides in I-cell fibroblasts. J. Lab. Clin. Med. 86:672, 1975.
67. Bach, G., Ziegler, M., et al.: Mucopolysaccharide accumulation in cultured skin fibroblasts derived from patients with mucolipidosis IV. Am. J. Hum. Genet. 29:610, 1977.
68. Barton, N. W., and Rosenberg, A.: Metabolism of glucosyl [^{3}H] ceramide by human skin fibroblasts from normal and glucosylceramidotic subjects. J. Biol. Chem. 250:3966, 1975.
69. Kudoh, T., and Wenger, D. A.: Diagnosis of metachromatic leukodystrophy, Krabbe disease and Farber disease after uptake of fatty acid-labeled ceramide sulfate into cultured skin fibroblasts. J. Clin. Invest. 70:89, 1982.
70. Wood, S.: Cultured fucosidosis fibroblasts: A simple technique demonstrating storage of tritiated-fucose labeled material. Clin. Genet. 10:183, 1976.
71. Kyriakides, E. C., Filippone, N., et al.: Lipid studies in Wolman's disease. Pediatrics 46:431, 1970.
72. Glew, R. H., and Peters, S. P. (eds.): *Practical Enzymology of the Sphingolipidoses*. New York, Alan R. Liss, Inc., 1977.
73. Ginsburg, V. (ed.): Complex Carbohydrates, Part C, Methods in Enzymology. Colowick, S. P., and Kaplan, N. O. (eds.), Vol. L, New York, Academic Press, 1978.
74. Kolodny, E. H.: General principles and techniques of case identification, carrier testing and prenatal diagnosis. In *Practical Enzymology of the Sphingolipidoses*. Glew, R. H., and Peters, S. P. (eds.), New York, Alan R. Liss, Inc., 1977, pp. 18–20.
75. Zlotogora, J., and Bach, G.: Heterozygote detection in Hunter syndrome. Am. J. Med. Genet. 17:661, 1984.
76. Neufeld, E. F., and Cantz, M. J.: Corrective factors for inborn errors of mucopolysaccharide metabolism. Ann. N.Y. Acad. Sci. 179:580, 1971.
77. DiFerrante, N., Nichols, B. L., et al.: Induced degradation of glycosaminoglycans in Hurler's and Hunter's syndromes by plasma infusion. Proc. Natl. Acad. Sci. USA 68:303, 1971.
78. Dekaban, A. S., Holden, K. R., et al.: Effects of fresh plasma or whole blood transfusions on patients with various types of mucopolysaccharidoses. Pediatrics 50:688, 1972.
79. Danes, B. S., Degnan, M., et al.: Plasma infusions in the Hurler syndrome. Influence during the first year. Am. J. Dis. Child. 125:533, 1973.
80. Johnson, W. G., Desnick, R. J., et al.: Intravenous injection of purified hexosaminidase A into a patient with Tay-Sachs disease. In *Enzyme Therapy in Genetic Diseases*. Bergsma, D. (ed.), Baltimore, Williams & Wilkins, 1973, pp. 120–124.
81. Brady, R. O., Pentchev, P. C., et al.: Replacement therapy for inherited enzyme deficiency. Use of purified glucocerebrosidase in Gaucher's disease. New Engl. J. Med. 291:989, 1974.
82. Knudson, A. G., Jr., DiFerrante, N., et al.: Effect of leukocyte transfusion in a child with Type II mucopolysaccharidosis. Proc. Natl. Acad. Sci. USA 68:1738, 1971.
83. Jolly, R. D., Thompson, K. G., et al.: Enzyme replacement therapy—an experiment of nature in a chimeric mannosidosis calf. Pediatr. Res. 10:219, 1976.
84. Finkelstein, M., and Weissmann, G.: The introduction of enzymes into cells by means of liposomes. J. Lipid Res. 19:289, 1978.
85. Ihler, G. M., Glew, R. H., et al.: Enzyme loading of erythrocytes. Proc. Natl. Acad. Sci. USA 70:2663, 1973.
86. Groth, C. G., Blomstrand, R., et al.: Metabolic changes following splenic transplantation in a case of Gaucher's disease. In *Sphingolipids, Sphingolipidoses and Allied Disorders*. Volk, B. W., and Aronson, S. M. (eds.), New York, Plenum Press, 1972, pp. 633–639.
87. Desnick, S. J., Desnick, R. J., et al.: Renal transplantation in type II Gaucher disease. In *Enzyme Therapy in Genetic Diseases*. Bergsma, D. (ed.), Baltimore, Williams & Wilkins, 1973, pp. 109–119.
88. Daloze, P., Delvin, E. E., et al.: Replacement therapy for inherited enzyme deficiency: Liver orthotopic transplantation in Niemann-Pick disease type A. Am. J. Med. Genet. 1:229, 1977.
89. Dean, M. F., Stevens, R. L., et al.: Enzyme replacement therapy by fibroblast transplantation. J. Clin. Invest. 63:138, 1979.
90. Dean, M. F., Muir, H., et al.: Enzyme replacement therapy by HLA-compatible fibroblasts in Sanfilippo A syndrome. Pediatr. Res. 15:959, 1981.
91. Hobbs, J. R., Hugh Jones, K., et al.: Reversal of clinical features of Hurler's disease and biochemical improvement after treatment by bone marrow transplantation. J. Inher. Metab. Dis. 5(Suppl):59, 1982.
92. Adinolfi, M., and Brown, S.: Strategies for the correction of enzymatic deficiencies in patients with mucopolysaccharidoses. Develop. Med. Child Neurol. 26:401, 1984.
93. Pearson, A. D. J., Hobbs, J. R., et al.: Graft vs. host disease following bone marrow transplantation for lysosomal storage disease. Intern. Soc. Exp. Hematol. Abst. 1984.
94. Barranger, J. A.: Marrow transplantation in genetic disease. New Engl. J. Med. 311:1629, 1984.
95. Gaucher, P. C. E.: De l'epithelioma primitif de la rate. Thése, Paris, 1882.
96. Kozower, M., Kaplan, M. M., et al.: Esophageal varices in a 60 year old man with Gaucher's disease. Am. J. Dig. Dis. 19:565, 1974.
97. Boklan, B. F., and Sawitsky, A.: Factor IX deficiency in Gaucher disease. Arch. Intern. Med. 136:489, 1976.
98. Kolodny, E. H., Ullman, M. D., et al.: Phenotypic manifestations of Gaucher disease: clinical features in 48 biochemically verified type 1 patients and comment on

type 2 patients. In *Gaucher Disease: A Century of Delineation and Research*. Desnick, R. J., Gatt, S. and Grabowski, G. A. (eds.), New York, Alan R. Liss, Inc., 1982, pp. 33–65.
99. Schoenfeld, Y., Berliner, S., et al.: The association of Gaucher's disease and dysproteinemias. Acta Haematol. 64:241, 1980.
100. Ruestow, P. C., Levinson, D. J. et al.: Coexistence of IgA myeloma and Gaucher's disease. Arch. Intern. Med. 140:1115, 1980.
101. Krause, J. R., Bures, C., and Lee, R. E.: Acute leukemia and Gaucher's disease. Scand. J. Haematol. 23:115, 1979.
102. Bruckstein, A. H., Karanas, A., and Di Re, J. J.: Gaucher's disease associated with Hodgkin's disease. Am. J. Med. 68:610, 1980.
103. Lieberman, I., and Beutler, E.: Elevation of serum angiotensin converting enzyme in Gaucher's disease. New Engl. J. Med. 294:1442, 1976.
104. Gilbert, H. S., and Weinreb, N.: Increased circulating levels of transcobalamin II in Gaucher's disease. New Engl. J. Med. 295:1096, 1976.
105. Svennerholm, L., Hakansson, G., et al.: Chemical differentiation of the Gaucher subtypes. In *Gaucher Disease: A Century of Delineation and Research*. Desnick, R. J., Gatt, S., and Grabowski, G. A. (eds.), New York, Alan R. Liss, Inc., 1982, pp. 231–252.
106. Silverstein, E., Friedland, J., et al.: Marked elevation of serum angiotensin-converting enzyme and hepatic fibrosis containing long-spacing collagen fibrils in type 2 acute neuronopathic Gaucher's disease. Am. J. Clin. Pathol. 69:467, 1978.
107. Grover, W. D., Tucker, S. H., et al.: Clinical variation in two related children with neuronopathic Gaucher's disease. Ann. Neurol. 3:281, 1978.
108. Miller, J. D., McCluer, R., et al.: Gaucher's disease: Neurologic disorder in adult siblings. Ann. Intern. Med. 78:883, 1973.
109. Ginns, E. I., Tegelaers, F. P. W., et al.: Determination of Gaucher's disease phenotypes with monoclonal antibody. Clin. Chim. Acta 131:283, 1983.
109a. Bayever, E., Ladisch, S., et al.: Bone-marrow transplantation for metachromatic leukodystrophy. Lancet 2:471, 1985.
110. Niemann, A.: Ein unbekanntes Krankheitsbild. Jb. Kinderheilkd. 79:1, 1914.
111. Pick, L.: Zur pathologischen Anatomie des Morbus Gaucher. Med. Klin. 18:1408, 1922.
112. Pick, L.: Uber die lipoidzellige Splenohepatomegalie Typus Niemann-Pick als Stoffwechselerktankung. Med. Klin. 23:1483, 1927.
113. Crocker, A. C.: The cerebral defect in Tay-Sachs disease and Niemann-Pick disease. J. Neurochem. 7:69, 1961.
114. Breen, L., Morris, H. H., et al.: Juvenile Niemann-Pick disease with vertical supranuclear ophthalmoplegia. Arch. Neurol. 38:388, 1981.
115. Semeraro, L., Riely, C., et al.: Niemann-Pick variant lipidosis presenting as "neonatal hepatitis." J. Pediatr. Gastroenterol. Nutr. 5:492, 1986.
116. Schneider, E. L., Ellis, W. G., et al.: Prenatal Niemann-Pick disease: biochemical and histological examination of a 19-gestational week fetus. Pediatr. Res. 6:720, 1972.
117. Farber, S., Cohen, J., et al.: Lipogranulomatosis. A new lipoglycoprotein "storage" disease. J. Mt. Sinai Hosp. 24:816, 1957.
118. Moser, H. W., and Chin, W. W.: Ceramidase deficiency: Farber's lipogranulomatosis. In *The Metabolic Basis of Inherited Disease*. Stanbury, J. B., Wyngaarden, J. B., et al. (eds.), New York, McGraw-Hill, 1983, p. 820.
119. Antonarakis, S. E., Valle, D., et al.: Phenotypic variability in siblings with Farber disease. J. Pediatr. 104:406, 1984.
120. Ng Ying Kin, N. M. K., and Wolfe, L. S.: Characterization of oligosaccharides and glycopeptides excreted in the urine of G_{M1}-gangliosidosis patients. Biochem. Biophys. Res. Commun. 66:123, 1975.
121. Raghavan, S., Gajewski, A., et al.: G_{M1}-ganglioside β-galactosidase in leukocytes and cultured fibroblasts. Clin. Chim. Acta 81:47, 1977.
122. Matalon, R., Deanching, M., and Omura, K.: Hurler, Scheie, and Hurler-Scheie "compound": Residual activity of α-L-iduronidase toward natural substrates suggesting allelic mutations. J. Inher. Metab. Dis. 6(Suppl. 2):133, 1983.
123. Fortuin, J. J. H., and Kleijer, W. J.: Hybridization studies of fibroblasts from Hurler, Scheie, and Hurler/Scheie compound patients: Support for the hypothesis of allelic mutants. Hum. Genet. 53:155, 1980.
124. Jensen, O. A., Pedersen, C., et al.: The Hurler/Scheie phenotype in children from a consanguineous marriage: case report with electronmicroscopy of the conjunctiva and ERG. Metabolic Pediatric. Ophthal. 4:133, 1980.
125. Kaibara, H., Eguchi, H., et al.: Hurler-Scheie phenotype: A report of two pairs of inbred sibs. Hum. Genet. 53:37, 1979.
126. Kleijer, W. J., Thompson, E. J., et al.: Prenatal diagnosis of the Hurler syndrome: Report on 40 pregnancies at risk. Prenat. Diag. 3(3):179, July 1983.
127. Shapiro, L. J., Hall, C. W., et al.: The relationship of α-L-iduronidase and Hurler corrective factor. Arch. Biochem. Biophys. 172:156, 1976.
128. Tinessen, T., Gultler, F., and Lykkelund, C.: Reliability of the use of fructose 1-phosphate to detect Hurler cells in fibroblast cultures of obligate carriers of the Hunter syndrome. Hum. Genet. 64:371, 1983.
129. Gatt, R., Borrone, C., et al.: Sanfilippo disease: clinical findings in two patients with a new variant of mucopolysaccharidosis III. Eur. J. Pediatr. 138:168, 1983.
130. Sly, W. S., Quinton, B. A., et al.: Beta glucuronidase deficiency: report of clinical, radiologic, and biochemical features of a new mucopolysaccharidosis. J. Pediatr. 82:249, 1973.
131. Irani, D., Kim, H. S., et al.: Postmortem observations on beta-glucuronidase deficiency presenting as lethal hydrops fetalis. Ann. Neurol. 14:486, 1983.
132. Poenaru, L., Castelnau, L., et al.: Prenatal diagnosis of a heterozygote for mucopolysaccharidosis type VII (β-glucuronidase deficiency). Prenat. Diag. 2:251, 1982.
133. Spranger, J. W. and Wiedemann, H. R.: The genetic mucolipidoses: Diagnosis and differential diagnosis. Hum. Genet. 9:113, 1970.
134. Goldstein, M. L., Kolodny, E. H., et al.: Macular cherry-red spot, myoclonic epilepsy and neurovisceral storage in a 17 year old girl. Trans. Am. Neurol. Assoc. 99:110, 1974.
135. Durand, P., Gatti, R., et al.: Sialidosis (mucolipidosis I). Helv. Paediatr. Acta 32:391, 1977.
136. Rapin, I., Goldfischer, S., et al.: The cherry-red spot–myoclonus syndrome. Ann. Neurol. 3:234, 1978.
137. Thomas, G. H., Tipton, R. E., et al.: Sialidase (α-N-acetylneuraminidase) deficiency: The enzyme defect in an adult with macular cherry-red spots and myoclonus without dementia. A new autosomal recessive disorder. Clin. Genet. 13:369, 1978.
138. Laver, J., and Fried, K., et al.: Infantile lethal neuraminidase deficiency (sialidosis). Clin. Genet. 23:97, 1983.
139. Kelly, T. E., and Graetz, G.: Isolated acid neuraminidase deficiency: a distinct lysosomal storage disease. Am. J. Med. Genet. 1:31, 1977.
140. Spranger, J., Gehler, J., et al.: Mucolipidosis I: A sialidosis. Am. J. Med. Genet. 1:21, 1977.
141. Cantz, M., Gehler, J., et al.: Mucolipidosis I: Increased sialic acid content and deficiency of α-N-acetylneuraminidase in cultured fibroblasts. Biochem. Biophys. Res. Commun. 74:732, 1977.

142. Michalski, J. C., Strecker, G., et al.: Structures of sialyloligosaccharides excreted in the urine of a patient with mucolipidosis I. FEBS Lett. 79:101, 1977.
143. Gravel, R. A., Lowden, J. A., et al.: Infantile sialidosis: A phenocopy of Type I G_{M1} gangliosidosis distinguished by genetic complementation and urinary oligosaccharides. Am. J. Hum. Genet. 31:669, 1979.
144. Matsuo, T., and Egawa, I., et al.: Sialidosis type 2 in Japan. J. Neurol. Sci. 58:45, 1983.
145. Sakuraba, H., Suzuki, Y., et al: β-Galactosidase-neuraminidase deficiency (galactosialidosis): Clinical, pathological, and enzymatic studies in a postmortem case. Ann. Neurol. 13:5:497, 1983.
146. D'Azzo, A., Hoogeveen, A., et al.: Molecular defect in combined β-galactosidase and neuraminidase deficiency in man. Proc. Natl. Acad. Sci. USA 79:4535, 1982.
147. Suzuki, Y., Sakuraba, H., et al.: β-Galactosidase-neuraminidase deficiency: Restoration of β-galactosidase activity by protease inhibitors. J. Biochem. 90:271, 1981.
148. Hoogeveen, A., d'Azzo, A., et al: Correction of combined β-galactosidase/neuraminidase deficiency in human fibroblasts. Biochem. Biophys. Res. Commun. 103:292, 1981.
149. Leroy, J. G., and DeMars, R. I.: Mutant enzymatic and cytological phenotypes in cultured human fibroblasts. Science 157:804, 1967.
150. Leroy, J. G., Spranger, J. W., et al.: I-cell disease: A clinical picture. J. Pediatr. 79:360, 1971.
151. Spitz, R. A., Doughty, R. A., et al.: Neonatal presentation of I-cell disease. J. Pediatr. 93:954, 1978.
152. Hasilik, A., Waheed, A., and von Figura, K.: Enzymatic phosphorylation of lysosomal enzymes in the presence of UDP-N-acetylglucosamine. Absence of activity in I-cell fibroblasts. Biochem. Biophys. Res. Commun. 98:761, 1981.
153. Kelly, T. E., Thomas, G. H., et al.: Mucolipidosis III (pseudo-Hurler polydystrophy): Clinical and laboratory studies in a series of 12 patients. J. Hopkins Med. J. 137:156, 1975.
154. Hasilik, A., Waheed, A., et al.: Impaired phosphorylation of lysosomal enzymes in fibroblasts of patients with mucolipidosis III. Europ. J. Biochem. 122:119, 1982.
155. Merin, S., Livni, N., et al.: Mucolipidosis IV: ocular, systemic and ultrastructural findings. Invest. Ophthalmol. 14:437, 1975.
156. Crandall, B. F., Philippart, M., et al.: Review article: Mucolipidosis IV. Am. J. Med. Genet. 12:301, 1982.
157. Berman, E. R., Livni, N., et al.: Congenital corneal clouding with abnormal systemic storage bodies: A new variant of mucolipidosis. J. Pediatr. 84:519, 1974.
158. Tellez-Nagel, I., Rapin, I., et al.: Mucolipidosis IV. Clinical, ultrastructural, histochemical, and chemical studies of a case, including a brain biopsy. Arch. Neurol. 33:828, 1976.
159. Goutieres, F., Arsenio-Nunes, M. L., et al.: Mucolipidosis IV. Neuropaediatr. 10:321, 1979.
160. Bach, G., Zeigler, M., et al.: Mucolipidosis type IV: ganglioside sialidase deficiency. Biochem. Biophys. Res. Commun. 90:1341, 1979.
161. Kohn, G., Livni, N., et al.: Prenatal diagnosis of mucolipidosis IV by electron microscopy. J. Pediatr. 90:62, 1977.
162. Alhadeff, J. A., and O'Brien, J. S.: Fucosidosis. In *Practical Enzymology of the Sphingolipidoses*. Glew, R. H., and Peters, S. P. (eds.), New York, Alan R. Liss, Inc., 1977.
163. Kousseff, B. G., and Beratis, N. G.,: Fucosidosis type 2. Pediatrics 57:205, 1976.
164. Loeb, H., Tondeur, M., et al.: Biochemical and ultrastructural studies in a case of mucopolysaccharidosis "F" (fucosidosis). Helv. Pediatr. Acta 24:519, 1969.
165. Libert, J., Van Hoef, F., and Tondeur, M.: Fucosidosis: Ultrastructural study of conjunctiva and skin and enzyme analysis of tears. Invest. Ophthalmol. 15:626, 1976.
166. Tsay, G. C., and Dawson, G.: Oligosaccharide storage in brains from patients with fucosidosis, G_{M1}-gangliosidosis, and G_{M2}-gangliosidosis (Sandhoff's disease). J. Neurochem. 27:733, 1976.
167. Strecker, G., Fournet, B., et al.: Structure de 9 oligosaccharides et glycopeptides riches en fucose excretes dans l'urine de deux sujets atteints de fucosidose. C. R. Acad. Sci., Ser. D 284:85, 1977.
168. Goss, S. J., and Harris, H: Gene transfer by means of cell fusion II. The mapping of 8 loci on human chromosome 1 by statistical analysis of gene assortment in somatic cell hybrids. J. Cell Sci. 25:39, 1977.
169. Turner, B. M., Turner, V. S., et al.: Polymorphism of human α-fucosidase. Am. J. Hum. Genet. 27:651, 1975.
170. Turner, B. M., Beratis, N. G., et al.: Silent allele as genetic basis for fucosidosis. Nature 257:391, 1975.
171. Ng W. G., Donnell, G. N., et al.: Biochemical and genetic studies of plasma and leukocyte α-L-fucosidase. Am. J. Hum. Genet. 28:42, 1976.
172. Durand, P., Gatti, R., et al.: Detection of carriers and prenatal diagnosis for fucosidosis in Calabria. Hum. Genet. 51:195, 1979.
173. Kjellman, B., Gamstorp, I., et al.: Mannosidosis: A clinical and histopathologic study. J. Pediatr. 75:366, 1969.
174. Desnick, R. J., Sharp, H. L., et al.: Mannosidosis: Clinical, morphologic, immunologic, and biochemical studies. Pediatr. Res. 10:985, 1976.
175. Kistler, J. P., Lott, I. T., et al.: Mannosidosis. New clinical presentation, enzyme studies and carbohydrate analysis. Arch. Neurol. 34:45, 1977.
176. Halperin, J. J., Landis, D. M. D., et al.: Communicating hydrocephalus and lysosomal inclusions in mannosidosis. Arch. Neurol. 41:777, 1984.
177. Sung, J. H., Hayano, M., et al.: Mannosidosis: pathology of the nervous system. J. Neuropathol. Exp. Neurol. 36:807, 1977.
178. Masson, P. K., and Lundblad, A.: Mannosidosis: Detection of the disease and of heterozygotes using serum and leucocytes. Biochem. Biophys. Res. Comm. 56:296, 1974.
179. Poenaru, L., Gerard, S., et al.: Antenatal diagnosis in three pregnancies at risk for mannosidosis. Clin. Genet. 16:428, 1979.
180. Champion, M. J., and Shows, T. B.: Mannosidosis: Assignment of the lysosomal α-mannosidase B gene to chromosome 19 in man. Proc. Natl. Acad. Sci. USA 74:2969, 1977.
181. Burditt, L. J., Phillips, N. C., et al.: Characterization of the mutant α-mannosidase in bovine mannosidosis. Biochem. J. 175:1013, 1978.
182. Jones, M. Z., and Laine, R. A.: Caprine oligosaccharide storage disease: Accumulation of β-mannosyl (1→ 4) β-N-acetylglucosaminyl (1→ 4) β-N-acetylglucosamine in brain. J. Biol. Chem. 256:5181, 1981.
183. Dorling, P. R., Huxtable, C. R., and Vogel, P.: Lysosomal storage in Swainsona SPP toxicoses: An induced mannosidosis. Neuropath. Appl. Neurobiol. 4:285, 1978.
184. Hultberg, B., and Masson, P. K.: Activation of residual acidic α-mannosidase activity in mannosidosis tissues by metal ions. Biochem. Biophys. Res. Commun. 67:1473, 1975.
185. Dickersin, G. R., Lott, I. T., et al.: A light and electron microscopic study of mannosidosis. Hum. Pathol. 11:245, 1980.
186. Jenner, F. A., and Pollitt, R. J.: Large quantities of α-acetamido-1-(beta-L-aspartamido)-1,2-dideoxy-glucose in the urine of mentally retarded siblings. Biochem. J. 103:48P, 1967.
187. Autio, S., Aspartylglycosaminuria (AGU). In *Population Structure and Genetic Disorders*. Erikson, A. W., Forsius, H. R., et al. (eds.), New York, Academic Press, 1980, pp. 577–582.

188. Isenberg, J. N., and Sharp, H. L.: Aspartylglucosaminuria: psychomotor retardation masquerading as a mucopolysaccharidosis. J. Pediatr. *86:*713, 1975.
189. Humbel, R., and Marchal, C.: Screening test for aspartylglucosaminuria. J. Pediatr. *84:*456, 1974.
190. Maury, C. P. J., and Palo, J.: N-acetylglucosamine-asparagine levels in tissues of patients with aspartylglycosaminuria. Clin. Chim. Acta. *108:*293, 1980.
191. Lundblad, A., Masson, P. K., et al.: Structural determination of three glycoasparagines isolated from the urine of a patient with aspartylglycosaminuria. Eur. J. Biochem. *67:*209, 1976.
192. Aula, P., Raivio, K., et al.: Enzymatic diagnosis and carrier detection of aspartylglucosaminuria using blood samples. Pediatr. Res. *10:*625, 1976.
193. Crocker, A. C., Vawter, G. F., et al.: Wolman's disease: Three new patients with a recently described lipidosis. Pediatrics *35:*627, 1965.
194. Coates, P. M., Cortner, J. A., et al.: Prenatal diagnosis of Wolman disease. Am. J. Med. Genet. *2:*397, 1978.
195. Christomanou, H., and Cap, C.: Prenatal monitoring for Wolman's disease in a pregnancy at risk: first case in the Federal Republic of Germany. Hum. Genet. *57:*440, 1981.
196. Kyriakides, E. C., Paul, B., and Balin, J. A.: Lipid accumulation and acid lipase deficiency in fibroblasts from a family with Wolman's disease, and their apparent correction in vitro. J. Lab. Clin. Med. *80:*810, 1972.
197. Kelly, S., and Bakhru-Kishore, R.: Fluorimetric assay of acid lipase in human leukocytes. Clin Chim Acta *97:*239, 1979.
198. Beaudet, A. L., Ferry, G. D., et al.: Cholesterol ester storage disease: clinical, biochemical, and pathological studies. J. Pediatr. *90:*910, 1977.
199. Hoeg, J. M., Demosky, S. J., Jr., et al.: Cholesterol ester storage disease and Wolman disease: phenotypic variants of lysosomal acid cholesteryl ester hydrolase deficiency. Am. J. Hum. Genet. *36:*1190, 1984.
200. Wolfe, L. S., Ng Ying Kin, N. M. K., et al.: Dolichols in brain and urinary sediment in neuronal ceroid lipofuscinosis. Neurology *33:*103, 1983.
201. Ng Ying Kin, N. M. K., and Wolfe, L. S.: Presence of abnormal amounts of dolichols in the urinary sediment of Batten disease patients. Pediatr. Res. *16:*530, 1982.
202. Barlow, C. F., Williams, R., et al.: Juvenile cerebromacular degeneration, with neuronal ceroid-lipofuscinosis (Batten's disease). Case records of the Massachusetts General Hospital. New Engl. J. Med. *299:*189, 1978.
203. Pilz, H., Goebel, H. H., et al.: Isoelectric enzyme patterns of leukocyte peroxidase in normal controls and patients with neuronal ceroid-lipofuscinosis. Neuropadiatrie *7:*261, 1976.
204. Schwerer, B., and Bernheimer, H.: Leucocyte PPD-peroxidase activity with polyunsaturated fatty acid hydroperoxides: normal values in Batten's disease. J. Neurochem. *31:*457, 1978.
205. Wolfe, L. S., Ng Ying Kin, N. M. K., et al.: Batten disease and related disorders: New findings on the chemistry of the storage material. In *Lysosomes and the Lysosomal Storage Diseases.* Callahan, J., Lowden, J. (eds.), New York, Raven Press, 1981, pp. 315-330.
206. Finkel, R. S., Bresnan, M. G., et al.: Neuronal ceroid-lipofuscinosis: A diagnostic approach. Ann. Neurol. *14:*366, 1983.
207. Pullarkat, R. K., and Reha, H.: Accumulation of dolichols in brains of the elderly. J. Biol. Chem. *257:*5991, 1982.
208. Wolfe, L. S., Ng Ying Kin, N. M. K., et al.: Raised levels of cerebral cortex dolichols in Alzheimer's disease. Lancet *2:*99, 1982.
209. Santavuori, P., Haltia, M., et al.: Infantile type of so-called neuronal ceroid-lipofuscinosis. I. A clinical study of 15 patients. J. Neurol. Sci. *18:*257, 1973.
210. Palo, J., Elovaara, I., et al.: Infantile neuronal ceroid-lipofuscinosis: isolation of storage material. Neurology *32:*1035, 1982.
211. Armstrong, D., Wehling, C., et al.: Diagnosis of Batten disease from urinary sediment: A brief report. Pathology *9:*39, 1977.
212. Goebel, H. H., Zeman, W., et al.: Significance of muscle biopsies in neuronal ceroid-lipofuscinoses. J. Neurol. Neurosurg. Psychiatr. *38:*985, 1975.
213. Goebel, H. H., Zeman, W., et al.: Ultrastructural investigations of peripheral nerves in neuronal ceroid-lipofuscinoses (NCL). J. Neurol. *213:*295, 1976.
214. Haltia, M., Rapola, J., et al.: Infantile type of so-called neuronal ceroid-lipofuscinosis. II. Morphological and biochemical studies. J. Neurol. Sci. *18:*269, 1973.
215. Lyon, B. B.: Peripheral nerve involvement in Batten-Spielmeyer-Vogt's disease. J. Neurol. Neurosurg. Psychiatr. *38:*175, 1975.
216. Zeman, W.: Studies in the neuronal ceroid-lipofuscinoses. J. Neuropathol. Exp. Neurol. *33:*1, 1974.
217. Boehme, D. H., Cottrell, J. C., et al.: A dominant form of neuronal ceroid-lipofuscinosis. Brain *94:*745, 1971.

COAGULATION

CHAPTER 39
Physiology of Coagulation: The Fluid Phase

ROBERT D. ROSENBERG

INTRODUCTION 1248
THE GENERATION OF THROMBIN 1249
 The Intrinsic Coagulation Cascade
 The Extrinsic Coagulation Cascade
 The Common Pathway
 Kinetic Relationships Among the Cascades and the Common Pathway of Thrombin Generation
 The Protein C–Thrombomodulin Mechanism
FORMATION OF THE FIBRIN CLOT 1257
THE FIBRINOLYTIC MECHANISM 1258
LIMITING REACTIONS 1262
 Antithrombin
 Antiplasmin
 α_2-Macroglobulin
 New Protease Inhibitors of the Hemostatic System

INTRODUCTION

A complex series of events is set into motion when the vascular endothelium is damaged. Subendothelial structures are exposed to the blood. These attract platelets and induce them to aggregate reversibly (1, 2). Thrombin is then formed on the surface of this mass of loosely interacting platelets. Once this enzyme is produced, it generates insoluble crosslinked fibrin and causes the platelets to aggregate irreversibly (3, 4). The resultant platelet-fibrin meshwork is an effective barrier against the egress of blood from the vascular system and also serves as a scaffold for repair of the damaged endothelium. Simultaneously, various limiting reactions are brought into play that confine hemostatic system activity to the site of injury (5, 6). After regeneration of the vascular endothelium has occurred, there is a gradual dissolution of the platelet-fibrin meshwork (7, 8).

The prototype transformations of the hemostatic mechanism are depicted in Figure 39–1. An enzyme precursor, or zymogen, is normally present in the blood but exhibits minimal biologic activity (9). This substance is transformed into a trypsin-like protease (serine protease) either by conformation alteration or by a converting enzyme that scissions peptide bonds (10). The rate of this reaction may be accelerated by non-enzymatic cofactors that are able to either alter zymogen conformation or bind the scissioning enzyme and zymogen close together on an appropriate surface. Once generated, the serine protease is free to act upon its natural substrate or substrates and transform them into biologically potent species. However, the enzyme may encounter plasma components that neutralize its activity. These inhibitory substances contain peptide sequences similar to those present within the natural substrate (11). When the enzyme interacts with these unique regions, bond hydrolysis is hindered rather than facilitated, as in the natural substrate, and a stable protease-protease inhibitor complex is formed. Thus, similar biochemical mechanisms are responsible for the generation and suppression of hemostatic system activity.

During the evolutionary process, homologous sets of zymogens, converting enzymes, cofactors, and inhibitors arose, owing to gene duplication and mutation. This has resulted in the development of a linked series of reactions in which a zymogen is converted into a serine protease that then catalyzes the subsequent precursor-protease transition. This complex, multistage system per-

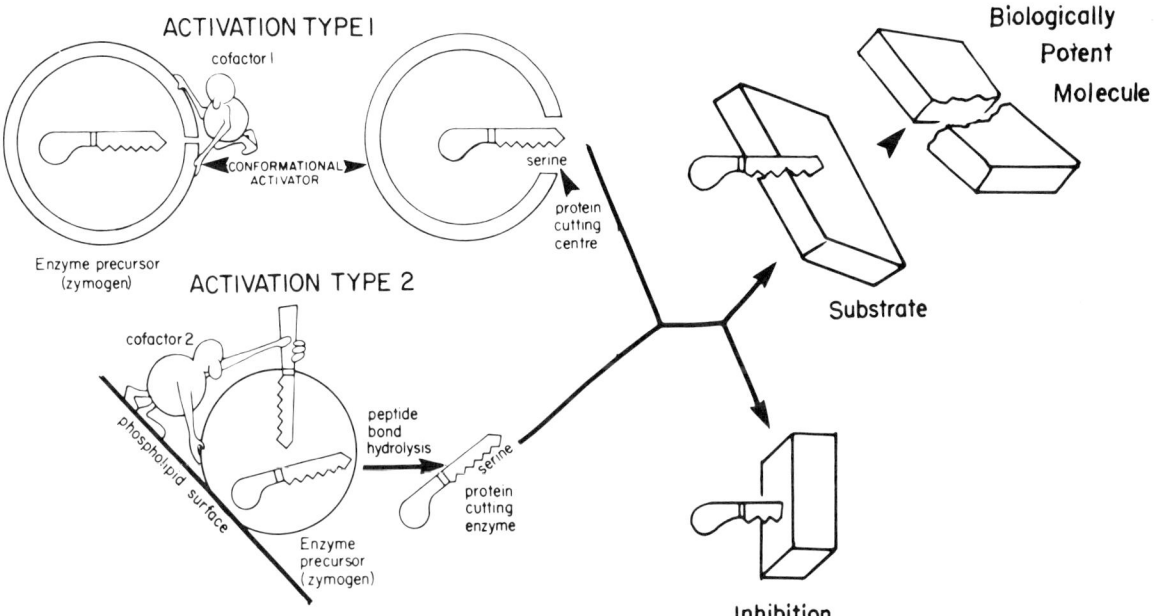

Figure 39–1. Activation mechanisms for zymogens of the hemostatic mechanism.

mits both amplification and modulation of the initial stimulus that sets the hemostatic mechanism into action. Table 39–1 lists the various components of this system, summarizes their roles within the hemostatic mechanism, and indicates their sites of synthesis.

In the following sections, we shall outline the detailed biochemistry of the hemostatic process. In particular, we shall describe the pathways of thrombin generation, the formation of the fibrin clot, the action of the fibrinolytic system, and the nature of the limiting reactions. Platelets play a critical function in these interactions, but the role of these cellular elements will not be considered since they are discussed in Chapter 40 and 42.

THE GENERATION OF THROMBIN

The generation of thrombin can be subdivided into two major sets of reaction sequences. The first phase involves the activation of Factor X, whereas the second phase is concerned with the subsequent conversion of prothrombin to thrombin.

The transformation of Factor X to its corresponding serine protease, Factor Xa, is accomplished via two distinct pathways termed the intrinsic and extrinsic coagulation cascades (12, 13). Activation of each pathway is initiated when blood comes in contact with damaged vascular endothelium and sequestered subendothelium components are able to interact with the specific plasma proteins of both coagulation cascades. It is essential that both these systems function in a normal fashion if adequate amounts of Factor Xa are to be generated under in vivo conditions.

The rapid conversion of prothrombin to thrombin is catalyzed by the serine protease Factor Xa and a cofactor, Factor V. This series of reactions takes place on phospholipid surfaces such as platelets or lipoproteins. The sequence of transformations is termed the common pathway (14).

The Intrinsic Coagulation Cascade

The activation of the intrinsic coagulation cascade is sparked by the exposure of collagen, basement membrane, or microfibrillar substance to the blood (15, 16). Factor XII (Hageman factor) is a zymogen having a single polypeptide chain of molecular weight 80,000 daltons that is present in plasma at a concentration of approximately 29 μg per ml (17, 18). This component is able to bind to the subendothelial structures listed previously and appears to undergo a conformational transition to Factor XIIa, which contains an active serine center (19) (Fig. 39–2). Alternatively, Factor XII can be converted to Factor XIIa by proteolytic cleavages that produce a diverse spectrum of products with molecular weights that range from 25,000 to 75,000 daltons (20). Once formed, this enzyme is able to hydrolyze prekallikrein and Factor XI as well as plasminogen and thus activate the kinin-generating, coagulation, and fibrinolytic mechanisms.

Prekallikrein (Fletcher factor) is a zymogen that possesses a single polypeptide chain of molecular weight 85,000 daltons and is present in plasma at a concentration of 15 to 45 μg per ml (21, 22). It circulates in the blood as a 1:1 stoichiometric complex with a cofactor termed high-molecular-

Table 39–1. COMPONENTS OF THE HEMOSTATIC MECHANISM

Component	Sites of Synthesis
Zymogens	
Coagulation components:	
Factor II (prothrombin)	Liver
Factor VII (SPCA)	Liver
Factor IX (Christmas factor)	Liver
Factor X (Stuart factor)	Liver
Factor XI (plasma thromboplastin antecedent)	Liver
Factor XII (Hageman factor)	Liver
Factor XIII (fibrinoligase or Laki-Lorand factor)	Liver or platelets
Prekallikrein (Fletcher factor)	Liver
Protein C	Liver
Fibrinolytic components:	
Plasminogen	Liver
Plasminogen activators	Endothelial cells and lysosomes of organs
Cofactors	
Factor V (labile factor)	Liver, endothelial cells and platelets
Factor VIII (von Willebrand factor)	Endothelial cells and platelets
High-molecular-weight kininogen	Liver
Proteins	Liver
Plasma Inhibitors	
Antithrombin (antithrombin III or heparin cofactor)	Liver
α_2-Plasmin inhibitor (antiplasmin)	Liver
α_2-Macroglobulin	Liver
Protein C inhibitor	Liver
Plasminogen activator inhibitor	Endothelial cells and platelets

weight kininogen (Fitzgerald-Williams-Flaujeac factor) of approximate molecular weight 120,000 daltons (23). Factor XIIa is able to cleave the prekallikrein zymogen and convert it into the serine protease kallikrein. The latter enzyme possesses both a heavy and a light polypeptide chain of approximate molecular weight 52,000 daltons and 33,000 daltons, respectively (24). The presence of high-molecular-weight kininogen cofactor is essential to bind prekallikrein to a negatively charged surface in close proximity to Factor XIIa and thereby allow rapid generation of kallikrein from prekallikrein (25). Once formed, this enzyme is able to scission the single polypeptide chain of the high-molecular-weight kininogen and release the decapeptide bradykinin from the center of the molecule (26). This polypeptide is a potent substance that lowers blood pressure, increases capillary permeability, and acts as a vasodilator. Kallikrein itself has been shown to exhibit chemotactic activity for human neutrophils and monocytes (27) and to induce aggregation and stimulate oxygen consumption by these cellular elements (27a), thereby acting to recruit and activate these blood cells at the sites of tissue injury.

Factor XI (plasma thromboplastin antecedent) is a zymogen whose structure is formed by two identical polypeptide chains of molecular weight 80,000 daltons connected by S-S bridges (28). This protein is present in plasma at a concentration of approximately 7 µg per ml and circulates as a 1:1 stoichiometric complex with high molecular-weight kininogen (29). Factor XIIa is able to convert the Factor XI zymogen into the serine protease Factor XIa. The transformation is accomplished by the scissioning of specific bonds within each of the polypeptide chains of the zymogen. This results in the formation of two sets of 50,000-dalton and 30,000 dalton fragments held together by S-S bridges (30). Thus, the structure of Factor XIa appears to be that of a "two-headed" dimeric enzyme. High-molecular-weight kininogen must be present if Factor XI is to be bound to a negatively charged surface in close proximity to Factor XIIa and thereby allow significant quantities of Factor XIa to be rapidly generated (31). Once formed, this enzyme is able to initiate activation of the remainder of the intrinsic coagulation cascade with resultant formation of Factor Xa.

Plasminogen is a zymogen normally found in the blood that is also activated by Factor XIIa to

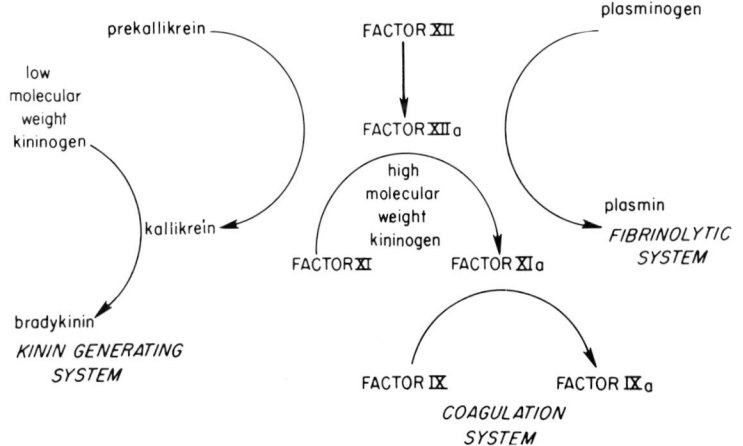

Figure 39–2. The consequences of Factor XII activation.

form the serine protease plasmin (32). This latter enzyme is able to lyse the fibrin clot (see later section on Fibrinolysis for details). Since Factor XIIa is capable of converting plasminogen to plasmin, it can initiate systemic fibrinolysis (33). At the present time, it is unclear whether Factor XIIa can directly activate plasminogen or whether this is indirectly accomplished via generation of kallikrein as well as Factor XIa, both of which subsequently cleave the zymogen.

It is of considerable interest that kallikrein, plasmin, and Factor XIa, all of which are generated by Factor XIIa, can, in turn, produce additional Factor XIIa by proteolytic cleavage of the Factor XII zymogen (34). High-molecular-weight kininogen is a critical cofactor in this process (35). These multiple pathways autocatalytically magnify the initial stimulus for activating Factor XII and result in the production of greater amounts of enzyme. However, the species generated is a low-molecular-weight form of Factor XIIa, which cannot bind to surfaces and is relatively impotent in activating the coagulation mechanism. This type of Factor XIIa is a powerful mobilizer of the fibrinolytic as well as the kinin-generating system. Thus, the amplification process described previously orients the hemostatic mechanism toward clot resolution and kinin formation as opposed to fibrin deposition.

Once Factor XIa has been generated, it is able to interact with a zymogen termed Factor IX (Christmas factor) and convert it to the serine protease Factor IXa (36) (Fig. 39–3). The Factor IX zymogen is present in plasma at a concentration of about 4 to 5 µg per ml. It is a single polypeptide chain of approximate molecular weight 55,000 daltons (37). The initial step in the activation mechanism involves a scission of a specific bond within the zymogen to form an inactive two-chain disulfide-linked intermediate. This species possesses heavy and light chains of molecular weight 38,000 daltons and 16,000 daltons, respectively. In a subsequent step, a polypeptide of approximate molecular weight 9000 daltons is split from the newly formed N-terminal of the heavy chain. The resultant molecule is the serine protease Factor IXa (38).

The preservation of the original N-terminal region of the zymogen within the structure of this enzyme appears to be a critical feature of the activation mechanism. This area contains a number of γ-carboxyglutamic acid residues whose presence is attributable to a vitamin K–dependent postribosomal modification (39). As will be noted, these unique amino acid moieties are responsible for the binding of Factor IXa to phospholipid and/or specific receptors on the endothelial cell surface (39a). Therefore, these residues are essential for the subsequent surface-dependent activation of Factor X (see Figure 39–2). The maintenance of these γ-carboxyglutamic acid moieties within Fac-

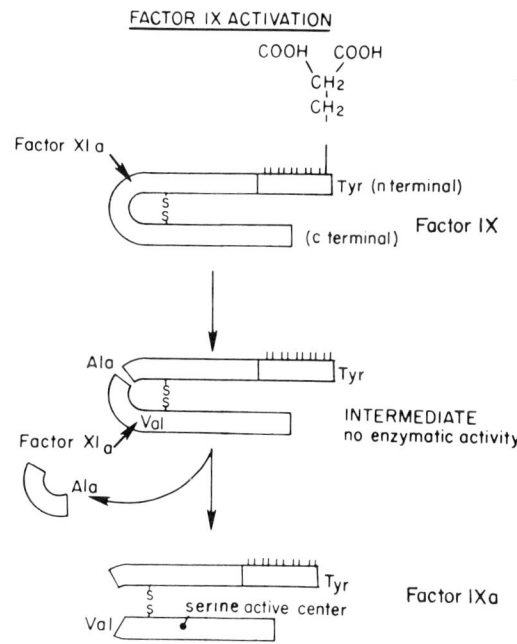

Figure 39–3. The activation of Factor IX.

tor IXa can be compared with the situation that occurs when prothrombin is transformed to thrombin. In the latter case, these residues are absent from the enzymatic end product (40). It has been suggested that these γ-carboxyglutamic acid residues in Factor IXa localize this enzyme to the area of hemostatic injury and allow it to interact with Factor X (Stuart factor) bound to the same surface. The absence of the same residues in thrombin facilitates diffusion of the enzyme from this locale and permits it to act upon platelets as well as fibrinogen at some distance from the site of hemostatic system activation.

When Factor IXa is formed, it converts the Factor X zymogen to the serine protease Factor Xa (41). Factor X is found in plasma at a concentration of approximately 10 µg per ml and exhibits a molecular weight of 55,000 daltons. It appears to circulate as a two-chain species whose primary structure is quite homologous to that of the Factor IX intermediate (42). The site at which the newly synthesized single-chain Factor X is scissioned to form this two-chain zymogen is unknown. The mechanism of activation of this latter component is virtually identical to the second step of Factor IX conversion depicted in Figure 39–3 (43). Additional scissions at the C-terminal of the heavy chain of Factor Xa can occur when high levels of reactants are utilized, but this represents a biologically unimportant set of side reactions (44).

In vivo, the activation of Factor X by Factor IXa must occur at a rapid rate and yet be localized to the site of hemostatic injury. This is accomplished by the action of a cofactor termed Factor VIII (antihemophilic factor) in association with Ca^{++}

ions and a specific receptor on a biologic surface. Factor VIII has recently been isolated in purified form, and the structure of the gene that encodes this component has been elucidated (45a, 45b). These studies have demonstrated that the above cofactor is a protein of about 330,000 daltons that circulates in plasma at a concentration of about 50 ng per ml. The overall structure of Factor VIII is depicted in Figure 39–4. It is readily apparent that the native cofactor, which has little procoagulant activity, consists of cysteine-rich N-terminal and C-terminal domains as well as a carbohydrate-rich central core. The polypeptide chain of Factor VIII can be scissioned by thrombin at two or more sites, which releases the original central core and generates Factor VIIIa, a two-chain species that possesses significant amounts of biologic activity. Both the overall structure of Factor VIII and its mechanism of activation are extraordinarily similar to that of Factor V (see below). The formation of the Factor IXa–Factor VIIIa–Factor X–Ca^{++}–interaction product is thought to require specific receptors located on endothelial cells and perhaps platelets (39a). The interactions that lead to the generation of the above complex are poorly understood but must be similar to those required for stabilization of the analogous Factor Xa–Factor Va–prothrombin–Ca^{++}–platelet receptor complex (see Figure 9–1). Based upon data available for Factor Va, it appears likely that the N-terminal arm of Factor VIIIa functions by binding to Factor IXa and to a specific receptor on the relevant biologic surface, whereas the C-terminal arm of Factor VIIIa is involved in interacting with Factor X. The gamma-carboxyglutamic acid residues of both Factor IXa and Factor Xa are also important in the formation of the above interaction product. The acceleration of Factor X activation is probably achieved by close approximation of enzyme and substrate on the surface as well as by a conformational change in Factor X that renders it more susceptible to enzymatic attack. Localization of Factor Xa generation is attained by formation of the multimolecular complex only at sites of injury and by the presence of gamma-carboxyglutamic acid residues on the enzyme. These structures are responsible for binding Factor Xa to the biologic surface via Ca^{++} ions and prevent it from diffusing away from this locale.

Factor VIII circulates within the blood complexed to von Willebrand's factor. The latter substance is present in plasma at a level of about 10 μg per ml and exhibits a multimeric structure with molecular weights that range up to 5 million daltons. The stable protomeric unit of this multimeric structure is a dimer that consists of disulfide-bonded polypeptide chains of approximate molecular weight 240,000 daltons. This species is able to assemble into larger aggregates via labile disulfide bridges that exhibit rapid interchange (46). These protomeric units also bear oligosaccharide chains similar in structure to blood group substance. As expected, these structures possess galactose and sialic acid groups as penultimate and ultimate residues (47).

Von Willebrand's factor functions by binding to specific platelet receptors such as glycoprotein Ib and perhaps glycoproteins IIb/IIIa. This interaction is thought to mediate the adhesion of platelets to subendothelial structures. A similar interaction between this plasma protein and glycoprotein Ib is required for the ristocetin-induced aggregation of these cellular elements (48). The larger multimeric forms of von Willebrand's factor are essential for its biologic action upon platelets. This appears to be due to the high affinity of this form of the protein for glycoprotein Ib as well as its subsequent ability to bridge the distance between these cellular elements and induce platelet association (48). The lower-molecular-weight forms of von Willebrand's factor exhibit this ability to only a minimal extent (48). The oligosaccharide chains attached to the protomeric unit are also critical with respect to platelet interactions. Removal of the terminal sialic acid and galactose residues dramatically reduces the activity of the von Willebrand's factor (49). Furthermore, the desialyated form of the protein has a very short survival within the circulation, which is due to its removal by a specific hepatic receptor (49). It is of interest that individuals with a congenital decrease in von Wil-

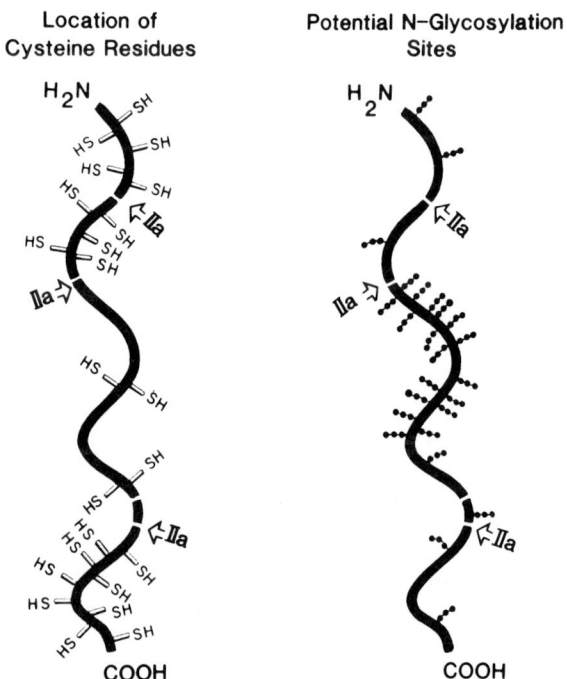

Figure 39–4. Structural features of human Factor VIII:C, showing schematically the location of cysteine residues and potential N-glycosylation sites (Asn-X-Ser/Thr) with respect to thrombin cleavage domains (IIa).

lebrand's factor (von Willebrand's disease) exhibit reductions in the multimeric forms of this protein and may also possess incomplete forms of the oligosaccharide chains (50, 50a). This may, in part, explain the clinical abnormalities of platelet function that are an integral part of von Willebrand's disease.

It is particularly revealing to contrast the abnormalities noted in von Willebrand's disease with those that occur in Factor VIII deficiency (classic hemophilia). Patients with the former disorder suffer abnormalities in platelet function as well as reductions in Factor VIII activity. Patients with the latter abnormality have normal platelet function but exhibit defects in the intrinsic coagulation cascade. These findings support the experimental data that indicate that von Willebrand's factor is a carrier of Factor VIII. These claims are further strengthened by the observation that transfusion of plasma from individuals with severe Factor VIII deficiency into those with von Willebrand's disease promptly normalizes the latter's Factor VIII activity. This is accomplished by providing a source of endogenous von Willebrand's factor that can associate with endogenous Factor VIII. Fragmentary experimental data indicate that the site of association may be either within the endothelial cell or within the liver (51).

The Extrinsic Coagulation Cascade
(Fig. 39–5)

The activation of the extrinsic coagulation cascade is initiated by the exposure to the blood of a membrane-bound glycoprotein termed tissue factor (52). This latter component is present on the surfaces of various somatic cells, especially smooth muscle cells and fibroblasts in subendothelial locations (55). Surfaces of cells that are customarily in contact with blood, such as endothelial cells or leukocytes, also possess tissue factor, but this species is inaccessible unless proteolytic enzymes or membrane damage makes it available.

Tissue factor is able to form a stable complex with a plasma protein termed Factor VII (serum proconvertin accelerator) (54). The phospholipid component of tissue factor appears critical for this interaction. Factor VII is present in plasma at a level of about 1 µg per ml and is composed of a single polypeptide chain of approximate molecular weight 60,000 daltons (55). This zymogen is structurally homologous to prothrombin, Factor IX, and Factor X (56). Unlike the other proteins, however, Factor VII is thought to possess intrinsic enzymatic activity.

A conformational alteration in Factor VII to form Factor VIIa appears to occur when it complexes with tissue factor. This interaction increases the affinity of Factor VII for Factor X and also dramatically augments the ability of this protein

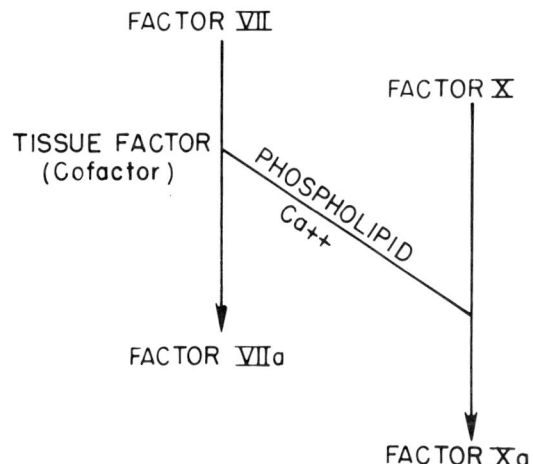

Figure 39–5. The extrinsic coagulation cascade.

to proteolyze Factor X. Subsequently, Factor X is bound to the Factor VII-tissue factor complex partially via the phospholipid–Ca^{++} γ-carboxyglutamic acid residue interactions similar to those described for Factor IXa. It is rapidly converted to Factor Xa via proteolytic cleavages identical to those occurring during the intrinsic activation of Factor X.

The extrinsic coagulation cascade exhibits both positive and negative control mechanisms. For example, generation of Factor Xa initially results in the specific cleavage of Factor VII to form a disulfide-linked two-chain daughter species. This component binds more tightly to tissue factor and has 80-fold greater potency with respect to Factor X activation. As larger quantities of Factor Xa are produced, additional peptide cleavage of the two-chain form of Factor VII renders it inactive (57).

The Common Pathway

Prothrombin is a single-chain zymogen (M.W.~65,000 daltons) that is present in plasma at a level of about 100 µg per ml (53). As shown in Figure 39–6, this protein possesses two triple-loop structures termed kringles within its N-terminal region. The kringles divide this area of the prothrombin molecule into two semi-independent domains termed the F_1 and F_2 regions (59). The F_1 region contains 10 unique gamma-carboxyglutamic residues, of which 6 are present in pairs (60). These moieties are formed by a vitamin K–dependent postribosomal process in which pre-existing specific glutamic acid residues are gamma-carboxylated (61). The various sets of these unique sites have a great avidity for Ca^{++} ions and are critically involved in the interaction of the zymogen with the phospholipid or activated platelet surface (61). During coumarin ingestion, prothrombin is synthesized without a full complement of these unique residues. As expected, the zymo-

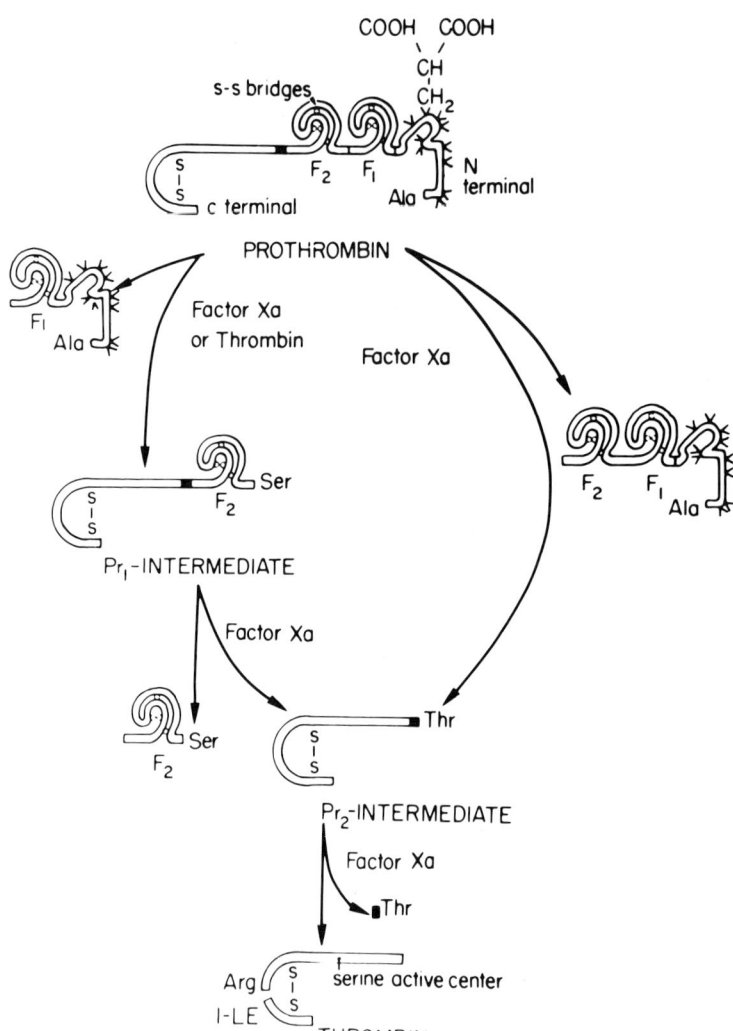

Figure 39–6. The common pathway of thrombin generation.

gen cannot bind tightly to appropriate surfaces and is unable to be rapidly activated to thrombin (62). Similar functional defects are noted with Factors VII, IX, X, and protein C synthesized during the same time period. The F_2 region contains a Factor Va binding site that allows prothrombin to interact with the activated cofactor that binds the zymogen to the surface of the activated platelet (see below) (63).

Once the intrinsic and extrinsic coagulation cascades have generated sufficient amounts of Factor Xa, this enzyme can convert prothrombin to the disulfide-linked two-chain serine protease thrombin. This is accomplished by scissioning Arg_{273}-Thr_{274} and/or Arg_{155}-Ser_{156} and releasing the N-terminal polypeptide F_{1+2} or F_1 and F_2 (64, 64a). In a subsequent step of the activation mechanism, Factor Xa cleaves Arg_{322}-Ile_{323} in the C-terminal region of prothrombin and generates a two-chain component with enzymatic activity. Release of a 13 amino acid polypeptide from the N-terminal of the latter species may also occur (64, 64a).

Under in vitro conditions, this sequence of events proceeds slowly with many hours needed for thrombin generation. In vivo, the process is dramatically accelerated by the action of a cofactor termed Factor V/Va (labile factor or Ac globulin) in conjunction with Ca^{++} ions and an activated platelet surface. Factor V is a glycoprotein that consists of a single polypeptide chain (M.W.~330,000 daltons) that is present in plasma at a concentratrion of about 10 μg per ml (64b, 64c). Factor V represents a minimally active form of this coagulation protein. Several investigators have demonstrated that the addition of relatively low concentrations of thrombin to Factor V dramatically augments the ability of the cofactor to function in the conversion of prothrombin to thrombin (65, 65a). Definitive biochemical studies of this process have revealed that the activation of

Factor V, shown in Figure 39–7, is initiated by a cleavage of the single polypeptide chain with the formation of a component that possesses two separate polypeptide chains of molecular weight 280,000 (A) and 105,000 (D). This molecular species has minimal amounts of biologic activity. In addition, a second bond is scissioned, within polypeptide chain A_1, with the generation of a component that exhibits two polypeptide chains of molecular weight 71,000 (B) and 220,000 (C) respectively. This molecular species has significant amounts of cofactor activity. Subsequently, two additional bonds can be cleaved within polypeptide C to produce a molecule that consists of two polypeptide chains of molecular weight 150,000 (E) and 71,000 (F), with only a small additional increment in biologic activity. This stable form of Factor Va is held together by noncovalent interactions in the presence of calcium ions (Fig. 39–7).

Factor Va consists of a hydrophobic light chain that binds to a specific protein within the platelet membrane (in order to provide a receptor for Factor Xa) and a heavy chain that is available to bind to prothrombin (66). The interactions of Factor Xa with Factor Va and the platelet surface also occur via gamma-carboxyglutamic acid residues. It is important to note that platelet activation is not required to bind the Factor Va–Factor Xa complex to the platelet surface, but it is essential for the binding of prothrombin to these cellular elements (67). The net effect of all of the above interactions leads to two separate sets of events. On the one hand, there is a significant local concentration of enzyme and substrate near to or on the platelet surface. On the other hand, there is evidence for a profound increase in the turnover rate of the bound Factor Va–Factor Xa enzyme as compared with free Factor Xa. The co-concentration of reagents and the elevated catalytic efficiency of the prothrombinase complex appear to be sufficient to account for the 300,000-fold acceleration in the rate of conversion of prothrombin to thrombin so that this process can take place in a matter of seconds (68).

To sum up, it is apparent that several critical events must take place if prothrombin is to be converted to thrombin on the platelet surface. Intially, Factor Va must bind tightly to a specific protein on the platelet membrane so that this complex can form the receptor needed for recruiting Factor Xa. This set of interactions is not greatly altered by platelet activation. Subsequently, prothrombin must be able to bind to the above enzyme complex in a configuration that permits the zymogen to be rapidly converted to thrombin. This latter process can be dramatically enhanced by the addition of platelet agonists. It would appear that the stimulatory effect is manifested by either an exposure of an accessory prothrombin binding site adjacent to the Factor Va / Factor Xa complex or by the mobilization of platelet-bound prothrombin so that the zymogen is made available to the prothrombinase complex. Thus, the rate of thrombin generation is tightly linked to the extent of platelet activation.

Kinetic Relationships Among the Cascades and the Common Pathway of Thrombin Generation

We have considered various control mechanisms that may operate within each of the three discrete elements of the coagulation mechanism. However, certain specific interactions among the intrinsic cascade, the extrinsic cascade, and the common pathway are also critical in modulating the action of this system.

The first intersystem control mechanism is based on the ability of thrombin to increase dramatically the potency of Factor VIII. Indeed, without prior thrombin activation, this protein is virtually unable to act as a cofactor in the Factor IXa–dependent conversion of Factor X to Factor Xa (69).

The second intersystem control mechanism depends on the capacity of the Factor VII–tissue factor complex to convert Factor IX to Factor IXa and subsequently Factor X to Factor Xa (70). This is accomplished at about half the rate of direct transformation of Factor X to Factor Xa under the conditions normally present in blood.

The third intersystem control mechanism involves the interaction between Factor Xa and Factor IX. Factor Xa can proteolyze Factor IX and convert it into a serine protease (71). The capacity of the extrinsic cascade to bypass the earliest phases of the intrinsic cascade may explain the minimal hemorrhagic complications noted in Factor XI deficiency.

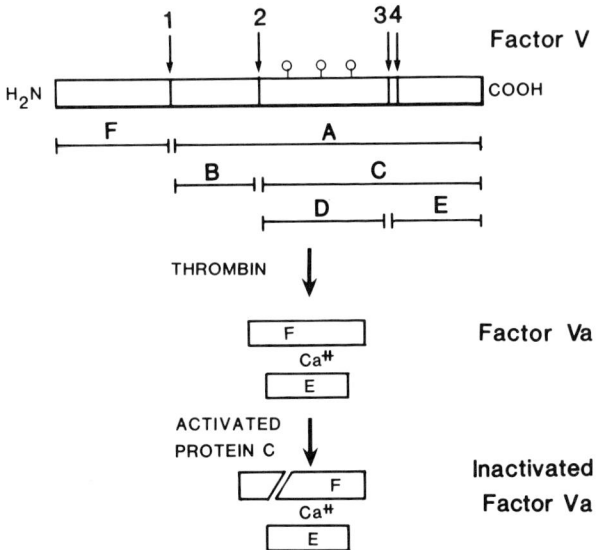

Figure 39–7. The activation of Factor V.

These three intersystem control mechanisms allow the extrinsic cascade to activate the more complex and slower-acting intrinsic cascade. This would permit the intrinsic cascade to produce additional thrombin.

The fourth intersystem control mechanism depends on the proteolysis of Factor VII by Factor XIIa. This results in the production of a disulfide-linked two-chain form of Factor VII with increased affinity for tissue factor and an enhanced potency as an activator of Factor X. Thus, activation of the intrinsic cascade can augment the thrombin-generating ability of the extrinsic cascade.

The existence of these multiple intersystem control mechanisms indicates that the three major elements of the coagulation mechanism are linked in a complex kinetic fashion. These interactions appear to be essential for the generation of adequate amounts of thrombin under in vivo conditions. This surmise is supported by the clinical observation that patients with an isolated congenital defect in either cascade may exhibit profound bleeding diatheses.

The Protein C–Thrombomodulin Mechanism

The protein C–thrombomodulin mechanism also appears to be critically involved in regulating the activity of the intrinsic cascade and the common pathway of thrombin generation (Fig. 39–8). Protein C is a vitamin K–dependent glycoprotein that consists of a heavy chain of 41,000 daltons and a light chain of 21,000 daltons, the two chains being joined by a single disulfide bridge (72a, 72b). In order to perform its biologic function, protein C must be converted to the serine protease protein Ca. This process involves the scissioning of a single Arg^{12}-Leu^{13} bond at the amino-terminal end of the heavy chain of the zymogen, with release of an activation peptide of molecular weight ~1400. Both protein C and protein Ca possess gamma-carboxyglutamic acid residues, located in their light chains, which are required for the binding of either protein to calcium ions and cell membranes. Thrombin is the only physiologically relevant serine protease that can convert protein C to protein Ca. The rate of this reaction is quite slow when blood is allowed to clot under in vitro conditions. This observation raised a serious question about the biologic role of protein C within the human body. However, it has been possible to demonstrate that perfusion of protein C and thrombin through the vascular tree of animals resulted in a 20,000-fold increase in the rate of conversion of zymogen to serine protease (73). Given that this process could be saturated with either excess protein C or thrombin, it seemed likely that a receptor was present on the endothelium that could dramatically accelerate the reaction.

This hypothesis was substantiated by isolating the putative receptor—a protein of molecular weight ~74,000—from rabbit lungs (74). The addition of thrombin to this receptor, termed thrombomodulin, leads to the formation of a 1:1 stoichiometric complex of enzyme and cofactor that is able to rapidly activate protein C in the presence of calcium ions. It should be noted that thrombin attached to thrombomodulin can be neutralized by antithrombin at a rate equivalent to that of free enzyme (see below). However, the thrombin-thrombomodulin complex exhibits a diminished ability to clot fibrinogen, to activate Factor V, or to trigger platelet activation.

Once evolved, protein Ca is known to function as a potent inhibitor of the Cofactors V–Va and VIII–VIIIa (75a, 75b). Its first site of action is located at the surface of the platelet, where Factor V–Va bound to specific sites on these cellular elements acts as a receptor for Factor Xa. This multimolecular prothrombinase complex is able to rapidly convert prothrombin to thrombin. Protein Ca functions as a naturally occurring anticoagulant

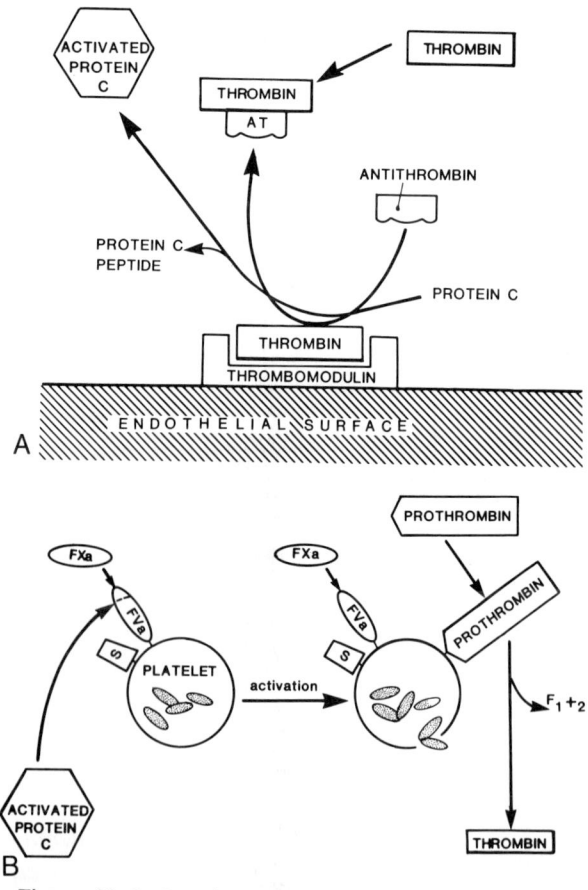

Figure 39–8. Protein C–thrombomodulin mechanism. *A*, The activation of protein C and its inhibition by protein C inactivator. *B*, The action of activated protein C on Factor Va.

by specifically scissioning the heavy chain of Factor V or Factor Va, which is required for the binding of prothrombin to the surface of the platelet. Factor Va seems to be particularly sensitive to destruction by protein Ca, especially under in vivo conditions, in which the levels of this enzyme are exceedingly low. Thus, protein Ca possesses the requisite specificity to prevent assembly of the prothrombinase complex, and it thereby suppresses the production of thrombin. This inhibitory effect of protein Ca appears to be modulated by a variety of additional interactions. On the one hand, a slow rate of cleavage of Factor V–Va will allow Factor Xa to bind to the unaffected cofactor and thereby protect this protein against any subsequent action of protein Ca. On the other hand, various plasma proteins appear to be involved in the protein Ca–dependent destruction of Factor V–Va on the platelet surface. For example, protein S is able to enhance the binding of protein Ca to phospholipid-containing membranes and to accelerate the cleavage of Factor Va by this serine protease (76a). The complement component, C4b binding protein, is known to complex with protein S and may be involved in regulating the function of the latter protein (76b). Thus, it seems likely that a variety of interactions are responsible for determining the rate of translocation of protein Ca from its site of production on the endothelium to the surface of the platelet. Of course, one might expect that small amounts of protein Ca remain bound to the endothelial cell surface via gamma-carboxyglutamic acid residues on this serine protease. In this manner, protein Ca could also regulate the Factor Va–dependent thrombin generation that is known to occur on the endothelial cell surface in a fashion analogous to that described for the platelet membrane.

The second site of action of protein Ca occurs at a locale where Factor VIIIa regulates the interaction between Factors IXa and X. At the present time, little is known concerning the biochemical details of the protein Ca–dependent cleavage of this cofactor or of the biologic surface where these events take place. However, recent studies would suggest that a specific binding site for Factor IXa, VIIIa, and X exists on the endothelium (39a). If this supposition is correct, protein Ca could be involved in limiting the generation of Factor Xa at the endothelial surface and thereby preventing the production of thrombin at either the endothelial locale or perhaps on the platelet surface itself.

Clinical observations indicate that the protein C–thrombomodulin mechanism functions under in vivo conditions to suppress hemostatic system activity. Several families have been described with congenital reductions of about 50 per cent in the antigenic levels of protein C; members of these families exhibit repeated thrombotic episodes (76c,d,e). It is of interest to note that other kindreds have been reported in which individuals who are heterozygous for protein C deficiency have minimal symptoms whereas those who are homozygous for this trait die in infancy with massive venous thrombosis and purpura fulminans (76e). These data suggest that other factors—such as the density of thrombomodulin on the endothelium, the levels of protein S within the blood, and the amounts of Factor V–Va present on the platelet surface — are likely to modulate the effects of protein C deficiency. Indeed, several families have recently been investigated in whom inherited reductions in the concentrations of protein S appear to be related to the development of thrombotic events (76g).

FORMATION OF THE FIBRIN CLOT

Fibrinogen is a protein of molecular weight 340,000 daltons that is present in plasma at a concentration of about 3 mg per ml (77). It is composed of three pairs of polypeptide chains, designated α, β, and γ of molecular weights 64,000 daltons, 56,000 daltons, and 47,000 daltons, respectively (78). The six chains are held together by 29 disulfide bridges, with the N-terminal regions of all polypeptides maintained in a rigid symmetrical configuration at one end of the molecule (79) (Fig. 39–9A). This area is referred to as the N-terminal disulfide knot (N-DSK) and is part of a larger nodular structure termed the E domain that is made up of the six intertwined polypeptide chains. These chains emerge from this region to form two lateral bundles, each containing single α, β, and γ polypeptides. Subsequently, the bundles intertwine to form two nodular structures termed D domains. The carboxy terminal regions of the α and γ chains are in a particularly exposed position within the D domains and represent sites for fibrin-fibrin interactions (80).

Once thrombin is evolved, it attacks the two sets of α and β chains within the N-DSK region and thereby converts fibrinogen to fibrin (81) (Fig. 39–9A). Initially, the enzyme cleaves the Arg_{16}-Gly_{17} bond in the two α chains and releases a pair of acidic polypeptides (fibrinopeptide A) (82). Thrombin must have a particularly high affinity for structures in the α chain to account for the observed rapid release of fibrinopeptide A. This specificity is dependent upon a fairly limited amino acid sequence associated with the cleaved bond. Indeed, all the elements needed for recognition by thrombin are contained within the first 51 residues of the α chain (83). After a lag phase, a second scission of the Arg_{14}-Gly_{15} bond in the two β chains becomes apparent, and a second set of acidic polypeptides (fibrinopeptide B) is liberated (84). Release of fibrinopeptide A induces a conformational change within the fibrin molecule that makes the Arg_{14}-Gly_{15} bond in the Bβ chains accessible to the action of thrombin.

The liberation of fibrinopeptide A from fibrinogen initiates fibrin polymerization. Snake venoms, such as reptilase, release only fibrinopeptide A from fibrinogen but are still capable of generating a fibrin clot (85). This venom has been utilized to assay fibrinogen in the presence of heparin since it cannot be rapidly neutralized by the mucopolysaccharide-antithrombin complex. Fibrinopeptide B release is also of some importance in promoting fibrin polymerization, and its liberation is thought to favor a more compact clot structure (86). Sensitive radioimmunoassays for both types of fibrinopeptides are gradually coming into clinical use (87). These two species may represent important markers for thrombotic phenomena.

Release of these fibrinopeptides unmasks a specific set of sites within the E domain. This transformation permits the E domain to interact with the D domains of other molecules of fibrin or fibrinogen (Fig. 39–9B). Two options are available once fibrin has been generated. On the one hand, it may bind to fibrinogen and form soluble fibrin–fibrinogen complexes (SFC). Patients with hyperactive coagulation systems may exhibit elevated levels of SFC as quantitated by a variety of assays. These include methods based upon (a) immunologic identification of soluble fibrinogen-like material at molecular weights that are multiples of 340,000, (b) the discharge of fibrin from SFC by the addition of protamine sulfate or ethanol, or (c) cryoprecipitation with resultant polymerization of this protein into fine strands (88, 89). Unfortunately, these procedures are variable and not entirely satisfactory for the detection of disseminated intravascular coagulation or thrombotic phenomena. On the other hand, interactions may occur between fibrin molecules. The resultant polymers may gradually grow in size and become insoluble. This fibrin meshwork is held together by hydrophobic as well as electrostatic interactions between D and E domains (90) (Fig. 39–9B). This staggered array of fibrin polymers can easily be disrupted by the addition of agents such as urea or monochloracetic acid. In a subsequent step of the coagulation mechanism (to be discussed), covalent crosslinks are introduced between polymerized fibrin molecules, and the "vulcanized" clot structure is no longer susceptible to the action of these denaturants.

The covalent crosslinking of loosely associated fibrin polymers is attained by a transpeptidation reaction catalyzed by Factor XIIIa. The precursor of this enzyme, Factor XIII, is found in plasma at a concentration of about 6 μg per ml or on platelet surfaces (91). Plasma Factor XIII is a tetramer composed of two pairs of identical subunits termed "a" and "b" of molecular weights 75,000 daltons and 80,000 daltons, respectively. Platelet Factor XIII is a dimer containing two "a" subunits (92). When thrombin is formed, it hydrolyzes the Arg_{36}-Gly_{37} bond within the N-terminal region of the "a" chains of both forms of Factor XIII and liberates a pair of polypeptides of molecular weight approximately 4500 daltons (93). In the presence of calcium ions, the thrombin-activated subunits termed "a^1" undergo a conformational alteration that permits them to dissociate from "b" subunits, if present. This transition also induces the exposure of a single SH group per two "a^1" subunits, which constitutes the active center of the enzyme ("half of sites reactivity") (94). Thus, a calcium-induced form of the "a^1" dimer represents Factor XIIIa. The "b" subunits present in plasma zymogen are thought to be important for secretion of the protein at its site of synthesis and for prolonged survival of this component within the circulation.

Once Factor XIIIa is generated, it binds to fibrin molecules and covalently joins the side chains of specific lysyl donor sites with the side chains of specific glutamyl acceptor regions. It is thought that four to six such ε-(γ-glutamyl) lysine bonds are formed between sets of fibrin monomers (95). The critical areas crosslinked are within the C-terminal region of the α and γ chains in the D domains of these molecules (96). Initially, these bonds are formed between pairs of γ chains, and, subsequently, cross-links are placed between multiple sets of α chains (97). These areas are brought into close proximity during fibrin polymerization. It is of considerable interest that these regions are relatively inaccessible to Factor XIIIa unless fibrinogen is converted to fibrin. Thus, as shown in Figure 39–10, thrombin must convert fibrinogen to fibrin as well as activate Factor XIII if a stable clot is to be formed. This crosslinked structure is mechanically stronger and better able to withstand the brunt of collisional events within the vascular system. It is also more slowly dissolved by the fibrinolytic mechanism. The physiologic importance of fibrin cross-linking is emphasized by the occurrence of bleeding disorders in patients with defects in this process (98).

THE FIBRINOLYTIC MECHANISM

The fibrinolytic mechanism is primarily responsible for the dissolution of fibrin deposited on the vascular endothelium. A pivotal component of this mechanism is the zymogen plasminogen. This molecular species is present in plasma at a concentration of about 200 μg per ml and exhibits a molecular weight of approximately 81,000 daltons (99). A schematic representation of the structure of plasminogen is provided in Figure 39–11. A major section of the N-terminal region of this protein is composed of a series of five triple loop structures

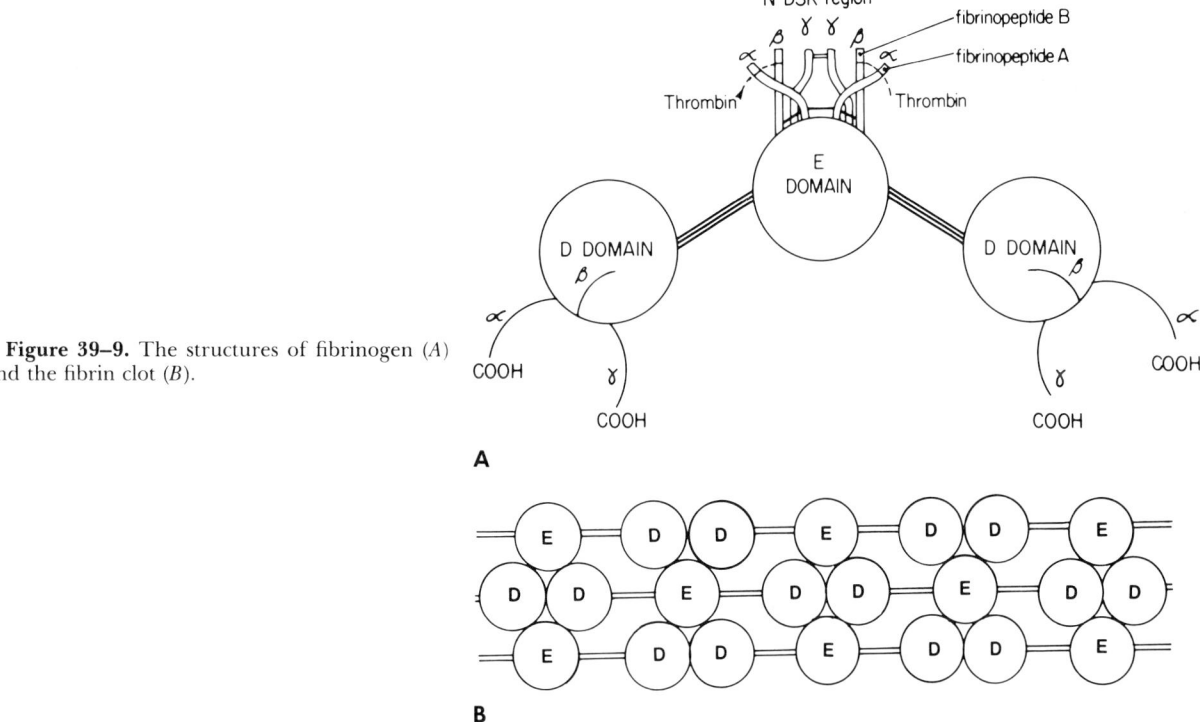

Figure 39–9. The structures of fibrinogen (A) and the fibrin clot (B).

termed kringles that are homologous to those found on the nonthrombin portion of prothrombin (see earlier section) (100). These unique features appear to represent specific binding sites on plasminogen that permit this zymogen to interact with the fibrin meshwork and become concentrated within this locale (101). Furthermore, antifibrinolytic amino acids such as ϵ-aminocaproic acid bind to these areas of plasminogen. This interaction causes a marked conformational alteration in plasminogen that significantly limits the ability of this zymogen to be converted to active enzyme. This alteration is most probably due to the dissociation of noncovalent interactions between a specific site on the preactivation peptide (to be discussed) and one of the kringle structures (102).

The central event in the fibrinolytic system is the transformation of the single-chain plasminogen to the enzymatically potent two-chain serine protease plasmin. This conversion is accomplished by scission of the zymogen at the Arg_{360}-Val_{561} bond as depicted in Figure 39–11 (103). The initial generation of plasmin frequently permits this enzyme to act upon plasminogen and induce several additional proteolytic cleavages within the zymogen at Lys_{77}-Lys_{78}, Arg_{68}-Met_{69}, and so forth prior to its activation. These auxiliary scissions result in the release of a fragment of approximate molecular weight 10,000 daltons that has been termed the preactivation peptide. However, this series of additional bond cleavages takes place to a minimal extent when plasminogen is converted to plasmin in the presence of protease inhibitors such as

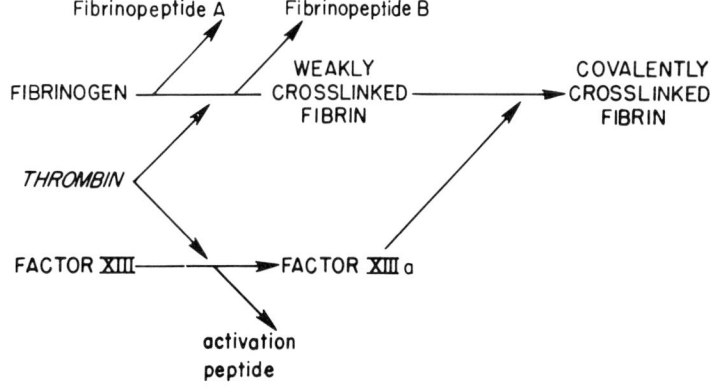

Figure 39–10. The formation of the crosslinked fibrin clot.

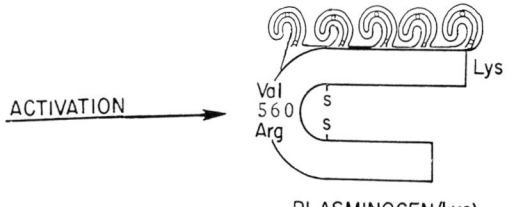

Figure 39–11. The structure of plasminogen and its mechanism of activation.

antiplasmin or antithrombin (104). Thus, the physiologically relevant pathway of plasminogen to plasmin conversion probably requires only a scission of the Arg_{560}-Val_{561} bond. The serine protease generated by this process still possesses the five kringle structures. These binding sites are critical for the interaction of plasmin with its natural substrate fibrin as well as for the rapid neutralization of this enzyme by antiplasmin (to be discussed).

The activation of plasminogen can occur by either an intrinsic or an extrinsic pathway. The intrinsic activation process is dependent upon substances that are normally present in the blood but remains poorly defined as compared with the coagulation cascade. Plasminogen conversion, in part, appears to be dependent upon the direct or indirect action of Factor XIIa. Thus, events that trigger clot formation via activation of Factor XII simultaneously set in motion a mechanism for their ultimate resolution. It has also been reported that a plasminogen activation pathway independent of Factor XII exists and that this process is responsible for about 50 per cent of the intrinsic zymogen-converting potential of blood (105).

The extrinsic activation pathway is triggered by two major classes of serine proteases that are found in various tissues and organs. The first major class is composed of tissue-type plasminogen activator and urokinase, which are immunologically distinct and are synthesized by venous endothelium as well as in capillary endothelium (106). Lower levels of these components are also generated by similarly designated cells on the arterial side of the circulation. Tissue-type plasminogen activator exhibits a molecular weight of approximately 70,000, possesses a high affinity for fibrin (which it employs as a cofactor during the conversion of plasminogen to plasmin), and appears to be involved in the generation of the latter enzyme on fibrin polymers as well as within the interstices of the clot structure (106a). Urokinase exhibits a molecular weight of about 54,000, transforms plasminogen to plasmin in the absence of a cofactor, and may be responsible for the continuous fluid phase generation of the latter enzyme (106b).

Thrombin has been reported to bind to endothelial cells and to inhibit the synthesis of urokinase as well as stimulate the production of tissue-type plasminogen activator (106 c,d). Both plasminogen activators are readily released into the blood by physiologic stimuli such as exercise, epinephrine, or bradykinin (107,108), as well as by pharmacologic components such as hypoglycemic drugs (sulfonylureas or biguanides), vasodilators (nicotinic acid or aminophylline), diuretics (furosemide) (109, 110) or semi-specific effector agents such as DDAVP, and pathologic stimuli such as hypotensive shock or infection. It appears highly likely that both tissue-type plasminogen activator and urokinase are partially responsible for keeping the microcirculation open and free of fibrin deposits.

Highly purified preparations of urokinase are commercially available and have been employed in the treatment of pulmonary emboli and coronary thrombosis, as well as other thrombotic disorders (111, 112). This product appears to have some advantage with respect to immunogenicity and reproducibility of action when compared with the previously used preparations of streptokinase. This latter protein is isolated from cultures of beta-hemolytic streptococci and has a molecular weight of 48,000 daltons. It is able to form a 1:1 complex with plasminogen that can subsequently activate large amounts of free uncomplexed zymogen (113). The use of tissue-type plasminogen activator has recently been advocated in the place of urokinase or streptokinase, since the former macromolecule could be infused into a peripheral vein and would be expected to specifically dissolve fibrin clots, but should not induce a systemic fibrinolytic state with potential hemorrhagic consequences (see below). The cloning of the tissue-type plasminogen activator gene is likely to make this form of therapy a practical reality within the next few years (113a,b).

The second major group of extrinsic plasminogen activators are located within a variety of organs such as the lungs, heart, adrenal glands, lymph nodes, and ovaries. These substances are relatively insoluble and can be extracted only with difficulty. However, several have been purified to near homogeneity (114). Current evidence suggests that these components are serine proteases with trypsin-like specificities and a narrowly restricted proteolytic activity directed toward plasminogen. The relationship between the activators described previously and related substances found within the lysosomal fractions of cells of numerous tissues is not yet fully understood. It is thought that this group of components has little physiologic significance with respect to plasminogen activation. However, these activators can be released into the blood at times of extensive organ damage and may be responsible for the frequent occurrence of systemic fibrinolysis in patients with widespread trauma.

Under normal conditions, fibrinolysis is a carefully regulated process (115). It is initiated by the incorporation of plasminogen within the fibrin clot as these polymers are deposited onto the vascular endothelium. This is due to the specific interaction of the kringle structures of the zymogen with the fibrin meshwork. In this locus, plasminogen is sequestered away from protease inhibitors normally present in the blood and in direct proximity to the fibrin substrate. Diffusion of plasminogen activators from the blood or endothelium into the clot transforms the zymogen into plasmin. The resultant enzyme remains bound to its substrate by interaction of the kringle structures with the fibrin strands and therefore can only be slowly neutralized by antiplasmin (to be discussed). In this manner, a gradual but effective lysis of the clot occurs. Leukocytes incorporated into the clot also elaborate proteases that may directly hydrolyze the fibrin meshwork (116). Outside the area of the clot, activators of the fibrinolytic system are relatively impotent. This is due, in large measure, to the presence of antiplasmin, which can rapidly neutralize plasmin as it is formed. Thus, fibrinolytic activity is restricted to the region of the resolving clot. However, in disease states excessive release of activators occurs, and large amounts of plasmin are generated. This gradually overwhelms the capacity of antiplasmin to limit the fibrinolytic process, and free enzyme, as well as plasmin-α_2-macroglobulin complexes, is found within the circulation. These two entities induce systemic fibrinolysis with proteolysis as well as inactivation of proteins such as Factor V, Factor VIII, and fibrinogen (117).

The degradation of the fibrinogen molecule by plasmin has been extensively investigated (118–120). This process has proved to be of considerable interest since the cleaved fibrinogen species induce the hemorrhagic phenomena observed in disseminated intravascular coagulation and represent the basis for a variety of tests utilized in detecting systemic fibrinolysis. Figure 39–12 depicts the sequential proteolysis of the fibrinogen molecule. In the first step of this pathway, exposed C-terminal regions of the α chains of fibrinogen within the D domains are cleaved. The N-terminal segments of the α chains containing fibrinopeptide A sites remain intact. Simultaneously, but at a slower rate, the N-terminal of the β chains are scissioned and a fragment containing fibrinopeptide B is released. This family of degradation components of approximate molecular weight 250,000 daltons has been termed fragment X. The limited degree of proteolysis exhibited by these molecular species appears to occur continuously in normal individuals, since about 25 per cent of the circulating fibrinogen molecules are in this form. In the

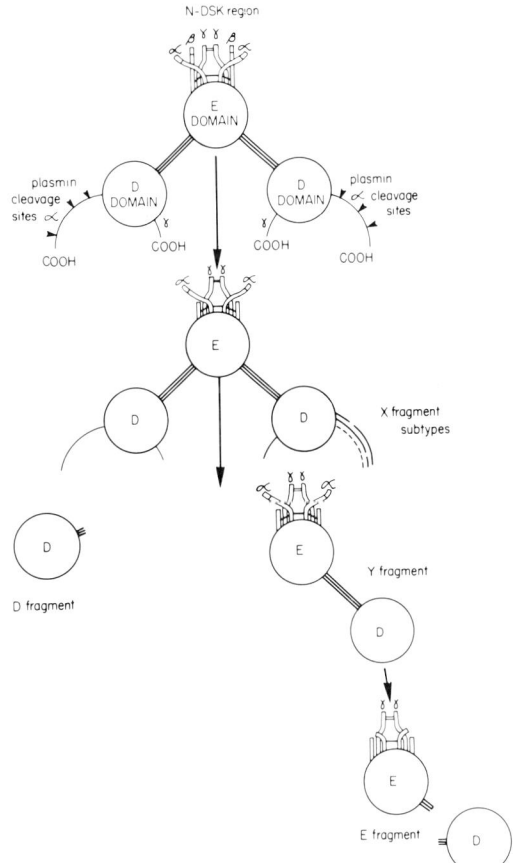

Figure 39–12. Degradation of fibrinogen.

second step of this process, plasmin cleaves one of the two polypeptide bundles that connect the D and E domains, with liberation of the D domain fragment of approximate molecular weight 100,000 daltons and a binodular structure termed fragment Y of approximate molecular weight 155,000 daltons. This latter component still contains both fibrinopeptide A sites in its N-terminal region. In the third step of the degradation, plasmin is able to clip the second of the two bundles connecting the D and E domains within fragment Y and liberate the nodules as individual species termed fragments D and E. During or immediately after this event, fragment E loses some of its fibrinopeptide A sites. Further degradation proceeds more slowly and results in the trimming of these latter fragments to a somewhat smaller molecular size.

The products obtained by plasmin degradation of fibrin clots are slightly different from those just described. In most instances, the earliest components are fragments of fibrin polymers, and their sizes are considerably larger than those of fibrinogen. At a later point in the degradation process, species similar to fragments Y, D, and E but without fibrinopeptide sites have been isolated. If the fibrin clots have been extensively crosslinked by Factor XIIIa, the D fragments obtained are dimeric in structure (121).

The various products of fibrinogen degradation have characteristic biologic properties. Fragment X can be converted by thrombin to form fibrin. However, this process takes place at a much slower rate than with normal fibrinogen. Fragments Y, D, and E cannot be clotted by thrombin. Indeed, the transformation of fibrinogen to fibrin as well as the subsequent polymerization of the latter species is slowed by these fragments. This phenomena is due to the ability of these components to competitively inhibit the action of thrombin on fibrinogen as well as their capacity to form a soluble complex with fibrin polymers (122). High concentrations of these degradation products can also inhibit platelet adhesion, aggregation, and release (123). The pathophysiologic significance of these latter findings remains in question. It has been suggested that a part of their effort may be due to the contamination of fibrinogen degradation products with plasmin-digested von Willebrand's factor (124). Various other biologic actions have been ascribed to the fragments X, Y, D, and E, including potentiation of the hypotensive effect of bradykinin (125), chemotactic properties with respect to monocytes as well as neutrophils (126), and an ability to impair the immunologic mechanism (127).

Several investigators have reported families with congenital abnormalities of the fibrinolytic mechanism who exhibit multiple episodes of venous thromboembolic disease. These have included functional defects in the plasminogen molecule (127a) and reductions in the release of plasminogen activator (127b), as well as alterations in the structure of fibrinogen (127c). It has been tacitly assumed that thrombotic phenomena observed in these patients are due to their reduced ability to lyse small fibrin clots and prevent extension. More recently, it has been suggested that plasmin may serve as a natural anticoagulant within the hemostatic mechanism and that the defects outlined above may also occur at an earlier stage in the coagulation system.

It is widely appreciated that thrombin is able to cleave a set of Arg_{16}-Gly_{17} bonds within the A-alpha chains of fibrinogen with release fibrinopeptide A and concomitant conversion of this macromolecule to fibrin I monomer. Subsequently, thrombin can scission a second set of Arg_{14}-Gly_{15} bonds within the B-beta chains of fibrin I monomer with liberation of fibrinopeptide B and concomitant generation of fibrin II monomer, which is capable of rapidly polymerizing to form a thrombus. Plasmin is also known to proteolyze a set of Arg_{42}-Ala_{43} bonds within the B-beta chains of fibrin I, releasing B-beta 1–42 and thereby converting fibrin I monomer to fragment X, which is further degraded to form soluble cleavage products (see above).

Several investigators have used radioimmunoassays for fibrinopeptide A, fibrinopeptide B, and B-beta 1–42 to investigate the pathophysiology of intravascular coagulation and venous thrombosis (127d). These physicians have examined patients receiving hypertonic saline to terminate pregnancy and have shown that immediately after intrauterine infusion, fibrin I monomer was generated by thrombin-mediated proteolysis of fibrinogen. Thereafter, fibrin I monomer was either cleaved by thrombin to liberate fibrinopeptide B or proteolyzed by plasmin to release B-beta 1–42. These data suggest that the relative rates at which thrombin and plasmin scission the B-beta chain of fibrin I monomer could determine the occurrence of thrombosis (127e). These techniques have been applied to study naturally occurring venous thrombosis. The results obtained indicate that individuals who developed thrombi, when compared with those who do not suffer from this complication, exhibited levels of fibrinopeptide A that were considerably greater than the concentration of B-beta 1–42 during the 4 days preceding the onset of this disorder (127f). These observations lend credence to the hypothesis that a sustained imbalance between the procoagulant effects of thrombin and the anticoagulant actions of plasmin upon fibrin I monomer may lead to the development of thrombotic disorders in humans (127f). The precise molecular defects responsible for these phenomena are currently unknown but most likely include abnormalities in the regulatory mechanisms that govern the release of plasminogen activators or their inhibitors from cellular sites.

LIMITING REACTIONS

As previously described, the hemostatic mechanism consists of a series of linked proteolytic reactions that sequentially generate a variety of serine proteases. The kinin-forming and complement mechanisms operate in similar fashion. When these three systems are activated at sites of injury, it is essential to localize their actions in order to avoid propagation of their effects throughout the vascular system. If protective mechanisms did not exist, minimal endothelial damage might lead to widespread thrombosis, systemic fibrinolysis, and profound changes in vascular permeability.

Diverse controls have been developed to prevent such an explosive outcome. These include the dilution of activated components by the rapid flow of blood, the clearance of circulating serine proteases by the hepatic system (128), and the physical localization of enzyme generation because of the sequential formation of multimolecular complexes. Of greater importance is a family of discrete plasma proteins that are able to directly inhibit various activated components of the coagulation, fibrinolytic, and kinin-generating systems. These include antithrombin (antithrombin III), antiplasmin (α_2-plasmin inhibitor). α_2-macroglobulin, Protein C inhibitor, plasminogen activator inhibitor, α_1-antitrypsin, and C1 inactivator. Inherited deficiencies of four of these proteins are known to result in human disease: (a) antithrombin deficiency is found in patients with severe thrombotic disease (129); (b) antiplasmin deficiency has been observed in a family with a bleeding diathesis, presumably secondary to unrestricted local fibrinolysis (130); (c) C1 inactivator deficiency is associated with hereditary angioneurotic edema; and (d) α_1-antitrypsin deficiency is present in patients with severe emphysema and liver disease. Inherited deficiencies of the other protease inhibitors are not strongly correlated with overt clinical disorders.

Based upon the pathophysiologic consequences of inherited deficiencies as well as a variety of biochemical data, it has become apparent that antithrombin, antiplasmin, and α_2-macroglobulin constitute critical modulators of the hemostatic mechanism. The structure and function of these three components will be discussed in considerable detail in the following sections. Protein C inhibitor as well as plasminogen activator inhibitor are also probably of physiologic importance to the regulation of the hemostatic system and will be briefly considered. The remaining plasma proteins—α_1-antitrypsin and C1 inactivator—are of greater importance in the inhibition of complement, kinin-generating, and leukocyte-derived serine proteases and will not be discussed further.

Antithrombin

The major inhibitor of the coagulation cascade is antithrombin. This molecular species is present in plasma at a concentration of 150 μg per ml (131). It exhibits a molecular weight of approximately 56,000 daltons and is also the essential cofactor for the action of heparin (132). The latter substance is a naturally occurring sulfated mucopolysaccharide of molecular weight 5000 to 50,000 daltons that is employed clinically as an anticoagulant. This polymer is composed of alternating residues of hexosamine and hexuronic acid. The hexosamine residues are glucosamines that may be N-sulfated, N-acetylated, or ester-sulfated. Alternatively, they may have no substituents at one or more of these positions. The hexuronic acid residues can be glucuronic acid, iduronic acid, or ester-sulfated iduronic acid (133). Thus, a great variety of possible hexosamine-uronic acid sequences may exist within a given heparin molecule.

It is known that the monosaccharide sequence iduronic acid — N-sulfate or N-acetyl glucosamine 6-O-sulfate—glucuronic acid—N-sulfated glucosamine 3,6-O-sulfate—iduronic acid 2-O-sulfate—N-sulfated glucosamine 3-O-6-O-sulfate represents the major antithrombin binding site on heparin (134a–d). Heparin has been isolated from a variety of organs and is also found in mast cells (135). Heparin-like species with the essential sequence of monosaccharides required to bind to antithrombin and accelerate hemostatic enzyme–protease inhibitor complex formation have recently been shown to be synthesized by endothelial cells of the macrovascular and microvascular system (135a–c). Furthermore, these components have been located on the luminal surface of the vascular tree, where they can modulate the function of the antithrombin and thereby regulate the activity of the hemostatic mechanism (136, 136a) (see below).

In the absence of heparin, antithrombin neutralizes the activity of thrombin by slowly forming a 1:1 complex of enzyme and inhibitor (137). In the presence of the sulfated mucopolysaccharide, the rate of complex formation is increased 2000- to 10,000-fold and neutralization of thrombin is virtually instantaneous. Formation of an enzyme-inhibitor complex in the presence and absence of heparin is dependent on the active serine center of thrombin. If this residue is blocked, interaction between thrombin and antithrombin is inhibited. The reactive site of the inhibitor, which binds the active serine center of thrombin, contains an arginine residue. Modification of this group on antithrombin virtually eliminates the ability of the protein to inhibit thrombin in the presence or absence of heparin (137).

In view of the highly acidic nature of heparin, one would expect that positive groups on antithrombin (e.g., ϵ-aminolysyl residues) form the binding site for this negatively charged anticoagulant. Chemical alteration of these residues prevents binding of heparin to this protein and suppresses the acceleration of inhibitor action by the anticoagulant. However, the slow, progressive neutralization of thrombin by antithrombin is not appreciably affected (138).

Furthermore, it has been demonstrated that heparin functions as a catalyst in this reaction. Relatively small amounts of this mucopolysaccharide are able to dramatically accelerate the interaction of considerably larger amounts of thrombin and antithrombin. This occurs because of the displacement of heparin from antithrombin during formation of the thrombin-antithrombin complex. Thus, the mucopolysaccharide is available to bind to free inhibitor and cyclically promote subsequent rounds of interactions (139).

In summary, antithrombin neutralizes the activity of thrombin by complex formation via a reac-

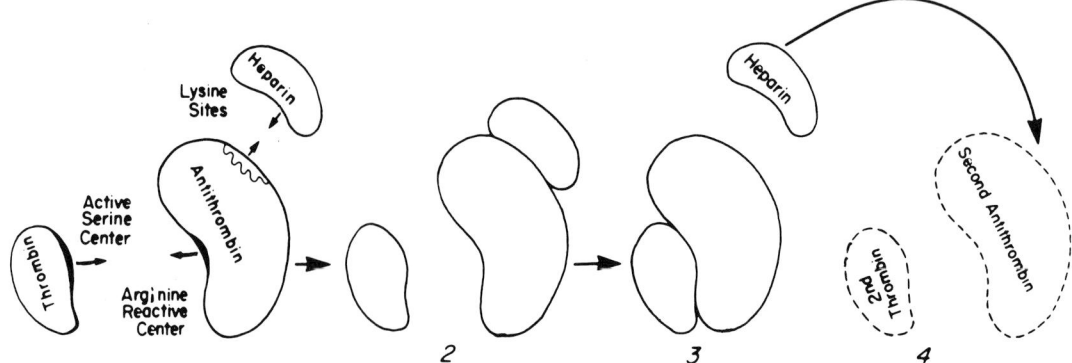

Figure 39–13. The mechanism of heparin action.

tive site (arginine)–active center (serine) interaction. If small amounts of heparin are added to the system, it preferentially binds to the lysyl residues on antithrombin. The resulting heparin-antithrombin complex rapidly inactivates thrombin. This most probably is due to a heparin-dependent conformational alteration of the inhibitor, which renders the reactive site arginine more accessible to the active serine center of thrombin. Once thrombin-antithrombin complex formation has occurred, heparin is released and is again available for binding to free inhibitor. Thus, the mucopolysaccharide is capable of catalyzing numerous subsequent rounds of thrombin–antithrombin complex formation (Fig. 39–13).

This mechanism of inhibitor action implies that antithrombin might neutralize all the serine proteases of the coagulation cascade and that heparin would accelerate each of these interactions. This hypothesis has been shown to be valid with respect to Factor IXa, Factor Xa, Factor XIa, and Factor XIIa (Fig. 39–14) (140–143). These heparin-dependent acceleratory interactions, with the possible exception of Factor XIIa, also take place in whole blood. The behavior of the remaining serine proteases of the hemostatic system—i.e., Factor VIIa and protein Ca—is anomalous with regard to the heparin-antithrombin system (144). The activities of these enzymes are not greatly affected by the protease inhibitor in the presence or absence of the mucopolysaccharide. Similarly designated enzymes generated in physiologic systems that are separate from but linked to the hemostatic mechanism (e.g., complement system, kallikrein system, and so forth) are only minimally affected by this inhibitory process.

The availability of heparin-like substances on endothelium would permit antithrombin to be selectively activated at blood-surface interfaces where enzymes of the hemostatic mechanism are generated. Thus, the plasma protease inhibitor would be critically placed to neutralize these enzymes and thereby protect natural surfaces against thrombus formation.

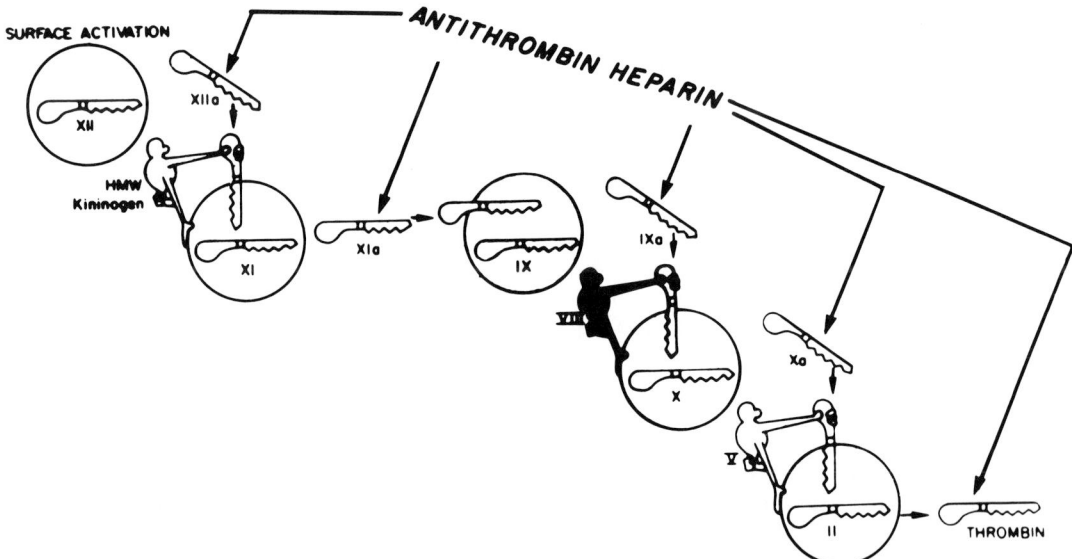

Figure 39–14. The site of action of antithrombin and heparin within the coagulation cascade.

Furthermore, the catalytic nature of heparin would ensure the continual regeneration of the nonthrombogenic properties of these natural surfaces. Once the antithrombin bound to platelet surface or vessel wall mucopolysaccharide has complexed with enzyme, the enzyme-inhibitor complex would be liberated into circulation. The heparin-like materal would again be available to recruit free antithrombin and thereby continually renew the ability of the surface to resist the attack of serine proteases of the hemostatic mechanism.

Antiplasmin

The principal inhibitor of the fibrinolytic mechanism is a plasma protein termed antiplasmin (145). Two forms of this component have been isolated that have slightly different physiochemical properties, but the biologic significance of this microheterogeneity remains unclear (146). Antiplasmin is normally present in the blood at a concentration of about 70 μg per ml and exhibits a molecular weight of approximately 67,000 daltons (147). Plasmin is rapidly neutralized by this plasma protein via formation of a 1:1 stoichiometric complex of enzyme and inhibitor (148). The mechanism appears to be similar to that discussed for the thrombin-antithrombin reaction and involves an interaction between the serine active center of plasmin and a reactive site on antiplasmin. However, accessory areas on the plasmin molecule such as the kringles are also critical for the rapid formation of enzyme-inhibitor complexes. The addition of low-molecular-weight ligands such as ε-aminocaproic acid that bind to the regions of plasmin can reduce the rapid rate of this interaction by 10- to 50-fold (149). Antiplasmin has also been observed to inactivate Factors XIa and XIIa, albeit at a relatively slow rate. Thus, this protease inhibitor may be partially involved in suppressing plasminogen-to-plasmin conversion as well as opposing the action of the enzyme when formed.

Sufficient levels of this protease inhibitor are normally present to inactivate half the plasmin that can theoretically be generated within the blood. Provided that this level of zymogen conversion is not exceeded in the fluid phase, plasmin neutralization is rapid, as well as complete, and systemic fibrinolysis is prevented. As previously noted, plasmin formed within the fibrin clot structure is sequestered from the action of protease inhibitors. This appears to be due to the interaction of the enzyme with the fibrin strands via its kringle structures. Under these conditions, plasmin can only be slowly neutralized by antiplasmin and is capable of gradually lysing the fibrin meshwork (see earlier discussion).

In pathologic states such as disseminated intravascular coagulation or during infusion of urokinase for therapeutic purposes, considerably more than half the circulating plasminogen may be converted to plasmin. Once the capacity of antiplasmin has been exceeded, excess proteolytic enzyme is bound to α_2-macroglobulin (150). Since a small percentage of the plasmin bound within this complex remains active, systemic fibrinolysis is able to take place. Thus, antiplasmin appears to be the major barrier against the action of the fibrinolytic system.

α_2-Macroglobulin

The proteolytic inhibitor α_2-macroglobulin is capable of neutralizing a wide variety of proteolytic enzymes such as plasmin, trypsin, thrombin, kallikrein, elastase, collagenase, cathepsins, and others (151). However, the rates of inactivation are relatively modest as compared with the other protease inhibitors. The α_2-macroglobulin is normally present in the blood at a concentration of about 2.5 mg per ml. However, its level in infants is approximately 2.5 times greater than the adult values just cited (152).

This plasma protein is composed of two equivalent half molecules of 360,000 daltons that are held together by noncovalent interactions. Each half molecule consists of two peptide chains of molecular weight 180,000 daltons that are linked by disulfide bridges (153). Current evidence suggests that the various endopeptidases are inactivated by formation of either 1:1 or 2:1 stoichiometric complexes of enzyme and inhibitor (154). The intial phase of this process most probably requires an interaction between the active center of the protease and a reactive site on α_2-macroglobulin. Thereafter, a complex alteration in the spacing of the four subunits that make up the protease is apparent (155).

This latter transition has two major consequences. First, enzyme molecules trapped within α_2-macroglobulin are able to function in a limited fashion as proteases (156). Indeed, if tested with small synthetic substrates, bound plasmin, trypsin, or kallikrein is almost fully active. However, if the physiologically relevant larger protein substrates are employed, only a small fraction of their activity is manifest (157). It is thought that the larger substrate molecules penetrate to the site of the bound enzyme with considerable difficulty. Second, the endopeptidases bound to the α_2-macroglobulin are protected against the action of other circulating protease inhibitors that would completely inactivate these enzymes (158). The enzyme–α_2-macroglobulin complexes are cleared by the reticuloendothelial system over the course of 15 to 30 minutes (159). It has been suggested that the primary in vivo function of this inhibitor is to preserve a portion of the biologic activity of bound enzyme within the circulatory system and to allow this bound enzyme to express its activity for a specified period of time in the presence of other plasma inhibitors. For example, plasmin bound to α_2-macroglobulin may play a critical role in the normal process of fibrinolysis whereas thrombin bound to this inhibitor may be important in activating small amounts of cofactors such as Factor V or Factor VIII. Thus, these sequestered enzymes may be capable of maintaining coagulation–fibrinolytic system activity at some basal level and thus of keeping the hemostatic system poised and ready for action.

New Protease Inhibitors of the Hemostatic System

Two new protease inhibitors of the hemostatic system have recently been described. The first of these macromolecules exhibits a molecular weight of about 57,000 and is able to slowly inactivate protein Ca generated within the blood (160). It is unclear whether alterations in the levels of this component can alter the function of the protein C–thrombomodulin mechanism. The second of these macromolecules exhibits a molecular weight of about 40,000, is produced by endothelial cells as well as platelets, and can rapidly neutralize the action of urokinase or tissue-type plasminogen activator (161). It has been suggested that congenital elevations in the latter protease inhibitor lead to thrombotic episodes in humans.

References

1. Wilner, G. D., Nossel, H. L., et al.: Activation of Hageman factor by collagen. J. Clin. Invest. 47:2608, 1968.
2. Zucker, M. D., and Borelli, J.: Platelet clumping produced by connective tissue suspensions and by collagen. Proc. Soc. Exp. Biol. Med. 109:779, 1962.
3. Mustard, J. F., and Packham, M. A.: Factors influencing platelet function. Pharmacol. Rev. 22:97, 1970.
4. Holmsen, H., and Day, H. L.: Thrombin-induced platelet release reaction and platelet lysosomes. Nature 219:760, 1968.
5. Rosenberg, R. D.: Biologic action of heparin. Semin. Hematol. 14:427, 1977.
6. Deykin, D., Cochios, F., et al.: Hepatic removal of activated factor X by the profused rabbit liver. Am. J. Physiol. 214:414, 1968.
7. Astrup, T.: Fibrinolysis in the organism. Blood 11:781, 1956.
8. Sherry, S., Alkjaersig, N., et al.: Fibrinolysis and fibrinolytic activity in man. Physiol. Rev. 39:343, 1959.
9. Neurath, H.: Limited proteolysis and zymogen activation. In *Proteases and Biologic Control*. Vol. 2, Reich, E., Rifkin, D. B., et al. (eds.), Cold Spring Harbor Conference on Cell Proliferation, 1975, pp. 51–64.
10. Walsh, K. A.: Unifying concepts among proteases. In *Proteases and Biologic Control*. Vol. 2. Reich, E., Rifkin, D. B., et al. (eds.), Cold Spring Harbor Conference on Cell Proliferation, 1975, pp. 1–12.
11. Huber, R., Kukla, D., et al.: Structure of the complex formed by bovine trypsin and bovine pancreatic trypsin inhibitor. *Proc. Vth Bayer Symposia V on Protease Inhibitors.* Fritz, H. (ed.), Berlin, Springer-Verlag, 1974, pp. 497–512.
12. Davie, E. W., and Ratnoff, O. D.: Waterfall sequence for intrinsic blood clotting. Science 145:1310, 1964.
13. McFarlane, R. G.: An enzyme cascade in the blood clotting mechanism and the function as a biochemical amplifier. Nature 202:498, 1964.
14. Magnusson, S.: Thrombin and prothrombin. In *The Enzymes*. Vol. 3. Boyer, P. D. (ed.), New York, Academic Press, 1970, p. 277.
15. Niewiarowski, S., Bankowski, E., et al.: Studies on the absorption and activation of Factor XII. Thromb. Diath. Haemorrh. 14:387, 1965.
16. Griffin, J. H., Harper, A., et al.: Studies on the activation of human blood coagulation Factor XII by soluble collagen. Fed. Proc. 34:860, 1975.
17. Revak, S. D., Cochrane, C. G., et al.: Structural changes accompanying enzymatic activation of Hageman Factor. J. Clin. Invest. 54:619, 1974.
18. Griffin, J. H., and Cochrane, C. G.: Human Factor XII. *Methods in Enzymology*. Lorand, L. (ed.). New York, Academic Press, 1976, pp. 56–65.
19. McMillan, C. R., Saito, H., et al.: The secondary structure of human factor XII and its alteration by activating agents. J. Clin. Invest. 54:1312, 1974.
20. Kaplan, A. P., and Austen, K. F.: A prealbumin activator of prekallikrein from active Hageman Factor by digestion with plasmin. J. Exp. Med. 133:672, 1971.
21. McConnel, D. J., and Mason, B.: The isolation of human plasma prekallikrein. Br. J. Pharmacol. 38:490, 1970.
22. Weupper, K. D., and Cochrane, C. G.: Isolation and mechanism of activation of components of the plasma kinin forming system. In *Biochemistry of the Acute Allergic Reactions. Second Int. Symp.* Austen, K. F., and Becker, E. L. (eds.), Oxford, Blackwell Scientific Publishers, 1971, pp. 299–320.
23. Mandel, R., Jr., Colman, R. W., et al.: Identification of prekallikrein and high molecular weight kininogen as a circulating complex in human plasma. PNAS 73:4179, 1976.
24. Mandell, R., and Kaplan, A. P.: Human plasma prekallikrein: Mechanism of activation by Hageman Factor and participation in Hageman Factor-dependent fibrinolysis. J. Biol. Chem. 252:6097, 1977.
25. Kaplan, A. P.: Initiation of the intrinsic coagulation and fibrinolytic pathways of man. In *Progress in Hemostasis and Thrombosis*. Vol. 4. Spaet, T. H. (ed.), New York, Grune and Stratton, 1978, pp. 127–175.
26. Kato, H., Han, H. Y., et al.: Isolation and characterization of the polypeptide fragments produced by plasma and tissue kallikreins. In *Kinins — Pharmacodynamics on Biological Roles*. Sicuteri, F., and Back, V. (eds.), New York, Plenum Press, 1975, pp. 135–150.
27. Gallin, J. I., and Kaplan, A. P.: Mononuclear cell chemotactic activity of kallikrein and plasminogen activator and its inhibition by Ci INH and α_2-macroglobulin. J. Immunol. 113:1928, 1974.
27a. Schapira, M., Despland, E., et al: Purified human plasma kallikrein aggregates human blood neutrophils. JCI 69:1199, 1982.
28. Weupper, K. D.: Biochemistry and biology of components of the plasma kinin-forming system. In *Inflammation: Mechanisms and Control*. Lepow, I. H., and Ward, P. A. (eds.), New York, Academic Press, 1972, pp. 93–117.
29. Thompson, R., Mandle, R., et al.: Interaction of Factor XI and kallikrein with high molecular weight kininogen. Thromb. Hemostatis. 38:13, 1977.
30. Kaode, T., Hermodson, M. A., et al.: Active site of bovine Factor XI. Nature 260:729, 1977.
31. Schiffman, S., and Lee, P.: Partial purification and characterization of contact activation cofactor. J. Clin. Invest. 56:1082, 1975.

32. Pechet, L.: Fibrinolysis. New Engl. J. Med. *273*:966, 1966.
33. Goldsmith, G., Saito, H., et al.: The activation of plasminogen by Hageman factor and Hageman factor fragments. Clin. Res. *25*:340, 1977.
34. Kaplan, A. P., Meier, H. L., et al.: Hageman factor and its substrates. In *Chemistry and Biology of the Kallikrein-Kinin System in Health and Disease*. Pisano, J. J., and Austen, K. F. (eds.), Fogarty International Center Proceedings. No. 27, Washington, D.C., U.S. Government Printing Office, 1974, pp. 237–254.
35. Meier, H. L., Pierce, F. V., et al.: Activation and functioning of human Hageman factor. J. Clin. Invest. *60*:18, 1977.
36. Ratnoff, O. E., and Davie, E. W.: The activation of factor IX by activated factor XI. Biochemistry *1*:677, 1962.
37. Thompson, A.: Personal communication.
38. Fujikawa, K., Coan, M. G., et al.: The mechanism of activation of bovine factor IX by bovine factor XIa. Biochemistry *13*:5290, 1974.
39. Bucher, D., and Thomsen, J.: Identification of α-carboxyglutamic acid residues in bovine factors IX and X and in a new vitamin K-dependent protein. FEBS Letters *68*:293, 1976.
39a. Stern, D. M., Nawroth, P. P., et al.: The binding of Factor IXa to cultured bovine aortic endothelial cells: induction of a specific site in the presence of Factors VIII and X. J. Biol. Chem. *260*:6717, 1985.
40. Magnusson, S., Peterson, T. E., et al.: Complete primary structures of prothrombin and regulation of prothrombin activation by thrombin. In *Proteases and Biologic Control*. Vol. 2. Reich, E., Rifkin, D. B., et al. (eds.), Cold Spring Harbor Conference on Cell Proliferation, 1975, pp. 123–149.
41. Osterud, B., and Rapaport, S. I.: Synthesis of intrinsic factor X activator. Biochemistry *9*:1854, 1975.
42. Fujikawa, K., Legaz, M. E., et al.: Bovine Factor X and Xa. Biochemistry *11*:4882, 1972.
43. Titani, K., Hermodson, M. A., et al.: Bovine Factor Xa. Biochemistry *11*:489, 1972.
44. Jesty, J., Spencer, A.K., et al.: The mechanism of activation of Factor X. J. Biol. Chem. *249*:5614, 1974.
45. Howard, J. B., and Nelsestuen, G. L.: Isolation and characterization of vitamin-K dependent region of bovine blood clotting Factor X. PNAS *72*:1281, 1975.
45a. Toole, J. J., Knopf, J. L., et al.: Molecular cloning of a cDNA encoding human antihaemophilic factor. Nature *212*:342, 1984.
45b. Vehar, G. A., Keyt, B., et al.: Structure of human factor VIII. Nature *312*:337, 1984.
46. Counts, R. B., Paskell, S. T., et al.: Disulfide bonds and the quaternary structure of Factor VIII, von Willebrand factor. J. Clin. Invest. *62*:702, 1978.
47. Sodetz, J. M., Pizzo, S. V., et al.: Relationship of sialic acid to function and in vivo survival of human Factor VIII/Von Willebrand's protein. J. Biol. Chem. *252*:5538, 1977.
48. Okumura, T., and Jamieson, G. A.: Platelet glycocalicin. Thromb. Res. 8701, 1976.
48a. Zimmerman, T. S., Abilgaard, C. L. F., et al.: Multiple molecular forms of Factor VIII-related antigen in normal plasma. Clin. Res. *24*:444A, 1976.
49. Ashwell, G., and Morell, A. G. The role of surface carbohydrates in the hepatic recognition and transport of circulating glycoproteins. Adv. Enz. Relat. Areas Mol. Biol. *41*:99, 1974.
50. Zimmerman, T. S., Ruggeri, Z. M., et al.: Factor VIII/Von Willebrand factor. In *Progress in Hematology*. Brown, E. B. (ed.), New York, Grune & Stratton, 1983, p. 279.
50a. Gralnick, H. R., Coller, B. S., et al.: Carbohydrate deficiency of the Factor VIII/Von Willebrand Factor protein in the Von Willebrand's disease variants. Science *192*:56, 1976.
51. Owen, C. A., Bowie, E. J. W., et al.: Generation of Factor VIII coagulant activity of isolated perfused neonatal pig livers and adult rat livers. Br. J. Haematol. *43*:307, 1979.
52. Nemerson, Y., and Pitlick, F. A.: The tissue factor pathway of blood coagulation. In *Progress in Hemostasis and Thrombosis*. Vol. l, Spaet, T. H. (ed.), New York, Grune & Stratton, 1972, p. l.
53. Maynard, J. R., Heckman, C. A., et al.: Assocation of tissue factor activity with the surface of cultured cells. J. Clin. Invest. *55*:814, 1975.
54. Osterud, B., Berre, A., et al.: Activation of the coagulation factor VII by tissue thromboplastin and calcium. Biochemistry *11*:2853, 1972.
55. Radcliffe, R. D., and Nemerson, Y.: Activation and control of factor VII by activated factor X and thrombin. J. Biol. Chem. *250*:388, 1975.
56. Fujikawa, K., Coan, M. H., et al.: A comparison of bovine prothrombin, Factor IX, and Factor X. PNAS *71*:427, 1974.
57. Osterud, B., and Schiffman, D.: Gel filtration properties of Factors II, VII, IX, IXa and X. Thromb. Diath. Haemorrh. *28*:317, 1972.
58. Suttie, J. W., and Jackson, C. M.: Prothrombin structure, activation and biosynthesis. Physiol. Rev. *57*:1, 1977.
59. Magnusson, S., Sottrup-Jensen, L., et al.: Homologous kringle structures common to plasminogen and prothrombin. In *Proteolysis and Physiological Regulation*. Ribbons, D. W., and Brew, K. (eds.), New York, Academic Press, 1976, p. 203.
60. Stenflo, J.: Vitamin K, prothrombin and γ-carboxyglutamic acid. New Engl. J. Med. *296*:624, 1977.
61. Stenflo, J., and Suttie, J. W.: Vitamin K dependent formation of γ-carboxyglutamic acid. Ann. Rev. Biochem. *46*:157, 1977.
62. Stenflo, J.: Vitamin K and the biosynthesis of prothrombin. J. Biol. Chem. *249*:5527, 1974.
63. Hemker, H. C., and Reekers, P. P. M.: Isolation and purification of proteins induced by vitamin K absence. Thromb. Diath. Haemorrh. *57*(Suppl.):83, 1974.
64. Stenn, K. A., and Blout, E. R.: Mechanism of bovine prothrombin activation by an insoluble preparation of bovine factor Xa. Biochemistry *11*:4502, 1972.
64a. Esmon, C. T., and Jackson, C. M.: The conversion of prothrombin to thrombin. J. Biol. Chem. *249*:7782, 1974.
64b. Nesheim, M. E., Myrmel, K. H., et al.: Isolation and characterization of single chain bovine Factor V. J. Biol. Chem. *254*:508, 1979.
64c. Kane, W. H., and Majerus, P. W.: Purification and characterization of human coagulation Factor V. J. Biol. Chem. *256*:1002, 1981.
65. Esmon, C. T.: The subunit structure of thrombin-activated Factor V. J. Biol. Chem. *254*:954, 1979.
65a. Suzuki, K., Dahlback, B., et al.: Thrombin catalyzed activation of human coagulation Factor V. J. Biol. Chem. *257*:6556, 1982.
66. Higgins, D. L., and Mann, K. G.: The interaction of bovine Factor V and Factor V–derived peptides with phospholipid vesicles. J. Biol. Chem. *258*:6503, 1983.
67. Nesheim, M. E., Eid, S., et al.: Assembly of the prothrombinase complex in the absence of prothrombin. J. Biol. Chem. *256*:9874, 1981.
68. Miletich, J. P., Jackson, C. M., et al.: Interaction of coagulation factor Xa with human platelets. Proc. Natl. Acad. Sci. USA *74*:4033, 1977.
69. Hultin, M. B., and Nemerson, Y.: Activation of Factor X by Factor Xa and Factor 8. Blood *52*:928, 1978.
70. Osterud, B., and Rapaport, S. I.: Activation of factor IX by the reaction product of factor VII and tissue factor. PNAS *74*:5260, 1977.
71. Kalousek, F., and Konigsberg, W., et al.: Activation of Factor IX by activated Factor X. FEBS Letters *50*:382, 1975.

72. Jackson, C. M., Esmon, C. T., et al.: Prothrombin activation. In *Protease and Biologic Control*. Vol. 2, Reich, E., Ritkin, D. B., et al. (eds.), Cold Spring Harbor Conference on Cell Proliferation, 1975, pp. 95–109.
72a. Kisiel, W.: Human plasma protein C: Isolation, characterization, and mechanism of activation by alpha-thrombin. J. Clin. Invest. *64*:761, 1979.
72b. Stenflo, J. and Fernlund, P.: Amino acid sequence of bovine protein C. J. Biol. Chem. *257*:12170, 1982.
73. Esmon, C. T., and Owen, H. G.: Identification of an endothelial cell cofactor for thrombin-catalyzed activation of protein C. Proc. Natl. Acad. Sci. USA *78*:2249, 1981.
74. Owen, W. G., and Esmon, C. T.: Functional properties of an endothelial cell cofactor for thrombin-catalyzed activation of protein C. J. Biol. Chem. *256*:5532, 1981.
75a. Walker, F. J., Sexton, P. W. et al.: The inhibition of blood coagulation by activated protein C through the selective inactivation of activated factor V. Biochem. Biophys. Acta *571*:333, 1979.
75b. Vehar, G. A., and Davie, E. W.: Preparation and properties of bovine factor VIII (antihemophilic factor). Biochemistry *19*:410, 1980.
76a. Walker, F. J.: Regulation of activated protein C by protein S: The role of phospholipid in factor Va inactivation. J. Biol. Chem. *256*:11128, 1981.
76b. Dahlback, B.: Purification of human vitamin K–dependent protein S and its limited proteolysis by thrombin. Biochem. J. *209*:837, 1983.
76c. Griffin, J. H., Evatt, B. et al.: Deficiency of protein C in congenital thrombotic disease. J. Clin. Invest. *68*:1370, 1981.
76d. Broekmans, A. W., Veltkamp, J. J., et al.: Congenital protein C deficiency and venous thromboembolism: a study of three Dutch families. New Engl. J. Med. *309*:340, 1983.
76e. Horellou, M. H., Samama, M., et al.: Protein C deficiency in 3 unrelated French patients with venous thrombosis. Thromb. Haemost. *50*:351, 1983 (Abstr.).
76f. Seligsohn, U., Berger, A., et al.: Homozygous protein C deficiency manifested by massive venous thrombosis in the newborn. New Engl. J. Med. *310*:559, 1984.
76g. Comp, P. C., Nixon, R. R., et al.: Familial protein S deficiency is associated with recurrent thrombosis. J. Clin. Invest. *24*:202, 1984.
76h. Schwarz, H. P., Fischer, M., et al.: Plasma protein S deficiency in familial thrombotic disease. Blood *65*:1297, 1984.
77. Wilner, G. D.: Molecular basis for measurement of circulating fibrinogen derivatives. In *Progress in Hemostasis and Thrombosis*. Vol. 4. Spaet, T. (ed.), New York, Grune and Stratton, 1978, pp. 211–248.
78. Blomback, B., and Blomback, M.: The molecular structure of fibrinogen. Ann. N.Y. Acad. Sci. *202*:77, 1972.
79. Blomback, B., Blomback, M., et al.: N-terminal disulfide knot of human fibrinogen. Nature (Lond.) *218*:130, 1968.
80. Blomback, B.: Naturally occurring inhibitors of fibrinolysis. In *Fibrinolytics and Antifibrinolytics*. Markwardt, F. (ed.), New York, Springer-Verlag, 1978.
81. Lorand, L.: "Fibrinopeptide." Nature *167*:992, 1951.
82. Doolittle, R. F.: Structural aspects of the fibrinogen to fibrin conversion. Adv. Prot. Chem. *27*:1, 1973.
83. Scheraga, H. A.: Active site mapping of thrombin. In *Chemistry and Biology of Thrombin*. Lundblad, R. L., Fenton, J. W., et al. (eds.), Ann Arbor, Mich., Ann Arbor Science Publ., 1977, pp. 145–158.
84. Blomback, B.: Selectional trends in the structure of fibrinogen of different species. In *The Hemostatic Mechanism in Man and Animals*. MacFarland, R. G. (ed.), New York, Academic Press, 1970, pp. 167–179.
85. Stocker, K., and Barlow, G. H.: The coagulation enzyme from Bothrops atrox venom. Meth. Enz. *45*:214, 1976.
86. Laurent, T. C., and Blomback, B.: On the significance of the release of two different peptides from fibrinogen during clotting. Acta Chem. Scand. *12*:1875, 1958.
87. Nossel, H. L., Yudelman, I., et al.: Measurement of fibrinopeptide A in human blood. J. Clin. Invest. *54*:43, 1974.
88. Fletcher, A. P., and Alkjaersig, N.: Blood hypercoagulability, intravascular coagulation and thrombosis. New diagnostic concepts. Thromb. Diath. Haemorrh. *45* (Suppl.):389, 1971.
89. Niewiarowski, S., and Gurewich, V.: Laboratory identification of intravascular coagulation. J. Lab. Clin. Med. *77*:665, 1971.
90. York, L. L., and Blomback, B.: Interaction of fragments of fibrinogen with insolubilized fibrin monomer. Thromb. Res. *8*:607, 1976.
91. Schwartz, M. L., Pizzo, S. V., et al.: The subunit structures of human plasma and platelet Factor XIII. J. Biol. Chem. *246*:5837, 1971.
92. Schwartz, M. L., Pizzo, S. V., et al.: Human Factor XIII from plasma and platelets. Molecular weights, subunit structure, proteolytic activation, and crosslinking of fibrinogen and fibrin. J. Biol. Chem. *248*:1395, 1970.
93. Takagi, T., and Doolittle, R. F.: Amino acid sequence studies on Factor XIII and the peptide released during its activation by thrombin. Biochemistry *13*:750, 1974.
94. Folk, J. E., and Chung, S.: Blood coagulation Factor XIII: Relationship to some biologic properties to subunit structure. In *Proteases and Biological Control*. Vol. 2, Reich, E., Rifkin, D. B., et al. (eds.), Cold Spring Harbor Conference on Cell Proliferation. 1975, pp. 157–170.
95. Posano, J. J., Bronzert, T. J., et al.: ε-(δ-Glutamyl) lysine cross–links. Determination in fibrin from normal and factor XIII deficient individuals. Ann. N.Y. Acad. Sci. *202*:98, 1972.
96. Fretto, L. J., and McKee, P. A.: Structure of α-polymer from in vitro and in vivo highly crosslinked human fibrin. J. Biol. Chem. *253*:6614, 1978.
97. McKee, P. A., Mattock, P., et al.: Subunit structure of human fibrinogen, soluble fibrin and crosslinked insoluble fibrin. PNAS *66*:738, 1970.
98. Rosenberg, R. D., Colman, R. W., et al.: A new haemorrhagic disorder with defective fibrin stabilization and cryofibrinogenaemia. Br. J. Haematol. *26*:269, 1974.
99. Barlow, G. H., Summaria, L., et al.: Molecular weight studies on human plasminogen and plasmin at the microgram level. J. Biol. Chem. *244*:1138, 1969.
100. Scottrup-Jensen, L., Claeys, H., et al.: Isolation of two lysine binding fragments and one "mini"-plasminogen. In *Progress in Chemical Fibrinolysis and Thrombosis*. Vol. 3. Davidson, J. F., Rowan, R. M., et al (eds.), New York, Raven Press, 1970, pp. 191–209.
101. Wiman, B.: Biochemistry of the plasminogen to plasmin conversion. In *Fibrinolysis: Current Fundamental and Clinical Concepts*. Gaffney, P. J., and Balkuv-Ukitin, S. (eds.), New York, Academic Press, 1970, pp. 47–60.
102. Wiman, B., and Wallen, P.: Structural relationship between "glutamic acid" and "lysine" forms of human plasminogen and their interaction with the NH_2-terminal activation peptide as studied by affinity chromatography. Eur. J. Biochem. *50*:489, 1975.
103. Robbins, K. C., and Summaria, L.: Human plasminogen and plasmin. In *Methods in Enzymology*. Vol. 19. Perlman, G. E., and Lorand, L. (eds.), New York, Academic Press, 1970, pp. 184–199.
104. Summaria, L., Boreisha, I. G., et al.: Activation of human glu-plasminogen to glu-plasmin by urokinase in the presence of plasmin inhibitors. J. Biol. Chem. *252*:3945, 1977.
105. Schreiber, A., and Austen, K. F.: Hageman Factor: Independent fibrinolytic pathway. Clin. Exp. Immunol. *17*:587, 1974.
106. Todd, A. S.: Localization of fibrinolytic activity in tissues. Br. Med. Bull. *20*:210, 1964.

106a. Rijken, D. C., and Collen, D.: Purification and characterization of the plasminogen activator secreted by human melanoma cells in culture. J. Biol. Chem. 256:7035, 1981.
106b. Wun, T.-C., Schleuning, W.-D., et al.: Isolation and characterization of urokinase from human plasma. J. Biol. Chem. 257:3276, 1982.
106c. Loskutoff, D. J.: Effect of thrombin on the fibrinolytic activity of cultured bovine endothelial cells. J. Clin. Invest. 64:329, 1979.
106d. Levin, Eugene G.: Latent tissue plasminogen activator produced by human endothelial cells in culture: evidence for an enzyme-inhibitor complex. Proc. Natl. Acad. Sci. USA 80:6804, 1983.
107. Schor, J. M., Steinberger, V., et al.: Studies with the synthetic fibrinolytic compound EN 1661. In *Chemical Control of Fibrinolysis-Thrombolysis*. Schor, J. M. (ed.), New York, Wiley Interscience, 1970, pp. 113–134.
108. Neri, S., Rossi, G. G., et al.: Effects of bradykinin on coagulation and fibrinolysis. Thromb. Diath. Haemorrh. 14:508, 1965.
109. Meneghini, P., and Piccinini, F.: Attivazione fibrinolytica del sangue da acida alcaol nicotinico. Arch. E. Maragliano Pat. Clin. 14:69, 1958.
110. Bruhn, H. D.: Activation of fibrinolysis by furosemide. Thromb. Diath. Haemorrh. 33:672, 1975.
111. White, W. F., Barloo, G. H., et al.: The isolation and characterization of plasminogen activators from human urine. Biochemistry 5:2160, 1966.
112. Editorial Committee: Urokinase-pulmonary embolism trial. Circulation 47(Suppl. 2):1, 1973.
113. Schick, L. A., and Castellino, F. J.: Direct evidence for the generation of an active site in the plasminogen moiety of the streptokinase-human plasminogen activator complex. BBRC 57:47, 1974.
113a. The TMI Study Group. Special Report: The Thrombolysis in Myocardial Infarction (TIMI) Trial. Phase I findings. New Engl. J. Med. 312:932, 1985.
113b. Collen, D., Rijken, D. C., et al.: Purification of human tissue-type plasminogen activator in centigram quantities from human melanoma cell culture fluid and its conditioning for use in vivo. Thromb. Haemost. 48:294, 1982.
114. Jijikata, A., Fujimoto, K., et al.: Some properties of the tissue plasminogen activator from the pig heart. Thromb. Res. 4:731, 1974.
115. Alkjaersig, N., Fletcher, A. P., et al.: The mechanism of clot dissolution by plasmin. J. Clin. Invest. 38:9086, 1959.
116. Plow, E. F., and Edgington, T. S.: An alternate pathway for fibrinolysis. J. Clin. Invest. 56:30, 1975.
117. Alkjaersig, N., Fletcher, A. P., et al.: Pathogenesis of the coagulation defect developed during pathologic plasma proteolytic states. J. Clin. Invest. 41:917, 1962.
118. Marder, V. J., and Budzynski, A. Z.: Data for defining fibrinogen and its plasmic degradation products. Thromb. Diath. Haemorrh. 33:199, 1975.
119. Furlan, M., Kemp, G., et al.: Plasmic degradation of fibrinogen. Biochem. Biophys. Acta 400:95, 1975.
120. Gaffney, P. J., and Dobos, P.: A structural aspect of human fibrinogen suggested by its plasmin degradation. FEBS Letters 15:13, 1971.
121. Pizzo, S. V., Schwartz, M. L., et al.: The effort of plasmin as the subunit structure of human fibrin. J. Biol. Chem. 248:4574, 1973.
122. Arnesen, H.: The effect of purified products D and E on the conversion of fibrinogen to fibrin as studied by N-terminal amino acid analysis. IV Int. Cong. on Thromb. Diath. Haemorrh. Abstract 253, Vienna, 1973.
123. Kopec, M., Wegrzynowicz, A., et al.: Interaction of fibrinogen degradation products with platelets. Exp. Biol. Med. 3:73, 1968.
124. Cullasso, D. E., Donati, M. B., et al.: Inhibition of human platelet aggregation by plasmin digest of human and bovine fibrinogen preparations: role of contaminating factor VIII related material. Blood 44:169, 1974.
125. Buluk, K., and Malofiegen, M.: The pharmacologic properties of fibrinogen degradation products. Br. J. Pharmacol. 35:79, 1969.
126. Richardson, D. L., Pepper, D. S., et al.: Chemotaxis for human monocytes by fibrinogen degradation peptides. Br. J. Haematol. 32:507, 1976.
127. Girman, G., Pees, H., et al.: Immunosuppression by micromolecular fibrin-fibrinogen degradation products in cancer. Nature 259:399, 1976.
127a. Acki, N., Moroi, M., et al.: Abnormal plasminogen: a hereditary molecular abnormality found in a patient with recurrent thrombosis. J. Clin. Invest. 62:1186, 1978.
127b. Johansson, L., Hedner, U., et al.: A family with thromboembolic disease associated with deficient fibrinolytic activity in vessel wall. Acta Med. Scand. 203:477, 1978.
127c. Carroll, N., Gabriel, P. A., et al.: Hereditary dysfibrinogenemia in a patient with thrombotic disease. Blood 62:439, 1983.
127d. Nossel, H. L.: Relative proteolysis of the fibrinogen B-beta chain by thrombin and plasmin as a determinant of thrombosis. Nature 291:165, 1981.
127e. Nossel, H. L., Wasser, J. et al.: Sequence of fibrinogen proteolysis and platelet release after intrauterine infusion of hypertonic saline. J. Clin. Invest. 64:1371, 1979.
127f. Owen, J., Kyam, D., et al.: Thrombin and plasmin activity and platelet activation in the development of venous thrombosis. Blood 61:476, 1983.
128. Deykin, D., Cochios, F., et al.: An hepatic inhibitor of activated factor X. Biochem. Biophys. Res. Commun. 34:325, 1969.
129. Egeberg, O.: Inherited antithrombin deficiency causing thrombophilia. Thromb. Diath. Haemorrh. 13:516, 1965.
130. Siato, H., Kamiya, T., et al.: Congenital deficiency of α_2-plasmin inhibitor associated with severe bleeding tendency. Blood 52:194, 1978 (Abstr.).
131. Murano, G., Williams, L., et al.: Some properties of antithrombin III and its concentration in human plasma. Thromb. Res. 18:259, 1980.
132. Abildgaard, U.: Highly purified antithrombin III with heparin cofactor activity prepared by disc electrophoresis. Scand. J. Clin. Lab. Invest. 21:89, 1968.
133. Danishefsky, I., Steiner, H., et al.: Investigations on the chemistry of heparin. J. Biol. Chem. 244:1741, 1969.
134. Rosenberg, R. D., and Lam, L. H.: A correlation between the structure and function of heparin. PNAS 76:1218, 1979.
134a. Rosenberg, R. D., Armand, G., et al.: Structure-function relationship of heparin species. Proc. Natl. Acad. Sci. USA 75:3065, 1978.
134b. Rosenberg, R. D., and Lam, L. H.: Correlation between structure and function of heparin. Proc. Nat. Acad. Sci. USA 76:1218, 1979.
134c. Leder, I. G.: A novel 3–0 sulfatase from human urine acting on methyl-2-deoxy-2-sulfamino-&-D-glucopyranoside-3-sulfate. Biochem. Biophys. Res. Commun. 94:1183, 1980.
134d. Lindahl, U., Backstrom, G., et al.: Structure of the antithrombin-binding site of heparin. Proc. Natl. Acad. Sci. USA 76:3198, 1979.
135. Metcalfe, D. P., Lewis, R. A., et al.: Isolation and characterization of heparin from human lung. J. Clin. Invest. 64:1537, 1979.
135a. Marcum, J. A., Fritze, L., et al.: Microvascular heparin-like species with anticoagulant activity. Am. J. Physiol. 245:H725, 1983.
135b. Marcum, J. A., and Rosenberg, R. D.: Anticoagulantly active heparin-like molecules from vascular tissue. Biochemistry 23:1730, 1984.
135c. Marcum, J. A., and Rosenberg, R. D.: Heparinlike molecules with anticoagulant activity are synthesized by cul-

tured endothelial cells. Biochem. Biophys. Res. Commun. *126*:365, 1985.
136. Marcum, J. A., McKenney, J. B., et al.: The acceleration of thrombin-antithrombin complex formation in rat hindquarters via heparin-like molecules bound to the endothelium. J. Clin. Invest. *74*:1, 1984.
136a. Stern, D., Nawroth, P., et al.: Interaction of antithrombin III with bovine aortic segments: role of heparin in binding and enhanced anticoagulant activity. J. Clin. Invest. *75*:272, 1985.
137. Rosenberg, R. D., and Damus, P. S.: The purification and mechanism of action of human antithrombin-heparin cofactor. J. Biol. Chem. *248*:6490, 1973.
138. Rosenberg, R. D.: Actions and interactions of antithrombin and heparin. New Engl. J. Med. *292*:146, 1975.
139. Jordan, R., Beeler, D., et al.: Fractionation of low molecular weight heparin species and their interaction with antithrombin. J. Biol. Chem. *254*:2902, 1979.
140. Seegers, W. H., Cole, E. R., et al.: Neutralization of autoprothrombin C activity with antithrombin. Can. J. Biochem. *42*:359, 1964.
141. Damus, P. S., Hicks, M., et al.: A generalized view of heparin's anticoagulant action. Nature (Lond.) *246*:355, 1973.
142. Rosenberg, J. S., McKenna, P., et al.: The inhibition of human factor Oxa by human antithrombin-heparin cofactor. J. Biol. Chem. *250*:8883, 1975.
143. Stead, N., Kaplan, A. P., et al.: The inhibition of activated Factor XII by antithrombin-heparin cofactor. J. Biol. Chem. *251*:6481, 1976.
144. Godal, H. C., Rygh, M., et al.: Progressive inactivation of purified factor VII by heparin and antithrombin III. Thromb. Res. *5*:773, 1974.
145. Aoki, N., and Norsi, M.: Distinction of serum inhibitor of activator-induced clot lysis from α_1–antitrypsin. Proc. Soc. Exp. Biol. Med. *146*:567, 1974.
146. Clemnenson, I.: Different molecular forms of α_2-antiplasmin. In *The Physiological Inhibitors of Blood Coagulation and Fibrinolysis*. Collen, D., Wiman, B., et al. (eds.), Amsterdam and New York, North Holland Biomedical Press, 1979, pp. 131–136.
147. Moroi, M., and Aoki, N.: Isolation and characterization of α_2-plasmin inhibitor from human plasma. J. Biol. Chem. *251*:5956, 1976.
148. Moroi, N., and Aoki, N.: Inhibition of proteases in coagulation, kinin-forming and complement systems by α_2-plasmin inhibitor. J. Biol. Chem. *82*:969, 1977.
149. Wiman, B., and Collen, D.: On the kinetics of the reaction between antiplasmin and plasmin. Eur. J. Biochem. *84*:573, 1978.
150. Highsmith, R. F., Weirich, C. J., et al.: Protease inhibitors and human plasmin: Interaction in a whole plasma system. Biochem. Biophys. Res. Commun. *79*:648, 1977.
151. Starkey, P. M., and Barrett, A. J.: α_2-Macroglobulin: a physiological regulator of protease activity. In *Proteases in Mammalian Cells and Tissues*. Barrett, A. J. (ed.), Amsterdam and New York, North Holland Publishing Company, 1977, pp. 663–696.
152. Harpel, P. H.: Human α_2-macroglobulin. In *Methods in Enzymology: Proteolytic Enzymes*. Vol. 45. Lorand, L. (ed.), New York, Academic Press, 1975, pp. 639–652.
153. Jones, J. M., Creeth, J. M., et al.: Thiol reduction of human α_2-macroglobulin. Biochem. J. *127*:187, 1972.
154. Starkey, P. M.: α_2-Macroglobulin: A review. In *The Physiologic Inhibitors of Blood Coagulation and Fibrinolysis*. Collen, D., Wiman, B., et al. (eds.), Amsterdam and New York, North Holland Biomedical Press, 1979, pp. 221–230.
155. Jacquot-Umand, Y., and Krebs, G.: The interaction of naphthalene dye with α_2-macroglobulin, free or bound to trypsin. Biochem. Biophys. Acta *303*:128, 1973.
156. Barrett, A. J., and Starkey, P. M.: The interaction of α_2-macroglobulin with proteases. Biochem. J. *133*:709, 1973.
157. Harpel, P. C., and Mossesson, M. W.: Degradation of human fibrinogen by plasma α_2-macroglobulin-enzyme complexes. J. Clin. Invest. *52*:2175, 1973.
158. Barrett, A. J., Starkey, P. M., et al.: The unique nature of the interaction of α_2-macroglobulin with proteases. *Proc. Vth Bayer Symposium on Protease Inhibitors*. Fritz, H. (ed.), Berlin, Springer-Verlag, 1974, pp. 72–77.
159. Ohlsson, K., and Laurell, C. B.: The disappearance of enzyme-inhibitor complexes from the circulation of man. Clin. Sci. Mol. Med. *51*:87, 1976.
160. Suzuki, K., Nishioka, J., et al.: Protein C inhibitor: Purification from human plasma and characterization. J. Biol. Chem. *258*:163, 1983.
161. Levin, E. G.: Latent tissue plasminogen activator produced by human endothelial cells in culture: evidence for an enzyme-inhibitor complex. Proc. Natl. Acad. Sci. USA *80*:6804, 1983.

COAGULATION

CHAPTER 40
Physiology of Coagulation: The Platelet

ROBERT I. HANDIN

INTRODUCTION 1271
DEVELOPMENT AND KINETICS OF
  MEGAKARYOCYTES AND PLATELETS 1272
PLATELET MORPHOLOGY AND GRANULE
  SECRETION 1276
PLATELET ENERGY METABOLISM 1277
PLATELET–ENDOTHELIAL CELL INTERACTIONS 1278
MEMBRANE STRUCTURE AND FUNCTION 1279
Glycoprotein Ib
Glycoproteins IIb and IIIa
PLATELET ADHESION TO SUBENDOTHELIUM 1282
PLATELET AGGREGATION 1283
PLATELET SIGNAL TRANSDUCTION AND
  INTRACELLULAR MESSENGERS 1284
ARACHIDONIC ACID TRANSFORMATION IN
  PLATELET AND ENDOTHELIAL CELLS 1285
PLATELET COAGULANT ACTIVITY 1287
SUMMARY 1287

INTRODUCTION

Hemostasis is an important homeostatic mechanism that limits blood loss following vascular injury. The platelet provides the first line of defense in this process by immediately adhering to and forming aggregates at sites of vascular injury. The platelet does not function alone in this regard because effective hemostasis requires carefully regulated interactions among platelets, plasma proteins, and components of the vessel wall. Although Bizzozero recognized the blood platelet as a discrete cellular element and accurately described its role in hemostasis over 100 years ago, our understanding of platelet physiology has lagged behind that of other components of the hemostatic system, such as the coagulation proteins (1). In the past few years, however, the field has exploded and a plethora of new information regarding platelet physiology has been published. The function of several platelet membrane proteins has been established, so that several platelet abnormalities can be firmly linked to a reduction or absence of specific membrane proteins (2). Our understanding of platelet signal transduction has been advanced by the observation that two phospholipid metabolites, inositol triphosphate and diacylglycerol, regulate platelet signal transduction (3, 4). The role of plasma adhesive glycoproteins in mediating platelet adhesion and aggregation also has been established (5). This chapter will provide an up-to-date review of normal platelet physiology and a conceptual framework for analysis of quantitative and qualitative platelet disorders. Although some of the clinical aspects of these disorders will be briefly discussed here because they help illustrate principles of platelet physiology, a detailed review of these aspects will be presented in Chapter 42.

The circulating platelet is a small, anuclear cell fragment with several important functions. During its 10-day life span, it traverses miles of blood vessels, helping maintain the integrity of the vascular endothelial lining and searching out potential vascular damage. When a break in the vascular endothelial lining is encountered, platelets immediately adhere to exposed subendothelium. The activated adherent platelets then generate various mediators, including the potent vasoconstrictor and platelet agonist thromboxane A_2, and secrete granule stores of ADP. ADP activates circulating platelets so that they bind to the adherent platelet monolayer to form a hemostatic plug.

The activated platelet surface also serves as a catalyst for plasma coagulation reactions and accelerates thrombin generation and fibrin formation. Thrombin causes additional platelets to secrete and aggregate, which adds to the size of the growing hemostatic plug. This temporary plug is then strengthened by the interposition of fibrin strands, converting it into a permanent barrier to the loss of body fluids—the definitive, or secondary, hemostatic plug.

It is not well appreciated that platelet secretory products may increase vascular permeability, act as chemotactic agents, and modulate vessel wall repair. In fact, there is abundant evidence that repeated cycles of vessel injury, platelet secretion, and vascular smooth muscle proliferation produce the myointimal thickening that is the harbinger of the atherosclerotic plaque.

The complex process of platelet plug formation, which has just been briefly described, is referred to as primary hemostasis and involves three basic platelet reactions—*adhesion, degranulation or release, and aggregation*. The events that generate fibrin and strengthen the hemostatic plug are collectively referred to as secondary hemostasis. These are, of course, somewhat arbitrary divisions, since both processes are intertwined and depend on interactions between platelet, plasma proteins, and components of the vessel wall. Both pathways are simultaneously activated following injury.

It is clear from many clinical and experimental observations that there are many more platelets in the circulation than are needed to effect primary hemostasis. Thus, most platelets complete their life span without being consumed in the hemostatic process. Bleeding occurs only when the number of circulating platelets is drastically reduced or the platelets are defective and cannot complete the sequence of reactions needed to generate a stable hemostatic plug. Quantitative and qualitative (5a) platelet disorders are common causes of mild to moderate hemorrhage in pediatric patients. Many commonly prescribed drugs as well as some metabolic disorders of childhood may secondarily perturb platelet production or function. In addition, there are a number of inherited disorders of platelet function that present in the pediatric age group.

DEVELOPMENT AND KINETICS OF MEGAKARYOCYTES AND PLATELETS

The intramedullary development of megakaryocytes and platelets follows the general schema described for other blood cells in Chapter 6. Some unique features deserve emphasis here. A committed megakaryocyte progenitor gives rise to colony-forming units (CFU-MK or CFU-Meg), which subsequently proliferate and differentiate (6). Unlike other marrow constituents, megakaryocytes mature by a process of nuclear endoreduplication that is not accompanied by cell division (7). This produces the extremely large polyploid cells recognized as mature megakaryocytes in bone marrow aspirates and biopsies. They have been classified into three developmental stages according to the extent of nuclear lobulation and granule content (8). Stimuli that increase megakaryocyte production, such as increased peripheral platelet destruction or hemorrhage, increase both the number and ploidy of marrow megakaryocytes (9).

One can fractionate mature megakaryocytes and their committed progenitors by density gradient centrifugation (10) or velocity sedimentation (11) and identify them using antibodies to specific membrane proteins present on megakaryocytes and platelets (12). Stage I to III megakaryocytes can be maintained for 24 to 48 hours in short-term liquid cultures (13), whereas long-term clonal assays utilizing soft agar or methylcellulose are needed to produce megakaryocytic colonies from committed progenitor cells (14). The CFU-MK is a small lymphoid cell. The early colonies derived from it are recognized only because they express megakaryocyte-specific antigens. Although it is now possible to grow human as well as murine megakaryocytes, much of our information regarding megakaryocyte development is derived from the murine system (15). A tentative scheme of murine megakaryocyte development is outlined in Figure 40–1.

As shown in the figure, optimal differentiation and proliferation of megakaryocytic precursors requires two humoral factors: megakaryocyte colony-stimulatating factor (CSF-MK or CSF-Meg), which in the mouse is identical with the lymphokine interleukin 3 (IL-3), and a less well defined megakaryocytic potentiator (10, 16–18). Although megakaryocytic colonies develop following the addition of purified IL-3 to murine progenitors in soft agar or methylcellulose, more colonies develop when fractions containing the megakaryocytic potentiator also are included in the culture. Increased human CSF-Meg activity, which may be identical to GM-CSF (see Chapter 6), is found in the urine of some thrombopenic individuals (18a).

A third humoral agent, thrombopoietin, also may regulate megakaryocyte development (19, 20). Thrombopoietin has not yet been purified but can be operationally defined by the infusion of plasma from thrombocytopenic animals to their normal counterparts. Plasma fractions enriched in thrombopoietin increase the number and ploidy of marrow megakaryocytes (21). However, fractions rich in thrombopoietin by bioassay have no effect on CFU-MK development in vitro, suggesting that it is distinct from MK-CSA and IL-3 (22). It is likely that thrombopoietin, like erythropoietin, induces the terminal differentiation of committed cells within megakaryocytic colonies to form Stages I to IV megakaryocytes. This process of differentiation then secondarily increases the number of

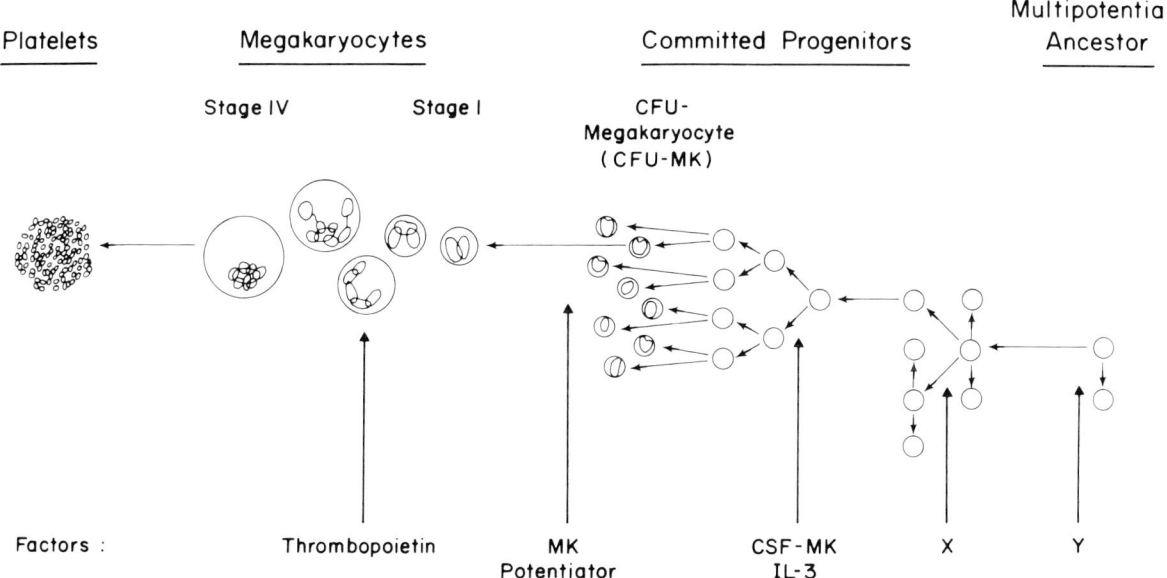

Figure 40–1. An outline of the current scheme for megakaryocyte development. X and Y are as yet unidentified early regulatory factors that may act on pluripotential stem cells. In the mouse, colony-stimulating factor megakaryocyte (CSF-MK) is identical to interleukin-3 (IL-3). MK potentiator and thrombopoietin are separate factors. Stages I to IV refer to the degree of differentiation of recognizable megakaryocytes.

committed progenitors that enter the megakaryocytic pathway of development (23). Greenberg and colleagues have identified and purified a protein from sheep plasma that induces megakaryocyte differentiation in vitro (24) and that may, in fact, be identical with thrombopoietin.

Although the development of megakaryocyte fractionation techniques and in vitro colony assays has improved our understanding of megakaryocyte development, these techniques are of limited utility in evaluating patients with quantitative platelet disorders. In order to study these clinical problems, Harker quantified megakaryocytopoiesis in vivo using the ferrokinetic model developed by Finch (Fig. 40–2) (25). He estimated megakaryocyte number on ultrathin histologic sections of marrow and related this to the number of nucleated red cells in the same sections. The total red cell mass was derived from isotopic measurements and, coupled with this ratio, was used to calculate total megakaryocyte mass. Although this technique is clearly too arduous for routine clinical

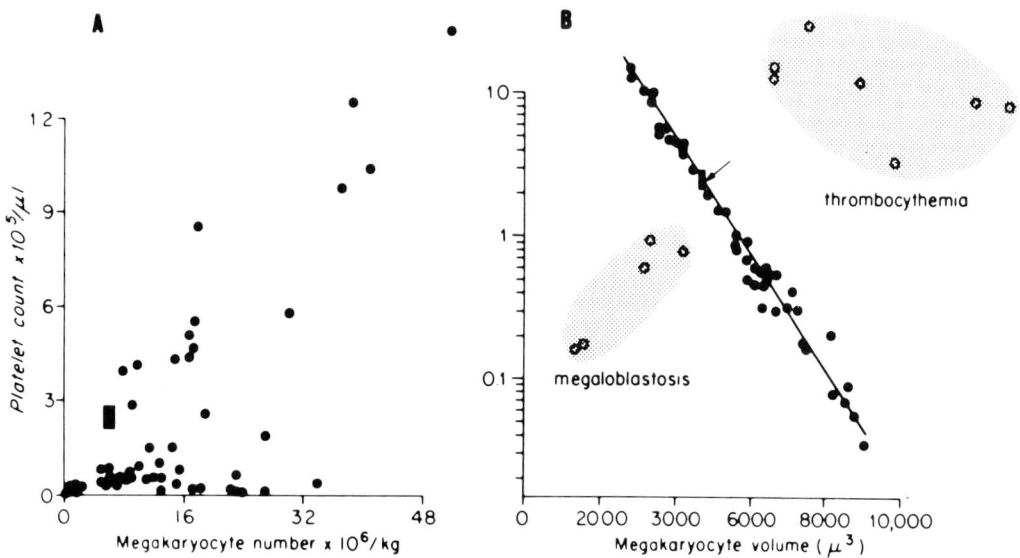

Figure 40–2. The relationship between platelet count and megakaryocyte number and megakaryocyte volume. As shown here, the megakaryocyte volume and, hence, the number of platelets produced increase as the platelet count falls. The only exceptions are patients with disorders that result in ineffective thrombopoiesis such as megaloblastic anemias or essential thrombocythemia. (From Harker, L. A., and Finch, C. A.: J. Clin. Invest. 48:972, 1969.)

use, an estimate of relative megakaryocyte number in marrow biopsy sections or aspirates, coupled with measurement of platelet life span and splenic size, provides a clinically useful way to classify patients with thrombocytopenia. For example, patients with decreased megakaryocyte number, normal platelet life span, and normal splenic size have a marrow production defect, whereas patients with shortened platelet survival and an increased number of megakaryocytes have peripheral platelet destruction. Patients who have an increased number of megakaryocytes in the marrow and normal survival of circulating platelets due to ineffective thrombopoiesis also have been identified (25).

Stimulation of megakaryocytopoiesis has important effects on peripheral platelet morphology and function. Following stimulation, the marrow releases larger platelets (26). These large platelets, or megathrombocytes, are said to be the equivalent of the red cell reticulocyte and to represent the influx of a young platelet population produced in response to hematopoietic stress (26). This concept, however, has been challenged by Thompson and colleagues (27). There is agreement that large platelets contain a higher concentration of glycolytic enzymes and may be more effective in hemostasis (28, 29).

Although the presence of megathrombocytes in thrombocytopenic patients is not disputed, their significance, as already noted (27), is not clear. The increased effectiveness of megathrombocytes has been used to explain the diminished incidence of bleeding in individuals with thrombocytopenia due to excess platelet destruction. There is, in fact, evidence that these "stress platelets" remain large and accumulate in the blood because of an inability to undergo appropriate remodeling (30). In addition, large platelets may not be younger but may arise solely because of changes in the pattern of megakaryocyte development and fragmentation that occurs during stressed megakaryocytopoiesis (31–33).

There are several hematologic disorders in which stem cell defects lead to dysplastic megakaryocyte development and thrombocytopenia (34). Ineffective thrombopoiesis, coupled with abnormal megakaryocyte and platelet morphology, has been described in patients with "preleukemia" and in individuals with myeloproliferative syndromes (35–37). These patients have smaller than normal megakaryocytes with a lower ploidy value and only one or two nuclear lobes. A number of membrane defects have been noted in the platelets of patients with these syndromes, including a decrease in certain membrane glycoproteins, loss of alpha$_2$-adrenergic and prostaglandin receptors, and abnormalities in arachidonic acid metabolism (38–40). These syndromes occur most often in middle-aged and elderly adults and are extremely rare in the pediatric age group.

A number of other stem cell disorders, including aplastic anemia, paroxysmal nocturnal hemoglobinuria, congenital thrombocytopenia with the May-Heggin anomaly, and Down's syndrome, are examples of conditions in which platelets as well as red cell and white cell abnormalities are present (34). There also is a group of inherited disorders in which platelet development is more selectively perturbed (34a). These include the Wiskott-Aldrich syndrome (41), the familial thrombocytopenias with abnormally large or small platelets (42), functional platelet defects like Glanzmann's thrombasthenia and the Bernard-Soulier syndrome (2), and the gray platelet syndrome (42a).

When platelets leave the marrow, they circulate for approximately 10 days. During this time, they decrease in size and increase in density, primarily because of the loss of plasma membrane. Studies in which platelets are radiolabeled with membrane and cytoplasmic markers have demonstrated preferential loss of membrane label (43). This selective loss of membrane was inhibited by the administration of drugs such as acetylsalicylic acid (ASA) and dipyridamole, which are known to inhibit platelet aggregation and release (44). This suggests that platelets lose membrane during reversible hemostatic encounters. There also are complementary studies demonstrating that platelets degranulate without losing their ability to circulate (45). These studies make it clear that platelets are not necessarily "consumed" during hemostasis and may participate in multiple hemostatic reactions and still live out their full life span.

Although much effort has been expended on the development of techniques to analyze platelet kinetics, there is no ideal label to estimate platelet production and turnover. Selenomethionine is a potentially useful cohort label (46). However, it is incorporated into a number of plasma proteins as well as proteins in other blood cells and has not been extremely useful. Radiolabeled di-isofluorophosphate (DFP^{32}) has been used to label membrane phospholipids, and ^{14}C-serotonin has been used to label the dense granule pool (47, 48). Both these labels are reutilized following platelet destruction, and this perturbs the survival curve. Although it has several limitations, the most widely used and successful platelet label is ^{51}Cr, which binds to cytoplasmic proteins (49). Only a small fraction of the added ^{51}Cr is taken up by the platelet because of competition by plasma proteins. In addition, one must label 2 to 5 × 10^{10} platelets to obtain satisfactory levels of circulating radioactivity, which requires withdrawal of 200 to 500 ml of blood. This is a potential problem when kinetic studies are needed for infants and small children.

Despite these practical limitations, ^{51}Cr is frequently used to estimate the intravascular recovery and life span of the platelet (Fig. 40–3). Interpretation of survival curves is complicated by the presence of a splenic platelet pool that is in equilibrium with the circulating platelets and that normally contains one third of the platelet mass. There is some intriguing evidence that the spleen preferentially sequesters young platelets following their release from the marrow and then releases them after 2 or 3 days of splenic "maturation" (50). The increase in platelet count that accompanies incidental or post-traumatic splenectomy in normal individuals is related to the removal of this sequestration site. In some pathologic states with splenic hypertrophy, the splenic pool can be enormous and may contain more than 90 per cent of the total platelet mass (51). Although the platelet count does not usually fall below 50,000 per mm^3, massive splenic pooling can cause severe thrombocytopenia and hemorrhage in occasional patients and must be corrected by splenectomy.

Although the platelet normally circulates for 10 days, its life span can be reduced by hypoxia or passage of blood through diseased vascular beds or prosthetic surfaces (47, 52, 53). The presence of immune complexes, viral or bacterial pathogens, or activated coagulation factors in the circulation also will reduce survival. Experimental infection of platelets with certain paramyxovirus strains, which contain neuraminidase, can reduce platelet sialic acid content sufficiently to shorten their survival (54). This raises the possibility that the thrombocytopenia and rapid platelet destruction that accompany certain viral infections may be direct effects of the virus rather than the host immune response. Although extremely useful in selected cases, platelet survival studies must be interpreted in light of the many environmental changes that can shorten survival.

As shown in Figure 10–3, the pattern of disappearance of labeled platelets in normal individuals is slightly curvilinear. This is not due to elution of the ^{51}Cr label, which occurs at a rate of 1.5 per cent each day, and therefore would not be detected during the 10-day survival study. There are several explanations for this curvilinear pattern, including a basal level of platelet consumption with some random destruction. To support this, there are studies that show age-related changes in platelet survival and a rough correlation between shortened survival and the presence of vascular diseases such as diabetes mellitus and atherosclerosis (55). However, even in pediatric patients with little or no vascular disease, some curvilinearity is seen. Murphy and colleagues have proposed a "random hit" model based on probability statistics that, they believe, best explains the survival patterns obtained with various isotopes, including ^{51}Cr (56).

A ^{51}Cr survival study can be used to detect the accelerated random destruction pattern seen in immunologic disorders such as idiopathic thrombocytopenic purpura (ITP) (see Chapter 42) as well as to assess the survival of platelets in inherited forms of thrombocytopenia (57). The technique can also compare the survival of normal and abnormal platelets in a single individual. An excellent example of such a study is that of Murphy and associates, who analyzed platelet kinetics in several families with congenital thrombocytopenia (42). Unfortunately, such studies require cross-transfusion and should not be performed because of the risk of transmitting hepatitis or AIDS. Individuals with mild thrombocytopenia (greater than 50,000 platelets per mm^3) should have an autologous platelet survival. If platelet survival is shortened or if the count is less than 50,000 platelets per mm^3, giving allogeneic platelets from a donor who is free of any clinical or laboratory evidence of hepatitis virus or HTLV-III infection may be justified if such a transfusion also is needed to improve hemostasis.

Investigators have estimated the degree of splenic sequestration by comparing the accumulation of radioactivity over the spleen and liver with that of the blood pool using point-counting techniques. Although theoretically appealing, liver:spleen and spleen:heart ratios are not reliable indices of organ sequestration despite some promising initial reports (58). The work of Aster and Keene, pointing out that the degree of splenic sequestration varies considerably after repeat study of patients with immune thrombocytopenia, has been reproduced in other laboratories (59). Unfortunately, differential platelet sequestration has not proved a useful way of predicting the clinical response to splenectomy in patients with immune platelet destruction.

Platelets have now been successfully labeled with gamma-emitting isotopes that have higher energy emission spectra and are suitable for direct imag-

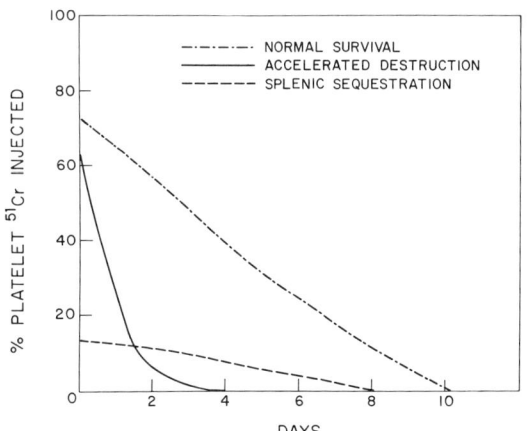

Figure 40–3. Clearance of ^{51}Cr-labeled platelets in normal individuals and patients with clinical disorders. Normally 70 per cent of the infused platelet radioactivity is recovered initially, with a slightly curvilinear 10-day life span. This pattern can be altered by splenomegaly, which reduces initial recovery or a variety of immune or nonimmune disorders that shorten subsequent platelet life span.

ing. Isotopes such as ^{111}In and ^{99m}Tc are currently being evaluated (60, 61). These studies may provide a useful way of rapidly labeling small quantities of blood that, in turn, may simplify kinetic studies. Their utility is still undefined, although platelet thrombi have been visualized within larger vessels, such as the carotid, iliac, and femoral arteries (62–64).

PLATELET MORPHOLOGY AND GRANULE SECRETION

The unactivated platelet circulates as a smooth-surfaced disc that is best demonstrated in scanning electron micrographs (Fig. 40–4). When activated, the platelet undergoes a dramatic morphologic transformation. It spheres, extends pseudopods, rearranges granules to the center of the cell, and discharges granule contents via the surface-connected canalicular system. Following pseudopod formation, the majority of the platelet cytosol is redistributed in these cellular extensions (65). A scanning electron micrograph of a platelet aggregate nicely illustrates both the extent of pseudopod formation and the interdigitation of platelets that accompanies aggregate formation (Fig. 40–5). These dramatic morphologic changes are effected by contractile and microtubular proteins distributed in the platelet cytosol.

A submembranous ring of microtubules is a prominent feature on transmission electron micrographs (Fig. 40–6). It functions as a "cytoskeleton" and maintains the discoid shape of the unactivated circulating platelet (66). Manipulations that depolymerize microtubules produce an irregular, spherical platelet (67). Examples include incubation in the cold and exposure to drugs such as vinblastine and vincristine (68, 69). In a similar manner, following platelet activation and pseudopod formation, there is a loss of visible cytoskeleton, thought to be due to microtubular depolymerization.

Actin, the most abundant platelet contractile protein, forms an extensive microfilamentous network that is distributed throughout the platelet cytosol (70). Although there is some disagreement, the majority of resting platelets have few formed actin microfilaments (71, 72). An actin-rich network of filaments forms during platelet activation by the assembly of actin molecules into filaments and bundles. Actin assembly is regulated by a series of proteins that control the rate of filament assembly and the branching and bundling of microfilaments (65). A second class of regulatory protein, gelsolin, in conjunction with calcium, inhibits actin filament assembly and depolymerizes already-formed filaments, providing a way to regulate both the extent and the location of the microfilament network (73). Although actin-rich filaments predominate, the platelet also contains myosin and associated regulatory proteins that link it to actin. Force generation by actomyosin is carefully regulated by multiple factors including the extent of phosphorylation of myosin light chains, which is increased during platelet activation (74).

The movement and secretion of granules are other important events thought to be mediated by contractile proteins. As previously discussed, during activation, granules move toward the center of the platelet and are then discharged into the surface-connected canalicular system, which delivers granule contents into the plasma and the vessel wall. Early studies postulated actomyosin as generating the contractile force that propels the granules centripetally (75). More recently, an alternative and equally attractive hypothesis has been put forward. Detailed studies of actin filament distribution suggest that the actin-rich filamentous network in the center of the platelet may be selectively

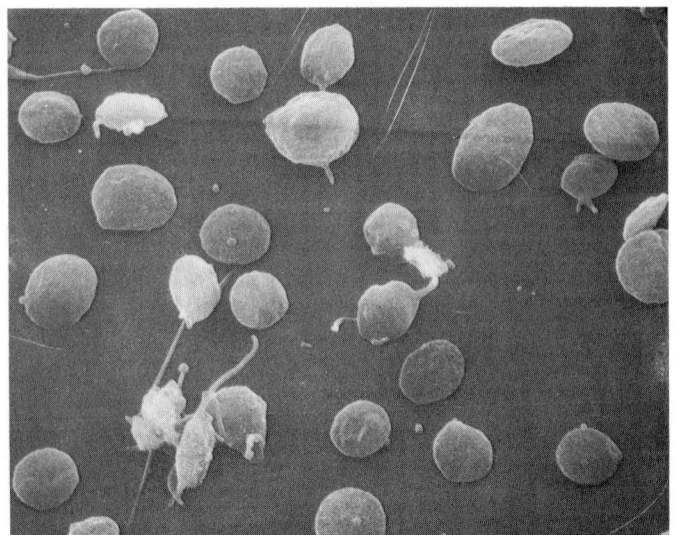

Figure 40–4. Scanning electron micrograph of platelets on a siliconized glass coverslip. Most of the platelets are smooth discs with occasional pseudopod formation. Final magnification ×5140. (Photograph courtesy of Dr. Kathleen Curwen, Department of Pathology, Brigham and Women's Hospital.)

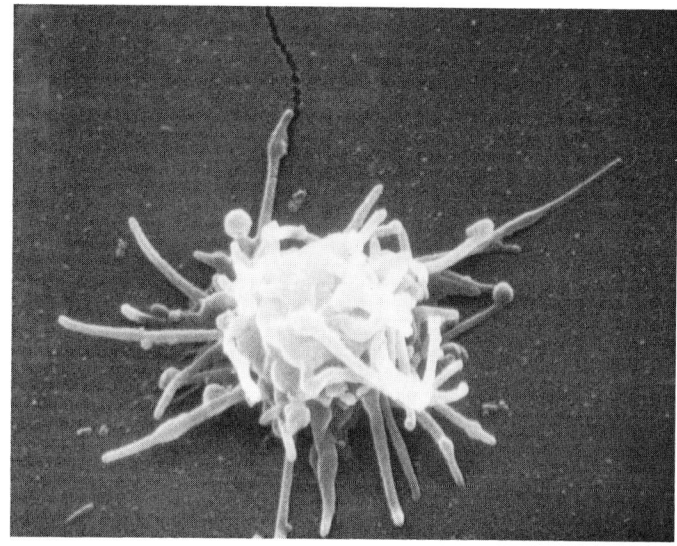

Figure 40–5. Scanning electron micrograph that demonstrates the extent of platelet pseudopod formation during aggregation. Final magnification ×9700. (Photography courtesy of Dr. Kathleen Curwen, Department of Pathology, Brigham and Women's Hospital.)

dissolved by gelsolin and calcium, permitting the granules to move toward the cell center (65, 76).

Transmission electron micrographs of the platelet demonstrate membrane-bound granules of varied electron density and size (see Figure 40–6). In addition to having lysosomal vesicles, which are common to many cells, the platelet contains two unique classes of secretable granules. The most electron-dense granules contain ADP, calcium, and serotonin (77). The less electron-dense alpha-granules, the absence of which results in the gray platelet syndrome (34a), contain platelet stores of several "plasma" proteins such as fibrinogen (78), fibronectin, von Willebrand's factor (79), and Factor V (80). These proteins are synthesized within megakaryocytes and are not adsorbed or pinocytized from plasma.

The alpha-granules contain several "platelet-specific" proteins as well. Platelet factor 4 is a 7800-dalton polypeptide that binds to and inactivates heparin and may modulate heparin-dependent coagulation reactions (81, 82). These granules contain a potent mitogen as well, the platelet-derived growth factor (PDGF), which stimulates smooth muscle proliferation and migration (83, 84). This factor may be important in normal wound-healing as well as in the pathogenesis of atherosclerosis (85, 86). "PDGF" may be a misnomer, as it is homologous with the oncogene product of simian sarcoma virus (v-sis) (87). In addition, PDGF transcripts have been discovered in endothelial cells (88), suggesting that it may be a more widely distributed growth factor.

Because many of the granule constituents promote aggregation, granule secretion is an important amplifying mechanism that promotes growth of the hemostatic plug. One of the most common causes of mild bleeding is a defect in this positive feedback loop. This defect is usually due to a failure to generate the biochemical messages needed to induce granule secretion. This failure is most commonly due to the ingestion of drugs, such as aspirin, that inhibit thromboxane synthesis (89). A second group of patients with "storage pool disease" cannot transport and package constituents in the dense or alpha-granule pool (90). Despite a normal release mechanism, platelets from these patients do not aggregate fully because of this lack of secreted material.

PLATELET ENERGY METABOLISM

The platelet has a complex metabolic system that enables it to produce the energy needed for vital reactions and to renew some cellular constituents. It can generate adenosine triphosphate (ATP) from aerobic and anaerobic glucose metabolism, synthesize and metabolize fatty acids and phospholipids, and both synthesize and break

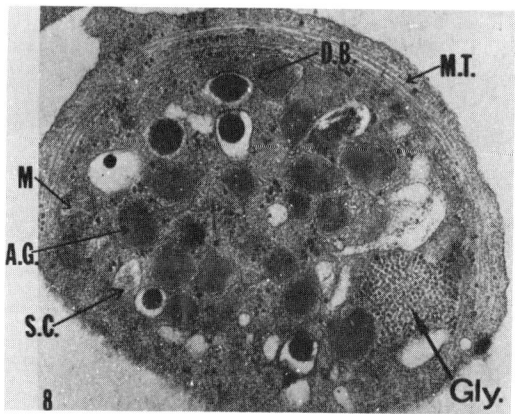

Figure 40–6. Transmission electron micrograph of a platelet to demonstrate subcellular structure. M.T., microtubes; M, mitochondria; A.G., alpha or nondense granules; S.C., surface canalicular system; D.B., dense body; and Gly., glycogen stores. (Electron micrograph courtesy of Dr. James White, Department of Pediatrics, University of Minnesota School of Medicine.)

down glycogen. Although the platelet contains traces of RNA, it is not capable of de novo protein synthesis.

The platelet normally accumulates glucose from plasma and degrades it to lactate. The platelets also have functional mitochondria, a hexose monophosphate shunt, and abundant glycogen stores. When platelets are stimulated, there is a four- to five-fold rise in lactate production (91, 92) as well as stimulation of glycogenolysis. Glycogen breakdown provides up to 40 per cent of the glucose needed for anaerobic carbohydrate metabolism (93). Increments in hexose monophosphate shunt and citric acid cycle activity accompany platelet activation but make a minor contribution to total platelet energy metabolism (94). These pathways do play some role, as it is necessary to block both glycolysis and citric acid cycle activity to completely inhibit platelet aggregation and release (95).

Studies of the correlation between glycolytic enzyme activity and platelet function have not been very fruitful because no glycolytic abnormalities have been identified in any of the qualitative platelet disorders. Patients with severe glucose-6-phosphate dehydrogenase (G6PD) deficiency have chronic hemolysis and a reduced level of platelet enzyme without a change in platelet life span or function (96). Furthermore, in tissue enzyme defects such as Type I glycogen storage disease, platelet glycogen stores are not increased despite a functional defect (97). The platelet defect in these patients is corrected by hyperalimentation, which reverses plasma acidosis, hypoglycemia, and hyperlipemia.

The best example of a glycolytic defect that impairs platelet function is seen in patients with the Wiskott-Aldrich syndrome. Because the usual small increment in citric acid cycle activity that accompanies platelet activation does not occur in these individuals, defective platelet aggregation and release result (98). A mild abnormality is present in carriers of this recessive disorder that can be brought out by treatment of their platelets with inhibitors of glycolysis, such as sodium fluoride (99). This may not be the sole abnormality in these patients, as Parkman and associates have described a membrane protein defect in platelets and lymphocytes from these patients that disappears following successful bone marrow transplantation (100).

PLATELET–ENDOTHELIAL CELL INTERACTIONS

Platelets do not normally adhere to endothelial cells lining blood vessels, although they help maintain the integrity of the vascular lining. When animals are made thrombocytopenic, gaps appear between endothelial cells, permitting the egress of red cells and plasma proteins (101). This red cell leakage into the dermis causes the pinpoint petechiae that are freqently associated with severe thrombocytopenia. The infusion of a small number of platelets eliminates the gaps and restores endothelial morphology to normal (Fig. 40–7) (102). The endothelial gaps can be partially eliminated by administration of high doses of corticosteroids (103). These studies demonstrate the importance of the platelet in maintaining vascular integrity as well as the efficacy of platelet transfusion for severely thrombocytopenic patients. In addition, the studies provide a rationale for the administration of corticosteroids in the treatment of vascular fragility associated with thrombocytopenia.

As expected from in vivo studies, platelets do not adhere to cultured endothelial cells. Platelets will adhere following treatment with thrombin or

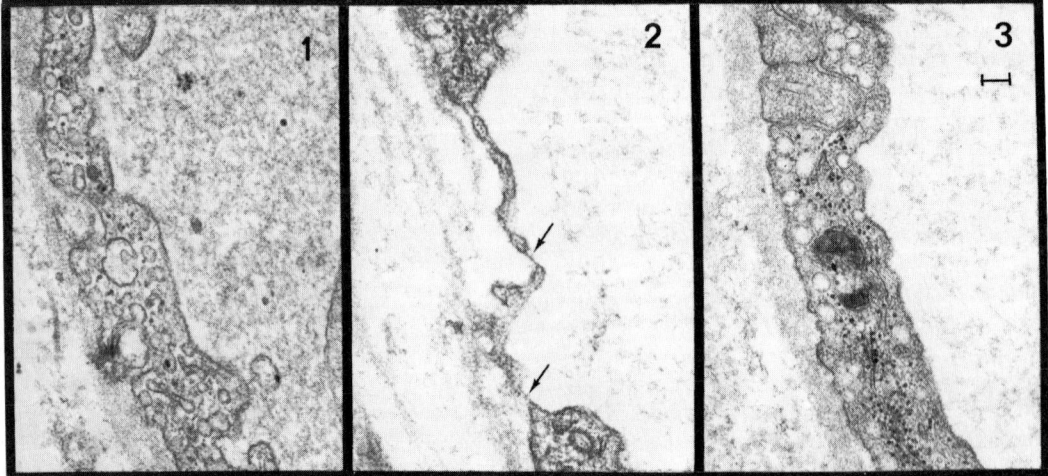

Figure 40–7. Effects of thrombocytopenia and prednisone therapy on endothelial cell morphology. (From Kitchens, C. S.: J. Clin. Invest. *60*:1129, 1977.) (Photograph montage courtesy of Dr. Craig Kitchens, University of Florida.)

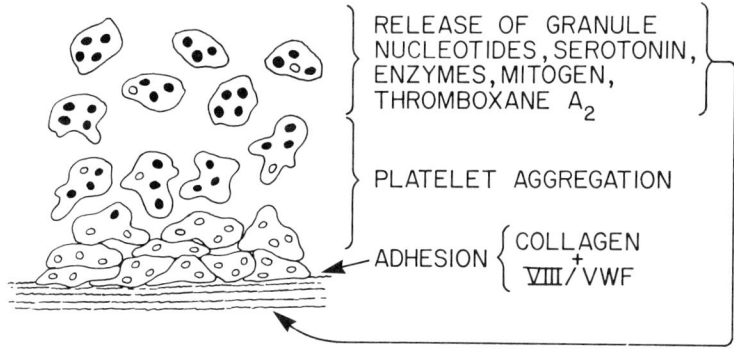

Figure 40-8. Platelet adhesion and aggregation on a damaged vessel wall. Adhesion is enhanced by plasma VIII/VWF, the von Willebrand's protein. Following adhesion, platelets degranulate, and the released mediators, primarily ADP and thromboxane A_2, induce aggregate formation.

after transformation of the endothelial cells. Although hemostasis is usually initiated by the removal of endothelium, which exposes platelets to subendothelial structures (Fig. 40-8), these studies suggest that platelets might adhere to endothelial cells in certain pathologic states in which endothelial cells are damaged. There is evidence that damaged endothelial cells bind fibrin and that they express increased amounts of tissue factor on their surface (104). In addition, endothelial cells modulate coagulation reactions on their surface and release proteins that regulate fibrinolysis. Both processes may secondarily affect the platelet (105, 106).

MEMBRANE STRUCTURE AND FUNCTION

The platelet membrane, like that of other mammalian cells, is a complex mixture of phospholipids, cholesterol, and proteins. The biogenesis of a typical membrane bilayer has been clarified by basic biochemical studies of model membrane systems. In an aqueous environment, phospholipids, which contain polar or hydrophilic head groups and lipophilic fatty acid side chains, spontaneously arrange themselves into a closed circular bilayer. They orient their hydrophobic fatty acid side chains internally and their polar head groups on the outside of the bilayer. This tightly packed phospholipid array provides the backbone or membrane skeleton in which other membrane constituents—primarily proteins—are embedded. The familiar fluid mosaic membrane model, originally proposed by Singer, still provides the best picture of general membrane organization (107). The platelet has some unique additional features. As previously discussed, portions of the platelet plasma membrane invaginate to form the surface-connected canalicular system. These deep channels greatly increase the surface area of the platelet. In addition, they connect the platelet membrane with the cytosol and provide a route for the exocytosis of secreted granule material.

Phospholipids are asymmetrically distributed in the platelet membrane, with the majority of the phosphatidyl serine (PS) and phosphatidyl choline (PC) restricted to the external leaflet of the bilayer and the bulk of the phosphatidyl inositol (PI) found in the cytoplasmic leaflet (108). This may be of physiologic significance, as PI metabolites regulate platelet signal transduction via regulatory enzymes in the platelet cytosol (109). Membrane lipids are in constant motion and can diffuse rapidly within the plane of each leaflet of the bilayer but rarely move across the bilayer. Proteins embedded in the membrane also are mobile. Because they are much larger, they diffuse more slowly than lipids. In addition, they are constrained by interactions with components of the submembranous cytoskeleton, which forms a lattice just beneath the cytoplasmic face of the platelet membrane.

An equimolar concentration of cholesterol is interspersed among the tightly packed fatty acid side chains. The ratio of cholesterol to phospholipid also regulates the rate of protein and phospholipid diffusion by changing membrane fluidity. Using fluorescence polarization techniques, Shattil and coworkers demonstrated that incubation of platelets with cholesterol-rich liposomes increases membrane microviscosity and lowers the platelet threshold for aggregating agents such as epinephrine and ADP (110, 111). This may be clinically important because the increase in plasma cholesterol seen in familial hypercholesterolemia also enhances platelet responses to aggregating agents by perturbing platelet cholesterol:phospholipid ratios.

Proteins embedded in the phospholipid bilayer serve cellular recognition, receptor, and transport functions and define some of the unique antigenic and functional properties of the platelet. They can be classified on the basis of their size, function, and orientation within the lipid bilayer. Antigens and receptor proteins project from the exterior of the membrane to facilitate interaction with antibodies or potential ligands. Many receptor proteins also span the bilayer to allow the transmission of information about receptor occupancy and activation to regulatory enzymes within the cell. Other proteins—for example, those constituting transport channels for ions such as sodium and calcium or small molecules such as serotonin—also span the bilayer. Membrane-bound enzymes such as adenylate cyclase and its associated regulatory proteins are localized on the cytoplasmic side of the membrane.

Specific membrane proteins can be identified by functional or enzymatic assays, specific radiolabeled ligands, or monospecific or monoclonal antibodies. Radioligand binding techniques are particularly useful for identifying biologically distinctive molecules that are present in scant numbers. Platelet prostaglandin, alpha$_2$-adrenergic, ADP, thrombin, and serotonin receptors have been identified with these techniques. More abundant membrane proteins as well as those with no distinctive function can be identified with more general membrane-labeling techniques that covalently tag either the polypeptide or carbohydrate portions of these glycoproteins (112, 113). Radiolabeled proteins are then solubilized and separated on the basis of their net electrical charge or molecular weight by one- and two-dimensional SDS-polyacrylamide gel electrophoresis (SDS-PAGE) or by a combination of isoelectric focusing and SDS-PAGE (114). A diagram of the major platelet membrane glycoproteins and their functions is shown in Figure 40–9. Although more than 20 platelet membrane proteins have been identified with these techniques, only a few of the most abundant proteins have been thoroughly studied. Three of these—glycoproteins Ib, IIb, and IIIa—constitute the bulk of the externally oriented membrane proteins (115).

Glycoprotein Ib

Glycoprotein Ib (GpIb) is a heavily glycosylated integral membrane protein containing two polypeptide subunits that are linked by disulfide bonds. The larger alpha-chain of GpIb has an estimated molecular weight of 150,000, and the molecular weight of the smaller beta-chain is approximately 20,000 (114). Fifty per cent of the alpha-chain mass is carbohydrate, consisting of aproximately 50 repeating hexasaccharide chains that are distributed along the polypeptide backbone. GpIb is the major component of the platelet glycocalyx and the major source of platelet sialic acid. Because of its extremely high carbohydrate content, the protein stains intensely with ruthenium red, a standard glycocalyx, or outer surface marker. GpIb also interacts with two other integral membrane proteins. It forms an equimolar complex with a 20,000-Mr protein identified as glycoprotein IX and is closely associated with GpV (116, 117). The alpha-chain of GpIb is readily attacked by circulating proteases and by an intraplatelet calcium-dependent protease (calpain) that is liberated when platelets are damaged (118). The carbohydrate-rich fragment cleaved from GpIb by enzymes such as calpain, trypsin, and plasmin is called glycocalicin (119, 120).

The best-defined function of GpIb is as a receptor for von Willebrand's factor (vWF) (121, 122). This interaction is critically important in hemostasis because it facilitates platelet adhesion to vascular subendothelium under the conditions of high shear stress that exist in the microcirculation. In fact, patients with the Bernard-Soulier syndrome, who lack GpIb, do not bind vWF to their platelets and have markedly impaired adhesion and a severe bleeding disorder (123). vWF binds to GpIb in vitro following incubation of vWF and platelets with the cationic antibiotic ristocetin. The receptor site for vWF is on the alpha-chain of GpIb and is retained by glycocalicin after its cleavage from the membrane (124, 125). Monoclonal antibodies directed against epitopes on GpIb and glycocalicin block vWF binding, ristocetin-induced platelet agglutination, and platelet adhesion in ex vivo perfusion systems. vWF binding is also inhibited by

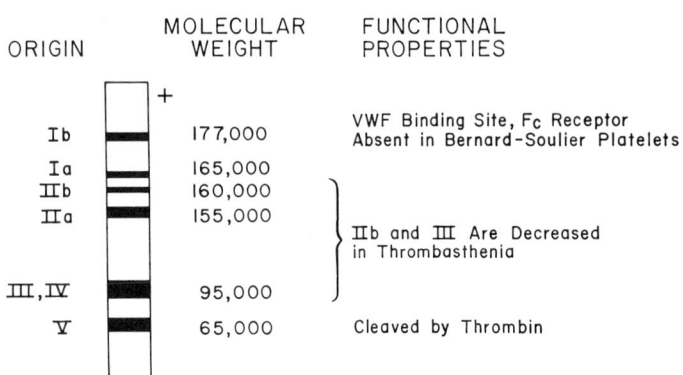

Figure 40–9. Platelet membrane glycoproteins. The left-hand section depicts a polyacrylamide gel electrophoresis pattern in the presence of SDS and reducing agent.

enzymatic digestion of the oligosaccharide chains on GpIb and glycocalicin (125). Although the physiologic stimulus that initiates vWF binding to GpIb has not been completely defined, there is evidence suggesting that one product of coagulation, fibrin monomer, can substitute for ristocetin and initiate vWF binding to GpIb (126).

GpIb and its proteolytic fragment, glycocalicin, bind thrombin also and may function as the platelet thrombin receptor (127, 128). Early radioligand-binding studies by Tollefson and co-workers demonstrated a reversible, saturable, high-affinity binding site on the platelet that binds either proteolytically active or DFP-treated (inactive) thrombin (129). Later studies by Larsen and Simons, who used photoaffinity-labeled derivatives of thrombin, confirmed the presence of a 170,000-Mr thrombin receptor that they solubilized and purified from platelet membranes (130). Jamieson and Okumura as well as others have shown that thrombin binds to GpIb and glycocalicin (128); Berndt and Philips have reported that thrombin cleaves GpV from the platelet surface and that this step is necessary for thrombin-induced platelet activation (131). Thrombin-induced platelet aggregation and secretion are reduced in patients with the Bernard-Soulier syndrome who lack GpIb (132), GpV, and GpIX. Although it is clear from all these studies that platelet activation requires proteolytically active thrombin, it is not yet clear whether there is a single thrombin receptor or whether signal transduction is a direct result of receptor occupancy or a secondary effect of GpV cleavage.

The mobility of GpIb within the plane of the platelet membrane is reduced following platelet activation by the interaction of the cytoplasmic tail of the alpha-chain with a submembranous cytoskeletal latticework containing actin and actin-binding protein. Solum and co-workers first detected this interaction by examining the mobility of detergent-solubilized platelet proteins by crossed immunoelectrophoresis (133). Subsequently, the composition of platelet cytoskeletal fractions produced by incubation of activated and unactivated platelets with a nonionic detergent (Triton X100) has been examined by SDS-PAGE (134). With this technique, GpIb can be solubilized and readily separated from the cytoskeleton of unactivated platelets but remains bound to triton-insoluble cytoskeletal components (platelet ghosts) following platelet activation. When platelets are incubated with radioactive phosphorus (^{32}P), the alpha-chain is selectively phosphorylated (135). Although it is tempting to link alpha-chain phosphorylation with the GpIb cytoskeletal interaction, the reaction is not regulated. For example, the degree of phosphorylation is not affected by incubation with either activators or inhibitors of platelet aggregation and release. This cytoskeletal interaction and the accompanying change in protein mobility may facilitate the binding of macromolecules such as thrombin and vWF to the platelet or may stabilize their interaction. However, there is evidence that purified GpIb binds vWF following insertion into artificial membrane vesicles (liposomes) that do not contain any cytoskeletal components (136). In addition, thrombin binds to solubilized, purified glycocalicin.

Glycoproteins IIb and IIIa

Glycoproteins IIb and IIIa form a noncovalent, calcium-dependent complex of 260,000 Mr (137). There are 50,000 copies of this heterodimer complex on each platelet, making it the most abundant platelet membrane protein (138). The complex contains cryptic receptor sites for several adhesive macromolecules, including fibrinogen, fibronectin, thrombospondin, and vWF, and is a major site for calcium binding. These latent receptors bind appropriate ligands following platelet activation.

The GpIIb subunit consists of an alpha-chain of 116,000 and a smaller beta-chain of 23,000 that are linked together by disulfide bonds. GpIIIa is a single chain polypeptide of 108,000 Mr that contains several intrachain disulfide bonds (137). Each of the two protein subunits contains 15 per cent carbohydrate arranged as a series of N-linked oligosaccharides. The subunits can be dissociated by calcium chelators such as EDTA that also inhibit receptor function. Although GpIIb/IIIa was originally thought to be a platelet-specific protein, molecules with immunologic cross-reactivity have now been detected in endothelial cells and several cultured hematopoietic cell lines (139, 140).

The most well defined function of GpIIb/IIIa is facilitation of platelet–platelet interactions (platelet aggregation) by provision of binding sites for multivalent ligands such as fibrinogen. The binding of fibrinogen occurs via specific sites on its alpha and gamma-chains (141). A tripeptide sequence, arg-gly-asp-ser, first described in the cellular adhesive domain of fibronectin, also is present in the alpha-chain of fibrinogen and near the carboxy terminus of vWF. It is responsible for the binding of all three adhesive proteins to the platelet IIb/IIIa site. In addition, fibrinogen has a second dodecapeptide sequence on the gamma-chain that also binds to GpIIb/IIIa. Following platelet aggregation, IIb/IIIa molecules become associated with the platelet cytoskeleton as determined by analysis of triton-insoluble ghosts (142).

In addition to its function as a binding site for adhesive proteins, the IIb/IIIa complex contains important platelet alloantigens. A 17,000-dalton fragment of GpIIIa contains the Pl[A1] antigen responsible for neonatal isoimmune thrombocytopenia and post-transfusion purpura (143). In addition, the Bak[a] antigen has been localized to

GpIIIa, and the Lek^a antigen has been shown to be on GpIIb (144). In addition to these alloantigens, there is evidence that the target antigens for the majority of the autoantibodies present in patients with ITP can be localized to GpIIIa (145). This specificity has been most convincingly demonstrated by the technique of Western blotting, in which platelet membranes are solubilized and proteins are separated by SDS-PAGE, transferred to nitrocellulose membranes, and overlaid with antiserum followed by a suitably labeled anti-immunoglobulin reagent (145).

Patients with Glanzmann's thrombasthenia have a striking reduction or a complete absence of GpIIb/IIIa. As expected, their platelets do not bind fibrinogen on the other adhesive glycoproteins, and they have a severe hemorrhagic disorder characterized by totally absent platelet aggregation. Because platelet binding of vWF to the GpIb site is not impaired, platelet adhesion is normal.

PLATELET ADHESION TO SUBENDOTHELIUM

As previously discussed, platelet adhesion to collagen in vascular subendothelium is critically important because it initiates hemostasis. Since collagen is readily extracted and purified from connective tissues, its reaction with platelets has been studied in great detail. The nature of the platelet–collagen interaction is being debated, although there are some areas of general agreement. With one notable exception, collagen from any source must form fibrils before it will promote platelet adhesion (146). Early studies suggested that collagen oligosaccharides were glycosylated by a platelet membrane enzyme and that this enzyme–substrate interaction provided a molecular basis for platelet adhesion (147, 148). Subsequent studies demonstrated that conditions used to remove carbohydrate from collagen also inhibited fibril formation. In addition, collagen that totally lacks detectable carbohydrate can still promote platelet adhesion (149). Several platelet membrane proteins have been proposed as collagen receptors, although none completely satisfies the criteria for a functional receptor. A patient with a hemostatic defect characterized by decreased adhesion to collagen has recently been described. This patient is missing a high-Mr platelet protein, GpIa, which may be a physiologically relevant collagen receptor site (150).

Collagen subtypes vary in their ability to induce adhesion and aggregation (151). Type III collagen is the most potent subtype (152). In addition, subtypes are asymmetrically distributed within the vascular subendothelium with an increase in Type III collagen near the intimal surface. These observations that collagen structure may influence platelet reactivity may help explain reports that patients with certain connective tissue disorders such as Marfan's syndrome and pseudoxanthoma elasticum have impaired hemostasis. Collagen derived from these patients does not induce normal platelet adhesion (153).

Many studies of the platelet–collagen interaction rely on platelet aggregation as an end-point. This may be inappropriate because only a small number of platelets adhere to the collagen fibrils. Aggregation results from the generation of mediators and the secretion of ADP from adherent platelets, which then activate nonadherent platelets. This technique is not a convenient way to simulate flow and standardize shear forces. Adhesion has been more closely stimulated by the technique developed by Baumgartner and colleagues, which involves the perfusion of de-endothelialized segments of blood vessels or collagen-coated surfaces with anticoagulated whole blood (154). As shown in Figure 40–8, platelets from the perfused blood initially form a monolayer that carpets the exposed subendothelium. These platelets then recruit additional pletelets from the flowing blood and build a platelet plug on top of the adherent monolayer. This system permits straightforward measurements of the percentage of vessel surface covered by platelets and the extent of platelet aggregate formation.

This perfusion model has been used to study blood from patients with hemostatic defects and to make clinical correlations. It has also provided a way to study the effects of flow and adhesive glycoproteins on platelet adhesion. For example, when blood from patients with von Willebrand's disease is perfused through the vessel segments, platelet adhesion is normal at low flow rates and decreases as flow rates and shear forces approach those seen in the microvasculature. Defective platelet adhesion at high shear forces can be completely corrected by the addition of a source of purified vWF or the addition of cryoprecipitate (155). In addition, platelets from patients with the rare Bernard-Soulier defect who lack GpIb and cannot bind vWF to this critical receptor do not adhere at high shear forces despite the presence of adequate plasma vWF.

In contrast, platelets perfused through matrix-coated chambers in the absence of fibronectin have reduced adhesion at all flow rates, suggesting a distinct function for this protein (156). These studies confirm earlier observations that fibronectin has a role in platelet adhesion and spreading. They also emphasize the idea that the formation of a stable union between platelets and the vessel wall requires structurally normal collagen, a normal platelet membrane, and the participation of several adhesive glycoproteins. The role of the two plasma glycoproteins that regulate platelet plug formation is diagrammed in Figure 40–10.

The most clinically relevant protein in the proc-

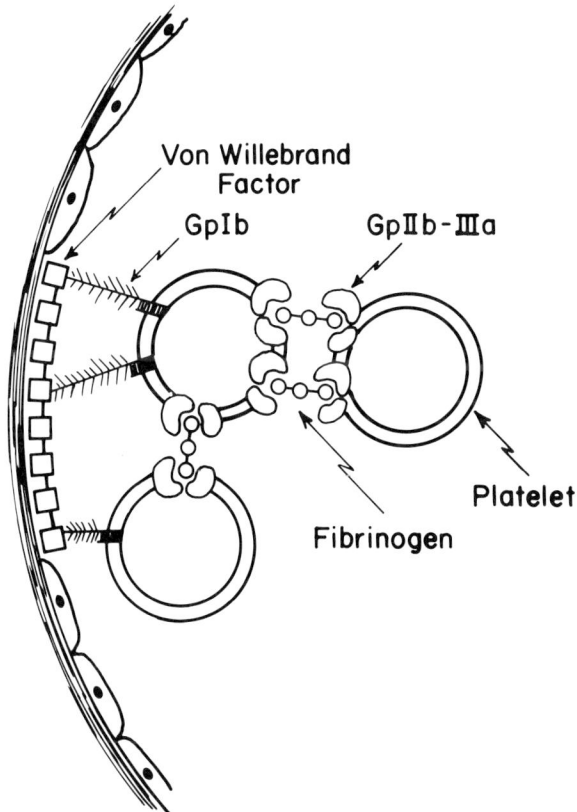

Figure 40–10. The role of adhesive proteins and platelet receptors in platelet adhesion and aggregation. (Adapted from Handin, R. I.: Bleeding and thrombosis. In *Harrison's Principles of Internal Medicine*. Braunwald, E., Isselbacher, K. J., et al. (eds.), New York, McGraw-Hill [in press].

ess of platelet adhesion is vWF, as deficiency or dysfunction of this molecule is a common cause of postoperative or spontaneous skin or mucous membrane bleeding. The cloning of vWF cDNA has provided new information about the structure and biosynthesis of this molecule and may provide tools to dissect the genetics of von Willebrand's disease (157). vWF is synthesized as a 300,000-kilodalton subunit polypeptide that is subsequently glycosylated, sulfated, and joined together into disulfide-linked dimers. A large (80,000-dalton) propolypeptide is cleaved from each subunit, and the resulting dimers are assembled into a heterogeneous series of multimers (158). vWF multimers are both continuously released from endothelial cells and stored in secretory granules (Weibel-Palade bodies) for later release (159).

As previously discussed, vWF facilitates platelet adhesion by bridging platelet membrane receptors and vascular subendothelium. The GpIb and collagen binding sites have been localized to a region in the amino terminal portion of the molecule, and the GpIIb/IIIa binding site has been found to be an arg-gly-asp sequence near the carboxyl terminus (160). Although each vWF subunit has the necessary collagen and platelet binding sites, it is clear from abundant clinical studies that vWF multimers of high molecular weight are needed for in vivo hemostasis.

PLATELET AGGREGATION

The process of platelet aggregation follows adhesion and converts the adherent platelet monolayer into a multicellular hemostatic plug (5a). Analysis is complicated because adhesion, granule secretion, and aggregate formation are closely related and each influences the other. In addition, aggregation requires blood flow for promotion of platelet contact. The platelet collisions required for aggregation induce platelets to release, and the released products in turn evoke new waves of aggregation.

One can conveniently quantify aggregation by observing and recording the change in light transmission of a platelet suspension following the addition of aggregating agents (161). A typical series of aggregation tracings is shown in Figure 40–11. High doses of ADP induce rapid and complete aggregation, incorporating virtually all the platelets in the suspension and causing a large monophasic aggregation tracing. Lower doses of ADP induce aggregation in two phases. The first phase results from a direct effect of ADP on the platelet membrane, and the second is caused by the release of granule ADP stores from the activated platelets. Collagen fibrils promote adhesion as previously described. The adherent platelets then release ADP and generate thromboxane A_2, both of which promote aggregation of all the platelets. This is reflected by a broad monophasic aggregation tracing with a long lag phase. The lag results from the time required for fibril formation and platelet adhesion, which do not affect light transmission. Epinephrine, which binds to platelet alpha$_2$-adrenergic receptors, causes a biphasic aggregation pattern, with initial aggregation due to receptor occupancy followed by a second wave generated by released ADP.

Although ADP is clearly an important mediator of aggregation, it acts synergistically with other agents such as thromboxane A_2. Attempts to block thromboxane production and to trap released ADP do not completely inhibit aggregation by potent agonists such as thrombin and collagen fibrils (162). Following its release, ADP binds to a distinct receptor site that then, as previously discussed, initiates fibrinogen binding to a latent receptor on the GpIIb/IIIa complex. Fibrinogen is a bivalent molecule that bridges adjacent platelets to form aggregates. Although there are both alpha- and gamma-chain binding sites, the gamma-chain dodecapeptide completely inhibits ADP-induced aggregation (141). In addition, incubation of platelets with a nucleotide analogue that competes for ADP binding sites, fluorosulfonylben-

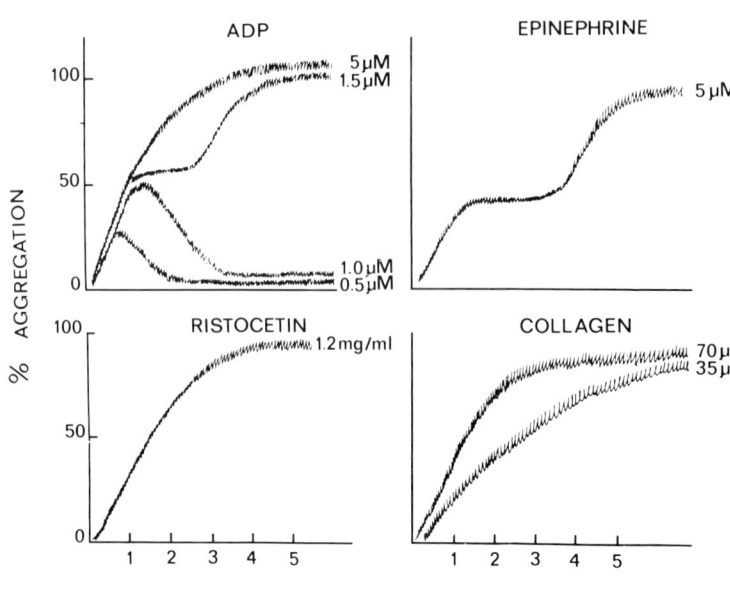

Figure 40–11. Normal platelet aggregation patterns. The amount of light transmitted through platelet-rich plasma suspensions following addition of aggregating agents is depicted. The samples are stirred continuously and warmed to 37°C.

zoyladenosine (FSBA), completely inhibits ADP-induced fibrinogen binding and platelet aggregation (163).

PLATELET SIGNAL TRANSDUCTION AND INTRACELLULAR MESSENGERS

All the major hemostatic reactions depend on appropriate "activation" of the platelet following the occupancy of platelet receptors by an appropriate ligand. This process of signal transduction is quite complex and involves the concerted action of phospholipid mediators such as inositol triphosphate and diacylglycerol, regulatory enzymes such as adenylate cyclase and protein kinase C, transient changes in intraplatelet ionized calcium levels, and selective phosphorylation of critical intracellular proteins. Our knowledge of these reactions has grown enormously, and the platelet has played a critical role as a model cell in studies of signal transduction.

Exposure of platelets to any of the agents that induce aggregation and release activates an intraplatelet enzyme, phospholipase C, which rapidly hydrolyzes a minor phospholipid species, phosphoinositol 4,5 bisphosphate (PIP_2), located predominantly within the inner leaflet of the platelet membrane, to produce inositol triphosphate (IP_3) and diacylglycerol (DAG) (Fig. 40–12). IP_3 can function as a calcium ionophore, mobilizing intraplatelet calcium stores (164). DAG specifically activates a second enzyme, protein kinase C, which phosphorylates a number of critical intracellular proteins that control platelet shape change, granule secretion, and aggregation (165). The requirement for receptor activation and PIP_2 hydrolysis can be bypassed and the platelet directly activated with appropriate experimental reagents. For example, oleylacylglycerol (OAG), a derivative of DAG and IP_3, can enter platelets that have become permeable and directly raise calcium stores and activate protein kinase C (166). In addition, protein kinase C can be directly activated by a lipid-soluble phorbol ester such as phorbol myristate

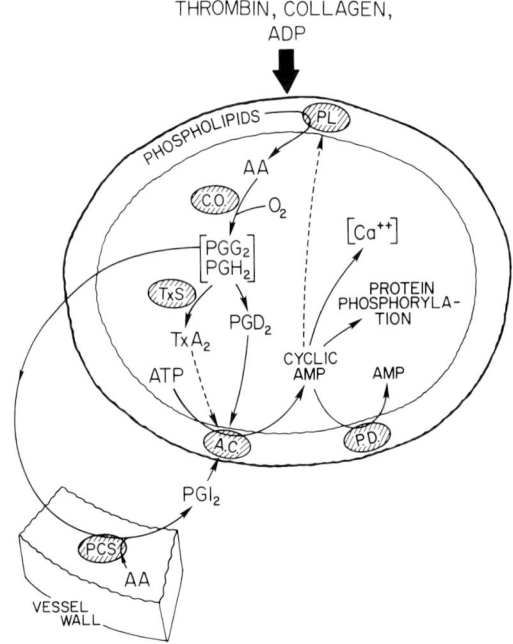

Figure 40–12. The metabolism of arachidonic acid into prostaglandins and related compounds is depicted. *PL*, phospholipase; *CO*, cyclo-oxygenase; *TxS*, thromboxane synthetase; *A.C.*, adenylate cyclase; *P.D.*, phosphodiesterase; *PCS*, prostacyclin synthetase.

acetate (PMA), which then induces platelet activation and secretion (176). Although the critical intracellular phosphorylation steps are not fully defined, two prominent phosphorylated products have been identified: the light chain of the contractile protein myosin and a 47,000-dalton protein of uncertain function (168). There is recent evidence that the 47,000-dalton protein is a phosphatase that inactivates IP_3 and thereby limits platelet aggregation and secretion. Phosphorylation of these two proteins correlates closely with secretion and aggregation.

The second major intracellular messenger is cyclic AMP (cAMP), which also regulates the phosphorylation of intracellular proteins via protein kinase A and the calcium calmodulin complex (169). Binding of an appropriate stimulatory or inhibitory ligand to its receptor activates a stimulatory or inhibitory GTP-dependent regulatory protein (G_s and G_i proteins), which then stimulate or inhibit adenylate cyclase. The extent to which all agonists regulate adenylate cyclase is uncertain because many agonists such as thrombin and ADP have little effect on enzyme activity in membrane preparations. However, it is clear that the system plays an important role in limiting the extent of platelet aggregation and secretion. Platelet PGI_2 and PGD_2 receptors are coupled to G_s proteins. Receptor activation then stimulates adenylate cyclase and inhibits platelet aggregation and release. Occupancy of the alpha$_2$ adrenergic receptor by epinephrine couples it to a G_i protein, which then inhibits adenylate cyclase activity. Inhibition of adenylate cyclase activity correlates with platelet activation and secretion. Although some of the details regarding these two intracellular messenger systems are still incomplete, it is clear that they are of major importance and control function in a wide variety of cells, including the platelet.

ARACHIDONIC ACID TRANSFORMATION IN PLATELET AND ENDOTHELIAL CELLS

Arachidonic acid is an essential polyunsaturated fatty acid that is present in very high concentrations in platelet membrane and granule phospholipids (170). When platelets are activated, they liberate large quantities of arachidonic acid. The arachidonic acid is then peroxidized and transformed into a number of biologically active compounds (171). There are two major sources of arachidonic acid for biotransformation. Some of the DAG liberated by phospholipase C is rapidly hydrolyzed by a diglyceride lipase to liberate arachidonic acid (172). A second enzyme, phospholipase A_2, which acts more slowly, releases additional arachidonic acid from the two other major phospholipids, PC and PS (173). The pathways for biotransformation of arachidonic acid and the function of various products are outlined in Figure 40–13.

A portion of the liberated arachidonic acid is converted by the enzyme cyclo-oxygenase to the unstable prostaglandin endoperoxide PGG_2. PGG_2 is subsequently converted to the nonprostaglandin derivative, thromboxane A_2, which induces platelet aggregation and secretion (174, 175), and is a

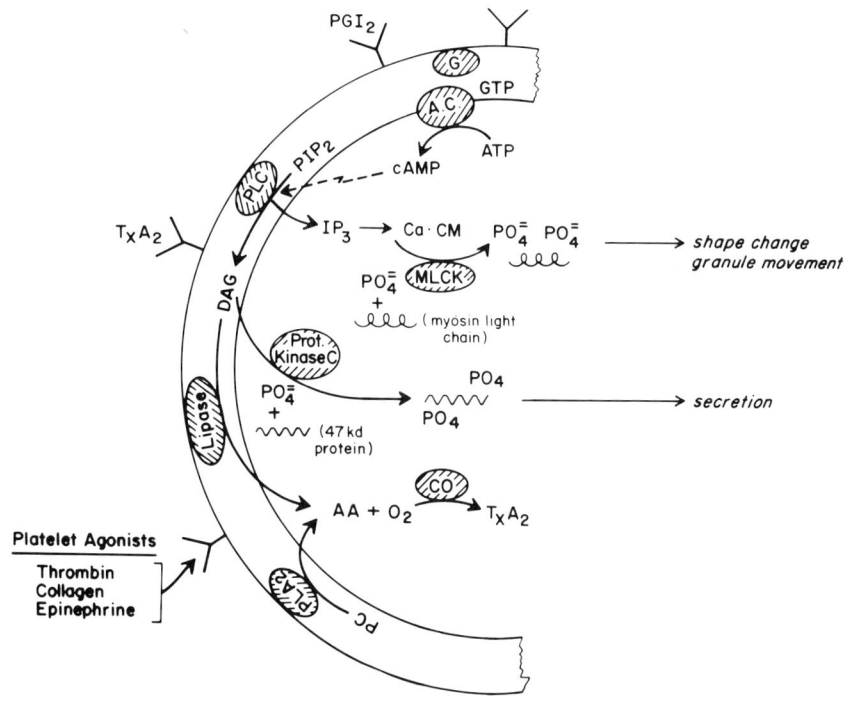

Figure 40–13. The role of phospholipid metabolites in platelet function is depicted. AC, adenylate cyclase; G, regulatory nucleotide binding proteins; PLC, phospholipase C; lipase, diglyceride lipase; PLA_2, phospholipase A_2; MLCK, myosin light chain kinase; CM, calmodulin. (Adapted from Handin, R. I.: Bleeding and thrombosis. In Harrison's Principles of Internal Medicine. Braunwald, E., Isselbacher, K. J., et al. (eds.), New York, McGraw-Hill. In press.)

potent vasoconstrictor (176). Some of the endoperoxide spontaneously breaks down to produce an inactive 17-carbon hydroxy fatty acid (HHT) and malondialdehyde, and a minor fraction forms stable prostaglandins such as PGD_2, which may inhibit platelet reactivity (177).

A second major pathway, controlled by the enzyme lipoxygenase, converts arachidonic acid to a 12-OH fatty acid (HETE). Neither HHT nor HETE have any effect on platelets but may be chemotactic for neutrophils and play a role in inflammation (178). The generation of these mediators by activated platelets may explain the close association of neutrophils and platelets in hemostatic plugs.

Clearly, thromboxane A_2 and, to a lesser extent, PGG_2 and PGH_2 can induce platelet aggregation and release (179, 180). The relative importance of the arachidonic acid metabolites in platelet function is a subject of some debate. However, it should be apparent that this is one of several pathways that lead to induction of platelet activation (181). Furthermore, total suppression of endoperoxide-thromboxane production by cyclo-oxygenase inhibitors such as aspirin and indomethacin will produce only a mild hemostatic defect. Platelets from an individual who has ingested sufficient aspirin to suppress thromboxane production totally will readily aggregate when exposed to slightly higher concentrations of collagen and thrombin and react normally to high concentrations of ADP. This is also reflected in the modest prolongation of the bleeding time—a good measure of in vivo hemostasis that accompanies aspirin ingestion. The most logical conclusion is that arachidonic acid derivatives amplify platelet responses but are not solely responsible for platelet secretion and aggregation.

In addition, the possibility that thromboxane A_2 functions primarily as a local vasoconstrictor cannot be overlooked. Thromboxane A_2 causes constriction of coronary and cerebral arterial strips in vitro (182, 183) and may be responsible for the vasoconstriction and vessel "retraction" that accompany injury. In certain situations, thromboxane A_2 may contribute to tissue ischemia by causing vascular spasm. This inappropriate or excessive vasoconstriction may contribute to clinical episodes of coronary and cerebral arterial ischemia.

Studies of the biogenesis and metabolism of prostaglandins and thromboxanes have helped clarify the nature of several congenital platelet disorders as well as the nature of the defects induced by nonsteroidal anti-inflammatory drugs. A single dose of aspirin inhibits platelet function for 5 to 7 days by irreversibly acetylating a serine residue near the active site of platelet cyclo-oxygenase (184). This impairs subsequent endoperoxide and thromboxane synthesis for the life of the platelet because the cell cannot synthesize new enzyme. Cyclo-oxygenase activity in other tissues recovers more rapidly because nucleated cells synthesize new enzyme. This relatively selective antiplatelet effect has been utilized to develop aspirin as an antithrombotic agent. Although the results have been mixed, there is evidence that aspirin may reduce the incidence of secondary strokes and myocardial infarcts (185, 186). It is less effective in preventing venous thromboembolism, in which platelets play a smaller role. Finally, there is some evidence that the antithrombotic action of aspirin may reduce the incidence of obstructive lesions and thrombosis in children with Kawasaki's syndrome (187).

A number of patients who have lifelong histories of easy bruising and mild bleeding actually have defects in platelet aggregation and release that resemble those of patients who have received aspirin (189). Several different defects have been described, including congenital deficiency of cyclo-oxygenase (189) and a loss of platelet receptors for thromboxane A_2 (190). It also is of interest that the administration of dietary supplements containing highly unsaturated fatty acids, such as eicosapentanoic acid (20:5), may exert their beneficial antithrombotic and anti-inflammatory effects by competing with arachidonic acid and producing biologically inactive derivatives (191). This procedure may provide an interesting new way to prevent the development of vascular atherosclerotic lesions and may partially explain the beneficial effects of diets rich in fish products.

Vascular endothelial cells produce a unique prostaglandin—PGI_2, or prostacyclin—which inhibits platelet aggregation and release and is a potent vasodilator (192). Mechanical injury and exposure to agonists such as thrombin and bradykinin can induce endothelial production of PGI_2. The substrate for PGI_2 can be either endogenous endothelial cell arachidonate or exogenous endoperoxide derived from activated platelets (193). Secretion of PGI_2 by endothelial cells may provide a way to regulate the rate and extent of platelet plug formation on adjacent subendothelium. Prostacyclin infusion has been used as a pharmacologic means to reduce platelet consumption and heparin requirements during cardiopulmonary bypass and as a substitute for heparin during hemodialysis (194, 195).

These studies suggest also that there may be a normal balance between platelet and endothelial cell arachidonic acid metabolism that produces compounds that stimulate and inhibit platelet aggregation and vessel constriction. Any illness or therapy that disturbs this balance may produce a hemostatic or thrombotic defect. For example, agents that decrease thromboxane A_2 production cause mild bleeding, and manipulations that increase vascular production of PGI_2 should have a similar effect. There are some data suggesting that

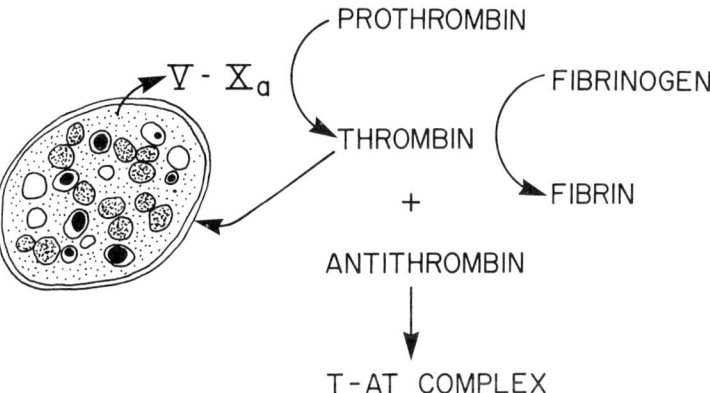

Figure 40–14. The role of platelets in coagulation. Platelets secrete an active form of Factor V that then acts as a receptor for Factor Xa. Following binding to the platelet surface, Factor Xa accelerates the conversion of prothrombin to thrombin. Thrombin can then bind to the platelet and induce further secretion or convert fibrinogen to fibrin. Antithrombin, in plasma, inactivates thrombin by formation of a thrombin-antithrombin complex. Thrombin bound to the platelets may be relatively resistant to inhibition by antithrombin.

uremic individuals who have defective platelet function in vivo and clinical bleeding may have an increase in vascular prostacyclin (196). Conversely, maneuvers that decrease PGI_2 production or increase thromboxane production might provoke thrombosis. Platelets from patients with diabetes and vascular disease produce increased quantities of prostaglandins (197). These studies point out the possibility that defects within the vessel wall may perturb normal platelet function and must be considered when either bleeding or thrombotic episodes are being analyzed.

PLATELET COAGULANT ACTIVITY

The idea that activated platelets accelerate plasma coagulation reactions has evolved over several decades. However, the precise nature of the platelet constituents responsible for the activity remains unclear. There is some evidence that if a platelet phospholipoprotein is exposed or modified during platelet activation, coagulation reactions may be promoted. This platelet property has been referred to as platelet factor 3 (PF-3) activity. It is important to note that no specific lipid fraction has been identified that is responsible for PF-3 activity and that such activity appears to be a general property of many cell membranes (198). In addition, platelet granule fractions are particularly rich in PF-3 activity (199).

Most previous work on platelet coagulant activity has focused on the lipid-dependent coagulation reactions, such as the interaction of Factors VIII, IX, and X and the interaction of Factors X, V, and prothrombin (200). Walsh proposed that activated platelets also catalyzed several early coagulation reactions such as the activation of Factors XII and XI (201). However, the precise nature of this platelet property has not been defined.

Some information has appeared that demonstrates that platelets can directly bind activated Factor X and then rapidly convert prothrombin to thrombin (Fig. 40–14) (202). Work from several laboratories has suggested that the Factor Xa binding site on platelets may actually be a form of Factor V, secreted after platelet activation (203). The binding reaction has been extensively studied and quantified, and binding has been precisely correlated with prothrombin conversion. These studies provide a new mechanism for so-called PF-3 activity and suggest that this activity may not reside solely in platelet lipid but may also involve the participation of secreted proteins such as Factor V.

SUMMARY

This chapter has focused primarily on the role of platelets in hemostasis—hemostasis being the process by which blood is prevented from leaving damaged blood vessels. Although the emphasis has been on intraluminal platelet plug formation, it should be clear that the platelet extends its influence beyond the hemostatic plug. It generates molecules that can regulate vascular tone and the inflammatory response and secretes proteins that accelerate plasma coagulation reactions and stimulate vessel wall repair. Viewed in this way, the platelet becomes a multifunctional cell with many important biologic roles.

The entire subject of the role of the platelet in atherosclerotic vascular disease and thromboembolism has been avoided because these are not major pediatric problems. It should be emphasized, in closing, that this other facet of the hemostatic system is of great interest to physicians who deal with adults and that it may receive increasing attention in the pediatric literature as physicians focus on the prevention of vascular disease, which actually begins to develop shortly after birth.

References

1. Bizzozero, G.: Sulla funzione ematopoietica del midollo delle osse. Seconda communicazione preventia. Zentrabl. Med. Wissenschr. *10*:149, 1869.
2. George, J. N.: Molecular defects in interactions of platelets with the vessel wall. New Engl. J. Med. *311*:1084, 1984.

3. Nishizuka, Y.: The role of protein kinase C in cell surface signal transduction and tumor promotion. Nature 308:693, 1984.
4. Berridge, M. J., and Irvine, R. F.: Inositol triphosphate, a novel second messenger in cellular signal transduction. Nature 312:315, 1984.
5. Plow, E. F., Srouji, A. H., et al.: Evidence that three adhesive proteins interact with a common recognition site on activated platelets. J. Biol. Chem. 259:5388, 1984.
5a. Day, H. J., and Rao, A. K.: Platelets and megakaryocytes. V. Evaluation of platelet function. Semin. Hematol. 23:89, 1986.
6. Nakahata, T., and Ogawa, M.: Clonal origin of murine hemopoietic colonies with apparent restriction to granulocyte-macrophage-megakaryocyte (GMM) differentiation. J. Cell. Physiol. 111:239, 1982.
7. Levine, R. F., Bunn, P. A., Jr., et al.: Flow cytometric analysis of megakaryocyte ploidy. Blood 56:210, 1980.
8. Levine, R. F.: Old and new aspects of megakaryocyte development and function. In *Megakaryocyte Development and Function*. Levine, R. F., Williams, N., et al. (eds.), New York, A. R. Liss, 1986, pp. 1–20.
9. Harker, L. A.: Control of platelet production. Ann. Rev. Med. 25:383, 1974.
10. Ishibashi, T., and Burstein, S. A.: Separation of megakaryocytes on continuous gradients of Percoll: evidence that maturity is inversely related to density. Thromb. Hemost. 54:279, 1985.
11. Levine, R. F., and Fedorko, M. E.: Isolation of intact megakaryoctes from guinea pig femoral marrow. J. Cell Biol. 69:159, 1976.
12. Rabellino, E. M., Nachman, R. L., et al.: Human megakaryocytes. II. Expression of platelet proteins in early marrow megakaryocytes. J. Exp. Med. 149:1273, 1979.
13. Nachman, R., Levine, R., Jaffe, E. A.: Synthesis of factor VIII antigen by cultured guinea pig megakaryocytes. J. Clin. Invest. 60:914, 1977.
14. Williams, N., Jackson, H., et al.: Regulation of megakaryocytopoiesis in long-term marrow cultures. Blood 51:245, 1978.
15. Williams, N., McDonald, T. P., et al.: Maturation and regulation of megakaryocytopoiesis. Blood Cells 5:43, 1979.
16. Williams, N., Eger, R. R., et al.: Two-factor requirement for murine megakaryocyte colony formation. J. Cell. Physiol. 110:101, 1982.
17. Quesenberry, P. J.: The effect of interleukin 3 and GM-CSA-2 on megakaryocyte and myeloid cloned colony formation. Blood 62:214, 1985.
18. Burstein, S. A.: Interleukin-3 is sufficient to promote murine megakaryocyte differentiation in vitro. In *Megakaryocyte Development and Function*. Levine, R. F., Williams, N., et al. (eds.), New York, A. R. Liss, 1986, pp. 247–252.
18a. Kawakita, M., Yamamota, S., et al.: Human urinary megakaryocyte colony-stimulating factor in thrombopoietic disorders. Br. J. Haematol. 62:715, 1986.
19. Evatt, B. L., Levin, J., et al.: Partial purification of thrombopoietin from the plasma of thrombocytopenic rabbits. Blood 54:377, 1979.
20. Miyake, T., Kawakita, M., et al.: Partial purification and biological properties of thrombopoietin extracted from the urine of aplastic anemia patients. Stem Cells 2:129, 1982.
21. Shreiner, D. P., and Levin, J.: Detection of thrombopoietic activity in plasma by stimulation of suppressed thrombopoiesis. J. Clin. Invest. 49:1709, 1970.
22. Williams, N., Jackson, H., et al.: The role of erythropoietin, thrombopoietic stimulating factor, and myeloid colony-stimulating factors on murine megakaryocyte colony formation. Exp. Hematol. 12:734, 1984.
23. Burstein, S. A., Adamson, J. A., et al.: Megakaryocytopoiesis in the mouse: response to varying platelet demand. J. Cell. Physiol. 109:333, 1981.
24. Greenberg, S. M., Kuter, D. J., et al.: In vitro stimulation of megakaryocyte maturation by megakaryocyte stimulating factor. J. Biol. Chem. In press.
25. Harker, L. A., and Finch, C. A.: Thrombokinetics in man. J. Clin Invest. 48:963, 1969.
26. Garg, S. K., Amorosi, E., et al.: Use of the megathrombocyte as an index of megakaryocyte number. New Engl. J. Med. 284:11, 1971.
27. Thompson, C. B., Love, D. G., et al.: Platelet size does not correlate with platelet age. Blood 62:487, 1983.
28. Karpatkin, S.: Heterogeneity of human platelets. I. Metabolic and kinetic evidence suggestive of young and old platelets. J. Clin. Invest. 48:1073, 1969.
29. Karpatkin, S.: Heterogeneity of human platelets. II. Functional evidence suggestive of young and old platelets. J. Clin. Invest. 48:1083, 1969.
30. Paulus, J. M.: Platelet size in man. Blood 46:321, 1975.
31. Evatt, B. L., Levin, J.: Measurement of thrombopoiesis in rabbits using [75]selenomethionine. J. Clin. Invest. 48:1615, 1960.
32. Penington, D. G., and Olsen, T. E.: Megakaryocytes in states of altered platelet production: cell numbers, size, and DNA content. Br. J. Haematol. 18:447, 1970.
33. Paulus, J. M., Bury, J., et al.: Control of platelet territory development in megakaryocytes. Blood Cells 5:59, 1979.
34. Ebbe, S.: Biology of megakaryocytes. In *Progress in Hemostasis and Thrombosis*, vol. 3. Spaet, T. H. (ed.), New York, Grune & Stratton, 1976, pp. 211–228.
34a. Rao, A. K., and Homser, H.: Congenital disorders of platelet function. Semin. Hematol. 23:102, 1986.
35. Harker, L. A.: The role of the spleen in thrombokinetics. J. Lab. Clin. Med. 77:247, 1970.
36. Maldonado, J. E., Pintado, T., et al.: Dysplastic platelets and circulating megakaryocytes in chronic myeloproliferative diseases. I. The platelet: ultrastructure and peroxidase reaction, Blood 43:797, 1974.
37. Lagerlöf, B., and Franzén, S.: The ultrastructure of megakaryocytes in polycythemia vera and chronic granulocytic leukemia. Acta Pathol. Microbiol. Scand. (A) 80:71, 1972.
38. Bolin, B. B., Okumara, T., et al.: Changes in distribution of membrane glycoproteins in patients with myeloproliferative disorders. Am. J. Hematol. 3:63, 1977.
39. Kaywin, P. M., McDonough, P., et al.: Platelet function and essential thrombosthenia. New Engl. J. Med. 299:505, 1978.
40. Keenan, J. P., Wharton, J., et al.: Defective lipid peroxidation in myeloproliferative disorders: a possible defect of prostaglandin synthesis. Br. J. Haematol. 35:275, 1977.
41. Corash, L., Shafer, B., et al.: Platelet-associated immunoglobulin, platelet size and effect of splenectomy in the Wiskott-Aldrich syndrome. Blood 65:1439, 1985.
42. Murphy, S., Oski, F. A., et al.: Platelet size and kinetics in hereditary and acquired thrombocytopenia. New Engl. J. Med. 286:499, 1972.
42a. Kohler, M., Hellstern, P., et al.: Gray platelet syndrome: selective alpha-granule deficiency and thrombocytopenia due to increased platelet turnover. Blut 50:331, 1985.
43. George, J. N., Lewis, P. C., et al.: Studies on platelet plasma membranes. II. Characterization of surface proteins of rabbit platelets in vitro and during circulation in vivo using diazotized (^{125}I)-diiodo sulfanilic acid as a label. J. Lab. Clin. Med. 88:247, 1976.
44. George, J. N., and Lewis, P. C.: Studies on platelet plasma membranes. III. Membrane glycoprotein loss from circulating platelets in rabbits: inhibition by aspirin-dipyridamole and acceleration by thrombin. J. Lab. Clin. Med. 91:301, 1978.
45. Reimers, J. J., Packham, M. A., et al.: Effect of repeated treatment of rabbit platelets with low concentrations of

thrombin on their function, metabolism and survival. Br. J. Haematol. 25:675, 1973.
46. Dassin, E., and Najean, Y.: The use of ^{75}Se-methionine as a tracer of thrombopoiesis I. In vivo incorporation of the tracer into platelet proteins: a biochemical study. Acta Haematol. 61:61, 1979.
47. Mustard, J. F., Rowsell, H. C., et al.: Platelet economy (platelet survival and turnover). Br. J. Haematol. 12:1, 1966.
48. Heyssel, R. M.: Determination of human platelet survival utilizing C-14-labelled serotonin. J. Clin. Invest. 40:2134, 1961.
49. Aas, K. A., and Gardner, F.: Survival of blood platelets labeled with chromium[51]. J. Clin. Invest. 37:1257, 1958.
50. Shulman, N. R., Watkins, S. P., Jr., et al.: Evidence that the spleen retains the youngest and hemostatically most effective platelets. Trans. Assoc. Am. Phys. 81:302, 1968.
51. Jandl, J. H., and Aster, R. H.: Increased splenic pooling and the pathogenesis of hypersplenism. Am. J. Med. Sci. 253:383, 1967.
52. Harker, L. A., and Slichter, S. J.: Studies of platelet and fibrinogen kinetics in patients with prosthetic heart valves. New Engl. J. Med. 287:1302, 1970.
53. Harker, L. A., and Slichter, S. J.: Platelet and fibrinogen consumption in man. New Engl. J. Med. 287:999, 1972.
54. Scott, S., Reimers, H. J., et al.: Effect of viruses on platelet aggregation and platelet survival in rabbits. Blood 52:47, 1978.
55. Abrahamsen, A. F.: Platelet survival studies in man. Scand. J. Haematol. 3(Suppl.):7, 1968.
56. Murphy, E. A., and Francis, M. E.: The estimation of blood platelet survival. II. The multiple hit model. Thromb. Diath. Haemorrh. 25:53, 1971.
57. Abrahamsen, A. F.: Survival of ^{51}Cr labeled autologous and isologous platelets as differential diagnostic aid in thrombocytopenic states. Scand. J. Haematol. 7:525, 1970.
58. Najean, Y., Ardailous, N., et al.: The platelet destruction site in thrombocytopenic purpuras. Br. J. Haematol. 13:409, 1967.
59. Aster, R. H., and Keene, W. R.: Sites of platelet destruction in idiopathic thrombocytopenic purpura. Br. J. Haematol. 16:61, 1969.
60. Scheffel, U., McIntyre, P. A., et al.: Evaluation of Indium-III as a new high photon yield gamma-emitting "physiological" platelet label. Johns Hopkins Med. J. 140:285, 1977.
61. Wiston, B. W., Grossman, Z. D., et al.: Labelling of platelets with oxine complexes of Tc-99m and In-III. J. Nucl. Med. 19:483, 1978.
62. Ezekowitz, M. D., Pope, C. F., et al.: Indium[111] platelet scintigraphy for the diagnosis of acute venous thrombosis. Circulation 73:668, 1986.
63. Finklestein, S., Miller, A., et al.: Imaging of acute arterial injury with 111-In–labelled platelets: a comparison with scanning electron micrographs. Radiology 145:155, 1982.
64. Powers, W. J.: In[111] platelet scintigraphy: carotid atherosclerosis and stroke. J. Nucl. Med. 25:626, 1984.
65. Lind, S. E., and Stossel, T. P.: The microfilament network of the platelet. In Progress in Hemostasis and Thrombosis. Spaet, T. H. (ed.), New York, Grune & Stratton, 1982, pp. 63–84.
66. White, J. G., and Gerrard, J. M.: Interaction of microtubules and microfilaments in platelet contractile physiology. Meth. Achiev. Exp. Pathol. 9:1, 1979.
67. Zucker, M. B., and Borelli, J.: Reversible alterations in platelet morphology produced by anticoagulants and by cold. Blood 9:602, 1954.
68. White, J. G., and Krivit, W.: An ultrastructural basis for the shape changes induced in platelets by chilling. Blood 30:625, 1967.
69. White, J. G.: Effects of colchicine and vinca alkaloids on human platelets. III. Influence on primary internal contraction and secondary aggregation. Am. J. Pathol. 54:467, 1969.
70. Zucker-Franklin, D.: Microfibrils of blood platelets: their relationship to microtubules and the contractile protein. J. Clin. Invest. 48:165, 1969.
71. Zucker-Franklin, D., and Grusky, G.: The actin and myosin filaments of human and bovine blood platelets. J. Clin. Invest. 51:419, 1972.
72. Nachmias, V. T.: Cytoskeleton of human platelets at rest and after spreading. J. Cell Biol. 86:795, 1980.
73. Yin, H. L., and Stossel, T. P.: Control of cytoplasmic actin gel-sol transformation by gelsolin, a calcium-dependent regulatory protein. Nature 218:583, 1979.
74. Adelstein, R. S., and Conti, M. A.: Phosphorylation of platelet myosin increases actin-activated myosin ATPase activity. Nature 256:597, 1975.
75. White, J. G.: Electron microscopic studies of platelet secretion. In Progress in Hemostasis and Thrombosis, vol. 2. Spaet, T. H. (ed.), New York, Grune & Stratton, 1974, pp. 49–98.
76. Ling, S. E., Yin, H. L. Stossel, T. P.: Human platelets contain gelsolin, a regulator of actin filament length. J. Clin. Invest. 69:1384, 1982.
77. Holmsen, H.: Platelet secretion. In Mechanism of Hemostasis and Thrombosis. Mielke, C. H. (ed.), Miami FL, Symposia Specialists, 1978, pp. 73–109.
78. Broekman, H. J., Handin, R. I., et al.: Distribution of fibrinogen and platelet factors 4 and XIII in subcellular fractions of human platelets. Br. J. Haematol. 31:51, 1974.
79. Nachman, R. L., and Jaffe, E. A.: Subcellular platelet factor VIII. J. Exp. Med. 141:1101, 1975.
80. Østerud, B., Rapaport, S. I., et al.: Factor V activity of platelets: evidence for an activated factor V molecule and for a platelet activator. Blood 49:819, 1977.
81. Handin, R. I., and Cohen, H. J.: Purification and binding properties of human platelet factor four. J. Biol. Chem. 251:4273, 1976.
82. Handin, R. I.: Clinical significance of platelet factor four. In Mechanism of Hemostasis and Thrombosis. Mielke, C. H. (ed.), Miami FL, Symposia Specialists, 1978, pp. 183–202.
83. Antoniades, H. N., and Scher, C. D.: Radioimmunoassay of a human serum growth factor for Balb/c 3T3 cells: derivation from platelets. Proc. Natl. Acad. Sci. U. S. A. 74:1973, 1977.
84. Friedman, R. J., Stemerman, M. B., et al.: The effect of thrombocytopenia on experimental arteriosclerotic lesion formation in rabbits. Smooth muscle cell proliferation and reendothelialization. J. Clin. Invest. 60:1191, 1977.
85. Ross, R., and Glomset, J.: The pathogenesis of atherosclerosis. New Engl. J. Med. 295:369, 402, 1976.
86. Deuel, T. F., and Huang, J. S.: Platelet-derived growth factor. Structure, function and roles in normal and transformed cells. J. Clin. Invest. 74:669, 1984.
87. Graves, D. T., Owen, A. J., et al.: Detection of c-sis transcripts and synthesis of PGDF-like proteins by human osteosarcoma cells. Science 226:972, 1984.
88. Collins, T., Ginsburg, D., et al.: Cultured human endothelial cells express platelet-derived growth factor B chain: cDNA cloning and structural analysis. Nature 316:748, 1985.
89. Needleman, P., Minkes, M., et al.: Cardiac and coronary prostaglandin synthesis and function. New Engl. J. Med. 298:1122, 1978.
90. Holmsen, H., and Weiss, H. J.: Further evidence for a deficient storage pool of adenine nucleotides in platelets from some patients with thrombocytopathia—"storage pool disease." Blood 39:197, 1972.
91. Warshaw, A. L., Laster, L., et al.: The stimulation by thrombin of glucose oxidation in human platelets. J. Clin. Invest. 45:1923, 1966.

92. Detwiler, T. C.: Control of energy metabolism in platelets. The effects of thrombin and cyanide on glycolysis. Biochem. Biophys. Acta 256:163, 1972.
93. Chaudry, A. A., Sagone, A. L., et al.: Relationship of glucose oxidation to aggregation of human platelets. Blood 41:249, 1973.
94. McElroy, F. A., Kinlough-Rathbone, R., et al.: The effect of aggregating agents or oxidative metabolism of rabbit platelets. Biochem. Biophys. Acta 253:64, 1971.
95. Murer, E. H., Hellem, H. J., et al.: Energy metabolism and platelet function. Scand. J. Clin. Invest. 19:280, 1960.
96. Miller, D. R., and Wollman, M. R.: A new variant of glucose-6-phosphate dehydrogenase deficiency hereditary hemolytic anemia, G6PD Cornell: erythrocyte, leukocyte and platelet studies. Blood 44:323, 1974.
97. Czapek, E. E., Deyskin, D., et al.: Platelet dysfunction in glycogen storage disease. Type I. Blood 41:235, 1971.
98. Kuramoto, A., Steiner, M., et al.: Lack of platelet response to stimulation in the Wiskott-Aldrich syndrome. New Engl. J. Med. 82:475, 1970.
99. Shapiro, R. S., Perry, G. S., et al.: Wiskott-Aldrich syndrome: detection of carrier state by metabolic stress of platelets. Lancet 1:121, 1978.
100. Parkman, R., Remold, E., et al.: Surface protein abnormality in lymphocytes and platelets from patients with Wiskott-Aldrich syndrome. Lancet 2:1387, 1981.
101. Kitchens, C. S., and Weiss, L.: Ultrastructural changes of endothelium associated with thrombocytopenia. Blood 46:567, 1975.
102. Wojcik, J. D., and Van Horn, D. L.: Mechanism whereby platelets support the endothelium. Transfusion 9:324, 1969.
103. Kitchens, C. S.: Amelioration of endothelial abnormalities by prednisone in experimental thrombocytopenia in the rabbit. J. Clin. Invest. 60:1129, 1977.
104. Bevilacqua, M. P., Pober, J. S., et al.: Interleukin 1 (IL-1) induces biosynthesis and cell surface expression of procoagulant activity in human vascular endothelial cells. J. Exp. Med. 160:618, 1984.
105. Stern, D. M., Nawroth, P. P., et al.: A coagulation pathway on bovine aortic segments leading to generation of factor Xa and thrombin. J. Clin. Invest. 74:1910, 1984.
106. Loskutoff, D. J., and Mussoni, L.: Interactions between fibrin and the plasminogen activators produced by cultured endothelial cells. Blood 62:62, 183.
107. Bretscher, M. S., and Raff, M. C.: Mammalian plasma membranes. Nature 258:43, 1971.
108. Rothman, J.E., and Lenard, J.: Membrane asymmetry. Science 195:743, 1977.
109. Berridge, M. J., and Irvine, R. F.: Inositol triphosphate, a novel second messenger in cellular signal transduction. Nature 312:315, 1984.
110. Shattil, S. J., Anaya-Galindo, R., et al.: Platelet hypersensitivity induced by cholesterol incorporation. J. Clin. Invest. 55:636, 1975.
111. Shattil, S. J., and Cooper, R. A.: Membrane microviscosity and human platelet function. Biochemistry 15:4832, 1976.
112. Nachman, R. L., Hubbard, A., et al.: Iodination of the human platelet membrane. Studies on the major surface glycoprotein. J. Biol. Chem. 248:2928, 1973.
113. Gahmberg, C. G., and Andersson, L. C.: Selective radioactive labeling of cell surface sialoglycoproteins by periodate-tritiated borohydride. J. Biol. Chem., 252:5888, 1977.
114. Phillips, D. R., and Agin, P. P.: Platelet membrane glycoproteins. Evidence for the presence of non-equivalent disulfide bonds using nonreduced-reduced two dimensional electrophoresis. J. Biol. Chem. 252:2121, 1977.
115. Berndt, M. C., and Caen, J. P.: Platelet glycoproteins. In Progress in Thrombosis and Hemostasis, vol. 7. Spaet, T. H. (ed.), New York, Grune & Stratton, 1984, pp. 111–150.
116. Berndt, M. C., Gregory, C., et al.: Additional glycoprotein defects in Bernard-Soulier's syndrome. Confirmation of genetic basis by parental analysis. Blood 62:800, 1983.
117. Berndt, M. C., and Phillips, D. R.: Purification and preliminary physicochemical characterization of human platelet membrane glycoprotein V. J. Biol. Chem. 256:59, 1981.
118. Clemetson, K. J., Wicki, A., and Luscher, E. F.: Cleavage of platelet membrane glycoprotein Ib by calcium-activated protease. Thromb. Hemost. 50:187, 1983.
119. Clemetson, K. J., Naim, H. Y., Luscher, E. F.: Relationship between glycocalicin and glycoprotein Ib of human platelets. Proc. Natl. Acad. Sci. U. S. A. 78:2712, 1981.
120. Yoshida, N., Weksler, B., et al.: Purification of human platelet calcium-activated protease: effect on platelet and endothelial function. J. Biol. Chem. 258:7168, 1983.
121. Kao, K. J., Pizzo, S. V., et al.: Demonstration and characterization of specific binding sites for factor VIII/von Willebrand factor on human platelets. J. Clin. Invest. 63:656, 1979.
122. Morisato, D. K., and Gralnick, H. R.: Selective binding of factor VIII/von Willebrand factor protein to human platelets. Blood 55:9, 1980.
123. Weiss, H. J., Tschopp, T. B., et al.: Decreased adhesion of giant (Bernard-Soulier) platelets to subendothelium. Further implications on the role of von Willebrand factor in hemostasis. Am. J. Med. 57:920, 1974.
124. Coller, B. S., Peerschke, E. I., et al.: Studies with a murine monoclonal antibody that abolishes ristocetin-induced binding of von Willebrand factor to platelets: additional evidence in support of GpIb as a platelet receptor for von Willebrand factor. Blood 61:99, 1983.
125. Michelson, A. D., Loscalzo, J., et al.: Partial characterization of a binding site for von Willebrand's factor on glycocalicin. Blood 67:19, 1986.
126. Loscalzo, J., and Handin, R. I.: van Willebrand protein facilitates platelet incorporation into polymerizing fibrin. J. Clin. Invest. In press.
127. Cooper, H. A., Bennett, W. P., et al.: Hydrolysis of human platelet membrane glycoprotein with a *Serratia marcescens* metalloprotease: effect on response to thrombin and von Willebrand factor. Proc. Natl. Acad. Sci. U. S. A. 79:1433, 1982.
128. Jamieson, G. A., and Okumura, T.: Reduced thrombin binding and aggregation in Bernard-Soulier platelets. J. Clin. Invest. 61:681, 1978.
129. Tollefson, D. M., Feagler, J. R., et al.: The binding of thrombin to the surface of human platelets. J. Biol. Chem. 249:2646, 1974.
130. Larsen, N. E., and Simons, E. R.: Preparation and application of a photoreactive thrombin analogue: binding of human platelets. Biochemistry 20:4141, 1981.
131. Berndt, M. C., and Phillips, D. R.: Interaction of thrombin with platelets. Purification of the thrombin substrate. Ann. N. Y. Acad. Sci. 370:87, 1981.
132. Okumura, T., and Jamieson, G. A.: Platelet glycocalicin: a single receptor for platelet aggregation induced by thrombin and ristocetin. Thromb. Res. 8:701, 1976.
133. Solum, N. O., Hagen, I., et al.: Platelet glycocalicin: its membrane association and solubilization in aqueous media. Biochim. Biophys. Acta 597:235, 1980.
134. Fox, J. E.: Linkage of a membrane skeleton to integral membrane glycoproteins in human platelets. Identification of one of the glycoproteins as glycoprotein Ib. J. Clin. Invest. 76:1673, 1985.
135. Clemetson, K. J., Bienz, D., et al.: Distribution of platelet glycoproteins and phosphoproteins in hydrophobic and hydrophilic phases in Triton X-114 phase partition. Biochim. Biophys. Acta 778:463, 1984.
136. Sie, P., Gillois, M., et al.: Reconstitution of liposomes bearing platelet receptors for human von Willebrand factor. Biochem. Biophys. Res. Comm. 97:135, 1980.

137. Jennings, L. K., and Phillips, D. R.: Purification of glycoproteins IIb and III from human platelet plasma membranes and characterization of a calcium-dependent glycoprotein IIb-III complex. J. Biol. Chem. 257:10458, 1982.
138. Coller, B. S., Peerschke, E. I., et al.: A murine monoclonal antibody that completely blocks the binding of fibrinogen to platelets produces a thrombasthenia-like state in normal platelets and binds to glycoprotein IIb and or IIIa. J. Clin. Invest. 72:25, 1983.
139. Burckhardt, J. J., Anderson, W. H. K., et al.: Human blood monocytes and platelets share a cell surface component. Blood 60:767, 1982.
140. Fitzgerald, L. A., Charo, I., et al.: Human and bovine endothelial cells synthesize membrane proteins similar to human platelet glycoproteins IIb and IIIa. J. Biol. Chem. 260:10893, 1985.
141. Kloczewiak, M., and Timmons, S., et al.: Platelet receptor recognition site on human fibrinogen. Synthesis and structure-function relationship of peptides corresponding to the carboxy terminal segment of the gamma chain. Biochemistry 23:1767, 1984.
142. Phillips, D. R., Jennings, L. K., et al.: Identification of membrane proteins mediating the interaction of human platelets. J. Cell Biol. 86:77, 1980.
143. Newman, P. J., and Martin, L. S.: Studies on the nature of the human platelet alloantigen P^{A1}: localization of a 17,000 dalton polypeptide. Mol. Immunol. 22:719, 1985.
144. Kieffer, N., Boizard, B., et al.: Immunochemical characterization of the platelet-specific alloantigen Leka: a comparative study with PLA^1 alloantigen. Blood 64:1212, 1984.
145. Beardsley, D. S., Spiegel, J. C., et al.: Platelet membrane glycoprotein IIIa contains target antigens that bind antiplatelet antibodies in immune thrombocytopenia. J. Clin. Invest. 74:1701, 1984.
146. Brass, L. F., and Bensusan, H. B.: The role of collagen quaternary structure in the platelet:collagen interaction. J. Clin. Invest. 54:1480, 1974.
147. Jamieson, G. A., Urban, C. L., et al.: Enzymatic basis for platelet collagen adhesion as the primary step in hemostasis. Nature (New Biol.) 234:5, 1971.
148. Chesney, C., Harper, E., et al.: Critical role of carbohydrate side chains of collagen in platelet aggregation. J. Clin. Invest. 51:2693, 1972.
149. Puett, D., Wusserman, B. K., et al.: Collagen-mediated platelet aggregation. Effects of collagen modification involving the protein and carbohydrate moieties. J. Clin. Invest. 52:2495, 1973.
150. Nieuwenhuis, H. K., Akkerman, J. W., et al: Human blood platelets showing no response to collagen fail to express surface glycoprotein Ia. Nature 318:470, 1985.
151. Balleiser, L., Gay, S., et al.: Comparative investigations on the influence of human and bovine collagen types I, II and III on the aggregation of human platelets. Klin. Wochenschr. 53:903, 1975.
152. Gay, S., Balleisen, L., et al.: Immunohistochemical evidence for the presence of collagen type III in human arterial walls, arterial thrombosis and in leukocytes incubated with collagen in vitro. Klin. Wochenschr. 53:899, 1975.
153. Estes, J. W.: Platelet abnormalities in heritable disorders of connective tissue. Ann. N. Y. Acad. Sci. 201:445, 1972.
154. Baumgartner, H. R., and Muggli, R.: Adhesion and aggregation: morphological demonstration and quantitation in vivo and in vitro. In Platelet in Biology and Pathology. Gordonet, J. L. (ed.), Amsterdam, North Holland Publishing Company, 1976, pp. 23–60.
155. Weiss, H. J., Tschopp, T. B., et al.: Impaired interaction (adhesion-aggregation) of platelets with the subendothelium in storage pool disease and after aspirin ingestion: a comparison with von Willebrand's disease. New Engl. J. Med. 293:619, 1975.
156. Houdijk, P., de Groot, P. G., et al.: Subendothelial proteins and platelet adhesion. von Willebrand factor and fibronectin, not thrombospondin, are involved in platelet adhesion to extracellular matrix of human vascular endothelial cells. Arteriosclerosis 6:24, 1986.
157. Ginsburg, D., Handin, R. I., et al.: Human von Willebrand factor (vWF): isolation of complementary DNA (cDNA) clones and chromosomal localization. Science 228:1401, 1985.
158. Fay, P. J., Kawai, Y., et al.: The propolypeptide of von Willebrand factor circulates in blood and is identical to von Willebrand antigen II. Science 232:995, 1986.
159. Wagner, D., and Olmsted, J. B.: Immunolocalization of von Willebrand protein in Weibel-Palade bodies of human endothelial cells. J. Cell Biol. 95:355, 1982.
160. Bockenstedt, P., Greenberg, J., et al.: Structural basis of von Willebrand's factor binding to platelet glycoprotein Ib and collagen. Effects of disulfide reduction and limited proteolysis on polymeric vWF. J. Clin. Invest. 77:743, 1986.
161. Born, G. V. R., and Cross, M. J.: The aggregation of blood platelets. J. Physiol. (Lond.) 168:178, 1963.
162. Claesson, H. E., and Malmsten, C.: On the inter-relationship of prostaglandin endoperoxide G_2 and cyclic nucleotides in platelet function. Eur. J. Biochem. 76:277, 1977.
163. Bennett, J. S., Vilaire, G., et al.: Identification of the fibrinogen receptor on human platelets by photoaffinity labelling. J. Biol. Chem. 257:8049, 1982.
164. Berridge, M. J.: Inositol triphosphate and diacylglycerol as second messengers. Biochem. J. 220:345, 1984.
165. Rittenhouse, S. E.: Human platelets contain phospholipase C that hydrolyzes polyphosphoinositides. Proc. Natl. Acad. Sci. U. S. A. 80:417, 1983.
166. Chaffoy de Courcelles, D., Roevens, P., et al.: 1-Oleyl-2-acetyl-glycerol (OAG) stimulates the formation of phosphatidylinositol 4-phosphate in intact human platelets. Biochem. Biophys. Res. Commun. 123:589, 1984.
167. Zavoico, G. B., Helenda, S. P., et al.: Phorbol myristate acetate inhibits thrombin-stimulated Ca^{2+} mobilization and phosphatidylinositol 4,5-bisphosphate hydrolysis in human platelets. Proc. Natl. Acad. Sci. U. S. A. 82:3859, 1985.
168. Lyons, R. M., Stanford, N., Majerus, P. W.: Thrombin-induced protein phosphorylation in human platelets. J. Clin. Invest. 56:924, 1975.
169. Jones, H. P.: Calmodulin and platelet function. In The Platelets: Physiology and Pharmacology. Longenecker, G. L. (ed.), New York, Academic Press, 1985, pp. 221–235.
170. Marcus, A. J.: The role of lipids in platelet function: with particular reference to the arachidonic acid pathway. J. Lipid Res. 19:793, 1978.
171. Rittenhouse-Simmons, S., and Deykin, D.: The mobilization of arachidonic acid in platelets exposed to thrombin or ionophore A23187. J. Clin. Invest. 60:495, 1977.
172. Rittenhouse, S. E.: Activation of phospholipase C in human platelets. Adv. Prost. Thromb. Leuk. Res. 15:113, 1985.
173. Longenecker, G. L.: Platelet arachidonic acid metabolism. In The Platelets: Physiology and Pharmacology. Longenecker, G. L. (ed.), New York, Academic Press, 1985, pp. 159–185.
174. Hamberg, M., Svensson, J., et al.: Isolation and structure of two prostaglandin endoperoxides that cause platelet aggregation. Proc. Natl. Acad. Sci. U. S. A. 71:345, 1974.
175. Hamburg, M., Svensson, J., et al.: Thromboxanes: a new group of biologically active compounds derived from prostaglandin endoperoxides. Proc. Natl. Acad. Sci. U. S. A. 72:2994, 1975.
176. Needleman, P., Minkes, M., et al.: Thromboxanes: selec-

177. Velz, O., Delz, R., et al.: Biosynthesis of prostaglandin D$_2$. 1. Formation of prostaglandin D$_2$ by human platelets. Prostaglandins *13*:225, 1977.
178. Turner, J. R., Tainer, J. A., et al.: Biogenesis of chemotactic molecules by the arachidonate lipoxygenase system of platelets. Nature *257*:680, 1975.
179. Smith, J. B., Ingerman, C. M., et al.: Effects of arachidonic acid and some of its metabolites on platelets. In *Prostaglandins in Hematology*. Silver, M. J., Smith, J. B., et al. (eds.), New York, Spectrum Publications, 1977, pp. 277–292.
180. Packham, M. A., and Mustard, J. F.: Clinical pharmacology of platelets. Blood *50*:555, 1977.
181. Packham, M. A., Kinlough-Rathbone, R. L., et al.: Mechanisms of platelet aggregation independent of adenosine diphosphate. In *Prostaglandins in Hematology*. Silver, M. J., Smith, J. B., et al. (eds.), New York, Spectrum Publications, 1977.
182. Ellis, E. F., Oelz, O., et al.: Coronary arterial smooth muscle contraction by a substance released from platelets: evidence that it is thromboxane A$_2$. Science *193*:1135, 1976.
183. Oelz, O., and Oates, J. A.: Cerebral arterial smooth muscle contraction by thromboxane A$_2$. Science *194*:1087, 1976.
184. Weiss, H. J.: Antiplatelet drugs—a new pharmacologic approach to the prevention of thrombosis. Am. Heart J. *92*:86, 1976.
185. Mustard, J.F., Kinlough-Rathbone, R., et al.: Aspirin in the treatment of cardiovascular disease: a review. Am. J. Med. *74*:43, 1983.
186. Hirsh, J.: Selection and results of antiplatelet therapy in the prevention of stroke and myocardial infarction. Arch. Intern. Med. *14*:311, 1981.
187. Koren, G., Rose, V., et al.: Probable efficacy of high-dose salicylates in reducing coronary involvement in Kawasaki disease. J. A. M. A. *254*:767, 1985.
188. Weiss, H. J., and Rogers, J.: Thrombocytopathia due to abnormalities in platelet release reaction—studies on six unrelated patients. Blood *39*:187, 1972.
189. Lagarde, M., Byron, P. A., et al.: Impairment of thromboxane A$_2$ generation and of the platelet release reaction in two patients with congenital deficiency of platelet cyclo-oxygenase. Br. J. Haematol. *38*:251, 1978.
190. Wu, K. K., Le Breton, G. C., et al.: Abnormal platelet response to thromboxane A$_2$. J. Clin. Invest. *67*:1801, 1981.
191. Knapp, H. R., Reilly, I. A., et al.: In vivo indexes of platelet and vascular function during fish-oil administration in patients with atherosclerosis. New Engl. J. Med. *314*:937, 1986.
192. Weksler, B. B., Marcus, A. J., et al.: Synthesis of prostaglandin I$_2$ (prostacyclin) by cultured human and bovine endothelial cells. Proc. Natl. Acad. Sci. U. S. A. *74*:3422, 1977.
193. Marcus, A. J., Weksler, B. B., et al.: Enzymatic conversion of prostaglandin endoperoxide H$_2$ and arachidonic acid to prostacyclin by cultured human endothelial cells. J. Biol. Chem. *253*:7138, 1978.
194. Longmore, D. B., Bennet, G., et al.: Prostacyclin: a solution to some problems of extracorporeal circulation. Experiments in greyhounds. Lancet *1*:1002, 1979.
195. Remuzzi, G., Cavenashi, A. E., et al.: Prostacyclin (PGI$_2$) and bleeding time in uremic patients. Thromb. Res. *11*:919, 1977.
196. Remuzzi, G., Benigni, A., et al.: Reduced platelet thromboxane formation in uremia. Evidence for a functional cyclooxygenase defect. J. Clin. Invest. *71*:762, 1983.
197. Halushka, P. V., Lurie, D., et al.: Increased synthesis of prostaglandin-E like material by platelets from patients with diabetes mellitus. New Engl. J. Med. *297*:1306, 1977.
198. Marcus, A. J.: The platelet as a source of phospholipid. In *Platelets, Drugs and Thrombosis*. Hirsch, J., Cade, J. F., et al. (eds.), Basel, S. Karger, 1975, pp. 49–53.
199. Broekman, M. J., Handin, R. I., et al.: Distribution of phospholipids, fatty acids and platelet factor 3 activity among subcellular fractions of platelets. Blood *47*:963, 1976.
200. Papahadjopoulos, D., and Hanahan, D. J.: Observations on the interaction of phosholipids and certain clotting factors in prothrombin activator formation. Biochem. Biophys. Acta *90*:436, 1964.
201. Walsh, P. N.: Platelet coagulant activities and hemostasis. A hypothesis. Blood *43*:597, 1974.
202. Miletich, J. P., Jackson, C. N., et al.: Interaction of coagulation factor Xa with human platelets. Proc. Natl. Acad. Sci. U. S. A. *74*:4035, 1977.
203. Miletich, J. P., Majerus, D. W., et al.: Patients with congenital factor V deficiency have decreased factor X binding site on their platelets. J. Clin. Invest. *62*:824, 1978.

COAGULATION

CHAPTER 41
Diseases of Coagulation: The Fluid Phase

JEANNE M. LUSHER

DIAGNOSIS 1293
History
Physical Examination
Laboratory Evaluation
  Overall Screening Tests
  Tests of Platelet Function
  Coagulation Tests
TREATMENT OF HEMOSTATIC ABNORMALITIES 1300
Blood Component Therapy
Other Agents
Avoidance of Drugs That Can Induce Platelet Dysfunction
HEREDITARY COAGULATION DISORDERS 1305
The Hemophilias
  Treatment
  Inhibitors
  Carrier Detection
  Prenatal Diagnosis
Von Willebrand's Disease
  Diagnosis
  Classification
  Incidence, Inheritance, and Clinical Expression
  Treatment
  Pseudo- (Platelet-Type) Von Willebrand's Disease
Other Hereditary Coagulation Disorders
  Fibrinogen Abnormalities
  Congenital Deficiencies and Abnormalities of Prothrombin, Factor V, Factor VII, and Factor X
  Factor XIII Deficiency
  Contact Factor Deficiencies
  Alpha$_2$-Antiplasmin Deficiency (Miyasato's Disease)
  Deficiencies Associated With Thrombotic Disease
ACQUIRED COAGULATION DISORDERS AND ASSOCIATED ABNORMALITIES 1326
Liver Disease
Vitamin K Deficiency
Congenital Heart Disease
Renal Failure
Amyloidosis
Anticoagulants
Disseminated Intravascular Coagulation (DIC)
  Etiology
  Diagnosis and Treatment
Snakebite

DIAGNOSIS

Optimal management of bleeding disorders requires accurate diagnosis. A careful history, complete physical examination, and appropriate laboratory tests are needed to establish a diagnosis; the role of each will be described in detail. In each aspect of the diagnostic approach it is helpful to relate the symptom, physical finding, or laboratory result to the overall hemostatic mechanism (Fig. 41–1). Details of the platelet and coagulation phases of normal hemostasis are described in Chapters 39 and 40. Although the emphasis of this chapter will be on disorders of coagulation, some mention will be made of platelet abnormalities in regard to diagnostic screening tests.

History

A careful history provides a valuable screening measure for the detection of mild bleeding disorders and can guide one to the most efficient use of the laboratory in evaluating all patients with bleeding manifestations (1, 2). In searching for evidence of an underlying bleeding disorder, one must ask specific questions regarding the patient and other family members. The following symptoms, listed in relative chronologic order of occurrence, may be useful: any bleeding during the neonatal period; bleeding after circumcision; delayed bleeding from the umbilical stump (a finding particularly suggestive of Factor XIII deficiency); deep hematoma formation after intramuscular injections, such as immunizations; easy bruising from handling (under the arms) or after minor injuries; epistaxis; bleeding into joints; prolonged bleeding from lacerations; excessive bleeding following any operative procedure, including tooth extraction and tonsillectomy; menorrhagia; hematuria; and any unexplained gastrointestinal bleeding. Any cyclic or episodic aspect of the bleeding or any unusual distribution of hemorrhagic skin lesions should be noted; in some cases, these findings may lead to suspicion of child abuse.

Nosebleeds are a common complaint during childhood, and if they occur in the absence of any other bleeding manifestation in the patient or family members, an underlying hemorrhagic disorder is unlikely. In this situation, further studies are not indicated unless the nosebleeds have been particularly severe or recurrent or both. Also, it is important that one note whether epistaxis is always from one or from both nostrils. Unilateral epistaxis almost always results from a local lesion rather than from a coagulation disorder. It is important,

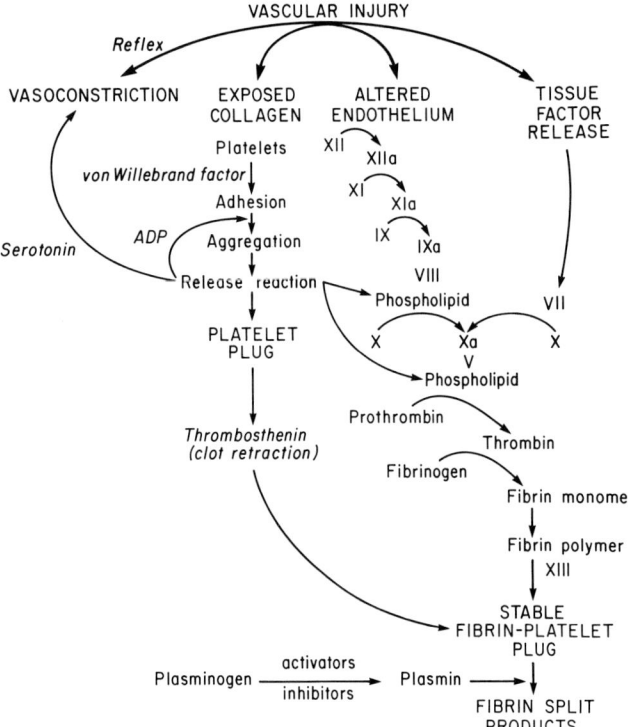

Figure 41–1. Diagrammatic representation of the hemostatic mechanism.

however, to investigate fully any excessive postoperative bleeding, which may be the first manifestation of mild hemophilia or von Willebrand's disease. These recommendations, made by Schulman in 1959, continue to be a useful guide to the selection of children with nosebleeds for laboratory evaluation (3).

Another important factor in the history is the use of or exposure to drugs that may influence the incidence and degree of bleeding or the results of laboratory studies or both. This is particularly true of aspirin and aspirin-containing medications but also applies to anticoagulant drugs. Heparin-containing solutions used to flush indwelling venous or arterial catheters can be administered in amounts adequate to induce an anticoagulant effect in the patient. Infants and small children or patients with poor renal function are particularly susceptible to this potential iatrogenic bleeding disorder.

The presence of primary conditions that may be associated with bleeding should be determined. Examples are lupus erythematosis, nephrosis, hypothyroidism, and sepsis. If bleeding manifestations seem to be acquired acutely (rather than being chronic or lifelong), one should search for a possible causative factor (e.g., antecedent illness prior to thrombocytopenic purpura). Anaphylactoid purpura (Henoch-Schönlein purpura) is not associated with an underlying generalized hemorrhagic tendency but does have a characteristic distribution of hemorrhagic skin lesions, which is often diagnostic. The rash is variable but usually starts as urticarial lesions that progress to hemorrhagic maculopapules with gradual fading, leaving a brownish discoloration. The sequence may take only 2 to 3 days. The lesions have a characteristic distribution involving the buttocks, posterior thighs and legs, extensor surfaces of the arms, and occasionally the tips of the ears, with sparing of the face and trunk. There may be associated gastrointestinal bleeding, colicky abdominal pain, hematuria, arthralgia, or edema of the scalp (in infants). Platelet function and coagulation studies are normal in this disorder and are not helpful diagnostic criteria.

A functional classification of hemorrhagic disorders (including platelet-related problems) is provided in Table 41–1.

Physical Examination

A complete physical examination is important in the evaluation of any child with a bleeding disorder. As previously indicated, the nature of the bleeding manifestation can provide a clue to the etiology, and the presence of other abnormalities (enlargement of the liver or spleen, lymphadenopathy, icterus, rash, etc.) may indicate an underlying disease with secondary bleeding. Any abnormality of the skin, mucous membranes, fundi, soft tissues, and joints should be noted (petechiae, ecchymosis, deep hematoma, mucous membrane bleeding, subconjunctival or retinal

Table 41–1. FUNCTIONAL CLASSIFICATION OF BLEEDING DISORDERS

Due to abnormal structure or function of blood vessels
  Hereditary hemorrhagic telangiectasia
  Cutis hyperelastica (Ehlers-Danlos syndrome)
  Idiopathic pulmonary hemosiderosis
  Scurvy
  Septic or toxic vasculitis
  Anaphylactoid purpura (Henoch-Schönlein syndrome)

Due to abnormality of platelet hemostatic mechanism
  Thrombocytopenia
    Due to decreased platelet production
      Secondary to marrow replacement (leukemia, tumors)
      Secondary to marrow damage by drugs, chemicals, or radiation
      Aplastic and hypoplastic anemias
      Congenital amegakaryocytic thrombocytopenia
    Due to increased platelet destruction or sequestration
      Idiopathic thrombocytopenic purpura
      Neonatal thrombocytopenic purpura (maternal ITP or isoimmunization)
      Familial thrombocytopenic purpura
      Immunologic drug purpura
      Intravascular coagulation
      Splenomegaly
      Cyanotic congenital heart disease (may be decreased production?)
      Giant hemangioma
      Wiskott-Aldrich syndrome
  Abnormal platelet function
    Von Willebrand's disease (lack of plasma factor necessary for platelet adhesiveness)
    Hereditary disorders of platelet function
      Storage pool disease
      Thrombasthenia (Glanzmann's disease)
      Bernard-Soulier syndrome
    Acquired disorders of platelet function (drugs, uremia)

Due to abnormal coagulation
  Congenital deficiencies
    Hemophilia
      Factor VIII deficiency (classic hemophilia; hemophilia A)
      Factor IX deficiency (Christmas disease; hemophilia B)
    Other congenital disorders
      Afibrinogenemia and hypofibrinogenemia
      Dysfibrinogenemia
      Hypoprothrombinemia
      Factor V deficiency
      Factor VII deficiency
      Factor X deficiency
      Factor XI deficiency
      Coagulation factor deficiencies not associated with bleeding
        Factor XII deficiency (Hageman trait)
        Prekallikrein deficiency (Fletcher factor)
        High-molecular-weight kininogen deficiency
      Combined coagulation factor deficiencies
      Hemorrhagic disease of the newborn (transient combined deficiencies of prothrombin and Factors VII, IX, X)
  Acquired deficiencies
    Liver disease (prothrombin and Factors V, VII, IX, X)
    Coumarin-induced (prothrombin and Factors VII, IX, X)
    Vitamin K deficiency (prothrombin and Factors VII, IX, X)
    Associated with congenital heart disease (variable factors)
    Associated with nephrosis (Factor IX and/or Factors XI and XII)
    Associated with amyloidosis (Factors IX and X)
    Anticoagulants
      In lupus erythematosus
      Against specific coagulation factors (usually Factor VIII)
      Heparin (extrinsic, intrinsic)
    Fibrinolysis
      Primary (extremely uncommon)
      Secondary (disseminated intravascular coagulation)
    Disseminated intravascular coagulation with consumption of coagulation factors

hemorrhage, and any joint abnormalities, including warmth, swelling, tenderness, or limitation of motion).

Laboratory Evaluation

OVERALL SCREENING TESTS

To evaluate a child with a *negative* history for bleeding (as in preoperative screening), a battery of tests must be performed so that all phases of hemostasis are covered. For this purpose the basic screening tests should include the following: platelet count (or careful evaluation of a blood smear for the presence of platelets); bleeding time (by a sensitive, reproducible method); activated partial thromboplastin time; and prothrombin time. Normal screening test findings in a child with a negative history should rule out the presence of a significant underlying bleeding disorder. If a patient with negative screening tests bleeds during or after an operative procedure, the studies should be repeated, and it may be necessary to perform additional tests. One rare disorder that this combination of screening tests will not detect is Factor XIII (fibrin stabilizing factor) deficiency, for which a specific test is required that measures the solubility of a plasma clot in 1 per cent monochloracetic acid or 5 M urea. Another patient who can escape detection by this combination of laboratory tests is one with mild von Willebrand's disease, in whom the bleeding time can occasionally be normal (usually such a patient has a positive history of bleeding as well as a positive family history).

Additional tests required to establish a specific diagnosis in patients with abnormal screening test results and in patients with a positive history of bleeding are considered in detail in the following sections.

TESTS OF PLATELET FUNCTION

In order to evaluate the platelet phase of hemostasis, one must document the presence of an adequate number of platelets and assess their function by performing a sensitive bleeding time. Additional tests of platelet function necessary to define specific abnormalities are described in Chapters 40 and 42. Because the bleeding time is essential to the diagnosis and management of von Willebrand's disease, a description of available bleeding time methods follows.

A variety of techniques are in general clinical use, but most are based on the Duke or Ivy methods. The first bleeding time was described by Duke in 1910, which he performed by making a small cut in the ear lobe with a spring lancet (4). This method is less sensitive than the Ivy method as a diagnostic test, and bleeding may be difficult to control in a patient with abnormal hemostasis.

In 1935, Ivy described a bleeding time method that he performed on the forearm using a spring lancet, with a blood pressure cuff on the upper arm inflated to 40 mm Hg (5). This method is more reproducible and more sensitive as a diagnostic test, and it allows prolonged bleeding to be easily controlled with pressure. One performs the Ivy bleeding time by making two or three punctures in the skin of the patient's forearm with a sterile no. 11 blade. For improved reproducibility, a piece of paper tape can be folded across the blade 3 mm from the tip so that the depth of the puncture can be controlled. Punctures are made, with superficial veins avoided, and the blood is absorbed on filter paper until bleeding ceases. The upper limit of normal for this method is 8 minutes. The greater sensitivity of the Ivy method makes it preferable to the Duke bleeding time as a diagnostic test (6).

Template Bleeding Time Methods. A modification of the Ivy bleeding time was described by Borchgrevink and Waaler in 1958, in which a superficial incision 1 mm deep by 10 mm long was made in the skin of the forearm with a sterile blade (7). The normal range for this test was 3½ to 11½ minutes. Subsequently, Mielke and colleagues modified the test using a template with a slit 11 mm long (providing an incision 9 mm long) and a scalpel guard, which let the blade protrude 1 mm through the template (8). A number of other modifications of this type of bleeding time have been developed and are usually referred to as "template" bleeding times (9–11). These modifications of the Ivy method have greatly improved the sensitivity and reliability of the test. Nonetheless, it is important that one realize that the reproducibility of the bleeding time depends on many variables, including the experience of the person performing the test, the skin temperature, and the direction, length, and depth of the incision (11). Disposable template devices are now available commercially for similar tests, and their use has no doubt improved the reproducibility of the template bleeding time among laboratories.* When performing the bleeding time, one must avoid disturbing the wound when absorbing the blood with filter paper, and patients should be warned that the test may leave a small scar. Normal values vary with the method used and should be determined by the laboratory performing the test.

Because recent ingestion of aspirin (within 5 to 7 days) may cause some prolongation of the bleeding time in normal individuals, the test may be difficult to interpret under such circumstances and probably should be deferred (9, 12). The observation that there may be an exaggerated prolon-

---

*Disposable bleeding time devices are available from General Diagnostics, Morris Plains, NJ, and from Hemakit, Malden, MA.

gation of the bleeding time after aspirin ingestion in patients with von Willebrand's disease (as well as in those with uremia and platelet function abnormalities) led some authors to recommend this maneuver as a diagnostic test (12, 13). However, the great variability of the effect of aspirin on the bleeding time and the lack of specificity of this test detract from its usefulness, and more specific and sensitive tests for von Willebrand's disease will be described.

The finding of a prolonged bleeding time with a normal platelet count in a patient with a positive history requires further evaluation. If von Willebrand's disease is ruled out by appropriate tests, additional platelet function studies are indicated (see Chapter 42).

COAGULATION TESTS

Screening Tests. Coagulation tests range from global screening tests, which are affected by nearly all coagulation factors, to specific assays for individual factors. The global screening tests vary in sensitivity. Although the whole blood clotting time (WBCT) is a global test, it is not a sensitive screening test. The presence of only 1 to 2 per cent Factor VIII will result in a normal clotting time (less than 10 minutes if done at 37° C.); therefore, the WBCT is no longer used for the purpose of screening (10). The activated clotting time (ACT) is a modification of the WBCT, in which blood is drawn into a tube containing celite for maximum contact activation (14). The normal range is approximately 1 minute 20 seconds to 2 minutes 20 seconds. Although the ACT is more sensitive than the WBCT, it is not an adequate screening test for mild hemophilia. However, the ACT has been useful for monitoring heparin therapy and has the advantage (or disadvantage) of being performed at the bedside (15).

Most other coagulation tests are performed on plasma obtained by centrifugation of citrated whole blood. Accurate coagulation tests are dependent on careful collection of specimens with clean veni-puncture (and/or "two-syringe" collection), prompt centrifugation, separation of plasma, and appropriate storage (if testing is delayed). One should re-evaluate any unexpected or unexplained abnormal result using a repeat blood sample to avoid problems secondary to faulty sample collection, processing, or storage. With the increased use of heparin to maintain intravenous lines, it should be ascertained that blood samples obtained for coagulation studies do not contain this drug. Use of such samples may lead to significant confusion because heparin will affect most studies dependent on clot formation.

Most clotting tests done on plasma are modifications of the plasma recalcification time that one performs by adding calcium to plasma and timing the formation of a clot (normal: less than 180 seconds). Although this test is relatively insensitive, its modifications are quite useful. The most sensitive global screening test is the activated partial thromboplastin time (APTT) (1, 16), which involves incubation of plasma with an inert activating agent (kaolin, celite, or bentonite) for maximum contact and a partial thromboplastin (cephalin, inosithin) as a platelet substitute, followed by addition of calcium. The APTT is sensitive to deficiencies of all the significant coagulation factors associated with bleeding except Factor VII and Factor XIII (Fig. 41–2).

Most APTT methods have an upper limit of normal from 35 to 45 seconds, but this depends on the specific reagents and method used. Because many different reagents are available and the sensitivity varies depending on the method employed, it is important to know the normal range and sensitivity of the specific APTT method used to study a patient. Properly performed, the APTT should be sensitive to levels of Factor VIII below 40 per cent and Factor IX below 20 to 30 per cent (17). A markedly prolonged APTT result that corrects to normal with 10- to 15-minute incubation in an asymptomatic individual leads to the presumptive diagnosis of Fletcher factor (prekallikrein) deficiency, a nonbleeding condition (18).

The prothrombin time (PT) involves addition of tissue factor (a complete thromboplastin) to plasma with subsequent (or simultaneous) recalcification (1, 19). The normal PT is approximately 11 to 12 seconds and has a narrow range of normal (in contrast to the APTT, which has a wider range of normal values). The PT is sensitive to deficiencies of prothrombin and Factors V, VII, X, and fibrinogen (Fig. 41–3). The prothrombin time is sensitive to three of the five factors in the "prothrombin complex" (Factors II, VII, IX, and X and protein C—the vitamin K-dependent coagulation factors), all of which are produced in the liver. The interrelationship of these categories is defined in Table 41–2.

The results of the APTT and PT tests may differentiate defects of the intrinsic versus extrinsic coagulation pathways, as illustrated in Figures 41–2 and 41–3. The combination of an abnormal APTT and a normal PT suggests a defect in the early intrinsic pathway; a normal APTT with an abnormal PT suggests an isolated deficiency of Factor VII. Abnormal results of both tests indicate a disorder of one or more of the factors involved in the common pathway. Because both the APTT and PT are screening tests, additional studies are required for specific diagnosis when abnormal results are observed.

One can make a presumptive diagnosis by determining the corrective effect on an abnormal APTT or PT by normal plasma compared with plasmas deficient in single coagulation factors. The use of specific deficient plasmas as reagents for

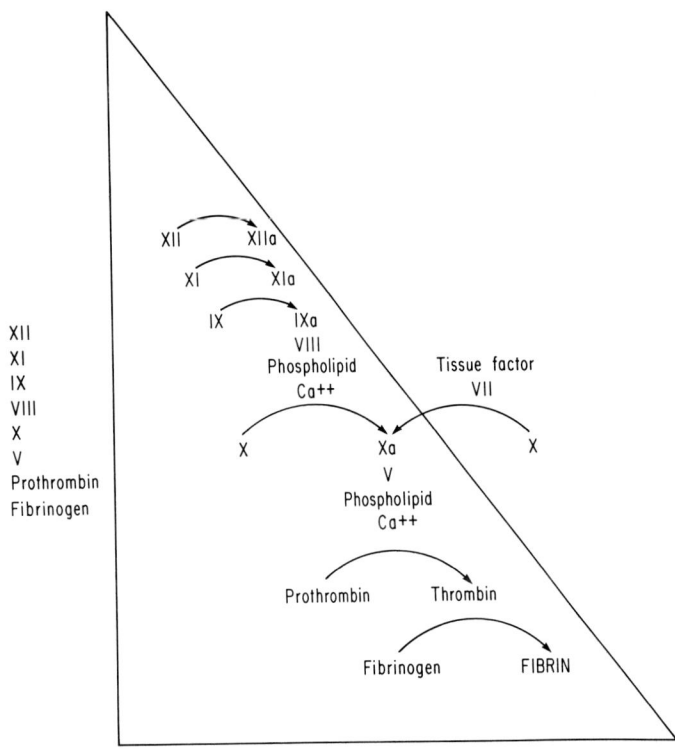

Figure 41–2. Activated partial thromboplastin time (APTT). The portion of the coagulation mechanism measured by the APTT is enclosed within the triangle, with the clotting factor to which the APTT is sensitive listed to the left.

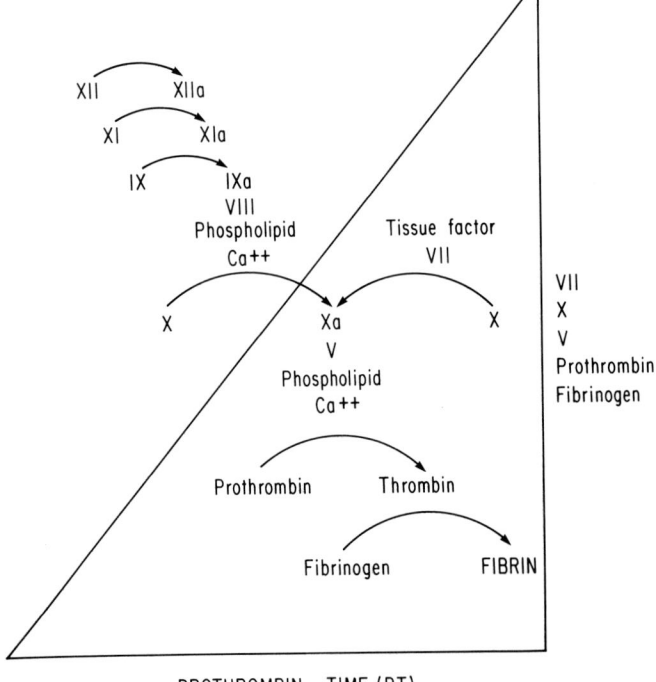

Figure 41–3. Prothrombin time (PT). The portion of the coagulation mechanism measured by the PT is enclosed within the triangle, with the clotting factors to which the PT is sensitive listed to the right.

Table 41–2. DEFINITION OF FACTORS MEASURED BY THE PROTHROMBIN TIME, COAGULATION FACTORS PRODUCED IN THE LIVER, AND THE PROTHROMBIN COMPLEX

Factors Measured by Prothrombin Time	Factors Produced in the Liver	Prothrombin Complex (Vitamin K–Dependent Factor)
Prothrombin (Factor II)	Prothrombin (Factor II)	Prothrombin (Factor II)
Factor V	Factor V	
Factor VII	Factor VII	Factor VII
	Factor IX	Factor IX
Factor X	Factor X	Factor X (and protein C)
Fibrinogen	Fibrinogen	
	Factor XI	
	Factor XII	
	Prekallikrein	
	High–molecular weight kininogen	
	Factor XIII	
	Protein C	
	AT III	

correction studies is preferable to use of adsorbed plasma and serum because serum can lead to nonspecific correction of the APTT and erroneous interpretation of results.

Additional screening tests for coagulation abnormalities include the prothrombin consumption test (serum prothrombin activity) and the thromboplastin generation test. Although both can detect abnormalities of the intrinsic pathway, the prothrombin consumption test is not adequately sensitive to mild defects, and the thromboplastin generation test is a time-consuming, cumbersome study. As a result, neither test is widely used at the present time.

Specific Assays. Recognition of Factor XIII deficiency requires a specific test in which the solubility of a plasma clot in 1 per cent monochloracetic acid or in 5 M urea is determined. All other coagulation screening tests are normal in plasma that is deficient in Factor XIII.

One assays individual coagulation factors by determining the ability of the plasma being tested to correct the clotting abnormality of plasma deficient in the factor being measured. Both the PT and APTT are used as the basis of specific assays. Some deficient substrate plasmas are prepared artificially, whereas others are obtained from patients with severe deficiencies (1, 19, 20).

Factor VIII can be measured by immunologic methods in which antibody to highly purified Factor VIII is used in an immunoelectrophoretic procedure or in a radioimmunoassay (21–23). These methods measure Factor VIII–related antigen (F VIIIR:Ag), which does not always correlate with Factor VIII coagulant activity (F VIII:C). In fact, most patients with severe hemophilia, who have less than 1 per cent Factor VIII coagulant activity, have normal amounts of Factor VIII–related antigen, a finding that suggests that such individuals have an abnormal Factor VIII molecule (or a molecule that lacks Factor VIII coagulant activity). F VIII:C and F VIIIR:Ag have approximately a 1:1 ratio in most normal women. A decreased ratio of F VIII:C to F VIIIR:Ag is found in most hemophilia carriers, and these measurements have improved the accuracy of carrier testing (see under Carrier Detection) (24).

F VIIIR:Ag is decreased in many patients with von Willebrand's disease, and this finding has proved diagnostically significant in this disorder (21).

Another valuable test in von Willebrand's disease depends on a factor in plasma needed for platelets to aggregate in response to ristocetin, an antibiotic that causes aggregation of normal platelets in vitro and in vivo (25). This property of normal plasma, termed ristocetin cofactor, is decreased in most patients with von Willebrand's disease. The amount of ristocetin cofactor in a patient's plasma can be measured with a platelet aggregometer or with tests dependent on visually timed macroscopic clumping (26, 27). There is a correlation of ristocetin cofactor with F VIIIR:Ag levels in most patients with classic (Type I) von Willebrand's disease.

Fibrinogen level may be estimated by tests based on the thrombin time (1) or by a simple heat precipitation test (28). The latter can be performed with a small amount of plasma, and, because this test is not affected by heparin, it has proved useful in following the course of infants and children with disseminated intravascular coagulation who are being treated with heparin (29). Fibrinogen is the only coagulation factor that is measured in absolute units (expressed as mg per dl), and there are several methods for assay (1, 20, 30).

Inhibitors of normal coagulation are recognized by the failure of normal plasma to correct the prolonged clotting time of an abnormal sample. Any plasma deficient in an individual coagulation factor (associated with a long PT and/or APTT, depending on the abnormality) should be corrected by the addition of an equal amount of normal plasma. Failure to obtain such correction suggests the presence of an inhibitor (circulating anticoagulant). Inhibitors can affect individual coagulation factors (as in hemophilia), can be directed against multiple factors, or have an antithrombin effect. Inhibitors against Factor VIII are usually time- and temperature-dependent, and incubation of the test mixture is required for detection of low levels of inhibitor activity. A standard method for quantitating Factor VIII inhibitor has been developed in the United States and is used widely (31). This assay is based on measurement of residual Factor VIII in a mixture of test plasma and normal plasma after incubation for 2 hours at 37° C. A decrease of 50 per cent greater than the control is defined as one Bethesda unit of inhibitor activity.

When evidence of a circulating anticoagulant is found in a hospitalized patient, one must test for the presence of heparin. Heparin prolongs the clotting time of all coagulation tests, but the thrombin time is the most sensitive test for its detection. Heparin is neutralized by protamine sulfate, and one can perform a rapid test to confirm the presence of heparin by adding protamine to the suspect plasma sample and repeating the thrombin time. A shortened clotting time indicates the presence of heparin. Protamine titration involving the thrombin time provides a guide to the dose of protamine required to neutralize heparin in vivo.

An additional test that may be useful in evaluating a plasma sample that contains heparin is the reptilase time. Reptilase is an enzyme that is not affected by heparin and will produce a normal clotting time when added to a normal plasma sample containing heparin. The combination of a long thrombin time and a normal reptilase time suggests the presence of heparin in the sample.

The action of thrombin on fibrinogen results in the splitting off of fibrinopeptides A and B, leaving fibrin monomer. Fibrin monomer forms soluble complexes and may complex with fibrin degradation products if the latter are present. Soluble fibrin monomer complexes may be detected in plasma by the protamine precipitation test (1, 32) or the ethanol gel test (33). One performs protamine test by adding 0.05 ml of 1 per cent protamine sulfate to 0.5 ml of plasma and observing for 15 minutes at 37° C for the formation of precipitate or fibrin strands. (The test can be done with only 0.1 ml of plasma and 0.01 ml of protamine). One performs the ethanol gel test by adding 0.15 ml of 70 per cent ethanol to 0.5 ml of plasma and observing for gel formation. A positive result by either of these "paracoagulation" tests indicates that thrombin has acted on fibrinogen. Both tests have been used in the diagnosis of disseminated intravascular coagulation.

Evidence of increased fibrinolysis can be obtained by determination of fibrinolytic activity or the level of fibrin degradation products. Although specific tests of plasminogen, plasminogen activator, and plasmin are available, a simple screening test of fibrinolytic activity is the euglobulin clot lysis time (34). To perform this test, one prepares a euglobulin fraction of plasma, clots it with thrombin, and measures the time to lysis (normal: greater than 120 minutes). Inhibitors of fibrinolysis are removed in the euglobulin fraction. Fibrin degradation products (FDP) can be determined by a rapid screening test or by more difficult quantitative methods such as the tanned red cell hemagglutination inhibition test. For clinical purposes, the screening test based on agglutination of latex beads coated with antibody to fibrin degradation products is the most useful procedure (Burroughs Wellcome Thrombo-Wellco test for FDP).

Antithrombin III is a plasma protein that, under physiologic conditions, has a slow antithrombin effect. Heparin alters the structure of antithrombin III, converting it to a rapid-acting inhibitor (35). The action of heparin depends on the presence of antithrombin III, and deficiencies of antithrombin III can be associated with an increased incidence of thrombosis. Antithrombin III can be measured by tests based on coagulation, by the use of an artificial chromogenic substrate, and by immunologic methods. Tests based on function are most useful for clinical purposes because in some patients normal levels of antithrombin III by immunoassay can represent nonfunctional protein. In the functional tests, the plasma to be tested is incubated with a known amount of thrombin, and the degree of neutralization is determined by the clotting time or by the effect of the remaining thrombin on a chromogenic substrate material.

TREATMENT OF HEMOSTATIC ABNORMALITIES

Blood Component Therapy: Available Products

In general, if a person with a hereditary coagulation disorder is bleeding (or is to undergo a surgical procedure) he should receive an intravenous infusion of the deficient clotting factor. Through the early 1960's, whole plasma was used because there were no clotting factor concentrates available. Then, in 1965, Dr. Judith Pool developed and described a simple rapid method of preparing cryoprecipitates from fresh plasma (36, 37), and by 1970 methods had been developed to fractionate large volumes of fresh plasma into both Factor VIII concentrates and prothrombin complex concentrates. These more concentrated preparations quickly became the mainstay of treatment for hemophilia A, hemophilia B, and von Willebrand's disease.

Fresh Frozen Plasma (FFP). Fresh frozen plasma is still useful in several situations, despite the availability of more concentrated preparations. In the relatively rare hereditary deficiencies of prothrombin and Factors V, VII, X, XI, and XIII, bleeding can generally be controlled with FFP in a dosage of 10 ml per kg body weight because the hemostatic levels of most of these factors are relatively low. Once hemostasis has been achieved, repeat treatment for that episode is seldom required.

In addition, in persons with mild hemophilia B with infrequent bleeding episodes, FFP may be preferable to commercially prepared prothrombin complex concentrates, mainly because of exposure to far fewer donors. Although an estimated 15 per cent of clotting factor activity is lost in the process of freezing and thawing, an average 230-ml unit of FFP will still contain approximately 200 units of activity for each of the clotting factors. (One unit of clotting factor is defined as the amount present in 1 ml of fresh normal plasma.)

In the case of bleeding associated with severe hepatocellular disease, FFP is the treatment of choice. Also, in disseminated intravascular coagulation (DIC) with bleeding, if replacement therapy is indicated, FFP may be useful in providing depleted coagulation factors and antithrombin III.

Concentrated Preparations of Factor VIII. Cryoprecipitates. These concentrates, prepared from single units of donor plasma, contain approximately 50 per cent of the F VIII:C, von Willebrand factor activity, fibrinogen, and F XIII that was present in the starting unit of plasma. On the average, a single bag of cryoprecipitate contains approximately 100 units of F VIII:C, and 0.20 to 0.30 g fibrinogen in a volume of approximately 10 ml. Since their introduction in 1966, cryoprecipitates have generally been regarded as the treatment of choice for von Willebrand's disease (vWD) because they contain vW factor (vWF) in addition to F VIII:C. (Since becoming available in parenteral form, however, the synthetic agent desmopressin has become the treatment of choice for classic, or Type I, vWD, as discussed further on under Desmopressin Acetate.)

Cryoprecipitates can also be used for treatment of bleeding episodes in hemophilia A and in severe hypofibrinogenemia or afibrinogenemia. Many pediatric hematologists prefer to treat infants and young children who have severe hemophilia A with cryoprecipitates because these agents are prepared from single units of voluntarily donated plasma and thus are presumed to be associated with a lower risk of transmission of viral hepatitis than are the commercially prepared, lyophilized concentrates.

The main disadvantages of cryoprecipitates are that they must be stored in a deep freezer (at $-20°$ to $-30°$ C), they are somewhat difficult to reconstitute and administer at home, and bags of cryoprecipitate vary considerably in their F VIII:C content. For purposes of calculation, one should assume that one bag contains 100 units of F VIII:C; however, in view of their variability in this regard, one should always give a minimum of three bags. In general, the recommended dosage for treatment of hemophilia or vWD is one bag of cryoprecipitate per 6 kg. Somewhat larger doses are needed for treatment of afibrinogenemia (38).

Commercially Prepared Factor VIII Concentrates. These concentrates are now produced by several manufacturers in the United States and have become the mainstay of treatment for hemophilia A. Each lot of concentrate is produced from a large volume of starting plasma that has been obtained by plasmapheresis of as many as 22,000 donors. Although these concentrates are excellent sources of F VIII:C activity, most do not contain enough vWF or fibrinogen to warrant their use in vWD or hypofibrinogenemia. Advantages of Factor VIII concentrates include their ease of storage, reconstitution, and infusion and the fact that each bottle is labeled with the number of Factor VIII units contained. Disadvantages relate to exposure of the recipient to very large numbers of donors and include viral hepatitis (particularly non-A, non-B hepatitis) (39–42) and, in concentrates prepared between 1977 and 1984, a risk of developing AIDS (43). However, primarily because of extreme concern about AIDS, in early 1983 all producers of clotting factor concentrates began screening potential donors much more thoroughly than before in an attempt to eliminate those who belonged to so-called high-risk groups for AIDS. In addition, following the identification (by Broder and Gallo in 1984) of the presumed AIDS virus (44), methods for screening blood for antibody to HTLV-III were developed, and by mid 1985 all blood and plasma collected in the United States was being screened for antibody to HTLV-III. Originally because of the hepatitis risk but then spurred on by extreme concern about AIDS, all manufacturers began producing *heat-treated concentrates* in an attempt to reduce the virus load of these products (see next discussion).

Heat-Treated Factor VIII Concentrates. All American manufacturers of Factor VIII concentrates are now producing heat-treated (or otherwise virus-attenuated) Factor VIII concentrates—and have ceased producing "standard," non–heat-treated concentrates—in an attempt to decrease the viral load of the concentrates. Although heat-treated products offer certain theoretical advantages, to date there are no data that indicate that heat treatment accomplishes the aim of eliminating the risk of hepatitis. Results of a European trial in which newly diagnosed, previously untreated hemophiliacs received a heat-treated product only (Hyland's Hemofil T) indicated that all remained HTLV-III seronegative, but 84 per cent developed elevations of liver enzymes (of at least twice upper limits of normal) within the first 6 months of the trial (45). This is not surprising because plasma coagulation proteins cannot withstand heat capable of inactivating hepatitis viruses ($60°$ C for 10 hours) (42). Thus, agents must be added to stabilize clotting factors to heating. Some investigators have speculated that such stabilizing agents may protect the virus as well as the clotting factors. At any rate, although in vitro testing has demonstrated a substantial diminution of virus in purposely virus-contaminated concentrates that have been heated, (46) these products are not virus-free and may still transmit hepatitis.

In contrast, the presumed AIDS virus, HTLV-

III, appears to be extremely heat-sensitive (47). In view of this plus the rapid rise in the number of confirmed cases of AIDS among hemophiliacs during 1984 and 1985, the National Hemophilia Foundation's Medical and Scientific Advisory Council recommended in the spring of 1985 that heat-treated (or otherwise virus-inactivated) concentrates be used for all severe hemophiliacs (48).

Despite the potential benefits of heat-treated products, however, some investigators are still concerned about potential long-term deleterious effects. Some worry that there may be an increased likelihood of inhibitor development if heat treatment alters the Factor VIII molecule slightly, rendering it more antigenic. It should be noted, however, that to date no such effects have been demonstrated.

Porcine Factor VIII Concentrates. These concentrates, prepared by Speywood Laboratories in the United Kingdom (trade name, HYATE:C), are useful in the management of persons (hemophiliacs as well as nonhemophiliacs) with Factor VIII inhibitors (49–51). Advantages include no risk of hepatitis or AIDS and the fact that one can follow response to therapy with Factor VIII assays. This newer, highly purified porcine Factor VIII preparation does not cause severe thrombocytopenia (which was a problem with older porcine preparations); however, allergic and, rarely, anaphylactic reactions may still occur. Such undesirable side effects can be eliminated or minimized by administration of 100 mg hydrocortisone with the first dose. HYATE:C is still considered investigational in the United States, but licensure for use in inhibitor patients is expected by late 1986.

Prothrombin Complex Concentrates (PCCs). These concentrates, which contain the vitamin K-dependent clotting factors—II, VII, IX, and X—as well as protein C, are currently produced by several American manufacturers. PCCs produced by different manufacturers vary somewhat in their content of Factor VII; for example, Hyland's Proplex SX contains very little Factor VII. In addition to nonactivated Factors II, VII, IX and X, some activated clotting factor is contained in variable amounts in PCCs. The presence of activated clotting factor occasionally results in DIC or thromboembolic problems and presumably accounts for the beneficial effects of PCC in controlling bleeding in hemophiliacs with Factor VIII or Factor IX inhibitors.

The main indication for use of PCCs is in the treatment of bleeding episodes in persons with severe hemophilia B. As is true of Factor VIII concentrates, PCCs offer certain advantages over FFP. They provide Factor IX in a concentrated form, thus permitting achievement of high levels of Factor IX in the recipient without danger of fluid overload. They can be stored for prolonged periods in an ordinary refrigerator ($-4°C$) and are easy to reconstitute and administer, and thus they are ideal for home use. In addition, each bottle is labeled with the number of Factor IX units contained. However, one must also be aware of the potential adverse effects of PCCs. As is true of Factor VIII concentrates, PCCs have associated risks, including those related to exposure to plasma from very large numbers of donors. Another concern is that PCCs may occasionally result in serious, even life-threatening, thromboembolic complications. Because PCCs contain some activated clotting factors (principally Factors IXa and Xa) (58), disseminated intravascular coagulation or thromboembolic phenomena or both may occur in persons receiving large repeated doses over a period of several days, especially if they are immobile following, for example, an orthopedic surgical procedure, crush injury, or extensive trauma (during which thromboplastic materials may be released into the circulation) or extensive muscle hemorrhage. The risk of thrombogenicity is also increased in patients with hepatocellular disease, presumably owing to low levels of antithrombin III and decreased capacity to clear clotting intermediates from the circulation (52–58). In 1975, Kasper surveyed coagulation specialists and reported a large number of previously unreported thromboembolic complications associated with PCCs in patients with hepatocellular disease, in neonates, and in persons with hemophilia B undergoing surgical procedures (54). However, the denominator in such reports is not known, and the collection of source plasma in plastic bags is thought to have decreased the thrombogenicity of PCCs somewhat since the mid 1970's. Many have followed the 1975 recommendation made by the International Committee on Thrombosis and Haemostasis to add heparin to reconstituted PCC just before use (5 units per ml of reconstituted PCC) (59), especially in orthopaedic surgical situations, and greater overall awareness of potential thrombogenicity has resulted in greater care in the use of PCCs. Thus, although the incidence of thromboembolism associated with the use of PCCs is not known, it is probably lower than it was in the early 1970's. Because neonates and individuals with liver disease are especially prone to thrombosis with PCCs, such patients should be managed with FFP rather than with PCCs whenever possible.

Another potential complication of PCCs is acute myocardial infarction. To date, myocardial infarction has been reported in four young men (ages 15 to 22 years) who were receiving large, repeated doses of PCCs (60–63). All were patients with hemophilia A and Factor VIII inhibitor. It is noteworthy that in two of the three who died, there was no autopsy evidence of thromboembolus as a primary cardiac event. The major pathologic feature in both patients was massive transmural ventricular hemorrhage. These observations raise the possibility that some other effect of PCCs on the coronary vasculature or myocardium might be involved. Because high-molecular-weight kininogens are present in PCCs, it has been proposed that release of bradykinin may lead to vascular leakage and myocardial injury (62). Although the exact etiology and pathogenesis of myocardial infarction in these subjects remain unknown, each individual had received large doses of PCCs (at least 200 Factor IX units per kg per day) for at least 4 consecutive days.

It seems at least theoretically possible that a similar problem may occur with activated PCCs. Myocardial infarction has been reported in a 40-year-old hemophiliac who was receiving an activated PCC, FEIBA, for 7 consecutive days (64), and Tabor and Votaw have described fatal myocardial infarction in a 29-year-old man who had received both standard and activated PCCs (65).

Activated Prothrombin Complex Concentrates (APCCs). Purposely activated PCCs are produced by two manufacturers (Hyland Laboratories, Glendale, CA, and Immuno, Vienna, Austria). These products are for use *only* in inhibitor patients. Both Hyland's Autoplex and Immuno's FEIBA contain more activated clotting factor than the "standard" PCC. They were developed in an attempt to bypass the need for Factor VIII (or Factor IX) in persons with Factor VIII (or Factor IX) inhibitors.

APCCs are reportedly more effective than "standard" PCCs in controlling bleeding episodes in inhibitor patients, especially in serious, or "open," types of bleeding. However, although some published anecdotal reports claim excellent responses to either Autoplex or FEIBA, other reports indicate that these products are not predictably effective (66, 67). To date, one controlled trial has been conducted with each of the two activated products. Sjamsoedin and colleagues found a 64 per cent response rate to FEIBA, in contrast to 52 per cent for nonactivated PCC (68). Lusher and colleagues found no difference in response rate between a single dose of Autoplex and a single dose of the nonactivated PCC, Proplex, in the control of acute hemarthrosis (67). Additional trials incorporating two doses of each unknown product and a longer period of observation would be of interest.

Disadvantages of APCCs include cost. Both APCCs are very expensive (Autoplex is currently 89 cents per "Factor VIII correctional unit" [FECU]; at the recommended dose of 50 to 100 FECU per kg, a single dose for a 70-kg adolescent costs 3000 to 6000 dollars. FEIBA, at 75 cents per FEIBA unit, is only slightly less costly). In addition, as is the case with nonactivated PCCs, there is no means of laboratory monitoring for effectiveness in the recipient, and APCCs are not always effective in achieving hemostasis. Also, as is true of all clotting factor concentrates, the hepatitis risk is quite high.

Heat-Treated PCCs and APCCs. All American manufacturers of clotting factor concentrates are now producing heat-treated PCCs, and both Hyland and Immuno are now producing heat-treated APCCs in an attempt to decrease the virus load of the concentrates. (For theoretical benefits and risks, see previous comments regarding heat-treated Factor VIII concentrates.)

Coagulation Factor IX. The American Red Cross has described a method of preparing a Factor IX concentrate that is essentially free of Factors II, VII, and X and that is thought to be less thrombogenic than PCCs (69); however, this product is not currently licensed for use in the United States.

Antithrombin III (AT III) Concentrates. Several varieties of AT III concentrates have been available, either for investigational use (in Europe and the United States) or commercially (in Europe only at present, available from Kabi Vitrum AB as Antithrombin 500 IV). Antithrombin is the main physiologic inhibitor of blood coagulation. It is the heparin cofactor and is essential to effective heparin therapy. In addition to neutralizing thrombin, antithrombin is the main physiologic inhibitor of activated Factor X (Factor Xa). It inhibits a variety of other serine proteases (activated coagulation factors) as well, including kallikrein, plasmin, C_1 esterase and Factors IXa, XIa, XIIa (70–72). AT III concentrates have been recommended for use in the following situations: (1) congenital deficiency states involving acute thrombosis, (2) congenital deficiency states before surgery or during late pregnancy, (3) acquired deficiencies with acute thrombosis or DIC, particularly if heparin is contraindicated because of bleeding sites (e.g., trauma or surgery) (73).

It should be noted that FFP will provide limited replacement of antithrombin if AT III concentrates are not available. (It is anticipated that AT-III concentrates will soon be licensed for use in the United States) AT III concentrates, like Factor VIII concentrates and PCCs, are categorized as high-risk plasma derivatives in terms of potential transmission of viral hepatitis (42).

Production of Factor VIII From Cloned DNA. F VIII:C has been successfully cloned (74), and efforts are underway to produce coagulation factor concentrates by such recombinant DNA technology. However, it will probably be at least 1988 before a safe, effective, and clinically tested product is available for use. To date, the expression of F VIII:C in mammalian cells has been very low, and it is probable that more effective vectors or host-cell systems will have to be devised. Also, effective large-scale tissue culture and purification methods must be developed. F IX:C also has been cloned. However, in addition to technical obstacles, there has been little commercial interest in developing it.

Other Agents

Antifibrinolytics. Epsilon amino caproic acid (EACA) and tranexamic acid are antifibrinolytic agents that act by inhibiting plasminogen activation. Such drugs are useful adjuncts in certain specific situations in which one wishes to prevent lysis of a clot that has already formed as a result of specific factor replacement therapy. Their greatest use in hemophilia and other hereditary clotting disorders has been in the management of bleeding in the oral cavity (e.g., tongue and mouth lacerations, extraction of permanent teeth, and other oral surgical procedures). In such situations, EACA is given in a dosage of 75 mg per kg four times daily for a period of 7 to 10 days or until wound healing is complete. The dosage of tranexamic acid is less, being approximately 25 mg per kg per dose. At least from a theoretical standpoint, the concomitant administration of antifibrinolytic agent and PCC may be hazardous, since PCC contains some activated clotting factors. If one decides to use both these agents (as in a child with hemophilia B who has a mouth laceration), they should probably be spaced at intervals of at least 4 hours between doses of PCC and doses of EACA or tranexamic acid.

Desmopressin Acetate. Desmopressin acetate (1-deamino-8-d-arginine vasopressin; DDAVP), is a synthetic analogue of the naturally occurring antidiuretic hormone, 8-arginine vasopressin. This drug, which is almost totally devoid of the unpleasant side effects of other vasopressin derivatives, results in a transient threefold increase in all components of the Factor VIII system and in an increase in plasminogen activator. It is ideally suited for raising the Factor VIII level in persons with mild to moderate hemophilia A or classic (Type I) von Willebrand's disease. Although its mechanism of action is not known with certainty, it has been postulated that desmopressin acts centrally, causing release of a second, as yet unidentified messenger from the CNS that stimulates release of Factor VIII from its endothelial cell storage sites (75). The rise in Factor VIII following intravenous desmopressin occurs so rapidly that increased synthesis is unlikely to account for it, and the endogenous release of Factor VIII appears much more likely. In addition, utilizing a human umbilical vein model, Barnhart and colleagues have demonstrated that the drug has a direct effect on the vessel wall as well, as evidenced by increased platelet adhesion and platelet spreading at injury sites (76).

Clinico-pharmacologic studies done by Mannucci and co-workers have demonstrated that the optimal intravenous dose for increasing Factor VIII with desmopressin is 0.3 µg per kg (77). Although individuals vary somewhat in their degree of Factor response, on the average this dosage will result in a threefold increase in F VIII:C and a twofold increase in F VIIIR:Ag and F VIIIR:Cof (half-life, 8 to 10 hours) (77). The response is quite rapid, with peak values being reached between 15 and 30 minutes post infusion. Although repeated doses can be given at 12 to 24-hour intervals, many individuals will have a suboptimal response to such repetitive doses by the second, third, or fourth day, reflecting a transient depletion of the storage sites (77, 78).

Side effects of desmopressin acetate are minimal but include facial flushing, facial warmth, and, occasionally, transient headache or nausea or both. One can minimize side effects by mixing the drug with 30 to 50 ml normal saline solution and injecting it slowly, over a period of 15 to 30 minutes. Rare side effects include hypertension, bleeding from increased fibrinolysis, and hyponatremia and water intoxication. Although there have been only a few reports of the latter, most cases have occurred in persons who were receiving repeated doses of desmopressin along with large amounts of intravenous fluids postoperatively (79, 80). Thus, in such situations, it is probably wise for one to monitor serum electrolytes and osmolality.

Danazol. Danazol, an attenuated androgen that stimulates protein synthesis, was reported in one study to increase plasma levels of both F VIII:C and F IX:C in persons with moderately severe hemophilia A or B when given daily for several weeks (81). Dosage was 600 mg/day orally in three divided doses. Athough Gralnick and co-workers reported a low incidence of side effects with such daily administration of danazol, others have observed a greater degree of undesirable side effects (e.g., hepatocellular dysfunction, generalized pruritic rashes, and an increase in bleeding manifestations). More important, several other groups have found no clinical benefit when using the same regimen as that reported by Gralnick's group, and, in each of two separate controlled, double-blind, crossover studies in which danazol was being compared with a placebo, no beneficial effects were noted in individuals with hemophilia A or B (82, 83). However, this agent may eventually prove to be useful in other situations (e.g., to increase fibrinolysis or to increase antithrombin III levels).

Avoidance of Drugs That Can Induce Platelet Dysfunction

Aspirin and aspirin-containing compounds as well as certain other drugs (84, 85) can cause platelet dysfunction, which can aggravate bleeding in persons who have an underlying coagulation defect. Thus, these drugs should be avoided in persons with a coagulation disorder.

Joint or soft-tissue hemorrhage in hemophilia or other coagulopathy is often painful. If aspirin or an aspirin-containing compound is taken to relieve the pain, the bleeding tendency may worsen because aspirin inhibits platelet aggregation. This effect is mediated by inhibition of prostaglandin synthesis and is due to irreversible inhibition of platelet cyclo-oxygenase. Acetaminophen is recommended as an alternative to aspirin for relief of mild pain or temperature elevation.

Among other drugs that interfere with platelet function are the antihistamines, phenothiazines, penicillin compounds in high concentration, and nonsteroidal antiinflammatory drugs such as indomethacin (84).

HEREDITARY COAGULATION DISORDERS

The Hemophilias

Hemophilia A (Factor VIII deficiency) and hemophilia B (Factor IX deficiency) are bleeding disorders that are inherited as X-linked recessive traits. Thus, both affect males almost exclusively. The two disorders are clinically indistinguishable but can easily be differentiated by Factor VIII and Factor IX activity assays. In hemophilia A, the Factor VIII procoagulant moiety (F VIII:C) is deficient or abnormal, but other components of the Factor VIII system (Factor VIII–related antigen and von Willebrand's factor) are normal. In general, the severity of bleeding manifestations correlates well with the F VIII:C value, with assay values of less than 0.03 units per ml (3 per cent) being associated with spontaneous hemorrhage into joints and soft tissues.

Hemophilia B (Factor IX deficiency; Christmas disease) is characterized by subnormal Factor IX activity, which may reflect a quantitative or qualitative abnormality in the Factor IX molecule. Although the Factor VIII complex has a molecular weight of about 1.5 million daltons, the human Factor IX molecule is much smaller, having a molecular weight of 60,000 daltons. As in hemophilia A, a Factor IX assay value of less than 0.03 units per ml is generally associated with spontaneous bleeding into joints and soft tissue.

Both hemophilia A and hemophilia B are heterogeneous conditions. At least six different subtypes of hemophilia B have been described (86). Although all are characterized by low levels of Factor IX coagulant activity, the degree of the deficiency varies, and in several of the subtypes there is laboratory evidence of qualitative abnormalities of the Factor IX molecule (86). Within a given kindred, however, there does not appear to be heterogeneity. Of the two types of hemophilia, hemophilia A is far more common, occurring in one in 10,000 males in the United States. In contrast, the incidence of hemophilia B is 0.25 in 10,000 males. In both types of hemophilia, clinical severity varies considerably. Because the minimal level of Factor VIII or Factor IX needed for effective hemostasis is approximately 0.30 units per ml (30 per cent), persons with mild hemophilia A or B (with Factor VIII or Factor IX levels of 8 to 20 per cent) often lead fairly normal lives and have excessive bleeding only after significant trauma or surgery. In contrast, those with severe hemophilia (with Factor VIII or Factor IX levels of <3 per cent) generally have spontaneous bleeding into joints and soft tissues beginning at an early age. In moderate hemophilia A (with levels of 3 to 8 per cent), spontaneous hemorrhage is infrequent, but relatively minor trauma may precipitate acute hemarthrosis or soft-tissue bleeding.

The male infant who inherits a gene for severe hemophilia is born with a severe deficiency of Factor VIII or Factor IX activity because neither factor can cross the placenta. Thus, first-born affected males occasionally develop large cephalhematomas (Fig. 41–4), especially if there is a long, difficult labor or forceps delivery. (The latter should be avoided if it is known that the mother is a "carrier" and thus that her male infant is at risk, as intracranial hemorrhage occasionally can result.)

The diagnosis can be made at birth (and, in fact, prenatally in highly specialized centers) with assays of the infant's blood for F VIII:C or F IX:C. If circumcision is planned, the appropriate assay should always precede the procedure. For a pregnant woman who is a known or even a possible carrier for hemophilia A or B, the physician should make arrangements to obtain a cord blood sample at the time of delivery if the infant is a boy. The cord blood sample should be collected in citrate (standard "blue top tube") and should be delivered to the coagulation laboratory as soon as possible.

If not traumatized during or immediately following delivery, the infant with hemophilia generally has few problems during the first year of life. Excessive bruising may be noted, but joint bleeding is uncommon. During the toddler years, when the child is learning to walk and is frequently falling and bumping into things or falling and biting his tongue, bleeding episodes requiring treatment begin to occur. Tongue and mouth lacerations are often seen in toddlers and are often perplexing to treat (see further on). Acute hemarthroses, secondary to trauma or spontaneous, begin to occur when the child is approximately 1 to 2 years of age, and then continue on an episodic basis throughout the hemophiliac's life.

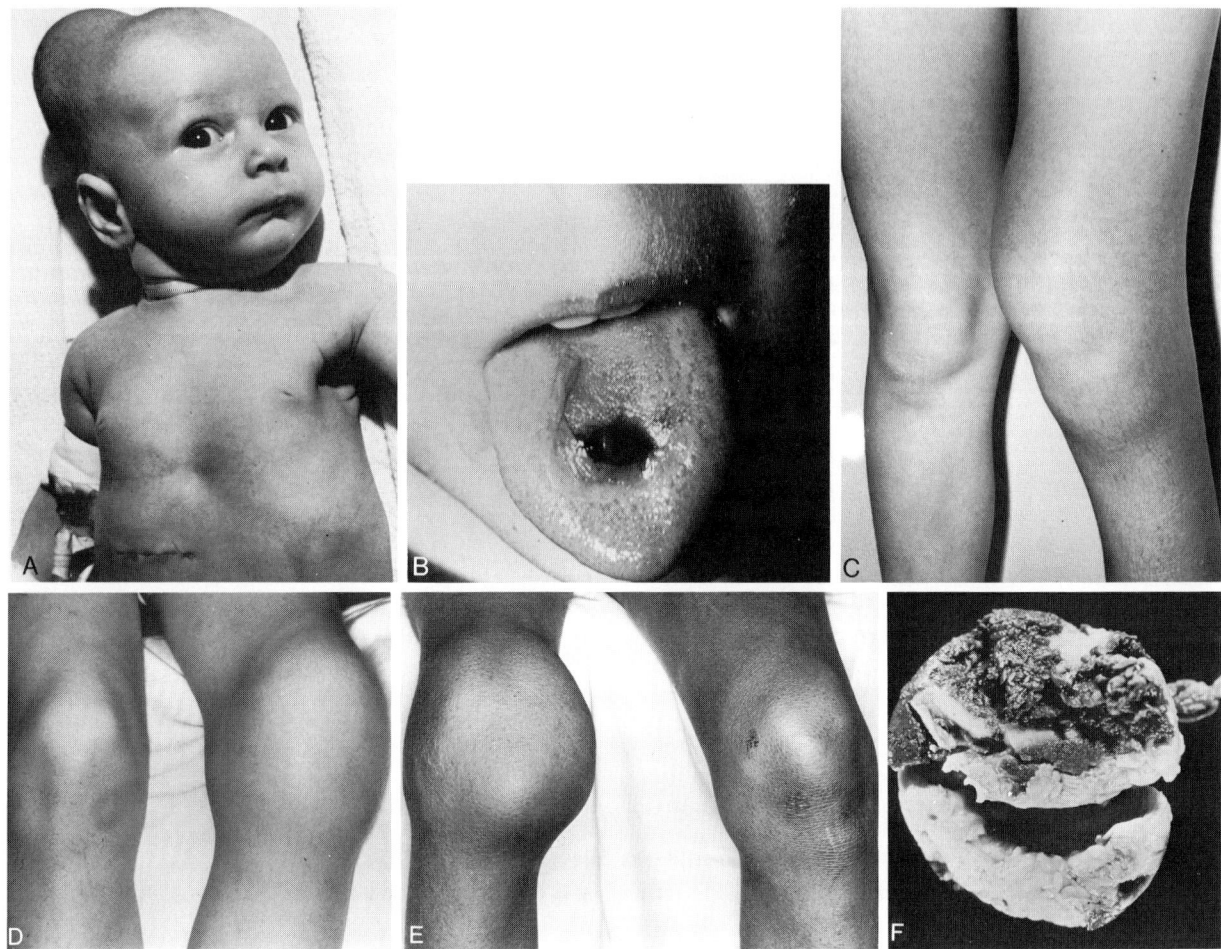

Figure 41-4. In hemophilia A or B a variety of bleeding manifestations may be seen. *A*, A large cephalhematoma in an infant with severe hemophilia A who was born to a gravida 1 mother. Neither Factor VIII nor Factor IX crosses the placenta, and thus male infants who inherit a gene for hemophilia lack Factor VIII or Factor IX at birth. *B*, Bleeding from a small tongue laceration in a 2-year-old child with hemophilia. *C*, Suprapatellar hemorrhage in a boy with hemophilia B. *D*, Extreme swelling of left knee from acute hemarthrosis in a boy with severe hemophilia A. Such extreme swelling is now unusual, as it is recommended that patients be treated at the first indication of bleeding into a joint so that chronic joint disease is avoided. *E*, Chronically swollen right knee resulting from proliferative synovitis and recurrent bleeding into joint. *F*, Synovium removed from knee shown in *E*. Note hemosiderin deposits and thickened, irregular synovium.

Before cryoprecipitates and clotting factor concentrates became available, chronic joint disease had developed in all boys with severe hemophilia by an early age (10 to 12 years), resulting from recurrent bleeding into joints. Many who survived into adult life were severely disabled and often confined to wheel chairs. Many died at an early age, most often from intracranial hemorrhage or hemorrhage following dental extractions or other surgical procedures.

Since the 1960's, the availability of concentrated preparations of Factor VIII and Factor IX has greatly improved the lives of hemophiliacs. Not only has the life expectancy for these individuals doubled but also the quality of life has become vastly better. The availability of cryoprecipitates and lyophilized Factor VIII and Factor IX concentrates has made many things possible, including outpatient treatment (rather than hospitalization for minor bleeding episodes, which was routinely used when only plasma was available), home treatment (see further on), and elective surgery.

Despite these advances, however, many problems remain. Hemophilia is a multifaceted disorder that can potentially affect many organ systems. There are complications of treatment, some of which are quite serious and sometimes fatal. Many aspects of the lives of the hemophiliac and his family are greatly affected by the disease. Therefore, a team approach to comprehensive care for hemophiliacs is necessary.

TREATMENT
Regional Comprehensive Care

In 1975, Congress established the Hemophilia Diagnostic and Treatment Center Program, for which 3 million dollars per year in federal funds were allocated. There is now a network of regional comprehensive hemophilia diagnostic and treatment centers across the United States that are partially subsidized by federal or state grants or both (87). At each center, a team of experts provides comprehensive periodic assessment of each individual seen and makes recommendations to the patient and his family and to his local health care providers. The team should include, in addition to a pediatric hematologist and an internist, an orthopedic surgeon, a physical therapist, a dentist, a dental hygienist, a hemophilia nurse, a social worker, a genetic counselor, and a vocational rehabilitation counselor. With such a multifaceted approach, the broader needs of the hemophiliac and his family can be met. Patient education, home treatment training, vocational planning, genetics, and prophylaxis are stressed, including exercises and attention to dental hygiene.*

Home Infusion Program

Since the early 1970's, the concept of "home care" for hemophilia has steadily gained in popularity and acceptance. Essentially all hemophilia centers in the United States now have programs for teaching the hemophiliac and his family not only the techniques of self-infusion but also when to treat, how to calculate the proper dosage of concentrate, when to call center personnel (e.g., call immediately in the case of head injury!), and how to dispose of used needles and syringes. The National Hemophilia Foundation has produced an excellent home treatment training module that is utilized by many hemophilia centers. The many advantages of home treatment include (1) prompt treatment for acute bleeding episodes, (2) decreased time lost from work for parent and from school for child, (3) an increased sense of independence, and (4) decreased health care costs. The prompt treatment of acute hemarthroses made possible by home infusion has no doubt lessened the incidence of chronic joint disease and should make it possible for affected individuals to lead much more productive lives. In many states, those on home treatment must complete and return "home treatment log sheets" that include the date, site of bleeding, brand, lot number and dosage of concentrate used, perceived effectiveness, and any untoward side effects noted.

Although a few hemophilia centers still prescribe cryoprecipitates for home infusion, most use commercially prepared (heat-treated) lyophilized concentrates because these agents are much easier to store, reconstitute, and administer at home. Children 11 or 12 years of age can usually learn to self-infuse, and a parent of a child 3 years of age or older can generally be taught to start and administer the child's infusion.

Hemophilia A (Factor VIII Deficiency). In general, replacement therapy with cryoprecipitates of Factor VIII concentrates is used only for acute bleeding episodes. The most common indications for treatment are acute joint hemorrhage (acute hemarthrosis) and bleeding into a muscle mass. Such bleeding episodes should be treated as a medical emergency! Prompt treatment not only will stop the bleeding, but also will often lessen the total amount of clotting factor needed to treat the episode and, more important, prevent the gradual development of crippling musculoskeletal deformities. Treatment consists of Factor VIII replacement therapy with either cryoprecipitates or Factor VIII concentrates and rest of the affected part.

Because of its presumed lower risk of transmitting viral hepatitis, cryoprecipitate is preferred by some, especially in the treatment of infants and small children, and in persons of any age who have had infrequent exposure to blood products. Most prefer heat-treated lyophilized Factor VIII concentrates for the management of children over 4 years of age with severe hemophilia A, mainly because of the ease of storage, reconstitution, and administration of these products.

Dosage of Factor VIII. In calculating the dosage of Factor VIII (see Table 41–3), one can assume that one unit of Factor VIII (defined as the amount of Factor VIII contained in 1 ml of normal fresh plasma) per kg will raise the recipient's Factor VIII level by 0.02 units per ml (2 per cent). Thus, if a severe hemophiliac whose baseline Factor VIII is less than 0.01 units per ml (<1 per cent) is given an infusion of 20 units per kg, his F VIII:C would be expected to rise to 0.40 units per ml (40 per cent). The half-life of infused Factor VIII is 8 to 12 hours but may be shorter if the patient has an extensive bleeding episode or is febrile.

When using commercial concentrates, one will find the number of Factor VIII units contained in each bottle printed on its label. Any excess in the bottle (i.e., excess over calculated amount) should be given rather than discarded. If using cryoprecipitates, one should assume, for purpose of calculation, that each bag of cryoprecipitate contains approximately 100 units Factor VIII. However, in view of the bag-to-bag variability in Factor VIII content, it is recommended that a minimum of three bags be given even if calculations for a very small child indicate that one or two bags would be sufficient.

Acute Hemarthroses. Acute bleeding into joints is the most common type of bleeding requiring treatment in hemophiliacs. Acute hemarthroses should

---

*A booklet listing the hemophilia centers that provide comprehensive care can be obtained from the National Hemophilia Foundation, The Soho Building, Suite 406, 110 Greene St., New York, NY 10012. The Foundation also maintains a number of current educational booklets for hemophiliacs and their families and health care providers. Topics include genetics, musculoskeletal problems, inhibitors, financial planning, and psychosocial issues.

Table 41–3. RECOMMENDED DOSAGES OF FACTOR VIII FOR HEMOPHILIA A*

Type of Bleeding	Initial Dosage (U/kg)	Repeat Dosage (U/kg)	Other Treatment
Acute hemarthrosis†			
Early	10	Seldom necessary	
Late	20	20 q 12h	Ice packs, non–weight bearing; sling or light-weight splint may be helpful; rarely, joint aspiration (see text)
Intramuscular hemorrhage†	20–30	20 q 12h; often, several days of treatment required for extensive hemorrhages	Non–weight bearing; complete bed rest for iliopsoas hemorrhage

Life-threatening situations‡
  Intracranial hemorrhage
  Major surgery
  Major trauma
  Tongue or neck bleeding with potential airway obstruction
	50	25–30 q 8–12h
		or
		Preferably, bolus dose of 25 U/kg followed by continuous infusion, 3–4 U/kg/hour	

Severe abdominal pain‡	20–40	20–25 q 12h	
Tongue and mouth lacerations‡	20	20 q 12h	An antifibrinolytic agent (tranexamic acid or EACA), sedation, NPO in small child; local application of orahesive gauze may be beneficial for gum bleeding
Extractions of permanent teeth‡	20	20 q 12h; however, often not necessary in uncomplicated extractions	Antifibrinolytic agent beginning 1 day pre-op; continue 7–10 days
Painless spontaneous gross hematuria	None		Increased PO fluids; corticosteroids and/or Factor VIII are used by some

*Refers to heat-treated or otherwise virus-attenuated Factor VIII.
†In infants and children under 4 years of age, some still prefer to use cryoprecipitates rather than virus-attenuated lyophilized Factor VIII concentrates (see text). In individuals who have mild hemophilia A, it is preferable to use desmopressin rather than lyophilized Factor VIII concentrates.
‡These cases should be treated in a comprehensive hemophilia center. If a case is first seen in another hospital, the hemophilia center should be contacted and the patient transferred after emergency treatment is given at the local hospital.
(Reprinted with permission from Lusher, J. M.: Hemophilia. Hematol. Rev. Commun. *1*:1–34, 1986.)

be considered an emergency and should be treated promptly. *Prompt treatment is of the utmost importance!* Early treatment will often obviate the need for repeated doses of concentrate and will lessen the likelihood of gradual development of chronic debilitating joint disease.

Each episode of joint bleeding results in synovial inflammation. Synovitis becomes chronic if repeated joint hemorrhages are not promptly treated. Chronic synovitis leads to increased proliferation of the inflamed synovium, which is very vascular, making frequent recurrent joint hemorrhages likely. There is then gradual destruction of cartilage and resorption of bone with cyst formation. This leads to joint instability, which in turn leads to more frequent bleeding into the joint and surrounding soft tissue, chronic joint pain and subsequent disuse atrophy of surrounding muscles, and thus even greater instability of the joint (88, 89). Acute hemarthroses most often involve the elbow, knee, and ankle, although hemarthroses of the shoulder, wrist, hip, and finger joints also occur. Acute joint bleeding may be spontaneous or may result from trauma. Recurrent episodes of bleeding in a particular "target joint" may occur without trauma, presumably because of synovial proliferation and increased vascularity (or more advanced changes) that followed earlier hemorrhages into that joint.

Although pain, swelling, and limitation of joint motion are the hallmarks of acute hemarthrosis, one should begin treatment before these symptoms occur. Many patients describe an unusual sensation, tingling, or minimal discomfort when they are beginning to bleed into a joint, prior to obvious swelling and pain. This is the optimal time to treat. In the management of acute hemarthrosis a good motto is, "when in doubt, treat!"

The recommended dose of Factor VIII is shown in Table 41–3. In general, the earlier an acute hemarthrosis is treated, the less clotting factor is required (e.g., if a patient is on home treatment and treats himself at the earliest indication of joint bleeding, he can usually use one half the amount that would be required if several hours had elapsed and the joint had become painfully distended). Rest of the affected part during the acute phase of bleeding also is important. For an elbow hemorrhage, a sling may be helpful. For an extensive knee hemorrhage in a small child, a lightweight splint may help protect the joint from repeated use during the acute phase. Immobilization is generally not necessary for early hemarthroses, however, because response to clotting factor concentrates is usually quite rapid. When immobilization is used, it should not be continued for more than a few days because muscle atrophy may result. Ice packs also may provide temporary symptomatic relief from pain associated with an acute hemarthrosis (90, 91).

Acute distended, painful joints (see Fig. 41–4) are seen much less often now because most acute hemarthroses are being treated promptly. However, if bleeding has progressed to the extent that a joint is extremely distended and excruciatingly painful, the joint should be aspirated. When joint aspiration is indicated, it should be done with careful attention to aseptic technique and only after infusion of clotting factor concentrate. A single intravenous dose of narcotic analgesic (e.g., meperidine) may be necessary for control of excruciating pain resulting from such an acutely distended joint prior to aspiration.

As already described, frequent recurrent hemarthroses may result in disuse muscle atrophy; therefore, physical therapy is quite important. Isometric exercises often help prevent atrophy of the quadriceps group, thus lessening the chance of reinjury to the knee. High-top padded hiking boots can provide ankle stability and lessen the chances of ankle injury. Swimming is an excellent form of exercise for improving and maintaining muscle tone. The hemophilia team's physical therapist is often an excellent resource person for instructing and providing follow-up on appropriate exercises.

Muscle Hemorrhage. Intramuscular hemorrhage is the second most common indication for replacement therapy with clotting factor concentrates. Intramuscular hemorrhage is usually associated with pain, swelling, and limitation of motion of the affected area. Although a single dose of clotting factor will often suffice for early joint bleeding, repeated doses are usually needed for treatment of intramuscular hemorrhage. Clotting factor should be given twice daily until the muscle mass begins to soften and pain subsides.

Although intramuscular bleeding into such areas as the calf, forearm, and thigh is quite visible, with tense swelling and tenderness, iliopsoas bleeding is not. The symptoms and signs of an iliopsoas hemorrhage are generally limited to ill-defined discomfort in the groin and flexion of the thigh with resistance of extension. On roentgenographic examination, one characteristically sees obliteration of the psoas shadow on the affected side. A large iliopsoas hemorrhage may result in displacement of the kidney and ureter, anemia secondary to contained hemorrhage, and neurologic evidence of femoral nerve compression. Management should consist of hospitalization or bed rest at home, with clotting factor concentrate given every 12 hours for several days.

Head Injury. Head trauma in a hemophiliac is an indication for immediate treatment with large doses of clotting factor concentrate (see Table 41–3), careful neurologic examination, and close observation. If head injury occurs at or near home in a child who is on home treatment, a dose of clotting factor should be given before he is brought to the emergency room. In those who are not on home treatment and in those for whom the trip to the hospital would be quicker than infusing at home, clotting factor should be given immediately on arrival in the emergency room. Unless the head injury is judged to be trivial, the child should then be seen by a neurosurgeon, have a CT scan, and be hospitalized for observation and further treatment (91). Subsequent doses of clotting factor should be given every 8 to 12 hours or, preferably, as a continuous infusion. In giving Factor VIII concentrate by continuous infusion, one should first give a bolus dose of 40 to 50 units per kg, which will raise the patient's Factor VIII level to 80 to 100 per cent. The continuous infusion should then be given at a rate of 3 to 4 units per kg per hour with the subsequent rate being determined by the patient's Factor VIII level. In general, a rate of 2 units per kg per hour will result in a Factor VIII level of 25 per cent; 3 units per kg per hour will result in a 50 per cent level; and 4 units per kg per hour will result in a 75 per cent level. One should not, however, merely assume that these levels will be achieved, and daily monitoring of the patient's Factor VIII level is recommended so that the infusion rate can be readjusted to and maintained at the desired level. Such continuous infusion therapy produces reliable therapeutic levels and is ideally suited for situations such as intracranial hemorrhage and major surgery, in which one needs to maintain a high level of Factor VIII for a prolonged period (92, 93).

If intracranial hemorrhage has been demonstrated, one should maintain Factor VIII levels at 50 per cent by providing continuous infusion for a minimum of 14 days, followed by 30 units per kg per day for another week. In view of the high incidence of spontaneous recurrent CNS hemorrhages within a few months of the first episode, some recommend 2 to 12 months of alternate-day prophylaxis with Factor VIII concentrates (94).

Oral Bleeding. Tongue and mouth lacerations usually occur in toddlers but are occasionally seen in older children. Although clotting factor concentrate should be given to all hemophiliacs with these injuries, ancillary management depends on the age of the patient and the site and extent of intraoral injury. An infusion of clotting factor concentrate will result in local clot formation, but it is difficult to maintain an intact clot, particularly on the tongue of a small child (see Fig. 41–4). Because the clot will almost always be dislodged in this age group, all infants and small children with tongue or mouth lacerations should be hospitalized. Management should consist of cryoprecipitates given every 12 hours; 75 mg per kg of the antifibrinolytic agent, epsilon aminocaproic acid (EACA), given every 6 hours; heavy sedation; and maintenance of the child on parenteral nutrition, with nothing given by mouth. If this regimen is followed without interruption, healing is usually complete within 4 or 5 days. Although ineffective on tongue lacerations, an orahesive gauze (e.g., Squibb's Stomahesive) is often quite helpful when firmly placed over gum lacerations. The orahesive gauze sheets can be cut to the desired size, with the cut piece then placed firmly over the wound.

In an older child or adolescent with a similar lesion, outpatient management consists of clotting factor replacement, local use of an orahesive gauze, administration of an antifibrinolytic agent (EACA), and continued attention to preventing dislodgement of the clot. Cold liquids followed by a soft diet are recommended. EACA should be continued for 7 to 10 days or until wound healing is complete.

When performing tooth extractions in hemophiliacs, it is essential that one provide, in addition to a pre-extraction dose of clotting factor concentrate, careful local attention to the extraction site to prevent hemorrhage. Microcrystalline collagen, a platelet-aggregating agent that is placed directly into the socket of the extracted tooth, is often quite effective, especially when used in combination with EACA or tranexamic acid. The latter agents should be given for 7 to 10 days.

Hematuria. Gross hematuria may result from trauma or a blow to the kidney, in which case clotting factor concentrate is indicated. However, painless gross hematuria most often occurs spontaneously. Especially in children, one should rule out other possible causes of painless gross hematuria, such as acute glomerulonephritis. If other underlying causes are excluded, no specific treatment is indicated. It has been our practice to allow the patient to continue his usual activities and to have him drink extra fluids until hematuria stops (usually within 2 to 7 days). If gross hematuria persists beyond a week, one or two doses of clotting factor concentrate may be tried, but EACA should be avoided because ureteropelvic obstruction by clots may occur with its use. Although some routinely use clotting factor concentrates or corticosteroids or both at the onset of gross hematuria, there is currently no evidence that these result in more rapid cessation of hematuria than no treatment. A multicenter-controlled blinded trial is currently being conducted by Gomperts and colleagues, in which prednisone is being compared to a similar-appearing placebo. It is hoped that the results of this trial will determine whether or not prednisone plays a useful role in this situation.

Surgical Procedures. If the patient with hemophilia A does not have an inhibitor (see section on inhibitors further on), surgery can generally be accomplished without problems as long as management is carefully planned in advance and synchronized with close cooperation among medical, surgical, and laboratory personnel. Preoperative planning is essential, even for emergency procedures. Whenever time allows, this should include testing the patient's plasma for an inhibitor (antibody against Factor VIII) because inhibitors can occur at any time and make management extremely difficult. In addition to performing an inhibitor assay, many also recommend giving a test dose of Factor VIII a day or so before surgery in order to determine the half-life of infused Factor VIII. This is thought to be a more sensitive means of detecting a low-level inhibitor (95). One should always ensure that an adequate supply of clotting factor concentrate is on hand, not only for the day of surgery but also for the entire postoperative period. If the patient is blood type A, B, or AB and a prolonged period of replacement therapy is anticipated, one can begin with routinely available Factor VIII concentrates if necessary but should order and give blood type–specific concentrates as soon as they are available in order to prevent hemolysis due to anti-A and anti-B isoagglutinins, which are present in lyophilized Factor VIII (and Factor IX) concentrates.

Clotting factor replacement therapy should begin 15 to 60 minutes before surgery, with a Factor VIII bolus dose of 40 to 50 units per kg. Replacement therapy should then continue every 12 hours or, preferably, as a continuous infusion for 7 to 10 days postoperatively for most major surgical procedures (92, 93) (see previous section on head injury for details). A longer period of treatment (often 4 to 6 weeks) is required for extensive orthopaedic surgical procedures. Continuous infusion of clotting factor will result in a more constant Factor VIII level and is generally regarded as the preferred method of postoperative replacement therapy. When administering Factor VIII at a rate of 3 units per kg per hour, one can expect to maintain a level of approximately 0.50 units per ml (50 per cent); however, it is recommended that daily assays be performed so that maintenance of appropriate levels can be ensured.

Surgery in a hemophiliac should be undertaken only in a hospital in which there is a hemophilia center, a reliable around-the-clock coagulation laboratory, a major blood bank, and an appropriate rehabilitative team for postoperative management. The patient's chart should include a prominent notation that no intramuscular injections should be given and that all aspirin-containing compounds must be avoided.

ORAL SURGERY. For oral surgical procedures, including extraction of permanent teeth, EACA should be given in a dosage of 75 mg per kg every 6 hours, begun 1 day before surgery and continued for 7 to 10 days thereafter. Alternatively, tranexamic acid can be given in a dosage of 25 mg per kg. As for other surgical procedures, preoperative screening for inhibitors is essential! Clotting factor concentrates should be given 15 to 60 minutes before surgery and every 12 hours thereafter for 1 or 2 days, depending on the nature and extent of the oral surgery and the appearance of the local lesion.

Desmopressin Acetate in Mild to Moderate Hemophilia A. In individuals with mild or moderate hemophilia A (as well as in low-level "carriers") whose baseline F VIII:C values are 0.08 to 0.2 units per ml (8 to 20 per cent), desmopressin will be useful whenever it is judged that a transient threefold increase in Factor VIII will be sufficient to control bleeding (96, 97). This synthetic agent, which is remarkably free of side effects, is now regarded as the treatment of choice for minor bleeding episodes, teeth extractions, and certain other surgical procedures in persons with mild to moderate hemophilia and in those with classic von Willebrand's disease (see further on). As already noted (see discussion of other agents used to treat hemostasis), the main advantage of desmopressin is the fact that it is a synthetic agent rather than a blood derivative and thus does not transmit hepatitis or AIDS. Recommended dosage is 0.03 µg per kg per dose, given intravenously. Repeated responses can be obtained; however, if the drug is given every 12 or 24 hours (e.g., following surgical procedures), one must be aware of the possibility of a diminished, suboptimal response by the second, third, or fourth day due to depletion of Factor VIII stores (77). Although not all persons exhibit this tachyphylaxis phenomenon, many do. Thus, if a sustained elevation of Factor VIII is desired following a surgical procedure, F VIII:C levels must be monitored, and supplementation with cryoprecipitates may be necessary.

Several European groups have also used desmopressin intranasally (77, 98). However, even though the intranasal preparation available in Europe is much more concentrated than that available in the United States, the rise in Factor VIII is less, and is less predictable, than when the drug is given intravenously (77, 98). Nonetheless, should a more concentrated intranasal form eventually become available in the United States, it could potentially be quite useful for home treatment of minor bleeding episodes.

Danazol. Although Gralnick and co-workers reported a high percentage of beneficial responses when danazol was given daily to patients with hemophilia A and B, with sustained increase in plasma levels of Factor VIII or Factor IX (81), other groups have been unable to reproduce these results and in addition have noted a high incidence of undesirable side effects (82, 83, 99).

Hemophilia B (Factor IX Deficiency)

Many of the principles of treatment for hemophilia A are applicable to hemophilia B, with Factor IX concentrates being substituted for Factor VIII. However, the dosage calculation is different. Factor IX is a smaller molecule than Factor VIII. It diffuses from intravascular to extravascular sites, and thus a larger dose is required in order to achieve the same circulating level. Even though a dosage of 1 unit of Factor VIII per kg body weight will raise the circulating Factor VIII by 0.02 units per ml (2 per cent), the same dosage of Factor IX will raise the circulating Factor IX by only 1 per cent. Although the Factor IX level required for hemostasis will depend somewhat on the type and extent of bleeding, in general the hemostatic level appears to be less than that for Factor VIII. A circulating Factor IX level of 20 per cent is sufficient for most bleeding episodes, although higher levels will be required for extensive injuries and surgical situations (Table 41–4).

In persons with mild hemophilia B with baseline Factor IX values of 10 to 20 per cent, fresh frozen plasma rather than commercial Factor IX concentrates should be used whenever possible so that the greater hepatitis risk associated with the latter is avoided.

Surgery. Some hemophilia centers avoid all elective surgical procedures in persons with hemophilia B in view of the risk of thromboembolic complications when repeated doses of PCC are given to an immobile postoperative patient. Although this risk seems to be greatest in adult patients who undergo extensive orthopaedic surgical procedures, it is not limited to such cases. If a major surgical procedure is planned, certain measures can be taken in an attempt to minimize the risk of disseminated intravascular coagulation and thromboembolism. It is recommended that heparin be added to the reconstituted PCC in a dosage of 5 units per ml of reconstituted material (59). It also may be useful to infuse a unit of FFP as a source of antithrombin III prior to the initial dose of PCC if prolonged intensive use of PCC is anticipated. Close cooperation among surgical, medical, and laboratory personnel is essential.

For oral surgical procedures, when PCC is given pre- and postoperatively, an antifibrinolytic agent (EACA or tranexamic acid) should not be given concurrently with PCC. It is recommended that such antifibrinolytic drugs be withheld for approximately 6 hours after the last dose of PCC so that thromboembolic complications are avoided.

Danazol. See previous comments in the discussion of therapy for hemophilia A.

Table 41–4. RECOMMENDED DOSAGES OF FACTOR IX FOR HEMOPHILIA B

Type of Bleeding	Initial Dosage and Source of Factor IX (U/kg)*	Repeat Dosage and Source of Factor IX (U/kg)*	Other Treatment
Acute hemarthrosis†	15 (FFP)	None	
In individual with mild hemophilia B			
Early, in severe hemophilia B	20 (PCC)	None	Seldom necessary
Late (pain, swelling, limitation of motion) in severe hemophilia B	30 (PCC)	20–25 (PCC) q12h	Ice packs; non–weight bearing; a sling may be useful; rarely, joint aspiration
Intramuscular hemorrhage†	15 (FFP)	10–15 (FFP) q12h	
In individual with mild hemophilia B			
In severe hemophilia B	30–40 (PCC)	30 (PCC) q12h; several days of treatment may be required for extensive intramuscular hemorrhage	Non–weight bearing; complete bed rest for iliopsoas hemorrhage
Life-threatening situations‡	50 (PCC)	20–25 (PCC) q12h *or* Bolus dose followed by continuous infusion	AT III concentrate or 300 ml FFP as a source of AT III; add heparin to reconstituted PCC (see text)
Intracranial hemorrhage			
Major trauma			
Tongue or neck bleeding with potential airway obstruction			
Severe abdominal pain‡			
In mild hemophilia B	15 (FFP)	10 (FPP) q12h	
In severe hemophilia B	40 (PCC)	20 (PCC) q12h	
Tongue and mouth laceration‡			
Extraction of permanent teeth			
In mild hemophilia B	15 (FFP)	10 (FFP) q12h	An antifibrinolytic agent (EACA or tranexamic acid)
In severe hemophilia B	30 (PCC)	20 (PCC) q12h; however, may not be necessary in uncomplicated extractions	An antifibrinolytic agent begun day after PCC is stopped; orahesive gauze may be helpful for gum bleeding
Painless spontaneous gross hematuria	None		Increased PO fluids; corticosteroids and/or PCC used by some

*FFP = fresh frozen plasma; PCC = heat-treated or otherwise virus-attenuated prothrombin complex concentrate. As soon as a nonthrombogenic Factor IX concentrate is licensed and available, it would become the preferred product for most of the above situations.

†In infants and children under 4 years of age, some physicians still prefer to use FFP rather than PCC, even in those patients with moderately severe hemophilia B (see text).

‡These cases should be treated in a comprehensive hemophilia center. If a case is first seen in another hospital, the hemophilia center should be contacted and the patient transferred after emergency treatment is given at the local hospital.

(Reprinted with permission from Lusher, J. M.: Hemophilia. Hematol. Rev. Commun. 1:1–34, 1986.)

INHIBITORS

Inhibitors (antibodies) develop in approximately 15 per cent of individuals with severe hemophilia A and in 1 to 2 per cent of those with hemophilia B (100). Since the 1960's, a great deal has been learned about the nature of Factor VIII and Factor IX inhibitors, and various therapeutic approaches have been tried. However, to date none of these approaches has worked as well as Factor VIII does in a noninhibitor patient, and management of bleeding episodes in hemophiliacs with inhibitors is still a major problem.

Most inhibitors occur in severe hemophiliacs (i.e., those with less than 1 per cent Factor VIII activity) (100). These inhibitors are IgG antibodies, and, of those characterized, most have been monoclonal antibodies with kappa light chains (101). Factor VIII inhibitors act specifically against Factor VIII procoagulant activity, rarely interfering with other activities of the Factor VIII system (e.g., vWF activity). There is some degree of species specificity, with human Factor VIII being neutralized to a much greater extent than Factor VIII from other species (e.g., porcine and bovine Factor VIII), an observation that has potential therapeutic implications.

The development of an inhibitor is clearly related to some exposure to Factor VIII, although the amount is quite variable. Some hemophiliacs have developed inhibitors after as little as 8 or 10 days of exposure to Factor VIII, whereas others have had several hundred exposures over a period of many years before the appearance of an inhibitor. Interestingly, nearly one third of all inhibitors are detected by 5 years of age, and two thirds are detected by age 20 (102). However, some inhibitors develop much later in life, and there is probably no age or number of exposure days at which a hemophiliac is safe from developing an inhibitor.

Although the reasons for inhibitor development are far from clear, genetic predisposition appears to play a role. The United States Inhibitor Study Group found a higher incidence of inhibitors in black hemophiliacs (21 per cent) and in brother pairs (100); Shapiro found, in an analysis of HLA types and complement haplotypes, that HLA_1 was underrepresented in hemophiliacs with inhibitors, whereas the complement haplotypes C_4A_4 and C_4B_2 were twice as common in inhibitor patients (103).

Hemophiliacs with inhibitors can be categorized as "high" or "low" responders, depending on the degree of anamnestic response that they exhibit (Fig. 41–5). Most are high responders, having a marked increase in inhibitor concentration following infusion of any Factor VIII–containing material (102). Others are low responders, forming antibodies in low concentration only, even after repeated antigenic challenge. Bleeding episodes in low responders are relatively easy to treat because human Factor VIII concentrates in slightly higher dosage can be used effectively. However, with repeated infusions of Factor VIII, some low responders eventually become high responders (100, 102). In other low responders, the inhibitor may disappear spontaneously and not reappear on subsequent rechallenge with Factor VIII (102). In contrast, spontaneous disappearance of high-titer antibodies rarely occurs.

A variety of methods can be used to detect and quantitate inhibitors. For the routine 6 months' screening of hemophiliacs not suspected of having an inhibitor, the APTT test is recommended (95).

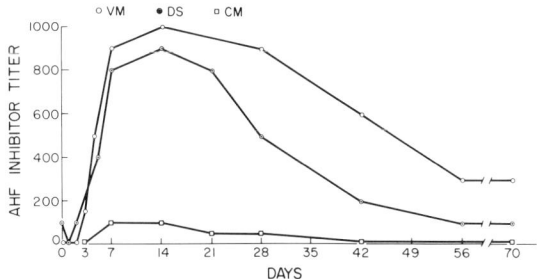

Figure 41–5. Graph showing anamnestic rise in inhibitor titer in three severe hemophiliacs with Factor VIII inhibitors following infusion of Factor VIII at time zero. Patients VM and DS are "high responders," exhibiting a marked increase in inhibitor titer, whereas CM is a "low responder." Bleeding episodes in low responders can usually be managed with Factor VIII concentrates.

If elective surgery is being planned, some recommend that in addition to the APTT screening test an in vivo Factor VIII recovery and survival study be done preoperatively because the latter is an even more sensitive method for detecting an unsuspected, weak inhibitor (95). For assaying known inhibitors, the method of Kasper and colleagues is recommended, in which the inhibitor concentration is expressed in Bethesda units (95, 104).

Management

Management of high responder inhibitor patients remains frustrating and controversial. Although the presence of an inhibitor does not increase the frequency of bleeding, it does make treatment of bleeding episodes difficult. Since the 1960's, various therapeutic approaches have been tried with variable but often disappointing results. Therapeutic options in current use will be briefly described, along with the author's preference in various situations. Because there is currently no completely reliable form of management, some clinicians prefer one therapeutic modality, whereas others prefer another. Most would agree, however, that the choice of treatment for a particular situation depends on several variables—the patient's current inhibitor concentration, whether he is a high or low responder, the nature and extent of the bleeding episode, product availability, and the experience of the medical personnel involved.

Factor VIII Concentrates. Human Factor VIII concentrates in large amounts are preferred by some, particularly for acute surgical emergencies and other life-threatening bleeding episodes, especially if the patient's inhibitor concentration is less than 10 Bethesda units or can be lowered to that by plasmapheresis (105, 106). Factor VIII should be given in high dosage (e.g., for an adolescent patient, 5000 units of Factor VIII should be given as a bolus, immediately followed by a constant infusion of 500 to 1000 units per hour. Dosage should then be adjusted, depending on the patient's Factor VIII level (106). If Factor VIII activity is undetectable 2 to 3 hours after the start of such a regimen, further treatment with Factor VIII will probably be ineffective.

Porcine Factor VIII Concentrates. A relatively new highly purified porcine Factor VIII preparation, Hyate:C, is produced by Speywood Laboratories in the United Kingdom. Although this product is still considered investigational in the United States (i.e., it has not been licensed by the United States Office of Biologics), it has proved quite effective in controlling serious bleeding episodes in inhibitor patients whose Factor VIII inhibitor does not significantly cross-react with porcine Factor VIII. Hyate:C lacks the tendency to provoke thrombocytopenia, which was one of the major disadvantages of the earlier porcine preparations. However, both allergic and anamnestic reactions may occur. Kernoff and colleagues in the United Kingdom have had extensive experience with this product and report excellent clinical results, with a less than 10 per cent incidence of side effects. They have found that side effects are minimized by administration of 100 mg of hydrocortisone with the first dose. Although it has been recommended that patients be selected on the basis of in vitro testing for cross-reactivity of their inhibitor to Hyate:C, Kernoff has found a very good to excellent response to Hyate:C in almost all subjects whose inhibitor level to human Factor VIII is less than 50 Bethesda units (51). The recommended starting dose of Hyate:C is 50 to 100 units per kg; subsequent doses are determined by the patient's F VIII:C level. In addition to being used in Europe, Hyate:C has been employed in several United States hemophilia centers for surgical emergencies and other life- or limb-threatening bleeding episodes with excellent results (50, 105). Advantages of this product include the fact that one can measure the Factor VIII response in the recipient and the fact that porcine Factor VIII does not transmit hepatitis or AIDS. As is the case with human Factor VIII concentrates, treatment with Hyate:C often (but not always) stimulates an anamnestic rise in the patient's Factor VIII inhibitor concentration.

Prothrombin Complex Concentrates (PCC). So-called standard or not purposely activated PCCs have been extensively used in inhibitor patients since 1972. Although their precise mechanism of action in "bypassing" the need for Factor VIII is still not known, PCCs do seem to be moderately effective in controlling bleeding in hemophiliacs with inhibitors. To date, three controlled studies have been done in which PCCs have been evaluated. It is noteworthy that in each of the three controlled, double-blind studies (two in the United States and one in Europe) (67, 68, 107), a single dose of nonactivated PCC was found to be effective in controlling acute hemarthrosis in approximately 50 per cent of episodes (108). Thus, for lack of a clearly superior product at present, many feel that PCCs are appropriate for treatment of acute hemarthroses in high responder inhibitor patients. Recommended dosage is 75 Factor IX units per kg. Although this dose can be repeated in 12 hours if necessary, one should avoid giving more than three or four doses in succession. Not only is the repetitive administration of such high doses of PCCs potentially hazardous (see earlier discussion of complications of PCCs) and expensive, but also it is unlikely that additional doses will be beneficial if the patient's bleeding has failed to respond to three or four doses.

Two purposely activated PCCs also are available for use in inhibitor patients. One of these, FEIBA Immuno, has been extensively used in Europe since the mid 1970's and was licensed for use in inhibitor patients in the United States in 1982. The other, Hyland's Autoplex, was licensed for use in the United States in early 1980. Both these products are costly (currently Autoplex is 89 cents per unit and FEIBA is 75 cents per unit). Although these activated products have been used fairly extensively in some parts of the United States, many hemophilia centers have used them very little or not at all because of their cost. At a dosage of 50 to 100 FECU* per kg, which is recommended on the package insert for Autoplex, a single dose for an adolescent weighing 70 kg would cost 3000 to 6000 dollars. Often, more than one dose is needed, thus doubling or tripling this cost. Particularly in areas of the United States in which state hemophilia programs provide a certain amount of money for clotting factor concentrates, the cost of activated PCCs was thought to be too high to justify their use except in unusual circumstances (life-threatening or other serious bleeding episodes), and in such situations many (but not all) observers were impressed with the effectiveness of these activated products (66).

Although numerous anecdotal reports have suggested that the activated products, FEIBA Immuno and Autoplex, are superior to standard, nonactivated PCCs, there have been only two controlled, double-blind studies in which activated products were directly compared with nonactivated PCCs. FEIBA was found to be somewhat more effective than nonactivated PCC (64 per cent versus 52 per cent) in the Dutch trial (68), whereas in an American multicenter trial in which a single dose of Autoplex was compared with a single dose of nonactivated PCC, no difference was found between the two products (67).

Hemophilia B patients with inhibitors should be treated with Factor IX concentrates (PCCs) in a dosage of 75 Factor IX units per kg body weight. In general, one or two (but sometimes three) doses will suffice for treatment of an acute hemarthrosis or soft-tissue bleeding. However, as in the case of hemophilia A patients with inhibitors, response to treatment is not as good as in noninhibitor patients. For severe open bleeding, central nervous system hemorrhage, or acute surgical emergency, an activated PCC (Autoplex or FEIBA Immuno) should be used.

CARRIER DETECTION

In cases of hemophilia A (Factor VIII deficiency), one can identify over 90 per cent of female carriers of the hemophilia gene by determining the ratio of F VIII:C to F VIIIR:Ag in their plasma. Although many obligate carriers have levels of F VIII:C that are below the normal range, many others do not. Because the levels of F VIII:C depend on chromosome X function, extreme in-

---

*Factor Eight Correction Units

activation of the hemophilic-bearing chromosome X in somatic cells can result in F VIII:C values within the normal range, thus making these carriers unidentifiable by this method alone. However, levels of autosomally controlled F VIIIR:Ag are normal or increased in males with hemophilia A and are also normal or increased in obligate carriers, with relatively less F VIII:C. In contrast, normal control women have roughly equal amounts of F VIII:C and F VIIIR:Ag. One can thus distinguish over 90 per cent of carriers by determining the ratio of these two Factor VIII components. In general, F VIII:C/VIIIR:Ag ratios of less than 0.6 indicate the carrier state. More complex methods of analysis are used by some geneticists, and laboratory results combined with family history data can be used to calculate a probability figure for the individual subject. It is important to remember that some carriers will be indistinguishable from normal, and it is thus unwise to assure a possible carrier that she is normal.

Oberle and associates have described a new method of screening for hemophilia A in families at risk for the disease. They have used a DNA probe, St 14, which detects a very polymorphic region on the human X chromosome that is closely linked to hemophilia A. These investigators claim that the DNA probe can be used in conjunction with biologic assays for Factor VIII to detect carriers with an accuracy of 96 per cent or greater (109).

In the case of hemophilia B (Factor IX deficiency), carrier detection is a more complicated matter owing to the greater heterogeneity of hemophilia B (86). Although the average level of F IX:C in heterozygotes is 50 per cent of normal, only one fourth of all heterozygotes have levels low enough to be identified with confidence by this means. If a possible carrier does not have a subnormal F IX:C level, one should probably consult a hemophilia center with special interest and capability in this area. If an affected male relative can be classified according to subtype of hemophilia B (86), one may be able to select tests that may be of help in carrier detection. However, for some subtypes of hemophilia B and for situations in which an affected male relative is not available for study, the only possible means of identifying carriers is by detection of a low F IX:C value.

PRENATAL DIAGNOSIS

If a known or possible carrier of the hemophilia A gene is pregnant and wishes to know whether or not her fetus will have hemophilia, the sex of the fetus can be determined by amniocentesis. This procedure is generally carried out between the twelfth and fourteenth weeks of pregnancy. In a few highly specialized centers it is now possible, if the fetus is male, to determine whether or not the fetus will have hemophilia A. A sample of fetal blood is obtained via fetoscopy, and F VIII:C antigen (F VIII:CAg) is measured by immunoradiometric assay (89).

Detection of fetuses with hemophilia B is not possible at present but no doubt will eventually be so, at least in the case of CRM-negative families, in whom F IX:CAg assays of fetal blood could be used (89).

Von Willebrand's Disease

The hereditary bleeding disorder referred to as von Willebrand's disease (vWD) was first described in 1926 by Dr. Erik von Willebrand, in inhabitants of the Åland Islands in the Gulf of Bothnia (110). Affected individuals had excessive bruising and mucous-membrane bleeding and prolonged bleeding times despite normal platelet counts. The disorder appeared to be transmitted in an autosomal dominant fashion, and the hemostatic defect was attributed to a platelet abnormality (111).

For a number of years thereafter, the only diagnostic criteria for vWD were a prolonged bleeding time with normal platelet count and an autosomal dominant mode of inheritance. However, as new coagulation tests were developed and applied to individuals with vWD, it became apparent that Factor VIII activity was reduced in this disorder (112, 113). It was also noted that infusions of plasma, Factor VIII concentrates, or even hemophiliac plasma often resulted in a secondary, sustained rise in Factor VIII activity (113–115), a phenomenon referred to by some as "de novo synthesis." Subsequently, however, it was shown that simple correction of Factor VIII procoagulant activity (F VIII:C) does not necessarily correct the bleeding time defect or produce adequate hemostasis (116).

In the 1960's and 1970's, other laboratory abnormalities were detected in vWD. It was noted that levels of Factor VIII–related antigen (VIIIR:Ag) were reduced (117). Platelet retention in a glass bead column was found to be reduced (118), and platelet adhesion to exposed subendothelial connective tissue (119) or injured vessel wall (120) also was reduced. It was also noted that persons with vWD often had reduced levels of a plasma factor needed for platelet agglutination by the antibiotic ristocetin (121).

Although each of these observations improved our understanding of the defects in vWD, the three tests that proved most applicable to routine diagnostic purposes were the assays of plasma F VIII:C, F VIIIR:Ag, and ristocetin cofactor activity (F VIIIR:Cof). Thus, routine diagnostic testing for suspected vWD now includes the performance of a template bleeding time, and assays of the patient's plasma for F VIII:C, F VIIIR:Ag, and F VIIIR:Cof.

The multimeric structure of Factor VIII–von

Willebrand factor (F VIII/vWF) has been extensively studied, and it has become apparent that the larger multimers are associated with unique antigenic and functional characteristics. Absence of the larger multimers from the plasma of some individuals with vWD has led to the recognition of a number of vWD variants (122, 123). Table 41–5 lists both the old and new nomenclature proposed by the International Committee on Thrombosis and Haemostasis for describing the various properties of F VIII/vWF.

DIAGNOSIS

In most patients in whom vWD is suspected, the diagnosis can be made on the basis of the clinical picture, autosomal inheritance, and relatively simple tests. In "classic" (or what is now referred to as "Type I") vWD, all three components of the Factor VIII system are proportionately decreased, and the bleeding time is prolonged. However, it is now apparent that vWD is an extremely heterogeneous condition, and in some individuals it may be difficult to make—or to exclude—the diagnosis on the basis of laboratory testing done on one or two occasions.

There is considerable variation in clinical and laboratory manifestations not only among families but also among affected members of the same family (124), and some individuals vary considerably when tested at different times (125). Once the diagnosis of vWD has been entertained, one cannot exclude this possibility on the basis of a single set of normal coagulation studies. However, although important from a genetic standpoint, such diagnostically difficult cases generally involve very mild disease.

Diagnostic criteria for vWD include a prolonged bleeding time associated with quantitative or qualitative abnormalities of F VIIIR:Ag and usually decreased F VIIIR:Cof. F VIII:C is usually low but may be normal (126).

The bleeding time is always prolonged at some time in the course of the disease, especially in severe (Type III) and variant (Type II) vWD. The bleeding time is more variable in Type I, and repeated testing may be necessary to document prolongation.

F VIIIR:Ag can be quantitated by a variety of methods (Laurell electroimmunoassay [127], radioquantitative immunoelectrophoresis [128], and enzyme assay or radioimmunoassay [129]). In Type I vWD, levels of F VIIIR:Ag are usually decreased proportionately to levels of F VIII:C and F VIIIR:Cof. In Type II vWD levels of F VIIIR:Ag may be normal or decreased, and F VIIIR:Cof is often, but not always, undetectable. In Type III vWD, in which the affected individual has inherited a gene for vWD from each parent, F VIIIR:Ag is present in only minute amounts.

CLASSIFICATION (Table 41–6)

It has been shown that von Willebrand's factor exists in normal plasma as a series of multimers that range in size from approximately 800,000 daltons to over 14 million daltons (123). Functional properties of the polymers are related to their size. The largest multimers show the greatest platelet-related activities and appear to have a major role in primary hemostasis.

Type I vWD is transmitted as an autosomal dominant trait and is characterized by proportionately decreased levels of the entire Factor VIII complex (F VIIIR:Ag, F VIIIR:Cof, and F VIII:C). The bleeding time is usually prolonged but may be normal. The F VIII–WF appears to be normal in composition, as evidenced by a normal pattern on crossed immunoelectrophoresis and the presence of all the different-sized multimers on SDS gels (123).

Mannucci and colleagues have described three subtypes of vWD Type I, defined according to platelet content of F VIIIR:Ag and F VIIIR:Cof. These subtypes are referred to as "platelet normal," "platelet discordant," and "platelet low" (130).

Type II vWD also is transmitted as an autosomal

Table 41–5. FACTOR VIII–vWF NOMENCLATURE

Designation		Definition
Old	New*	
F VIII:C	Same	Procoagulant activity that corrects the clotting abnormality of hemophilia A plasma
F VIII:C Ag	VIII:Ag	Factor VIII:C antigen, which reacts with homologous antibodies appearing in hemophilia A
F VIIIR:vWF	vWF	Von Willebrand's factor, bleeding time factor, the activity necessary for formation of a platelet plug; decreased or absent in von Willebrand's disease (vWD)
F VIIIR:Cof	Same	Ristocetin-cofactor activity; the activity necessary for ristocetin-induced platelet aggregation
F VIIIR:Ag	vWF:Ag	Von Willebrand's antigen I, which reacts with heterologous antisera prepared against F VIII/vWF
F vW AG II	Same	Von Willebrand's antigen II, immunologically distinct from vWF:Ag; absent in severe vWD and present in variable amounts in other forms of the disease

*"New" refers to revised nomenclature adopted by International Committee on Thrombosis and Haemostasis, July, 1985. Thrombos. Haemostas. 54:871, 1985.

Table 41–6. SUBTYPES OF VON WILLEBRAND'S DISEASE AND EXPECTED RESPONSE TO DESMOPRESSIN

Type	Subtype	Characteristic Laboratory Abnormalities	Clinical Response to Desmopressin
I ("classic" vWD)		Subnormal levels of all components of F VIII system; normal pattern on crossed immunoelectrophoresis of plasma F VIIIR:Ag	Good; there is usually complete correction of bleeding time*
II		Abnormal pattern on crossed immunoelectrophoresis (increased anodal migration); Types IIA and IIB can be distinguished by platelet aggregometry with varying concentrations of ristocetin	
	IIA	Subnormal platelet aggregation with ristocetin	Slight, partial correction of bleeding time
	IIB	Enhanced aggregation with very low levels of ristocetin	Desmopressin is contraindicated, as it will precipitate in vivo and result in aggregation and thrombocytopenia
	IIC	Normal F VIII:C, F VIIIR:Ag levels but decreased VIIIR:Cof; most striking abnormality (can only be seen on SDS gels) is aberrant multimeric structure of vWF; a doublet, rather than the usual repeating triplet, is found	F VIIIR:Cof increases, but bleeding time may not be corrected
	IID	Similar to those of IIC; but multimeric analysis on 3% agarose gel demonstrates different subbands	Not known, but probably same as in IIC
III		Extremely low or undetectable levels of all components of F VIII system	None, as there is nothing to be released from storage sites

*Although most individuals with vWD Type I have at least a transient correction of the bleeding time, some do not. Mannucci and colleagues have described "platelet-low" and "platelet-discordant" subtypes of Type I vWD, in which the bleeding time does not correct following desmopressin (130).

dominant trait but is characterized by an absence of the large forms of F VIII–WF. This results in an abnormal pattern on crossed immunoelectrophoresis of the patient's plasma, with increased anodal migration (126).

Several subtypes of Type II vWD have been described. Subtype IIA is characterized by a marked deficiency or absence of F VIIIR:Cof, and levels of F VIII:C, F VIIIR:Ag, and F VIIIR:Cof are usually discrepant, with F VIII:C often being normal or only slightly decreased and F VIIIR:Ag being moderately decreased (5 to 45 per cent) (123, 126). In this subtype, the large and intermediate-sized multimers are absent from plasma and platelets (123).

Subtype IIB exhibits the same crossed immunoelectrophoresis abnormality as that demonstrated by IIA; however, this subtype is characterized by an increased sensitivity of F VIII–WF to ristocetin. Platelet aggregation and F VIIIR:Ag binding to normal platelets occur at very low concentrations of ristocetin (less than that required for normal individuals). This enhanced platelet aggregation with low concentrations of ristocetin is in distinct contrast to that seen in subtype IIA. Also, F VIIIR:Cof levels are normal or only slightly reduced in subtype IIB vWD (126). In this subtype, the larger multimers are absent from plasma but are present in platelets in normal amounts.

Subtypes IIC and IID have been identified and reported in a very few individuals. These subtypes have aberrant multimeric patterns on SDS gels (123). Subtype IIC is inherited as an autosomal recessive trait (123), whereas subtype IID is autosomal dominant (131).

Type III vWD, the severe form, represents homozygous or doubly heterozygous vWD. Fortunately, this form is relatively uncommon. The bleeding time is consistently prolonged, and all components of the Factor VIII complex are present in only minute amounts.

From a practical standpoint, it is important to determine the patient's subtype because treatment options vary according to the subtype (see further on). Type III vWD can be easily distinguished by the severity of the patient's bleeding manifestations and laboratory abnormalities. However, one cannot differentiate between Types I and II by evaluating clinical manifestations or by merely assaying the components of the Factor VIII system. Because relatively few centers have multimeric analysis by SDS gels available for routine diagnostic testing, it is fortunate that Types I and II can usually be distinguished by crossed immunoelectrophoresis. Patients with Type I vWD will have a normal pattern, whereas those with Type II disease will have an abnormal pattern with increased anodal migration (126) (Fig. 41–6). One can then further classify Type II vWD into Subtypes IIA and IIB by performing platelet aggregation with various concentrations of ristocetin. Although platelet aggregation with ristocetin is reduced in subtype IIA disease, platelets in subtype IIB are hyperreactive to very low concentrations of ristocetin (Fig. 41–7) (132).

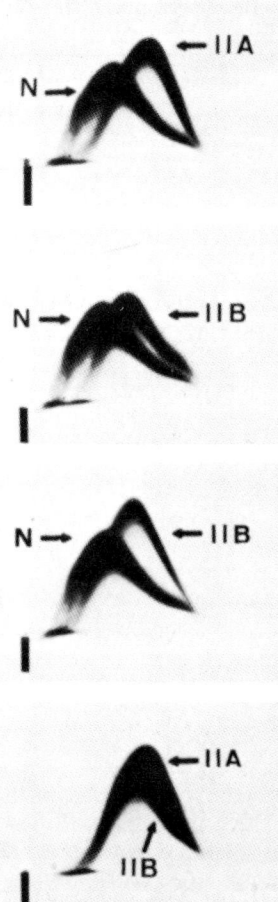

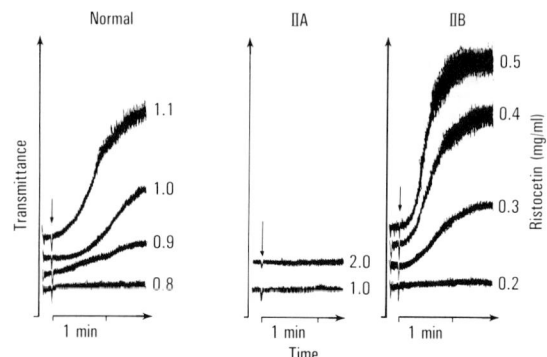

Figure 41-7. Ristocetin-induced platelet aggregation in von Willebrand's disease subtypes. In Type IIA, no aggregation occurred at any concentration of ristocetin. In Type IIB, aggregation was already maximal at concentrations of ristocetin that were too low for any response in the normals. (From Ruggeri, Z. M., Pareti, F. I., et al.: New Engl J Med 302:1047, 1980.)

Figure 41-6. Crossed immunoelectrophoresis of von Willebrand's factor in normal plasma (N) and Types IIA and IIB von Willebrand's disease. The first-dimension sample well is indicated by the vertical black line. The anode (direction of electrophoresis) is to the right in the first dimension and to the top in the second. The patterns from the different plasmas have been overlaid for comparison. Patterns of von Willebrand's factor from two different patients with Type IIB von Willebrand's disease are shown. The asymmetric pattern in normal plasma results from the different migration rates of different-sized multimers. In Types IIA and IIB von Willebrand's disease, the largest multimers (slowest migrating and therefore least anodic) are missing. No difference between Types IIA and IIB is evident with this technique, although the difference is easily seen with SDS-agarose electrophoresis. (From Ruggeri, Z. M., Pareti, F. I., et al.: New Engl J Med 302:1047, 1980.)

INCIDENCE, INHERITANCE, AND CLINICAL EXPRESSION

This heterogeneous condition is thought to be the most common of the hereditary disorders of hemostasis. However, its true incidence is difficult to determine because mild cases often go undiagnosed. When one family member is found to have vWD, it is not uncommon to find that many relatives have laboratory abnormalities consistent with this diagnosis. Often such persons who are diagnosed as part of a family study have a history of mild mucocutaneous bleeding, somewhat excessive bruising, or bleeding following surgical intervention. However, others give completely "negative" histories for unusual bleeding.

In contrast to hemophilia A and hemophilia B, vWD is transmitted as an autosomal trait. Two types of inheritance have been recognized, dominant and recessive (133).

In severe (homozygous or doubly heterozygous) vWD, the onset of bleeding occurs in infancy or early childhood and tends to decrease somewhat with age. However, in this form, affected individuals may have acute hemarthroses and intramuscular bleeding (as is seen in hemophilia) in addition to mucocutaneous bleeding (134). In the usual heterozygous forms of vWD, both mucosal bleeding and cutaneous bleeding occur (epistaxis, menorrhagia, gingival bleeding, melena, bruising). Excessive bleeding following surgery or dental extractions is common if preoperative treatment has not been given and, in fact, may often lead to the diagnosis. Postpartum bleeding is relatively uncommon and may be restricted to Type II vWD, in which the Factor VIII increase in late pregnancy is that of an abnormal molecular form that does not correct the bleeding tendency.

TREATMENT

Treatment depends on the severity and type of vWD and the nature of the bleeding. In milder forms of the disorder, often no specific treatment is necessary. Local measures (pressure, application of cold compresses, nasal packing, etc.) may suffice for control of epistaxis. However, for moderate or severe forms of vWD, treatment is often indicated prior to and following surgery or for control of spontaneous or traumatic bleeding. Since their introduction in the late 1960's until recently, cryoprecipitates were regarded as the treatment of choice for all types of vWD. Cryoprecipitates, like fresh frozen plasma, contain the entire Factor VIII complex and all multimers of F VIII–WF; in contrast, lyophilized high-purity Factor VIII concentrates lack the largest multimers (123, 126). Infusion of cryoprecipitates (1 bag per 5 kg body weight) will thus provide normal F VIII–WF in a relatively small volume of material. The need for follow-up doses and the frequency and duration of such treatment depend on the severity of the patient's vWD and the nature and extent of the bleeding (126). It should be noted, however, that correction of the bleeding time lasts only a few hours, probably because the larger forms of vWF are cleared more rapidly from the circulation.

Although cryoprecipitates remain the treatment of choice for Type III vWD, and for the Type II variants when treatment is judged indicated, *desmopressin* is now regarded as the treatment of choice for Type I vWD (Tables 41–6 to 41–9). This synthetic agent results in a rapid increase in all components of the Factor VIII system. This increase, which is approximately threefold, results from endogenous release of the Factor VIII complex from its storage sites. Individuals with Type I vWD have subnormal levels of structurally and functionally normal F VIII–WF, and administration of desmopressin results in rapid release of normal Factor VIII components and transient correction of the bleeding time. The bleeding time correction usually lasts 3 or 4 hours, then returns to baseline values.

Although most persons with Type I vWD will have correction of the bleeding time following infusions of desmopressin, some do not. Mannucci and co-workers have shown that those who do not have subnormal amounts of platelet F VIIIR:Ag and F VIIIR:Cof (130).

Desmopressin is clinically ineffective in Type III vWD because individuals with this severe disease have nothing to be released from the stores. In Type II vWD, Factor VIII moieties will be released, but they will be the abnormal forms that will not correct the bleeding time or improve hemostasis. Desmopressin is contraindicated in subtype IIB vWD because the abnormal forms released have a heightened affinity for platelets, resulting in in vivo platelet aggregation and a transient drop in platelets (see Table 41–6) (130). Thus, it is extremely important to determine the patient's subtype so that the most appropriate

Table 41–7. EFFECTS OF DESMOPRESSIN ON TESTS OF HEMOSTASIS

Transient increase in
  F VIII:C (approximately threefold)
  F VIIIR:Ag (approximately twofold)
  F VIIIR:Cof (approximately twofold)
  Plasminogen activator (approximately three- to fourfold)
In addition, in most subjects with von Willebrand's disease Type I ("classic" vWD), there is transient correction of bleeding time

Table 41–8. PERSONS LIKELY TO BENEFIT FROM DESMOPRESSIN

1. Those with mild hemophilia A (whose baseline F VIII:C values are 5 to 20 per cent) and those with "classic" (Type I) vWD, whenever a transient threefold increase in F VIII would be sufficient treatment. (*Note:* If frequent repetitive doses are planned, as following major surgery, one must keep in mind the possibility of tachyphylaxis.)
2. Although still considered investigational for other purposes, desmopressin has also resulted in a transient correction of the bleeding time in persons with renal failure who were undergoing renal biopsy and in persons with some types of platelet function defects.

therapy can be selected. As discussed earlier, the recommended dose of desmopressin is 0.3 μg per kg (mixed in 50 ml normal saline solution and infused over a period of 15 to 20 minutes). In vWD, it is particularly important that one give a test dose at least several days before elective surgery or dental extractions in order to ensure that the patient has a good response to the drug with transient correction of the bleeding time (97, 135).

If desmopressin is to be used repetitively over a relatively short period of time (e.g., following surgery), one must be aware of a possible diminution in response by day 2, 3, or 4. If this occurs, one must be prepared to give cryoprecipitates (97).

Antifibrinolytic Agents. Regardless of whether one is using cryoprecipitates or desmopressin, an antifibrinolytic agent, tranexamic acid, or epsilon aminocaproic acid (EACA) is a useful adjunct for management of bleeding in the oral cavity (see earlier comments). As is true for all hereditary bleeding disorders, aspirin and all aspirin-containing compounds should be rigorously avoided (136).

PSEUDO- (PLATELET-TYPE) VON WILLEBRAND'S DISEASE

In pseudo-vWD (123, 137–139), the underlying defect is in the platelets. The heightened affinity of platelets for vWF is responsible for the absence of the largest multimers from the plasma of patients with this disease. The enhanced interaction between platelets and vWF is thought to account for the thrombocytopenia that is observed in these patients. Pseudo-vWD should not be confused with subtype IIB vWD, in which the heightened vWF–platelet interaction results from abnormal vWF rather than from abnormal platelets.

Table 41–9. ADVANTAGES AND SIDE EFFECTS OF DESMOPRESSIN

Advantages
  No transmission of viral hepatitis or AIDS
  Easy to mix and administer
  Cost usually less than that of blood products
Side effects
  Common: facial flushing, facial warmth
  Less common: transient headache, nausea
  Rare: hypertension, fluid and electrolyte problems

Other Hereditary Coagulation Disorders

Although far less common than hemophilia and vWD, hereditary deficiencies and abnormalities of other clotting factors also exist. Although some of these (e.g., deficiencies of Factor XII, Fletcher factor, and Fitzgerald factor) are not associated with a bleeding tendency, congenital deficiencies or abnormalities of fibrinogen, prothrombin, and Factors V, VII, X, XIII, and sometimes XI are associated with bleeding. Most of these rare conditions are inherited in an autosomal recessive manner (Table 41–10).

FIBRINOGEN ABNORMALITIES

Congenital disorders of fibrinogen synthesis include those associated with deficient synthesis (afibrinogenemia and hypofibrinogenemia) and those associated with defective synthesis (the dysfibrinogenemias). In afibrinogenemia there is absence of circulating fibrinogen, whereas in hypofibrinogenemia there is a reduced level of apparently normal fibrinogen. In the dysfibrinogenemias, the circulating fibrinogen may be in normal or reduced amounts but exhibits abnormal characteristics.

Afibrinogenemia. Congenital afibrinogenemia is a rare disorder of fibrinogen synthesis associated with abnormal bleeding that may be manifested in the first few days of life as melena, hematemesis, mucosal bleeding, hematomas, or umbilical cord hemorrhage. Other lifelong bleeding problems associated with this disease may include easy bruising, bleeding after minor trauma, menorrhagia, hemarthrosis, and cerebral hemorrhage. Despite the complete lack of fibrinogen in the most severely affected patients, bleeding manifestations in these individuals may be relatively mild, and spontaneous hemorrhage is uncommon. Variability of bleeding occurs with time, and periods relatively free of bleeding are noted, even though the fibrinogen defect is constant.

Congenital afibrinogenemia probably represents the homozygous state of hypofibrinogenemia because parents of individuals with this disease have lower than normal levels of fibrinogen. The heterozygous hypofibrinogenemic individuals are asymptomatic. More than 100 cases of congenital afibrinogenemia have been reported, but the incidence of asymptomatic hypofibrinogenemia is not known (140–142).

Because the substrate for fibrin formation is lacking in afibrinogenemia, all coagulation tests based on fibrin formation are abnormal (whole-blood clotting time, plasma recalcification time, partial thromboplastin time, prothrombin time, thrombin time, and snake venom clotting times). Addition of normal plasma or purified fibrinogen will correct the abnormality in all these tests. The diagnosis of afibrinogenemia or hypofibrinogenemia is confirmed by quantitative measurement of fibrinogen, including methods based on precipitation, coagulation, and immunologic techniques. The most sensitive of these, the immunologic methods, will demonstrate trace levels of fibrinogen in most homozygous afibrinogenemic patients, even when no fibrinogen is detected by precipitation or coagulation techniques. Heterozygous in-

Table 41–10. FREQUENCY AND MODE OF TRANSMISSION OF INHERITED DISORDERS OF HEMOSTASIS

Deficiency	Frequency	Inheritance
Fibrinogen		
Afibrinogenemia	Rare (more than 100 cases)	Autosomal recessive
Hypofibrinogenemia	Rare (more than 100 cases)	Autosomal recessive
Dysfibrinogenemia	Rare (more than 100 cases)	Autosomal recessive or autosomal dominant
Prothrombin	Rare (less than 50 cases)	Autosomal recessive
Factor V	Rare (less than 100 cases)	Autosomal recessive
Factor VII	Rare (less than 100 cases)	Autosomal recessive (incomplete)
Factor VIII	Most common hemophilia (one in 20,000 individuals)	X-linked recessive
Factor IX	Less common hemophilia	X-linked recessive
Factor X	Rare (less than 100 cases)	Autosomal recessive (incomplete)
Factor XI	Rare (100 cases)	Autosomal recessive (primarily in Ashkenazi Jews)
Factor XII	Rare (more than 100 cases)	Autosomal recessive
Factor XIII	Rare (more than 100 cases)	Autosomal recessive
Fletcher factor (prekallikrein)	Rare (less than 50 cases)	Autosomal recessive
High-molecular-weight kininogen	Rare (less than 50 cases)	Autosomal recessive
Von Willebrand's disease		
Type I ("classic")	Relatively common (greater frequency than hemophilia)	Autosomal dominant
Type II	Incidence not known, but less common than Type I	Autosomal dominant (Type IIC recessive)
Type III (severe)	Rare	Affected individuals are doubly heterozygous or homozygous for vWD

dividuals are hypofibrinogenemic by all methods (141). Additional abnormalities that have been observed in afibrinogenemia include mild to moderate thrombocytopenia and prolonged bleeding time. Because the latter abnormality is not a constant finding, it is not possible to explain the role of fibrinogen in the production of the primary hemostatic platelet plug.

Bleeding in afibrinogenemia can be treated with whole blood, plasma, or cryoprecipitate. Fibrinogen levels of 50 to 100 mg per dl are adequate for hemostasis. Because fibrinogen has a long half-life, repeated infusions may not be required, depending on the nature of the bleeding. When fibrinogen is needed, hemostatic levels may be maintained by infusions every 4 to 5 days. Because of the significantly greater risk of hepatitis associated with their use, fibrinogen concentrates should not be used for replacement therapy (143).

Dysfibrinogenemias. The dysfibrinogenemias are qualitative abnormalities of the fibrinogen molecule. When reviewed by Mammen in 1974, 26 different abnormalities in families (including 103 affected individuals) had been described (140). Now more than 130 abnormal fibrinogens are known, and the precise structural defect has been identified in 23 of them. This group of disorders has also been reviewed by Flute (141), Beck (142), Morse (144), and Galanakis (145). The abnormal fibrinogens have been named according to the cities in which they were recognized (fibrinogen Parma, fibrinogen Detroit, etc.). In contrast to those with congenital afibrinogenemia, less than half the families with dysfibrinogenemia had even mild bleeding tendencies, and many individuals with this disorder have been discovered as a result of routine screening tests. Symptoms have included easy bruising, prolonged bleeding after minor trauma, menorrhagia, and wound dehiscence. Excessive bleeding is more commonly observed in patients with defective fibrinopeptide release than in those in whom the major defect is one of fibrin polymerization (143).

Abnormal fibrinogens appear to be transmitted as autosomal dominant traits. Homozygotes have all abnormal fibrinogen, whereas heterozygotes have a mixture of normal and abnormal fibrinogen.

The laboratory abnormalities in dysfibrinogenemia vary with the severity of the defect. The whole-blood clotting time, prothrombin time, and partial thromboplastin time may be normal or prolonged, but the thrombin time is almost always abnormal. In addition, the reptilase time (Bothrops snake venom time) is prolonged. Reptilase releases only fibrinopeptide A, and the reptilase time is not prolonged in heparin therapy, a useful distinction in differential diagnosis (143).

Quantitative fibrinogen determinations based on precipitation and immunologic methods should be normal, but those based on coagulation and thrombin clotting time techniques are often decreased. Other coagulation tests are normal, as is the bleeding time. Addition of normal plasma to patient's plasma has a variable effect on the thrombin time, with an inhibitory effect being observed in some types of abnormal fibrinogens.

Most patients with dysfibrinogenemia do not require treatment for bleeding, but the infusion of plasma or cryoprecipitates appears to be reasonable if uncontrolled bleeding occurs.

CONGENITAL DEFICIENCIES AND ABNORMALITIES OF PROTHROMBIN, FACTOR V, FACTOR VII, AND FACTOR X

Hypoprothrombinemia and Dysprothrombinemia. These are very rare disorders that may be associated with relatively mild bleeding problems. Easy bruising, menorrhagia, and prolonged bleeding after injuries, dental extractions, or surgery may occur. Both disorders are transmitted as autosomal recessive traits and are associated with slight to moderate prolongation of the one-stage prothrombin time. Congenital hypoprothrombinemia was described first in 1941, and very few additional cases have been reported (146). In a 1978 review, Owen and colleagues described 24 affected families. Of these, 11 seemed to represent true deficiencies of prothrombin (hypoprothrombinemia), and seven appeared to represent the inheritance of abnormal molecular variants of prothrombin (dysprothrombinemia) (147). Additional kindreds with hypoprothrombinemia have been described by Gill and associates (148) and Montgomery and colleagues (149), and a few additional prothrombin variants have been reported by Bloom (150). In hypoprothrombinemia, the level of prothrombin is found to be decreased when one- or two-stage assay methods are used, but some activity is present even in homozygous individuals. Congenital hypoprothrombinemia must be differentiated from acquired disorders, including vitamin K–deficient states, although this distinction may be difficult in the neonatal period.

Bloom has summarized the characteristics of the reported dysprothrombinemias (150). In these conditions, prothrombin measured by one- or two-stage methods utilizing tissue extract is always reduced, but levels measured with the use of other activators may be variable (150). Immunologic prothrombin assay provides normal results.

Although the mild bleeding manifestations of these disorders may not require treatment, significant bleeding can be treated with normal plasma. Because prothrombin is stable, the plasma does not have to be fresh, and prothrombin is present in the supernatant plasma from cryoprecipitate. However, fresh frozen plasma may be the most convenient form of treatment, and a dose of 10 to 20 ml per kg should provide a hemostatic level of prothrombin. Because of prothrombin's long half-life, repeat treatment may be necessary only every 2 to 3 days. In the face of serious bleeding requiring repeated infusions, the use of prothrombin complex concentrate may prevent plasma overload. Vitamin K is of no value in the treatment of congenital prothrombin deficiency or dysprothrombinemia.

Factor V Deficiency (Parahemophilia). This is a mild bleeding disorder first described by Owren in 1947 (151). Factor V deficiency is an uncommon disorder. In a 1972 review, Seeler found and described 58 reported cases. She also noted that there was often an association with congenital anomalies (renal, cardiovascular, and skeletal) (152). Bleeding manifestations usually involve the mucous membranes or skin, and menorrhagia may be severe. Significant bleeding may occur after injury or surgery. The disorder is transmitted as an autosomal trait, with homozygotes manifesting a complete lack of the protein, indicated by functional assay as well as by the failure of such plasma to neutralize antisera against Factor V (153). Abnormal results are noted with both the prothrombin time and the partial thromboplastin time. The diagnosis is confirmed by use of a specific assay for Factor V.

Because of the instability of Factor V, fresh frozen plasma (preferably less than 1 month old) or freshly drawn plasma must be used for treatment of bleeding. Doses of 10 to 20 ml per kg should provide hemostatic levels, but daily infusions are required to maintain hemostasis for surgical procedures.

Inhibitors to transfused Factor V have been reported in patients with congenital Factor V deficiency (153, 154).

Combined deficiency of Factors V and VIII has been described in several families (155, 156) and in some, but not all, of these appears to be due to the hereditary lack of an inhibitor of activated protein C, which is present in normal plasma (155, 156).

Factor VII Deficiency. This is a rare bleeding disorder with variable symptoms, depending on the severity of the defect. It was described first in 1951 by Alexander and associates (157) and is inherited as an autosomal recessive trait. By 1964, an additional 40 cases had been described (158). Heterozygotes have Factor VII levels from 16 to 42 per cent of normal and have been reported to have bleeding episodes. Some affected homozygotes have a nonfunctional protein in their plasma that is detectable by immunologic methods, whereas others have no detectable Factor VII by either functional or immunologic tests (159). Girolami and colleagues have reported a number of apparent variants of Factor VII in defined areas of Northern Italy (160). These have been summarized by Bloom (150). Factor VII deficiency has been reported in association with Gilbert's disease (congenital hyperbilirubinemia) (161) and Dubin-Johnson syndrome (162), but the conditions are not necessarily related (150).

Bleeding symptoms, including serious intracranial hemorrhage, may occur in the newborn. Mucous membrane bleeding is most common, and nosebleeds and menorrhagia may be troublesome.

The results of the prothrombin time (which is significantly prolonged) and the partial thromboplastin time (which is normal) provide a presumptive diagnosis of Factor VII deficiency because this combination of findings occurs only in this disorder. Russell's viper venom time is normal. The diagnosis is confirmed by specific Factor VII assay.

Treatment for bleeding can be provided with fresh frozen plasma in a dose of 10 to 20 ml per kg or by an appropriate amount of prothrombin complex concentrate. Because the half-life of Factor VII is only 4 to 6 hours, frequent infusions may be required to maintain a hemostatic level after severe injury or surgery. In this situation, use of prothrombin complex concentrate may prevent plasma overloading; however, one must keep in mind the potential complications of the use of PCC, particularly viral hepatitis. Vitamin K is of no value in the treatment of congenital Factor VII deficiency.

Factor X Deficiency. This is a very rare coagulation disorder that is associated with mucous membrane bleeding, prolonged bleeding after trauma, easy bruising, and menorrhagia. Neonatal bleeding may occur intracranially or from the gastrointestinal tract or vagina. The disorder was described in 1956 in a family named Prower (163) and in 1957 in a family named Stuart (164), and Factor X is therefore sometimes referred to as the Stuart-Prower factor. During the 5 years after the initial case reports, a number of Factor X–deficient patients were studied (165–168). Several extensive family studies were undertaken, and it was determined that Factor X deficiency is inherited as a highly penetrant, incompletely recessive autosomal characteristic (169). Approximately 58 cases of hereditary Factor X deficiency have now been reported (170). In addition to these, a number of abnormal variant Factor X deficiency states have been described (150, 170, 171). If one includes the variant forms of Factor X deficiency, approximately 70 cases have been reported (170). Several types of abnormal Factor X molecules have been recognized (150). One type has abnormal function but does cause neutralization of an antibody to Factor X (171); a second type has abnormal function and antibody-neutralizing ability but can be activated by Russell's viper venom (172); and a third type has no coagulant activity but does cause partial neutralization of antibody to Factor X

(173). Heterozygotes may have Factor X levels reduced to the point that abnormal bleeding can occur with surgery or trauma.

Factor X deficiency is associated with prolongation of both the prothrombin time and the partial thromboplastin time. The Russell's viper venom time may be normal, as in the Factor X Friuli defect (150), and thus is not a good screening test for Factor X deficiency. The diagnosis can be confirmed by specific assay of Factor X.

The need for factor replacement is dependent on the severity of Factor X deficiency. Fresh frozen plasma is the preferred therapeutic agent. However, in life-threatening bleeding situations and in cases of severe Factor X deficiency, prothrombin complex concentrates are indicated. A Factor X level of 10 to 40 per cent is considered adequate for hemostasis. This can usually be achieved by administration of 10 ml plasma per kg body weight, followed by 3 to 6 ml per kg every 12 hours (170). Vitamin K is of no value in congenital Factor X deficiency.

Acquired isolated Factor X deficiency has been described in a number of cases of primary systemic amyloidosis and appears to be due to specific adsorption of Factor X to amyloid fibrils (see further on). Such patients are refractory to treatment with vitamin K, fresh frozen plasma, or prothrombin complex concentrates (170, 174).

FACTOR XIII DEFICIENCY

Congenitial deficiency of Factor XIII is a rare hereditary bleeding disorder first described in 1960 by Duckert (175). Factor XIII (fibrin-stabilizing factor) had been recognized as being necessary for normal clot solubility long before its congenital deficiency was known (176–178). The clinical bleeding disorder may result from lack of the protein or the presence of a nonfunctional protein (175, 178). Over 100 patients with the deficiency have now been described (179), and genetic, biochemical, and immunologic studies have revealed considerable heterogeneity of both the Factor XIII molecule and its disorders (180). Heterozygous individuals may have decreased levels of Factor XIII activity in some families.

In severe Factor XIII deficiency, the bleeding manifestations begin in infancy, and delayed bleeding from the umbilical cord is a strikingly common symptom. Easy bruising, hematoma formation following trauma, and poor wound healing also are common manifestations in children and persist throughout life. Although bleeding may occur directly following trauma, it is characteristically delayed for several hours or days. Healing is thus delayed, probably because the clot is unstable and susceptible to fibrinolysis and does not support the proper growth of fibroblasts (181).

Plasma Factor XIII, when activated by thrombin, forms an enzyme (transamidase) that in the presence of calcium ions catalyzes the formation of crosslinks between fibrin monomers. Deficiency of Factor XIII renders clots unstable. They lack elasticity, are more susceptible to digestion by plasmin, and are soluble in 5 M urea or 1 per cent monochloracetic acid. All routine coagulation tests are normal in patients with Factor XIII deficiency, but the diagnosis may be suspected as a result of a friable clot. One can screen for severe Factor XIII deficiency by testing the solubility of a plasma clot in 5 M urea or 1 per cent monochloracetic acid. Normal plasma clots remain insoluble for 24 hours. This screening test may not detect heterozygous subjects, however. The diagnosis can be confirmed by specific biochemical or immunologic assays (150), which are needed to detect carriers. Factor XIII deficiency must be differentiated from dysfibrinogenemia and afibrinogenemia, in which there may be similar symptoms of wound dehiscence.

Significant bleeding may be treated by small amounts of fresh or fresh frozen plasma. A single infusion of 5 to 10 ml per kg should provide effective therapy for most bleeding episodes because the level required for hemostasis is only 2 to 3 per cent of normal, and the half-life is 6 days.

Factor XIII levels are low in normal newborn infants but reach adult levels by 1 month after delivery (182). Acquired deficiency of Factor XIII has been described in a number of conditions, including liver disease, malignancies, collagen diseases, and disseminated intravascular coagulation (183).

CONTACT FACTOR DEFICIENCIES

The intrinsic pathway of blood coagulation is activated when plasma is exposed to a variety of negatively charged materials, such as glass, celite, kaolin, certain collagen and connective tissue preparations, and endotoxin. Factor XII (Hageman factor) is the enzyme that is central to this pathway. Activated Factor XII (XIIa) activates Factor XI, which in turn activates Factor IX. Factor XIIa also triggers the kinin-forming pathway, plasminogen activation, conversion of Factor VII to Factor VIIa, and conversion of prorenin to renin (184).

Four plasma proteins are involved in normal contact activation reactions: Factor XI, Factor XII, plasma prekallikrein, and high-molecular-weight kininogen. A deficiency in any one of the contact activation proteins is inherited as an autosomal recessive trait (185). Interestingly, an inherited deficiency in any one of the contact activation proteins except Factor XI is not associated with a bleeding tendency (185).

Factor XI (PTA) Deficiency. This occurs mainly in Jewish persons of Ashkenazi descent (who have emigrated from Eastern Europe). Seligsohn has calculated that 0.1 to 0.3 per cent of Ashkenazi Jews in Israel are homozygous for this trait and that 5.5 to 11 per cent are heterozygous (186). In contrast, Factor XI deficiency is rare in Oriental and Sephardic Jews and in other population groups.

The hemorrhagic tendency is usually mild, even in homozygotes, and is not necessarily related to the level of Factor XI coagulant or antigen (187). Manifestations include excessive bruising, menorrhagia, epistaxis, and postoperative bleeding.

The prothrombin time is normal, whereas the activated or nonactivated partial thromboplastin time is prolonged. One can make the diagnosis by performing a Factor XI assay, using either severe Factor XI–Deficient plasma from a patient or an artificially prepared substrate (188). Because tests of contact activation factors can be influenced by freezing and thawing, such testing should be done on fresh plasma (150).

Factor XII (Hageman Factor), Prekallikrein (Fletcher Factor), and High-Molecular-Weight Kininogen Deficiencies. These rare disorders are not associated with bleeding but are usually discovered as an incidental finding. In nearly every case, the abnormality was recognized because of prolonged coagulation screening tests done for routine purposes. The main clinical importance of recognizing individuals with these disorders is to avoid denying them necessary surgical procedures because of their abnormal laboratory findings. Because most people with these deficiencies demonstrate no symptoms (e.g., they do not have abnormal bleeding), there seem to be alternative mechanisms. These deficiency states have also stimulated considerable interest because of the interrelationships of the contact factors with the coagulation, fibrinolytic, kinin-generating, and complement systems (189).

Factor XII (Hageman factor) deficiency was first described by Ratnoff and Colopy in 1955 in a patient named Hageman who underwent routine preoperative coagulation testing. Despite a prolonged clotting time, the patient had no hemorrhagic symptoms and, in fact, later died from thromboembolic disease (190). Over 100 cases of Hageman factor deficiency have now been described. As is true of all the contact factor deficiency states, Factor XII deficiency is inherited as an autosomal recessive trait, with most heterozygotes having 30 to 60 per cent activity, whereas homozygotes lack Factor XII (191). Most persons with Hageman trait are asymptomatic, but rarely there may be a mild tendency to bleed (192).

Tests related to the initial phase of coagulation are abnormal in Factor XII deficiency (whole-blood clotting time, partial thromboplastin time), although the prothrombin time is normal. The clotting abnormality can be corrected by the effect of normal plasma on a glass test tube, but the diagnosis is established by specific assay for Factor XII.

Prekallikrein (Fletcher Factor) deficiency was first described by Hathaway and colleagues in 1965. The abnormality was recognized in asymptomatic siblings (one of whom underwent routine preoperative coagulation screening) who were born to consanguineous parents (193). Subsequently, a number of other cases have been described, many in black individuals (194). Heterozygotes have Fletcher factor levels of 40 to 72 per cent, and homozygotes have levels of 1 per cent or less (195). None of the individuals reported to have Fletcher factor deficiency has had any abnormal bleeding.

As in Factor XII deficiency, plasma lacking Fletcher factor causes grossly abnormal test results related to the initial phase of coagulation, but the prothrombin time is normal. A unique feature of Fletcher factor–deficient plasma is the decrease in the partial thromboplastin time (PTT) observed after one increases the incubation with kaolin to 10 to 20 minutes (from the usual 3- to 5-minute incubation used in most PTT methods). This corrective effect on the clotting time of the PTT due to increased incubation does not occur in other coagulation factor deficiencies, and this phenomenon provides a presumptive test for Fletcher factor deficiency. Definitive coagulation studies depend on cross-correction with known deficient plasma or chromogenic assay for plasma prekallikrein (150).

Fletcher factor–deficient plasma lacks prekallikrein, with resulting abnormalities of both bradykinin generation and fibrinolysis. Despite the multisystem abnormalities related to this deficiency, none of the individuals with prekallikrein deficiency has been shown to have any significant clinical manifestations.

High-molecular-weight kininogen deficiency is another asymptomatic condition that has been recognized in a few families as the result of detection of abnormal coagulation tests on routine screening. The reported individuals have been free of bleeding manifestations. The first subject described was an asymptomatic 71-year-old man named Fitzgerald. He was found to have an unexpectedly prolonged activated partial thromboplastin time that did not shorten with prolonged incubation with kaolin (196). Subjects with similar abnormalities were independently reported, and their surnames were used to describe their respective defects: Fleaujeac (197), Williams (198), and Reid (199). However, these plasmas are not mutually corrective, and subsequent studies have shown that they are deficient in components of the kininogen system. Fitzgerald factor–deficient plasma lacks high-molecular-weight kininogen, and defective kinin production is not corrected by addition of purified kallikrein. The Reid defect appears to be similar; however, in the Williams and Fleaujeac traits, there is a deficiency of both high- and low-molecular-weight kininogens.

Plasmas deficient in prekallikrein, high-molecular-weight kininogen, or Factor XII show not only impaired generation of kinin molecules but also reduced ability to generate fibrinolytic activity when exposed to negatively charged surfaces (189).

The *Passavoy defect* is somewhat similar to Fletcher factor deficiency in that affected individuals have a prolonged partial thromboplastin time that is corrected by prolonged incubation with kaolin. However, the defect is associated with a mild bleeding tendency and in that respect seems to be distinct from Fletcher factor deficiency (200, 201).

ALPHA$_2$-ANTIPLASMIN DEFICIENCY (MIYASATO'S DISEASE)

A severe hemorrhagic defect resembling hemophilia has been reported in one patient in association with a severe deficiency of α_2-antiplasmin deficiency (202). The affected individual was the product of a consanguineous marriage; both parents had intermediate levels of α_2-antiplasmin. The euglobulin lysis time was abnormally short, and excessive bleeding responded to treatment with tranexamic acid, an antifibrinolytic agent (203).

DEFICIENCIES ASSOCIATED WITH THROMBOTIC DISEASE

Current evidence suggests that two plasma proteins play critical roles in the regulation of blood coagulation. Antithrombin III (AT III) is the most widely recognized; however, it has been shown that protein C also is an important regulatory protein. Deficiencies of AT III and of protein C are associated with recurrent thrombosis, and both AT III and protein C are consumed during coagulation in vivo. Although they differ in their mechanism of action, these two anticoagulant and antithrombotic proteins share many properties.

Antithrombin III Deficiency. AT III is the main physiologic inhibitor of blood clotting. It is the heparin cofactor and is thus essential to effective heparin therapy. As its name implies, antithrombin neutralizes thrombin. It is also the main physiologic inhibitor of activated Factor X (Xa) and may control all serine proteases in the coagulation sequence (204). Antithrombin is responsible for 50 to 80 per cent of the inhibitory capacity of plasma, with the rest being provided by α_2-macroglobulin, α_1-antitrypsin, and possibly C$_1$-esterase inhibitor.

AT III is synthesized in the liver and has a biologic half-life of approximately 2 to 5 days, which is decreased during heparin treatment. Normal full-term infants have mean AT III levels of 45 to 60 per cent by clotting activity methods and 40 to 87 per cent by immunologic methods (205).

Congenital AT III deficiency is associated with a high risk of thromboembolic disorders. Beyond infancy, spontaneous thrombosis may occur at levels of 50 to 60 per cent of normal. In 1965, Egeberg described a Norwegian family with a high incidence of venous thromboembolic disease, often occurring in association with trauma, surgery, inflammation, or pregnancy. Affected family members were found to have low levels (about 50 per cent of normal) of antithrombin, as measured by both biologic and immunologic methods. Egeberg concluded that antithrombin deficiency could cause a severe tendency to thrombosis (206). Numerous other families have now been reported. Although both qualitative (functional) and quantitative abnormalities have been described, the most common variant appears to be characterized by low levels of functionally normal antithrombin (204).

The frequency of congenital AT III deficiency in the population is in the range of one per 2000 to one per 5000 (207, 208). In persons with hereditary AT III deficiency, the initial thrombotic event usually occurs between the ages of 10 and 30 years. Family history often reveals that one or more relatives have died suddenly of thromboembolic disease. Events that predispose to thrombosis include surgery, trauma, infection, and pregnancy. Patients who experience such events often appear to be heparin-resistant because of their AT III deficiency and require very large amounts of heparin to prolong the APTT (209). Although low levels of AT III are lifelong, it is unusual to see thrombotic problems during the first decade. Shapiro has speculated that the increased levels of α_2-macroglobulin documented in infancy (210) may provide protection against thrombotic events in this age group (208).

Antithrombin deficiency can be diagnosed by specific assay. Such assays are based on immunologic, enzymatic, or clotting properties (204, 211). The principal of the clotting assays of antithrombin is that a constant amount of thrombin or Factor Xa is added to various dilutions of plasma, and, after a defined incubation time, the residual enzyme concentration is measured. Without heparin, the antithrombin concentration can be measured in terms of the initial rate or the total amount neutralized (204). Antithrombin can also be measured immunologically with monospecific antisera. However, the presence of an abnormal molecule can be missed by such immunologic assays that measure the concentration of protein, not its biologic activity. Chromogenic assay methods for antithrombin also are available (204).

In patients with antithrombin deficiency, either congenital or acquired, the tendency to thrombosis can be controlled by oral anticoagulant therapy (204). Purified preparations of human antithrombin are now becoming available for clinical use;

however, they are not yet licensed in the United States, and clinical trials demonstrating therapeutic benefits have not yet been reported. European investigators who have used AT III concentrates recommend an initial dose of 50 IU per kg. One should then attempt to keep the patient's AT III level over 80 per cent. These investigators recommend the use of antithrombin concentrates in patients with congenital deficiency of antithrombin who have acute thrombosis, who are about to undergo a surgical procedure, or who are in the third trimester of pregnancy (73, 207, 211–215).

Another therapeutic approach that has been tried is daily administration of danazol, an attenuated androgen that stimulates protein synthesis. Eyster and colleagues found an increase in AT III levels in two congenitally deficient patients following danazol therapy (216).

Protein C Deficiency. Protein C also is an important regulatory protein. Activated protein C is a potent anticoagulant, a vitamin K–dependent serine protease that was originally identified in 1960 by Mammen and co-workers, who termed it autoprothrombin IIa (217). In 1976, Stenflo described what later was shown to be the same protein and named it protein C (218).

Activated protein C functions by inactivating the cofactor proteins, Factors V and VIII. Inactivation of the activated forms of the cofactors, Va and VIIIa, is much more rapid than that of the precursors (219–221). In addition to having anticoagulant function, activated protein C indirectly facilitates clot lysis (220, 222).

The clinical picture of protein C deficiency, like AT III deficiency, is that of venous thromboses in adolescents or young adults. In 1981, the first study of human protein C in patients was published, with the description of hereditary venous thrombosis associated with protein C deficiency (223). Since the initial report, more than 25 families have been identified in which thromboembolic disease was associated with protein C deficiency (156). Thrombophlebitis or recurrent pulmonary emboli or both often appear in late adolescence, sometimes following trauma. Protein C deficiency is inherited as an autosomal dominant trait. It appears that heterozygotes, who generally have protein C levels of approximately 50 per cent, are at risk for thromboembolic disease. The homozygous state has been associated with recurrent purpura fulminans (156, 224), and most homozygous protein C–deficient individuals die of thrombotic complications during infancy (156). However, one infant has been successfully maintained on periodic infusions of prothrombin complex concentrates (which contain protein C) (224), despite the inherent risk of enhancing the thrombotic tendency with PCC. More highly purified and specific protein C concentrates are needed but are not currently available.

In 1980, Marlar and Griffin reported that the plasma of patients with combined Factor V and Factor VIII deficiency lacked protein C inhibitory activity. They postulated that the uninhibited activity of protein C, which inactivates Factors V and VIII, accounted for the clinical state of combined Factor V and Factor VIII deficiency (155). This hypothesis was challanged by some (222), and Gardiner and Griffin have demonstrated that extreme care must be used in handling and storing plasma samples that are to be assayed for protein C inhibitor (225). These investigators confirmed the presence of protein C inhibitor in plasmas deficient in Factor V and Factor VIII and showed that freezing and thawing significantly reduced the ability of both normal plasmas and those with this combined deficiency to inhibit activated protein C. Thus, conflicting literature reports probably reflect this artifactual lowering of protein C inhibitory activity.

Protein C now can be assayed by both functional and immunologic methods (156, 220), although the latter were developed first and have been used more commonly. Protein C can be detected in plasma by Laurell rocket immunoelectrophoresis, and one can improve the sensitivity of the assay by using either radiolabeled or peroxidase-labeled antibodies to detect the immunoprecipitate (220).

Protein S Deficiency. Protein S, another vitamin K–dependent plasma protein, serves as a cofactor for the expression of the anticoagulant activity of activated protein C. Hereditary deficiency of protein S has been shown to be associated with recurrent venous thrombosis. Heterozygotes have plasma levels of protein S of 35 to 50 per cent of normal and have recurrent venous thrombotic disease beginning in adolescence or early adulthood (226).

ACQUIRED COAGULATION DISORDERS AND ASSOCIATED ABNORMALITIES

Liver Disease

The liver is the site of synthesis of most coagulation factors (fibrinogen, prothrombin, prekallikrein, high-molecular-weight kininogen, and Factors V, VII, IX, X, XI, XII, and XIII. It is also the site of synthesis of plasminogen, regulators of coagulation (AT III; proteins C and S), and inhibitors of fibrinolysis (antiplasmin and α_1-antitrypsin). The liver is also involved in the clearance of activated coagulation factors and activators of fibrinolysis from the circulation (227–229). As a result, hepatocellular damage is frequently associated with multiple hemostatic defects that can predispose to clinical bleeding. Hepatic failure can also lead to disseminated intravascular coagulation as the result of decreased synthesis of AT III and decreased hepatic clearance of activated coagulation factors.

Most patients with acute viral or toxic hepatitis do not demonstrate marked abnormalities on coagulation tests. In contrast, in those with fulminant hepatitis (of either infectious or toxic etiology), hemostatic abnormalities are more pronounced and are often associated with hemorrhagic symptoms, and the extent of the hemostatic abnormalities does have prognostic significance (230, 231). The level of Factor VII decreases early in the course of acute liver failure, and a later increase in Factor VII is usually an early sign of recovery. Factor VII values of less than 10 per cent are associated with an unfavorable prognosis (230). In patients with fulminant hepatitis or acute liver necrosis, disseminated intravascular coagulation also may occur (231).

In chronic liver disease, coagulation test results vary. Factor VII does not appear to have the same prognostic value as it does in patients with fulminant hepatitis, and it appears that no specific factor assays are more likely to predict the risk of bleeding any more reliably than do the screening tests (231). Other hemostatic abnormalities may include thrombocytopenia (often resulting from hypersplenism), increased fibrinolysis, and disseminated intravascular coagulation.

Treatment of the coagulation abnormalities in liver disease depends on the specific clinical circumstance, with the nature and site of the bleeding (e.g., gastrointestinal bleeding, bleeding from biopsy site, or generalized bleeding in a child with fulminant hepatitis) taken into account. Parenteral vitamin K may be beneficial if the coagulation defect is associated with malabsorption. If the degree of parenchymal liver disease is severe and there is no response to parenteral vitamin K, fresh frozen plasma may control bleeding. Fresh frozen plasma contains all the coagulation factors and is thus theoretically the treatment of choice for correction of the multiple defects found in liver disease. However, correction of the hemostatic defects may be difficult to achieve with fresh frozen plasma because of the large volumes required, particularly to correct Factor VII (231).

Prothrombin complex concentrates, which contain high concentrations of Factors II, VII, IX, and X, may be useful in certain situations (e.g., preparation for liver biopsy), either alone or in combination with fresh frozen plasma. However, their use is not without hazard. Risks include transmission of viral hepatitis and thromboembolic disease. The risk of thromboembolic episodes and disseminated intravascular coagulation is much greater in the presence of hepatocellular disease (52–58); therefore, use of prothrombin complex concentrates should be limited to patients who require liver biopsy and to those in whom other methods of controlling bleeding have failed (231).

Platelet concentrates are seldom indicated in patients with liver disease, even when severe thrombocytopenia exists. Thrombocytopenia is usually not the cause of bleeding in these patients, and transfused platelets are rapidly sequestered in the spleen (231).

The hemostatic abnormalities in liver disease may be similar to those found in disseminated intravascular coagulation, and, as mentioned previously, the latter disorder may occur in patients with liver disease. Differentiating the abnormalities due to liver disease from those due to disseminated intravascular coagulation may be difficult, if not impossible, and use of heparin in a patient with severe liver disease may be unwise (232).

Vitamin K Deficiency

Deficiency of vitamin K results in the failure of the vitamin K–dependent coagulation factors to develop calcium-binding sites essential to their function in the coagulation process (233). In the absence of vitamin K, the polypeptide chains of vitamin K–dependent factors are produced normally, but the carboxylation step (gamma carboxylation of the amino terminal glutamic acid residues) does not take place. The acarboxy forms of Factors II, VII, IX, and X cannot bind calcium and thus cannot participate in the coagulation sequence (234). Whether due to dietary deficiency, failure of absorption, or specific drug antagonism of vitamin K, the unavailability of vitamin K renders the circulating molecules of prothrombin, Factor VII, Factor IX, and Factor X ineffective in coagulation.

In infants beyond the newborn period, vitamin K is absorbed from the colon, and synthesis by bacterial flora provides a major source. Vitamin K is not absorbed from the colon in older children or adults but is absorbed from the ileum (234). The daily requirement of this fat-soluble vitamin is probably about 1 µg per kg of body weight (234), which is supplied easily in most normal diets, particularly those containing green, leafy vegetables. After absorption from the upper small intestine, vitamin K is stored in the liver.

The "physiologic" decrease in activities of the vitamin K–dependent coagulation factors that may lead to hemorrhagic disease of the newborn in its most severe form is discussed in Chapter 5. Beyond the newborn period, a "delayed" form of this condition has been described in infants in whom several concomitant factors resulted in significant bleeding (235). The combination of gastrointestinal infection with diarrhea, prolonged antibiotic therapy, and milk-substitute formulas not supplemented with vitamin K has led to hemorrhagic symptoms due to vitamin K deficiency. Because this complication has been recognized and milk-substitute formulas have been supplemented with vitamin K, the problem has become rare (236).

Conditions associated with malabsorption of vitamin K that may result in a hemorrhagic state include cystic fibrosis, biliary atresia, chronic hemolytic anemia with secondary cholelithiasis and obstructive jaundice, and disorders leading to upper small intestine dysfunction (234). In the absence of marked dietary deficiency of vitamin K, malabsorption due to alteration of gastrointestinal bacterial flora by antibiotic therapy is rare (237).

An additional source of hemorrhagic symptoms due to vitamin K deficiency may be secondary to ingestion (accidental or deliberate) of coumarin compounds. These vitamin K antagonists are the most commonly used oral anticoagulant agents and may induce serious deficiencies of the vitamin K–dependent coagulation factors. Because the effect of vitamin K antagonism on the efficacy of the vitamin K–dependent clotting factors is related to the synthesis and longevity of these factors, bleeding complications following coumarin ingestion may be delayed for 2 or 3 days and should be preventable by administration of vitamin K, if given early.

The hemorrhagic symptoms of vitamin K deficiency are nonspecific and may range from easy bruising to massive ecchymoses, serious mucous membrane hemorrhage, or posttraumatic bleeding. Significant central nervous system hemorrhage may occur, but hemathrosis is rare. Laboratory findings include prolonged PT and PPT with normal thrombin time. Assays of individual coagulation factors provide confirmation of the diagnosis, but reversal of abnormal PT and PTT following vitamin K therapy also confirms the diagnosis if assays are not available.

The immediate treatment of vitamin K deficiency is intravenous administration of 5 to 10 mg of vitamin K_1. Because clinical improvement of bleeding symptoms should occur within a few hours and significant improvement of vitamin K–dependent coagulation factors (as well as PT and PTT) should be noted within 24 hours, replacement therapy usually is not necessary. If serious bleeding is present, however, fresh frozen plasma (10 ml per kg) should be given immediately because of the delay in response to vitamin K therapy.

Congenital Heart Disease

Variable laboratory abnormalities of hemostasis, including platelet dysfunction (see Chapter 42) and coagulation factor deficiencies, have been described in children with congenital heart disease (cyanotic and acyanotic), but significant bleeding is rarely a problem in such patients (238).

Children with cyanotic congenital heart disease who are very polycythemic often have multiple hemostatic defects, including thrombocytopenia, poor clot retraction, low levels of certain plasma coagulation factors, and elevated levels of fibrin degradation products. Although the precise etiology of these abnormalities remains uncertain, it seems likely that a common denominator is impaired hepatic synthesis of clotting factors and impaired platelet production resulting from chronic hypoxia, increased blood viscosity, and poor perfusion (239). In a few individuals, there also may be an element of low-grade disseminated intravascular coagulation (239).

The preoperative correction of elevated hematocrit levels in polycythemic children with cyanotic congenital heart disease may decrease blood viscosity and improve overall cardiac function by decreasing peripheral vascular resistance and increasing stroke volume, systemic blood flow, and oxygen transport (240). This is achieved by alternate removal of whole blood and replacement with fresh frozen plasma or 5 per cent human albumin in saline in 30- to 50-ml aliquots until the hematocrit value is reduced to the desired level (between 55 and 75 per cent, depending on the initial hematocrit level).

Evaluation of hemostasis in children with congenital heart disease should be individualized in relation to the history and physical findings. Blood obtained from children with cyanotic heart disease must be added to an appropriate volume of citrate anticoagulant so that overdilution of the plasma and the effects of excess citrate on the coagulation test are avoided (Fig. 41–8) (239). Evaluation should include a platelet count, PT, PTT, tests for fibrinolytic activity, and specific coagulation factor assays if indicated by abnormal screening tests. Except for reduction of excessively high hematocrit levels, preoperative preparation is usually not required. However, replacement of significantly depleted coagulation factors or suppression of excessive fibrinolytic activity with ε-aminocaproic acid may be advisable in some patients.

A variety of hemostatic abnormalities may occur in patients following cardiopulmonary bypass operations for correction of congenital heart defects. These abnormalities include thrombocytopenia, functional platelet defects, plasma coagulation factor deficiencies, disseminated intravascular coagulation, excessive fibrinolysis, and heparin-induced defects. Meaningful evaluation of postoperative bleeding in such patients requires a battery of laboratory tests (usually including thrombin time, PT, PTT, reptilase time, and platelet count) (225, 242) and requires that blood specimens used be free of any contamination with heparin. Conservative replacement therapy with platelets and fresh or fresh frozen plasma should be given unless laboratory findings document the need for more specific agents (e.g., heparin for disseminated intravascular coagulation or ε-ami-

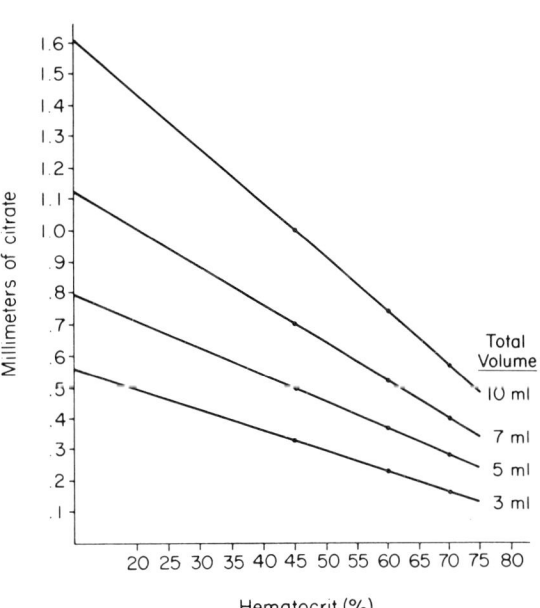

Figure 41–8. Nomogram for correction of amount of anticoagulant based on hematocrit. Correction should be made in the anticoagulant:whole blood ratio if the hematocrit is unusually high (e.g., in newborn infants or in children with cyanotic congenital heart disease) so that the appropriate citrate:plasma ratio can be maintained. (From Lusher, J. M., and Barnhart, M. I. (eds.); *Acquired Bleeding Disorders in Children: Platelet Abnormalities and Laboratory Methods.* New York, Masson Publ., 1981, p. 111.)

nocaproic acid for excessive fibrinolysis). Prothrombin complex concentrates should *not* be used to treat bleeding associated with cardiovascular surgery. In this setting, the potential risks far outweigh the possible benefits of their use (52, 57, 58).

Renal Failure

Isolated or multiple hemostatic defects may occur in renal disease (243, 244). Platelet function abnormalities and thrombocytopenia are often seen in patients with chronic renal failure and uremia (245, 246) (see Chapter 42). In the acute phase of renal disease, during allograft rejection, and in chronic renal insufficiency, laboratory evidence of disseminated intravascular coagulation is often found. It is often impossible to determine whether these abnormalities result from local changes in the kidney or arise as a result of uremic and metabolic effects leading to disseminated intravascular coagulation. In hemolytic-uremic syndrome, acute damage to glomerular capillaries often leads to thrombocytopenia, although the precise pathogenesis of this disorder remains unclear (see Chapter 42).

Occasionally, children with the nephrotic syndrome develop a deficiency of Factor IX or, more commonly, of Factors XI and XII (243). These deficiencies are usually recognized because of an abnormal coagulation screening test result (PTT), not because of hemorrhagic symptoms. The primary significance of recognizing such abnormalities is that if the patient needs a renal biopsy, a deficiency of Factor XII does not constitute a problem, whereas a significantly low level of Factor IX (if uncorrected) is a contraindication to biopsy. The mechanism responsible for decreased levels of Factor IX and/or Factors XI and XII is thought to be related to loss of these proteins in the urine. Levels of the decreased coagulation factors return to normal when proteinuria subsides, whether due to spontaneous remission or response to steroid therapy.

In addition to the aforementioned factors, other plasma proteins of molecular weight similar to that of albumin can be excreted in the urine in the nephrotic syndrome. AT III and plasminogen have been found in the urine of children with the nephrotic syndrome (247, 248), and it has been postulated that thrombosis in patients with severe proteinuria may result in part from urinary loss of AT III (249).

Amyloidosis

In generalized amyloidosis, a variety of coagulation factor deficiencies have been reported.

These are often associated with excessive bleeding, particularly after surgical biopsies. Deficiencies of Factors V, VII, IX, and X and of fibrinogen as well as altered antithrombin activity have been reported (250, 251). The combined deficiency of Factor IX and Factor X, resulting from adsorption onto the amyloid, often results in a severe bleeding disorder (251).

Anticoagulants

Acquired inhibitors due to antibodies to a variety of coagulation factors have been recognized in individuals without pre-existing coagulation factor deficiencies (252, 253). Many of these individuals have had lupus erythematosus or other collagen disorders. Acquired anticoagulants are rare in children, except for those occurring in hemophilia.

Acquired inhibitors to Factor VIII are the most common, and more than 100 cases have been reported (101, 254). Patients have included at least 30 postpartum women and a similar number of patients with collagen vascular disease, chronic bowel disorders, or chronic skin disease. Several acquired Factor VIII inhibitors have occurred in association with penicillin or other drug therapy, and at least 25 cases have been observed in healthy individuals (usually elderly) with no apparent cause. The management of bleeding episodes in such patients has been similar to that of hemophiliacs with Factor VIII inhibitors; however, some have recommended the use of porcine Factor VIII (Hyate:C) rather than lyophilized concentrates of human Factor VIII or prothrombin complex concentrates because of the hepatitis risk associated with the latter (105). The use of corticosteroids or immunosuppressive drugs or both in eradicating acquired Factor VII inhibitors has been more successful than in hemophilia, but this is difficult to evaluate in view of the wide variety of underlying conditions and the greater tendency for spontaneous remission.

Acquired von Willebrand's disease has been reported in a few individuals, but not all have had evidence of an inhibitor or an anticoagulant (252). Inhibitors to fibrinogen, Factor V, Factor IX, Factor XI, and fibrin-stabilizing factor (Factor XIII) have been reported in a small number of individuals, with and without relationship to underlying conditions, surgery, or drugs.

A small number of patients with systemic lupus erythematosus develop a nonspecific anticoagulant that causes prolongation of the PT and PTT in mixtures of patient and normal plasma (252). The "lupus anticoagulant" does not cause bleeding manifestations. However, specific inhibitors (e.g., inhibitors directed against Factor VIII, Factor IX, or von Willebrand's factor) may occur in the same patient, and assays should be performed if screening tests suggest the presence of an anticoagulant.

The "lupus anticoagulant" has also been found in persons with other immunologic disorders, in psychiatric patients receiving high doses of phenothiazines, and in individuals without underlying disease (252).

Disseminated Intravascular Coagulation (DIC)

ETIOLOGY

Disseminated intravascular coagulation (DIC) is not a disease but a process that is triggered by a wide variety of stimuli. It is an acquired coagulopathy that occurs when there is generalized in vivo activation of the coagulation mechanism resulting in the transformation of fibrinogen to fibrin. Potential causes of DIC in children are listed in Table 41–11. The spectrum of DIC ranges from clinically insignificant states, in which the turnover of platelets and fibrinogen is increased without apparent fibrin deposition or fibrinogen and platelet depletion, to fulminant disorders resulting in massive fibrin deposition and necrosis of vital organs or consumption of platelets and coagulation factors with subsequent serious hemorrhage.

The generalized Shwartzman reaction (GSR) in the rabbit has served as a useful model for study of the process of DIC, and there are human counterparts to the end stage of the GSR in the rabbit (i.e., bilateral renal cortical necrosis) (255). The GSR is induced in young rabbits weighing

Table 41–11. CONDITIONS ASSOCIATED WITH DISSEMINATED INTRAVASCULAR COAGULATION (DIC) IN CHILDREN

Disorders of the Newborn
  Intrauterine infections
  Maternal toxemia
  Abruptio placentae
  Severe respiratory distress syndrome
  Necrotizing enterocolitis

Infections
  Bacterial sepsis with shock
  Parasitic (malaria)
  Mycotic
  Rickettsial
  Viral (disseminated)

Other Conditions
  Leukemia and other disseminated malignancies
  Intravascular hemolysis
  Giant hemangioma (Kasabach-Merritt syndrome)
  Purpura fulminans
  Hemorrhagic shock
  Massive trauma
  Burns
  Heat stroke
  Hypothermia
  Postoperative states
  Intracranial injuries
  Acute anaphylaxis
  Snakebite
  Hemolytic uremic syndrome (?)
  Thrombotic thrombocytopenic purpura (?)

approximately 1 kg by two properly spaced (24 hours) intravenous doses of bacterial endotoxin. It is generally accepted that the initial dose of endotoxin triggers intravascular coagulation, which is reversible if no further endotoxin is given but which impairs the effectiveness of the reticuloendothelial system in clearing activated coagulation products from the circulation. As a result of the administration of this preparation, the second dose of endotoxin triggers more severe intravascular coagulation, which results in fibrin deposition in the glomerular capillaries as well as in other small blood vessels throughout the body. Rabbits that develop bilateral renal cortical necrosis as the result of fibrin deposition ultimately die from renal failure. The dynamic nature of DIC is illustrated in this animal model by the fact that, at the time that fatal renal cortical necrosis is progressing, the levels of circulating coagulaton factors have returned to normal. This aspect of the phenomenon makes diagnosis difficult, but it is important that one be aware of the rapidly changing pattern of the laboratory manifestations of DIC.

A number of factors influence the susceptibility of the rabbit to the development of the GSR. The phenomenon can be triggered by a single dose of endotoxin in pregnant rabbits and in those in which the reticuloendothelial system has been impaired. Intravenous administration of antigen-antibody complexes can trigger the GSR in rabbits prepared with a single dose of endotoxin. Administration of heparin or depletion of neutrophils protects rabbits from endotoxin-triggered DIC. Although it is not known whether all these observations can be applied to human forms of DIC, they illustrate the multifactorial nature of the process.

As can be seen from the variety of causes of DIC in children, there are many potential stimuli of this disorder. The mechanism of DIC in states in which known thromboplastic materials are released into the circulation is readily understood—for example, intravascular hemolysis following a mismatched transfusion with release of red cell membrane contents and the release of thromboplastic contents from acute promyelocytic leukemia cells or tumor cells into the circulation. The activation of blood coagulation in vivo can also result from diffuse endothclial damage or from tissue injury in which procoagulant materials enter the circulation. Injury to the vascular endothelium, such as occurs in certain viral illnesses and in bacterial endotoxemia, exposes underlying collagen and basement membrane. Factor XII is thus activated, and platelets adhere to the damaged endothelium, aggregate, undergo shape changes, and release phospholipids. The intrinsic pathway of coagulation is activated by Factor XIIa, leading to intravascular fibrin formation. In addition, Factor XIIa activates fibrinolysis and kinin formation (256). DIC resulting from activation of Factor XII is almost always accompanied by hypotension, which is due in part to bradykinin release, which results from prekallikrein activation by Factor XIIa. Hypotension is a unique feature of DIC-associated Factor XII activation and distinguishes it from DIC associated with tissue injury (257).

Obstetric causes of DIC include abruptio placentae, amniotic fluid embolism, and retained dead fetus. Necrotizing enterocolitis, which occurs in approximately 5 per cent of premature infants, may trigger DIC through release of tissue procoagulant substances from the damaged, necrotic bowel. The occurrence of DIC in such infants is a poor prognostic sign (256).

Because the phenomenon of DIC occurs as a relatively rare complication of many of the conditions listed in Table 41–11, it seems likely that host factors also are important. When a triggering event initiates DIC, it appears that factors such as the amount of clot-promoting material, the functional capability of the reticuloendothelial system, vascular flow, and the levels of naturally occurring inhibitors (e.g., AT III) are critical to the determination of the rate, duration, and extent of DIC.

The most common causes of DIC in infancy and childhood are fulminant bacterial septic shock (e.g., meningococcemia and *Hemophilus influenzae* sepsis), severe neonatal respiratory distress syndrome, disseminiated viral diseases, and massive head injuries. In contrast to the situation in bacterial septicemia, children with disseminated viral diseases or rickettsial diseases may develop DIC in the absence of shock. This probably reflects severe endothelial damage, which may accompany these disease states. Neonates with severe respiratory distress syndrome (RDS) regularly have DIC, whereas those with less severe RDS do not. Shock states, severe crush injury, and full-thickness burns also may be accompanied by DIC. Massive head injury, as from gunshot wounds, can cause the release of large amounts of thromboplastic material into the systemic circulation, resulting in DIC. Hemolytic transfusion reactions due to major blood group incompatibility (fortunately now a rarity) also can initiate DIC by a similar mechanism. Regardless of the underlying primary disease, the clinical picture in children with DIC can be predominantly that of bleeding or of thrombosis. The clinical manifestations of DIC may be minimal until consumption of platelets and coagulation factors leads to bleeding or the tissue damage secondary to fibrin thrombi becomes apparent. Bleeding manifestations range from easy bruising and oozing from venipuncture sites to massive purpura and mucous membrane bleeding or localized hemorrhagic gangrenous skin lesions

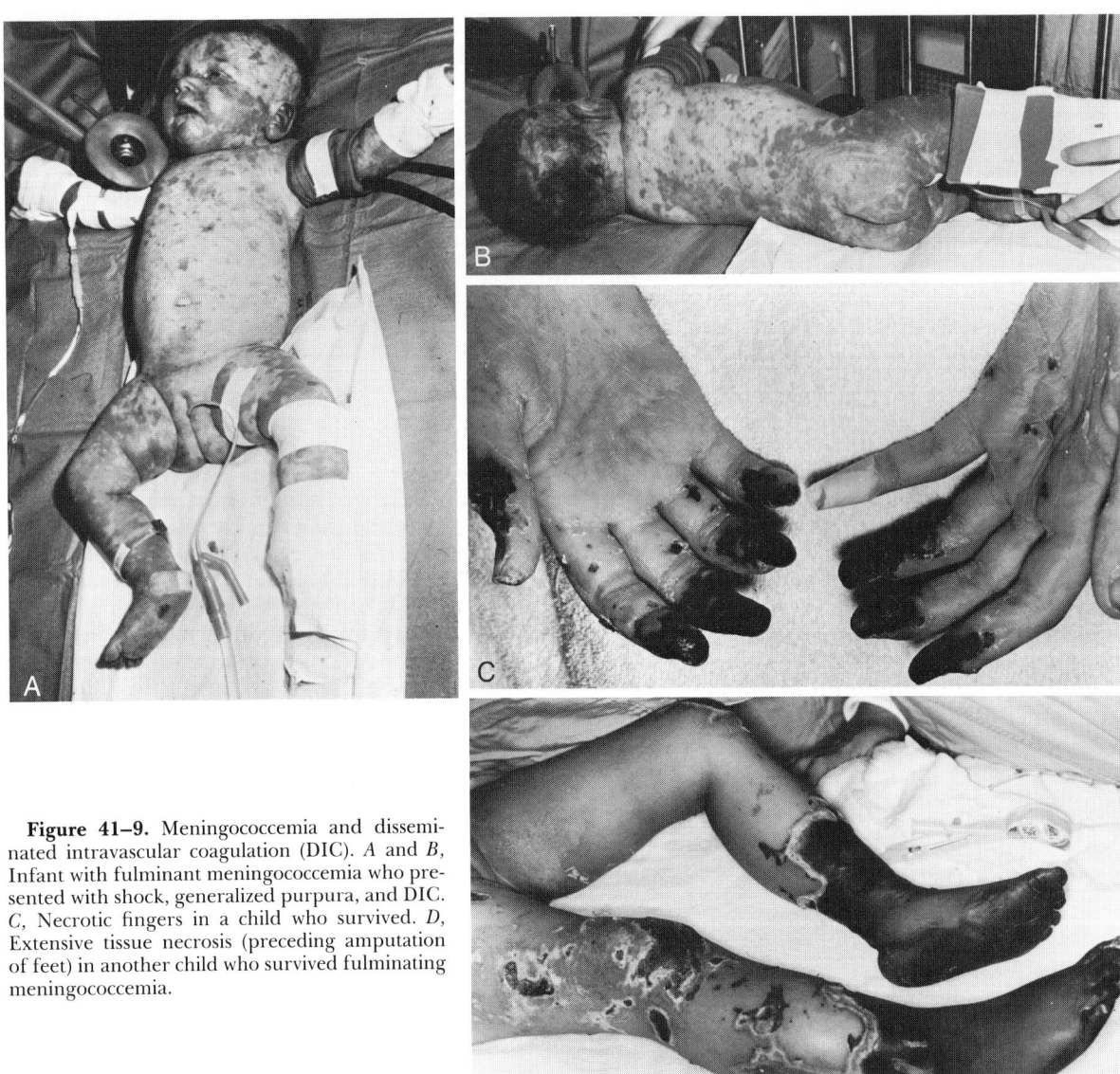

Figure 41–9. Meningococcemia and disseminated intravascular coagulation (DIC). *A* and *B*, Infant with fulminant meningococcemia who presented with shock, generalized purpura, and DIC. *C*, Necrotic fingers in a child who survived. *D*, Extensive tissue necrosis (preceding amputation of feet) in another child who survived fulminating meningococcemia.

(as in purpura fulminans). Thrombotic manifestations such as renal cortical necrosis may occur with minimal hemorrhagic symptoms.

Children with bacterial septicemia who are not in shock rarely, if ever, develop DIC. The classic picture of DIC associated with bacteremia is that of a child with fulminant meningococcemia who is rushed to the emergency room in shock, with massive cutaneous purpura and a very short history of illness (Fig. 41–9).

DIAGNOSIS AND TREATMENT

If DIC is suspected because of either clinical symptoms or the presence of a condition known to predispose to DIC, a battery of laboratory studies should be done. As listed in Table 41–12, several practical tests are readily available that help one detect the presence of DIC. Red cell fragmentation indicative of microangiopathic hemolytic anemia does not occur in all instances of DIC, but its presence should suggest the possibility of this diagnosis. Thrombocytopenia and abnormal coagulation screening tests indicate consumption of both platelets and coagulation factors. Depletion of fibrinogen can be detected readily by rapid semiquantitative screening tests (see earlier section on laboratory evaluation, under "Diagnosis" at the beginning of this Chapter). The presence of soluble fibrin monomer as detected by one of the "paracoagulation" tests (protamine or ethanol gel) indicates the action of thrombin in the circulation and, if performed properly, may provide a useful clue to the occurrence of DIC. In almost all significant episodes of DIC, there is secondary trig-

Table 41–12. LABORATORY TESTS USEFUL IN THE EVALUATION OF SUSPECTED DISSEMINATED INTRAVASCULAR COAGULATION (DIC)

Immediate
- Examination of blood smear for evidence of red cell fragmentation and/or thrombocytopenia
- Platelet count
- Prothrombin time
- Partial thromboplastin time
- Thrombin time
- Fibrinogen screening test
- Fibrin degradation products (screening test)
- Paracoagulation tests for fibrin monomer
    - Protamine test
    - Ethanol gel test

Later (optional)
- Specific coagulation factor assays
    - Fibrinogen
    - Factor V
    - Factor VIII
- Platelet and/or fibrinogen survival studies

---

gering of fibrinolysis with resultant fibrin degradation products in the circulation that can be detected readily by a screening test.

Quantitative measurements of fibrinogen, Factor V, and Factor VIII may help one confirm the suspicion of DIC, but because these tests are often not immediately available they are not useful when a rapid diagnosis is needed. Although platelet and fibrinogen survival studies may provide the most sensitive index of the occurrence of DIC, they are rarely practical for diagnostic purposes (258).

Purpura fulminans is a relatively rare disorder that usually occurs in children, most often following a viral infection (varicella is a common antecedent illness). The condition is associated with striking hemorrhagic skin lesions that rapidly become gangrenous and usually are located on the extremities bilaterally. Typical laboratory findings of DIC are present. Prior to the recognition of this aspect of the disorder and its treatment with heparin, the condition was often fatal or associated with the loss of one or more extremities. The etiology remains unknown.

The typical findings are described in the following case report of an infant with purpura fulminans. The patient was a 1-month-old girl who was hospitalized with a 24-hour history of intermittent loose stools, refusal of all fluids, and an oral intake limited to cereal. She had poor skin turgor, sunken eyes, and gray, cyanotic, cold extremities, and she was extremely lethargic. The infant improved following administration of intravenous fluids, but the abnormal color of her extremities fluctuated during the first day. Initial laboratory findings included the following: white blood cell count, 10,300 per mm^3; hemoglobin, 9.4 g per dl; platelets decreased on smear; serum sodium, 186 mEq/liter; and blood urea nitrogen, 204 mg per dl. Despite her initial improvement after intravenous fluid therapy, the following day her fingers and toes appeared quite abnormal with ecchymotic discoloration (Color Plate III), and repeat laboratory studies revealed the following: hemoglobin, 7.4 g per dl; platelets, 7000 per mm^3; abnormal red cell morphology (Color Plate III); PT and PTT, greater than 200 seconds; no measurable fibrinogen; serum sodium, 157 mEq/liter; and blood urea nitrogen, 102 mg per dl.

The abnormal platelet and coagulation studies combined with the rapidly progressive gangrenous lesions of the patient's toes led to the diagnosis of purpura fulminans, and intravenous heparin was started (400 units per kg every 4 hours). As shown in Figure 41–10, there was rapid improvement in the fibrinogen level (normal within 3 to 4 days), and platelet values rose to normal by approximately 1 week. Serum sodium and blood urea nitrogen levels returned to normal over the next few days. Both platelets and fibrinogen rose to supernormal levels by 2 weeks. This overresponse is characteristic of patients recovering from DIC, whether spontaneously or in response to heparin therapy. Although the lesions of the infant's fingers were completely reversible, gangrene persisted in both feet, with ultimate autoamputation of several toes (Color Plate III). There was no extension of the gangrenous involvement of the feet from the time heparin therapy was started.

This case description is representative of purpura fulminans, and the laboratory evidence of DIC is similar to that found in children with a variety of conditions complicated by this phenomenon. Because of its often fatal or serious course, most authorities recommend that purpura fulminans be treated with heparin, and a 2- to 3-week course is usually required (259–261). Premature cessation of heparin therapy may lead to progression of necrotic skin lesions. The reason for the thrombotic gangrenous involvement of the skin in this disorder is not known, but similar lesions may occur in meningococcemia.

Although heparin therapy is of primary importance in purpura fulminans, there is less agreement regarding its use in other conditions complicated by DIC in children (262–266). General supportive measures (fluid replacement, treatment of shock, etc.) are always indicated, and specific treatment of the underlying triggering condition (if it is identified) is of major importance and may be all that is needed. The decision to block further intravascular coagulation with heparin is a clinical judgement, influenced by the patient's condition, the severity of laboratory abnormalities, the potential effectiveness of available therapy for the basic condition, and the likelihood of serious problems from either the hemorrhagic or the thrombotic manifestations of DIC. Anticoagulant therapy may not be needed in patients with minimal laboratory

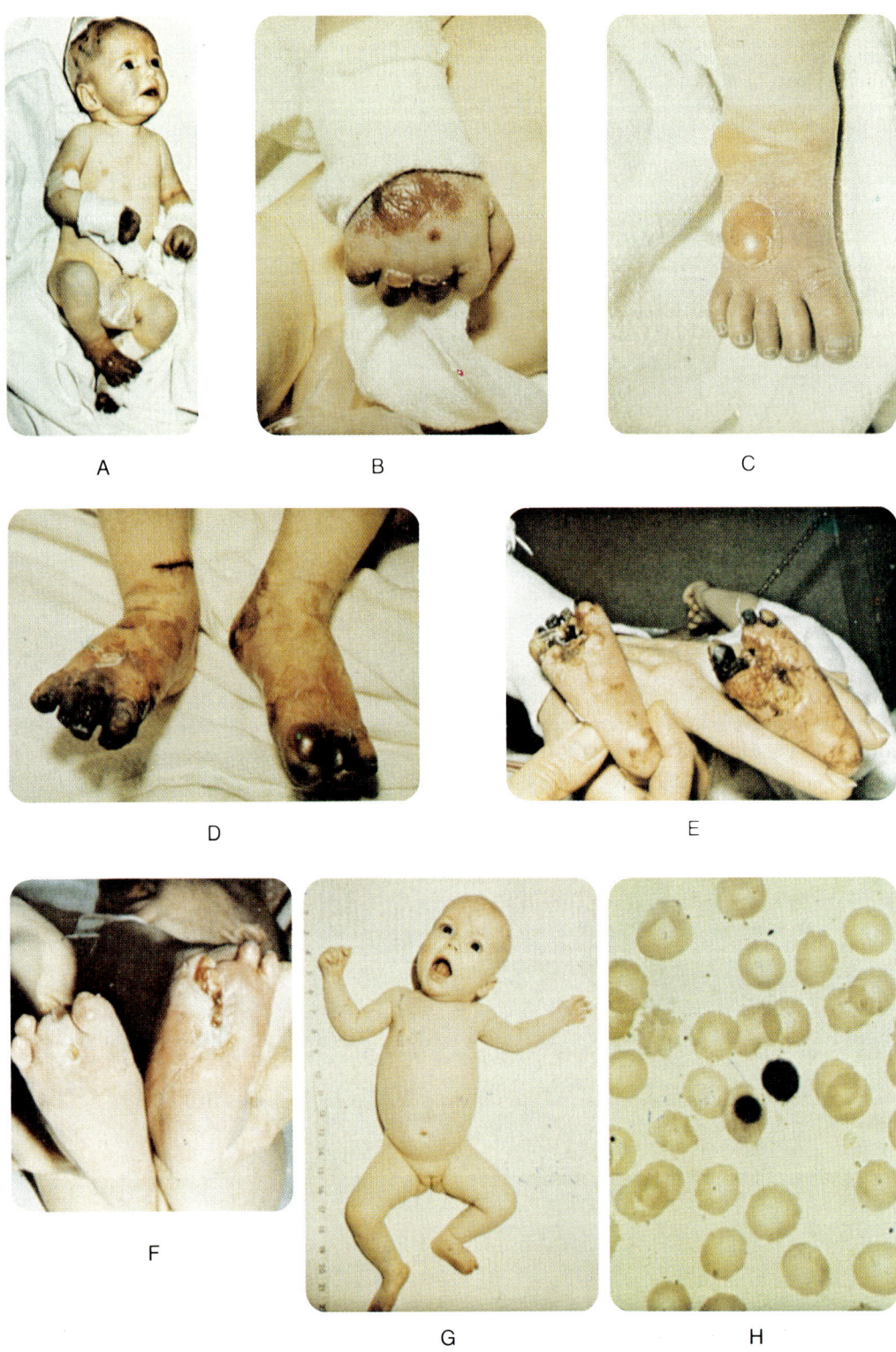

Color Plate III. Serial changes in infant with purpura fulminans. *A, B, C*, Day 2; *D*, day 11; *E*, day 19; *F, G*, day 57; *H*, peripheral blood smear on day 2 with burr cells and nucleated red blood cells.

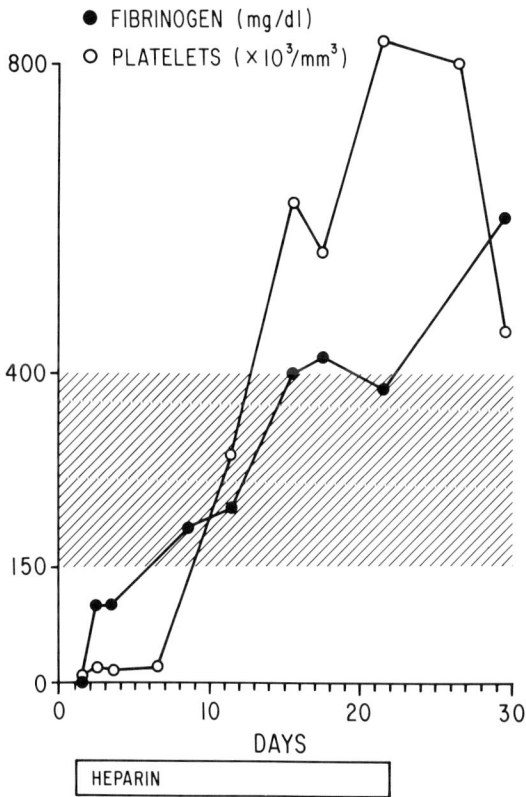

Figure 41–10. Results of serial platelet and fibrinogen levels in infant with purpura fulminans on heparin therapy. Heparin was given intravenously in a dose of 100 units/kg. every 4 hours for 21 days.

evidence of DIC and no hemorrhagic or thrombotic manifestations, whose underlying condition can be treated effectively. In those with mild to moderate hemorrhagic manifestations, replacement of platelets and coagulation factors (with platelet concentrates and cryoprecipitate) combined with treatment or removal of the stimulus for DIC may be adequate. Patients with serious hemorrhagic manifestations or potential thrombotic complications (skin, renal, etc.) may benefit from the addition of heparin to these measures (263).

Because of the fulminant nature of meningococcemia and the potential for serious thrombotic complications, it may be wise to initiate heparin therapy in critically ill or hypotensive patients as soon as blood is obtained for laboratory studies. If no evidence of DIC is detected, discontinuation of heparin is simple. In those with DIC, a 24- to 48-hour course of heparin may prevent serious thrombotic complications. Despite the rapid return to normal of coagulaton studies reported in some children with DIC secondary to sepsis who were treated with antibiotics and supportive measures alone, at least one child with serious thrombotic complications (with partial loss of feet) has been reported (266), and the author is aware of others (see Figure 41–9). Expectant therapy with heparin may avoid thrombotic problems in such patients.

Prompt use of heparin may also prevent serious complications following a major transfusion reaction with intravascular hemolysis. The decision to use heparin to treat DIC following major trauma or operative procedures is difficult and must be individualized. Although still considered investigational in the United States, the use of AT III concentrates may ultimately have a role in such situations in which heparin might be judged contraindicated (see further on).

The use of heparin in conditions such as the hemolytic uremic syndrome is controversial and thought to be of little or no value by some investigators. Because recognition of the hemolytic uremic syndrome is frequently delayed, the opportunity to use heparin may be missed by the time the condition is recognized. If this condition represents an example of localized intravascular coagulation primarily involving the kidney, the damage by fibrin deposition may occur early. If so, the use of heparin would be effective only if given early in the course of the disorder, and the time of recognition of the condition may influence the decision to use this agent. The value of supportive therapy and the use of peritoneal dialysis for azotemia are generally recognized in the management of the hemolytic uremic syndrome.

If heparin is used for DIC, a bolus dose of 100 units per kg should be given, followed by continuous intravenous administration of 100 units per kg per 6 hours. A smaller dose (50 units per kg per 4 hours) or a larger dose (200 units per kg per 4 hours) may be required, depending on the condition being treated, the response to therapy, and the level of AT III in the patient. If the AT III level is significantly depressed, heparin may be ineffective unless this level is elevated by infusion of fresh frozen plasma or by AT III concentrates. However, whether AT III infusions will restore responsiveness to heparin is not known at present. AT III concentrates are not currently licensed for use in the United States; however, they have been used instead of or in addition to heparin to treat DIC in Europe and in Japan (215, 269–272). Several nonrandomized trials suggested that DIC improved after AT III concentrates when the pretreatment level of AT III was low. An advantage of AT III concentrates in acute DIC is that they can be used in settings in which heparin might be contraindicated because of bleeding sites (e.g., trauma and surgery) (267, 268).

Heparin is excreted primarily by the kidneys, and the presence of poor renal function may lead to accumulation of this agent, with resultant bleeding. If severe renal disease is present, it may be wise to start with a lower dose of heparin (50 units per kg per 4 hours).

The most useful test for evaluating the effect of

heparin is the fibrinogen level (which can be done by the semiquantitative screening test mentioned in the earlier section on laboratory evaluation, under "Diagnosis" at the beginning of this Chapter). Even in the presence of severe defibrination, the fibrinogen level may rise to a normal or near normal level within 24 hours of initiation of effective heparin therapy. The PT and PTT are of little value in monitoring heparin therapy in DIC because both tests are prolonged in the presence of heparin. Although the platelet count is not affected by heparin, return to normal may take several days (as illustrated in the purpura fulminans case), and it does not provide an early guide to the efficacy of heparin therapy. The exacerbation of bleeding manifestations following initiation of heparin therapy should lead to discontinuation of heparin and re-evaluation of the need for replacement of platelets and coagulation factors in addition to heparin. Heparin may be neutralized by the administration of intravenous protamine sulfate (1 mg for each 100 units of heparin), but this is rarely necessary because heparin has a relatively short half-life.

The duration of heparin therapy for DIC may vary from 12 to 24 hours in conditions in which the underlying triggering condition can be treated effectively, to 2 to 3 weeks (or longer) in conditions such as purpura fulminans or leukemia.

DIC usually elicits a secondary fibrinolytic response that removes fibrin and prevents thrombotic complications. Because of this important protective effect, the fibrinolytic mechanism should not be blocked unless ongoing DIC is under control. In very rare instances, the fibrinolytic response may be excessive, with resultant destruction of fibrinogen, Factor V, and Factor VIII and inhibition of fibrin formation by fibrin degradation products. In such cases, use of ϵ-aminocaproic acid or tranexamic acid to block the fibrinolytic mechanism may be indicated, but only as an adjunct after heparin has been started.

Primary forms of excessive fibrinolysis are extremely rare in children but may occur during or immediately following cardiopulmonary bypass (273–275).

Snakebite

Snake venoms are complex peptide mixtures (276) and are likely to cause damage to several body systems. Snakebite by certain species, especially the vipers and rattlesnakes, can produce hypofibrinogenemia with or without thrombocytopenia. The syndrome resembles DIC (277). In the United States, the most common snakebite encountered is that of the rattlesnake. The venom of the rattlesnake contains not thrombin but thrombin-like material. Thus, although hypofibrinogenemia may be seen, the thrombin-like material will not be eliminated by heparin. Antivenom is the treatment of choice (277).

References

1. Bloom, A. L., and Thomas, D. P. (eds): *Haemostasis and Thrombosis.* London, Churchill-Livingstone, 1981.
2. Ingram, G. I. C.: Investigation of a long-standing bleeding tendency. Br. Med. Bull. *33:*261, 1977.
3. Schulman, I.: The significance of epistaxis in childhood. Pediatrics *24:*489, 1959.
4. Duke, W. W.: The relation of blood platelets to hemorrhagic disease. J. A. M. A. *55:*1185, 1910.
5. Ivy, A. C., Shapiro, P. F., et al.: The bleeding tendency in jaundice. Surg. Gynecol. Obstet. *60:*781, 1935.
6. Nilsson, I. M., Magnusson, S., et al.: The Duke and Ivy methods for determination of the bleeding time. Thromb. Diath. Haemorrhag. *10:*223, 1963.
7. Borchgrevink, C. F., and Waaler, B. A.: The secondary bleeding time: a new method for the differentiation of hemorrhagic disease. Acta Med. Scand. *162:*362, 1958.
8. Mielke, C. H., Jr., Kaneshiro, M. M., et al.: The standardized normal Ivy bleeding time and its prolongation by aspirin. Blood *34:*204, 1969.
9. Abildgaard, C. F., Simone, J. V., et al.: Von Willebrand's disease: a comparative study of diagnostic tests. J. Pediatr. *73:*355, 1968.
10. Harker, L. A., and Slichter, S. J.: The bleeding time as a screening test for evaluation of platelet function. New Engl. J. Med. *287:*155, 1972.
11. Nieuwenhuis, H. K., and Sixma, J. J.: Bleeding time measurements. In *Measurements of Platelet Function.* Harker, L., and Zimmerman, T. S. (eds.), New York, Churchill-Livingstone, 1983, p. 26.
12. Sahud, M. A., and Cohen, R. J.: Aspirin-induced prolongation of the Ivy bleeding time. Its diagnostic usefulness. Calif. Med. *115:*10, 1971.
13. Stuart, M. J., Miller, M., et al.: The post-aspirin bleeding time: a screening test for evaluating a hemostatic disorder. Br. J. Haematol. *43:*649, 1979.
14. Hattersly, P. G.: Activated coagulation time of whole blood. J. A. M. A. *166:*436, 1966.
15. Hattersly, P. G.: Progress report: the activated coagulation time of whole blood (ACT). Am. J. Clin. Pathol. *66:*899, 1976.
16. Proctor, R. R., and Rapaport, S. I.: The partial thromboplastin time with kaolin. Am. J. Clin. Pathol. *36:*212, 1961.
17. Hillman, C. R. L., and Lusher, J. M.: Determining sensitivity of coagulation screening reagents: a simplified method. J. Lab. Med. *13:*162, 1982.
18. Abildgaard, C. F., and Harrison, J.: Fletcher factor deficiency: family study and identification. Blood *43:*641, 1974.
19. Quick, A. J.: *Hemorrhagic Diseases and Thrombosis,* 2nd ed. Philadelphia, Lea and Febiger, 1966.
20. Biggs, R. (ed.): *Human Blood Coagulation, Haemostasis and Thrombosis.* Oxford, Blackwell Scientific Publications, 1972.
21. Zimmerman, T. S., Ratnoff, O. D., et al.: The immunologic differentiation of classic hemophilia (Factor VIII deficiency) and von Willebrand's disease with observations on combined deficiencies of antihemophilic factor and proaccelerin (Factor V) and on an acquired anticoagulant against antihemophilic factor. J. Clin. Invest. *40:*224, 1971.
22. Gralnick, H. R., Abrell, E., et al.: Immunological studies of Factor VIII (antihemophilic globulin) in hemophilia A. Nature *230:*16, 1971.
23. Bloom, A. L., and Peake, I. R.: Molecular genetics of Factor VIII and its disorders. Semin. Hematol. *14:*319, 1977.

24. Zimmerman, T. S., Ratnoff, O. D., et al.: Detection of carriers of classic hemophilia using an immunologic assay for antihemophilic factor (Factor VIII). J. Clin. Invest. *50:*235, 1971.
25. Howard, M. A., and Firkin, B. G.: Ristocetin—a new tool in the investigation of platelet aggregation. Thromb. Diath. Haemorrhag. *26:*362, 1971.
26. Weiss, H. J., Rogers, J., et al.: Defective ristocetin-induced platelet aggregation in von Willebrand's disease and its correction by Factor VIII. J. Clin. Invest. *52:*2697, 1973.
27. Allain, J. P., Cooper, H. A., et al.: Platelets fixed with paraformaldehyde: a new reagent for assay of von Willebrand factor and platelet aggregating factor. J. Lab. Clin. Med. *85:*318, 1975.
28. Searcy, R. L., Simms, N. M., et al.: A simple method for rapid detection of hypofibrinogenemia. Am. J. Med. Tech. *33:*326, 1967.
29. Abildgaard, C. F.: Recognition and treatment of disseminated intravascular coagulation. J. Pediatr. *74:*163, 1969.
30. Ratnoff, O. D., and Menzie, C.: A new method for the determination of fibrinogen in small samples of plasma. J. Lab. Clin. Med. *37:*316, 1950.
31. Kasper, C. K., Aledort, L. M., et al.: A more uniform measurement of Factor VIII inhibitors. Thromb. Diath. Haemorrhag. *34:*871, 1975.
32. Kidder, W. R., Logan, L. J., et al.: The plasma protamine paracoagulation test: clinical and laboratory evaluation. Am. J. Clin. Pathol. *58:*675, 1972.
33. Godal, H. C., and Abildgaard, U.: Gelation of soluble fibrin in plasma by ethanol. Scand. J. Haematol. *3:*342, 1966.
34. Buckell, M.: The effect of citrate on englobulin methods of estimating fibrinolytic activity. J. Clin. Pathol. *11:*403, 1958.
35. Rosenberg, R. D.: Actions and interactions of antithrombin and heparin. New Engl. J. Med. *292:*146, 1975.
36. Pool, J. G., and Shannon, A. E.: production of high potency concentrates of antihemophilic globulin in a closed bag system; assay in vitro and in vivo. New Engl. J. Med. *273:*1443, 1965.
37. Hershgold, E. J., Pool, J. G., and Pappenhagen, A. R.: The potent antihemophilic globulin concentrate derived from a cold insoluble fraction of human plasma: characterization and further data on preparation and clinical trial. J. Lab. Clin. Med. *67:*23, 1966.
38. Lewis, J. H., Spero, J. A., et al.: Transfusion support for congenital clotting deficiencies other than haemophilia. Clin. Haematol. *13:*119, 1984.
39. Sugg, U., Schnaidt, M., et al.: Clotting factors and non-A, non-B hepatitis. New Engl. J. Med. *303:*943, 1980.
40. Norkrans, G., Widell, A., et al.: Acute hepatitis non-A, non-B following administration of Factor VIII concentrates. Vox Sang. *41:*129, 1981.
41. Gerety, R. J., and Eyster, M. E.: Hepatitis among hemophiliacs. In *Non-A, Non-B hepatitis.* Gerety, R. J. (ed), New York, Academic Press, 1981, pp. 97–117.
42. Gerety, R. J., and Aronson, D. L.: Plasma derivatives and viral hepatitis. Transfusion *22:*347, 1982.
43. CDC Update: Acquired immunodeficiency syndrome (AIDS) in persons with hemophilia. M. M. W. R. *33:*589, 1984.
44. Broder, S., and Gallo, R. D.: A pathogenic retrovirus (HTLV-III) linked to AIDS. New Engl. J. Med. *311:*1292, 1984.
45. Colombo, M., Mannucci, P. M., et al.: Transmission of non-A, non-B hepatitis by heat-treated Factor VIII concentrate. Lancet *2:*1, 1985.
46. Dolana, G., Tse, D. C., et al.: Hepatitis risk reduced in hemophilia: a heat-treated Factor VIII preparation (abstr.). Blood *60* (suppl. 1): 210A, 1980.
47. Levy, J. A., Mitra, G., and Mozen, M. M.: Recovery and inactivation of infectous retroviruses from Factor VIII concentrates. Lancet *2:*722, 1984.
48. National Hemophilia Foundation Medical and Scientific Advisory Council: Recommendations concerning AIDS and therapy of hemophilia (revised March 1, 1985). New York, National Hemophilia Foundation, 1984.
49. Gatti, L., and Mannucci, P. M.: Use of porcine Factor VIII in the management of seventeen patients with Factor VIII antibodies. Thromb. Haemost. *51:*379, 1984.
50. Boylen, A. L., Ewing, N. P., and Kasper, C. K.: Porcine VIII:C provided effective surgical hemostasis despite anamnestic response. In *Factor VIII Inhibitors.* Hoyer, L. (ed.), New York, Alan R. Liss, 1984, p. 378.
51. Kernoff, P. B. A.: Porcine factor VIII: preparation and use in treatment of inhibitor patients. In *Factor VIII Inhibitors.* Hoyer, L. (ed.), New York, Alan R. Liss, 1984, p. 207.
52. Blatt, P. M., Lundblad, R. L., et al.: Thrombogenic materials in prothrombin complex concentrates. Ann. Intern. Med. *81:*766, 1974.
53. Cederbaum, A. L., Blatt, P. M., and Roberts, H. R.: Intravascular coagulation with use of human prothrombin complex concentrates. Ann. Intern. Med. *84:*683, 1976.
54. Kasper, C. K.: Clinical use of Factor IX concentrates: report on thromboembolic complications. Thromb. Diath. Haemorrhag. *33:*642, 1975.
55. Kasper, C. K.: Postoperative thrombosis in hemophilia B. New Engl. J. Med. *289:*610, 1973.
56. Menache, D., and Guillin, M. C.: The use of Factor IX concentrates in hemophilia B patients and in liver disease. In *Treatment of Bleeding Disorders with Blood Components.* Mammen, E., Barnhart, M. I., Lusher, J. M. (eds.), Westbury, CN, PJD Publ. Ltd., 1980, p. 183.
57. Menache, D.: Prothrombin complex concentrates: clinical use. Ann. N. Y. Acad. Sci. *370:*747, 1981.
58. White, G. C., Lundblad, R. L., and Kingdon, H. S.: Prothrombin complex concentrates: preparation, properties and clinical uses. In *Current Topics in Hematology,* vol. 2. Piomelli, S., and Yachnin, S. (eds.), New York, Alan R. Liss, 1979, p. 204.
59. Menache, D., and Roberts, H. R.: Summary report and recommendations of task force members and consultants. Thromb. Diath. Haemorrhag. *33:*645, 1975.
60. Fuerth, J. H., and Mahrer, P.: Myocardial infarction after Factor IX therapy. J. A. M. A. *245:*1455, 1981.
61. Agrawal, B. L., Zelkowitz, L., and Hletko, P.: Acute myocardial infarction in a young hemophiliac patient during therapy with Factor IX concentrate and epsilon aminocaproic acid. J. Pediatr. *98:*93, 1981.
62. Gruppo, R. A., Bove, K. E., and Donaldson, V. H.: Fatal myocardial necrosis associated with prothrombin complex concentrate therapy in hemophilia A (letter). New Engl. J. Med. *309:*242, 1983.
63. Sullivan, D. W., Purdy, L. J., et al.: Fatal myocardial infarction following therapy with prothrombin complex concentrates in a young man with hemophilia A. Pediatrics *74:*279, 1984.
64. Schimpf, K. L., Zeltsch, C. H., and Zeltsch, P.: Myocardial infarction complicating activated prothrombin complex concentrate substitution in a patient with hemophilia A. Lancet *2:*1043, 1982.
65. Tabor, D. C., and Votaw, M. L.: Fatal myocardial infarction in hemophilia A after factor IX and Autoplex therapy (abstr.). Blood *62:*278A, 1983.
66. Lusher, J. M.: The role of prothrombin complex concentrates in the treatment of hemophiliacs with Factor VIII inhibitors. Scand. J. Haematol. *33*(suppl. 40):195, 1984.
67. Lusher, J. M., Blatt, P. M. et al.: Autoplex vs. Proplex: A controlled, double-blind study of effectiveness in acute hemarthroses in hemophiliacs with inhibitors to Factor VIII. Blood *62:*1135, 1983.
68. Sjamsoedin, L. J., Heisnen, L., et al.: The effect of activated prothrombin complex concentrate (FEIBA) on joint and muscle bleeding in patients with hemophilia A

and antibodies to Factor VIII. A double-blind clinical trial. New Engl. J. Med. *305*:717, 1981.
69. Menache, D., Behre, H. E., et al.: Coagulation Factor IX concentrate. Method of preparation and assessment of potential in vivo thrombogenicity in animal models. Blood *64*:1220, 1984.
70. Brandt, J. T.: The role of natural inhibitors in hemostasis. Clin. Lab. Med. *4*:245, 1984.
71. Odegaard, O., and Abildgaard, U.: Antithrombin III. Critical review of assay methods: significance of variations in health and disease. Haemostasis *7*:127, 1978.
72. Abildgaard, U.: Antithrombin and related inhibitors of coagulation. In *Recent Advances in Blood Coagulation*, No. 3. Poller, L. (ed.), Edinburgh, Churchill-Livingstone, 1981, p. 745.
73. Sherman, L. A.: New plasma components. Clin Haematol *13*:17, 1984.
74. Wood, W. I., Capon, D. J., et al.: Expression of active human Factor VIII from recombinant DNA clones. Nature *312*:330, 1984.
75. Mannucci, P. M., Aberg, M., et al: Mechanism of plasminogen activator and factor VIII increase after vasoactive drugs. Br. J. Haematol. *30*:81, 1975.
76. Barnhart, M. I., Chen, S., and Lusher, J. M.: DDAVP: Does the drug have a direct effect on the vessel wall? Thromb. Res. *31*:239, 1983.
77. Mannucci, P. M., Canciani, M. L., et al.: Response of Factor VIII/von Willebrand factor in healthy subjects and patients with hemophilia A and von Willebrand's disease. Br. J. Haematol. *47*:283, 1981.
78. Mariani, G.: Evaluation of the effectiveness of DDAVP in surgery and bleeding episodes in mild and moderate hemophilia A (abstr. 139). Presented at XVI Internatl. Congr. World Fed. Hemophilia, Rio de Janeiro, August 24–28, 1984.
79. Lowe, G., Pettigrew, A., et al.: DDAVP in hemophilia (letter). Lancet *2*:614, 1977.
80. Ratnoff, O. D.: Personal communication.
81. Gralnick, H. R., and Rick, M. E.: Danazol increases Factors VIII and IX in classic hemophilia and Christmas disease. New Engl. J. Med. *308*:1393, 1983.
82. Nugent, B. D., Bray, G. et al.: Double blind crossover study using Danazol in patients with hemophilia A and B (abstr.). Blood *64* (suppl. 1):258A, 1984.
83. Lega, B., Saidi, P., et al.: Effect of Danazol in Factor VIII and IX levels, bleeding frequency and immune parameters in hemophiliacs. A randomized double blind crossover study (abstr.). Blood *64* (suppl. 1):257A, 1984.
84. Hillman, C., Barnhart, M. I., and Lusher, J. M.: Drugs or conditions that alter platelet function. In *Acquired Bleeding Disorders in Children. Platelet Abnormalities and Laboratory Testing*. Lusher, J. M., and Barnhart, M. I. (eds.), New York, Masson Publishing U. S. A., 1981, p. 171.
85. Deykin, D.: Hemorrhagic complications of drugs. In *Hemostasis and Thrombosis. Basic Principles and Clinical Practice*. Colman, R. W., Hirsh, J., et al. (eds.), Philadelphia, J. B. Lippincott Co., 1982, p. 602.
86. Kasper, C. K., Osterud, B., et al.: Hemophilia B: characterization of genetic variants and detection of carriers. Blood *50*:351, 1977.
87. Aledort, L. M.: Current concepts in diagnosis and management of hemophilia. Hosp. Pract. *17*:77, 1982.
88. Mainardi, C. L., Levine, P. H., et al: Proliferative synovitis in hemophilia. Arthritis Rheum. *21*:137, 1978.
89. Forbes, C. D.: Clinical aspects of the hemophilias and their treatment. In *Disorders of Hemostasis*. Ratnoff, O. D., and Forbes, C. D. (eds.), New York, Grune & Stratton, 1984, p. 177.
90. Lusher, J. M.: Hemophilia and related conditions. In *Conn's Current Therapy*. Conn, H. F. (ed.), Philadelphia, W. B. Saunders Co., 1981, p. 278.
91. Lusher, J. M.: Hemophilia and related disorders. In *Current Emergency Medical Therapy—1984*. Edlich, R. F. (ed.), Norwalk, CT, Appleton-Century-Crofts, 1984, p. 519.
92. Hathaway, W. E., Christian, M. J., et al.: Comparison of continuous and intermittent Factor VIII concentrate therapy in hemophilia A. Am. J. Hematol. in press.
93. Hilgartner, M. W., Lachiewicz, P., and Delson, E. S.: Continuous concentrate infusion with the autosyringe for hemostasis in the patient with hemophilia (abstr.). Blood *62*:274A, 1983.
94. Hilgartner, M. W., and Gendelman, S.: Central Nervous System bleeding: new methods of diagnosis and management (abstr. 182). Presented at XVI Internatl. Congr. World Fed. Hemophilia, Rio de Janeiro, August 24–28, 1984.
95. Kasper, C. K.: Measurement of Factor VIII inhibitors. In *Factor VIII Inhibitors*. Hoyer, L. (ed.), New York, Alan R. Liss, 1984, p. 87.
96. Lusher, J. M.: Use of desmopressin acetate in disorders of hemostasis (mild hemophilia A and classical von Willebrand's disease). Am. Soc. Clin. Pathol. Check Sample. Thromb. Haemost. No. Th. 84–85, 1984.
97. Lusher, J. M.: Desmopressin acetate as an alternative to blood products for surgical hemostasis in hemophilia and von Willebrand's disease. Amsterdam, Excerpta Medica 1985.
98. Streit, A., Furlan, M., and Beck, E. A.: Home self-care with intranasally administered DDAVP in mild hemophilia and von Willebrand's disease (abstr. 141). Presented at XVI Internatl. Congr. World Fed. Hemophilia, Rio de Janeiro, August 24–28, 1984.
99. Kasper, C. K., and Boylen, A. L.: Poor response to Danazol in hemophilia. Blood *65*:211, 1985.
100. Gill, F. M., Shapiro, S. S., et al.: The natural history of Factor VIII inhibitors in patients with hemophilia A: a national cooperative study. I. Characteristics of the population. Blood, in press.
101. Shapiro, S. S.: Antibodies to blood coagulation factors. Clin. Haematol. *8*:207, 1979.
102. McMillan, C. W., Shapiro, S. S., et al.: The natural history of Factor VIII inhibitors in patients with hemophilia A: a national cooperative study. II. Observations on the initial development of Factor VIII inhibitors. Blood, in press.
103. Shapiro, S. S.: Genetic predisposition to inhibitor formation. In *Factor VIII Inhibitors*. Hoyer, L. (ed.), New York, Alan R. Liss, 1984, p. 45.
104. Kasper, C. K., Counts, R., et al.: A more uniform measurement of Factor VIII inhibitors. Thromb. Diath. Haemorrhag. *34*:869, 1975.
105. Lusher, J. M., Eyster, E., et al.: Panel discussion. In *Factor VIII Inhibitors*. Hoyer, L. (ed.), New York, Alan R. Liss, 1984, p. 323.
106. Blatt, P. M., White, G. C., II, et al.: Treatment of anti–Factor VIII antibodies. Thromb. Haemost. *38*:514, 1977.
107. Lusher, J. M., Shapiro, S. S., et al.: Efficacy of prothrombin complex concentrates in hemophiliacs with antibodies to factor VIII. A multicenter therapeutic trial. New Engl. J. Med. *303*:421, 1980.
108. Lusher, J. M.: Controlled clinical trials with prothrombin complex concentrates. In *Factor VIII Inhibitors*. Hoyer, L. (ed.), New York, Alan R. Liss, 1984, p. 277.
109. Oberle, I., Camerino, D., et al.: Genetic screening for hemophilia A (classic hemophilia) with a polymorphic DNA probe. New Engl. J. Med. *312*:682, 1985.
110. von Willebrand, E. A.: Hereditäre pseudohemofili. Finska Läk. Sällsk. Handl. *68*:87, 1926.
111. von Willebrand, E. A., and Jurgens, R.: Uber ein neues verebbares blutangsubel: die constitutionelle thrombopathy. Deutsch. Arch. Klin. Med. *175*:453, 1933.
112. Jurgens, R., Lehmann, W., et al: Mitterlung uber den

Mangel an antihämophein globulin (Factor VIII) bei der Aaländischen Thrombopathie (v.Willebrand-Jurgens). Thromb. Diath. Haemorrhag. *1:*257, 1957.
113. Nilsson, I. M., Blombäck, M., and von Francken, I.: On an inherited autosomal haemorrhagic diathesis with antihaemophilic globulin (AHG) deficiency and prolonged bleeding time. Acta Med. Scand. *159:*35, 1957.
114. Nilsson, I. M., Blombäck, M., and Blombäck, B.: von Willebrand's disease in Sweden. Its pathogenesis and treatment. Acta Med. Scand. *164:*3, 1959.
115. Cornu, P., Larrieu, M. J., et al.: Transfusion studies in von Willebrand's disease: effect on bleeding time and Factor VIII. Br. J. Haematol. *9:*189, 1963.
116. Green, D., and Potter, E. V.: Failure of AHF concentrate to control bleeding in von Willebrand's disease. Am. J. Med. *60:*357, 1976.
117. Zimmerman, T. S., Ratnoff, O. D., and Powel, A. E.: Immunologic differentiation of classic hemophilia (Factor VIII deficiency) and von Willebrand's disease. J. Clin. Invest. *5:*244, 1971.
118. Salzman, E. W.: Measurement of platelet adhesiveness. A simple in vitro technique demonstrating an abnormality in von Willebrand's disease. J. Lab. Clin. Med. *62:*724, 1963.
119. Tschopp, T. P., Weiss, H. J., and Baumgartner, H. R.: Decreased adhesion of platelets to subendothelium in von Willebrand's disease. J. Lab. Clin. Med. *83:*296, 1974.
120. Barnhart, M. I., Wilkins, R. M., and Lusher, J. M.: Platelet-vessel wall interactions: experience with von Willebrand platelets. Ann. N. Y. Acad. Sci. *370:*154, 1981.
121. Howard, M. A., and Firkin, B.: Ristocetin—a new tool in the investigation of platelet aggregation. Thromb. Diath. Haemorrhag. *26:*362, 1971.
122. Ruggeri, Z. M., Mannucci, P. M., et al.: Multimeric composition of Factor VIII/von Willebrand factor following administration of DDAVP: Implications for pathophysiology and therapy of von Willebrand's disease subtypes. Blood *59:*1272, 1982.
123. Zimmerman, T. S., and Ruggeri, Z. M.: von Willebrand's disease. Clin. Haematol. *12:*175, 1983.
124. Hoyer, L. W.: The assessment of von Willebrand's disease. In *The Hemophilias.* Bloom, A. L. (ed), London, Churchill-Livingstone, 1982, p. 106.
125. Abildgaard, C. F., Suzuki, Z., et al.: Serial studies in von Willebrand's disease: variability versus "variants." Blood *56:*712, 1980.
126. Meyer, D., and Zimmerman, T. S.: von Willebrand's disease. In *Hemostasis and Thrombosis.* Colman, R., Hirsh, J., et al. (eds.), Philadelphia, J. B. Lippincott Co., 1982, pp. 64–74.
127. Zimmerman, T. S., Hoyer, L. W., et al.: Determination of the von Willebrand's disease antigen (Factor VIII–related antigen) in plasma by quantitative immunoelectrophoresis. J. Lab. Clin. Med. *86:*152, 1975.
128. Koutts, J., Walsh, P. N., et al.: Active release of human platelet Factor VIII–related antigen by adenosine diphosphate, collagen and thrombin. J. Clin. Invest. *62:*1255, 1979.
129. Ruggeri, Z. M., Mannucci, P. M., et al.: Immunoradiometric assay of Factor VIII–related antigen with observations in 32 patients with von Willebrand's disease. Br. J. Haematol. *33:*221, 1976.
130. Mannucci, P. M., Lombardi, R., et al.: Evidence for an abnormal von Willebrand factor (vWF) in a subgroup of patients with type I von Willebrand's disease. Thromb. Haemost. *54:*171, 1985.
131. Kinoshita, S., Harrison, J., et al.: A new variant of dominant type II von Willebrand's disease with aberrant multimer pattern of Factor VIII–related antigen (type IID). Blood *63:*1369, 1984.
132. Ruggeri, Z. M., Pareti, F. I., et al.: Heightened interaction between platelets and Factor VIII/von Willebrand factor in a new subtype of von Willebrand's disease. New Engl. J. Med. *302:*1047, 1980.
133. Wahlberg, T. B., Blombäck, M., and Ruggeri, Z. M.: Differences between heterozygous dominant and recessive von Willebrand's disease type I expressed by bleeding symptoms and combinations of Factor VIII variables. Thromb. Haemost. *50:*864, 1983.
134. Lusher, J. M., and McMillan, C. W.: Severe Factor VIII and Factor IX deficiency in females. Am. J. Med. *65:*637, 1978.
135. Abildgaard, C. F.: Progress and problems in hemophilia and von Willebrand's disease. In *Advances in Pediatrics,* vol. 31. Barness, L. (ed.), Chicago, Year Book Medical Publishers, 1984, p. 137.
136. Levine, P. H., and Zeltzer, L.: Control of Pain. New York, National Hemophilia Foundation, 1985.
137. Miller, J. L., and Castella, A.: Platelet type von Willebrand's disease: characterization of a new bleeding disorder. Blood *60:*790, 1982.
138. Miller, J. L.: Platelet-type von Willebrand's disease. Clin. Lab. Med. *4:*319, 1984.
139. Takahashi, H., Nagayama, R., et al.: Platelet aggregation induced by DDAVP in platelet-type von Willebrand's disease. New Engl. J. Med. *310:*722, 1984.
140. Mammen, E. F.: Congenital abnormalities of the fibrinogen molecule. Semin. Thromb. Hemost. *1:*184, 1974.
141. Flute, P. T.: Disorders of plasma fibrinogen synthesis. Br. Med. Bull. *33:*253, 1977.
142. Beck, E. A.: Congenital abnormalities of fibrinogen. Clin. Haematol. *8:*169, 1979.
143. Cash, J.: Blood replacement therapy. In *Haemostasis and Thrombosis.* Bloom, A. L., and Thomas, D. P. (eds.), London, Churchill-Livingstone, 1981, p. 472.
144. Morse, E. E.: The fibrinogenopathies. Ann. Clin. Lab. Sci. *8:*234, 1978.
145. Galanakis, D. K.: Dysfibrinogenemia. A current perspective. Clin. Lab. Med. *4:*395, 1984.
146. Rhoads, J. E., and Fitzgerald, T., Jr.: Idiopathic hypoprothrombinemia—an apparently unrecorded condition. Am. J. Med. Sci. *202:*662, 1941.
147. Owen, C. A., Henriksen, R. A., et al.: Prothrombin Quick: a newly identified dysprothrombinemia. Mayo Clin. Proc. *53:*29, 1978.
148. Gill, F. M., Shapiro, S. S., and Schwartz, E.: Severe congenital hypoprothrombinemia. J. Pediatr. *93:*264, 1978.
149. Montgomery, R. R., Otsaku, A., and Hathaway, W. E.: Hypoprothrombinemia: case report. Blood *51:*299, 1978.
150. Bloom, A. L.: Inherited disorders of blood coagulation. In *Haemostasis and Thrombosis.* Bloom, A. L., and Thomas D. P. (eds.), London, Churchill-Livingstone, 1981, p. 321.
151. Owren, P. A.: Coagulation of blood: investigation of a new clotting factor. Acta Med. Scand. *194* (suppl.):1, 1947.
152. Seeler, R. A.: Parahemophilia, Factor V deficiency. Med. Clin. North Am. *56:*119, 1972.
153. Feinstein, D. I., Rapaport, S. I., et al.: Factor V anticoagulants: clinical, biochemical and immunological observations. J. Clin. Invest. *49:*1578, 1970.
154. Fratantoni, J. C., Hilgartner, M. W., et al.: Nature of the defect in congenital Factor V deficiency. Study in a patient with an acquired circulatory anticoagulant. Blood *39:*751, 1972.
155. Marlar, R. A., and Griffin, J. H.: Deficiency of protein C inhibitor in combined Factor V/VIII deficiency disease. J. Clin. Invest. *66:*1186, 1980.
156. Griffin, J. H.: Clinical studies of protein C. Semin. Thromb. Hemost. *10:*162, 1984.
157. Alexander, B., Goldstein, R., et al.: Congenital SPCA deficiency: a hitherto unrecognized coagulation defect with hemorrhage rectified by serum and serum fractions. J. Clin. Invest. *30:*596, 1951.

158. Marder, V. J., and Shulman, N. R.: Clinical aspects of congenital factor VIII deficiency. Am. J. Med. 37:182, 1964.
159. Glueck, H., and Sutherland, J. M.: Inherited Factor VII defect in a Negro family. Pediatrics 27:204, 1961.
160. Girolami, A., Cattarozzi, G., et al.: Factor VII Padua 2: another Factor VII abnormality with defective ox brain thromboplastin activation and a complex hereditary pattern. Blood 54:46, 1979.
161. Seligsohn, U., Shani, M., and Ramot, B.: Gilbert syndrome and Factor VII deficiency. Lancet 1:1398, 1970.
162. Seligsohn, U., Shani, M., et al.: Dubin-Johnson syndrome in Israel. II. Association with Factor VII deficiency. Q. J. Med. 39:569, 1970.
163. Telfer, T. P., Denson, K. W., et al.: A "new" coagulation defect. Br. J. Haematol. 2:308, 1956.
164. Hougie, C., Barrow, E. M., et al.: Stuart clotting defect. I. Segregation of an hereditary hemorrhagic state from the heterogeneous group heretofore called "stable factor" (SPCA, proconvertin, Factor VII deficiency). J. Clin. Invest. 36:485, 1957.
165. Bachmann, F. F., Duckert, F., et al.: Über einen neuartigen kongenitalen gerinnungsdefects (Mangel an Stuart faktor). Thromb. Diath. Haemorrhag. 1:87, 1957.
166. Gonyea, L. M., and Krivit, W.: Congenital coagulation deficiency of Stuart factor activity. J. Lab. Clin. Med. 51:398, 1958.
167. Roos, J., Van Arkel, C., et al.: A "new" family with Stuart-Prower deficiency. Thromb. Diath. Haemorrhag. 3:59, 1959.
168. Rabiner, S. F., and Kretchmer, N.: The Stuart-Prower factor: utilization of clotting factors obtained by starch-block electrophoresis for genetic evaluation. Br. J. Haematol. 7:99, 1961.
169. Graham, J. B., Barrow, E. M., and Hougie, C.: Stuart clotting defect. II. Genetic aspects of a new hemorrhagic state. J. Clin. Invest. 36:497, 1957.
170. Triplett, D. A.: Spectrum of Factor X deficiency. Am. Soc. Clin. Pathol. Check Sample. Thromb. Haemost. 5:1, 1983.
171. Denson, K. W. E., Lurie, A., et al.: The Factor X defect: recognition of abnormal forms of Factor X. Br. J. Haematol. 18:317, 1970.
172. Girolami, A., Molaro, G., et al.: "New" congenital hemorrhagic condition due to presence of an abnormal Factor X (Factor X Friuli): Study of a large kindred. Br. J. Haematol. 19:179, 1970.
173. Prydz, H., and Gladhaug, A.: Factor X. Immunologic studies. Thromb. Diath. Haemorrhag. 25:157, 1971.
174. Furie, B.: Acquired coagulation disorders and dysproteinemias. In Hemostasis and Thrombosis: Basic Principles and Clinical Practice. Colman, R. W., Hirsh, J., et al. (eds.), Philadelphia, J. B. Lippincott Co., 1982, p. 577.
175. Duckert, F.: Le Facteur XIII et la proteine XIII. Nouv. Rev. Fr. Hematol. 10:685, 1960.
176. Robbins, K. C.: A study on the conversion of fibrinogen to fibrin. Am. J. Physiol. 152:581, 1944.
177. Laki, K., and Lorand, L.: On the solubility of fibrin clots. Science 108:280, 1948.
178. Lorand, L., Urayama, T., et al.: Inheritance of deficiency of the fibrin stabilizing factor (Factor XIII). Am. J. Hum. Genet. 22:89, 1970.
179. Girolami, A., Burul, A., et al.: Studies on Factor XIII antigen in congenital Factor XIII deficiency. A tentative classification of the disease into two groups. Folia Haematol. (Leipz) 105:131, 1978.
180. Lorand, L., Losowsky, M. S., and Miloszewski, K. J. M.: Human factor XIII: fibrin stabilizing factor. Progr. Hemost. Thromb. 5:245, 1980.
181. Beck, E. A., Duckert, F., and Ernst, M.: The influence of fibrin stabilizing factor on the growth of fibroblasts in vitro and wound healing. Thromb. Diath. Haemorrhag. 6:485, 1961.
182. Bouhasin, J., and Altay, C.: Factor XIII deficiency: concentrations in relatives of patients and in normal infants. J. Pediatr. 72:336, 1968.
183. Losowsky, M. S., and Miloszewski, K. J. A.: Factor XIII. Br. J. Haematol. 37:1, 1977.
184. Griffin, J. H.: The contact phase of blood coagulation. In Haemostasis and Thrombosis. Bloom, A. L., and Thomas, D. P. (eds.), London, Churchill-Livingstone, 1981, p. 84.
185. Ratnoff, O. D., and Saito, H.: Surface-mediated reactions. In Current Topics in Hematology, vol. 2. New York, Allen R. Liss, 1979, p. 1.
186. Seligsohn, U.: High gene frequency of Factor XI (PTA) deficiency in Ashkenazi Jews. Blood 51:1223, 1978.
187. Rimon, A., Schiffman, S., et al.: Factor XI activity and Factor XI antigen in homozygous and heterozygous Factor XI deficiency. Blood 48:165, 1976.
188. Giddings, J. C.: Preparation and use of a new artificial system for Factor XI assay. Med. Lab. Tech. 28:284, 1971.
189. Bennett, B., and Ogston, D.: Role of complement, coagulation, fibrinolysis and kinins in normal haemostasis and disease. In Haemostasis and Thrombosis. Bloom, A., and Thomas, D. P. (eds.), London, Churchill-Livingstone, 1981, p. 236.
190. Ratnoff, O. D., and Colopy, J. E.: A familial hemorrhagic trait associated with a deficiency of a clot-promoting fraction of plasma. J. Clin. Invest. 34:602, 1955.
191. Ratnoff, O. D., and Steinberg, A. G.: Further studies on the inheritance of Hageman trait. J. Lab. Clin. Med. 59:980, 1962.
192. Ratnoff, O. D.: The surface-mediated initiation of blood coagulation and related phenomena. In Haemostasis: Biochemistry, Physiology and Pathology. Ogston, D., and Bennett, B. (eds.), London, John Wiley & Sons, 1977, p. 25.
193. Hathaway, W. E., Bechasen, L. P., et al.: Evidence for a new plasma thromboplastin factor. Blood 26:521, 1965.
194. Hattersley, P. G., and Hayse, D.: Fletcher factor deficiency; a report of three unrelated cases. Br. J. Haematol. 18:411, 1970.
195. Abildgaard, C. F., and Harrison, J.: Fletcher factor deficiency: family study and detection. Blood 43:661, 1974.
196. Waldman, R., Abraham, J. P., et al.: Fitzgerald factor: a hitherto unrecognized coagulation factor. Lancet 1:949, 1975.
197. Lacombe, M., Varet, B., and Levy, J.: A hitherto undescribed plasma factor acting at the contact phase of blood coagulation (Fleaujeac factor): case report and coagulation studies. Blood 46:761, 1975.
198. Colman, R. W., Bagdasarian, A., et al.: Williams trait: human kininogen deficiency with diminished levels of plasminogen proactivator and prekallikrein associated with abnormalities of the Hageman factor–dependent pathways. J. Clin. Invest. 56:1650, 1975.
199. Lutcher, C. L.: Reid trait: a new expression of high molecular weight kininogen deficiency. Clin. Res. 24:440, 1967.
200. Hougie, C.: McPherson, R. A., and Aronson, L.: Passavoy factor; a hitherto unrecognized factor necessary for hemostasis. Lancet 2:290, 1975.
201. Hougie, C.: Hemophilia and related conditions—congenital deficiencies of prothrombin (Factor II), Factor V and Factors VII to XII. In Hematology, 2nd ed. Beutler, E., Erslev, A., and Rundles, R. (eds.), New York, McGraw-Hill, 1977, p. 1404.
202. Koie, K., Kamiya, T., et al.: α_2-plasmin–inhibitor deficiency (Miyasato's disease). Lancet 2:1334, 1978.
203. Aoki, N., Saito, H., et al.: Congenital deficiency of α FC-plasmin inhibitor associated with severe hemorrhagic tendency J. Clin. Invest. 63:877, 1979.
204. Barrowcliffe, T., and Thomas, D. P.: Antithrombin III and heparin. In Haemostasis and Thrombosis. Bloom, A. L., and Thomas, D. P. (eds.), London, Churchill-Livingstone, 1981, p. 712.

205. Hathaway, W. E., and Bonnar, J.: *Perinatal Coagulation.* New York, Grune & Stratton, 1978, p. 68.
206. Egeberg, O.: Inherited antithrombin deficiency causing thrombophilia. Thromb. Diath. Haemorrhag. *13*:516, 1965.
207. Ødegard, O. R., and Abildgaard, U.: Antifactor Xa activity in thrombophilia. Studies in a family with AT III deficiency. Scand. J. Haematol. *18*:86, 1977.
208. Shapiro, S. S., and Anderson, D. B.: Thrombin inhibition in normal plasma. In *Chemistry and Biology of Thrombin.* Lundblad, R., Fenton, J., Mann, K. (eds.), Ann Arbor, MI, Ann Arbor Sci. Publ., 1977, p. 361.
209. Filip, D. J., Eckstein, J. D., and Veltkamp, J. J.: Hereditary antithrombin III deficiency and thromboembolic disease. Am. J. Hematol. *2*:343, 1976.
210. Tunstall, A. M., Merriman, J. M. L., et al.: Normal and pathological serum levels of α_2-macroglobulins in men and mice. J. Clin. Pathol. *28*:133, 1975.
211. Brandt, P.: Observations during the treatment of antithrombin III deficient women with heparin and antithrombin concentrate during pregnancy, parturition and abortion. Thromb. Res. *22*:15, 1981.
212. Blomback, M.: Personal communication.
213. Laharrague, P., Bierme, R., et al.: Antithrombin III: Substitutive treatment of the hereditary deficiency. Thromb. Haemost. *1*:72, 1980.
214. Schander, K., Niesen, M., et al.: Diagnosis and therapy of a congenital antithrombin III deficency during the newborn period. Blut *40*:68, 1980.
215. Thaler, E., Niessner, H., et al.: Antithrombin III replacement therapy in patients with congenital and acquired antithrombin III deficiency. Thromb. Haemost. *42*:327, 1979.
216. Eyster, M. E., and Parker, M. E.: Treatment of familial antithrombin-III deficiency with Danazol. Haemostasis *15*:119, 1985.
217. Mammen, E. F., Thomas, W. R., and Seegers, W. H.: Activation of purified prothrombin to autoprothrombin I or autoprothrombin II (platelet cofactor III) or autoprothrombin II-A. Thromb. Diath. Haemorrhag. *5*:218, 1960.
218. Stenflo, J.: A new vitamin K–dependent protein. Purification from bovine plasma and preliminary characterizations. J. Biol. Chem. *251*:355, 1976.
219. Esmon, C. T.: Protein C: biochemistry, physiology, and clinical implications. Blood *62*:1155, 1983.
220. Esmon, C. T.: The functions of protein C. Contemp. Hematol./Oncol. *3*:137, 1984.
221. Stenflo, J.: Structure and function of protein C. Semin. Thromb. Hemost. *10*:109, 1984.
222. Gardiner, J. E., and Griffin, J. H.: Human protein C and thromboembolic disease. Progr. Hematol. *13*:265, 1983.
223. Griffin, J. H., Evatt, B., et al.: Deficiency of protein C in congenital thrombotic disease. J. Clin. Invest. *68*:1370, 1981.
224. Marciniak, E., Wilson, H. D., and Marlar, R.: Neonatal purpura fulminans as expression of homozygosity for protein C deficiency (abstr.). Blood *62*:303A, 1983.
225. Gardiner, J. E., and Griffin, J. H.: Studies on human protein C inhibitor in normal and Factor V/VIII–deficient plasmas. Thromb. Res. *36*:197, 1984.
226. Schafer, A. I.: The hypercoagulable states. Ann. Intern. Med. *102*:814, 1985.
227. Owen, C. A., Jr.: Coagulation disorders associated with hematocellular disease. In *Acquired Bleeding Disorders in Children.* Lusher, J. M., and Barnhart, M. I. (eds.), New York, Masson Publishing U. S. A., 1981, p. 41.
228. Rock, W. A., Jr.: Laboratory assessment of coagulation disorders in liver disease. Clin. Lab. Med. *4*:419, 1984.
229. Roberts, H. R., and Cederbaum, A. I.: The liver and blood coagulation: physiology and pathology. Gastroenterology *63*:297, 1972.
230. Dymock, I. W., Tucker, J. S., et al.: Coagulation studies as a prognostic index in acute liver failure. Br. J. Haematol. *29*:385, 1975.
231. Mannucci, P. M., and Forman, S. P.: Hemostasis and liver disease. In *Hemostasis and Thrombosis: Basic Principles and Clinical Practice.* Colman, R. W., Hirsh, J., et al. (eds.), Philadelphia, J. B. Lippincott Co., 1982, p. 595.
232. Straub, P. W.: Diffuse intravascular coagulation in liver disease. Semin. Thromb. Hemost. *4*:29, 1977.
233. Prydz, H.: Vitamin K–dependent clotting factors. Semin. Thromb. Hemost. *4*:1, 1977.
234. Olson, R. E.: Vitamin K. In *Hemostasis and Thrombosis: Basic Principles and Clinical Practice.* Colman, R. W., Hirsh, J., et al. (eds.), Philadelphia, J. B. Lippincott Co., 1982, p. 582.
235. Goldman, H. I. and Deposito, F.: Hypoprothrombinemic bleeding in young infants. Am. J. Dis. Child. *111*:430, 1966.
236. Committee on Nutrition, American Acadamy of Pediatrics: Vitamin K supplementation for infants receiving milk substitute infant formulas and for those with fat malabsorption. Pediatrics *48*:483, 1972.
237. Frick, P. G., Riedler, G., et al.: Response and minimal daily requirement for vitamin K in man. J. Appl. Physiol. *23*:387, 1967.
238. Maurer, H. M.: Hematologic effects of cardiac disease. Pediatr. Clin. North Am. *19*:1083, 1972.
239. Warrier, A. I.: The hemorrhagic diathesis associated with cyanotic congenital heart disease. In *Acquired Bleeding Disorders in Children: Abnormalities of Hemostasis.* Lusher, J. M., and Barnhart, M. I. (eds.), New York, Masson Publishing U. S. A., 1981, p. 91.
240. Rosenthal, A., Nathan, D. G., et al.: Acute hemodynamic effects of red cell volume reduction in polycythemia of cyanotic congenital heart disease. Circulation *42*:297, 1970.
241. Hillman, C. R., and Lusher, J. M.: Tests of blood coagulation: technical points of clinical relevance. In *Acquired Bleeding Disorders in Children: Platelet Abnormalities and Laboratory Methods.* Lusher, J. M., and Barnhart, M. I. (eds.), New York, Masson Publishing U. S. A. 1981, p. 91.
242. Fekete, L. F., and Bick, R. L.: Laboratory modalities for assessing hemostasis during cardiopulmonary bypass. Semin. Thromb. Hemost. *3*:83, 1976.
243. Lazerson, J.: Hemostatic defects associated with renal failure. In *Acquired Bleeding Disorders in Children: Abnormalities of Hemostasis.* Lusher, J. M., and Barnhart, M. I. (eds.), New York, Masson Publishing U. S. A. 1981, p. 83.
244. Frumin, A. M.: Platelet function, coagulation, and fibrinolysis. In *Hematologic Problems in Renal Disease.* Jepson, J. H. (ed.), Reading, MA, Addison-Wesley, 1979, p. 193.
245. Rabiner, S. F.: Uremic bleeding. In *Progress in Thrombosis and Hemostasis.* Spaet, T. H. (ed.), New York Grune & Stratton, 1972, p. 233.
246. Hardisty, R. M.: Disorders of platelet function. Br. Med. Bull. *33*:207, 1977.
247. Thaler, E., Balzar, E., et al.: Acquired antithrombin III deficiency in patients with glomerular proteinuria. Haemostasis *7*:257, 1978.
248. Lau, S. O., Tkachuck, J. Y., et al.: Plasminogen and antithrombin III deficiencies in childhood nephrotic syndrome associated with plasminogenuria and antithrombinuria. J. Pediatr. *96*:390, 1980.
249. Kauffmann, R. H., Veltkamp, J. J., et al.: Acquired antithrombin III deficiency and thrombosis in the nephrotic syndrome. Am. J. Med. *65*:607, 1978.
250. Forbes, C. D., and Prentice, C. R. M.: Vascular and non-thrombocytopenic purpuras. In *Haemostasis and Thrombosis.* Bloom, A. L., and Thomas, D. P. (eds.), London, Churchill-Livingstone, 1981, p. 268.

251. McPherson, R. P., Oustad, J. W., et al.: Coagulopathy in amyloidosis: combined deficiency of Factor IX and X. Am. J. Hematol. *3:*225, 1977.
252. Feinstein, D. I.: Acquired inhibitors against Factor VIII and other clotting proteins. In *Hemostasis and Thrombosis: Basic Principles and Clinical Practice.* Colman, R. W., Hirsh, J., et al. (eds.), Philadelphia, J. B. Lippincott, 1982, p. 563.
253. Lusher, J. M., and Hillman, C. R. L.: The effect of inhibitors on coagulation factor assays. In *Blood Coagulation.* Triplett, D. (ed.), American College of Pathologists, 1986, Chapter 7.
254. Shapiro, S. S., and Hultin, M.: Acquired inhibitors to the blood coagulation factors. Semin. Thromb. Hemost. *1:*336, 1975.
255. McKay, D. G.: Disseminated intravascular coagulation. New York, Harper & Row, Hoeber Medical Division, 1965.
256. Colman, R. W., and Marder, V. J.: Disseminated intravascular coagulation (DIC): pathogenesis, pathophysiology and laboratory abnormalities. In *Hemostasis and Thrombosis: Basic Principles and Clinical Practice.* Colman, R. W., Hirsh, J., et al.: Philadelphia, J. B. Lippincott, 1982, p. 654.
257. Mason, J. W., and Colman, R. W.: The role of Hageman factor in disseminated intravascular coagulation induced by septicemia, neoplasia or liver disease. Thromb. Diath. Haemorrhag. *26:*325, 1971.
258. Harker, L. A., and Slichter, S. J.: Platelet and fibrinogen consumption in man. N. Engl. J. Med. *287:*999, 1972.
259. Little, J. R.: Purpura fulminans treated successfully with anticoagulation. J. A. M. A. *169:*104, 1959.
260. Allen, D. M.: Heparin therapy of purpura fulminans. Pediatrics *38:*211, 1966.
261. Hjort, P. F., Rapaport, W. I., et al.: Purpura fulminans: report of a case successfully treated with heparin and hydrocortisone: review of 50 cases from literature. Scand. J. Haematol. *1:*169, 1964.
262. Willoughby, M. L. N.: *Pediatric Haematology.* Edinburgh, Churchill-Livingstone, 1977.
263. Heene, D. L.: Disseminated intravascular coagulation: evaluation of therapeutic approaches. Semin. Thromb. Hemost. *3:*291, 1977.
264. Haneberg, B., Gutteberg, T. J., et al.: Heparin for infants and children with meningococcal septicemia. Results of a randomized therapeutic trial. NIPH Ann. *6:*43, 1983.
265. Corrigan, J. J., Jr.: Heparin therapy in bacterial septicemia. J. Pediatr. *91:*695, 1977.
266. Corrigan, J. J., Jr., Jordan, C. M., et al.: Disseminated intravascular coagulation in septic shock. Report of three cases not treated with heparin. Am. J. Dis. Child. *126:*629, 1974.
267. Hellgren, M., Javelin, L., et al.: Antithrombin III concentrate as adjuvant in DIC treatment. A pilot study in 9 severely ill patients. Thromb. Res. *35:*459, 1984.
268. Blauhut, B., Necek, S., et al.: Therapy with an antithrombin III concentrate in shock and DIC. Thromb. Res. *27:*271, 1982.
269. Sakata, Y., Yoshida, N., et al.: Treatment of DIC with antithrombin III concentrates. Bibl. Haematologica *49:*307, 1983.
270. Thaler, E., and Lechner, K.: Substitutions therapie mit antithrombin III—konzentrat. Deutsch Med. Wochenschr. *107:*147, 1982.
271. Thaler, E., and Lechner, K.: Antithrombin III deficiency and thromboembolism. Clin. Haematol. *10:*369, 1981.
272. Schipper, H. G., Jenkins, C. S., et al.: Antithrombin III transfusion in disseminated intravascular coagulation. Lancet *1:*854, 1978.
273. Bloom, A. L.: Changes in the blood after using an extracorporeal circulation. Br. Med. J. *2:*16, 1961.
274. Gralnick, H. R., and Fisher, R. D.: The hemostatic response to open heart operations. J. Thorac. Cardiovasc. Surg. *61:*909, 1971.
275. Kalter, R. D., Saul, C. M., et al.: Cardiopulmonary bypass. Associated hemostatic abnormalities. J. Thorac. Cardiovasc. Surg. *77:*427, 1979.
276. Russell, F. E.: Pharmacology of animal venoms. Clin. Pharmacol. Ther. *8:*849, 1967.
277. Reid, H. A.: Clinical hemostatic disorders caused by venoms. In *Disorders of Hemostasis.* Ratnoff, O. D., and Forbes, C. D. (eds.), New York, Grune & Stratton, 1984, p. 511.
278. Montgomery, R. W., and Hathaway, W. E.: Acute bleeding emergencies. Pediatr. Clin. North Am. *27:*327, 1980.

COAGULATION

CHAPTER 42
The Platelet: Quantitative and Qualitative Abnormalities

MARIE J. STUART
JOHN G. KELTON

I. Quantitative Abnormalities

II. Qualitative Abnormalities

I. QUANTITATIVE ABNORMALITIES 1344
INTRODUCTION AND OVERVIEW OF PLATELET FUNCTION 1344
QUANTITATIVE PLATELET ABNORMALITIES 1345
Spurious Thrombocytosis and Thrombocytopenia
General Approach to the Thrombocytopenic Patient
DESTRUCTIVE THROMBOCYTOPENIA 1348
IMMUNE THROMBOCYTOPENIAS 1348
Pathogenesis
Idiopathic Thrombocytopenic Purpura of Childhood
Chronic Idiopathic Thrombocytopenic Purpura
Drug-Induced Thrombocytopenia
Infection-Induced Thrombocytopenia
Post-Transfusion Purpura
Neonatal Immune Thrombocytopenia
Thrombocytopenia Associated with Allergy and Anaphylaxis
Thrombocytopenia Associated with Transient Rejection
Immune Thrombocytopenia Associated with Other Disorders
DESTRUCTIVE THROMBOCYTOPENIAS ASSOCIATED WITH NONIMMUNOLOGIC MICROANGIOPATHIC PROCESSES 1383
Chronic Microangiopathic Hemolytic Anemia and Thrombocytopenia
Hemolytic-Uremic Syndrome and Thrombotic Thrombocytopenic Purpura
Thrombocytopenia Caused by Catheters, Prostheses, and Cardiopulmonary Bypass
Thrombocytopenia Secondary to Congenital Heart Disease
Thrombocytopenia Secondary to Acquired Heart Disease
DESTRUCTIVE THROMBOCYTOPENIA WITH CONSUMPTION OF PLATELETS AND FIBRINOGEN 1385
Disseminated Intravascular Coagulation
Thrombocytopenia Associated with Giant Hemangioma (Kasabach-Merritt Syndrome)
Other Causes of Local Consumption Coagulopathy
DESTRUCTIVE THROMBOCYTOPENIA DUE TO MISCELLANEOUS CAUSES 1388
Thrombocytopenia in Glomerular Disease
Thrombocytopenia in Preeclampsia

Thrombocytopenias Peculiar to the Neonate
Fatty Acid–Induced Thrombocytopenia
CONGENITAL AND HEREDITARY THROMBOCYTOPENIAS DUE TO IMPAIRED OR INEFFECTIVE PRODUCTION 1390
Thrombocytopenia Absent Radii (TAR) Syndrome
Other Congenital Thrombocytopenias with Megakaryocyte Hypoplasia
Fanconi's Aplastic Anemia
Bernard-Soulier Syndrome
May-Hegglin Anomaly
Wiskott-Aldrich Syndrome
Miscellaneous Hereditary Thrombocytopenias
ACQUIRED THROMBOCYTOPENIAS DUE TO IMPAIRED OR INEFFECTIVE PRODUCTION 1393
Thrombocytopenia due to Aplastic Anemia or Marrow Infiltration
Drug- and Radiation-Induced Thrombocytopenia as Part of Total Marrow Suppression
Drug-Induced Thrombocytopenia with Platelet-Specific Suppression
Thrombocytopenia Associated with Nutritional Deficiency States
THROMBOCYTOPENIA DUE TO PLATELET SEQUESTRATION 1394
Hypersplenism
Hypothermia
DIAGNOSTIC APPROACH TO THE THROMBOCYTOPENIC PATIENT 1395
THROMBOCYTOSIS 1395
APPENDIX 1399
Techniques Used to Measure Platelet Antibodies
II. QUALITATIVE ABNORMALITIES 1429
PLATELET STRUCTURE–FUNCTION RELATIONSHIPS 1429
Platelet Adhesion
Platelet Aggregation
Interaction of the Coagulation Proteins with Platelets
CONGENITAL DISORDERS OF PLATELET FUNCTION 1432
Inherited Disorders of Platelet Surface Glycoproteins
Bernard-Soulier Syndrome
Glanzmann's Thrombasthenia
Platelet-Type von Willebrand's Disease
Platelet Granule Defects
Alpha-Granule Deficiency (Gray Platelet Syndrome)
Dense Granule Deficiencies (Storage Pool Deficiency)
Defects in Platelet Arachidonic Acid Metabolism
Miscellaneous Secretion Defects
Defective Platelet Metabolic Adenine Nucleotide Metabolism
Defects in Platelet Procoagulant Activity
Miscellaneous Disorders
Diagnosis and Management of a Patient with a Congenital Disorder of Platelet Function
PHYSIOLOGIC QUALITATIVE ABNORMALITIES 1444
Neonatal Platelet Function
ACQUIRED QUALITATIVE PLATELET ABNORMALITIES 1445
Uremia
Liver Disease
Qualitative Platelet Defects Following Cardiopulmonary Bypass and in Children with Congenital or Acquired Cardiac Defects
Myeloproliferative Disorders
Preleukemia and Acute Leukemia
Miscellaneous Disorders

DRUG–INDUCED PLATELET DYSFUNCTION 1447
Nonsteroidal Anti-Inflammatory Agents
Platelet-Mediated Thrombotic Disorders and the Use of
 Antiplatelet Agents
Antibiotic-Related Dysfunction
Membrane-Active Drugs
Miscellaneous Drugs
Treatment of Drug-Induced Platelet Dysfunction
HYPERCOAGULABILITY 1455
Presence of Prosthetic Devices in the Circulation
Diabetes Mellitus
Homocystinuria
Nephrotic Syndrome
Kawasaki Syndrome
VASCULAR PURPURAS 1459
Allergic Purpura (Schönlein-Henoch Purpura)
APPENDIX: TECHNIQUES USED TO STUDY PLATELET
 MEMBRANE GLYCOPROTEINS 1461
Gel Electrophoresis
Radioimmunoprecipitation
Immunoblotting

I. Quantitative Abnormalities

INTRODUCTION AND OVERVIEW OF PLATELET FUNCTION

The role of platelets in physiology and pathophysiology is only now being defined. Platelets play a pivotal role in hemostasis, interacting directly or indirectly with the other limbs of the hemostatic system—the coagulation factors and the vessel wall. Platelets also participate in the repair process following vascular injury, a function that is vitally important for maintaining patent vessels. But it is also the platelets, in conjunction with other cellular and plasma factors, that can lead to a proliferative response in the vessel wall that is manifest pathologically as atherosclerosis. Platelets can directly cause ischemic tissue damage if a platelet-fibrin thrombus is dislodged from its attachment to the vessel wall, occluding a distal vessel. Thus platelets are important not only in normal hemostasis but also in the pathogenesis of atherosclerosis and the complications of this disorder, strokes and myocardial infarction. In this chapter we will briefly discuss the role of platelets in normal hemostasis and describe certain disorders of platelet number and function.

Platelets are anuclear cytoplasmic fragments that originate from the megakaryocytes of the bone marrow. They circulate as biconcave discs remaining in the circulation for 7 to 10 days before being removed by the cells of the reticuloendothelial system. The anatomy of platelets is unique among cells, reflecting the complexity of platelet function (1). The platelet wall invaginates to form the open canalicular system, which allows the rapid movement of the platelet's intracytoplasmic granular contents to the external milieu of the platelet. The platelet membrane is made up of a typical lipid bilayer, but on the outside of this coat is a glycoprotein surface termed the glycocalyx. Below the lipid bilayer are several fiber systems in various states of polymerization that maintain platelet shape both at rest and during platelet secretion. Platelets also contain a number of organelles, including electrodense structures termed dense granules, which contain calcium, serotonin, and the nonmetabolic pool of adenine nucleotides ADP and ATP; and alpha granules, which contain the platelet-specific proteins (including β-thromboglobulin, and platelet factor 4), coagulation factors, and various cationic proteins (including platelet-derived growth factor). Recently, glycoprotein G (also termed thrombospondin), a high-molecular-weight glycoprotein, has been identified in platelet α-granules (2, 3). It is suggested that glycoprotein G is the platelet endogenous lectin and that fibrinogen is the lectin receptor (4). Lysosomes and mitochrondria are also dispersed in the platelet cytoplasm. One other platelet system of importance is the dense tubular system, which not only is the site of cyclooxygenase activity but also sequesters much of the mobilizable calcium contained in the platelet (1).

Platelets are crucial for hemostasis: they form a primary hemostatic plug when the vessel wall is damaged or transected; they release vasoactive factors that result in vasoconstriction of the vessel wall; and they function as a surface upon which many of the coagulation reactions occur. Because platelets participate in all three limbs of the hemostatic system, a reduction in the platelet count can result in bleeding, the severity of which is related to both platelet quantity and function.

The participation of platelets in hemostasis can be considered in several sequential steps. Platelets do not adhere to the endothelial lining of the blood vessel wall, but if that lining is damaged, platelets adhere to the subendothelial layers, in particular collagen (Fig. 42–1). This platelet-collagen adhesion reaction requires a plasma component, (Factor VIII:von Willebrand factor (VIII:vWF), and a specific part of the platelet membrane, termed glycoprotein Ib. Individuals with abnormalities of either of these components will manifest abnormal platelet adhesion. This includes patients with the rare Bernard-Soulier syndrome who have reduced or absent platelet glycoprotein Ib, and individuals with the much more common inherited bleeding disorder called von Willebrand's disease, who have a deficiency (common) or a functional abnormality (uncommon) of Factor VIII:vWF.

As platelets adhere to collagen, they release platelet-reactive compounds into the circulation that in turn recruit nearby platelets into the primary platelet plug in a process termed platelet aggregation. Platelet aggregation, like platelet adhesion, depends upon a plasma coagulation factor, fibrinogen, and the platelet glycoprotein com-

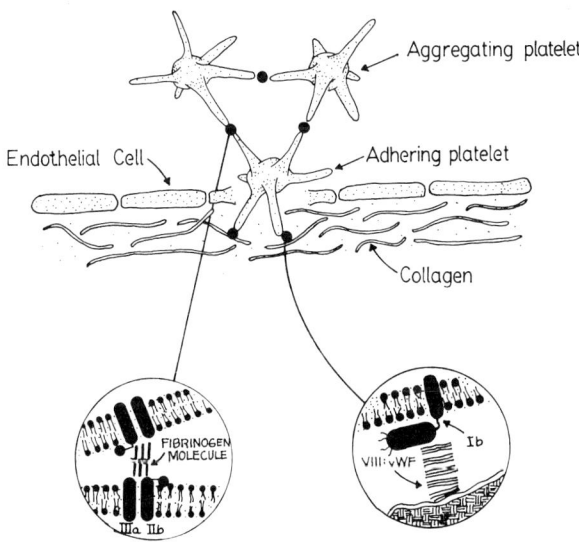

Figure 42–1. A schematic representation of platelet adhesion and aggregation demonstrating how each of these functions requires a specific platelet glycoprotein and plasma coagulation factor.

plex, IIb-IIIa (Fig. 42–1). Platelet glycoproteins IIb-IIIa are absent or greatly reduced in platelets from patients with Glanzmann's thrombasthenia. Besides serving as functionally important sites for cell-cell interaction, some platelet glycoproteins also carry platelet-specific antigens. For example, the Pl^{A1} antigen is found on glycoprotein IIIa, and the Bak^a antigen (also known as Lek^a) is located on glycoprotein IIb.

Platelet aggregation is initiated by the interaction of a specific agonist with a platelet membrane receptor. The interaction results in the transfer of a signal to the interior of the platelet and this in turn initiates aggregation. A number of physiologic substances induce platelet aggregation, with the most important being adenosine diphosphate (ADP), collagen, and thrombin (5). ADP binds to a specific ADP receptor on the platelet membrane and causes the platelet to undergo shape change, followed by reversible and subsequently irreversible (secondary wave) aggregation. In vitro, the secondary wave of aggregation and the release of platelet granule contents induced by ADP occur only in a low calcium medium and are entirely dependent upon the prostaglandin pathway. Certain drugs such as aspirin inhibit the rate-limiting enzyme of the prostaglandin pathway, cyclooxygenase, and block the secondary wave of ADP-induced aggregation. Collagen is a more potent agonist than ADP, and although low concentrations of collagen induce aggregation through the prostaglandin pathway, higher concentrations also induce aggregation via the direct release of platelet ADP. Thrombin, the most potent physiologic aggregating agent, activates both of these pathways plus other as yet undefined mechanisms of aggregation (5).

QUANTITATIVE PLATELET ABNORMALITIES

Spurious Thrombocytosis and Thrombocytopenia

In the neonate, child, and adult, the normal platelet count ranges from 150,000 to 450,000 cells per mm^3. In most laboratories, platelet counts now are determined using electronic particle counters because of lower costs and greater reliability. For example, electronic counters have a better reproducibility (coefficient variation (CV) = 4 per cent) compared with conventional manual techniques (CV = 16 to 23 per cent). However, automated platelet counters do have one major drawback—their potential to over- or underestimate the actual number of platelets in certain clinical situations. The reason for this lies in the method used to perform the platelet count. Electronic counters measure the number of platelets (and other cells) by counting the number of particles of a certain size. Particles that lie within this size distribution but are not platelets are counted as platelets, leading to an overestimation of the actual number of platelets. For example, microspherocytes, Pappenheimer bodies, red cell fragments, leukocyte fragments, and bacteria all can cause spuriously high platelet counts (6–10).

A more serious potential error for the patient is an incorrectly low platelet count, a phenomenon called pseudothrombocytopenia which can result in unnecessary tests and inappropriate treatment (11–13). Pseudothrombocytopenia, once a laboratory curiosity, is now assuming greater importance as clinicians put more reliance on electronic particle counting. For this reason, it is imperative that the blood film of every individual with a purported decrease in the platelet count be examined carefully to ensure that the patient does not have pseudothrombocytopenia. Platelet clumps should be sought in the tail of the blood smear and platelet-leukocyte aggregates looked for throughout the film.

A spuriously low platelet count will occur if a clot has formed in the collection tube due to improper blood collection or inadequate or inactive anticoagulants. Usually this technical problem is obvious because blood clots are present in the anticoagulated blood sample, but in contrast to other causes of pseudothrombocytopenia, thrombocytopenia is not present when the platelet count is repeated. Occasionally, pseudothrombocytopenia is first noted because of apparent leukocytosis, which is actually caused by the particle counter's classifying platelet clumps as neutrophils (14). The usual causes for a spuriously low platelet count include:

EDTA-Dependent Platelet Clumping. This is the most common cause of pseudothrombocytopenia and is a regular finding in virtually every large hematology laboratory. This artifact was first described by Gowland and co-workers in 1969 (15) and subsequently has been observed by many other investigators (14–19). The precise frequency of EDTA-dependent pseudothrombocytopenia is uncertain but it has been reported to range from a low of 0.9 per cent to a high of 2 per cent (11, 20) with the frequency being highest in ill, hospitalized patients.

The characteristic features of EDTA-dependent platelet clumping have been well studied. The clumping depends upon EDTA, but occasionally other anticoagulants can produce this phenomenon, although less vigorously. In some patients, EDTA-induced pseudothrombocytopenia occurs at virtually any temperature, but in most clumping is greatest at or below room temperature. The clumping is dependent upon a plasma factor and is independent of the source of the platelets. Most investigators have reported that the platelet clumping is due to either an IgG or an IgM EDTA-dependent antiplatelet antibody (17, 18, 21). In one report, platelets from a patient with Glanzmann's thrombasthenia were nonreactive, suggesting that the antibody binds to glycoprotein IIb or IIIa.

Although in many cases, EDTA-dependent platelet clumping is a laboratory artifact, sometimes it accompanies a true autoimmune thrombocytopenia, making the accurate estimate of the platelet count difficult (21, 22). This laboratory artifact usually is easy to diagnose because of the large number of platelet clumps noted on the stained blood film. An accurate platelet count can usually be obtained by performing the count either on a warmed specimen, with a different anticoagulant such as sodium citrate, or by lowering the pH of the anticoagulated blood. Sometimes an accurate platelet count can be obtained only by performing a phase contrast platelet count on a finger prick blood sample.

Platelet Cold Agglutinins. Pseudothrombocytopenia caused by platelet cold agglutinins is similar to EDTA-dependent platelet agglutination except that the agglutination reaction occurs with any anticoagulant (23). In fact in some patients, the clumping is so dramatic that it is impossible to obtain a reliable platelet count. This laboratory artifact is far less common than EDTA-dependent pseudothrombocytopenia, but it too is due to an antibody, often IgG (24–27). An accurate platelet count can be obtained by a phase contrast count using blood obtained from a finger prick specimen. Some investigators have suggested that reducing the pH to below 5.5 will prevent clumping and allow an accurate estimate of the platelet count (27).

Platelet Satellitism. This is the least common cause of pseudothrombocytopenia and is characterized by platelets adhering to the outer membranes of neutrophils or monocytes. As with other types of platelet clumping, the clumping is maximal at room temperature or lower and is most frequently observed when EDTA is the anticoagulant (28–37).

General Approach to the Thrombocytopenic Patient

The thrombocytopenic patient most frequently seeks attention because of characteristic thrombocytopenic bleeding—petechiae and purpura. Sometimes the thrombocytopenia is discovered during the routine laboratory investigation of another suspected abnormality. When this occurs, or when thrombocytopenia is not accompanied by any clinical evidence of bleeding, it is especially important that pseudothrombocytopenia be excluded.

Assuming that the thrombocytopenia is "real," the physician must address two interrelated issues. The first is paramount: is the patient sufficiently hemostatically impaired to require therapy? As will be emphasized subsequently, many patients with moderate thrombocytopenia will not have any hemostatic impairment and hence aggressive therapy may result in greater morbidity than that caused by the thrombocytopenia itself. The second issue the clinician must resolve is identifying the mechanism of the thrombocytopenia. Defining the cause of the thrombocytopenia is necessary before intervention is initiated because treatment undertaken without knowing the mechanism of the disorder is arbitrary and seldom successful. For example, patients with an aregenerative thrombocytopenia such as aplastic anemia will have a transient rise in their platelet count following platelet transfusion whereas patients with consumptive thrombocytopenia will almost never respond to random donor platelets.

The first step in defining the cause of the thrombocytopenia is a careful history. For example, if the patient has thrombocytopenia that follows the ingestion of any medication, then the diagnosis of drug-induced thrombocytopenia is a strong possibility. Unlike coagulation disorders, thrombocytopenia is much more likely to be acquired than congenital, and although a careful review of the family history for bleeding is helpful, it is less likely to be positive than in patients with a coagulation defect.

As outlined in Table 42–1, there are certain characteristic physical findings that help the clinician to differentiate platelet and vascular defects from those due to plasma coagulation factor abnormalities. Platelet or vascular defects give rise

Table 42–1. CLINICAL FEATURES OF THE TWO MAIN GROUPS OF HEMOSTATIC DISEASE

Clinical Findings	Platelet or Vascular Defects	Plasma Coagulation Defects
Common hemorrhagic symptoms	Epistaxis, petechiae, purpura, ecchymoses, gastrointestinal hemorrhage, and menorrhagia	Deep tissue hemorrhages, especially hemarthroses and intramuscular bleeds
Bleeding from superficial cuts and abrasions	Often profuse and prolonged	Usually mild
Bleeding from deep cuts, lacerations, dental extractions	Onset immediate; often permanently arrested with local pressure; seldom rebleeds	Onset often delayed; not permanently controlled by local pressure; rebleeding likely to occur several hours after removal of local pressure
Spontaneous bleeding	Usually superficial; small and multiple loci of involvement	Usually a single locus; large and deep-seated hematomas or hemarthroses

to multiple superficial skin and mucosal hemorrhages that occur immediately upon injury and can be controlled by local pressure. The hallmark of bleeding due to a low platelet count or platelet dysfunction is the presence of tiny subcutaneous collections of red cells termed petechiae. In contrast, the deficiency of a plasma coagulation factor causes deep tissue and joint hemorrhages that usually occur at a single site and are less likely to be controlled by local pressure. Bleeding is also more commonly seen in a patient with a coagulation factor deficiency. Sometimes there is both a platelet defect and a coagulation abnormality such as occurs in disseminated intravascular coagulation, or hemophilia A complicated by idiopathic thrombocytopenic purpura (38, 39). As might be predicted, the combination of these hemostatic defects produces hemorrhagic manifestations characteristic of both platelet and coagulation factor impairment.

After the clinical impression of thrombocytopenia is confirmed by laboratory testing, it is important for the clinician to determine the mechanism responsible for the thrombocytopenia. Three general categories of thrombocytopenia exist:

1. *Destructive thrombocytopenia.* An increased rate of platelet destruction overwhelms the ability of the bone marrow to produce platelets.

2. *Aregenerative thrombocytopenia.* The production of platelets by the bone marrow is so reduced that it is unable to keep up with normal platelet turnover.

3. *Platelet Sequestration.* The platelets are trapped within an increased vascular bed, almost always the spleen.

In practice it is relatively easy to distinguish among these three different causes. For example, since the red and white cells originate from the same precursor stem cells as platelets, aregenerative thrombocytopenia almost always involves all three cell lines. In contrast, disorders of platelet consumption usually result in isolated thrombocytopenia. Thrombocytopenia due to splenic sequestration is easily identified, because a normal-sized spleen precludes the diagnosis. The vast majority of thrombocytopenic disorders are caused by an increased rate of platelet destruction, most commonly immune related.

The determination of the average platelet size, termed the mean platelet volume (MPV), can help distinguish among the various causes of thrombocytopenia. Today, almost every laboratory performs blood counts using automated counters. These particle counters not only determine platelet number, but also give the mean (and sometimes median) platelet volume in femtolitres (1 fL = 10^{-15} L). Consumptive thrombocytopenic disorders are almost always associated with larger than average platelets with volume usually increased to greater than 10 fL. In contrast, disorders of platelet sequestration and underproduction usually are characterized by mean platelet volumes within the normal range.

There are two hypotheses that seek to explain platelet size and age relationships: One hypothesis proposes that the youngest platelets are large and contain many granules. As the platelets mature in the circulation, they gradually become smaller, presumably because of loss of membrane and granular contents. The other hypothesis suggests that when the platelet count is low, larger than average and reactive platelets, termed stress platelets, are preferentially produced (40–46). Irrespective of which hypothesis proves correct, disorders of chronically increased platelet turnover almost always are characterized by large platelets, whereas disorders of underproduction or sequestration are characterized by normal or small platelets (47). The size-age relationship also explains why at any given platelet count, a patient with aregenerative thrombocytopenia is more likely to bleed than a patient with thrombocytopenia due to increased platelet turnover.

In summary, by taking a careful history, performing a physical examination, and noting the platelet count and size, the clinician can deduce the probable mechanism of the thrombocytopenia before other more complex tests such as bone marrow examination or platelet survival studies are performed.

DESTRUCTIVE THROMBOCYTOPENIA

Destructive, or consumptive, thrombocytopenia is defined as a thrombocytopenia due to an increased rate of platelet destruction that overwhelms the ability of the patient's own megakaryocytes to produce more platelets. Because the marrow is producing platelets at maximal capacity, the number of megakaryocytes in the bone marrow usually is increased in patients with a destructive thrombocytopenia. By definition, a patient with a destructive thrombocytopenia will have an increased rate of platelet destruction, which sometimes can be proven only by the performance of an autologous platelet survival.

In this test, patient platelets are isolated and labeled with a gamma emitting radioactive substance (^{51}chromium or ^{111}indium). The platelets are reinfused into the individual and blood samples collected over the next week. By measuring the rate of loss of the radioactive tracer from the blood stream, an accurate estimate of platelet lifespan can be determined. Although not every hospital is technically equipped to perform this test, for many patients with obscure thrombocytopenic disorders this evaluation may prove extremely useful.

When thrombocytopenia is due to increased platelet destruction, immune mechanisms are usually operative, although thrombin-induced platelet consumption like that occurring with disseminated intravascular coagulation may be another etiologic consideration. A combination of immune and nonimmune mechanisms (e.g., the thrombocytopenia of sepsis) may also result in platelet consumption.

IMMUNE THROMBOCYTOPENIAS

Pathogenesis

Immune thrombocytopenia is characterized by an increased rate of platelet destruction, which can be proved by a shortened autologous platelet survival, plus the demonstration of sensitization of the platelets by IgG or complement or both (activated by IgG or IgM). Most cases of immune thrombocytopenia are caused by humoral mechanisms (i.e., IgG alone) or, less commonly, IgM plus complement. To date, there has never been convincing evidence that cell-mediated platelet destruction can cause immune thrombocytopenia. Immune thrombocytopenia is almost always characterized by increased amounts of IgG on the platelets (termed platelet-associated IgG [PAIgG]). It is now known that this PAIgG causes the thrombocytopenia, although there is not always a direct relationship between the amount of IgG on the platelets and the severity of the thrombocytopenia. This is not unexpected: it should be remembered that the severity of any cytopenia depends upon the final equilibrium that is achieved between the rate of cell production and the rate of cell destruction (Fig. 42–2). Consequently, two patients with precisely the same rate of platelet destruction caused by autoantibodies will have very different degrees of thrombocytopenia if they have different rates of platelet production. Furthermore, the rate of cell destruction is related not only to the amount and characteristics of the autoantibody but also to the functional activity of the reticuloendothelial cell system. Consequently, it is not surprising to find that the measurement of a single variable in the equation (in this case platelet-associated IgG) will not necessarily predict the result of the equation, that is, the severity of the thrombocytopenia. We will briefly describe the two most important determinants of platelet destruction: the IgG on the platelet surface and the functional activity of the Fc-dependent reticuloendothelial cell system.

IgG. IgG is the most important antibody for host defense. IgG molecules act as bridges between soluble and particle-bound antigens and the reticuloendothelial cells that ultimately will remove these antigens from the circulation. This is a highly efficient and effective process in which tiny molecules (IgG) with virtually unlimited specificity can recognize many thousands of different particles. The cell- or particle-bound IgG is in turn recognized by the effector limb of the immune system—the monocytes and macrophages of the reticuloendothelial (RE) system.

IgG is a symmetrical molecule made of two heavy and two light polypeptide chains (Fig. 42–

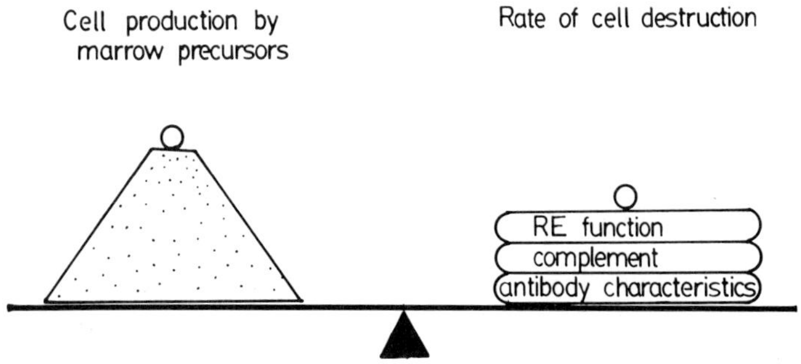

Figure 42–2. A schematic illustration of the factors determining the severity of an immune cytopenic disorder. There is a balance between cell production and destruction. A cytopenia develops if this balance is altered. (From Kelton, J. G.: *Current Concepts in Transfusion Therapy*. Arlington, Virginia, American Association of Blood Banks, 1985.)

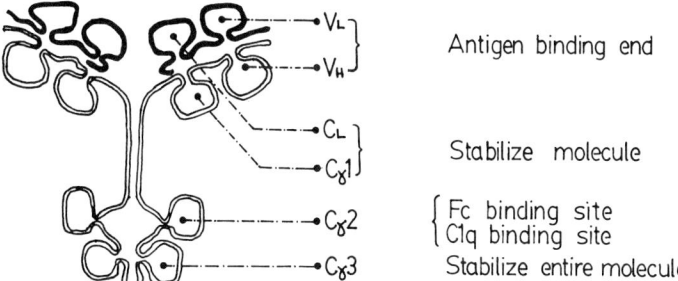

Figure 42–3. A schematic representation of the IgG molecule relating structure to function.

3) (48). The two identical Fab regions are joined to one Fc region by a flexible hinge. Antigens bind to the variable portion of the Fab terminus, which is the aminoterminus of the molecule. The effector region is termed the Fc (fragment crystallizable) portion and each set of antibodies with a common Fc structure is termed a class. The predominant immunoglobulin class is IgG, which is present in the body in high concentrations (about 20 per cent of all plasma proteins). The heavy and light chains are divided into regions termed domains, and certain functions are located within certain domains. The VH and VL domains on the Fab portion of IgG act as the antigen-binding part of the molecule and by necessity this region is extremely variable. In contrast, the domains on the heavy chains of IgG differ only slightly, but based on these differences IgG is divided into four subclasses. The Cγ1 domains, which are located on the Fab arm, not only stabilize the antigen binding part of the molecule but also act as spacers between the functional part of the molecule and the effector part of the molecule. The Cγ2 domain is the major effector portion of the IgG molecule and binds the first component of complement (C1q) as well as Fc receptors of monocytes and macrophages. The Cγ3 region is located at the C terminal end of IgG and stabilizes the entire molecule.

The Reticuloendothelial System. Retinculoendothelial (RE) cells are mesenchyme-derived cells distributed through the body, with the highest concentrations found in the spleen, lungs, liver, and bone marrow. There are several reasons why the RE cells within the spleen are the most important cellular elements for the clearance of IgG-sensitized cells such as platelets. First, the spleen has a very high concentration of monocytes and macrophages. Second, because of its unique circulation, the plasma is skimmed away from the platelets, bringing them into intimate contact with the RE elements in the red pulp of the spleen. The removal of the plasma from these cells in the spleen has the effect of removing the inhibitory effect of monomeric IgG, and as a result the IgG-sensitized platelets are cleared by the RE system.

For phagocytosis to occur, the RE cells must recognize cell-bound IgG and distinguish it from the uncomplexed (monomeric) IgG that is present in the plasma at concentrations that greatly exceed that of the complexed IgG. Increasing evidence suggests that the RE cells cannot distinguish between complexed IgG that is bound to a cell and uncomplexed (monomeric) IgG that is free in the plasma. However, when IgG binds to a cell such as the platelet in immune thrombocytopenia, the multiple antibody binding sites on the platelet surface act to concentrate the IgG and increase the relative concentration of IgG that is presented to the Fc receptors of the RE cells (49, 50). Consequently, a cell with large amounts of IgG bound to its surface is cleared because it overcomes the inhibitory concentration of free monomeric IgG in the plasma.

Recent advances in the understanding of how IgG-sensitized cells interact with Fc receptors and the influence of monomeric and complexed IgG on this interaction have provided a better understanding of the biological relevance of some of our laboratory tests, such as assays that measure platelet-associated IgG. Perhaps more importantly, the understanding of the determinants of cell clearance has offered the therapeutic potential of manipulating these factors, as for example, in treatment with intravenous IgG (IV1gG).

Several groups of investigators have reported that occasionally patients with elevated levels of platelet-associated IgG may not be thrombocytopenic nor do they have a shortened platelet lifespan, thus bringing into question the biologic relevance of elevated PAIgG on platelets (51–53). There are two possible explanations for this: either the IgG on the cells is not recognized by the Fc receptors of the RE cells, or reticuloendothelial function is impaired in these individuals, making the RE cells unable to clear sensitized platelets. Fc-dependent reticuloendothelial cell function can be measured by determining the rate of clearance of ^{51}chromium-labelled autologous red cells sensitized with a precise amount of anti-D alloantibody. The advantage of this technique is that the patient's RE cell system is presented with autologous red cells sensitized with a known amount of antibody. More importantly, the spatial orientation of the binding of the IgG to the red cell antigens is known; i.e., Fab binding makes the Fc region available for binding to the Fc receptors of the RE cells. When these tests are performed in individuals with elevated PAIgG but normal autologous platelet survivals, they show that reticuloendothelial function is significantly impaired (54). Subsequent investigations in these and similar patients have shown that the mechanism responsible for the impaired Fc-dependent RE function was a disease-related increase in the level of monomeric IgG in the plasma (Fig. 42–4, hypothesis A). Thus, these patients represent a naturally occurring "model," which explains why some patients with ITP will often have a resolution of their thrombocytopenia following treatment with intravenous IgG. Our understanding of the interrelationships between plasma IgG, RE cell function, and IgG-sensitized platelets also explains why patients with congenital agammaglobulinemia often have very severe thrombocytopenia. These individuals lack monomeric IgG that can compete for monocyte/macrophage Fc receptors with IgG-sensitized platelets.

RE cells do not carry receptors for IgM and therefore cells sensitized only by IgM will not be cleared any more quickly than normal cells. The binding of IgG to platelets with subsequent clearance by the RE cells represents the major mechanism of platelet destruction in immune thrombocytopenia. Complement can be activated on the platelet surface, causing platelet clearance via complement receptors, but unlike complement-mediated red cell destruction, there is little evidence that the complement cascade is "completed" resulting in intravascular platelet lysis. Rather, immune thrombocytopenia almost always is caused by an increased rate of platelet destruction by RE cells, which is mediated by IgG.

It is also theoretically possible that some episodes of immune thrombocytopenia are in part due to a relative underproduction of platelets. Some antiplatelet antibodies that result in an increased rate of platelet destruction can also damage megakaryocytes and in this way limit the ability of these cells to produce platelets (55–57). It should be emphasized however that this is a relatively uncommon occurrence and that the primary mechanism of immune thrombocytopenia is an increased rate of platelet destruction.

Immune thrombocytopenia can be divided into several categories according to the mechanism responsible for the binding of the IgG to platelets (Fig. 42–5). The orientation of binding of IgG to the platelet membrane is slowly being defined. For example, children and adults with chronic idiopathic thrombocytopenic purpura (ITP) have increased binding of IgG to their platelets that is caused by the specific binding of antiplatelet autoantibodies to platelet-specific epitopes on glycoproteins Ib, IIb, and IIIa (58–60). These autoantibodies lead to thrombocytopenia by causing an increased rate of platelet destruction. Occasionally, the binding of the IgG to the platelet will also result in platelet dysfunction. IgG can likewise bind to platelet-specific alloantigens as occurs in alloimmune neonatal thrombocytopenia. The majority of these cases are caused by the binding of an IgG alloantibody to a platelet-specific antigen, which is located on glycoprotein IIIa and has been termed PL^{A1}.

IgG can also bind to an antigen adsorbed onto platelets from plasma. It is likely that this represents an important cause of increased PAIgG as occurs in acute childhood ITP, drug-induced thrombocytopenia, and the thrombocytopenia of bacterial septicemia and viremia. To date, however, the only condition clearly demonstrated to be caused by the binding of IgG to a platelet-bound antigen is malaria-induced thrombocytopenia (61).

Finally, as also illustrated in Figure 42–5, platelets carry Fc receptors and hence IgG alone, or after being complexed to an antigen, can bind through its Cγ2 domain to the platelet Fc receptor. Once this mechanism was felt to be responsible for many episodes of thrombocytopenia associated with "immune complex diseases," such as systemic lupus erythematosus, and some cases of drug-induced thrombocytopenia. However, studies by one group of investigators have demonstrated that

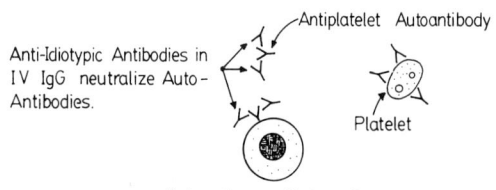

Figure 42–4. Two different hypotheses proposed to explain the efficacy of intravenous IgG as a treatment for idiopathic thrombocytopenic purpura.

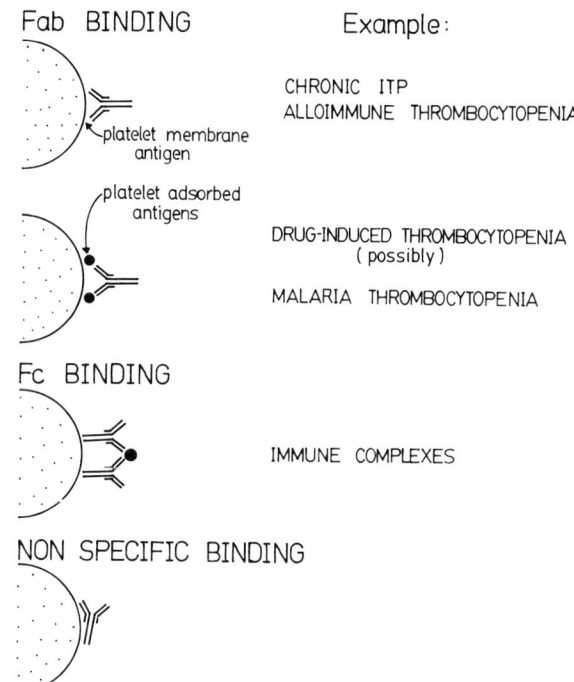

Figure 42-5. A schematic representation of the possible mechanisms responsible for the binding of IgG to platelets.

the binding affinity of the platelet Fc receptor for complexed IgG is so low as to make it unlikely that immune complexes can overcome the inhibitory concentration of monomeric plasma IgG and bind to the platelet Fc receptors (62).

Idiopathic Thrombocytopenic Purpura of Childhood

Idiopathic thrombocytopenic purpura (ITP) of childhood is an acute, usually self-limited disorder, characterized by peripheral thrombocytopenia (platelet count less than 100,000 cells per mm^3), concomitant with increased platelet production and a decrease in platelet life span. The name itself is somewhat of a misnomer: the illness is not idiopathic but is caused by the binding of IgG to platelets, which results in their destruction by the reticuloendothelial system. Whether or not the IgG represents a true autoantibody bound to a platelet-specific antigen or an IgG-viral complex remains uncertain. Acute childhood ITP can be considered to be the mirror image of the ITP that occurs in adults. Approximately 90 per cent of children with acute ITP make an uneventful recovery, the platelet count returning to normal within a few weeks to months, whereas 80 to 90 per cent of adults will continue to have active disease and thrombocytopenia (63-75). The term "chronic idiopathic thrombocytopenic purpura" is reserved for those children in whom thrombocytopenia persists for longer than 6 months. In some patients, initial recovery of the platelet count to normal levels is followed by a recrudescence of thrombocytopenia. This relatively infrequent third pattern of childhood ITP is termed recurrent idiopathic thrombocytopenia.

CLINICAL FEATURES

Age, Sex, and Race. Immune thrombocytopenia in the neonate (less than 4 months of age) is excluded from this discussion since it is a different entity, which will be described fully in Chapter 5. The annual incidence of clinically symptomatic childhood ITP is approximately 4 per 100,000 children (76, 77), but it is possible that the incidence is even higher because of undetected cases. The age of onset is variable. In a survey of 305 consecutive newly diagnosed cases of ITP, the peak age was between 2 and 5 years (Fig. 42-6), a period which is also the peak age for childhood viral infections. The age of onset is much more variable in children whose thrombocytopenia ultimately proves chronic. However, in general, the older the child, the more likely that the ITP will become chronic. There is no sex predilection in acute childhood ITP, in contrast to the adult form of the disease in which there is a 3:1 predominance in women. However, those children in whom TP ultimately becomes chronic are predominantly female. There is no obvious peak seasonal incidence.

Clinical Manifestations. A composite analysis of the clinical manifestations of ITP in 1438 children is shown in Table 42-2. In the majority of children the onset is acute. Typically, a previously well child suddenly develops easy bruising and petechial bleeding 1 to 3 weeks after a viral illness. Bleeding into the skin is the hallmark of ITP, with petechiae and purpura being present at diagnosis in nearly every case. Epistaxis, the next most frequent symp-

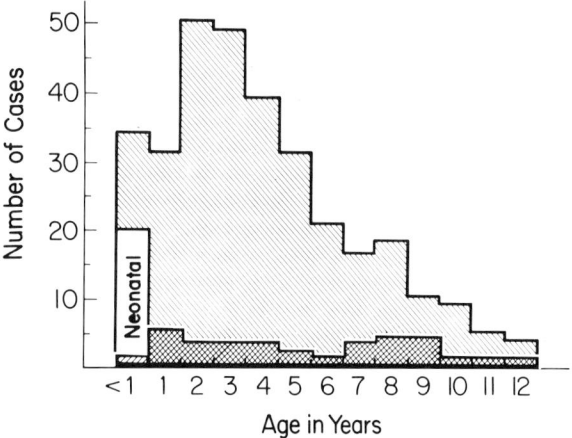

Figure 42-6. Age of onset in 305 consecutive cases of ITP seen at the Children's Hospital of Michigan. The heavy crosshatching indicates age of onset in 32 children whose course became chronic. (From Lusher, J. M., and Iyer, R.: Semin. Thromb. Hemostas. 3:175, 1977.)

Table 42–2. CLINICAL MANIFESTATIONS OF CHILDHOOD ITP—A COMPILATION OF DATA ON 1438 PATIENTS

Factors	Walker and Walker (64, 75)†	Lusher et al. (66, 73, 74)	Choi and McClure (67, 68)	Benham and Taft (100)	Simons et al. (71)	Lammi and Lovric (69)
Number of patients evaluable	181	465	413	132	95	152
Skin bleeding (petechiae and purpura)			Close to 100%			
Epistaxis	24%	27%	32%	26%	20%	NA*
Gastrointestinal hemorrhage or melena	4%	NA	8%	NA	2%	NA
Hematuria	NA	5%	8%	NA	7%	NA
Gum or oral mucosal bleeding	4%	NA	7%	NA	7%	NA
Splenomegaly	20%	7.5%	10%	17%	NA	NA

*NA = Data not available.
†Indicates chapter reference.

tom, is present in 20 to 30 per cent of children. Hematuria, and oral and gastrointestinal bleeding are seen less commonly. The incidence of minimal splenomegaly is approximately that present in normal children, i.e., 5 to 10 per cent. Hence, marked enlargement of either the liver or the spleen should warn the physician to consider alternative diagnoses.

LABORATORY EVALUATION AND DIFFERENTIAL DIAGNOSIS

The platelet count is less than 40,000 cells per mm^3 in approximately 80 per cent of children with ITP. Among those children whose thrombocytopenia ultimately proves to be chronic, platelet counts are often slightly higher when first seen (20,000 to 75,000 cells per mm^3). With the introduction of automated instruments, new information on platelet volume measurements have become available and may prove helpful in the differential diagnosis of the thrombocytopenic states (78). Although thrombocytopenia is evident on peripheral blood smear and is often accompanied by bizarrely shaped or giant forms (Fig. 42–7), the mean platelet volume (MPV) may not always be elevated in acute ITP. In a study of thrombocytopenia in childhood, Tomita and associates demonstrated that although in chronic ITP both MPV and per cent large platelets were significantly increased over control values, these parameters remained essentially unchanged in the acute form (79). It should however be remembered that reproducibility is less optimal in the low platelet range (80–82). In contrast to the findings in ITP, the presence of a low or normal MPV suggests an aregenerative thrombocytopenia: i.e., bone marrow suppression or a marrow infiltrative process (83). The degree of platelet heterogeneity, effectively measured by the platelet distribution width (PDW), may be more discriminating than the MPV in the detection of a compensated thrombolytic state (78).

The total leucocyte count is usually normal, although a mild to moderate lymphocytosis is not uncommon (73). Mild peripheral eosinophilia may occur in 20 per cent of children but this finding bears no relationship to prognosis. Atypical lymphocytes may be noted, suggesting a concomitant viral infection. The hemoglobin is usually normal in a child with acute ITP; rarely, children with ITP, especially those with the chronic form, will manifest a coexisting autoimmune hemolytic anemia. Leukoerythroblastic or microangiopathic

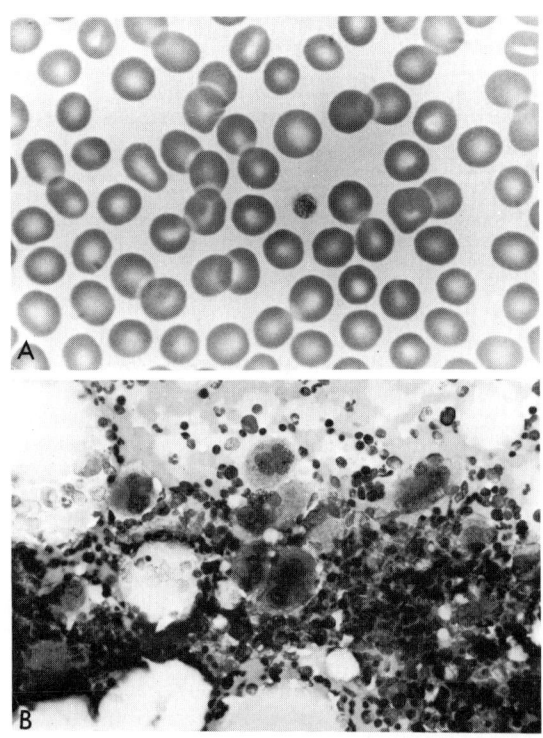

Figure 42–7. *A*, Peripheral blood smear from a child with ITP, showing a single large platelet. *B*, Smear from a bone marrow aspirate from a child with ITP. Megakaryocytes are present in increased numbers.

changes do not occur in ITP, and their presence should alert the physician to other diagnoses, such as marrow infiltrative disease, the hemolytic uremic syndrome, or thrombotic thrombocytopenic purpura.

The typical presentation of ITP is sufficiently clear that a bone marrow evaluation is redundant. Usually this presentation involves the acute onset of bruising in a previously healthy youngster following a viral infection and the appearance of megathrombocytes on the peripheral blood smear. However bone marrow examination may be necessary to rule out aplastic anemia in cases of thrombocytopenia of a more insidious onset. Marrow examination has also been advised prior to the initiation of corticosteroid therapy for presumed ITP, since the use of the latter drug could potentially mask the presence of acute lymphoblastic leukemia. In a recently published survey, 74 per cent of practicing pediatric hematologists-oncologists performed a bone marrow evaluation for classic-onset ITP while 26 per cent did not (84). Besides the reasons enumerated previously, another important consideration (given by 46 per cent) was to allay parental anxiety regarding the possibility of a more sinister underlying condition. It is, however, extremely unlikely that a child with acute leukemia would present with isolated thrombocytopenia and a completely normal physical examination (85).

Bone marrow aspirate should reveal a normocellular marrow with normal erythroid and myeloid maturation. Megakaryocytes are easily identified and are present in usually increased, but at least normal, numbers (Fig. 42-7). It is debatable whether megakaryocyte morphology is helpful in the diagnosis—some investigators report that in ITP megakaryocytes are more basophilic and less mature (68). It should be noted that examination of the marrow will not distinguish ITP from other forms of platelet destruction, including drug-induced and other immune-mediated thrombocytopenic disorders.

Coagulation tests (prothrombin time, partial thromboplastin time, thrombin time, and assays for fibrin degradation products) are normal in ITP. These tests are not necessary in straightforward cases, although they may be appropriate if microangiopathic processes (hemolytic-uremic syndrome or disseminated intravascular coagulation) are being seriously considered in the differential diagnosis of ITP. The bleeding time is prolonged in a child with petechiae and purpura and consequently measurement of it is seldom indicated in a child with the acute illness. However in some relatively asymptomatic patients with thrombocytopenia, a bleeding time can be of help in making management decisions. Rarely, patients with mild chronic ITP manifest antibody-induced platelet dysfunction (86, 87). These individuals will have markedly prolonged bleeding times despite near normal platelet counts. In such individuals the near normal count could convey a sense of false security, and a bleeding time estimation would be of benefit in assessing the need for future therapeutic intervention. In contrast, patients with a normal bleeding time and no clinical evidence of hemostatic impairment probably do not need treatment irrespective of their platelet count.

The measurement of platelet-associated IgG (PAIgG) is described in detail in the appendix at the end of this chapter. Measurement of platelet-associated IgG can be a useful adjunct in the investigation of a patient with suspected acute ITP. The test is positive in approximately 85 per cent of thrombocytopenic children with ITP (88). However, it should be remembered that PAIgG is also elevated in many other immune thrombocytopenic disorders and hence the specificity of the test for ITP is low—less than 50 per cent. As noted in the appendix, this low specificity should *not* be interpreted to indicate that PAIgG is a nonspecific findings. Rather, PAIgG is elevated in many different thrombocytopenic states. The *diagnostic* implications are thus disappointing—to date there is no diagnostic laboratory test for ITP. However, the *biologic* implications of the demonstration of elevated PAIgG in many thrombocytopenic disorders are exciting and imply that immune mechanisms contribute to many more thrombocytopenic disorders than hitherto appreciated. In summary, measurement of platelet-associated IgG can be helpful in the diagnosis of ITP: a positive test is consistent with but not diagnostic of ITP; a negative test makes the diagnosis much less likely.

Over the past 5 years, platelet survival studies using the radioisotope ^{111}indium (^{111}In) have become available. Previously, ^{51}chromium was the isotope used for platelet radiolabeling, but it had several major disadvantages including a very low labeling efficiency (less than 5 per cent), a low percentage of gamma photon emissions, and a long half-life (27.8 days). In contrast, ^{111}In produces a large amount of gamma emissions (greater than 100 per cent), has a short half-life (2.8 days), and most importantly, has a very high labeling efficiency. Consequently, an autologous platelet survival can be performed using platelets collected from thrombocytopenic children.

There are characteristic patterns of platelet recovery and survival that allow one to classify the thrombocytopenic disorders. For example, an immune thrombocytopenic disorder such as acute ITP is characterized by a near normal platelet recovery but a very short platelet survival; hypersplenism is characterized by a markedly reduced platelet recovery with a near normal platelet survival; aregenerative thrombocytopenia is characterized by a near normal platelet recovery with a near normal platelet survival (89–93). Although not routinely performed in acute ITP, a homologous platelet survival may be extremely useful in the case of insidious-onset thrombocytopenia where differentiation of chronic ITP from a hereditary thrombocytopenic disorder is difficult. Concomitant with the decrease in platelet survival in ITP, there is a corresponding increase in platelet production by the bone marrow. Whether this increase in platelet production is entirely effective, or whether there is a component of ineffective production or intramedullary destruction is a matter of debate. While some investigators have reported that platelet turnover is approximately five times normal in ITP (94), others have noted that platelet turnover may be normal to only twice normal (93, 95–97). Impairment of platelet production may be related to antibody cytotoxic effects (57).

The collection of acute and convalescent sera samples for measurement of viral titres can be helpful in retrospectively knowing whether a viral infection precipitated the ITP. Viruses most frequently associated with ITP are rubella, rubeola, varicella, mumps, infectious mononucleosis, hepatitis, and cytomegalovirus. Serologic studies for rubella should be obtained even in the absence of characteristic clinical manifestations of this viral infection (98). Because the monospot test may give a false negative result in a young child, Epstein-Barr titers should be obtained if infectious mononucleosis is suspected (99).

In a small percentage (about 3 per cent) of cases of childhood ITP, the thrombocytopenia is the first sign of an autoimmune disorder that can manifest itself months to years later. Autoimmune disorders that follow childhood ITP include systemic lupus erythematosus, autoimmune hemolytic anemia, hyperthyroidism, rheumatoid arthritis, and nephritis (68). Consequently, if the ITP is atypical and has an insidious onset, or develops in an older child, other investigations should be performed including the direct and indirect antiglobulin tests, antinuclear antibody and other tissue autoantibody measurements, quantitative immunoglobulins, and thyroid function studies. Isohemagglutinins are easily evaluated and may provide an initial differentiating feature in the rare case of Wiskott-Aldrich syndrome that masquerades as chronic ITP.

PROGNOSIS AND MANAGEMENT

Natural History. A rational approach to therapy in ITP has to be based on a knowledge of the natural history of the disease in childhood, and any intervention can be made only after balancing the risks of treatment against the risks of no treatment. This is an especially important consideration for childhood ITP because most children who present with this illness will have a complete remission without therapy and without sequelae. Table 42–3 is a summary of data available on the course of this disorder in 1123 children after varying periods of observation (67, 69, 71, 73–75, 100). Between 70 and 90 per cent of children with ITP will achieve a complete and permanent recovery in the absence of any specific therapy. In fact, if one excludes from analysis children with clinically established chronic ITP at the time of initial evaluation, the rate of complete recovery approximates 90 per cent. Of the patients who recover, 55 to 75 per cent do so within the first month of their illness, and 80 to 90 per cent do so within 4 to 6 months (Table 42–3). In contrast, children who present with chronic ITP are less likely to remit. Walker and co-workers (75) reported that only about a third of these children will remit spontaneously, the remissions usually occurring late in the course of the illness (81 per cent remitted between 1 and >10 years after presentation) (Table 42–3).

The diagnosis of chronic ITP is reserved for those patients who continue to have a platelet count of less than 100,000 cells per mm^3 6 months or more after the onset of their illness. From Table 42–3 it will be seen that (depending on the period of follow-up achieved in an individual patient cohort) of the children who ultimately recover spontaneously, 10 per cent do so between 6 months and more than 10 years after diagnosis. This observation is an important one in planning therapy since hitherto it has been a commonly held assumption that spontaneous recovery after the initial 6 month period was rare. Following the return of the platelet count to normal levels, recurrent episodes of thrombocytopenia occur in 1 to 4 per cent of patients (Table 42–3). Recurrence may follow episodes of presumed viral infection and usually remit spontaneously. In general, children with a history of illness within 6 weeks prior to the onset of purpura have a shorter clinical course, and it has been suggested that children whose purpura follows a known viral exanthem almost never develop chronic ITP (73).

Mortality in all recent series has been in the 0 to 1 per cent range with an overall frequency of 0.43 per cent. Deaths have resulted primarily from intracranial hemorrhage, gastrointestinal bleeding, or postsplenectomy sepsis. Although the initial weeks after diagnosis of acute ITP are the period of greatest risk for hemorrhagic complications, serious bleeding is not confined to this interval and can occur at any time after disease onset in the face of persistent thrombocytopenia of less than 20,000 cells per mm^3.

Intracranial Hemorrhage. Intracranial hemorrhage (ICH) is the most devastating complication of childhood ITP. Although it is extremely rare, (recent studies place the risk at less than 1 per cent), the grave implications of this side effect require a detailed discussion. It is likely that the

Table 42–3. NATURAL COURSE OF CHILDHOOD ITP—A COMPILATION OF DATA ON 1123 EVALUABLE PATIENTS

Factors	Lusher et al. (66, 73, 74)	Choi & McClure (67, 68)		Benham & Taft (100)		Simons et al. (71)	Lammi & Lovric (69)	Walker & Walker (64, 75)
		Treated[b]	Untreated	Treated	Untreated			
Patients in survey	465	239		132		95	177	181
Patients evaluable	453	161		96		84	152	177
Patients with chronic ITP at initial evaluation excluded	Yes	NA[a]		NA		No	NA	No (onset acute in 132 and chronic in 45)
Patients treated with steroids	35 (all prior to 1972)	80		75		27	40	47 (acute cases)
Untreated patients	418	20		21		20	112	63 (acute cases)
Recovery:	Median time to recovery was 3 weeks in the untreated and 4 weeks in the treated group	64%	75%	54%	63%	By day 9 a significantly greater number in the treated group had a platelet count of >25,000	Mean duration of illness was 46.5 days and 46 days in untreated and treated groups respectively	92% acute
0–1 mo								75% in 3 mo
1–4 mo		26%	15%	23%	26%			12% in 3–6 mo
>4 mo		10%	10%	23%	11%			5% in 6–12 mo
								8% in 1 to >10 yr
								36% chronic / 19% in 3 mo
								81% in 1 to >10 yr
Recovery rate (usually a platelet count >100,000 within 6 mo of onset)	85%	65 to 75%[c]		74%		60%[d]	70%	78%
Chronicity (platelet count <100,000 at 6 mo)	11%	21 to 30%[c]		26%		36%[d]	4% (remissions occurred >6 mo from diagnosis)	22%[e]
Longest interval before spontaneous recovery	<6 mo	5 yr		NA		NA	3½ yr	>10 yr
Recurrence	18/453 (4%)	6/161 (3.8%)		NA		3/84 (3.6%)	2/152 (1.3%)	NA
Patients splenectomized	NA	27		17		11	8	32
Splenectomy response (complete and partial)	81%	17/22 (77%)		78% at 1 yr / 50% at 4 yr		9/11 (82%)	7/8 (88%)	24/32 (75%)
Postsplenectomy infections	NA	0/22 (0%)		0/17 (0%)		0/11 (0%)	NA	1/32 (3%)
Predictive value of response to steroids in determining success of splenectomy	None	NA		±		None	NA	None
Mortality from ITP	0/453 (0%)[f]	1/161 (0.6%)		0/132 (0%)		1/84 (1.2%)	1/152 (0.7%)	2/177 (1.1%)

[a]NA = data not available or not evaluable.
[b]Treated = group treated with corticosteroid therapy; untreated = group without corticosteroid therapy.
[c]Patients who recovered quickly were lost to follow-up. A more realistic figure for acute cases would be closer to 180/239 (75%). Similarly, the percentage of chronic cases would be closer to 49/239 (21%).
[d]Lower remission figures and increased rate of chronic ITP are due to the fact that patients with clinically established chronic ITP at the time of initial evaluation were included in analysis.
[e]In the Walker study, interval between diagnosis and follow-up is from 3 to 35 years (mean 16.4 years). Only 8% are persistently thrombocytopenic.
[f]In this survey, 3 children with intracranial hemorrhage were excluded from the final analysis.

high frequency of ICH reported in the early studies was due to the incorrect diagnosis of other disorders such as disseminated intravascular coagulation, hemolytic uremic syndrome, and thrombotic thrombocytopenic purpura as ITP (63, 64).

Table 42–4 presents an analysis of all reported cases of ICH in childhood ITP (67–71, 73–75, 100–104). All of these children had a platelet count of less than 20,000 cells per mm^3 at the time of hemorrhage. Eight children were receiving corticosteroid therapy while fourteen were not. Additional risk factors beyond the thrombocytopenia could be identified in many of the children. For example, in three of the children on steroid therapy the intracranial hemorrhage followed head trauma; one child had severe hypertension, possibly induced by high-dose corticosteroid therapy for a prolonged period of time. Injudicious high-dose steroids for long intervals could prove to be more of a liability than an asset. Other children had recently ingested aspirin, a medication that inhibits platelet function and consequently increases the risk of bleeding (103). There is no obvious "high risk time" for intracranial hemorrhage. Although eight of the reported cases occurred during the first month following diagnosis, an equal number presented 1 to 6 months later and another episode occurred 5 years later.

Estimates of Clinical Severity. Some authors have attempted to estimate the clinical severity of ITP. However the therapeutic relevance of such a classification is uncertain. Although one group of investigators (70) reported that five of six patients who subsequently developed ICH had hematuria, epistaxis, and/or gastrointestinal bleeding, it should be noted that the vast majority of children with these hemostatic finding do not have an intracranial bleed. Nonetheless, the physician should recognize that the child with a trivial hemostatic impairment such as rare cutaneous petechiae will have a lower risk of serious bleeding than the patient who presents with petechiae, purpura, hematuria, and retinal hemorrhages. Approximately 3 to 4 per cent of children with ITP fall into this latter category (73).

Treatment of the Acute Phase

Defensive Management. During the initial period following the onset of ITP, restriction of physical activity and complete avoidance of all contact sports and playground activities are indicated, particularly in the older child. In the younger child, especially one less than 5 years of age, some physicians advise hospitalization and bed rest for the first few days of the illness until the bleeding manifestations subside (73, 74). This policy is not standard practice at many institutions including our own, since there is no indication that the hospital is a safer place than home for the thrombocytopenic child (105). All medications with antiplatelet activity should be avoided including aspirin, antihistamines, phenothiazines, and glyceryl guaiacolate. Vaccinations, especially those using live viruses, and intramuscular injections should not be given during the period of thrombocytopenia. Recent reports suggest that an increase in hematocrit to above 30 per cent shortens the bleeding time in patients with defective platelet function (106, 107). Thus, in any patient with ITP in whom bleeding has caused a drop in hemoglobin to below 9 to 10 g per dl, a replacement packed red cell transfusion may be indicated.

Corticosteroid Therapy

Although acute ITP is a common condition, with the average pediatrician seeing several cases per year, it is surprising that the decision whether or not to intervene therapeutically with corticosteroids has never been entirely resolved. Indeed, this has been, and continues to be, an area of considerable debate with knowledgeable clinicians reviewing the same information and reaching opposite conclusions. For example, within the past few years one of two groups of workers reviewing the same literature concluded that corticosteroids were indicated (108) while the other decided they were not (74). The following section presents a brief review of various theoretical observations on the effects of corticosteroids on platelet-vascular and antigen-antibody interactions. Later, the clinical trials that have been performed will be summarized (Table 42–5).

Theoretical Basis for Corticosteroid Therapy. Corticosteroids have many different effects and their predominant mechanism of action remains uncertain. They have been shown to increase the platelet life span in ITP (96), an effect that could be due to dissociation of antibody from the platelets or to blocking of reticuloendothelial cell function. Corticosteroids have been demonstrated in vitro to inhibit the phagocytosis of antibody-sensitized platelets by splenic macrophages (109). However, it is likely that the major effect of corticosteroids is to suppress antibody production by B lymphocytes and bone marrow (110a, b). There are other, more theoretical effects of corticosteroid therapy including the potential benefit on capillary integrity (111–114). It has been suggested that platelets perform an "endothelial supporting function" (115). One group of investigators (116) reported endothelial thinning in experimental thrombocytopenia resulting in increased vascular permeability. They also reported the presence of abnormal pores and fenestration in capillary endothelium from thrombocytopenic animals and suggested that corticosteroids could reverse these endothelial abnormalities (117). However, other investigators have been unable to confirm endothelial ultrastructural differences between experimentally induced thrombocytopenic animals and controls (118, 119). Thinning of capillary endothelium has

Table 42–4. AN ANALYSIS OF THE REPORTED CASES OF INTRACRANIAL HEMORRHAGE (ICH) IN CHILDHOOD ITP

Factors	Walker & Walker (75)[a]	Lusher et al. (66, 73, 74)	Choi & McClure (66, 68, 101)	Benham & Taft (100)	Simons et al. (71)	Lammi & Lovric (69)	Zerella et al. (70)	Lightsey et al. (102)	Woerner et al. (103)	Imbach et al. (104)
Numbers of children with ICH	1/181 (0.5%)	0/465 (0%)[b]	6/413 (1.4%)	2/132 (1.5%)	1/95 (1.1%)	1/152 (0.7%)	6/183 (3.3%)	1	3[c]	1/108 (0.9%)
Numbers of children evaluated	Cases of ITP seen 1950–1980	Consecutive newly diagnosed cases from 1961–1982	Cases of ITP seen 1950–1975	Cases of ITP seen 1958–1966	Consecutive cases of ITP from 1956–1973	Consecutive cases of ITP from 1963–1973	All cases of ITP admitted to Cincinnati Children's Hospital	None	None	Prospective evaluation of all cases of acute ITP from 28 European centers. All children randomized to corticosteroid or IV IgG
Platelet count at onset of symptoms	<20,000 (1)		<20,000 (5) NA (1)[d]	NA	<20,000 (1)	NA	<20,000 (6)	<20,000 (1)	<20,000 (3)	NA
Antecedent history of trauma		None	1/6	0/2	0/1	0/1	2/6	None	1/3	None
Numbers of patients receiving corticosteroids when ICH occurred		1/1	0/6	1/2[e]	0/1	0/1	4/6	1/1	1/3	0/1
Interval between diagnosis of ITP and ICH		<1 mo (1)	<1 mo (2) 1–6 mo (3) >6 mo (1)	NA (1) 1–6 mo (1)	<1 mo (1)	>6 mo (1)	<1 mo (2) 1–6 mo (3) >6 mo (1)	1–6 mo (1)	<1 mo (2) >6 mo (1)	<1 mo (1)
Mortality due to ICH		0/1	2/6	0/2	1/1	1/1	2/6	0/1	1/3	1/1

[a]Indicates chapter reference.
[b]Three children with ICH excluded from analysis (#1 moribund on admission; #2 a 13-year-old girl with vasculitis later diagnosed as lupus; #3 a child with chronic ITP).
[c]Two of three children reported by Woerner had ingested acetylsalicylic acid within 48 hours prior to their ICH.
[d]NA = data not available.
[e]Inappropriate use of steroids, 60 mg per day for 2 months, with ? steroid-related hypertension.

Table 42-5. SUMMARY OF CLINICAL TRIALS EVALUATING CORTICOSTEROID THERAPY IN ACUTE CHILDHOOD ITP

First Author and Year Study Reported (Reference)	Study Design	Entry Criteria	Mean Entry Platelet Count	Duration of ITP Before Treatment	Entrants and Treatment Allocation	Corticosteroid Treatment	Outcome and Comments
Sartorius 1984 (123)	Prospective; double-blind	Age 6 mo to 16 years Platelet count <100,000 per mm^3 Exclusion of other causes for thrombocytopenia	14,600 cells per mm^3	Not stated	73 evaluable entrants Prednisolone, n = 42 Placebo, n = 31	Prednisolone, 60/mg/m^2/day for 21 days	The treatment group had a significantly faster rise in platelets to safe levels. Ninety % of corticosteroid-treated compared to 45% of placebo-treated children attained a "safe" platelet count of 30,000 cells per mm^3 within 10 days. The treated group also demonstrated more rapid improvement in platelet/vessel interaction as tested by a negative Rumpel-Leede test. The large percentage (22%) of nonevaluable entrants is of concern.
Buchanan and Holtkamp 1984 (124)	Prospective; double-blind	Age <10 years Illness of <7 days duration	10,000 cells per mm^3	<7 days	27 entrants Prednisone, n = 13 Placebo, n = 14	Prednisone, 2 mg/kg/day for 14 days, then tapered over 7 days	The treatment group had a trend towards higher platelet counts and reduced bleeding (normal bleeding time) from day 1 to 2 that reached statistically significant levels by day 7. It is possible that larger numbers of entrants may have allowed a significant difference in the treatment group to be demonstrated even earlier in therapy.
McWilliams and Mauer 1979 (72,125)	Prospective; randomized	Illness of <14 days	About 20,000 cells per mm^3	<14 days	27 entrants Prednisone, n = 13 Placebo, n = 14	Prednisone, 2 mg/kg/day for 3 weeks	The treatment group had a significantly shorter time to normalization (>150,000 cell per mm^3) of the platelet count (n = 21 days) compared with the control group (n = 60 days).
Lusher et al. 1966, 1984 (66, 74)	Retrospective, but included consecutive patients	Not stated	Usually below 20,000 cells per mm^3	Not stated	No corticosteroids, n = 276; Corticosteroids, n = 35	Varying doses, usually 2–3 mg per kg per day.	The median and mean interval from onset of therapy (or no therapy) to a normal platelet count was very similar for both the corticosteroid and the untreated group (median of 3 to 4 weeks). However, information is not provided as to whether there is a difference in the interval by which time the patient had achieved a *safe* platelet count (≥30,000 cells per mm^3).

Benham and Taft 1972 (100)	Retrospective, analysis of 132 cases	Age 6 mo to 14 yr	Median platelet count of 30,000 cells per mm^3 in corticosteroid group and 35,000 cells per mm^3 in nonsteroid group	89 patients (67%) had symptoms for <1 mo	No corticosteroids, n = 19 (evaluable cases) Corticosteroids (started within 4 days of diagnosis), n = 76	Not stated	Four of 19 untreated patients had a platelet count rise to above 100,000 cells per mm^3 within 7 days, and 12 had the platelets rise to 100,000 cells per mm^3 within 1 month. Eight of 76 patients given corticosteroids had a platelet count rise to above 100,000 cells per mm^3 within 7 days, and in 36 it occurred within 1 month. In the untreated group cessation of bleeding manifestations took 5 days, compared to 3.5 days in those given corticosteroids.
Lammi and Lovric 1973 (69)	Retrospective, but included consecutive patients	Platelet count <100,000 cells per mm^3. Age 4 mo to 13 yr	Usually <50,000 cells per mm^3	Not stated	No corticosteroids, n = 112 Corticosteroids, n = 40	Not stated	There was no difference in the duration of the thrombocytopenia or the rate of amelioration of acute bleeding manifestations in the corticosteroid compared to the nontreated group. Irrespective of the therapy, approximately 70% of all children recovered within 6 months. Most of the other children had a spontaneous recovery within the next few years. However, this study is difficult to evaluate because of missing data.
Walker and Walker 1984 (75)	Retrospective, with matched historical controls	Unexplained thrombocytopenia Age 4 mo to 15 yr	Not stated	Not stated	No corticosteroids, n = 63 Corticosteroids, n = 47	Not stated	Eighty-five per cent of the prednisone-treated patients recovered spontaneously compared with 92% of the untreated patients. The time for recovery was the same for both groups. Data allowing for a careful analysis of the results were not provided.
Simons et al. 1975 (71)	Retrospective, but including consecutive patients	Illness of <14 days Children <10 years	Not stated	<14 days	No corticosteroids, n = 20 Prednisone, n = 27	Varying dosage and preparations	The treatment group had a trend towards higher platelet counts from day 2 to 3 that achieved significance by day 9. The report is difficult to evaluate because of varying steroid doses and missing data. There was no difference between treated and untreated children in eventual outcome.

recently been confirmed in human thrombocytopenic states, with reversal following steroid therapy (119a). Other potential effects of corticosteroids include the normalization or reduction of the prolonged bleeding time in the thrombocytopenic animal model, a finding probably related to the inhibition of vascular prostacyclin synthesis by corticosteroids (120, 121).

Clinical Trials. First, it should be emphasized that statistically it is not possible to perform a randomized trial in which the endpoint is the reduction of death due to intracranial hemorrhage. For example, Krivit and associates (122) estimated that if the true frequency of intracranial hemorrhage was approximately 1 per cent and corticosteroids were 50 per cent effective in preventing ICH, then a randomized trial of corticosteroids versus placebo would require some 14,000 patients to demonstrate efficacy. Hence, one cannot criticize a study that does not demonstrate a reduction in intracranial hemorrhage. But that is not to say that treatment with corticosteroids could not prevent the ICH; it says only that statistically it would be virtually impossible to demonstrate this effectiveness. Consequently, one must use as endpoints the rate of return of the platelet count to safe (>20,000 to 30,000 cells per mm^3) or normal levels, or alternatively the correction of a hemostatic test such as the bleeding time. Another important principle is that if a study contains only small numbers of entrants, then often a statistically significant difference cannot be demonstrated, not because of lack of efficacy of the treatment but merely because of limited numbers.

In considering the data for and against corticosteroids, the studies will be ranked in order of reliability—i.e., in ability to give the "truth." For example, a double-blind randomized trial is more likely to be correct than a nonblinded randomized trial since the former eliminates physician and patient bias. Similarly, a prospective study is more likely to give the "truth" than a retrospective study. This is especially true for an illness such as acute ITP, since there is a tendency for physicians to intervene with therapy (in this case corticosteroids) in patients with more severe disease. Hence, any retrospective study is almost always biased in that those patients with the most severe disease are more likely to receive treatment, and as a result, this group may have a less positive outcome, not because they received the treatment but because they had more severe disease prior to therapy.

Prospective Studies

DOUBLE-BLIND RANDOMIZED TRIALS. There have been two double-blind randomized trials (123, 124; Table 42–5). In the first, 73 children less than 16 years of age with acute ITP were randomized to receive prednisolone (60 mg per m^2 for 21 days) (n=42), or placebo (n=31). The platelet count at entry was identical in both groups (15,000 cells per mm^3) and the groups were otherwise comparable. The group that received corticosteroid therapy had a significantly faster rise in platelet count and a significantly faster return of hemostasis to normal, as assayed by the Rumpel-Leede test. This study (123) is open to criticism because of the large number of entrants who did not complete the study (of 93 initial entrants only 73 were evaluable).

The second double-blind prospective study was performed by Buchanan and associates (124). In this study, 27 children younger than 10 years of age with acute ITP of less than 7 days' duration were randomized to prednisone (2 mg per kg per day for 2 weeks, then tapered over the third week) (n=13) or an identical placebo in the same dosage schedule (n=14). It is important to note that bleeding times were performed in this study. The investigators demonstrated that a significant decrease in bleeding time and an increase in the platelet count occurred only at day 7 for the corticosteroid-treated children. However, it is of interest that there was a consistent but nonsignificant trend to a higher platelet count and shorter bleeding times in the corticosteroid group compared with the placebo group during the first 2 weeks. Thus, it is possible that had the study group been larger, a more significant difference would have been obtained.

NONBLINDED RANDOMIZED STUDIES. McWilliams (72, 125) reported a nonblinded study of children with acute ITP (duration of disease < 14 days) who were randomized to receive prednisone at a dose of 2 mg per kg per day for 3 weeks (13 children) or no therapy (14 children). The median time to the normalization of the platelet count (defined as a rise to >150,000 cells per mm^3) was significantly shorter in the corticosteroid group (day 21) compared with the control group (day 60). Unfortunately, not enough details are given about the study, the method of randomization, or the interval taken to achieve a "safe" platelet count to allow a critical analysis of the results.

SUMMARY. Two of the three prospective studies demonstrated a significantly more rapid return to normal of the platelet count and/or platelet function. The third study, while not demonstrating a consistently significant difference, demonstrated a clear trend toward benefit in the corticosteroid group. The results of all three studies were therefore similar.

Retrospective Studies

RETROSPECTIVE STUDIES OF CONSECUTIVE CASES. Simons and co-workers (71) described the outcome of 104 consecutive patients with ITP seen over a 7-year period. A total of 47 children less than 10 years of age who presented with ITP of less than 2 weeks' duration were given either corticosteroids (27 patients) or no corticosteroids (20 patients). It should be emphasized that this was not a random allocation. The corticosteroid group achieved a significantly higher platelet count earlier than did the group who did not receive the therapy. Although there was a trend toward a higher platelet count in the corticosteroid group from day 2, a significant difference was achieved only at day 9 following treatment.

In a second study, Lammi and associates (69) described 152 consecutive cases of ITP managed by them over a 10-year period. Inclusion criteria included thrombocytopenia and an age of 4 months to 13 years. Forty children were treated with corticosteroids (neither the dose nor the preparation described) and 112 observed without therapy. The duration of thrombocytopenia was essentially identical in each group, and these investigators were unable to demonstrate that the corticosteroid therapy either shortened the duration of the disease or ameliorated the acute bleeding manifestations. The authors concluded that corticosteroid therapy did not influence the course, duration, or prognosis of the illness.

OTHER RETROSPECTIVE STUDIES. In 1966 and 1984, Lusher and colleagues (66, 74) reviewed their experience of children with ITP and noted that 35 had received corticosteroids whereas 276 had not. The control group took 3 weeks (median) from onset of thrombocytopenia to recovery, whereas the treated group took slightly longer at 4 weeks. The authors concluded that there was no apparent advantage to using corticosteroids. However, the very large difference in the size of the two groups suggests that there may have been some degree of selection; i.e., the more severely affected patients might have been more likely to receive corticosteroids. Also, information is not provided as to whether there was a difference in the time taken for the platelet count to reach a relatively safe level (>20,000 to 30,000 cells per mm^3), since as previously discussed (Table 42–4) it is at levels of less than 20,000 cells per mm^3 that serious bleeding is most likely to occur.

Benham and Taft (100) analyzed 19 evaluable children not given corticosteroids and compared their outcomes to those of 76 who were given corticosteroids within 4 days of diagnosis. Fifty-four per cent of the group who received corticosteroids had a platelet count above 100,000 cells per mm^3 within 1 month compared to 63 per cent of the group who received no therapy, a nonsignificant difference. However, these authors reported that the average time from diagnosis to cessation of bleeding manifestations was 4.9 days in the control group versus 3.5 days in those children treated with corticosteroid.

In 1984, Walker and Walker (75) described the outcome and follow-up in 181 children (ages 4 months to 15 years) who presented with unexplained thrombocytopenia. They obtained follow-up data on 177 children of whom 75 per cent were subsequently demonstrated to have acute disease. Forty-seven acute patients were treated with corticosteroids and their results were compared with those of 63 matched controls. Per cent recovery of the treated and untreated groups were similar (85 per cent versus 92 per cent), as was the time taken to recover.

SUMMARY. A careful analysis (Table 42–5) of these studies provides the following information: In those studies least likely to be affected by observer bias, patient selection, and negative reporting bias, there can be little doubt that corticosteroids restored the platelet count to safe levels more rapidly than did no treatment. None of the studies demonstrated a significant reduction in the development of chronic ITP nor prevention of intracranial hemorrhage through the use of corticosteroids. But as noted previously, because of the low frequency of this latter event, it would be statistically impossible to demonstrate efficacy given the sample sizes in all of the studies. Hence, one must conclude that corticosteroids will more rapidly raise the platelet count, and because severe thrombocytopenia represents a risk factor for intracranial hemorrhage, corticosteroids presumably may prevent this event. The clinician must then balance the risks of treatment against the benefits. Only a few of the studies specifically address the issue of whether corticosteroids themselves produce morbidity, and in those studies that did, few or no adverse effects were reported. But even the proponents of corticosteroids acknowledge that a transient recurrence of thrombocytopenia may occur in 20 to 25 per cent of children following discontinuation of therapy.

We favor a *selective* approach to therapy; i.e., the child, not the platelet count, should be treated (66). In children who present with a mild illness, no therapy other than purely defensive management appears necessary. We treat the child with severe thrombocytopenia and generalized petechiae and purpura, the patient with fundal or mucosal hemorrhage, and the active younger child (especially those less than 3 to 4 years of age). We use either steroids during the initial 2 to 3 weeks of the illness or intravenous IgG (see next section). Most proponents of steroid therapy administer prednisone at a dose of 2 mg per kg per day for 2 weeks followed by a taper over the third week. As the corticosteroids are being decreased, some patients will have a drop in their platelet count, but this is usually transitory and is generally not an indication for increasing the dose of steroids to previous levels. In the very severe clinical form of the disease an initial 4- to 5-day period of prednisone, at 4 mg per kg per day, may be tried, followed by a reduction in dosage thereafter to more conventional levels.

Steroid therapy *should not be given for long periods of time*. Sustained high-dose corticosteroids may themselves suppress platelet formation (126, 127). More importantly, long-term corticosteroids can have severe cosmetic effects and can limit growth, especially in the young child. Other adverse effects include pancreatitis, hyperglycemia, hypertension, fluid and electrolyte disturbances, and psychosis (128–130).

Intravenous Immunoglobulin

Immune serum globulin (ISG) has long been the treatment of choice for patients with hypogammaglobulinemia. In recent years, IgG has been used not only as an immune replacement, but also as an immune suppressant. Before summarizing some of the recent studies of this blood product as a treatment for acute ITP, we will highlight several issues concerning its use.

Development of Intravenous Preparations. All IV IgG preparations begin as immune serum globulin (ISG) prepared by Cohn fractionation. Immune serum globulin is a remarkably pure blood product, containing 95 to 98 per cent IgG and only 1 to 2 per cent IgA and IgM (131). There are other trace contaminants, including components of kallikrein-kinin and coagulation systems, but these are unimportant compared to the most important "contaminant"—IgG that has self-aggregated into immune complexes. The IgG–immune complexes probably are the reason why ISG produces severe anaphylactoid side effects when it is administered by the intravenous route (132). Over the past several years, techniques capable of removing the immune complexes from the ISG or preventing their formation have become available, and currently three such IV IgG preparations are licensed in North America. These include IgG preparations in which: (1) the IgG aggregates are prevented from forming by partial enzymatic digestion by pepsin (Sandoglobulin); (2) the IgG is partially digested with pepsin and the complexes removed by polyethylene glycol precipitation (Iveegam); and (3) immune complexes are prevented from forming by alteration of the IgG molecule by gentle reduction and alkalation (Gamimune). All of these preparations are essentially free (less than 10 per cent) of dimeric immune complexes and contain less than 1 per cent oligomeric complexes. These IgG preparations are well tolerated and large amounts can be given intravenously, allowing the serum concentration of IgG to be raised rapidly to normal or supernormal levels.

Adverse Effects. Side effects of IV IgG are of two types: those that are unique to IV IgG, and those that are common to any blood product. Adverse effects unique to ISG and IV IgG are side effects that are caused by the presence of IgG aggregates within the preparations. Indeed, the large amount of IgG–oligomeric complexes within ISG is the reason why this product produces severe anaphylactoid reactions typical of complement activation when infused intravenously (132). The modification of ISG to remove IgG–immune complexes has greatly reduced the frequency of these side effects. Although some investigators have suggested that vasoactive contaminants within the IV IgG preparations could contribute to these reactions (133, 134), increasing evidence suggests that the IgG complexes within the IV IgG preparations are themselves responsible for the adverse effects (135).

Because of their subjective nature, it is difficult to define the precise frequency of many of the side effects of IV IgG, but a reasonable estimate is that approximately 5 to 20 per cent of patients treated with IV IgG will have some type of reaction including headache, nausea, and occasionally fever. The side effects are more likely to occur in hypogammaglobulinemic patients and appear to be dose dependent (135). Fatal thrombotic events have been described in two elderly patients treated with intravenous immunoglobulin for autoimmune thrombocytopenia (135a).

Side effects of IV IgG that are common to the infusion of any blood product include the risk of infection. However, it should be emphasized that the risk of transmitting a viral infection via IV IgG is extremely low. Gammaglobulin is prepared from pooled plasma that is treated with ethanol, and viral antigens tend not to be recovered during this fractionation (136–139). Nonetheless, hepatitis B can be transmitted by ISG and, theoretically, by IV IgG (140–147). Non-A, non-B hepatitis also can be transmitted by IV IgG, but again the risk is very low (148, 149). However, it might be higher than the risk of transmitting hepatitis B infection because the general population has little viral neutralizing antibody against non-A, non-B hepatitis (149). Other side effects include the passive transmission of anti–red cell alloantibodies (150, 151).

Mechanism of Action. There is no doubt that the administration of IV IgG produces an initial rapid response in the majority (75 per cent) of children with acute or chronic ITP. However, there is debate as to the mechanism of efficacy of IV IgG in raising the platelet count. Increasing evidence suggests that IV IgG preparations are effective in immune thrombocytopenic disorders because they compete with the IgG-sensitized platelets for the Fc binding sites on the monocytes and macrophages. For IgG-sensitized platelets to be cleared by the cells of the reticuloendothelial system, unoccupied Fc binding sites on the RE cells must bind to the Fc portion of the IgG molecules. The attachment of a number of platelet-IgG molecules to the Fc binding sites on the RE cells results in the ingestion of the IgG-sensitized platelet by the RE cells. Following the infusion of high doses of IV IgG, there is an immediate rise in the serum concentration of IgG to two to three times normal levels. Consequently, the IgG-sensitized platelets cannot be cleared by the RE cells because the Fc receptors on the RE cells are already saturated by monomeric IgG (Fig. 42–4).

Another theory that has been proposed to explain the efficacy of IV IgG as an immunosuppressant is the anti-idiotypic theory. An IgG molecule binds to a specific antigen by its Fab terminus. The extreme variability of this terminus produces a unique three dimensional shape that not only allows it to bind to one single antigen but also allows this part of the antibody itself to act as an antigen, a property termed the antibody's idiotype. An antibody directed against the antigen-combining portion of another immunoglobulin molecule is said to have anti-idiotypic activity. The production of anti-antibodies (anti-idiotypes) is considered to be one method by which individuals control their immune response. For example, following stimulation by an antigen, an antibody is formed that binds specifically to that particular antigen. It has been suggested that the immune system then produces an anti-idiotypic antibody that is directed against the initial antibody, and this second antibody functions to suppress idiotype-bearing B lymphocytes either directly or through inactivation of idiotype-bearing T lymphocytes. The anti-idiotype then triggers the generation of a subsequent anti–anti-idiotype, which in turn inactivates the anti-idiotypic T and B cells. Thus "concentric waves" of suppression-regulation occur, each wave becoming weaker until the immune system has been calmed. The anti-idiotypic theory of efficacy of IV IgG suggests that within the large amount of IgG that is administered to a patient during treatment, specific anti-idiotypic antibodies are found. These anti-idiotypes bind to, inactivate, and suppress the formation of antiplatelet autoantibodies. This hypothesis is illustrated schematically in Figure 42–4. Although this is an attractive model for explaining the efficacy of IV IgG, it remains at this time entirely hypothetical. Several other theories of efficacy of IV IgG have been proposed and are reviewed elsewhere (135).

Treatment Modalities. For a number of years, different investigators have suggested that plasma or IgG could raise the platelet count in patients with immune thrombocytopenia (152–154). It was suggested initially that this effect might be due to antiviral antibodies within the IgG preparation that would clear the viruses that might be triggering the ITP (155). Although this effect is unlikely in light of our present knowledge, the effectiveness of IV IgG in acute and chronic ITP is now apparent. Over the last several years, Imbach and co-workers have used this therapy in the treatment of children with acute or chronic ITP. In their initial report (156), they administered IV IgG (0.4 grams per kg per day for 5 days) to six children with acute ITP, inducing a "complete remission," defined as a platelet count of greater than 100,000 cells per mm^3 in four of the six patients within 3 weeks. Since 55 to 75 per cent of the children with acute ITP who recover do so within the first month of their illness, this reported response could have occurred independent of IgG usage. However, perusal of a more recent, detailed account of these six children (159) reveals that in all children in whom daily platelet counts were obtained during the initial 5-day infusion period, a rise in count to 30,000 to 180,000 cells per mm^3 (i.e., a safe range) was noted within 1 to 2 days following initiation of IgG therapy. Since the major goal in the treatment of the acute illness is to restore the platelet count to a relatively safe level as soon as possible, this study suggested that intravenous IgG might be useful in the treatment of acute ITP.

Subsequently, Bussel and co-workers (160) treated 25 children less than 16 years of age with acute ITP using IV IgG. Fifteen of the children were previously untreated, and ten had received prior corticosteroids without response. The children received an initial treatment of 1 gram per kg IV IgG daily up to a total of three consecutive daily doses followed by maintenance infusions as necessary. The response to the IV IgG was very rapid. A mean platelet count of 68,000 (range 8000 to 240,000 cells per mm^3) was attained within 24 hours of therapy.

Recently, Imbach and associates (104) described a randomized multicenter trial in which IV IgG was compared with oral corticosteroids in 94 children with untreated acute ITP. The children were randomized to receive corticosteroids (prednisone 60 mg per m^2 daily for 21 days), or IV IgG (0.4 grams per kg intravenously daily for 5 days). If the platelet count did not rise within the first 7 days, or fell below 30,000 cells per mm^3 during the following 14 days, the patient was crossed over to the other treatment arm. Forty-seven children received corticosteroids and 47 received IV IgG. The mean age (6 years) and the mean platelet count at presentation (9000 to 10,000 cells per mm^3) were the same for each group. Approximately 80 per cent of patients in each group responded to the therapy with a mean time to the peak platelet count of 12 days in the corticosteroid group versus 9 days for IV IgG. Thus, the effects of corticosteroids and IV IgG were identical for children who responded rapidly to treatment (62 per cent of all children). However, for individuals requiring more than an initial treatment, there was a better response if the child received IV IgG. (One fatality occurred: an 11-year-old girl with ITP who was treated with IV IgG for 3 days and then switched to corticosteroids when the platelet count did not rise.) Approximately 20 per cent of the children treated with IV IgG had some type of reaction including headache, fever, vomiting, and fatigue, but in most children, these reactions were trivial. Approximately 77 per cent of the children who received corticosteroids had increased body weight, acne, or some other side effect.

In summary, for many patients with acute ITP, IV IgG does not offer a major advantage over corticosteroids. However, there appears to be a subset of individuals who respond more rapidly to IV IgG. Unfortunately, to date there is no way to predict which child is best treated initially with this preparation.

There is one more factor that must be considered before IV IgG is used—its cost. The cost for a 5-day course of administration for a 20-kg child is approximately $4000 versus $10 for oral corticosteroids.

The Emergency Management of Bleeding

Fortunately, life-threatening bleeding in a child with ITP is rare. Bleeding is most serious when a vital organ such as the brain is the site of hemorrhage. Again it should be emphasized that the actual frequency of intracranial hemorrhage is very low, less than 1 per cent. However, when the patient presents with life-threatening bleeding, either externally or in a vital cavity, urgent treatment is needed to raise the platelet count as quickly as possible.

Initially, *general measures* should be directed at raising the platelet count. Since the antiplatelet antibody in ITP is directed against both autologous and homologous platelets, the *routine* use of platelet transfusions in acute ITP is not indicated, as the transfused platelets will have a very short life span in the recipient's circulation. Platelet transfusions, however, do play a limited role in this emergency situation, and a bolus infusion of 6 to 12 units (depending upon the size of the child) should be administered immediately, as they may exert hemostatic benefit before being cleared by the RE cells. Large doses of corticosteroids should also be started by the intravenous route (4 mg per kg per day of prednisone or its equivalent).

At one time, life-threatening bleeding was an indication for an emergency splenectomy. However, it is now possible to perform a "medical splenectomy" by the infusion of IV IgG. As noted in the previous section, IV IgG at a dose of 2 grams per kg administered intravenously over 2 days usually results in a very rapid rise in the platelet count. Nevertheless, due to the immediacy of the clinical situation, and since occasional patients may fail to respond to IV IgG within the first 24 hours (160, 161), some clinicians may still prefer to perform an emergency splenectomy because they believe that this surgical procedure may produce a more rapid rise in the platelet count than can be obtained with IV IgG. Preferences as to which therapy is better are based on clinical bias rather than reliable data.

The management of the patient who fails to respond to splenectomy or IV IgG is more difficult. Removal of the antibody by plasma exchange should be considered at this juncture. Although plasma exchange will produce a rise in the platelet count in some patients it is not always successful and consequently should not be undertaken as a first line of therapy.

Specific measures instituted will depend on the site of the hemorrhage. For example, a patient with a suspected intracranial hemorrhage should have emergency computed tomography to localize the site of bleeding. Neurosurgical consultation should be sought immediately since some lesions can be treated by surgical evacuation. One group of investigators have stressed that a conservative approach to posterior fossa hematomas may not be appropriate even in the patient who appears neurologically stable (103). They suggested that edema around such lesions could quite suddenly obliterate the fourth ventricle leading to acute hydrocephalus and brain stem compression. Other considerations in the management of the patient with ICH should include intravenous mannitol and intubation with hyperventilation if neurologic deterioration is precipitous and associated with a mass effect.

Since some cases of ICH have followed the use of aspirin (103), care should be taken to warn against the use of this drug in children with ITP.

Chronic Idiopathic Thrombocytopenic Purpura

Chronic ITP is defined as a platelet count that persists below 100,000 cells per mm^3 for 6 months or more. Depending upon the age and the sex of the child, as many as 10 to 20 per cent of all children with ITP will continue to remain thrombocytopenic, thus falling into this category (Table 42–3). Although the majority of these patients have persistent disease, a recent study indicated that approximately 20 per cent of patients with chronic ITP will ultimately make a spontaneous recovery (75). Unfortunately, it is not possible in the individual child to identify with certainty the factors that predict chronicity or spontaneous recovery.

Chronic ITP in children is similar to ITP in adults and is caused by autoantibodies against platelets (67, 73, 162, 163). The risk of chronicity is much greater in children who are over 10 years of age at diagnosis than in younger children, although ITP that will ultimately prove to be chronic can present at any age (71). Also, in contrast to acute ITP, in which there is often a history of antecedent viral infections, children with chronic ITP are much more likely to have an insidious onset of bruising without an antecedent infection. Although acute ITP affects both sexes equally, the majority of patients with chronic ITP are female (66–69, 71, 73, 100). Other factors distinguishing these two disorders are less certain.

For example, it has been suggested that the platelet count is slightly higher at presentation in chronic ITP (73–74). Also, a lower level of serum IgA at the time of onset of the ITP has been reported to be seen more often in the chronic disease (164). Finally, some investigators have reported that the level of platelet-associated IgG may help to differentiate children with acute versus chronic ITP (162, 163). Recent studies, however, suggest that this is extremely unlikely (165).

PATHOGENESIS

ITP is caused by an increased rate of platelet destruction by the cells of the RE system, especially the monocytes and macrophages of the spleen, bone marrow, and lungs, the histiocytes of the marrow, and the Kupffer cells of the liver. The "signal" for the platelet destruction by the RE cells is the increased amounts of IgG autoantibody on the platelet surface. Studies* by several groups of investigators have identified the platelet membrane targets of this autoantibody.

In 1951, Harrington and co-workers demonstrated that ITP was caused by an antiplatelet antibody in the serum of patients with this disorder (166, 167). These investigators showed that thrombocytopenia developed rapidly in healthy subjects following the infusion of plasma from patients with ITP. This study convincingly demonstrated that the platelet consumption was due to a serum factor and was not cell mediated. Subsequent investigators used in vitro techniques to show that the serum factor was IgG (these evaluations are summarized in the appendix at the end of this chapter). The origin of the IgG antiplatelet antibody was unknown until the studies of McMillan (168, 169) and Karpatkin (170), which demonstrated that splenic lymphocytes from patients with ITP produced an IgG autoantibody that bound to the platelet membrane.

The next issue to be defined was the target on the platelet membrane of the antiplatelet antibody. For example, theoretically the IgG antiplatelet antibody could bind to a plasma-adsorbed antigen or a platelet glycoprotein or might even bind as an immune complex. Part of this question was resolved by the studies of McMillian and associates (171) who demonstrated that the $F(ab^1)_2$ fraction of IgG (that component lacking the Fc portion) bound equally well to platelets and intact IgG. In other words, immune complex binding did not occur.

A short time later, several groups of investigators independently showed that the IgG antiplatelet antibody in patients with ITP was a specific antibody and was not due to IgG binding to circulating bacterial, viral, or plasma antigens that were adsorbed to the platelet surface. This was accomplished by demonstrating in direct binding assays that sera from patients with chronic ITP bind to specific platelet membrane glycoproteins, including IIb/IIIa and Ib (58–60, 172–175). While Beardsley and co-workers (60) found by immunoblot analysis that sera from most patients with chronic ITP contained antibodies that bound to glycoprotein IIIa, no similar finding was noted when the sera of eight children with acute ITP were concomitantly tested. This observation suggests that acute ITP probably has a different pathophysiology than chronic disease.

Although there is now virtually complete agreement that both childhood and adult chronic ITP are caused by the production of an antiplatelet antibody that binds to a specific glycoprotein on the platelet surface, many other questions remain unresolved. For example, why do certain patients produce this antiplatelet antibody whereas others do not? Predictably, investigators have looked for an HLA class 1 or class 2 association in patients with chronic ITP, since certain alloantigens may predispose a patient to either chronic infection or an abnormal immune response to a viral or bacterial antigen. However, an increased association of ITP with specific A, B, or C haplotypes (class 1 antigens) has not been convincingly demonstrated (176, 178). A report associating chronic ITP with the HLA-DRw2 alloantigen (179) has also been questioned (178, 180).

A variety of other lymphocytic or immunologic abnormalities have been described in patients with ITP (181–189). Some of the immediate family members of children with chronic ITP may also manifest a variety of immunologic deficits, including decreased T cell numbers, autoantibody formation, and abnormal in vitro responses to phytohemagglutinin (183–184). Similar findings and defective numbers or function of immunoregulatory lymphocytes have been observed in patients with active and chronic ITP (185–188). Finally, although there is considerable variability in the various lymphocyte subsets (OKT^4, OKT^8, OKT^3), mean values for mononuclear cells bearing these markers lie within the normal range (189). In essence, while the abnormalities of the humoral limb of ITP have been well defined, questions remain concerning the biologic relevance of the various abnormalities of the cellular limb of the immune response that have been observed to date.

Other aspects of the pathophysiology of chronic ITP remain unresolved; i.e., not all of the increased IgG on platelets from patients with chronic ITP is antiplatelet autoantibody (see the appendix to this chapter). Once it was thought that these results could be due in part to assay artifacts, but now it is known that these concerns were un-

---

*Some studies cited in this section are of adult chronic ITP; their data and conclusions are relevant to this discussion because adult and childhood chronic ITP appear to be the same disease.

founded, and one is left with the difficult-to-explain finding that not all of the elevated platelet-associated IgG represents true autoantibody. One hypothesis to explain this observation is that the binding of antiplatelet antibody to the platelet membrane produces abnormalities of the membrane that result in the secondary binding of plasma proteins.

Finally, the role of IgM antiplatelet antibodies and complement activation in the destruction of platelets from patients with ITP remains unresolved. Several groups have demonstrated increased platelet-bound IgM and complement in patients with chronic ITP. It is likely that just as a subset of cases of autoimmune hemolytic anemia are caused by IgM anti-red cell antibodies, some cases of ITP are caused by IgM antibody. The issue may be of considerable practical significance since complement-mediated cell clearance occurs primarily via the liver. Hence, splenectomy may not be successful in patients with IgM (complement)-mediated cell destruction.

DIAGNOSIS AND MANAGEMENT

Chronic ITP by definition is ITP that has persisted for over 6 months. Hence the diagnostic tests used for chronic ITP are similar to those used for the diagnosis of the acute illness. Several tests deserve special emphasis: First, in a patient in whom the diagnosis is uncertain, a platelet survival is very helpful since a normal ^{111}In or ^{51}chromium labeled autologous or homologous platelet survival excludes the diagnosis of chronic ITP (190–192). Other tests that should be performed include a complete blood count, platelet sizing, bone marrow examination, measurement of platelet-associated IgG, measurement of antinuclear and other autoantibody, and thyroid function studies. Some children present with thrombocytopenia of insidious onset and the clinician may be uncertain whether the patient has chronic ITP or another thrombocytopenic disorder such as a hereditary platelet abnormality. A description of the laboratory and clinical aspects of these various hereditary disorders is included later in this chapter.

The management strategies for children and adults with chronic ITP are changing. Once the platelet count was the main focus of attention, but in recent years, the emphasis has changed to include the overall impact of both *platelet count and function* on hemostasis. The strategy of treatment is to administer the least amount of therapy that will prevent bleeding. The emphasis upon hemostasis rather than the platelet count results from the recognition that the platelet count is but one measure of the contribution of platelets to overall hemostasis. The other, and equally important, aspect is platelet function. Some patients can have marked thrombocytopenia yet normal or near normal hemostasis because of better than expected platelet function. In fact, this is the rule rather than the exception for patients with ITP. The reason is that ITP is characterized by an increased proportion of "young," functionally active platelets. As a result, some patients with ITP can have no symptoms or signs of a bleeding disorder, a normal bleeding time, and no manifestations of excessive bleeding while remaining markedly thrombocytopenic (193, 194). In such patients, it would be difficult to justify aggressive therapy that itself could result in morbidity when they have no measurable defect with the exception of a low platelet count. On the other hand, there is a subgroup of patients (possibly as many as 5 per cent of all patients with chronic ITP) who have impaired platelet function presumably as a result of antibody-induced platelet dysfunction (195). In 1972, one group of investigators reported that platelets from certain patients with ITP had defective in vitro aggregation with restoration of normal function when the ITP remitted (196). Similar findings have been noted by other investigators not only in ITP but also in a variety of other secondary immune thrombocytopenic disorders, especially systemic lupus erythematosus (197–203).

Recently the platelet function defect has been studied in detail both in vitro and in vivo in a group of children with chronic ITP (86). Three of these patients had trivial thrombocytopenia (platelet count 89,000–136,000 cells per mm^3) with a marked prolongation of their bleeding time and an increased bleeding tendency. All patients demonstrated impaired biosynthesis of platelet thromboxane B$_2$. The reason for this defect in the cyclooxygenase pathway is not known, but it could be due to IgG-mediated steric inhibition of an agonist binding site or to the induction of partial platelet release by antiplatelet antibody. In another study, two individuals were described with chronic ITP, mild thrombocytopenia, yet markedly prolonged bleeding times (87). These patients had an IgG antiplatelet antibody that bound to platelet glycoprotein IIIa and interfered with the fibrinogen binding site on the IIb-IIIa glycoprotein complex.

In summary, although the platelet count is an important parameter to follow in patients with ITP, it does not give information about overall platelet function. We recommend the performance of the template bleeding time in all patients with chronic ITP prior to a decision regarding the necessity for further therapeutic intervention.

In the next section, the various therapeutic modalities that can be used in the management of chronic ITP are listed and some of their advantages and disadvantages described. Again, it should be emphasized that the goal of therapy is to provide the least amount of treatment that will result in a safe platelet count for a particular patient. The endpoint of therapy should not necessarily be the restoration of a normal platelet count. Some thrombocytopenic patients with chronic ITP thus may not require any intervention.

Intravenous Immunoglobulin G

The use of intravenous IgG preparations have revolutionized the initial therapeutic approach to the child with chronic ITP. Where splenectomy was once the mainstay of such treatment, IgG has now become the initial therapy of choice in most cases, preventing or postponing splenectomy.

As can be seen from Table 42–6, high-dose gamma globulin is effective for *temporarily* raising the platelet count in approximately 70 to 80 per cent of children with chronic ITP (156, 159, 204–208). The usual dose is 2 grams per kg given intravenously over 2 to 5 days. The platelet count rises within 1 to 3 days following therapy and usually peaks within a week. However for both children and adults with chronic ITP, IV IgG usually does not result in a cure; permanent remission occurred in only a minority of children evaluated (0 to 20 per cent; Table 42–6). Refractoriness to infusions became apparent on continued usage in approximately 25 per cent. In the remainder, effectiveness gradually declined over 2 to 4 weeks following infusion as the plasma concentration of IgG fell to normal levels. A safe count of >40,000 cells per mm^3 may however be achieved with periodic booster doses in this subgroup. Children who later proved refractory to IgG appeared to respond suboptimally to their initial 5-day course of therapy (peak platelet response of <100,000 cells per mm^3). Although splenectomy still continues to be the most effective treatment for patients with chronic ITP, surgery puts the patient at risk for postsplenectomy septicemia (209). Intravenous IgG on the other hand has only a few generally minor side effects.

Splenectomy

It must be reiterated that for a child with chronic ITP whose platelet count remains in a relatively safe range and whose bleeding time is fairly normal, no therapy would appear warranted except defensive management. Some of these children will spontaneously remit even 10 to 20 years post-diagnosis if followed for prolonged intervals of time (75). However, for the child with bleeding symptoms whose count remains precariously low (<40,000 cells per mm^3) and who has proven to be nonresponsive or refractory to intravenous IgG, splenectomy remains the only viable alternative.

The rationale for splenectomy includes the fact that the spleen is the most important site for the destruction of antibody-coated platelets and is one of the major loci of antibody production (168–170). The response rate to splenectomy in children varies between 65 and 88 per cent (Table 42–3).

There is no definite test by which one can predict this response. Although the earlier literature suggested a correlation between an initial response to prednisone and a subsequent response to splenectomy, most recent studies do not demonstrate any such predictive relationship (210, 211) (Table 42–3). Some researchers have advocated the use of thrombokinetic studies in chronic ITP in an attempt to select those patients who would benefit most from splenectomy. Other authors, however, do not feel that this is a necessary prerequisite since hepatic sequestration does not preclude significant improvement in platelet survival and platelet count after splenectomy (68, 191).

Only a single case has been reported in which excessive bleeding occurred during elective splenectomy for chronic ITP (73). Having platelet concentrates in the operating room is unnecessary if such products are readily available. At the time of splenectomy, the surgeon should look carefully for an accessory spleen since leaving any functional splenic tissue in the abdomen can result in a relapse of the ITP after surgery.

In many patients with chronic ITP, the platelet count starts to rise immediately following surgery, with levels reaching greater than 300,000 cells per mm^3 in the immediate postoperative period. Peak platelet levels occur within the first 1 to 2 weeks, remaining at high levels for several more weeks, and then gradually dropping to normal values by 4 to 8 months (67, 73). In general, the higher the initial platelet response, the higher the ultimate equilibrium, with individuals whose postoperative counts reached 500,000 cells per mm^3 and greater having the best likelihood of achieving a permanent remission (67).

Platelet counts of 1 to 2 million can occur after splenectomy. Since there have been no reported cases of thrombosis at these very high platelet levels, we do not routinely administer antiplatelet agents to children postsplenectomy for the period of transient thrombocytosis (211a).

Occasionally, children with a poor initial platelet rise will eventually achieve a complete or partial response to splenectomy, but this pattern is the exception, not the general rule (64). Finally, it is important to recognize that splenectomy should be considered successful if in its aftermath the platelet count achieved allows normal activity and symptomatic control, regardless of whether a normal platelet count results from the procedure. For instance a rise from 5000 to 25,000 platelets per mm^3 may alleviate symptoms and reduce the risk of bleeding.

Examination of the spleen following surgery reveals striking phagocytosis by splenic macrophages and monocytes, with numerous lipid-laden histiocytes in some patients. The origin of these "foam cells" is uncertain but may be related to the breakdown products of platelets (67). Using scan-

Table 42-6. AN ANALYSIS OF THE RESPONSE TO INTRAVENOUS IgG IN CHILDREN WITH CHRONIC ITP

	References					
	Imbach et al. (156, 159)	Bussel et al. (204)	Bussel et al. (205)	Mori et al. (206)	Warrier and Lusher (207)	Uchino et al. (208)
Number of children (<17 yr)	7	8	12	25	6	102 (? all chronic)*
Pre-/postsplenectomy	4/3	6/2	12/0	23/2	4/2	NA
Period of observation	18 to 27 mo	≥6 mo	4 to 9 mo	4 to 12 mo	NA	NA
Product used	Sandoglobulin (Sandoz)	Sandoglobulin (Sandoz)	Sandoglobulin (11) Endobulin (1)	Endobulin (Immuno-Vienna)	Gamimmune (Cutter Biological)	Venilon (Teijin Ltd.)
Pretherapy platelet counts (cells per mm³)	<20,000 in all patients	10 to 65,000	3 to 70,000	23,000 ± 12,000 (mean ± SD)	3 to 100,000	26,000 ± 26,000 (mean ± SD)
Peak Platelet Response (cells per mm³)						
>150,000	7	5	7	8 (↑196,000 ± 11,000)	0	51 (↑100,000, sustained)
100,000 to 150,000	0	0	3	8 (↑103,000 ± 32,000)	2	23 (↑100,000, unsustained)
30,000 to 100,000	0	3	0	4 (↑42,000 ± 9,000)	1	18 (<100,000)
0 to 30,000	0	0	2	5 (no change)	3	10 (no rise)
Time to occurrence of maximum effect	In 10 days	In 10 days	In 10 days	In 7 days	In 12 days	In 7 days
Duration of response	NA†	63 days (average)	NA	1 to 4 weeks	2 to 3 weeks	NA
Outcome						
Remission	2 (>150,000)	2 (100,000 to 300,000)	1	4 (100,000 to 210,000)	0	NA
Stable (no periodic boosters)	0	2 (40,000 to 70,000)	4 (>40,000)	0	1 (initial boosters—now stable)	
Periodic boosters necessary	4 (every 2 to 6 weeks)	3 (every 2 to 10 weeks)	4 (every 4 to 10 weeks)	16 (? all on booster Rx)	2	
Refractory	1	1	3 (1/1 responded to splenectomy)	5 (all unresponsive from start of therapy)	3 (2/2 responded to splenectomy)	
Miscellaneous		The refractory patient and those requiring frequent boosters responded poorly to initial IgG therapy	In the 3 refractory patients initial platelet response to IgG was <100,000			Previous exposure to steroids and/or splenectomy did not affect response to IgG

*67/102 children had ITP of <1 year's duration. However, the study does not delineate how many of these were newly diagnosed cases of acute ITP (of importance in evaluating therapeutic response).
†NA = Not available.

ning electron microscopy, one group of workers (212) reported the presence of lymphocytes and plasma cells with many membrane projections and microvillae. This observation is consistent with active secretory cells being present in the spleens of patients with ITP, a finding that may represent the intense antiplatelet antibody formation by the spleens of these patients. Occasionally, histologic examination of the spleen will produce evidence of another disease masquerading as ITP, such as sarcoidosis or a lymphoproliferative disorder like Hodgkin's disease. The pathologist should be alerted to look for such disorders.

Postsplenectomy Septicemia. Concern about the potential hazard of postsplenectomy septicemia is the reason why most pediatricians are hesitant about rapidly proceeding to a splenectomy in a child with chronic ITP. While this often fatal complication deserves concern, occasionally this results in the splenectomy's being deferred for such a long time that the patient develops other serious complications due to therapy. Indeed, it is possible that with the use of appropriate vaccinations and antibiotics, the risk of this complication can be reduced.

There is general agreement that the incidence of postsplenectomy sepsis is highest when the splenectomy is associated with a serious underlying disorder, such as thalassemia major, sickle cell disease, or Hodgkin's disease. The risk of infection is much lower in those children who do not have an underlying disease, or have only a mild disorder such as hereditary spherocytosis (209, 213–217). The risk of postsplenectomy septicemia is also related to the age of the child (218) The risk of severe infection is greatest in infancy and early childhood, and most deaths that occur happen within the first 2 to 3 years following splenectomy (218–220). However, the risk persists into adult life, and death from overwhelming pneumococcal septicemia has been reported in individuals 30 years following splenectomy.

Patients who develop overwhelming postsplenectomy septicemia have an acute onset of fever, nausea, vomiting, and confusion that leads to coma and death within hours (221–226). In children initial symptoms may be more subtle. The case fatality rate is about 50 per cent, and many patients have evidence of disseminated intravascular coagulation, hypoglycemia, electrolyte imbalance, and shock. These patients can have such large numbers of pneumococci in their peripheral blood that they are visible on the stained blood film. At autopsy many of the patients have adrenal hemorrhage (Waterhouse-Friderichsen syndrome). The parents of children who have undergone splenectomy should be instructed to bring their child to immediate medical attention for any febrile illness. Family physicians in hospital emergency rooms should be instructed that these patients are at risk and that prompt antimicrobial therapy should be initiated for suspected bacteremia. Following appropriate cultures, a loading dose of intravenous ampicillin (50 mg per kg) plus chloramphenicol (25 mg per kg) or a third generation cephalosporin (for example, Cefuroxime at 50 mg per kg) should be administered. Unless the signs and symptoms suggest a full-blown postsplenectomy septicemia, the patient can be observed for several hours in the emergency room. Buffy coat smears of the peripheral blood can aid in the positive identification of known pathogens. As emphasized by Pearson (215), perhaps the most important part of the approach to the asplenic patient is the education of the parents and child to be alert for signs of infection and to follow instructions carefully. The family should also be cognizant of the urgency in seeking medical attention from physicians familiar with the treatment of the postsplenectomy syndrome.

PREVENTION. Once the decision is made to perform a splenectomy in a child with ITP, polysaccharide pneumococcal vaccine should be administered at least 2 weeks before surgery. The current vaccine contains antigens for 23 pneumococcal sera types and replaces the 14-valent polysaccharide vaccine licensed in the United States in 1977. This new vaccine includes capsular antigens representing 88 per cent of the types causing adult disease and nearly 100 per cent of the types causing childhood bacteremia and meningitis (227, 228). The timing of vaccine administration relative to splenectomy appears from most studies not to be a critical determinant of antibody response (229). However, a few reports indicate that antibody response may be suboptimal after splenectomy, and these authors have suggested that whenever possible pneumococcal vaccine should be administered prior to surgery (230). Firm recommendations about the need for and timing of booster shots with the new vaccine have not yet been established because the duration of protection from primary vaccination has not been determined. Revaccinated patients may experience a severe reaction (227). For patients who received the previously available 14-valent vaccine, revaccination at 1 to 2 years after initial immunization is recommended with the newer vaccine (231). Vaccination does not protect the splenectomized individual against other encapsulated organisms such as *H. influenzae* and meningococci that can cause post-splenectomy infection. Immunizations against these latter pathogens is however also becoming available. It should be noted that vaccines are of variable efficacy in children below the age of 2 years, whose immune responses against encapsulated bacteria are suboptimal. Many physicians recommend that high-risk children (<4 years of age) who undergo splenectomy should also receive continuous antibiotic prophylaxis. However, no data exist in humans to prove that this antimicrobial prophylaxis is effective; indeed, it is possible that prophylaxis could instill a false sense of security. Nonetheless, we recommend several years of antibiotic prophylaxis in the very young child following splenectomy. The rationale for this approach is twofold. As previously discussed, the risk of postsplenectomy pneumococcal septicemia is highest in the first several years following surgery. As the child ages, the risk will progressively drop.

The decision for therapeutic (IgG) or surgical intervention (splenectomy) is particularly difficult in the older child with chronic ITP and mild bleeding symptoms. In such children disruption of life style brought about by curtailment of activity and the inability to engage in contact sports or other peer group activities can lead to significant duress for both patient and physician. In selecting the best management under such circumstances, the physician must take into consideration the fact that for the most part chronic ITP is a benign disease with the distinct possibility of late spontaneous remission (75).

Nonsteroidal Immunosuppressive Therapy

For the children with severe chronic ITP who respond to either intravenous IgG or splenectomy no further therapy is necessary. However, a small number (<2 per cent) will not respond to either treatment and will continue to have a bleeding tendency with platelet counts of less than 20,000 to 40,000 cells per mm^3. In these children the use of immunosuppressive therapy is the only alternative. Nonsteroidal immunosuppressive agents used in the adult have primarily included azathioprine, 6-mercaptopurine, cyclophosphamide, vincristine, and vinblastine (232–234).

Data from adults with chronic ITP suggest that the splenectomized patient is more sensitive to the effects of immunosuppressive agents than the nonsplenectomized individual. Approximately 20 per cent of splenectomized adults will have a complete and lasting remission following a course of immunosuppression and will require no maintenance therapy. Another 10 to 20 per cent will have a partial response but will relapse at a later date (232).

The vinca alkaloids act more quickly, but cyclophosphamide has a more lasting effect. Immunosuppressive agents act by suppressing the antigen-processing cell (the major component of the afferent limb of the immune response), the lymphocyte (the major component of the efferent limb), or the ingesting macrophage. The vinca alkaloids are administered intravenously either as vincristine (0.025 mg per kg; total dose per injection not to exceed 2 mg) or vinblastine (0.125 mg per kg; total dose less than 10 mg) once weekly for a total of three to four doses.

Ahn and associates (235) suggested a modification of this treatment by attempting to selectively enhance delivery of chemotherapy to the macrophage, the cell responsible for platelet destruction in ITP. These investigators incubated platelets with an excess of vinblastine, which became bound to the platelet. Following incubation, the excess alkaloid was removed and the platelets were infused into adults with chronic ITP who were refractory to all measures, including the intravenous administration of the vinca alkaloids. This novel approach should theoretically have resulted in the targeted delivery of the drug to the effector cells, i.e., the macrophages. However, the use of vinca-loaded platelets has not fulfilled its early promise, being less than uniformly successful (236). Furthermore, the demonstration that the binding of vinblastine to platelets is easily reversible (237) suggests that the delivery of vinblastine to the macrophages will depend on the platelets' being phagocytized very rapidly, i.e., before the drug elutes from the cell. Further studies using this approach should be directed at methods to maintain the drug within the platelet or possibly the use of vincristine, which binds more tightly to the platelet (236). Recently, a constant infusion of vincristine has been suggested in adult chronic ITP in lieu of a bolus infusion (238). The overall advantage of this method of administration has not been established. Other agents used in the adult with chronic ITP include frentizole, an immunosuppressive phenylurea (239), or colchicine (240, 241).

Azathioprine, cyclophosphamide, and vincristine have been used infrequently in the treatment of childhood ITP refractory to splenectomy. The reported studies using azathioprine show marked variations in the rate of remission (71, 242–246). A problem in interpreting the results of the study with the highest remission rate is that treatment with azathioprine was often instituted during the first 6 months after the onset of ITP. Consequently, some of the responses could have been spontaneous rather than a direct result of immunosuppression (245). If one excludes from analysis all children treated within the first 6 months of their illness, the remission rate would be approximately 20 to 30 per cent. Trials of vincristine in childhood chronic ITP also show great variations in remission rates (247–250).

Nonsteroidal immunosuppressives should be used with great caution in children. Since alkylating agents are known to be mutagenic, and vincristine can be neurotoxic (especially in the young child), vinblastine may be the "safest" of this class of agents for use in children. Close monitoring of the patient (including white counts and differentials) should be instituted if immunosuppressive therapy is undertaken. The parents of the child should be informed that treatment with certain immunosuppressants (such as cyclophosphamide) could increase the child's risk of subsequent malignancy.

Corticosteroids

The majority of patients with chronic ITP will have a rise in the platelet count following the administration of corticosteroids. However, the dose or duration of therapy or both can result in unacceptable side effects, including impairment of growth, steroid myopathy, hyperglycemia, osteoporosis, hirsutism, weight gain, and acne. In these patients, the adverse effects of the steroids outweigh their benefits. Occasionally, a patient with chronic ITP can be managed successfully with low-dose corticosteroids (i.e., 5 mg every second or third day) or pulse-doses of methylprednisolone (251) such that continued corticosteroid therapy may represent the safest approach in these patients. But in general, because of the serious complications associated with long-term corticosteroid therapy, these drugs should play only a small role in the management of children with chronic ITP. Rarely, sustained high-dose corticosteroid therapy can itself result in thrombocytopenia and in these patients, reduction of the dose can alleviate the thrombocytopenia (126, 127).

Miscellaneous Treatment Approaches

Danazol. The use of the nonvirilizing synthetic androgen danazol either as a single agent in chronic ITP or to decrease the need for glucocorticoids (and thus offset their undesirable antianabolic effects) has been advocated by some (252). The exact indication for the use of danazol in childhood chronic ITP and its efficacy is yet to be established.

Plasma Infusions. In 1960, Schulman and associates reported the case of a child with "chronic ITP" in whom periodic infusions of plasma regularly induced increments in the platelet count (253). Since this initial report, several groups (254–256) have infused plasma into a total of 43 children with acute ITP in dosages varying from 10 to 30 ml per kg over a 24-hour period. Administration was followed by a dramatic elevation in platelet count within 72 hours in more than 50 per cent of the children. It is likely that at least some of the responders would have had a spontaneous rise in platelet count at about the same time that the plasma was given because of the natural evolution of acute childhood ITP. However, some demonstrated only a temporary platelet elevation, with a drop in counts to original levels after a few days. This second type of response makes it appear possible that a cause and effect relationship did exist in some of the children so treated. No definite explanation for the apparent effectiveness of plasma is yet available. Whether success in these cases is due to an unknown "plasma factor" or to mechanisms analogous to those operative during IV IgG therapy is not known. Plasma infusions, although of theoretical interest, are not recommended for routine use in childhood ITP, and this therapy must be considered to be experimental.

Plasmapheresis. Using plasma as an exchange medium has resulted in a transient rise in the platelet count in some patients with ITP but rarely induces a long-lasting remission (257–261).

Long-Term Drug Therapy. It is important that the clinician managing a child with refractory ITP periodically reduce or withdraw the drugs used to maintain the patient in remission, since these children may spontaneously enter remission many years after their initial diagnosis (75, 262, 263).

NATURAL HISTORY OF ITP

Among children presenting with acute ITP, approximately 10 to 20 per cent will ultimately develop the chronic form. Of these, most will remit following IV IgG therapy, splenectomy or both. Of the remaining children (1 to 2 per cent) with moderate to severe thrombocytopenia, approximately half to one third should be able to maintain platelet counts in the relatively safe range by periodic booster IV IgG infusions. Even in "nonresponders," the long-term outcome for children with chronic ITP is good (75, 262, 263). The long-term follow-up by Walker and associate (75) showed that four patients with severe thrombocytopenia for periods of 12 to 27 years managed fairly well with minimal symptoms. Two underwent major surgical procedures without steroid or platelet cover and did not experience undue bleeding. These authors feel that given the benign course of their patients, long-term immunosuppressant therapy is not warranted.

A similar benign course has been described in other natural history studies of chronic childhood ITP (262, 263). It may be timely to reflect that if the need for treatment in all children with persistent thrombocytopenia is accepted uncritically, there is a real danger that some could eventually suffer more from their treatment than from their disease (77). As opposed to the essentially benign self-limited course of childhood ITP in the United States and western Europe, childhood ITP in the Middle East may manifest a greater tendency toward chronicity (264).

RECURRENT ITP

In 1 to 4 per cent of children with ITP (Table 42–3) return of the platelet count to normal levels is followed months or years later by a recrudescence of thrombocytopenia, often following a viral infection. Recurrent episodes are usually multiple in a given patient and occur with a characteristically sudden onset. Each recurrence of thrombocytopenia is followed by a return of the platelet count to normal levels (73, 265). Accelerated rates of platelet destruction have been demonstrated during these recurrences. Some patients with recurrent ITP show normal interim platelet life spans (265); others, however, may demonstrate a compensated thrombocytolytic state, with periods of remission and relapse that are dependent on variable rates of compensatory platelet production by the bone marrow. Recurrent ITP should not be confused diagnostically with the syndromes of recurrent thrombocytopenia and hemolysis due to absence of plasma factors (266, 267).

In a few patients, thrombocytopenia recurs after a long period of clinical improvement. Recurrences may be due either to exacerbations of indolent chronic disease or to hypertrophy of accessory splenic tissue (268, 269). This latter, relatively rare phenomenon can easily be demonstrated by the absence of Howell-Jolly bodies on peripheral blood smears or the absence of "pitting" of the red cells by Nomarski optics in a splenectomized patient who has previously had these characteristic signs of asplenia (269–271). Further documentation of accessory splenic tissue can be performed by radioactive imaging studies, including standard technetium 99m sulfur colloid imaging. Because accessory splenic tissue may not always be visualized by this method, more sensitive tests including imaging with [111]indium-labeled platelets or a double dose of heat damaged red cells may be necessary (272, 273).

LONG-TERM FOLLOW-UP

It has been reported that approximately 0.5 to 3 per cent of children with childhood ITP will eventually develop an autoimmune disease (68, 76). A recent follow-up study of 177 children with ITP suggests however that the risk is much lower (75). Nonetheless it is reasonable to continue to periodically evaluate the older female with chronic ITP for evidence of concomitant autoimmune disease (68, 184–187).

One report in the literature suggests that children with chronic ITP are more likely to have short attention spans, poor memory, behavior problems, and learning difficulties (274). No other recent studies have followed up on this observation.

MANAGEMENT OF THE PREGNANT ADOLESCENT

The majority of children and young adults with chronic ITP are women. Some of these patients will become pregnant, and because the IgG antiplatelet antibody is actively transported across the placenta, it can produce thrombocytopenia in the woman's offspring. The management of the pregnant patient with ITP is difficult since the physician must treat not only the mother, whose platelet count is readily measurable, but also her infant, whose platelet count cannot be measured until delivery.

Until recently, the impact of ITP on the pregnant mother and her unborn child was overestimated by reports in the literature that suggested a perinatal mortality rate of 6 to 17 per cent (275). Several recent prospective studies have indicated that the true risk is actually far lower (276). When the results of these prospective studies are compiled, a more accurate picture of the impact of ITP on mother and child emerges. For example, although 5 of 99 conceptions in 95 pregnancies died, these deaths probably were not preventable as they occurred in utero between 18 and 28 weeks of gestation. Fifty-one per cent of the live-born infants were thrombocytopenic, but the postdelivery infant morbidity was low. Only 10 of the 94 infants had any evidence of bleeding, and only 6 had serious bleeding (3 developed gastrointestinal blood loss and 1 each had hematuria, periumbilical bleeding, and intracranial hemorrhage). However, it is important for the pediatrician to note that often the infant's platelet count continues to fall for several days after delivery.

The optimal management of both mother and infant continues to be uncertain. Management decisions concerning the pregnant mother with severe ITP are not difficult because she requires therapy to render her hemostatically competent. Most physicians would give corticosteroids or intravenous IgG to restore her platelet count to safe levels. Seldom is splenectomy either indicated or justified during a pregnancy.

The optimal management of the asymptomatic pregnant patient with either mild ITP or a past history of ITP is much more difficult because the therapy is directed at the infant rather than the mother. The central issue is that it is very difficult to predict which infants will be thrombocytopenic. For example, about one half of the infants born to mothers with a present or past history of ITP will be thrombocytopenic, but the maternal platelet count is of no value in predicting whether the infant will be affected (276, 277). Measurement of either bound or unbound antiplatelet antibody on the mother's platelets or in her serum increases the physician's ability to predict whether her infant will be thrombocytopenic (278, 279). However, the test is neither totally sensitive nor specific, and therefore we do not believe that management decisions concerning delivery should be based solely upon the measurement of maternal platelet-associated IgG levels.

Because infants of mothers with ITP can be thrombocytopenic at birth, some physicians recommend delivering all infants by cesarean section. The rationale for this approach is that delivery by cesarean section may be a more gentle maneuver for a thrombocytopenic infant than would vaginal delivery. Although this makes intuitive sense, there is neither animal nor clinical data to support this viewpoint. Perhaps more importantly, the delivery of every mother with ITP by cesarean section will result in many unnecessary cesarean deliveries.

We recommend the performance of a fetal scalp platelet count immediately after the membranes have ruptured or following amniotomy (277, 280). To perform this test, the fetal scalp is punctured and a few drops of blood are collected into an EDTA-anticoagulated capillary tube for measurement of the fetal scalp platelet count. If the infant is severely thrombocytopenic (platelets less than 50,000 per mm^3), an immediate cesarean section is performed. However, if the infant is not thrombocytopenic, or is only mildly thrombocytopenic, spontaneous vaginal delivery is allowed to occur. It should be emphasized that because a severely thrombocytopenic infant could bleed excessively from even a small cut on the scalp, the physician should be ready to proceed to an immediate cesarean section if the scalp platelet count is very low.

Karpatkin and co-workers have recommended administering corticosteroids to pregnant ITP patients (prednisone, 10 to 20 mg p.o. daily) for the last 2 to 6 weeks of pregnancy. The rationale for this approach is that steroids might lower the amount of antiplatelet antibody and consequently prevent thrombocytopenia in the infant (281). Although corticosteroids are favored by some, other investigators have questioned this approach since it does not always prevent neonatal thrombocytopenia. Theoretically, steroids could also worsen the quantitative platelet defect by displacing maternal antiplatelet antibody from platelets to maternal serum and hence into the fetal circulation. Others have suggested that corticosteroids could increase the risk of preeclampsia (282–286). Hence, firm recommendations concerning the usefulness of corticosteroids for pregnant women with ITP must await the performance of randomized clinical trails evaluating both risks and benefits.

Finally, some investigators have used IV IgG in these patients in hopes of blockading both the maternal and fetal RE systems and thereby raising the fetal platelet count (286–291). Although IgG freely crosses the placenta, transfer to fetus may be slow, and equilibration may take up to 3 weeks (292). Infusions may therefore have to be repeated over time to achieve IgG levels in the fetus that would be associated with RE blockade. Although case reports suggest success in some cases, the benefits and risks of this therapy remain unknown.

Because the platelet count in infants born to mothers with ITP can continue to fall for several days after delivery (281), all infants should be carefully monitored. If the count falls to very low levels, the infant should be treated with corticosteroids or IV IgG (293, 294). Seldom is exchange transfusion required.

In girls who spontaneously recover from acute ITP of childhood, long-term follow-up suggests that their offspring will be without quantitative platelet abnormalities at birth (75). A safe approach in such cases may be to evaluate asymptomatic mothers with a previous history of childhood ITP for platelet antibody production, rather than to assume that their offspring will run no risk of thrombocytopenia at birth.

Drug-Induced Thrombocytopenia

Thrombocytopenia is a common and potentially serious complication of drug therapy. In the hospitalized patient, most episodes of thrombocytopenia are due to drug-induced suppression of the bone marrow megakaryocytes by chemotherapeutic agents given for malignant disorders. This type of thrombocytopenia is diagnosed easily because the reduced platelets are accompanied by suppression of other cell lines, especially the leukocytes. A less common, but often clinically more important, cause of thrombocytopenia is idiosyncratic drug-induced thrombocytopenia due to peripheral destruction of platelets by immune mechanisms. Finally, certain drugs produce isolated platelet destruction by nonimmune mechanisms. The best example of this is the antibiotic ristocetin, a drug no longer used to treat patients. The general mechanisms of drug-induced thrombocytopenia are shown in Table 42–7. Also shown in this table are some of the laboratory findings that can help categorize the general mechanism of the drug-induced thrombocytopenia.

IDIOSYNCRATIC DRUG-INDUCED IMMUNE THROMBOCYTOPENIA

Idiosyncratic drug-induced thrombocytopenia is a common cause of unexpected thrombocytopenia in a hospitalized patient. The term "idiosyncratic" implies that not every patient who receives a particular drug will become thrombocytopenic. In fact, even the most immunogenic drug seldom causes thrombocytopenia.

Two other aspects of idiosyncratic drug-induced thrombocytopenia deserve emphasis. First, the thrombocytopenia is almost always due to immune mechanisms, although as will be noted subsequently, it can be difficult to demonstrate a drug-antibody-platelet interaction. Second, because immune mechanisms are responsible for most episodes of idiosyncratic drug-induced thrombocytopenia, there is a lag between the administration of the drug and the development of thrombocytopenia in the patients. This lag can range from days to weeks or months. If the patient has previously received the drug, thrombocytopenia can develop on the first day of administration.

Idiosyncratic drug-induced thrombocytopenia is caused by an increased rate of platelet consump-

Table 42–7. GENERAL MECHANISMS AND LABORATORY FINDINGS IN DRUG-INDUCED THROMBOCYTOPENIAS

General and Specific Mechanisms	Example	Relative Frequency	Peripheral Blood Findings	Bone Marrow	Platelet Life Span	Platelet Associated IgG	Drug-Dependent Binding of IgG to Platelets in vitro
Underproduction							
Nonimmune (stem cell suppression)	Chemotherapeutic agents	Common	Pancytopenia	Hypocellular	Near normal	Near normal	Negative
Immune	Quinidine-induced immune marrow aplasia	Very uncommon	Pancytopenia	Hypocellular	Near normal	Near normal	Negative
Increased destruction							
Nonimmune	Ristocetin	Very uncommon	Isolated thrombocytopenia	Increased megakaryocytes	Reduced	Near normal	Negative
Immune							
Autoimmune	Methyldopa Interferon	Uncommon	Isolated thrombocytopenia	Increased megakaryocytes	Reduced	Elevated	Negative
Drug-dependent	Quinidine Heparin	Common	Isolated thrombocytopenia	Increased megakaryocytes	Reduced	Elevated	Positive

tion due to drug-induced binding of antibodies to the platelet membrane. Although it is theoretically possible that some drugs could produce thrombocytopenia by injuring the megakaryocyte, this has not yet been shown. This pathologic condition can be divided into two general categories. Rarely, drugs can induce true autoantibodies that bind to platelets without the requirement that the drug be present. The prototype of this mechanism is methyldopa-induced antiplatelet antibodies, but other drugs including procainamide and interferon can cause platelet destruction by the induction of true antiplatelet autoantibodies (295–297). The second, and more common, general mechanism of idiosyncratic drug-induced thrombocytopenia is drug-dependent antiplatelet antibody formation.

PATHOPHYSIOLOGY

Why only certain drugs in certain individuals initiate drug-induced immune thrombocytopenia is not known. Also unknown is the explanation for the specificity of the reaction; i.e., why upon exposure to the same drug, platelets are the target cell in some patients, whereas others have hemolytic anemia or develop drug-induced leukopenia. Increasing information concerning the antibody and the orientation of its binding to the platelet surface is becoming available. There is general consensus about some of the data, while other aspects remain unresolved. First, the areas of agreement: Most investigators find that almost every patient with drug-induced immune thrombocytopenia has increased IgG on the platelet surface. Most clinicians also believe that the IgG is responsible for the thrombocytopenia. Uncertainty remains, however, about the spatial orientation of the IgG that is bound to the platelet surface. Two models have been proposed to explain the orientation of binding of IgG to the platelets.

Immune Complex Binding. This model, illustrated schematically in Figure 42–8A suggests that a drug-IgG complex binds to the platelet by the platelet Fc or C3b receptor. Shulman studied quinidine-induced thrombocytopenia in vitro and concluded that the drug did not act as a hapten in combination with the platelet membrane, because drug-dependent platelet lysis and complement fixation could not be inhibited by the addition of excess drug (300, 309, 310). Consistent with this model are the studies by Christie and co-workers, who used radiolabeled quinidine to study the binding of IgG to platelets (311). These investigators provided evidence that the drug and antibody initially interacted in solution and then bound to a platelet receptor. There are problems however with the immune complex model as an explanation for the drug-dependent binding of IgG to platelets. For example, it is now clear that immune complex–Fc interactions are antigen independent, and hence one would expect that immune complexes would bind to any cell with Fc receptors (312). Thus, those cells with the highest affinity for Fc receptors (such as monocytes and macrophages whose affinity for the Fc portion of IgG is approximately a thousand times higher than that of platelets) would preferentially bind to the IgG complexes (312). The study of Karas and co-investigators also argues against immune complex interactions as the explanation for the binding of IgG to platelets in drug-induced immune thrombocytopenia (313). These authors demonstrated that the binding affinity of immune complexes to platelets was so low that it did not withstand an aqueous washing step.

The Binding of IgG Antidrug Antibody to a Drug-Platelet Complex. This model, illustrated schematically in Figure 42–8B proposes that IgG binds to platelet-bound drug by its Fab terminus. Although two groups of workers were unable to demonstrate the drug-dependent binding of F(ab')2 to platelets, such studies are difficult to perform (314, 315). Recently, one group of investigators provided evidence suggesting that this model is responsible for at least some episodes of drug-induced thrombocytopenia. These authors studied whether platelets that had interacted with quinidine-dependent antiplatelet antibodies would form rosettes around immobilized staphylococcus protein A (316). The rationale for this approach was that if the interaction of the IgG with the platelets was via its Fc

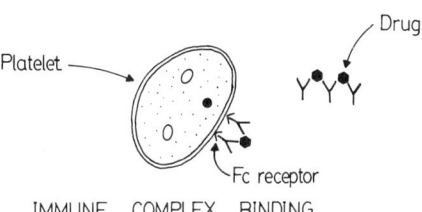

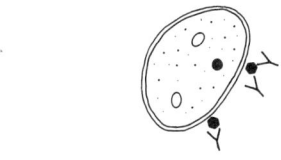

Figure 42–8. A schematic diagram illustrating possible mechanisms by which immune drug-induced thrombocytopenia occurs. Model A suggests that a drug-IgG complex binds to a platelet by the platelet Fc or C3b receptor. Model B proposes that IgG binds to platelet-bound drug by its Fab terminus.

terminus (i.e., immune complex binding), then the Fc receptor would not be available to interact with protein A. The results of these studies strongly support the binding of drug-dependent IgG to a drug-platelet complex via the Fab terminus of the IgG molecule.

DIAGNOSIS

In some patients the diagnosis of drug-induced thrombocytopenia is obvious; e.g., the patient with isolated, severe thrombocytopenia who is receiving a drug such as trimethoprim-sulfamethoxazole or quinidine. But in others, the diagnosis can be difficult. Many seriously ill children who have other medical and surgical complications such as infections, or are in the postoperative stage, often pose diagnostic difficulties because there are several potential causes for the thrombocytopenia including septicemia, disseminated intravascular coagulation, or a variety of medicinal agents. At present, there is no entirely sensitive or specific diagnostic test for any of these thrombocytopenic disorders, and hence, the physician is usually required to make decisions based on diagnostic probabilities.

It is useful to measure platelet-associated IgG (PAIgG) in a case of suspected drug-induced thrombocytopenia, because almost every patient will have markedly elevated levels. However, the low specificity of this finding limits its diagnostic usefulness. In particular, many of the conditions that are confused with drug-induced thrombocytopenia, including thrombocytopenia due to bacterial infections, are also characterized by elevated levels of PAIgG. Our approach in these children is to exclude the possibility of disseminated intravascular coagulation (DIC) by the appropriate laboratory investigations and identify all other potential causes for the thrombocytopenia.

To be certain that a patient unequivocally has a drug-induced decrease in platelet count, a number of criteria must be satisfied (298). First, the thrombocytopenia must develop while the patient is receiving the suspected drug and resolve following its discontinuation. The thrombocytopenia also cannot be initially observed while the patient is not taking the medication. The second criterion for the diagnosis of drug-induced thrombocytopenia is that other causes of thrombocytopenia be excluded, including other causes of immune thrombocytopenia such as bacterial or viral infections or other autoimmune diseases. Simultaneously with these investigations, all medications that the patient has been receiving should be stopped or substituted with others. Perhaps the only way one can be totally certain that the patient has had an episode of drug-induced immune thrombocytopenia is to demonstrate a recurrence of the thrombocytopenia following readministration of the drug. Although this is the most direct way to confirm the diagnosis, this approach exposes the patient to some degree of risk since patients can have serious bleeding after being rechallenged with the drug (299, 300). Hence, the physician seldom is justified in confirming the diagnosis by an in vivo rechallenge. In vitro techniques should always be used to insure patient safety (298, 301).

In Vitro Techniques for Confirming the Diagnosis. As previously discussed the diagnosis of drug-induced thrombocytopenia can be difficult to make on clinical grounds if the patient has other co-morbid conditions that could cause thrombocytopenia. Consequently, it would be useful to have an in vitro test that could be used to diagnose an immune drug-induced decrease in the platelet count. Although a number of techniques are available, there has not been sufficient experience with any method to allow an accurate assessment of their sensitivity and specificity. The original (Phase 1) assays all measured a platelet-dependent endpoint (301–308). The more recent (Phase 2) methods measure the drug-dependent binding of patient IgG, IgM, or complement to control platelets (298).

Phase 1 Tests. All of these tests use the same basic principle: a measurable endpoint is induced in normal platelets following the mixture of patient serum with the drug. For a positive result to occur, the proper concentration of immunoglobulin in patient serum must interact with a precise concentration of drug or its metabolite and the test platelets. A negative result will therefore indicate that the patient does not have drug-induced thrombocytopenia, or it may be a false negative result. As is summarized in the appendix to this chapter, all of these assays have predictable drawbacks in that complement usually must be activated to give a positive result. Hence, those drug-antibody-platelet reactions that do not activate complement will give negative test results. Secondly, because a "nonspecific" endpoint of platelet reactivity is measured, such tests have problems of specificity because positive results can be caused by nonimmunologic stimuli. Some of the techniques that in the past have been used to test for drug-dependent antiplatelet antibodies include clot retraction inhibition (317–319); platelet migration inhibition (320, 321); platelet aggregation or agglutination (322–324); platelet lysis (325); complement activation (326); platelet factor III availability (327, 328); and serotonin release (329, 330). The only tests still used today are platelet lysis (^{51}Cr release) and serotonin release.

Phase 2 Tests. Several years ago, a group of investigators reported that many patients with drug-induced thrombocytopenia had drug-dependent binding of IgG to platelets in vitro (331). These investigators documented drug-dependent binding of patient IgG to normal platelets using patient sera from individuals with the clinical diagnosis of thrombocytopenia induced by quinidine, gold, trimethoprim, sulfamethoxazole, ampicillin, cimetidine, or penicillin. Although such tests have a high specificity, problems remain with their sensitivity, with false-negative results a particular problem. It is likely that such techniques will be modified further and will become the method of choice for diagnosis.

A list of the various medications reported to cause drug-induced immune thrombocytopenia and the results of studies used to confirm the diagnosis are shown in Table 42–8. It should be emphasized that virtually any drug can be associated with the development of idiosyncratic drug-induced thrombocytopenia and that this possibility should always be considered in a patient on drug therapy.

Heparin-Induced Thrombocytopenia

Heparin-induced thrombocytopenia is probably the most common idiosyncratic drug reaction. However, until recently, it has not been well understood because clinicians tended to "lump" a variety of heparin-platelet interactions under this designation. Heparin can interact with platelets in a nonidiosyncratic, nonimmune fashion to cause heparin-induced platelet aggregation, heparin-induced augmentation of aggregation, and heparin-induced prolongation of the bleeding time. These reactions depend primarily upon the characteristics of the heparin preparation. For example, high molecular weight heparin fractions induce or augment platelet aggregation irrespective of its antithrombin III affinity. Of the low molecular weight heparin fractions, those that have low antithrombin III affinity are more likely to induce or augment platelet aggregation than preparations with high antithrombin III affinity (434–437). Heparin also prolongs the bleeding time in some individuals. However, it should be emphasized that all of these reactions of heparin with platelets are non-immune and of uncertain clinical relevance. In contrast, heparin can induce an idiosyncratic thrombocytopenia in some individuals, a complication of great clinical importance.

Frequency. A number of prospective studies comprising over 1500 patients have investigated the frequency of heparin-induced thrombocytopenia, and based on these studies, one can make several conclusions.

First, the estimated frequency of this condition has declined from 20 to 25 per cent to the current figure of approximately 5 per cent (438–449). The earlier studies may have overestimated the true frequency of this complication since many of these investigations included ill patients in the postoperative phase who may have been thrombocytopenic due to other causes. Second, the studies indicate that the frequency of heparin-induced thrombocytopenia is independent of the dose and route of administration. In some patients, the thrombocytopenia may even resolve while the patient continues to receive the same dosage and preparation of heparin. This unexpected finding has never been explained. Finally, the risk of heparin-induced thrombocytopenia is related to the type of preparation used. In prospective studies evaluating the frequency of thrombocytopenia in patients treated with bovine or porcine heparin, an increased frequency of thrombocytopenia has been seen whenever the bovine preparation has been used (450–454). Pooling the results of all studies, a reasonable estimate of the frequency of heparin-induced thrombocytopenia in children or adults is 3 to 5 per cent for the porcine versus 5 to 10 per cent for the bovine preparation.

Heparin-Induced Thrombocytopenia plus Acute Arterial Thrombosis. Heparin-induced thrombocytopenia typically occurs on day 8 to 11 of therapy. Although most patients will not experience major complications that are directly attributable to their thrombocytopenia, a *small* subset of patients will have a serious complication directly attributable to the heparin effect: acute arterial thrombosis. This rare and potentially devastating complication is unique among all types of drug-induced thrombocytopenia in that it is peculiar to heparin and usually occurs concurrently with the episode of thrombocytopenia. The frequency of heparin-induced thrombocytopenia plus acute arterial thrombosis is not known, but the risk is far lower than the risk of thrombocytopenia alone. For example, there has not been a single patient in any of the prospective studies (of over 1500 individuals) who has developed acute arterial thrombosis (455). Nonetheless, the seriousness of this disorder should not be underestimated. Approximately 20 per cent of patients with heparin-induced arterial thrombosis will experience a major morbidity including limb amputation, stroke, myocardial infarction, or death (456–472).

Pathophysiology. Heparin-induced thrombocytopenia was initially thought to be pathophysiologically different from heparin-induced thrombocytopenia plus acute arterial thrombosis. Although earlier studies suggested that the thrombocytopenia might be caused or contributed to by the presence of disseminated intravascular coagulation, it is now known that the majority of patients do not have any laboratory evidence of DIC. Although an IgG antiheparin antibody is responsible for the thrombocytopenia (465, 474), it remains unknown whether the antibody binds as an IgG-heparin immune complex or whether the IgG antiheparin antibody binds to a heparin-platelet complex. Also unknown is why some patients have transient and reversible thrombocytopenia while continuing on the same heparin preparation and dosage, while others have thrombocytopenia and acute arterial thrombosis.

Diagnosis. The diagnosis of heparin-induced

Table 42–8. A RETROSPECTIVE ANALYSIS OF DRUGS REPORTED TO CAUSE IMMUNE THROMBOCYTOPENIA

Drug	Compatible Clinical History	In Vivo Test Dose Rechallenge	Confirmation of the Drug Responsible Using In Vitro Testing		References
			1st Generation Tests (Drug-Dependent Platelet Reactions)	2nd Generation Tests (Drug-Dependent Binding of IgG to Platelets)	
Acetaminophen	Yes	Yes	Yes		318, 332–335
Acetazolamide	Yes		Yes		336, 337
Acetylsalicylic acid	Yes		Yes		338, 339
Actinomycin D	Yes				340
Allylisopropylcarbamide	Yes	Yes	Yes		341, 342
Alprenolol	Yes	Yes			343
Amrinone	Yes				344–347
Antazoline	Yes	Yes			348
Benzodiazepine	Yes	Yes	Yes	Yes	349
Bleomycin	Yes				350
Carbamazepine	Yes		Yes		351–353
Cephalothin	Yes	Yes	Yes		354–355
Chlorothiazide	Yes	Yes	Yes		319, 351, 356, 357
Chlorpropamide	Yes				358
Cimetidine	Yes	Yes	Yes	Yes	359–363
Clinoril					364
Clonazepam	Yes				365
Co-trimoxazole	Yes		Yes		366–368
Desipramine	Yes		Yes		369
Diazepam	Yes		Yes		325
Digitoxin	Yes	Yes	Yes		370–372
Digoxin	Yes	Yes	Yes	Yes	331, 373, 374
Diphenylhydantoin	Yes		Yes		325, 375, 376
Fenoprofen	Yes				377, 378
Heparin	Yes	Yes	Yes	Yes	379
Heroin	Yes	Yes			380–382
Hydrochlorothiazide	Yes				356, 383, 384
Isoniazid	Yes				385
Levamisole	Yes	Yes			386
Levodopa	Yes				387
Meprobamate	Yes				351
Methicillin	Yes	Yes	Yes		388
Methyldopa	Yes	Yes	Yes		389–391
Minoxidil		Yes			392
Morphine	Yes		Yes		393
Nitroprusside					394
Novobiocin	Yes	Yes	Yes		395
Organic arsenicals	Yes	Yes			396
Oxphenbutazone	Yes				397
Oxprenolol	Yes	Yes			398, 399
Para-aminosalicylic acid	Yes	Yes	Yes		400–402
Penicillin	Yes		Yes	Yes	331, 403
Procainamide	Yes	Yes			404
Quinidine	Yes	Yes	Yes	Yes	327, 330, 331, 351, 375, 405–413
Quinine	Yes	Yes	Yes	Yes	324, 375, 411, 413–416
Rifampicin	Yes	Yes	Yes		417
Spironolactone	Yes		Yes		351
Stibophen	Yes	Yes	Yes		418, 419
Sulfamethazine	Yes		Yes		411
Sulfamethoxypyridazine	Yes				420–422
Sulfisoxazole	Yes	Yes	Yes		325, 423–426
Sulfonamide					427
Tolbutamide					428
Trimethoprim-sulfamethoxazole	Yes		Yes	Yes	331, 429–431
Valproic acid	Yes		Yes		479
Vancomycin	Yes				432
Xylocaine	Yes	Yes	Yes		433

thrombocytopenia alone or with arterial thrombosis was initially one of exclusion. A number of investigators have reported a heparin-dependent platelet aggregating factor in the serum of these patients (440, 443, 450, 457–459). An earlier prospective study designed to evaluate the sensitivity and specificity of testing for the heparin-dependent platelet aggregating factor found the test to be neither sensitive nor specific (473). However, recent test modifications measuring platelet release rather than aggregation have improved its diagnostic capability (474).

Management. Management depends, in part, on the severity of the thrombocytopenia. In a patient with heparin-induced thrombocytopenia plus acute arterial thrombosis, the heparin must be immediately discontinued and alternative antithrombotic therapy instituted. The acute arterial occlusion should be treated whenever feasible. Because aspirin inhibits the heparin-dependent platelet aggregating factor, some clinicians recommend its administration, although the efficacy of this approach remains uncertain (467, 468). Patients with severe heparin-induced thrombocytopenia but without arterial occlusion should have their heparin discontinued as quickly as possible. Again, depending upon the nature, location, and duration of treatment of the underlying thrombosis, other antithrombotic intervention may be required. It is debatable whether the majority of patients with heparin-induced thrombocytopenia who have a mild to moderate decrease in their platelet count require any intervention. In many of these individuals, the thrombocytopenia will neither worsen nor be complicated by arterial thrombosis. Indeed, in some patients the thrombocytopenia will resolve completely without clinical sequelae while the patient continues on heparin therapy. Consequently, the risks of immediate discontinuation of the heparin (with the requirement of alternative antithrombotic therapy) must be balanced against the risk of continuing the heparin for the minimum duration required for oral anticoagulants to become effective.

Valproic Acid–Induced Thrombocytopenia

Valproic acid is an effective antiepileptic that has a unique chemical structure—a branched chain carboxylic acid with structural similarity to fatty acid constituents of cell membranes. A number of case reports have demonstrated thrombocytopenia in patients receiving valproic acid, and in several prospective studies thrombocytopenia was documented in a large proportion (greater than 20 per cent) of the patients treated with this drug (475–479). Often, the thrombocytopenia is mild and will spontaneously reverse (475–479). In the patients in whom it has been studied, the thrombocytopenia is associated with elevated levels of platelet-associated immunoglobulin, indicating that the thrombocytopenia is due to immune mechanisms (479, 480). Because the thrombocytopenia in many patients will resolve spontaneously, we favor continuing the medication with careful monitoring of the platelet count except in those patients in whom the thrombocytopenia is severe.

TREATMENT OF IDIOSYNCRATIC DRUG-INDUCED IMMUNE THROMBOCYTOPENIA

Except for unusual circumstances, the most important aspect in managing this condition is to stop the drug as quickly as possible. If another agent is required to treat the underlying disorder, a chemically unrelated drug should be substituted. Although there have been no studies designed to test the efficacy of corticosteroids in drug-induced thrombocytopenia, many physicians administer these agents (prednisone, 1 to 2 mg per kg) in symptomatic patients. Intravenous IgG now offers a more rapid treatment for such individuals (481), and we favor the administration of IV IgG (1 to 2 grams per kg over 2 to 3 days) as the therapy for severe drug-induced immune thrombocytopenia. Platelet transfusions should also be considered in a patient who has a very low platelet count (platelets less than 10,000 to 20,000 cells per mm^3) and bleeding manifestations. Although the platelets will have a markedly reduced survival, in some patients a rise in count will follow the platelet transfusion and this improvement may last for several hours. Furthermore, because the amount of drug in the body is the limiting factor in the resolution of the thrombocytopenia, the infusion of platelets that bind to a drug-antibody complex may increase the rate of clearance of the drug and in doing so hasten recovery.

The majority of patients will have a return of their platelet count to normal limits within days of stopping the drug. Rarely the thrombocytopenia can persist for weeks following the discontinuation of the drug—well beyond the time it would take for the drug to be cleared from the circulation. This suggests that in some patients a transient autoimmune destruction of platelets may be precipitated. Gold-induced thrombocytopenia is an exception to the generalization that the majority of patients will have a rapid and complete recovery of their platelet count following discontinuation of the drug. The chronicity of gold-induced thrombocytopenia is due to the fact that this metal remains in the body for long periods and is slowly released into the circulation.

Once an individual has been identified as having a drug-induced thrombocytopenia, it is important to make the patient's family aware of this allergy, since re-exposure to the offending agent could have serious consequences. We recommend a medical identification bracelet indicating that the individual is allergic to a particular drug.

Infection-Induced Thrombocytopenia

Bacterial, viral, and parasitic infections are often associated with hemostatic changes, especially thrombocytopenia.

BACTERIAL-INDUCED HEMOSTATIC ABNORMALITIES

Thrombocytopenia is an early sign of bacterial infection and usually indicates that the infection has become systemic. The precise frequency of thrombocytopenia during bacterial septicemia is uncertain, but it may be as high as 20 to 30 per cent (482–488). The thrombocytopenia is usually not severe, but in some patients the platelet count can fall below 10,000 cells per mm^3 with concomitant hemorrhagic manifestations.

It was initially thought that the thrombocytopenia of septicemia was probably due to suppression of the megakaryocytes by infecting organisms. The demonstration of a reduced survival of transfused platelets, increased numbers of megakaryocytes in the bone marrow, and the presence on peripheral smear of larger than average size platelets, however, all indicate that the primary reason for the thrombocytopenia is usually platelet consumption (488).

The mechanism of the thrombocytopenia in septicemia has only recently been systematically investigated. Early reports suggested that some patients with thrombocytopenia and septicemia had disseminated intravascular coagulation, an observation consistent with the possibility that the thrombocytopenia was due to the action of thrombin on platelets (489–494). However, more recent studies indicate that the majority of thrombocytopenic bacteremic patients do not have laboratory evidence of DIC. Kreger and associates performed coagulation studies in 222 patients with bacteremia or bacterial septicemic syndromes, and although thrombocytopenia occurred in 56 per cent of the patients, disseminated intravascular coagulation (defined by laboratory parameters) occurred in only 11 per cent (495). Indeed, even when sensitive indicators of thrombin activation, including the radioimmunoassay for fibrinopeptide A and the measurement of fibrin-fibrinogen multimers by fibrinogen gel chromatography are performed in septicemic thrombocytopenic patients, only a minority have evidence of thrombin activation (488). Thus, although thrombin can contribute to the thrombocytopenia, in most patients thrombin-independent mechanism are responsible for the decrease in the platelet count.

Although bacterial-induced DIC is uncommon, its pathophysiology can be studied by administering repetitive sublethal injections of bacteria to animals to produce the generalized Shwartzman reaction (496). Such studies have demonstrated the pivotal role of the leukocytes in inducing endotoxin and bacterial-induced DIC (497, 498). The interaction of bacteria with certain leukocytes, especially the monocytes, results in the synthesis of a procoagulant material with tissue factor activity, which in turn activates coagulation Factor X in the presence of calcium and Factor VII (499–507). Bacteria can also activate Factor XII, increase the biosynthesis of kallikrein, and reduce levels of antithrombin III (508–511). Together all of these factors contribute to the development of DIC.

Increasing evidence indicates that the thrombocytopenia of septicemia is caused, or contributed to, by immune platelet destruction. PAIgG is elevated in the majority of thrombocytopenic patients with both gram-negative and gram-positive sepsis (487, 412, 513). A number of potential mechanisms could be responsible for the increase in PAIgG documented in bacterial septicemia, including the binding of IgG to platelet-bound antigens; the binding of immune complexes consisting of bacterial antigens and IgG to platelets; and the nonspecific binding of IgG to platelet membranes that have been injured by bacteria. One group of investigators suggested that in some patients with a bacteria-associated elevation of PAIgG, evidence of a true autoantibody was present, best detected when EDTA was used as the anticoagulant (514). They suggested that bacteria could induce the exposure of a neoantigen on the platelet membrane, resulting in the formation of antiplatelet autoantibodies. These investigators could not find any correlation between the level of PAIgG and the severity of the thrombocytopenia. Another group noted that the likelihood of finding elevated levels of PAIgG was related to the time of blood sampling. For example, if PAIgG was measured during recovery (when the platelet count was rising), then levels were invariably normal. However, if measured during the time of maximum thrombocytopenia, PAIgG was elevated (515). This latter study also strongly supports the contention that PAIgG is causally related to the development of the thrombocytopenia during septicemic episodes.

Other factors probably also contribute to the consumptive thrombocytopenia that occurs. These include the binding of platelets to subendothelial layers exposed by the bacterial infection (508, 516–520) as well as the direct interaction between bacteria and platelets (521–523). Figure 42–9 schematically represents the various mechanisms that may be operative in the thrombocytopenia of bacterial infections.

Certain bacterial infections are also associated with specific syndromes. For example, meningococcemia characteristically produces hemorrhagic manifestations that range in severity from petechial skin lesions (524) to the hemorrhagic necrosis of the adrenal glands known as the Waterhouse-Friderichsen syndrome (525). Although this com-

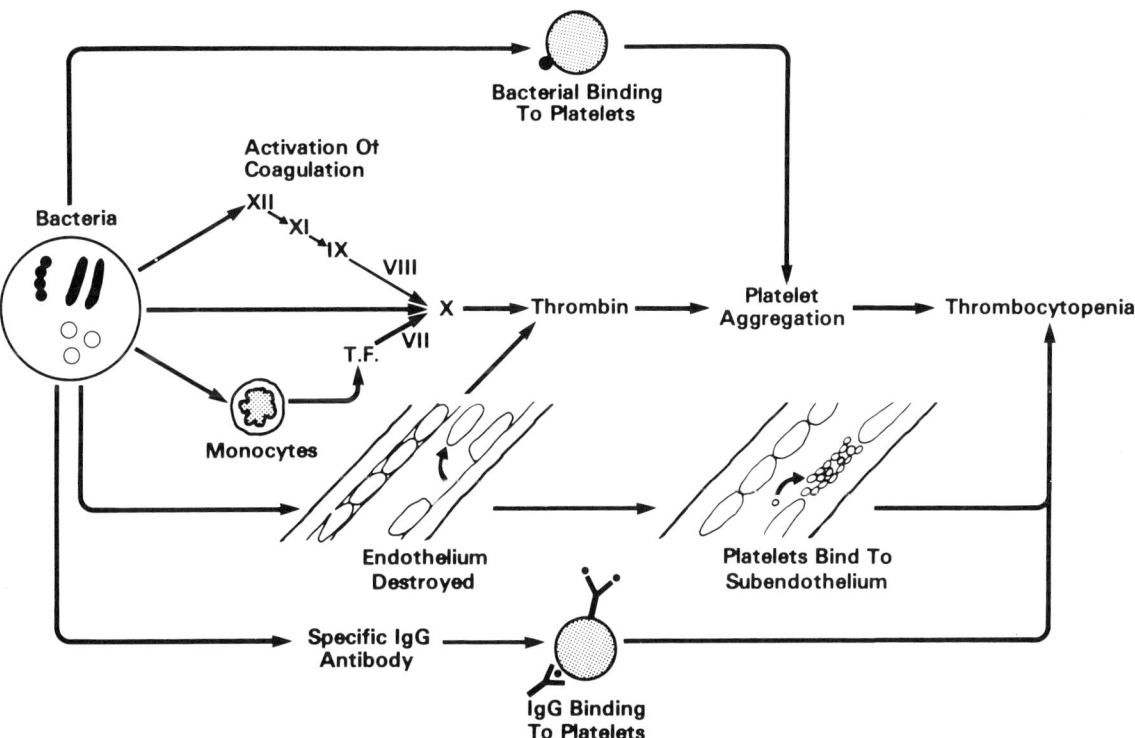

Figure 42–9. A schematic representation of the various mechanisms that may be operative in the thrombocytopenia associated with bacterial infections.

plication of meningococcemia is uncommon (3 to 10 per cent of patients), its early recognition is important since it often is fatal (526).

VIRAL-INDUCED THROMBOCYTOPENIA

Isolated thrombocytopenia is a common complication of viral infections, but its precise frequency and mechanism remain uncertain. Although a few case reports have described patients with decreased numbers of megakaryocytes in the bone marrow following a viral infection or vaccination (527–530), most investigators have found normal to increased numbers of megakaryocytes (531, 532). More importantly, platelet survival studies have demonstrated a decrease in platelet life span, and PAIgG levels are often elevated, suggesting that immune destruction is probably the primary cause of the thrombocytopenia (531, 532). Infectious mononucleosis, for example, is frequently associated with thrombocytopenia; platelet survival is reduced and levels of PAIgG are invariably found to be elevated (533–539). Consistent with this model are the reports that the thrombocytopenia of infectious mononucleosis responds to corticosteroid therapy (533–535, 537). Viruses can directly interact with platelets, and this effect may also contribute to the thrombocytopenia. For example, when platelets are incubated with live influenza virus, a shortened in vivo platelet survival results (540, 541a). In most infants with congenital or acquired viral infection, the thrombocytopenia is self limited with a return to a normal platelet count in 1 to 4 months. A more prolonged period of thrombocytopenia can occasionally occur (541b, c, d).

Protozoal (Malaria)-Induced Bleeding. Malaria is one of the most important and serious infectious disease in the world today. The risk of developing thrombocytopenia during malarial infections has been well studied. Two prospective studies have demonstrated that thrombocytopenia complicates virtually every case of malaria. In one study, healthy individuals were infected with malaria and their platelet counts followed longitudinally. Every patient became thrombocytopenic (542). In another study of naturally acquired malaria, 32 of 33 patients developed thrombocytopenia (543). The decrease in platelet count is due to increased platelet consumption (544, 545). As was the case with bacterial-induced thrombocytopenia, earlier investigators suspected that disseminated intravascular coagulation was responsible for most episodes of malaria-induced thrombocytopenia. These conclusions were based mostly upon case reports describing DIC complicating malarial infections (546–549). Although DIC can occur, recent prospective studies have demonstrated that this complication is extremely uncommon (61, 546).

The mechanism of the thrombocytopenia of malaria is due to the binding of antimalarial antibodies to platelets. Indeed, the precise orientation of the binding has been worked out (61). Malaria antigens are released from red cells during red cell lysis, and these antigens bind to specific malaria binding sites on the platelet. IgG antimalarial antibody in turn binds to the platelet-bound malaria antigen, and the IgG-parasite-platelet complex is removed by the phagocytic cells of the reticuloendothelial system (61).

Post-Transfusion Purpura

Post-transfusion purpura is a rare but important disorder that has been carefully studied but remains poorly understood. Although this entity has not yet been described in children, it is important because it is caused by antibodies against platelet-specific antigens, in particular the PL^{A1} antigen. The disease almost always occurs in middle-aged or older women who have had a previous pregnancy (550–554). Women are primarily affected because they are sensitized to the PL^{A1} or other platelet-specific antigens during pregnancy. Typically, post-transfusion purpura follows the transfusion of any blood product by an interval of 2 to 14 days (553). The thrombocytopenia is very severe with the occurrence of cutaneous and mucous membrane bleeding that can last from 1 to 8 weeks (550–553). In some patients, the thrombocytopenia is life-threatening. Effective treatment includes exchange transfusion (550, 553, 555) and plasmapheresis (553, 556). Although corticosteroids have been claimed to be effective in some patients (557, 558), other studies have reported no beneficial effect (553). A recent report describes successful treatment with intravenous IgG (559).

Although the pathogenesis of post-transfusion purpura remains uncertain, the syndrome has one unique feature: autologous platelets are destroyed, presumably by allo- or autoantibodies. Several theories have been proposed to explain the mechanism of destruction of the patients' own platelets. They include the generation of antiplatelet autoantibody (551) and the adsorption of antigen-antibody complexes comprised of PL^{A1} platelet antigens and anti-PL^{A1} antibody to the platelet surface (550). It is possible that just as platelets adsorb ABO antigens from plasma, the PL^{A1}-negative platelets adsorb PL^{A1}-positive antigens from the blood product, and the patients' anti-PL^{A1} antibodies in turn destroy their own platelets. Following an episode of post-transfusion purpura, these individuals should not receive further transfusions from PL^{A1} positive donors, since this would cause a recurrence of the thrombocytopenia. If blood products from individuals of an unknown PL^{A1} type must be given, they should be washed extensively prior to being transfused.

Neonatal Immune Thrombocytopenia

Immune thrombocytopenia can be acquired in the neonate by the transplacental passage of antiplatelet autoantibodies (if the mother has idiopathic thrombocytopenic purpura) or alloantibodies. Although these disorders differ in regard to the platelet reactivity of the antibody, they share one important feature—the transplacental passage of an antiplatelet antibody. Thus the thrombocytopenia of each disorder is transient, resolves completely, and will not recur once the antiplatelet antibody is cleared from the infant's circulation. These conditions are discussed in Chapter 5 and have therefore been omitted from this review.

Thrombocytopenia Associated with Allergy and Anaphylaxis

A decrease in the platelet count following the ingestion of various foods can be observed in certain patients with food allergies (578, 579). Thrombocytopenia has also been observed following the intracutaneous injection of an antigen to which previous sensitization has been documented (580) and in anaphylactic shock (581). Specific food antigens have been detected in immune complexes formed after eating in food-allergic patients (582, 583), and it is possible that the platelet destruction is due to the interaction between the Fc receptor on the platelet and the circulating immune complexes (581, 584, 585). Recently, Little and co-workers (586) observed an acute fall in serotonin levels in platelet-rich plasma following a food challenge in patients with food allergy. These authors suggest that immune complex–mediated release of platelet serotonin may occur following an acute food challenge in patients considered to be food allergic.

Thrombocytopenia Associated with Transplant Rejection

The participation of platelets in hyperacute and acute rejection of heterografts and allografts in the presensitized animal model has been documented (587, 588). In human kidney allotransplantation, hyperacute and acute rejections are accompanied by thrombocytopenia and an accumulation of platelets in the rejected organ (589, 590). The introduction of ^{111}indium oxine as a platelet label has made a new approach to the study of platelet kinetics possible. This isotope allows the imaging of the distribution of labeled platelets within the body, permitting quantitative in vivo studies of sites of platelet accumulation and redistribution (591). With this technique, platelets can be shown to accumulate within the kidneys in patients with acute rejection (592, 593). Nephrectomy of the nonfunctioning kidney usually will serve to return the platelet count to normal.

In chronic renal transplant rejection, although a moderate shortening in platelet survival occurs, evidence for deposition of ^{111}In-labeled platelets in the kidney is not always present (593, 594). Thrombocytopenic episodes may also occur in patients with well-functioning renal allografts. The cause of these episodes is unclear but could be related to the use of immunosuppressive agents, the presence of platelet antibodies, or both (595, 596a). Recently Foegh and associates demonstrated that in human cardiac and renal allograft transplant recipients, and in the animal cardiac heterograft model, increased levels of urinary thromboxane B_2 were observed as one of the earlier signs of rejection. The use of thromboxane synthetase inhibitors also appeared to increase allograft survival (596b). These studies suggest that whatever the mechanism of the platelet destruction, platelet metabolites produced during aggregation (including those formed via the cyclooxygenase pathway) may serve to potentiate the rejection process.

Severe thrombocytopenia can occur following allogeneic and autologous bone marrow transplantation even in patients with demonstrable megakaryocyte engraftment (597). The incidence of this complication may be as high as 20 to 30 per cent (597a). Antibodies against circulating (donor origin) platelets have been demonstrated in such patients, the severity of the thrombocytopenia depending on the ability of the engrafted marrow to compensate for the rate of antibody-mediated platelet destruction. Immunologic mechanisms also contribute to the thrombocytopenia observed following antilymphocyte globulin therapy (598).

Immune Thrombocytopenia Associated with Other Disorders

Immune thrombocytopenia can occur in a variety of collagen-vascular disorders and in patients with lymphoid and other malignancies (560–570). It may also be present in a variety of other conditions including immunodeficiency syndromes, rheumatoid arthritis, nephritis, atrophic gastritis, myasthenia gravis, hemophilia, thyroid disease, and sarcoidosis (38, 39, 183, 570–577).

DESTRUCTIVE THROMBOCYTOPENIAS ASSOCIATED WITH NONIMMUNOLOGIC MICROANGIOPATHIC PROCESSES

Chronic Microangiopathic Hemolytic Anemia and Thrombocytopenia

In 1960, Schulman and associates described an 8-year-old girl with chronic thrombocytopenia and microangiopathic hemolytic anemia unresponsive to corticosteroid therapy or splenectomy (266). The platelet count transiently rose to normal levels following the infusion of fresh plasma, fresh frozen plasma, or whole blood. Subsequently, the child developed nephritis, hypertension, and microangiopathic hemolytic anemia (599). The authors postulated that thrombocytopenia could be due to a congenital deficiency of "thrombopoietin" necessary for megakaryocytic maturation and platelet release.

In 1978, Upshaw described a similar patient whose episodes of thrombocytopenia and microangiopathic hemolytic anemia were triggered by viral infections (267). During asymptomatic periods, although the platelet count and hemoglobin level were near normal, radiolabeled platelet and red cell survival studies demonstrated reduced life spans of both these cellular elements. This disorder is remarkably similar to both thrombotic thrombocytopenic purpura and hemolytic uremic syndrome (both of which are described in detail in Chapter 16). In particular, some of these latter patients have a factor in their serum that induces the agglutination of normal platelets (600). When their platelet count is normal, these individuals may also have abnormally large factor VIII: von Willebrand factor multimers in their plasma. During acute exacerbations of their illness, the largest multimers are lost (601, 602). Patients respond to fresh frozen or stored plasma and factor VIII concentrates, but not to purified albumin (602).

Hemolytic-Uremic Syndrome and Thrombotic Thrombocytopenic Purpura

(These entities are discussed in Chapter 16.)

Thrombocytopenia Caused by Catheters, Prostheses, and Cardiopulmonary Bypass

Selective platelet consumption, usually without an increase in fibrinogen turnover, is observed in patients in whom arterial catheters, arteriovenous silastic cannulas, ventriculojugular shunts, Swan-Ganz catheters, prosthetic heart valves, dacron vascular prostheses, or aortofemoral grafts are introduced into the circulation (603–613). Platelet-dense-body adenine nucleotide levels, as well as β-thromboglobulin content of platelet α-granules, have been shown to be decreased in some of these patients, indicating in vivo activation and release of granule constituents (614, 615). In most adults, despite kinetic evidence of platelet consumption, compensatory increases in platelet production are adequate to maintain platelet counts. Platelet consumption slows down (although it may not normalize) months after the implantation, presumably due to progressive endothelial coverage of the foreign surface that occurs after implantation (616). Recent use of heterograft valves and modern nonfabric valves, as well as changes in the coating of artificial valves, has reduced the likelihood of platelet consumption on these artificial devices (612, 617).

Catheter placement in the neonate is more likely to be complicated by thromboses, thromboembolic phenomena, thrombocytopenia, or consumption coagulopathy (618–620). Blood sampling through such access lines may provide erroneous information on the state of the patient's hemostatic mechanisms. Blood obtained, especially via long catheters, may be "activated" during the sampling procedure and display a lower platelet count, abnormalities of fibrinogen and factor V, and evidence for platelet activation (including increased plasma levels of β-thromboglobulin and platelet factor 4), when compared to simultaneously obtained venous blood (621, 622).

Cardiopulmonary bypass is associated with complex derangements of hemostasis, including the occurrence of thrombocytopenia, which may result from a variety of causes (including consumption coagulopathy, dilution, sequestration and destruction of platelets in the oxygenator, and fibrinolysis) (623–625). Platelet destruction under these circumstances is presumably secondary to aggregation and release caused by the large foreign surfaces in the oxygenator and by thrombin formed either in the pump or at the surgical site. In spite of the predictable decreases in coagulation factors associated with bypass, abnormal bleeding following extracorporeal circulation is generally not due to a reduction in coagulation factors since patients usually maintain levels considered to be relatively hemostatic. Clinical bleeding appears to be related primarily to defective platelet function (625, 626) and possibly primary fibrinolysis (625, 627).

Harker and associates have demonstrated that following the onset of bypass the usual relationship between platelet numbers and the bleeding time becomes increasingly disparate, with markedly prolonged bleeding times occurring at relatively normal platelet counts of greater than 100,000 cells per mm^3. This platelet dysfunction has been referred to as an "acquired storage pool disease," with various investigators demonstrating either a selective loss of platelet α-granular contents (615, 626) or a combination of α-granule and dense granule abnormalities (628). Platelet transfusion successfully normalizes the bleeding time in these patients and controls the hemorrhagic manifestations (626).

Similar findings (i.e., increased plasma levels of platelet factor 4 and β-thromboglobulin) together with increases in thromboxane B_2 have been observed during simulated extracorporeal circulation in vitro (629). In this model, inhibition of cyclooxygenase activity by aspirin completely inhibits the rise in plasma thromboxane following bypass but only partially blocks platelet PF4 release. The inadequacy of aspirin alone in preventing platelet activation during in vitro simulation of the extracorporeal circulation contrasts with the demonstrated efficacy of prostacyclin and PGE_1, which provide a more effective degree of platelet inhibition (630–632). Although some in vivo studies in man have demonstrated a similar beneficial effect of prostacyclin and PGE_1 in significantly reducing platelet activation during cardiopulmonary bypass (633–635), others have shown that thrombocytopenia was not prevented and that the bleeding time abnormality remained (636, 637). Furthermore, the hypotension caused by PGE_1 or prostacyclin therapy when used in high enough doses to produce a platelet sparing effect may limit the usefulness of these agents. Recently, desmopressin (DDAVP) has been used to reduce blood loss in patients undergoing complex cardiac surgery (628a).

Thrombocytopenia Secondary to Congenital Heart Disease

Thrombocytopenia with an increased bleeding tendency is frequently seen in patients with cyanotic congenital heart disease (CHD). It occurs most frequently in patients whose mean oxygen saturation is below 60 per cent and in those in whom hematocrit levels are above 60 per cent (638, 639). At hematocrits above 60 per cent, small increments can produce large changes in viscosity (640), and since hyperviscosity and vascular stasis can trigger the process of intravascular coagulation, various workers have looked for this syndrome in patients with cyanotic congenital heart disease. The results of coagulation studies, however, are inconsistent. Most demonstrate a variable number of abnormalities in coagulation screening tests and factor assays, but the hemostatic alterations do not indicate a pattern of intravascular consumption (639, 641–644). A few studies have presented evidence for consumption (645–647), whereas others have described the presence of increased fibrinolytic activity (648–650) or a decrease in clotting factors synthesized in the liver (651, 652). It is possible that at least some of the reported coagulation abnormalities are artifacts, due to excessive in vitro anticoagulation due to the high hematocrit (653).

Platelet kinetic measurements in children with cyanotic CHD have demonstrated a decrease in platelet life span both in those with normal platelet counts and those with thrombocytopenia (654, 655). While intense systemic arterial unsaturation (oxygen saturation values <60 per cent) and erythrocytosis (hematocrits >71 per cent) are always associated with an abnormal platelet half-life, the presence of relatively normal values does not preclude the presence of a thrombolytic state (655).

Platelet aggregation abnormalities have been described in approximately one quarter to one half of children with cyanotic CHD (656–661), although no correlation between the platelet functional defect and the bleeding time has been noted (656, 657, 662). Clinically, no relationship between the preoperative platelet functional defect and intra- or postoperative blood loss has been observed (658). These findings, plus the observation that platelet aggregation abnormalities have been found to correct themselves very quickly following red cell volume reduction (662), make it likely that some studies have reported on an in vitro artifact due to concomitant polycythemia (663) or the size of the needle used to collect the blood sample. In fact, in a recent study in polycythemic adults with cyanotic CHD, elevations of fibrinopeptide A, plasma β-thromboglobulin, and PF4 occurred when a 21- or 22-gauge needle was used for blood collection. Blood sampling through a larger caliber needle appeared to lessen the problem (664). The platelet functional defect may not be related to concomitant polycythemia in all cases, since two types of acyanotic heart disease (ventricular septal defect and pulmonic stenoses) not associated with high hematocrits have also been shown to have platelet functional abnormalities.

Preoperatively, bleeding time, platelet count, and coagulation screening tests should be performed in all patients scheduled for cardiac surgery. The amount of anticoagulant should be adjusted for the hematocrit to reduce the likelihood of abnormal test results (663, 665). Recommendations for preoperative therapeutic maneuvers will depend on the results of the evaluation. Preoperative phlebotomy with plasma replacement may be used in a patient with cyanotic CHD and extreme thrombocytopenia, coagulation deficits, or a markedly prolonged bleeding time in an attempt to improve hemostatic mechanisms (652, 662). As previously discussed, postoperative bleeding in these patients is due to an "acquired platelet storage pool disease" caused by platelet activation during cardiopulmonary bypass and is controlled by platelet transfusion (615, 626, 628). In addition to their bleeding tendency, children with cyanotic CHD and polycythemia are also paradoxically prone to thrombosis of major cerebral vessels. This complication appears to occur mainly in those patients who have concomitant iron deficiency (666, 667).

Thrombocytopenia Secondary to Acquired Heart Disease

A mild consumptive thrombocytopenia is present in some patients with valvular heart disease, including left ventricular outflow obstruction and mitral valve disease. In addition, microangiopathic hemolytic anemia is usually present (668, 669). Platelet activation with resultant acquired platelet storage pool disease has been reported to occur in patients with severe rheumatic (mitral) valvular disease (628), presumably due to platelet activation during flow over the damaged heart valve.

DESTRUCTIVE THROMBOCYTOPENIAS WITH CONSUMPTION OF PLATELETS AND FIBRINOGEN

Disseminated Intravascular Coagulation

The term "disseminated intravascular coagulation" (DIC) was used by Rodriguez-Erdmann (670) to describe a variety of clinical circumstances in which thrombin is formed and the conversion of plasma fibrinogen to fibrin is accelerated. DIC is described in detail in Chapter 41, and will be only briefly summarized here.

DIC reflects the multiple actions of thrombin on fibrinogen, prothrombin, Factors V, VIII, XIII, and platelets, resulting in decreased levels of Factors I, II, V, VIII, XIII and thrombocytopenia, concomitant with the formation of fibrin thrombi. There is usually simultaneous activation of the fibrinolytic system, which causes plasmin generation with lysis of local deposits of fibrin, resulting in the accumulation of fibrinogen-fibrin degradation products in the circulation (671).

Colman and co-workers have proposed a set of widely accepted criteria for the diagnosis of this entity (672, 673). Etiologic factors in which various hypothetical mechanisms are seen to activate the coagulation system are shown in Table 42–9 and include injury to endothelial cells resulting in activation of the intrinisic coagulation system, extrinsic activation through tissue injury, acceleration of blood clotting due to the release of red blood cell or platelet procoagulant phospholipids, and a decrease in the clearance of activated coagulation factors. Injury to vascular endothelium exposes basement membrane collagen, which alone or in combination with proteoglycans activates Factor XII (674, 675). A specific Factor XII activator has also been shown to be localized in endothelial cells (676). Thus endothelial cell damage is related to activation of the intrinsic clotting system. Recently, endothelial cells under certain conditions have also been demonstrated to possess tissue factor activity and to act as cofactors with Factor VII in the activation of Factor X (677, 678).

Therapy for DIC is directed toward the primary underlying condition that triggered the process. Most physicians replace the depleted hemostatic factors and platelets but heparin or fibrinolytic agents are seldom used (see Chapter 41). The studies of Harker (603) indicate that antiplatelet therapy is not effective in situations in which consumption of both platelets and fibrinogen occurs. The presence of platelets also does not ap-

Table 42–9. ETIOLOGIC FACTORS FOR DISSEMINATED INTRAVASCULAR COAGULATION

I. *Injury to endothelial cells and/or activation of intrinsic system*
  Gram-negative sepsis (672, 673, 684)*
    Escherichia coli
    Haemophilus influenzae
    Klebsiella spp.
    Neisseria meningococcus and *gonococcus*
    Proteus mirabilis
    Pseudomonas aeruginosa
    Salmonella spp.
    Serratia spp.
  Gram-positive sepsis (672, 673, 685)
    Staphylococcus aureus and *albus*
    Streptococcus spp.
    Pneumococcus pneumoniae
  Rocky mountain spotted fever (686)
  Fungal infections (672, 673)
    Aspergillus sepsis
    Disseminated *Candida albicans*
    Toxoplasmosis
  Protozoa (672, 673, 687)
  Viruses (673, 688)
    Arbovirus
    Cytomegalovirus
    Disseminated herpes simplex
    Hemorrhagic fevers (Korean, Thai)
    Influenza
    Rubella
    Varicella
  Angiography (673)
  Prolonged hypotension from any cause (689, 690)
  Severe acidosis (690, 691)
  Diabetic ketoacidosis (692, 693)
  Hypoxemia or asphyxia (690, 691)
  Systemic vasculitis (672)
  Hypothermia (694)
  Polycythemia and stasis (695)
  Intrauterine growth retardation (696)
  Cavernous hemangioma (737–744)
  Lymphangioma (697, 698)

II. *Tissue injury with liberation of tissue thromboplastic activity and activation of extrinsic system*
  Obstetric complications (672, 673, 699)
    Abruptio placentae
    Amniotic fluid embolism
    Dead twin fetus
    Eclampsia and preeclampsia
  Brain injury (700)
  Surgical procedures; cardiopulmonary bypass (701–703)
  Trauma (672, 704, 705)
  Extensive burns (704, 706)
  Heat stroke (707, 708)
  Rhabdomyolysis due to various causes (709, 710)
  Drowning (673)
  Necrotizing enterocolitis (711, 712)
  Neoplasms (672, 673, 713–721)
    Acute promyelocytic leukemia
    Rarely, acute and chronic granulocytic leukemia, acute lymphatic leukemia, or lymphoma
    Pediatric solid tumors (Ewing's sarcoma, neuroblastoma, rhabdomyosarcoma, Wilms' tumor)

III. *Direct activation of Factor II or Factor X*
  Snake bite (procoagulant venoms) (722, 723)
  Mucin-secreting adenocarcinomas of the adult, and protease-secreting tumors (673, 724)

IV. *Red blood cell, platelet, or immunologic injury*
  Intravascular hemolysis (691, 725, 726)
    Incompatible red blood cell transfusions
    Severe erythroblastosis fetalis
  Antigen-antibody reactions (672, 673)
    Renal transplant rejection

V. *Reticulendothelial system injury with decreased clearance of activated coagulation factors*
  Reticuloendothelial hypofunction (672, 673)
  Hepatic diseases (672, 673, 727)

VI. *Miscellaneous*
  Congenital deficiency of anticoagulants; e.g., protein C deficiency (728, 729)
  Types II and IV hyperlipidemias (730)
  Exposure to 100 per cent oxygen in the experimental animal (731)
  Factor IX replacement therapy (673)

*Indicates chapter references.

pear to be a critical determinant for the occurrence of DIC, since the syndrome can be induced in the presence of thrombocytopenia (679–683).

Thrombocytopenia Associated with Giant Hemangioma (Kasabach-Merritt Syndrome)

The association between giant cavernous hemangiomas in infancy and thrombocytopenia was described by Kasabach and Merritt in 1940 (732). Since their original observation, numerous other cases have been reported, with Shim describing 74 such cases (733).

Clinical Presentation. The incidence of thrombocytopenia in the presence of a hemangioma is difficult to estimate but may be in the range of 1 to 2 cases of thrombocytopenia per 300 to 700 infants with hemangiomas (733). Since the hemangiomas are congenital, bleeding manifestations secondary to thrombocytopenia usually occur in the first days or weeks of life with a median age at presentation of 5 weeks (733). Occasionally, bleeding may be delayed for months or years. The hemangiomas can be superficial and solitary, associated with bone or with certain viscera, including the tongue, thorax, liver, and spleen. Subcutaneous and visceral lesions rarely coexist. The majority of the hemangiomas occur on the limbs or on a portion of the trunk with involvement of the proximal adjacent limb (733). Emphasis has previously been placed on the "giant" quality of the lesions that are associated with thrombocytopenia. Large size, however, is not a prerequisite for the occurrence of thrombocytopenia. Several cases have been documented in which a decrease in the platelet count was associated with lesions that were no larger than 5 to 6 cm in diameter (733).

In many cases, development of hemorrhagic complications is preceded by changes in the hemangioma itself, which may acutely increase in size, change its consistency, or develop a purplish hue. The vascular mass may become tense and woody in texture, with overlying taut, shiny, discolored skin. In some instances, such an appearance has mistakenly suggested cellulitis. Initially, petechiae and ecchymoses may occur in the skin overlying and adjacent to the lesion, then spread to other areas. A further complication of hemangiomatous lesions, particularly those of the liver, is congestive heart failure due to arteriovenous shunts within the tumor (733–735).

Laboratory Findings and Pathogenesis. A localized intrahemangioma consumption coagulopathy with increased turnover of both platelets and fibrinogen is characteristic of the Kasabach-Merritt syndrome (737–743). Using the ^{111}In oxine label, platelet localization in the hemangioma has been unequivocally demonstrated (743). Occasionally, localized platelet consumption progresses to a disseminated process, with the consumption of coagulation factors typical of DIC, i.e., thrombocytopenia, microangiopathic changes on the peripheral blood smear, and a decrease in Factors I, V, and VIII with an elevation in titer of fibrin degradation products (FDP). Rarely, these changes may be detected only in blood taken directly from the tumor (744). Occasionally a state of chronic consumption may be present, with normal or even elevated levels of coagulation factors due to compensatory coagulation protein synthesis. Increased fibrinolytic activity has rarely been demonstrated in cavernous hemangiomas (740). Whether this is primary or secondary to intravascular consumption, however, is unclear. A platelet functional defect associated with a prolonged bleeding time and a normal count has been described in this syndrome, presumably reflecting in vivo platelet activation within the tumor (741).

Treatment. Capillary and cavernous hemangiomas in infancy and childhood are fairly common. Estimates as to their frequency vary from 1 to 8 per cent in children below the age of 1 year. Most hemangiomas rapidly enlarge during the first 6 to 12 months of life, then spontaneously regress between 1 and 5 years (733). Monitoring of the hemangioma, together with the periodic evaluation of platelet counts, appears to be appropriate initial management. If moderate thrombocytopenia occurs in the absence of any significant hemorrhagic manifestations, corticosteroids can be used to help shrink the lesion. If the hemangioma is enlarging rapidly and the platelet count is in a steep decline, prednisone therapy at a dosage of 2 to 4 mg per kg per day may prevent further growth and effectively palliate the condition (733, 745). Several authors have doubted the efficacy of systemic corticosteroids, but in many instances an inadequate dose for too brief a period had been employed (746). Generally a 2- to 4-week period of a relatively high dose is necessary for an adequate trial (745). In an occasional case, relapse may occur following steroid discontinuation (747, 748) or this therapeutic modality may prove to be relatively ineffective (745).

Recent studies by Folkman have given us an insight into the possible mechanism of action of corticosteroids in causing hemangioma regression (749). He has shown that the growth of new capillaries occurs in a series of sequential steps, which include the degradation of basement membrane in a parent venule and the migration of endothelial cells towards an "angiogenic stimulus." This phase is followed by one of cellular proliferation and the alignment of cells with each other to form a vascular sprout which canalizes and elongates with continued directional migration of its endothelial cells. Finally, two or more vascular sprouts join to form a newly fledged capillary loop. This process of neovascularization is seen in many physiologic processes including wound healing, and in pathologic states including hemangiomatous lesions, tumor angiogenesis, and the retinopathy that accompanies various diseases. Most recently Folkman and his co-workers have shown that a combination of corticosteroids and heparin prevents many types of embryonic, inflammatory, and tumor-mediated angiogenic growth (750). Thus the use of corticosteroids and heparin for the treatment of patients with hemangiomas may have a sound theoretical basis.

If the patient continues to deteriorate despite the use of large doses of corticosteroids, with persistence or worsening of the coagulation defects, heparin (100 u per kg every 4 to 6 hours by continuous infusion) appears indicated in an attempt to control the bleeding. The platelet count, fibrinogen concentration, and partial thromboplastin time should be monitored during the heparin therapy (745, 751, 752). As discussed above, the work of Folkman suggests that corticosteroids may potentiate the action of heparin for the treatment of this condition (750). Replacement therapy with packed red cells, fresh frozen plasma, or platelet concentrates may also be necessary.

The presence of lesions in areas that could compromise vital functions, e.g., enlargement of hemangiomas of the neck or thorax, calls for more aggressive management. Such measures include surgical removal, radiation, or the combined use of steroids and embolization (753–754). In choosing one of these modalities, the physician must take into account their risks and benefits and the skills and experience of the radiotherapist and surgeon. In particular, the long-term effects of radiation therapy on the young infant must be kept in mind. Damage to secondary ossification centers and severe growth retardation may follow such treatment (754–757).

Lesions of the liver (cavernous hemangiomas, infantile hemangioendotheliomas, or vascular hamartomas) may present with congestive heart failure (733–735). Successful management of severe congestive heart failure resulting from arteriovenous shunting within the tumor has been accomplished by tumor resection (734), ligation of the hepatic artery (735), or low-dose radiation to part of the tumor (736).

Additional therapeutic maneuvers, of unproven efficacy, include the use of antiplatelet drugs or treatment with antifibrinolytic agents. Aspirin (20 mg per kg per day) and dipyridamole (1.5 to 2.5 mg per kg per day) was used by Koerper and associates in two children with the Kasabach-Merritt syndrome (758). In both infants, drug therapy was associated with a prompt rise in platelet count and cessation of clinical bleeding. Others have not shown any benefit from such therapy (759). Although the fibrinolytic component is usually considered to be secondarily activated in patients with this syndrome, plasminogen activators are present in arterial and venous endothelial cells, and not only could they initiate localized fibrinolysis and plasmin production within the hemangioma but they also appear necessary for neovascularization. Thus some patients may benefit from antifibrinolytic therapy including tranexamic and aminocaproic acids (760, 761).

About 20 per cent of the reported cases proved fatal due to hemorrhage, airway obstruction, or infection. Mortality among unselected cases is probably much lower, and the Kasabach-Merritt syndrome is basically a self-limited condition (733, 745). The specific management chosen in the individual child is dependent on the patient's clinical status and hematologic evaluation, but whenever possible, expectant observation is the safest approach. Aggressive therapy with drugs, surgical extirpation, or radiation may however be necessary in the management of the symptomatic child.

Other Causes of Local Consumption Coagulopathy

Thrombocytopenia has been observed with choranangioma (762–763), hemangioendotheliomas of the liver (764, 765), hemangiomatous transformation of the spleen (766), and diffuse angiomatosis (767, 768). Rare cases of localized consumption with lymphangiomas also exist (697, 698). In some of these patients the hemostatic abnormality may progress to a more disseminated form of intravascular coagulation.

DESTRUCTIVE THROMBOCYTOPENIA DUE TO MISCELLANEOUS CAUSES

Thrombocytopenia in Glomerular Disease

In most forms of glomerulonephritis (but not systemic lupus erythematosus, in which immunologic thrombocytopenia may occur), the platelet count remains in the normal range. However, occasional cases of thrombocytopenia associated with glomerulonephritis have been reported in the pediatric literature (769). In contrast to the platelet count, platelet life span measurements have shown a reduced half-life in acute proliferative glomerulonephritis (770–772), with evidence for platelet activation (773–775) and only minimal decreases in fibrinogen and plasminogen survival (771). Platelet consumption in specific cases has been attributed to immunologic mechanisms, the presence of a plasma factor that can agglutinate platelets, hypoalbuminemia, and hypercholesterolemia (776, 777). Examination of renal biopsies for platelets within glomerular lesions has on the whole proved disappointing, although occasional investigators have demonstrated their presence (778, 779).

Platelets may act as important mediators in renal disease. They can facilitate immune complex deposition, augment the inflammatory response, and cause proliferation of vascular smooth muscle and endothelial cells by releasing permeability and growth promoting factors (780). Since platelets may participate either primarily or secondarily in glomerular disease, a number of studies involving the use of antiplatelet agents have been performed with or without concomitant immunosuppressive therapy (776, 781–784). Donadio and co-workers (784) have recently reported on a controlled, double-blind study in which the antiplatelet agents aspirin and dipyridamole were shown to positively alter the natural course of Type I membranoproliferative glomerulonephritis, thus providing evidence for the role of platelets in glomerular pathology.

Thrombocytopenia in Preeclampsia

Both platelet count and life span remain within normal limits during the uncomplicated pregnancy (785–789). Most studies that have evaluated platelet numbers in women with preeclampsia reveal that approximately 15 to 20 per cent develop thrombocytopenia early in their illness (790), with a return of the count to normal within a week after delivery. The drop in platelet count is caused by increased peripheral platelet destruction as shown by the presence of a shortened platelet survival and an increase in bone marrow megakaryocytes and mean platelet volume (789–791). Although in a small percentage of patients the thrombocytopenia of preeclampsia may be thrombin mediated (790, 792–794), in most, other factors appear responsible for the platelet destruction (790, 795, 796). Mechanisms that could contribute to the thrombocytopenia include platelet adherence to damaged vascular endothelial surfaces, elevations in platelet-associated IgG levels (which occur in approximately 50 per cent of the thrombocytopenic patients), and decreased vascular prostacyclin formation (790, 797–800). As a result of these various pathologic processes, circulating platelets undergo partial release, are less responsive to aggregating agents, and demonstrate a decrease in their adenine nucleotide and serotonin content. Increases in the plasma levels of platelet granule constituents including β-thromboglobulin are concomitantly seen (799, 801, 802).

The platelet activation that can occur in vivo may be the reason why some women with preeclampsia have a disproportionate prolongation of their bleeding time even at relatively normal platelet counts, suggesting that the activated platelets of preeclampsia may not be functional (803). It is unclear whether platelet activation is an initiating or secondary event in the pathogenesis of preeclampsia. Although uncontrolled studies purport to show that antiplatelet therapy (aspirin and dipyridamole) given to high-risk mothers from the third month of gestation onward may protect against the occurrence of the disease and improve fetal outcome (804, 805), more rigorous clinical trials need to be done before the efficacy of these agents can be established.

Preeclamptic mothers with platelet counts of less than 50,000 cells per mm^3 often give birth to thrombocytopenic infants (806, 807). Causes of the quantitative platelet defects in these infants include mechanisms similar to those operative in the mother, i.e., consumptive coagulopathy, immunologic mechanisms, and a decrease in vascular prostacyclin production (790, 808, 809).

Thrombocytopenias Peculiar to the Neonate

The platelet counts of normal full-term and premature infants are within the adult normal range of 150,000 to 450,000 cells per mm^3 (810). However, neonates, especially prematures in the intensive care setting, appear to be peculiarly susceptible to thrombocytopenia. A recent study (811) observed that approximately 30 per cent of such infants became thrombocytopenic in the first week of life, with resolution usually occurring by day 10. The thrombocytopenia is caused by an increased rate of platelet destruction as shown by an increase in mean platelet volumes, shortened ^{111}indium platelet survivals, and increased numbers of megakaryocytes. In the majority of neonates (80 per cent), the thrombocytopenia could be attributed to disseminated intravascular coagulation, immune mechanisms, or exchange transfusions. This interesting study provided the first insights into the mechanisms of thrombocytopenia so commonplace in the sick neonate. Other workers have also documented that a decrease in the neonatal platelet count is most often associated with infection, with evidence in some studies for an immunologic cause for the platelet destruction (812, 813).

Thrombocytopenia also occurs more frequently in premature infants with respiratory distress syndrome, meconium aspiration, persistent pulmonary hypertension, necrotizing enterocolitis, hyperbilirubinemia and polycythemia and in those receiving phototherapy or having an umbilical catheter in place (814).

Phototherapy. Phototherapy in the neonate has been reported to be associated with mild thrombocytopenia (815). Phototherapy shortens platelet life span in rabbits, and in vitro, blue fluorescent light induces biochemical and morphologic changes in human platelets with a concomitant decrease in aggregatory ability.

Thrombocytopenia, Pulmonary Hypertension, and the Perinatal Aspiration Syndromes. Platelets may be important in the pathogenesis of persistent pulmonary hypertension (PPH) complicating the perinatal aspiration syndromes (816). In these neonates, it is postulated that either hypoxia or amniotic fluid aspiration or both induce abnormal platelet aggregation, with the release into the pulmonary vascular bed of prostaglandins, thromboxane A$_2$, or both causing an increase in pulmonary vascular tone (817). In support of this hypothesis is the observation that the pulmonary microcirculation is blocked by platelet aggregates at necropsy in some neonates with PPH (817). Increased production of thromboxane B$_2$, the stable end product of proaggregatory thromboxane A$_2$, has also been observed in these neonates (818). A similar syndrome has been reported by Favara and co-workers, who described platelet thrombi on atrioventricular valves and pulmonary arteries at necropsy in neonates with thrombocytopenia and severe respiratory distress (819). Although an association with persistent pulmonary hypertension was not described in the original paper, subsequent reports have noted this association (820, 821).

Thrombocytopenia Associated with Rhesus Alloimmunization and Following Exchange Transfusion. Moderate thrombocytopenia occurs frequently in infants with Rh erythroblastosis fetalis. Disseminated intravascular coagulation, hypersplenism, and alloimmune cell destruction have all been suggested as the cause for this finding, but the precise mechanism remains unknown. Thrombocytopenia has also been observed following exchange transfusion or massive replacement blood transfusion. This phenomenon is probably due to the dilution of neonatal blood by the transfused blood products, since neither plasma nor stored red cells contain viable platelets (822). The platelet count can usually be restored to normal by the use of platelet transfusions in patients with severe thrombocytopenia.

Recently, one group of physicians reported that 60 per cent of neonates given exchange transfusions with irradiated blood developed a transient maculopapular rash with eosinophilia, lymphopenia, and thrombocytopenia (823). These infants had been given both intrauterine and postnatal exchange transfusions for erythroblastosis fetalis.

Hematologic abnormalities resolved within several weeks and no patient progressed to acute or chronic graft-versus-host disease.

Polycythemia. The thrombocytopenia observed in polycythemic neonates commonly occurs at venous hematocrits of greater than 70 per cent (824–826). Postulated mechanisms for the quantitative decrease in the platelet count include a thrombocytolytic state due to DIC or to platelet consumption on an abnormal microvascular surface induced by stasis and hypoxia. Hemodilution, preferably with plasma, is advocated in the symptomatic neonate (827).

Miscellaneous Causes. Inherited metabolic disorders associated with thrombocytopenia include methylmalonic acidemia, ketotic glycinemia, and holocarboxylase synthetase deficiency (828, 829). The cause of the thrombocytopenia is unknown.

Isovaleric acidemia is a rare inherited disorder of metabolism that may also be associated with neonatal thrombocytopenia (830, 831). Homologous platelets survived normally in two neonates with this disorder. The thrombocytopenia was associated with anemia and leukopenia, with the bone marrow demonstrating early erythroid and myeloid forms. Pancytopenia is thought to be caused by an abnormality of cell maturation due to the abnormal elevation in serum isovaleric acid levels (831).

Fatty Acid–Induced Thrombocytopenia

In vivo and in vitro, platelet aggregation and thrombocytopenia can be caused by certain fatty acids (832). Arachidonic acid aggregates human platelet-rich plasma in vitro, and when injected into an animal can cause sudden death associated with occlusion of the pulmonary microcirculation by platelet aggregates. Pretreatment of the animals with aspirin protects against this effect (833). Similar abnormalities can be induced by the intravenous infusion of oleic acid, with the development of hypoxemia, thrombocytopenia, and hemorrhagic pulmonary injury, and the demonstration of ^{111}indium platelet localization in the lung (834). Because of the physiologic similarities between fatty acid–induced pulmonary injury and the abnormalities (including thrombocytopenia and a reduction in platelet survival) seen in the adult respiratory distress syndrome (ARDS), this injury model has been used to evaluate the pathophysiology of the latter condition (834–836). It is possible that syndromes associated with increased pulmonary vascular resistance of the adult and neonate (e.g., ARDS and PPH), may have in common the direct involvement of platelet activation.

Hypertriglyceridemia has been reported in association with thrombocytopenia (837), and hypercholesterolemia has been demonstrated to reduce platelet survival (838–840). Various fat emulsions have been used for parenteral nutrition in humans; the preparation of choice appears to be the soybean lipid emulsion Intralipid. In adults, Intralipid has not been demonstrated to reduce either the platelet count or the platelet life span (841), although it has been associated with hemolytic episodes, reticuloendothelial cell blockade, and abnormalities in cellular immune function (842–844). In general, thrombocytopenia has not been found to occur in children receiving hyperalimentation with this compound. However, one case report involved a neonate with thrombocytopenia that bore a temporal relationship to Intralipid on more than one occasion, and no other cause for the low platelet count could be discerned (845). Since arachidonic acid binding to plasma is decreased in the hypoalbuminemic premature infant, especially in those receiving Intralipid (846), theoretical reasons exist for the cautious use of this compound in neonates with preexisting pulmonary hypertension. Intimal lipid deposits have also been described within the small pulmonary arteries of neonates supported by intravenous Intralipid infusions (847–849). In the neonate, a pump-assisted continuous infusion is preferred to an infusion over a shorter period of time.

CONGENITAL AND HEREDITARY THROMBOCYTOPENIAS DUE TO IMPAIRED OR INEFFECTIVE PRODUCTION

Thrombocytopenia Absent Radii (TAR) Syndrome

This inherited disorder is characterized by neonatal thrombocytopenia, striking forearm abnormalities (including hypoplastic or absent radii and ulnae), a high incidence of transient leukemoid reactions, and cardiac lesions in approximately one third of the neonates. This entity is probably inherited in an autosomal recessive fashion. A review of 40 cases indicates that the first year of life is the period of highest risk for bleeding. Ninety per cent of all deaths from hemorrhage occur during this time (850), with an overall mortality rate of about 35 per cent in the first year of life. The first 4 months of life in particular are the most hazardous for major bleeding episodes. Platelet counts are usually in the 15,000 to 30,000 cells per mm^3 range. White cell counts may show a leukocytosis (>100,000 cells per mm^3), often with a shift to the left. Anemia may develop as a result of blood loss. Bone marrow examination usually reveals an absence of megakaryocytes, often with concomitant myeloid hyperplasia. Occasionally, megakaryocytes may be present, appearing small and immature (851, 852) or even normal in number (853).

Abnormalities in platelet survival, aggregation,

dense granule content, and ultrastructure (suggestive of a storage pool defect) have been reported in some individuals with the TAR syndrome (851, 853–855). In one report, the father of the affected infant also showed abnormal platelet function (856). Discrepancies in platelet function studies may reflect platelet heterogeneity or the difficulty of interpreting platelet studies in thrombocytopenic individuals. Bone marrow culture studies evaluating thrombopoiesis have provided conflicting results (857, 858).

Many affected children develop failure to thrive, diarrhea, and other symptoms of milk allergy in early life (859). The platelet count slowly begins to rise after the first year and life expectancy normalizes. Occasional patients may never have episodes of bleeding severe enough to warrant hematologic investigation until their adult years (860). During the first year of life, it is important to avoid surgery and stress since these events can precipitate hemorrhagic episodes. A variety of orthopedic procedures are usually necessary to correct the skeletal anomalies, but these should be postponed until after infancy.

In symptomatic patients, treatment is generally supportive with platelet and blood transfusions as necessary. Since refractoriness to platelet transfusion will eventually occur, platelet transfusions should be given only to infants with serious or recurrent hemorrhages. Corticosteroids and splenectomy have not proved effective.

Genetic counseling should be provided to mothers with previously affected children since the risk of recurrence for future offspring approximates 25 per cent. In a study of six pregnancies at risk for the TAR syndrome, the demonstration of absent radii by fetal radiography at 16 to 20 weeks gestation correctly identified two affected fetuses (861). Accurate identification of the limb anomaly is also possible by ultrasonography, obviating the risks associated with fetal radiography (862, 863). If diagnosis of the TAR syndrome is made in the prenatal period and the mother elects to continue her pregnancy, consideration should be given to a cesarean delivery to minimize birth trauma.

Other Congenital Thrombocytopenias with Megakaryocyte Hypoplasia

In addition to the recognizable entity of the TAR syndrome, there have been reports of other congenital thrombocytopenias associated with hypoplasia of megakaryocytes. Congenital thrombocytopenia has been associated with phocomelia (864, 865), chromosomal abnormalities including trisomies 13 and 18 (866–868), and microcephaly (869, 870). Other reports have described thrombocytopenia accompanied by elevated levels of fetal hemoglobin (871), or preceding the syndrome of dyskeratosis congenita (872). Recently Gardner and associates described a syndrome of congenital amegakaryocytic thrombocytopenia, multiple malformations (with a grossly normal appendicular skeleton), and neurologic dysfunction (873). Amegakaryocytic thrombocytopenia in the neonatal period has also been observed to precede the onset of aplastic anemia. The congenital malformations of Fanconi's anemia have not been seen in these children. Treatment with androgens or bone marrow transplantation has been attempted in some cases (874). A familial form of thrombocytopenia associated with platelet antibodies and chromosomal changes resembling those seen in Fanconi's anemia has also been described recently (875).

Fanconi's Aplastic Anemia

In this form of congenital megakaryocytic hypoplasia (876), thrombocytopenia occurs together with a depression of both myeloid and erythroid elements and is associated with a broader pattern of congenital abnormalities than that which occurs in the TAR syndrome, discussed earlier. Symptoms usually do not occur in early infancy.

Bernard-Soulier Syndrome

This hereditary form of thrombocytopenia is associated with important defects in platelet function and will be discussed in Section II of this chapter, which deals with inherited qualitative platelet abnormalities.

May-Hegglin Anomaly

The May-Hegglin anomaly is a rare disorder inherited in an autosomal dominant fashion. It is characterized by the presence of giant platelets and Döhle bodies (basophilic inclusions; see below) in the leukocytes (877). About one third of the patients described have associated thrombocytopenia. The majority of individuals do not have bleeding manifestations, the disease entity usually being discovered as an incidental finding. Occasionally, severe thrombocytopenia associated with a hemorrhagic tendency has been reported (852).

The most striking finding noted on the peripheral blood smear is the presence of basophilic patches of cytoplasm devoid of normal granulation in leukocytes. These patches of RNA are called Döhle bodies and probably represent a defect in the maturation of normal leukocyte granules. Platelets vary in size and shape, with the presence of occasional elongated forms that are 20 μ or greater in size. Platelet ultrastructural studies may be normal or reveal hypergranularity (852). A significant increase in giant granules has been observed by some authors (878, 879), although an indirect estimation of alpha granule number by measuring β-thromboglobulin has been found to be normal when expressed per platelet mass (880). Bone marrow evaluation reveals normal numbers of megakaryocytes. The primary abnormality has been suggested to be abnormal megakaryocyte fragmentation (881). A decrease in platelet survival was noted in earlier reports (882, 883), although most recent studies have shown that platelet survival in this disorder is normal (879, 881). Platelet aggregation and release and platelet membrane glycoproteins are normal (852, 879, 884). In occasional kindreds, variable clinical manifestations of the syndrome may occur with some individuals exhibiting the classic triad of giant platelets, Döhle bodies, and thrombocytopenia. Other family members may present only with giant platelets (885). Hereditary nephritis has also been reported in conjunction with this anomaly (886).

Wiskott-Aldrich Syndrome

Wiskott-Aldrich Syndrome (WAS), inherited as an X-linked recessive trait, is characterized by eczema, thrombocytopenia (platelet count usually below 50,000 cells per mm^3), and an increased susceptibility to infections. Bleeding commonly occurs in the first 6 months of life and may abate thereafter (852). The clinical course is often fatal, with death due to infection, hemorrhage, or lymphoreticular malignancy. Immunologic abnormalities include defects of both cellular and humoral systems: dysgammaglobulinemia, low or absent concentrations of isohemagglutinins, lymphopenia, and an impaired delayed-type hypersensitivity are frequently present. Patients with WAS are also usually anergic to various antigens, have poor lymphocyte blast transformation in response to antigenic stimulation, and fail to make specific antibodies to polysaccharide antigenic challenge. Accelerated catabolism of serum immunoglobulins and depressed monocyte-mediated antibody-dependent cellular cytotoxicity are also present (887). T cells exhibit a progressive decline in number and function such that a profound lymphopenia becomes manifest at about 6 years of life, and the mixed lymphocyte response becomes increasingly depressed. Examination of lymph nodes reveals reticular hyperplasia, the absence of germinal centers, and depletion of the T cell–dependent areas.

The thrombocytopenia of the Wiskott-Aldrich syndrome may be multifactorial. Ineffective thrombopoiesis (888) and deceased autologous platelet survival (889, 890) have been demonstrated, although not always to a degree sufficient to account for the thrombocytopenia. Allogeneic platelet survival is reported to be comparable to that of patients with bone marrow failure (888, 889, 891, 892). Lum and associates (893) have suggested that in some cases the thrombocytopenia may be secondary to the abnormal coating of platelets by IgG molecules.

Although an acquired thrombocytolytic state is often characterized by the presence of megathrombocytes, this is not the case in the Wiskott-Aldrich syndrome (894). In the eusplenic patient with WAS, although platelet size may be broadly distributed, overlapping the normal range, mean platelet volume is decreased (894, 895). Following splenectomy, platelet size increases toward normal (895). The elevated levels of PAIgG also normalize if the platelet count rises postsplenectomy (895). In contrast, in individuals who relapse following the removal of their spleen, thrombocytopenia recurs, and PAIgG levels become elevated, although platelet size may continue to be normal (895). Thus, splenic function clearly plays a role in the production of the microthrombocyte seen in WAS. Besides the change in platelet size, lymphocyte size also appears to increase postsplenectomy, with improvement in T cell function.

Bone marrow megakaryocytes are abnormal with either decreased numbers or abnormal appearance of storage organelles (852). Ultrastructural studies of the WAS platelet usually reveal a reduction in the number of dense bodies and mitochondria, although in occasional cases normal numbers of organelles may be seen (878, 896). Defective aggregation to ADP, collagen, and epinephrine with a normal thrombin response also has been reported (889, 890). One report has described the absence of a 115,000 dalton glycoprotein on lymphocytes from patients with WAS, and a reduction in glycoprotein Ib on platelets from these individuals (898, 899). Since these abnormalities are not observed in every patient, their relationship to pathogenesis remains uncertain.

Treatment of this disease with allogeneic bone marrow transplantation is curative (900, 901). If this is not feasible, splenectomy is useful in alleviating the thrombocytopenia but carries a serious risk of infection (893, 897). Postsplenectomy antibiotic coverage is mandatory. Corticosteroids are not effective in the treatment of this disease (891). In the presence of severe bleeding manifestations, platelet transfusions will cause a temporary elevation in the platelet count with cessation of bleeding.

A sensitive and specific test for carriers is not yet available. One group (902) reported that carriers of the Wiskott-Aldrich syndrome could be identified by a metabolic stress test in which 2-deoxy-D-glucose completely inhibited the second wave of platelet aggregation. Subsequent investigators have not confirmed these results (903). Other abnormalities in carriers include impaired production of platelet metabolic ADP (904). The measurement of platelet size in fetuses using fetoscopic blood samples may prove useful for the intrauterine diagnosis of this condition (903).

Miscellaneous Hereditary Thrombocytopenias

A heterogeneous group of familial thrombocytopenias has been described with either X-linked or autosomal modes of inheritance. However, data on marrow findings, platelet kinetics, and platelet function often are incomplete. A number of kindreds have been described with X-linked thrombocytopenia as a solitary abnormality or together with partial manifestations of the Wiskott-Aldrich syndrome. Most of these patients do not present with bleeding manifestations in early infancy and have a better prognosis than that seen in Wiskott-Aldrich syndrome. These individuals may benefit from steroids or splenectomy (905–909). A kindred with X-linked thrombocytopenia, platelet dysfunction, imbalanced globin chain synthesis, and hemolysis also has been described (910).

Hereditary thrombocytopenias can occur without other associated defects and may closely simulate acquired chronic ITP. The defect is usually transmitted as an autosomal dominant trait, although a few families have been described in which the mode of inheritance was autosomal recessive (911–919). No consistent pattern of megakaryocytopoiesis has been described, although recently developed in vitro culture techniques may ultimately aid in their categorization. Platelet function may be normal or impaired. Platelet survival of autologous platelets is often decreased, whereas homologous platelets survive normally. The bleeding tendency is mild, and steroids or splenectomy may be of benefit (914, 916).

A moderate degree of thrombocytopenia associated with the presence of megathrombocytes is described in large numbers of people of Mediterranean ancestry (920, 921). Total circulating platelet mass does not differ from normal, and this morphologic variant is not associated with a bleeding tendency.

ACQUIRED THROMBOCYTOPENIAS DUE TO IMPAIRED OR INEFFECTIVE PRODUCTION

Thrombocytopenia due to Aplastic Anemia or Marrow Infiltration

Thrombocytopenia in association with depression of both myeloid and erythroid elements occurs in aplastic anemia and various marrow infiltrative disorders including leukemia, lymphomas, solid tumors, myelofibrosis, reticuloendothelioses, osteopetrosis, storage diseases, and granulomatous disorders. When marrow replacement occurs, the blood picture usually suggests a leukoerythroblastic reaction, with the peripheral blood smear showing red cell abnormalities, including anisocytosis, poikilocytosis, tear drop forms, basophilia, and nucleated red cells. Immature myeloid forms and circulating megakaryocytic nuclei may also be seen. Splenomegaly and hypersplenism may complicate the picture.

Drug- and Radiation-Induced Thrombocytopenia as Part of Total Marrow Suppression

Chloramphenicol. This drug, which is being used with increasing frequency to combat resistant *Haemophilus influenzae* infections, can cause either a dose-dependent reversible bone marrow suppression or an idiosyncratic dose-independent, often irreversible marrow aplasia. Thrombocytopenia related to the dose-dependent effect of chloramphenicol is preceded by evidence of suppression of erythropoiesis, such as reticulocytopenia and an elevated serum iron level (922). Although cases of isolated thrombocytopenia developing in patients receiving chloramphenicol have been reported (923, 924), it is difficult to exclude other causes of thrombocytopenia in such instances. In a patient being treated with chloramphenicol, the appearance of moderate to severe thrombocytopenia related to dose-dependent drug toxicity requires withdrawal of the drug.

Cancer Chemotherapeutic Agents. Most antimetabolites and DNA-intercalating agents are marrow toxic, and in the doses given for chemotherapeutic effects will induce a suppressive thrombocytopenia. In most instances, this suppression is followed by marrow recovery. There appears to be a differential sensitivity of the marrow cell lines to the various chemotherapeutic agents. For instance, the particular antimegakaryocytic activity of hydroxyurea or cytosine arabinoside has been used to control thrombocytosis in the myeloproliferative disorders.

Cyclophosphamide and 6-mercaptopurine (925, 926) are less likely to cause thrombocytopenia, and thrombocytosis can follow the use of vinca alkaloids, methotrexate, 5-fluorouracil, and azathioprine (927, 928). During myelosuppression, mean platelet volume and megakaryocyte ploidy are decreased. The recovery phase is heralded first by an increase in ploidy, followed 1 to 2 days later by an increase in the mean platelet volume (929). Of the three marrow cell lines, megakaryocytes may be the least susceptible to the effects of ionizing radiation (930).

Drug-Induced Thrombocytopenia with Platelet-Specific Suppression

Although the use of certain drugs has been associated with thrombocytopenia concomitant with presumed bone marrow depression, studies to date have been unsatisfactory in specifically delineating this effect (929). Since in vitro cultures evaluating megakaryocytopoiesis have recently become feasible, it is possible that these techniques will provide new information concerning drug-induced marrow toxicities.

Alcohol. Chronic excessive ingestion of alcohol is frequently associated with thrombocytopenia, even in the absence of concomitant nutritional deficiency (931–933). Marrow megakaryocytes are either normal or reduced in number. A direct toxic effect of alcohol on the marrow and a reduction in platelet life span are probably responsible for the thrombocytopenia (934, 935). Increased platelet pooling in the spleen may play an added role in a few cases. Following alcohol withdrawal the platelet count rises in 3 to 5 days, and may be followed by a rebound thrombocytosis during recovery (929). No prospective information on the incidence of thrombocytopenia in infants born to alcoholic mothers is available.

Estrogens. The administration of pharmacologic doses of estrogenic hormones may result in thrombocytopenia associated with normal or reduced numbers of marrow megakaryocytes (936, 937). The exact mode of action remains unclear.

Thiazide Diuretics. There are at least two mechanisms by which these drugs can induce thrombocytopenia in the adult, namely, an effect on thrombopoiesis (929, 938, 939) or, rarely, drug-dependent antibody formation (940). Thrombocytopenia with hemorrhagic complications was previously reported in neonates of mothers who had received one of the thiazide drugs prior to delivery (941). Subsequent prospective, controlled studies have refuted this claim, however (942, 943). In the initial report, the observed neonatal thrombocytopenia probably occurred as a complication of maternal preeclampsia rather than thiazide ingestion.

Miscellaneous Drugs. Neonatal thrombocytopenia has been described in three infants born to mothers who were treated with hydralazine for hypertension during the last trimester of pregnancy (944). Since the hypertensive disorders of pregnancy themselves may be associated with neonatal thrombocytopenia (806, 807), a drug-induced fall in platelet count is difficult to substantiate under these circumstances. An analagous situation occurred in an infant with neonatal thrombocytopenia following tolbutamide ingestion in a diabetic mother (945). A rare case of prednisone-associated marrow suppression has also been described (126, 946, 947).

Thrombocytopenia Associated with Nutritional Deficiency States

In patients with either vitamin B_{12} or folic acid deficiency, a mild to moderate thrombocytopenia may occur. There is, however, a discrepancy between the usually mild degree of thrombocytopenia observed in these patients and the marked prolongation in bleeding time, apparently caused by a platelet qualitative abnormality (948, 949). Impaired or ineffective thrombopoiesis is seen in the megaloblastic anemias. Although megakaryocyte mass is increased, platelet turnover is markedly reduced, with only approximately 10 per cent of the expected platelet production occurring (950). Those platelets that are released into the circulation may also not survive normally (951). A decrease in the mean platelet volume (MPV) has been observed in patients with megaloblastic anemia accompanied by an increased heterogeneity in platelet size (952, 953). These abnormalities revert to normal following therapy.

Although thrombocytosis is frequently observed in iron deficiency anemia, thrombocytopenia has also been reported in profound iron deficiency, with a rise in the platelet count to normal levels following iron therapy (954–958). Increased numbers of bone marrow megakaryocytes have been observed in patients with iron deficiency associated with normal or increased platelet counts (91, 959), whereas a decrease in megakaryocyte numbers has been observed in those patients who are thrombocytopenic (955). Platelet life span is normal. It has been suggested that iron is necessary for the initiation of platelet protein synthesis and that in severe iron deficiency anemia platelet production is therefore impaired (960, 961). Mean platelet volume remains in the normal range in iron deficiency anemia (962).

THROMBOCYTOPENIA DUE TO PLATELET SEQUESTRATION

Hypersplenism

A moderate degree of thrombocytopenia may accompany splenomegaly due to diverse causes. Platelet counts usually range between 50,000 and 100,000 cells per mm^3 and rarely result in hemorrhagic manifestations. A platelet count of less than 20,000 cells per mm^3 suggests that the thrombocytopenia may be due to mechanisms other than hypersplenism alone. Bone marrow megakaryocytes are present in normal or increased numbers. The decrease in the platelet count sometimes, but not always, is associated with anemia, leukopenia, or both.

The thrombocytopenia associated with hypersplenism is caused by splenic "pooling." Under normal circumstances, approximately one third of the platelet mass is present in the spleen. Thus, in a normal person the transfusion of ^{51}Cr-labeled platelets will result in a platelet recovery rate of 60 to 75 per cent. In hypersplenic individuals, up to 90 per cent of the platelet mass may be present within the spleen, and the percentage of ^{51}Cr-labeled platelets that can be recovered from the peripheral circulation following platelet transfusion is decreased to approximately 10 to 30 per cent. In contrast, in asplenic individuals, 90 to 100 per cent of transfused platelets can be recovered (963). It must be emphasized that the platelet "pooling" observed in hypersplenism is not analogous to the situation seen in immune thrombocytopenias, in which destruction of immunologically altered platelets occurs in the spleen. In hypersplenism, normal platelets are delayed in their passage through the enlarged organ. Platelet survival curves are characteristic in this disorder, demonstrating low recovery with a normal or only minimally decreased platelet life span (90).

Since the decrease in the platelet count is not severe, hemorrhagic manifestations are seldom seen. Splenectomy therefore is more often performed for concomitant anemia associated with increasing transfusion requirements or for problems resulting from the splenomegaly per se, rather than for thrombocytopenia alone. Removal of the spleen is followed by restoration of the platelet count to either normal or elevated levels.

Hypothermia

The lowering of the body temperature to levels below 25°C can be associated with a fall in the platelet count (964, 965). This process is usually reversible following restoration of body temperature to normal (966, 967). Splenic and hepatic sequestration appears to be the main mechanism by which the peripheral thrombocytopenia occurs (966). It may also be due in part to clumping and the formation of in vivo platelet aggregates (964). Thrombocytopenia has also been found to accompany neonatal cold injury (968, 969). A worsening of the thrombocytopenia during the initial period of warming may occur in the neonate prior to restoration of the platelet count to normal levels (969).

DIAGNOSTIC APPROACH TO THE THROMBOCYTOPENIC PATIENT

An approach to the evaluation of a child with a platelet count of less than 150,000 cells per mm^3 is outlined in Figure 42–10. The particular considerations pertaining to the neonate are reviewed in Chapter 5 and are not discussed here.

In history taking, particular attention should be paid to drug ingestions, previous illnesses, operations, or immunizations; exposure to exanthema; and a family history of easy bruising, autoimmune disorders, or splenectomy. Physical findings to be noted include the presence or absence of associated anomalies, as well as the presence of conditions predisposing the patient to disseminated intravascular coagulation (see Table 42–9), jaundice, or hepatosplenomegaly.

Laboratory investigation should initially consist of the evaluation of a well-prepared peripheral blood smear. In a "sick" child the initial studies should also include a coagulation screen (PT, PTT, TT, and fibrinogen). The presence of an increased MPV is strongly suggestive of an acquired thrombocytolytic state. The examination of the bone marrow is often helpful in the further delineation of the cause of the thrombocytopenia. A marrow biopsy is the procedure of choice in the infant or child in whom confirmation of a marrow infiltrative process is being sought. A biopsy should also be performed in patients in whom megakaryocyte hypoplasia is considered, since a spurious decrease in the numbers of these cells may be encountered in a dilute aspirate specimen. Using the relatively simple approach outlined in Figure 42–10 and Table 42–10 together with appropriate ancillary tests, the evaluation of the thrombocytopenic child should prove an exciting diagnostic challenge.

THROMBOCYTOSIS

An elevation in the platelet count above the normal range of 450,000 cells per mm^3 is defined as thrombocytosis. This elevation may be the result of a primary hematologic disease (e.g., part of a myeloproliferative disorder) or secondary to a coexisting physiologic or pathologic process, in which case it is termed reactive. Table 42–11 lists the various conditions in which an elevation of the platelet count may be observed in infants and children. In a child with a normally functioning spleen, thrombocytosis is usually secondary to iron deficiency, chronic inflammation, a hematologic disorder, or neoplastic disease. This type of thrombocytosis usually is asymptomatic and disappears following therapy or remission of the primary disorder (970). Primary thrombocytosis is a disease of adult life and is extremely rare in children (971–978).

At least two humoral regulators are important in the control of normal human megakaryocytopoiesis (979, 980). The first regulator, megakaryocyte colony-stimulating activity (Meg-CSA) exerts its effect on the megakaryocyte colony-forming unit (CFU-M), causing these cells to proliferate and undergo partial maturation. Another regulator, termed thrombopoietin, does not support CFU-M growth in vitro but stimulates megakaryocyte differentiation.

In vitro studies of megakaryocytopoiesis may help to differentiate primary from reactive thrombocytoses (981). The CFU-M unit is quantitatively and qualitatively normal, and levels of Meg-CSA are not elevated in reactive thrombocytosis. In primary thrombocytosis on the other hand, the intrinsic stem cell defect affects the CFU-M, resulting in an expanded stem cell pool with increased proliferative capacity (981). These in vitro

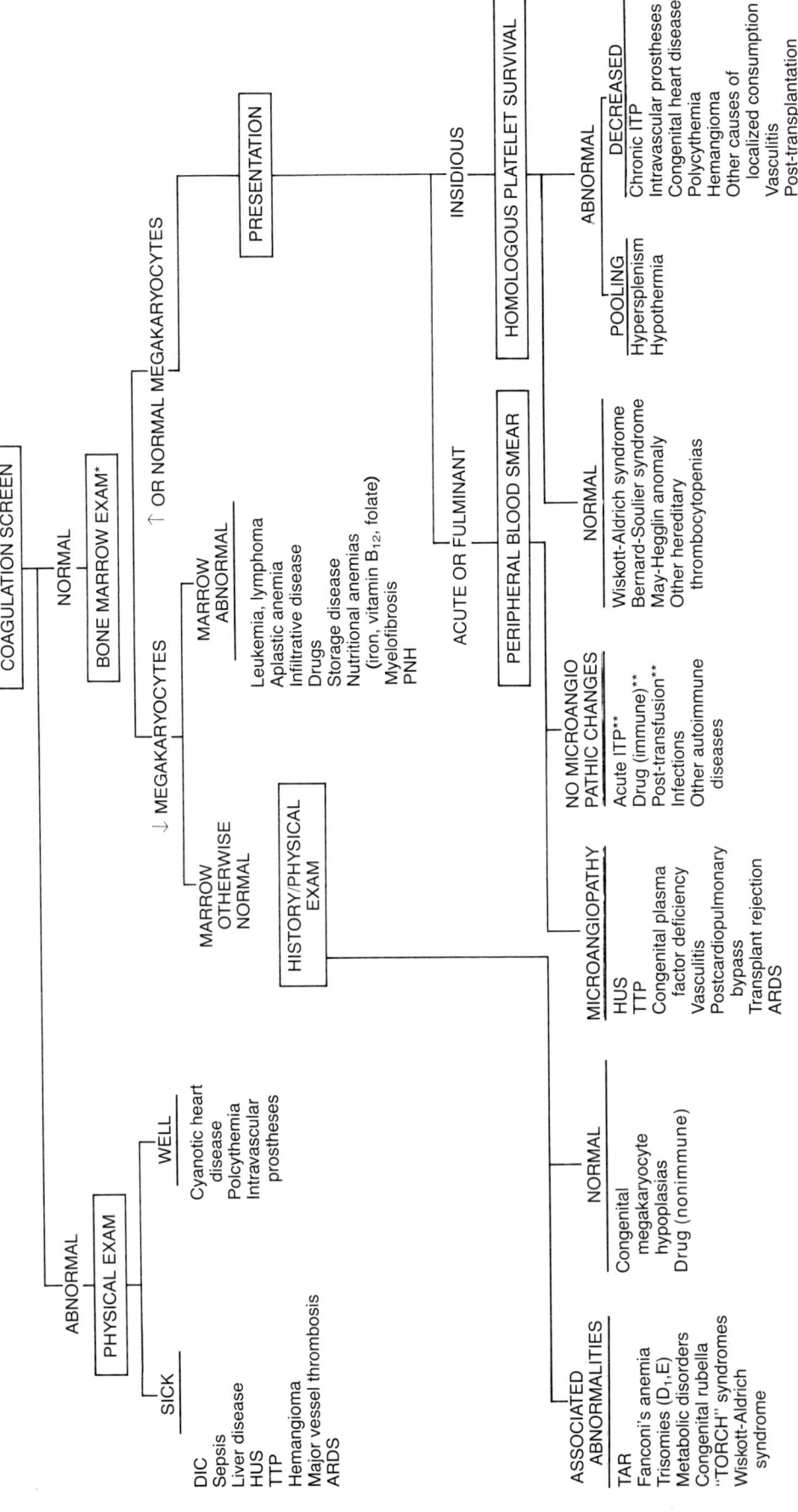

Figure 42–10. An evaluation of thrombocytopenia in children. (The neonate is excluded from this analysis.)

Table 42–10. DIFFERENTIAL DIAGNOSIS OF THROMBOCYTOPENIA IN CHILDREN

I. *DESTRUCTIVE THROMBOCYTOPENIAS*
   Primary Platelet Consumption Syndromes

      Immunologic
- Idiopathic thrombocytopenic purpura
- Drug-induced thrombocytopenia
- Infection-induced thrombocytopenia
- Post-transfusion purpura
- Autoimmune or lymphoproliferative disorders
- Neonatal immune thrombocytopenias
- Allergy and anaphylaxis
- Post-transplant thrombocytopenia

      Nonimmunologic
- Chronic microangiopathic hemolytic anemia and thrombocytopenia
- Hemolytic uremic syndrome
- Thrombotic thrombocytopenic purpura
- Catheters, prostheses, or cardiopulmonary bypass
- Congenital or acquired heart disease

   Combined Platelet and Fibrinogen Consumption Syndromes
      Disseminated intravascular coagulation
      Kasabach-Merritt syndrome
      Other causes of local consumption coagulopathy

   Miscellaneous Causes

      Specific to the neonate
- Phototherapy
- Perinatal aspiration syndromes
- Persistent pulmonary hypertension
- Rhesus alloimmunization
- Post-exchange transfusion
- Polycythemia
- Metabolic disorders

      Glomerular disease
      Pre-eclampsia
      Fatty acid–induced thrombocytopenia

II. *IMPAIRED OR INEFFECTIVE PRODUCTION*
   Congenital and Hereditary Disorders

      Primary Hematologic Processes
- TAR syndrome
- Other congenital thrombocytopenias with megakaryocytic hypoplasia
- Fanconi's aplastic anemia
- Bernard-Soulier syndrome*
- May-Hegglin anomaly*
- Wiskott-Aldrich syndrome*
- Miscellaneous hereditary thrombocytopenias (X-linked or autosomal)*
- Mediterranean thrombocytopenia

      Associated with Trisomy 13 or 18

      Metabolic Disorders
- Methylmalonic acidemia
- Ketotic glycinemia
- Holocarboxylase synthetase deficiency
- Isovaleric acidemia

   Acquired Disorders
      Aplastic anemia
      Marrow infiltrative processes
      Drug- or radiation-induced
      Nutritional deficiency states (iron, folate, or vitamin B_{12})

III. *SEQUESTRATION*
   Hypersplenism
   Hypothermia

*These hereditary thrombocytopenias can be associated with normal or increased bone marrow megakaryocytes.

Table 42–11. DIFFERENTIAL DIAGNOSIS OF THROMBOCYTOSIS* IN INFANCY AND CHILDHOOD

I. *Primary or Autonomous Thrombocytosis*
    Myeloproliferative syndromes
        Essential thrombocythemia
        Polycythemia vera
        Chronic myelogenous leukemia
        Myeloid metaplasia
        5q− syndrome
        Idiopathic sideroblastic anemia
II. *Secondary or Reactive Thrombocytosis*
    Inflammatory Diseases
        Acute infections
        Acute rheumatic fever
        Rheumatoid arthritis
        Ankylosing spondylitis
        Ulcerative colitis
        Regional enteritis
        Celiac sprue
        Tuberculosis
        Sarcoid
        Chronic hepatitis
        Chronic osteomyelitis
    Drug-induced
        Epinephrine
        Vinca alkaloids
        Therapy for iron deficiency or vitamin B_{12} deficiency
        Passively addicted neonates
    Immune disorders
        Collagen vascular disorders
        Graft-versus-host disease
        Nephrotic syndrome
    Hematologic disorders
        Iron deficiency
        Vitamin E deficiency
        Chronic hemolytic anemias and hemoglobinopathies
        "Rebound" following thrombocytopenia
    Neoplasms
        Lymphomas
        Hodgkin's disease
        Neuroblastoma
        Hepatoblastoma
        Other childhood solid tumors
        Carcinomas
    Surgical or functional asplenia
    Miscellaneous
        Following hemorrhage or gastrointestinal blood loss
        Following surgery
        Following exercise
        Caffey's disease
        Kawasaki syndrome

*Spurious thrombocytosis may be caused by the presence of microspherocytes, Pappenheimer bodies, red cell and leukocyte fragments, or bacteria (6–10, 982).

studies, although important in elucidating the etiology of the increased megakaryocyte mass and platelet numbers, will not help in the clinical differentiation of these disorders since they are not available in most laboratories.

In reactive thrombocytosis the platelet count seldom exceeds 600,000 cells per mm³ and platelet function is normal. As seen in Table 42–11, the primary cause for the increase in platelet numbers will become evident on further investigation. No specific therapy directed at the platelet count per se is necessary in these children.

In adults with primary thrombocytosis, the increase in platelet numbers and megakaryocytic mass may be associated with a generalized myeloproliferative disorder such as polycythemia rubra vera, chronic myelogenous leukemia, myeloid metaplasia, or other myelodysplastic syndromes. Recently, diagnostic criteria for primary thrombocytosis have been outlined (983, 984). These include a platelet count of greater than 1 million per mm³; normal red cell mass; the absence of the Ph^1 karyotype, and rigorous exclusion of the causes for reactive thrombocytosis.

Platelets in myeloproliferative disease have a multitude of defects (983). Although mean platelet volume may be normal, there usually is a wide distribution of size with increased numbers of both small and large platelets. Surface membrane function is abnormal with decreased numbers of α-adrenergic and prostaglandin D_2 receptors (985–987). Alterations in the amounts of platelet membrane glycoproteins have been observed (988, 989), as has the presence of an additional platelet protein which appears to be a modified form of the normal subunit of platelet-glycoprotein G (thrombospondin) found in platelet α-granules (990). Deficiencies in platelet adhesiveness and serotonin uptake have been reported (991, 992). Variable defects in platelet arachidonic acid metabolism (including cyclooxygenase and lipoxygenase metabolism) may also be present (993–997). Ultrastructural abnormalities include both qualitative and quantitative defects in platelet organelles, microtubules, and the dense tubular system (979, 983). Platelet aggregation abnormalities include spontaneous aggregation as well as a reduction in platelet response to epinephrine, collagen, and ADP (983, 996, 998–1002).

The bleeding time is rarely prolonged in primary thrombocytosis or polycythemia vera, although it is often abnormal in myeloid metaplasia (983). In this disorder, long-term follow-up has shown that hemorrhagic or thrombotic complications may occur in approximately one quarter to one third of the patients, although such abnormalities are rare in the young adult and child (971, 1003–1006). Complications are not generally predictable by platelet function studies.

No bone marrow suppressive therapy is advocated for children with primary thrombocytosis. Mutagenic agents are especially contraindicated since this form of treatment has been shown to increase the incidence of leukemia in adults with polycythemia vera (983). In the rare event that the child with primary thrombocytosis has to be prepared for elective surgery or develops an acute thrombotic or hemorrhagic complication, the platelet count can be quickly lowered by plateletpheresis (1007). As primary thrombocytosis is an extremely rare childhood disease, the long-term prognostic implications of this disorder are unknown. One such child, diagnosed at age 11 years, has progressed on to myelofibrosis (1008). As a growth factor released by platelet and megakaryocytes has been suggested to stimulate the proliferation of fibroblasts (1009), this long-term sequela is not unexpected.

APPENDIX

Techniques Used to Measure Platelet Antibodies

The interaction of antibodies or complement with platelets can be measured either directly or indirectly. Indirect assays were the first techniques used to measure IgG-platelet interactions, but they have largely been supplanted by direct binding assays. All indirect assays use the same general approach: test patient serum is incubated with normal platelets and a platelet-related endpoint is measured. A large number of different platelet endpoints have been used, including inhibition of platelet migration, platelet lysis, and platelet release. Although indirect techniques offer the advantage of simplicity of collection and storage of test samples, these assays are both insensitive and nonspecific. The insensitivity of all indirect assays is predictable: the antibody must measurably damage or activate the target platelets to be detected. Although certain antiplatelet antibodies are capable of inducing a measurable platelet endpoint, many are not, and such antibodies cannot be detected using indirect techniques. The other problem with indirect assays is their low specificity, which is likewise predictable: many other nonimmune stimuli also cause platelet aggregation, release, or lysis, and consequently produce false-positive results.

We will briefly summarize the indirect assays according to the endpoint measured. These assays are schematically represented in Figure 42–11.

INDIRECT ASSAYS THAT MEASURE THE INTERACTION OF ANTIBODY-SENSITIZED PLATELETS WITH OTHER CELLS

These techniques measure biologic "signals" sent from platelets to other cells.

Lymphocyte Transformation. Control platelets are incubated with patient serum to allow sensitization by the antibody. The platelets are then incubated with autologous or control lymphocytes and the reactivity of the lymphocytes measured by the uptake of radiolabeled thymidine (182, 1010).

Leukocyte Phagocytosis. Radiolabeled control platelets are incubated with test serum and mixed with granulocytes. The platelet/granulocyte interaction (phagocytosis) is measured following the separation of the platelets bound to granulocytes from the unphagocitized platelets (1011).

Complement Fixation. Control platelets and patient serum are incubated with a source of complement. The amount of complement bound to the platelets is quantitated by measuring the lysis of sheep red cells in the presence of antisheep red cell antibody (326, 1012).

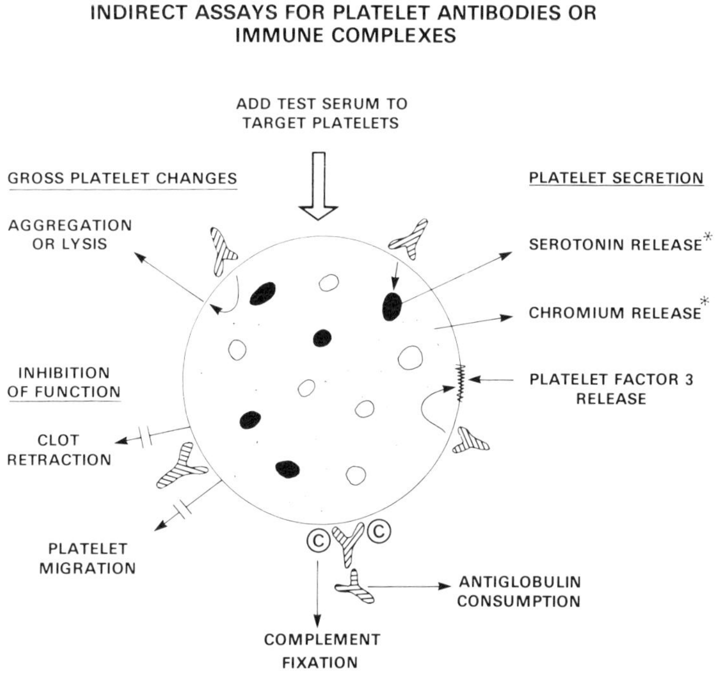

Figure 42–11. A schematic representation of indirect techniques for measuring platelet immune interactions. (From Kelton, J. G.: Progr. Hematol. *13*:163, 1983.)

INDIRECT ASSAYS THAT MEASURE THE INHIBITION OF PLATELET FUNCTION

All of these assays measure antibody-dependent inhibition of a measurable aspect of platelet function. Like the previously described assays, these techniques provide biologically interesting information but have neither sufficient sensitivity nor specificity to be useful as diagnostic tests.

Clot Retraction Inhibition. Platelets participate in clot retraction, and this reaction can be inhibited by certain antiplatelet antibodies. Test serum is mixed with freshly collected whole blood plus complement. Clot retraction is assessed by measuring the volume of serum expressed from the clot (1013).

Platelet Migration Inhibition. Platelets can migrate toward substances such as collagen, and this movement can be inhibited by antibodies. To perform this test, viable platelets are isolated from whole blood and the platelet-rich plasma is incubated with test serum. The platelet migration that occurs over the next 24 hours is measured in a migration chamber (320, 321).

INDIRECT ASSAYS THAT MEASURE ANTIBODY-INDUCED PLATELET AGGREGATION OR DAMAGE

Of all the indirect tests, these assays have proved the most useful for antiplatelet allo- and autoantibodies.

Platelet Aggregation; Serotonin or Adenine Release. These tests are all basically the same. Target platelets are incubated with test patient serum with or without complement, and the endpoint of the reaction measured. Initially, platelet aggregation was measured, then in an attempt to increase the sensitivity of these assays, the release of radiolabeled serotonin or adenine was assessed (322–324, 329–330).

Platelet Lysis. Patient serum plus control platelets are incubated together and complement is added. Antibody-induced platelet lysis is measured either in an aggregometer or by measuring the release of radiolabeled chromium from the platelets. This technique is still used as a test for drug-dependent antiplatelet antibodies (325, 1014, 1015).

Platelet Factor 3 Release. The endpoint of this test is antibody-induced exposure of the platelet procoagulant, platelet factor 3. Heat-inactivated patient serum plus platelet-rich plasma are incubated together, and the time required for clot formation after the addition of a contact factor activator and calcium is measured (1016–1018).

THE DIRECT MEASUREMENT OF PLATELET-BOUND IgG AND COMPLEMENT

Assays that measure the binding of IgG and/or IgM and complement to platelets are now used by many laboratories to investigate patients with suspected immune thrombocytopenia. These assays have dramatically increased our understanding of the pathogenesis of a variety of thrombocytopenic disorders. However, like many investigative tools, they have raised as many questions as they have answered.

Although techniques capable of measuring IgG on red cells have been available for some 40 years, it has only been within the past decade that assays that could measure IgG on platelets have been developed. There are a number of reasons why it has been so difficult to measure IgG on platelets. It is technically difficult to isolate a relatively pure population of platelets from a thrombocytopenic patient; in contrast, even in a patient with severe hemolytic anemia, it is not difficult to obtain enough red cells for testing. Second, there is a narrow "window" between the amount of IgG present on platelets from a patient with ITP as compared with a normal control. Although the precise amount of IgG on normal platelets remains uncertain, one group of investigators using the same assay to measure IgG on red cells and platelets found that washed red cells from a normal individual carried approximately 25 to 50 molecules of IgG per red cell (1019). In contrast, a patient with autoimmune hemolytic anemia with a + or ++ direct antiglobulin test had 500 to 1000 molecules of IgG per red cell (a 50- to 100-fold difference). The situation for platelets was entirely different: normal platelets carried from 500 to 2000 molecules of IgG per platelet, while platelets from patients with immune thrombocytopenia typically had 4000 to 6000 molecules of IgG per cell, only a ten-fold increase (1020). Thus not only is the "baseline" level of IgG much higher on platelets as compared with red cells, but the difference in IgG between ITP platelets and control platelets is much smaller when compared with red cells from controls versus patients with immune hemolytic anemia (1019, 1020).

Another reason why it has been difficult to develop sensitive and specific tests for immune thrombocytopenia is that platelets nonspecifically bind plasma proteins. The problem of nonspecific binding of test reagents to the target cells can complicate virtually any assay; however, this is a major problem in the measurement of IgG on platelets. A simple example illustrates the problem. Assume that a very pure anti-IgG preparation contains 100 protein molecules of which 10 per cent are specifically anti-IgG. During the labeling procedure all proteins are labeled and consequently the nonspecific binding of a labeled protein other than anti-IgG to the platelet cannot be distinguished from specific binding of the labeled anti-IgG. If all labeled anti-IgG binds to the platelet membrane, plus 10 per cent of nonimmune proteins, then 50 per cent of the label on the platelets is not the anti-IgG. Consequently, it can be difficult to differentiate a normal from an abnormal result.

The IgG measured on or in the test platelets is termed platelet-associated IgG (PAIgG), because there is no way of knowing whether the IgG is bound through its Fab terminus (recognizing a platelet-specific antigen); via its Fc portion (as an immune complex); or nonspecifically. No assay can differentiate among these different types of binding. More importantly, there is no evidence that the monocytes or macrophages of the reticuloendothelial system recognize any of these IgG-platelet interactions in a different fashion.

Various techniques capable of measuring IgG on washed platelets from patients with suspected immune thrombocytopenia have been reported. Although there are some 20 to 30 different assays, all are modifications of three basic techniques: (1) 2-stage assays; (2) direct binding assays; and (3) assays that measure platelet-IgG following lysis of the test platelets. All of these assays use an immunologic "probe" to measure the platelet-associated IgG because the amount of IgG present per platelet is very small (i.e., 1 to 5 fg [1 fg = 10^{-15} g]) and the IgG is "masked" by other platelet proteins present in much higher concentrations.

Two-Stage Assays. Dixon and colleagues described the first assay that measured IgG on platelets from patients with idiopathic thrombocytopenic purpura (1021). The general principle of this and all subsequent two-stage assays has been the same: antiserum (anti-IgG) in excess of the amount of IgG on the platelets is incubated with varying dilutions of washed test platelets. The unbound anti-IgG is then separated from the platelets and quantified. A standard curve is performed simultaneously, except that known concentrations of IgG standards are substituted for the washed test platelets. The amount of IgG per platelet is calculated by relating the number of platelets that inhibit 50 per cent of the lysis of sheep red cells by the anti-IgG plus complement to that concentration of IgG standard producing an equal amount (50 per cent) of inhibition of lysis. In the original technique the investigators measured the unbound anti-IgG using a biological endpoint—the lysis of IgG-sensitized sheep cells in the presence of complement (1021).

Several different groups subsequently have modified the original two-stage assay to increase its reproducibility. In the immunoradiometric assay (IRMA) (Fig. 42–12), varying dilutions of washed test platelets or known amounts of IgG standard are incubated with a fixed concentration of radiolabeled (^{125}I) anti-IgG (1020). After the ^{125}I–anti-IgG has bound to the IgG on the test platelets, the unbound ^{125}I–anti-IgG is then quantified by measuring its binding to IgG attached to a solid phase (agarose beads). The amount of ^{125}I–anti-IgG that has bound to the IgG beads (solid phase) is measured radioactively. This assay, like all two-stage assays, measures ^{125}I–anti-IgG that is not bound to IgG on the platelets.

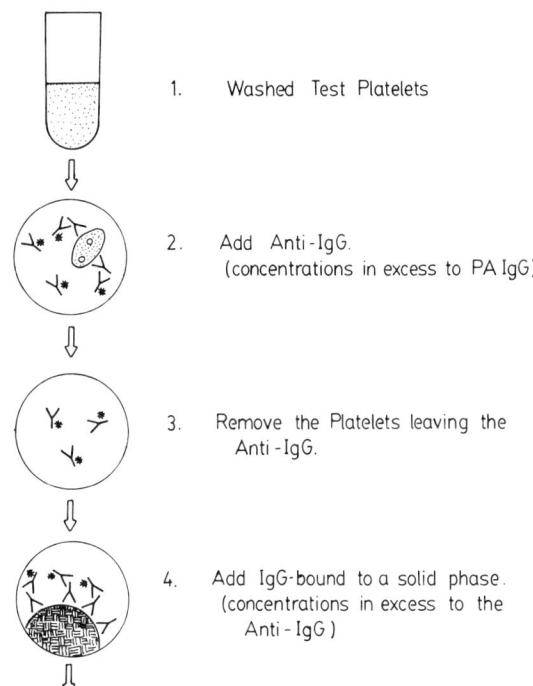

Figure 42–12. A schematic representation of a typical two-stage assay. Test platelets are washed, and then anti-IgG (in excess to the amount of IgG present) is added. The anti-IgG is labeled, using a radioisotope or a fluorescein conjugate. In step 3 the platelets are removed, leaving the unbound anti-IgG, which is then quantitated in step 4 by adding IgG bound to a solid phase. The standard curve is performed identically, except that IgG standard is substituted for the washed test platelets.

Other investigators have used other labels for anti-IgG, including fluorescein and enzymes (1022–1026). Two-stage assays have the advantage of simplicity in quantitating the results and can measure IgG on the surface of intact platelets or after lysis of the platelets. However, two-stage assays have one real and one theoretical disadvantage: First, they are complex techniques. Second, it has been suggested that two-stage assays may overestimate the amount of IgG present on platelets (1022). This latter consideration is more theoretical than practical as the precise amount of IgG on platelets is only of modest interest. It is the ability to distinguish the amount of IgG on normal platelets from that on platelets from patients with immune thrombocytopenia that is important, and two-stage assays can readily accomplish this.

Direct Binding Assays. Direct binding assays measure the binding of labeled antiserum, usually anti-IgG, to test platelets. These assays offer the advantage of simplicity, but they are difficult to quantitate. Furthermore, the nonspecific platelet binding of labeled proteins other than anti-IgG is a problem. Nonspecific binding can be reduced, but never completely eliminated, by diluting the labeled anti-IgG in unlabeled serum from the same species or by using an unlabeled protein as a "blocking agent." Although direct binding techniques have been used for many years, recently interest has been reawakened in these techniques with the availability of very pure and highly specific antiserum probes (monoclonal antibodies or staphylococcal protein A).

The principle of all direct binding assays is the same: the labeled probe, for example ^{125}I–anti-IgG, is incubated in antibody excess with washed test platelets (Fig. 42–13). Following this incubation, the anti-IgG that has bound to the IgG on the platelets is separated from the unbound anti-IgG by washing or by passage across a density gradient. The platelet-bound anti-IgG is then quantitated. By knowing both the specific activity of the anti-IgG and the platelet count in the test sample, the amount of anti-IgG binding to the IgG on the platelets can be calculated. This result is usually reported either qualitatively (per cent increase above the binding to normal platelets) or quantitatively on a weight basis.

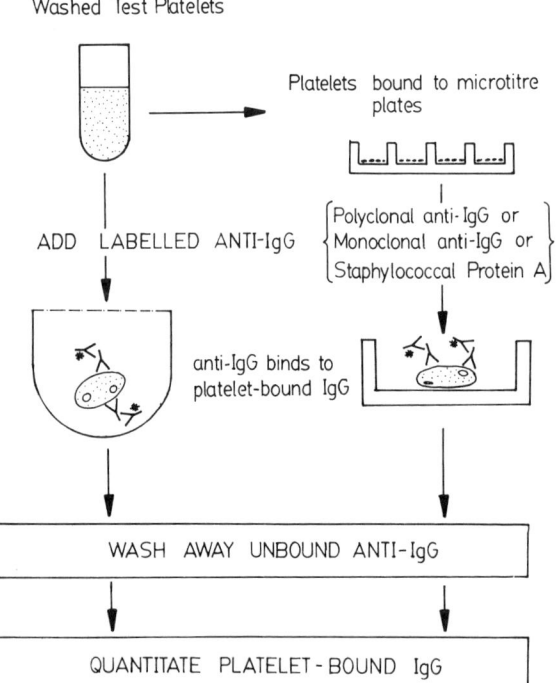

Figure 42–13. The principle of direct binding assay. Platelets are either maintained in a suspension or are bound to a microtiter plate. Labeled anti-IgG in excess to the amount of IgG on the test platelets is then added. The anti-IgG is labeled with either enzymes, fluorescein, or a radioactive label (polyclonal IgG, a monoclonal anti-IgG, or a staphylococcal protein A). After the anti-IgG has bound to the platelet-bound IgG, the unbound is washed away and the anti-IgG bound to the IgG is quantitated.

The first direct binding assays used polyclonal anti-IgG that was labeled with ^{125}iodine (1027), fluorescein (1028), or an enzyme (1029–1033). More recently, radiolabeled monoclonal anti-IgG or staphylococcal protein A have been used (1022, 1034, 1035).

Staphylococcal protein A (SpA) is a component of the cell wall of *Staphylococcus aureus* that binds with high affinity to human IgG subclasses 1, 2, and 4. Very pure SpA and monoclonal IgG are available and consequently much smaller amounts are needed to ensure that the anti-IgG is in excess of its target antigens (the platelet-bound IgG). Because the nonspecific binding of proteins to any cell is concentration dependent, the use of monoclonal anti-IgG or staphylococcal A lowers nonspecific binding of labelled proteins to the platelet membrane.

Measurement of IgG after Solubilization of the Platelets. Antibodies or IgG-immune complexes that bind to platelets probably are taken into the platelet's interior by the process of phagocytosis. This IgG will not be measured unless the platelet is disrupted, as for example by dissolving the lipid bilayer. The PAIgG measured following lysis of the platelet membrane includes the IgG on the surface of the platelet and the IgG within the platelet, i.e., the total PAIgG of the platelet. Measurement of the total PAIgG offers two technical advantages: First, there are no problems of nonspecific adsorption of proteins to the platelet membrane because the membrane is dissolved. Second, because far more IgG resides within the platelet than on its surface, it is technically easier to measure total PAIgG than surface PAIgG. The principle of the total PAIgG assays is the same: the washed test platelets are made soluble, usually by using low concentrations of a detergent (Fig. 42–14). The IgG is then measured using a radioprecipitation technique (1036–1038), nephelometry (1039), or radial immunodiffusion (1040). PAIgG is calculated by relating the number of test platelets to the amount of IgG measured. Not unexpectedly, the amount of platelet-associated IgG measured after platelet lysis is much higher than that measured on the surface of platelets. Yet all three general types of assays are equally sensitive in the diagnosis of immune thrombocytopenia (1041).

CONTROVERSIES CONCERNING THE MEASUREMENT OF PLATELET-ASSOCIATED IgG

The technical and theoretical aspects of assays that measure IgG on platelets have been scrutinized as few other laboratory tests (1042). In this section we will summarize some of the issues that have been raised about the measurement and biologic implications of platelet-associated IgG.

Potential Artifacts in the Measurement of Platelet-Associated IgG. The techniques used to measure platelet-associated IgG are sufficiently complex

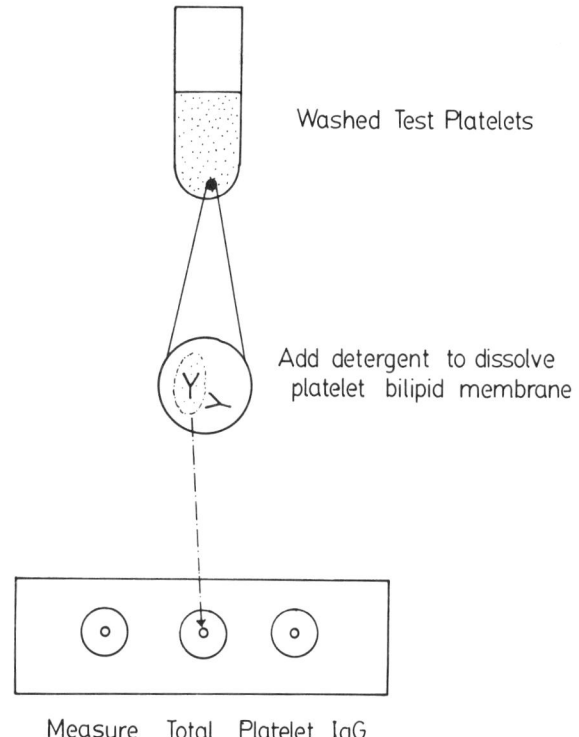

Figure 42–14. Measurement of total platelet-associated IgG. Washed test platelets are isolated and the lipid bilayer is dissolved, using a detergent. The total platelet-associated IgG, which consists of the IgG not only on the surface of the platelet but also in the interior of the platelet, is then measured using standard techniques (radioimmunodiffusion is shown here).

that the potential exists to incorrectly estimate the amount of IgG on platelets. For example, both EDTA and acid-citrate dextrose have been used as whole blood anticoagulants before isolation of platelets for measurement of platelet-associated IgG. However, if the whole blood sample is stored for longer than 1 day before platelet isolation, EDTA should not be used as an anticoagulant because the level of platelet-associated IgG artifactually rises. In contrast, ACD is an acceptable anticoagulant for specimens kept for several days before measurement of PAIgG (1043).

Other questions concerning the potential technical and theoretical problems in measuring platelet-associated IgG on platelets from patients with immune thrombocytopenia have been raised. For example, immune thrombocytopenia is characterized by increased platelet turnover and hence there is an increased population of larger than average-sized platelets. Consequently, it is theoretically possible that the increased platelet size in these disorders could passively contribute to elevated PAIgG; i.e., there could be increased IgG when measured per platelet, yet the amount of IgG per unit platelet surface area may not be increased. The question of the relationship of PAIgG to platelet size is difficult to resolve because the two variables could be related to a third. For example, there is an approximate relationship between the severity of the thrombocytopenia and the level of platelet-associated IgG (discussed subsequently). There also is an approximate correlation between the severity of the thrombocytopenia and the platelet size (1044, 1045). Hence, the platelet size and PAIgG level could be related to a third variable, such as the severity of the thrombocytopenia, and although correlated with each not be causally related.

In a recent study, platelets from healthy individuals were separated according to size and density. The results of this investigation indicated a slight correlation between platelet size and the level of platelet-associated IgG (1046). Together, these observations suggest that platelet size affects "physiologic" platelet IgG, that is IgG on platelets from healthy individuals. In contrast, in disorders of immune thrombocytopenia that may or may not be characterized by large platelets, the large amount of "pathologic" IgG not influenced by platelet size overwhelms the contribution of platelet size to IgG.

Platelet Fragments Contributing to PAIgG Results. The theoretical basis for this issue is as follows: The amount of IgG associated with test platelets is measured using the assays described previously. The result of IgG is divided by the platelet count to express the results as IgG per unit number of platelets. Hence the systematic underestimation of the number of platelets (or platelet fragments) in the test sample would artifactually increase the amount of PAIgG. There is biologic justification for this concern: platelet fragments and microvesicles are found in the plasma of healthy individuals and patients with ITP. Thus, if the platelet vesicles or fragments or both were present in the test specimen and their IgG measured, then the amount of IgG measured per platelet would appear to be higher than that actually present. Recent studies indicate that this measurement artifact does not occur. The apparent platelet fragments seen in electron microscopic sections of the washed test platelet sample probably represent artifacts—transected micropseudopods originating from intact platelets that lie above and below the plane of section (1047).

Although there is no doubt that platelet fragments are present in the circulation of patients with ITP, it is unlikely that they coprecipitate with intact platelets during platelet washing. Furthermore, when the results of the PAIgG assays are related to total platelet protein and not platelet count, there is no correlation (1020).

One can therefore be confident that the elevated levels of platelet-associated IgG observed on platelets from patients with immune thrombocytopenia as well as many other thrombocytopenic disorders are not due to artifacts of platelet collection, processing, or counting. However, it should also be emphasized that there is evidence that not all of the IgG on these platelets is "pathologic" IgG. This evidence comes from several sources. First, the amount of IgG on these platelets is probably higher than can be accounted for by the amount of "pathologic" antibody in the serum. Second, there is an approximate correlation between the amount of PAIgG and platelet-associated albumin on platelets from patients with immune thrombocytopenia (1048). Because the albumin presumably is nonspecifically bound to the platelet surface, one can assume that at least a proportion of the IgG is nonspecifically bound. However, this should not be interpreted as indicating that the increased IgG on platelets from patients with immune thrombocytopenia is a "nonspecific" finding. More importantly, it is likely that the IgG that binds to the platelet contributes to the shortened platelet life span.

In summary, current evidence indicates that technical explanations do not account for the markedly elevated levels of platelet-associated IgG in ITP and other immune thrombocytopenic disorders. There is also evidence that not all of the IgG on the platelet surface is "true autoantibody," but these observations do not indicate that the IgG is a "nonspecific" finding. More importantly, there is no evidence that the IgG (irrespective of how it binds to the platelet) does not result in an increased rate of platelet clearance by the reticuloendothelial system.

The Level of Platelet-Associated IgG on Washed Platelets from Healthy Individuals. Estimates of the amount of PAIgG on washed platelets from healthy, nonthrombocytopenic individuals vary from 150 to 4000 molecules of IgG per platelet (1021, 1024, 1034, 1035). It is now obvious that many of the first assays used to measure PAIgG overestimated the true amount. The real issue is one of calibration. There are two techniques that can be used. First, by relating the specific activity of the anti-IgG and calculating its binding ratio, it is possible to estimate the amount of PAIgG. Such a technique using radiolabeled staphylococcal protein A or monoclonal anti-IgG gives results of approximately 200 to 500 molecules of IgG per platelet (1034, 1035). Alternatively, the PAIgG can be quantitated as is done in the two-stage assays. The early reports using these assays gave measurements of PAIgG of approximately 2000 to 4000 fg per platelet (1021, 1024). It is likely that this represented an overestimate of the true amount of PAIgG. More recent experience with the same assays give results of approximately 1000 molecules of IgG per platelet. What the "true" amount of PAIgG is has not yet been entirely resolved, but it is interesting to note that all techniques report much higher levels of IgG on platelets than on red cells.

THE USE OF PAIgG MEASUREMENTS AS A DIAGNOSTIC TEST FOR IDIOPATHIC THROMBOCYTOPENIC PURPURA

Approximately 10 years ago, Dixon and coworkers (1021) used a two-stage assay (the antiglobulin consumption assay) as a technique for diagnosing idiopathic thrombocytopenic purpura. They found that the level of PAIgG was elevated in the majority of thrombocytopenic patients with ITP. Most investigators report similar findings, with PAIgG being elevated in approximately 85 to 90 per cent of patients (including children) with ITP (88). This finding of elevated PAIgG in immune thrombocytopenia is consistent whether one measures IgG using a direct binding assay or a two-stage assay or following platelet lysis. Do these findings indicate that elevated platelet-associated IgG is diagnostic of idiopathic thrombocytopenic purpura? To answer this question, one must examine not only the sensitivity but also the specificity of this diagnostic test. It should be remembered that when a clinician is faced with a thrombocytopenic patient, he or she does not know a priori if the thrombocytopenia is due to ITP or if it is secondary to a drug reaction, viral infection, collagen-vascular disease, or lymphoproliferative disorder. Therefore, to gain a proper prospective of the diagnostic usefulness of any test, one must relate the test results not only to patients with the disease but also to patients with similar diseases.

One group of investigators (1049) performed a 12-month prospective study relating a total of 859 patient diagnostic test procedures to the clinical diagnoses responsible for the thrombocytopenia in 169 different individuals. This prospective study confirmed that the measurement of platelet-associated IgG was highly sensitive for the diagnosis of ITP; however, the test was also positive in many other disorders, some of which, such as systemic lupus erythematosus and lymphoproliferative disorders, are traditionally considered to be due to immune mechanisms. The test however was also positive in other disorders generally not considered to be caused by immune mechanisms (Table 42–12). The study found that the specificity of a positive PAIgG assay for ITP was less than 50 per cent, indicating that PAIgG is not useful as a *single* diagnostic test for ITP. Similar results have been reported by other investigators (51). Nonetheless, PAIgG measurements can be used to help support the diagnosis of ITP.

Subsequent investigators have suggested that other assays, such as monoclonal PAIgG assays capable of measuring IgG, might have a higher specificity for ITP (1034). We feel that this is unlikely, since IgG on a cell is just that—IgG on a cell—and it will be most surprising if the spatial orientation of binding of the IgG to the cell surface affects whether a particular assay gives a positive

Table 42-12. RESULTS OF THE FIRST PLATELET-ASSOCIATED IgG DETERMINATION PERFORMED ON 169 DIFFERENT PATIENTS WITH THROMBOCYTOPENIA*

Disorder	Number of Patients With Elevated PAIgG	Total Number Tested	Percentage of Patients With Elevated PAIgG
Classic Immunologic Disorders			
Indiopathic thrombocytopenic purpura	62	68	91
Systemic lupus erythematosus and rheumatoid arthritis	10	11	91
Vasculitis	2	2	100
Drug-induced thrombocytopenia	9	10	90
Post-transfusion purpura	1	1	100
Neoplastic Disorders			
Multiple myeloma	2	4	50
Lymphoproliferative disorders	5	6	83
Carcinoma	5	5	100
Acute leukemia	9	16	56
Myeloproliferative disorders	4	5	80
Infective Disorders			
Bacterial septicemia	9	11	82
Malaria	2	2	100
Hepatic Disorders			
Cirrhosis, chronic active liver disease	4	9	44
Miscellaneous Disorders			
Preeclampsia toxemia	6	10	60
Hypersplenism	2	2	100
Thrombotic thrombocytopenic purpura	2	2	100
Amyloidosis	1	1	100
Disseminated intravascular coagulation	0	1	
Aplastic anemia	0	2	
Amegakaryocytic thrombocytopenia	0	1	

*Modified from Kelton, J. G., Powers, P. J., et al., Blood *60*:1050, 1982.

or negative result. Final resolution of this issue will require the completion of comparative prospective studies.

MEASUREMENT OF COMPLEMENT, IgM, AND OTHER IMMUNOGLOBULINS ON PLATELETS

Approximately 90 per cent of children and adults with acute or chronic ITP will have elevated levels of platelet-associated IgG (88). It is possible that complement-mediated platelet destruction is responsible for the 10 per cent of thrombocytopenic patients with normal levels of PAIgG. If this is the case, then it might be useful to have a laboratory test capable of identifying such patients. Furthermore, complement-mediated cell clearance occurs primarily through nonsplenic monocytes and macrophages, especially those within the liver, and therefore, splenectomy may not be expected to produce a remission in these patients.

Once a laboratory has developed an assay for measuring platelet-associated IgG, it is a small step to modify the technique so that it is capable of measuring platelet-associated complement, platelet-associated IgM, or any other protein bound to the platelet membrane. All that is required is to replace the anti-IgG for the antisera of interest, for example, anti-C3b (1050–1060). Although technically it is not difficult to measure such proteins on the platelet surface, to date the results from clinical studies using platelet-bound complement or IgM have not unequivocally demonstrated a need for such a test (1054, 1056, 1058, 1059).

Thus, at present, there is no convincing evidence that it is important for a laboratory to have a technique capable of measuring platelet-associated IgM or complement for the investigation or management of patients with immune thrombocytopenia.

OTHER CURRENT USES FOR ASSAYS CAPABLE OF MEASURING PLATELET-ASSOCIATED IgG

Confirmation of the Diagnosis of Alloimmune Neonatal Thrombocytopenia. Alloimmune neonatal thrombocytopenia is caused by antiplatelet alloantibodies directed against platelet-specific antigens on the infant's platelets. These antigens, lacking in the mother, are inherited from the father. The mother, upon exposure to the infant's platelets, produces IgG anti-platelet alloantibodies that cross the placenta and cause thrombocytopenia in the neonate. The diagnosis of alloimmune neonatal thrombocytopenia is made by demonstrating that the mother has an antiplatelet alloantibody in her serum that reacts against paternal or infant platelets but not her own. Most frequently, alloimmune neonatal thrombocytopenia is caused by antibodies against the platelet-specific alloantigen PL^{A1} (a component of platelet membrane glycoprotein IIIa). When screening for the presence of these antibodies, it is important to react maternal serum not only against maternal and paternal platelets but also against platelets from PL^{A1}-positive and PL^{A1}-negative donors. Because of the major implications of the diagnosis of alloimmune neonatal thrombocytopenia, i.e., future offspring could be affected, we believe it is important to confirm the diagnosis using a second test system such as a Western blot analysis. Once the diagnosis of alloimmune neonatal thrombocytopenia is confirmed, other family members (mother's sisters) should also be evaluated to identify whether their infants are also at risk.

The Diagnosis of Drug-Induced Thrombocytopenia. As noted earlier in this chapter, one is seldom justified in confirming the diagnosis of drug-induced immune thrombocytopenia by rechallenging the patient with the suspected drug. It is more appropriate to measure the drug-dependent binding of patient IgG to control platelets. In those patients in whom the test is positive, one can be confident that the drug was responsible for the thrombocytopenia. Some of the techniques used and the results obtained when testing for drug-induced thrombocytopenia are shown in Table 42–8.

Platelet Crossmatching. Just as red cells are selected by compatibility testing, it is likely that in the near future we will identify the optimal platelets for a particular patient by measuring platelet-bound IgG following the incubation of the recipient's serum with platelets from potential donors. To use platelet antibody techniques for a platelet crossmatch, a rapid test capable of assessing many different samples is needed, since the potential recipient's serum must be tested against a panel of potential donor platelets.

References to Part I (Quantitative Abnormalities)

1. White, J. G.: The ultrastructure and regulatory mechanisms of blood platelets. In *Blood Platelet Function and Medicinal Chemistry.* Lasslo, A. (ed.), New York, Elsevier Biomedical, 1984, p. 15.
2. Gerrard, J. M., Phillips, D. R., et al.: Biochemical studies of two patients with the gray platelet syndrome. Selective deficiency of platelet α-granules. J. Clin. Invest. 66:102, 1980.
3. Phillips, D. R., Jennings, I. K., et al.: Ca^{++}-mediated association of glycoprotein G (thrombin-sensitive protein, thrombospondin) with human platelets. J. Biol. Chem. 255:11629, 1980.
4. Jaffe, E. A., Leung, L. L. K., et al.: Thrombospondin is the endogenous lectin of human platelets. Nature (Lond.) 295:246, 1982.
5. Packham, M. A., and Mustard, J. F.: Normal and abnormal platelet activity. In *Blood Platelet Function and Medicinal Chemistry.* Lasslo, A. (ed.), New York, Elsevier Biomedical, 1984, p. 61.
6. Gloster, E. S., Strauss, R. A., et al.: Spurious elevated platelet counts associated with bacteremia. Am. J. Hematol. 18:329, 1985.
7. Akwari, A. M., Ross, D. W., et al.: Spuriously elevated platelet counts due to microspherocytosis. Am. J. Clin. Pathol. 77:220, 1982.
8. Morton, B. D., Orringer, E. P., et al.: Pappenheimer bodies. An additional cause for a spurious platelet count. Am. Soc. Clin. Pathol. 74:310, 1980.
9. Stass, S. A., Holloway, M. L., et al.: Cytoplasmic fragments causing spurious platelet counts in the leukemic phase of poorly differentiated lymphocytic leukemia. Am. J. Clin. Pathol. 71:125, 1979.
10. Armitage, J. O., Goeken, J. A., et al.: Spurious elevation of the platelet count in acute leukemia. J.A.M.A. 239:433, 1978.
11. Payne, B. A., and Pierre, R. V.: Pseudothrombocytopenia: a laboratory artifact with potentially serious consequences. Mayo Clin. Proc. 59:123, 1984.
12. Ansford, A. J., Findlay, A. B., et al.: Cold platelet agglutinins. Lancet 1:417, 1975.
13. Onder, O., Weinstein, A., et al.: Pseudothrombocytopenia caused by platelet agglutinins that are reactive in blood anticoagulated with chelating agents. Blood 56:177, 1980.
14. Savage, R. A.: Pseudoleukocytosis due to EDTA-induced platelet clumping. Am. J. Clin. Pathol. 81:317, 1984.
15. Gowland, E., Kay, H. E. M., et al.: Agglutination of platelets by a serum factor in the presence of EDTA. J. Clin. Pathol. 22:460, 1969.
16. Shreiner, D. P., and Bell, W. R. Pseudothrombocytopenia: manifestation of a new type of platelet agglutinin. Blood 42:541, 1973.
17. Veenhoven, W. A., van der Schans, G. S., et al.: Pseudothrombocytopenia due to agglutinins. Am. Soc. Clin. Pathol. 72:1005, 1979.
18. Mant, M. J., Doery, J. C. G., et al.: Pseudothrombocytopenia due to platelet aggregation and degranulation in blood collected in EDTA. Scand. J. Haematol. 15:161, 1975.
19. Girmann, G., Pees, H., et al.: Pseudothrombocytopenia and mexiletine. Ann. Intern. Med. 100:767, 1984.
20. Onder, O., Weinstein, A., et al.: Pseudothrombocytopenia caused by platelet agglutinins that are reactive in blood anticoagulated with chelating agents. Blood 56:177, 1980.
21. Pegels, J. G., Bruynes, E. C. E., et al.: Pseudothrombocytopenia: an immunologic study on platelet antibodies dependent on ethylene diamine tetra-acetate. Blood 59:157, 1982.
22. Forscher, C. A., Sussman, I., et al.: Pseudothrombocytopenia masking true thrombocytopenia. Am. J. Hematol. 18:313, 1985.
23. Watkins, S. P., and Shulman, R. N.: Platelet cold agglutinins. Blood 36:153, 1970.
24. Greipp, P. R., Didisheim, P., et al.: Platelet cold agglutinins. Lancet 2:814, 1975.
25. Ansford, A. J., Findlay, A. B., et al.: Cold platelet agglutinins. Lancet 2:417, 1975.
26. Cimo, P. L.: Cold agglutinins for platelets. New Engl. J. Med. 298:402, 1978.
27. Berning, H., and Stilbo, I. Pseudothrombocytopenia and the haematology laboratory. Lancet 2:1469, 1982.
28. Djaldetti, M., and Fishman, P. Satellitism of platelets to monocytes in a patient with hypogammaglobulinaemia. Scand. J. Haematol. 21:305, 1978.
29. McGregor, D. H., Davis, J. W., et al.: Platelet satellitism. Experimental studies. Lab. Invest. 42:343, 1980.
30. Casteli, D. O., and Farrell, R. L.: Granulocyte-platelet rosettes. New Engl. J. Med. 289:1146, 1973.
31. Kjeldsberg, C. R., and Swanson, J.: Platelet satellitism. Blood 43:831, 1974.
32. Greipp, P. R., and Gralnick, H. R.: Platelet to leukocyte adherence phenomena associated with thrombocytopenia. Blood 47:513, 1976.
33. Larson, J. H., and Pierre, R. V.: Platelet satellitism as a cause of abnormal hemalog D differential results. Am. J. Clin. Pathol. 68:758, 1977.
34. Liso, V., and Bonomo, L.: Platelet satellitism to basophils in a patient with chronic myelocytic leukaemia. Blut 45:347, 1982.
35. Skinnider, L. F., Musclow, C. E., et al.: Platelet satellitism—an ultrastructural study. Am. J. Hematol. 4:179, 1978.

36. Kjeldsberg, C. R., and Hershgold, E. J.: Spurious thrombocytopenia. J.A.M.A. *227:*628, 1974.
37. Cohen, A. M., Lewinski, U. H., et al.: Satellitism of platelets to monocytes. Acta Hematol. *64:*65, 1980.
38. Hruby, M. A.: Coexistent hemophilia A and idiopathic thrombocytopenic purpura. J. Pediatr. *90:*773, 1977.
39. Ratnoff, O. D., Meinitove, J. E., et al.: Coincident classic hemophilia and ITP in patients under treatment with concentrates of antihemophilic factor (Factor VIII). New Engl. J. Med. *308:*439, 1983.
40. Karpatkin, S.: Heterogeneity of human platelets. Functional evidence suggestive of young and old platelets. J. Clin. Invest. *48:*1083, 1969.
41. Pennington, D. G., Lee, N. L. Y., et al.: Platelet density and size: the interpretation of heterogeneity. Br. J. Haematol. *34:*365, 1976.
42. Karpatkin, S.: Heterogeneity of rabbit-platelets. Further resolution of changes in platelet density, volume, and radioactivity following cohort labelling with ^{75}Se-selenomethionine. Br. J. Haematol. *39:*459, 1978.
43. Mezzano, D., Hwang, K., et al.: Evidence that platelet buoyant density, but not size, correlates with platelet age in man. Am. J. Haematol. *11:*61, 1981.
44. Corash, L., and Shafer, B.: Use of asplenic rabbits to demonstrate that platelet age and density are related. Blood *60:*166, 1982.
45. Thompson, C. B., Love, D. G., et al.: Platelet size does not correlate with platelet age. Blood *62:*487, 1983.
46. Corash, L., Costa, J. L., et al.: Heterogeneity of human whole blood platelet subpopulations. Density-dependent differences in subcellular constituents. Blood *64:*185, 1984.
47. Bessman, J. D., Williams, L. J., et al.: Platelet size in health and hematologic disease. Am. J. Clin. Pathol. *78:*150, 1982.
48. Burton, D. R.: Immunoglobulin G: functional sites. Molec. Immunol. *22:*161, 1985.
49. Metzger, J.: The effect of antigen on antibodies: recent studies. In *Contemporary Topics in Molecular Immunology.* Reisfeld, R. A., and Inman, F. P. (eds.), New York, Plenum Press, 1978, pp. 119–152.
50. Kelton, J. G., Singer, J., et al.: The concentration of IgG in the serum is a major determinant of Fc-dependent reticuloendothelial cell function. Blood *66:*490, 1985.
51. Mueller-Eckhardt, C., Kayser, W., et al.: The clinical significance of PAIgG. A study of 298 patients with various disorders. Br. J. Haematol. *46:*123, 1980.
52. Mueller-Eckhardt, C., Mueller-Eckhardt, G., et al.: PAIgG, platelet survival and platelet sequestration in thrombocytopenic states. Br. J. Haematol. *52:*49, 1982.
53. Kelton, J. G., Carter, C. J., et al.: The relationship among PAIgG, platelet lifespan, and reticuloendothelial cell function. Blood *63:*1434, 1984.
54. Kelton, J. G.: Impaired reticuloendothelial function in patients treated with methyldopa. New Engl. J. Med. *313:*596, 1985.
55. McKenna, J. L., and Pisciotta, A. V.: Fluorescence of megakaryocytes in ITP stained with fluorescent antiglobulin serum. Blood *19:*664, 1962.
56. McMillan, R., Luiken, G. A., et al.: Antibody against megakaryocytes in ITP. J.A.M.A. *239:*2460, 1978.
57. Hoffman, R., ZaKnoen, S., et al.: An antibody cytotoxic to megakaryocyte progenitor cells in a patient with immune thrombocytopenic purpura. New Engl. J. Med. *312:*1170, 1985.
58. Woods, V. L., Oh, E. H., et al.: Autoantibodies against the platelet-glycoprotein IIb/IIIa complex in patients with chronic ITP. Blood *63:*368, 1984.
59. Woods, V. L., Kurata, Y., et al.: Autoantibodies against platelet glycoprotein Ib in patients with chronic ITP. Blood *64:*156, 1984.
60. Beardsley, D. S., Spiegel, J. E., et al.: Platelet membrane glycoprotein IIIa contains target antigens that bind antiplatelet antibodies in immune thrombocytopenias. J. Clin. Invest. *74:*1701, 1984.
61. Kelton, J. G., Keystone, J., et al.: Immune-mediated thrombocytopenia of malaria. J. Clin. Invest. *71:*832, 1983.
62. Karas, S. P., Rosse, W. F., et al.: Characterization of the IgG-Fc receptor on human platelets. Blood *60:*1277, 1982.
63. Komrower, G. M., and Watson, G. H.: Prognosis in idiopathic thrombocytopenic purpura of childhood. Arch. Dis. Child. *29:*502, 1954.
64. Walker, J. H., and Walker, W.: Idiopathic thrombocytopenic purpura in childhood. Arch. Dis. Child. *36:*649, 1961.
65. Schulman, I.: Diagnosis and treatment: management of idiopathic thrombocytopenic purpura. Pediatrics *33:*979, 1964.
66. Lusher, J. M., and Zuelzer, W. W.: Idiopathic thrombocytopenic purpura in childhood. J. Pediatr. *68:*971, 1966.
67. Choi, S. I., and McClure, P. D.: Idiopathic thrombocytopenic purpura in childhood. Can. Med. Assoc. J. *97:*562, 1967.
68. McClure, P. D.: Idiopathic thrombocytopenic purpura in children: diagnosis and management. Pediatrics *55:*68, 1975.
69. Lammi, A. T., and Lovric, V. A.: Idiopathic thrombocytopenic purpura: an epidemiologic study. J. Pediatr. *83:*31, 1973.
70. Zerella, J. T., Martin, L. W., et al.: Emergency splenectomy for idiopathic thrombocytopenic purpura in children. J. Pediatr. Surg. *13:*243, 1978.
71. Simons, S. M., Main, C. A., et al.: Idiopathic thrombocytopenic purpura in children. J. Pediatr. *87:*16, 1975.
72. McWilliams, N. B., and Maurer, H. M.: Acute idiopathic thrombocytopenic purpura in children. Am. J. Hematol. *7:*87, 1979.
73. Lusher, J. M., and Iyer, R.: Idiopathic thrombocytopenic purpura in children. Semin. Thromb. Hemostas. *3:*175, 1977.
74. Lusher, J. M., Enami, A., et al.: Idiopathic thrombocytopenic purpura in children. Am. J. Pediatr. Hematol. Oncol. *6:*149, 1984.
75. Walker, R. W., and Walker, W.: Idiopathic thrombocytopenia, initial illness and long term followup. Arch. Dis. Child. *59:*316, 1984.
76. Cohn, J.: Thrombocytopenia in childhood. An evaluation of 433 patients. Scand. J. Haematol. *16:*226, 1976.
77. Lilleyman, J. S.: Idiopathic thrombocytopenic purpura—where do we stand? Arch. Dis. Child. *59:*701, 1984.
78. Dumoulin-Lagrange, M., and Capelle, C.: Evaluation of automated platelet counters for the enumeration and sizing of platelets in the diagnosis and management of hemostatic problems. Semin. Thromb. Hemostas. *9:*235, 1983.
79. Tomita, E., Akatsuka, J., et al.: Differential diagnosis of various thrombocytopenias in childhood by analysis of platelet volume. Pediatr. Res. *14:*133, 1980.
80. Bessman, J. D., Williams, L. J., et al.: The inverse relation of platelet size and count in normal subjects and an artifact of other particles. Am. J. Pathol. *76:*289, 1981.
81. Dumoulin-Lagrange, M., and Samama, M.: Errors in platelet counts. Am. J. Clin. Pathol. *77:*511, 1982.
82. George, J. N., Thor, L. L., et al.: Isolation of human platelet membrane microparticles from plasma and serum. Blood *60:*834, 1982.
83. Gardner, F. H., and Bessman, J. D.: Thrombocytopenia due to defective platelet production. Clin. Hematol. *12:*23, 1983.

84. Dubansky, A. S., and Oski, F. A.: Controversies in the management of acute idiopathic thrombocytopenic purpura: a survey of specialists. Pediatrics 77:49, 1986.
85. McIntosh, N.: Is bone marrow investigation required in isolated childhood thrombocytopenia? Lancet 1:956, 1982 (Letter).
86. Stuart, M. J., Kelton, J. G., et al.: Abnormal platelet function and arachidonate metabolism in chronic ITP. Blood 58:326, 1981.
87. Beardsley, D. J., S. Timmons, S., et al.: Human antiplatelet autoantibodies which interfere with fibrinogen binding. Blood 64:845, 1984 (Abstract).
88. Cheung, N. V., Hilgartner, M. W., et al.: Platelet-associated IgG in childhood ITP. J. Pediatr. 102:366, 1983.
89. Aster, R. H., and Keene, W. R.: Sites of platelet destruction in idiopathic thrombocytopenic purpura. Br. J. Haematol. 16:61, 1969.
90. Cohen, P., Gardner, F. J., et al.: Reclassification of the thrombocytopenias by the ^{51}Cr-labelling method for measuring platelet life span. New Engl. J. Med. 264:1294, 1961.
91. Harker, L. A., and Finch, C. A.: Thrombokinetics in man. J. Clin. Invest. 48:963, 1969.
92. Najean, Y., and Ardaillou, N.: The sequestration site of platelets in idiopathic thrombocytopenic purpura: its correlation with the results of splenectomy. Br. J. Haematol. 21:153, 1971.
93. Branehög, I., Kutti, J., et al.: Platelet survival and platelet production in idiopathic thrombocytopenic purpura (ITP). Br. J. Haematol. 27:127, 1974.
94. Harker, L. A.: Thrombokinetics in idiopathic thrombocytopenic purpura. Br. J. Haematol. 19:95, 1970.
95. Branehög, I., Kutti, J., et al.: The relation of thrombokinetics to bone marrow megakaryocytes in idiopathic thrombocytopenic purpura (ITP). Blood 45:551, 1975.
96. Branehög, I., and Weinfeld, A.: Platelet survival and platelet production in idiopathic thrombocytopenic purpura (ITP) before and during treatment with corticosteroids. Br. J. Haematol. 12:69, 1974.
97. Ballem, P., Segal, C., et al.: Pathophysiology of ATP. Autoantibodies impair platelet production. Blood 64:844, 1984 (Abstract).
98. Ozsoylu, S., Kanra, G., et al.: Thrombocytopenic purpura related to rubella infection. Pediatrics 62:567, 1978.
99. Tamir, D., Benderly, A., et al.: Infectious mononucleosis and Epstein-Barr virus in childhood. Pediatrics 53:330, 1974.
100. Benham, E. S., and Taft, L. I.: Idiopathic thrombocytopenic purpura in children: results of steroid therapy and splenectomy. Aust. Pediatr. J. 8:311, 1972.
101. Humphreys, R. P., Hockley, A. D., et al.: Management of intracerebral hemorrhage in idiopathic thrombocytopenic purpura. J. Neurosurg. 45:700, 1976.
102. Lightsey, A. L., McMillan, R., et al.: Childhood idiopathic thrombocytopenic purpura. Aggressive management of life-threatening complications. J.A.M.A. 232:734, 1975.
103. Woerner, S. J., Abildgaard, C. F., et al.: Intracranial hemorrhage in children with idiopathic thrombocytopenic purpura. Pediatrics 67:453, 1981.
104. Imbach, P., Berchtold, W., et al.: Intravenous IgG versus oral corticosteroids in acute immune thrombocytopenic purpura of childhood. Lancet 2:464, 1985.
105. Buchanan, G. R.: Childhood ITPL: how many tests and how much treatment required. J. Pediatr. 106:928, 1985.
106. Livio, M., Marchesi, D., et al.: Uraemic bleeding: role of anemia and beneficial effect of red cell transfusion. Lancet 2:1013, 1982.
107. Editorial—The bleeding time and the haematocrit. Lancet 1:997, 1984.
108. Dunn, N. L., and Maurer, H. M. Prednisone treatment of acute ITP of childhood. Am. J. Pediatr. Hematol. Oncol. 6:159, 1984.
109. McMillan, R., Longmire, R. L., et al.: In vitro platelet phagocytosis by splenic leucocytes in idiopathic thrombocytopenic purpura. New Engl. J. Med. 290:249, 1974.
110a. Dixon, R., and Rosse, W.: Platelet antibody in autoimmune thrombocytopenia. Br. J. Haematol. 31:129, 1975.
110b. McMillan, R., Longmire, R., et al.: The effect of corticosteroids on human IgG synthesis. J. Immunol. 116:1592, 1976.
111. Robson, H. N., and Duthie, J. J. R.: Capillary resistance and adrenocortical activity. Br. Med. J. 2:971, 1950.
112. Labran, C.: Etude de l'action vaso-constrictrice de la prednisone. Rev. Franc. Etude Clin. Biol. 8:765, 1963.
113. Hutter, J. J., and Hathaway, W. E.: Prednisone-induced hemostasis in a platelet function abnormality. Am. J. Dis. Child. 129:641, 1975.
114. Alexander, M., van den Bogart, N., et al.: Le pronostic et le traitement du purpura thrombopénique idiopathique de l'enfant. Arch. Franc. Pediatr. 33:329, 1976.
115. Johnson, S. A.: Endothelial supporting function of platelets. In *The Circulating Platelet*. Johnson, S. A. (ed.), New York, Academic Press, 1971, p. 283.
116. Kitchens, C. S., and Weiss, L.: Ultrastructural changes of endothelium associated with thrombocytopenia. Blood 46:567, 1975.
117. Kitchens, C. S., and Weiss, L.: Amelioration of endothelial abnormalities by prednisone in experimental thrombocytopenia in the rabbit. J. Clin. Invest. 60:1129, 1977.
118. Shepro, D., Sweetman, H. E., et al.: Experimental thrombocytopenia and capillary ultrastructure. Blood 56:937, 1980.
119. Miles, R. G., and Hurley, J. V.: The effect of thrombocytopenia on the ultrastructure and reaction to injury of vascular endothelium. Microvasc. Res. 26:273, 1983.
119a. Kitchens, C. S., and Pendergast, J. F.: Human thrombocytopenia is associated with structural abnormalities of the endothelium that are ameliorated by glucocorticoid administration. Blood 67:203, 1986.
120. Senyi, A., Blajchman, M. A., et al.: The experimental corrective effect of hydrocortisone on the bleeding time in thrombocytopenic rabbits. American Society of Hematology, 18th Annual Meeting, 1975, p. 80 (Abstract).
121. Blajchman, M. A., Senyi, A. F., et al.: Shortening of the bleeding time in rabbits by hydrocortisone caused by inhibition of prostacyclin generation by the vessel wall. J. Clin. Invest. 63:1026, 1979.
122. Krivit, W., Tate, D., et al.: Idiopathic thrombocytopenic purpura and intracranial hemorrhage. Pediatrics 67:570, 1981.
123. Sartorius, J. A.: Steroid treatment of idiopathic thrombocytopenic purpura in children. Preliminary results of a randomized cooperative study. Am. J. Pediatr. Hematol. Oncol. 6:165, 1984.
124. Buchanan, G. R., and Holtkamp, C. A.: Prednisone therapy for children with newly diagnosed idiopathic thrombocytopenic purpura. A randomized clinical trail. Am. J. Pediatr. Hematol. Oncol. 6:355, 1984.
125. Dunn, N. L., and Maurer, H. M.: Prednisone treatment of acute idiopathic thrombocytopenic purpura of childhood. Am. J. Pediatr. Hematol. Oncol. 6:159, 1984.
126. Cohen, P., and Gardner, F. H.: The thrombocytopenic effect of sustained high-dosage prednisone therapy in thrombocytopenic purpura. New Engl. J. Med. 265:611, 1961.
127. Giles, A. H. B., and Shellshear, I. D.: Unwanted corticosteroid effects in childhood bone marrow failure, renal failure and brain damage—case report. N.Z. Med. J. 539:424, 1975.
128. David, D. S., Grieco, H., et al.: Adrenal glucocorticoids

after twenty years. A review of their clinically relevant consequences. J. Chronic Dis. *22*:637, 1970.
129. Melby, J. C.: Drug spotlight program: systemic corticosteroid therapy, pharmacology, and endocrinologic considerations. Ann. Intern. Med. *81*:505, 1974.
130. Streck, W. F., and Lockwood, D. H.: Pituitary adrenal recovery following short term suppression with corticosteroids. Am. J. Med. *66*:910, 1979.
131. Finlayson, J. S.: Immune globulins. Semin. Thromb. Hemostas. *6*:44, 1979.
132. Barandun, S., Kistler, P., et al.: Intravenous administration of human γ-globulin. Vox Sang. *7*:157, 1962.
133. Alving, B. M., Tankersley, D. L., et al.: Contract-activated factors: contaminants of immunoglobulin preparations with coagulant and vasoactive properties. J. Lab. Clin. Med. *96*:334, 1980.
134. Aronson, D. L., and Finlayson, J. S.: Historical and future therapeutic plasma derivatives. Semin. Thromb. Hemostas. *6*:121, 1980.
135. Kelton, J. G.: The interaction of IgG with reticuloendothelial cells: biological and therapeutic implications. In *Current Concepts in Transfusion Therapy.* Garratty, G. (ed.), Arlington, VA, American Association of Blood Banks, 1985.
135a. Woodruff, R. K., and Griggs, A. P.: Fatal thrombotic events during treatment of autoimmune thrombocytopenia with IV IgG in elderly patients. Lancet *2*:217, 1986.
136. Schroeder, D. D., and Mozen, M. M.: Australia antigen: distribution during Cohn ethanol fractionation of human plasma. Science *168*:1462, 1970.
137. Hoofnagle, J. H., Gerety, R. J., et al.: Antibody to the hepatitis B surface antigen in immune serum globulin. Transfusion *15*:408, 1975.
138. Hoofnagle, J. H., Gerety, R. J., et al.: The prevalence of hepatitis B surface antigen in commercially prepared plasma products. J. Lab. Clin. Med. *88*:102, 1976.
139. Barker, L. F., and Hoofnagle, J. H.: Transmission of viral hepatitis, type B, by plasma derivatives. Dev. Biol. Stand. *27*:178, 1974.
140. Morgado, A. F., and daFonte, J. G.: An outbreak of hepatitis attributable to inoculation with contaminated gamma globulin. Bull. Pan Am. Health Org. *13*:177, 1979.
141. Petrilli, F. L., Crovari, P., et al.: Hepatitis B in subjects treated with a drug containing immunoglobulins. J. Infect. Dis. *135*:252, 1977.
142. Nakamura, S., and Sato, T.: Acute hepatitis B after administration of gammaglobulin. Lancet *1*:478, 1976.
143. John, J. T., Ninan, G. T., et al.: Epidemic hepatitis B caused by commercial human immunoglobulin. Lancet *1*:1074, 1979.
144. DeSilva, L. C., Sette, H., et al.: Commercial gammaglobulin (CGG) as a possible vehicle of transmission of HBsAg in familial clustering. Rev. Inst. Med. Trop. Sao Paulo *19*:352, 1977.
145. Meneghetti, F., Pornaro, E., et al.: HBsAg investigation in commercial preparations containing gamma globulins. G. Mal. Infett. *29*:1027, 1977.
146. Dioguardi, N., and de Franchis, R.: Hepatitis-B surface antigen in commercial gamma-globulin. Lancet *2*:816, 1975.
147. Tabor, E., and Gerety, R. J.: Transmission of hepatitis B by immune serum globulin. Lancet *2*:1293, 1979.
148. Lane, R. S.: Non-A, non-B hepatitis from intravenous immunoglobulin. Lancet *2*:974, 1983.
149. Lever, A. M. L., Brown, D., et al.: Non-A, non-B hepatitis occurring in agammaglobulinaemic patients after intravenous immunoglobulin. Lancet *2*:1062, 1984.
150. Lang, G. E., and Veldhuis, B.: Immune serum globulin—a cause of anti-Rh(D) passive sensitization. Am. J. Clin. Pathol. *60*:205, 1973.
151. Oberman, H. A., and Beck, M. L.: Red blood cell sensitization due to unexpected Rh antibodies in immune serum globulin. Transfusion *11*:382, 1971.
152. Grassi, A., and Brogi, M.: Le gammaglobuline nella terapia della trombocitopenia. Minerva Pediatr. *29*:1227, 1977.
153. Masson, P. L.: The therapeutic use of human immunoglobulin selected on the basis of their antibody activity against circulating antigens. In *Plasma Protein Pathology.* Peters, H, and Wright, P. (eds.), Oxford, Pergamon Press, 1979.
154. Bondolfi, R., Hirt, A., et al.: Autoimmunehaemolytische Anamie bei congenitaler Agammaglobulinaemie. Behandlungserfolg durch Immunglobulin-Substitution. Schweiz Med. Wochenschr. *110*:1950, 1980.
155. Masson, P. L.: The therapeutic use of human immunoglobulin selected on the basis of their antibody activity against circulating antigens. In *Plasma Protein Pathology.* Peters, H., and Wright, P. (eds.), Oxford, Pergamon Press, 35–44, 1979, pp. 35–44.
156. Imbach, P., d'Apuzzo, V., et al.: High-dose intravenous gammaglobulin for idiopathic thrombocytopenic purpura in childhood. Lancet *1*:1228, 1981.
157. Imbach, P., and Jungi, T. W.: Possible mechanism of intravenous immunoglobulin treatment in childhood idiopathic thrombocytopenic purpura. Blut *46*:117, 1983.
158. Gaedicke, G., Imbach, P., et al.: The place of intravenous immunoglobulin (IgG) therapy in thrombocytopenia. Blut *48*:409, 1984.
159. Imbach, P., Barandun, S., et al.: Intravenous immunoglobulin for idiopathic thrombocytopenic purpura (ITP) of childhood. Am. J. Pediatr. Hematol. Oncol. *6*:171, 1984.
160. Bussel, J. B., Goldman, A., et al.: Treatment of acute ITP of childhood with intravenous infusions of 1 gram per kg per day of gammaglobulin. J. Pediatr. *106*:886, 1985.
161. Schmidt, B., and Forster, R.: Increased platelet associated IgG in a child on high dose gammaglobulin for ITP. Lancet *2*:39, 1982 (Letter).
162. Luiken, G. A., McMillan, R., et al.: Platelet-associated IgG in immune thrombocytopenic purpura. Blood *50*:317, 1977.
163. Lightsey, A. L., Koenig, H. M., et al.: Platelet-associated immunoglobulin G in childhood idiopathic thrombocytopenic purpura. J. Pediatr. *94*:201, 1979.
164. Khalifa, A. S., Lusher, J. M., et al.: Immunoglobulins in idiopathic thrombocytopenic purpura in childhood. Acta Haematol. *56*:205, 1976.
165. McMillan, R.: Immune thrombocytpenia. Clin. Haematol. *12*:69, 1983.
166. Harrington, W. J., Minnich, V., et al.: Demonstration of a thrombocytopenic factor in the blood of patients with thrombocytopenic purpura. J. Lab. Clin. Med. *38*:1, 1951.
167. Harrington, W. J., Sprague, C. C., et al.: Immunologic mechanisms in idiopathic and neonatal thrombocytopenic purpura. Ann. Intern. Med. *38*:433, 1953.
168. McMillan, R., Longmire, R. L., et al.: Immunoglobulin synthesis in vitro by splenic tissue in idiopathic thrombocytopenic purpura. New Engl. J. Med. *286*:681, 1972.
169. McMillan, R., Longmire, R. L., et al.: Quantitation of platelet-binding IgG produced in vitro by spleens from patients with ITP. New Engl. J. Med. *291*:812, 1974.
170. Karpatkin, S., Strick, N., et al.: Detection of splenic antiplatelet antibody synthesis in idiopathic autoimmune thrombocyopenic purpura (ATP). Br. J. Haematol. *23*:167, 1972.
171. McMillan, R., Tani, P., et al.: The demonstration of antibody binding to platelet-associated antigens in patients with immune thrombocytpenic purpura. Blood *56*:993, 1980.

172. van Leeuwen, E. F., van der Ven, J. T. M., et al.: Specificity of autoantibody in autoimmune thrombocytopenia. Blood 59:23, 1982.
173. Woods, V. L., and McMillan, R.: Platelet antiantigens in chronic ITP. Br. J. Haematol. 57:1, 1984.
174. Mason, D., and McMillan, R.: Platelet antigens in chronic ITP. Br. J. Haematol. 56:529, 1984.
175. Anderson, M. J., Woods, V. L., et al.: Autoantibodies to platelet glycoprotein IIb/IIIa and to the acetylcholine receptor in a patient with chronic ITP and myasthenia gravis. Ann. Intern. Med. 100:829, 1984.
176. Mohanty, D., Quadri, M. I., et al.: HLA and idiopathic thrombocytopenic purpura (ITP). Br. J. Haematol. 42:329, 1979.
177. Veenhoven, W. A., Sijpesteijn, J. A. K., et al.: HLA antigens in idiopathic thrombocytopenic purpura. Acta Haematol. 62:153, 1979.
178. Gratama, J. W., D'Amaro, J., et al.: The HLA system in immune thrombocytopenic purpura: its relation to the outcome of therapy. Br. J. Haematol. 56:287, 1984.
179. Karpatkin, S., Fotino, M., et al.: Association of HLA-DRW2 with autoimmune thrombocytopenic purpura. J. Clin. Invest. 63:1085, 1979.
180. Mayr, W. R., Muller-Eckhardt G., et al.: HLA-DR in chronic ITP. Tissue Antigens 18:56, 1981.
181. Wybran, J., and Fudenberg, H. H.: Cellular immunity in idiopathic thrombycytopenic purpura. Blood 40:856, 1972.
182. Clancy, R. L.: Cellular immunity to autologous platelets and serum blocking factors in ITP. Lancet 1:6, 1972.
183. Clancy, R. L., Muller, H. K., et al.: Immunodeficiency and grouping with thyrogastric autoimmune disease in patients with chronic idiopathic thrombocytopenic purpura. Aust. N.Z. J. Med. 4:243, 1974.
184. Stuart, M. J., Tomar, R. H., et al.: Chronic idiopathic thrombocytopenic purpura—a familial immunodeficiency syndrome? J.A.M.A. 239:938, 1978.
185. McIntosh, S., Johnson, C., et al.: Immunoregulatory abnormalities in children with thrombocytopenic purpura. J. Pediatr. 99:525, 1981.
186. Laster, A. J., Conley, C. L., et al.: Chronic immune thrombocytopenic purpura in monozygotic twins. Genetic factors predisposing to ITP. New Engl. J. Med. 307:1495, 1982.
187. Lippman, S. M., Arnett, F. C., et al.: Genetic factors predisposing to autoimmune diseases. Am. J. Med. 73:827, 1982.
188. Warrier, I., and Moore, E.: Immunologic studies in childhood ITP. 18th Congress of the International Society of Hematology, Montreal, 1980. Abstract #1493, p. 275.
189. Shannon, K. M., Buchanan, G. R., et al.: Lymphyocyte populations in childhood ITP. Am. J. Dis. Child. 138:64, 1984.
190. Murphy, S., Oski, F. A., et al.: Platelet size and kinetics in hereditary and acquired thrombocytopenia. New Engl. J. Med. 286:499, 1972.
191. Murphy, S., and Gardner, F. H.: Platelet survival and sequestration studies in idiopathic thrombocytopenic purpura. Ann. Intern. Med. 80:786, 1974.
192. Buchanan, G. R., Scher, C. S., et al.: Use of homologous platelet survival in the differential diagnosis of chronic thrombocytopenia of childhood. Pediatrics 59:49, 1977.
193. Harker, L. A., and Slichter, S. J.: The bleeding time as a screening test for evaluation of platelet function. New Engl. J. Med. 287:155, 1972.
194. Malpass, T. W., and Harker, L. A.: Acquired disorders of platelet function. Semin. Haematol. 17:242, 1980.
195. Cortelazzo, S., Viero, P., et al.: Bleeding in patients with autoimmune thrombocytopenic purpura and normal platelet counts. Scand. J. Haematol. 32:403, 1984.
196. Clancy, R., Jenkins, E., et al.: Qualitative platelet abnormalities in idiopathic thrombocytopenic purpura. New Engl. J. Med. 286:622, 1972.
197. Heyns, A., Fraser, J., et al.: Platelet aggregation in chronic idiopathic thrombocytopenic purpura. J. Clin. Pathol. 31:1239, 1978.
198. Clancy, R., and Firkin, B.: Antibody-induced thrombocytopathy. Thromb. Res. 3:375, 1973.
199. Regan, M. G., Lackner, H., et al.: Platelet function and coagulation profile in lupus erythematosus. Ann. Intern. Med. 81:462, 1974.
200. Karpatkin, S., and Lackner, H. L.: Association of antiplatelet antibody with functional platelet disorders. Am. J. Med. 59:599, 1975.
201. Lackner, H. L., and Karpatkin, S.: On the "easy bruising" syndrome with normal platelet count. A study of 75 patients. Ann. Intern. Med. 83:190, 1975.
202. Zahavi, J., and Marder, V. J.: Acquired "storage pool disease" of platelets associated with circulating antiplatelet antibodies. Am. J. Med. 56:883, 1974.
203. Weiss, H. J., Rosove, M. H., et al.: Acquired storage pool deficiency with increased platelet-associated IgG. Report of 5 cases. Am. J. Med. 69:711, 1980.
204. Bussel, J. B., Kimberly, R. P., et al.: Intravenous gammaglobulin treatment of chronic ITP. Blood 62:480, 1983.
205. Bussel, J. B., Schulman, I., et al.: I.V. IgG in the treatment of chronic immune thrombocytopenic purpura as a means to defer splenectomy. J. Pediatr. 103:651, 1983.
206. Mori, P. G., Mancuso, G., et al.: Chronic ITP treated with immunoglobulin. Arch. Dis. Child. 58:851, 1983.
207. Warrier, I., and Lusher, J. M.: I.V. IgG treatment for chronic ITP in children. Am. J. Med. 76:193, 1984.
208. Uchino, H., Yasunaga, K., et al.: A cooperative clinical trial of high dose I.V. IgG in 177 cases of ITP. Thromb. Hemostas. 51:182, 1984.
209. Dickerman, J. D.: Splenectomy and sepsis: a warning. Pediatrics 63:938, 1979.
210. Weinblatt, M. E., and Ortega, J. A.: Steroid responsiveness: a predictor of the outcome of splenectomy in children with chronic ITP. Am. J. Dis. Child. 136:1064, 1982.
211. Steinherz, R., and Zaizov, R.: Steroid responsiveness. Am. J. Dis. Child. 137:1129, 1983.
211a. Boxer, M. A., Braun, J., et al.: Thromboembolic risk of postsplenectomy thrombocytosis. Arch. Surg. 113:808, 1978.
212. Barnhart, M. I., and Lusher, J. M.: Splenic structural physiology in chronic idiopathic thrombocytopenic purpura. In *Platelets, Recent Advances in Basic Research and Clinical Aspects.* Ulutin, O. N. (ed.), Amsterdam, Excerpta Medica, 1974, p. 462.
213. Eraklis, A. J., Kevy, S. V., et al.: Hazard of overwhelming infection after splenectomy in childhood. New Engl. J. Med. 276:1225, 1967.
214. Krivit, W.: Overwhelming postsplenectomy infection. Am. J. Hematol. 2:193, 1977.
215. Pearson, H. A.: Splenectomy: its risks and its roles. Hosp. Pract. August, 1980, p. 85.
216. Heier, H. E. Splenectomy and serious infection. Scand. J. Haematol. 24:5, 1980.
217. Krivey, N., and Tatarski, I.: Infections after splenectomy. New Engl. J. Med. 298:165, 1978.
218. Singer, D. B.: Postsplenectomy sepsis. Perspect. Pediatr. Pathol. 1:285, 1973.
219. Gwaltney, J. M., Jr., Sande, M. A., et al.: Spread of Streptococcus pneumoniae in families. II. Relation of transfer of S. pneumoniae to incidence of colds and serum antibody. J. Infect. Dis. 132:62, 1975.
220. Schur, P. H., Rosen, F., et al.: Immunoglobulin subclasses in normal children. Pediatr. Res. 13:181, 1979.

221. Posey, D. L., and Marks, C.: Overwhelming postsplenectomy sepsis in childhood. Am. J. Surg. *145:*318, 1983.
222. Hague, A. U., and Min, K. W.: Postsplenectomy pneumococcemia in adults. Arch. Pathol. Lab. Med. *104:*258, 1980.
223. Krivit, W.: Overwhelming postsplenectomy infection. Surg. Clin. North Am. *59:*223, 1979.
224. Schwartz, P. E., Sterioff, S., et al.: Postsplenectomy sepsis and mortality in adults. J. A. M. A. *248:*2279, 1982.
225. Kingston, M. E., and MacKenzie, C. R.: The syndrome of pneumococcemia, disseminated intravascular coagulation and asplenia. Can. Med. Assoc. J. *121:*57, 1979.
226. Whitaker, A. N.: Infection and the spleen: association between hyposplenism, pneumococcal sepsis and disseminated intravascular coagulation. Med. J. Aust. *1:*1213, 1969.
227. Brunell, P. A., Bass, J. W., et al.: American Academy of Pediatrics—Recommendations for using pneumococcal vaccine in children. Pediatrics *75:*1153, 1985.
228. Klein, J. O.: The epidemiology of pneumococcal disease in infants and children. Rev. Infect. Dis. *3:*S246, 1981.
229. Giebink, G. S., Foker, J. E., et al.: Serum antibody and opsonic response to pneumococcal capsular polysaccharide vaccination in normal and splenectomized children. J. Infect. Dis. *141:*404, 1980.
230. Pedersen, F. K., Henricksen, J., et al.: Antibody response to vaccination with pneumococcal capsular polysaccharides in splenectomized children. Acta Paediatr. Scand. *71:*451, 1982.
231. Giebink, G. S., Chap, T. L., et al.: Decline of serum antibody in splenectomized children after vaccination with pneumococcal capsular polysaccharides. J. Pediatr. *105:*576, 1984.
232. Caplan, S. N., and Berkman, E. M.: Immunosuppressive therapy of idiopathic thrombocytopenic purpura. Med. Clin. North Am. *60:*971, 1976.
233. Ahn, Y. S., and Harrington, W. J.: Treatment of idiopathic thrombocytopenic purpura (ITP). Ann. Rev. Med. *28:*299, 1977.
234. Kelton, J. G., and Gibbons, S.: Autoimmune platelet destruction: idiopathic thrombocytopenic purpura. Semin. Thromb. Hemostas. *8:*83, 1982.
235. Ahn, Y. S., Byrnes, J. J., et al.: The treatment of idiopathic thrombocytopenic purpura with vinblastine-loaded platelets. New Engl. J. Med. *298:*1101, 1978.
236. Rosse, W. F.: Whatever happened to vinca-loaded platelets? New Engl. J. Med. *310:*1051, 1984.
237. Kelton, J. G., McDonald, J. W. D., et al.: The reversible binding of vinblastine to platelets: implications for therapy. Blood *57:*431, 1981.
238. Ahn, Y. S., Harrington, W. J., et al.: Slow infusion of vinca alkaloids in the treatment of idiopathic thrombocytopenic purpura. Ann. Intern. Med. *100:*192, 1984.
239. O'Duffy, J. D., Colgan, J. P., et al.: Frentizole therapy of thrombocytopenia in systemic lupus erythematosus refractory ITP. Mayo Clin. Proc. *55:*601, 1980.
240. Melo, J., Harrington, W. J., et al.: Colchicine therapy of ITP. Blood *58*(Suppl. 1):200a, 1981 (Abstract).
241. Strother, S. V., Zuckerman, K. S.: Colchicine therapy of refractory immune thrombocytopenia. Blood *60*(Suppl. 1):193a, 1982 (Abstract).
242. Kuzemko, J. A., and Keidan, S. E.: Treatment of chronic ITP with azathioprine and prednisolone. A clinical trial with three children. Clin. Pediatr. *7:*216, 1968.
243. Lo, S. S., Hitzig, W. H., et al.: Management of chronic ITP in children, with particular reference to immunosuppressive therapy. Acta Haematol. *41:*1, 1969.
244. Hilgartner, M. W., Lanzkowsky, P., et al.: The use of azathioprine in refractory idiopathic thrombocytopenic purpura in children. Acta Paediatr. Scand. *59:*409, 1970.
245. Saenz, A., Tussell, J., et al.: treatment of idiopathic thrombocytopenic purpura in children with steroids and azathioprine: results in 120 cases. In *Platelets, Recent Advances in Basic Research and Clinical Aspects.* Ulutin, O. N. (ed.), Amsterdam, Excerpta Medica, 1975, p. 499.
246. Marmont, A. M., Damasio, E. E.: Clinical experiences with cytotoxic immunosuppressive treatment of ITP. Acta Haematol. *46:*74, 1971.
247. Hicsonmez, G., and Ozsoylu, S.: Vincristine for treatment of chronic thrombocytopenia in children. New Engl. J. Med. *296:*454, 1977 (Letter).
248. Massimo, L., Genova, R., et al.: More on vincristine in treatment of ITP in children. New Engl. J. Med. *297:*397, 1977 (Letter).
249. Tangun, Y., and Atamer, T.: More on vincristine in treatment of ITP. New Engl. J. Med. *297:*894, 1977.
250. Seip, M.: Vincristine in the treatment of postinfectious and neonatal thrombocytopenia. Acta Paediatr. Scand. *69:*253, 1980.
251. Menichelli, A., Del Principe, D., et al.: Intravenous pulse methyl prednisolone in chronic ITP. Arch. Dis. Child. *59:*777, 1984.
252. Ahn, Y. S., Harrington, W. J., et al.: Danazol for the treatment of idiopathic thrombocytopenic purpura. New Engl. J. Med. *308:*1396, 1983.
253. Schulman, I., and Currimabhoy, Z.: Platelet stimulating properties of human plasma with observation on the role of the spleen in the pathogenesis and treatment of ITP. Am. J. Dis. Child. *100:*747, 1960.
254. Schulman, I., Abildgaard, C. F., et al.: Studies on thrombopoiesis. II. Assay of human plasma thrombopoietic activity. J. Pediatr. *66:*604, 1965.
255. Berglund, G.: Plasma transfusion treatment in six children with ITP. Acta Pediatr. *51:*523, 1962.
256. Reiquam, C. W., and Prosper, J. C.: Fresh plasma transfusions in the treatment of acute thrombocytopenic purpura. J. Pediatr. *68:*880, 1966.
257. Novak, R., and Williams, J.: Plasmapheresis in catastrophic complications of idiopathic thrombocytopenic purpura. J. Pediatr. *92:*434, 1978.
258. Branda, R. F., McCullough, J. J., et al.: Plasma exchange in the treatment of fulminant ITP. Lancet *1:*688, 1978.
259. Weir, A. B., Poon, M., et al.: Plasma exchange in ITP. Arch. Intern. Med. *140:*1101, 1980.
260. Blanchette, V. S., Hogan, V. A., et al.: Intensive plasma exchange therapy in ten patients with ITP. Transfusion *24:*388, 1984.
261. Brooks, B. D., Steane, E. A., et al.: Therapeutic plasma exchange in the immune hemolytic anemias and immunologic thrombocytpenic purpura. In *Therapeutic Apheresis and Plasma Perfusion.* Aster, R. (ed.), New York, A. R. Liss, 1982, pp. 317–329.
262. Ramos, M. E. G., Newman, A. J., et al.: Chronic thrombocytopenia in children. J. Pediatr. *92:*584, 1978.
263. Den Otholander, G. J., Gratama, J. W., et al.: Long term follow up study of 168 patients with immune thrombocytopenia. Implications for therapy. Scand. J. Haematol. *32:*101, 1984.
264. Afifi, A. M.: Childhood ITP in Egypt and the neighboring Arab countries. 18th Congress of the International Society of Hematologists, Montreal, 1980, Abstract #1489, p. 275.
265. Dameshek, W., Ebbe, S., et al.: Recurrent acute idiopathic thrombocytopenic purpura. New Engl. J. Med. *269:*647, 1963.
266. Schulman, I., Pierce, M., et al.: Studies on thrombopoiesis. I. A factor in normal human plasma required for platelet production; chronic thrombocytopenia due to its deficiency. Blood *16:*943, 1960.
267. Upshaw, J. D.: Congenital deficiency of a factor in normal plasma that reverses microangiopathic hemolysis and thrombocytopenia. New Engl. J. Med. *298:*1350, 1978.
268. Aspnes, G. T., Pearson, H. A., et al.: Recurrent idiopathic thrombocytopenic purpura with "accessory" splenic tissue. Pediatrics *55:*131, 1975.

269. Verheyden, C. N., Beart, R. W., et al.: Accessory splenectomy in management of recurrent idiopathic thrombocytopenic purpura. Mayo Clin. Proc. 53:442, 1978.
270. Thorek, P., Gradman, R., et al.: Recurrent primary thrombocytopenic purpura with accessory spleens: review of the literature. Ann. Surg. 128:304, 1948.
271. Pearson, H. A., Johnston, D., et al.: The born-again spleen: return of splenic function after splenectomy for trauma. New Engl. J. Med. 298:1389, 1978.
272. Davis, H. H., Varki, A., et al.: Detection of accessory spleens with Indium lll-labeled autologous platelets. Am. J. Hematol. 8:81, 1980.
273. Voet, D., Afschrift, M., et al.: Sonographic diagnosis of an accessory spleen in recurrent ITP. Pediatr. Radiol. 13:39, 1983.
274. Matoth, Y., Zaizov, R., et al.: Minimal cerebral dysfunction in children with chronic thrombocytopenia. Pediatrics 47:698, 1971.
275. Territo, M., Finklestein, J., et al.: Management of autoimmune thrombocytopenia in pregnancy and in the neonate. Obstet. Gynecol. 41:579, 1973.
276. Kelton, J. G.: Management of the pregnant patient with ITP. Ann. Intern. Med. 99:796, 1983.
277. Scott, J. R., Cruikshank, D. P., et al.: Fetal platelet counts in the obstetric management of immunologic thrombocytopenic purpura. Am. J. Obstet. Gynecol. 136:495, 1980.
278. Cines, D. B., Dusak, B., et al.: Immune thrombocytopenic purpura and pregnancy. New Engl. J. Med. 306:826, 1982.
279. Kelton, J. G., Inwood, M. J., et al.: The prenatal prediction of thrombocytopenia in infants of mothers with clinically diagnosed immune thrombocytopenia. Am. J. Obstet. Gynecol. 144:449, 1982.
280. Ayromlooi, J. A.: A new approach to the management of immunologic thrombocytopenic purpura in pregnancy. Am. J. Obstet. Gynecol. 130:235, 1978.
281. Karpatkin, M., Porges, R. F., et al.: Platelet counts in infants of women with autoimmune thrombocytopenia: effects of steroid administration to the mother. New Engl. J. Med. 305:936, 1981.
282. Logaridis, T. E., Doran, T. A., et al.: The effect of maternal steroid administration on fetal platelet count in immunologic thrombocytopenic purpura. Am. J. Obstet. Gynecol. 145:147, 1983.
283. Murray, J. M., and Harris, R. E.: The management of the pregnant patient with ITP. Am. J. Obstet. Gynecol. 126:449, 1976.
284. Scharfman, W. B., Babcock, R. B., et al.: New Engl. J. Med. 306:745, 1982 (Letters).
285. Laros, R. K. and Sweet, R. L.: Management of ITP during pregnancy. Am. J. Obstet. Gynecol. 122:182, 1975.
286. Handin, R. I.: Neonatal immune thrombocytopenia—the doctor's dilemma. New Engl. J. Med. 305:951, 1981.
287. Morgenstern, G. R., Measday, B., et al.: Autoimmune thrombocytopenia in pregnancy: new approach to management. Br. Med. J. 287:584, 1983.
288. Newland, A. C., Boots, M. A., et al.: Intravenous IgG for ITP in pregnancy. New Engl. J. Med. 310:261, 1984 (Letter).
289. Mizunuma, H., Taguchi, H., et al.: A new approach to ITP during pregnancy by high-dose IgG. Am. J. Obstet. Gynecol. 148:218, 1984.
290. Tchernia, G., Dreyfus, M., et al.: Management of immune thrombocytopenia in pregnancy. Response to infusion of IgG. Am. J. Obstet. Gynecol. 148:225, 1984.
291. Besa, E. C., MacNab, M. W., et al.: High dose intravenous IgG in the management of pregnancy in women with ITP. Am. J. Haematol. 18:373, 1985.
292. Mollison, P. L.: *Blood Transfusion in Clinical Medicine*, 7th ed. Oxford, Blackwell Scientific Publications, 1983.
293. Karpatkin, M.: Corticosteroid therapy in thrombocytopenic infants of women with autoimmune thrombocytopenia. J. Pediatr. 105:623, 1984.
294. Chirico, G., Duse, M., et al.: High dose IgG for passive immune neonatal thrombocytopenia. J. Pediatr. 103:654, 1983.
295. Shalev, O, and Brezis, M.: Methyldopa-induced thrombocytopenia in chronic lymphocytic leukemia. New Engl. J. Med. 297:1471, 1977.
296. Rosenstein R, Kosfeld, R. E., et al.: Procainamide-induced thrombocytopenia. Am. J. Hematol. 16:181, 1984.
297. Bernard, A. H., and Schoenker, A. H.: Thrombocytopenia after use of methyldopa. Lancet 2:292, 1965.
298. Hackett, T., Kelton, J. G., et al.: Drug-induced platelet destruction. Semin. Thromb. Hemostas. 8:116, 1982.
299. Weifuse, L., Spear, P. W., et al.: Quinidine-induced thrombocytopenic purpura. Am. J. Med. 17:414, 1954.
300. Shulman, N. R.: Immunoreactions involving platelets. IV. Studies on the pathogenesis of thrombocytopenia in drug purpura using test doses of quinidine in sensitized individuals; their implications in idiopathic thrombocytopenic purpura. J. Exp. Med. 107:711, 1958.
301. Kelton, J. G., Meltzer, D., et al.: Drug-induced thrombocytopenia is associated with increased binding of IgG to platelets both in vivo and in vitro. Blood 58:524, 1981.
302. Cimo P. L., Pisciotta, A. V., et al.: Detection of drug-dependent antibodies by the ^{51}Cr platelet lysis test: documentation of immune thrombocytopenia induced by diphenylhydantoin, diazepam, and sulfisoxazole. Am. J. Hematol. 2:65, 1977.
303. David J. W., and Wilson, S. J.: Quinidine effect on platelet uptake and release of serotonin. Blood 24:841, 1964.
304. Deykin D., and Hellerstein, L. K.: The assessment of drug-dependent and isoimmune antiplatelet antibodies by the use of platelet aggregometry. J. Clin. Invest. 51:3142, 1972.
305. Duquesnoy, R. J., Lorentzen, D. F., et al.: Platelet migration inhibition: a new method for detection of platelet antibodies. Blood 45:741, 1975.
306. Hirschman R. J., and Shulman, N. R.: The use of platelet serotonin release as a sensitive method for detecting anti-platelet antibodies and a plasma anti-platelet factor in patients with idiopathic thrombocytopenic purpura. Br. J. Haematol. 24:793, 1973.
307. Horowitz, H. I., Rappaport, H. I., et al.: Change in platelet factor 3 as a means of demonstrating immune reactions involving platelets: its use as a test for quinidine-induced thrombocytopenia. Transfusion 5:336, 1965.
308. Karpatkin, M., and Siskind, G. W., et al.: The platelet factor 3 immunoinjury technique re-evaluated. Development of a rapid test for antiplatelet antibody. Detection in various clinical disorders, including immunologic drug-induced and neonatal thrombocytopenias. J. Lab. Clin. Med. 89:400, 1977.
309. Shulman, N. R.: Immunoreactions involving platelets. I. A steric and kinetic model for formation of a complex from a human antibody, quinidine as haptene, and platelets; and for fixation of complement by the complex. J. Exp. Med. 107:665, 1958.
310. Shulman, N. R.: Immunoreactions involving platelets. III. Quantitative aspects of platelet agglutination, inhibition of clot retraction and other reactions caused by the antibody of quinidine purpura. J. Exp. Med. 107:697, 1958.
311. Christie, D. J., Kunicki, T. J., et al.: Characterization of the binding of quinine and quinidine-dependent antibodies with human platelets by an electroimmunoassay (ABST). Transfusion 21:640, 1981.
312. Burton, D. R.: Immunoglobulin G: functional sites. Molec. Immunol. 22:161, 1985.
313. Karas S. P., Rosse, W. F., et al.: Characterization of the

IgG-Fc receptor on human platelets. Blood 60:1277, 1982.
314. van Leeuwen E. F., Englefrieft, C. P., et al.: Studies on quinine-and quinidine-dependent antibodies against platelets and their reaction with platelets in the Bernard-Soulier syndrome. Br. J. Haematol. 51:551, 1982.
315. Lerner, W., Faig, D., et al.: Mechanisms of drug-induced immunologic thrombocytopenic purpura. Blood 60(Suppl. 1):188a, 1982.
316. Christie, D. J., Mullen, P. C., et al.: Fab-mediated binding of drug-dependent antibodies to platelets in quinidine-and quinine-induced thrombocytopenia. J. Clin. Invest. 75:310, 1985.
317. Ackroyd, J. R.: The mechanism of the reduction of clot retraction by Sedormid in the blood of patients who have recovered from Sedormid purpura. Clin. Sci. 8:235, 1949.
318. Kornberg, A., and Polliak, A.: Paracetamol-induced thrombocytopenia and haemolytic anaemia [Letter]. Lancet 2:1159, 1978.
319. Nordqvist P., Cramer, G., et al.: Thrombocytopenia during chlorothiazide treatment. Lancet 1:272, 1959.
320. Duquesnoy R. J., Lorentzen, D. F., et al.: Platelet migration inhibition: a new method for detection of platelet antibodies. Blood 45:741, 1975.
321. Nathan, P.: The migration of human platelets in vitro. Thromb. Diath. Haemorrh. 30:173, 1973.
322. Ackroyd, J. F.: Seminars on blood coagulation. Allergic purpura, including purpura due to foods, drugs and infections. Am. J. Med. 14:605, 1953.
323. Deykin, D., and Hellerstein, L. J.: The assessment of drug-dependent and isoimmune antiplatelet antibodies by the use of platelet aggregometry. J. Clin. Invest. 51:3142, 1972.
324. Grandjean, L. C.: A case of purpura haemorrhagica after administration of quinine with specific thrombocytolysis demonstrated in vitro. Acta Med. Scand. 131(Suppl. 213):165, 1948.
325. Cimo, P. L., Pisciotta, A. V., et al.: Detection of drug-dependent antibodies by the ^{51}Cr platelet lysis test: documentation of immune thrombocytopenia induced by diphenylhydantoin, diazepam, and sulfisoxazole. Am. J. Hematol. 2:65, 1977.
326. Aster, R. H., Cooper, H. E., et al.: Simplified complement fixation test for the detection of platelet antibodies in human serum. J. Lab. Clin. Med. 63:161, 1964.
327. Horowitz, H. I., Rappaport, H. I., et al.: Change in platelet factor 3 as a means of demonstrating immune reactions involving platelets: its use as a test for quinidine-induced thrombocytopenia. Transfusion 5:336, 1965.
328. Karpatkin, M., Siskind, G. W., et al.: The platelet factor 3 immunoinjury technique re-evaluated. Development of a rapid test for antiplatelet antibody. Detection in various clinical disorders, including immunologic drug-induced and neonatal thrombocytopenias. J. Lab. Clin. Med. 89:400, 1977.
329. Davis, J. W., and Wilson, S. J.: Quinidine effect on platelet uptake and release of serotonin. Blood 24:841, 1964.
330. Hirschman, R. J., and Shulman, N. R.: The use of platelet serotonin release as a sensitive method for detecting anti-platelet antibodies and a plasma anti-platelet factor in patients with idiopathic thrombocytopenic purpura. Br. J. Haematol. 24:793, 1973.
331. Kelton, J. G., Meltzer, D., et al.: Drug-induced thrombocytopenia is associated with increased binding of IgG to platelets both in vivo and in vitro. Blood 58:524, 1981.
332. Scheinberg, I. H.: Thrombocytopenic reaction to aspirin and acetaminophen [Letter]. New Engl. J. Med. 300:678, 1979.
333. Schoenfeld, Y., Shaklai, M., et al.: Thrombocytopenia from acetaminophen [Letter]. New Engl. J. Med. 303:47, 1980.
334. Eisner, E. V., and Shahidi, N. T.: Immune thrombocytopenia due to a drug metabolite. New Engl. J. Med. 287:376, 1972.
335. Kornberg, A., and Polliack, A.: Paracetamol-induced thrombocytopenia and hemolytic anemia. Lancet 2:1159, 1978.
336. Bertino, J. R., Rodman, T., et al.: Thrombocytopenia and renal lesions associated with acetazolamide (Diamox) therapy. Arch. Intern. Med. 99:1006, 1957.
337. Reisner, E. H., and Morgan, M. C.: Thrombocytopenia following acetazolamide (Diamox) therapy. J. A. M. A. 160:206, 1956.
338. Nieweg, H. O., Bouma, H. G. D., et al.: Hematological side effects of some antirheumatic drugs. Ann. Rheum. Dis. 22:440, 1963.
339. Garg, S. K., and Sarker, C. R.: Case report. Aspirin-induced thrombocytopenia on an immune basis. Am. J. Med. Sci. 267:129, 1974.
340. Hodder, F. S., Kempert, P., et al.: Immune thrombocytopenia following actinomycin-D therapy. J. Pediatr. 107:611, 1985.
341. Ackroyd, J. F.: The pathogenesis of thrombocytopenic purpura due to hypersensitivity to Sedormid (allyl-isopropylacetylcarbamide). Clin. Sci. 7:249, 1949.
342. Lowey, F. E.: Thrombopenic haemorrhagic purpura. Due to idosyncrasy towards the hypnotic sedormid allergotoxic effect. Lancet 1:845, 1934.
343. Magnusson B., and Rodjer, S.: Alprenolol-induced thrombocytopenia. Acta Med. Scand. 207:231, 1980.
344. Rubin, S. A., Lee, S., et al.: Thrombocytopenia and fever in a patient taking amrinone [Letter]. New Engl. J. Med. 301:1185, 1979.
345. Ansell, J., Tiarks, C., et al.: Amrinone-induced thrombocytopenia. Arch. Intern. Med. 144:949, 1984.
346. Rubin, S., Lee, S., et al.: Thrombocytopenia and fever in a patient taking amrinone. New Engl. J. Med. 301:1185, 1979.
347. Kinney, E. L., Ballard, J. O., et al.: Amrinone-mediated thrombocytopenia. Scand. J. Haematol. 31:376, 1983.
348. Ackroyd, J. F.: Thrombocytopenic purpura due to hypersensitivity to the antihistaminic drug antazoline (2-N-phenyl-N-benzyl-amino-methyl imidazoline). Sang 26:115, 117, 1955 (Abstr.).
349. Conti, L., and Gandolfo, G. M.: Benzodiazepine-induced thrombocytopenia. Acta Haematol. 70:386, 1983.
350. Hilgard, P., and Hossfeld, D. K.: Transient bleomycin-induced thrombocytopenia. A clinical study. Eur. J. Cancer 14:1261, 1978.
351. Karpatkin, S.: Drug-induced thrombocytopenia. Am. J. Med. Sci. 262:69, 1971.
352. Pearce, J., and Ron, M. A.: Thrombocytopenia after carbamazepine [Letter]. Lancet 2:223, 1968.
353. Kornberg, A., and Kobrin, I.: IgG antiplatelet antibodies due to carbamazepine. Acta Haematol. 68:68, 1982.
354. Gralnick, H. R., McGinniss, M., et al.: Thrombocytopenia with sodium cephalothin therapy. Ann. Intern. Med. 77:401, 1972.
355. Sheiman, L., Spielvogel, A. R., et al.: Thrombocytopenia caused by cephalothin sodium. Occurrence in a penicillin-sensitive individual. J. A. M. A. 203:601, 1968.
356. Ball, P.: Thrombocytopenia and purpura in patients receiving chlorothiazide and hydrochlorothiazide. J. A. M. A. 173:663, 1960.
357. Jaffe, M. O., and Kierland, R. R.: Purpura due to chlorothiazide (Diuril). J. A. M. A. 168:2264, 1958.
358. FitzPatrick, W. J.: Thrombocytopenia occurring during chlorpropamide therapy. Diabetes 12:457, 1963.
359. Isaacs, A. J.: Cimetidine and thrombocytopenia. Br. Med. J. 280:294, 1980.

360. Yates, V. M., and Kerr, R. E. I.: Cimetidine and thrombocytopenia [Letter]. Br. Med. J. *280:*1453, 1980.
361. McDaniel, J. L., and Stein, J. J.: Thrombocytopenia with "cimetidine therapy" [Letter]. New Engl. J. Med. *300:*864, 1979.
362. Mar, D. D., Brandstetter, R. D., et al.: Cimetidine-induced immune mediated leukopenia and thrombocytopenia. South. Med. J. *75:*1283, 1982.
363. Glotzbach, R. E.: Cimetidine-induced thrombocytopenia. South. Med. J. *75:*232, 1982.
364. Stambaugh, J. E., Gordon, R. L., et al.: Leucopenia and thrombocytopenia secondary to clinoril [Letter]. Lancet *2:*594, 1980.
365. Veall, R. M., and Hogarth, H. C.: Thrombocytopenia during treatment with clonazepam. Br. Med. J. *4:*462, 1975.
366. Claas, F. H., van der Meer, J. W. M., et al.: Immunological effect of co-trimoxazole on platelets. Br. Med. J. *2:*898, 1979.
367. Mohan, P.: Thrombocytopenia and agranulocytosis following Septrin. Practitioner *202:*553, 1969.
368. Barr, A. A., and Whineray, M.: Case report. Immune thrombocytopenia induced by cotrimoxazole. Aust. N. Z. J. Med. *10:*54, 1980.
369. Rachmilewitz, E. A., Dawson, R. B., Jr., et al.: Serum antibodies against desipramine as a possible cause for thrombocytopenia. Blood *32:*525, 1968.
370. Berger, H.: Thrombopenic purpura following use of digitoxin. J. A. M. A. *148:*282, 1952.
371. Young, R. C., Nachman, R. L., et al.: Thrombocytopenia due to digitoxin. Demonstration of antibody and mechanisms of action. Am. J. Med. *41:*605, 1966.
372. Hess, S., Riesen, W., et al.: Digoxin intoxication with severe thrombocytopenia: reversal by digoxin-specific antibodies. Eur. J. Clin. Invest. *13:*159, 1983.
373. Pirovino, M., Ohnhaus, E. E., et al.: Digoxin-associated thrombocytopenia. Eur. J. Clin. Pharmacol. *19:*205, 1981.
374. Pirovino, M., Ohnhaus, E. E., et al.: Digoxin-associated thrombocytopenia. Eur. J. Clin. Pharmacol. *19:*205, 1981.
375. Weintraub, R. M., Pechet, L., et al.: Rapid diagnosis of drug-induced thrombocytopenic purpura. J. A. M. A. *180:*528, 1962.
376. Fincham, R. W., Hamilton, H. E., et al.: Late-onset thrombocytopenia with phenytoin therapy. Ann. Neurol. *6:*370, 1979.
377. Simpson, R. E., Goldstein, D. J., et al.: Acute thrombocytopenia associated with fenoprofen. New Engl. J. Med. *298:*629, 1978.
378. Katz, M. E., and Wang, P.: Fenoprofen-associated thrombocytopenia. Ann. Intern. Med. *92:*262, 1980.
379. King, D. J., and Kelton, J. G.: Heparin-associated thrombocytopenia. Ann. Intern. Med. *100:*535, 1984.
380. Moss, R. A., and Okun, D. B.: Heroin-induced thrombocytopenia. Arch. Intern. Med. *139:*752, 1979.
381. Ryan, D. H.: Heroin and thrombocytopenia [Letter]. Ann. Intern. Med. *90:*852, 1979.
382. Fishman, A. J.: Thrombocytopenia and heroin [Letter]. Ann. Intern. Med. *94:*280, 1981.
383. Gesink, M. H., and Bradford, H. A.: Thrombocytopenic purpura associated with hydrochlorothiazide therapy. J.A.M.A. *172:*556, 1960.
384. Eisner, E. V., and Crowell, E. B.: Hydrochlorothiazide-dependent thrombocytopenia due to IgM antibody. J.A.M.A. *215:*480, 1971.
385. Hansen, J. E.: Hypersensitivity to isoniazid with neutropenia and thrombocytopenia. Am. Rev. Respir. Dis. *83:*744, 1961.
386. El-Ghobarey, A. F., and Capell, H. A.: Levamisole-induced thrombocytopenia. Br. Med. J. *2:*555, 1977.
387. Wanamaker, W. M., Wanamaker, S. J., et al.: Thrombocytopenia associated with long-term levodopa therapy. J. A. M. A. *235:*2217, 1976.
388. Schiffer, C. A., Weinstein, H. J., et al.: Methicillin-associated thrombocytopenia. Ann. Intern. Med. *85:*338, 1973.
389. Manohitharajah, S. M., Jenkins, W. J., et al.: Methyldopa and associated thrombocytopenia. Br. Med. J. *1:*494, 1971.
390. Shalev, O., and Brezis, M.: Methyldopa-induced thrombocytopenia in chronic lymphocytic leukemia [Letter]. New Engl. J. Med. *297:*1471, 1977.
391. Benraad, A. H., and Schoenaker, A. H.: Thrombocytopenia after use of methyldopa [Letter]. Lancet *2:*292, 1965.
392. Peitzman, S. J., and Martin, C.: Thrombocytopenia and Minoxidil [Letter]. Ann. Intern. Med. *92:*874, 1980.
393. Cimo, P. L., Hammond, J. J., et al.: Morphine-induced immune thrombocytopenia associated with a platelet antibody cross-reactive with other opiates. Clin. Res. *27:*744A, 1979.
394. Mehta, P., Mehta, J., et al.: Nitroprusside lowers platelet count [Letter]. New Engl. J. Med. *299:*1134, 1978.
395. Day, H. J., Conrad, F. G., et al.: Immunothrombocytopenia induced by novobiocin. Am. J. Med. Sci. *236:*475, 1958.
396. Falconer, E. H., Epstein, N. N., et al.: Purpura haemorrhagica due to arsphenamines. Arch. Intern. Med. *66:*319, 338, 1940.
397. Armstrong, F. B., and Scherbel, A. L.: Review of toxicity of oxyphenebutazone. Report of a case of thrombocytopenic purpura. J. A. M. A. *175:*614, 1961.
398. Hare, D. L., and Hicks, B. H.: Thrombocytopenia due to oxprenolol [Letter]. Med. J. Aust. *2:*259, 1979.
399. Dodds, W. N., and Davidson, R. J. L. Thrombocytopenia due to slow release oxprenolol [Letter]. Lancet *2:*683, 1978.
400. Hayes, R. H., and Weiss, M.: Hypersensitivity reactions to oral para-aminosalicylic acid. Dis. Chest *23:*645, 1953.
401. Wurzel, H. A., and Mayock, R. L.: Thrombocytopenia induced by sodium para-amino-salicylic acid. Report of a case. J. A. M. A. *153:*1094, 1953.
402. Eisner, E. V., and Kasper, K.: Immune thrombocytopenia due to a metabolite of para-aminosalicylic acid. Am. J. Med. *53:*790, 1972.
403. Salamon, D. J., Nusbacher, J., et al.: Red cell and platelet bound IgG penicillin antibodies in a patient with thrombocytopenia. Transfusion *24:*395, 1984.
404. Rosenstein, R., Kosfeld, R. E., et al.: Procainamide-induced thrombocytopenia. Am. J. Hematol. *16:*181, 1984.
405. Barkham, P., and Tocantins, L. M.: Observations on the thrombocytopenia due to hypersensitivity to quinidine. Blood *9:*134, 1954.
406. Bigelow, F. S., and Desforges, J. F.: Platelet agglutination by an abnormal plasma factor in thrombocytopenic purpura associated with quinidine ingestion. Am. J. Med. Sci. *224:*274, 1952.
407. Shulman, N. R.: Immunoreactions involving platelets. IV. Studies on the pathogenesis of thrombocytopenia in drug purpura using test doses of quinidine in sensitized individuals; their implications in idiopathic thrombocytopenic purpura. J. Exp. Med. *107:*711, 1958.
408. Larson, R. K.: The mechanism of quinidine purpura. Blood *8:*16, 1953.
409. Bolton, F. G., and Dameshek, W.: Thrombocytopenic purpura due to quinidine clinical studies. Blood *11:*527, 1956.
410. Weisfuse, L., Spear, P. W., et al.: Quinidine-induced thrombocytopenic purpura. Am. J. Med. *17:*414, 1954.
411. Bolton, F. G., and Young, R. V.: Observations on cases of thrombocytopenic purpura due to quinine, sulphamethazine, and quinidine. J. Clin. Pathol. *6:*320, 1953.

412. Alperin, J. B., deGroot, W. J., et al.: Quinidine induced thrombocytopenia with pulmonary hemorrhage. Arch. Intern. Med. *140*:266, 1980.
413. Christie, D. J., and Aster, R. H.: Drug-antibody-platelet interaction in quinine and quinidine-induced thrombocytopenia. J. Clin. Invest. *70*:989, 1982.
414. Helmly, R. B., Bergin, J. J., et al.: Quinine-induced purpura. Arch. Intern. Med. *120*:59, 1967.
415. Steinkamp, R., Moore, C. V., et al.: Thrombocytopenic purpura caused by hypersensitivity to quinine. J. Lab. Clin. Med. *45*:18, 1955.
416. Mauer, A. M., DeVaux, W., et al.: Neonatal and maternal thrombocytopenic purpura due to quinine. Pediatrics *19*:84, 1957.
417. Blajchman, M. A., Lowry, R. C., et al.: Rifampicin-induced immune thrombocytopenia. Br. Med. J. *3*:24, 1970.
418. Kahn, H. R., and Brod, R. C.: Thrombocytopenia due to stibophen. Arch. Intern. Med. *108*:496, 1961.
419. Rivera, J. V., Rodriguez, H. F., et al.: Thrombocytopenic purpura due to faudin (Stibophen). Am. J. Trop. Med. Hyg. *5*:863, 1956.
420. Thomas, T. F.: Thrombocytopenic purpura secondary to sulfamethoxypridazine. NY State J. Med. *63*:2554, 1963.
421. Schwartz, M. J., and Norton, W. S.: Thrombocytopenia and leukopenia associated with use of sulfamethoxypridazine. J.A.M.A. *167*:457, 1958.
422. Green, I., and Finkel, M.: Thrombocytopenic purpura associated with sulfamethoxypyridazine administration. NY State J. Med. *59*:2034, 1959.
423. Green, T. W., and Early, J. Q.: Thrombocytopenic purpura resulting from sulfisoxazole (Gantrisin) therapy. Report of two cases. J. A. M. A. *161*:1563, 1956.
424. Geiger, J.: Thrombocytopenic purpura induced by sulfisoxazole (Gantrisin) therapy. Report of a case controlled by platelet transfusion. J. A. M. A. *149*:1219, 1952.
425. Hamilton, H. E., and Sheets, R. F.: Sulfisoxazole-induced thrombocytopenic purpura: immunologic mechanism as cause. J. A. M. A. *239*:2586, 1978.
426. Hurd, R. W., and Jacox, R. F.: Thrombocytopenic purpura developing as a complication of sulfathiazole and sulfadizine therapy. J. A. M. A. *122*:296, 1943.
427. Kracke, R. R., and Townsend, E. W.: The effect of sulfonamide drugs on the blood platelets. Report of two cases of thrombopenic purpura and experimental studies on patients receiving sulfonamide drugs. J. A. M. A. *122*:168, 1943.
428. Jost, F.: Blood dyscrasias associated with tolbutamide therapy. J. A. M. A. *169*:1468, 1959.
429. Hagen, M. D., and White, R. D.: Thrombocytopenia secondary to trimethoprim-sulfamethoxazole. South. Med. J. *74*:503, 1981.
430. Schwartz, R. H., Rodriguez, W. J., et al.: Thrombocytopenia associated with PF_3 antiplatelet activity against the sulfa component of trimethoprim-sulfamethoxazole. South. Med. J. *74*:640, 1981.
431. Bradley, P. P., Warden, G. D., et al.: Neutropenia and thrombocytopenia in renal allograft recipients treated with trimethoprim-sulfamethoxazole. Ann. Intern. Med. *93*:560, 1980.
432. Walker, R. W., and Heaton, A.: Thrombocytopenia due to Vancomycin. Lancet *1*:932, 1985.
433. Stefanini, M., and Hoffman, M. N.: Case report. Studies on platelet. XXVIII. Acute thrombocytopenic purpura due to lidocaine (Xylocaine^R) mediated antibody. Report of a case. Am. J. Med. Sci. *275*:365, 1978.
434. Mims, J. A., Sarji, K. E., et al.: Heparin-induced platelet aggregation in burn patients. Thromb. Res. *1*:291, 1977.
435. Salzman, E. W., Rosenberg, R. D., et al.: Effect of heparin and heparin fractions on platelet aggregation. J. Clin. Invest. *65*:64, 1980.

436. Thomson, C., Forbes, C. D., et al.: The potentiation of platelet aggregation and adhesion by heparin in vitro and in vivo. Clin. Sci. Molec. Med. *45*:485, 1973.
437. Carter, C. J., Kelton, J. G., et al.: The relationship between the hemorrhagic and antithrombotic properties of low molecular weight heparin in rabbits. Blood *59*:1239, 1982.
438. Bell, W. R., Tomasulo, P. A., et al.: Thrombocytopenia occurring during the administration of heparin: a prospective study in 52 patients. Ann. Intern. Med. *85*:155, 1976.
439. Eika, C., Godal, H. C., et al.: Low incidence of thrombocytopenia during treatment with hog mucosa and beef lung heparin. Scand. J. Haematol. *25*:19, 1980.
440. Nelson, J. C., Lerner, R. G., et al.: Heparin-induced thrombocytopenia. Arch. Intern. Med. *138*:548, 1978.
441. Malcolm, I. D., Wigmore, T. A., et al.: Heparin-associated thrombocytopenia: low frequency in 104 patients treated with heparin of intestinal mucosa origin. Can. Med. Assoc. J. *120*:1086, 1979.
442. Powers, P. J., Cuthbert, D., et al.: Thrombocytopenia found uncommonly during heparin therapy. J.A.M.A. *241*:2396, 1979.
443. Gallus, A. S., Goodall, K. T., et al.: Heparin associated thrombocytopenia: case report and prospective study. Aust. NZ J. Med. *10*:25, 1980.
444. Holm, H. A., Eika, C., et al.: Thrombocytes and treatment with heparin from porcine mucosa. Scand. J. Haematol. *36*(Suppl.):81, 1980.
445. Olin, J., and Graor, R.: Heparin-associated thrombocytopenia [Letter]. New Engl. J. Med. *304*:609, 1981.
446. Kelton, J. G., and Power, P. J.: Heparin-associated thrombocytopenia: an immune disorder. In *Chemistry and Biology of Heparin*. Lundblad, R. L., Brown, W. V., et al. (eds.), New York, Elsevier-North Holland, Inc., 1981, p. 365.
447. Economopoulos, T. C., Payayannis, A. G., et al.: Postoperative platelet function in patients on small subcutaneous doses of heparin. Acta Haematol. *57*:266, 1977.
448. Ayars, G. H., and Tikoff, G.: Incidence of thrombocytopenia in medical patients on "mini-dose" heparin prophylaxis [Letter]. Am. Heart J. *99*:816, 1980.
449. Johnson, R.A., Lazarus, K. H., et al.: Heparin-induced thrombocytopenia: a prospective study. Am. J. Hematol. *17*:349, 1984.
450. Kin, D.: Heparin-induced thrombocytopenia: a prospective study. Thromb. Haemostas. *43*:61, 1980.
451. Bell, W. R., and Royall, R. M.: Heparin-associated thrombocytopenia: a comparison of three heparin preparations. New Engl. J. Med. *303*:902, 1980.
452. Kwaan, H. C., Kampmeier, P. A., et al.: Incidence of thrombocytopenia during therapy with bovine lung and porcine gut mucosal heparin preparations. Thromb. Haemostas. *46*:680A, 1981.
453. Powers, P. J., Kelton, J. G., et al.: Studies on the frequency of heparin-associated thrombocytopenia. Thromb. Res. *33*:439, 1984.
454. Ansell, J., Slepchuk, N., Jr., et al.: Heparin induced thrombocytopenia: a prospective study. Thromb. Haemostas. *43*:61, 1980.
455. King, D. J., and Kelton, J. G.: Heparin-associated thrombocytopenia. Ann. Intern. Med. *100*:535, 1984.
456. Weismann, R. E., and Tobin, R. W.: Arterial embolism occurring during systemic heparin therapy. Arch. Surg. *76*:219, 1958.
457. Rhodes, G. R., Dixon, R. H., et al.: Heparin-induced thrombocytopenia with thrombotic and hemorrhagic manifestations. Surg. Gynecol. Obstet. *136*:409, 1973.
458. Cimo, P. L., Moake, J. L., et al.: Heparin-induced thrombocytopenia: association with a platelet aggregating factor and arterial thrombosis. Am. J. Hematol. *6*:125, 1979.
459. Hussey, C. V., Bernhard, V. M., et al.: Heparin-induced

platelet aggregation: *in vitro* confirmation of thrombotic complications associated with heparin therapy. Ann. Clin. Lab. Sci. *9:*487, 1979.
460. Kapsch, D. N., Adelstein, E. H., et al.: Heparin-induced thrombocytopenia, thrombosis, and hemorrhage. Surgery *86:*148, 1979.
461. Towne, J. B., Bernhard, V. M., et al.: White clot syndrome: peripheral vascular complications of heparin therapy. Arch. Surg. *114:*372, 1979.
462. Kaupp, H. A., and Roberts, B.: Arterial embolization during subcutaneous heparin therapy: case report. J. Cardiovasc. Surg. *13:*210, 1972.
463. Baird, R. A., and Convery, F. R.: Arterial thromboembolism in patients receiving systemic heparin therapy: a complication associated with heparin-induced thrombocytopenia. J. Bone Joint Surg. *59A:*1061, 1977.
464. Rhodes, G. R., Dixon, R. H., et al.: Heparin-induced thrombocytopenia: eight cases with thrombotic-hemorrhagic complications. Ann. Surg. *186:*752, 1977.
465. Cines, D. B., Kaywin, P., et al.: Heparin-associated thrombocytopenia. New Engl. J. Med. *303:*788, 795, 1980.
466. Babcock, R. B., Dumper, C. W., et al.: Heparin-induced immune thrombocytopenia. New Engl. J. Med. *295:*237, 1976.
467. Chong, B. H., Grace, C. S., et al.: Heparin-induced thrombocytopenia: effect of heparin platelet antibody on platelets. Br. J. Haematol. *49:*531, 1981.
468. Green, D., Harris, K., et al.: Heparin immune thrombocytopenia: evidence for a heparin-platelet complex as the antigenic determinant. J. Lab. Clin. Med. *91:*167, 1978.
469. White, P. W., Sadd, J. R., et al.: Thrombotic complications of heparin therapy: including six cases of heparin-induced skin necrosis. Ann. Surg. *190:*595, 1979.
470. Van Aken, W. G.: Thrombocytopenia (and consumption coagulopathy) induced by heparin: a case report. Scand. J. Haematol. *36*(Suppl.):85, 1980.
471. Tobelem, G., Michel, H., et al.: Purpura thrombocytopenique lors d'une héparinothérapie. Nouv. Presse Med. *8:*649, 1979.
472. Klein, H. G., and Bell, W. R.: Disseminated intravascular coagulation during heparin therapy. Ann. Intern. Med. *80:*477, 1974.
473. Kelton, J. G., Sheridan, D., et al.: Clinical usefulness of testing for a heparin-dependent platelet aggregating factor in patients with suspected heparin-associated thrombocytopenia. J. Lab. Clin. Med. *103:*606, 1984.
474. Sheridan, D., Carter, C. J., et al.: A diagnostic test for heparin-induced thrombocytopenia. Blood *67:*27, 1986.
475. Covanis, A., Gupta, A. K., et al.: Sodium valproate: monotherapy and polytherapy. Epilepsia *23:*693, 1982.
476. Eastham, R. D., and Jancar, J.: Sodium valproate and platelet counts. Br. Med. J. *280:*186, 1980.
477. Neophytides, A. M., Nott, J. G., et al.: Thrombocytopenia associated with sodium valproate treatment. Ann. Neurol. *5:*389, 1979.
478. Morris, N., Barr, R. D., et al.: Valproic acid and thrombocytopenia. Can. Med. Assoc. J. *125:*63, 1981.
479. Barr, R. D., Copeland, S. A., et al.: Valproic acid and immune thrombocytopenia. Arch. Dis. Child. *57:*681, 1982.
480. Sandler, R. M., Emberson, C., et al.: IgM platelet autoantibody due to sodium valproate. Br. Med. J. *2:*1683, 1978.
481. Mueller-Eckhardt, C., Kuenzlen, E., et al.: Cyclophosphamide-induced immune thrombocytopenia in a patient with ovarian carcinoma successfully treated with intravenous IgG. Blut *46:*165, 1983.
482. Riedler, G. F., Straub, P. W., et al.: Thrombocytopenia in septicemia. A clinical study for the evaluation of its incidence and diagnostic value. Helv. Med. Acta *36:*23, 38, 1971.
483. Beller, F. K., and Douglas, G. W.: Thrombocytopenia indicating gram-negative infection and endotoxemia. Obstet. Gynecol. *41:*521, 1973.
484. Corrigan, J. J.: Thrombocytopenia: a laboratory sign of septicemia in infants and children. J. Pediatr. *85:*219, 1974.
485. Milligan, G. F., MacDonald, J. A. E., et al.: Pulmonary and hematologic disturbances during septic shock. Surg. Gynecol. Obstet. *138:*43, 1974.
486. Oppenheimer, L., Hryniuk, W. M., et al.: Thrombocytopenia in severe bacterial infections. J. Surg. Res. *20:*211, 1976.
487. Kelton, J. G., Neame, P. B., et al.: Elevated platelet-associated IgG in the thrombocytopenia of septicemia. New Engl. J. Med. *300:*760, 1979.
488. Neame, P. B., Kelton, J. G., et al.: Thrombocytopenia in septicemia: the role of disseminated intravascular coagulation. Blood *56:*88, 1980.
489. Dalldorf, F. G., Carney, C. N., et al.: Pulmonary capillary thrombosis in septicemia due to gram-positive bacteria. J. A. M. A. *206:*583, 1968.
490. Evans, R. W., Glick, B., et al.: Fatal intravascular consumption coagulopathy in meningococcal sepsis. Am. J. Med. *46:*910, 1969.
491. Gerjarusak, P., Hinthorn, D. R., et al.: Hyposplenism and disseminated intravascular coagulation (DIC) in fulminant pneumoccal sepsis. South. Med. J. *70:*995, 1977.
492. Haurani, F. I., Regan, J., et al.: Thrombocytopenia secondary to intravascular thrombosis. Am. J. Med. Sci. *248:*260, 1964.
493. Jewitt, J. F.: Coagulopathy syndrome due to streptococci. New Engl. J. Med. *289:*43, 1973.
494. Komp, D. M., and Donaldson, M. H.: Sepsis in leukemia and the Shwartzman reaction. Am. J. Dis. Child. *119:*114, 1970.
495. Kreger, B. E., Craven, D. E., et al.: Gram-negative bacteremia. IV. Re-evaluation of clinical features and treatment in 612 patients. Am. J. Med. *68:*344, 1980.
496. Hjort, P. F., and Rapaport, S. I.: The Shwartzman reaction: pathogenetic mechanisms and clinical manifestations. Ann. Rev. Med. *16:*135, 1965.
497. Thomas, L., and Good, R. A.: Studies on the generalized Shwartzman reaction. I. General observations concerning the phenomenon. J. Exp. Med. *96:*605, 1952.
498. Horn, R. G., and Collins, R. D.: Studies on the pathogenesis of the generalized Shwartzman reaction. Lab. Invest. *18:*101, 1968.
499. Edwards, R. L., Rickles, F. R., et al.: Mononuclear cell tissue factor. Cell of origin and requirements for activation. Blood *54:*359, 1979.
500. Lerner, R. G., Goldstein, R., et al.: Stimulation of human leukocyte thromboplastic activity by endotoxin. Proc. Soc. Exp. Biol. Med. *138:*145, 1971.
501. Lerner, R. G., Goldstein, R., et al.: Production of thromboplastin (tissue factor) and thrombi by polymorphonuclear neutrophilic leukocytes adhering to vein walls. Thromb. Res. *11:*11, 1977.
502. Muhlfelder, T. W., Khan, I., et al.: Factors influencing the release of procoagulant tissue factor activity from leukocytes. J. Lab. Clin. Med. *92:*65, 1978.
503. Niemetz, J.: Coagulant activity of leukocytes. Tissue factor activity. J. Clin. Invest. *51:*307, 1972.
504. Niemetz, J., and Fani, K.: Thrombogenic activity of leukocytes. Blood *42:*47, 1973.
505. Niemetz, J., and Marcus, A. J.: The stimulatory effect of platelets and platelet membranes on the procoagulant activity of leukocytes. J. Clin. Invest. *54:*1437, 1974.
506. Rivers, R. P. A., Hathaway, W. E., et al.: The endotoxin-

506. induced coagulation activity of human monocytes. Br. J. Haematol. *30:*311, 1975.
507. Thiagarajan, P., and Niemetz, J.: Procoagulant-tissue factor activity of circulating peripheral blood leukocytes. Results of in vivo studies. Thromb. Res. *17:*891, 1980.
508. Morrison, D. C., and Cochrane, C. G.: Direct evidence for Hageman factor (factor XII) activation by bacterial lipopolysaccharides (endotoxins). J. Exp. Med. *140:*797, 1974.
509. Walker, R. I., Porvaznik, M., et al.: Hageman factor activation and tight junction disruption in mice challenged with attenuated endotoxin. Experientia *35:*759, 1979.
510. Marcel, G. A., Casper, C., et al.: Significance of kaolin-induced arginine esterase in human plasma during septic shock: depletion in prekallikrein and prekallikrein activator. Thromb. Res. *3:*281, 1973.
511. Schipper, H. G., Roos, J., et al.: Antithrombin III deficiency in surgical intensive care patients. Thromb. Res. *21:*73, 1981.
512. Duedari, N., George, C., et al.: Platelet-associated IgG in septicemia. New Engl. J. Med. *301:*271, 1979.
513. Tate, D. Y., Carlton, G. T., et al.: Immune thrombocytopenia in severe neonatal infections. J. Pediatr. *98:*449, 1981.
514. van der Leli, J., van der Plas-van Dalen, C. M., et al.: Platelet autoantibodies in septicaemia. Br. J. Haematol. *58:*755, 1984.
515. Poskitt, T. R., and Poskitt, P. K.: Thrombocytopenia of sepsis: the role of circulating IgG-containing immune complexes. Arch. Intern. Med. *145:*891, 1985.
516. Gaynor, E., Bouvier, C., et al.: Vascular lesions: possible pathogenetic basis of the generalized Shwartzman reaction. Science *170:*986, 1970.
517. McGrath, J. M., and Stewart, G. J.: The effect of endotoxin on vascular endothelium. J. Exp. Med. *129:*833, 1969.
518. Cohen, P. S., O'Brien, T. F., et al.: The risk of endothelial infection in adults with salmonella bacteremia. Ann. Intern. Med. *89:*931, 1978.
519. Sotto, M. N., Langer, B., et al.: Pathogenesis of cutaneous lesions in acute meningococcemia in humans. Light, immunofluorescent and electron microscopic studies of skin biopsy specimens. J. Infect. Dis. *133:*506, 1976.
520. Margaretten, W., Nakai, H., et al.: Significance of selective vasculitis and the "bone marrow" syndrome in pseudomonas septicemia. New Engl. J. Med. *265:*773, 1961.
521. Clawson, C. C., White, J. G.: Platelet interaction with bacteria. I. Reaction phases and effects of inhibitors. Am. J. Pathol. *65:*367, 1971.
522. MacIntyre, D. E., Allen, A. P., et al.: Endotoxin-induced platelet aggregation and secretion. I. Morphological changes and pharmacological effects. J. Cell Sci. *28:*211, 1977.
523. Nagayama, M., Zucker, M. B., et al.: Effects of a variety of endotoxins on human and rabbit platelet function. Thromb. Diath. Haemorrh. *26:*467, 1971.
524. Davis, C. E., and Arnold, K.: Role of meningococcal endotoxin in meningococcal purpura. J. Exp. Med. *140:*159, 1974.
525. Fox, B.: Disseminated intravascular coagulation and the Waterhouse syndrome. Arch. Dis. Child. *46:*680, 1971.
526. De Voe, I. W.: The meningococcus and mechanisms of pathogenicity. Microbiol. Rev. *46:*162, 1982.
527. Bierman, H. R., and Nelson, E. R.: Hematodepressive virus diseases of Thailand. Ann. Intern. Med. *62:*867, 1965.
528. Nelson, E. R., and Bierman, H. R. Dengue fever: a thrombocytopenia disease? J. A. M. A. *190:*99, 1964.
529. Cooper, L. Z., Green, R. H., et al.: Neonatal thrombocytopenic purpura and other manifestations of rubella contracted in utero. Am. J. Dis. Child. *110:*416, 1965.
530. Oski, F. A., and Naiman, J. L.: Effect of live measles vaccine on the platelet count. New Engl. J. Med. *275:*352, 1966.
531. Feusner, J. H., Slichter, S. J., et al.: Mechanisms of thrombocytopenia in varicella. Am. J. Hematol. *7:*255, 1979.
532. Morse, E. E., Zinkham, W. H., et al.: Thrombocytopenic purpura following rubella infection in children and adults. Arch. Intern. Med. *117:*573, 1966.
533. Andrews, M. V., and Bart, J. B.: Thrombocytopenic purpura in infectious mononucleosis—a rare complication? South. Med. J. *68:*94, 1975.
534. Clark, B. F., and Davies, S. H.: Severe thrombocytopenia in infectious mononucleosis. Am. J. Med. Sci. *248:*703, 1964.
535. Freeman, T., and Wakefield, G. S.: Platelet-agglutinating factor in glandular fever complicated by jaundice and thrombocytopenia. Lancet *2:*883, 1958.
536. Goldstein, E., and Porter, D. Y.: Fatal thrombocytopenia with cerebral hemorrhage in mononucleosis. Arch. Neurol. *20:*533, 1969.
537. Radel, E. G., and Schorr, J. B.: Thrombocytopenic purpura with infectious mononucleosis. Report of 2 cases and a review of the literature. J. Pediatr. *63:*46, 1963.
538. Smith, D. S., Abell, J. D., et al.: Auto-immune haemolytic anemia and thrombocytopenia complicating infectious mononucleosis. Br. Med. J. *1:*1210, 1963.
539. Boyd, J. F., and Reid, D.: Bone marrow in infectious mononucleosis [Letter]. Br. Med. J. *2:*176, 1973.
540. Scott, S., Reimers, H. J., et al.: Effect of viruses on platelet aggregation and platelet survival in rabbits. Blood *52:*42, 1978.
541a. Terada, H., Baldini, M., et al.: Interaction of influenza virus with blood platelets. Blood *28:*213, 1966.
541b. Cooper, L. Z., Green, P. H., et al.: Neonatal thrombocytopenic purpura and other manifestations of rubella contracted in utero. Am. J. Dis. Child. *110:*416, 1965.
541c. Zinkham, W. H., Medearis, D. N., et al.: Blood and bone marrow findings in congenital rubella. J. Pediatr. *71:*512, 1967.
541d. Chesney, P. J., and Shahidi, N. T.: Acute viral-induced thrombocytopenia: a review of human disease, animal models and in vitro studies. In *Acquired Bleeding Disorders in Children*. Lusher, J. M., and Barnhart, M. I. (eds.), New York, Masson Publishers, 1981, pp. 65–81.
542. Hill, G. J., Knight, V., et al.: Thrombocytopenia in vivax malaria. Lancet *1:*240, 1964.
543. Beale, P. J., Cormack, J. D., et al.: Thrombocytopenia in malaria with immunoglobulin (IgM) changes. Br. Med. J. *1:*345, 1972.
544. Horstmann, R. D., Dietrich, M., et al.: Malaria-induced thrombocytopenia. Blut *42:*157, 1981.
545. Skudowitz, R. B., Katz, J., et al.: Mechanisms of thrombocytopenia in malignant tertian malaria. Br. Med. J. *2:*515, 1973.
546. Butler, T., Tong, M. J., et al.: Blood coagulation studies in plasmodium falciparum malaria. Am. J. Med. Sci. *265:*63, 1973.
547. Jaroonvesama, N.: Intravascular coagulation in falciparum malaria. Lancet *1:*221, 1972.
548. Reid, H. A., and Nkrumah, F. K.: Fibrin-degradation products in cerebral malaria. Lancet *1:*218, 1972.
549. Srichaikul, T., Puwasatien, P., et al.: Complement changes and disseminated intravascular coagulation in plasmodium falciparum malaria. Lancet *1:*770, 1975.
550. Shulman, N. R., Aster, R. H., et al.: Immunoreactions involving platelets. V. Post-transfusion Purpura due to

a complement-fixing antibody against a genetically controlled platelet antigen. A proposed mechanism for thrombocytopenia and its relevance in "autoimmunity." J. Clin. Invest. 40:1597, 1961.
551. Pegels, J. G., Bruynes, E. C. E., et al.: Post transfusion purpura: a serological and immunochemical study. Br. J. Haematol. 49:521, 1981.
552. Howard, J. E., Glassberg, A. B., et al.: Post-transfusion thrombocytopenic purpura: a case report. Am. J. Hematol. 1:339, 1976.
553. Mueller-Eckhardt, C., Lechner, K., et al.: Post-transfusion thrombocytopenic purpura: immunological and clinical studies in two cases and review of the literature. Blut 40:249, 1980.
554. Dunstan, R. A., and Rosse, W. F.: Posttransfusion purpura. Report of a case with anti-PL[A1] masked by HLA antibodies. Transfusion 25:219, 1985.
555. Mueller-Eckhardt, C., Kuenzlen, E., et al.: High-dose intravenous immunoglobulin for post-transfusion purpura. New Engl. J. Med. 308:287, 1983.
556. Abramson, N., Eisenberg, P. D., et al.: Post-transfusion purpura: immunologic aspects and therapy. New Engl. J. Med. 291:1163, 1974.
557. Weisberg, L. J., and Linker, C. A.: Prednisone therapy of post-transfusion purpura. Ann. Intern. Med. 100:76, 1984.
558. Seidenfeld, A. M., Owen, J., et al.: Post-transfusion purpura cured by steroid therapy in a man. Can. Med. Assoc. J. 118:1285, 1978.
559. Becker, T., Panzer, S., et al.: High-dose intravenous immunoglobulin for post transfusion purpura. Br. J. Haematol. 61:149, 1985.
560. Sacks, P. V.: Autoimmune hematologic complications in malignant lymphoproliferative disorders. Arch. Intern. Med. 134:781, 1974.
561. Jones, S.: Autoimmune disorders and malignant lymphomas. Cancer 31:1092, 1973.
562. Cohen, J.: Idiopathic thrombocytopenic purpura in Hodgkin's disease. Cancer 41:743, 1978.
563. Fink, K., and Al-Mondhiry, H.: Idiopathic thrombocytopenic purpura in lymphoma. Cancer 37:1999, 1976.
564. Colman, R. W., Osterland, C. K., et al.: A unique lymphoproliferative disorder associated with an IgM platelet agglutinin, diffuse hypergammaglobulinemia, amyloid deposition and excessive urinary excretion of IgG fragments. Am. J. Med. 45:607, 1968.
565. Carey, R. W., McGinnis, A., et al.: Idiopathic thrombocytopenic purpura complicating chronic lymphocytic leukemia. Arch. Intern. Med. 136:62, 1976.
566. Harvey, A. M., Shulman, L. E., et al.: Systemic lupus erythematosus: review of the literature and clinical analysis of 138 cases. Medicine 33:291, 1954.
567. Rabinowitz, Y., and Dameshek, W.: Systemic lupus erythematosus after "idiopathic" thrombocytopenic purpura. A review: a study of systemic lupus erythematosus occurring after 78 splenectomies for "idiopathic" thrombocytopenic purpura with a review of the pertinent literature. Ann. Intern. Med. 52:1, 1960.
568. Papadopoulos, C., Jiji, R., et al.: Lupus erythematosus and hyperthyroidism. Am. J. Dis. Child. 118:621, 1969.
569. Budman, D. R., and Steinberg, A. D.: Hematologic aspects of systemic lupus erythematosus. Current concepts. Ann. Intern. Med. 86:220, 1977.
570. Clark, W. F., Lewis, M. L., et al.: Intrarenal platelet consumption in the diffuse proliferative nephritis of systemic lupus erythematosus. Clin. Sci. Mol. Med. 49:247, 1975.
571. Blanchette, V. S., Hallett, J. J., et al.: Abnormalities of the peripheral blood as a presenting feature of immunodeficiency. Am. J. Hematol. 4:87, 1978.
572. Pont, J., Dieterlan, M., et al.: Hemolytic anemia with autoantibodies, thrombopenia, atrophic gastritis, with anti-stomach antibodies in a 12 year old child. Fr. Pediatr. 27:417, 1972.
573. Segal, B. M., and Weintraub, M. I.: Hashimoto's thyroiditis, myasthenia gravis, idiopathic thrombocytopenic purpura [Letter]. Ann. Intern. Med. 85:761, 1976.
574. Takeda, R., Funaza, T., et al.: Idiopathic thrombocytopenic purpura associated with hyperthyroidism. South. Med. J. 66:553, 1973.
575. Chintu, C., and McClure, P.: Idiopathic thrombocytopenic purpura in two children with Graves' disease. Am. J. Dis. Child. 129:101, 1975.
576. Remuzzi, G., Misiani, R., et al.: Possible role of HLA-B8 antigen as a genetic marker of autoimmune thrombocytopenia in a patient with myasthenia gravis. Thromb. Haemostas. 38:593, 1977.
577. Dickerman, J. D., Holbrook, P. R., et al.: Etiology and therapy of thromboytopenia associated with sarcoidosis. J. Pediatr. 81:758, 1972.
578. Squier, T. L., and Madison, F. W.: Thrombocytopenic purpura due to food allergy. J. Allergy 8:143, 1937.
579. Caffrey, E. A., Sladen, G. E., et al.: Thrombocytopenia caused by cow's milk [Letter]. Lancet 2:361, 1981.
580. Storck, H., Hoigne, R., et al.: Thrombocytes in allergic reactions. Int. Arch. Allergy 6:372, 1955.
581. Muller-Eckhardt, C. H.: Immune reactions of platelets and their clinical significance. Klin. Wochenschr. 53:889, 1975.
582. Paganelli, R., Levinsky, R., et al.: Immune complexes containing food proteins in normal and atopic subjects after oral challenge and effect of sodium cromoglycate on antigen absorption. Lancet 1:1270, 1979.
583. Paganelli, R., Levinsky, R., et al.: Detection of specific antigen within circulating immune complexes. Validation of the assay and its application to food antigen-antibody complexes formed in healthy and food allergic subjects. Clin. Exp. Immunol. 46:44, 1981.
584. Jobin, F., LaPointe, F., et al.: Platelet reactions and immune processes. VI. The effect of immunoglobulins and other plasma proteins on platelet surface interactions. Thromb. Diath. Hemorrh. 25:86, 1971.
585. Israels, E. D., Nisli, G., et al.: Platelet Fc receptor as a mechanism for Ag-Ab complex–induced platelet injury. Thromb. Diath. Hemorrh. 29:434, 1973.
586. Little, C. H., Stewart, A. G., et al.: Platelet serotonin release in rheumatoid arthritis: a study in food-intolerant patients. Lancet 2:297, 1983.
587. Rosenburg, J. C., Hawkins, E., et al.: Mechanism of immunologic injury during antibody-mediated hyperacute rejection of renal heterografts. Transplantation 11:151, 1971.
588. Sharma, H. M., Rosenzweig, J., et al.: Platelets in hyperacute rejection of heterotopic cardiac allografts in presensitized dogs. Am. J. Pathol. 70:155, 1973.
589. Porter, K. A., Dossetor, J. B., et al.: Human renal transplants. I. Glomerular changes. Lab. Invest. 16:153, 1967.
590. Pillary, V. K. G., Kurtzman, N. A., et al.: Selective thrombocytopenia due to localized microangiopathy of renal allografts. Lancet 2:988, 1973.
591. Thakur, M. L., Welch, M. J., et al.: Indium-111-labelled platelets: studies on preparation and evaluation of in vitro and in vivo functions. Thromb. Res. 9:345, 1976.
592. Fenech, A., Nicholls, A., et al.: Indium 111-labelled platelets in the diagnosis of renal transplant rejection. Preliminary findings. Br. J. Radiol. 54:325, 1981.
593. Heyns, A. P., Lotter, M. G., et al.: A quantitative study of Indium-111-oxine platelet kinetics in acute and chronic renal transplant rejection. Clin. Nephrol 18:174, 1982.
594. Leithner, C., Sinzinger, H., et al.: Indium-111 labelled

platelets in chronic kidney transplant rejection. Lancet 2:213, 1980.
595. Landis, T. F., von Felten, A., et al.: Thrombocytopenic episodes in patients with well functioning renal allografts. Acta Haematol. 61:2, 1979.
596a. Felten, A., and Kuster, J.: Antiplatelet autoantibodies with new specificities detected in patients after renal allotransplantation. Transplantation 22:531, 1976.
596b. Foegh, M. L., Alijani, M. R., et al.: Thromboxane and leukotrienes in clinical and experimental transplant rejection. Adv. Prostaglandin Thromboxane Leukotriene Res. 13:209, 1985.
597. Minchinton, R. M., Waters, A. H., et al.: Autoimmune thrombocytopenia after autologous bone marrow transplantation. Lancet 2:391, 1982.
597a. First, L. R., Smith, B. R., et al.: Isolated thrombocytopenia after allogeneic bone marrow transplantation: existence of transient and chronic thrombocytopenic syndromes. Blood 65:368, 1985.
598. Gratama, J. W., Brand, A., et al.: Factors influencing platelet survival during antilymphocyte globulin treatment. Br. J. Haematol. 57:5, 1984.
599. Abildgaard, C. F., Simone, J. V., et al.: Chronic thrombocytopenia due to thrombopoietin deficiency: a progress report. Blood 30:546, 1967 (Abstr.).
600. Kelton, J. G., Moore, J., et al.: Detection of a platelet-agglutinating factor in thrombotic thrombocytopenic purpura. Ann. Intern. Med. 101:589, 1984.
601. Moake, J. L., Rudy, C. K., et al.: Unusually large plasma factor VIII: von Willebrand factor multimers in chronic relapsing thrombotic thrombocytopenic purpura. New Engl. J. Med. 307:1432, 1982.
602. Miura, M., Koizumi, S., et al.: Efficacy of several plasma components in a young boy with chronic thrombocytopenia and hemolytic anemia who responds repeatedly to normal plasma infusions. Am. J. Hematol. 17:307, 1984.
603. Harker, L. A., and Slichter, S. J.: Platelet and fibrinogen consumption in man. New Engl. J. Med. 287:999, 1972.
604. Harker, L. A., and Slichter, S. J.: Studies of platelet and fibrinogen kinetics in patients with prosthetic heart valves. New Engl. J. Med. 283:1302, 1970.
605. Weily, H. S., Steele, P. P., et al.: Platelet survival in patients with substitute heart valves. New Engl. J. Med. 290:534, 1974.
606. Stuart, R. K., McDonald, J. W., et al.: Platelet survival in patients with prosthetic heart valves. Am. J. Cardiol. 33:840, 1974.
607. Stuart, M. J., Stockman, J. A., et al.: Shortened platelet life span in patients with hydrocephalous and ventriculojugular shunts: preliminary attempts at correction. J. Pediatr. 80:21, 1972.
608. Harker, L. A., Slichter, S. J., et al.: Platelet consumption by arterial prostheses: the effects of endothelialization and pharmacologic inhibition of platelet function. Ann. Surg. 186:594, 1977.
609. Meuleman, D. G., Vogel, G. M. T., et al.: Effect of intra-arterial cannulation on blood platelet consumption in rats. Thromb. Res. 20:45, 1980.
610. Harker, L. A., Hanson, S. R., et al.: Experimental arterial thromboembolism in baboons. Mechanism, quantitation and pharmacologic prevention. J. Clin. Invest. 64:559, 1979.
611. Packham, M. A., and Mustard, J. F.: Normal and abnormal platelet activity. In *Blood Platelet Function and Medicinal Chemistry*. Lasslo, A. (ed.), New York, Elsevier Biomedical, 1984, p. 61.
612. Baier, R. E., and Meyer, A. E.: Surface chemistry and physics relevant to platelet interactions with prosthetic devices and other biomaterials. In *Blood Platelet Function and Medicinal Chemistry*. Lasslo, A. (ed.), New York, Elsevier Biomedical, 1984, p. 175.

613. Richman, K. A., Kim, Y. L., et al.: Thrombocytopenia and altered platelet kinetics associated with prolonged pulmonary-artery catheterization in the dog. Anesthesiology 53:101, 1980.
614. Savage, B., Malpass, T. W., et al.: Platelet adenine nucleotide levels in patients with dacron vascular prostheses. Thromb. Res. 32:365, 1983.
615. Pumphrey, C. W., and Dawes, J.: Platelet α-granule depletion in patients with prosthetic heart valves and following cardiopulmonary bypass surgery. Thromb. Res. 30:257, 1983.
616. Stratton, J. R., Thiele, B. L., et al.: Natural history of platelet deposition on dacron aortic bifurcation grafts in the first year after implantation. Am. J. Cardiol. 52:371, 1983.
617. Harker, L. A.: Platelet survival time: its measurement and use. Progr. Hemostas. Thromb. 4:321, 1978.
618. Tyson, J. E., and deSa, D. J.: Thromboatheromatous complications of umbilical arterial catheterization in the newborn period. Arch. Dis. Child. 51:744, 1976.
619. Henriksson, P., Wesström, G., et al.: Umbilical artery catheterization in newborns. Acta Paediatr. Scand. 68:719, 1979.
620. Oski, F. A.: Blood coagulation and its disorders in the newborn. In *Hematologic Problems in the Newborn*. Oski, F. A., and Naiman, J. L., (eds.), Philadelphia, W. B. Saunders Co., 1982, p. 137.
621. Jacobsson, B., and Nilsson, I. M.: Effect of vascular catheterization on blood coagulation. Acta Chir. Scand. 136:369, 1970.
622. Mant, M. J., Kappagoda, C. T., et al.: Platelet activation caused by cardiac catheter blood collection, and its prevention. Thromb. Res. 33:177, 1984.
623. Salzman, E. W.: Blood platelets and extracorporeal circulation. Transfusion 3:272, 1963.
624. Burstein, S. A., and Harker, L. A.: Quantitative platelet disorders. In *Haemostasis and Thrombosis*. Bloom, A. L., and Thomas, D. P. (eds.), Edinburgh, Churchill Livingstone, 1981, p. 279.
625. Bick, R. L.: Hemostasis defects associated with cardiac surgery, prosthetic devices and other extracorporeal circuits. Semin. Thromb. Hemostas. 11:249, 1985.
626. Harker, L. A., Malpass, T. W., et al.: Mechanisms of abnormal bleeding in patients undergoing cardiopulmonary bypass: acquired transient platelet dysfunction associated with selective α-granule release. Blood 56:824, 1980.
627. Bachmann, F., Mckenna, R., et al.: The hemostatic mechanism after open-heart surgery. I. Studies on plasma coagulation factors and fibrinolysis in 512 patients after extracorporeal circulation. J. Thorac. Cardiovasc. Surg. 70:76, 1975.
628. Beurling-Harbury, C., and Galvan, C. A.: Acquired decrease in platelet secretory ADP associated with increased postoperative bleeding in post-cardiopulmonary bypass patients and in patients with severe valvular heart disease. Blood 52:13, 1978.
628a. Salzman, E. W., Weinstein, M. J., et al.: Treatment with desmopressin acetate to reduce blood loss after cardiac surgery. New Engl. J. Med. 314:1402, 1986.
629. Addonizio, V. P., Smith, J. B., et al.: Thromboxane synthesis and platelet protein release during simulated extracorporeal circulation. Blood 54:371, 1979.
630. Addonizio, V. P., Macarak, E. J., et al.: Preservation of human platelets with PGE_1 during in vitro simulation of cardiopulmonary bypass. Circ. Res. 44:350, 1979.
631. Addonizio, V. P., Macarak, E. J., et al.: Effects of prostacyclin and albumin on platelet loss during in vitro simulation of extracorporeal circulation. Blood 53:1033, 1979.
632. Addonizio, V. P., Strauss, J. F., et al.: Preservation of platelet number and function with prostaglandin E_1

during total cardiopulmonary bypass in rhesus monkeys. Surgery 83:619, 1978.
633. Longmore, D. B., Bennett, J. G., et al.: Prostacyclin administration during cardiopulmonary bypass in man. Lancet 1:800, 1981.
634. Longmore, D. B., Bennett, J. G., et al.: Prostacyclin, a solution to some problems of extracorporeal circulation. Lancet 1:1002, 1979.
635. Aren, C., Feddersen, K., et al.: Effects of prostacyclin infusion on platelet activation and postoperative blood loss in coronary bypass. Ann. Thorac. Surg. 36:49, 1983.
636. Malpass, T. W., Amory, D. W., et al.: The effect of prostacyclin infusion on platelet hemostatic function in patients undergoing cardiopulmonary bypass. J. Thorac. Cardiovasc. Surg. 87:550, 1984.
637. van den Dungen, J. J. A., Karliczek, G. F., et al.: The effect of prostaglandin E₁ in patients undergoing clinical cardiopulmonary bypass. Ann. Thorac. Surg. 35:406, 1983.
638. Gross, S., Keefer, V., et al.: The platelets in cyanotic congenital heart disease. Pediatrics 42:651, 1968.
639. Wedemeyer, A. L., Edson, J. R., et al.: Coagulation in cyanotic congenital heart disease. Am. J. Dis. Child. 124:656, 1972.
640. Kontras, S. B., Bodenbender, J. G., et al.: Hyperviscosity in congenital heart disease. J. Pediatr. 76:214, 1970.
641. Johnson, C. A., Abildgaard, C. F., et al.: Absence of coagulation abnormalities in children with cyanotic congenital heart disease. Lancet 2:660, 1968.
642. Ekert, H., and Gilchrist, G. S.: Coagulation studies in congenital heart disease. Lancet 2:280, 1968.
643. Iølster, N. J.: Blood coagulation in children with cyanotic congenital heart disease. Acta Paediatr. Scand. 59:551, 1970.
644. Ekert, H., Gilchrist, G. S., et al.: Hemostasis in cyanotic congenital heart disease. J. Pediatr. 76:221, 1970.
645. Dennis, L. H., Stewart, J. L., et al.: Heparin treatment of haemorrhagic diathesis in cyanotic congenital heart disease. Lancet 1:1088, 1967.
646. Komp, D. M., and Sparrow, A. W.: Polycythemia in cyanotic heart disease—a study of altered coagulation. J. Pediatr. 76:231, 1969.
647. Ihenacho, H. N. C., Fletcher, D. J., et al.: Consumption coagulopathy in congenital heart disease. Lancet 1:231, 1973.
648. Brodsky, I., Gill, D. N., et al.: Fibrinolysis in congenital heart disease. Am. J. Clin. Pathol. 51:51, 1969.
649. Gralnick, H. R.: ε-Aminocaproic acid in preoperative correction of haemostatic defects in cyanotic congenital heart disease. Lancet 1:1204, 1970.
650. Eckert, H., and Sheers, M.: Pre and postoperative studies of fibrinolysis and prothrombin in cyanotic congenital heart disease. Haemostasis 3:158, 1974.
651. Henriksson, P., Varendh, G., et al.: Haemostatic defects in cyanotic congenital heart disease. Br. Heart J. 41:23, 1979.
652. Wedemeyer, A. L., and Lewis, J. H.: Improvement in hemostasis following phlebotomy in patient with cyanotic heart disease. J. Pediatr. 83:46, 1973.
653. Naiman, J. L.: Clotting and bleeding in cyanotic congenital heart disease. J. Pediatr. 75:333, 1970.
654. Goldschmidt, B., Sarkadi, B., et al.: Platelet production and survival in cyanotic congenital heart disease. Scand. J. Haematol. 13:110, 1974.
655. Waldman, J.D., Czapek, E.E., et al.: Shortened platelet survival in cyanotic heart disease. J. Pediatr. 87:77, 1975.
656. Maurer, H.M., McCue, C.M., et al.: Impairment in platelet aggregation in congenital heart disease. Blood 40: 207, 1972.
657. Ekert, H., and Dowling, S. V.: Platelet release abnormality and reduced prothrombin levels in children with cyanotic congenital heart disease. Aust. Paediatr. J. 13:17, 1977.
658. Ekert, H., and Sheers, M.: Preoperative and postoperative platelet function in cyanotic congenital heart disease. J. Thorac. Cardiovasc. Surg. 67:184, 1974.
659. Goldschmidt, B.: Platelet functions in children with congenital heart disease. Acta Paediatr. Scand. 63:271, 1974.
660. Alagille, D., Heims deBalsae, R., et al.: Les thrombopathies associées aux cardiopathies congénitales; étude de l'hémostase dans cinquante cas. Rev. Franc. Clin. Biol. 3:322, 1958.
661. Maurer, H. M., McCue, C. M., et al.: Impairment in platelet aggregation in congenital heart disease. Blood 40:207, 1972.
662. Maurer, H. M., McCue, C. M., et al.: Correction of platelet dysfunction and bleeding in cyanotic congenital heart disease by simple red cell volume reduction. Am. J. Cardiol. 35:831, 1975.
663. Kelton, J. G., Powers, P., et al.: Sex-related differences in platelet aggregation: influence of hematocrit. Blood 56:38, 1980.
664. Rosove, M. H., Hocking, W. G., et al.: Studies of B-thromboglobulin, platelet factor 4, and fibrinopeptide A in erythrocytosis due to cyanotic congenital heart disease. Thromb. Res. 29:225, 1983.
665. Hathaway, W. E.: Coagulation and hemostasis: general considerations. In *Perinatal Coagulation*. Hathaway, W. E., and Bonnar, J. (eds.), New York, Grune & Stratton, 1978.
666. Martelle, R. R., and Linde, L. M.: Cerebrovascular accidents with tetralogy of Fallot. Am. J. Dis. Child. 101:206, 1961.
667. Cottrill, C. M., and Kaplan, S.: Cerebral vascular accidents in cyanotic congenital heart disease. Am. J. Dis. Child. 125:484, 1973.
668. Jacobson, R. J., Rath, C. E., et al.: Intravascular hemolysis and thrombocytopenia in left ventricular outflow obstruction. Br. Heart J. 35:849, 1973.
669. Steele, P. P., Weily, H. S., et al.: Platelet survival in patients with rheumatic heart disease. New Engl. J. Med. 290:537, 1974.
670. Rodriguez-Erdmann, F.: Bleeding due to increased intravascular blood coagulation; hemorrhagic syndromes caused by consumption of blood clotting factors (consumptive coagulopathies). New Engl. J. Med. 273:1370, 1965.
671. McKay, D. G.: *Disseminated Intravascular Coagulation*. New York, Harper & Row, 1965.
672. Colman, R. W., Robboy, S. J., et al.: DIC: an approach. Am. J. Med. 52:679, 1972.
673. Colman, R. W., Robboy, S. J., et al.: DIC: a reappraisal. Ann. Rev. Med. 30:359, 1979.
674. Niewiarowski, S., Stuart, R. K., et al.: Activation of intravascular coagulation by collagen. Proc. Soc. Exp. Biol. Med. 123:196, 1966.
675. Wilner, G. D., Nossel, H. L., et al.: Activation of Hageman factor by collagen. J. Clin. Invest. 47:2608, 1968.
676. Wiggins, R. C., Loskutoff, D. J., et al.: Activation of rabbit Hageman factor by homogenates of cultured rabbit endothelial cells. J. Clin. Invest. 65:197, 1980.
677. Rodgers, G. M., Broze, G. J., et al.: The number of receptors for factor VII correlates with the ability of cultured cells to initiate coagulation. Blood 63:434, 1984.
678. Drake, T. A., Rodgers, G. M., et al.: Tissue factor is a major stimulus for vegetation formation in enterococcal endocarditis in rabbits. J. Clin. Invest. 73:1750, 1984.
679. Müller-Berghaus, G., Goldfinger, D., et al.: Platelet factor 3 and the generalized Shwartzman reaction. Thromb. Diath. Haemorrh. 18:726, 1967.
680. Evensen, S. A., and Jeremic, M.: Platelets and the

triggering mechanism of intravascular coagulation. Br. J. Haematol. *19:*33, 1970.
681. Margaretten, W., and McKay, D. G.: The role of the platelet in the generalized Shwartzman reaction. J. Exp. Med. *129:*585, 1969.
682. Müller-Berghaus, G., Bolin, E., et al.: Activation of intravascular coagulation by endotoxin: the significance of granulocytes and platelets. Br. J. Haematol. *33:*213, 1976.
683. Lipinski, B., and Gurewich, V.: The effect of leucopenia versus thrombocytopenia on endotoxin-induced intravascular coagulation. Thromb. Res. *8:*403, 1976.
684. Whaun, J. M., and Oski, F. A.: Experience with disseminated intravascular coagulation in a children's hospital. Can. Med. Assoc. J. *107:*963, 1972.
685. Rytel, M. W., Dee, T. H., et al.: Possible pathogenic role of capsular antigen in fulminant pneumococcal disease with DIC. Am. J. Med. *5:*889, 1974.
686. Craybill, J. R., Hawiger, J., et al.: Complement and coagulation in Rocky Mountain spotted fever. South. Med. J. *66:*410, 1973.
687. Blount, E. R., Hartmann, R., et al.: Kala-azar as a cause of DIC. Clin. Pediatr. *19:*139, 1980.
688. McKay, D. G., and Margaretten, W.: Disseminated intravascular coagulation in virus disease. Arch. Intern. Med. *120:*129, 1967.
689. Corrigan, J. J., Ray, W. L., et al.: Changes in the blood coagulation system associated with septicemia. New Engl. J. Med. *279:*851, 1968.
690. Lascari, A. D., and Wallace, P. D.: Disseminated intravascular coagulation in the newborn. Survey and appraisal as exemplified in 2 case histories. Clin. Pediatr. *10:*11, 1971.
691. Chessells, J. M., and Wigglesworth, J. S.: Hemostatic failure in babies with rhesus isoimmunization. Arch. Dis. Child. *46:*38, 1971.
692. Timperley, W. R., Preston, F. E., et al.: Cerebral intravascular coagulation in diabetic ketoacidosis. Lancet *1:*952, 1974.
693. Cooper, M. R., Turner, R. A., et al.: Diabetic ketoacidosis complicated by DIC. South. Med. J. *66:*653, 1973.
694. Chadd, M. A., and Gray, O. P.: Hypothermia and coagulation defects in the newborn. Arch. Dis. Child. *47:*819, 1972.
695. Rivers, R. P. A.: Coagulation changes associated with a high hematocrit in the newborn infant. Acta Paediatr. Scand. *64:*449, 1975.
696. Perlman, A., and Dvilansky, A.: Blood coagulation status of small-for-dates and postmature infants. Arch. Dis. Child. *50:*424, 1975.
697. Morphis, L. G., Arcinae, E. L., et al.: Generalized lymphangioma in infancy with chylothorax. Pediatrics *46:*566, 1970.
698. Dietz, W. H., and Stuart, M. J.: Splenic consumptive coagulopathy in a patient with disseminated lymphangiomatosis. J. Pediatr. *90:*421, 1977.
699. Verstraete, M., and Vermylen, J.: Acute and chronic defibrination in obstetrical practice. Thromb. Diath. Haemorrh. *20:*444, 1968.
700. Drayer, B. P., and Poser, C. M.: Disseminated intravascular coagulation and head trauma. J.A.M.A. *231:*174, 1975.
701. Soulier, J. P., Mathey, J., et al.: Syndrome hemorrhagiques mortèles avec incoagulabilité totale par défibrination et avec fibrinolyse. I. Au cours des exérèses pulmonaires. Rev. Hématol. *7:*30, 1952.
702. Gans, H., Siegal, D. L., et al.: Problems in hemostasis during open-heart surgery. II. On the hypercoagulability of blood during cardiac bypass. Ann. Surg. *156:*19, 1962.
703. Gans, H., and Castaneda, A. R.: Problems in hemostasis during open-heart surgery. VII. Changes in fibrinogen concentration during and after cardiopulmonary bypass with particular reference to the effect of heparin neutralization on fibrinogen. Ann. Surg. *165:*551, 1967.
704. Eeles, G. H., and Sevitt, S.: Microthrombosis in injured and burned patients. J. Pathol. Bacteriol. *93:*275, 1967.
705. Sarnaik, A. P., Stringer, K. D., et al.: DIC with trauma: treatment with exchange transfusion. Pediatrics *63:*337, 1979.
706. Holder, I. A., Malin, L. L., et al.: Hypercoagulability after thermal injuries. Surgery *54:*316, 1963.
707. Sohal, R. S., Sun, S. C., et al.: Heat stroke. An electron microscopic study of endothelial cell damage and disseminated intravascular coagulation. Arch. Intern. Med. *122:*43, 1968.
708. Bachmann, F.: Evidence for hypercoagulability in heat stroke. J. Clin. Invest. *46:*1033, 1967.
709. Koppes, G. M., Daly, J. J., et al.: Exertion-induced rhabdomyolysis with acute renal failure and disseminated intravascular coagulation in sickle cell trait. Am. J. Med. *63:*313, 1977.
710. Fischer, S. P., Lee, J., et al.: Disseminated intravascular coagulation in status epilepticus. Thromb. Haemostas. *38:*909, 1977.
711. Hutter, J. J., Hathaway, W. E., et al.: Hematologic abnormalities in severe neonatal necrotizing enterocolitis. J. Pediatr. *88:*1026, 1976.
712. Patel, C. C.: Hematologic abnormalities in acute necrotizing enterocolitis. Ped. Clin. North Am. *24:*579, 1977.
713. Gralnick, H. R., and Abrell, E.: Studies of the procoagulant and fibrinolytic activity of promyelocytes in acute promyelocytic leukemia. Br. J. Haematol. *24:*89, 1973.
714. Al-Mondhiry, H.: Hypofibrinogenemia associated with vincristine and prednisone therapy in lymphoblastic leukemia. Cancer *35:*144, 1975.
715. Poechedly, C., Miller, S. P., et al.: 'Hypercoagulable state' in children with acute leukemia or disseminated solid tumors. Oncology *28:*517, 1973.
716. Sills, R. H., Stockman, J. A., et al.: Consumptive coagulopathy: a complication of therapy of solid tumors in childhood. Am. J. Dis. Child. *132:*870, 1978.
717. McMillan, C. W., Gandry, C., et al.: Coagulation defects and metastatic neuroblastoma. J. Pediatr. *72:*347, 1968.
718. Wang, A. H.: Wilms' tumor associated with venous thrombosis and consumption coagulopathy. Am. J. Dis. Child. *123:*599, 1972.
719. Merskey, C.: Pathogenesis and treatment of altered blood coagulability in patients with malignant tumors. Ann. NY Acad. Sci. *230:*289, 1974.
720. Hathaway, W. E., and Hays, T.: Hypercoagulability in childhood cancer. J. Pediatr. Surg. *10:*893, 1975.
721. Bick, R. L.: DIC and related syndromes: etiology, pathophysiology, diagnosis and management. Am. J. Hematol. *5:*265, 1978.
722. Warrell, D. A., Pope, H. M., et al.: Disseminated intravascular coagulation caused by carpet viper (*Echis carinatus*). Trial of heparin. Br. J. Haematol. *33:*335, 1976.
723. Simon, T. L., and Grace, T. G.: Envenomation coagulopathy in wounds from pit vipers. New Engl. J. Med. *305:*443, 1981.
724. Pinev, G. F., Brain, M. C., et al.: Tumors, mucus production, and hypercoagulability. Ann. NY Acad. Sci. *230:*262, 1974.
725. Rabiner, F., and Friedman, A.: Role of intravascular haemolysis and the reticuloendothelial system in the production of a hypercoagulable state. Br. J. Haematol. *14:*105, 1968.
726. Bick, R. L., Schmalhorst, W. R., et al.: Disseminated intravascular coagulation and blood component therapy. Transfusion *16:*361, 1976.
727. Tygat, G. N., Colleen, D., et al.: Metabolism of fibrinogen in cirrhosis of the liver. J. Clin. Invest. *50:*1690, 1971.
728. Branson, H. E., Marble, R., et al.: Inherited protein C deficiency and coumarin-responsive chronic relapsing

purpura fulminans in a newborn infant. Lancet 2:1165, 1983.
729. Seligsohn, U., Berger, A., et al.: Homozygous protein C deficiency manifested by massive venous thrombosis in the newborn. New Engl. J. Med. 310:559, 1984.
730. Carvalho, A. C., Lees, R. S., et al.: Intravascular coagulation in hyperlipidemia. Thromb. Res. 8:843, 1976.
731. Kiesow, L. A., Shapiro, S., et al.: Oxygen-induced consumptive coagulopathy and its enhancement by lead acetate. Thromb. Haemostas. 37:170, 1977.
732. Kasabach, H. H., and Merritt, K. K.: Hemangioma with extensive purpura. Am. J. Dis. Child. 59:1063, 1940.
733. Shim, W. K. T.: Hemangiomas of infancy complicated by thrombocytopenia. Am. J. Surg. 116:896, 1968.
734. Linderkamp, O., Hopner, F., et al.: Solitary hepatic hemangioma in a newborn infant complicated by cardiac failure, consumption coagulopathy, microangiopathic hemolytic anemia, and obstructive jaundice. Case report and review of the literature. Eur. J. Pediatr. 124:23, 1976.
735. Laird, W. P., Friedman, S., et al.: Hepatic hemangiomatosis. Am. J. Dis. Child. 130:657, 1976.
736. Rotman, M., John, M., et al.: Radiation treatment of pediatric-hepatic hemangiomatosis and coexisting cardiac failure. New Engl. J. Med. 302:852, 1980.
737. Brizel, H. E., and Raccuglia, G.: Giant hemangioma with thrombocytopenia. Radioisotopic demonstration of platelet sequestration. Blood 26:751, 1965.
738. Propp, P. P., and Scharfman, W. B.: Hemangioma thrombocytopenia syndrome associated with microangiopathic hemolytic anemia. Blood 28:623, 1966.
739. Kontas, S. B., Green, O. C., et al.: Giant hemangioma with thrombocytopenia. Am. J. Dis. Child. 105:188, 1963.
740. Henriksson, P., Nilsson, I. M., et al.: Giant hemangioma with a disorder of coagulation. Acta Paediatr. Scand. 60:227, 1971.
741. Khurana, M. S., Lian, E. C., et al.: "Storage Pool Disease": association with multiple congenital cavernous hemangiomas. J.A.M.A. 244:169, 1980.
742. Straub, P. W., Kessler, S., et al.: Chronic intravascular coagulation in Kasabach-Merritt syndrome. Arch. Intern. Med. 129:475, 1972.
743. Schmidt, R. P., and Lentle, B. C.: Hemangioma with consumptive coagulopathy. Detection by Indium-111-oxine labeled platelets. Clin. Nucl. Med. 9:389, 1984.
744. Inceman, S., and Tangun, Y.: Chronic defibrination syndrome due to a giant hemangioma associated with microangiopathic hemolytic anemia. Am. J. Med. 46:997, 1969.
745. Esterly, N. B.: Kasabach-Merritt syndrome in infants. J. Am. Acad. Dermatol. 8:504, 1983.
746. Brown, S. H., Neerhout, R. C., et al.: Prednisone therapy in the management of the large hemangiomas in infants and children. Surgery 71:168, 1972.
747. Fost, N. C., and Esterly, N. B.: Successful treatment of juvenile hemangiomas with prednisone. J. Pediatr. 72:351, 1968.
748. Lasser, E. A., and Stein, A. F.: Steroid treatment of hemangiomas in children. Arch. Dermatol. 108:565, 1973.
749. Folkman, J.: Toward a new understanding of vascular proliferative disease in children. Pediatrics 74:850, 1984.
750. Folkman, J., Langer, R., et al.: Angiogenesis inhibition and tumor regression caused by heparin or a heparin fragment in the presence of cortisone. Science 221:719, 1983.
751. Verstraet, M., Amery, A., et al.: Heparin treatment of bleeding [Letter]. Lancet 1:446, 1963.
752. Hillman, R. S., and Phillips, L. L.: Clotting and fibrinolysis in a cavernous hemangioma. Am. J. Dis. Child. 113:649, 1967.
753. Argenta, L. C., Bishop, E., et al.: Complete resolution of a life-threatening hemangioma by embolization and corticosteroids. Plast. Reconstr. Surg. 70:739, 1982.
754. Orenstein, D. M., Yonas, H., et al.: Hemangioma thrombocytopenia syndrome. Am. J. Dis. Child. 131:680, 1977.
755. Nordberg, U. B., and Sundberg, J.: Indications and methods for radiotherapy of cavernous hemangiomas. Acta Radiol. 1:257, 1963.
756. Duncan, W., and Halnan, K. E.: Giant hemangioma with thrombocytopenia. Clin. Radiol. 15:224, 1964.
757. Margileth, A. M.: Treatment of giant hemangioma [Letter]. J. Pediatr. 92:1030, 1978.
758. Koerper, M. A., Addiego, J. E., et al.: Use of aspirin and dipyridamole in children with platelet trapping syndromes. J. Pediatr. 102:311, 1983.
759. Hagerman, L. J., Czapek, E., et al.: Giant hemangioma with consumption coagulopathy. J. Pediatr. 87:766, 1975.
760. Henriksson, B. A. P., Nilsson, I. M., et al.: Regression of hemangioma-thrombocytopenia syndrome. Acta Obstet. Gynecol. Scand. 61:479, 1982.
761. Neidhart, J. A., and Roach, R. W.: Successful treatment of skeletal hemangioma and Kasabach-Merritt syndrome with aminocaproic acid. Am. J. Med. 73:434, 1982.
762. Froelich, L. A., and Housler, M.: Neonatal thrombocytopenia and chorangioma. J. Pediatr. 78:516, 1971.
763. Bauer, C. R., Fojaco, R., et al.: Microangiopathic hemolytic anemia and thrombocytopenia in a neonate associated with a large placental chorangioma. Pediatrics 62:574, 1978.
764. Al-Rashid, R. A.: Cyclophosphamide and radiation therapy in the treatment of hemangioendothelioma with disseminated intravascular clotting. Cancer 27:364, 1971.
765. Jackson, C., Greene, H. L., et al.: Hepatic hemangioendothelioma. Angiographic appearance and apparent prednisone responsiveness. Am. J. Dis. Child. 131:74, 1977.
766. Shanberge, J. N., Tanaka, K., et al.: Chronic consumption coagulopathy due to hemangiomatous transformation of the spleen. Am. J. Clin. Pathol. 56:723, 1971.
767. Dadash-Zadeh, M., Czapek, E. E., et al.: Skeletal and splenic hemangiomatosis with consumption coagulopathy: response to splenectomy. Pediatrics 57:803, 1976.
768. Koblenzer, P. J., and Bukowski, M. J.: Angiomatosis (hamartomatous hemangio-lymphangiomatosis). Report of a case with diffuse involvement. Pediatrics 28:65, 1961.
769. Kaplan, B. S., and Esseltine, D.: Thrombocytopenia in patients with acute post-streptococcal glomerulonephritis. J. Pediatr. 93:974, 1978.
770. Carruthers, J. A., Ralfs, I., et al.: Platelet survival in acute proliferative glomerulonephritis. Clin. Sci. Mol. Med. 47:507, 1974.
771. George, C. R. P., Slichter, S. J., et al.: A kinetic evaluation of hemostasis in renal disease. New Engl. J. Med. 291:1111, 1974.
772. Clark, W. F., Lewis, M. L., et al.: Intrarenal platelet consumption in the diffuse proliferative nephritis of systemic lupus erythematosus. Clin. Sci. Mol. Med. 49:247, 1975.
773. Parbtani, A., and Cameron, J. S.: Platelet involvement in glomerulonephritis. In Hemostasis, Prostaglandins and Renal Disease. Remuzzi, G., Mecca, G., et al. (eds.), New York, Raven Press, 1980, p. 45.
774. Clark, W. F., Friesen, M., et al.: The platelet as a mediator of tissue damage in immune complex glomerulonephritis. Clin. Nephrol. 6:287, 1976.
775. George, C. R. P., Clark, W. F.: The role of platelets in glomerulonephritis. Adv. Nephrol. 5:19, 1975.
776. Cameron, J. S.: Platelets in glomerular disease. Ann. Rev. Med. 35:175, 1984.

777. Kasai, N., Parbtani, A., et al.: Platelet-aggregating immune complexes in glomerulonephritis. Clin. Exp. Immunol. 43:64, 1981.
778. Duffy, J. L., Clinque, T., et al.: Intraglomerular fibrin, platelet aggregation and subendothelial deposits in lipoid nephrosis. J. Clin. Invest. 49:251, 1970.
779. Richman, A. V., and Kashic, G.: Endothelial and platelet reactions in the idiopathic nephrotic syndrome. Hum. Pathol. 13:548, 1982.
780. Hayslett, J. P.: Role of platelets in glomerulonephritis. New Engl. J. Med. 310:1457, 1984.
781. Cameron, J. S.: The treatment of severe glomerulonephritis with combined immunosuppression and anticoagulation. Proceedings, 6th International Congress of Nephrologists, Montreal. Basel, Karger, 1982, p. 419.
782. Futrakul, P., Poshyachinda, M., et al.: Focal sclerosing glomerulonephritis: a kinetic evaluation of hemostasis, and the effect of anticoagulant therapy—a controlled study. Clin. Nephrol. 10:180, 1978.
783. Robson, A. M., Cole, B. R., et al.: Severe glomerulonephritis complicated by coagulopathy: treatment with anticoagulant and immunosuppressive drugs. J. Pediatr. 90:881, 1979.
784. Donadio, J. V., Anderson, C. F., et al.: Membranoproliferative glomerulonephritis. A prospective clinical trial of platelet inhibitor therapy. New Engl. J. Med. 310:1421, 1984.
785. Sejeny, S. A., Eastham, R. D., et al.: Platelet counts during normal pregnancy. J. Clin. Pathol. 28:812, 1975.
786. Fay, R. A., Hughes, A. O., et al.: Platelets in pregnancy: hyperdestruction in pregnancy. Obstet. Gynecol. 61:238, 1983.
787. Fenton, V., and Saunders, K.: The platelet count in pregnancy. J. Clin. Pathol. 30:68, 1977.
788. Wallenburg, H. C. S., and Van Kessel, P. H.: Platelet life span in normal pregnancy as determined by a nonradioisotopic technique. Br. J. Obstet. Gynaecol. 85:33, 1978.
789. Rakoczi, R., Tallian, S., et al.: Platelet lifespan in normal pregnancy and preeclampsia as determined by a nonradioisotopic technique. Thromb. Res. 15:553, 1979.
790. Gibson, B., Hunter, D., et al.: Thrombocytopenia in preeclampsia and eclampsia. Semin. Thromb. Hemostas. 8:234, 1982.
791. Giles, C., and Inglis, T.C.M.: Thrombocytopenia and macrothrombocytosis in gestational hypertension. Br. J. Obstet. Gynecol. 88:1115, 1981.
792. Bonnar, J., McNicol, G. P., et al.: Coagulation and fibrinolysis in preeclampsia and eclampsia. Br. Med. J. 2:12, 1971.
793. Howie, P. W., and McNicol, G. P.: Coagulation, fibrinolysis and platelet function in preeclampsia, essential hypertension and placental insufficiency. J. Obstet. Gynecol. Br. Commonw. 78:992, 1971.
794. Gordon, Y. B., Ratky, S. M., et al.: Circulating levels of fibrin-fibrinogen degradation fragment E measured by RIA in preeclampsia. Br. J. Obstet. Gynecol. 83:287, 1976.
795. Condie, R. G.: A serial study of coagulation factors XII, XI, and X in plasma in normal pregnancy and in preeclampsia. Br. J. Obstet. Gynecol. 83:636, 1976.
796. Pritchard, J. A., Cunningham, F. G., et al.: Coagulation changes in eclampsia: their frequency and pathogenesis. Am. J. Obstet. Gynecol. 124:855, 1976.
797. Remuzzi, G., Marchesi, D., et al.: Reduced umbilical and placental vascular prostacyclin in severe preeclampsia. Prostaglandins 20:105, 1980.
798. Rote, N. S., Lau, R. J., et al.: Immunologic mechanism of maternal and fetal thrombocytopenia in pregnancy induced hypertension. Am. J. Reprod. 5:95, 1984.
799. Borok, Z., Weitz, J., et al.: Fibrinogen proteolysis and platelet alpha granule release in preeclampsia. Blood 63:525, 1984.
800. Vassalli, P., Morris, R. H., et al.: The pathogenic role of fibrin deposition in the glomerular lesions of toxemia of pregnancy. J. Exp. Med. 118:467, 1963.
801. Whigham, K. A. E., Howie, P. W., et al.: Abnormal platelet function in preeclampsia. Br. J. Obstet. Gynecol. 85:28, 1978.
802. Redman, C. W. G., Allington, M. J., et al.: Plasma β-thromboglobulin in preeclampsia [Letter]. Lancet 2:248, 1977.
803. Kelton, J. G., Hunter, D. J., et al.: A platelet function defect of pre-eclampsia. Obstet. Gynecol. 65:107, 1985.
804. Goodlin, R. C., Haesslein, H. O., et al.: Aspirin for the treatment of recurrent toxaemia [Letter]. Lancet 2:51, 1978.
805. Beaufils, M., Donsimoni, R., et al.: Prevention of preeclampsia by early antiplatelet therapy. Lancet 1:840, 1985.
806. Kleckner, H. B., Giles, H. R., et al.: The association of maternal and neonatal thrombocytopenia in high risk pregnancies. Am. J. Obstet. Gynecol. 128:235, 1977.
807. Brazy, J. E., Grimm, J. K., et al.: Neonatal manifestations of severe maternal hypertension occurring before the thirty-sixth week of pregnancy. J. Pediatr. 100:265, 1982.
808. Nielsen, N. C.: Influence of preeclampsia on coagulation and fibrinolysis in women and their newborn infants immediately after delivery. Acta Obstet. Gynecol. Scand. 48:523, 1969.
809. Stuart, M. J., Sunderji, S., et al.: Decreased prostacyclin production: a characteristic of chronic placental insufficiency syndromes. Lancet 1:1126, 1981.
810. Stuart, M. J.: Bleeding in the newborn and pediatric patient. In *Hemostasis and Thrombosis: Basic Principles and Clinical Practice.* Colman, R., Hirsh, J., et al. (eds.), Philadelphia, J. B. Lippincott, 1986.
811. Castle, V., Andrew, M., et al.: Frequency and mechanism of neonatal thrombocytopenia. J. Pediatr. 108:749, 1986.
812. Zipursky, A., Palko, J., et al.: The hematology of bacterial infections in premature infants. Pediatrics 57:839, 1976.
813. Tate, D., Carlton, G. T., et al.: Immune thrombocytopenia in severe neonatal infections. J. Pediatr. 98:449, 1981.
814. Mehta, P., Vasa, R., et al.: Thrombocytopenia in the high risk infant. J. Pediatr. 97:791, 1980.
815. Maurer, H. M., Fralkin, M., et al.: Effect of phototherapy on platelet counts in low birth weight infants, and on platelet production and life span in rabbits. Pediatrics 57:506, 1976.
816. Segall, M. L., Goetzman, B. W., et al.: Thrombocytopenia and pulmonary hypertension in the perinatal aspiration syndromes. J. Pediatr. 96:727, 1980.
817. Levin, D. L., Weinberg, A. F., et al.: Pulmonary microthrombi syndrome in newborn infants with unresponsive persistent pulmonary hypertension. J. Pediatr. 102:299, 1983.
818. Hammerman, C., Strates, E., et al.: Thromboxane B_2 labels in neonates with persistent fetal circulation. Fed. Proc. 325A:1377, 1984 (Abstr.).
819. Favara, B. E., Franciosi, R. A., et al.: Disseminated intravascular and cardiac thrombosis of the neonate. Am. J. Dis. Child. 127:197, 1974.
820. Morrow, W. R., Haas, J. E., et al.: Nonbacterial endocardial thrombosis in neonates: Relationship to persistent fetal circulation. J. Pediatr. 100:117, 1982.
821. Krous, H. F.: Neonatal nonbacterial thrombotic endocarditis. Arch. Path. Lab. Med. 103:76, 1979.

822. Jackson, D. P., Krevans, J. R., et al.: Mechanism of the thrombocytopenia that follows multiple blood transfusions. Trans. Assoc. Am. Phys. 69:155, 1956.
823. Chudwin, D. S., Ammann, A. J., et al.: Post-transfusion syndrome. Am. J. Dis. Child. 136:612, 1982.
824. Gross, G. P., Hathaway, W. E., et al.: Hyperviscosity in the neonate. J. Pediatr. 82:1004, 1973.
825. Mentzer, W. C.: Polycythemia and the hyperviscosity syndrome in newborn infants. Clin. Haematol. 7:63, 1978.
826. Katz, J., Rodriguez, E., et al.: Normal coagulation findings, thrombocytopenia, and peripheral hemoconcentration in neonatal polycythemia. J. Pediatr. 101:99, 1982.
827. Henricksson, P.: Hyperviscosity of the blood and haemostasis in the newborn infant. Acta Paediatr. Scand. 68:701, 1979.
828. Naiman, J. L.: Disorders of platelets. In *Hematologic Problems in the Newborn*. Oski, F. A., Naiman, J. L. (eds.), Philadelphia, W. B. Saunders Co, 1982, p. 175.
829. Morrow, G., Barness, L. A., et al.: Observation on the coexistence of methylmalonic acidemia and glycinemia. J. Pediatr. 74:680, 1969.
830. Allen, D. W., Necheles, T. F., et al.: Reversible neonatal pancytopenia due to isovaleric acidemia. Soc. Pediatr. Res. Atlantic City, 1969, p. 156 (Abstr.).
831. Kelleher, J., Yudkoff, M.: Hematologic findings in isovaleric acidemia. Pediatr. Res. 12:466, 1978 (Abstr.).
832. Hoak, J. C., Warner, E. D., et al.: Platelets, fatty acids, and thrombosis. Circ. Res. 20:11, 1967.
833. Silver, M. J., Hoch, W., et al.: Arachidonic acid causes sudden death in rabbits. Science 183:1085, 1974.
834. Spragg, R. G., Abraham, J. L., et al.: Pulmonary platelet deposition accompanying acute oleic acid–induced pulmonary injury. Am. Rev. Resp. Dis. 126:553, 1982.
835. Katzenstein, A. A., Bloor, C. M., et al.: Diffuse alveolar damage. The role of oxygen, shock and related factors. Am. J. Pathol. 85:210, 1976.
836. Schneider, R. C., Zapol, W. M., et al.: Platelet consumption and sequestration in severe acute respiratory failure. Am. Rev. Resp. Dis. 122:445, 1980.
837. Romics, L. Hypertriglyceridemia associated with thrombocytopenia and lipoprotein lipase deficiency. Ann. Intern. Med. 95:660, 1981.
838. Ross, R., and Harker, L. A.: Hyperlipidemia and atherosclerosis. Chronic hyperlipidemia initiates and maintains lesions by endothelial cell desquamation and lipid accumulation. Science 193:1094, 1976.
839. Corash, L., Andersen, J., et al.: Platelet function and survival in patients with severe hypercholesterolemia. Arteriosclerosis 1:443, 1981.
840. Wanless, I. R.: The effect of dietary cholesterol on platelet survival in the rabbit. A study using ^{14}C-serotonin and ^{51}chromium double labelled platelets. Thromb. Haemostas. 52:85, 1984.
841. Grottum, K. A., Nordoy, A., et al.: Lipid infusions in man. Blood platelet uptake of lipid and effects on platelet functions. Thromb. Diath. Haemorrh. 29:701, 1973.
842. Gibson, J. C., Simons, L. A., et al.: Haematological and biochemical abnormalities associated with intralipid hyperalimentation. Anaesth. Intensive Care 4:350, 1975.
843. McGrath, K. M., Zalcberg, J. R., et al.: Intralipid induced hemolysis [Letter]. Brit. J. Haematol. 50:376, 1982.
844. Berken, A., and Bennacerraf, B. J.: Depression of reticuloendothelial system phagocytic function by ingested lipids. Proc. Soc. Exp. Biol. Med. 128:793, 1968.
845. Lipson, A. H., Pritchard, J. et al.: Thrombocytopenia after intralipid infusion in a neonate [Letter]. Lancet 2:1462, 1974.
846. Sadowitz, P. D., Walenga, R. W., et al.: Differential binding of arachidonic acid by neonatal and adult plasma. Pediatr. Res. 18:145A, 1984 (Abstr. No. 295).
847. Levene, M. I., Wigglesworth, J. S., et al.: Pulmonary fat accumulation after intralipid infusion in the preterm infant. Lancet 2:815, 1980.
848. Dahms, B. B., and Halpin, T. C.: Pulmonary arterial lipid deposit in newborn infants receiving intravenous lipid infusion. J. Pediatr. 97:800, 1980.
849. Wakely, P. E., and Hug, G.: Intralipid vasculopathy. Lancet 2:1416, 1981.
850. Hall, J. G., Levin, L., et al.: Thrombocytopenia with absent radius (TAR). Medicine 48:411, 1969.
851. Sultan, Y., Scrobohaci, M. L., et al.: Abnormal platelet function, population, and survival time in a boy with congenital absent radii and thrombocytopenia [Letter]. Lancet 2:653, 1972.
852. Lusher, J. M., and Barnhart, M. I.: Congenital disorders affecting platelets. Semin. Thromb. Hemostas. 4:123, 1977.
853. Armitage, J. O., Hoak, J. C., et al.: Syndrome of thrombocytopenia and absent radii. Scand. J. Haematol. 20:25, 1978.
854. Day, H. J., and Holmsen, H.: Platelet adenine nucleotide "storage pool deficiency" in TAR syndrome. J.A.M.A. 221:1053, 1972.
855. Juhan, I., Bayle, J., et al.: Thrombopenie et aplasie radiale. Pathol. Biol. 27:473, 1979.
856. Zahavi, J., Gale, R., et al.: Storage pool disease in an infant with TAR. Haemostas. 10:121, 1981.
857. Lui, V. K., Ragab, A. H., et al.: Bone marrow cultures in children with Fanconi anemia and TAR. J. Pediatrics 91:952, 1977.
858. Linch, D. C., Stewart, J. W., et al.: Blood and bone marrow cultures in a case of TAR. Clin. Lab. Haematol. 4:313, 1982.
859. Whitefield, M. F., and Barr, D. G. D.: Cow's milk allergy in the syndrome of thrombocytopenia with absent radius. Arch. Dis. Child. 51:337, 1976.
860. Fayen, W. T., and Harris, J. W.: Case report: Thrombocytopenia with absent radii. Am. J. Med. Sci. 280:95, 1980.
861. Luthy, D. A., and Hall, J. G.: Prenatal diagnosis of TAR. Clin. Genet. 15:495, 1979.
862. Luthy, D. A., Mack, L., et al.: Prenatal ultrasound diagnosis of thrombocytopenia with absent radii. Am. J. Obstet. Gynecol. 141:350, 1981.
863. Filkins, K., Russo, J., et al.: Prenatal diagnosis of TAR using ultrasound and fetoscopy. Prenatal Diag. 4:139, 1984.
864. Dignan, P. S., Mauer, A. M., et al.: Phocomelia with congenital hypoplastic thrombocytopenia and myeloid leukemoid reactions. J. Pediatr. 70:561, 1967.
865. Cherstvoy, E., Lazjuk, G., et al.: Syndrome of multiple congenital malformations including phocomelia, thrombocytopenia, encephalocele, and urogenital abnormalities. Lancet 2:485, 1980.
866. Markenson, A. J., Hilgartner, M. W., et al.: Transient thrombocytopenia in 18-trisomy. J. Pediatr. 87:834, 1975.
867. Christodoulou, C., and Werner, B.: A girl with 18-trisomy and thrombocytopenia. Acta Genet. 17:77, 1967.
868. Rabinowitz, J. G., Moseley, J. E., et al.: Trisomy 18, esophageal atresia, anomalies of the radius and congenital hypoplastic thrombocytopenia. Radiology 89:488, 1967.
869. Eisenstein, E. M.: Congenital amegakaryocytic thrombocytopenic purpura. Clin. Pediatr. 5:143, 1966.
870. Hoyeraal, H. M., and Lamvik, J.: Thrombocytopenia and cerebral malformations. Acta Pediatr. Scand. 59:185, 1970.
871. Van Oostrom, C. G., and Wilms, R. H. H.: Congenital thrombocytopenia associated with raised concentrations of hemoglobin F. A case report. Helv. Paediatr. Acta 33:59, 1978.

872. DeBoeck, K., Degreef, H., et al.: Thrombocytopenia as the first symptom in a patient with dyskeratosis congenita. Pediatrics 67:898, 1981.
873. Gardner, R. J. M., Morrison, P. S., et al.: A syndrome of congenital thrombocytopenia with multiple malformations and neurologic dysfunction. J. Pediatr. 102:600, 1983.
874. Alter, B. P., Potter, N. U., et al.: Classification and etiology of the aplastic anemias. Clin. Haematol. 7:431, 1978.
875. Helmerhorst, F. M., Heaton, D. C., et al.: Familial thrombocytopenia associated with platelet autoantibodies and chromosome breakage. Hum. Genet. 65:252, 1984.
876. Fanconi, G: Familial constitutional panmyelopathy. Semin. Hematol. 4:233, 1967.
877. Hegglin, R.: Gleichzeitige Konstitutionelle veranderungen an neutrophilen und thrombozyten. Helv. Med. Acta 12:439, 1945.
878. White, J. G., Gerrard, J. M.: Ultrastructural features of abnormal blood platelets. A Review. Am. J. Pathol. 83:589, 1976.
879. Hamilton, R. W., Shaikh, B. S., et al.: Platelet function, ultrastructure and survival in the May-Hegglin anomaly. Am. J. Clin. Pathol. 74:663, 1980.
880. Fabris, F., Casonato, A., et al.: Plasma and platelet beta-thromboglobulin levels in the May-Hegglin anomaly. Am. J. Clin. Pathol. 74:663, 1980.
881. Godwin, H. A., and Ginsburg, A. D.: May-Hegglin anomaly. A defect in megakaryocyte fragmentation? Br. J. Haematol. 26:117, 1974.
882. Najean, Y.: Survival of radiochromium-labeled platelets in thrombocytopenias. Blood 22:718, 1963.
883. Davis, J. W., and Wilson, S. J.: Platelet survival in the May-Hegglin anomaly. Br. J. Haematol. 12:61, 1966.
884. Coller, B. S., and Zarrabi, M. H.: Platelet membrane studies in the May-Hegglin anomaly. Blood 58:279, 1981.
885. Rosenberg, T., Arad, E., et al.: May-Hegglin anomaly. Israel J. Med. Sci. 7:1073, 1971.
886. Brivel, F., Girot, R., et al.: Hereditary nephritis associated with May-Hegglin anomaly. Nephron 29:59, 1981.
887. Blaese, R. M., Strober, W., et al.: Immunodeficiency in the Wiskott-Aldrich syndrome. In *Immunodeficiency in Man and Animals*. Bergsma, D., Good, R. A., et al. (eds.), Boston, Sinauer, 1975, p. 250.
888. Ochs, H. D., Slichter, S. J., et al.: The Wiskott-Aldrich syndrome—studies of lymphocytes, granulocytes, and platelets. Blood 55:243, 1980.
889. Grottum, K. A., Hovig, T., et al.: Wiskott-Aldrich syndrome: qualitative defects and short platelet survival. Br. J. Haematol. 17:373, 1969.
890. Baldini, M. G.: Nature of the platelet defect in the Wiskott-Aldrich syndrome. Ann. N.Y. Acad. Sci. 201:437, 1972.
891. Pearson, H. A., Shulman, N. R., et al.: Platelet survival in Wiskott-Aldrich syndrome. J. Pediatr. 68:755, 1966.
892. Krivit, W., Yunis, E., et al.: Platelet survival studies in Aldrich syndrome. Pediatrics 37:339, 1966.
893. Lum, L. G., Tubergen, D. G., et al.: Splenectomy in the management of the thrombocytopenia of the Wiskott-Aldrich syndrome. New Engl. J. Med. 302:892, 1980.
894. Murphy, S., Oski, F. A., et al.: Platelet size and kinetics in hereditary and acquired thrombocytopenia. New Engl. J. Med. 286:499, 1972.
895. Corash, L., Shafer, B., et al.: Platelet associated IgG, platelet size, and the effect of splenectomy in the Wiskott-Aldrich syndrome. Blood 65:1439, 1985.
896. Trung, P. H., and Griscelli, C.: Ultrastructure des plaquettes sanguines dans le syndrome de Wiskott-Aldrich. Pathol. Biol. 23:57, 1975.
897. Nathan, D. G.: Splenectomy in the Wiskott-Aldrich syndrome. New Engl. J. Med. 302:916, 1980.
898. Parkman, R., Kenney, D. M., et al.: Surface protein abnormalities in lymphocytes and platelets from patients with Wiskott-Aldrich syndrome. Lancet 2:1387, 1981.
899. O'Donnell, E. R., Kenney, D. M., et al.: Characterization of a human lymphocyte surface sialoglycoprotein that is defective in Wiskott-Aldrich Syndrome. J. Exp. Med. 159:1705, 1984.
900. August, C. S., Hathaway, W. E., et al.: Improved platelet function following bone marrow transplantation in an infant with Wiskott-Aldrich syndrome. J. Pediatr. 82:58, 1973.
901. Parkman, R., Rappeport, J., et al.: Complete correction of the Wiskott-Aldrich syndrome by allogeneic bone marrow transplantation. New Engl. J. Med. 298:921, 1978.
902. Shapiro, R. S., Gerrard, J. M., et al.: Wiskott-Aldrich syndrome. Detection of carrier state by metabolic stress of platelets. Lancet 1:121, 1978.
903. Holmberg, L., Gustavili, B., et al.: A prenatal study of fetal platelet count and size with application to fetus at risk for Wiskott-Aldrich syndrome. J. Pediatr. 102:773, 1983.
904. Akkerman, J. W. N., van Brederode, W., et al.: The Wiskott Aldrich syndrome: Studies on a possible defect in mitochondrial ATP resynthesis in platelets. Br. J. Haematol. 51:561, 1982.
905. Canales, L., and Mauer, A. M.: Sex-linked hereditary thrombocytopenia as a variant of Wiskott-Aldrich syndrome. New Engl. J. Med. 277:899, 1967.
906. Chiaro, J. J., Dharmkrong-at, A., et al.: X-linked thrombocytopenic purpura. Am. J. Dis. Child. 123:565, 1972.
907. Moore, J. R.: X-linked "idiopathic" thrombocytopenia. Clin. Genet. 5:344, 1974.
908. Cohn, J., Hauge, M., et al.: Sex-linked hereditary thrombocytopenia with immunological defects. Hum. Hered. 25:309, 1975.
909. Weiden, P. L., and Blaese, R. M.: Hereditary thrombocytopenia: Relation to Wiskott-Aldrich syndrome with special reference to splenectomy. J. Pediatr. 80:276, 1972.
910. Thompson, A. R., Wood, W. G., et al.: X-linked syndrome of platelet dysfunction, thrombocytopenia and imbalanced globin chain synthesis with hemolysis. Blood 50:303, 1977.
911. Roberts, M. H., and Smith, M. H.: Thrombopenic purpura. Report of 4 cases in one family. Am. J. Dis. Child. 79:820, 1950.
912. Bithell, T. C., Didisheim, P., et al.: Thrombocytopenia inherited as an autosomal dominant trait. Blood 25:231, 1965.
913. Mullyla, G., Pelkonen, R., et al.: Hereditary thrombocytopenia. Report of 3 families. Scand. J. Haematol. 4:441, 1967.
914. Cullum, C., Cooney, D. P., et al.: Familial thrombocytopenic thrombocytopathy. Br. J. Haematol. 13:147, 1967.
915. Kurstjens, R., Bolt, C., et al.: Familial thrombopathic thrombocytopenia. Br. J. Haematol. 15:305, 1968.
916. Murphy, S., Oski, F. A., et al.: Hereditary thrombocytopenia with an intrinsic platelet defect. New Engl. J. Med. 281:857, 1969.
917. Murphy, S.: Hereditary thrombocytopenia. Clin. Haematol. 1:359, 1972.
918. Law, I. V., Deveny, A., et al.: Case report. Familial thrombocytopenia in seven members of three generations. Postgrad. Med. 63:136, 1978.
919. Danielsson, L., Jelf, E., et al.: A new family with inherited thrombocytopenia. Scand. J. Haematol. 24:427, 1980.

920. Von Behrens, W. E.: Mediterranean macrothrombocytopenia. Blood 46:199, 1975.
921. Von Behrens, W. E.: Splenomegaly, macrothrombocytopenia, and stomatocytosis in healthy Mediterranean subjects. Scand. J. Haematol. 14:258, 1975.
922. Yunis, A. A.: Chloramphenicol-induced bone marrow suppression. Semin. Hematol. 10:225, 1973.
923. Poulton, E. M.: Thrombocytopenic purpura during chloramphenicol therapy. Br. Med. J. 2:106, 1955.
924. Friedman, A.: An evaluation of chloramphenicol therapy in typhoid fever in children. Pediatrics 14:28, 1954.
925. Ellison, R. R., Holland, J. D., et al.: Arabinosyl cytosine: A useful agent in the treatment of acute leukemia in adults. Blood 32:507, 1968.
926. Karnofsky, D. A.: Cancer chemotherapeutic agents. Cancer 18:80, 1968.
927. Robertson, J. H., and McCarthy, G. M.: Periwinkle alkaloids and the platelet count. Lancet 2:353, 1969.
928. Ogston, D., Dawson, A. A. et al.: Methotrexate and the platelet count. Br. J. Cancer 22:244, 1968.
929. Gardner, F. H., and Bessman, J. D.: Thrombocytopenia due to defective platelet production. Clin. Haematol. 12:23, 1983.
930. Adelstein, S. J., and Dealy, J. B., Jr.: Hematologic responses to human whole body irradiation. Analytic approaches to biologic dosimetry. Am. J. Roentgenol. 93:927, 1965.
931. Sullivan, L. W.: Effect of alcohol on platelet production. In *Platelet Kinetics*. Paulus, J. M. (ed.), Amsterdam, North-Holland Publishing Co, 1972, p. 247.
932. Lindenbaum, J., and Lieber, C. S.: Hematologic effects of alcohol in man in the absence of nutritional deficiency. New Engl. J. Med. 281:333, 1969.
933. Post, R. M., and Desforges, J. F.: Thrombocytopenia of severe alcoholism. Ann. Intern. Med. 68:1230, 1968.
934. Cowan, D. H.: Thrombokinetic studies in alcohol related thrombocytopenia. J. Lab. Clin. Med. 81:64, 1973.
935. Cowan, D. H., and Graham, R. C.: Studies on the platelet defect in alcoholism. Thrombos. Diath. Haemorrh. 33:310, 1975.
936. Watson, C. J., Schultz, A. L., et al.: Purpura following estrogen therapy with particular reference to hypersensitivity to (diethyl) stilbestrol and with a note on the possible relationship of purpura to endogenous estrogens. J. Lab. Clin. Med. 32:606, 1947.
937. Cooper, B. A., and Bigelow, F. W.: Thrombocytopenia associated with the administration of diethylstilbestrol in man. Ann. Intern. Med. 52:907, 1960.
938. Weinfeld, A., and Kutti, J.: Inverkan av moderna diuretika pa blodbilden. MSD Symposium, "Diuretika och o Demterapi," 1966.
939. Kutti, J., and Weinfeld, A.: The frequency of thrombocytopenia in patients with heart disease treated with oral diuretics. Acta Med. Scand. 183:245, 1968.
940. Eisner, E. V., and Crowell, E. B.: Hydrochlorothiazide-dependent thrombocytopenia due to IgM antibody. J.A.M.A 215:480, 1971.
941. Rodriguez, S. U., Leiken, S., et al.: Neonatal thrombocytopenia associated with antepartum-administration of thiazide drugs. New Engl. J. Med. 270:881, 1964.
942. Merenstein, G. B., O'Loughlin, E. P., et al.: Effects of maternal thiazides on platelet counts of newborn infants. J. Pediatr. 76:766, 1970.
943. Jerkner, J., Kutti, J., et al.: Platelet counts in mothers and their newborn infants with respect to antepartum administration of oral diuretics. Acta Med. Scand. 194:473, 1973.
944. Winderlöv, E., Karlman, I., et al.: Hydralazine-induced neonatal thrombocytopenia [Letter]. New Engl. J. Med. 303:1235, 1980.
945. Schiff, D., Aranda, J. V., et al.: Neonatal thrombocytopenia and congenital malformations associated with administration of tolbutamide to the mother. J. Pediatr. 77:457, 1970.
946. Lisciandro, R. C., and Twomey, J. J.: Adrenocorticosteroid-induced thrombocytopenia. Pac. Med. Surg. 75:33, 1967.
947. Cohen, P., and Gardner, F. H.: The effect of massive triamcinolone administration in blunting the erythropoietic response to phenylhydrazine hemolysis. J. Lab. Clin. Med. 65:88, 1965.
948. Levine, P. H.: A qualitative platelet defect in severe vitamin B_{12} deficiency. Ann. Intern. Med. 78:533, 1966.
949. Ingelberg, S., and Stoffersen, E.: Platelet dysfunction in patients with vitamin B_{12} deficiency. Acta Haematol. 61:75, 1979.
950. Slichter, S. J., and Harker, L. A.: Thrombocytopenia: Mechanisms and management of defects in platelet production. Clin. Haematol. 7:523, 1978.
951. Kotilainen, M.: Platelet kinetics in normal subjects in haematological disorders. Scand. J. Haematol. 5(Suppl):5, 1969.
952. Bessman, J. D., Williams, L. J., et al.: Platelet size in health and disease. Am. J. Clin. Pathol. 78:150, 1982.
953. Dzik, W. H.: Platelet size in megaloblastic anemia. Am. J. Clin. Pathol. 79:274, 1983.
954. Gross, S., Keefer, V., et al.: The platelets in iron deficiency anemia. I. The response to oral and parenteral iron. Pediatrics 34:315, 1964.
955. Lopas, H., and Rabiner, S. F.: Thrombocytopenia associated with iron deficiency anemia. I. The response to oral and parenteral iron. Clin. Pediatr. 5:609, 1966.
956. Sonneborn, D.: Thrombocytopenia and iron deficiency. Ann. Intern. Med. 80:111, 1974.
957. Scher, H., and Silber, R.: Iron responsive thrombocytopenia [Letter]. Ann. Intern. Med. 84:571, 1976.
958. Dincol, K., and Aksoy, M.: On the platelet levels in chronic iron deficiency anemia. Acta Haematol. 41:135, 1969.
959. Garg, S. K., Amorosi, E. L., et al.: Use of the megathrombocyte as an index of megakaryocyte number. New Engl. J. Med. 284:11, 1971.
960. Karpatkin, S., Garg, S. K., et al.: Role of iron as a regulator of thrombopoiesis. Am. J. Med. 57:521, 1974.
961. Freedman, M. L., and Karpatkin, S.: Requirement of iron for platelet protein synthesis. Biochem. Biophys. Res. Commun. 54:475, 1973.
962. Levin, J., and Bessman, J. D.: The inverse relation between platelet volume and platelet number. J. Lab. Clin. Med. 101:295, 1983.
963. Aster, R. H.: Pooling of platelets in the spleen. Role in the pathogenesis of "hypersplenic" thrombocytopenia. J. Clin. Invest. 45:645, 1966.
964. Bjork, V. O., and Hultqvist, G.: Brain damage in children after deep hypothermia for open heart surgery. Thorax 15:284, 1969.
965. Bunker, J. P., and Goldstein, R.: Coagulation during hypothermia in man. Proc. Soc. Exp. Biol. Med. 97:199, 1958.
966. Villalobos, T. J., Adelson, E., et al.: A cause of thrombocytopenia and leukopenia that occurs in dogs during deep hypothermia. J. Clin. Invest. 37:1, 1958.
967. Pina-Cabral, J. M., Amaral, I., et al.: Hepatic and splenic sequestration during deep hypothermia in the dog. Haemostasis 2:235, 1974.
968. Racine, J., and Jarjoui, E.: Severe hypothermia in infants. Helv. Paediatr. Acta 37:317, 1982.
969. Cohen, I. J., Amir, J., et al.: Thrombocytopenia of neonatal cold injury. J. Pediatr. 104:620, 1984.
970. Addiego, J. E., Mentzer, W. C., et al.: Thrombocytosis in infants and children. J. Pediatr. 85:805, 1974.
971. Spach, M. S., Howell, D. A., et al.: Myocardial infarction and multiple thromboses in a child with primary thrombocytosis. Pediatrics 31:268, 1963.

972. Thieffrey, S., Buhot, S., et al.: Une observation de thrombocythemie essentielle. Sang 28:264, 1957.
973. Ozer, F. L., Truax, W. E., et al.: Primary hemorrhagic thrombocythemia. Am. J. Med. 28:807, 1960.
974. Lumley, S. E.: Essential thrombocythemia in childhood. Proc. Roy. Soc. Med. 64:22, 1971.
975. Freedman, M. H., Olivares, R. S., et al.: Primary thrombocythemia in a child. J. Pediatr. 83:163, 1973.
976. Koide, R., Tsunematsu, Y., et al.: Ultrastructural abnormal changes of megakaryocytes in an infant with primary thrombocythemia. Jpn. J. Clin. Haematol. 15:1255, 1974.
977. Wundisch, G. F., Steidle, C., et al.: Elektronenmikroskopische and Gerinnungsunter-suchungen einem Fall von primarer thrombozythamie in Kindersalter. Klin. Wochenschr. 55:995, 1977.
978. Barnhart, M. I., Kim, T. H., et al.: Essential thrombocythemia in a child: Platelet ultrastructure and function. Am. J. Hematol. 8:87, 1980.
979. Williams, N., McDonald, T. P., et al.: Maturation and regulation of megakaryocytopoiesis. Blood Cells 5:43, 1979.
980. Nakeef, A.: Colony forming unit, megakaryocyte (CFU-M). Its use in elucidating the kinetics of humoral control of the megakaryocytic committed progenitor cell compartment. In *Experimental Haematology Today*. Baum, S. J., and Ledney, G. D. (eds.), New York, Springer-Verlag, 1977, p. 111.
981. Gewirtz, A. M., Bruno, E., et al.: In vitro studies of megakaryocytopoiesis in thrombotic disorders of man. Blood 61:384, 1983.
982. Gilmer, P. R., Williams, L. J., et al.: Spuriously elevated platelet counts due to microspherocytes. Am. J. Clin. Pathol. 78:259, 1982.
983. Murphy, S. Thrombocytosis and thrombocythemia. Semin. Haematol. 12:89, 1983.
984. Iland, H. J., Laszlo, J., et al.: Essential thrombocythemia: Clinical and laboratory characteristics at presentation. Trans. Assoc. Am. Phys. 96:165, 1983.
985. Kaywin, P., McDonough, M., et al.: Platelet function in essential thrombocythemia. New Engl. J. Med. 299:505, 1978.
986. Cooper, B., Schafer, A. I., et al.: Platelet resistance to PGD_2 in patients with myeloproliferative disorders. Blood 52:618, 1978.
987. Cooper, B., and Ahern, D.: Characterization of the platelet PGD_2 receptor. J. Clin. Invest. 64:586, 1979.
988. Bolin, R. B., Okumura, T., et al.: Changes in distribution of platelet membrane glycoproteins in patients with myeloproliferative disorders. Am. J. Hematol. 3:63, 1977.
989. Eche, N., Sie, P., et al.: Platelets in myeloproliferative disorders. III. Glycoprotein profile in relation to platelet function and density. Scand. J. Haematol. 26:123, 1981.
990. Booth, W. J., Berndt, M. C., et al.: An altered platelet granule glycoprotein in patients with essential thrombocythemia. J. Clin. Invest. 73:291, 1984.
991. Boneu, B., Nouvel, C., et al.: Platelets in myeloproliferative disorders. I. A comparative evaluation with certain platelet function tests. Scand. J. Haematol. 25:214, 1980.
992. Pareti, F. I., Gugliotta, L., et al.: Biochemical and metabolic aspects of platelet dysfunction in chronic myeloproliferative disorders. Thromb. Haemostasis 47:84, 1982.
993. Schafer, A. I.: Deficiency of platelet lipoxygenase activity in myeloproliferative disorders. New Engl. J. Med. 306:381, 1982.
994. Keenan, J. P., Wharton, J., et al.: Defective platelet lipid peroxidation in myeloproliferative disorders—a possible defect of prostaglandin synthesis. Br. J. Haematol. 35:275, 1977.
995. Okuma, M., and Uchino, H.: Altered arachidonate metabolism by platelets in patients with myeloproliferative disorders. Blood 54:1258, 1979.
996. Gerrard, J., Stoddard, S., et al.: Platelet storage pool deficiency and prostaglandin synthesis in chronic granulocytic leukemia. Br. J. Haematol. 40:597, 1978.
997. Cunietti, E., Gandini, R., et al.: Defective platelet aggregation and increased platelet turnover in patients with myelofibrosis and other myeloproliferative diseases. Scand. J. Haematol. 26:339, 1981.
998. McClure, P. D., Ingram, G. I. C., et al.: Platelet function tests in thrombocythaemia and thrombocytosis. Br. J. Haematol. 12:478, 1966.
999. Zucker, S., and Mielke, C. H.: Classification of thrombocytosis based on platelet function tests: Correlation with hemorrhagic and thrombotic complications. J. Lab. Clin. Med. 80:385, 1972.
1000. Neemeh, J. A., Bowie, E. J. W., et al.: Quantitation of platelet aggregation in myeloproliferation disorders. Am. J. Clin. Pathol. 57:336, 1972.
1001. Ginsberg, A. D.: Platelet function in patients with high counts. Ann. Intern. Med. 82:506, 1975.
1002. Wu, K. K.: Platelet hyperaggregability and thrombosis in patients with thrombocythemia. Ann. Intern. Med. 88:7, 1978.
1003. Hoagland, H. C., and Silverstien, M. N.: Primary thrombocythemia in the young patient. Mayo Clin. Proc. 53:578, 1978.
1004. Kessler, C. M., Klein, H. G., et al.: Uncontrolled thrombocytosis in chronic myeloproliferative disorders. Br. J. Haematol. 50:157, 1982.
1005. Sanyal, S. K., Yules, R. B., et al.: Thrombocytosis, central nervous system disease, and myocardial infarction pattern in infancy. Pediatrics 38:629, 1966.
1006. Huttenlocher, P. R., and Smith, D. B. Acute infantile hemiplegia associated with thrombocytosis. Develop. Med. Child. Neurol. 10:621, 1968.
1007. Panlilio, A. L., and Reiss, R. F.: Therapeutic plateletpheresis in thrombocythemia. Transfusion 19:147, 1979.
1008. Amato, D., and Freedman, M.: Eleven year follow-up of primary thrombocythemia in a child. J. Pediatr. 104:639, 1984.
1009. Castro-Malaspina, H., Rabellino, E. M. et al.: Human megakaryocyte stimulation of proliferation of bone marrow fibroblasts. Blood 57:781, 1981.
1010. Piessens, W. F., Wybran, J., et al.: Lymphocyte transformation induced by autologous platelets in a case of thrombocytopenic purpura. Blood 36:421, 1970.
1011. Handin, R. I., and Stossel, T. P.: Phagocytosis of antibody-coated platelets by human granulocytes. New Engl. J. Med. 290:989, 1974.
1012. Shulman, N. R., Aster, R. H., et al.: Immunoreactions involving platelets. VI. Reactions of maternal isoantibodies responsible for neonatal purpura. Differentiation of a second platelet antigen system. J. Clin. Invest. 41:1059, 1962.
1013. Freedman, A. L., Barr, P. S., et al.: Hemolytic anemia due to quinidine: Observations on its mechanism. Am. J. Med. 20:806, 1956.
1014. Aster, R. H., and Enright, S. E.: A platelet and granulocyte membrane defect in paroxysmal nocturnal hemoglobinuria: Usefulness for the detection of platelet antibodies. J. Clin. Invest. 48:1199, 1969.
1015. Cimo, P. L., and Gerber, S. A.: AET-treated platelets: Their usefulness for platelet antibody detection and an examination of their altered sensitivity to immune lysis. Blood 54:1101, 1979.
1016. Karpatkin, S., Strick, N., et al.: Detection of splenic antiplatelet antibody synthesis in idiopathic autoimmune thrombocytopenic purpura (ATP). Br. J. Haematol. 23:167, 1972.
1017. Karpatkin, S., and Siskind, G. W.: Studies on the specificity of anti-platelet autoantibodies. Proc. Soc. Exp. Biol. Med. 147:715, 1974.

1018. Mueller-Eckhardt, C., and Mersch-Baumert, K.: The problem of platelet autoantibodies. I. Evaluation of the platelet factor 3 availability test for their detection. Vox Sang 33:221, 1977.
1019. Jeje, M. O., Blajchman, M. A., et al.: Quantitation of red cell–associated IgG using an immunoradiometric assay. Transfusion 24:473, 1984.
1020. Kelton, J. G., Denomme, G., et al.: The measurement of platelet-associated IgG using an immunoradiometric assay. J. Immunoassay 4:65, 1983.
1021. Dixon, R., Rosse, W., et al.: Quantitative determination of antibody in idiopathic thrombocytopenic purpura. Correlation of serum and platelet-bound antibody with clinical response. New Engl. J. Med. 292:230, 1975.
1022. Rosse, W. F., Devine, D. V., et al.: Reactions of immunoglobulin G binding ligands with platelets and PAIgG. J. Clin. Invest. 73:489, 1984.
1023. Hedge, U. M., Gordon-Smith, E. C., et al.: Platelet antibodies in thrombocytopenic patients. Br. J. Haematol. 35:113, 1977.
1024. Kelton, J. G., Neame, P. B., et al.: The direct assay for platelet-associated IgG (PAIgG): Lack of association between antibody level and platelet size. Blood 53:73, 1979.
1025. McGrath, K. M., Stuart, J. J., et al.: II. Correlation between serum IgG, platelet membrane IgG, and platelet function in hypergammaglobulinemic states. Br. J. Haematol. 42:585, 1979.
1026. Nel, J. D., and Stevens, K.: A new method for the simultaneous quantitation of platelet-bound immunoglobulin (IgG) and complement (C3) employing an enzyme-linked immunoabsorbent assay (ELISA) procedure. Br. J. Haematol. 44:281, 1980.
1027. Cines, D. B., and Schreiber, A. D.: Immune thrombocytopenia. Use of a Coombs antiglobulin test to detect IgG and C3 on platelets. New Engl. J. Med. 300:106, 1979.
1028. Von dem Borne, A., Verheugt, F., et al.: A simple immunofluorescence test for the detection of platelet antibodies. Br. J. Haematol. 39:195, 1978.
1029. Tate, D. Y., Sorenson, R. L., et al.: An immunoenzyme histochemical technique for the detection of platelet antibodies from the serum of patients with idiopathic (autoimmune) thrombocytopenic purpura (ITP). Br. J. Haematol. 37:265, 1977.
1030. Kahane, S., Dvilansky, A., et al.: Detection of antiplatelet antibodies in patients with idiopathic thrombocytopenic purpura (ITP) and in patients with rubella and herpes group viral infections. Clin. Exp. Immunol. 44:49, 1981.
1031. Leporrier, M., Dighiero, G., et al.: Detection and quantification of platelet-bound antibodies with immunoperoxidase. Br. J. Haematol. 42:605, 1979.
1032. Schmidt, G. M., Bross, K. J., et al.: Detection of platelet-directed immunoglobulin G in sera using the peroxidase-antiperoxidase (PAP) slide technique. Blood 55:299, 1980.
1033. Gudino, M., and Miller, W. V.: Application of the enzyme linked immunospecific assay (ELISA) for the detection of platelet antibodies. Blood 57:32, 1981.
1034. LoBuglio, A. F., Court, W. S., et al.: Immune thrombocytopenic purpura. Use of a ^{125}I-labeled antihuman IgG monoclonal antibody to quantify platelet-bound IgG. New Engl. J. Med. 309:459, 1983.
1035. Shaw, G. M., Axelson, J., et al.: Quantification of platelet-bound IgG by ^{125}I-staphylococcal protein A in immune thrombocytopenic purpura and other thrombocytopenic disorders. Blood 63:154, 1984.
1036. McMillan, R., Smith, R. S., et al.: Immunoglobulins associated with human platelets. Blood 37:316, 1971.
1037. Luiken, G. A., McMillan, R., et al.: Platelet-associated IgG in immune thrombocytopenic purpura. Blood 50:317, 1977.
1038. McMillan, R., Tani, P., et al.: The demonstration of antibody binding to platelet-associated antigens in patients with immune thrombocytopenic purpura. Blood 56:993, 1980.
1039. Morse, B. S., Giuliani, D., et al.: A rapid quantitation of platelet-associated IgG by nephelometry. Am. J. Hematol. 12:271, 1982.
1040. Morse, B. S., Giuliani, D., et al.: Quantitation of platelet-associated IgG by radial immunodiffusion. Blood 57:809, 1981.
1041. Kelton, J. G., Denomme, G., et al.: Comparison of the measurement of surface or total platelet-associated IgG in the diagnosis of immune thrombocytopenia. Am. J. Hematol. 18:1, 1985.
1042. Kelton, J. G.: The measurement of platelet-bound immunoglobulins: An overview of the methods and the biologic relevance of PAIgG. Progr. Hematol. 13:163, 1983.
1043. Gibbons, S., and Kelton, J. G.: Assessment of the optimal anticoagulant solution for storage of whole blood samples prior to measurement of platelet-associated IgG. Transfusion 22:295, 1982.
1044. Kelton, J. G., Neame, P. B., et al.: The direct assay for platelet-associated IgG. Lack of association between antibody level and platelet size. Blood 53:527, 1979.
1045. Pfueller, S. L., Cosgrove, L., et al.: Relationship of raised PAIgG in thrombocytopenia to total platelet protein content. Br. J. Haematol. 49:293, 1981.
1046. Kelton, J. G., Denomme, G.: The quantitation of platelet-associated IgG on cohorts of platelets separated from healthy individuals by buoyant density centrifugation. Blood 60:136, 1982.
1047. Kelton, J. G.: Platelet fragments do not contribute to elevated levels of platelet-associated IgG. Br. J. Haematol. (in press).
1048. Kelton, J. G., and Steeves, K.: The amount of platelet-bound albumin parallels the amount of IgG on washed platelets from patients with immune thrombocytopenia. Blood 62:924, 1983.
1049. Kelton, J. G., Powers, P. J., et al.: A prospective study of the usefulness of the measurement of platelet-associated IgG for the diagnosis of ITP. Blood 60:1050, 1982.
1050. Sandvik, T., Endresen, G. K. M., et al.: Studies on the binding of complement factor C4 in human platelets. Int. Arch. Allergy Appl. Immunol. 74:152, 1984.
1051. Myers, T. J., Kim, B. Y., et al.: Platelet-associated complement C3 in immune thrombocytopenic purpura. Blood 59:1023, 1982.
1052. Kayser, W., Mueller-Eckhardt, C., et al.: Platelet-associated complement C3 in thrombocytopenic states. Br. J. Haematol. 54:353, 1983.
1053. McMillan, R., and Martin, M.: Fixation of C3 to platelets in vitro by antiplatelet antibody from patients with immune thrombocytopenic purpura. Br. J. Haematol. 47:251, 1981.
1054. Hauch, T. W., and Rosse, W. F.: Platelet-bound complement (C3) in immune thrombocytopenia. Blood 50:1129, 1977.
1055. Kayser, W., Mueller-Eckhardt, C., et al.: Complement-fixing platelet autoantibodies in autoimmune thrombocytopenia. Am. J. Haematol. 11:213, 1981.
1056. Nel, J. D., Stevens, K., et al.: Platelet-bound IgM in autoimmune thrombocytopenia. Blood 61:119, 1983.
1057. Kernoff, L. M., and Malan, E.: Complement (C3) binding to platelets in autoimmune thrombocytopenia. Clin. Lab. Haematol. 5:1, 1983.
1058. Pawha, J., Giuliani, D., et al.: Platelet-associated IgM levels in thrombocytopenia. Vox Sang 45:97, 1983.
1059. Hegde, U. M., Bowes, A., et al.: Platelet-associated complement (PAC_{3c} and PAC_{3d}) in patients with autoimmune thrombocytopenia. Br. J. Haematol. 60:49, 1985.
1060. Cines, D. B., Wilson, S. B., et al.: Platelet antibodies of the IgM class in immune thrombocytopenic purpura. J. Clin. Invest. 75:1183, 1985.

II. Qualitative Abnormalities

In Part I of this chapter we discussed disorders of platelet number, with particular emphasis on a group of common platelet abnormalities, all of which are characterized by reduced numbers of platelets. In Part II, Qualitative Abnormalities, the discussion will focus upon disorders of platelet function. It is pertinent to re-emphasize that platelets are unique blood cells whose functional role is more complex, for instance, than that of the red cell. Whereas in red cells, the quantitative estimation of hemoglobin allows one to generally predict the clinical impact of this cellular element on pathophysiology, the issues for platelets are far more complicated. For normal hemostasis, platelet functional activity is as crucial as platelet number. Yet, none of the basic or specialized in vitro tests of platelet function developed to date (Table 42–3) provides a good correlation with an individual subject's bleeding or thrombotic risk.

To date, the best predictive test of a patient's bleeding risk is the in vivo bleeding time. There is general agreement that a normal bleeding time in an asymptomatic patient indicates that the individual is at a low risk for serious bleeding. Similarly, a marked bleeding time prolongation suggests that the patient could bleed excessively during a major hemostatic challenge. Predictably the test has neither total sensitivity nor specificity. Some patients with a normal bleeding time may bleed excessively at surgery, while others may demonstrate no abnormal surgical blood loss even in the presence of a greatly prolonged bleeding time.

It is appropriate in this chapter to briefly review certain aspects of platelet function, and in particular, recent advances in the understanding of platelet membrane glycoproteins. A more detailed discussion is available in Chapter 40, but for purposes of continuity, we will highlight certain aspects of the platelet's structure-function relationship before discussing the inherited disorders of platelet function.

PLATELET STRUCTURE–FUNCTION RELATIONSHIPS

Platelets are anuclear cells with very specialized functions, and play a pivotal role in hemostasis. Like all circulating blood cells, platelets originate from common stem cells and share certain characteristics with both the red cell and the leukocyte. Like white cells, platelets are capable of undergoing dramatic changes in shape; are able to phagocytize particles; and can release a variety of chemical substances when stimulated. Like red cells, platelets do not have nuclei, and consequently, enzymes that are lost or inactivated cannot be regenerated. As will be discussed later in this chapter, the inability of platelets to regenerate inactivated enzymes has therapeutic implications when drugs such as aspirin are administered.

Platelets can be considered as carriers of vasoactive chemicals. When these chemicals are released into the circulation, they can cause both acute and long-term changes in the adjacent vessel walls and platelets. However, in order to release the chemical mediators, the platelet must receive "signals." These signals, termed platelet agonists, can be hormones, enzymes, proteins, or chemical compounds. The binding of these substances to receptors on the platelet surface results in a series

Table 42–13. EVALUATION OF A PATIENT WITH A SUSPECTED PLATELET DISORDER

History and Physical Exam
1. Detailed evaluation of bleeding tendencies—onset, frequency, duration and severity, transfusion requirement, and characteristic sites of involvement
2. Bleeding associated with surgery or trauma, tonsillectomy, tooth extractions, and circumcisions
3. Drug history, including multi-ingredient formulations that may contain aspirin or other known antiplatelet agents
4. Family history—inheritance pattern and severity of bleeding
5. Complete physical exam, including signs of recent bleeding (petechiae, ecchymoses, purpura, etc.), restricted joint mobility, and findings associated with particular congenital abnormalities (absent radii, albinism, telangiectasia, and inherited connective tissue disorders)

Coagulation and Fibrinolytic Evaluation
Screening and, if indicated, more definitive tests in order to detect abnormalities not related to platelets

Bleeding Time

Basic Studies of Platelets
1. Peripheral blood smear—numbers, size, appearance, clumping tendency
2. Electronic platelet count, including platelet sizing
3. Platelet aggregation (and simultaneous ATP release when firefly luciferin-luciferase reaction utilized) on platelet-rich plasma in response to collagen, ADP, epinephrine, ristocetin, arachidonic acid, and calcium ionophore (A23187)

Specialized Studies of Platelets (Membrane- and Granule-Related)
1. Surface membrane glycoprotein characterization
2. Platelet-ligand binding studies—fibrinogen, thrombin, vWF
3. Platelet adhesiveness
4. Studies of uptake and release of radioactive serotonin
5. Analysis of intracellular constituents—ATP, ADP, serotonin, platelet fibrinogen, platelet factor 4, β-thromboglobulin, platelet-derived growth factor, α-actinin, and lysosomal enzymes

Specialized Studies of Platelets (Miscellaneous)
1. Platelet morphology by electron microscopy
2. Evaluation of arachidonic acid metabolism through the cyclo-oxygenase and lipoxygenase pathways, and endoperoxide-induced aggregation
3. Ca^{++} mobilization using Fura 2 or quin 2.
4. Studies of platelet phosphatidylinositol hydrolysis
5. Platelet survival
6. Platelet-associated antibody
7. Evaluation of platelet coagulant activities

of both energy-dependent and energy-independent events within the platelet.

The platelet consists of a bilipid layer supported by a protein skeleton. Scattered over the surface of the lipid bilayer and penetrating it at various points are proteins. Some surface proteins carry antigens that help identify the cell as being "self." Other proteins serve as channels to allow the passage of nutrients and other substances in and out of the platelet. Still other proteins serve as specific binding sites or receptors that mediate certain platelet functions. Over the past several years, our knowledge of the structure and function of these membrane proteins has increased dramatically. The techniques used to study these proteins are summarized in the appendix at the end of this chapter.

Platelet Adhesion

When the endothelial lining of the blood vessel is damaged, the subendothelial layers are exposed. Platelets bind to these layers, a process termed *platelet adhesion*. Adhesion has been studied at high and low rates of blood flow (termed high and low shear rates), and in general, results obtained under conditions of high shear rate most closely simulate what happens in vivo (1,2).

Platelet adhesion requires the participation of one particular platelet glycoprotein, termed platelet glycoprotein Ib (GP Ib) plus a plasma coagulation factor, von Willebrand factor (1–3). If either component is absent because of an inherited deficiency, a hemorrhagic diathesis results, which is characterized by cutaneous bleeding and a prolonged bleeding time. The autosomal dominant bleeding disorder known as von Willebrand's disease is caused by a deficiency of the von Willebrand factor (described in detail in Chapter 41). The autosomal recessive disorder, Bernard-Soulier syndrome, is characterized by deficient glycoprotein Ib plus deficiencies in platelet glycoproteins V and IX. It is, however, the deficiency of Ib that produces bleeding in these patients. This entity is described in greater detail subsequently in this chapter.

Glycoprotein Ib. As shown in Figure 42–15, glycoprotein Ib is made of two chains (Ib_α, M_r 135 kD; and Ib_β, M_r 25 kD) (4). The subunits are covalently joined by disulfide bonds and are also linked, in a noncovalent fashion, with glycoprotein IX, a small protein of 22 kD. Most of the Ib_α chain is located outside the lipid bilayer and is called glycocalicin. Glycocalicin contains large amounts of carbohydrate (60 per cent by weight) and can be cleaved from the rest of the Ib_α chain by a calcium-dependent protease located within the platelet (5,6). Plasmin can also cleave glycocalicin. Glycoprotein Ib is an integral membrane protein and is bound to the actin skeleton within the

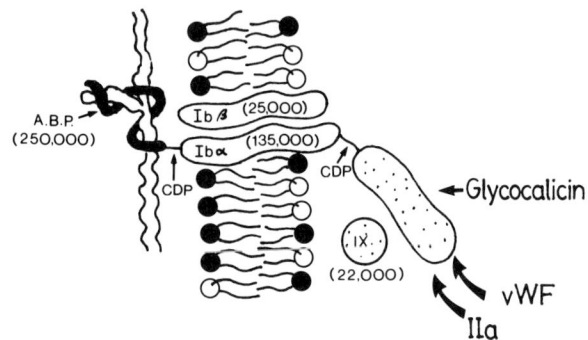

Figure 42–15. A schematic representation of the glycoprotein Ib-IX complex. Glycoprotein Ib (25,000 copies per platelet; M_r 170,000) is made of two components, Ib_α and Ib_β, with much of the Ib_α lying outside the bilipid layer and termed glycocalicin. Glycocalicin can be cleaved from the rest of Ib by the action of a calcium-dependent protease (CDP). CDP also can cleave Ib_α from actin-binding protein (ABP), which binds the glycoprotein Ib complex to the platelet cytoskeleton. Glycoprotein IX, a small peripheral glycoprotein, is closely but not covalently associated with the glycoprotein Ib complex.

platelet by an actin-binding protein (7). Because it is anchored to the platelet, its lateral mobility across the platelet membrane is limited. However, the anchor site on Ib is cleaved by the calcium-dependent protease, allowing it to be mobile. The calcium-dependent protease itself is activated by a variety of aggregating agents (8,9).

Glycoprotein Ib has several very important functions. First, the von Willebrand factor (vWF) binds to the glycocalicin part of Ib. This bridging function of the vWF molecule between glycocalicin on Ib and the subendothelial layers is responsible for platelet adhesion. Another important function of the glycoprotein Ib molecule is that it is the platelet binding site for thrombin. Thrombin binds to the glycocalicin portion of Ib, but at a site distinct from that of von Willebrand factor (10).

Platelet Aggregation

After platelets adhere to the subendothelial lining of blood vessels, they rapidly spread over the surface and release their contents. Vasoactive substances contained or generated in the platelet include the adenine nucleotides ADP and ATP and the following arachidonic acid metabolites: thromboxane A_2 and the cyclical endoperoxides PGG_2 and PGH_2. All of these substances can activate adjacent platelets in the circulation and induce them to undergo a change in shape. The activated platelets bind to each other and to the adherent platelets in a process termed platelet aggregation. Platelet aggregation, like platelet adhesion, requires a particular platelet glycoprotein complex termed IIb/IIIa, plus fibrinogen (3,10–13). Patients deficient in either of these "components" will have a bleeding disorder. Patients with the autosomal recessive disorder Glanzmann's thrombasthenia lack the glycoprotein IIb/IIIa complex. This rare but important bleeding disorder will be discussed subsequently.

Glycoprotein IIb/IIIa Complex. Glycoproteins IIb and IIIa are the most abundant surface glycoproteins on the platelet, there being approximately 50,000 copies of each per platelet (Fig. 42–16) (14,15). These glycoproteins bind to each other in a 1:1 ratio in the presence of calcium, and only when complexed are they functional. Glycoprotein IIb has a molecular weight of 140 kD and is made up of two disulfide-linked subunits, GP IIb$_\alpha$ and GP IIb$_\beta$, whereas glycoprotein IIIa has an M_r of 90 kD and is a single polypeptide chain (4,16). Glycoproteins IIb and IIIa are integral membrane glycoproteins, although most of the complex is above the lipid bilayer, with only a small amount embedded within it. The IIb/IIIa complex binds not only fibrinogen but also a variety of molecules capable of causing platelet-platelet interactions, including von Willebrand factor and fibronectin (17–20). However, the much higher concentration of fibrinogen, compared with that of either of the other two molecules, means that under most physiologic circumstances fibrinogen is the dominant plasma protein responsible for platelet aggregation.

Glycoproteins IIb and IIIa also carry certain platelet-specific alloantigens. The Bak^a antigen is found on IIb, and the Pl^{A1} antigen is on IIIa (21–23). The IIb/IIIa complex is present on the surface of unstimulated platelets, but it is likely that IIb/IIIa will bind fibrinogen and other filamentous molecules only after the complex has undergone conformational changes initiated by platelet activation.

The other platelet glycoproteins have not been as well characterized, primarily because congenital deficiencies of these glycoproteins have not been described. Consequently their physiologic role in platelet function is less certain.

Glycoprotein V. Glycoprotein V (M_r 82 kD) is a peripheral glycoprotein that can be eluted from the surface of platelets. Its precise role in platelet function remains uncertain, although this glycoprotein is the only platelet substitute for thrombin identified to date (24). In a recent report, it was suggested that glycoprotein V is a receptor for drug-dependent (quinidine) interactions (25).

Glycoprotein IX. Glycoprotein IX is a small (M_r 20 kD) glycoprotein that has recently been given considerable importance, as it was reported to be a binding site for quinine- and quinidine-induced thrombocytopenia (26). This small and probably peripheral glycoprotein is strongly, but not covalently, associated with the glycoprotein Ib complex (27). Perhaps not coincidentally, the platelet glycoprotein complexes of both Ib and IX are absent in patients with the congenital disorder Bernard-Soulier syndrome. This is probably the reason why early investigators studying drug-induced thrombocytopenia felt that the drug-dependent receptor was located on glycoprotein Ib. The relative importance of either glycoprotein V or glycoprotein IX remains uncertain.

The Platelet Fc Receptor. Recently, Rosenfeld and associates reported that the platelet binding site for the Fc portion of the IgG molecule was a 40-kD glycoprotein (28). Our own observations have confirmed these results, and in addition have demonstrated that the Fc binding site is an integral glycoprotein. The identification of the Fc receptor should facilitate the characterization of immune complex interactions involving platelets.

PLATELET AGGREGATION AND RELEASE

Studies defining pathways of platelet aggregation and release have not been as well studied as platelet membrane structure-function relationships. The main reason is that only recently have the immuno-biochemical techniques that were used to explore platelet structure and function been applied to the study of pathways of platelet aggregation. Platelet activation, aggregation, and secretion have been studied chemically, and also in patients who have defects in these various pathways.

Platelets carry three distinct classes of secretory granules: dense granules, α-granules, and lysozymes. In general, the release reaction and secretion of each type of granule is proportional to the strength of the stimulus. For example, weak stimuli induce release of the dense granules, which carry adenosine diphosphate (ADP), serotonin, calcium, pyrophosphate, and a small amount of adenosine triphosphate (ATP). Stronger stimuli result in the release not only of the dense granules but also of the α-granules. The α-granules contain proteins specific for platelets, including β-throm-

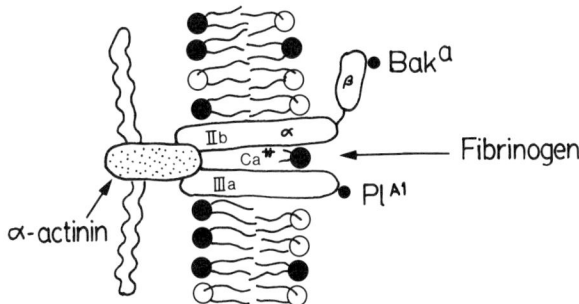

Figure 42–16. A schematic representation of the platelet glycoprotein IIb/IIIa complex. These glycoproteins are the most common glycoproteins in the platelet membrane (50,000 copies per platelet; IIb: M_r 140,000; IIIa: M_r 90,000) and are important for a number of reasons. First, they are the fibrinogen receptor and are required for platelet aggregation. Second, they carry the alloantigens (Pl^{A1} and Bak^a) as also autoantigens.

boglobulin, platelet factor 4, and platelet-derived growth factor; they also contain proteins that are homologues of plasma proteins, including fibrinogen, vWF, Factor V, high-molecular-weight kininogen, fibronectin, thrombospondin or glycoprotein G, albumin, and Factors D and B_1H-globulin of the complement system. The strongest stimuli cause the secretion of all granule contents, including the dense bodies, α-granules, and lysozymes.

ADP, adrenalin, and low concentrations of collagen and thrombin cause the release of arachidonic acid (AA) from the platelet membrane. The release of AA is mediated by the activation of several enzymes, including phospholipase A_2, and by the sequential activation of phospholipase C and diglyceride lipase (29,30–30a). Once arachidonic acid has been released, it is converted by a series of enzymes, including cyclo-oxygenase and thromboxane synthetase, into the potent platelet proaggregatory metabolite thromboxane A_2 (31–34). Thromboxane A_2, and to a lesser extent the cyclic endoperoxides PGG_2 and PGH_2, can cause platelet aggregation and secretion of the platelet dense granules (35, 36a).

Collagen and low concentrations of thrombin are examples of intermediate strength platelet agonists. These aggregating agents induce platelet aggregation through the prostaglandin pathway, but in addition they cause direct release of ADP even when the prostaglandin pathway is interrupted. The mechanism of this interaction remains undefined.

Thrombin is a potent stimulator of platelet aggregation. Thrombin activates the prostaglandin pathway, and also causes direct release of ADP from the dense bodies, as well as secretion of the α-granules and lysozomal contents.

Agonist-induced platelet aggregation and secretion are accompanied by rapid changes in phosphoinositide metabolism. While cytoplasmic Ca^{++} serves as a second messenger in the stimulus-response coupling for most platelet functions, recent studies of platelet activation suggest that other second messenger products of the phosphatidylinositol cycle (including diglyceride and inositoltriphosphate) may also act synergistically with calcium to mediate platelet responses (36b).

Interaction of the Coagulation Proteins with Platelets

The concept of platelets as cells whose primary function is to "plug holes" in damaged blood vessels is giving way to the realization that platelets are intimately involved in many aspects of hemostasis, not only in the arterial but also within the venous circulation. However, it should be emphasized that platelet thrombi are primarily restricted to the fast-flowing arterial circulation. One interpretation of platelet-coagulation interactions is that platelets act as a transport system to move coagulation factors to sites of vascular damage (37). In addition, coagulation factors are actively secreted from the platelet α-granules, increasing the relative concentration of coagulation factors at these sites. Finally, platelets have been shown to have specific binding sites for various clotting factors.

Within the platelet α-granules are fibrinogen, von Willebrand factor (vWF), Factor V, and high-molecular-weight kininogen, as well as a number of plasma proteinase inhibitors (38). The amount of vWF associated with platelets is very large and can represent approximately 25 per cent of all vWF present in the plasma (39–41). More important, the vWF within the platelet contains the largest vWF multimers, these latter multimers being the most reactive type of vWF. Whether or not platelet vWF is important for platelet adhesion and aggregation remains uncertain (38). It has, however, been proposed that this vWF not only participates in platelet adhesion but also binds to the platelet glycoprotein IIb/IIIa complex following platelet activation (39–42).

Platelets also carry in their α-granules a large amount of fibrinogen (approximately 10 per cent by weight of all platelet protein) (43). Most of this fibrinogen is released during platelet secretion and participates in platelet aggregation by crosslinking platelets at the glycoprotein IIb/IIa complex (44,45). Platelet fibrinogen may also participate in coagulation.

Coagulation Factor V is present in high concentrations in the platelet α-granules. Indeed, approximately 25 per cent of the plasma Factor V is platelet associated (46). Platelet Factor V has been postulated to act as the platelet binding site for activated Factor X (Xa) (47).

Platelets also carry high-molecular-weight kininogen (HMWK). HMWK, like the other coagulation factors, is located in the α-granules and is released during platelet secretion (48,49). Although the function of platelet high-molecular-weight kininogen is uncertain, it probably serves as the receptor for Factor XIa on the platelet surface (50).

Also present within platelets are fibronectin (51a) and thrombospondin (51b). Whereas platelet fibronectin may participate in platelet-platelet binding, thrombospondin has been suggested to play the role of an endogenous lectin, mediating platelet aggregation by binding to a specific receptor on other platelets.

CONGENITAL DISORDERS OF PLATELET FUNCTION

We will discuss the various congenital disorders of platelet function according to the type of the platelet functional abnormality involved (Table 42–14). It is important to emphasize that all of these disorders are very uncommon, and consequently, their investigation and management is not a major issue for the average pediatrician. Nonetheless, these disorders are important because the biochemical studies that have been undertaken to establish their etiology have increased our understanding of platelet structure and function relationships.

Inherited Disorders of Platelet Surface Glycoproteins

BERNARD-SOULIER SYNDROME

The Bernard-Soulier syndrome, initially described in 1948 by Bernard and Soulier (52), is a congenital bleeding disorder transmitted in an autosomal recessive fashion. It is characterized by the presence of unusually large platelets, absent aggregation to the antibiotic ristocetin, and a prolonged bleeding time. The defect is caused by an inherited deficiency of glycoprotein Ib.

Molecular Defects. Nurden and Caen were the first investigators to document a platelet membrane glycoprotein deficiency in patients with the Bernard-Soulier syndrome (53). These studies initially focused on the absence of glycoprotein Ib, but it is now recognized that patients with this syndrome also lack glycoproteins V and IX. Although it is most likely that all three glycoproteins are absent, it is also possible that the defect resides in post-translational glycosylation (54–56). As noted previously, glycoprotein Ib is one of the most common platelet glycoproteins (25,000 copies per platelet) and is made up of two subunits, a large Ib_α and a small Ib_β, which are covalently linked by disulfide bonds. The deficiency of glycoprotein Ib is responsible for most—and possibly all—of the laboratory abnormalities of the Bernard-Soulier syndrome. For example, the glycocalicin component of the Ib subunit is the site of the attachment of von Willebrand factor (Fig. 42–15). Consequently, the absence of this glycoprotein results in the profound defects of platelet adhesion, the prolonged bleeding time, and the bleeding manifestations that characterize this syndrome.

Glycoprotein Ib is an integral membrane glycoprotein, and is joined to the platelet cytoskeleton by an actin-binding protein. The attachment of Ib to the platelet skeleton may help keep the platelet in its characteristic discoid shape (Fig. 42–15). Consequently, its absence in the Bernard-Soulier syndrome may be responsible for the larger than average sized platelets that characterize this entity, and for their unusual deformability (57).

Following the demonstration that platelets from patients with the Bernard-Soulier syndrome lacked glycoprotein Ib, other glycoproteins were also demonstrated to be missing in these patients, including glycoprotein V (M_r 82 kD) and glycoprotein IX (M_r 20 kD) (54,55). An additional minor glycoprotein of M_r approximately 100 kD also has been shown to be absent. Sensitive and precise assays such as electroimmunoassay have shown the complete absence of GP Ib in patients with the Bernard-Soulier syndrome (58). Flow cytofluorimetry studies have demonstrated that the reduced Ib is not due to its absence on certain fixed populations of platelets but rather to its absence from all the platelets of an affected individual (59). Parents of patients of the Bernard-Soulier syndrome have approximately 50 per cent levels of glycoproteins Ib, IX, and V, yet exhibit entirely normal platelet function. This interesting finding indicates that even small amounts of these membrane glycoproteins are sufficient to permit normal platelet function (55).

A study by Moake and associates has demonstrated markedly reduced ristocetin-induced binding of von Willebrand factor to Bernard-Soulier platelets. It appears, therefore, that it is the defective attachment of vWF that prevents vWF-mediated agglutination in Bernard-Soulier platelets rather than impaired platelet-platelet interaction subsequent to vWF-platelet binding (60).

Laboratory Diagnosis. Patients described in the literature have been reported to have normal or reduced platelet counts. Whether in fact patients with Bernard-Soulier syndrome are actually thrombocytopenic or whether they merely appear to be as a result of counting difficulties remains unsolved. For example, because of the size and density of Bernard-Soulier platelets, it is almost impossible to count them; consequently, even carefully prepared platelet-rich plasma from these patients will lose many of the platelets as a result of co-precipitation with red cells. It has been suggested that platelets in this disorder may in fact be of normal size while in whole blood or platelet-rich plasma, but that they undergo increased spreading upon contact with a foreign surface (61). Although this property may partially contribute to their increased size, studies using electron-microscopy, micropipette aspiration, and a variety of sizing techniques have shown that Bernard-Soulier platelets are indeed increased in size, with the changes not due to increased amounts of internalized surface membrane (57). In addition, these platelets carry increased numbers of dense granules (62).

Every patient with the Bernard-Soulier syndrome will have a marked prolongation of the bleeding time. Our experience, using a commercial template-type bleeding time device, is that the bleeding time is invariably greater than 20 minutes in patients with this disease (normal <8 minutes). Tests of platelet adhesion are markedly abnormal, including the adhesion of platelets to de-endothelialized vessels (63). Diagnosis is strongly suspected by the characteristic pattern of platelet

Table 42–14. CHARACTERISTICS OF THE MAJOR CONGENITAL DISORDERS OF PLATELET FUNCTION

Disorder	Molecular Defect	Aggregation Pattern in Platelet-Rich Plasma	Release of ATP and Serotonin	Inheritance	Other Characteristic Abnormalities
Platelet Surface Membrane Glycoprotein Abnormalities					
Bernard-Soulier syndrome	Deficiency of GP Ib, V, and IX	Markedly decreased with ristocetin (without correction by von Willebrand factor); decreased with thrombin; normal response to other agents	Decreased with ristocetin	Autosomal	Markedly prolonged bleeding time with moderate thrombocytopenia; platelets appear large on blood smear; decreased adhesiveness to subendothelium
Glanzmann's thrombasthenia	Deficiency or abnormality of GP IIb/IIIa	Markedly decreased with all agents except ristocetin (which may show a reversible single phase)	Normal with thrombin, calcium ionophore, and ristocetin; may be decreased with collagen, ADP, and epinephrine	Autosomal recessive	Long bleeding time (but normal platelet count and morphology); clot retraction absent or markedly decreased; fibrinogen receptor, PL^{A1}, and Bak^a antigens decreased; α-actinin and intraplatelet fibrinogen may be decreased
Platelet Granule Defects					
Gray platelet syndrome	Absence of α-granules and their secreted proteins	Decreased with all agents	Decreased with all agents	Autosomal	Prolonged bleeding time with moderate thrombocytopenia; large pale-appearing agranular platelets on blood smear; both platelet-specific proteins and platelet coagulation proteins are severely deficient
Dense granule deficiencies (Hermansky-Pudlak, Chédiak-Higashi, Wiskott-Aldrich, and thrombocytopenia with absent radii syndromes, or as an isolated abnormality)	Absence or decreased numbers of platelet dense granules and their secreted metabolites	Decreased aggregation (particularly second phase) with weak agents; usually normal response to arachidonic acid, calcium ionophore, and high concentrations of weak agonists	Decreased	Autosomal (except for Wiskott-Aldrich syndrome, which is sex-linked)	Variably prolonged bleeding time; decreased dense granule content of ADP, ATP, 5-HT, and calcium; increased total platelet ATP:ADP ratio; oculocutaneous albinism and reticuloendothelial ceroid deposition in Hermansky-Pudlak syndrome; thrombocytopenia associated with Chédiak-Higashi, Wiskott-Aldrich, and TAR syndromes; decreased autologous platelet survival and an increase in platelet-associated IgG in Wiskott-Aldrich syndrome
Combined defects	Variable decrease in both platelet dense bodies and α-granules	Decreased	Decreased		Heterogeneity of granule deficiencies reported

Disorder			Inheritance
Defects of Platelet Arachidonic Acid (AA) Metabolism			
Impaired release of AA from platelet membrane phospholipids	Decreased with ADP, epinephrine, and collagen; normal with AA	Decreased with ADP, epinephrine, and collagen	Thromboxane production abnormal in response to ADP, epinephrine, and collagen; normal with AA. This abnormality may occur in combination with dense granule deficiency
Enzyme deficiencies (platelet cyclo-oxygenase or thromboxane synthetase)	Impaired with ADP, epinephrine, collagen and AA; normal response to the endoperoxide PGG_2 in cyclo-oxygenase deficiency; response impaired in patients with thromboxane synthetase deficiency		Variably prolonged bleeding time; platelet thromboxane production absent or markedly decreased in response to ADP, epinephrine, collagen, and AA; thromboxane production in response to PGG_2 is normal in platelet cyclo-oxygenase deficiency, but markedly decreased or absent in thromboxane synthetase deficiency; formation of lipoxygenase products from exogenous ^{14}C-AA appears to be normal
Defects in Platelet Procoagulant Activity			
Deficiency of coagulation Factor Va binding sites on the platelet surface	Normal	Normal	Normal bleeding time, platelet count, and morphology, but abnormal platelet procoagulant studies and decreased thrombin generation
Miscellaneous			
Isolated disorders of aggregation and/or release; as a concomitant finding in a variety of pathologic states, including Epstein syndrome, the May-Hegglin anomaly, inherited disorders of connective tissue, glycogen storage disease Type I, fructose 1:6-diphosphatase deficiency, Down's syndrome, and congenital heart disease	Variable	Variable	Heterogeneity of defects	Unknown
Platelet type (or pseudo-) von Willebrand's disease	Increased at low ristocetin concentrations—addition of cryoprecipitate by itself produces aggregation; normal response to other agonists	Cryoprecipitate by itself produces release; normal response to other agonists	Prolonged bleeding time; borderline thrombocytopenia; selective decrease of higher molecular weight plasma vWF multimers; increased platelet binding of normal vWF	Autosomal

aggregation responses. In particular, Bernard-Soulier platelets have normal to increased responsiveness to ADP (64,65), normal responses to the agonists epinephrine and collagen, and decreased aggregation to thrombin (66–69). Bernard-Soulier platelets also demonstrate essentially an absent response to the antibiotic ristocetin. This is because platelet agglutination by ristocetin requires intact platelet membrane glycoprotein Ib as one of its essential prerequisites. It should also be noted that an impaired response to ristocetin is also observed in patients with von Willebrand disease (Chapter 41). However, in this latter disease entity, abnormal ristocetin-induced platelet agglutination can usually be corrected in vitro by the addition of normal cryoprecipitate. Whereas patients with the Bernard-Soulier syndrome have normal levels of plasma von Willebrand factor, this circulating protein is abnormal in patients with von Willebrand disease. The diagnosis of Bernard-Soulier syndrome can be confirmed only by the demonstration of the complete absence of platelet membrane glycoprotein Ib (58). In contrast, this glycoprotein is present on platelets from patients with von Willebrand disease.

The Clinical Impact of the Bernard-Soulier Syndrome and Its Management. Virtually every patient described with this entity has a severe bleeding disorder. Almost all patients have easy bruising and may have severe hemorrhage following even minor trauma. There is no specific treatment for this disease. The physician should, insofar as possible, limit the patient's exposure to platelets until they are absolutely and urgently needed. Indeed, platelet transfusion can be lifesaving, but individuals with this disorder will be able to successfully receive only a few platelet transfusions during their entire lifetime. Since the absent platelet glycoproteins (Ib, V, and IX in Bernard-Soulier syndrome; and IIb/IIIa in Glanzmann's thrombasthenia) are potent immunogens, and since normal platelets carry these glycoproteins, individuals with either of these disease entities will, following platelet transfusion therapy, rapidly produce high-titer antiplatelet alloantibodies against the platelet glycoproteins that they lack. These alloantibodies can have two effects. First, they can result in the rapid destruction of any transfused normal platelets. Second, because these antibodies bind to platelet-specific alloantigens (in particular, Ib, IIb, or IIIa) they will also alter the functional activity of normal transfused platelets.

GLANZMANN'S THROMBASTHENIA

Thrombasthenia was the term used by Glanzmann in 1918 to describe a heterogeneous group of hemorrhagic disorders characterized by abnormal clot retraction but normal platelet numbers (70). The disorder is now well characterized, and has been given the name Glanzmann's thrombasthenia. This disease, like the Bernard-Soulier syndrome, is a very rare autosomal recessive inherited disorder of platelet function. As shown in Table 42–14, the platelet response in Glanzmann's thrombasthenia is almost the mirror image of the Bernard-Soulier syndrome. In particular, platelets from patients with Glanzmann's thrombasthenia respond with apparent normal aggregation (which in fact is actually platelet agglutination) to the antibiotic ristocetin; however, the platelets do not aggregate to any of the other agonists, including ADP, epinephrine, collagen, and thrombin (71,72).

Pathophysiology and Molecular Defects. A great deal of work has been performed in the area of defining the precise platelet glycoprotein abnormalities in Glanzmann's thrombasthenia. The reason for the lack of response of platelets from patients with this disease to various aggregating agents has provided new insight into normal platelet physiology. Platelets from these patients manifest normal adhesion to damaged vessel walls and collagen fibers (72,73). However, the platelets are incapable of binding to each other during the process of platelet aggregation. This defect is not because the aggregating agents do not bind to the platelet surface (74,75). Rather, it is the platelet-platelet interaction (platelet aggregation) that is defective. As noted previously, platelet aggregation is mediated by the bridging of platelets at the glycoprotein IIb/IIIa complex by long fibrillary molecules, usually fibrinogen (76,77). Thus, the inherited absence of these glycoproteins is responsible for the abnormalities of platelet aggregation in patients with Glanzmann's thrombasthenia (78–80). Glycoproteins IIb/IIIa are the most abundant glycoproteins on the platelet surface, with 50,000 copies each per platelet. These glycoproteins are both strong immunogens, and they also carry a number of platelet-specific alloantigens (PL^{A1} antigen on glycoprotein IIIa and Bak^a antigen on glycoprotein IIb) (21a,b;22). Of interest, glycoproteins IIb and IIIa are also carried on monocytes and other cells, although their function on these latter cells remains uncertain (81). In Glanzmann's thrombasthenia, intraplatelet fibrinogen may also be absent or present in decreased amounts, and does not bind to platelet-surface membranes (72,82–84).

Glanzmann's thrombasthenia has been subdivided into two categories: Type I, in which there appears to be a total lack of the glycoprotein IIb/IIIa complex (measured either by using crossed immunoelectrophoresis or by functional assays), as well as lack of a fibrinogen immunoprecipitate (85–88). Type II disease is caused by a partial deficiency (GP IIb/IIIa content varies from 5 to 20 per cent), and appreciable quantities of intraplatelet fibrinogen are usually present (86,88). Although it is possible that Type I disease is caused by a total absence of the genes for IIb and IIIa, whereas Type II represents only a partial absence, this concept has been recently called into question by a group of investigators who demonstrated that virtually all patients, even those with Type I disease, have small amounts of platelet IIb/IIIa (89). These observations suggest that total gene deletions are not the cause of the abnormalities of IIb/IIIa. The issue is even more complex, because in some patients the level of the glycoprotein IIb/IIIa complex may be at least 50 per cent (or higher) of the control values, indicating that in these individuals, the disease is probably caused by a functional deficiency of IIb/IIIa (90,91). Thus it is apparent that Glanzmann's thrombasthenia is a far more complex disorder than the Bernard-Soulier syndrome.

Platelets from patients with Glanzmann's disease may have other membrane glycoprotein defects besides the characteristic absent, reduced, or defective IIb/IIIa. Changes in the isoelectric point of glycoproteins Ib and IIIb, and abnormal periodic acid–Schiff reagent staining of other membrane glycoproteins, have been observed by one group. If confirmed, this finding would suggest that there may be a more general perturbation of platelet membrane glycoproteins than had been previously suspected (92). Some investigators have also suggested that platelet α-actinin is absent in patients with Glanzmann's disease, although this finding has not been confirmed by others (93, 94).

Laboratory Diagnosis. In most patients the diagnosis is not difficult. The patient has a life-long bleeding history, a markedly prolonged bleeding time (usually greater than 20 to 30 minutes), and absence of aggregation responses to all agonists except ristocetin. The diagnosis can be confirmed in most patients by the absence or marked decrease of platelet membrane glycoproteins IIb/IIIa, using standard techniques such as radioimmunoprecipitation and immunoblotting (described in the appendix to this chapter). Because most carriers of this disease have reduced amounts of IIb/IIIa, they can also be identified by means of either gel electrophoretic techniques or flow cytometry (95–97). As previously discussed, defective glycoprotein function may also produce the clinical manifestations of Glanzmann's thrombasthenia in some individuals (90,91). It should be emphasized, however, that this type of disease is very rare. Antenatal diagnosis of this condition has been described by examination of fetal blood samples at 22 weeks' gestation (98).

Clinical Features. Glanzmann's thrombasthenia is a very rare inherited disorder, with fewer than 200 cases described to date. Only two large series of patients have been described (99,100). Like most rare autosomal inherited disorders, consanguinity is common. Most of the patients have signs of cutaneous bleeding, including petechiae and purpura, as well as gum bleeding, epistaxis, and gastrointestinal bleeding. Almost always the women have menorrhagia (99). In some patients bleeding can be fatal.

Treatment is the same as that for patients with Bernard-Soulier syndrome. Again, one of the key aspects of therapy is the avoidance of alloimmunization by platelet transfusions. Platelet glycoproteins IIb and IIIa are potent immunogens, and although platelet transfusions can be lifesaving, *only the first few transfusions will prove successful, because of the subsequent development of immunization.*

PLATELET-TYPE VON WILLEBRAND'S DISEASE

A hemorrhagic disorder resembling von Willebrand's disease has been described in several families. Although plasma vWF is normal in these individuals, there appears to be an intrinsic platelet-membrane abnormality that creates a plasma vWF multimeric pattern like that of Type II von Willebrand's disease. This abnormality is apparently caused by increased platelet binding of normal vWF. This defect has been described in greater detail in Chapter 41.

Platelet Granule Defects

ALPHA-GRANULE DEFICIENCY (Gray Platelet Syndrome)

This syndrome, first described by Raccuglia (101), derives its name from the peculiar gray color of the platelets on Wright-stained blood smears. Other families have since been described with a similar platelet morphologic appearance that results from the absence or marked deficiency of platelet α-granules(102–108). Megakaryocytes obtained from affected patients also demonstrate a similar deficiency (105, 107, 108). Platelet dense bodies and lysozymes are present in normal amounts, and platelet membrane glycoproteins are normal (102–104, 106). As previously discussed, since α-granules contain platelet-specific proteins (β-thromboglobulin, platelet factor 4, platelet-derived growth factor) and the coagulation proteins (including fibrinogen, vWF, Factor V, high-molecular-weight kininogen, fibronectin, and thrombospondin), these platelet proteins are severely deficient in platelets in this disorder (102, 104, 106, 107).

Bleeding symptoms characteristic of a primary hemostatic defect (ecchymoses, petechiae, epistaxis) begin from early childhood. Symptoms suggesting a coagulation factor defect, including hemarthrosis and spontaneous hematomas, may also occur (101, 104). Laboratory investigations usually reveal moderate thrombocytopenia, large platelets, impaired platelet aggregation responses to collagen and thrombin and occasionally to ADP, and a prolonged bleeding time (102, 104, 108).

The syndrome provides evidence for the important role of platelet α-granule proteins in normal platelet-vascular function. Although many of the α-granule proteins are synthesized by other cells, including vascular endothelium, the secretion of these proteins locally by platelets into a developing platelet aggregate appears to be a critical factor in cell-cell interaction in primary hemostasis. The bleeding symptoms suggestive of a coagulation factor abnormality may be due to the deficiency in α-granule platelet coagulation Factor V, with resultant defects in thrombin and fibrin generation (109, 110).

Plasma levels of platelet factor 4 and β-thromboglobulin are increased in patients with this disorder, and may indicate that while megakaryocyte synthesis of these proteins is normal, their packaging and storage into α-granules is defective (102, 104) An increased amount of stainable marrow reticulin fibers in affected individuals could be due to increased levels of platelet-derived growth factor (PDGF), because this factor stimulates fibroblast proliferation (104, 105).

DENSE GRANULE DEFICIENCIES (Storage Pool Deficiency)

Several families have been studied with a mild to moderate bleeding diathesis and abnormalities in platelet aggregation associated with defects in secretion of platelet dense body constituents, including platelet serotonin and the adenine nucleotides ATP and ADP (111–117). The decreased amounts of platelet ATP and ADP are due specifically to deficiencies of granule-bound nucleotides, because the cytosolic nucleotides that participate in platelet metabolism are normal. This storage pool of granule-bound nucleotides is quite distinct from the metabolic pool of adenine nucleotides that are actively involved in platelet metabolism. The latter are labeled by incubation of platelets for relatively short periods of time with either ^{3}H- or ^{14}C-adenine. In contradistinction, the storage pool of adenine nucleotides remains unlabeled, participates only slowly in platelet metabolism, is granule-bound, and is packaged together with serotonin and calcium in the platelet dense granules.

The laboratory hallmark of storage pool deficiency is a decrease in the levels of both storage ADP and ATP. In normal platelets, ADP is more selectively concentrated in the dense granules than is ATP. Therefore, a deficiency of the storage pool adenine nucleotides has the effect of decreasing platelet ADP to a greater extent than ATP, resulting in an ATP:ADP ratio that is markedly greater than that in normal platelets (118). Following incubation of storage pool–deficient platelets with ^{3}H- or ^{14}C-adenine, uptake of radioactivity into the metabolic pool is normal. The measurement of the specific radioactivity of ADP and ATP reflects the proportion of nucleotides in the two pools. Since the nonlabeled storage pool is absent in this disorder, the determination of specific radioactivity of ADP and ATP is markedly increased (118).

Detailed studies in patients with this disorder have revealed considerable heterogeneity. While both electron microscopic and direct measurements indicate a paucity of dense granules (119) and decreased dense granule contents (adenine nucleotides, platelet serotonin, calcium, and pyrophosphate) (117, 120, 121), some of the patients studied also demonstrate a deficiency of platelet α-granule contents as well (122). Thus, the term storage pool deficiency now applies to families with isolated deficiencies of dense granules or deficiencies encompassing the α-granules as well. A number of other functional defects have been described in some patients with storage pool deficiency. These include abnormalities in arachidonic acid metabolism (abnormal arachidonate release and conversion to platelet proaggregatory thromboxane A_2, and abnormal aggregation responses to arachidonic acid) (123–127), as well as platelet lysozymal secretion abnormalities (128, 129).

As previously mentioned, this group of patients is extremely heterogeneous. In one family the defect was transmitted as an autosomal dominant trait. A platelet dysfunctional state also occurs in some individuals with the *Hermansky-Pudlak syndrome*, a rare autosomal recessive disorder characterized by oculocutaneous albinism with the accumulation of ceroid-like pigment in bone marrow macrophages (124, 125, 130, 131). Platelet storage pool disease has also been described in some patients with the *Wiskott-Aldrich* (112, 132, 133), *thrombocytopenia with absent radii* (134–136), and *Chédiak-Higashi* syndromes (137–139a,b). Thus, storage pool disease may be a common endpoint for a variety of different diseases or insults, and consequently clinical characteristics vary according to the underlying abnormality. Ultrastructural abnormalities also vary according to the primary disease. Dense bodies are virtually absent in the Hermansky-Pudlak syndrome (140), whereas in the other disease entities numerous dense bodies with markedly abnormal ultrastructural characteristics may be present (141). It is possible that the defect in the dense bodies occurs at some stage of precursor cell development (142).

Defects in Platelet Arachidonic Acid Metabolism

A mild to moderate bleeding diathesis has been described in various patients with presumed congenital deficiencies of platelet arachidonic acid (AA) metabolism. As described earlier in this chapter and in Figure 42–17, defects in this pathway may arise either at the stage of arachidonate release from platelet membrane phospholipids or as

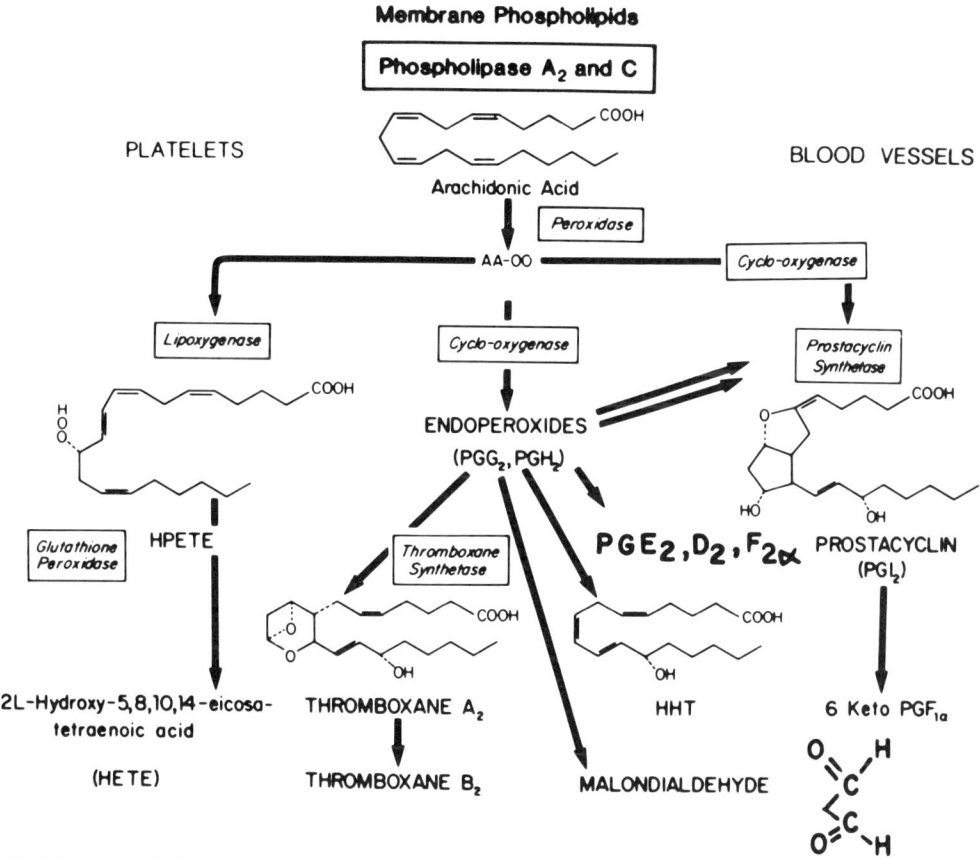

Figure 42-17. Schema depicting the pathways of arachidonic acid peroxidation and metabolite formation in the platelet and vessel wall. (Courtesy of G.H.R. Rao.)

a result of a deficiency of platelet cyclo-oxygenase or thromboxane synthetase.

Impaired release of AA from platelet membrane phospholipids, with concomitant abnormalities in platelet secretion, has been described (143). In the individuals studied, although granule contents were normal, platelet aggregation, secretion, and thromboxane B_2 production in response to the agonists ADP, epinephrine, and collagen were impaired. Arachidonic acid, however, elicited a normal response. Prelabeling of platelets with ^{3}H-AA, followed by thrombin stimulation, revealed impaired AA release, thus suggesting an abnormality of either phospholipase A_2 or phospholipase C activity. Since phosphorylation of platelet myosin light chain was found to be normal, a defect in mobilization of intracellular Ca^{++} appeared unlikely as the underlying cause of the defective AA release (phospholipase A_2 and phospholipase C are both calcium-dependent enzymes) (143). One other patient with abnormal platelet AA release due to impaired phospholipase A_2 activity has been described; this patient also demonstrated platelet storage pool deficiency (124).

Several patients have been described with an abnormality of platelet cyclo-oxygenase (144–151). Impaired aggregation to ADP, epinephrine, collagen, and arachidonic acid occurs, although a normal response to the platelet endoperoxide PGG_2 is seen. Following stimulation with ^{14}C-AA, platelets in these individuals produce normal lipoxygenase metabolites, including 12-HETE, although the formation of the platelet endoperoxide PGG_2 (the first intermediary of the cyclo-oxygenase pathway) is markedly diminished. Using a radioimmunoassay for cyclo-oxygenase, normal levels of enzyme have been found in some patients, suggesting that a functionally aberrant form of cyclo-oxygenase can occur in some individuals with this disorder (150). Whereas one patient had progressive arteriosclerosis in spite of his platelet cyclo-oxygenase deficiency (149), another manifested bleeding rather than a thrombotic tendency, despite deficiency of vascular cyclo-oxygenase and hence impairment of prostacyclin production (148).

Congenital defects affecting thromboxane synthetase have also been described (152–154). In these patients, the production of platelet thromboxane A_2 is decreased after stimulation with various agonists, including the cyclic endoperoxides. The disorder appears to be transmitted as an autosomal dominant trait (153, 154). Impaired responsiveness to normally synthesized platelet thromboxane A_2 has also been postulated to occur in some individuals with platelet dysfunction (155–157). Whether the defect involves the thromboxane A_2 platelet receptor or is due to a concomitant abnormality in ADP secretion has not been definitively established (158).

Miscellaneous Secretion Defects

This heterogeneous group of disorders includes individuals with mild to moderate platelet secretion defects usually involving the dense bodies and lysozymes. Platelets from these patients synthesize normal amounts of thromboxane A_2, and granule content is normal (159–161a). Since many platelet functions are calcium dependent, calcium mobilization in platelets has been evaluated in some of these cases in an attempt to elucidate the cause of the platelet dysfunction. Although an impairment in the platelet response to the calcium ionophore A23187 (which activates platelets by increasing levels of cytoplasmic Ca^{++}) is suggestive of a defect in Ca^{++} mobilization, this finding is not pathognomonic, since the platelet response to A23187 may be dependent on various other factors, including thromboxane synthesis. The recent availability of the fluorescent probes quin 2 and Fura 2 (which serve as indicators of cytoplasmic free Ca^{++}) should help to clarify whether defects in calcium mobilization are the cause of many of the hitherto unclassified platelet secretion abnormalities. To date, this latter investigative approach has been taken only in an occasional patient with a bleeding diathesis (161b).

Defective Platelet Metabolic Adenine Nucleotide Metabolism

A mild bleeding tendency has been observed in children with *glycogen storage disease Type I* (glucose-6-phosphatase deficiency) and *fructose 1:6 diphosphatase deficiency*. These patients also exhibit a prolongation in bleeding time, together with abnormalities in platelet aggregation and release. Although platelet nucleotides are deficient in both of these enzyme deficiency states, the ATP:ADP ratio is normal, suggesting that the metabolic pool is involved. Continuous glucose administration results in a gradual return of platelet nucleotide release and aggregation to normal, suggesting that the defect in platelet function in these hereditary disorders results from a failure of nucleotide synthesis secondary to hypoglycemia (162–164). In patients with the Lesch-Nyhan syndrome, because of the deficiency in hypoxanthine-guanine phosphoribosyl transferase (HGPRT), total platelet ATP levels are reduced to approximately 34 percent. Functional studies of these platelets have been normal, and the patients have no bleeding manifestations (165).

Defects in Platelet Procoagulant Activity

As previously discussed, platelets actively secrete, and specifically bind, various coagulation factors, providing the phospholipid surface on which the enzymatic reactions of blood coagulation occur (166). Platelets play a role in accelerating the initial reactions involving Factor XI and high-molecular-weight kininogen, and activated platelet coagulation Factor Va binds to specific plasma-membrane receptor sites, becoming, in turn, the surface receptor for Factor Xa, and thus enhancing the rate of prothrombin-to-thrombin conversion by 300,000-fold over that observed in the absence of platelets (167). Consequently, defects in platelet procoagulant activity could cause or contribute to bleeding. One of the oldest techniques used to evaluate the contribution made by platelets to the interactions of Factor Xa, Factor V, and calcium in prothrombin activation is the platelet factor 3 (PF3) assay. *Deficiency or decreased availability of PF3* has been reported in individuals who have a hemorrhagic diathesis (168–176). In these patients, platelet aggregation and secretion is generally normal, with only an occasional prolongation in bleeding time (174). Detailed studies performed on one such patient (171) revealed decreased binding of Factor Xa by the platelets, caused by a *deficiency of Factor Va binding sites* on the platelet surface (177). An interesting aspect of this case was that the bleeding diathesis resembled a plasma coagulation disorder rather than a defect in platelet function. The postsurgical maintenance of hemostasis in this individual with the use of platelet transfusions confirmed the role of platelets in this disorder. A similar defect due to a deficiency of Factor Va binding sites on the platelet surface has been described in a second individual (178).

Fibrinogen in both plasma and platelets is absent or severely decreased in patients with autosomal recessive *afibrinogenemia* (179–181a). Because of the absence of fibrinogen, primary platelet aggregation is markedly impaired, with bleeding manifestations in these individuals that resemble those of platelet defects. Spontaneous deep tissue hematomas and hemarthroses may also occur, although infrequently.

The association of a severe bleeding disorder with the *absence of platelet Factor V activity* has also been reported. This patient demonstrates that the platelet content of coagulation Factor V, and its subsequent release after platelet activation, is a critical determinant of the efficacy of the hemostatic process (181b).

Miscellaneous Disorders

The syndrome of macrothrombocytopathia, deafness, and nephritis occurs in association with a decrease in platelet count and has been termed *Epstein syndrome* (182–184a,b). Platelet functional abnormalities have been described in two of these reports, along with the morphologic finding of "Swiss-cheese" platelets. In one family, however, normal in vitro platelet function and ultrastructure were demonstrated in the presence of a clinical hemorrhagic tendency (183). This disorder, therefore, appears to be heterogeneous. The bleeding tendency is usually proportionate to the degree of thrombocytopenia.

Other macrothrombocytopathies include the *Montreal platelet syndrome*, first described by Lacombe and co-workers (185). This disorder is characterized by the appearance of giant platelets on peripheral smear, thrombocytopenia, abnormal shape change, spontaneous platelet aggregation, normal clot retraction, and a prolongation in bleeding time. Ristocetin-induced aggregation is normal, with abnormal or absent aggregation to thrombin (186a). The *May-Hegglin anomaly* is characterized by giant platelets, thrombocytopenia, and basophilic inclusions (Döhle bodies) in the leukocytes. Some patients with this disorder have a concomitant platelet functional defect. This entity is described in Part I of this chapter.

Other miscellaneous macrothrombocytopathies with thrombocytopenia and platelet ultrastructural defects have been described (186b).

A mild bleeding tendency may occur in patients with genetically determined *disorders of connective tissue*, including Ehlers-Danlos syndrome, pseudoxanthoma elasticum, osteogenesis imperfecta, and Marfan's syndrome (187–194). The bleeding time may be within the normal range or slightly prolonged. Other abnormalities include defects in platelet adhesion, platelet factor 3 release, and platelet aggregation in response to ADP, epinephrine, and collagen. Clot retraction and prothrombin consumption may also be abnormal. The platelet count is normal, although platelet size can be increased (190). Platelet ultrastructural abnormalities have also been reported in these disorders (188). Bleeding is most likely to result from the underlying connective tissue defect rather than from the mild platelet dysfunction.

Platelets from children with *Down's syndrome* have been shown to demonstrate a variety of biochemical alterations. These include low levels of platelet serotonin and decreased transport of this metabolite into platelets (195); an increased content of Na^+ and decreased content of K^+, with a decrease in ouabain-sensitive Na^+/K^+ ATPase activity (196, 197); and a decrease in platelet intracellular Ca^{++} content and uptake (198a). No bleeding diathesis, however, has been reported in these individuals.

Platelet functional abnormalities have also been described in Bartter's syndrome, adenosine deaminase deficiency, Duchenne muscular dystrophy, and idiopathic scoliosis (198b).

In *Bartter's syndrome*, abnormalities involve both aggregation and release, although the bleeding time is normal. Plasmatic factors cause the platelet abnormality, since the defect can be induced in normal platelets when resuspended in plasma from individuals with the disease (198c).

In *adenosine deaminase deficiency*, the abnormalities in platelet aggregation may be normalized by adding adenosine deaminase to the patient's platelet-rich plasma. No prolongation of bleeding time is noted in individuals with this abnormality (198b).

Duchenne muscular dystrophy is associated with impaired platelet serotonin transport and increased dense granule content of Ca^{++} (198b). No hemostatic abnormality has been observed.

In *idiopathic scoliosis*, abnormal platelet aggregation responses to the agonists ADP and epinephrine have been noted together with platelet ultrastructural abnormalities involving both the dense bodies and α-granules. No bleeding diathesis is known to occur in these individuals (198d).

Diagnosis and Management of a Patient with a Congenital Disorder of Platelet Function

The management of a patient with a congenital disorder of platelet function presupposes the ability to document that such a defect is present in the setting of clinical bleeding or history of a bleeding diathesis. Since hemostasis is dependent on vascular integrity, adequate numbers of functional blood platelets, and the presence of certain plasma factors that promote fibrin formation, evaluation of the patient will initially encompass a wide range of possible congenital or acquired abnormalities. The thorough, stepwise evaluation of a patient with a bleeding tendency generally leads to categorization of the defect and the ability to institute appropriate therapy.

Table 42–13 presents an overview of such an approach, with special emphasis being placed on the laboratory evaluation of platelet function. Successful diagnosis is aided by a thorough consideration of the patient's previous history of bleeding. Characteristic types of bleeding differentiate platelet and vascular defects from those due to plasma coagulation factor abnormalities. Platelet or vascular defects give rise to multiple superficial skin or mucosal hemorrhages that arise spontaneously or immediately following injury and which are often permanently arrested by local pressure. Deficiency of a plasma coagulation factor, on the other hand, causes deep tissue or joint hemorrhage that is difficult to control by local measures. The ingestion of one of the widely available drugs that affect platelet function (especially aspirin) in the 10 days prior to evaluation can lead to the erroneous interpretation of platelet function tests. A careful history and physical examination, as outlined in Table 42–13, will prevent the latter problem and also may provide valuable diagnostic clues to the type of disorder involved.

The approach to the management of bleeding in patients with congenital platelet disorders has not attained the degree of effectiveness available for the treatment of patients with congenital deficiencies of coagulation factors, such as hemophilia A or B. Since, with few exceptions, the specific lesion of the platelet cannot be remedied, the treatment must be more general. Our approach to the management of patients with congenital disorders of platelet function is outlined in Table 42–15. Of major importance in these patients is the avoidance of drugs that have been previously demonstrated to either increase the bleeding time or affect in vitro platelet function in normal people following their ingestion (see Table 42–18).

In women with severe menorrhagia, the regulation of menses by oral contraceptive therapy has been beneficial. Other prophylactic measures include maintenance of good oral hygiene, regular dental evaluations, and prevention of iron deficiency. In patients with a severe defect, the use of an identification bracelet stating the patient's blood type and specific diagnosis should be considered.

Table 42–15. MANAGEMENT OF PATIENTS WITH CONGENITAL DISORDERS OF PLATELET FUNCTION

Prophylactic Measures
  Avoidance of known antiplatelet drugs
  Anovulatory drugs for menorrhagia
  Good dental care
  Prevention of iron deficiency
  Identification bracelet to be considered in severe cases

Local Measures
  Amicar for intraoral bleeds
  Local pressure, packing, and topical thrombin
  Dental stents for gingival bleeds
  Salt pork, Avitene, or surgical nasal packs for epistaxis

Systemic Therapy
  Cryoprecipitate
  DDAVP
  Prednisone
  Platelet transfusion
  Volume expansion in cases of massive blood loss

Miscellaneous
  Splenectomy may be beneficial in Wiskott-Aldrich syndrome
  Bone marrow transplantation in Wiskott-Aldrich syndrome

LOCAL TREATMENT

In the event of bleeding, easily accessible sites may be treated by external measures, including local pressure (applied manually or by pressure dressings) and the use of topical thrombin. Dental stents for gingival bleeds, and salt pork nasal packs for epistaxis have also proved helpful in the management of patients with platelet disorders. Salt pork nasal packs are useful for bleeding in the posterior nares, an area not accessible to manual pressure. This local therapy is ideal in the neutropenic patient, since, unlike the case with regular nasal packs, bacterial contamination of the salt pork rarely occurs. Avitene or Surgicel nasal packs may also be used in the local treatment of epistaxis.

SYSTEMIC THERAPY

When local measures prove ineffectual or life-threatening internal hemorrhage occurs, platelet transfusions may be necessary to control blood loss. However, as previously discussed, patients with absence of the functional membrane glycoproteins Ib or IIb/IIIa—i.e., those with Bernard-Soulier syndrome or Glanzmann's thromboasthenia—will develop antiplatelet alloantibodies against the platelet glycoproteins that they lack following transfusion therapy. In addition to destroying the transfused platelets, these antibodies will also alter the functional activity of any remaining transfused platelets that may circulate.

Since Chapter 48 deals in depth with the administration of platelet concentrates, the details of platelet storage will not be discussed here. Suffice it to say that a unit of platelet concentrate should contain at least 5.5×10^{10} platelets. Following transfusion, approximately 50 to 70 per cent of the transfused platelets should be recovered from the recipient's circulation in the absence of conditions such as splenomegaly, infection, disseminated intravascular coagulation (DIC), or the presence of antiplatelet antibodies that cause a poor recovery. Dosage of platelet concentrates is calculated as follows: *adult*—1 unit of platelets increases the platelet count in a 70-kg adult by approximately 5000 cells per μl; *child*—1 unit of platelets increases the platelet count by approximately 10,000 cells per μl for each square meter of body surface area.

There are no definitive recommendations regarding the approach to patients requiring repeated platelet transfusions for serious hemorrhage. If platelet transfusions become necessary, we suggest the initial use of random single donor platelet concentrates (199). Since repeated transfusions are frequently complicated by a refractory state that is associated with alloimmunization primarily due to HLA incompatibility, an HLA-identical donor (if available) should be used for subsequent transfusions once refractoriness develops.

Such donors are most commonly available among siblings who have a 25 per cent chance of being HLA identical. When the patient is negative for the HLA-A2 antigen (50 per cent of the general population), prolonged platelet support may be provided by avoiding HLA-A2-positive donors. If an HLA-identical sibling is not available, the probability of a nonrelated donor being HLA identical is much less than 1 in 1000. If a complete HLA match is not available, a close match may prove better than a random match. It should be noted that, in patients with congenital disorders of platelet function, an added complication exists in the assessment of response to platelet concentrates—that is, the presence usually in the recipient of a normal or near-normal platelet count prior to transfusion. Thus, the response to a transfusion is mainly assessed by its clinical efficacy in the bleeding patient and by correction of a prolonged bleeding time. Irradiation of concentrates may be indicated to prevent graft-versus-host disease in selected recipients (e.g., patients with Wiskott-Aldrich syndrome in whom bone marrow transplantation may be contemplated). In patients who are refractory to platelet transfusions, the use of high-dose intravenous IgG to induce reticuloendothelial Fc blockade and increase the level of transfused platelets in the circulation has been attempted with success in some (200–202), but not all (203), reported cases. However, this therapy will not affect alloantibodies that bind to platelets and impair their function. Plasmapheresis followed by the administration of platelet concentrates may be necessary in the event of a major hemorrhagic episode.

An intriguing observation is the use of infusions of cryoprecipitate to temporarily decrease the bleeding time in patients with congenital storage pool deficiency (204). Instead of platelet transfusions, prophylactic administration of cryoprecipitate was used prior to surgery in these patients, to prevent intraoperative bleeding. Although no corroborative information on the use of cryoprecipitate by others is available at this time, this approach clearly warrants further investigation in patients with congenital disorders of platelet function. If temporary hemostasis can be achieved, cryoprecipitate may prove preferable to platelet transfusions, since it will obviate the problem of platelet alloimmunization. Recently, Kobrinsky and co-workers (205) reported the successful use of 1-desamino-8-D-arginine vasopressin (DDAVP) in shortening the bleeding time in patients with congenital and acquired platelet dysfunctions. An advantage of this agent is that, since it is not a blood product, it carries no risk of either alloimmunization or infection. However, other investigators have not been able to achieve a shortening of the bleeding time in patients with storage pool deficiency who were given DDAVP (206). The use of DDAVP in patients with qualitative platelet defects has therefore yet to be definitively established.

A short course (3 to 5 days) of oral prednisone (40 mg per m^2) may be used for specific problems when local measures have not successfully controlled bleeding and when the degree of blood loss does not compel the immediate institution of platelet replacement therapy. Although steroids have not been shown to normalize platelet function under these circumstances, they may help to maintain hemostasis by a possible endothelial supportive role (207), and by decreasing prostacyclin production by vascular endothelium (208).

The fibrinolytic blocking agent epsilon-aminocaproic acid (Amicar) has also been used successfully in the management of oral cavity bleeds in patients with hemophilia A and B. We have used Amicar for 5 to 7 days for oral lacerations and for intraoral dental procedures in patients with qualitative platelet defects, with or without the use of other systemic measures, depending on the magnitude of the bleeding. Potent fibrinolytic activators that disrupt preformed clots or inhibit hemostatic clot formation are normally present in saliva. Following oral ingestion, Amicar is secreted into saliva, inhibiting fibrinolysis. It is given as a syrup or tablet at an initial dose of 200 mg per kg, followed by 100 mg per kg every 4 to 6 hours. The maximum adult dose is 24 g per day (209). Amicar is contraindicated in the presence of liver disease or hematuria. It has also been reported that Amicar can interfere with platelet function by inhibiting platelet-fibrinogen binding (210).

An occasional individual has been treated with bone marrow transplantation, with correction of the congenital platelet defect (Glanzmann's thrombasthenia [211]) or of both the platelet and immune abnormalities (Wiskott-Aldrich syndrome [212, 213]). Splenectomy has also been performed in some patients with congenital disorders of platelet function and concomitant thrombocytopenia, including Bernard-Soulier disease and the Wiskott-Aldrich syndrome. In the former entity, although a transient increase in platelet count has been demonstrated after splenectomy, no lasting clinical benefit is apparent. Splenectomy may be of benefit in the management of some patients with the Wiskott-Aldrich syndrome by producing a sustained rise in platelet count and an improvement in hemostatic function (214). However, because some patients not taking prophylactic antibiotics post splenectomy can die of sepsis, the advantages and disadvantages of splenectomy must be carefully weighed in the individual patient.

In summary, this group of disorders is heterogeneous both in the nature of the defects involved and in the variability in severity of the bleeding manifestations. The hemorrhagic diathesis is variable not only among the various congenital platelet disorders but often even among individually affected family members. Our plan of management, which employs prophylactic, local and systemic modalities of therapy, has to be tailored to the individual needs of the patient, and should be tried in every patient prior to the use of platelet replacement therapy. If these measures fail, or in the event of life-threatening hemorrhage, the use of platelet transfusion will become necessary. The benefits of such therapy should be carefully balanced against its potential risk—i.e., alloimmunization, especially in Bernard-Soulier syndrome and Glanzmann's thrombasthenia. Indeed, it has been our experience that the management of a severely bleeding alloimmunized patient with an inherited disorder of platelet function is almost impossible. Platelet transfusions given to these patients are rapidly cleared or rendered ineffective by the alloantibody. It is possible that by concomitantly administering intravenous IgG one can reduce the rate of clearance of these platelets, but this treatment will not affect alloantibodies that bind to platelets and impair their function.

PHYSIOLOGIC QUALITATIVE ABNORMALITIES

Neonatal Platelet Function

A variety of qualitative abnormalities have been observed in the neonatal platelet. Defects in adhesion have been shown by some investigators (215), but not by others (216). Abnormalities in platelet aggregation to low doses of adenosine diphosphate (ADP), collagen, epinephrine, and thrombin have been demonstrated by most investigators who have conducted systematic studies of platelet aggregation in normal neonates in whom maternal drug ingestion of antiplatelet agents was ruled out (217–221).

Most marked is the abnormality in aggregation using epinephrine as the stimulus. This impairment is probably related to the deficiency in α-adrenergic receptor sites that has been demonstrated on the neonatal platelet membrane. Corby and O'Barr (222) showed that platelets from the neonate exhibit normal affinities for ^{3}H-dihydroergocryptine (DHE; an α-adrenergic antagonist) and epinephrine, but bound less than one-half the amount of DHE bound by maternal platelets. Reduced binding was not due to in vivo occupancy of platelet α-adrenergic receptors by circulating endogenous catecholamines. The impaired aggregation response of the neonatal platelet to the other agonists could be due to a deficiency of secretable products, including nonmetabolic nucleotides stored within the platelet (i.e., storage pool deficiency), or the abnormality could reside in the stimulus-response coupling cascade necessary for normal platelet function.

Studies to elucidate a neonatal platelet storage pool deficiency have yielded conflicting results. Corby and Zuck (218) found a slightly decreased total ADP and ATP content in newborn platelets, with decreased release of storage (nonmetabolic) ADP and ATP following stimulation with collagen. They further demonstrated normal values for specific radioactivities of platelet ATP and ADP following incubation of platelets with ^{3}H- or ^{14}C-adenine. One of their findings (decreased total nucleotides) suggested a storage-pool deficiency, whereas the other (normal values for specific radioactivities) suggested that the abnormality was not a storage pool type defect. Since their observed decrease in total nucleotides was minimal when compared with that seen in true storage pool–deficient platelets, and since stimulation with suprathreshold concentrations of collagen resulted in the release of normal amounts of adenine nucleotides, these authors concluded that platelets in the newborn did not demonstrate a classic storage pool deficiency syndrome. Some minimal decrease in ADP and ATP content was present, however, in both the metabolic and nonmetabolic pools (218). In contrast to the previously described study, Whaun has reported that platelets from term infants contain normal amounts of total adenine nucleotides (223). However, following the prelabeling of platelet-rich plasma with ^{3}H-adenine, Whaun also demonstrated marked elevations of specific radioactivity of ADP and ATP in resting neonatal platelets, a finding suggestive of storage pool disease. It is possible that the conflicting results of Corby versus Whaun may be due to differences in procurement of the blood samples, since platelets from cord blood (unless meticulously collected) could have undergone partial activation and release, resulting in an in vitro artefactual storage pool–like deficiency. Since no marker of platelet release was concomitantly evaluated (plasma platelet factor 4 activity), platelet activation in the cord blood samples prior to testing cannot be ruled out in the latter study.

Studies of arachidonic acid metabolism in the platelet of the neonate have provided evidence that the neonatal platelet defect is not "aspirin-like" in nature (224–226). Using platelet malonyldialdehyde formation as an indicator of platelet endoperoxide synthesis, neonatal platelets were found to produce arachidonate metabolites in amounts sufficient to cause irreversible aggregation when mixed with platelets from adult donors who had recently ingested aspirin (224). Follow-up studies have provided evidence that endogenous thromboxane production in neonatal platelet-rich plasma in response to thrombin and collagen is similar to that observed in platelets from adults (225). Impaired thromboxane production was observed in response to epinephrine stimulation, an observation in keeping with previous findings that neonatal platelets respond with markedly impaired aggregation and nucleotide release to this cathecholamine. Studies of exogenous arachidonate metabolism in the neonatal platelet have provided evidence of enhanced arachidonic acid release from platelet membrane phospholipids following thrombin stimulation, coupled with a decrease in cyclo-oxygenase activity (226). Another interesting observation is the heightened response in thromboxane production by neonatal platelet-rich plasma in response to exogenous arachidonic acid (225), a finding that may be due to significant differences in the binding capacities for arachidonic acid between neonatal and adult plasmas (227).

Other miscellaneous investigations have shown a fairly normal ultrastructure for platelets from term neonates (221), abnormalities in platelet factor 3 content and release (215), low serotonin content and release (228), and normal release of platelet α-granule products (platelet factor 4)(220). Aggregation of neonatal platelet-rich plasma in response to ristocetin is increased, although the cause of this phenomenon has not been ascertained (221). Evidence also suggests that membrane glycoproteins in platelets from newborns are similar to those from adults (229, 230). Thus, investigation of neonatal platelet function has not conclusively identified the cause of the impairment in platelet aggregation and release. Unequivocal evidence for storage pool deficiency has not been obtained by either study using platelets prelabeled with ^{3}H-adenine, and neonatal platelet ultrastructural findings do not support an abnormality in dense body formation. Differences in membrane receptors may be responsible for some of the impaired platelet responses, although unequivocal evidence for such differences have been shown only in the case of the α-adrenergic sites. The relationship of the mild platelet secretion defect to changes in intracellular Ca^{++} mobilization and other second messenger product formation has not been studied. Although of interest, the in vitro platelet functional abnormalities do not find a counterpart in the most crucial test of in vivo platelet-vascular interactions—the bleeding time. Both term and preterm infants have been documented to possess normal bleeding times (216, 231), and the healthy term infant does not suffer from an enhanced bleeding tendency. Both the term and the premature infant, however, demonstrate a bleeding tendency when their hemostatic mechanisms are stressed—for example, by maternal drug ingestion prior to delivery (386a, b).

ACQUIRED QUALITATIVE PLATELET ABNORMALITIES

An impairment in the ability of the platelet to perform its crucial role in primary hemostasis may be the consequence of a temporary defect induced by the ingestion of various types of drugs. A functional platelet defect may also arise secondary to a more persistent defect caused by a variety of systemic disease states that may interfere with platelet function by producing either intrinsically defective platelets or plasma metabolites that can interfere with platelet function.

Uremia

The bleeding tendency associated with uremia is in part due to a defect in platelet function. The picture may also be complicated by the presence of coagulation abnormalities and thrombocytopenia. The platelet qualitative abnormalities include a decrease in platelet adhesion, impaired platelet factor 3 availability, defective platelet aggregation, and a prolongation in the bleeding time (232–238a, b) The platelet dysfunction, as well as the bleeding tendency, can be corrected within 24 to 48 hours following hemodialysis or peritoneal dialysis (233). The abnormality therefore appears to be due to a plasma factor or to the presence of retained metabolites. Both guanidinosuccinic acid and phenolic acid have been implicated in the impairment in platelet function (238a, 239). Investigators have also separated uremic serum by gel filtration using Sephadex G-15 and have shown that several peaks of the middle molecular range inhibit normal platelet function (240–243a). Other investigators have suggested that secondary hyperparathyroidism and elevated plasma levels of parathormone could cause some of the abnormalities observed in platelet aggregation and secretion (243b). Abnormalities in the balance between platelet and vascular prostaglandin synthesis have also been described. A decrease in platelet proaggregatory thromboxane synthesis due to a functional deficiency of cyclo-oxygenase has been observed (244, 245), as well as an increase in plasma factor(s) that stimulate prostacyclin release from vascular endothelium (246, 247).

Platelet transfusions do not control bleeding in patients with uremia. Besides dialysis, two other recent therapeutic modalities have been successfully used in the acute management of such patients: cryoprecipitate (248) and the use of 1-desamino-8-D-arginine vasopressin (DDAVP) (249). A temporary correction of the bleeding time without correction of platelet abnormalities occurs following either of these therapies. Since levels of both Factor VIII:C and ristocetin cofactor, as well as the larger multimeric forms of VWF, are normal in patients with uremia, the reason why this treatment corrects a prolonged bleeding time is unknown. Correction could be related to a hitherto unrecognized effect on platelets (250), to a local effect of the drug on the vessel wall (251a, b), or to a decrease in vascular prostacyclin production (252). The last possibility is unlikely to be the major mechanism for the DDAVP effect on bleeding time, since bleeding time correction also occurs after aspirin ingestion in normal volunteers (253). In the daily management of these individuals, correction of concomitant anemia appears to lessen the bleeding tendency and the prolongation in bleeding time (254, 255). Other modalities that have been used to normalize the bleeding time include the use of a conjugated estrogen preparation (256). A shortening of the bleeding time for up to 10 days was observed following discontinuation of the drug.

Liver Disease

The hemostatic defects observed in liver disease are so complex that the contribution of platelet functional abnormalities to the overall bleeding tendency is difficult to assess. A deficiency of plasma coagulation factors, the occurrence of diffuse intravascular coagulation, enhanced fibrinolysis, dysfibrinogenemia, and thrombocytopenia all lead to a hemorrhagic tendency (257, 258).

Qualitative platelet abnormalities have also been described and include impaired in vivo adhesiveness, defects in platelet aggregation, and a decrease in platelet factor 3 availability (259–263). Since the dialysate from patients with cirrhosis can inhibit normal platelet aggregation, these abnormalities probably are the result of a plasma factor (262, 264). Fibrinogen degradation products (FDP) are well known to interfere with platelet aggregation and to contribute to the hemostatic failure that results from disseminated intravascular coagulation (265, 266). Thomas has suggested that the presence of FDP in patients with liver failure may be the cause of the platelet functional abnormality, an effect due to the binding of FDP to the platelet-fibrinogen receptor, with resulting impairment in the aggregation response (264). However, the abnormality in aggregation is observed at FDP levels that are not sufficiently elevated to cause impaired platelet function in vivo (267). The dysfibrinogenemia of liver disease is also unlikely to be the cause of the abnormalities in platelet function (268). Inconsistent abnormalities in platelet membrane glycoproteins have been described in patients with cirrhosis (269). A thorough evaluation of the roles of both coagulation and platelet mechanisms should be undertaken in an individual patient prior to starting appropriate replacement therapy. Recently, the use of DDAVP to temporarily shorten the bleeding time in individuals with liver disease has been advocated to prepare these individuals for surgical procedures and liver biopsies (253, 270). However, the effect is relatively short-lived, and since complex hemostatic derangements are usually present, the sole use of this agent may not be sufficient to prevent hemorrhage. As in patients with uremia, individuals with liver disease have normal or high baseline levels of vWF, and the multimeric structure of their vWF is similar to the pattern observed in healthy subjects. Thus, the definitive mechanism of the bleeding time correction by DDAVP is unknown. A shortening of the partial thromboplastin time and prothrombin time, together with an increase in various intrinsic coagulation factor activities, has also been noted after DDAVP administration in patients with hepatic dysfunction (253, 271).

Qualitative Platelet Defects Following Cardiopulmonary Bypass and in Children with Congenital or Acquired Cardiac Defects

Hemorrhage occurs following cardiopulmonary bypass surgery in approximately 10 to 25 per cent of patients. It is crucial that nonsurgical hemorrhage be readily distinguished from surgical bleeding in these individuals, so that appropriate measures can be instituted. Bleeding can result from vascular tears and lacerations, inadequate heparin neutralization, consumption or dilution of coagulation factors, and hyperfibrinolysis, as well as from defined and clinically significant qualitative platelet defects (272, 273). In fact, platelet dysfunction probably is the major cause of bleeding after bypass surgery. Platelet dysfunction following cardiopulmonary bypass surgery and in children with acquired heart disease has been extensively reviewed in Part I of this chapter and will not be discussed here.

Myeloproliferative Disorders

It is well recognized that patients with essential thrombocythemia, polycythemia rubra vera, chronic myelogenous leukemia, and myelofibrosis can suffer from a bleeding tendency in the presence of a normal or increased platelet count. In general, whereas individuals with polycythemia rubra vera are prone to thrombosis, those with myeloid metaplasia and essential thrombocythemia tend to be more prone to bleeding (274). Bleeding and/or thrombosis occurs least frequently in chronic myelogenous leukemia. The risk of complications also increases significantly with age, young adults with essential thrombocythemia being remarkably free of thrombohemorrhagic symptoms (275). The types of bleeding observed are characteristic of platelet-vascular dysfunction, with ecchymoses, epistaxis, and mucosal hemorrhages commonly noted, occasionally occurring in paradoxical association with thromboses (deep venous, pulmonary embolism, coronary, cerebrovascular, and peripheral). In essential thrombocythemia, two characteristic microvascular patterns of thromboses can occur: (a) digital ischemia and (b) involvement of the cerebral circulation with neurologic manifestations (276, 277).

A variety of platelet defects have been observed in patients with myeloproliferative syndromes and these are outlined in Table 42–16. Theoretically, some of the abnormalities should cause thromboses (spontaneous aggregation, loss of PGD_2 receptors, increased coagulant activity, increased Fc receptors), whereas others should potentiate bleeding (loss of α-adrenergic receptors, storage pool disease, decreased arachidonate release); however, there is no correlation in any individual between the in vitro findings and the patient's clinical course. The abnormalities are also only infrequently accompanied by a prolongation in bleeding time (268, 274, 278). An occasional case of an abnormal bleeding time and acquired von Willebrand's disease has also been documented in the myeloproliferative syndromes (279a).

In patients with polycythemia rubra vera, thrombotic complications are correlated with changes in hematocrit (279b). There is, however, no clear-cut correlation between the platelet count and the frequency of either hemorrhage or thrombosis (279b–281). Thus, in the asymptomatic young patient, no therapy is usually indicated, even when the platelet count is >1 million per μl (274). Alkylating agents are especially contraindicated, since this form of treatment has been shown to increase the risk of leukemia (282). In patients with active bleeding or thromboses, measures to reduce the level of the platelet count with chemotherapeutic agents such as hydroxyurea and thrombocytophoresis may be appropriate. Antiplatelet therapy has not been shown to prevent thromboses in patients with polycythemia rubra vera randomized prospectively to either placebo therapy or aspirin (300 mg tid) and persantine (75 mg tid) (283). In fact, the use of aspirin has been associated with bleeding in individuals with myeloproliferative disorders (281). Its use should therefore be reserved for only those situations in which symptoms suggestive of microvascular arterial thrombi are present (284).

Preleukemia and Acute Leukemia

Bleeding diatheses have occurred in individuals with leukemia in the presence of a normal platelet count. Although most of the patients identified with such qualitative platelet defects are those with acute granulocytic leukemia, this complication has also been noted in individuals with preleukemia, myelomonocytic leukemia, lymphocytic leukemia, and hairy-cell leukemia (285–290). Morphologic abnormalities include giant platelets with disorganized microtubules and decreased storage organelles (291). Functional defects include abnormalities in aggregation and secretion suggestive of both storage pool deficiency and primary secretory defects. Abnormalities in platelet coagulant activity, thromboxane synthesis, and thrombin binding sites have also been reported (285, 286, 288–290, 292). Clinically, platelet transfusions are indicated in such individuals for bleeding symptoms that may occur at platelet counts above the level of 20,000 to 30,000 per μl.

Miscellaneous Disorders

Acquired defects in platelet function may be associated with a variety of conditions; these are listed in Table 42–17. Acquired platelet storage pool deficiency occurs in many of these disorders, often as a result of thrombin- or antibody-mediated platelet activation and partial release.

DRUG–INDUCED PLATELET DYSFUNCTION

Although drug-induced platelet dysfunction can contribute to bleeding, drug ingestion under most circumstances does not give rise to spontaneous hemorrhage. However, if the patient's hemostatic mechanisms are impaired by pre-existing qualitative or quantitative abnormalities affecting the platelets, clotting factors, or vascular integrity, administration of a drug that impairs platelet function may cause serious hemorrhage.

Table 42–16. PLATELET ABNORMALITIES IN PATIENTS WITH MYELOPROLIFERATIVE SYNDROMES*

Morphologic
1. Heterogeneous, with increased size distribution
2. Decreased numbers of dense bodies
3. Disorganization of microtubules
4. Hypertrophy of dense tubular and open canalicular systems

Functional
1. Abnormal adhesion
2. Abnormal aggregation responses (complete absence of response to epinephrine; abnormalities with ADP and collagen, and occasional spontaneous aggregation)
3. Storage-pool deficiency (dense bodies ± α-granules)
4. Defective serotonin uptake
5. Receptor abnormalities (loss of α-adrenergic and PGD_2 receptors; increased Fc receptors)
6. Abnormalities in arachidonate metabolism (defective arachidonic acid release from membrane phospholipids; usually normal cyclo-oxygenase activity; decreased lipoxygenase activity)
7. Variable platelet coagulant activities
8. Alterations in platelet membrane glycoproteins

*Individual references for the abnormalities noted are listed at the end of the chapter (refs. 268, 274, and 278).

Table 42–17. OTHER ACQUIRED DISORDERS ASSOCIATED WITH IMPAIRMENT IN PLATELET FUNCTIONS

Acidosis (293, 294)*
Antibody (ITP, lupus, toxemia) (295–299a,b,c)
Atopic states (300)
Crises in sickle cell anemia (301–306)
Disseminated intravascular coagulation (307)
Dysproteinemias (268, 308)
Essential fatty acid deficiency (309)
Hemangioma (310)
Hyperbilirubinemia (311, 312)
Hypothyroidism (313, 314)
Intralipid infusion (315)
Infections (316)
Inflammatory bowel disease (317)
Nutritional (feeding of omega-3-polyunsaturated fatty acids, vitamin E administration, megaloblastic anemias) (318a–n, 319, 320)
Postoperative states (321, 322)
Phototherapy (323)
Renal transplant rejection (324)
Replacement therapy in hemophilia (325)
Scurvy (326–328)
Stress (329–331)
Stored platelets (332, 333)
Thermal injury (334)
Thrombotic thrombocytopenic purpura/hemolytic uremic syndrome (324, 335, 336)

*Numbers refer to references at end of chapter.

Since many of the important drug-related effects are due to inhibition of platelet cyclo-oxygenase activity, a summary of platelet arachidonic acid metabolism (Fig. 42–17) will precede the discussion of specific drug-related effects. Following the exposure of platelets to a variety of agonists (ADP, epinephrine, low-dose collagen, or thrombin), arachidonic acid (AA) is released from platelet membrane phospholipid by the activation of several enzymes, including phospholipase A_2 and the sequential activation of phospholipase C and diglyceride lipase (29, 30–30d). In intact platelets, loss of AA through the phospholipase A_2 pathway occurs primarily from phosphatidylcholine. Platelet cyclo-oxygenase catalyzes the synthesis from AA of the labile endoperoxides PGG_2 and H_2. Thromboxane A_2, which is produced from PGH_2 by the enzyme thromboxane synthetase, is a potent platelet aggregating and vasoconstrictor agent with a very short half-life (31–34). While thromboxane A_2 is the major AA product in activated platelets, conversion of PGH_2 to PGD_2, PGE_2 and $PGF_2\alpha$ via endoperoxide isomerases and reductase occurs, although this conversion is minimal in stimulated platelets.

Incubation of AA with human platelet suspensions has also led to the isolation and identification of additional transformation products from PGH_2; 12L-hydroxy-heptadecatrienoic acid (HHT) and a three-carbon fragment, malonaldehyde (31). HHT stimulates leukocyte chemotaxis (31) and also has recently been shown to stimulate endothelial cell prostacyclin synthesis by an effect on vascular cyclo-oxygenase (337). Prostacyclin synthetase, an enzyme present in the innermost lining of human arteries and veins, catalyzes the synthesis of vascular prostacyclin (PGI_2) from the labile platelet endoperoxides or directly from endogenously released vascular arachidonic acid. Prostacyclin is a potent physiologic inhibitor of platelet aggregation and secretion (338, 339). It has been suggested that a balance between the formation of proaggregatory thromboxane synthesized by the platelets and antiaggregatory prostacyclin synthesized by the endothelial cells plays a critical role in the modulation of hemostasis (340–342). Figure 42–17 shows that arachidonic acid can also be converted via the platelet lipoxygenase pathway to 12-hydroperoxy-eicosatetraenoic acid (HPETE), a fatty acid that is then reduced to the final product 12L-hydroxy-eicosatetraenoic acid (HETE). Significant amounts of 12-HETE are formed after platelet stimulation, although no definitive functional role has been assigned to this pathway. Platelet 12-HPETE inhibits prostacyclin synthetase in the animal model, and low concentrations also inhibit human platelet thromboxane production (343).

Nonsteroidal Anti-Inflammatory Agents

ACETYLSALICYLIC ACID (ASPIRIN)

Aspirin ingestion was identified as early as 1945 as a possible etiologic factor in postoperative hemorrhage (344). However, the effects of this compound on platelet function were not evaluated for another two decades. The ubiquity of aspirin in over-the-counter and prescription preparations is exemplified by a list of such drugs made in 1976 (345).

Mode of Action. Acetylsalicylic acid was the first agent identified as an inhibitor of cyclo-oxygenase (346a, b), causing a time-dependent inactivation of the enzyme (347). The mechanism of this inactivation has been well characterized. Roth and co-workers demonstrated that in human platelets, acetylsalicylic acid transfers its acetate moiety to a serine residue at the active site of the cyclo-oxygenase molecule (348, 349). This finding has been confirmed by others (350). Although the resultant enzyme is devoid of catalytic activity, it does not undergo extensive conformational alteration, since monoclonal antibodies against native cyclo-oxygenase are equally reactive toward the aspirin-acetylated enzyme (351). Since the covalent modification of cyclo-oxygenase by aspirin is not reversible, and since platelets cannot synthesize new enzyme, the defect persists for the lifetime of the platelet. As a result of this inhibition, aspirin prevents the generation of the labile endoperoxides PGG_2 and PGH_2 from arachidonic acid, with consequent inhibition of the synthesis of the proaggregatory compound thromboxane A_2 (352–355). The inhibitory effect of aspirin on secondary platelet aggregation and dense body release induced by ADP and epinephrine, as well as the inhibition of collagen-induced aggregation, is in keeping with the inhibition of thromboxane A_2 synthesis, since secondary aggregation with these agents is mediated via the arachidonate pathway. Primary ADP-induced aggregation is independent of the arachidonate pathway and is not inhibited by aspirin. Thrombin has other modes of action by which it induces platelet aggregation and release independent of the arachidonate pathway. Aspirin is therefore a very weak inhibitor of thrombin-induced aggregation and release (356a). Aspirin also does not inhibit α-granule or lysozomal release (356b), or platelet adhesion at physiologic rates of flow (356c).

The synthesis of PGI_2 in cultured human endothelial cells and arterial smooth muscle cells is also inhibited by aspirin (357, 358). The actions of aspirin on prostaglandin synthesis therefore can be a double-edged sword, since it prevents the synthesis of both vascular prostacyclin (a potent vasodilator and platelet inhibitor), and platelet thromboxane A_2 (a potent proaggregatory metabolite).

Evaluation of the dosage of aspirin required to produce an optimal antithrombotic effect has therefore been seen by many investigators as a matter of therapeutic interest. It was initially suggested that a differential sensitivity of platelet versus vascular cyclo-oxygenase might exist, so that an ideal dose of aspirin (that would block platelet thromboxane while leaving vascular prostacyclin production relatively intact) could be made available. Indeed, initial animal studies (359, 360) suggested that vascular prostacyclin production was inhibited only by large dosages of aspirin (150 mg per kg of body weight). However, studies in humans have not shown a clear-cut differential sensitivity between the vascular and platelet enzymes at conventional aspirin doses. In normal controls, aspirin at a dosage of 1 to 4 mg per kg of body weight was enough to block both platelet thromboxane and vascular prostacyclin activity (361–364). Prostacyclin production by normal venous tissue was inhibited by a single 300 mg dose of aspirin, and was partially inhibited by 80 mg (362, 365). Although in two reports a single low dose of 40 mg of aspirin inhibited platelet thromboxane without a marked concomitant inhibition of vascular prostacyclin (365, 366), in a third study this dose when given daily for 4 days caused inhibition of both prostacyclin and thromboxane synthesis (367).

Comparison of such in vivo studies is complicated not only by differences between single-versus-multiple dosage therapy but also by the possible differing sensitivities of arterial-versus-venous cyclo-oxygenase, as well as the sensitivities of normal-versus-atheromatous vessels to aspirin-induced prostacyclin inhibition (366). Some of these problems have been resolved in a study by Fitzgerald and co-workers (368), who measured the urinary metabolites 2,3-dinor-6-keto-$PGF_1α$ and 2,3-dinor-TXB_2 (the major urinary metabolites of prostacyclin and thromboxane A_2 respectively) in normal subjects following continuing aspirin administration. This study of urinary prostaglandin metabolites provides us with important data on the inhibition of *microvascular* prostacyclin synthesis, and reflects the contribution of microvascular endothelium, which composes approximately 95 per cent of the vascular surface. Fitzgerald and colleagues demonstrated that although thromboxane formation is highly susceptible to aspirin inhibition, prostacyclin biosynthesis was less markedly affected over a daily dosage range of 20 to 2600 mg aspirin. Although the urinary excretion of the thromboxane B_2 metabolite was significantly reduced at aspirin dosages of 80 mg per day and above, the inhibition of the dinor-6-keto product attained significance only at aspirin doses >160 mg per day. Relatively similar results were achieved by Patrignani and associates (364). It is possible that the use of thromboxane synthetase inhibitors in combination with very low doses of aspirin may permit an antiplatelet effect with endothelial "sparing" (369). Although some investigators have suggested that high doses of aspirin (which totally abolishes prostacyclin synthesis) can shorten the bleeding time in humans or animals, this is not a universal finding (370, 371). More important, aspirin is clinically effective at doses that abolish vascular prostacyclin biosynthesis (372), since at these relatively higher doses multicenter trials have shown a reduction in cardiac death and the prevention of myocardial reinfarction, stroke, or transient ischemic attacks (372, 373). In some but not all studies, aspirin was also more effective in males than in females, but the reasons for the sex difference in antithrombotic activity are unknown (373–377a, b).

It is possible that some of the antithrombotic effects of aspirin are mediated via alternate mechanisms. For example aspirin reduces the activity of the vitamin K–dependent coagulation factors, probably as a result of inhibition of gamma carboxylation (378a). Aspirin also enhances whole blood fibrinolytic activity (378b), enhances the conversion of ADP to antiaggregatory adenosine (372), and rechannels released arachidonic acid toward the formation of lipoxygenase metabolites (374).

Thus, although a theoretical case has been made for use of low-dose aspirin by proponents of the thromboxane A_2-prostacyclin "balance" theory, other evidence seems to point to the possibility that this "balance" has been overestimated, and that a rigorous search for possible other effects of aspirin on hemostasis should be actively pursued.

Clinical and Diagnostic Implications. In normal individuals the ingestion of ≤1 g aspirin produces a slight prolongation of the bleeding time without a marked bleeding tendency. However, this is not the case in individuals in whom the aspirin-induced platelet dysfunction is superimposed either on pre-existing deficiencies in the fluid phase of coagulation or on qualitative or quantitative platelet abnormalities. In hemophilias A and B, bleeding times following aspirin ingestion have been demonstrated to be markedly prolonged (10 minutes to greater than 40 minutes in some cases) (379). Quick described marked prolongation of the bleeding time and proposed the use of the "aspirin tolerance test" as an ancillary diagnostic tool in the identification of patients with von Willebrand's disease (380). This observation has been confirmed by others (381–382). The "aspirin-tolerance test" has also been shown to identify patients with "intermediate" syndromes of platelet dysfunction (382, 383). In pathologic disease states associated with platelet dysfunction, the ingestion of aspirin can markedly prolong bleeding times and exacerbate the existing clinical hemostatic abnormalities (380, 384).

Aspirin ingestion can also alter clinical hemostasis in the neonate. In 1970, Bleyer and Breckenridge (385) demonstrated that aspirin ingestion was associated with an increased incidence of clinical bleeding in the full-term neonate. We have been able to confirm this observation (386a). In our study, we used the inhibition of platelet malonyldialdehyde formation by aspirin to document aspirin ingestion by mothers in the week prior to delivery. Clinical abnormalities in hemostasis were present in neonates whose mothers had ingested aspirin within 5 days of delivery. The hemostatic abnormalities consisted mainly of bleeding into the skin and mucous membranes, with major manifestations that included a cephalhematoma, bleeding from a circumcision site for greater than 24 hours, and profuse petechiae over the presenting part. Other workers have also suggested that the rate of intracranial hemorrhage is higher in premature infants whose mothers had ingested aspirin in the week prior to delivery (386b).

Aspirin can induce small amounts of gastrointestinal bleeding, which usually is occult. Such bleeding is the result of hemostatic alterations plus the effects of aspirin on local prostaglandin synthesis (387–389). PGE_2 protects against mucosal injury and prevents the aspirin-induced fall in gastric transmucosal potential difference induced by aspirin. Anecdotal reports have linked aspirin ingestion to gastrointestinal hemorrhage, but given the high prevalence of aspirin ingestion in the normal population, these reports are difficult to assess (390, 391).

The effect of aspirin on platelets also has been used as a diagnostic tool in the determination of platelet life span. This technique takes advantage of the fact that the formation of the platelet endoperoxides PGG_2 and PGF_2 and their by-product malonyldialdehyde (Fig. 42–17) is permanently inhibited by the ingestion of a single dose of aspirin (392a). Malonyldialdehyde formation gradually returns to baseline values over a 10-day period, thereby permitting the calculation of platelet life span by this nonradioisotope technique. Using the specific inhibition of platelet cyclo-oxygenase by aspirin, Burch and co-workers (392b) have also shown that the enzyme activity returns to normal with a time course that reflects platelet turnover (life span 8.2 ± 2 days). Although this technique has been used to document a shortened platelet survival in pathologic states associated with pregnancy (in which radioactive platelet should be avoided), under certain assay conditions it may not parallel a radiolabeled platelet life span study (392c).

Several other compounds that have anti-inflammatory, analgesic, or antipyretic properties can be safely used when the aspirin-associated inhibition of platelet function is contraindicated. Sodium salicylate (393a–393c) and salicylate choline (Arthropan) (393d) do not induce a platelet dysfunction and can be safely prescribed for patients with arthritis. Acetaminophen (Tylenol), propoxyphene (Darvon), or codeine and pentazocine (Talwin) can be substituted when an antipyretic or analgesic effect comparable to aspirin is desired, since the former drugs have not been demonstrated to induce hemostatic abnormalities, even in patients with pre-existing disorders of intrinsic clotting (393c–f).

INDOMETHACIN

Indomethacin has been characterized in vitro as a time-dependent irreversible inhibitor of cyclo-oxygenase, yet its effects on human platelets in vivo have been found to be reversible (347, 394a, b, c). Unlike aspirin, which forms a covalent bond with cyclo-oxygenase, no linkage is formed in the case of indomethacin (394a, b, c). In vivo, the platelet population recovers cyclo-oxygenase activity after indomethacin ingestion more rapidly than can be accounted for by new platelet protein synthesis (394c–397). In vitro, platelets regain cyclo-oxygenase activity following their removal from a milieu containing indomethacin with a half-time of less than 3 hours. The in vivo inhibitory effect of indomethacin on platelet aggregation is undetectable 6 hours after ingestion. In adults, the ingestion of a single dose of indomethacin (50 mg) was not associated with a prolongation in the bleeding time. However, multiple doses (25 mg three times daily for 3 days) resulted in significant bleeding time prolongation (398). The recent use of this drug in the premature neonate to facilitate ductal closure has been associated with a prolongation in bleeding time (399). However, no correlation was observed between the indomethacin-induced platelet dysfunction and the occurrence or progression of intraventricular hemorrhage (399, 400). One case report of bleeding possibly associated with indomethacin has been reported (401). The half-life of the drug may be prolonged in the neonate, especially in the premature infant, and any hematologic effects could be proportionately increased (401). Sulindac, an isostere of indomethacin, is approximately 10 times less potent than the parent compound and does not prolong the bleeding time in humans (402).

SULFINPYRAZONE

Sulfinpyrazone was introduced as a uricosuric agent and was fortuitously noted to lengthen a shortened platelet survival (403). Subsequently, it was shown to have antiplatelet activity. This drug does not affect coagulation (403), and it has no effect upon platelet adhesion in pharmacologic concentrations (404). Like aspirin, it is an inhibitor of cyclo-oxygenase (405). However, unlike aspirin, sulfinpyrazone is a competitive inhibitor of the enzyme, and consequently cyclo-oxygenase activity returns to normal as the concentration of sulfinpyrazone declines. It is possible, however, that a metabolite of sulfinpyrazone may produce prolonged inhibition of platelet functions (406). Sulfinpyrazone does not prolong the bleeding time (407a).

Sulfinpyrazone is rapidly absorbed orally, with peak plasma concentrations occurring at 1 to 2 hours following ingestion (407b). The major side effect of this drug is dyspepsia, which occurs in 10 to 15 per cent of patients and is dose related. Less commonly, hypersensitivity reactions such as a rash can occur.

Unlike aspirin, which has no effect upon the shortened platelet life span in patients with prosthetic heart valves and arteriovenous shunts, sulfinpyrazone can lengthen a shortened platelet survival (408, 409).

DIPYRIDAMOLE

Dipyridamole is a pyrimido-pyrimidine compound that was initially introduced as a vasodilator and was subsequently shown to have antiplatelet activity. This agent has no effect on platelet adhesion under physiologic conditions. Unlike the antiplatelet activities of aspirin and sulfinpyrazone, which are mediated via inhibition of the prostaglandin pathway, the major effect of dipyridamole is through inhibition of platelet phosphodiesterase activity (the enzyme responsible for breaking down cyclic AMP) (410). Inhibition of phosphodiesterase results in an elevated level of cyclic AMP, which in turn causes the level of intracytoplasmic free Ca^{++} to fall, thus inhibiting platelet aggregation and secretion. Dipyridamole may also potentiate the platelet antiaggregatory activity of prostacyclin, thereby acting synergistically to increase platelet cyclic AMP levels through activation of platelet adenyl cyclase (411). This suggestion has not been confirmed by others, either in human studies or in cultured human endothelial cells (412, 413). In vivo dipyridamole does not prolong the bleeding time (414).

Dipyridamole is rapidly absorbed following oral administration, and the antiplatelet dose (100 to 400 mg per day in an adult) has relatively little vasodilatory effect. In some patients, higher doses (greater than 60 mg per kg) have been associated with headaches. Other side effects include gastrointestinal upset.

Dipyridamole can reduce the amount of thrombus formation on vascular catheters, on the membranes used for hemodialysis and cardiopulmonary bypass, and in patients with prosthetic heart valves (415). In patients with prosthetic heart valves and decreased platelet survival, dipyridamole alone or in combination with aspirin lengthens a shortened platelet life span (416–418). A reduction in the risk of thromboembolic complications in patients with prosthetic heart valves has also been reported when dipyridamole was used in combination with anticoagulants (419, 420). In experimentally induced homocystinemia, dipyridamole prevents the decrease in platelet life span that occurs as a concomitant to endothelial injury, and it also markedly reduces homocystine-induced atherosclerosis (421a, b). In combination with aspirin it has been shown to preserve renal function in patients with membranoproliferative glomerulonephritis (422).

TICLOPIDINE

This drug has potent antiplatelet activity, although its mode of action is not known. It is neither a prostaglandin synthesis inhibitor nor a cyclic AMP–phosphodiesterase inhibitor. Several studies suggest that ticlopidine may act on the platelet membrane to alter its reactivity to agonist stimulation (423). This agent inhibits the aggregation induced by various agonists, including epinephrine, collagen, thrombin, arachidonic acid, thromboxane A_2, and the endoperoxides PGG_2 and PGH_2. It also enhances the platelet inhibitory effect of PGI_2, and prolongs the bleeding time. Ticlopidine is unusual not only in that its effects on platelet function are manifested 24 to 48 hours after administration but also because these effects last for several days following discontinuation of the drug.

Platelet-Mediated Thrombotic Disorders and the Use of Antiplatelet Agents

Platelet-mediated thrombotic events occur primarily in the fast-flowing arterial circulation. One explanation for this is that in the arterial circulation, the rapid rate of blood flow results in centripetal streaming of the blood. Platelets, because of their density, are found at the margins of flow, where they come into close proximity with the arterial wall. Consequently, if the arterial wall is damaged, platelets adhere to the damaged endothelium, undergo aggregation, and form a platelet thrombus. The platelet thrombus, whose function is to prevent blood loss from the damaged vessel, may also have a negative impact on the well being of the individual. For example, a number of platelet secretory products, including platelet-derived growth factor, diffuse into the damaged vessel wall and initiate the repair process by stimulating smooth muscle and fibroblast proliferation. However, over time, the repair process can become self-sustaining, with the production of atherosclerotic lesions (424–426) In addition, the embolization of platelet thrombi from the damaged vessel wall can result in acute thrombotic disorders such as strokes and heart attacks.

In contrast to the situation in the arterial circulation, thrombi that form within the venous circulation primarily consist of red cells passively trapped within a fibrin network. In the venous circulation, abnormalities of the vessel wall, coagulation factors, or impaired blood flow usually precipitate thrombus formation, with platelets being only minor participants in its evolution. Consequently, antiplatelet agents for the most part are ineffective for venous thrombi. The thrombi that occur in vascular implants, including arteriovenous shunts, grafts, and prosthetic heart valves, are composed of both platelets and fibrin strands. Thus, the combination of an antiplatelet agent plus an anticoagulant is most effective in the treatment of thromboembolic disease due to such implants.

The selection of optimal antiplatelet agents has proved difficult. This difficulty arises because our understanding of platelet-mediated acute and chronic thrombotic events is still at a relatively primitive level. Consequently, the in vitro demonstration of antiplatelet activity does not necessarily translate into in vivo effectiveness. In fact, there is no agreement on the optimal test (or tests) of antiplatelet efficacy. For example, both aspirin and dipyridamole are effective in the treatment of certain platelet-mediated thrombotic disorders. Yet aspirin prolongs the bleeding time, whereas dipyridamole does not affect this parameter. Aspirin does not normalize a reduced platelet life span, although dipyridamole does. The issue is even more complicated by the demonstration that some antiplatelet agents that are effective in certain situations are not effective in others.

Most antiplatelet agents are initially evaluated using an in vitro test, and then are assessed in clinical trials. Unfortunately, since these trials are extremely expensive, they are usually limited to only the most promising antiplatelet agents. Thus, although many different agents have been tested for their in vitro efficacy, only a few have been evaluated for their antithrombotic effectiveness in vivo. These drugs include aspirin, dipyridamole, sulfinpyrazone, and ticlopidine.

ACTIVITY OF ANTIPLATELET AGENTS IN THROMBOTIC DISORDERS

Most platelet-mediated thrombotic disorders take many years to develop and consequently are not usually manifested in the pediatric population. Nonetheless, atherosclerosis begins at an early age, and although the clinical endpoints—such as strokes and heart attacks—are not seen until midlife, it is appropriate to summarize some of the studies of antiplatelet agents in this section. Readers interested in more information are referred to some of the recent review articles in which the various trials are discussed in detail (427–430).

Myocardial Infarction. As initial myocardial infarction represents the final endpoint of many years of atherosclerosis, it is difficult for any medication to have a therapeutic impact. The reason is that the medication is required for many years, and as is the case for virtually all chronic medications, compliance becomes a problem. Also, the relative effectiveness of any antiplatelet agent is limited. A large number of prospective and retrospective studies have suggested that aspirin ingestion is associated with a reduced risk of heart attacks in high-risk populations, but because of design flaws in the studies reported, none have been ideally performed. The issue thus remains open (431–435).

It is much simpler to perform a study designed to test whether an antiplatelet agent can prevent the recurrence of a further myocardial infarction or prevent death following myocardial infarction (secondary prevention studies). Six double-blind randomized trials have investigated the effect of aspirin in preventing reinfarction or death following myocardial infarction. When the results of these studies were pooled, aspirin was shown to be effective in preventing death and reinfarction (436–441). Sulfinpyrazone has been investigated in two large multicenter trials, both of which showed the drug to be beneficial, although one demonstrated a reduction in reinfarction rate whereas the other showed a reduction in sudden death (442, 443). Dipyridamole has not been convincingly shown to be effective (437). Aspirin has been shown to prevent patients with unstable angina from having a subsequent myocardial infarction or death (444, 445).

Cerebrovascular Disease. Platelets have been implicated as causing or contributing to strokes, and antiplatelet agents have been tried in a number of studies. Aspirin has been demonstrated in several different studies to significantly reduce the risk of stroke in patients with transient cerebral ischemia (446–448).

Embolization from Prosthetic Heart Valves. Recent technical advances in prosthetic heart valves have significantly reduced the risk of systemic embolization. The risk, however, still remains considerable, being as high as 5 per cent per year in some individuals. Antiplatelet agents alone are not effective in preventing systemic embolization, but their use in conjunction with an oral anticoagulant has proved effective (418–420, 449–451). However, when aspirin is added to an oral anticoagulant, there is also an increased risk of bleeding (418).

Arteriovenous Shunts. Thrombosis of an arteriovenous shunt terminates its usefulness. Aspirin and sulfinypyrazone have both been shown to reduce the risk of shunt thrombosis (452–454).

Ventriculojugular Shunts. Aspirin and persantine have been shown to lengthen shortened platelet survivals in patients with these shunts (455).

Antibiotic-Related Dysfunction

The *semisynthetic derivatives of penicillin* affect hemostasis by causing a time- and dose-related defect in platelet aggregation, the most sensitive indicator of platelet dysfunction being an abnormality in ADP aggregation (456, 457). The in vitro effects are associated with prolongations in the bleeding time that vary according to the drug dosages involved and the duration of therapy (456, 458–460). Platelet secretion and adhesion to subendothelium and collagen-coated surfaces are also inhibited (459, 465). Both penicillin G and carbenicillin have been shown to inhibit the binding of various agonists, including epinephrine, dihydroergocryptine (an α-adrenergic antagonist), 5'-p-fluoro-sulfonylbenzoyl adenosine (an ADP affinity label) and vWF to the platelet membrane receptors (457). Thus these drugs appear to exert an effect on various platelet membrane functions.

The severity of the hemostatic defect is variable, although it is usually more predictable and profound with carbenicillin, ticarcillin, and nafcillin than with piperacillin, mezlocillin, ampicillin, and apalcillin (456–458, 460–464). In normal volunteers, prolongation of the bleeding time was present at dosages of carbenicillin of 600 mg per kg per day. In patients receiving therapy with carbenicillin, mucosal hemorrhages have occurred at lower doses (300 to 400 mg per kg per day). A bleeding tendency has been noted with use of penicillin G at doses greater than 20 million units per day and with ticarcillin at doses of 300 mg per kg per day (458, 466). If semisynthetic penicillin is required for a patient at high risk for bleeding—e.g, a patient with septicemia plus thrombocytopenia—as low a dose as possible should be used. Ticarcillin offers some advantage over carbenicillin, since lower doses of ticarcillin can be used because of its greater antibacterial potency.

The cephalosporins, which are closely related in chemical structure to the penicillins, have also been reported to cause platelet dysfunction (467–469). Recent studies suggest that temocillin has the least effect on platelet functions (bleeding time and ADP-induced primary aggregation remain unchanged) when compared with other semisynthetic β-lactam compounds such as moxalactam (470, 471).

The potential for bleeding with these antibiotics is higher in patients with renal failure, in whom platelet function may be defective before antibiotic therapy and in whom very high blood concentrations of the drug may be reached.

Membrane-Active Drugs

Drugs of several different classes have been thought to stabilize biologic membranes. The tricyclic antidepressants (imipramine, desmethylipramine, amitriptyline, and nortriptyline), the phenothiazines (chlorpromazine and promethazine), and the antihistamines (diphenhydramine) all inhibit aggregation induced by ADP, epinephrine, and collagen in vitro (472–474). In patients with disorders of intrinsic coagulation (severe Factor VIII or IX deficiency), ingestion of multiple doses of chlorpromazine (thorazine) impaired platelet aggregation but was not associated with abnormalities in the template bleeding time (475). Diphenhydramine hydrochloride (Benadryl) in single or multiple doses has not been found to cause abnormalities either in bleeding time or platelet aggregation (398, 476, 477). The use of chlorpheniramine maleate (Chlor-Trimeton) or a combination of pseudoephedrine hydrochloride and triprolidine hydrochloride (Actifed) also produced no abnormalities in platelet aggregations or bleeding time (476, 477).

Tertiary amine local anesthetics also modify a variety of platelet membrane–related functions, including adhesion, secretion, fibrinogen-mediated platelet aggregation, and vWF-mediated platelet agglutination (478, 479). They have also been shown to dissolve platelet cytoskeletal components and to inhibit protein kinase C and phospholipase A_2 activity (480–482). Some of their effects on cellular membrane functions have been attributed to the ability of local anesthetics to perturb membrane phospholipid organization, fluidity, and protein conformation (483). Effects on cellular calcium metabolism have also been described (484). However, the clinical impact of these agents on overall platelet function remains uncertain. These agents are more likely to be used as laboratory tools, because of their widespread membrane effects.

Miscellaneous Drugs

Dextran. Dextran is a macromolecular compound with mild antithrombotic activity. It has been shown to inhibit a variety of platelet responses, including adhesion, aggregation, and platelet coagulant activity (485–487). A prolongation in bleeding time also occurs (488). Dextran has been used after surgery, to prevent venous thromboembolism (489). Its effects on coagulation include abnormalities of fibrin polymerization. Effects appear to be dose related and are most pronounced with the high-molecular-weight dextrans (490).

Ethyl Alcohol. The concentrations that produce both inebriation and platelet inhibition are similar. At concentrations greater than 200 mg per 100 ml, alcohol induces abnormalities in the secondary wave of aggregation with ADP and epinephrine and causes inhibition of collagen-induced aggregation. These findings are associated with a decrease in platelet factor 3 availability, together with subnormal release of platelet adenine nucleotides and a prolongation in bleeding time (491–493). A decrease in platelet life span has also been observed, as discussed in Part I of this chapter. The concomitant ingestion of aspirin accentuates the platelet dysfunction caused by ethanol.

Glyceryl Guaiacolate. This drug is an integral component of many antitussives used commonly in pediatric practice. In vitro studies have demonstrated that glyceryl guaiacolate produces impairment both in platelet adhesion and in platelet aggregation with ADP and epinephrine (398, 494, 495). However, no abnormalities in bleeding time occur either in normal controls or in hemophiliacs given this medication (398, 475, 477).

Heparin. Bleeding complications in patients receiving heparin are usually related to the effect of heparin on blood coagulation. Heparin, however, can inhibit platelet adhesion, aggregation, and secretion (356a, 496). Parenteral administration of heparin (100 to 200 units per kg) may also prolong the bleeding time in normal subjects (497). Certain heparin fractions, especially those of higher molecular weight, can aggregate platelets in vitro (498, 499).

Nitrofurantoin. This urinary antiseptic can inhibit primary ADP and collagen-induced platelet aggregation. In humans, a prolongation of the bleeding time has been reported in the presence of high blood levels of this drug (500).

Vinca Alkaloids. Vincristine and vinblastine are known to affect microtubules in several cell systems. Exposure of human platelets in vitro to large doses of these drugs results in loss of microtubules and the discoid shape of the platelet (501). Reduction in adhesiveness and inhibition of the secondary wave of platelet aggregation have also been demonstrated (502). Steinherz and associates (503), in their study of a pediatric population with various malignancies treated with vincristine, found abnormalities in platelet adhesion and in the secondary wave of platelet aggregation with ADP and epinephrine. The bleeding time following vincristine therapy remained normal, however, and no change was seen in serotonin uptake and release, clot retraction, platelet factor 3 release, or collagen-induced platelet aggregation.

Other Chemotherapeutic Agents. Mithramycin therapy has been associated with abnormalities in platelet aggregation and with prolongation of the template bleeding time (504). It has been suggested that the effect of this agent may be mediated by an alteration of the calcium influx into platelets (505). Although platelet aggregation has been demonstrated to be abnormal following cytoxan or actinomycin D therapy, no clinical bleeding tendency was apparent (506). Cytosine arabinoside has not been observed to cause changes in platelet function (507).

Sodium Valproate. This drug appears to affect both qualitative and quantitative platelet function (508–510). Following the ingestion of sodium valproate, abnormalities of platelet aggregation and adhesion have been reported in some patients. Bleeding time tests have given variable results in patients receiving this drug. Thrombocytopenia has also been documented. Prolongation in the bleeding time is, however, usually seen in the absence of thrombocytopenia.

Treatment of Drug-Induced Platelet Dysfunction

If a drug is suspected to be contributing to bleeding, it should be discontinued. Unless the bleeding is severe, platelet transfusions are not indicated, since platelet function rapidly returns to normal after the drug is stopped.

No one-to-one correlation has been reported between the development of a clinically significant bleeding tendency and any of the in vitro laboratory tests of platelet function. Even the bleeding time, our best measure of in vivo platelet adhesion and aggregation, will not predict with accuracy which patient will bleed. Two lists of drugs that inhibit platelet function are included in this chapter. The first (Table 42–18) summarizes reported abnormalities in platelet function, including the bleeding time, which have been observed to occur

Table 42–18. DRUGS THAT INHIBIT PLATELET FUNCTIONS FOLLOWING INGESTION[1]

Amicar*
Antibiotics (ampicillin,* apalcillin, carbenicillin*, cephalosporins,* mezlocillin, methicillin,* nafcillin,* penicillin G,* piperacillin, ticarcillin*)
Anti-inflammatory nonsteroidal agents (aspirin,* indomethacin,* naproxen,* phenylbutazone, sulindac, sulfinpyrazone)
β-Blockers (propranolol)
Chemotherapeutic agents (actinomycin D, cytoxan, mithramycin,* vinca alkaloids)
Clofibrate
Ethyl alcohol*
Dextran*
Glyceryl guaiacolate
Heparin*
Mo-Er or black fungus*
Macromolecules (dextran)*
Nitrofurantoin*
Omega-3-polyunsaturated fatty acids (eicosapentaenoic acid)*
Onion and garlic extracts
Phenothiazines (chlorpromazine)
Pyrimido-pyrimidine compounds (dipyridamole)
Prostaglandin I_2, D_2, E_1
Tricyclic antidepressants (amitriptyline, desmethylimipramine, imipramine, nortriptyline)
Ticlopidine*
Thromboxane synthetase inhibitors (imidazole, levamisole)
Valproate sodium*
Vitamin E

[1] Following administration, these drugs have been demonstrated to affect in vitro platelet function. Those drugs marked by an asterisk (*) have also been shown to cause a prolongation in bleeding time.

following in vivo ingestion of the agent. Drug ingestion in such cases may be accompanied by a clinically apparent bleeding tendency. The second (Table 42–19) is a list of various drugs that have been found to affect platelet function mainly in vitro. Most of these agents have been administered to humans without measurably impairing platelet function, and it is unlikely that they cause or contribute to bleeding.

HYPERCOAGULABILITY

"Hypercoagulability" is a hypothetical concept implying that prethrombotic changes can be detected in blood, and that these changes could contribute to the development of thrombosis (511). The studies cited in the literature purporting to document a "hypercoagulable" state are often unsatisfactory. Although certain laboratory tests and diseases can be associated with thrombosis, usually there is no evidence of a cause-and-effect relationship. In fact, relatively few conditions have been causally linked to thrombosis. These include the inherited deficiencies of antithrombin III, protein C, and protein S. In general, etiologic factors associated with and possibly predisposing to thrombosis include those associated with decreased blood flow or increased blood viscosity, alterations in plasma coagulation factor levels (including deficiencies of the normally present inhibitors of activated clotting factors), decreased fibrinolytic activity, impaired clearance mechanisms, and the presence of platelets that are hyperfunctional or abnormally activated in vivo. Table 42–20 is a list of the clinical conditions in which a transient or a more persistent hypercoagulable state may exist. Several reviews of the hypercoagulable state are currently available (511–516). Although most of the disorders listed in Table 42–20 are adult diseases, a few are particularly pertinent to pediatrics. Since the thrombotic tendencies associated with cancer, the hemolytic uremic syndrome, thrombotic thrombocytopenic purpura, disseminated intravascular coagulation, and the infusion of clotting factors are discussed elsewhere in this text, the remaining associations relevant to the pediatrician will be summarized.

Table 42–19. DRUGS THAT INHIBIT PLATELET FUNCTION (WHEN ADDED TO PLATELETS IN VITRO)*

Adenosine
Alpha-adrenergic blocking agents (dihydroergotamine, phentolamine)
Anesthetics, local (cocaine, dibucaine, nupercaine, procaine, lidocaine)
Anesthetics, general (cyclopropane diethyl ether, halothane, nitrous oxide, methoxyglurane)
Anti-inflammatory agents, nonsteroidal (flufenamic acid, ibufenac, ibuprofen, meclofenamic acid, mefenamic acid, phenoprofen, solufenum)
Antihistamines (chlorpheniramine maleate, diphenhydramine)
Atropine
Barbituric acid derivatives (sodium pentobarbital)
Cis-unsaturated fatty acids
Chelating agents
Chemotherapeutic agents (azathioprine, BCNU, melphalan)
Chloroquine compounds
Colchicine
Contrast agents used in diagnostic radiology
Diuretics (furosemide)
Halofenate
Histamine
Isoprenaline
Methyl xanthines (aminophylline, caffeine, theophylline, papaverine)
Mercurial diuretics (meralluride, mersalyl)
Nicotinic acid
Nitroprusside
Pseudoephedrine hydrochloride
Reserpine
Serotonin antagonists (cyproheptadine, promethazine, suloctidil, metergoline)
Steroids (hydrocortisone, methyl prednisolone)
Vasodilators (papaverine, quazodine, suloctidil)
Vitamin C, Vitamin B_6

*These drugs have been demonstrated to affect platelet function when added to platelets in vitro. Most of these agents have been administered to humans without measurably impairing platelet function, and it is unlikely that they cause or contribute to bleeding.

Table 42-20. CLINICAL CONDITIONS OR DISEASES THAT MAY BE ASSOCIATED WITH A "HYPERCOAGULABLE" STATE

Acute peripheral arterial insufficiency
Aging
Antithrombin III deficiency
Angina pectoris and coronary artery disease
Arteriovenous shunts
Atherosclerosis
Behçet's disease
Buerger's disease
Cancer
Catheters
Cardiomyopathy, atrial fibrillation, mitral valve prolapse
Chronic valvular heart disease
Cigarette smoking
Contraceptive therapy (estrogens)
Crohn's disease
Deep vein thrombosis
Diabetes mellitus
Diet high in saturated fats
Disseminated intravascular coagulation
Dysfibrinogenemia
Factor XII deficiency
Glomerular disease
Hemolytic uremic syndrome
Heparin therapy
Homocystinuria
Hypercholesterolemia
Hyperbetalipoproteinemia Type II
Hypothermia
Intravenous therapy with clotting factors (especially in Factor IX deficiency)
Kawasaki syndrome
Liver disease
Lupus anticoagulant
Myeloproliferative syndromes
Nephrotic syndrome
Nutritional deficiencies (Vitamin E deficiency; selenium deficiency)
Oxygen toxicity
Paroxysmal nocturnal hemoglobinuria
Placental insufficiency syndromes
Plasminogen and plasminogen activator abnormalities
Post myocardial infarction
Postoperative states (especially cardiopulmonary and orthopedic)
Post streptokinase or coumarin therapy
Prosthetic devices in the circulation
Prostacyclin or plasma prostacyclin regenerating factor deficiencies
Protein C and S deficiencies
Pregnancy
Preeclampsia
Renal allograft rejection
Sickle cell anemia
Snake venoms
Stasis
Thrombotic thrombocytopenic purpura
Transient cerebral ischemic attacks
Ulcerative colitis
Vasculitis
Ventriculojugular shunts

Presence of Prosthetic Devices in the Circulation

Prosthetic heart valves, arterial grafts, arteriovenous shunts, ventriculojugular shunts, and silastic catheters can lead to thrombosis or thromboembolic phenomena. Following prosthetic heart valve replacement, a decrease in platelet life span is found in some patients, and it has been suggested that these patients are at higher risk for thromboembolic complications (511). Antiplatelet agents in combination with anticoagulant therapy will reduce the risk of thromboembolism.

Shunting of cerebrospinal fluid from the lateral ventricles to the right atrium via a ventriculojugular shunt is accompanied by an increased risk of thromboembolic phenomena (517). Clot formation in or about the distal end of the shunt represents a leading cause of shunt dysfunction. We found that 5 of 12 children with ventriculojugular shunts had shortened platelet life spans (455). Two children from the group with shortened platelet survivals were treated for a 2-week period with oral dipyridamole (1.5 mg per kg per day) and aspirin (10 mg per kg per day), which returned the shortened platelet life span to normal.

Diabetes Mellitus

Studies on hemostasis in patients with diabetes mellitus have been undertaken by numerous workers in an attempt to correlate a "hypercoagulable" state with the well-recognized long-term vascular complications of this disease. Patients with diabetes mellitus have increased levels of coagulation Factors I, V, VIIIC, and vWF (518, 519). Studies of platelet function in diabetes mellitus have shown the following: increased platelet adhesion (which may be related to the elevated levels of vWF) (518, 519); increase in platelet factor 3 availability (520); increased plasma concentrations of β-thromboglobulin (521, 522); platelet hyperaggregability in response to the aggregating agents ADP, epinephrine, and collagen; and the occurrence of circulating platelet aggregates (519, 520, 522–527). In general, although platelet function abnormalities occur in patients with vascular complications, these abnormalities may also be observed in prediabetes and in latent diabetes (523–526). This hypersensitivity of the platelet to aggregating agents may be related to a plasma factor (or factors) present in this disorder (527).

Platelets from diabetics synthesize increased amounts of platelet thromboxane A_2* when compared with control platelets (528–533). A similar finding has been observed in both the spontaneously diabetic BB Wistar rat, and in rats with streptozocin-induced disease (534–536). The increase in platelet thromboxane* production is due to the combined effect of the higher percentage of arachidonic acid (AA) in platelet phospholipids of subjects with diabetes and the increased AA

---

*The terms thromboxane A_2 and thromboxane are used interchangeably.

release from the platelet membrane (532, 536, 537). Other authors have also suggested that conversion of AA via cyclo-oxygenase may be increased, since increased thromboxane A_2 synthesis was observed following the addition of exogenous AA to platelets, thus bypassing the release step (519, 529, 538). Platelets obtained from diabetic subjects may also be less sensitive to the antiaggregatory effects of thromboxane synthetase inhibitors and prostacyclin (530, 533, 539). A positive correlation between the plasma glucose level and platelet thromboxane production has been observed (530). Such platelet changes may, however, arise equally as well from other causes, such as increased plasma cholesterol levels, since platelets rich in cholesterol are hyperaggregable and produce more thromboxane than do normal platelets (540, 541).

In contrast to the increased platelet thromboxane synthesis, blood vessels from diabetic humans and from the animal model of diabetes appear to synthesize less prostacyclin when these vessels are evaluated in vitro (519, 534, 536, 542–544). This abnormality appears to be due to decreased vascular prostacyclin synthetase activity (536). It is difficult to explain both increased platelet thromboxane A_2 and decreased vascular prostacyclin production on the basis of changes in cyclo-oxygenase activity. However, our recent finding that 15-hydroxyeicosatetraenoic acid (a product found in human vessels but not in platelets) inhibits vascular cyclo-oxygenase activity and is increased in vessels from the diabetic milieu may help to resolve this issue (545).

A decrease in platelet life span and the presence of megathrombocytes have also been noted in patients with diabetes mellitus (519, 527, 546, 547). This suggests that these patients could have increased platelet turnover as a result of abnormal platelet–vessel wall interactions. It is possible that the increased risk of atherosclerosis in diabetes could be due in part to platelet hyperaggregability, increased thromboxane formation, and decreased prostacyclin synthesis. No data are available on the use of either antiplatelet therapy or other therapeutic modifiers of platelet arachidonate metabolism in diabetes mellitus. However, normalization of glucose homeostasis may be important in reducing the contribution of platelets to the development of diabetic vascular disease, since platelet hypersensitivity is abolished by optimal plasma glucose control (548).

Maternal diabetes is an important etiologic factor in the pathogenesis of both arterial and venous thromboses that occur in the infant during the neonatal period. Oppenheimer and Esterly (549), in a review of 4000 infants who died in the first 2 weeks of life, noted that 15.8 per cent of those neonates with a history of maternal diabetes showed evidence of thromboses at autopsy, whereas similar lesions were found in only 0.8 per cent of autopsied infants of nondiabetic mothers. The thrombi discovered in the infants of diabetic mothers were formed earlier and exhibited organization and calcification, strongly suggestive of in utero development. Although renal vein thrombosis is reported most frequently in these infants, arterial thrombus formation may also occur (550, 551).

The pathogenesis of this complication in the infant of the diabetic mother is speculative at best. Dehydration and polycythemia with local stasis of blood have been suggested as causative factors, and disseminated intravascular coagulation has been found to be present in an occasional patient. None of these factors, however, has been implicated in the majority of patients with thrombosis in the neonatal period.

Platelet hyperaggregability and changes in both platelet and vascular arachidonate metabolism have been seen in infants of diabetic mothers. The changes observed are similar to those seen in adults with diabetes, and occur only in infants born to mothers with abnormal glucose homeostasis. The abnormalities include increased platelet endoperoxide formation (552) and decreased vascular prostacyclin biosynthesis (545, 553, 554). Decreased prostacyclin formation may be due to inhibition of vascular cyclo-oxygenase. The inverse correlation observed between vascular 15-hydroxyeicosatetraenoic acid and prostacyclin levels suggests that elevated levels of this hydroxyacid may be in part responsible for the decreased prostacyclin production by an inhibitory effect on vascular cyclo-oxygenase (545). Since neonatal changes reflect maternal glucose homeostasis, the best method of protection against the potential adverse effects of these platelet-vascular arachidonate abnormalities appears to be good maternal diabetic control.

Homocystinuria

The homocystinurias occur as a result of genetically determined defects in the metabolism of homocysteine (555). The most common cause, cystathionine-B-synthase deficiency, results in a decrease in the rate of conversion of homocysteine to cystathionine and is generally accompanied by hypermethioninemia. Deficiencies in the remethylation of homocysteine to methionine cause homocystinemia accompanied by hypomethioninemia, but are much less common than cystathionine-B-synthase deficiency. In all these disorders, accumulated homocysteine is oxidized to homocystine, which is found in excessive amounts in blood and urine.

Cystathionine-B-synthase deficiency is characterized by dislocated lenses, skeletal deformities, central nervous system abnormalities, and a high frequency of thromboembolic disease. Atherosclerosis and occlusion of major vessels, such as the myocardial, cerebral, renal, and pulmonary arteries and veins, can occur as early as the first decade, often with a fatal outcome (555, 556). Vascular lesions are similar to those seen in classic atherosclerosis and are characterized by intimal thickening, medial disorganization, and fibrosis with loss of elastic tissue, hyperplasia of smooth muscle cells, and mural or occlusive thrombi (556). The atherothrombotic complications in cystathionine-B-synthase deficiency are not considered to be adequately explained either by a structural abnormality in collagen (557) or by abnormalities in the fluid phase of coagulation, although homocystine in vitro causes activation of Factor XII (557, 558).

Studies of platelet survival and reactivity in patients with homocystinuria have yielded variable results (559–564). One group of investigators reported shortened platelet life span studies in patients with homocystinuria, with lengthening of survivals following dipyridamole administration (561). These same investigators demonstrated that the chronic infusion of L-homocysteine into primates caused a shortening of platelet survival associated with vascular endothelial damage and the development of lesions similar to those observed in atherosclerosis. The concurrent administration of dipyridamole partially blocked the development of these abnormalities (565). Other investigators, however, have not found a shortened platelet survival in patients with homocystinuria (563, 564). These differences remain unexplained and do not appear to be due to genetic heterogeneity or to differences in plasma homocystine concentration (566).

The possibility of changes in platelet thromboxane–vascular prostacyclin balance have also been raised by the in vitro findings that homocystine and homocysteine increase platelet thromboxane production (567). A decrease in vascular prostacyclin production may also occur in vitro (568). Since no assessment of in vivo thromboxane-prostacyclin biosynthesis has been reported, the relevance of these in vitro findings to the atherosclerotic tendency in homocystinuria remains uncertain. Dipyridamole and aspirin have been recommended as therapeutic agents in patients with homocystinuria in whom elevated plasma concentrations of homocystine persist despite pyridoxine therapy (566).

Most recently, a strong case has been made that heterozygosity for cystathionine-B-synthase deficiency and other partial impairments of homocysteine metabolism are risk factors for peripheral and cerebrovascular arterial disease (569–572).

Nephrotic Syndrome

Although a deficiency of Factors IX, XI, and XII can occur in the nephrotic syndrome, owing to the urinary loss of these protein molecules (573–576), thrombosis, rather than bleeding, is a well-recognized complication of this disease entity. Thrombosis may be either arterial or venous, with renal vein, deep venous, and primary arterial thrombosis occurring in both adults and children during the acute phase of their disease (577–585). In addition, patients with the nephrotic syndrome have been shown to have an increased risk and earlier onset of atherosclerotic vascular disease (586, 587). The cause of this clinical "hypercoagulable" state has been variously attributed to an increase in the levels of Factors I, V, VII, VIII, and X (582, 583, 588) or to a decrease in plasma antithrombin III levels (589, 590). Since a number of cases of idiopathic venous thromboses have been reported to occur in patients with familial antithrombin III deficiency, the presence of this abnormality may be important in the development of "hypercoagulability" in the nephrotic syndrome (591, 592).

Platelet abnormalities reported have been both quantitative and qualitative, with platelet hyperaggregability and spontaneous aggregation being demonsrated in many cases (593–596). Bang and associates (593) first documented the presence of enhanced platelet aggregation in patients with active glomerular disease, including the nephrotic syndrome. They found that the degree of platelet function abnormality was significantly correlated with the degree of proteinuria and the serum albumin level. Furthermore, they attributed the platelet hyperaggregability to the urinary losses of plasma proteins normally responsible for the inhibition of platelet aggregation. Others have shown that platelet hyperaggregability was normalized by the addition of albumin to the patient's platelet-rich plasma (594, 595). Hypercholesterolemia may also be responsible for the platelet dysfunction (540).

Increased platelet malonyldialdehyde formation, platelet hyperaggregability, and a decrease in platelet life span have been reported in children with nephrotic syndrome during the period of active disease (596). Platelet function returned to normal during remission. Since a reduction in platelet survival is associated with an increased risk of thromboembolism in a number of pathologic states, this finding appears to be of clinical significance and defines another parameter associated with the "hypercoagulable" state in the nephrotic syndrome. No data are available on the clinical use of antiplatelet agents in this disease.

Kawasaki Syndrome

Kawasaki disease (mucocutaneous lymph node syndrome) is an acute febrile vasculitis of early childhood (597). The most serious complications of this disorder include sudden death from coronary arteritis with thrombosis, and aneurysm formation (598). Coronary angiography demonstrates that approximately 20 per cent of patients unselectively examined manifest coronary artery abnormalities, which may either regress or persist for as long as 2 years following the development of the acute disease (599, 600). The pathogenesis of the coronary arteritis and aneurysm formation, however, remains unknown. Activation of both coagulation and platelets has been observed in this disease entity. Changes in coagulation during the acute phase of the illness (the first 3 weeks following onset of fever) have included elevations in Factor VIII:C and fibrinogen, with decreased levels of antithrombin III, and depletion of fibrinolytic activity as measured by a prolonged euglobulin lysis time (601).

Evidence for platelet activation has also been reported in this syndrome. Yamada and co-workers have found increased ADP, epinephrine and collagen-induced platelet aggregation in children up to 9 months after the onset of other illness (602). This finding has been confirmed by other investigators (603). Hyperaggregability could be suppressed by the administration of either aspirin (30 mg per kg per day) or by flubiprofen (602, 603). Other evidence supporting the presence of intravascular platelet activation includes increased plasma β-thromboglobulin levels (601), as well as increased biosynthesis of proaggregatory platelet thromboxane A_2 following the addition of arachidonic acid to platelet-rich plasma in vitro (604). The increase in plasma β-thromboglobulin levels during the acute illness was only seen in patients who subsequently developed coronary arterial aneurysms, and has thus been suggested as a possible marker for the development of this complication (601).

Aspirin has been used in the therapy of Kawasaki syndrome, both for its anti-inflammatory effect and for its inhibitory effect on platelet cyclooxygenase. Various dosage schedules from 3 to 150 mg/kg/day have been advocated (601, 603), but no data are available as to which dosage is most effective in the long-term outcome of children with this disease entity. The use of intravenous IgG, usually in combination with aspirin, has been shown to be highly effective when administered early in the course of Kawasaki syndrome (605, 606).

VASCULAR PURPURAS

Purpura is a disorder of hemostasis caused by extravasation of blood from the microcirculation. Characteristic lesions include petechiae (purpuric spots ≤3 mm) and purpura (larger extravasations of red cells into the cutaneous tissues). Purpura may be the presenting symptom of a wide variety of clinical conditions that vary from the trivial to life-threatening. Table 42–21 is a summary of some of the more common pathologic states associated with purpura that is primarily vascular in nature. Purpura may also be associated with disorders of coagulation (e.g., purpura fulminans), or with qualitative or quantitative platelet dysfunction. Since Schönlein-Henoch purpura is the common pediatric entity encountered under the category of vascular purpuras, review of this disease is appropriate.

Allergic Purpura (Schönlein-Henoch Purpura)

Heberden (607) and William (608) first described patients with severe purpura, abdominal pain, and edema of the hands and feet. Schönlein in 1837 (609) described the arthritic component associated with the purpura, and Henoch in 1874 (610) added his classic description of four children with skin lesions associated with colicky abdominal pain, gastrointestinal hemorrhage, and joint pain. Renal involvement in this disease entity has been demonstrated by Henoch and various other workers over the last century.

Clinical and Laboratory Findings. Schönlein-Henoch allergic or anaphylactoid purpura is a disease affecting primarily children, with most cases occurring between the second and seventh

Table 42–21. CAUSES OF VASCULAR PURPURA*

Allergic or Schönlein-Henoch purpura
Autoimmune, mainly collagen vascular
Autoerythrocyte sensitivity
Autosensitivity to DNA
Angiokeratoma
Amyloidosis
Antibody-mediated injury
Benign hyperglobulinemic purpura
Cushing's disease
Cryoglobulinemic purpura
Drug-induced
Embolic
Hereditary disorders of connective tissue (Ehlers-Danlos syndrome, Marfan's syndrome, osteogenesis imperfecta, pseudoxanthoma elasticum)
Hereditary familial purpura simplex
Hereditary hemorrhagic telangiectasia
Hypergammaglobulinemic purpura in cystic fibrosis
Infectious
Injury
Mechanical
Neoplastic (dysproteinemic states, such as multiple myeloma, Waldenström's macroglobulinemia; Kaposi's hemorrhagic sarcoma)
Osler-Weber-Rendu disease
Purpura simplex
Psychogenic
Scurvy
Senile purpura
Stasis

*Although purpura is primarily vascular in nature, coagulation and platelet abnormalities may occasionally be associated with purpura.

years of life (611–613). Males are affected most commonly, with the peak seasonal incidence occurring in spring or autumn (611). A definite history of an upper respiratory tract infection occurring 1 to 3 weeks prior to the onset of the symptoms of allergic purpura may be elicited in approximately two thirds of children (611).

Figure 42–18 summarizes the various signs and symptoms that occurred in 131 children with this entity described in the classic survey of Allen and associates in 1960 (611). The skin manifestations of allergic purpura are often urticarial at the onset. The urticaria fades, to be replaced by red macular or maculopapular lesions, which may remain small and discrete or which may coalesce. The initial reddish hue is replaced by a brown color, and ecchymotic areas may appear. Petechial lesions may also be observed. Involvement tends to be fairly symmetrical and usually includes the extensor aspects of the lower extremities, particularly the knees and feet, and the buttocks. The extensor surfaces of the arms, particularly the elbows, may also commonly be affected. Face, trunk, and mucous membrane involvement may also occasionally occur. Although the skin rash is present in all children, its appearance may sometimes be delayed, thus posing a problem in differential diagnosis, particularly in the child whose presenting symptoms may simulate an acute abdomen (611). It is not uncommon for patients to exhibit new crops of lesions throughout the initial 2 to 4 weeks of their illness.

Joint involvement occurs in about two thirds of children (611) and is usually characterized by nonmigratory polyarthralgias, most often affecting the ankles and knees. The wrists, elbows, and fingers are involved with much less frequency. Involvement is mainly periarticular, usually without any change in the actual joint space. Residual deformity does not occur. Localized edema of the subcutaneous tissues of the dorsum of the hands and feet, scalp, ears, or periorbital region may also be present in approximately half the patients (611). Painful swelling of the scalp or face is more frequently seen in children below the age of 3 years. Colicky abdominal pain associated with frank melena or guaiac-positive stools occurs in approximately half the children. This symptomatology is due to hemorrhage and edema into a segment of the small intestine, which may then serve as the lead point for an intussusception. It has been recommended that all children with allergic purpura and abdominal symptoms be hospitalized for close observation, since serious complications (i.e., massive gastrointestinal hemorrhage with shock or an irreducible intussusception with gangrene of the bowel) are potential complications that can occur with great rapidity (611, 614, 615).

Renal symptoms, including the presence of gross or microscopic hematuria often accompanied by proteinuria, may occur in 25 to 50 per cent of children in the second or third week of their illness (611). Hematuria is never the presenting feature of allergic purpura, usually following at least two of the other major manifestations of the disease. Males and older children are more prone to develop renal involvement than are the younger infant and child (611, 612, 616). Renal involvement may sometimes be accompanied by hypertension, with or without a transient diminution of renal function or renal failure.

Other rare symptoms include testicular hemorrhage and torsion (611). Neurologic symptoms such as transient paresis, convulsions, and cranial nerve palsies, including optic atrophy, may rarely develop because of involvement of the central nervous system (617).

Platelet numbers and function are normal in this disorder. Laboratory findings are not diagnostic for this syndrome of nonthrombocytopenic

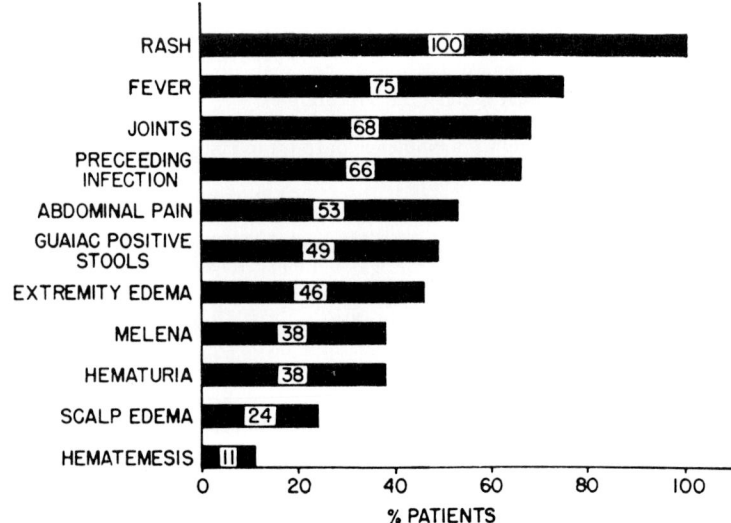

Figure 42–18. Occurrence of various signs and symptoms in 131 children with allergic purpura. (From Allen, D.M., Diamond, L. K., et al.: Am. J. Dis. Child. 99:833, 1960. Copyright © 1960, American Medical Association.)

purpura, except for histologic examination of the skin lesion, which reveals an aseptic vasculitis most marked in the vessels of the dermis. The small blood vessels in the dermis demonstrate perivascular cuffing, with varying numbers of polymorphonuclear leukocytes, lymphocytes, histiocytes, and eosinophils. Fibrinoid necrosis, platelet plugging of vessels, and interstitial edema, together with small areas of extravasated erythrocytes, may also be noted (611, 616). IgA, IgM, C3, C4, C5, and properdin may be found at the site of the inflammatory lesion, suggesting that the injury may be complement-mediated. A reduction in serum levels of properdin and properdin convertase may be present during the acute phase of allergic purpura, suggesting activation of the "alternative pathway" (618).

Vascular lesions similar to those present in the skin may occur in the submucosa of the bowel in patients with visceral involvement. Renal lesions are characterized by segmental glomerular proliferation and occlusion of capillaries by Schiff-positive fibrinoid material. Older lesions appear as segmented areas of organized hyaline material or as frank segmental scars of fibrous tissue (611). In contrast to the findings in glomerulonephritis, mesangial rather than basement membrane localization of fibrinogen, complement, and α-globulin has been demonstrated by fluorescent microscopy (619, 620). Immunofluorescent studies frequently reveal diffuse glomerular deposits that contain IgA in 90 per cent of reported cases. C3, fibrin, IgG, properdin, and IgM are also noted (621). Prognosis regarding renal function has been correlated with the findings on renal biopsy at the time of initial presentation—a poor prognosis being associated with diffuse renal involvement.

Pathogenesis and Treatment. Allergic purpura is a disorder manifested by widespread injury to multiple organ systems. Since the histopathologic changes observed resemble experimentally induced "immune complex" disease, it has been suggested that this mechanism may be responsible for the vasculitis and renal disease observed (622). Indeed, circulating IgA immune complexes have been described in Schönlein-Henoch purpura as well as in IgA nephropathy (621). The source of the IgA noted in both the circulating immune complexes and renal deposits is unknown (623). It is unclear whether the IgA originates from mucosa stimulated by upper respiratory tract infection or from peripheral blood lymphocytes (621). Although cases of allergic purpura have been associated with food allergy, insect bites, drugs, and bacterial infections (particularly β-hemolytic streptococci), conclusive proof is lacking for a cause-and-effect relationship between any of these inciting agents and the development of allergic vasculitis.

Prednisone therapy for children with abdominal involvement has been recommended in an attempt to reduce edema of the bowel wall and therefore reduce the possibility of the occurrence of an intussusception (611). Prednisone may also be used to reduce edema and provide relief from the pain associated with scalp edema or joint involvement. This drug, however, does not alter the course of renal involvement (611, 619) or modify the skin manifestations of allergic purpura. Approximately 50 per cent of children affected may experience one or more recurrences of their disease in the initial weeks, with the occurrence of fresh crops of skin lesions or abdominal pain heralding the recurrence. The ultimate prognosis is uniformly good, with long-term renal complications occurring in less than 15 per cent of patients who present initially with renal involvement (621, 624).

APPENDIX: TECHNIQUES USED TO STUDY PLATELET MEMBRANE GLYCOPROTEINS

Gel Electrophoresis

One of the first techniques used to study platelet membrane proteins was gel electrophoresis. In this procedure, the lipid bilayer is dissolved using a detergent, and after the platelet protein skeleton is removed (usually by centrifugation), the surface proteins are studied. These proteins include integral proteins (which penetrate the lipid bilayer) and peripheral proteins (located on the platelet surface). The proteins are separated from each other according to size, using sodium dodecyl sulfate polyacrylamide gel electrophoresis (SDS-PAGE). Following this procedure, the proteins are identified by staining. The sensitivity of gel electrophoresis can be increased by using two-dimensional electrophoresis. The platelet glycoproteins have been designated by roman numerals, with the largest protein being designated as I and the numbers increasing with the progressively smaller proteins. As more glycoproteins have been identified, alphabetical letters have been used to designate them, i.e. Ia, Ib, IIa, IIb, IIIa, etc. The proteins are identified by protein or carbohydrate staining or by autoradiography. The latter technique is accomplished by radiolabeling the platelet proteins, usually with ^{125}Iodine (which labels tyrosine and histidine) or ^{3}H-borohydride (which labels surface carbohydrates). Surface protein radiolabeling also allows the identification of immunologic reactions involving specific glycoproteins, and these techniques will be discussed in the next section.

Radioimmunoprecipitation

This technique is used to evaluate whether a ligand (usually an antibody) binds to a particular platelet surface glycoprotein. During the performance of this procedure, which is illustrated schematically in Figure 42–19, platelet proteins are surface radiolabeled, usually with ^{125}I. It should be emphasized that iodination labels only certain surface proteins.

After the ligand has reacted with the platelet proteins, the lipid bilayer is dissolved using a detergent. Alternatively, the antiserum can be added after the bilipid layer has been dissolved. A "catcher system" is then added to bring down all antibody. The catcher system usually is staphylococcal protein A (which has a high affinity for IgG), with the protein A bound to a solid matrix. The platelet protein–antibody/catcher system is pelleted and washed, and the radiolabeled platelet protein is then separated from the antibody. The platelet protein, which has bound to the ligand, is applied to an electrophoretic gel, and the proteins are separated according to size, with the radiolabeled protein identified by autoradiography. This technique has proved useful for studying a variety of platelet-ligand interactions.

Negative results using radioimmunoprecipitation may mean that the antibody of interest did not bind to any platelet proteins. Alternatively, the antibody may have bound, but the particular platelet protein was not radiolabeled and hence could not be detected.

Immunoblotting

The technique of immunoblotting, also termed Western blotting, is similar to radioprecipitation, with one important difference. The ligand (usually antiserum) is allowed to react with the platelet glycoproteins *after* they have been separated electrophoretically. This technique offers certain advantages over radioimmunoprecipitation, but has distinct disadvantages. Because the platelet glycoproteins are not radiolabeled, immunoblotting detects surface antigens that cannot be radiolabeled. However, the separation of the proteins on the gel before the immunologic reaction can modify the antigen binding sites on these glycoproteins, so that they are not detected by the antibody. This has proved a problem for certain monoclonal antibodies directed against platelet-specific glycoproteins.

To perform an immunoblot, platelets are solubilized by a detergent that dissolves the lipid bilayer (Fig. 42–20). The proteins are then separated according to size, using SDS-PAGE. Following the separation, the proteins are transferred onto a solid matrix (nitrocellulose), to which they strongly bind. Once bound to the nitrocellulose, the platelet glycoproteins are stable for long periods of time. The antibody of interest is then overlayed onto the nitrocellulose strip that carries the glycopro-

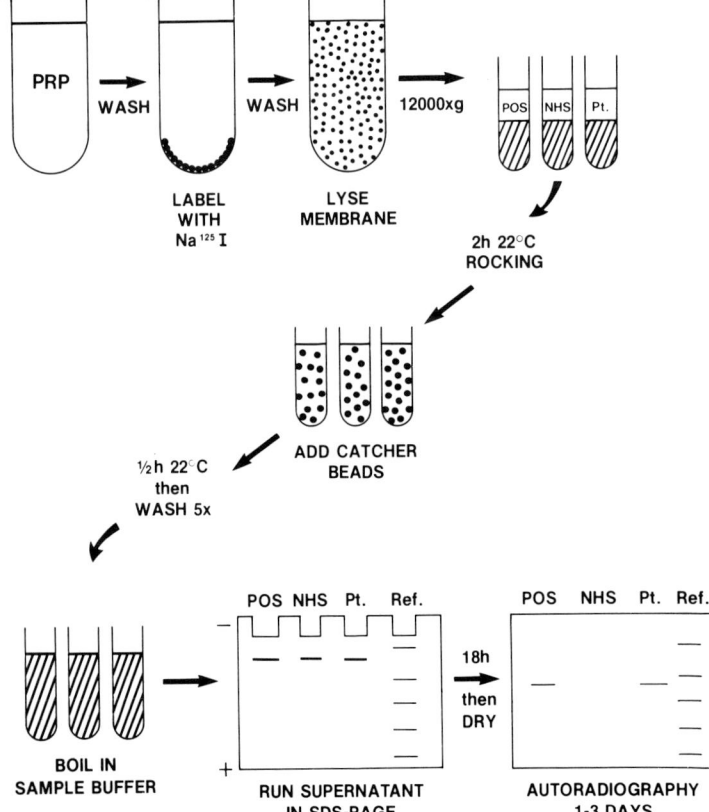

Figure 42–19. Schematic representation of the radioimmunoprecipitation technique used to study platelet proteins. Platelet-rich plasma (PRP) is washed and the surface proteins are radiolabeled, frequently by means of sodium ^{125}Iodine. After a further wash, the lipid bilayer is lysed (usually using a detergent). The soluble and radiolabeled proteins are then separated from the platelet skeleton by high-speed centrifugation. The various test seras are added to the radiolabeled platelet membrane (shown in the upper right hand corner of the diagram). POS indicates a positive control, NHS (normal human serum) represents the negative control, and PT represents the patient test serum of interest. This step allows the antibody of interest in the patient test serum to react with the surface-labeled glycoproteins. All of the antibody is recovered by the use of a "catcher" system, in this case staphylococcal beads, as shown in the center of the diagram. The beads (which now carry the antibody plus the radiolabeled glycoprotein that bound to the antibody) are pelleted and washed. Antibody bound to the staphylococcal protein A, and the platelet protein are separated from each other by boiling. The soluble protein is applied to an SDS-PAGE, and the protein is separated by electrophoresis and identified by radioautography.

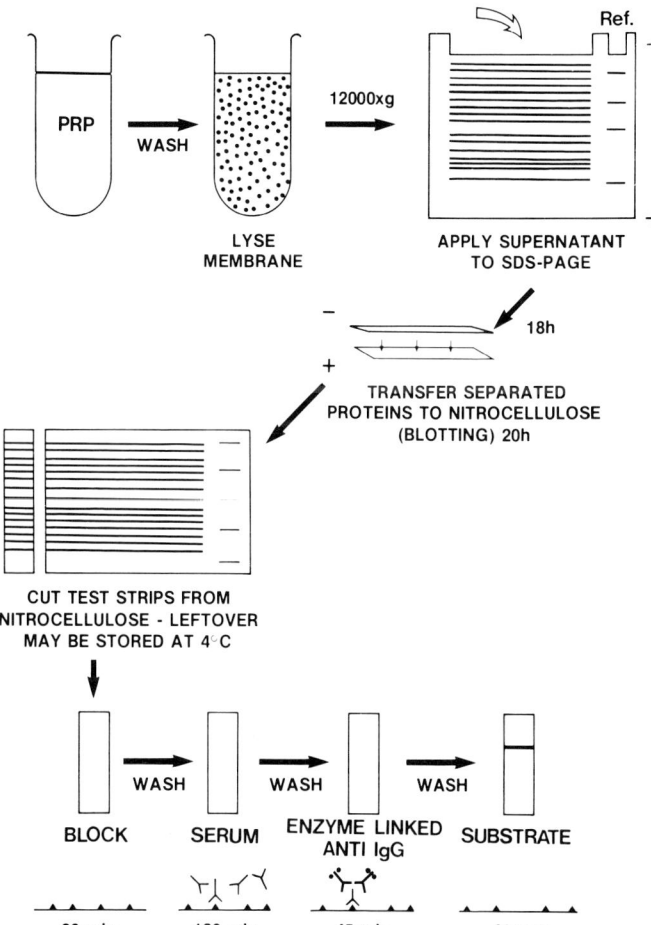

Figure 42–20. The principle of immunoblotting is represented. Platelet-rich plasma (PRP; upper left hand corner of the figure) is washed, and the lipid bilayer is solubilized (usually by the addition of detergent). The platelet skeleton is removed by high-speed centrifugation, and the platelet glycoproteins are separated according to size, using an SDS-PAGE (upper right hand corner of the figure). After separation, the platelet proteins are then transferred to a solid matrix (usually nitrocellulose) in the "blotting" part of the procedure. The efficiency of the blotting can be increased by using electrophoretic techniques for the protein transfer (shown in the center of this figure). The strips are then cut from the nitrocellulose and stored. A schematic representation of the actual technique used to study the various antisera of interest is shown at the bottom of the figure. The nitrocellulose strip is mixed with the test serum, and unbound test serum is then washed away. An enzyme-linked antiserum (usually anti-IgG) is then added, and, after a further wash, the binding of the enzyme-linked antiserum is detected by the addition of a substrate.

teins. After washing, an indicator system (usually an enzyme-labeled antibody against the test antibody) is added, so that the original antibody–platelet glycoprotein interaction can be detected.

References to Part II (Qualitative Abnormalities)

1. Weiss, H. J., Turitto, V. T., et al.: Effect of shear rate on platelet interaction with subendothelium in citrated and native blood. I. Shear rate-dependent decrease of adhesion in von Willebrand's disease and the Bernard-Soulier syndrome. J. Lab. Clin. Med. *92*:750, 1978.
2. Turitto, V. T., Weiss, H. J., et al.: Decreased platelet adhesion on vessel segments in von Willebrand's disease: a defect in initial platelet attachment. J. Lab. Clin. Med. *102*:551, 1983.
3. Zimmerman, T. S., and Ruggeri, Z. M.: von Willebrand's disease. Clin. Haematol. *12*:175, 1983.
4. Phillips, D. R., and Agin, P. P.: Platelet plasma membrane glycoproteins. Evidence for the presence of nonequivalent disulfide bonds using nonreduced-reduced two-dimensional gel electrophoresis. J. Biol. Chem. *252*:2121, 1977.
5. Okumura, T., Lombart, C., et al.: Platelet glycocalicin. II. Purification and characterization. J. Biol. Chem. *251*:5950, 1976.
6. Solum, N. O., Hagen, I., et al.: Platelet glycocalicin: its membrane association and solubilization in aqueous media. Biochim. Biophys. Acta *597*:235, 1980.
7. Fox. J. E. B., Baughan, A. K., et al.: Direct linkage of GP Ib to a M_r = 250,000 polypeptide in platelet cytoskeletons. Blood *62*:255a, 1983.
8. Tusznski, G. P., Daniel, J., et al.: Association of proteins with the platelet cytoskeleton. Semin. Hematol. *22*:303, 1985.
9. Fox, J. E. B., Reynolds, C. C., et al.: Calcium-dependent proteolysis occurs during platelet aggregation. J. Biol. Chem. *258*:9973, 1983.
10. Peerschke, E. I. B.: The platelet fibrinogen receptor. Semin. Hematol. *22*:241, 1985.
11. Nachman, R. L., and Leung, L.: Complex formation of platelet membrane glycoproteins IIb and IIIa with fibrinogen. J. Clin. Invest. *69*:263, 1982.
12. Bennett, J. S., Hoxie, J. A., et al.: Inhibition of fibrinogen binding to stimulated human platelets by a monoclonal antibody. Proc. Natl. Acad. Sci. USA *80*:2417, 1983.
13. Parise, L. V., and Phillips, D. R.: Reconstitution of the purified platelet fibrinogen receptor. Fibrinogen binding properties of the glycoprotein IIb-IIIa complex. J. Biol. Chem. *260*:10698, 1985.
14. McEver, R. P., Bennett, E. B., et al.: Identification of two structurally and functionally distinct sites on human platelet membrane glycoprotein IIb-IIIa using monoclonal antibodies. J. Biol. Chem. *258*:5269, 1983.
15. Pidard, D., Montgomery, R. R., et al.: Interaction of Ap-2, a monoclonal antibody specific for human platelet glycoprotein IIb-IIIa complex, with intact platelets. J. Biol. Chem. *258*:12582, 1983.
16. Solum, N. O.: Platelet membrane proteins. Semin. Hematol. *22*:289, 1985.
17. Marguerie, G. A., Thomas-Maison, N., et al.: The platelet

fibrinogen receptor. Evidence for proximity of the α-chain of fibrinogen to platelet membrane glycoproteins IIb/IIIA. J. Biol. Chem. *139*:5, 1984.
18. Fujimoto, T., and Hawiger, J.: Adenosine diphosphate induces binding of von Willebrand factor to human platelets. Nature *297*:154, 1982.
19. Nokes, T. J. C., Mahmoud, N. A., et al.: von Willebrand factor has more than one binding site for platelets. Thromb. Res. *34*:361, 1984.
20. Schullek, J., Jordan, J., et al.: Interaction of von Willebrand factor with human platelets in the plasma milieu. J. Clin. Invest. *73*:421, 1984.
21a. Kunicki, T. J., and Aster, R. H.: Deletion of the platelet-specific alloantigen Pl[Al] from platelets in Glanzmann's thrombasthenia. J. Clin. Invest. *61*:1225, 1978.
21b. Kunicki, T. J., and Aster, R. H.: Isolation and immunologic characterization of the human platelet alloantigen, Pl[Al]. Mol. Immunol. *16*:353, 1979.
22. Van Loeuwen, E. F., Kr von Dem Borne, A. E. G., et al.: Absence of platelet specific alloantigens in Glanzmann's thrombasthenia. Blood *57*:49, 1981.
23. Kieffer, N., Boizard, B., et al.: A new platelet alloantigen specific from membrane glycoprotein IIb. Blood (in press).
24. Berndt, M. C., and Phillips, D. R.: Purification and preliminary physiochemical characterization of human platelet membrane glycoprotein V. J. Biol. Chem. *256*:59, 1981.
25. Stricker, R. B., and Shuman, M. A.: Quinidine purpura: evidence that glycoprotein V is a target platelet antigen. Blood *67*:1377, 1986.
26. Chong, B. H., Berndt, M. C., et al.: Quinidine-induced thrombocytopenia and leukopenia—demonstration and characterization of distinct antiplatelet and antileucocyte antibodies. Blood *62*:1218, 1983.
27. Berndt, M. C., Gregory, C., et al.: Additional glycoprotein defects in Bernard-Soulier's syndrome: confirmation of genetic basis by parental analysis. Blood *62*:800, 1983.
28. Rosenfeld, S. I., Looney, R. J., et al.: Human platelet Fc receptor for immunoglobulin G. J. Clin. Invest. *76*:2317, 1985.
29. Bills, T. K., Smith, J. B., et al.: Metabolism of (^{14}C) arachidonic acid by human platelets. Biochem. Biophys. Acta *424*:303, 1976.
30. Bell, R. L., Kennerly, D. A., et al.: Diglyceride lipase: a pathway for arachidonate release from human platelets. Proc. Natl. Acad. Sci. USA *76*:3238, 1979.
30a. Smith, J. B., Danglemeyer, C., et al.: Measurement of arachidonic acid liberation in thrombin stimulated human platelets. Biochim. Biophys. Acta *835*:344, 1985.
30b. Holub, B.-J.: Diacylyglycerol lipase pathway is a minor source of released arachidonic acid in thrombin-stimulated, human platelets. Biochim. Biophys. Res. Comm. *134*:1327, 1986.
30c. Brookman, M. J., Ward, J. W., et al.: Phospholipid metabolism in stimulated human platelets. Changes in phosphatidylinositol, phosphatidic acid and lysophospholipids. J. Clin. Invest. *66*:275, 1980.
30d. Ballou, L. R., DeWitt, L. M., et al.: Substrate specific forms of human platelet phospholipase A_2. J. Biol. Chem. *261*:3107, 1986.
31. Marcus, A. J.: The role of lipids in platelet function: with particular reference to the arachidonic acid pathway. J. Lipid Res. *19*:793, 1978.
32. Granstrom, E., Dieztalusy, U., et al.: Thromboxane A_2: biosynthesis and effects on platelets. In *Prostaglandins and the Cardiovascular System*. Oates, J. A. (ed.), New York, Raven Press, 1982 p. 15.
33. Gerrard, J. M.: Arachidonic acid metabolizing enzymes and inhibitors. In *Prostaglandins and Leukotrienes*. Brinkhous, K. M. (ed.), New York, Marcel Dekker, 1985, p. 61.
34. Gerrard, J. M.: Blood platelets and arachidonic acid metabolism. In *Prostaglandins and Leukotrienes*. Brinkhous, K. M. (ed.), New York, Marcel Dekker, 1985, p. 77.
35. Charo, I. F., Feinman, R. D., et al.: Interrelations of platelet aggregation and secretion. J. Clin. Invest. *60*:866, 1977.
36a. Charo, I. F., Feinman, R. D., et al.: Prostaglandin endoperoxides and thromboxane A_2 can induce platelet aggregation in the absence of secretion. Nature *269*:66, 1977.
36b. Holmsen, H.: Platelet metabolism and activation. Semin. Hematol. *22*:219, 1985.
37. Adelson, E., Rheinbold, J. J., et al.: The platelet as a sponge: a review. Blood *17*:767, 1961.
38. Schmaier, A. H.: Platelet forms of plasma proteins: plasma cofactors/substrates and inhibitors contained within platelets. Semin. Hematol. *22*:187, 1985.
39. Howard, M. A., Montgomery, D. C., et al.: Factor VIII-related antigen in platelets. Throm. Res. *4*:617, 1974.
40. Hoyer, L. W., des Los Santo, R. P., et al.: Anti-hemophilic factor antigen localization in endothelial cells by immunofluorescent microscopy. J. Clin. Invest. *52*:2737, 1973.
41. Koutts, J., Walsh, P. N., et al.: Active release of human platelet factor VIII-related antigen by adenosine diphosphate, collagen and thrombin. J. Clin. Invest. *62*:1255, 1978.
42. Ruggeri, Z. M., Bader, R., et al.: High affinity interaction of platelet von Willebrand factor with distinct platelet membrane sites. Thromb. Haemost. *50*:35, 1983.
43. Nachman, R. L., Marcus, A. J., et al.: Immunologic studies of proteins associated with subcellular fractions of normal human platelets. J. Lab. Clin. Med. *69*:651, 1967.
44. Day, H. J., and Solum, N. O.: Fibrinogen associated with subcellular platelet particles. Scand. J. Haematol. *10*:136, 1973.
45. Kaplan, K. L., Broekman, J., et al.: Platelet alpha-granule proteins: studies on release and subcellular localization. Blood *53*:604, 1979.
46. Tracy, P. B., Eide, L. L., et al.: Radioimmunoassay of factor V in human plasma and platelets. Blood *60*:59, 1982.
47. Miletich, J. P., Majerus, D. W., et al.: Patients with congenital factor V deficiency have decreased factor Xa binding sites on their platelets. J. Clin. Invest. *62*:824, 1978.
48. Schmaier, A. H., Zuckerbert, A., et al.: High molecular weight kininogen. A secreted platelet protein. J. Clin. Invest. *71*:1477, 1983.
49. Schmaier, A. H., Smith, R. M., et al.: High molecular weight kininogen: localization in unstimulated and activated platelets, and activation by a platelet cysteine protease. Circulation *70*:II–352, 1984.
50. Sinha, D., Seaman, F. S., et al.: Blood coagulation factor XIa binds specifically to a site on activated human platelets distinct from that for factor XI. J. Clin. Invest. *73*:1550, 1984.
51a. Plow, E. F., Birdwell, C., et al.: Identification and quantification of platelet-associated fibronectin antigen. J. Clin. Invest. *63*:540, 1979.
51b. Phillips, D. R., Jennings, I. K., et al.: Ca^{++}-mediated association of glycoprotein G (thrombin-sensitive protein, thrombospondin) with human platelets. J. Biol. Chem. *255*:11629, 1980.
52. Bernard, J., and Soulier, J.: Sur une nouvelle variété de dystrophie thrombocytaire hemorragipare congenitale. Sem. Hop. Paris *24*:3217, 1948.
53. Nurden, A. T., and Caen, J. P.: Specific roles for platelet surface glycoproteins in platelet function. Nature *255*:720, 1975.
54. Clemetson, K. J., McGregor, J. L., et al.: Characterization of the platelet membrane glycoprotein abnormalities in Bernard-Soulier syndrome and comparison with normal

55. Berndt, M. C., Gregory, C., et al.: Additional glycoprotein defects in Bernard-Soulier's syndrome: confirmation of genetic basis by parental analysis. Blood 62:800, 1983.
56. Nurden, A. T.: Didry-Dupruis, D., et al.: Molecular defect of platelets in the Bernard-Soulier syndrome. Blood Cells 9:333, 1983.
57. White, J. G., Burris, S. M., et al.: Micropipette aspiration of human blood platelets: a defect in Bernard-Soulier's syndrome. Blood 63:1249, 1984.
58. Kristopeit, S. M., and Kunicki, T. J.: Quantitation of platelet membrane glycoproteins in Glanzmann's thrombasthenia and the Bernard-Soulier syndrome by electroimmunoassay. Thromb. Res. 36:133, 1984.
59. Johnston, G. I., Heptinstall, S., et al.: The expression of glycoproteins on single blood platelets from controls and from patients with congenital bleeding disorders. Biochem. Biophys. Res. Commun. 123:1091, 1984.
60. Moake, J. L., Olson, J. D., et al.: Binding of radioiodinated human vWF to Bernard-Soulier, thrombasthenic and vW disease platelets. Thromb. Res. 19:21, 1980.
61. Frojmovic, M. M., Milton, J. G., et al.: Platelets from giant platelet syndrome (BSS) are discocytes and normal sized. J. Lab. Clin. Med. 91:109, 1978.
62. Rendu, F., Nurden, A. T., et al.: Relationship between mepacrine-labeled dense body number, platelet capacity to accumulate ^{14}C-5HT and platelet density in the Bernard-Soulier and Hermansky-Pudlak syndromes. Thromb. Haemost. 42:694, 1979.
63. Weiss, H. J., Tschopp T. B., et al.: Decreased adhesion of giant (Bernard-Soulier) platelets to subendothelium. Further implications on the role of von Willebrand factor in hemostasis. Am. J. Med. 57:920, 1974.
64. Bithell, T. C., Parekh, S. J., et al.: Platelet function in the Bernard-Soulier syndrome. Ann. N.Y. Acad. Sci. 201:145, 1972.
65. Caen, J. P., Levy-Toledano, S., et al.: La dystrophie thrombocytaire hemorrhagipare (interaction des plaquettes et du facteur Willebrand). Nouv. Rev. Fr. Hematol. 13:595, 1973.
66. Howard, M. A., Hutton, R. A., et al.: Hereditary giant platelet syndrome: a disorder of a new aspect of platelet function. Br. Med. J. 2:586, 1973.
67. Weiss, H. J., Witte, L. D., et al.: Heterogeneity in storage pool deficiency: studies on granule-bound substances in 18 patients including variants deficient in α-granules, platelet factor 4, β-thromboglobulin, and platelet-derived growth factor. Blood 54:1296, 1979.
68. Walsh, P. N., Mills, D. C. B., et al.: Hereditary giant platelet syndrome: absence of collagen-induced coagulant activity and deficiency of factor XI binding to platelets. Br. J. Haematol. 29:639, 1975.
69. Caen, J. P., Nurden, A. T., et al.: Bernard-Soulier syndrome—a new platelet glycoprotein abnormality. Its relationship with platelet adhesion to subendothelium and with the factor VIII von Willebrand protein. J. Lab. Clin. Med. 87:586, 1976.
70. Glanzmann, E.: Hereditare haemorrhagische thromboasthenie, E in Beitrag zur pathologie der blut plattchen. Jahrb Kinderheilk 88:1, 1918.
71. Hardisty, R. M., Dormandy, K. M., et al.: Thrombasthenia: studies on three cases. Br. J. Haematol. 10:371, 1964.
72. Caen, J. P., Castaldi, P. A., et al.: Congenital bleeding disorders with long bleeding time and normal platelet count. I. Glanzmann's thrombasthenia (report of 15 patients). Am. J. Med. 41:4, 1966.
73. Baumgartner, H. R., and Muggli, R.: Adhesion and aggregation: morphological demonstration and quantitation in vitro and in vivo. In Platelets in Biology and Pathology. Gordon, J. L. (ed.), Amsterdam, Elsevier/North Holland, 1976, p. 23.
74. Legrand, C., and Caen, J. P.: Binding of ^{14}C-ADP by thrombasthenic platelet membranes. Haemostasis 5:231, 1976.
75. White, G. C. H., Workman, E. F. Jr., et al.: Thrombin binding to thrombasthenic platelets. J. Lab. Clin. Med. 91:76, 1978.
76. Born, G. V. R., and Cross, M. J.: Effects of inorganic ions and of plasma proteins on the aggregation of blood platelets by adenosine diphosphate. J. Physiol. (Lond.) 170:397, 1964.
77. Mustard, J. F., Packham, M. A., et al.: Fibrinogen and ADP-induced platelet aggregation. Blood 52:453, 1978.
78. Nurden, A. T., and Caen, J. P.: An abnormal platelet glycoprotein pattern in three cases of Glanzmann's thrombasthenia. Br. J. Haematol. 28:253, 1974.
79. Phillips, D. R., and Agin, P. P.: Platelet membrane defects in Glanzmann's thrombasthenia: evidence for decreased amounts of two major glycoproteins. J. Clin. Invest. 60:535, 1977.
80. Nurden, A. T., and Caen, J. P.: The different glycoprotein abnormalities in thrombasthenic and Bernard-Soulier platelets. Semin. Haematol. 16:235, 1979.
81. Gogstad, G., Hettand, O., et al.: Monocytes and platelets share the glycoproteins IIb, IIIa that are absent from both cells in Glanzmann's thrombasthenia type I. Biochem. J. 214:331, 1983.
82. Lee, H., Nurden, A. T., et al.: Relationship between fibrinogen binding and the platelet glycoprotein deficiencies in Glanzmann's thrombasthenia type I and type II. Br. J. Haematol. 48:47, 1981.
83. Mustard, J. F., Kinlough-Rathbone, R. E., et al.: Comparison of fibrinogen association with normal and thrombasthenic platelets on exposure to ADP or chymotrypsin. Blood 54:987, 1979.
84. Bennett, J. S., and Vilaire, G.: Exposure of platelet fibrinogen receptors by ADP and epinephrine. J. Clin. Invest. 64:1393, 1979.
85. Caen, J. P.: Glanzmann's thrombasthenia. Clin. Haematol. 1:383, 1972.
86. Hagen, I., Nurden, A. T., et al.: Immunochemical evidence for protein abnormalities in platelets from patients with Glanzmann's thrombasthenia and Bernard-Soulier syndrome. J. Clin. Invest. 65:722, 1980.
87. Shulman, S., and Karpatkin, S.: Crossed immunoelectrophoresis of human platelet membranes. Diminished major antigen in Glanzmann's thrombasthenia and Bernard-Soulier syndrome. J. Biol. Chem. 255:4320, 1980.
88. Kunicki, T. J., Nurden, A. T., et al.: Characterization of human platelet glycoprotein antigens giving rise to individual immunoprecipitates in crossed immunoelectrophoresis. Blood 58:1081, 1981.
89. Nurden, A. T., Didry, D., et al.: Residual amounts of glycoproteins IIb and IIIa may be present in the platelets of most patients with Glanzmann's thrombasthenia. Blood 65:1021, 1985.
90. Lightsey, A., Plow, E. F., et al.: Glanzmann's thrombasthenia in the absence of GP IIb and III deficiency. Blood 58:199, 1981, (abstr.).
91. Caen, J. P., Rosa, J. P., et al.: Thrombasthenia Paris, I variant, a model for the study of the platelet glycoprotein (GP) IIb–IIIa complex. Blood 62:25, 1983 (abstr.).
92. Clemetson, K. J., Capitanio, A., et al.: Additional platelet membrane glycoprotein abnormalities in Glanzmann's thrombasthenia: a comparison with normals by high resolution two-dimensional polyacrylamide gel electrophoresis. Thromb. Res. 18:797, 1980.
93. Ikeda, Y., Satoh, K., et al.: Altered cytoskeletal structures of thrombasthenic platelets. Thromb. Res. 30:113, 1983.

94. Langer, B. G., Gonnella, P. A., et al.: α-Actinin and vinculin in normal and thrombasthenic platelets. Blood 63:606, 1984.
95. Zonneveld, G. T. E., van Leeuwen, E. F., et al.: Detection of carriers in Glanzmann's thrombasthenia. Thromb. Haemost. 49:182, 1983.
96. Stomorken, H., Gogstad, G. O., et al.: Diagnosis of heterozygotes in Glanzmann's thrombasthenia. Thromb. Haemost. 48:217, 1982.
97. Jennings, L. K., Ashmun, R. A., et al.: Analysis of human platelet glycoproteins IIb–IIIa and Glanzmann's thrombasthenia in whole blood by flow cytometry. Blood 68:173, 1986.
98. Kaplan, C., Patereau, C., et al.: Antenatal PL^{A1} cell typing and detection of GP IIb–IIIa complex. Br. J. Haematol. 60:586, 1985.
99. Reichert, N., and Seligsohn, U.: Clinical and genetic aspects of Glanzmann's thrombasthenia in Israel—Report of 22 cases. Thromb. Diath. Haemorrh. 34:806, 1975.
100. Nurden, A. T., George, J. N., et al.: Platelet membrane glycoproteins: their structure, function and modification in disease. In *Biology of Platelets*. Phillips, D. R., and Shuman, M. A. (eds.), San Diego, Academic Press (in press).
101. Raccuglia, G.: Gray platelet syndrome. A variety of qualitative platelet disorders. Am. J. Med. 51:818, 1971.
102. Gerrard, J. M., Phillips, D. R., et al.: Biochemical studies of two patients with the gray platelet syndrome: selective deficiency of platelet α-granules. J. Clin. Invest. 66:102, 1980.
103. White, J. G.: Ultrastructural studies of the gray platelet syndrome. Am. J. Pathol. 95:445, 1979.
104. Levy-Toledano, S., Caen, J. P., et al.: Gray platelet syndrome: α-granule deficiency: its influence on platelet function. J. Lab. Clin. Med. 98:831, 1981.
105. Breton-Gorius, J., Vainchenker, W., et al.: Defective α-granule production in megakaryocytes from gray platelet syndrome: ultrastructural studies of bone marrow cells and megakaryocytes growing in culture from blood precursors. Am. J. Pathol. 102:10, 1981.
106. Nurden, A. T., Kunicki, T. J., et al.: Specific protein and glycoprotein deficiencies in platelets isolated from 2 patients with the gray platelet syndrome. Blood 59:709, 1982.
107. Berndt, M. C., Castaldi, P. A., et al.: Morphologic and biochemical confirmation of gray platelet syndrome in 2 siblings. Aust. N. Z. J. Med. 13:387, 1983.
108. Mori, K., Suzuki, S., et al.: Electron microscopic and functional studies on platelets in gray platelet syndrome. Tohoku J. Exp. Med. 143:261, 1984.
109. Chesney, C. M., Pifer, D., et al.: Subcellular localization and secretion of factor V from human platelets. Proc. Natl. Acad. Sci. USA 78:5180, 1981.
110. George, J. N., Nurden, A. T., et al.: Molecular defects in interactions of platelets with the vessel wall. New Engl. J. Med. 311:1084, 1984.
111. Caen, J. P., Sultan, Y., et al.: New familial platelet disease. Lancet 1:203, 1968.
112. Grottum, K. A., Hovig, T., et al.: Wiskott-Aldrich syndrome: qualitative platelet defects and short platelet survival. Br. J. Haematol. 17:373, 1969.
113. Hardisty, R. M., and Hutton, R. A.: Bleeding tendency associated with a new abnormality of platelet behaviour. Lancet 1:983, 1967.
114. Sahud, M. A., and Aggeler, P. M.: Platelet dysfunction: differentiation of a newly recognized primary type from that produced by aspirin. New Engl. J. Med. 280:453, 1969.
115. Weiss, H. J.: Platelet aggregation, adhesion and ADP release in thrombopathia. Am. J. Med. 43:570, 1967.
116. Weiss, H. J., Chervenick, P. A., et al.: A familial defect in platelet function associated with impaired release of ADP. New Engl. J. Med. 281:1264, 1969.
117. Holmsen, H., and Weiss, H. J.: Hereditary defect in the release reaction caused by a deficiency in the storage pool of platelet adenine nucleotides. Br. J. Haematol. 19:643, 1970.
118. Weiss, H. J.: Platelet physiology and abnormalities of platelet function. New Engl. J. Med. 293:531, 580, 1975.
119. Weiss, H. J., and Ames, R. P.: Ultrastructural findings in storage pool disease and aspirin-like defects of platelets. Am. J. Pathol. 71:447, 1973.
120. Holmsen, H., and Weiss, H. J.: Further evidence for a deficient storage pool of adenine nucleotides in platelets from some patients with storage pool disease. Blood 39:197, 1972.
121. Lages, B., Scrutton, M., et al.: Metal ion content of gel-filtered platelets from patients with storage pool disease. Blood 46:119, 1975.
122. Weiss, H. J., Witte, C. D., et al.: Heterogeneity in storage pool disease. Blood 54:1296, 1979.
123. Willis, A. L., and Weiss, H. J.: A congenital defect in platelet prostaglandin production associated with impaired hemostasis in storage pool disease. Prostaglandins 4:783, 1972.
124. Rendu, F., Breton-Goruis, J., et al: Studies on a new variant of the Hermansky-Pudlak syndrome: Qualitative, ultrastructural, and functional abnormalities of platelet dense bodies associated with a phospholipase A-defect. Am. J. Hematol. 4:387, 1978.
125. Malmsten, C., Kindahl, H., et al.: Thromboxane synthesis and the platelet release reaction in Bernard-Soulier syndrome, Glanzmann thrombasthenia and Hermansky-Pudlak syndrome. Br. J. Haematol. 35:511, 1977.
126. Gerrard, J. M., White, J. G., et al.: Labile aggregating stimulating substance (LASS): the factor from storage pool deficient platelets correcting defective aggregation and release of aspirin treated normal platelets. Br. J. Haematol. 29:657, 1975.
127. Weiss, H. J., and Lages, B.: Platelet malondialdehyde production and aggregation responses induced by arachidonate, PGG$_2$, collagen and epinephrine in 12 patients with storage pool deficiency. Blood 58:27, 1981.
128. Weiss, H. J.: Congenital disorders of platelet function. Semin. Hematol. 17:228, 1980.
129. Holmsen, H., Setkowsky, C. A., et al.: Content and thrombin-induced release of acid hydrolases in gel filtered platelets from patients with storage pool deficiency. Blood 46:131, 1975.
130. Hermansky, F., and Pudlak, P.: Albinism associated with hemorrhagic diathesis and unusual pigmented reticular cells in the bone marrow. Report of 2 cases with histochemical studies. Blood 14:162, 1959.
131. Maurer, H. M., Wolff, J. A., et al.: Impotent platelets in albinos with prolonged bleeding times. Blood 39:490, 1972.
132. Baldini, M. G.: Nature of the platelet defect in the Wiskott-Aldrich syndrome. Ann. N.Y. Acad. Sci. 201:437, 1972.
133. Trung, P. H., Griscelli, C., et al.: Ultrastructure des plaquettes sanguines dans le syndrome de Wiskott-Aldrich. Pathol. Biol. 23:57, 1975.
134. Sultan, Y., Scrobohaci, M. L., et al.: Abnormal platelet function, population, and survival time in a boy with congenital absent radii and thrombocytopenia [Letter]. Lancet 2:653, 1972.
135. Day, H. J., and Holmsen, H.: Platelet adenine nucleotide "storage pool deficiency" in TAR syndrome. J.A.M.A. 221:1053, 1972.
136. Zahavi, J., Gale, R., et al.: Storage pool disease of platelets in an infant with thrombocytopenic absent radii syndrome simulating Fanconi anemia. Thromb. Haemost. 38:283, 1977 (Abstr.).
137. Buchanan, G. R., and Handin, R. I.: Platelet function in the Chédiak-Higashi syndrome. Blood 47:941, 1976.
138. Bell, T. G., Meyers, K. M., et al.: Decreased nucleotide

and serotonin storage associated with defective function in Chédiak-Higashi syndrome. Cattle and human platelets. Blood 48:175, 1976.
139a. Boxer, G. J., Holmsen, H., et al.: Abnormal platelet function in Chédiak-Higashi syndrome. Br. J. Haematol. 35:521, 1977.
139b. Rendu, F., Breton-Gorius, J., et al.: Evidence that abnormal platelet function in human Chédiak-Higashi syndrome is the result of lack of dense bodies. Am. J. Pathol. 111:307, 1983.
140. White, J. G., Edson, J. R., et al.: Studies of platelets in a variant of the Hermansky-Pudlak syndrome. Am. J. Pathol. 63:319, 1971.
141. Davis, W. C., and Douglas, S. D.: Defective granule formation and function in the Chédiak-Hegashi syndrome in man and animals. Semin. Hematol. 9:431, 1972.
142. Novak, E. K., McGarry, M. P., et al.: Correction of hereditary platelet storage pool disease by marrow transplantation in four genetically distinct mouse models. Blood 64:218a, 1984.
143. Rao, A. K., Kolke, K., et al.: A platelet secretion defect associated with impaired liberation of arachidonic acid and normal myosin light chain phosphorylation. Blood 64:914, 1984.
144. Malmsten, C., Hamber, M., et al.: Physiological role of an endoperoxide in human platelets. Hemostatic defect due to platelet cyclooxygenase deficiency. Proc. Natl. Acad. Sci. USA 72:1446, 1975.
145. Weiss, H. J., and Lages, B. A.: Possible congenital defect in platelet thromboxane synthesis. Lancet 1:760, 1977.
146. Lagarde, M., Byron, P. A., et al.: Impairment of platelet thromboxane A_2 generation and of the platelet release reaction in 2 patients with congenital deficiency of platelet cyclooxygenase. Br. J. Haematol. 38:251, 1978.
147. Horellou, M. H., Lecompte, T., et al.: Familial and constitutional bleeding disorder due to platelet cyclooxygenase deficiency. Am. J. Hematol. 14:1, 1983.
148. Pareti, F. I., Mannucci, P. M., et al.: Congenital deficiency of thromboxane and prostacyclin. Lancet 1:898, 1980.
149. Rak, K., and Boda, Z.: Hemostatic balance in congenital deficiency of platelet cyclooxygenase. Lancet 2:44, 1980.
150. Roth, G. J., and Machuga, R.: Radioimmune assay of human platelet prostaglandin synthetase. J. Lab. Clin. Med. 99:187, 1982.
151. Rao, A. K., Koike, K., et al.: Bleeding disorder associated with albumin-dependent partial deficiency in platelet thromboxane production. Am. J. Clin. Pathol. 83:687, 1985.
152. Mestel, F., Oetliker, O., et al.: Severe bleeding associated with defective thromboxane synthetase. Lancet 1:157, 1980.
153. Defreyn, G., Machin, S. J., et al.: Familial bleeding tendency with partial platelet thromboxane synthetase deficiency. Reorientation of cyclic endoperoxide metabolism. Br. J. Haematol. 49:29, 1981.
154. Wu, K. K., Minkoff, I. M., et al.: Hereditary bleeding disorder due to a primary defect in the platelet release reaction. Br. J. Haematol. 47:241, 1981.
155. Lages, B., Malmsten, C., et al.: Impaired platelet response to thromboxane A_2 and defective calcium mobilization in a patient with a bleeding disorder. Blood 57:545, 1981.
156. Samama, M., Lecrubier, C., et al.: Constitutional thrombocytopathy with subnormal response to thromboxane A_2. Br. J. Hematol. 48:293, 1981.
157. Wu, K. K., LeBreton, G. C., et al.: Abnormal platelet response to thromboxane A_2. J. Clin. Invest. 67:1801, 1981.
158. Rao, A. K., Willis, J., et al.: A major role of ADP in thromboxane transfer experiments. J. Lab. Clin. Med. 104:116, 1984.
159. Kolke, K., Rao, A. K., et al.: Platelet secretion defect in patients with the attention deficit disorder and easy bruising. Blood 63:427, 1984.
160. Rao, A. K., and Holmsen, H.: Congenital disorders of platelet function. Semin. Hematol. 23:102, 1986.
161a. Takahashi, H., Hattori, A., et al.: A family with a platelet release mechanism abnormality with normal arachidonate metabolism and defective response to ionophore A23187. Blood Vessels 12:223, 1981.
161b. Hardisty, R. M., Machin, S. I., et al.: A new congenital defect of platelet secretion: impaired responsiveness of the platelets to cytoplasmic free calcium. Br. J. Haematol. 53:543, 1983.
162. Czapek, E. E., Deykin, D., et al.: Platelet dysfunction in glycogen storage disease type I. Blood 41:235, 1973.
163. Corby, D. G., Putnam, C. W., et al.: Impaired platelet function in glucose-6-phosphatase deficiency. J. Pediatr. 85:71, 1974.
164. Hutton, R. A., Macnab, A. J., et al.: Defective platelet function associated with chronic hypoglycemia. Arch. Dis. Child. 51:49, 1976.
165. Rivard, G. E., Izadi, P., et al.: Functional and metabolic studies of platelets from patients with Lesch-Nyhan syndrome. Br. J. Haematol. 31:245, 1975.
166. Zwaal, R. F. A., and Bevers, E. M.: Platelet phospholipid asymmetry and its significance in hemostasis. Subcell. Biochem. 9:299, 1983.
167. Miletich, J. P., Jackson, C. M., et al.: Properties of the factor Xa binding site on human platelets. J. Biol. Chem. 253:6908, 1978.
168. Zucker, S., Mielke, H., et al.: Oozing and bruising due to abnormal platelet function. Ann. Intern. Med. 76:725, 1971.
169. Weiss, H. J.: Platelet aggregation, adhesion, and ADP release in thrombopathia (platelet factor 3 deficiency). Am. J. Med. 43:570, 1967.
170. Hardisty, R. M., and Hutton, R. A.: Bleeding tendency associated with a "new" abnormality of platelet behavior. Lancet 1:983, 1967.
171. Weiss, H. J., Vicic, W. J., et al.: Isolated deficiency of platelet procoagulant activity. Am. J. Med. 67:206, 1979.
172. Clancy, R., and Firkin, B.: Bisalbuminemia and defective platelets. Aust. N.Z. J. Med. 4:182, 1974.
173. Kasturi, J., Saraya, A. K., et al.: A study of platelet function in primary thrombopathy. Indian J. Med. Res. 60:567, 1972.
174. Girolami, A., Brunetti, D., et al.: Congenital thrombocytopathy (PF3 defect) with prolonged bleeding time but normal platelet adhesiveness, and aggregation. Acta Haematol. 50:116, 1973.
175. Schwartz, J. P., Cooperberg, A. A., et al.: Platelet function studies in patients with glucose-6-phosphate dehydrogenase deficiency. Br. J. Haematol. 27:273, 1974.
176. Sultan, Y., Brouet, J. C., et al.: Isolated platelet factor 3 deficiency [Letter]. New Engl. J. Med. 294:1121, 1976.
177. Miletich, J. P., Kane, W. H., et al.: Deficiency of factor Xa-factor Va binding sites on the platelets of a patient with a bleeding disorder. Blood 54:1015, 1979.
178. Minkoff, I. M., Wu, K. K., et al.: Bleeding disorder due to an isolated platelet factor 3 deficiency. Arch. Intern. Med. 140:366, 1980.
179. Gugler, E., and Luscher, E. F.: Platelet function in congenital afibrinogenemia. Thromb. Diath. Haemorrh. 14:361, 1965.
180. Weiss, H. J., and Rogers, J.: Fibrinogen and platelets in the primary arrest of bleeding: studies in 2 patients with congenital afibrinogenemia. New Engl. J. Med. 285:369, 1971.
181a. Marguerie, G. A., Thomas-Maison, N., et al.: The interaction of fibrinogen with human platelets in a plasma milieu. Blood 59:91, 1982.
181b. Tracy, P. B., Giles, A. R., et al.: Factor V Quebec: a

bleeding diathesis associated with a qualitative platelet factor V deficiency. J. Clin. Invest. 74:1221, 1984.
182. Epstein, M. A., Sahed, M. A., et al.: Hereditary macrothrombocytopathia, nephritis, and deafness. Am. J. Med. 52:299, 1972.
183. Ekstein, J. D., Filip, D. J., et al.: Hereditary thrombocytopenia, deafness, and renal disease. Ann. Intern. Med. 82:639, 1975.
184a. Bernheim, J., Dechavanne, M., et al.: Thrombocytopenia, macrothrombocytopathia, nephritis and deafness. Am. J. Med. 61:145, 1976.
184b. Hansen, M. S., Behnke, O., et al.: Megathrombocytopenia associated with glomerulonephritis, deafness, and aortic cystic medianecrosis. Scand. J. Haematol. 21:197, 1978.
185. Lacombe, M., and D'Angelo, G.: Etudes sur une thrombopathie familiale. Nouv. Rev. Fr. Hematol. 3:611, 1963.
186a. Milton, J. G., and Frojmovic, M. M.: Shape-changing agents produce abnormally large platelets in a hereditary giant platelet syndrome (MPS). J. Lab. Clin. Med. 93:154, 1979.
186b. Vizcaino, G. J., and Diez-Ewald, M.: Thrombocytopenic purpura with giant platelets and ultrastructural platelet defects. Am. J. Hematol. 15:89, 1983.
187. Goodman, R. M., Levitsky, J. M., et al.: The Ehlers-Danlos syndrome and multiple neurofibromatoses in a kindred of mixed derivation, with special emphasis on hemostasis in the Ehlers-Danlos syndrome. Am. J. Med. 32:976, 1962.
188. Kashiwagi, H., Riddle, J. M., et al.: Functional and ultrastructural abnormalities of platelet in Ehlers-Danlos syndrome. Ann. Intern. Med. 63:249, 1965.
189. Estes, J. W., Carey, R. J., et al.: Marfan's syndrome. Hematological abnormalities in a family. Arch. Intern. Med. 116:889, 1965.
190. Estes, S.: Platelet abnormalities in heritable disorders of connective tissue. Ann. N.Y. Acad. Sci. 201:445, 1972.
191. Hathaway, W. E.: Bleeding disorders due to platelet dysfunction. Am. J. Dis. Child. 121:127, 1971.
192. Hathaway, W. E., Solomons, O. C., et al.: Platelet function and pyrophosphates in osteogenesis imperfecta. Blood 39:500, 1972.
193. Onel, D., Ulutin, S. B., et al.: Platelet defect in a case of Ehlers-Danlos syndrome. Acta Haematol. 50:238, 1973.
194. Evensen, S. A., Myhre, L., et al.: Hemostatic studies in osteogenesis imperfecta. Scand. J. Haematol. 33:177, 1984.
195. Lott, I. T., Chase, T. N., et al.: Down's syndrome: transport, storage and metabolism of serotonin in blood platelets. Pediatr. Res. 6:730, 1972.
196. McCoy, E. E., and Enns, L.: Sodium transport, ouabain binding and Na$^+$/K$^+$ ATPase activity in Down's syndrome platelets. Pediatr. Res. 12:685, 1978.
197. McCoy, E. E., and Enns, L.: Potassium uptake by platelets from Down's syndrome and normal subjects. Life Sci. 26:603, 1980.
198a. McCoy, E. E., and Sneddon, J. M.: Decreased calcium content and ^{45}Ca^{++} uptake in Down's syndrome platelets. Pediatr. Res. 18:914, 1984.
198b. Firkin, B. G.: Qualitative platelet disorders. In *The Platelet and its Disorders*. Firkin, B. G. (ed.): Lancaster, England, MTP Press Ltd, 1984.
198c. O'Regan, S., Rivard, G. E., et al.: A circulating inhibitor of platelet aggregation in Bartter's syndrome. Pediatrics 64:939, 1979.
198d. Yarom, R., Muhlrad, A., et al.: Platelet pathology in patients with idiopathic scoliosis. Lab. Invest. 43:208, 1980.
199. Gmiir, J., vonFelten, A., et al.: Delayed alloimmunization using random single donor platelet transfusions: a prospective study in thrombocytopenic patients with acute leukemia. Blood 62:473, 1983.
200. Kekomaki, R., Elfenbein, G., et al.: Improved response of patients refractory to random-donor platelet transfusions by intravenous gamma globulin. Am. J. Med. 76:(suppl):199, 1984.
201. Junghans, R. P., and Ahn, Y. S.: High dose intravenous IgG to suppress alloimmune destruction of donor platelets. Am. J. Med. 76(suppl):204, 1984.
202. Becton, D. L., Kinney, T. R., et al.: High dose intravenous IgG for severe platelet alloimmunization. Pediatrics 74:1120, 1984.
203. Schiffer, C. A., Hogge, D. E., et al.: High dose intravenous IgG in alloimmunized platelet transfusion recipients. Blood 64:937, 1984.
204. Gerritsen, S. W., Akkerman, JWN, et al.: Correction of the bleeding time in patients with storage pool deficiency by infusion of cryoprecipitate. Br. J. Haematol. 40:153, 1978.
205. Kobrinsky, N. L., Israels, E., et al.: Shortening of the bleeding time by 1-deamino-8D-arginine vasopressin in various bleeding disorders. Lancet 1:1145, 1984.
206. Mannucci, P. M., Vicente, V., et al.: The effect of DDAVP on prolonged bleeding time. A placebo controlled trial. Thromb. Haemost. 54:220, 1985.
207. Kitchens, C. S., and Pendergast, J. F.: Human thrombocytopenia is associated with structural abnormalities of the endothelium that are ameliorated by glucocorticosteroid administration. Blood 67:203, 1986.
208. Blajchman, M. A., Senyi, A. F., et al.: Shortening of the bleeding time in rabbits by hydrocortisone caused by inhibition of prostacyclin generation by the vessel wall. J. Clin. Invest. 63:1026, 1979.
209. Corrigan, J. J.: Oral bleeding in hemophilia: treatment with epsilon aminocaproic acid and replacement therapy. J. Pediatr. 80:124, 1972.
210. Green, D., and Ts'ao, C.: Epsilon-aminocaproic acid inhibits platelet binding of fibrinogen. Blood 58:194a, 1981.
211. Bellucci, S., Devergie, A., et al.: Complete correction of Glanzmann's thrombasthenia by allogeneic bone marrow transplantation. Br. J. Haematol. 59:635, 1985.
212. Parkman, R., Rappeport, J., et al.: Correction of the Wiskott-Aldrich syndrome by bone marrow transplantation. New Engl. J. Med. 298:921, 1978.
213. Kapoor, N., Kirkpatrick, D., et al.: Reconstitution of normal megakaryocytopoiesis and immunologic functions in Wiskott-Aldrich syndrome by bone marrow transplantation. Blood 57:692, 1981.
214. Lum, L. G., Tubergen, D. G., et al.: Splenectomy in the management of the thrombocytopenia of the Wiskott-Aldrich syndrome. New Engl. J. Med. 302:892, 1980.
215. Hrodek, O.: Blood platelets in the newborn. Acta Univ. Carol. [Med. Monogr.] 22, 1966.
216. Mull, M. M., and Hathaway, W. E.: Altered platelet function in newborns. Pediatr. Res. 4:229, 1970.
217. Corby, D. G., and Schulman, I.: The effects of antenatal drug administration on aggregation of platelets of newborn infants. J. Pediatr. 79:307, 1971.
218. Corby, D. G., and Zuck, T. F.: Newborn platelet dysfunction: a storage pool and release defect. Thromb. Haemost. 36:200, 1976.
219. Foley, M. E., Clayton, J. K., et al.: Haemostatic mechanisms in maternal, umbilical vein and umbilical artery blood at the time of delivery. Br. J. Obstet. Gynaecol. 84:81, 1977.
220. Whaun, J. M., Smith, G. R., et al.: Effect of prenatal drug administration on maternal and neonatal platelet aggregation and PF 4 release. Haemostasis 9:226, 1980.
221. Ts'ao, C., Green, D., et al.: Function and ultrastructure of platelets of neonates: enhanced ristocetin aggregation of neonatal platelets. Br. J. Haematol. 32:225, 1976.
222. Corby, D. G., and O'Barr, T. P.: Decreased alpha-adrenergic receptors in newborn platelets: cause of abnormal responses to epinephrine. Dev. Pharmacol. Ther. 2:215, 1981.
223. Whaun, J.: The platelet of the newborn infant—adenine

223. nucleotide metabolism and release. Thromb. Haemost. *43*:99, 1980.
224. Stuart, M. J.: The neonatal platelet: evaluation of platelet malonyldialdehyde formation as an indicator of prostaglandin synthesis. Br. J. Haematol. *39*:83, 1978.
225. Stuart, M. J., Dusse, J., et al.: Differences in thromboxane production between neonatal and adult platelets in response to arachidonic acid and epinephrine. Pediatr. Res. *18*:823, 1984.
226. Stuart, M. J., and Allen, J. B.: Arachidonic acid metabolism in the neonatal platelet. Pediatrics *69*:714, 1982.
227. Sadowitz, P., Walenga, R. W., et al.: Differential binding of arachidonic acid by neonatal and adult plasmas. Pediatr. Res. *18*:295, 1984 (Abstr.).
228. Whaun, J. M.: The platelet of the newborn infant. 5HT uptake and release. Thromb. Diath. Haemorrh. *30*:327, 1973.
229. Bendouma, M., McGregor, J. C., et al.: Proteins and glycoproteins of neonatal platelets. Thromb. Haemost. *50*:657, 1983 (Abstr)
230. Gruel, Y., Boizard, B., et al.: Determination of platelet antigens and glycoproteins in the human fetus. Blood *68*:488, 1986.
231. Feusner, J. H.: Normal and abnormal bleeding times in neonates and young children utilizing a fully standardized template technique. Am. J. Clin. Pathol. *74*:73, 1980.
232. Horowitz, H. I., Cohen, B. D., et al.: Defective ADP-induced platelet factor 3 activation in uremia. Blood *30*:331, 1967.
233. Stewart, J. H., and Castaldi, P. A.: Uraemic bleeding: a reversible platelet defect corrected by dialysis. Q. J. Med. *36*:409, 1967.
234. Salzman, E. W., and Neri, L. J.: Adhesiveness of blood platelets in uremia. Thromb. Diath. Haemorrh. *15*:84, 1966.
235. Rabiner, S. F., and Hrodek, O.: Platelet factor 3 in normal subjects and patients with renal failure. J. Clin. Invest. *47*:901, 1968.
236. Eknoyan, G., Wacksman, S. J., et al.: Platelet function in renal failure. New Engl. J. Med. *280*:677, 1969.
237. Joist, J. H., Pechan, J., et al.: Untersuchungen zur Natur und Atiologie der uramischen Thrombocytopathie. Verh. Dtsch. Ges. Inn. Med. *75*:476, 1969.
238a. Horowitz, H. I., Stein, I. M., et al.: Further studies on the platelet inhibitory effect of guanidino-succinic acid: its role in uremic bleeding. Am. J. Med. *49*:336, 1970.
238b. Castillo, R., Lozano, T., et al.: Defective platelet adhesion on vessel subendothelium in uremic patients. Blood *68*:337, 1986.
239. Rabiner, S. F.: Uremic bleeding. Prog. Hemost. Thromb. *1*:233, 1972.
240. Lindsay, R. M., Dennis, B. N., et al.: Platelet function as an assay for uremic toxins. Artif. Organs *4*:82, 1980.
241. Gallice, P., Fournier, N., et al.: In vitro inhibition of platelet aggregation by uremic middle molecules. Biomedicine *33*:185, 1980.
242. Contreras, P., Later, R., et al.: Molecules in the middle molecular weight range. Critical review of methods of separation from fluids of uremic patients. Nephron *32*:193, 1982.
243a. Bazilinski, N., Shaykh, M., et al.: Inhibition of platelet function by uremic middle molecules. Nephron *40*:423, 1985.
243b. Remuzzi, G., Dodesini, P., et al.: Parathyroid hormone inhibits human platelet function. Lancet *2*:1321, 1981.
244. Smith, M. C., and Dunn, M. J.: Impaired platelet thromboxane production in renal failure. Nephron *29*:133, 1981.
245. Remuzzi, G., Benigni, A., et al.: Reduced platelet thromboxane formation in uremia. Evidence for a functional cyclooxygenase defect. J. Clin. Invest. *71*:762, 1983.
246. Defreyn, G., Dauden, M. V., et al.: A plasma factor which stimulates prostacyclin release from cultured endothelial cells. Thromb. Res. *19*:695, 1980.
247. Remuzzi, G., Cavenaghi, A. E., et al.: Bleeding in uremic patients: prostacyclin-like activity and bleeding in renal failure. Lancet *2*:1195, 1977.
248. Janson, P. A., Jubelvier, S. J., et al.: Treatment of the bleeding tendency in uremia with cryoprecipitate. New Engl. J. Med. *303*:1318, 1980.
249. Mannucci, P., Remuzzi, G., et al.: Deamino-8-d-arginine vasopressin shortens the bleeding time in uremia. New Engl. J. Med. *308*:8, 1983.
250. Carvalho, A. C.: Bleeding in uremia—a clinical challenge. New Engl. J. Med. *308*:38, 1983.
251a. Barnhart, M. I., Chen, S., et al.: DDAVP: does the drug have a direct effect on the vessel wall? Thromb. Res. *31*:239, 1983.
251b. Sakariassen, K. S., Cattaneo, M., et al.: DDAVP enhances platelet adherence and platelet aggregate growth on human artery subendothelium. Blood *64*:229, 1984.
252. Stuart, M. J., Ganley, C., et al.: DDAVP inhibits prostacyclin formation: a potential mechanism for bleeding time correction in hemostatic disorders. Pediatr. Res. *19*:268A, Abstract #944, 1985.
253. Mannucci, P. M., Vicente, V., et al.: Controlled trial of desmopressin in liver cirrhosis and other conditions associated with a prolonged bleeding time. Blood *67*:1148, 1986.
254. Livio, M., Marchesi, D., et al.: Uraemic bleeding: role of anaemia and beneficial effect of red cell transfusions. Lancet *2*:1013, 1982.
255. Fernandez, F., Goudable, C., et al.: Low hematocrit and prolonged bleeding time in uraemic patients. Effects of red cell transfusion. Br. J. Haematol. *59*:139, 1985.
256. Liu, Y. K., Kosfeld, R. E., et al.: Treatment of uraemic bleeding with conjugated oestrogen. Lancet *2*:887, 1984.
257. Lechner, K., Niessner, H., et al.: Coagulation abnormalities in liver disease. Semin. Thromb. Hemost. *4*:40, 1977.
258. Straub, P. W.: Diffuse intravascular coagulation in liver disease. Semin. Thromb. Hemost. *4*:29, 1977.
259. Mandel, E. E., and Lazerson, J.: Thrombasthenia in liver disease. New Engl. J. Med. *265*:56, 1961.
260. Weiss, H. J., and Eichelberger, J. W.: Secondary thrombocytopathia: platelet factor 3 in various disease states. Arch. Intern. Med. *112*:827, 1963.
261. Cortet, P., Klepping, C., et al.: Le facteur plaquettaire au cours des cirrhoses alcooliques: Etude de l'adhesivité in vivo par le test de Borchgrevink. Arch. Mal. Appar. Digestif. *53*:1041, 1964.
262. Thomas, D. P., Ream, V. J., et al.: Platelet aggregation in patients with Laennec's cirrhosis of the liver. New Engl. J. Med. *276*:1344, 1967.
263. Ballard, H. S., and Marcus, A. J.: Platelet aggregation in portal cirrhosis. Arch. Intern. Med. *136*:316, 1976.
264. Thomas, D. P.: Abnormalities of platelet aggregation in patients with alcoholic cirrhosis. Ann. N.Y. Acad. Sci. *201*:243, 1972.
265. Jerushalmy, Z., and Zucker, M. B.: Some effects of fibrinogen degradation products (FDP) on blood platelets. Thromb. Diath. Haemorrh. *15*:413, 1966.
266. Kowalski, E.: Fibrinogen derivatives, and their biologic activities. Semin. Hematol. *5*:45, 1968.
267. Solum, N. O., Rigollot, C., et al.: A quantitative evaluation of the inhibition of platelet aggregation by low molecular weight degradation products of fibrinogen. Br. J. Haematol. *24*:419, 1973.
268. Rao, A. K., and Walsh, P. N.: Acquired qualitative platelet disorders. Clin. Haematol. *12*:201, 1983.
269. Ordinas, A., Maragall, S., et al.: A glycoprotein I defect in platelets of three patients with severe cirrhosis of the liver. Thromb. Res. *13*:297, 1978.

270. Burroughs, A. K., Matthews, K., et al.: Desmopressin and bleeding time in patients with cirrhosis. Br. Med. J. *291*:1377, 1985.
271. Agnelli, G., Berrettini, M., et al.: Desmopressin-induced improvement of abnormal coagulation in chronic liver disease. Lancet *1*:645, 1983.
272. Bick, R. L.: Hemostasis defects associated with cardiac surgery, prosthetic devices, and other extracorporeal circuits. Semin. Thromb. Hemost. *11*:249, 1985.
273. Mammen, E. F., Koets, M. H., et al.: Hemostasis changes during cardiopulmonary bypass surgery. Semin. Thromb. Hemost. *11*:281, 1985.
274. Schafer, A. I.: Bleeding and thrombosis in the myeloproliferative disorders. Blood *64*:1, 1984.
275. Hoagland, H. C., and Silverstein, M. N.: Primary thrombocythemia in the young patient. Mayo Clin. Proc. *53*:578, 1978.
276. Singh, A. K., and Wetherley-Mein, G.: Microvascular occlusive lesions in primary thrombocythaemia. Br. J. Haematol. *36*:553, 1977.
277. Jabaily, J., Iland H. J., et al.: Neurologic manifestations of essential thrombocythemia. Ann. Intern. Med. *99*:513, 1983.
278. Murphy, S.: Thrombocytosis and thrombocythaemia. Clin. Haematol. *12*:89, 1983.
279a. Budde, U., Schaefer, G., et al.: Acquired von Willebrand's diseases in the myeloproliferative syndrome. Blood *64*:981, 1984.
279b. Pearson, T. C., and Wetherley-Mien, G.: Vascular occlusive episodes and venous hematocrit in primary proliferative polycythaemia. Lancet *2*:1219, 1978.
280. Walsh, P. N., Murphy, S., et al.: The role of platelets in the pathogenesis of thrombosis and hemorrhage in patients with thrombocytosis. Thromb. Haemost. *38*:1085, 1977.
281. Kessler, C. M., Klein, H. G., et al.: Uncontrolled thrombocytosis in chronic myeloproliferative disorders. Br. J. Haematol. *50*:157, 1982.
282. Berk, P. D., Goldberg, J. D., et al.: Increased incidence of acute leukemia in polycythemia vera associated with chlorambucil therapy. New Engl. J. Med. *304*:441, 1981.
283. Tartaglia, A. P., Goldberg, J. D., et al.: Aspirin and persantine do not prevent thrombotic complications in patients with polycythemia vera treated with phlebotomy. Blood *58*:240a, 1981.
284. Preston, F. E.: Aspirin, prostaglandins and peripheral gangrene. Am. J. Med. *74*(Suppl.):55, 1983.
285. Freidman, I. A., Schwartz, S. O., et al.: Platelet function defects with bleeding: early manifestations of acute leukemia. Arch. Intern. Med. *113*:177, 1964.
286. Caen, J., Rendu, F., et al.: Platelet aggregation and populations in acute leukemia. Haemostasis *1*:61, 1972.
287. Sultan, Y., and Caen, J. P.: Platelet dysfunction in preleukemic states and in various types of leukemia. Ann. N.Y. Acad. Sci. *201*:300, 1972.
288. Cowan, D. H., and Haut, J. J.: Platelet function in acute leukemia. J. Lab. Clin. Med. *79*:893, 1972.
289. Cowan, D. H., Graham, R. C., et al.: The platelet defect in leukemia, platelet ultrastructure, adenine nucleotide metabolism, and the release reaction. J. Clin. Invest. *56*:188, 1975.
290. Russell, N. H., Keenan, J. P., et al.: Thrombocytopathy in preleukemia: association with a defect of thromboxane A_2 activity. Br. J. Haematol. *41*:417, 1979.
291. Maldonado, J. E., and Pierre, R. V.: The platelets in preleukemia and myelomonocytic leukemia. Ultrastructural cytochemistry and cytogenetics. Mayo Clin. Proc. *50*:573, 1975.
292. Ganguly, P., Sutherland, S. B., et al.: Defective binding of thrombin to platelets in myeloid leukemia. Br. J. Haematol. *39*:599, 1978.
293. Lamberth, E. L., Warriner, R. A., et al.: Effect of metabolic acidosis and alkalosis on human platelet aggregation induced by epinephrine and ADP. Proc. Soc. Exp. Biol. Med. *145*:743, 1974.
294. Foley, M. E., and McNicol, G. P.: An in vitro study of acidosis, platelet function, and perinatal cerebral intraventricular haemorrhage. Lancet *1*:1230, 1977.
295. Clancy, R., Jenkins, E., et al.: Qualitative platelet abnormalities in idiopathic thrombocytopenic purpura. New Engl. J. Med. *286*:622, 1972.
296. Stuart, M. J., Kelton, J. G., et al.: Abnormal platelet function and arachidonate metabolism in chronic idiopathic thrombocytopenic purpura. Blood *58*:326, 1981.
297. Zahavi, J., and Marder, V. J.: Acquired "storage pool disease" of platelets associated with circulating antiplatelet antibodies. Am. J. Med. *56*:883, 1974.
298. Weiss, H. J., Rosove, M. H., et al.: Acquired storage pool deficiency with increased platelet associated IgG. Report of 5 cases. Am. J. Med. *69*:711, 1980.
299a. Regan, M. G., Lackner, H., et al.: Platelet function and coagulation profile in lupus erythematosus. Ann. Intern. Med. *81*:462, 1974.
299b. Whigham, K. A. E., Howie, P. W., et al.: Abnormal platelet function in preeclampsia. Br. J. Obstet. Gynecol. *85*:28, 1978.
299c. Kelton, J. G., Hunter, D. J., et al.: A platelet function defect of pre-eclampsia. Obstet. Gynecol. *65*:107, 1985.
300. Solinger, A., Bernstein, I. L., et al.: The effect of epinephrine on platelet aggregation in normal and atopic subjects. J. Allergy Clin. Immunol. *51*:29, 1973.
301. Stuart, M. J., Stockman, J. A., et al.: Abnormalities of platelet aggregation in the vasoocclusive crisis of sickle cell anemia. J. Pediatr. *85*:629, 1974.
302. Gruppo, R. A., Glueck, H. I., et al.: Platelet function in sickle cell anemia. Thromb. Res. *10*:325, 1977.
303. Mehta, P., and Mehta, J.: Abnormalities of platelet aggregation in sickle cell disease. J. Pediatr. *96*:209, 1980.
304. Mehta, P., and Mehta, J.: Circulating platelet aggregates in sickle cell disease patients with and without vasoocclusion. Stroke *10*:464, 1979.
305. Buchanan, G. R., and Holtkamp, C. A.: Platelet aggregation, malondialdehyde generation and production time in children with sickle cell anemia. Thromb. Hemost. *46*:690, 1981.
306. Buchanan, G. R., and Holtkamp, C. A.: Evidence against enhanced platelet activity in sickle cell anemia. Br. J. Haematol. *54*:595, 1983.
307. Pareti, F. I., Capitanio, A., et al.: Acquired storage pool disease in platelets during DIC. Blood *48*:511, 1976.
308. Furie, B.: Acquired coagulation disorders and dysproteinemias. In *Thrombosis and Hemostasis: Basic Principles and Clinical Practice*. Colman, R. W., Hirsh, J., et al. (eds.), Philadelphia, J. B. Lippincott, 1982, p. 577.
309. Friedman, Z., Lamberth, E. L., et al.: Platelet dysfunction in the neonate with essential fatty acid deficiency. J. Pediatr. *90*:439, 1977.
310. Khurana, M. S., Lian, E. C., et al.: Storage pool disease of platelets—association with multiple congenital cavernous hemangiomas. J.A.M.A. *44*:169, 1980.
311. Maurer, H. M., and Caul, J.: Influence of bilirubin on human platelets. Pediatr. Res. *6*:136, 1972.
312. Suvansri, U., Cheung, W. H., et al.: The effect of bilirubin on the human platelet. J. Pediatr. *74*:240, 1969.
313. Edson, J. R., Fecher, D. R., et al.: Low platelet adhesiveness, and other hemostatic abnormalities in hypothyroidism. Ann. Intern. Med. *82*:342, 1975.
314. Nordoy, A., Vik-Mo, H., et al.: Haemostatic and lipid abnormalities in hypothyroidism. Scand. J. Haematol. *16*:154, 1976.
315. Grottum, K. A., Nordoy, A., et al.: Lipid infusions in man. Blood platelet uptake of lipid and effects on platelet function. Thromb. Diath. Haemorrh. *29*:701, 1973.
316. Clancy, R., Jenkins, E., et al.: Platelet defect of infectious mononucleosis. Br. Med. J. *4*:646, 1971.
317. Lake, A. M., Stauffer, J. Q., et al.: Hemostatic alterations

in inflammatory bowel disease. Response to therapy. Am. J. Dig. Dis. 23:897, 1978.
318a. Siess, W., Scherer, B., et al.: Platelet membrane fatty acids, platelet aggregation and thromboxane formation during a mackerel diet. Lancet 1:441, 1980.
318b. Renaud, S., and Nordoy, A.: α-Linolenic and eicosapentaenoic acid in man. Lancet 1:1169, 1983.
318c. Eskimo diets and disease [Editorial]. Lancet 1:1139, 1983.
318d. Lorenz, R.: Platelet function, thromboxane formation and blood pressure control during supplementation of the Western diet with cod liver oil. Circulation 67:504, 1983.
318e. Fischer, S., Weber, P. C., et al.: Prostaglandin I$_3$ is formed in vivo in man after dietary eicosapentaenoic acid. Nature 307:165, 1984.
318f. Gloset, J. A.: Fish, fatty acids and human health. New Engl. J. Med. 314:1253, 1985.
318g. Knapp, H. R., Reilly, I. A. G., et al.: In vivo indexes of platelet and vascular function during fish oil administration in patients with atherosclerosis. New Engl. J. Med. 314:937, 1986.
318h. Fong, J. S. C.: Inhibition of platelet aggregation by α-tocopherol. Fed. Proc. 35:761, 1976.
318i. Machlin, L. G., Filipski, R., et al.: Influence of vitamin E on platelet aggregation and thrombocythemia in the rat. Proc. Soc. Exp. Biol. Med. 149:275, 1975.
318j. Lake, A. M., Stuart, M. J., et al.: Vitamin E deficiency and enhanced platelet function; reversal following vitamin E supplementation. J. Pediatr. 90:722, 1977.
318k. Steiner, M., and Anastasi, J.: Vitamin E: an inhibitor of the platelet release reaction. J. Clin. Invest. 57:732, 1976.
318l. Cox, A. C., Rao, G. H. R., et al.: The influence of vitamin E Quinone on platelet structure, function and biochemistry. Blood 55:907, 1980.
318m. Steiner, M.: Effect of α-tocopherol administration on platelet function in man. Thromb. Haemost. 49:73, 1983.
318n. Ali, M., Gubranson, G., et al.: Inhibition of human platelet cyclooxygenase by α-tocopherol. Prostaglandins Med. 4:79, 1980.
319a. Bello, A., Dorantes, S., et al.: Physical and biochemical characteristics of platelets in severely malnourished children with purpura. Scand. J. Haematol. 8:321, 1971.
319b. Levine, P. H.: A qualitative platelet defect in severe B$_{12}$ deficiency. Ann. Intern. Med. 78:533, 1973.
320. Ingeberg, S., and Stoffersen, E.: Platelet dysfunction in patients with vitamin B$_{12}$ deficiency. Acta Haematol. 61:75, 1979.
321. O'Brien, J. R., Etherington, M., et al.: Refractory state of platelet aggregation with major operations. Lancet 2:741, 1971.
322. O'Brien, J. R., Tulevski, V. G., et al.: Platelet function studies before and after operation and the effect of postoperative thrombosis. J. Lab. Clin. Med. 83:342, 1974.
323. Maurer, H. M., Haggins, J. C., et al.: Platelet injury during phototherapy. Am. J. Hematol. 1:89, 1976.
324. Pareti, F. I., Capitanio, A., et al.: Acquired dysfunction due to circulation of exhausted platelets. Am. J. Med. 69:235, 1980.
325. Hathaway, W. E., Mahasendana, C., et al.: Paradoxical bleeding in intensively tranfused hemophiliacs. Alteration of platelet function. Transfusion 13:6, 1973.
326. Wilson, P., McNicol, G. P., et al.: Platelet abnormality in human scurvy. Lancet 1:975, 1967.
327. Purcell, I. M., and Constantine, J. W.: Platelets and experimental scurvy. Nature 235:389, 1972.
328. Ihle, B. U., and Gillies, M.: Scurvy and thrombocytopathy in a chronic hemodialysis patient. Aust. N. Z. J. Med. 13:523, 1983.
329. Arkel, Y. S., Haft, J. I., et al.: Alteration in second phase platelet aggregation associated with an emotionally stressful activity. In Platelet Function Testing. Day, J. H., and Holmsen, H. (eds.), DHEW Publication No (NIH) 78–1087, Washington, D.C. 1978, p. 705.
330. Eriksson, K. A., Sigvaldason, A., et al.: Platelet activation in response to phlebotomy. An experimental study of healthy blood donors. Acta Med. Scand. 212:121, 1982.
331. Andrén, L., Wadenvik, H., et al.: Stress and platelet activation. Acta Haematol. 70:302, 1983.
332. Rao, A. K., Niewiarowski, S., et al.: Acquired granular pool defect in stored platelets. Blood 57:203, 1981.
333. Rao, A. K., and Murphy, S.: Secretion defect in platelets stored at 4°C. Thromb. Haemost. 47:221, 1982.
334. Eurenius, K., and Rothenberg, J.: Platelet aggregation after thermal injury. J. Lab. Clin. Med. 83:355, 1974.
335. Kaplan, B. S., and Fong, J. S. C.: Reduced platelet aggregation in haemolytic uremic syndrome. Thromb. Haemost. 43:154, 1980.
336. Fong, J. S. C., and King-Hrycaj, B. D.: Impaired and exhausted platelets in modified generalized Shwartzman reaction: an analogue of hemolytic uremic syndrome associated with endotoxemia. J. Lab. Clin Med. 102:847, 1983.
337. Sadowitz, P. D., and Stuart, M. J.: Platelet HHT stimulates prostacyclin production by human endothelial cells. Blood 68:326A, Abstract #1182, 1986.
338. Moncada, S., Gryglewski, R., et al.: An enzyme isolated from arteries transforms prostaglandin endoperoxides to an unstable substance that inhibits platelet aggregation. Nature 263:663, 1976.
339. Moncada, S., Higgs, E. A., et al.: Human arterial and venous tissues generate prostacyclin (prostaglandin X) a potent inhibitor of platelet aggregation. Lancet 1:18, 1977.
340. Marx, J. L.: Blood clotting. The role of prostaglandins. Science 196:1072, 1977.
341. Moncada, S., and Vane, J.: Arachidonic acid metabolites and the interactions between platelets and blood-vessel walls. New Engl. J. Med. 300:1142, 1979.
342. Gerrard, J. M.: Hemostasis, thrombosis, and atherosclerosis. The response of blood cells to vessel wall injury. In Prostaglandins and Leukotrienes. Brinkhous, K. M. (ed.), New York, Marcel Dekker, 1985, p. 217.
343. Siegel, M. I., McConnell, R. T., et al.: Regulation of arachidonate metabolism via lipoxygenase and cyclooxygenase by 12-HPETE, the product of human platelet lipoxygenase. Biochem. Biophys. Res. Commun. 89:1273, 1979.
344. Singer, R.: Acetylsalicylic acid, a probable cause for secondary post-tonsillectomy hemorrhage. Arch. Otolaryngol. 42:19, 1945.
345. Cohen, L. S.: Clinical pharmacology of acetylsalicylic acid. Semin. Thromb. Hemost. 2:146, 1976.
346a. Vane, J. B.: Inhibition of prostaglandin synthesis as a mechanism of action of aspirin-like drugs. Nature 231:232, 1971.
346b. Smith, J. M., and Willis, A. L.: Aspirin selectively inhibits prostaglandin production in human platelets. Nature 231:235, 1971.
347. Rome, L. H., and Lands, W. E. M.: Structural requirements for time-dependent inhibition of prostaglandin synthesis by anti-inflammatory drugs. Proc. Natl. Acad. Sci. USA 72:4863, 1975.
348. Roth, G. J., and Majerus, P. W.: The mechanism of the effect of aspirin on human platelets. Acetylation of a particulate fraction protein. J. Clin. Invest. 56:624, 1975.
349. Roth, G. J., Stanford, N., et al.: Acetylation of prostaglandin synthase by aspirin. Proc. Natl. Acad. Sci. USA 72:3073, 1975.
350. Van Der Ouderaa, F. J., Buytenhek, M., et al.: Acetylation of prostaglandin endoperoxide synthetase with acetylsalicylic acid. Eur. J. Biochem. 109:1, 1980.
351. Dewitt, D. L., Day, J. S., et al.: Monoclonal antibodies

against prostaglandin synthase: an immunoradiometric assay for quantitating the enzyme. Methods Enzymol. 86:229, 1982.
352. Hamberg, M., Svensson, J., et al.: Thromboxanes: a new group of biologically active compounds derived from prostaglandin endoperoxides. Proc. Natl. Acad. Sci. USA 72:2994, 1975.
353. Hamberg, M., Svensson, J., et al.: Isolation and structure of two prostaglandin endoperoxides that cause platelet aggregation. Proc. Natl. Acad. Sci. USA 71:345, 1974.
354. Willis, A. L., Vane, F. M., et al.: An endoperoxide aggregator (LASS) formed in platelets in response to thrombotic stimuli: purification, identification and unique biological significance. Prostaglandins 8:453, 1974.
355. Smith, J. B., Ingerman, C., et al.: Formation of an intermediate in prostaglandin biosynthesis and its association with the platelet release reaction. J. Clin. Invest. 53:1468, 1974.
356a. Packham, M. A., and Mustard, J. F.: Clinical pharmacology of platelets. Blood 50:555, 1977.
356b. Holmsen, H., Setkowsky, C. A., et al.: Content and thrombin-induced release of acid hydrolases in gel-filtered platelets from patients with storage pool disease. Blood 46:131, 1975.
356c. Baumgartner, H. R., Tshopp, T. B., et al.: Platelet interaction with collagen fibrils in flowing blood. Thromb. Haemost. 37:17, 1977.
357. Baenziger, M. L., Dillender, M. J., et al.: Cultured human skin fibroblasts and arterial wall produce a labile platelet inhibitory prostaglandin. Biochem. Biophys. Res. Commun. 78:294, 1977.
358. Burch, J. W., Baenzinger, N. L., et al.: Sensitivity of fatty acid cyclooxygenase from human aorta to acetylation by aspirin. Proc. Natl. Acad. Sci. USA 75:5181, 1978.
359a. Kelton, J. G., Hirsh, J., et al.: Thrombogenic effect of high dose aspirin in rabbits; relationship to inhibition of vessel wall synthesis of prostaglandin I_2-like activity. J. Clin. Invest. 62:892, 1978.
359b. Shaikh, B. S., Bott, S. J., et al.: The differential inhibition of prostaglandin synthesis in response to aspirin. Prostaglandins Med. 4:439, 1980.
360. Wu, K. K., Chen, Y. C., et al.: Differential effects of two doses of aspirin on platelet-vessel wall interaction in vivo. J. Clin. Invest. 68:382, 1981.
361. Pareti, F. I., D'Angelo, A., et al.: Platelets and the vessel wall: how much aspirin? Lancet 1:371, 1980.
362. Preston, F. E., Whipps, S., et al.: Inhibition of prostacyclin and platelet thromboxane A_2 after low dose aspirin. New Engl. J. Med. 304:76, 1981.
363. Masotti, G., Galanti, G., et al.: Differential inhibition of prostacyclin production and platelet aggregation by aspirin. Lancet 2:1213, 1979.
364. Patrignani, P., Filabozzi, P., et al.: Selective cumulative inhibition of platelet thromboxane production by low dose aspirin in healthy subjects. J. Clin. Invest. 69:1366, 1982.
365. Hanley, S. P., and Bevan, J.: Differential inhibition by low dose aspirin of human venous prostacyclin synthesis and platelet thromboxane synthesis. Lancet 1:969, 1981.
366. Weksler, B. B., Pett, S. B., et al.: Differential inhibition by aspirin of vascular and platelet prostaglandin synthesis in atherosclerotic patients. New Engl. J. Med. 308:800, 1983.
367. Preston, F. E., and Greaves, M.: Low dose aspirin inhibits platelet and venous cyclooxygenase in man. Thromb. Res. 27:477, 1982.
368. Fitzgerald, G. A., and Oates, J. A.: Endogenous biosynthesis of prostacyclin and thromboxane and platelet function during chronic administration of aspirin in man. J. Clin. Invest. 71:676, 1983.
369. Bertelé, V., Falnaga, A., et al.: Platelet thromboxane synthetase inhibitors with low doses of aspirin: possible resolution of the aspirin dilemma. Science 220:517, 1983.
370. Rajah, S. M., and Penny, A.: Aspirin and bleeding time. Lancet 2:1104, 1978.
371. Buchanan, M. R., Blajchman, M. A., et al.: Shortening of the bleeding time in thrombocytopenic rabbits after exposure of the jugular vein to high aspirin concentrations. Prostaglandins Med. 3:333, 1979.
372. Aspirin: what dose? [Editorial] Lancet 1:592, 1986.
373. Marcus, A. J.: Aspirin as an antithrombotic medication. New Engl. J. Med. 309:1515, 1983.
374. Marcus, A. J.: The aspirin dilemma revisited. New Engl. J. Med. 310:1326, 1984.
375. McKenna, R., Bachmann, F., et al.: Prevention of venous thromboembolism after total knee replacement by high dose aspirin or intermittent calf and thigh compression. Br. Med. J. 280:514, 1980.
376. Harris, W. H., Salzman, E. W., et al.: Aspirin prophylaxis of venous thromboembolism after total hip replacement. New Engl. J. Med. 297:1246, 1977.
377a. Kelton, J. G., Hirsh, J., et al.: Sex differences in the antithrombotic effects of aspirin. Blood 52:1073, 1978.
377b. Buchanan, M. R., Rischke, J. A., et al.: The sex-related differences in aspirin pharmacokinetics in rabbits and man and its relationship to antiplatelet effects. Thromb. Res. 29:125, 1983.
378a. Loew, D., and Vinazzer, H.: Dose-dependent influence of acetylsalicylic acid on platelet functions and plasmatic coagulation factors. Haemostasis 5:239, 1976.
378b. Moroz, L.: Increased blood fibrinolytic activity after aspirin ingestion. New Engl. J. Med. 296:525, 1977.
379. Kaneshiro, M. M., Mielke, C. H., et al.: Bleeding time after aspirin in disorders of intrinsic clotting. New Engl. J. Med. 281:1039, 1969.
380. Quick, A. J.: Salicylates and bleeding. The aspirin tolerance test. Am. J. Med. Sci. 252:265, 1966.
381. Sahud, M. A., and Cohen, R. J.: Aspirin-induced prolongation of the Ivy bleeding time: its diagnostic usefulness. Calif. Med. 115:10, 1971.
382. Stuart, M. J., Miller, M. L., et al.: The post-aspirin bleeding time: a screening test for evaluating hemostatic disorders. Br. J. Haematol. 43:649, 1979.
383. Czapek, E. E., Deykin, D., et al.: Intermediate syndrome of platelet dysfunction. Blood 52:103, 1978.
384. Adams, T., Schutz, L., et al.: Platelet function abnormalities in the myeloproliferative disorders. Scand. J. Haematol. 13:215, 1974.
385. Bleyer, W. A., and Breckenridge, R. T.: Studies on the detection of adverse drug reactions in the newborn. II. The effects of prenatal aspirin on newborn hemostasis. J.A.M.A. 213:2049, 1970.
386a. Stuart, M. J., Gross, S. J., et al.: The effect of prenatal acetylsalicylic acid ingestion on maternal and neonatal hemostasis. New Engl. J. Med. 307:909, 1982.
386b. Rumack, C. M., Guggenheim, M. A., et al.: Neonatal intracranial hemorrhage, and maternal use of aspirin. Obstet. Gynecol. 58(Suppl.):52S, 1981.
387. Grossman, M. I., Matsumoto, K. K., et al.: Fecal blood loss produced by oral and intravenous administration of various salicylates. Gastroenterology 40:383, 1961.
388. Cook, A. R., and Goulstun, K.: Failure of intravenous aspirin to increase gastrointestinal blood loss. Br. Med. J. 3:330, 1969.
389. Leonards, J. R., and Levy G.: Aspirin induced occult gastrointestinal blood loss: local versus systemic effects. J. Pharm. Sci. 59:1511, 1970.
390. Mills, D. G., Borda, I. T., et al.: Effects of in vitro aspirin on blood platelets of gastrointestinal bleeders. Clin. Pharmacol. Ther. 15:187, 1974.
391. Naiman, J. L., Bergman, G., et al.: Severe gastrointestinal hemorrhage after therapeutic doses of aspirin in normal children. J. Pediatr. 88:501, 1976.
392a. Stuart, M. J., Murphy, S., et al.: A simple nonradioisotope technique for the determination of platelet life-span. New Engl. J. Med. 292:1310, 1975.

392b. Burch, J. W., Stanford, N., et al.: Inhibition of platelet prostaglandin synthetase by oral aspirin. J. Clin. Invest. *61*:314, 1978.
392c. Catalano, P. M., Smith, J. B., et al.: Platelet recovery from aspirin inhibition in vivo: differing patterns under various assay conditions. Blood *57*:99, 1981.
393a. Weiss, H. J., Aledort, L. M., et al.: The effect of salicylates on the hemostatic properties of platelets in man. J. Clin. Invest. *47*:2169, 1968.
393b. O'Brien, J. R.: Effects of salicylates on human platelets. Lancet *1*:779, 1968.
393c. Sutor, A. H., Bowie, E. J. W., et al.: Effect of aspirin, sodium salicylate and acetaminophen on bleeding. Mayo Clin. Proc. *46*:178, 1971.
393d. Binder, R. A., Durocher, J., et al.: Treatment of pain in hemophilia. Effect of drugs on bleeding time. Am. J. Dis. Child. *127*:371, 1974.
393e. Mielke, C. H., and Britten, A. F. H.: Use of aspirin or acetaminophen in hemophilia [Letter]. New Engl. J. Med. *282*:1270, 1970.
393f. Kasper, C. K., and Rapaport, S. I.: Bleeding times and platelet aggregation after analgesics in hemophilia. Ann. Intern. Med. *77*:189, 1972.
394a. Stanford, N., Roth, G. J., et al.: Lack of covalent modification of prostaglandin synthetase (cyclooxygenase) by indomethacin. Prostaglandins *13*:669, 1977.
394b. Kulmacz, R. J., and Lands, W. E. M.: Stoichiometry and kinetics of the interaction of prostaglandin H synthetase with anti-inflammatory agents. J. Biol. Chem. *260*:12572, 1985.
394c. Walenga, R. W., Wall, S. F., et al.: Time dependent inhibition of platelet cyclooxygenase by indomethacin is slowly reversible. Prostaglandins *31*:625, 1986.
395. Rane, A. O., Oelz, J. C., et al.: Relation between plasma concentration of indomethacin and its effect on prostaglandin synthesis and platelet aggregation in man. Clin. Pharmacol. Ther. *23*:658, 1978.
396. Huijgens, P. C., Van den Berg, C. A. M., et al.: Sulphinpyrazone and indomethacin for inhibition of platelet prostaglandin synthesis. Thromb. Res. *24*:267, 1981.
397. Livio, M. A., Del Maschio C., et al.: Indomethacin prevents the long-lasting inhibitory effect of aspirin on human platelet cyclooxygenase activity. Prostaglandins *23*:787, 1982.
398. Buchanan, G. R., and Martin, V.: The effects of "antiplatelet" drugs on bleeding time and platelet aggregation in normal human subjects. Am. J. Clin. Pathol. *68*:355, 1977.
399. Corozza, M. S., Davis, R. F., et al.: Prolonged bleeding time in preterm infants receiving indomethacin for patent ductus arteriosus. J. Pediatr. *105*:292, 1984.
400. Gersony, W. M., Peckham, G. J., et al.: Effects of indomethacin in premature infants with PDA: results of a national collaborative study. J. Pediatr. *102*:895, 1983.
401. Friedman, Z., Whitman, V., et al.: Indomethacin disposition in premature infants: bleeding due to platelet dysfunction after single doses of indomethacin. Pediatr. Res. *12*:405, 1978.
402. Green, D., Given, K. M., et al.: The effects of a new nonsteroidal anti-inflammatory agent, sulindac, on platelet function. Thromb. Res. *1*:283, 1977.
403. Smythe, H. A., Ogryzlo, M. A., et al.: The effect of sulphinpyrazone (anturan) on platelet economy and blood coagulation in man. Can. Med. Assoc. J. *92*:818, 1965.
404. Davies, J. A., Essien, E., et al.: The influence of red blood cells on the effects of aspirin or sulphinpyrazone on platelet adherence to damaged rabbit aorta. Br. J. Haematol. *42*:283, 1979.
405. Ali, M., and McDonald, J. W. D.: Effects of sulphinpyrazone on platelet prostaglandin synthesis and platelet release of serotonin. J. Lab. Clin. Med. *89*:868, 1977.
406. Buchanan, M. R., Rosenfeld, J., et al.: The prolonged effect of sulphinpyrazone on collagen-induced platelet aggregation in vivo. Thromb. Res. *13*:883, 1978.
407a. Winchester, J. F., Forbes, C. D., et al.: Effect of sulphinpyrazone and aspirin on platelet adhesion to activated charcoal and dialysis membranes in vitro. Thromb. Res. *11*:443, 1977.
407b. Dieterle, W., and Faigle, J. W.: Biotransformation and pharmacokinetics of sulphinpyrazone (anturan) in man. Eur. J. Clin. Pharmacol. *9*:135, 1975.
408. Steele, P., Carroll, J., et al.: Effect of sulphinpyrazone on platelet survival time in patients with transient cerebral ischemic attacks. Stroke *8*:396, 1977.
409. Weily, H. S., and Genton, E.: Altered platelet function in patients with prosthetic mitral valves. Effects of sulphinpyrazone therapy. Circulation *42*:967, 1970.
410. Mills, D. C. B., and Pareti, F. I.: Platelet aggregation and the adenylate cyclase system. Plate. Thromb. *10*:63, 1977.
411. Moncada, S., and Korbut, R.: Dipyridamole and other phosphodiesterase inhibitors act as antithrombotic agents by potentiating endogenous prostacyclin. Lancet *1*:1286, 1978.
412. DiMinno, G., Villa, S., et al.: Dipyridamole as an antithrombotic agent: an intricate mechanism of action. In *Diet and Drugs in Atherosclerosis*. Noseda, G., Lewis, B., et al. (eds.): New York, Raven Press, 1980, p. 121.
413. Brotherton, A. F. A., Hoak, J. C., et al.: Role of Ca^{++} and cyclic AMP in the regulation of the production of prostacyclin by vascular endothelium. Proc. Natl. Acad. Sci. USA *79*:495, 1982.
414. Weston, M. J., Rubin, M. H., et al.: Effects of sulphinpyrazone and dipyridamole on capillary bleeding time in man. Thromb. Res. *10*:833, 1977.
415. Weiss, H. J.: Antiplatelet drugs: a new pharmacologic approach to the prevention of thrombosis. Am. Heart. J. *92*:86, 1976.
416. Harker, L. A., and Slichter, S. J.: Studies of platelet and fibrinogen kinetics in patients with prosthetic heart valves. New Engl. J. Med. *282*:1302, 1970.
417. Harker, L. A., and Slichter, S. J.: The bleeding time as a screening test for evaluation of platelet function. New Engl. J. Med. *287*:155, 1972.
418. Dale, J., Myhre, E., et al.: Effects of dipyridamole and acetylsalicylic acid on platelet functions in patients with aortic ball-valve prostheses. Am. Heart J. *89*:613, 1975.
419. Sullivan, J. M., Harken, D. E., et al.: Pharmacologic control of thromboembolic complications of cardiac-valve replacement. New Engl. J. Med. *284*:1391, 1971.
420. Kashara, T.: Clinical effects of dipyridamole ingestion after prosthetic heart valve replacement. Nippon Kyobu Geka Gakki Zasshi *25*:1007, 1977.
421a. Harker, L. A., Ross, R., et al.: Homocystine-induced arteriosclerosis. The role of endothelial injury and platelet response in its genesis. J. Clin. Invest. *58*:731, 1976.
421b. Harker, L. A., Wall, R. T., et al.: Sulfinpyrazone prevention of homocysteine-induced endothelial cell injury and arteriosclerosis. Clin. Res. *26*:554, 1978.
422. Donadio, J. V., Jr., Anderson, J. C., et al.: Membranoproliferative glomerulonephritis. A prospective clinical trial of platelet-inhibition therapy. New Engl. J. Med. *310*:1421, 1984.
423. O'Brien, J. P.: Ticlopidine. Haemostasis *13*(Suppl. 2):1, 1983.
424. Ross, R., and Glomset, J. A.: The pathogenesis of atherosclerosis. New Engl. J. Med. *295*:369, 420, 1976.
425. Gryglewski, R. J.: Prostaglandins, platelets and atherosclerosis. CRC Crit. Rev. Biochem. *7*:291, 1980.
426. Ross, R.: The pathogenesis of atherosclerosis. An update. New Engl. J. Med. *314*:488, 1986.
427. Kelton, J. G.: Antiplatelet agents: rationale and results. Clin. Haematol. *12*:311, 1983.
428. Kistler, J. P., Ropper, A. H., et al.: Therapy of ischemic cerebral vascular disease due to atherothrombosis. New Engl. J. Med. *311*:27, 1984.

429. Sherry, S.: Clinical aspects of antiplatelet therapy. Semin. Hematol. 22:125, 1985.
430. Harker, L. A.: Antiplatelet drugs in the management of patients with thrombotic disorders. Semin. Thromb. Hemost. 12:134, 1986.
431. Craven, L. L.: Experiences with aspirin (acetylsalicylic acid) in the nonspecific prophylaxis of coronary thrombosis. Miss. Valley Med. J. 75:38, 1963.
432. Linos, A. J.,Worthington, J. W., et al.: Effect of aspirin on prevention of coronary and cerebrovascular disease in patients with rheumatoid arthritis. Mayo Clin. Proc. 53:581, 1978.
433. Heikinheimo, R., and Jarvinen, K.: Acetylsalicylic acid and arteriosclerotic-thromboembolic diseases in the aged. J. Am. Geriatr. Soc. 19:403, 1971.
434. Hammond, E. C., and Garfinkel, L.: Aspirin and coronary heart disease: findings of a prospective study. Br. Med. J. 2:269, 1975.
435. Hennekens, C. H., Karlson, L. K., et al.: A case-control study of regular aspirin use and coronary deaths. Circulation 58:35, 1978.
436. Elwood, P. C., Cochrane, A. L., et al.: A randomized controlled trial of acetylsalicylic acid in the secondary prevention of mortality from myocardial infarction. Br. Med. J. 1:436, 1974.
437. Persantine-Aspirin Reinfarction Study Research Group. Persantine and aspirin in coronary heart disease. Circulation 62:449, 1980.
438. Coronary Drug Project Research Group. Aspirin in coronary heart disease. J. Chronic. Dis. 29:625, 1976.
439. Elwood, P. C., and Sweetnam, P. M.: Aspirin and secondary mortality after myocardial infarction. Lancet 2:1313, 1979.
440. Breddin, K., Lowe, D., et al.: Secondary prevention of myocardial infarction: a comparison of acetylsalicylic acid, placebo and phenprocoumon. Haemostasis 9:325, 1980.
441. Aspirin Myocardial Infarction Study Research Group. A randomized, controlled trial of aspirin in persons recovered from myocardial infarction. J.A.M.A. 243:661, 1980.
442. Anturane, Reinfarction Italian Study. Sulphinpyrazone in post-myocardial infarction. Lancet 1:237, 1982.
443. Anturane Reinfarction Trial Research Group. Sulphinpyrazone in the prevention of sudden death after myocardial infarction. New Engl. J. Med. 302:250, 1982.
444. Lewis, H. D. Jr., Davis, J. W., et al.- Protective effects of aspirin against acute myocardial infarction and death in men with unstable angina. Results of a Veterans Administration cooperative study. New Engl. J. Med. 309:396, 1983.
445. Cairns, J., Gent, M., et al.: Study of aspirin and/or sulfinpyrazone in unstable angina. Circulation 70:411, 1984.
446. Fields, W. S., Lemak, N. A., et al.: Controlled trial of aspirin in cerebral ischemia. Stroke 8:877, 1977.
447. Canadian Cooperative Study Group. A randomized trial of aspirin and sulphinpyrazone in threatened stroke. New Engl. J. Med. 299:53, 1978.
448. Bousser, M. G., Eschwege, E., et al.: "AICLA" controlled trial of aspirin and dipyridamole in the secondary prevention of athero-thrombotic cerebral ischemia. Stroke 14:5, 1983.
449. Taguchi, K., Matsumura, H., et al.: Effect of antithrombogenic therapy, especially high dose therapy of dipyridamole, after prosthetic valve replacement. J. Cardiovasc. Surg. 16:8, 1975.
450. Arrants, J. E., and Hairston, P.: Use of persantine in preventing thromboembolism following valve replacement. Am. Surg. 38:432, 1972.
451. Altman, R., Boullon, F., et al.: Aspirin and prophylaxis of thromboembolic complications in patients with substitute heart valves. J. Thorac. Cardiovasc. Surg. 72:127, 1976.
452. Adrassy, K., Malluche, H., et al.: Prevention of postoperative clotting of arteriovenous fistulae with acetylsalicylic acid: results of a prospective double blind study. Klin. Wochenschr. 52:348, 1974.
453. Kaegi, A., Pineo, G. F., et al.: Arteriovenous-shunt thrombosis. Prevention by sulfinpyrazone. New Engl. J. Med. 290:304, 1974.
454. Harter, H. R., Burch, J. W., et al.: Prevention of thrombosis in patients on hemodialysis by low-dose aspirin. New Engl. J. Med. 301:577, 1979.
455. Stuart, M. J., Stockman, J. A., et al.: Shortened platelet life-span in patients with hydrocephalous and ventricular jugular shunts. Results of preliminary attempts at correction. J. Pediatr. 80:21, 1972.
456. Brown, C. H. E., III, Natelson, E. A., et al.: The hemostatic defect produced by carbenicillin. New Engl. J. Med. 291:265, 1974.
457. Shattil, S. J., Sanford, J. S., et al.: Carbenicillin and penicillin G inhibit platelet function in vitro by impairing the interaction of agonists with the platelet surface. J. Clin. Invest. 65:329, 1980.
458. Brown, C. H., III, Bradshaw, M. W., et al.: Defective platelet function following the administration of penicillin compounds. Blood 47:949, 1976.
459. Cazenave, J. P., Guccione, M. A., et al.: Effects of cephalothium and penicillin G on platelet function in vitro. Br. J. Haematol. 35:135, 1977.
460. Natelson, E. A., Siebert, W. T., et al.: Combined effects of ticarcillin and cefazolin on blood coagulation and platelet function. Am. J. Med. Sci. 278:217, 1980.
461. Copelan, E. A., Kusumi, R. K., et al.: A comparison of the effects of mezlocillin and carbenicillin on hemostasis in volunteers. J. Antimicrob. Chemother. 11(Suppl. C):43, 1983.
462. Gentry, L. O., Jemsek, J. G., et al.: Effects of sodium piperacillin on platelet functions in normal volunteers. Antimicrob. Agents Chemother. 19:532, 1981.
463. Gentry, L. O., and Wood, B. A.: Effects of apalcillin on platelet function in normal volunteers. Antimicrob. Agents Chemother. 27:683, 1985.
464. Alexander, D. P., Russo, M. E., et al.: Nafcillin-induced platelet dysfunction and bleeding. Antimicrob. Agents Chemother. 23:59, 1983.
465. Cazenave, J. P., Packham, M. A., et al.: Effects of penicillin G on platelet aggregation, release, and adherence to collagen. Proc. Soc. Exp. Biol. 142:159, 1973.
466. Brown, C. H., III, Natelson, E. A., et al.: Study of the effects of ticarcillin on blood coagulation and platelet function. Antimicrob. Agents Chemother. 7:652, 1975.
467. Natelson, E. A., Brown, C. H., III, et al.: Influence of cephalosporin antibiotics on blood coagulation and platelet function. Antimicrob. Agents Chemother. 9:91, 1976.
468. Quintiliani, R.: Bleeding disorders associated with newer cephalosporins. Clin. Pharmacokinet. 2:360, 1983.
469. Smith, C. R., and Lipsky, J. J.: Hypoprothrombinemia and platelet dysfunction caused by cephalosporin and oxalactam antibiotics. J. Antimicrob. Chemother. 11:496, 1983.
470. Bang, N. U., Tessler, S. S., et al.: Effects of moxalactam on blood coagulation and platelet function. Rev. Infect. Dis. 4:S546, 1982.
471. Nunn, B., Baird, A., et al.: Effect of temocillin and moxalactam on platelet responsiveness and bleeding time in normal volunteers. Antimicrob. Agents Chemother. 27:858, 1985.
472. Mills, D. C. B., and Roberts, G. C. K.: Membrane active drugs and the aggregation of human blood platelets. Nature (Lond). 213:35, 1967.
473. Thomson, C., Forbes, C. D., et al.: A comparison of the effects of antihistamines on platelet function. Thromb. Diath. Haemorrh. 30:547, 1973.
474. Warlow, C., Ogston, D., et al.: The effects of chlorpromazine and antihistamines on human blood platelets in

vitro and in vivo. 7th European Conference on Microcirculation. Part II (Bibl. Anat. No. 12), 1973, p. 249.
475. Buchanan, G. R., and Handin, R. I.: Impairment of hemostasis in patients with severe hemophilia. Failure of diphenhydramine, chlorpromazine, and guaifenesin. J.A.M.A. 240:2173, 1978.
476. Ungaro, P. C., Beck, T. M., et al.: The in vivo and in vitro effect of antihistamines on platelet aggregation. Thromb. Diath. Haemorrh. 30:597, 1973.
477. Champion, L. A. A., Schwartz, A. D., et al.: The effects of four commonly used drugs on platelet function. J. Pediatr. 89:653, 1976.
478. Coller, B. S.: Effects of tertiary amine local anesthetics on vWF dependent platelet functions: alteration of membrane reactivity and degradation of GPIb by a calcium dependent protease. Blood 60:731, 1982.
479. Feinstein, M. B., Fiekers, J., et al.: An analysis of the mechanism of local anesthetic inhibition on platelet aggregation and secretion. J. Pharmacol. Exp. Ther. 197:215, 1976.
480. Nachmias, V., Sullender, J., et al.: Shape and cytoplasmic filaments in control and lidocaine-treated human platelets. Blood 50:39, 1977.
481. Mori, T., Takai, Y., et al.: Inhibitory action of chlorpromazine, dibucaine and other phospholipid interacting drugs on calcium dependent protein kinase. J. Biol. Chem. 255:8378, 1980.
482. Vanderhoek, J. Y., and Feinstein, M. B.: Local anesthetics, chlorpromazine and propranolol inhibit stimulus-activation of phospholipase A_2 in human platelets. Mol. Pharmacol. 16:171, 1979.
483. Seeman, P.: The membrane actions of anesthetics and tranquilizers. Pharmacol. Rev. 24:583, 1972.
484. Peerschke, E.: Platelet membrane alterations induced by the local anesthetic Dibucaine. Blood 68:463, 1986.
485. Ewald, R. A., Eichelberger, J. W., et al.: The effect of dextran on platelet factor 3 activity: in vitro and in vivo studies. Transfusion 5:109, 1965.
486. Bygdeman, S., and Eliasson, R.: Effect of dextrans on platelet adhesiveness and aggregation. Scand. J. Clin. Lab. Invest. 20:17, 1967.
487. Evans, R. J., and Gordon, J. D.: Mechanisms of the antithrombotic action of dextran. New Engl. J. Med. 290:748, 1974.
488. Langdell, R. D., Adelson, E. A., et al.: Dextran and prolonged bleeding time. J.A.M.A., 166:346, 1958.
489. Clagett, G. P., and Salzman, E. W.: Prevention of venous thromboembolism in surgical patients. New Engl. J. Med. 290:93, 1974.
490. Weiss, H. J.: The effect of clinical dextran on platelet aggregation, adhesion, and ADP release in man: in vivo and in vitro studies. J. Lab. Clin. Med. 69:37, 1967.
491. Thomas, D. P.: Abnormalities of platelet aggregation in patients with alcoholic cirrhoses. Ann. N.Y. Acad. Sci. 201:243, 1972.
492. Haut, M. J., and Cowan, D. H.: The effect of ethanol on the hemostatic properties of human blood platelets. Am. J. Med. 56:22, 1974.
493. Cowan, D. H.: Effects of alcoholism on hemostasis. Semin. Hematol. 17:137, 1980.
494. Eastham, R. D., and Griffiths, E. P.: Reduction of platelet adhesiveness and prolongation of coagulation time of activated plasma by glyceryl guaiacolate. Lancet 1:795, 1966.
495. Silverman, J. L., and Wurzel, H. A.: The effect of glyceryl guaiacolate on platelet function and other coagulation factors in vivo. Am. J. Clin. Pathol. 51:35, 1969.
496. Besterman, E. M., and Gillett, M. P.: Heparin effects on irreversible platelet aggregation. Lancet 2:282, 1972.
497. Heiden, D., Mielke, C. H., et al.: Impairment by heparin of primary haemostasis and platelet (^{14}C) 5-hydroxytryptamine release. Br. J. Haematol. 36:427, 1977.
498. Eika, C.: The platelet aggregating effect of eight commercial heparins. Scand. J. Haematol. 9:480, 1972.
499. Salzman, E. W., Rosenberg, R. D., et al.: Effect of heparin and heparin fractions on platelet aggregation. J. Clin. Invest. 65:64, 1980.
500. Rossi, E. C., and Levin, N. W.: Inhibition of primary ADP induced platelet aggregation in normal subjects after administration of nitrofurantoin (Furadantin). J. Clin. Invest. 52:2457, 1973.
501. White, J. G.: Effects of colchicine and vinca alkaloids on human platelets. I. Influence on platelet microtubules and contractile function. Am. J. Pathol. 53:281, 1968.
502. White, J. G.: Effects of colchicine and vinca alkaloids on human platelets. III. Influence on primary internal contraction and secondary aggregation. Am. J. Pathol. 54:467, 1969.
503. Steinherz, P. G., Miller, D. R., et al.: Platelet dysfunction in vincristine treated patients. Br. J. Haematol. 32:439, 1976.
504. Ahr, D. J., Scialla, S. J., et al.: Acquired platelet dysfunction following mithramycin therapy. Cancer 41:448, 1978.
505. Chas, F. C., and Tullis, J. L.: The in vitro effects of mithramycin on the aggregation and the calcium uptake of human platelets. Thromb. Diath. Haemorrh. 29:712, 1973.
506. Hicsönmez, G., and Buyukpamukcu, M.: Effect of cancer chemotherapy drugs on platelet aggregation in children. Acta Haematol. 58:312, 1977.
507. Gagliano, R. G., Terrebonne, A. M., et al.: The effect of cytosine arabinoside on platelet aggregation. Cancer 38:2247, 1976.
508. Pinder, R. M., Brogden, R. N., et al.: Sodium valproate: a review of its pharmacological properties and therapeutic efficacy in epilepsy. Drugs 13:81, 1977.
509. Eastham, R. D., and Jamcar, J.: Sodium valproate and platelet counts. Br. Med. J. 280:186, 1980.
510. Barr, R. D., Copeland, S. A., et al.: Valproic acid and immune thrombocytopenia. Arch. Dis. Child. 57:681, 1982.
511. Hirsh, J.: Hypercoagulability. Semin. Hematol. 14:409, 1977.
512. Breddin, K.: Detection of prethrombotic states in patients with atherosclerotic lesions. Semin. Thromb. Hemost. 12:110, 1986.
513. Stewart, G. J.: The role of hypercoagulability in thrombosis. Br. J. Haematol. 40:359, 1978.
514. Penner, J. A.: Hypercoagulation and thrombosis. Med. Clin. North Am. 64:743, 1980.
515. Ratnoff, O. D.: Thrombosis and atherogenesis: the role of hemostatic mechanisms. Clin. Haematol. 10:261, 1981.
516. Kitchens, C. S.: Concept of hypercoagulability: a review of its development, clinical application and recent progress. Semin. Thromb. Hemost. 11:293, 1985.
517. Talner, N. S., Liu, H., et al.: Thromboembolism complicating the Holter valve shunt. Am. J. Dis. Child. 101:602, 1961.
518. Colwell, J. A., and Halushka, P. V.: Platelet function in diabetes mellitus. Br. J. Haematol. 44:521, 1980.
519. Colwell, J. A., Winocour, P. D., et al.: New concepts about the pathogenesis of atherosclerosis in diabetes mellitus. Am. J. Med. 75(Suppl. 5B):67, 1983.
520. Nordoy, A., and Rodset, J. M.: Platelet phospholipids and their function in patients with juvenile diabetes and maturity onset diabetes. Diabetes 19:698, 1970.
521. Burrows, A. W., Chavin, S. I., et al.: Plasmathromboglobulin concentrations in diabetes mellitus. Lancet 1:235, 1978.
522. Preston, F. E., Ward, J. D., et al.: Elevated β-thromboglobulin levels and circulating platelet aggregates in diabetic microangiopathy. Lancet 1:238, 1978.
523. O'Malley, B. C., Ward, J. D., et al.: Platelet abnormalities in diabetic peripheral neuropathy. Lancet 2:1274, 1975.

524. Kwaan, H. C., Colwell, J. A., et al.: Increased platelet aggregation in diabetes mellitus. J. Lab. Clin. Med. 80:236, 1972.
525. Dobbie, J. G., Kwaan, H. C., et al.: The role of platelets in the pathogenesis of diabetic retinopathy. Trans. Am. Acad. Ophthalmol. Otolaryngol. 77:43, 1973.
526. Sagel, J., Colwell, J. A., et al.: Increased platelet aggregation in early diabetes mellitus. Ann. Intern. Med. 82:733, 1975.
527. Colwell, J. A., Sagel, J., et al.: Correlation of platelet aggregation, plasma factor activity, and megathrombocytes in diabetic subjects with and without vascular disease. Metabolism 26:279, 1977.
528. Halushka, P. V., Lurie, D., et al.: Increased synthesis of PGE-like material by platelets from patients with diabetes mellitus. New Engl. J. Med. 297:1306, 1977.
529. Ziboh, V. A., Maruta, H., et al.: Increased biosynthesis of TxA$_2$ by diabetic platelets. Eur. J. Clin. Invest. 9:223, 1979.
530. Halushka, P. V., Rogers, R. C., et al.: Increased platelet thromboxane synthesis in diabetes mellitus. J. Lab. Clin. Med. 97:87, 1981.
531. Butkus, A., Skrinska, V. A., et al.: Thromboxane production and platelet aggregation in diabetic subjects with clinical complications. Thromb. Res. 19:211, 1980.
532. Largarde, M., Burtin, M., et al.: Increase of platelet TXA$_2$ formation and its plasmatic half-life in diabetes mellitus. Thromb. Res. 19:823, 1980.
533. Davi, G., Rini, G. B., et al.: TXB$_2$ formation and platelet sensitivity to prostacyclin in insulin dependent and independent diabetics. Thromb. Res. 26:359, 1982.
534. Subbiah, M. T. R., and Deitemeyer, D.: Altered synthesis of prostaglandins in platelet and aorta from spontaneously diabetic Wistar rats. Biochem. Med. 23:231, 1980.
535. Landgraf-Leurs, M. M. C., Landgraf, R., et al.: Aggregation and thromboxane formation by platelets, and vascular prostacyclin production from BB rats; an animal model for type I diabetes. Prostaglandins 24:35, 1982.
536. Gerrard, J. M., Stuart, M. J., et al.: Alterations in the balance of prostaglandin and thromboxane synthesis in diabetes. J. Lab. Clin. Med. 95:950, 1980.
537. Morita, I., Takahashi, R., et al.: Increased arachidonic acid content in platelet phospholipids from diabetic patients. Prostaglandins Leukotrienes Med. 11:33, 1983.
538. McDonald, J. W. D., Dupre, J., et al.: Comparison of platelet thromboxane synthesis in diabetics on conventional insulin therapy and continuous insulin infusions. Thromb. Res. 28:705, 1982.
539. Betteridge, D. J., Tahir, K. E. H., et al.: Platelets from diabetic subjects show decreased sensitivity to prostacyclin. Eur. J. Clin. Invest. 12:395, 1982.
540. Shattil, S. V., and Analya-Galindo, R.: Platelet hypersensitivity induced by cholesterol incorporation. J. Clin. Invest. 55:636, 1975.
541. Stuart, M. J., Gerrard, J. M., et al.: Effect of cholesterol on production of TXB$_2$ by platelets in vitro. New Engl. J. Med. 302:6, 1980.
542. Johnson, M., Harrison, H. E., et al.: Vascular prostacyclin may be reduced in diabetes in man. Lancet 1:325, 1979.
543. Silberbauer, K., Schernthaner, G. G., et al.: Decreased prostacyclin in juvenile onset diabetes [letter]. New Engl. J. Med. 300:366, 1979.
544. Harrison, H. E., and Johnson, M.: Vascular prostacyclin release and metabolic derangement in diabetes. Horm. Metab. Res. 11(Suppl. 1):43, 1981.
545. Setty, B. N. Y., and Stuart, M. J.: 15-Hydroxy-5,8,11,13-eicosatetraenoic acid inhibits human vascular cyclooxygenase. Potential role in diabetic vascular disease. J. Clin. Invest. 77:202, 1986.
546. Abrahamsen, A. F.: Platelet survival. Scand. J. Haematol. 3(Suppl.):53, 1968.
547. Jones, R. L., Paradise, C., et al.: Platelet survival in patients with diabetes mellitus. Diabetes 30:486, 1981.
548. Mustard, J. F., and Packham, M. A.: Platelets and diabetes mellitus. New Engl. J. Med. 311:665, 1984.
549. Oppenheimer, E. H., and Esterly, J. R.: Thrombosis in the newborn: comparison between infants of diabetic and nondiabetic mothers. J. Pediatr. 67:549, 1965.
550. Avery, M. E., Oppenheimer, E. H., et al.: Renal vein thrombosis in newborn infants of diabetic mothers: report of 2 cases. New Engl. J. Med. 256:1134, 1957.
551. Takeuchi, A., and Benirschke, K.: Renal vein thrombosis of the newborn, and its relation to maternal diabetes. Report of 16 cases. Biol. Neonate 3:237, 1961.
552. Stuart, M. J., Elrad, H., et al.: Increased synthesis of platelet malonyldialdehyde and platelet hyperfunction in infants of mothers with diabetes mellitus. J. Lab. Clin. Med. 94:12, 1979.
553. Stuart, M. J., Sunderji, S. G., et al.: Decreased prostacyclin production in the infant of the diabetic mother. J. Lab. Clin. Med. 98:412, 1981.
554. Stuart, M. J., Sunderji, S. G., et al.: Abnormalities in vascular arachidonic acid metabolism in the infant of the diabetic mother. Br. Med. J. 290:1700, 1985.
555. Mudd, S. H., and Levy, H. L.: Disorders of transsulfuration. In *The Metabolic Basis of Inherited Disease*. Stanbury, J. B., Wyngaarden, J. B., et al. (eds.), New York, McGraw-Hill, 1978, p. 458.
556. McCully, K. S.: Homocysteine theory of arteriosclerosis: development and current status. Atherosclerosis Rev. 11:157, 1983.
557. Davis, J. W., Flournoy, L. D., et al.: Aminoacids and collagen-induced platelet aggregation: lack of effect of three aminoacids that are elevated in homocystinuria. Am. J. Dis. Child. 129:1020, 1975.
558. Ratnoff, O. D.: Activation of Hageman factor by L-homocystine. Science 162:1007, 1964.
559. Cline, J. W., Goyer, R. A., et al.: Adult homocystinuria with ectopia lentis. South. Med. J. 64:613, 1971.
560. Harker, L. A., Slichter, S. J., et al.: Homocystinemia: vascular injury and arterial thrombosis. New Engl. J. Med. 291:537, 1974.
561. Harker, L. A., and Slichter, S. J.: Homocystinemia: vascular injury and arterial thrombosis. New Engl. J. Med. 291:537, 1974.
562. McDonald, L., Bray, C., et al.: Homocystinuria, thrombosis and the blood platelets. Lancet 1:745, 1964.
563. Uhlemann, E. R., TenPas, J. H., et al.: Platelet survival and morphology in homocystinuria due to cystathionine synthase deficiency. New Engl. J. Med. 295:1283, 1976.
564. Hill-Zobel, R. L., Pyeritz, R. E., et al.: Kinetics and distribution of ^{111}In-labeled platelets in patients with homocystinuria. New Engl. J. Med. 307:781, 1982.
565. Harker, L. A., and Ross, R.: Homocystine-induced arteriosclerosis: the role of endothelial cell injury and platelet response in its genesis. J. Clin. Invest. 58:731, 1976.
566. Harker, L. A., and Scott, C. R.: Platelets in homocystinuria [letter]. New Engl. J. Med. 296:818, 1977.
567. Graeber, J. E., Slott, J. A., et al.: Effect of homocysteine and homocystine on platelet and vascular arachidonic acid metabolism. Pediatr. Res. 16:490, 1982.
568. Silver, M. J., Sedar, A. W., et al.: Homocysteine damages endothelial cells in situ and causes diminished prostacyclin production by arteries. Blood 58(Suppl. 1):239a, 1981.
569. Boers, G. H. J., Smals, A. G. H., et al.: Heterozygosity for homocystinuria in premature peripheral and cerebral occlusive arterial disease. New Engl. J. Med. 313:709, 1985.
570. Wilcken, D. E. L., Reddy, S. G., et al.: Homocysteinemia, ischemic heart disease, and the carrier state for homocystinuria. Metabolism 32:363, 1983.
571. Brattstrom, L. E., Hardebo, J. E., et al.: Moderate ho-

mocysteinemia—a possible risk factor for arteriosclerotic cerebrovascular disease. Stroke 15:1012, 1984.
572. Mudd, S. H.: Vascular disease and homocysteine metabolism. New Engl. J. Med. 313:751, 1985.
573. Handley, D. A., and Lawrence, J. R.: Factor IX deficiency in the nephrotic syndrome. Lancet 1:1079, 1967.
574. Natelson, E. A., Lynch, E. C., et al.: Acquired factor IX deficiency in the nephrotic syndrome. Ann. Intern. Med. 73:373, 1970.
575. Honig, G. R., and Lindley, A.: Deficiency of Hageman factor (Factor XII) in patients with nephrotic syndrome. J. Pediatr. 78:633, 1971.
576. Lange, L. G., Carvalho, A., et al.: Activation of Hageman factor in the nephrotic syndrome. Am. J. Med. 56:565, 1974.
577. Gootman, N., Gross, J., et al.: Pulmonary artery thrombosis. Pediatrics 34:861, 1964.
578. Pollak, V. E., Kark, R. M., et al.: Renal vein thrombosis and the nephrotic syndrome. Am. J. Med. 21:496, 1956.
579. Levin, S. E., Zamit, R., et al.: Thrombosis of the pulmonary arteries and the nephrotic syndrome. Br. Med. J. 1:153, 1967.
580. Lieberman, E., Heuser, E., et al.: Thrombosis, nephrosis, and corticosteroid therapy. J. Pediatr. 73:320, 1968.
581. Goldbloom, R. B., Hillman, D. A., et al.: Arterial thrombosis following femoral venipuncture in edematous nephrotic children. Pediatrics 40:450, 1967.
582. Kanfer, A., Kleinknecht, D., et al.: Coagulation studies in 45 cases of nephrotic syndrome without uremia. Thromb. Diath. Haemorrh. 24:562, 1970.
583. Kendall, A. G., Lohmann, R. C., et al.: Nephrotic syndrome: a hypercoagulable state. Arch. Intern. Med. 127:1021, 1971.
584. Llach, F., Arieff, A. I., et al.: Renal vein thrombosis and nephrotic syndrome. Ann. Intern. Med. 83:8, 1975.
585. Clarkson, A. R., and Seymour, A. E.: Coagulation and renal disease. Med. J. Aust. 1:573, 1976.
586. Porro, G. B., and Bianchessi, M.: Ischaemic heart disease complicating the nephrotic syndrome. Lancet 2:804, 1969.
587. Curry, R. C., and Roberts, W. C.: Status of the coronary arteries in the nephrotic syndrome. Am. J. Med. 63:183, 1977.
588. Thomson, C., Forbes, C. D., et al.: Changes in blood coagulation and fibrinolysis in the nephrotic syndrome. Q. J. Med. 43:499, 1974.
589. Kauffmann, R. H., deGraeff, J., et al.: Unilateral renal vein thrombosis and nephrotic syndrome. Report of a case with protein selectivity and antithrombin III clearance studies. Am. J. Med. 60:1048, 1976.
590. Kauffmann, R. H., Veltkamp, J. J., et al.: Acquired antithrombin III deficiency and thrombosis in the nephrotic syndrome. Am. J. Med. 65:607, 1978.
591. Jorgensen, K. A., and Stoffersen, E.: Antithrombin III and the nephrotic syndrome. Scand. J. Haematol. 22:442, 1979.
592. Kauffman, R. H., Veltkamp, J. J., et al.: Acquired antithrombin III deficiency and thrombosis in the nephrotic syndrome. Am. J. Med. 65:607, 1978.
593. Bang, N. U., Trygstad, C. W., et al.: Enhanced platelet function in glomerular disease. J. Lab. Clin. Med. 81:651, 1973.
594. Yoshida, N., and Aoki, N.: Release of arachidonic acid from human platelets. A key role for the potentiation of platelet aggregability in normal subjects as well as in those with nephrotic syndrome. Blood 52:969, 1968.
595. Remuzzi, G., Mecca, G., et al.: Thrombosis and the nephrotic syndrome. Blood 52(Suppl.):288, 1978 (Abstr.).
596. Stuart, M. J., Spitzer, R. E., et al.: Nephrotic syndrome: increased platelet malonyldialdehyde formation, hyperaggregability and reduced platelet life span. Reversal following remission. Pediatr. Res. 14:1078, 1980.
597. Kawasaki, T., Kosaki, F., et al.: A new infantile acute febrile mucocutaneous lymph node syndrome prevailing in Japan. Pediatrics 54:271, 1974.
598. Tanaka, N., Naoe, S., et al.: Pathological study on autopsy cases of mucocutaneous lymph node syndrome in childhood, particularly in relation with periarteritis nodosa-like arteritis. Med. J. Jpn. Red Cross Central Hospital 1:85, 1971.
599. Kato, H., Koike, S., et al.: Coronary heart disease in children with Kawasaki disease. Jpn. Circ. J. 43:469, 1979.
600. Sasaguri, Y., and Kato, H.: Regression of aneurysms in Kawasaki disease: a pathological study. J. Pediatr. 100:225, 1982.
601. Burns, J. C., Glode, M. P., et al.: Coagulopathy and platelet activation in Kawasaki syndrome: identification of patients at high risk for development of coronary artery aneurysms. J. Pediatr. 105:206, 1984.
602. Yamada, K., Fukumoto, T., et al.: The platelet functions in acute febrile mucocutaneous lymph node syndrome. A trial of prevention for thrombosis by antiplatelet agents. Acta Haematol. Jpn. 41:113, 1978.
603. Yokoyama, T., Kato, H., et al.: Aspirin treatment and platelet function in Kawasaki disease. Kurume Med. J. 27:57, 1980.
604. Hidaka, T., Nakano, M., et al.: Increased synthesis of thromboxane A_2 by platelets from patients with Kawasaki disease. J. Pediatr. 102:94, 1983.
605. Furusho, K., Kamiya, T., et al.: High dose intravenous gammaglobulin for Kawasaki disease. Lancet 2:1055, 1984.
606. Newburger, J. W., Takahashi, M., et al.: The treatment of Kawasaki syndrome with intravenous gamma globulin. New Engl. J. Med. 315:341, 1986.
607. Heberden, W., cited by Rook, A.: William Heberden's cases of anaphylactoid purpura. Arch. Dis. Child. 33:271, 1958.
608. William, R.: *On Cutaneous Disease.* London, J. Johnson, 1808.
609. Schönlein, J.: Allgemeine und specielle pathologie und therapie, Vol. 2, 3rd ed. Herisau, Lit. Compt., 1837, p. 48.
610. Henoch, E.: Uber eine eigenthiinliche form von purpura. Berl. Klin. Wochenschr. 11:641, 1874.
611. Allen, D. M., Diamond, L. K., et al.: Anaphylactoid purpura in children (Schonlein-Henoch syndrome). Am. J. Dis. Child. 99:833, 1960.
612. Lewis, I. C.: The Schonlein-Henoch syndrome compared with certain features of nephritis and rheumatism. Arch. Dis. Child. 30:212, 1955.
613. Wedgewood, R., and Klaus, M. H.: Anaphylactoid purpura: a long term follow-up study with special reference to renal involvement. Pediatrics 16:196, 1955.
614. Harvey, J. G., and Colditz, P. B.: Henoch-Schonlein purpura—a surgical review. Aust. Pediatr. J. 20:13, 1984.
615. Martinez-Frontanilla, L. A., Haase, G. M., et al.: Surgical complications in Henoch-Schonlein purpura. J. Pediatr. Surg. 19:434, 1984.
616. Gairdner, D.: The Schonlein-Henoch syndrome (anaphylactoid purpura). Q. J. Med. 17:95, 1948.
617. Gottlieb, A. J.: Allergic purpura. In *Hematology.* Williams, W. J., Beutler, E., et al. (eds.), New York, McGraw-Hill, 1977, p. 1393.
618. Spitzer, R. E., Urmson, J. R., et al.: Alteration of the complement system in children with Henoch-Schonlein purpura. Clin. Immunol. Immunopathol. 11:52, 1978.
619. Urizar, R. E., Michael, A., et al.: Anaphylactoid purpura. II. Immunofluorescent and electron microscopic studies of the glomerular lesions. Lab. Invest. 119:437, 1969.
620. Heaton, J. M., and Turner, D. R.: Localization of glo-

merular deposits in Henoch-Schonlein purpura. Histopathology *1*:93, 1977.
621. Austin, H. A., and Balow, J. E.: Henoch-Schonlein nephritis: prognostic features and the challenge of therapy. Am. J. Kidney Dis. *11*:512, 1983.
622. Cochrane, C. G., and Weigle, W. O.: The cutaneous reaction to soluble antigen-antibody complexes: a comparison with the Arthus phenomenon. J. Exp. Med. *108*:591, 1958.
623. Batlle, D. C.: IgA glomerulonephritis, asymptomatic hematuria, and systemic disease. Arch. Intern. Med. *141*:1264, 1981.
624. Sterky, G., and Thilen, A.: A study on the onset and prognosis of acute vascular purpura (the Schonlein-Henoch syndrome) in children. Acta Paediatr. *49*:217, 1960.

GENETICS

CHAPTER 43
Chromosomal Abnormalities in Childhood Tumors

JANET D. ROWLEY

INTRODUCTION 1479
METHODS 1480
CHRONIC MYELOGENOUS LEUKEMIA (CML) 1480
Chronic Phase
Acute Phase
Juvenile CML and Other Chronic Myelodysplasias
ACUTE NONLYMPHOCYTIC LEUKEMIA (ANLL) DE NOVO 1483
Chromosome Gain and Loss
Structural Rearrangements
   The 8;21 Translocation in Acute Myeloblastic Leukemia (AML-M2)
   The 15;17 Translocation in Acute Promyelocytic Leukemia (APL-M3)
   Inv(16) and Del(16q) in Acute Myelomonocytic Leukemia (AMMoL-M4)
   Structural Alterations of 11q in Acute Monocytic Leukemia (AMoL-M5)
   Differences in Frequency of Aberrations Between Children and Adults
   Correlation of Karyotype and Survival
ACUTE LYMPHOBLASTIC LEUKEMIA (ALL) 1487
Structural Rearrangements
   The 8;14 Translocation
   The 4;11 Translocation
   The Ph^1 Chromosome
   The 1;19 Translocation
   Structural Rearrangements in T Cell ALL
   Near-haploid ALL
   Hyperdiploidy with 50 to 60 Chromosomes
EMBRYONIC TUMORS 1490
Retinoblastoma
Wilms' Tumor
Neuroblastoma
Ewing's Sarcoma
THE BIOLOGIC SIGNIFICANCE OF CONSISTENT CHROMOSOMAL ABNORMALITIES 1492
When Do Chromosomal Rearrangements Occur?
Defining the Critical Recombinant Chromosome
CONCLUSIONS 1494

INTRODUCTION

Cytogenetic analysis of human tumors is one of the most rapidly progressing and exciting areas of cancer research. Major advances in our understanding of the specificity of some of the abnormalities observed have occurred within the last 10 years, as a result of the application of chromosome banding techniques and improved methods of cell culture. Thus, the hypothesis put forward by Boveri at the turn of the century, namely, that an abnormal chromosome pattern was intimately associated with the malignant phenotype of the tumor cell, can now be tested with the substantial hope of obtaining a valid answer (1).

Although most of the information regarding the chromosome patterns in human tumors has been obtained for adults, sufficient data are available for the acute leukemias to compare the frequency of various abnormalities in children and adults. As will become apparent in the specific sections, the frequency varies considerably, and the differences undoubtedly have biologic significance, although it is not understood at present.

In some instances, the tumors are unique to children (the tumors of embryonic cell origin, for example), and these have already provided new insights into some of the chromosomal mechanisms related to malignant transformation. The emphasis in this chapter will be on childhod malignant diseases, but these will be viewed in the context of what is known in general about the chromosome pattern for each particular disease.

The factors that are associated with chromosome aberrations, and especially the recurring structural rearrangements, are poorly understood. It is clear that the chromosome breakage syndromes, such as Bloom's Syndrome, Fanconi's anemia, and ataxia-telangiectasia, are genetic disorders associated with both an increased frequency in chromosome breaks in all cells and an increased incidence of cancer and leukemia (1a). Cytotoxic agents, both chemicals and x-rays, are also associated with the development of malignant diseases. More recently, it has been suggested that fragile sites may be a factor that predisposes cells to chromosome rearrangements (1b, 1c). Fragile sites may be heritable or "constitutive". The heritable variety involves fewer than 20 chromosome bands at present; these sites are relatively rare, and they have a clearly defined pattern of inheritance (1d). The constitutive fragile sites, on the other hand, are ubiquitous. Both types require special culture conditions to induce their expression (1e). The remarkable concordance of the location of heritable fragile sites and the breakpoints in consistent chromosome rearrangements has been noted: In the author's laboratory, 10 of 11 patients with an inversion of chromosome No. 16 in acute myelomonocytic leukemia had a fragile site at 16q22, which is one of the breakpoints in the inversion (LeBeau, unpublished observations). Given the rarity of the fragile sites in the general population, this increased incidence in patients whose leukemic cells have a break in the same band implies an important relationship. It must be emphasized, however, that any chromosome rearrangement, whatever the cause, will not lead to a clonal proliferation unless it provides the particular cell type with a proliferative advantage at some stage in the differentiation of that cell type.

METHODS

Cytogenetic analyses in malignant disease must be based upon the study of the tumor cells themselves. In leukemia, the specimen is usually a bone marrow aspirate either processed immediately (direct preparation) or cultured for 24 to 48 hours (2). When a bone marrow aspirate cannot be obtained, a bone marrow biopsy (bone core specimen) can often be successfully processed. Alternatively, in patients with a white blood cell count higher than 15,000 cells per mm^3, with about 10 per cent immature myeloid or lymphoid cells, a sample of peripheral blood can be cultured without adding phytohemagglutinin (PHA). The karyotype of the dividing cells will be similar to that obtained from the bone marrow. Mitogens such as PHA are not routinely added to the peripheral blood cultures in acute leukemia, since stimulation of division of normal lymphoid cells may interfere with the analysis of spontaneously dividing malignant cells. The use of amethopterin or fluorodeoxyuridine to synchronize dividing cells enables one to obtain elongated chromosomes that have an increased number of bands (3). This may provide enhanced resolution.

In this chapter, chromosomal abnormalities are described according to the International System for Human Cytogenetic Nomenclature (4). The criteria initially suggested by Rowley and Potter (5) and accepted at the First International Workshop on Chromosomes in Leukemia (6) are used for the identification of abnormal clones. Following these criteria, observation of at least two "pseudodiploid" (e.g., translocations, deletions, inversions) or hyperdiploid cells, or three hypodiploid cells, each showing the same abnormality, is considered evidence for the presence of an abnormal clone. Even one cell with a normal karyotype is considered evidence for the presence of a normal cell line. Patients whose cells show no alteration, or in whom the alterations involve different chromosomes in different cells, are considered normal. Isolated changes such as chromosome loss may be due to technical artifacts or to random mitotic errors. Some malignant diseases, such as Hodgkin's disease or multiple myeloma, continue to show a high frequency of normal karyotypes. These diseases are characterized by malignant cells with a low mitotic index, and therefore it is likely that the dividing cells studied do not represent the malignant cells.

A variety of different chromosome changes have been observed in neoplastic cells, and these often occur in combination. This seriously impedes precise identification of the individual abnormalities. The simplest changes are either a gain or a loss of a whole chromosome. Common structural alterations are *translocations*, which involve the exchange of material between two or more chromosomes, and *deletions*, which involve the loss of DNA from a chromosome and thus from the affected cell. Chromosome *inversions* have also been observed; in this rearrangement, a single chromosome is broken in two places, and the central portion is inverted and rejoined to the ends of the chromosome. A series of international meetings over the last 25 years has led to the establishment of a universally accepted system for chromosome nomenclature; that standard nomenclature will be used here. Each chromosome band is numbered (4). The total chromosome number is followed by the sex chromosomes; gains and losses of whole chromosomes are identified by a + or − *before* the chromosome number. A gain or loss of part of a chromosome is identified by a + or − *after* the chromosome number; p and q represent the short and long arm, respectively. Translocations are indicated by t; the chromosomes involved are noted in the first set of brackets, and the breakpoints in the second set of brackets. For example, the karyotype of the leukemic clone in a woman with Ph^1 = positive chronic myeloid leukemia would be: 46, XX, t(9;22)(q34; q11); the translocation involves chromosomes 9 and 22 with a break in the long arm of No. 9 in band q34, and in the long arm of No. 22 in band q11. Other abnormalities will be defined when they are first described.

CHRONIC MYELOGENOUS LEUKEMIA (CML)

Chronic Phase

Chronic myelogenous leukemia is a particularly important subtype of leukemia because it was in this disease that the first consistent chromosomal abnormality in a malignant disease was noted (Table 43–1). This abnormality, the Philadelphia or Ph^1 chromosome, was first described in 1960 by Nowell and Hungerford (7) as a deletion of part of the long arm of a G-group chromosome, and

Table 43–1. COMMON CHROMOSOME CHANGES IN LEUKEMIA

Type	Gains	Losses	Rearrangements
CML			
Chronic Phase	—	—	t(9;22)
Blast Crisis	+8, +Ph¹	Rare; −7	t(9;22), i(17q)
ANLL			
AML-M2	+8	−7; less frequently, −5	t(8;21)
APL	—	—	t(15;17)
AMMoL	+8	−7	inv(16)
AMoL	—	—	t(11q) or del(11q)
CLL			
B cell	+12	—	14q+
T cell	—	—	inv(14)
ALL			
Null	+21; +6	Rare; −9	t(9;22), t(4;11)
B cell	—	—	t(8;14)
Pre–B cell	—	—	t(1;19)
T cell	—	—	t(11;14)

later with the use of quinacrine fluorescence banding techniques as a 22q−. The nature of the chromosome aberration was clarified in 1973, when Rowley (8) reported that the Ph¹ chromosome resulted from a translocation rather than a deletion as many investigators had previously assumed. In each of 9 patients, pale fluorescent material was added to the end of the long arm of chromosome 9 [t(9;22)(q34; q11)]. The reciprocal nature of this translocation was established only recently, when the Abelson oncogene, c-*abl*, normally located on No. 9, was identified on the Ph¹ chromosome (9) (Fig. 43–1). Other studies with chromosomal polymorphisms and enzyme markers have shown that the CML cells originated from a single cell and were therefore clonal in origin (9a).

Historically, about 85 per cent of all patients diagnosed as having CML were found to have the Ph¹ chromosome (10). Identification of patients as Ph¹+ or Ph¹− was found to be clinically significant in that Ph¹+ patients had a better prognosis than those with Ph¹− CML (42- vs. 15-month survival) (10). However, in a recent study by Pugh and coworkers (11) of patients who were initially diagnosed as having CML and whose cells lacked the Ph¹ chromosome, it was shown that most of the 25 Ph¹− patients did *not* have CML, but instead had some type of myelodysplasia, most commonly chronic myelomonocytic leukemia or refractory anemia with excess blasts. Thus Ph¹− CML may not exist. Studies of a few patients with various myelodysplastic syndromes have shown that the red cells, granulocytes, and megakaryocytes are derived from the same clone (11a).

The karyotypes of many Ph¹ patients with CML have been examined with banding techniques, and, in a recent review of 1129 Ph¹+ patients, the

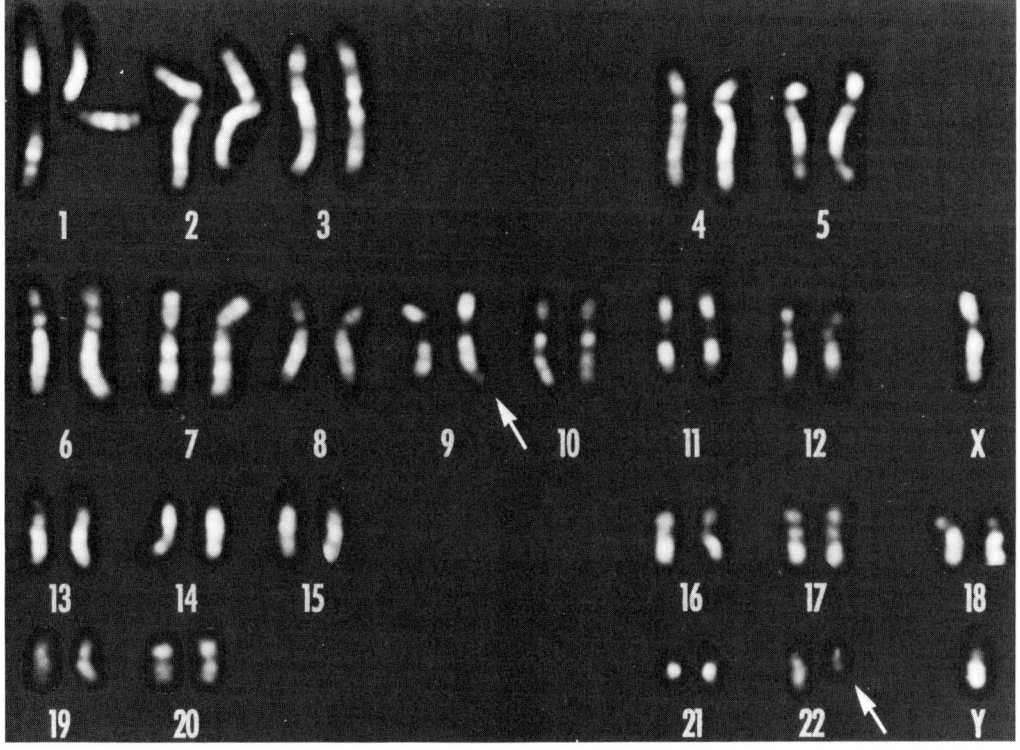

Figure 43–1. Karyotype of a metaphase from the bone marrow of a male patient with CML. The metaphase was stained with quinacrine mustard (Q-banding) and examined with ultraviolet fluorescence. The arrows indicate the translocation between the long arm of chromosome 9 and the long arm of chromosome 22 [46,XY,t(9;22)(q34; q11)].

9;22 translocation was identified in 1036 (92 per cent) (12). Variant translocations have been discovered, however, in addition to the typical t(9;22) karyotype. Until very recently, these were thought to be of two kinds: one appeared to be a simple translocation involving No. 22 and some chromosome other than No. 9 (42 patients, 3.7 per cent), and the other was a complex translocation involving three or more chromosomes, two of which were No. 9 and No. 22 (46 patients; 4.1 per cent). Although the data are limited, the frequency of variant translocations appears to be similar in children and adults. Recent data clearly demonstrate that No. 9 is affected in the simple as well as the complex translocations, and that its involvement had previously been overlooked (13). The genetic consequence of the standard t(9;22) karyotype or the complex translocations involving at least three chromosomes is the movement of the c-abl gene on No. 9 next to a gene on No. 22 whose identity is currently unknown (Fig. 43–2).

Acute Phase

When patients with CML enter the terminal acute phase (blast crisis), about 20 per cent appear to retain the 46,Ph^1+ cell line unchanged, whereas 80 per cent show karyotypic evolution (12). It is now recognized that the blast cells of some patients in the acute phase of CML have lymphoid rather than myeloid characteristics. At present, the data are insufficient to determine whether a particular karyotype is associated with the lymphoid or with the myeloid type of blast crisis (12).

Bone marrow chromosomes from 392 patients with Ph^1+ CML in the acute phase, analyzed with banding techniques, were reviewed by Rowley and Testa (12). Eighty-nine (22 per cent) showed no change in their karyotype, whereas 303 patients had additional chromosomal abnormalities. The most common changes—gain of No. 8, No. 19, a second Ph^1, and i(17q)—frequently occur in combination to produce modal chromosome numbers of 47–50. When patients had only a single new chromosome change, this most commonly involved the gain of a second Ph^1, and i(17q), or a +8, in descending order of frequency. Chromosome loss occurs only rarely; that most often seen was −7, which occurred in only 3 per cent of patients. Very little information is available about the karyotype in children in blast crisis. However, there is no evidence that it differs from that seen in adult patients.

Juvenile CML and Other Chronic Myelodysplasias

Chronic myeloproliferative diseases are rare in children; for example, CML accounts for less than 5 per cent of all cases of childhood leukemia. CML occurs in two forms, one that is similar to that seen in adults, with the leukemic cells containing a Ph^1 chromosome, and the other, so-called juvenile CML, which is really a misnomer. The latter is characterized by monocytosis rather than granulocytosis, an increase in fetal hemoglobin, and a rapidly fatal course, with death usually resulting from complications of bone marrow failure rather than from acute progression. As in the chronic myeloproliferative diseases in adults, the Ph^1− juvenile form is a collection of heterogeneous disorders. Using the FAB classification of the myelodysplasias, we were able to show that, except for one patient, all of the adults with Ph^1− CML whom we studied could be reclassified as having one of the myelodysplastic syndromes (11). The chromosome pattern in juvenile CML appears to be variable with many patients having a normal karyotype; other patients have relatively common changes such as +8 or a −7 (14).

There have been several reports on the chromosome pattern in childhood preleukemia (15). Clinically, these children have a chronic myeloproliferative disorder that appears similar to juvenile CML. Recurrent infections are a prominent feature; these patients generally do not have an elevated fetal hemoglobin and, as the name implies, they generally progress to ANLL. Sieff and colleagues (16) reported on 6 boys, ages 5½ months to 8 years, median 10 months, who had a myeloproliferative disorder associated with −7. These 6 were among 15 children with marrow dysplasia seen within a 3-year period. Three patients died of ANLL, one developed myelofibrosis, one died of complications of anemia, and one was

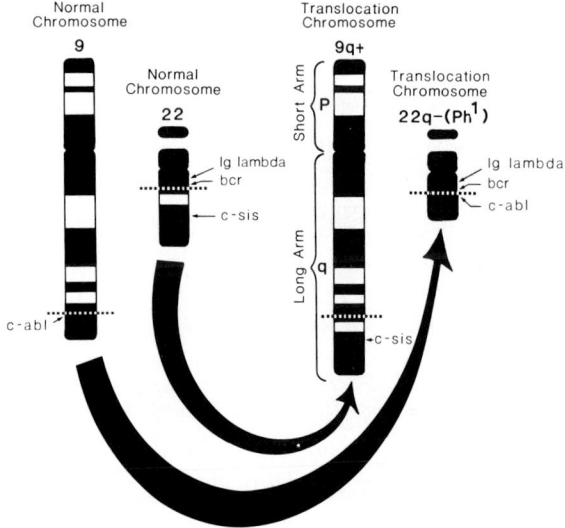

Figure 43–2. Diagrammatic representation of the Ph^1 translocation.

stable 17 months after diagnosis. Of the 11 patients reviewed by Sieff, 8 died of ANLL.

In the future, a careful assessment of children with chronic myelodysplasia will result in a more biologically valid classification. This assessment should clearly include detailed cytogenetic analysis as well as review of the marrow slides for morphology and various markers.

ACUTE NONLYMPHOCYTIC LEUKEMIA (ANLL) DE NOVO

Numerous reports on cytogenetic analyses, with banding techniques, of relatively large series of unselected patients with ANLL have been reported (12, 17, 18, 19). On the basis of results of the earlier series, as well as of data from the Fourth International Workshop on Chromosomes in Leukemia (20), it appeared that about 50 per cent of patients studied at diagnosis had an abnormal karyotype. It is clear that these studies substantially underestimate the frequency of clonal abnormalities. In a recent summary, Yunis and his associates (19) reported that 92 of 99 patients (93 per cent) had an abnormality; the author's laboratory has observed clonal abnormalities in over 80 per cent of patients whose cells have been studied in the last 2 years. The change in frequency is the result of several factors. First, techniques of marrow culture and the use of amethopterin to achieve longer chromosomes has led to a substantial improvement in the quality of banding and therefore has allowed us to identify some of the subtle rearrangements that were previously overlooked. Second, we know that for some types of myeloid leukemia, a period of culture increases the percentages of metaphase cells with a clonal abnormality. Berger and his colleagues (21) have evidence that in some patients the normal metaphase cells observed in direct preparations are derived from erythroblasts and that these disappear on culture, to be replaced by dividing leukemic myeloblasts or monoblasts.

Chromosome Gain and Loss

Although the karyotypes of patients with ANLL may be variable, both the nonrandom gain and loss of chromosomes and their involvement in structural rearrangement are evident. The number of chromosomes gained or lost in 354 patients with a clonal abnormality studied at the Fourth Workshop (20) is shown in Figure 43–3. With the exceptions of chromosome 16, which was never observed as a gain, and chromosome 1, which was never lost, each of the autosomes and sex chromosomes contributed to the numerical changes. A gain of No. 8, the most frequent abnormality seen in ANLL, was found in 47 patients (13.3 per cent). Loss of No. 7, another frequent numerical change,

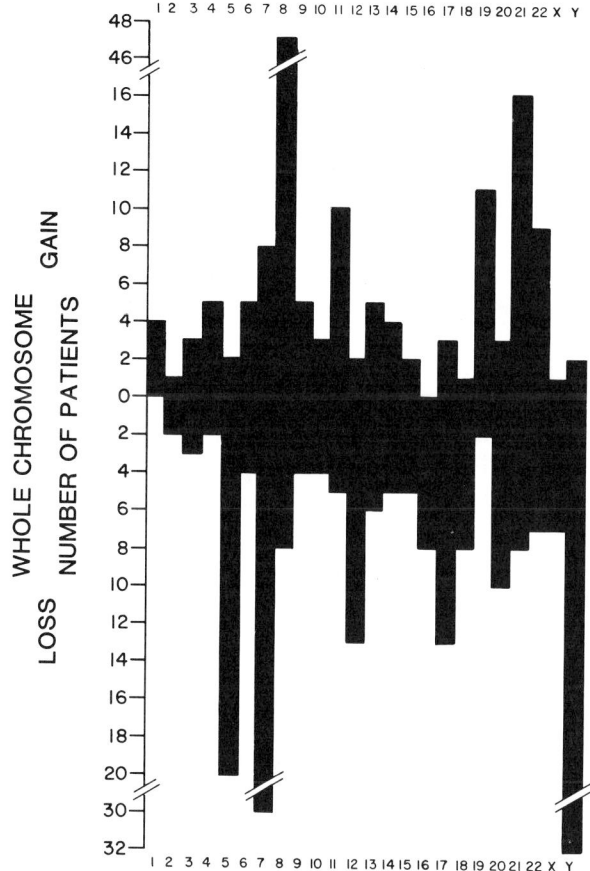

Figure 43–3. Histogram illustrating the frequency of whole chromosome gain and loss in 660 patients with acute nonlymphocytic leukemia de novo studied at the Fourth International Workshop on Chromosomes in Leukemia (1984). (From LeBeau, M. M., and Rowley, J. D.: Chromosomal abnormalities in leukemia and lymphoma: clinical and biological significance. In *Advances in Human Genetics*, Vol. 15. Harris, H., and Hirschhorn, K. H. (eds.), New York, Plenum Publishing Corp., 1986, pp. 1–54.)

was observed in 30 (8.5 per cent) patients, and loss of one No. 5 was noted in 20 patients (5.6 per cent). When gains or losses of these chromosomes are analyzed by the age of the patient, it is clear that there are remarkable differences in frequency between children and adults; these will be detailed below. Gains or losses of the other autosomes seldom occurred as the sole abnormality. Thus, abnormalities of the other autosomes were likely to represent secondary events occurring in clonal evolution, rather than primary chromosomal changes. Losses of the Y chromosome (the second most frequent numerical change in this summary) and of the X chromosome often occurred in association with 8;21 translocation.

Structural Rearrangements

The distribution of chromosomes involved in structural rearrangements in the patients studied at the Fourth Workshop is illustrated in Figure 43–4. Translocation and deletions account for most of the rearrangements observed. The most frequently rearranged chromosome was No. 17; abnormalities of this chromosome were noted in 53 patients, 43 of whom had the t(15;17) pattern. Likewise, the majority of cases with rearrangements of chromosomes 8, 15, or 21—the three next most frequently altered chromosomes—resulted from the two specific translocation, t(8;21) and t(15;17). A deletion of 5q was identified in 25 patients, and rearrangements of 11q, primarily translocations, were also frequent. As will become apparent, all of these specific abnormalities (except 5q−) are proportionately more common in children compared with adults.

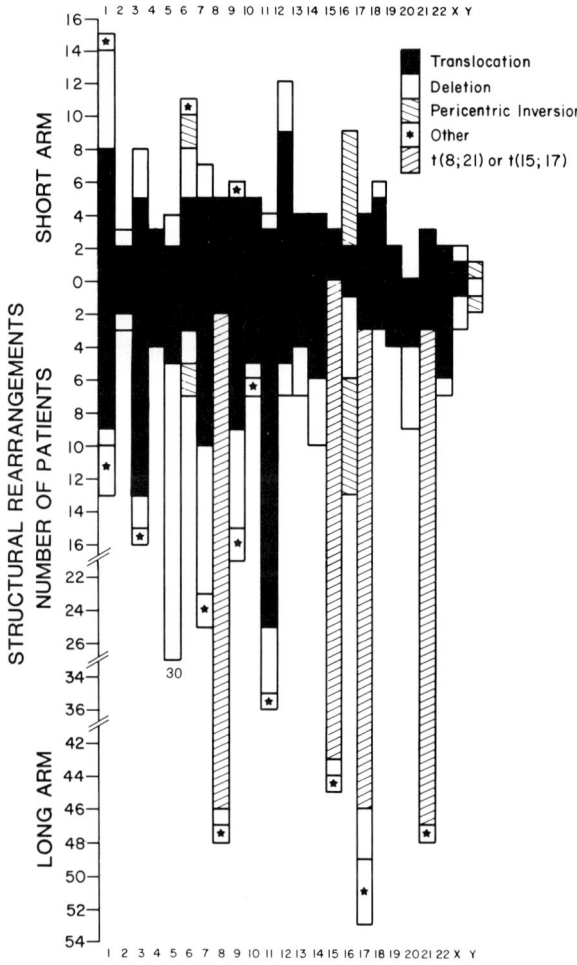

Figure 43–4. Histogram illustrating the frequency of structural rearrangements in 660 patients with acute nonlymphocytic leukemia de novo (Fourth International Workshop on Chromosomes in Leukemia, 1984). (From LeBeau, M. M., and Rowley, J. D.: Chromosomal abnormalities in leukemia and lymphoma: clinical and biological significance. In *Advances in Human Genetics*, Vol. 15. Harris, H., and Hirschhorn, K. H. (eds.), New York, Plenum Publishing Corp., 1986, pp. 1–54.)

THE 8;21 TRANSLOCATION IN ACUTE MYELOBLASTIC LEUKEMIA (AML-M2)

In 1973, the author (22) described a balanced translocation between chromosomes 8 and 21 [t(8;21)(q22; q22)]. The frequency appears to vary from one laboratory to another, but 25 of 249 (10 per cent) abnormal cases reviewed by Rowley and Testa (12) had this arrangement. In this review, the t(8;21) was found to be the most frequent abnormality in children with ANLL, being reported in 17 per cent (10 of 60) of karyotypically abnormal cases. When only patients with AML-M2 are considered, 18 per cent (41 of 226) of all patients and 33 per cent (11 of 32) of patients under 20 years in the Fourth Workshop had a t(8;21) pattern (20).

The abnormality initially appeared to be restricted to patients with a diagnosis of M2 leukemia (acute myeloblastic leukemia with maturation) according to the FAB classification. However, 7 per cent (3 of 44) of patients analyzed at the Fourth Workshop whose cells had a t(8;21) and adequate bone marrow material available for cytologic review had a diagnosis of M4 leukemia (acute myelomonocytic leukemia).

The 8;21 translocation is of particular interest for several other reasons. First, chromosomes 8 and 21 can participate in three-way rearrangements similar to those involving chromosomes 9 and 22 in CML. Second, the t(8;21) is often accompanied by the loss of a sex chromosome; of the patients reviewed at the Second Workshop, 32 per cent of the males with t(8;21) were −Y, and 36 per cent of the females were missing one X. These figures were found to be higher at the Fourth Workshop, with 28 of 33 (85 per cent) males being −Y and 8 of 11 (73 per cent) females, −X. This association is particularly noteworthy because sex chromosome abnormalities are otherwise rarely observed in ANLL. Third, this translocation has never been reported as a constitutional abnormality or in other malignant diseases (Rowley, unpublished observations). Thus, it may be lethal in all cells except granulocytes.

THE 15;17 TRANSLOCATION IN ACUTE PROMYELOCYTIC LEUKEMIA (APL-M3)

A structural rearrangement involving the long arm of chromosomes No. 15 and No. 17 in APL-M3 was first recognized by Rowley and co-workers (23). The precise breakpoints involved in this translocation have been difficult to determine; however, with the use of elongated chromosomes, the rearrangement has been defined as t(15;17) (q22; q21) (20, 24). The frequency of this translocation has appeared to vary among different laboratories. Present evidence suggests that at least some of the variation is related to suboptimal processing; the frequency of t(15;17) cells increases with culture compared with direct processing of the marrow sample. Thus, of the 80 patients with APL who were reviewed at the Second Workshop (25), 33 (41 per cent) had a t(15;17), either alone (23 cases) or with other abnormalities (10 cases; 7 had other types of chromosomal changes; and 40 had a normal karyotype. With improved techniques, including widespread use of bone marrow culture, only 15 of 61 patients (25 per cent) analyzed at the Fourth Workshop had a normal karyotype. Forty-three patients (70 per cent) had a t(15;17) karyotype, and 3 patients had other abnormalities. In our laboratory, every one of 27 patients with APL had a t(15;17), as reported by Larson and co-workers (24). The rearrangement was not found in patients with any other type of leukemia or other solid tumor.

INV(16) AND DEL(16Q) IN ACUTE MYELOMONOCYTIC LEUKEMIA (AMMoL-M4)

Another clinical-cytogenetic association recently identified involves myelomonocytic (M4) leukemia with abnormal eosinophils. Arthur and Bloomfield (26) described 5 cases (3 with AML-M2 and 2 with AMMoL-M4 leukemia) in which the bone marrow contained an excess of eosinophils (8 to 54 per cent); all 5 patients had a deleted chromosome 16 [del(16)(q22)]. Le Beau and co-workers (2) have reported on a related entity in 18 patients, all of whom had M4 leukemia with eosinophils that showed alterations in morphology, cytochemical reactions, and ultrastructure, including the presence of large and irregular basophilic granules, and a positive reaction with periodic-acid–Schiff and chloroacetate esterase. Many of these patients did not have an increased percentage of marrow eosinophils; one third had fewer than 5 per cent eosinophils. All patients had an inversion of chromosome 16, inv(16)(p13q22), and in three patients a del(16)(q22) was noted in the homolog (Fig. 43–5). The breakpoint in the long arm for the del(16) and for the inv(16) is the same. Among the M4 patients studied in our laboratory, 23 per cent have an inv(16). Tantravahi and colleagues (26a) noted an inv (16) in 3 of 18 children with ANLL; all had the characteristic abnormalities of eosinophils just described. Those patients with inv(16) had a good response to intensive therapy; 13 of 17 (76 per cent) treated patients entered a complete remission (CR). Although the median survival has not yet been reached (median follow-up 65 weeks), this value is well over the 29-week survival realized by treated AMMoL patients who do not have this chromosomal rearrangement (CR, 34 per cent) (17). It must be emphasized, however, that with different treatment programs, such a prognostic finding could become less important.

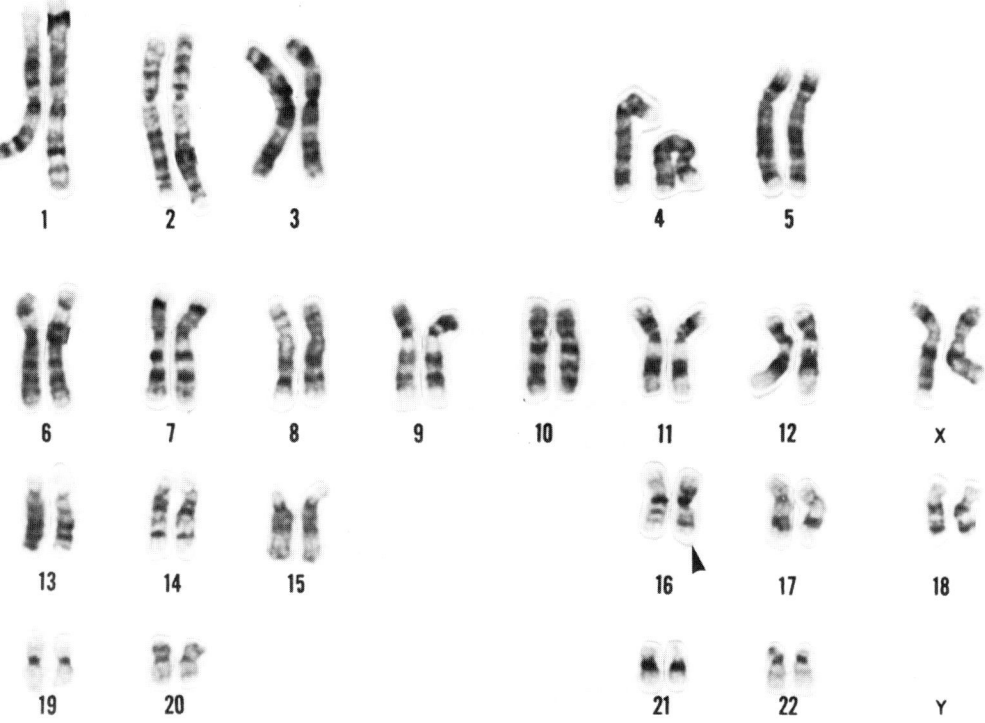

Figure 43–5. G-banded metaphase cell from a female patient with AMMoL whose eosinophils show distinctive morphologic and cytochemical abnormalities. The karyotype illustrates the inversion of chromosome 16 (arrowhead), which is seen in the leukemic cells. The breakpoints occur in the middle of the short arm and between the two distal dark bands in the long arm, with inversion of the intervening segment. The karyotype is 46,XX, inv (16) (p13q22). (From LeBeau, M. M., and Rowley, J. D.: Chromosomal abnormalities in leukemia and lymphoma: clinical and biological significance. In *Advances in Human Genetics*, Vol. 15. Harris, H., and Hirschhorn, K. H. (eds.), New York, Plenum Publishing Corp., 1986, pp. 1–54.)

STRUCTURAL ALTERATIONS OF 11Q IN ACUTE MONOCYTIC LEUKEMIA (AMoL-M5)

In addition to these consistent rearrangements, a new chromosome-morphology relationship has recently been described. Berger and co-workers (27) presented 10 cases of acute monocytic leukemia (AMoL-M5) that had an unexpectedly high incidence of rearrangements of the long arm of chromosome 11. They recently reported on 34 patients, 24 of whom had type M5a, or poorly differentiated monocytic leukemia, and 10 of whom had type M5b, or well-differentiated monocytic leukemia (28). Thirteen of the 34 appeared to have a normal karyotype, 9 had various abnormalities, and 12 had aberrations involving 11q. Following a review of these findings, the author suggested that abnormalities of 11q were particularly frequent in children with poorly differentiated leukemia (type a). Specifically, 6 of 8 children and 5 of 16 adults with M5a leukemia studied by Berger and colleagues had 11q abnormalities. Of 10 patients with well-differentiated monocytic leukemia, 1 of 3 children and 0 of 7 adults had 11q abnormalities.

This association of 11q abnormalities and AMoL was confirmed at the Fourth Workshop (20). Of 33 patients with de novo ANLL and an abnormality of 11q, 21 patients (64 per cent) had AMoL, and the great majority were M5a. Correlation of the morphologic classification and breakpoint of 11q revealed that in 86 per cent of M5 patients with an abnormal 11q, the breakpoint was in q23 or q24. Overall, 78 per cent of the rearrangements involving 11q23 occurred in M5 patients.

Aberrations of 11q differ from the t(8;21) and t(15;17) in three ways. First, the breakpoint in 11q usually involves band 11q23 to q24, but it can also occur in 11q13 to q14. Second, the other chromosome involved in the translocation is variable, although 9p is the one affected most often. A specific translocation between chromosomes 9 and 11 [t(9;11)(p26; q23)] has been described by a number of investigators (29, 30). Finally, 11q aberrations have been reported in patients with acute leukemia other than AMoL M5. In a series of children reported by Kaneko et al. (30) a translocation involving 11q was seen in a patient with AML-M2, although the cytochemical reaction of the leukemic cells was of the monocytic type. It may be that the chromosome analyses have revealed a spectrum of morphologic features in AMoL not heretofore suspected.

DIFFERENCES IN FREQUENCY OF ABERRATIONS BETWEEN CHILDREN AND ADULTS

The frequency of certain specific abnormalities in children and adults has been discussed in the preceding sections. An overview is presented here. The data used are those from the Fourth Workshop, but they are compatible with a review of 503 patients published earlier (31). The Workshop data have the advantage that both the karyotypes and the bone marrow slides were reviewed, so that the classification by FAB type is uniform. The data are presented in Table 43–2, and they include the karyotypic abnormality and the number and proportion of each abnormality that was seen in two groups of children. Each patient was classified only once, so a patient with a t(8;21) and a +8 would be listed as t(8;21). Of the 660 patients with ANLL de novo, 24 (3.6 per cent) were under the age of 2, and 78 (11.8 per cent) were ages 2 to 19 years. The most significant increases with regard to the proportion of patients are the great excess in infants of 11q aberrations, and of +21 and t(8;21) in the 2 to 19 age group. Although −7 is a feature of some children with a preleukemia syndrome, it is clear from these data that abnormalities of chromosome 7 are relatively rare in children.

Thus, no infants and only 1 patient in the 2 to 19 age group had a −7; only 1 in each group had a 7q−. None of the children had a −5, and 2 had a 5q−. Overall, combining all aberrations of chromosomes 5 and 7, only 5 of 102 patients under the age of 20 had these aberrations, compared with 73 of 558 patients over the age of 20. The author has commented previously on the possible biologic significance of these differences (31, 32). Two points should be emphasized: one is that the median age for all of the consistent rearrangements is much younger than for AMLL overall, and this is especially true for the aberrations involving 11q23. The second is that, based on the study of various subsets of adults with ANLL, those who had previous exposure to mutagens either as the result of treatment or because of occupation have a higher incidence of deletions of chromosomes 5 and/or 7 than would be expected (33–35).

Table 43–2. PROPORTION OF PATIENTS 0–2 YEARS AND 2–19 YEARS WITH PARTICULAR CHROMOSOMAL PATTERNS

Karyotype	Total Number	Age of Patients	
		<2 Years	2–19 Years
Normal	306	7 [2.3]*	36 [11.7]
−5	11	0	0
5q−	18	0	2 [11.1]
−7	18	0	1 [5.6]
7q−	10	1 [10]	1 [10]
5 & 7 abn	21	0	0
+8	36	1 [2.8]	2 [5.6]
+21	12	0	4 [33]
t(15;17)	43	1 [2.3]	7 [16.3]
t(18;21)	44	0	12 [27.3]
11q	30	8 [26.7]	3 [10]
Other	111	6 [5.4]	10 [9]
TOTAL:	660	24 [3.6]	78 [11.8]

*Number in brackets is percentage of total number with each abnormality.

CORRELATION OF KARYOTYPE AND SURVIVAL

The Children's Cancer Study Group has recently reported on its studies correlating survival with the chromosome analysis of 195 patients with ANLL who were less than 18 years of age (36). As with many earlier studies, they found that only 49 per cent of patients had clonal abnormalities. The most common abnormalities were: +8 (18 patients); t(8;21) (11 patients, 5 of whom had loss of a sex chromosome); t(15;17) (7 patients); -7 (7 patients); and pH^1 chromosome (up to 4 patients). A t(9;22) was identified in only 1 patient, the other 3 having a 22q- chromosome. No patient had a -5. It was noted that t(8;21) was associated significantly with children over 4 years, whereas -7 and 11q aberrations were associated with younger children.

The study noted no difference in the rate of remission induction, which was 75 per cent in patients with or without a clonal abnormality. Successful remissions were induced in 89 per cent or more of the patients with +8, t(8;21), inv(16), and 11q aberrations, whereas patients with -7 did poorly. These results are comparable to those reported for children and adults at the Fourth Workshop.

ACUTE LYMPHOBLASTIC LEUKEMIA (ALL)

It has been reported that the most useful prognostic indicators in ALL, the most frequent leukemia in children, are age, WBC count, and immunologic markers. Patients who are between 3 and 7 years of age, with WBC count of less than 10,000 cells per mm^3, and whose leukemic cells have non-T, non-B surface membrane markers have the best prognosis. Metaphase chromosomes from ALL patients are often of poor morphology with indistinct bands, thus making an accurate analysis difficult. For this reason, there have been fewer reports of chromosome patterns in ALL than in ANLL. Remarkable improvements, however, have been made in recent years, and it is now possible to correlate the karyotype with other recognized prognostic factors. It was rigorously demonstrated for the first time at the Third Workshop (37) that the karyotype is an important independent prognostic factor in ALL when certain therapeutic programs are utilized. It should be clear from the preceding discussion of ANLL that various structural rearrangements are specifically associated with particular subtypes based on the FAB classification. I have no doubt that the same correlation will be established in ALL when we can define subsets of patients with ALL on the basis of certain genetic (chromosome) changes and then can relate these changes to various functional and immunologic studies. In this way, we will gain a much more sophisticated and accurate understanding of the interrelationships of the various subsets of lymphoid cells.

A number of laboratories have presented karyotypic data on small series of patients (12, 38). In the earlier studies, about 50 per cent of patients had clonal abnormalities. More recently, Williams and co-workers (39) reported 67 per cent and Kaneko and colleagues (40) reported 70 per cent abnormal karyotypes. The study of 330 ALL patients (173 adults, 157 children) at the Third Workshop (37) also revealed that a higher proportion, 65 per cent, of the patients had clonal abnormalities. As in ANLL, the proportion of chromosomally abnormal clones will certainly increase with continued improvement in techniques. Of the 213 aneuploid patients, 35 per cent were pseudodiploid, 25 per cent were hyperdiploid, and only 7 per cent were hypodiploid. In the report of Williams and co-workers, 41 of 136 children had a hyperdiploid model number greater than 50, and 18 others had 47 to 50 chromosomes in the leukemic cells. Although a number of karyotypic changes, many of which are complex, have been observed in patients with ALL, certain abnormalities recur. Those abnormalities observed most frequently are described in the following sections.

Structural Rearrangements

THE 8;14 TRANSLOCATION

A reciprocal translocation involving the long arm of chromosomes 8 and 14 has been detected in a high proportion of Burkitt's tumors of both African and non-African origin, independent of whether they are Epstein-Barr virus positive or negative (41). An apparently identical translocation [t(8;14)(q24;q32)] has been observed in ALL patients whose leukemic cells have B cell markers, and in patients with L3-type leukemic cells, indicating that Burkitt's lymphoma and most B cell ALL of the L3 type are probably different manifestations of the same disease (42) (Fig. 43–6a). About 15 per cent of patients with B-ALL or Burkitt's lymphoma have one of two variant translocations; each one involves chromosome 8, with breaks in 8q24 and one of the bands carrying the light chain gene of the immunoglobulin locus, either lambda on 2p12–13 or kappa on 22q11 (Fig. 43–6b).

Sixteen patients with the t(8;14) rearrangement (7.4 per cent of all patients with abnormalities) were studied at the Third Workshop. In this group there was an excess of males over females, and of adults over children. Thus, 6 of the 16 patients with a t(8;14) were children (median age 10 years), all of whom were males. Except for one child, all had splenomegaly and, as would be expected, none had a mediastinal mass. Cells from 5 children had B cell markers and were classified as L3; in the exceptional patient, the leukemic cells had a pre-

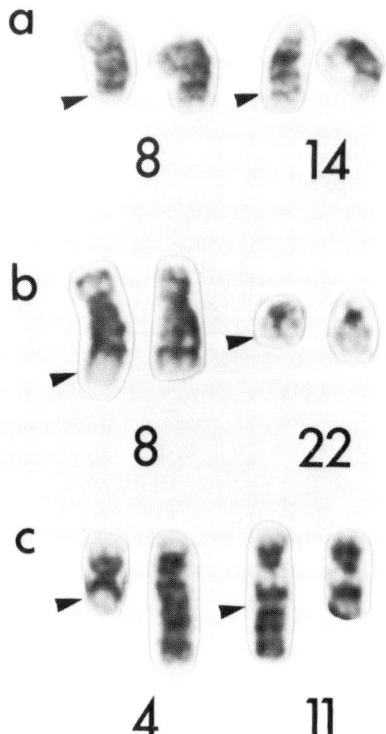

Figure 43-6. Partial karyotype of metaphase cells from three patients with ALL; the chromosomes were treated to give trypsin-Giemsa banding.

A, Patient with B cell ALL and a t(8;14) (q24; q32). The end band of No. 8 is translocated to No. 14. *B*, Patient with B cell ALL and a t(8;22)(q24; q11). The distal portion of No. 22 is translocated to No. 8. Both No. 8's are broken in the same band and in fact in the same gene, namely c-*myc*. *C*, Patient with non-B, non-T ALL and a t(4;11)(q21; q23). There is a reciprocal exchange between the end of Nos. 4 and 11. The breakpoints in the involved chromosomes are indicated with arrows. (From LeBeau, M. M., and Rowley, J. D.: Chromosomal abnormalities in leukemia and lymphoma: clinical and biological significance. In *Advances in Human Genetics*, Vol. 15. Harris, H., and Hirschhorn, K. H. (eds.), New York, Plenum Publishing Corp., 1986, pp. 1–54.)

B cell phenotype. This group of patients had a poorer prognosis (CR rate for children was 83 per cent; for adults, 44 per cent; median survival was 5 months) than did any other group of patients classified according to chromosome patterns.

THE 4;11 TRANSLOCATION

A translocation involving the long arms of chromosomes 4 and 11 [t(4;11)(q21;q23)] has been observed in a small percentage of patients with ALL, especially those with congenital leukemia (43–45) (Fig. 43–6c). Of 216 ALL patients with chromosomal abnormalities studied at the Third Workshop, 18 (8.3 per cent) had this rearrangement. One-half of these patients were adults and the other half were children, most of whom were less than 1 year old; thus the median age for children was 1 year. Three of the 9 children were males. The association of the 4;11 translocation with neonatal or early-childhood ALL is particularly interesting in view of the low incidence of ALL in this age group (acute leukemias in this age group are usually of the myeloid type). Children with a t(4;11) karyotype had very high leukocyte counts (median WBC, 214,000 cells per mm^3), which is considered to be a poor prognostic factor. Of the 8 patients for whom data were available, the leukemic cells were L1 type in 5 patients, L2 type in 2 patients, and L3 type in 1 patient; all patients in whom immunologic markers were tested had non-T, non-B ALL. These patients had a very poor prognosis; the complete remission rate was 88 per cent, and the median survival was 10 months.

Two different groups of investigators have described more detailed studies of patients with a t(4;11) karyotype; although the morphology of some of the cells often appears lymphoid, other features are more suggestive of a monocytic leukemia. This heterogeneity is also present when the cells are studied with monoclonal antibodies and with ultrastructural cytochemistry. Recent data described by Strong and colleagues (46) reaffirm that the nature of the t(4;11) leukemic cell is a puzzle. A cell line containing this translocation was studied very extensively. The significant features are that the cells contain rearranged heavy and light chain (κ) genes that provide strong evidence for B cell differentiation. However, the cells are basically negative for cytoplasmic immunoglobulin, and thus they are in a very early stage of B cell differentiation. On the other hand, a proportion of cells both from the patient and the cell line show monocytic features. In response to culture with the phorbol ester TPA, a monocyte-like phenotype was induced. Thus these cells appear to be very early precursor cells that have dual lineage capabilities.

THE Ph^1 CHROMOSOME

The Ph^1 chromosome, resulting from a reciprocal translocation between chromosomes 22 and 9, is seen in patients with ALL as well as in patients with CML. Thirty-nine Ph^1-positive patients (18 per cent of patients with abnormalities) were evaluated at the Third Workshop; 30 were adults and 9 were children. The incidence of Ph^1-positive patients with ALL was 5.7 per cent for children and 17.3 per cent for adults. Thus, the Ph^1 chromosome is the most frequent rearrangement in adult ALL. Thirty-six patients had the typical t(9;22) karyotype, and the remaining 3 had variant translocations [one was a child with t(6;22)(p23;q11)]. The incidence of the variant form was 8 per cent, which is similar to that observed in CML patients. About one half of the patients showed abnormalities in addition to the Ph^1 chromosomes. These additional changes were quite variable, and the usual changes seen in the acute blastic phase of CML were absent except for +8 in one case.

As a group, the 9 children with a Ph[1] chromosome had the second highest median leukocyte count (75,000 cells per mm^3); all had non-T, non-B ALL, and all except one had L1 morphology. The median survival for the children was 14 months, indicating a poor prognosis for these patients. By identifying this chromosomal abnormality, one can detect individuals in the non-T, non-B category who have a poor prognosis.

THE 1;19 TRANSLOCATION

The t(1;19) abnormality was not identified in the Third Workshop as a recurring change, although individual patients had been reported previously (40). Three laboratories published data simultaneously suggesting that this abnormality was a frequent occurrence among patients in whom leukemic cells had a pre-B phenotype (47–49). The designated breakpoints differ somewhat in the three series and in the patient reported by Kaneko and co-workers (40), although it appears likely that the same translocation has been observed by all investigators. Regarding the breakpoint in chromosome 19, analysis of longer chromosomes from patients studied in our laboratory, as well as from one cell line (reference 49a), showed that the break is in 19p13. Regarding chromosome 1, two of the four laboratories place the break in 1q21, whereas the others place it in 1q23. These discrepancies will be resolved when well-defined molecular probes are available; a provisional designation, t(1;19)(q23;p13), will be used here. The karyotype also shows some variation with regard to the specific abnormalities of the t(1;19). Thus, of the 16 patients reported, 6 appear to have a balanced translocation involving chromosomes 1 and 19, whereas 9 have an unbalanced translocation. The latter patients have two normal No. 1 chromosomes, plus the long arm of No. 1 translocated to 19q, leading to trisomy for 1q. One other patient has a balanced translocation, t(1;19), with duplication of the No. 19 chromosome containing 1q, which also leads to trisomy for 1q. Two of the series reported only on children; of those with a pre-B phenotype (CALLA+ and CIg+), 11 of 40 patients had the t(1;19) karyotype. We studied a 3-year-old female with a non-T, non-B phenotype (40), and 3 of the 4 patients (2 children and 2 adults) reported by Michael and co-workers (49) also were CALLA+. Specific clinical data for individual patients are not provided in two series; however, Carroll and colleagues (48) state that their patients with a t(1;19) appeared to be older (mean age 11 years) than those with a pre-B phenotype who lacked the t(1;19) karyotype (6 years). Also, the mean WBC was 12,000 in the former compared with 88,000 in the latter group. They also noted that those pre-B patients with the t(1;19) karyotype had a shorter duration of the first remission (34 weeks) than did those lacking the translocation (66 weeks). Michael and co-workers, however, noted that their patients appeared *not* to have a poorer survival, with two of them alive at 17 and 21 months after diagnosis. Our patient survived 829 days. The data are not sufficient to assign prognostic significance.

STRUCTURAL REARRANGEMENTS IN T CELL ALL

T cell ALL is a less common form of ALL and it has been more difficult to identify any chromosome abnormalities specifically related to T cell ALL until recently. Thus, of patients with T-ALL reported at the Third Workshop (37), only 39 per cent had a clonal abnormality compared with 70 per cent of non-T, non-B ALL and 100 per cent of B-ALL. Williams and co-workers (47) reported that 4 of 16 patients with T-ALL had a translocation involving the proximal part of chromosomes 11 and 14 [t(11;14)(p13;q13)]; a 4-year-old patient with a similar aberration and T-ALL had previously been reported on by Kaneko and colleagues (40). These patients are of particular interest because of the breakpoint in 14q13. Kaiser-McCaw and colleagues (50) described a variety of translocations in peripheral T lymphocytes obtained from patients with ataxia-telangiectasia with breaks in this band. This study has been extended by Aurias (51), who found similar results. In a survey of the chromosome aberrations involving No. 14 in patients with various types of T cell malignant diseases, bands 14q11 to q13 were frequently involved, whereas this region is rarely affected by structural rearrangements in B cells (52) (Fig. 43–7). In 1975, Kaiser-McCaw and colleagues (50) proposed that genes in this region provided malignant T lymphocytes with a proliferative advantage. The author's laboratory (52a), as well as Croce and co-workers (52b), have localized the alpha-chain gene for the T cell receptor to 14q11. Moreover, the author's laboratory has shown that this gene is translocated to another chromosome in two cell lines established from patients with T cell leukemia. Thus, it appears that the alpha chain gene in T cells acts in a manner similar to the heavy chain gene of the Ig locus in B cells.

There are now two reports linking deletions of the short arm of chromosome 9 (9p−) with an unusual form of ALL associated with T cell markers, a high leukocyte count, and short survival (53, 54). We also noted that these patients usually had a mediastinal mass as well as lymphadenopathy (54). Kowalczyk and Sandberg (53) found 7 of 70 patients (all children) with either a deletion of 9p (5 cases) or a missing No. 9 (2 cases). We have reported that 8 of 65 patients with ALL had features of lymphomatous ALL (L-ALL). Six of these, all under 20 years of age, had a 9p− chromosome (5 cases) or loss of No. 9. In both

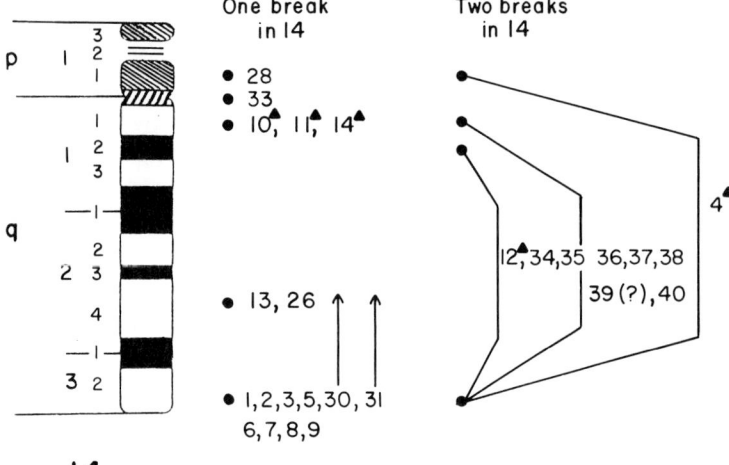

Figure 43–7. Diagrammatic representation of the breakpoints involving chromosome 14 in the patients with T cell malignant diseases. The numbers in the diagram refer to the case numbers in reference 52. Breakpoints in patients with only a single break are shown on the left, and those with two breaks are represented by the connected lines on the right. The ▲ indicates patients whose breakpoints were inferred from the published karyotype because they were not defined in the report. The vertical lines for patients 30 and 31 indicate uncertainty in the breakpoints in these patients. (Reprinted, with permission, from Ueshima, Y., Rowley, J. D., et al.: Cytogenetic studies on patients with chronic T cell leukemia/lymphoma. Blood 63:1028, 1984.)

series band 9p21 appeared to be missing in every patient.

NEAR-HAPLOID ALL

The occurrence in ALL of leukemic cells with a near-haploid number of chromosomes is rare; seven such cases have been reported (12). Of these 7 cases, 4 were males and 3 were females. Five patients were children or adolescents, and 2 were adults. These 7 patients had a remarkably consistent chromosome pattern. The chromosome number of the near-haploid clone ranged from 26 to 36 (median, 28). In addition to a haploid set, +21 was seen in all patients; +10 and +18 in 6; +X or +Y in 5; +6 in 4; and +1, +19 and +22 in 3. Four patients had a variable percentage of cells that contained double the number of chromosomes of the near-haploid line. Of the 2 patients for whom immunologic markers were tested, both had non-T, non-B ALL and one was identified as having common ALL. The median survival for these 7 patients was 9 months. Thus, ALL with near haploidy may be a unique subgroup of ALL, with a prognosis that is poor compared with that for other types of non-T, non-B ALL.

HYPERDIPLOIDY WITH 50 TO 60 CHROMOSOMES

The leukemic cells of some patients with ALL are characterized by a gain of many chromosomes and few structural abnormalities. Chromosome numbers usually range from 50 to 60, and a few patients may have up to 65 chromosomes. Although identical karyotypes are unusual, certain additional chromosomes are commonly seen. Among 30 hyperdiploid patients (14 per cent of patients with abnormalities), including 22 children and 8 adults evaluated at the Third Workshop, +21 was seen in 22; +6 in 15; +18 in 14; +14 in 11; and +4 or +10 each in 10 patients (37). It is interesting that some of these chromosomes, particularly Nos. 10, 18, and 21, are also seen as additional chromosomes in patients with near-haploidy.

The median age of the 22 children with this abnormality was 3 years, and that of all 30 patients was 5 years, which was less than that of patients with other abnormalities. The WBC count in patients with hyperdiploidy was low, with a median of 6000 cells per mm^3, and 64 per cent of all children had counts of less than 10,000 cells per mm^3. The L1 and L2 types of leukemic cells were seen in 65 and 35 per cent of patients, respectively, and all patients had non-T, non-B ALL. The complete remission rate for the 22 children was 91 per cent. The median survival had not been reached at over 2 years. Thus, in patients who have hyperdiploidy with more than 49 chromosomes, all of the previously recognized factors, including age between 3 and 7 years, low WBC count, and non-T, non-B markers, that indicate a good prognosis are present. It should also be emphasized that the median survival of the hyperdiploid patients, including both children and adults, is longer than that of patients with a normal karyotype. This has been the experience of other groups as well (39).

EMBRYONIC TUMORS

The study of the chromosome pattern of children with embryonic tumors has provided some remarkable insights into (1) the chromosomal location of genes that may be important in the development of these tumors, and (2) the variety of chromosomal mechanisms that can lead to genetic changes in tumor cells, many of which are undetectable at the cytogenetic level.

Retinoblastoma

This tumor is important because analysis of the pattern of its inheritance led Knudson (55) in 1971 to develop his "two-hit" hypothesis. He noted that patients with bilateral retinoblastoma were first diagnosed at a significantly earlier age than those with unilateral disease. Moreover, there was a positive family history in the majority of patients with bilateral tumors; this has been shown to have an autosomal dominant pattern of inheritance. Therefore, he postulated that in the bilateral hereditary form, the first mutation was of germinal origin, and the second mutation was a somatic mutation in the retinoblast. This requirement for a single new mutation in the hereditary form, compared with the necessity for two independent mutations to affect the same cell in the unilateral, nonhereditary form, explains the difference in age of diagnosis. About 30 per cent of patients have the bilateral and 70 per cent of patients have the unilateral form of retinoblastoma. A number of patients have been identified whose somatic cells show a constitutional deletion of chromosome 13 always including band 13q14. The frequency of the constitutional deletion in patients with retinoblastoma is not clear, but it appears to involve a minority. Sparkes and co-workers localized the retinoblastoma gene (Rb) to band 13q14 and showed that it was closely linked to the locus of esterase D (56).

Murphree and Benedict (57) recently reviewed the chromosome pattern in the tumor cells reported by three laboratories. In addition to obvious changes in 13q leading to deletion of part or all of the chromosome, other abnormalities also recur. These include an isochromosome for the short arm of No. 6 (iso6p), which was noted in a variable proportion of patients with either unilateral or bilateral tumors. In Benedict's series, an iso6p was noted in 6 of 20 tumors; it was noted in 9 of 17 patients reported by Squire and co-workers (58) and in 7 of 10 reported by Kusnetsova and co-workers (59). The other chromosome change is an extra copy of the long arm of chromosome 1 (+1q). Squire and Phillips found trisomy 1q in 11 of 17 tumors, including triplication of bands 1q25 to 1q32. This region has also been implicated in various hematologic malignant diseases (60). Benedict also noted trisomy 1q in 7 of 20 tumors analyzed in his laboratory.

The genetic analysis of these tumor cells can now be extended from the level of light microscopy to the molecular level. This work was described by Cavanee and co-workers (61), who first used polymorphic cDNA probes localized to different parts of chromosome 13 to compare the pattern in the normal somatic cells of the patient with the pattern in the tumor cells. These investigations provided evidence that a variety of chromosomal mechanisms could lead to expression at the recessive allele, rb, on chromosome 13. These include loss of one No. 13 chromosome carrying the normal Rb gene, loss of the normal chromosome 13 and reduplication of the No. 13 carrying rib, and mitotic recombination as a result of somatic crossing over. There is also evidence for inactivation of the Rb gene as the result of an X;13 translocation.

Wilms' Tumor

Studies of patients with Wilms' tumors yield results analogous to those discussed for retinoblastoma. Wilms' tumor, too, is present in a hereditary and a nonhereditary form. Only about 5 to 10 per cent of patients have bilateral tumors, and the average age at diagnosis is 15 months, as compared with 3 to 4 years for the unilateral form. A few patients (about 1 in 80) have aniridia. It was discovered by Miller and co-workers (62) that patients who have sporadic aniridia have a 1 in 3 risk of developing Wilms' tumor. Some of these patients have a constitutional deletion of the short arm of chromosome 11 (11p−), always including 11p13 (63).

Chromosome studies have been completed on cells from many fewer Wilms' tumors than from retinoblastomas. The author's laboratory has recently reported on the karyotype of nine Wilms' tumors analyzed with chromosome banding techniques (64). Peripheral lymphocytes had a normal karyotype in all six analyzed cases. Cultured cells from one tumor had a normal karyotype; however, they appeared to be fibroblasts. A chromosome 11 deletion, del(11)(p13p14), similar to that seen in patients with sporadic aniridia, was found as the sole abnormality in cells from one tumor. Abnormalities of chromosome 1 resulting in trisomy for the long arm (q21–q32) were found in five cases. Two of them had a translocation involving 1q and 16q, although the breakpoints in each chromosome appeared to differ in the two cases. Two patients had an isochromosome of the long arm, i(1q), and a fifth case had a duplication of the long arm as a result of karyotypic evolution. Chromosome 16 abnormalities were found in three cases, resulting in the partial monosomy of the long arm, sharing q22 as a common deletion. The same three cases also had trisomy 1q, caused by an unbalanced translocation of 1q or an i(1q). Trisomy for both chromosomes 9 and 12 was present in three cases. Our data show that although an 11p deletion can occur as a mutation confined to tumor cells, the most common changes are trisomy for 1q, and less often a deletion of 16q. Chromosome analyses of only five Wilms' tumors have been reported by others; these were primarily reports of single cases, and in each instance an abnormality of 11p was described.

Although it appeared initially that the deletion of 11p13 might involve the proto-oncogene homologue for the Harvey rat sarcoma virus (c-Ha-ras-1), subsequent studies showed that this was not the case (65, 66). More recently, polymorphic DNA probes have been used by a number of laboratories, and these have shown that, as in retinoblastoma, homozygosity for distal loci on 11p can be found in tumor tissue, although these same loci are heterozygous in unaffected cells from the same individuals (67–70). Unfortunately, only two of these tumor cells have been karyotyped, and thus it is not possible at present to correlate the cytogenetic and molecular genetic data.

Neuroblastoma

Neuroblastoma is another childhood tumor that has similarities to retinoblastoma. A deletion of the short arm of chromosome 1 distal to 1p32 has been described by Brodeur and co-workers (71) in 70 per cent of both primary neuroblastomas and tumor-derived cell lines. Another common cytogenetic finding has been the presence of large numbers of double minute chromosomes (DM) or a homogeneously staining region (HSR). These have been shown to represent two related forms of amplification of genes. The circumstances that lead to one cytologic form of amplification rather than another are not understood. It appears that HSRs are more stable, since they are integrated into the chromosome, whereas DM, which lack centromeres and which appear to "hitch-hike" on the telomeres of other chromosomes during cell division, assort randomly in mitosis between the daughter cells.

It has recently been shown that one of the proto-oncogenes, N-*myc*, is amplified in untreated neuroblastoma cells as well as in cell lines (72). The amplified N-*myc* sequences have been mapped to HSRs on three different chromosomes in three neuroblastoma cell lines by in situ hybridization. Moreover, Brodeur and his associates in the Children's Cancer Center Study Group have recently shown that N-*myc* was amplified in neuroblastoma tissue from 24 of 63 untreated patients (73). This amplification was found only in patients with stage 3 and stage 4 disease. Thus N-*myc* amplification is associated with a poor prognosis. The N-*myc* gene is located on 2p, which is not obviously involved in chromosome aberrations in cell from neuroblastomas.

Ewing's Sarcoma

Ewing's sarcoma is another embryonic tumor that has been found to show consistent aberrations. Two independent laboratories reported that cells from fresh tumors or from established cell lines had a recurring translocation, t(11;22)(q24;q12). Thus, the t(11;22) was seen in two of four fresh tumors; a third tumor had a complex translocation involving chromosomes 2, 11, and 1; and the fourth tumor also involved chromosome 22 as well as Nos. 9 and 20 (74). Four of five cell lines examined by Turc-Carel and colleagues (75) also had the t(11;22) karyotype. This translocation was not mentioned in a report (abstract) of 8 patients in whom a deletion of 1p or 3p was the recurring aberration (76). Complete karyotypes of five cell lines were published by Turc-Carel and colleagues (77); all were established from treated patients in relapse. The t(11;22) pattern was observed in four cell lines (two were from one patient). Histologic material was not available for the exceptional patient, who may therefore not have a Ewing's sarcoma. The karyotypes of all cell lines were very complex, and it is difficult to determine how much of the complexity is related to prior therapy or to changes in vitro. All cell lines had HSRs, and often several HSRs were seen on different chromosomes in the same cell line; the short arm of chromosome 7 was involved in three of the five cell lines. As in the other embryonic tumors, trisomy for 1q21 to 1q31 was common, as well as trisomy for 8q24 and monosomy 2p, 10q25 to the end, and 17p.

It is, of course, of great interest that another proto-oncogene homologous to the simian sarcoma virus, c-*sis*, was localized to 22q12. However, a more recent paper has reported that c-*sis* is neither rearranged on Southern blots nor activated as determined by Northern blot analysis (78). Its role, if any, in Ewing's sarcoma is therefore unclear.

THE BIOLOGIC SIGNIFICANCE OF CONSISTENT CHROMOSOMAL ABNORMALITIES

When Do Chromosomal Rearrangements Occur?

Some of the mechanisms leading to chromosome rearrangements were discussed briefly in the Introduction and in a detailed review (79). An equally important question is, when in the process of malignant transformation of a particular cell do translocations or other chromosomal aberrations occur? All available evidence from the study of carcinogenesis suggests that this is a multistage process. As is best illustrated by the blast crisis of CML, some chromosome changes occur as part of the further evolution of the malignant phenotype; they are, therefore, relatively late events. But what about the occurrence of the t(9;22) in CML, for example? In an individual patient, does the Ph[1] occur in a single normal cell that becomes the progenitor of the leukemic clone (translocation as a primary or sole event in pathogenesis of CML)? Alternatively, is there expansion of a clone, possibly a preleukemic one, in which a translocation occurs in one of these already abnormal cells (translocation as one of several events), or is the translocation a secondary or unrelated event, occurring in an already malignant cell? Because of the lack of independent markers for the leukemic cell (79a), this question is not easily resolved. Fialkow and colleagues (80) recently presented additional evidence supporting the concept that the Ph[1] translocation occurs in a chromosomally normal cell that is initiated or "preleukemic." They have evidence from two other patients with ANLL or myelodysplasia that supports this hypothesis (81). The data from these three patients imply that the initial event is expansion of a chromosomally normal but altered clone, and that the chromosome abnormality occurs in a cell belonging to this clone. What is required for resolution of this issue is a reliable marker for leukemic cells, or for preleukemic "initiated" cells, that is, cells that are independent of the karyotype. One could then correlate the karyotype with this marker to determine how many cells with a normal karyotype were positive for the marker.

Defining the Critical Recombinant Chromosome

It is now apparent that the sites of consistent translocations pinpoint chromosome segments that contain genes critically involved in malignant transformation. Isolation and analysis of these segments of DNA have a high research priority; the evidence in various lymphomas and CML is exciting and clearly points the way for future research in this area.

There are two recombinant chromosomes in each translocation, and it would appear useful to determine which is the critical recombinant—that is, which of the two chromosomes contains the essential gene rearrangement (82). As has been indicated earlier, each of the three common translocations in myeloid leukemia, t(9;22), t(8;21), and t(15;17), also occurs in a variant form in a limited number of patients, and one can use these variants to determine whether one recombinant chromosome is constant in these variant forms. Based on the available data, the critical event leading to malignant transformation in these types of myeloid leukemia is related to the movement of 9q next to 22q in CML, that of 21q to 8q in AML, and that of the end of 17q to 15q in APL. The findings, in a patient with AMMoL and eosinophilia, of an inv(16) as well as a translocation of chromosome No. 1 to the same No. 16 [t(1;16;16)(q32;p13;q22)] suggest that the movement of 16p13 to band 16q22 (rather than the complementary recombinant) is the critical gene re-

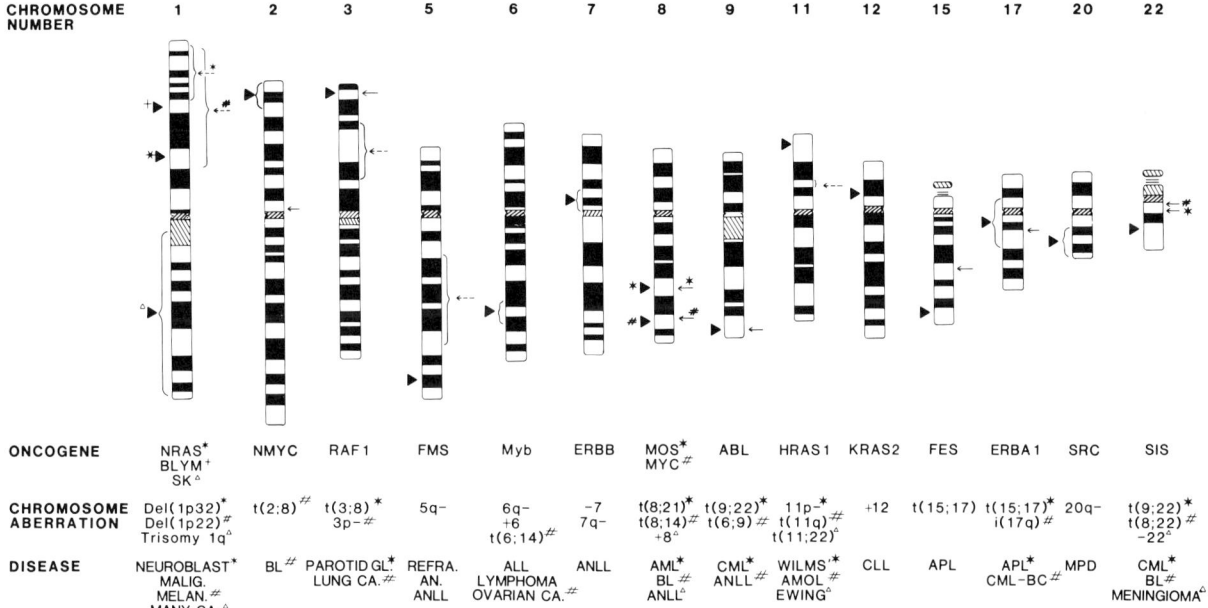

Figure 43–8. Diagram of chromosomes containing known cellular oncogenes; the number is above each chromosome, and the oncogenes, karyotypic aberrations, and neoplastic diseases associated with these aberrations are indicated below the chromosomes. The arrowhead (▶) to the left of each chromosome indicates the band carrying the cellular oncogene; the arrows to the right of the chromosome identify specific bands involved in consistent translocation (←) or deletions (←--) observed in patients having the disorders listed. Under No. 1, *Blym* has been localized to 1p32 (+▶); the deletions distal to 1p32 and 1p22 are associated with neuroblastoma and malignant melanoma, respectively. For chromosome No. 6, *myb* has been localized to 6q22–24 (▶). The t(6;14) is found in ovarian cancer. Under No. 8, * indicates the c-*mos* and the t(8;21) in AML-M2, and # indicates c-*myc* and t(2;8), t(8;14), or t(8;22) in Burkitt's lymphoma (BL). In chromosome 12, the *ras*-K-2 shows two regions of homology with in situ hybridization. Other notations are defined as follows: *Refra. an.*, refractory anemia; *CLL*, chronic lymphocytic leukemia; *MPD*, myeloproliferative disorders; *p* indicates the short arm and *q* the long arm of the chromosome. (Reprinted, with permission, from Rowley, J. D.: Biological implications of consistent chromosome rearrangements in leukemia and lymphoma. Cancer Res. 44:3159, 1984.)

arrangement (83). The patient reported by Yunis (84) with a t(6;6;9)(p23;q23q25;q34) translocation indicates that the movement of 9q34 to 6p23 is the relevant gene arrangement. A similar analysis of a variant translocation involving three chromosomes in B cell ALL indicates that the important change is the movement of 8q to 14q (40).

CONCLUSIONS

The evidence presented in this chapter clearly demonstrates the remarkable specificity of certain chromosome rearrangements for particular subtypes of leukemia or lymphoma. The mechanism or mechanisms by which this specificity is achieved are unknown. In an earlier consideration of this problem, Rowley noted that the specificity implied that a particular rearrangement provided a proliferative advantage only to a particular cell lineage, and only at a particular stage in differentiation within that lineage (60).

Since the initial description of the Ph^1 chromosome some 25 years ago, cytogenetic research has moved from a cellular to a molecular level. In some cases, breakpoints in chromosome bands can now be associated with specific genes. The identification of cellular oncogenes at or adjacent to these breakpoints raises many still unanswered questions regarding the role of these transforming genes in human neoplasia (85). In both BL and CML, evidence is accumulating that cellular oncogenes are critically involved in the specific chromosome translocations and that the resultant alterations in these oncogenes is one essential step in the multistep process of malignant transformation (Fig. 43-8). Given the rapidity with which this area of investigation is progressing, the answers to many of these questions will become clear within the next few years.

References

1. Boveri, R.: Zur Frage der Entstehung Maligner Tumoren. Jena, Fischer, 1914.
1a. German, L. (ed.): *Chromosome Mutation and Neoplasia.* New York, A. R. Liss, 1983, p. 135.
1b. de la Chapelle, A., and Berger, R.: Human gene mapping 7. Report of the Committee on Neoplasia and on Fragile Sites. Cytogenet. Cell Genet. *37*:274, 1984.
1c. LeBeau, M. M., and Rowley, J. D.: Heritable fragile sites in cancer. Nature *308*:607, 1984.
1d. Sutherland, G. R., Jasky, P. B., et al.: Heritable fragile sites on human chromosomes. XI. The folate insensitive fragile sites at 10q25, 16q22, and 17p12. Am. J. Hum. Genet. *36*:110, 1984.
1e. Yunis, J. J., and Soreng, A. L.: Constitutive fragile sites and cancer. Science *226*:1199, 1984.
2. LeBeau, M. M., Larson, R. A., et al.: Association of inv(16)(p13q22) with abnormal marrow eosinophils in acute myelomonocytic leukemia: a unique cytogenetic-clinicopathologic association. New Engl. J. Med. *309*:630, 1983.
3. Yunis, J. J.: Comparative analysis of high-resolution chromosome techniques for leukemic bone marrows. Cancer Genet. Cytogenet. 7:43, 1982.
4. ISCN: An international system for human cytogenetic nomenclature. In *Birth Defects: Original Article Series*, Vol. 14, No. 8. Cell Genet. *21*:309, 1978.
5. Rowley, J. D., and Potter, D.: Chromosomal banding patterns in acute leukemia. Blood *47*:705, 1976.
6. First International Workshop on Chromosomes in Leukemia: Chromosomes in acute nonlymphocytic leukaemia. Br. J. Haematol. *39*:311, 1978.
7. Nowell, P., and Hungerford, D. A.: A minute chromosome in human chronic granulocytic leukemia. Science *132*:1197, 1960.
8. Rowley, J. D.: A new consistent chromosomal abnormality in chronic myelogenous leukemia identified by quinacrine fluorescence and Giemsa staining. Nature *243*:290, 1973.
9. de Klein, A., Geurts van Kessel, A. H. M., et al.: A cellular oncogene is translocated to the Philadelphia chromosome in chronic myelocytic leukemia. Nature *300*:765, 1982.
9a. Fialkow, P. J., Martin, P. J., et al.: Evidence for a multistep pathogenesis of chronic myelogenous leukemia. Blood *58*:158, 1981.
10. Whang-Peng, J., Canellos, G. P., et al.: Clinical implications of cytogenetic variants in chronic myelocytic leukemia (CML). Blood *32*:755, 1968.
11. Pugh, W. C., Pearson, M. G., et al.: Ph^1-negative CML: a morphologic reassessment. Br. J. Haematol. *60*:457, 1985.
11a. Fialkow, P. J., and Singer, J. W.: Tracing development and cell lineages in human hemopoietic neoplasia. In *Leukemia: Dahlem Konferenzen*. Weissman, I. L. (ed.), Berlin, Heidelberg, New York, Tokyo: Springer-Verlag, 1985, p. 203.
12. Rowley, J. D., and Testa, J. R.: Chromosome abnormalities in malignant hematologic diseases. Adv. Cancer Res. *36*:103, 1982.
13. Hagemeijer, A., Bartram, C. R., et al.: Is the chromosomal region 9q34 always involved in variants of the Ph^1 translocation? Cancer Genet. Cytogenet. *13*:1, 1984.
14. Blank, J., and Lange, B.: Preleukemia in children. J. Pediatr. *98*:565, 1981.
15. Nowell, P., Wilmoth, D., et al.: Cytogenetics of childhood preleukemia. Cancer Genet. Cytogenet. *10*:261, 1983.
16. Sieff, C. A., Chessells, J. M., et al.: Monosomy in childhood: a myeloproliferative disorder. Br. J. Haematol. *49*:235, 1981.
17. Larson, R. A., Le Beau, M., et al.: The predictive value of initial cytogenetic studies in 148 adults with acute nonlymphocytic leukemia: a 12 year study (1970–1982). Cancer Genet. Cytogenetic. *10*:219, 1983.
18. Mitelman, F.: Catalogue of chromosome aberrations in cancer. Cytogenet. Cell Genet. *36*:1, 1983.
19. Yunis, J. J., Brunning, R. D., et al.: High-resolution chromosomes as an independent prognostic indicator in adult acute nonlymphocytic leukemia. N. Engl. J. Med. *311*:812, 1984.
20. Fourth International Workshop on Chromosomes in Leukemia: A prospective study of acute nonlymphocytic leukemia. Cancer Genet. Cytogenet. *11*:249, 1984.
21. Berger, R., Bernheim, A., et al.: Absences d'anomalie chromosomique et leucémie aigue. CR Acad. Sci. Paris *290*:1557, 1980.
22. Rowley, J. D.: Identification of a translocation with quinacrine fluorescence in a patient with acute leukemia. Ann. Genet. *16*:109, 1973.
23. Rowley, J. D., Golomb, H. M., et al.: 15/17 translocation, a consistent chromosomal change in acute promyelocytic leukemia. Lancet *1*:549, 1977.
24. Larson, R. A., Kondo, K., et al.: Evidence for a 15;17 translocation in every patient with acute promyelocytic leukemia. Am. J. Med. *76*:827, 1984.
25. Second International Workshop on Chromosomes in Leukemia. Cancer Genet. Cytogenet. *2*:89, 1980.
26. Arthur, D. C., and Bloomfield, C. D.: Partial deletion of

the long arm of chromosome 16 and bone marrow eosinophilia in acute nonlymphocytic leukemia: a new association. Blood *61*:994, 1983.
26a. Tantravahi, R., Schwenn, M., et al.: A pericentric inversion of chromosome 15 is associated with dysplastic marrow eosinophils in acute myelomonocytic leukemia. Blood *63*:800, 1984.
27. Berger, R., Bernheim, A., et al.: Cytogenetic studies on acute monocytic leukemia. Leuk. Res. *4*:119, 1980.
28. Berger, R., Bernheim, A., et al.: Acute monocytic leukemia chromosome studies. Leuk. Res. *6*:17, 1982.
29. Hagemeijer, A., Hahlen, K., et al.: Translocation (9;11)(p21;q23) in three cases of acute monoblastic leukemia. Cancer Genet. Cytogenet. *5*:96, 1982.
30. Kaneko, Y., Rowley, J. D., et al.: Chromosome pattern in childhood acute nonlymphocytic leukemia (ANLL). Blood *60*:389, 1982.
31. Rowley, J. D., Alimena, G., et al.: A collaborative study of the relationship of the morphologic type of acute nonlymphocytic leukemia with patient age and karyotype. Blood *59*:1013, 1982.
32. Rowley, J. D.: Chromosome changes in leukemic cells as indicators of mutagenic exposure. In *Chromosomes and Cancer: From Molecules to Man*. Rowley, J. D., and Ultmann, J. E. (eds.): New York, Academic Press, 1983, pp. 140–159.
33. Rowley, J. D., Golomb, H.M., et al.: Nonrandom chromosome abnormalities in acute leukemia and dysmyelopoietic syndrome in patients with previously treated malignant disease. Blood *58*:759, 1981.
34. Mitelman, F., Nilsson, P. G., et al.: Chromosome pattern, occupation, and clinical features in patients with acute nonlymphocytic leukemia. Cancer Genet. Cytogenet. *4*:197, 1981.
35. Golomb, H. M., Alimena, G., et al.: Correlation of occupation and karyotype in adults with acute nonlymphocytic leukemia. Blood *60*:404, 1982.
36. Children's Cancer Study Group: Correlation of chromosome abnormalities with patient characteristics, histologic subtype and induction success in children with acute nonlymphocytic leukemia (ANLL). J. Clin. Oncol. *3*:3, 1985.
37. The Third International Workshop on Chromosomes in Leukemia. Cancer Genet. Cytogenet. *4*:95, 1981.
38. Mitelman, F., and Levan, G.: Clustering of aberrations to specific chromosomes in human neoplasms. III. Incidence and geographic distribution of chromosome aberrations in 856 cases. Hereditas *89*:207, 1978.
39. Williams, D. L., Tsiatis, A., et al.: Prognostic importance of chromosome number in 136 untreated children with acute lymphoblastic leukemia. Blood *60*:864, 1982.
40. Keneko, Y., Rowley, J. D., et al.: Correlation of karyotype with clinical features in acute lymphoblastic leukemia (ALL). Cancer Res. *42*:2918, 1982.
41. Zech, L., Haglund, V., et al.: Characteristic chromosomal abnormalities in biopsies and lymphoid cell lines from patients with Burkitt and non-Burkitt lymphomas. Int. J. Cancer *17*:47, 1976.
42. Berger, R., Bernheim, A., et al.: t(8;14) translocation in Burkitt's type of lymphoblastic leukemia (L3). Br. J. Haematol. *43*:87, 1979.
43. Prigogina, E. L., Fleischman, E. W., et al.: Chromosomes in acute leukemia. Hum. Genet. *53*:5, 1979.
44. Van den Berghe, H., David, G., et al.: A new chromosome anomaly in acute lymphoblastic leukemia (ALL). Hum. Genet. *46*:173, 1979.
45. Parkin, J. L., Arthur, D. C., et al.: Acute leukemia associated with the t(4;11) chromosome rearrangement: ultrastructural and immunologic characteristics. Blood *60*:1321, 1982.
46. Strong, R. C., Korsmeyer, S. J., et al.: Human acute leukemia cell line with the t(4;11) chromosomal rearrangement exhibits B-lineage and monocytic characteristics. Blood *65*:21, 1985.

47. Williams, D. L., Look, A., et al.: New chromosomal translocations correlate with specific immunophenotypes of childhood acute lymphoblastic leukemia. Cell *36*:101, 1984.
48. Carroll, A. J., Christ, W. M., et al.: Pre-B cell leukemia associated with chromosome translocation 1;19. Blood *63*:721, 1984.
49. Michael, P. M., Levin, M. D., et al.: Translocation 1;19—a new cytogenetic abnormality in acute lymphocytic leukemia. Cancer Genet. Cytogenet. *12*:333, 1984.
49a. Jack, I., Seshadri, R., et al.: RCH-ACV: a lymphoblastic leukemia cell line with chromosome translocation 1;19 and trisomy 8. Cancer Genet. Cytogenet. *19*:261, 1986.
50. Kaiser-McCaw, B., Hecht, F., et al.: Somatic rearrangement of chromosome 14 in human lymphocytes. Proc. Natl. Acad. Sci. USA *72*:2071, 1975.
51. Aurias, A.: Analyse cytogénétique de 21 cas de l'ataxie-télangiectasie. J. Genet. Hum. *29*:235, 1981.
52. Ueshima, Y., Rowley, J. D., et al.: Cytogenetic studies on patients with chronic T cell leukemia/lymphoma. Blood *63*:1028, 1984.
52a. Shima, E. A., LeBeau, M. M., et al.: T-cell receptor genes move immediately downstream of c-*myc* in a chromosomal 8;14 translocation in a cell line from a human T-cell leukemia. Proc. Natl. Acad. Sci. USA *83*:3439, 1986.
52b. Croce, C. M., Isobe, M., et al.: The gene for the α-chain of the human T cell receptor is on the region of chromosome 14 involved in translocations and in inversions in T cell neoplasms. Science *227*:1044, 1985.
53. Kowalczyk, J., and Sandberg, A. A.: Possible subgroup of ALL with 9p−. Cancer Genet. Cytogenet. *9*:383, 1983.
54. Chilcote, R., Brown, E., et al.: Lymphoblastic leukemia with lymphomatous features (L-ALL) is associated with abnormalities of the short arm of chromosome 9. New Engl. J. Med. *313*:286, 1985.
55. Knudson, A. G.: Mutation and cancer: statistical study of retinoblastoma. Proc. Natl. Acad. Sci. USA *68*:820, 1971.
56. Sparkes, R. S., Murphree, A. L., et al.: Gene for hereditary retinoblastoma assigned to human chromosome 13 by linkage to esterase D. Science *219*:971, 1983.
57. Murphree, A. L., and Benedict, W. F.: Retinoblastoma: clues to human oncogenesis. Science *223*:1028, 1984.
58. Squire, J., Phillips, R. A, et al.: Isochromosome 6p, a unique chromosomal abnormality in retinoblastoma: verification by standard staining techniques, new densitometric methods, and somatic cell hybridization. Hum. Genet. *66*:46, 1984.
59. Kusnetsova, L. E., Prigogina, E. L., et al.: Similar chromosomal abnormalities in several retinoblastomas. Hum. Genet. *61*:201, 1982.
60. Rowley, J. D.: Mapping of human chromosomal regions related to neoplasia: evidence from chromosomes 1 and 17. Proc. Natl. Acad. Sci. USA *74*:5729, 1977.
61. Cavenee, W. K., and Dryja, T. P., et al.: Chromosomal mechanisms revealing recessive alleles in retinoblastoma. Nature *305*:779, 1983.
62. Miller, R. W., Fraumeni, J. F., Jr., et al.: Association of Wilms' tumor with aniridia, hemihypertrophy and other congenital malformations. New Engl. J. Med. *27*:922, 1964.
63. Riccardi, V. M., Sujansky, E., et al.: Chromosomal imbalance in the aniridia-Wilms' tumor association: 11p interstitial deletion. Pediatrics *61*:604, 1978.
64. Kondo, K., Chilcote, R., et al.: Chromosome abnormalities in tumor cells from patients with sporadic Wilms' tumor. Cancer Res. *44*:5376, 1984.
65. de Martinville, B., and Francke, U.: The c-Ha-*ras* 1, insulin and beta-globin loci map outside the deletion associated with aniridia-Wilms' tumor. Nature *305*:641, 1983.
66. Huerre, C., Despoisse, S., et al.: c-Ha-*ras* 1 is not deleted in aniridia-Wilms' tumor association. Nature *305*:638, 1983.
67. Koufos, A., Hansen, M. F., et al.: Loss of alleles at loci on human chromosome 11 during genesis of Wilms' tumor. Nature *309*:170, 1984.

68. Fearon, E. R., Vogelstein, B., et al.: Somatic deletion and duplication of genes on chromosome 11 in Wilms' tumours. Nature 309:176, 1984.
69. Orkin, S. H., Goldman, D. S., et al.: Development of homozygosity for chromosome 11p markers in Wilms' tumour. Nature 309:172, 1984.
70. Reeve, A. E., Housiaux, P. J., et al.: Deletion of a Harvey-ras allele occurs in Wilms' tumor. Nature 309:174, 1984.
71. Brodeur, G. M., Green, A. A., et al.: Cytogenetic features of human neuroblastomas and cell lines. Cancer Res. 41:4678, 1981.
72. Schwab, M., Alitalo, K., et al.: Amplified DNA with limited homology to *myc* cellular oncogene is shared by human neuroblastoma cell lines and a neuroblastoma tumor. Nature 305:245, 1983.
73. Brodeur, G. M., Seeger, R. C., et al.: Amplification of N-*myc* in untreated human neuroblastomas correlates with advanced disease stage. Science 224:1121, 1984.
74. Aurias, A., Rimbaut, C., et al.: Chromosomal translocations in Ewing's sarcoma. New Engl. J. Med. 309:496, 1983.
75. Turc-Carel, C., Philip, I., et al.: Chromosomal translocation in Ewing's sarcoma. New Engl. J. Med. 309:497, 1983.
76. Douglas, E., Green, A., et al.: Deletion of chromosomes 1 and 3 in Ewing's sarcoma. Am. Assoc. Cancer Res. 24:11, 1983.
77. Turc-Carel, C., Phillip, I., et al.: Chromosome study of Ewing's sarcoma cell lines. Consistency of a reciprocal translocation t(11;22)(q24; q12). Cancer Genet. Cytogenet. 12:1, 1984.
78. Bechet, J. M., Bornkamm, G. B., et al.: The c-*sis* oncogene is not activated in Ewing's sarcoma. New Engl. J. Med. 310:393, 1984.
79. Rowley, J. D.: Chromosome abnormalities in cancer. Cancer Genet. Cytogenet. 2:175, 1980.
79a. Reid, M. M., Tantravahi, R., et al.: Detection of leukemia related karyotypes in granulocyte colonies from a patient with myelomonocytic leukemia. New Engl. J. Med. 308:1324, 1983.
80. Fialkow, P. J., Martin, P. J., et al.: Evidence for a multistep pathogenesis of chronic myelogenous leukemia. Blood 58:158, 1981.
81. Fialkow, P. J., and Singer, J. W.: Tracing development and cell lineages in human hemopoietic neoplasia. In *Leukemia: Dahlem Konferenzen*. Weissman, I.L. (ed.), Berlin, Heidelberg, New York, Tokyo: Springer-Verlag, 1985 (in press).
82. Rowley, J. D.: Identification of the constant chromosome regions involved in human hematologic malignant disease. Science 216:479, 1982.
83. de la Chapelle, A., and Lahtinen, R.: Chromosome 16 and bone-marrow eosinophilia. New Engl. J. Med. 309:1394, 1983.
84. Yunis, J. J.: Recurrent chromosomal defects are found in most patients with acute nonlymphocytic leukemia. Cancer Genet. Cytogenet.11:125, 1984.
85. Rowley, J. D.: Biological implications of consistent chromosome rearrangements in leukemia and lymphoma. Cancer Res. 44:3159, 1984.

GENETICS

CHAPTER 44
Erythrocyte Blood Groups in Humans

W. LAURENCE MARSH

TECHNICAL PROCEDURES 1497
The Antiglobulin (Coombs') Test
Donor Blood Processing
Blood Transfusion Compatibility Tests
RECOGNITION OF BLOOD GROUP SYSTEMS 1498
BLOOD GROUP GENETICS 1499
CLINICAL IMPORTANCE OF BLOOD GROUPS 1500
Transfusion
Immune Hemolysis
Maturation of Blood Groups
Acquired Antigen Changes
Characteristics and Distribution of Blood Group Antigens
BLOOD GROUPS AND DISEASE 1502
The Rh_{null} Syndrome
The Duffy Blood Groups, Membrane Glycophorins, and Malaria
The P Blood Group and *E. coli* Infection
Kell Blood Groups and Chronic Granulomatous Disease
Associations Between Blood Group Frequency and Disease
THE BLOOD GROUPS 1504
The ABO System
The MN Groups
The P System
The Rh System
The Lutheran System
The Kell System
The Lewis System
Ii Blood Groups
The Duffy System
The Kidd Groups
The Xg Blood Groups
The En Blood Groups
The Gerbich Groups
Other Blood Group Systems
ACQUIRED AUTOIMMUNE HEMOLYTIC ANEMIA 1515
BLOOD TESTS IN DISPUTED PATERNITY 1516
CONCLUSIONS 1516

Knowledge of human blood groups contributes to genetics, anthropology, ethnology, forensic science, and the understanding of cell membrane structure. Most importantly, such information has also provided the basis for development of simple, largely uneventful procedures for blood transfusion. Without knowledge of blood groups, supportive blood transfusion therapy would not be possible.

Recognition of a blood group begins with discovery of an antibody. Such an antibody reacts in a recognizable manner with red cells carrying the appropriate antigen. Depending on the nature of the antibody and, to some extent, on the number and topography of antigen sites (called *receptors*) on the cell membrane, the reaction may be agglutination or hemolysis, or the reaction may fix complement components to the cell membrane without leading to hemolysis. If the antigen is in a soluble form, the result may be precipitation of insoluble antibody-antigen complexes. In human blood group grouping, most tests involve agglutination techniques.

TECHNICAL PROCEDURES

In the *saline agglutination test*, red cells are suspended in 0.9 per cent saline, and a few drops of the suspension are mixed with an equal volume of antiserum in a small test tube. After a short incubation period at the optimal reaction temperature for the antibody, the cells are examined for agglutination. Brief centrifugation at low speed encourages agglutination. Antibodies that react in this manner are often called *saline-reactive*, or *complete*, agglutinins. Most of them are immunoglobulin-M (IgM) proteins with a molecular weight of nearly 1 million daltons. Red cells have a negative charge. As a result, a repellent force exists between them that, under normal conditions, prevents them from touching. The large size of the IgM molecule and its multiple valency (each molecule has 10 antigen-combining sites) allow it to bridge the charge-induced gap between cells to produce agglutination.

Many blood group antibodies are IgG proteins. These are often called *incomplete* antibodies because, although they will attach to red cells suspended in saline, in most cases they do not cause the cells to agglutinate. The reason for this inability lies in the small size of the IgG molecule, which has a molecular weight of only 160,000 daltons. Molecules of IgG antibody have two antigen combining sites. Special procedures such as enzyme treatment of the red cells, suspension of the cells in albumin or a synthetic polymer, or use of the antiglobulin (Coombs') test are required to induce red cells coated with IgG antibody to agglutinate.

The Antiglobulin (Coombs') Test

The antiglobulin test has contributed more to understanding of the human blood groups than has any other procedure (1). Designed originally to demonstrate incomplete Rh antibodies, it has allowed recognition of most of the "new" blood group systems found since the mid 1940s. The test depends on two sequential antibody-antigen reactions. In the first, human blood group antibody combines with its specific antigen on the red cell membrane. In the second, antibody molecules on the cell react with rabbit immune serum (Coombs' serum) containing antibody to human IgG protein. Agglutination takes place in the second stage of the reaction. At the technical level, it is important to wash red cells sensitized with human antibody in order to remove free IgG globulin before antiglobulin serum is added. Inadequate washing results in neutralization of anti-IgG in the rabbit serum and a false-negative result. The antiglobulin test is sensitive: approximately 150 molecules of Rh antibody per cell are sufficient to give a positive result.

Two applications of the test are in common use. In the *direct* Coombs' test, the patient's red cells are washed and tested with Coombs' serum. A positive result indicates in vivo sensitization by antibody. Such an occurrence is seen following an incompatible blood transfusion, in newborn infants with hemolytic disease, in certain drug reactions, and in individuals with an autoimmune condition sometimes associated with malignancies. The *indirect* Coombs' test is used to detect IgG antibody in a sample of serum. After incubation with red cells of known blood type, the cells are washed and tested with Coombs' serum. A positive result is evidence of antibody in the serum sample. Compatibility tests involving use of the patient's serum usually include an indirect Coombs' test, which constitutes the major crossmatch. No single technical procedure is able to detect all known blood group antibodies, and in practice multiple techniques are used to ensure broad coverage.

Donor Blood Processing

The donor's red cells are typed with anti-A and anti-B, and the serum is tested against known A cells and B cells. If the serum "back-typing" does not confirm the results of cell typing, it is possible that a weakly reactive antigen is present on the donor's red cells or that an unexpected antibody is present in the donor's serum. The cells are tested with anti-D (Rh_o), and apparent D negatives are tested by a sensitive technique used to detect weak D (D^u) variants. The indirect Coombs' test is usually performed for this purpose, although some automated methods that combine the use of enzymes with a high-molecular-weight additive are sufficiently sensitive that the Coombs' test can be omitted. There is a good deal of evidence that low-grade D^u's are not immunogenic (2).

Routine testing of D-negative donor bloods for C or E antigens is unnecessary and a source of confusion. There is good evidence that C or E antigens on their own have very little immunogenicity and pose little threat to the recipient. Even when a rare D-negative person does develop anti-C or anti-E as a result of blood transfusion, the overwhelming majority of D-negative donor bloods are also C- and E-negative and will be compatible. No other blood group antigens have immunogenicity and frequency that justify further routine typing of donor red cells.

Blood Transfusion Compatibility Tests

An important part of a hospital admission routine is to establish patients' ABO and Rh types and check their serum for the presence of irregular blood group antibodies. Any blood grouping problems can then be resolved and a supply of compatible blood obtained in an orderly manner. Complex blood group studies performed at great speed in an attempt to provide compatible blood in an emergency situation are highly vulnerable to error. The direct compatibility test, in which the recipient's serum is tested against the donor's red cells, protects the patient from the consequences of mistakes in ABO typing and will also reveal active incompatibility involving other blood group systems. The direct compatibility test will reveal only active incompatibility caused by pre-existing blood group antibody. It does not reveal potential incompatibility, and it will not, for example, prevent the accidental transfusion of Rh-positive blood to a nonimmunized Rh-negative recipient.

Blood group antibodies in donor plasma present almost no hazard to the recipient. There is, therefore, no justification for including a "minor crossmatch," in which the recipient's red cells are tested for compatibility with the donor plasma, as part of a blood bank routine.

RECOGNITION OF BLOOD GROUP SYSTEMS

Discovery of an antibody is the starting point in the recognition of a blood group. Alloantibodies in human biology are antibodies produced by a person who lacks the corresponding antigen. They are active against the cells of different members of the same species. In some blood group systems, antibodies are found in sera as "naturally occurring" phenomena. In the ABO system, for example, anti-A and anti-B are found in the sera of all adult individuals who lack the antigens. Anti-P_1 may occur as a "natural" antibody in the serum of people who lack the P_1 antigen, although only a minority of these individuals have detectable antibody. On rare occasions, other blood group antibodies may be found that have apparent "natural occurrence" in serum from people who have not knowingly been exposed to the antigen.

A-like and B-like antigens are widely distributed in nature, being present on many microorganisms, and it is probable that immunization to bacterial A and B antigens is responsible for anti-A or anti-B in human serum. The origin of other natural blood group antibodies is still obscure. However, the demonstration that an example of natural anti-Kell in an infant followed enterocolitis that was caused by a pathogenic coliform organism having a Kell-like antigen (3) suggests that immunization by bacterial antigens may account for some other blood group antibodies. Some natural antibodies (e.g., anti-M^g) may be common, whereas individuals whose cells carry the reactive antigen are rare. Certain blood group antibodies are found only after immunization by blood transfusion or pregnancy. These include antibodies in the Rhesus, Duffy, and Kidd systems and the great majority of those in the Kell system.

BLOOD GROUP GENETICS

The conclusions of Jacob and Monod (4) about the mode of gene activation and regulation in *E. coli* seem to be tailor-made for the complex human blood groups. A genetic model for the Rh system based on the operon scheme has been described (5), and the concepts of regulators, operators, and structural genes can be invoked to explain observed phenomena in other blood groups.

A blood group system comprises a group of related antigens that are determined by a single gene; "gene," in this context, is defined as a DNA sequence short enough that linkage disequilibrium (i.e., divergence from random frequency) is apparent on analysis of populations in Hardy-Weinberg equilibrium. Chromosomal cross-overs that separate components of this DNA sequence are so uncommon that some combinations of antigens are more frequent than would otherwise be expected. Linkage disequilibrium is illustrated in the Rhesus blood group by the finding that a large percentage of D+ individuals are also C+, whereas most D− individuals are also C−.

About 400 antigenic specificities have been recognized on red cells. Most of these belong to one of approximately 20 systems. Not all the named systems have been shown to be independent of each other, and there is at present no means of establishing the exact number of blood group systems. No one has yet been identified, for example, who is positive for both Wright (Wr^a) and Diego (Di^a). However, the children of such a person would demonstrate whether Wr^a and Di^a segregate with independent systems. For genetic studies, maximal information would be provided by a blood typing reagent having a reaction frequency of 50 per cent. Anti-A, in the ABO system, comes close to this frequency (45 per cent positive). Many blood group antigens have frequencies of less than 1 per cent or greater than 99 per cent; these antigens provide little help in identifying genetic relationships within a population.

Most blood group genes are clearly expressed and seem to obey simple laws of mendelian inheritance. They thus provide excellent markers for use in genetic studies. There is usually an apparent one-to-one relationship between gene and antigen, with the synthesis of each antigen being ordered by one structural gene. On rare occasions, complex antigens arise by interaction of the products of more than one independent gene. Thus, Le^b in the Lewis system requires contributions by the *Le*, *H*, and *Se* (secretor) genes for formation of the Le^b antigenic configuration. In a similar manner, interaction between *I* and *ABO* genes produces hybrid antigens with IH, IA, or IB specificity, whereas the *I* and P_1 genes combine to produce IP_1 antigen. The Duffy-related antigen called Fy5 appears to result from interaction between Duffy and Rhesus gene products.

A blood group system may have genetically independent modifiers, with dominant or recessive inheritance, that interfere with proper expression of a blood group gene. Rarely, expression of a blood group gene is prevented by absence of an essential precursor structure that is involved in the biosynthetic pathway. Production of the precursor is itself determined by other independent genes. In a broad sense, genes controlling production of precursors may be viewed as modifiers of the blood group gene.

Genetic independence of different systems is most easily shown, when relevant data are available, by 2 × 2 contingency tables, although this does not rule out linkage. Independence of the ABO and Rhesus blood groups is shown by the observed frequencies listed in Table 44-1. The

Table 44–1. INDEPENDENCE OF THE ABO AND Rh SYSTEMS*

Individuals	A +	A −	Total
Rh +	347	494	841
Rh −	66	93	159
Total	413	587	1000*

*One thousand individuals were studied, and the frequency of Rh and A antigens in this population is shown in the 2 × 2 contingency table. The frequency of Rh-positive blood is almost identical in both A's and non-A's.

frequencies are so close to randomness that there is little room for doubt. Demonstration that the Rh gene is at the end of the short arm of chromosome 1 (6, 7), whereas the ABO locus is at the end of the long arm of chromosome 9 (8), has now put the stamp of cytogenetic authority on the independence of the two loci. This does not mean that there can be no relationship between the products of the two genes but only that the loci themselves are independent.

CLINICAL IMPORTANCE OF BLOOD GROUPS

Transfusion

With the increasing use of blood transfusions, a growing proportion of the population is becoming immunized to blood group antigens. Giblett (9), reporting data from a centralized transfusion service in 1977, found that the proportion of patients with immune blood group antibodies was one in 60.

Most clinical problems of blood transfusion are associated with antigens having high immunogenicity together with a fairly high incidence of negative (i.e., susceptible) individuals in the population. Antigens of high immunogenicity and high positive frequency do not commonly cause problems because few people have the capability of mounting an immune response to them. Thus, Tj^a, of the P system, is a good immunogen, but only about one person in 1 million is $Tj(a-)$. Supply of compatible blood to an immunized person having such a rare phenotype may, however, pose a great problem and require the resources of a large blood collection center for its resolution. Rare antigens of high immunogenicity present little clinical problem because the majority of donors will lack the antigen and be compatible.

Giblett (10) has estimated the "potency," or immunization potential, of various blood group antigens. Figures on the incidence of different antibodies found by several laboratories were used in the analysis. The evaluation allowed for variation in antigen frequency—and therefore for variation in the frequency of susceptible individuals—among different blood group systems. The study suggested that approximately 5 per cent of people receiving one unit of K-positive blood make anti-K and that K has 2.5 times greater immunogenicity than c of the Rh system, about 3 times greater than E, and about 20 times greater than any other moderately frequent blood group antigen, except, of course, for A, B, and D. Fortunately, K has a relatively low frequency (9 per cent), and there is no problem in locating compatible donors. Furthermore, the great majority of transfusions to K-negative patients will be made with K-negative blood.

Maternal immunization to paternal blood group antigens is the well-known cause of hemolytic disease in newborns. The possible involvement of different blood groups in this situation depends on four factors: (1) whether the antigen is developed on fetal red cells, (2) the immunogenicity of the particular antigen, (3) whether the maternal blood group antibody that results is a placenta-passing (IgG) protein and (4) whether the antibody is able to potentiate red cell destruction.

Immune Hemolysis

There is substantial evidence that formation of an antibody-antigen complex on the red cell membrane does not damage the cell (11). Destruction of antibody-sensitized red cells in vivo is achieved mainly by splenic and hepatic macrophages that have receptors for the Fc portion of IgG or for the C3b component of complement, which is bound by some antibodies. Of the four IgG subclasses, only IgG1 and IgG3 potentiate significant interaction with macrophages (12, 13). Antibodies that are IgG2 or IgG4 have little importance with respect to blood transfusion. Many antibodies to high-incidence antigens, such as Yk^a, Cs^a, JMH, Ch, and Rg, are in the nonhemolytic category, and serologically incompatible blood can be transfused to patients with these antibodies without adverse reactions or reduced red cell survival.

Maturation of Blood Groups

The erythrocytes of newborns are grossly deficient in I antigen and have greatly increased activity of an antithetical antigen called i (14). The cells lack Lewis antigens (15), with the characteristic phenotype at birth being $Le(a-b-)$, and they are also somewhat deficient in A and B antigens, Lutheran, P_1, and a few exotic antigens such as Sd^a and Bg. As would be expected, the I, Lewis, P_1 and Lutheran blood groups have not been incriminated as a cause of hemolytic disease in the newborn. Rhesus antigens and antigens of the Kell, Duffy, and Kidd systems appear to be comparable to those found on cells from adults.

Newborns seldom manufacture anti-A or anti-B on their own but usually develop these antibodies, depending on their ABO type, within about 6 months of birth. Among the other blood group systems, no antibodies occur as invariable natural phenomena in the serum of adults who lack an antigen. A very rare exception to this rule occurs in the P system, in which those with the rare p $(Tja-)$ phenotype almost always have antibodies to other P antigens.

Acquired Antigen Changes

All human sera from adults contain antibodies with capability of reaction against enzymatically changed red cells. The membrane of a normal red cell carries a number of hidden antigenic structures. The uncovering of such an antigen by an extracellular agent leaves the cell susceptible to agglutination by apparently inert human serum (16). This phenomenon is called *polyagglutination,* and many varieties are known. In the common form (T-activation), bacterial or viral neuraminidase splits *N*-acetyl–neuraminic acid (a sialic acid) from the cell membrane to expose an underlying T receptor. The activated cells are then agglutinable by anti-T present in all sera from normal adults. A useful and potent lectin anti-T can be prepared from peanuts *(Arachis hypogaea)* (17). T-activation may occur as an in vitro or in vivo phenomenon.

An interesting change of cellular antigenicity is that found in the acquired-B phenomenon (18). On rare occasions, group A individuals acquire a weak B antigen on their red cells as a temporary characteristic. They become, for a variable period of time, group AB. The change may occur in patients with infections or with lesions (especially cancer) of the intestinal tract. A few examples have also been found in healthy individuals. This form of weak B is not inherited and is believed to arise by the action of bacterial enzymes (19); an intestinal lesion possibly facilitates absorption of the bacterial enzymes. From the chemical viewpoint, A antigen specificity is determined by the immunodominant sugar *N*-acetylgalactosamine, whereas D-galactose gives B specificity. In vivo acquisition of a B-like antigen is believed to reflect activity of bacterial deacetylase, which converts *N*-acetylgalactosamine in the red cell membrane to galactosamine (20). This is sufficiently close to the structure of galactose that it cross-reacts with anti-B testing serum. If a blood transfusion is needed, group A individuals with the acquired-B phenomenon should be given group A blood.

Characteristics and Distribution of Blood Group Antigens

Blood group antigenicity may be a characteristic of a membrane protein, a sugar that is attached to a protein or to a lipid, or to a complex formed between protein and lipid. Estimates of the number of antigen receptors on erythrocytes can be obtained by immunoelectron microscopy, in which antibody molecules are coupled covalently with an electron-dense marker (usually ferritin), or by measurement of the uptake of antibody that has been labeled with radioactive iodine (^{125}I). Studies involving either or both of these techniques indicate that a single group A_1 red cell has between 810,000 and 1,170,000 A sites (21), an Rh-positive red cell of ordinary phenotype has between 6800 and 19,600 D sites (22), a Kell, or K-positive heterozygote cell has from 2100 to 5400 K sites (23), and a Duffy-positive red cell has between 10,000 and 14,500 Fy^a sites (24). Human red cell membranes have at least seven major polypeptide chains and an indeterminate number of minor components. The wide variation in the number of receptor sites for the blood groups suggests that the antigens mark different membrane components.

A, B, and H antigens are present on leukocytes, platelets, and most tissue cells and in plasma and gastric and salivary mucoids. Not all individuals have the ability to secrete A, B, or H antigens in a water-soluble form in their saliva. The characteristic is under genetic control, being ordered by inheritance of a secretor *(Se)* gene. The *Se* gene segregates independently of the *AB* or *H* genes, and about 77 per cent of random individuals are secretors (25).

Studies during the last few years have revealed that some other blood group antigens are not exclusive properties of the red cells. Lewis (Le^a) antigen (26) and Ii antigens are present on lymphocytes, and U antigen of the MNS system (27), Jk3 antigen of the Kidd system (28), and Gerbich and Scianna (Sc1) antigens are present on neutrophil leukocytes. Kx antigen, which is related to the Kell blood group system, is present on normal neutrophils and monocytes (29). Absence of this antigen is rare, but the deficiency is of more than genetic interest because Kx-negative leukocytes have a defect in their bactericidal function, and persons with such cells have chronic granulomatous disease (see the following section). These extended territorial claims are not restricted to red cell blood groupers because recent studies have shown that certain HLA antigens are also present on red cells, where they masquerade under other names (Table 44–2). In addition, Chido (Ch) is present in plasma, on red cells, and on lymphocytes. Studies have also shown that the Ch locus is closely linked to the HLA locus on chromosome 6 (30) and, more recently, that Chido and Rodgers antigens are markers on the C4 component of complement (31).

Table 44–2. SOME SHARED ANTIGENS OF LEUKOCYTES AND ERYTHROCYTES

System	Equivalent Nomenclature	
	Leukocytes	*Erythrocytes*
ABO	A,B	A,B
Lewis	Le^a	Le^a
Ii	I	I
HLA	HLA-B7	Bg^a (Ot)
HLA	HLA-B17	Bg^b (Ho)
HLA	HLA-A28	Bg^c (DBG)
Ch	Ch	Ch
MNSs	U	U
Kidd	Jk3	Jk3
Scianna	Sc1	Sc1
Kell	Kx	Kx

BLOOD GROUPS AND DISEASE

It is most unlikely that complex genes such as those of the blood groups would persist during evolution if their products did not have some advantageous functional influence on the cell. But, despite the fact that blood group studies have been conducted since the early 1900's, it has only recently been possible to assign functions to certain antigens.

The Rh$_{null}$ Syndrome

The Rhesus blood group system includes many subtly different variant antigens as well as the important D. In 1961 an Australian aboriginal woman was found who lacked all antigens of the Rhesus complex, a phenotype that was subsequently named Rh$_{null}$ (32). Other examples of this rare type have been found, as well as another rare phenotype called Rh$_{mod,}$ in which mere traces of red cell Rh antigens can be detected. Subsequent studies have established that lack of, or gross deficiency of, Rh antigens in these individuals is associated with changes in red cell morphology, in which stomatocytosis is the most prominent feature, and in vivo red cell survival is reduced (33, 34). These individuals have increased red cell osmotic fragility and the hematologic and biochemical changes expected of a hemolytic condition. Although Rh blood group characteristics may be the same in unrelated Rh$_{null}$ individuals, there is considerable variation in the severity of the associated hemolytic condition. Rh$_{null}$ red cells have an altered membrane permeability in which both passive and active K^+ and Na^+ transport are increased (35, 36). However, it does not appear that Rh antigen and the Na^+K^+ pump share common structural components of the red cell membrane, and the exact nature of the cellular defect in the Rh$_{null}$ syndrome is still unknown. Rh$_{null}$ red cells lack two thiol group–containing proteins of 32,000 and 34,000 daltons (37). It is possible that these are Rh proteins, but proof has not yet been obtained.

The Duffy Blood Groups, Membrane Glycophorins, and Malaria

Anthropologists have speculated for many years on reasons for the marked variations in frequency that occur with certain blood groups in different populations. Are they caused by random processes operating during prehistorical tribal migrations, or are they an effect of natural selection? If possession of a certain blood group phenotype confers an advantage or disadvantage in a particular environment, the antigenic structures or the antibodies that an individual can produce must have some functional importance. Many organisms share A, B, and H antigens, and it has been suggested that such shared antigenicity might adversely influence an ability to produce antibody against the microorganism. Thus, individuals of certain ABH blood types may have been better able to survive during great epidemics.

The first instance in which natural selection appears to favor a specific blood group phenotype is the association that has been recognized between the Duffy blood groups and benign tertian malaria. Almost all whites have Fy^a and/or Fy^b antigens of the Duffy system. However, 70 per cent of blacks in North America and an even higher percentage in West Africa lack both antigens, having the phenotype Fy(a–b–) (38). It has been known since the early 1960's that the great majority of blacks are resistant to infection by *Plasmodium vivax* (39), the parasite causing benign tertian malaria. The significance of these closely similar frequencies was recognized by Miller and colleagues (40, 41). *P. vivax* cannot be cultured in vitro, but *P. knowlesi*, a simian parasite that infects humans, can be grown. Repeated in vitro experiments revealed that the parasite would not invade red cells from Fy(a–b–) individuals but would invade Fy(a+) or Fy(b+) cells without difficulty (40). Furthermore, coating Fy(a+) red cells with specific anti-Fy^a serum largely protected them from invasion by the parasite. Retrospective studies revealed that six black volunteers who were Fy(a+) or Fy(b+) were all infected after exposure to mosquitoes carrying *P. vivax* malaria, whereas five volunteers who were Fy(a–b–) showed no evidence of infection during the 3 to 6 months that they were studied. A great deal of additional information has confirmed that possession of the Fy(a–b–) phenotype protects against benign tertian malaria and that a Duffy antigen or a membrane structure related to it must be a receptor utilized by the parasite during its penetration of the red cell membrane (41). Natural selection presumably accounts for the very high frequency of the Fy(a–b–) phenotype in West Africans.

P. falciparum, the parasite causing malignant malaria, does not utilize Duffy antigen for its invasion (42). In vitro studies have shown that red cells lacking a sialoglycoprotein, glycophorin A or glycophorin B, are less susceptible to invasion by the parasite (43). A good deal of supporting evidence has indicated that the recognition structure for the parasite is present on the glycophorins, close to the red cell membrane (44, 45). Interaction between the merozoite and red cell receptor does not appear to be a charge-related phenomenon associated with cell-membrane sialic acid but may depend on spatial conformation of clusters of oligosaccharides forming a specific receptor (43). The receptor can be blocked with specific antibody, preventing invasion by the parasite in vitro, which raises the possibility of a novel approach to therapy in this important disease.

The P Blood Group and *E. coli* Infection

Binding of *E. coli* to uroepithelial cells is important in the initiation of urinary tract infections. Bacterial virulence is related to the ability to bind to host cell membranes. Studies have shown that a specific receptor is involved in this interaction and that it is part of the P blood group (46–48). In vitro experiments have established that pyelonephritic strains of *E. coli* bind to uroepithelial cells and to red cells (causing agglutination) through a specific cell galactosyl-galactose structure that is part of the P antigen. Filamentous recognition structures on coliform organisms, called *fimbriae*, or *pili*, are involved in the interaction (46). P glycosphingolipids are present on many cell types, including urinary tract and kidney. Uroepithelial cells and red cells from rare type p people, who lack P antigen, are deficient in the binding structure and do not interact with these strains of *E. coli* (46, 47). Binding of pyelonephritic *E. coli* to P-positive cells is inhibited by a synthetic disaccharide with structure related to the P group. None of 30 individuals of p type had a history of recurrent urinary tract infection, but the number of subjects was too small for a meaningful statistical analysis (46). These various studies underscore the narrow specificity and the importance of cell receptors that are utilized by parasites intent on invasion.

Kell Blood Groups and Chronic Granulomatous Disease

The Kell groups have expanded into a blood group system of great complexity. Two rare phenotypes that are of particular interest in the system are K_0, in which all antigens produced by the Kell autosomal gene are missing (49), and McLeod, in which very weak forms of red cell Kell antigens are present (50). Most Kell variant phenotypes are inherited as autosomal dominant characteristics, but the McLeod phenotype has X-linked inheritance and has been found thus far only in men. About 50 examples of McLeod phenotype are known. Blood transfusions of common Kell type given to McLeod patients may stimulate production of an antibody, called anti-KL, that reacts with all blood samples except those having the McLeod phenotype (51). Anti-KL serum contains two separable antibodies, anti-Km and anti-Kx (29, 52).

Some boys with X-linked chronic granulomatous disease (CGD) have red cells of the McLeod phenotype (53). Only a few men are known who have the McLeod phenotype without CGD, and the findings in CGD cannot be due to coincidence.

Chronic granulomatous disease is characterized by high susceptibility to infections by low-grade pathogens (54). Antibody responses in these patients occur normally, but their phagocytic leukocytes have a defect in bactericidal activity (55).

The key to associating the Kell blood groups of erythrocytes with an X-linked defect of the phagocytic leukocytes proved to be anti-Kx. Normal leukocytes do not appear to have Kell antigens but do have readily detectable Kx. Phagocytic leukocytes from boys with X-linked CGD are Kx-negative. The exact nature of the biochemical lesion in CGD leukocytes is unknown, but it centers on a defect in activation of an oxidative substance in the plasma membrane (56, 57). It appears possible that Kx is a marker of a leukocyte membrane structure that is involved in oxidative enzyme activity.

Inheritance of the McLeod phenotype is X-linked. The normal allele, which produces Kx antigen, is called X^1k. Inheritance of variant alleles at the Xk locus is responsible for absence of Kx on leukocytes or red cells or both (58). Kx is related to the Kell system, but it is not a product of the Kell gene.

Although the blood group characteristics of the McLeod type were described in 1961, it was not realized until 1975 that the phenotype was associated with both striking changes in red cell morphology and a hemolytic condition. McLeod red cells show acanthocytosis and anisocytosis, and there is a concomitant reticulocytosis (59). Despite extensive biochemical studies, an explanation for the cell defect has not been obtained. The red cells have normal gross protein and lipid constitution, normal membrane Na^+ and K^+ transport, and normal intracellular glycolytic and nonglycolytic enzymes (60). The only changes recognized are a marked increase in phosphorylation of some membranes' components, notably band 3 protein and the β chain of spectrin (61), and an increase in intramembrane particle density when the cells are examined by freeze-fracture electron microscopy (62).

The Xk locus is inactivated by the Lyon phenomenon of X-chromosome inactivation, and female carriers of variant *Xk* alleles may have a double population of functional and nonfunctional leukocytes as well as McLeod acanthocytes and normal red cells of common Kell type (59). Whether the mosaicism involves one or both of these cell lines depends on the variant *Xk* allele that is involved.

Abnormalities of McLeod syndrome are not restricted to hemopoietic tissues. McLeod subjects have elevated serum creatine phosphokinase in the range 1000 to 2500 IU per liter (normal up to 180 IU per liter) (63), high levels of the muscle enzyme carbonic anhydrase III (64), and thereafter a slowly developing muscular dystrophic condition, although there are no associated symptoms until about the fifth decade (60, 65). Older men with McLeod syndrome have a progressive neurologic disorder with areflexia and choreiform movements and cardiomyopathy (60). Family studies show that these conditions are inherited together and they appear to be pleiotropic effects of one gene. The X-linked gene causing the McLeod red cell phenotype appears to be of considerable biologic importance in a number of tissues.

Associations Between Blood Group Frequency and Disease

Many apparent associations between blood group frequency and disease and between blood groups and many other human characteristics have been reported, but few have been confirmed. However, some positive associations do seem to exist, although the mechanisms by which they operate are unknown. Many studies have confirmed that group A individuals have approximately 20 per cent greater chance of developing cancer of the stomach than group O persons (66) and that the latter have about 20 per cent greater chance of developing duodenal ulcer than individuals of other ABO types (67). In addition, several confirmatory studies have shown that duodenal ulceration is about 50 per cent more likely to develop in people who are nonsecretors of ABH substances than in those who are secretors (68). It may be significant that these positive correlations involve lesions of the gastrointestinal tract, in which large quantities of secreted ABH substances may be present. Simple postulates that soluble blood group substances exert a protective effect are unlikely to be true, however, because ABH nonsecretors have about the same amount of secreted mucopolysaccharide as secretors, with the specificity difference reflecting only a variation in a few terminal sugars.

THE BLOOD GROUPS

Blood group notation has evolved since the early 1900's and, as might be expected in an evolutionary process, has produced some oddities. In the MN system, for example, M and N are regarded as products of alleles, but so also are S and s in the same system. Despite these terminologic inconsistencies, there is general agreement on the order of presentation, and blood group phenotypes are usually written in the sequence that the groups were discovered. This section will, therefore, follow the same order.

The ABO System

The ABO groups are still yielding secrets after many years of study. Two independent loci, ABO and H, and probably a third, Y, are involved in expression of ABO. The *O* allele at the ABO locus is believed to be an amorph, having no recognizable product. The ABO locus is known to be near the end of the long arm of chromosome 9 (8, 69), where it provides a useful cytogenetic marker, but the *H* gene has not yet been mapped. The gene called *Y* appears to be necessary for proper expression of *A* on red cells. Homozygosity for recessive *y* alleles results in marked depression of A antigenicity.

A, B, and H antigenicities are determined by specific sugars attached to a precursor structure. Two types of precursor chains, called type 1 and type 2, have slight structural differences, but both have acceptors for ABH sugars. The antigens cannot be direct gene products but reflect activity of products that are transferase enzymes, responsible for attachment of the sugars. The *H* gene produces an L-fucosyltransferase, which adds L-fucose to the precursor, whereas the *A* and *B* genes direct transferases, which add *N*-acetylgalactosamine and D-galactose, respectively, to the same structure. These transferases are present in various body fluids and can be demonstrated in plasma. The origin of plasma transferases is unknown, and they are not responsible for the AB and H antigens on red cells. Group O red cells do not have a specific O antigen, but the absence of A or B sugars leaves exposed a considerable amount of H substance.

An important development in transfusion medicine is the capability of modifying certain cell antigens in vitro without compromising subsequent cell viability in vivo. Goldstein and colleagues (70) have used a purified alpha-galactosidase to remove an immunodominant sugar and convert B red cells to O in vitro and have shown that such cells have normal survival when transfused.

Inheritance of the ABO groups is usually uncomplicated. An example of a common and informative family is shown in Figure 44–1. Family members have the following features: Parents are group A and group B, whereas children are group A, B, AB, or O. In such a family, it is obvious that the parents are *AO* and *BO* and that the four possible ABO types will occur with equal frequency among their offspring. A mating between O and AB persons produces only A or B children. An AB person does not, under normal circumstances, have an O child or an O parent.

On rare occasions, individuals have been found who are homozygous for a silent (*h*) allele at the H locus. The first example was recognized in

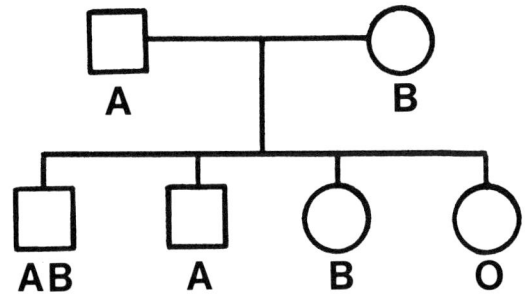

Figure 44-1. ABO types of a common and informative family. It is obvious that the A individuals must be of genotype *AO*, and the B's, *BO*.

India, which explains why the variant is called the Bombay phenotype (71). The H antigen structure is required for attachment of A or B sugars, and, because of this, red cells of Bombay phenotype are not agglutinated by anti-A, anti-B, or anti-H. At first, the cells appear to be group O, but further study shows that they are H-negative (an alternative term for the variant is O_h). People with these rare cells always have anti-A, anti-B, and anti-H in their sera, which are compatible only with blood of the Bombay phenotype, which must be used for transfusion. Because the ABO and H loci are independent, an *hh* person will have normal but unexpressed genes at the ABO locus (72). The children of an *hh* person usually inherit an *H* gene from the other parent, and an *A* or *B* gene inherited from the Bombay parent will be expressed normally, sometimes suggesting nonparentage. The specific sugars do not appear to be vital for integrity of the red cell membrane because Bombay cells have normal morphology and normal in vivo survival.

ABO antigens have been demonstrated in many tissues, which is important from the histocompatibility viewpoint. In malignancy, tissues lose their ABH antigens, a change that is believed to reflect dedifferentiation in malignant cells. It has been suggested that tests for tissue ABO antigens may be helpful in the diagnosis of certain cancers (73). On rare occasions, red cells from patients with leukemia or an allied condition show reduction in A, B, or H antigenicity. The magnitude of the antigenic change may fluctuate in parallel with the clinical course of the disease, and the antigens sometimes reappear during remission (74).

Reactions due to the accidental transfusion of ABO-incompatible blood may be mild and pass unnoticed, but they may be severe enough to lead to renal shutdown. The most severe reactions usually occur in recipients whose serum contains a reactive ABO antibody that has hemolytic properties when tested in vitro. ABO blood group incompatibility is a common cause of hemolytic disease of the newborn, with most of the mothers being group O and the children group A or B. In the great majority of cases, however, the hemolytic condition in the infant is mild and requires no treatment.

Many phenotypes characterized by weak A or B antigens have been described. Most of these arise by inheritance of variant alleles at the ABO locus, but some appear to result from interference, in which expression of a normal *A* or *B* gene is changed by an independent modifier. Both recessive (75) and dominant (76) types of modifying gene have been reported.

Cis-AB

A discovery of considerable theoretical importance, rejected by the scientific community for more than 40 years (77) and finally rediscovered in 1964 (78), was the finding that some AB individuals are able to transmit both *A* and *B* genes to a single child. In these cases, an AB parent married to an O partner may produce AB children. The A and B antigens in these cases are usually weaker than those of normal AB individuals. The phenomenon is very rare in whites but is more common in Japan and other countries of the East, where it has been estimated that this type is found in about one in 5000 people with group AB blood (79). The explanation may be a mutation at the AB locus, resulting in a gene that produces a transferase able to attach both *N*-acetylgalactosamine and D-galactose to the ABO precursor structure. Alternatively, it is possible that uneven chromosome cross-over has duplicated an ABO gene. Cytogenetic studies of *cis*-AB individuals have not shown any recognizable change of chromosome 9 (80), but current techniques for examining chromosomes are not sufficiently sensitive to reveal very small duplications. The importance of the phenotype lies in the belief that complex blood group genes have arisen during evolution by gene duplication as a result of uneven cross-over. Mutation of a duplicated gene then produces complexity, and further cross-over and mutation later continue the process. *Cis*-AB, with the possibility that *A* and *B* genes are both together on one chromosome, may be an example of this evolutionary phenomenon in progress.

The MN Groups

Human blood group antibodies may occur naturally or may be an immune response to blood transfusion or pregnancy. Some animals may be stimulated to produce new specificities by being injected with human red cells. An immune rabbit serum will contain powerful species antibodies that react with all human red cells, but specific antibodies may remain after absorption with selected human cell samples. Such a procedure resulted in discovery of the MN blood groups in 1926 (81). Two antibodies, named anti-M and anti-N, were made by rabbits that had been injected with red cells from different humans. Three cell types were defined: M+N+, M+N−, and M−N+. Tests of families indicated that M and N were inherited as codominant characters. Complications in the system began with the discovery of anti-S and anti-s, which define a second pair of alleles (82). Family studies showed that the *Ss* genes segregated with the *MN* genes. S is more often associated with M than with N, whereas s is found more often in company with N. This linkage disequilibrium is further evidence that Ss and MN loci are closely linked. Very rare examples of recombination between MN and Ss have been reported. From practical and genetic viewpoints, the loci are very close together. Approximately 1 per cent of blood from American blacks is S−s−. These individuals, if immunized, make an antibody called anti-U, which is compatible with other examples of the same phenotype (83). Anti-U was originally thought to be anti-S plus anti-s, but the discovery that some S−s− blood samples are U-positive established that U must be a separate specificity that nearly always accompanies S and s. The frequency of S−s−U− individuals varies in different African population groups, with the record at present being held by Congo Pygmies, in whom the phenotype frequency is about 35 per cent (84). The frequencies of some MN antigens are shown in Table 44–3.

More than 30 additional MN antigens have been described, with many being of low frequency. Human sera often contain naturally occurring antibody against one or more of the uncommon antigens, but the source of stimulation is unknown.

The MN antigens have very little clinical importance because, although they are good immunogens in rabbits, they have very little immunogenicity in humans. Anti-S and, less commonly, anti-s have been responsible for a few transfusion reactions. Anti-U is a rare antibody, found only in blacks of the S−s−U− type, but it is usually IgG, may be extremely powerful, and has been a cause of transfusion reactions and erythroblastosis fe-

talis. The main interest in the MN system is from the genetic viewpoint because, if the four antisera are used in family studies, the system is the most discriminating of all the red cell blood group systems. A pedigree illustrating inheritance of MN is shown in Figure 44–2.

Red cells treated with papain, ficin, bromelin, or neuraminidase lose their MN antigenicity. Sialic acid, which is split by these enzymes, forms a part of the glycoprotein antigenic determinant. Early studies had suggested that N might be a precursor of M (85). In this case N would not be produced by an allele of M, but would simply represent an excess of unconverted precursor left exposed by absence of an *M* gene. However, studies have shown that the MN genes put the stamp of specificity on the protein moiety of the membrane sialoglycoprotein glycophorin A (86, 87). The amino acid sequence of this 31,000-dalton glycoprotein has been established (88). When the structure has M specificity, amino acid residues at positions 1 and 5 of the amino terminus are serine and glycine, whereas leucine and glutamic acid are substituted at positions 1 and 5, respectively, when the specificity is N (89, 90). Oligosaccharides may represent important but nonspecific components of the immunodeterminants recognized by some anti-M sera. They may be present in different steric configurations on M or N glycoproteins as a result of the differences in amino acid sequences.

The P System

Like the antibodies in the MN system, the first antibodies in the P system were produced by injection of rabbits with human blood (91). Absorption of species antibodies from the immune rabbit serum left a new antibody that agglutinated about 78 per cent of human red cell samples. The reactive antigen was named P. Subsequent studies have shown that anti-P (now called anti-P_1) occurs in many animal sera and is not uncommon in human sera. Human anti-P_1 is nearly always a naturally occurring cold agglutinin with very little

Table 44–3. SOME ANTIGENS OF THE MN SYSTEM

Designation	Frequency of Antigens in Whites	Date of Discovery
M	0.78	1927
N	0.72	1927
Hu	<0.01	1934
Vw(Gr)	<0.01	1946
S	0.55	1947
s	0.89	1951
He	<0.01	1951
Mi[a]	<0.01	1951
U	>0.99	1953

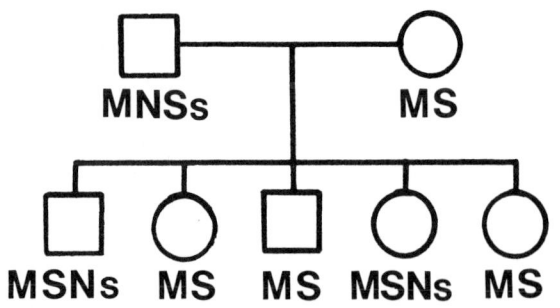

Figure 44–2. A representative pedigree showing inheritance of the MN blood groups. Genotypes are shown for the two MNSs children. The father must have the genotype *MSNs*, and s is segregating with N.

clinical significance. The P_1 antigen is not well developed on the red cells of infants at birth, and the antibody does not cause hemolytic disease.

Anti-Tj^a was discovered in 1951 (92) and reacts with an almost universal antigen. Several years after the discovery of Tj^a, it was realized that this antigen is part of the P system (93). Discussion of one rare and two common phenotypes must be included here for a basic level of understanding. The first, called p, or Tj(a−), is very rare, and sera from people with this phenotype almost always contain anti-P plus anti-P_1. P_2 (previously called P negative) occurs in approximately 22 per cent of people; sera from P_2 individuals may contain anti-P_1. These red cells have basic P antigen. The most common phenotype, P_1, occurs with a frequency of 78 per cent; sera from these individuals contain no P antibodies.

The reaction strength of P_1 red cells taken from different people varies widely. Some P_1 cell samples react only with very strong anti-P_1 sera. The variation in P_1 antigenicity is due in part to inheritance of a weak P_1 gene and in part to zygosity. (Heterozygous red cells in many blood groups are known to be less strongly reactive.) Serologic characteristics of the P system are summarized in Table 44–4.

Another complication of P was revealed by the discovery of P^k. The antigen is unusual in that it appears to have recessive inheritance because P^k-negative parents may have P^k-positive children (94). As will be seen in the next paragraph, however, biochemists have provided an explanation for this phenomenon.

Biochemical studies have shown that P system antigens are glycosphingolipids (95). In the biosynthetic pathway, lactosyl ceramide is converted to trihexosyl ceramide, resulting in a structure with P^k specificity (96, 97). This, in turn, is converted to globoside by addition of a nonreducing β-galactosaminyl residue. The substance that results has P activity. P^k erythrocytes are deficient in the transferase that adds the galactosaminyl residue, and, as a result, trihexosyl ceramide with P^k activity accumulates in the cells. In an alternative pathway, lactosyl ceramide is converted to paragloboside and then, by addition of α-linked galactose, to P_1 substance. In people with red cells of p type, a primary transferase deficiency blocks production of globoside and conversion of paragloboside into a P_1-active structure (98). Biochemists have changed our way of thinking of the P system, for with the two separate branches in the P pathway, the concept that P_1 and P (P_2) are allelic genes is no longer tenable. As would be expected, red cells of p type have only trace amounts of globoside.

P antigens are not restricted to red cells but have been demonstrated on fibroblasts (99), where it has been found that all cells were P^k-positive irrespective of the red cell type of the donor. The cold-reactive autohemolysin known as the Donath-Landsteiner antibody causes paroxysmal cold hemoglobinuria and usually has P specificity (100).

The Rh System

The Rhesus system (101, 102) is second only to the ABO system in terms of clinical importance because it is still the most commonly involved blood group in pregnancy-associated immunization. However, as a long-range result of Rh immune globulin prophylaxis, the incidence of anti-Rh(D) is steadily decreasing. The name "Rhesus" honors the monkey whose red cells stimulated the first antibodies when these cells were injected into rabbits and guinea pigs. Subsequent investigations have indicated that although the Rhesus monkey antigen is similar to the Rh(D) antigen of human cells, it is not identical. Human cells have both the monkey antigen and a separate, but related, Rh antigen. The name LW, which honors Landsteiner and Wiener, has been given to the antigen that is shared by human and monkey red cells.

Since the early 1940's, Rh has grown into a system of great complexity. More than 40 antibody specificities are known. The most important of these is still D, although it is now clear that D itself comprises a cluster of antigenically separate components. At least six categories are known, each lacking a different component of the D mosaic. Red cells lacking one of these components may have in its place an alternative antigen. Anti-Go^a and anti-D^w, for example, react with uncommon antigens that are substitutions for the missing D components in category IV and category V, respectively.

Table 44–4. PHENOTYPES IN THE P SYSTEM*

Phenotypes			Reactions with Sera			
Current Nomenclature	Former Nomenclature	Incidence	Anti-P_1	Anti-PP$_1$P^k (anti-Tj^a)	Anti-P	Anti-P^k
P_1	P+	0.75	+	+	+	0
P_2	P−	0.25	0	+	+	0
p	Tj (a−)	Very rare	0	0	0	0
P_1^k		Very rare	+	+	0	+
P_2^k		Very rare	0	+	0	+

*Modified from Race, R. R., and Sanger, R.: *Blood Groups in Man*, 6th ed. Philadelphia, F. A. Davis, 1975, p. 157.

Early studies suggested that three closely linked genes were responsible for three antigens called C, D, and E. Numerous alternatives have been identified at the C and E loci, but nothing corresponding to d has been identified. Most workers consider d to represent an absence of D. Much controversy has existed over the exact genetic mechanism that governs Rh, but whether one super-gene or three separate closely linked genes are involved is of no practical importance. The complexities that have become apparent in Rh may be viewed simplistically as variations on the basic three-gene theme. The concept of a single super-gene is more likely to be correct, however, and a genetic model for the Rh complex based on four operators, each with a structural gene, has been described (5). On the descriptive level, the C, D, and E theme has certain advantages. In an attempt to circumvent these ideologic quicksands, a numerical notation that corresponds only with phenotypic characteristics has been devised (103). Alternative notations for the more important Rh antigens are shown in Table 44–5.

From the practical viewpoint, Rh D is a strong immunogen and will provoke anti-D in about 50 per cent of D-negative people transfused with one unit of D-positive blood. Anti-E and anti-c are the next most frequently encountered Rh antibodies. Almost all antibody specificities in the Rh system have been responsible for erythroblastosis fetalis and for hemolytic transfusion reactions. It is sometimes a consoling thought that although transfusion of ABO-incompatible blood may cause severe hemolytic transfusion reactions and has a significant mortality, reactions due to incompatibility in other blood group systems, including Rh, are seldom fatal. Rh antibodies are usually IgG proteins, often with high titer, but they do not fix complement to the surface of the erythrocyte.

The Rh gene is located near the end of the short arm of chromosome 1 (6, 7). It is one of a linked group of genes that includes El_1, which determines a type of erythrocyte elliptocytosis, and genes for the enzymes 6-phosphogluconate dehydrogenase (6PDG), phosphoglucomutase-1 (PGM_1), and peptidase C (PEP C).

One of the most interesting and informative aspects of Rh has been the discovery of partially deleted and fully deleted phenotypes. Rare blood samples may lack all antigens of the C or E variety. These −D− samples have greatly increased amounts of D antigen.

People with such red cells are prone to make antibody (called anti-Rh 17), which is compatible with only −D− or Rh_{null} cells. Other partial deletions include cD− and $C^wD−$. There also are a number of other gene complexes with markedly depressed, but not quite aberrant, expression of parts of the Rh complex.

Rh_{null} cells lack all antigens produced by the Rh gene (32). The phenotype may arise by inheritance of independently segregating recessive modifying genes (called X^0r) that prevent expression of Rh (104) or by inheritance of silent alleles at the Rh locus itself (105). An important contribution to knowledge made by Rh_{null} individuals was that Rh protein is necessary for maintenance of red cell membrane integrity. Rh_{null} red cells are stomatocytes and have reduced in vivo survival. Further details on this were given in the earlier section on blood groups and disease. Rh antigen labels a protein component of the red cell membrane, but phospholipids in the membrane are required for manifestation of the antigenicity (106).

The Lutheran System

The Lutheran blood group system has undergone an expansion. For about 15 years the system contained only the antigen Lu^a, with a frequency of about 8 per cent in whites, and Lu^b, which reacts with more than 99 per cent of random blood samples (107, 108). In many of the blood group systems, discovery of a null phenotype has allowed advances in knowledge, and perhaps nowhere has this been more striking than in the Lutheran system. An antibody that reacts with almost all random blood samples but is compatible with Lu(a−b−) red cells must be associated with the Lutheran system. The key discovery of the Lu(a−b−) phenotype was made by the proposita herself when testing her own blood (109). Such cells are not agglutinated by anti-Lu^a or anti-Lu^b. Family studies were surprising because they revealed a dominant mode of inheritance. A child of the dominant Lu(a−b−) type always has an Lu(a−b−) parent. Many such families are known. Inheritance of an independently segregating dominant inhibitory gene prevents expression of the Lutheran genes (110). The inhibitor gene is not aimed exclusively at Lutheran because it also prevents proper expression of Auberger (Au^a), P_1, and some other antigens (117). The inhibitor gene was originally named In(Lu) (inhibitor of Lu-

Table 44–5. EQUIVALENT NOTATIONS FOR SOME Rh ANTIGENS

Wiener	Fisher-Race	Numerical	Frequency in Whites
Rh_o	D	Rh1	0.84
rh'	C	Rh2	0.70
rh''	E	Rh3	0.30
hr'	c	Rh4	0.80
hr''	e	Rh5	0.97
hr	ce(f)	Rh6	0.64
rh^{w1}	C^w	Rh8	0.01
rh^G	G	Rh12	0.85
	Total Rh	Rh29*	>0.99

*Anti-Rh29 is the antibody made by people of Rh_{null} type.

theran) (110), but with recognition of its wider impact on antigen synthesis a name change to SYN-1B has been proposed (112).

More recently, families have been found in which the Lu(a−b−) phenotype is inherited as a recessive characteristic through a silent allele at the Lutheran locus (113, 114). There are thus two genetic mechanisms that can give rise to the Lu(a−b−) type. Critical studies have revealed that the two kinds of Lu_{null} phenotype are subtly different. Red cells from the dominant inheritance forms have very small amounts of Lutheran antigens, detectable by special antibody absorption elution techniques. In contrast, the recessive form of Lu(a−b−) is devoid of Lutheran antigens. This difference has some importance. Individuals of dominant Lu(a−b−) type do not make Lutheran antibodies, but recessives may make an antibody called anti-Lu3 if they are transfused with blood of common Lutheran type. Anti-Lu3 is compatible only with red cells that are Lu(a−b−).

Discovery of anti-Lu4 in 1971 (115) was an event that triggered an explosion in the study of the Lutheran blood groups. In the ensuing surge of interest, anti-Lu5, anti-Lu6, anti-Lu7, anti-Lu8, anti-Lu11, anti-Lu12 (Much), and anti-Lu13 were identified (116–118). Each antibody reacts with a different high-incidence red cell antigen, but in each case Lu(a−b−) red cells are compatible. Two antibodies that react with low-frequency Lutheran antigens have given illuminating results. Anti-Lu9 (Mu11) reacts with about 2 per cent of random blood samples (119). Family studies established that the Lu^9 gene segregated with Lutheran. Further investigation revealed that Lu:−6 red cells were always reactive with anti-Lu9. Thus, there is convincing evidence that Lu^6 and Lu^9 are a second pair of alleles at the Lutheran locus. The other illuminating antibody is anti-Lu14, which has a reaction frequency of approximately 2.5 per cent (120). Serologic and genetic studies have shown that Lu^{14} is an allele of Lu^8; therefore, these constitute a third pair of Lutheran alleles. Table 44–6 shows antigenic and genetic relationships in the Lutheran system.

Although this expansion of the Lutheran blood group system is of considerable genetic interest, the antibodies involved are usually weak and do not cause hemolytic transfusion reactions or erythroblastosis fetalis.

The Kell System

Discovery of anti-Kell (anti-K) was an early bonus that followed the development and application of the antiglobulin test (1). The first antibody caused erythroblastosis fetalis, and other antibodies have subsequently been incriminated as a cause of hemolytic transfusion reactions. About 9 per cent of whites are K-positive. The antigen has strong immunogenicity. About 1 in 20 K-negative individuals transfused with K-positive blood will make anti-K.

Blood grouping tests of many families have shown that Kell is an autosomal trait inherited independently of ABO, MN, P, Rh, Lutheran, and many other loci.

The discovery of anti-k in 1949 allowed positive identification of the alternative antigen to K (121). The presence of anti-k in a patient's serum poses a serious logistic problem in terms of blood supply because only approximately one in 500 random donors is compatible.

The age of simplicity in the Kell system lasted an additional 8 years, but the recognition of Kp^a and Kp^b and the demonstration that they were controlled from the Kell locus established that the system was far from simple (122, 123). In an attempt to maintain consistency in notation, a numerical system of terminology was introduced, which has been expanded as new specificities have been recognized (124). In this notation, a positive phenotype is written K:1 and a negative phenotype is designated K:−1.

In 1957, a new phenotype that lacked K, k, Kp^a, and Kp^b was described (49). This null phenotype, called K_0, is now known to lack all antigens that are part of or are related to the Kell system, with the exception of Kx. The K_0 phenomenon is specific for Kell, with other blood group antigens being normal. Many examples of K_0 are now known, and family studies have established that these arise by homozygous inheritance of silent (K^0) genes at the Kell locus. It is useful to borrow the Jacob-Monod concept of gene regulation and imagine that K^0 represents mutation at the operator region of the Kell gene, whereas the many Kell antigens reflect different mutational sites in the structural gene. The antigens produced by the Kell gene do not appear to be essential to proper survival and appearance of red cells. Scanning

Table 44–6. ANTIGENS RELATED TO THE LUTHERAN BLOOD GROUP SYSTEM

Common antigens (frequency >99 per cent)	Lu^b	Lu6	Lu8	Lu4	Lu5	Lu7	Lu11	Lu12	Lu13
	↑	↑	↑						
		alleles							
	↓	↓	↓						
Uncommon antigens (frequency <8 per cent)	Lu^a	Lu9	Lu14						

electron microscopic examinations of K_0 red cells show them to be normal, and hematologic studies of K_0 individuals show nothing unusual. K_0 patients may pose difficulty if they are recipients of blood transfusions because the antibody they make, anti-Ku, is compatible only with other examples of the K_0 phenotype.

When anti-Js^a (Sutter) was discovered in 1958, it seemed at first to herald a new blood group system (125). Approximately 20 per cent of North American blacks were Js(a+), whereas tests of nearly 500 blood samples from whites did not reveal a single positive individual. Subsequent studies have confirmed that Js^a is common only in black populations, although a few Js(a+) blood samples from whites have been found. The antibody that defined the alternative antigen to Js^a was found 5 years later and, following accepted practice at that time, was named anti-Js^b (126). The discovery that K_0 red cells were Js(a−b−) suggested that Sutter belonged in the Kell system, and segregation studies in families subsequently confirmed that this was so.

A fourth pair of alleles has been defined in the Kell system. K11 (Côté) is a high-frequency antigen, whereas K17 (Wk^a) is rare (127). (The K17 phenotype frequency in whites is 0.3 per cent.) K_0 red cells, as would be expected, are K:−11,−17.

Kell antigens show marked associations with different populations. K and Kp^a are mainly characteristics in white populations, whereas Js^a is found in blacks. A rare exception to this is found in Bedouins of the Sinai Peninsula, in whom relatively high frequencies of both K and Js^a genes occur, presumably due to racial admixture. Ul^a is a rare antigen, except that it has been found in 2.5 per cent of Finnish people. Segregation studies show that it is probably part of the Kell complex. To date, no antibody with anti-Ul^b specificity has been found.

A number of other antibodies have been described that react with "public" (very common) antigens but are compatible with K_0 red cells. Anti-K12, anti-K13, anti-K14, anti-K18, anti-K19, and anti-K22 detect different antigens in this category (128). Although there is serologic evidence to associate these antigens with Kell, there is as yet no proof that they are controlled by the Kell gene complex. However, biochemical studies have now established that at least some of the antigens are on the same protein molecule as Kell (129). Evidence from several sources has suggested that Kell antigens are glycoproteins. The antigens have been separated from red cells by immunoprecipitation with Kell system antibodies and shown to be markers on a 93,000-dalton glycoprotein (129). In the cell membrane, Kell protein is complexed with other proteins, which may be components of the cell skeleton, and appears to be held in a folded configuration by intrachain disulfide bonds (130). Isolation of Kell protein from normal cells may be a first step in understanding the nature of the Kell group abnormality and the functional defect, present in red cells of McLeod phenotype. Table 44–7 lists antigenic specificities associated with Kell.

Investigations have shown that synthesis of Kell antigens occurs in two distinct stages (58). The first involves production of a precursor substance that carries an antigenic marker called Kx. In the second stage, the Kell gene orders attachment of Kell-specific substances to the Kx precursor. The Kx-producing gene, which is called X^1k, is X-linked, but the Kell gene itself is autosomal. Kell phenotypes thus reflect action and interaction of the products of these two independent loci.

The rare Kell variant called McLeod (named after the propositus) was found in 1961 (50). The red cells have markedly weakened forms of common Kell antigens. The phenotype arises by inheritance of a variant allele at the Xk locus that does not allow production of Kx precursor in red cells (59). Lack of Kx is associated with acanthocytic changes in red cell morphology and a hemolytic condition. Kx antigen is present on normal phagocytic leukocytes of the blood, including those cells of men with the McLeod type, but is absent from leukocytes of boys with X-linked chronic granulomatous disease. Individuals of McLeod phenotype also have a slowly progressive wasting disorder of skeletal muscles and a neurologic defect (60). Further details of these relationships are given in the earlier section on blood groups and disease.

The Lewis System

Lewis is usually considered an independent blood group system; however, two independent loci, H and secretor, play an important part in the

Table 44–7. ANTIGENS RELATED TO THE KELL BLOOD GROUP SYSTEM

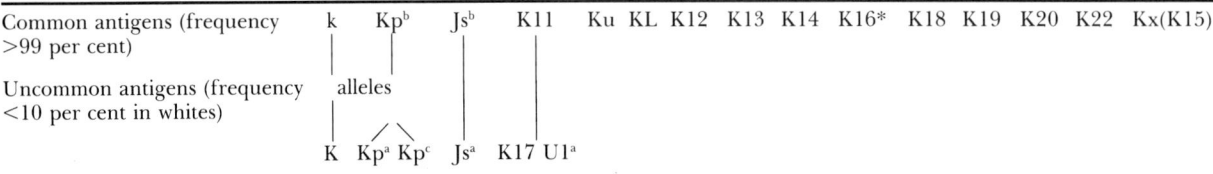

*K16 is a "k-like" antigen. Erythrocytes of McLeod type lack Kx, KL, and K16.

production of Lewis antigens. Furthermore, the sugars that determine Le^a and Le^b specificities are attached to the same precursors that are utilized for ABH antigenicity. There is good evidence that Ii antigens also have a biochemical interrelation with ABO and Lewis, and, from the conceptual viewpoint, it may be easier to consider AB, H, Lewis, and I as parts of one highly complex multigenic system. An important difference between Lewis and most other red cell antigens is that Lewis is not primarily a red cell antigen. Lewis substances are found in abundance in plasma and are passively adsorbed by any red cells that are present (131). As a result, red cells from an Le(a−) person transfused to an Le(a+) recipient become Le(a+) within about 72 hours. The classic experiment of nature was performed in a pair of chimeric twins (132). Each had a double population of red cells that differed in several blood group systems, and the twins were of different genetic Lewis types. However, all red cells in each twin were of the Lewis type of the host. Thus, inheritance must determine the type of plasma Lewis substance produced by an individual, but passive adsorption is responsible for its presence on red cells. Adsorption of plasma antigens to give positive red cell phenotypes is not peculiar to humans. Closely similar systems are known in cattle (J system) (133) and sheep (R system) (134).

Lewis antigens are present in saliva and some other body fluids, including plasma. Three independent genes are involved in production of Le^a and Le^b substances. The Lewis (*Le*) gene codes for an α-4-fucosyltransferase that attaches L-fucose to the AB precursor structure, but in a position different from the fucose added by the H gene enzyme (which is an α-2-fucosyltransferase). This Lewis-specified transferase gives Le^a specificity to the molecule. The secretor gene may be thought of as a regulator of the *H* gene in secretions. Inheritance of *Se* allows expression of *H*, and the double fucose that is then added gives a structure that has Le^b specificity. The three genes involved in this interaction, with their corresponding red cell and saliva phenotypes, are shown in Table 44–8. Le^a and Le^b antigens are not present on red cells of infants at birth because all newborns type Le(a−b−). However, within 10 days of birth the phenotype changes, and many infants become Le(a+). By approximately 2 years of age, the child's red cell and plasma antigens have settled into the pattern that will be maintained throughout life. Many examples of Lewis antisera react well only with red cells from O or A_2 individuals. About 22 per cent of adult group O persons are Le(a+b−), and 72 per cent are Le(a−b+). In whites, only approximately 6 per cent of random populations are Le(a−b−), but this proportion is much higher in blacks (up to 22 per cent).

Three additional antibodies in the Lewis system

Table 44–8. LEWIS PHENOTYPES AND THEIR GENETIC BACKGROUND*

Genes	Erythrocytes		Saliva		
	Le^a	*Le*^b	*ABH*	*Le*^a	*Le*^b
Le, Se, H	0	+	+	+	+
Le, se, H *Le, Se, h* *Le, se, h*	+	0	0	+	0
le, Se, H	0	0	+	0	0
le, se, H *le, Se, h* *le, se, h*	0	0	0	0	0

*Abbreviations: + = antigen present; 0 = antigen absent.

have been described. Anti-Le^x gives the reactions of anti-Le^a plus anti-Le^b, except that anti-Le^x reacts strongly with red cells from most newborn infants (135). Anti-Le^c is a rare antibody that reacts only with red cells of Le(a−b−) nonsecretor individuals (136). Anti-Le^d was made by injection of a goat with saliva from a group O Le(a−b+) person (137). The animal produced several antibodies. However, after the immune serum was absorbed with Le(a+b−) red cells, anti-Le^b and the new anti-Le^d remained; the latter reacted only with cells from Le(a−b−) secretors. The reactions of anti-Le^d are also explainable by the reactive antigen's being, on a type 1 ABH precursor chain, an H determinant that is taken up by red cells from plasma (138).

Anti-Le^a and anti-Le^b are mostly saline-reactive agglutinins, active over a wide thermal range but optimally at 12°C to 15°C. An IgG component is often present, and some sera have complement-binding and hemolytic properties.

Lewis antibodies do not cause erythroblastosis fetalis, but strong hemolytic anti-Le^a has been responsible for a transfusion reaction on rare occasions. No well-documented case of a transfusion reaction caused by anti-Le^b is known, although very large numbers of Le(b+) blood samples have been transfused to recipients with anti-Le^b. It has been demonstrated that transfusion of plasma from an Le(b+) person to such a recipient neutralizes the Lewis antibody and that Le(b+) red cells can subsequently be transfused safely (139). The fact that Lewis antigens are only passengers on red cells probably accounts, in part at least, for the effectiveness of this procedure. Transfused Le(b+) red cells soon lose their Le^b antigen and become Le(a−b−), like the cells of the recipient.

Because Lewis types reflect interaction among several independent genes, inheritance of phenotypes is somewhat complicated. Children who will be Le(a+) at maturity can be born to Le(a−) parents, and Le(b+) children can have Le(b−) parents. Le^a will be present in plasma and serum if *Le* is inherited, whereas *Le, Se,* and *H* must be inherited for Le[b] to appear.

Ii Blood Groups

"Nonspecific cold agglutinins" have been an accepted nuisance of blood group serologic studies for many years. These common cold-reactive antibodies agglutinate the individual's own red cells and all random red cell samples but are inactive at body temperature. It was assumed by early workers that some kind of universal, and possibly fundamental, receptor was involved. Studies since the early 1960's, however, have shown that these antibodies are part of a complex blood group called *I* (140) and that very rare individuals exist whose red cells are virtually lacking in I antigen. Cold autoagglutinins that cause hemolytic anemia nearly always have I specificity. These antibodies can be very powerful, some having titers exceeding 1 million. Their ability to induce in vivo hemolysis depends on reactivity at physiologic temperature and, most importantly, their ability to activate complement.

Soluble I substance is present in saliva, milk, and various cystic fluids and is inhibitory against some anti-I sera (141).

Anti-i, a cold agglutinin defining an antigen that is reciprocally related to I, was discovered in 1960 (14). Red cells that are rich in I have very little i and vice versa. Rare adults who are almost lacking in I have a large amount of i on their red cells, a phenotype called i adult.

Conventional genetic explanations, in which *I* and *i* are allelic genes, cannot be applied to the I system because at an early stage of fetal development only i exists. The i adult phenotype is an inherited characteristic, but we imagine that it arises by failure to inherit a common gene Z, which superimposes I specificity onto fetal i. Without this gene (i.e., genotype zz) the fetal status of Ii antigens persists for life. Strong anti-i may be found occasionally in patients with reticulosis and in those with a few other pathologic conditions, and weaker forms of the antibody are found commonly in patients with infectious mononucleosis (142). In each of these situations, anti-i may be of sufficient potency to cause hemolytic anemia. Unlike anti-I, anti-i has not been found as a natural antibody in a healthy person. Soluble i substance is present in secretions.

The red cells of newborn infants are markedly deficient in I antigen and, as would be expected, react strongly with anti-i. Red cells taken from umbilical cord blood can be used, therefore, as an aid in identifying Ii system antibodies.

Biochemical studies have shown that I and i specificities are carried on the same polypeptide backbone as the ABH- and Lewis-specific sugars (143). However, I antigen is heterogeneous and involves a group of sugars in various linkages. Blood group active glycosphingolipids having 20 to 60 sugar molecules attached to a ceramide residue also have been isolated from red cells and have a spectrum of I, together with A, B, and H, activity (144). Red cells taken from adults have a much greater proportion of branched oligosaccharide surface structures than red cells from newborns (145). The change from i to I antigen status appears to be a consequence of an increase in branched oligosaccharide chains that have I activity, with associated masking of straight chain structures that have i activity (146). The genetic basis for the I or i status of the individual lies in a gene that determines branching of these oligosaccharide chains.

I antigens have been identified not only on red cells but also on epithelial cells and on T and B lymphocytes (147, 148). Some primates, notably macaque monkeys, have very strong i antigens, and their red cells are useful in identifying weak examples of anti-i (149).

In adults, maturation of I antigen occurs during normal erythropoiesis. In hemolytic and hemorrhagic conditions and during recovery from aplastic anemia, all of which are associated with erythropoietic hyperplasia, marrow transit time of the maturing cells is reduced. Red cells from individuals with these conditions often have increased i antigenicity (150) as well as unused fetal hemoglobin. These are so-called F cells.

An uncommon cold-reactive autoantibody, not related to I, is anti-Sp_1, or Pr (151, 152). Sp_1 is well developed on the red cells of newborn infants. No nonreactive adult cell sample has been found, despite many thousands of random tests with anti-Sp_1. The Sp_1 (Pr) receptor is denatured by various proteolytic enzymes and by neuraminidase, showing that sialic acid is involved in its structure (152). This provides a means of distinguishing between the I and Sp_1 systems because Ii antibodies give enhanced reactions against enzyme-treated red cells.

The Duffy System

The first example of anti-Fy[a] was found in the serum of a patient named Duffy, a much-transfused hemophiliac (153). The notation "Fy" was chosen to avoid confusion with D of the Rh system. The antibody, which reacts with about 65 per cent of blood samples from white populations, is not uncommon in patients receiving multiple blood transfusions. Anti-Fy[b], which recognizes the product of an allele of *Fy*[a], is much rarer (154). The majority of blacks lack Fy[a] and Fy[b] antigens, having the phenotype Fy(a−b−) (38). This probably arises by natural selection because the Fy[a] and Fy[b] antigens appear to be associated with a receptor utilized by the merozoite of *Plasmodium vivax* malaria during its invasion of the red cells (41). Individuals of Fy(a−b−) type are resistant to this variety of malaria. Anti-Fy3 is found, on rare occasions, in the serum of Fy(a−b−) individuals (155). Fy3 antigen has, so far, always accompanied Fy^a or Fy^b, but there are good reasons for believing that Fy3 is a distinct entity and that anti-Fy3 is not simply anti-Fy^a plus Fy^b. Fy4 is present on Fy(a−b−) red cells and may be produced by an allele of *Fy3* (156). Fy5 resembles Fy3 except that Rh_{null} red cells (which lack Rh antigens) lack Fy5 as well. It has been suggested that Duffy and Rh genes interact to produce the membrane structure that has Fy5 specificity (157).

Duffy frequencies for black and white populations are given in Table 44–9. The only reported examples of anti-Fy4 have not been strong enough for meaningful genetic studies, and it is possible that although most "*Fy*" genes in blacks are really Fy^4, some may be *Fy*, a silent allele.

Duffy antibodies are almost always IgG proteins, reactive only by the antiglobulin test. They may cause a hemolytic reaction following a transfusion of incompatible blood and, on rare occasions, have been responsible for erythroblastosis fetalis. The red cell Fy^a and Fy^b antigens are denatured by treatment with the enzymes papain, bromelin, and ficin. The antigens are unaffected by neuraminidase, however, and the denaturing effect of the plant latex enzymes is a result of protease activity. Fy3, Fy4, and Fy5 antigens are not denatured by enzymes, a finding that supports the belief that they are structurally different from Fy^a and Fy^b. Although the biochemical basis for specificity in the Duffy group has not been established, the membrane structure carrying the antigens has been identified. The Fy^a antigen is present on a 35- to 43-kilodalton membrane protein (158). Fy^a antigenicity of this structure has remarkable resistance to a variety of chemical procedures used during isolation, but it is destroyed by certain proteases.

Duffy was the first human gene to be assigned to a specific autosome when, in 1968, it was shown to be closely linked to a structural marker of chromosome 1 (159). The locus is close to the centromere of chromosome 1, probably on the long arm.

Because of its role in benign tertian malaria, Duffy is a system of considerable importance. No other red cell blood group system makes such a great distinction among different sections of the world population.

The Kidd Groups

Antibodies in the Kidd system are often difficult to work with because, although they are IgG proteins, they may not react well in the antiglobulin test. The original anti-Jk^a caused erythroblastosis fetalis (160), and the antibody has subsequently been incriminated in many hemolytic transfusion reactions. In the same way, anti-Jk^b may be a cause of severe hemolytic reaction (161). In each case, a dramatic clinical effect from an antibody of apparently low potency is sometimes seen, as judged by in vitro tests. The hemolytic reactions sometimes occur several days to weeks after the sensitizing transfusion.

Kidd antigens are inherited in a straightforward manner as autosomal dominant characteristics. On rare occasions, individuals of the Jk(a−b−) phenotype have been found who appear to be homozygous for silent *Jk* genes (162). Transfusion of blood to these people may provoke anti-Jk3, which is compatible only with other examples of the Jk(a−b−) phenotype. Jk3 appears to be a distinct specificity because phagocytic leukocytes of the blood have Jk3 antigen but appear to lack Jk^a and Jk^b (28). Jk(a−b−) red cells are resistant to lysis by 2-M urea, but other red cells are lysed easily (163). This curious finding suggests that Kidd null red cells have a membrane anomaly, but its nature is unknown. Table 44–10 shows characteristics and frequencies in the Kidd blood group system.

The Xg Blood Groups

One of the most interesting and informative of the blood group antigens is X-linked Xg^a (164). Only one specificity, anti-Xg^a, has been found, but numerous examples of the antibody are known. Because females have two X chromosomes, they have twice the chance of inheriting an X chromosome carrying Xg^a, and, as would be expected, the phenotype Xg(a+) is more frequent in females than in males. No antibody defining an antithetical antigen has been found, and the Xg(a−) phenotype has been recognized only by the absence of Xg^a. Following usual genetic practice, this presently silent allele is called *Xg*. If an antibody is found that recognizes a product of this gene, *Xg* will become Xg^b.

Family studies have established that Xg^a obeys

Table 44–9. GENES AND ANTIGENS OF THE DUFFY BLOOD GROUP SYSTEM

Gene	Frequencies		Antigens Produced*			
	Whites	Blacks	Fy^a	Fy^b	Fy3	Fy4
Fy^a	0.425	0.064	+	0	+	0
Fy^b	0.557	0.113	0	+	+	0
Fy^x	0.016	Unknown	0	Weak	Weak	Unknown
Fy	0.002	0.823	0	0	0	+

*Fy5 antigen is produced by interaction between Duffy and Rh gene products.

the fairly complicated rules of inheritance for dominant X-borne characters. The acid test for X-linkage is used in a family in which the mother is negative, the father is positive, all sons are negative, and all daughters are positive.

Discovery of Xg^a, with its useful frequency, stimulated early hopes that linkages with other X-linked characters would follow quickly. The pasture is now seen to be rich, but the harvest has been slower growing than was anticipated. One of the reasons is that the X chromosome is much longer in terms of recombination units than was thought a few years ago. A number of prominent loci, including G6PD, hemophilia, Christmas disease, deutan and protan color blindness, and Duchenne's muscular dystrophy, are not linked to Xg^a, but the loci for ichthyosis, ocular albinism, and retinoschisis are (165). Another linkage is between Xg and Xk, the locus responsible for X-linked chronic granulomatous disease and the McLeod syndrome (166). (See section on blood groups and disease.) This association may provide a means of genetic counseling in CGD families in which the carrier mother is heterozygous at the Xg locus. Direct prenatal diagnosis for this condition has been reported (167).

One of the most useful applications of Xg^a has been to sex chromosome aneuploidy, in which an abnormal number of X chromosomes occur. The results in patients with XO Turner's syndrome, for example, show a male distribution of Xg^a (165), providing confirmation, if it were needed, that Xg^a is indeed X-linked. In individuals with an excess of X chromosomes, Xg^a typing may show whether the nondisjunction occurred during oogenesis or during spermatogenesis.

Xg^a is present on red cells of newborns, although it appears to be a little weaker than in adults. It has also been identified on cultured fibroblasts (168). The antigen, or at least one closely similar to it, is present in some gibbon red cell samples, in which again it appears to be X-linked (169).

The Xg^a locus is not inactivated by the Lyon phenomenon of X chromosome inactivation; females who are heterozygous at the Xg locus do not have a double population of $Xg(a+)$ and $Xg(a-)$ red cells (170).

The En Blood Groups

Anti-En^a reacts with almost all random blood samples and thus defines a "public" antigen (171). $En(a-)$ red cells are extremely rare and have remarkable properties, behaving as though they have been treated with proteolytic enzymes. The cells have a reduced sialic acid level, show changes in electrophoretic mobility, and can be agglutinated in a simple saline medium by certain IgG blood group antibodies (172).

$En(a-)$ red cells lack glycophorin A, the major membrane sialoglycoprotein, and thus do not have the M or N antigens that are normally present on this structure (173). Despite the absence of this membrane constituent (of which a normal cell has at least 500,000 copies), the marked reduction in membrane sialic acid, and the alteration in cell charge, $En(a-)$ red cells have normal appearance and normal in vivo survival. The expression $En(a-)$ is an umbrella term, and critical studies have shown that anti-En^a antibodies may recognize different epitopes on the same sialoglycoprotein (174). The name En stands for envelope, signifying the involvement of En^a with membrane structure. A number of blood samples with unusual MN system–related antigens are known. Biochemical studies on some of them have shown that the cells have hybrid forms of the MN and Ss sialoglycoproteins (174).

The Gerbich Groups

Almost all whites have the Gerbich (Ge) antigen on their red cells (175). Very rarely (frequency approximately one in 40,000), a Gerbich-negative person is encountered. Serum from such a person may contain naturally occurring or immune anti-Ge that creates a major problem in providing blood for transfusion. Siblings of a Ge-negative patient are the first people who should be tested in the search for compatible blood.

Cross-testing of different samples of anti-Ge and Ge-negative red cells has shown that rare variant Ge phenotypes exist (176). An astonishing finding was that a high proportion of the population of Papua/New Guinea (in some areas up to 50 per cent) is Ge-negative (177). Ovalocytic red cells also are present in a high proportion of this population. Individuals with these cells have depressed reactivity of a wide range of blood group antigens, a phenomenon that is believed to reflect the red cell membrane anomaly (178). Ovalocytic red cells from Melanesians are resistant to in vitro invasion by the parasite of malignant malaria (*Plasmodium falciparum*) (179). Biochemical studies are merging these various findings. Membranes from red cells of certain Ge-negative and Ge-variant phenotypes and from cells of individuals having melanesian ovalocytosis lack or have an atypical hybrid form of the minor sialoglycoprotein, glycophorin C (180).

Although Gerbich antigen variants are rare and of little importance in North America, the glycophorin C membrane component with which they are associated appears to be of considerable importance in parts of Southeast Asia.

Other Blood Group Systems

A large number of blood group antigens are known that cannot be fitted into any of the established systems. Many of these have an incidence of greater than 99 per cent, and, with such a high frequency, genetic relationships are difficult to recognize. However, use of various null phenotype red cells in the testing procedure is informative, allowing one to conclude that an antibody that reacts strongly with K_0 and Rh_{null} cells, for example, is unlikely to be part of the Kell or Rhesus system.

Diego and Scianna are two blood group systems that are well characterized. The Di^a antigen of Diego is mainly a Mongoloid characteristic. Up to 35 per cent of American Indian blood samples and a smaller number of Oriental samples are Di(a+), but only rarely has the antigen been found in blood from white populations (181). Anti-Di^b, which recognizes an antithetical antigen (182), can be made only by Di^aDi^a persons, and, as could be expected, such individuals have always been of American Indian or Oriental extraction. All blood samples from whites are Di(b+). Diego has no clinical importance in white populations. The main interest of Diego lies in the field of anthropology (183). Di^a is absent in Eskimos, and it is difficult to explain how the gene can be present in two widely separated areas of the Mongoloid world but absent in the region of the Bering Straits, which is believed to be the topographic link between the areas. There is evidence that Diego is independent of Lutheran and that Diego has cleared the last hurdle and achieved full status as an independent blood group system (184).

Scianna is the name given to a system that resulted from a "marriage" between a rare antigen called Bu^a that is found in approximately one in 130 blood samples from whites (185) and a very common antigen called Sm that has a frequency of greater than 99.9 per cent (186). The discovery that an Sm-negative person was Bu(a+) led to investigations that established that the antigens are controlled by allelic genes. In the new notation, Bu^a is called Sc2 and Sm is called Sc1 (187). The separate identity of Scianna is almost established. The last obstacle in this claim to independence will be difficult because it has yet to be shown that Scianna is not part of Diego. A null phenotype has been found and is called Sc: −1, −2 (188). The Sc locus is known to be on chromosome 1, which appears to be important from the blood group viewpoint because the genes of Scianna, Duffy, and Rhesus all are located on this chromosome.

Many other blood group antigens are known, but space does not allow their description. Table 44–10, however, presents a summary of the characteristics of some of them.

ACQUIRED AUTOIMMUNE HEMOLYTIC ANEMIA

The autoantibodies responsible for red cell autoimmune states may be broadly divided into those

Table 44–10. SOME OTHER BLOOD GROUP ANTIGENS

System	Frequencies in Whites*	
Kidd	Jk^a, 0.77 (0.52)	Jk^b, 0.73 (0.48)
Diego	Di^a, <0.01 (<0.005)	Di^b, >0.99 (>0.995)
Cartwright	Yt^a, 0.998 (0.959)	Yt^b, 0.08 (0.041)
Colton	Co^a, 0.998 (0.954)	Co^b, 0.09 (0.046)
Auberger	Au^a, 0.82 (0.58)	
Xg	Xg^a, Females 0.89 (0.67)	Males 0.67
Dombrock	Do^a, 0.65 (0.41)	Do^b, 0.82 (0.59)

*Numbers in parentheses are gene frequencies.

that are cold-reactive, in which maximum activity is seen at 0°C, and those that have a thermal optimum of 37°C.

Cold-reactive autoantibodies are frequently of very high titer, usually have specificity in the Ii system (140, 142) are active at temperatures as high as 34°C, and have strong complement-binding characteristics. They may occur spontaneously, may follow primary atypical pneumonia caused by *Mycoplasma pneumoniae*, and may be associated with infectious mononucleosis or lymphoma. Paroxysmal cold hemoglobinuria is a rare disorder associated with syphilis. Autoantibodies in these patients are usually nonreactive with rare p red cells; the antibody has P antigen specificity.

Warm autoantibodies usually lack recognizable blood group specificity; however, about 10 per cent can be identified. Specificity is often in the Rh system, with anti-e being seen most frequently. A not uncommon finding is that all random blood samples are reactive, but Rh_{null} cells are compatible, a conclusion that implies some kind of Rh-related specificity. Other Rh specificities such as anti-D, anti-c, anti-E, and anti-f are seen occasionally in autoimmune states, as are anti-LW, anti-U, anti-En^a, and anti-Kell. Rare examples of many other blood group antibodies also have been found.

Patients with warm-antibody autoimmune hemolytic anemia (AHA) have strongly positive direct Coombs' tests, but in many cases there is no free antibody in the patients' sera. Antibody eluted from patients' red cells should be tested for specificity as part of the laboratory investigation. When specific autoantibodies can be identified, it may be possible to give compatible blood if transfusion is required. In some cases, demonstration that the autoantibody is specific is of academic interest only, since compatible donor blood would be unobtainable because of its rarity.

The serologic investigation of patients with warm-antibody AHA should be directed toward establishing blood group specificity and the immunologic nature of the sensitizing proteins on the patient's red cells. It also should be borne in mind, however, that previous transfusions or pregnancies may have initiated an alloantibody response. Thus, the patient's serum may contain unbound autoantibody and blood group–specific alloantibody. Transfusions given to AHA patients with "nonspecific" antibodies are usually made by selection of the "least incompatible" donor units. It is doubtful, however, that this procedure has any value in terms of better in vivo survival of the transfused cells.

Not infrequently, apparently healthy people are found who have a positive direct Coombs' test. The autoantibodies in these people are of an IgG subclass that does not potentiate accelerated red cell destruction (189). Similarly, some drugs (notably α-methyldopa) will induce autoimmunity, but only in a minority of cases is this associated with in vivo hemolysis (190).

BLOOD TESTS IN DISPUTED PATERNITY

The rapid development of new genetic markers during the past 40 years has greatly enhanced our ability to identify particular people by testing their blood. The frequency of the most common combination of phenotypes (O, Rh_1rh, MNSs, P_1, HLA-1, 2, 8, 12, etc.) in whites is approximately one in 60 million if the 18 most commonly used red cell, leukocyte, and serum protein systems are employed. As more polymorphic markers are recognized and utilized, it will undoubtedly become clear that no two unrelated individuals are alike. Utilizing these 18 markers, nonfathers are convincingly excluded by blood tests in 99 per cent of paternity cases. Because of the large number of haplotypes, leukocyte HLA typing is the single most useful determination. The serum protein markers are discussed in Chapter 46.

Along with the ability to exonerate falsely accused men has come the ability to establish, with a high degree of confidence, that a man really is the father in most cases in which he is not excluded.

CONCLUSIONS

The endless fascination of the human blood groups stems partly from the intricacies of their inheritance and partly from their involvement in clinical medicine. Most of the mechanisms of inheritance have models in the blood groups because in different systems the effects of recessive genes, silent alleles, independent modifiers, and gene interaction all can be recognized. Although in most cases blood group genes obey simple mendelian laws, the existence of rare variants necessitates caution in the interpretation of family data in which there is a question of disputed parentage. Silent (null) genes are known in most of the blood group systems, but they tend to be overlooked during testing of families. For example, a situation in which putative parents are K+k+ and K−k+ and a child is K+k− may not be an exclusion of parentage because the K−k+ parent may carry a silent (K^0) gene. This amorphic allele is believed to have a gene frequency of about 0.01 in whites; therefore, approximately one in 50 people will have this gene at one of their two Kell loci. With the great increase in the number of genetic markers that can be used, it is unlikely that an exclusion of parentage needs to be based on only one marker. From the opposite viewpoint, blood group tests can now confirm, with reasonable assurance in most cases, that ostensible parents of a particular child are, in fact, the biologic parents.

If we test different populations for all available genetic markers, an almost infinite variety of permutations is seen. However, one could surely identify a population sample as African, Asian, or white. Even two neighboring tribes or townships would differ, although less strikingly. Such differences are of great genetic and anthropologic interest. The similarities between different peoples, however, are even more striking than the differences. The unity of the human species is strikingly shown by its blood groups. For example, in all races nearly everyone is of the Kell type k+, Kp(b+), Js(b+). No population has been found that lacks any of the blood group systems, even though some populations are quite monomorphic.

Reasons for population differences in blood group frequency are no longer entirely speculative, and in some cases plausible explanations can be provided. A Duffy antigen on the red cell membrane, or a structure related to it, is utilized by the parasite of benign tertian malaria during its penetration of the cell. The pressure of natural selection has presumably caused the near elimination of Fy^a and Fy^b antigens in African populations. The parasite of malignant malaria appears to utilize receptors associated with sialoglycoproteins (glycophorins) on the red cell membrane. The conclusion that the high frequency of U-negative phenotypes (abnormal glycophorin B) in certain African populations and the high frequency of Gerbich-negative phenotypes (abnormal glycophorin C) in some Melanesian populations is in some way associated with resistance to malignant malaria infection seems inescapable.

Microbial or parasitic agents that are largely host-specific for humans must surely be telling us that specific receptors on human cells are needed for their virulence. The studies with *Escherichia coli* have established that pyelonephritic strains bind to a P antigen structure associated with cell membrane globoside on uroepithelial cells and that the organism does not recognize rare human cells that lack this receptor. In vitro studies in all these areas show that when cell receptors are blocked by specific antibody they are not accessible to the parasite. These discoveries may eventually be seen as milestones in blood groups, since if Fab antibody fragments reproduce the blocking phenomenon in vivo new approaches to therapy will become a possibility.

Some other blood group antigens have a recognizable functional role. From a broad view it seems that lack of an antigen in which specificity is determined by an immunodominant sugar carried above the membrane does not compromise the cell (191). However, absence of an antigen that is a membrane protein may alter cell morphology and prevent proper function. Certainly, the Rh_{null} syndrome and the McLeod syndrome tell us what happens without Rh or X^1k (Kx) gene products. Some blood group genes are, after all, not neutral from the evolutionary viewpoint.

Localization of the Duffy gene to chromosome 1 marked the beginning of autosomal gene mapping. Many genes have now found such locations, and, in linkage studies, blood groups have an especially important place because of their potential value in genetic counseling. Of the erythrocyte blood group genes, Duffy, Rh, ABO, Scianna, P, Chido, Rodgers, Xg, and probably Colton have been mapped so far. It is encouraging that no other blood group genes are linked to them. This may mean that genes of other blood groups are widely spread over the autosomes to make a net that, in due course, will trap other linkages.

There seems to be no end to the number of different blood group specificities. Indeed, if gene duplication followed by mutation is responsible for the bewildering array of antigens that have been recognized, the process will continue. It is also possible that technical advances will lead to better methods for the detection of antibodies and allow further expansion in knowledge of blood group antigens.

Rare negatives (people lacking very common blood group antigens) are the most interesting and informative of all blood types. They are worth identifying at every opportunity, especially among siblings and cousins of rare propositi. Red cells of rare type may help one identify difficult antibodies, establish associations between other high-frequency antigens, and, of course, transfuse immunized recipients. When the in vitro culture of red cells becomes possible on a large scale, these will surely be the first to be produced.

This general overview of the human blood groups is only an appetizer, and more extensive authoritative texts will supply further details. A past and, it is hoped, obsolete view of a blood group researcher was of an individual dedicated to frustrating surgeons in their attempts to obtain unlimited supplies of blood. The horizon of blood group science spreads ever wider, and it is hoped that some of the fascination and excitement of the subject illuminates these pages.

References

1. Coombs, R. R. A., Mourant, A. E., et al.: In vivo isosensitization of red cells in babies with hemolytic disease. Lancet 1:264, 1946.
2. Schmidt, P. J., Morrison, E. G., et al.: The antigenicity of the D^u blood factor. Blood 20:196, 1962.
3. Marsh, W. L., Nichols, M. E., et al.: Naturally occurring anti-Kell stimulated by E. coli enterocolitis in a 20-day old child. Transfusion 18:149, 1978.
4. Jacob, F., and Monod, J.: Genetic regulatory mechanisms in the synthesis of proteins. J. Molec. Biol. 3:318, 1961.
5. Rosenfield, R. E., Allen, F. H., Jr., et al.: Genetic model for the Rh blood-group system. Proc. Nat. Acad. Sci. USA 70:1303, 1973.
6. Ruddle, F., Ricciuti, F., et al.: Somatic cell genetic assignment of peptidase C and the Rh linkage group to chromosome A-1 in man. Science 176:1429, 1972.
7. Marsh, W. L., Chaganti, R. S. K., et al.: Mapping human autosomes: evidence supporting assignment of Rhesus to the short arm of chromosome 1. Science 183:966, 1974.
8. Westerveld, A., Jongsma, A. P. M., et al.: Assignment of the AK_1:Np:ABO linkage group to chromosome 9. Proc. Nat. Acad. Sci. USA 73:895, 1976.
9. Giblett, E. R.: Blood group alloantibodies: an assessment of some laboratory practices. Transfusion 17:299, 1977.
10. Giblett, E. R.: A critique of the theoretical hazard of inter- vs. intraracial transfusion. Transfusion 1:233, 1961.
11. Mollison, P. L.: *Blood Transfusion in Clinical Medicine*, 7th ed. Oxford, Blackwell Scientific Publications, 1983, p. 257.
12. Abramson, N., Gelfrand, E. W., et al.: The interaction between human monocytes and red cells. Specificity for IgG subclasses and IgG fragments. J. Exp. Med. 132:1207, 1970.
13. Huber, H., Douglas, S. D., et al.: IgG subclass specificity of human monocyte receptor sites. Nature 229:419, 1971.
14. Marsh, W. L.: Anti-i: a cold antibody defining the Ii relationship in human red cells. Br. J. Haematol. 7:200, 1961.
15. Andresen, P. H.: Blood groups with characteristic phenotypical aspects. Acta Pathol. Microbiol. Scand. 24:616, 1948.
16. Friedenreich, V.: *The Thomsen Hemagglutination Phenomenon*. Copenhagen, Levin and Munksgaard, 1930, p. 128.
17. Bird, G. W. G.: Anti-T in peanuts. Vox Sang. 9:748, 1964.
18. Cameron, C., Graham, F., et al.: Acquisition of a B-like antigen by red blood cells. Br. Med. J. 2:29, 1959.
19. Marsh, W. L., Jenkins, W. J., et al.: Pseudo B: an acquired group antigen. Br. Med. J. 2:63, 1959.
20. Gerbal, A., Maslet, C., et al.: Immunological aspects of the acquired B antigen. Vox Sang. 28:398, 1975.
21. Economidou, J., Hughes-Jones, N. C., et al.: Quantitative measurements concerning A and B antigen sites. Vox Sang. 12:321, 1967.
22. Hughes-Jones, N. C., Gardner, B., et al.: Observations of the number of available c, D, and E antigen sites on red cells. Vox Sang. 21:210, 1971.
23. Hughes-Jones, N. C., and Gardner, B.: The Kell system studied with radioactively labelled anti-K. Vox Sang. 21:154, 1971.
24. Masouredis, S. P.: Red cell membrane blood group antigens. In *Membrane Structure and Function of Human Blood Cells*. San Francisco, American Association of Blood Banks Symposium, 1976, p. 43.
25. Schiff, F., and Sasaki, H.: Der Ausscheidungstypus, ein auf serologischem Wege nachweisbares mendelndes Merkmal. Kiln. Wochenschr. 11:1426, 1932. (Translated in *Secretion of Blood Group Substances and Lewis System*, Vol. II. Camp, F. R., and Ellis, F. R. (eds.), Fort Knox, U.S. Army Medical Research Laboratory, 1970, p. 336.)

26. Dorf, M. E., Eguro, S. Y., et al.: Detection of cytotoxic non-HL-A antisera. I. Relationship to anti-Le^a. Vox Sang. 22:447, 1972.
27. Marsh, W. L., Øyen, R., et al.: Studies of MNSsU antigen activity on leukocytes and platelets. Transfusion 14:462, 1974.
28. Marsh, W. L., Øyen, R., et al.: Kidd blood-group antigens of leukocytes and platelets. Transfusion 14:378, 1974.
29. Marsh, W. L., Øyen, R., et al.: Chronic granulomatous disease and the Kell blood groups. Br. J. Haematol. 29:247, 1975.
30. Middleton, J., Crookston, M. C., et al.: Linkage of Chido and HL-A. Tissue Antigens 4:366, 1974.
31. O'Neill, G. J., Yang, S. F., et al.: Chido and Rodgers are distinct antigenic components of complement C4. Fed. Proc. 37:1269, 1978.
32. Vos, G. H., Vos, D., et al.: A sample of blood with no detectable Rh antigens. Lancet 1:14, 1974.
33. Schmidt, P. J., Lostumbo, M. M., et al.: Aberrant U blood group accompanying Rh$_{null}$. Transfusion 7:33, 1967.
34. Sturgeon, P.: Hematological observations on the anemia associated with blood type Rh$_{null}$. Blood 36:310, 1970.
35. Lauf, P. K., and Joiner, C. H.: Increased potassium transport and ouabain binding in human Rh$_{null}$ red blood cells. Blood 48:457, 1976.
36. Lauf, P. K.: Blood group antigens and membrane permeability in erythrocytes of man and ruminants. In Human Blood Groups. 5th International Convocation Immunology, Buffalo, NY, 1976, p. 383 (Basel, Karger, 1977).
37. Ridgwell, K., Roberts, S. J., et al.: Absence of two membrane proteins containing extracellular thiol groups in Rh$_{null}$ erythrocytes. Biochem. J. 213:267, 1983.
38. Sanger, R., Race, R., et al.: The Duffy blood groups of New York Negroes: the phenotype Fy(a−b−). Br. J. Haematol. 1:370, 1955.
39. Young, M. D., Eyles, D. E., et al.: Experimental testing of the immunity of Negroes to Plasmodium vivax. J. Parasitol. 41:315, 1955.
40. Miller, L. H., Mason, S. J., et al.: Erythrocyte receptors for (Plasmodium knowlesi) malaria: Duffy blood group determinants. Science 189:561, 1975.
41. Miller, L. H., Mason, S. J., et al.: The resistance factor to Plasmodium vivax in Blacks. New Engl. J. Med. 295:302, 1976.
42. McGinniss, M. H., and Miller, L. H.: Malaria, erythrocyte receptors and the Duffy blood group system. In Cellular Antigens and Disease. Atlanta, American Association of Blood Banks, 1977, p. 74.
43. Pasvol, G., Jungery, M., et al.: Glycophorin as a possible receptor for Plasmodium falciparum. Lancet 2:947, 1982.
44. Breuer, W. V., Ginsburg, H., et al.: An analysis of malaria parasite invasion into human erythrocytes. The effects of chemical and enzymatic modification of erythrocyte membrane components. Biochim. Biophys. Acta 755:263, 1983.
45. Perkins, M.: Inhibitory effects of erythrocyte membrane proteins on the in vitro invasion of the human malarial parasite (Plasmodium falciparum) into its host cell. J. Cell Biol. 90:563, 1982.
46. Källenius, G., Svenson, S. B., et al.: Structure of carbohydrate part of receptor on human uroepithelial cells for pyelonephritogenic Escherichia coli. Lancet 2:604, 1981.
47. Källenius, G., Svenson, S. B., et al.: Occurrence of P-fimbriated Escherichia coli in urinary tract infections. Lancet 2:1369, 1981.
48. Väisänen, V., Tallgren, L. G., et al.: Mannose-resistant hemagglutination and P antigen recognition are characteristic of Escherichia coli primary pyelonephritis. Lancet 2:1366, 1981.
49. Chown, B., Lewis, M., et al.: A "new' Kell blood-group phenotype. Nature (Lond.) 180:711, 1957.
50. Allen, F. H., Krabbe, S. M. R., et al.: A new phenotype (McLeod) in the Kell blood-group system. Vox Sang. 6:555, 1961.
51. van der Hart, M., Szaloky, A., et al.: A "new' antibody associated with the Kell blood group system. Vox Sang. 15:456, 1968.
52. Marsh, W. L.: Revised notation for anti-KL in the Kell blood group system. Vox Sang. 36:375, 1979.
53. Giblett, E. R., Klebanoff, S. J., et al.: Kell phenotypes in chronic granulomatous disease: A potential transfusion hazard. Lancet 1:1235, 1971.
54. Bridges, R. A., Berendes, H., et al.: A fatal granulomatous disease of childhood. Am. J. Dis. Child. 97:387, 1959.
55. Quie, P. G., White, J. G., et al.: In vitro bactericidal activity of human polymorphonuclear leukocytes: diminished activity in chronic granulomatous disease of childhood. J. Clin. Invest. 46:668, 1967.
56. Baehner, R. L., and Nathan, D. G.: Leukocyte oxidase: defective activity in chronic granulomatous disease. Science 155:835, 1967.
57. Segal, A. W., and Peters, T. J.: Characterization of the enzyme defect in chronic granulomatous disease. Lancet 1:1363, 1976.
58. Marsh, W. L.: The Kell bloods and their relationship to chronic granulomatous disease. In Cellular Antigens and Disease. Atlanta, American Association of Blood Banks, 1977, p. 52.
59. Wimer, B. M., Marsh, W. L., et al.: Haematological changes associated with the McLeod phenotype of the Kell blood group system. Br. J. Haematol. 36:219, 1977.
60. Marsh, W. L.: Deleted antigens of the Rhesus and Kell blood groups: association with cell membrane defects. In Blood Group Antigens and Disease. Arlington, VA, American Association of Blood Banks, 1983, p. 173.
61. Tang, L. L., Redman, C. M., et al.: Biochemical studies on McLeod phenotype erythrocytes. Vox Sang. 40:17, 1981.
62. Glaubensklee, C., Evan, A. P., et al.: Structural and biochemical analysis of the McLeod erythrocyte membrane. Vox Sang. 42:262, 1982.
63. Marsh, W. L., Marsh, N. J., et al.: Elevated serum creatine phosphokinase in subjects with McLeod syndrome. Vox Sang. 40:403, 1981.
64. Swash, M., Schwartz, M. S., et al.: Benign X-linked myopathy with acanthocytes (McLeod syndrome). Its relationship to X-linked muscular dystrophy. Brain 106:717, 1983.
65. Schwartz, S. A., Marsh, W. L., et al.: New clinical features of McLeod syndrome. Transfusion 22:404, 1982.
66. Aird, I., Bentall, H. H., et al.: A relationship between cancer of the stomach and the ABO blood groups. Br. Med. J. 1:799, 1953.
67. Aird, I., and Bentall, H. H.: The blood groups in relation to peptic ulceration and carcinoma of colon, rectum, breast and bronchus: an association between the ABO groups and peptic ulceration. Br. Med. J. 2:315, 1954.
68. Clarke, C. A., Edwards, J. W., et al.: ABO groups and secretor character in duodenal ulcer. Population and sibship studies. Br. Med. J. 2:725, 1956.
69. Ferguson-Smith, M. A., Aitken, D. A., et al.: Localization of the human ABO:Np-1:AK-1 linkage group by regional assignment of AK-1 to 9q34. Hum. Genet. 34:35, 1976.
70. Goldstein, J., Siviglia, G., et al.: Group B erythrocytes enzymatically coverted to group O survive normally in A, B, and O individuals. Science 215:168, 1982.
71. Bhende, Y. M., Deshpande, C. K., et al.: A "new" blood-group character related to the ABO system. Lancet 1:903, 1952.
72. Levine, P., Robinson, E., et al.: Gene interaction resulting in suppression of blood group substance B. Blood 10:1100, 1955.
73. Davidsohn, I.: Early immunologic diagnosis and prognosis of carcinoma. Am. J. Clin. Pathol. 57:715, 1972.

74. Gold, E. R., Tovey, G. H., et al.: Changes in the group A antigen in a case of leukemia. Nature (Lond.) *183*:892, 1959.
75. Weiner, W., Lewis, H. B. M., et al.: A gene y, modifying the blood group antigen A. Vox Sang. *2*:25, 1957.
76. Rubinstein, P., Allen, F. H., Jr., et al.: A dominant suppressor of A and B. Vox Sang. *25*:377, 1973.
77. Hirszfeld, L.: Konstitutionsserologie and Blutgruppenforschung. Berlin, Springer Verlag, 1928, 235 pp. For translation into English, see *Selected Contributions to the Literature of Blood Groups and Immunology*, Vol. III (in two parts) Part 1–Constitutional Serology and Blood Group Research. Camp, F. R., and Ellis, F. R. (eds.), Blood Transfusion Division, U.S. Army Medical Research Laboratory, Fort Knox, Kentucky, 1969 (see especially p. 109).
78. Seyfried, H., Walewska, I., et al.: Unusual inheritance of ABO group in a family with weak B antigens. Vox Sang. *9*:268, 1964.
79. Yamaguchi, H.: A review of cis AB blood. Jpn. J. Hum. Genet. *18*:1, 1973.
80. German, J. L.: Personal communication, 1977.
81. Landsteiner, K., and Levine, P.: Further observations on individual differences of human blood. Proc. Soc. Exp. Biol. Med. *24*:941, 1927.
82. Race, R. R., and Sanger, R.: *Blood Groups in Man*, 6th ed. Philadelphia, F. A. Davis, 1975.
83. Wiener, A. S., Unger, L. J., et al.: Fatal hemolytic transfusion reaction caused by sensitization to a new blood factor, U. J.A.M.A. *153*:1444, 1953.
84. Fraser, G. R., Giblett, E. R., et al.: Population genetic studies in the Congo. III. Blood groups (ABO, MNSs, Rh, Js^a). Am. J. Hum. Genet. *18*:546, 1966.
85. Prokop, O., and Uhlenbruck, G.: Lehrbuch der menslichen Blut- und Serumgruppen. Leipzig, Thieme Publishers, 1963, p. 349.
86. Dahr, W., Uhlenbruck, G., et al.: Immunochemical aspects of the MNSs blood group system. J. Immunogenet. *2*:87, 1975.
87. Walker, M. E., Rubinstein, P., et al.: Biochemical genetics of MN. Vox Sang. *32*:111, 1977.
88. Tomita, M., and Marchesi, V. T.: Amino acid sequence and oligosaccharide attachment sites of human erythrocyte glycophorin. Proc. Natl. Acad. Sci. USA *72*:2964, 1975.
89. Waśniowska, K., Drzeniek, Z., et al.: The amino acids of M and N blood group glycopeptides are different. Biochem. Biophys. Res. Comm. *76*:385, 1977.
90. Dahr, W., Uhlenbruck, G., et al.: Different N-terminal amino acids in the MN-glycoprotein from MM and NN erythrocytes. Hum. Genet. *35*:335, 1977.
91. Landsteiner, K., and Levine, P.: Further observations on individual differences of human blood. Proc. Soc. Exp. Biol. N.Y. *24*:941, 1927.
92. Levine, P., Bobbitt, O. B., et al.: Iso immunization by a new blood factor in tumor cells. Proc. Soc. Exp. Biol. N.Y. *77*:403, 1951.
93. Sanger, R.: An association between the P and Jay systems of blood groups. Nature (Lond.) *176*:1163, 1955.
94. Matson, G. A., Swanson, J., et al.: A "new" antigen and antibody belonging to the P blood group system. Am. J. Hum. Genet. *11*:26, 1959.
95. Naiki, M., and Marcus, D. M.: Human erythrocyte P and P^k blood group antigens: identification as glycosphingolipids. Biochim. Biophys. Res. Commun. *60*:1105, 1974.
96. Voak, D., Anstee, D., et al.: The α-galactose specificity of anti-P^k. Vox Sang. *25*:263, 1973.
97. Marcus, D. M., Naiki, M., et al.: Abnormalities in the glycosphingolipid content of the human P^k and p erythrocytes. Proc. Nat. Acad. Sci. USA *73*:3263, 1976.
98. Marcus, D. M., Naiki, M., et al.: Immunochemical studies of the human blood group P system. In *Human Blood Groups*. 5th International Convocation Immunology, Buffalo, N.Y., 1976, p. 206 (Basel, S. Karger, Publisher, 1977).
99. Fellous, M., Gerbal, A., et al.: Studies on the biosynthetic pathway of human P erythrocyte antigens using somatic cells in culture. Vox Sang. *26*:518, 1974.
100. Levine, P., Celano, M. J., et al.: The specificity of the antibody in paroxysmal cold hemoglobinuria (PCH). Transfusion *3*:278, 1963.
101. Landsteiner, K., and Wiener, A. S.: An agglutinable factor in human blood recognized by immune sera for rhesus blood. Proc. Soc. Exp. Biol. Med. *43*:223, 1940.
102. Levine, P., and Stetson, R. E.: An unusual case of intragroup agglutination. J.A.M.A. *113*:126, 1939.
103. Rosenfield, R. E., Allen, F. H., et al.: A review of Rh serology and presentation of a new terminology. Transfusion *2*:287, 1962.
104. Levine, P., Celano, M. J., et al.: A second example of —/— or Rh$_{null}$ blood. Transfusion *5*:492, 1965.
105. Ishimori, T., and Hasekura, H.: A case of Japanese blood with no detectable Rh blood group antigen. Proc. Jpn. Acad. *42*:658, 1966.
106. Green, F. A.: Erythrocyte membrane lipids and Rh antigen activity. J. Biol. Chem. *247*:881, 1972.
107. Callender, S. T., and Race, R. R.: A serological and genetical study of multiple antibodies formed in response to blood transfusion by a patient with lupus erythematosus diffusus. Ann. Eugen. *13*:102, 1946.
108. Cutbush, M., and Chanarin, I.: The expected blood-group antibody, anti-Lu^b. Nature (Lond.) *178*:855, 1956.
109. Crawford, M. N., Greenwalt, T. J., et al.: The phenotype Lu(a−b−) together with unconventional Kidd groups in one family. Transfusion *1*:228, 1961.
110. Taliano, V., Guévin, R. M., et al.: The genetics of a dominant inhibitor of the Lutheran antigens. Vox Sang. *24*:42, 1973.
111. Crawford, M. N., Tippett, P., et al.: The antigens Au^a, i, and P$_1$ of cells of the dominant type of Lu(a−b−). Vox Sang. *26*:283, 1974.
112. Marsh, W. L., Johnson, C. L., et al.: Proposed new notation for the In(Lu) modifying gene. Transfusion *24*:371, 1984.
113. Darnborough, J., Firth, R., et al.: A "new" antibody, anti-Lu^{a}Lu^b, and two further examples of the genotype Lu(a−b−). Nature (Lond.) *198*:796, 1963.
114. Brown, F., Simpson, S., et al.: The recessive Lu(a−b−) phenotype: a family study. Vox Sang. *26*:259, 1974.
115. Bove, J. R., Allen, F. H., Jr., et al.: Anti-Lu4, a new antibody related to the Lutheran blood group system. Vox Sang. *21*:302, 1971.
116. Marsh, W. L.: Anti-Lu5, anti-Lu6, and anti-Lu7. Three antibodies defining high frequency antigens related to the Lutheran blood group system. Transfusion *12*:27, 1972.
117. Marsh, W. L.: Blood groups of human red cells. In *Clinical Practice of Blood Transfusion*. New York, Churchill Livingstone, 1981, p. 101.
118. Marsh, W. L.: Recent developments relating to the Duffy and Lutheran blood groups. In *Recent Advances in Immunohematology*. American Association of Blood Banks, 1973, p. 101.
119. Molthan, L., Crawford, M. N., et al.: Lu9, another new antigen of the Lutheran blood-group system. Vox Sang. *24*:468, 1973.
120. Judd, W. J., Marsh, W. L., et al.: Anti-Lu14: a Lutheran antibody defining the product of an allele at the Lu8 blood group locus. Vox Sang. *32*:214, 1977.
121. Levine, P., Backer, M., et al.: A new human hereditary blood property (Cellano) present in 99.8% of all bloods. Science *109*:464, 1949.
122. Allen, F. H., and Lewis, S. J.: Kp^a(Penney) a new antigen in the Kell blood group system. Vox Sang. *2*:81, 1957.

123. Allen, F. H., Lewis, S. J., et al.: Studies of anti-Kp^b, a new antibody in the Kell blood group system. Vox Sang. 3:1, 1958.
124. Allen, F. H., and Rosenfield, R. E.: Notation for the Kell blood group system. Transfusion 1:305, 1961.
125. Giblett, E. R.: Js, a "new" blood group antigen found in Negroes. Nature (Lond.) 181:1221, 1958.
126. Walker, R. H., Argall, C. I., et al.: Anti-Js^b, the expected antithetical antibody of the Sutter blood group system. Nature (Lond.) 197:295, 1963.
127. Sabo, B., McCreary, J., et al.: Confirmation of K^{11} and K^{17} as alleles in the Kell blood group system. Vox Sang. 29:450, 1975.
128. Marsh, W. L.: The expanding Kell blood group and its relation to chronic granulomatous disease. Infusionstherapie 3:320, 1976.
129. Redman, C. M., Marsh, W. L., et al.: Isolation of Kell-active protein from the red cell membrane. Transfusion 24:176, 1984.
130. Redman, C. M., and Marsh, W. L.: Unpublished observations, 1984.
131. Sneath, J. S., and Sneath, P. H. A.: Transformation of the Lewis group of human red cells. Nature (Lond.) 176:172, 1955.
132. Nicholas, J. W., Jenkins, W. J., et al.: Human blood chimeras: a study of surviving twins. Br. Med. J. 1:1458, 1957.
133. Ferguson, L. C., Stormont, C., et al.: On additional antigens in the erythrocytes of cattle. J. Immunol. 44:147, 1942.
134. Fendel, J., Sorensen, A. N., et al.: Evidence for epistatic action of genes for antigenic substances in sheep. Genetics 39:396, 1954.
135. Andresen, P. H., and Jordal, K.: An incomplete agglutinin related to the L(Lewis) system. Acta Pathol. Microbiol. Scand. 26:636, 1949.
136. Gunson, H. H., and Latham, V.: An agglutinin in human serum reacting with cells from Le(a−b−) non-secretor individuals. Vox Sang. 22:344, 1972.
137. Potapov, M. I.: Detection of the antigen of the Lewis system, characteristic of the erythrocytes of the secretory group Le(a−b−). Probl. Haematol. (Moscow) 11:45, 1970.
138. Graham, H. A., Hirsch, H. F., et al.: Genetic and immunochemical relationships between soluble and cell-bound antigens of the Lewis system. In *Human Blood Groups*. 5th International Convocation Immunology, Buffalo, NY, 1976, p. 257 (Basel, Karger, 1977).
139. Mollison, P. L., and Polley, M. J.: Temporary suppression of Lewis blood-group antibodies to permit incompatible transfusion. Lancet 1:909, 1963.
140. Wiener, A. S., Unger, L. J., et al.: Type-specific cold autoantibodies as a cause of acquired hemolytic anemia and hemolytic transfusion reactions. Biologic test with bovine red cells. Ann. Intern. Med. 44:221, 1956.
141. Dzierzkowa-Borodej, W., Seyfried, H., et al.: The recognition of water soluble I blood group substance. Vox Sang. 18:222, 1970.
142. Jenkins, W. J., Koster, H. G., et al.: Infectious mononucleosis: an unsuspected source of anti-i. Br. J. Haematol. 11:480, 1965.
143. Feizi, T., Kabat, E. A., et al.: Immunochemical studies on blood groups. The I antigen complex precursors in the A, B, H, Le^a and Le^b blood group system—hemagglutination inhibition studies. J. Exp. Med. 133:39, 1971.
144. Gardas, A., and Kościelak, J.: I-active antigen of human erythrocyte membrane. Vox Sang. 26:227, 1974.
145. Watanabe, K., and Hakamori, S.: Status of blood group carbohydrate chains in ontogenesis and oncogenesis. J. Exp. Med. 144:644, 1976.
146. Watanabe, K., Hakemori, S., et al.: Characterization of a blood group I-active ganglioside. J. Biol. Chem. 254:3221, 1979.
147. Shumak, K. H., Rachkewich, R. A., et al.: Antigens of the Ii system on lymphocytes. Nature (New Biol.) 231:148, 1971.
148. Thomas, D. B.: Antibodies specific for human T lymphocytes in cold agglutinin and lymphocytotoxic sera. Eur. J. Immunol. 3:824, 1973.
149. Wiener, A. S., Moor-Jankowski, J., et al.: The blood factors I and i in primates, including man, and in lower species. Am. J. Phys. Anthropol. 23:389, 1965.
150. Hillman, R. S., and Giblett, E. R.: Red cell membrane alteration associated with marrow stress. J. Clin. Invest. 44:1730, 1965.
151. Marsh, W. L., and Jenkins, W. J.: Anti-Sp$_1$: the recognition of a new cold auto-antibody. Vox Sang. 15:177, 1968.
152. Roelcke, D.: A review. Cold agglutination. Antibodies and antigens. Clin. Immunol. Immunopathol. 2:266, 1974.
153. Cutbush, M., Mollison, P. L., et al.: A new human blood group. Nature (Lond.) 165:188, 1950.
154. Ikin, E. W., Mourant, A. E., et al.: Discovery of the expected haemagglutinin anti-Fy^b. Nature (Lond.) 168:1077, 1951.
155. Albrey, J. A., Vincent, E. E. R., et al.: A new antibody, anti-Fy3, in the Duffy blood-group system. Vox Sang. 20:29, 1971.
156. Behzad, O., Lee, C. L., et al.: A new anti-erythrocyte antibody in the Duffy system: anti-Fy4. Vox Sang. 24:337, 1973.
157. Colledge, K. I., Pezzulich, M., et al.: Anti-Fy5, an antibody disclosing a probable association between the Rhesus and Duffy blood group genes. Vox Sang. 24:193, 1973.
158. Hadley, T., David, P., et al.: Identification of an erythrocyte component carrying the Duffy blood group Fy^a antigen. Science 223:597, 1984.
159. Donahue, R. P., Bias, W. B., et al.: Probable assignment of the Duffy blood group locus to chromosome 1 in man. Proc. Nat. Acad. Sci. USA 61:949, 1968.
160. Allen, F. H., Diamond, L. K., et al.: A new blood-group antigen. Nature (Lond.) 167:482, 1951.
161. Plaut, G., Ikin, E. W., et al.: A new blood group antibody: anti-Jk^b. Nature (Lond.) 171:431, 1953.
162. Pinkerton, F. J., Mermod, L. E., et al.: The phenotype Jk(a−b−) in the Kidd blood group system. Vox Sang. 4:155, 1959.
163. Heaton, D. C., and McLoughlin, K.: Jk(a−b−) red blood cells resist urea lysis. Transfusion 22:70, 1982.
164. Mann, J. D., Cahan, A., et al.: A sex linked blood group. Lancet 1:8, 1962.
165. Race, R. R., and Sanger, R.: *Blood Groups in Man*, 6th ed. Philadelphia, F. A. Davis Company, 1975.
166. Marsh, W. L.: Linkage relationship of the Xg and Xk loci. Cytogenet. Cell Genet. 22:53, 1978.
167. Newburger, P. E., Cohen, H. J., et al.: Prenatal diagnosis of chronic granulomatous disease. New Engl. J. Med. (In press.)
168. Fellous, M., Bengtsson, B., et al.: Expression of the Xg^a antigen on cells in culture and its segregation in somatic cell hybrids. Ann. Hum. Genet. 37:421, 1974.
169. Gavin, J., Noades, J., et al.: Blood group antigen Xg^a in gibbons. Nature (Lond.) 204:1322, 1964.
170. Race, R. R.: Is the Xg blood group locus subject to inactivation? Proceedings 4th International Congress Human Genetics. Amsterdam, Excerpta Medica, 1971, p. 311.
171. Darnborough, J., Dunsford, I., et al.: The En factor. A genetic modification of human red cells affecting their blood grouping reactions. Program British Society Haematology Meeting, 1965, p. 28.
172. Furuhjelm, U., Myllyla, G., et al.: The red cell phenotype En(a−) and anti-En^a: serological and physiochemical aspects. Vox Sang. 17:256, 1969.
173. Tanner, M. J. A., and Anstee, D. J.: The membrane change in En(a−) human erythrocytes. Biochem. J. 153:271, 1976.

174. Issitt, P. D.: The MN blood group system. Cincinnati, Montgomery Scientific Publications, 1981, p. 139.
175. Rosenfield, R. E., Haber, G. V., et al.: Ge, a very common red-cell antigen. Br. J. Haematol. 6:344, 1960.
176. Race, R. R., and Sanger, R.: *Blood Groups in Man,* 6th ed. Oxford, Blackwell Scientific Publications, 1975, p. 420.
177. Booth, P. B., and McLoughlin, K.: The Gerbich blood group system, especially in Melanesians. Vox Sang. 18:547, 1972.
178. Booth, P. B., Serjeantson, S., et al.: Selective depression of blood group antigens associated with hereditary ovalocytosis among Melanesians. Vox Sang. 32:99, 1977.
179. Kidson, C., Lamont, G., et al.: Ovalocytic erythrocytes from Melanesians are resistant to invasion by malaria parasites in culture. Proc. Natl. Acad. Sci. USA 78:5829, 1981.
180. Anstee, D. J., Ridgwell, K., et al.: Individuals lacking the Gerbich blood-group antigen have alterations in the human erythrocyte membrane sialoglycoproteins β and α. Biochem. J. 221:97, 1984.
181. Layrisse, M., Arends, T., et al.: Nuevo grupo sanguinèo encontrado en descendientes de Indios. Acta Med. Venez. 3:132, 1955.
182. Thompson, P. R., Childers, D. M., et al.: Anti-Di^b—first and second examples. Vox Sang. 13:314, 1967.
183. Mourant, A. E., Kopec, A., et al.: *The Distribution of the Human Blood Groups.* London, Oxford University Press, 1976, p. 145.
184. Buchanan, D. I., Makelki, D., et al.: Genetic independence of the Lutheran and Diego blood group loci. Transfusion 17:277, 1977.
185. Anderson, C., Hunter, J., et al.: An antibody defining a new blood group antigen, Bu^a. Transfusion 3:30, 1963.
186. Schmidt, R. P., Griffitts, J. J., et al.: A new antibody, anti-Sm, reacting with a high incidence antigen. Transfusion 2:338, 1962.
187. Lewis, M., Kaita, H., et al.: Scianna blood group system. Vox Sang. 27:261, 1974.
188. McCreary, J., Vogler, A. L., et al.: Another minus-minus phenotype: Bu(a−) Sm−, two examples in one family. Transfusion 13:350, 1973.
189. Engelfriet, C. P., von dem Borne, A. E. G. Kr., et al.: In vivo destruction of erythrocytes by complement-binding and non-complement-binding antibodies. In *Immunobiology of the Erythrocyte.* New York, A. R. Liss, 1980.
190. Carstairs, K. C., Worlledge, S., et al.: Methyl dopa and hemolytic anaemia. Lancet 1:201, 1966.
191. Levine, P., Tripodi, D., et al.: Hemolytic anemia associated with Rh$_{null}$ but not with Bombay blood. Vox Sang. 24:417, 1973.

GENETICS

CHAPTER 45
The HLA System

EDMOND J. YUNIS
BO DUPONT

INTRODUCTION 1522
GENETICS OF THE HLA COMPLEX 1524
  HLA Haplotypes, Genotypes, and Haplotype Segregation
  Other Genes Within the HLA Complex
  The MHC Linkage Group
  Genetic Polymorphism
    HLA Class I
    HLA Class II
    Genetic Linkage Disequilibrium
    HLA Class III
TISSUE DISTRIBUTION, BIOCHEMISTRY, AND MOLECULAR GENETICS OF HLA 1531
  Tissue Distribution
  Biochemistry
    HLA Class I Molecules
    HLA Class II Molecules
  Molecular Genetics
    Structure of MHC Genes
    Restriction Fragment Length Polymorphisms (RFLPs)
    Gene Families and Superfamilies
CLINICAL HISTOCOMPATIBILITY TESTING 1536
  Problems of Kidney Transplantation
    Histocompatibility Testing of Donor and Recipient
    Tests for Presensitization
    Blood Transfusions
    Immunologic Monitoring of Recipients
    Immunosuppression
  Problems of Allogeneic Bone Marrow Transplantation
    Donors With Genotypically Different HLA
    Ex Vivo T Lymphocyte Depletion of Bone Marrow Grafts Prior to Transplantation
    Immunosuppression
HLA-ASSOCIATED DISEASE 1542
  Linkage of Disease Genes to HLA
  Mechanisms in HLA-Associated Disease
    Mimicry and Receptor Hypothesis
    Ir Gene and Linked Locus Hypothesis
CONCLUSIONS 1544

INTRODUCTION

The immune system in animals is a complex network of amplifying and suppressing systems that function in an integrated fashion to produce an immune response. This immune network is regulated primarily by molecules that are encoded by genes, some of which are within the major histocompatibility complex. These genes (1) are mapped within the H-2 region of chromosome 17 in mice, and, in humans, in a region analogous to H-2, called HLA (abbreviation for human leukocyte antigen system A), which is located on the short arm of chromosome 6.

The term major histocompatibility complex (MHC) refers to the closely linked genes of H-2 or HLA responsible for very important aspects of regulation of the immune responses. In particular, the gene products of the MHC are involved in the recognition of foreign antigens by T lymphocytes. As defined by Klein (1), "the MHC is a group of genetic loci, the products of which restrict the specificity of antigen recognition by T lymphocytes." The term restrict refers to the crucial role of MHC products in the control of antigen recognition, antibody production, lymphocyte proliferation, and T cell effector functions such as cytotoxicity and T cell help and suppression (1–3). There are two kinds of antigen recognition: by antibody idiotype (i.e., B lymphocyte response) and by the T cell receptor (i.e., T lymphocyte response); the MHC, however, is directly involved only with T cell–mediated immune responses. Although the MHC contains many different genes (see section on HLA linkage group), one can for simplicity consider the MHC genes proper as composed of two sets of genes coding for cell surface antigens: MHC Class I genes and MHC Class II genes. The Class I genes (i.e., HLA-A, HLA-B, HLA-C and H-2K, H-2D, H-2L) encode cell surface antigens expressed on all nucleated cells, whereas Class II genes (i.e., HLA-D related genes or H-2I) encoded differentiation antigens primarily expressed on B-lymphocytes and macrophages. The regulation of immune responses mediated by the MHC can, in a simplified model, be divided into two phases: (1) T lymphocyte recognition of a foreign antigen that occurs when macrophages present the antigen to the T cell in the context of MHC Class II antigens, and (2) the T lymphocyte effector phase, in which the T cell recognizes the foreign antigen in the context of MHC Class I antigens. According to this model, both MHC Class I and Class II genes would be considered immune response genes. In brief, Class II genes are involved in the initial recognition phase of the T lymphocyte response, whereas the Class I genes are involved in the effector phase of the T cell response.

The immune response is primarily mediated by three types of cells: T lymphocytes, B lymphocytes, and macrophages. B lymphocytes respond to an antigen, by producing cells that generate antibody (i.e., plasma cells). T cells interact directly with other cells to regulate the immune response or to kill cells expressing the appropriate foreign antigen. (B cells bind foreign antigens, but most T cells see foreign antigens when they are presented at the surface of an accessory cell—e.g., macrophage, Langerhans cell—where they are recognized along with the MHC.) The two types of T cells, present in both lymphoid organs and in peripheral blood, are helper cells and cytotoxic/suppressor cells (4). These cell types are identifiable according to the presence of certain cell surface glycoproteins that can be determined by the use of monoclonal antibodies. The helper T cell phenotype is defined by a glycoprotein of molecular weight 55 kD, which in humans is called CD4[T,p55] and which can be detected by monoclonal antibodies such as anti-T4 or anti-Leu 3. (The corresponding cell surface antigen characteristic for murine T helper cells is called L3/T4.) The cytotoxic/suppressor T cell phenotype is defined by a glycoprotein of molecular weight 32 to 33 kD, which in humans is called CD8[T,p32-33] and which can be defined by monoclonal antibodies such as anti-T8 or anti-Leu 2a. (The equivalent murine T cell antigen is called Lyt 2) (5).

It has been demonstrated that the relationship between the two T lymphocyte subsets (i.e., T cells with helper cell phenotype and T cells with cytotoxic/suppressor phenotype) and restriction of immune response with regard to MHC Class I and Class II antigens can be simplified further. T cells with the T4, or helper, phenotype are involved in antigen recognition and are associated with T cell effector functions restricted by MHC Class II antigens, whereas T cells with the T8, or suppressor, phenotype are involved in T cell functions restricted by MHC Class I antigen (reviewed by Flomenberg and colleagues; see reference 6). Although the MHC Class I and Class II antigens are very important for the regulation of immune response, other non-MHC–linked genes also play an essential role in immunoregulation. The understanding of the importance of the MHC gene products for the regulation of immune response has evolved as a result of research performed since the mid 1960's (7–10). Much older than this knowledge, however, is the recognition of the existence of MHC genes and their gene products, derived from investigations of allotransplantation of tumors and normal tissues.

Early work showed that autografts taken from and returned to the same individual became vascularized and healed, whereas allografts exchanged between two genotypically dissimilar individuals of one species became vascularized initially but were later rejected. Rejection was a consequence of interaction between the immune system of the transplanted individual (recipient) and the histocompatibility antigens of the transplant (donor).

In studies facilitated by the use of pure inbred strains of mice (genetically identical animals produced by sequential brother–sister matings), transplantation of skin or tumors between two different strains established that the transplantation antigens are codominantly inherited, with the antigens of both parents being expressed in the progeny. Transplantation of tissues from a parent strain into the F2 generation only rarely results in engraftment (less than 1 per cent). From these observations, it has been calculated that more than 20 different genetic systems are involved in transplantation.

The first breakthrough in transplantation immunology, during the late 1930's, was the working out of the serology of alloantigens of the MHC by Peter Gorer (11–13). In the mouse, the genetic system identified by these alloantigens was found to include the most important antigens involved in tissue rejection and was designated the H-2 system (13, 14). The H-2 system of the mouse has been of special interest to immunogeneticists because it is an important model for the MHC of other mammals, especially humans. Antigens of the major histocompatibility complex are more immunogenic than any other transplantation antigens, so that matching for the MHC results in a delay of rejection of allografts (11, 12).

The extreme importance of this particular set of genes for the outcome of allotransplantation has been the reason that this genetic system continues to be called the major histocompatibility complex. The biologic role of the MHC lies in its involvement in regulation of immune responses.

In both humans and animals, the MHC has been found to consist of a number of closely linked genetic loci that constitute a genetic system. Because the MHC genes interact to perform many functions and are normally inherited as a block, they can be considered a genetic unit—a supergene. Each of the loci within the MHC is highly polymorphic and can express different forms (i.e., alleles).

The main functions of the MHC products can therefore be summarized as follows: They are markers of self in the recognition of non-self by T lymphocytes. Class I molecules function as markers of self for the T lymphocytes with the cytotoxic T cell phenotype (i.e., T8 or Lyt2), and Class II molecules are markers of self for T lymphocytes of the helper T cell phenotype (i.e., T4 or L3/T4). The biologic involvement of these MHC-controlled, T cell–mediated immune responses occurs normally when a foreign antigen interacts with the T cells in conjunction with self MHC gene products. The T cell response to nonself MHC molecules, termed alloreactivity, occurs only experimentally, as in transplantation.

The foregoing simplified description of the importance of MHC gene products in the regulation of immune responses has focused on the central role played by the T lymphocytes in both antigen recognition and effector functions. The immune response is, however, composed of a series of complex interactions among many different cells in the immune system. A classic T cell–mediated immune response is initiated when macrophages present a foreign antigen to the T helper cell in the context of the macrophage self MHC Class II antigen. The T lymphocytes then influence and regulate B lymphocyte responses (i.e., antibody production) via a complex network of regulatory helper and suppressor T cells.

An understanding of the genetic composition, inheritance patterns, and biologic role of the genes and gene products of the MHC has become important in clinical medicine in two major areas: (1) in clinical transplantation, and (2) in classification of disease in which HLA alleles or HLA-linked genetic markers are associated with disease entities and their subsets.

GENETICS OF THE HLA COMPLEX

The HLA complex is located on the short arm (p) of chromosome 6 (15) and constitutes approximately one thousandth of the total human genome. By analysis of families with intra-HLA recombinant chromosomes, it has been shown that the HLA complex is composed of three genetic loci coding for the HLA-A, HLA-B, and HLC-C Class I antigens, respectively, together with the HLA-D region, which is composed of a series of genes encoding the HLA Class II antigens (16).

The HLA-A, HLA-B, and HLA-C loci code for cell surface antigens that occur on most nucleated cells and that can be serologically detected on these cells. In addition, most of the same antigens are also expressed on platelets. One can identify these antigens on peripheral blood lymphocytes by means of the complement-dependent cytotoxicity test, using operationally monospecific anti-HLA antibodies. Many of these antigens have also been detected by murine monoclonal antibodies.

The HLA-D region codes for the genetic determinants responsible for stimulation in the in vitro mixed lymphocyte culture reaction (16, 17). HLA-D determinants are operationally defined by use of lymphocytes from HLA-D homozygous cell donors (17). The serologically detectable Class II antigens (i.e., HLA-DR and HLA-DQ) are cell surface antigens that can be detected on B lymphocytes in the peripheral blood. Some of these antigens are also expressed on monocytes and on immature hematopoietic bone marrow progenitor cells.

A third set of HLA Class II antigens, called HLA-DP determinants, has been described. These determinants were originally designated SB antigens and can be detected only in cellular in vitro transformation assays (i.e., primed lymphocyte typing, or PLT) (18).

HLA Haplotypes, Genotypes, and Haplotype Segregation

The HLA chromosomal region covers a very small segment of the short arm of chromosome 6, corresponding to approximately 2 centimorgans. This means that genetic recombination crossover of genetic material between homologous chromosomes during meiotic division occurs very infrequently (i.e., ≤ 2 per cent). Therefore, the HLA complex can be considered a single genetic unit that is inherited as a block of genes from a parent by a child. The genetic unit composed of the HLA alleles present on the HLA-A, HLA-B, HLA-C, and HLA-D loci on each of the two homologous chromosomes 6 is called an HLA haplotype. The two HLA haplotypes present in each individual constitute the HLA genotype (19, 20). The gene products of each of the HLA Class I and Class II loci are codominantly expressed as cell surface antigens. The HLA haplotypes are accordingly transmitted as a dominantly inherited mendelian trait, so that each child expresses one paternal and one maternal HLA haplotype. If the father's two haplotypes are labeled *a* and *b* and the mother's are *c* and *d*, there are four possible genotypes for their children: *ac, ad, bc,* and *bd* (Fig. 45–1). If the inheritance of HLA haplotypes is random, the different genotypes should be present in equal numbers in the offspring. The chance of any one sibling within a family being identical with another in this respect is 25 per cent because there are only four possible genotypes (i. e., assuming that genetic recombination within HLA has not occurred). The chance of identity between siblings for one HLA haplotype is 50 per cent, and the likelihood of their being totally different is 25 per cent.

The two HLA haplotypes inherited from the parents of any individual give rise to the combined set of HLA antigens as they are detected on the cell surface of an individual's nucleated cells. This means that each individual expresses two HLA-A antigens, two HLA-B antigens, two HLA-C antigens, and two sets of HLA-D region gene products. These HLA antigens constitute the person's HLA phenotype. In general, most people are HLA

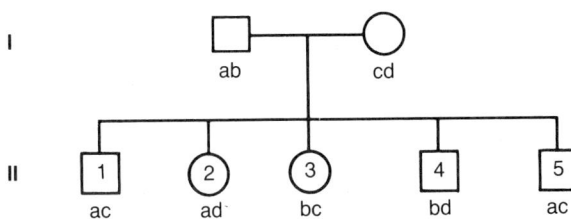

Figure 45–1. An example of a pedigree with the phenotyping and genotyping of HLA (A, B, C, and DR) alleles. Two haplotypes form one genotype. The father is ab genotype and the mother cd. Based on the phenotypes of the family, ac, ad, bc, and bd can be obtained. The siblings 1 and 5 are genotypically identical.

a: A1, B8, Cw8, DR3
b: A3, B7, Cw7, DR2
c: A2, B44, Cw3, DR4
d: A3, B35, Cw4, DR1

a, b, c, d: parental HLA haplotypes

ab; cd; ac; ad; bc; bd: HLA genotypes

A1,2; B8,44; Cw3,w8; DR3,4: HLA phenotype of siblings II.1 and II.5, who are HLA-identical with the HLA genotype A1, B8,Cw8,DR3/A2, B44, Cw3, DR4. Child II.4 is HLA-A3 homozygous.

heterozygous for each of the HLA locus determinants. Sometimes, however, a mother and father express the same HLA allele on one of their HLA haplotypes. A child who inherits these two haplotypes will then be homozygous for the corresponding HLA locus allele.

As already mentioned, genetic recombination within the HLA complex does sometimes occur during meiotic division. This produces a new, composite HLA haplotype that represents parts of each of the two HLA haplotypes from the parent in which the recombination has occurred. The new HLA recombinant haplotype can then be transmitted to a child (Fig. 45–2).

Other Genes Within the HLA Complex

In addition to the HLA Class I and Class II genes, Class III genes have been identified within the HLA complex. These consist of the structural genes for the serum complement components C2, Factor B (BF) (21), the two genes for serum complement C4 (i.e., C4A and C4B), and the two structural genes for adrenal cytochrome P450 21-hydroxylase (i.e., 21-OH,A and 21-OH,B). The identification of these genes within the HLA complex came from studies of autosomal recessive diseases involving these genes (22–24). Studies involving molecular genetic probes for the identification of the structural genes for these loci have established that the gene order within the HLA Class III region is as follows: C2; BF; C4A; 21OH,A; C4B; 21OH,B (see later section on molecular genetics of HLA genes). A map of the HLA region, shown in Figure 45–3, also demonstrates the major similarities between the genetic composition of the HLA complex and that of the murine H-2 complex.

The MHC Linkage Group

A substantial number of murine Class I genes are encoded for by genes located outside the H-2 complex. These genes are located telomeric to H-2D (see Figure 45–3). These are the TL genes, which control the antigenic determinants (TLa) expressed on thymocytes, in certain T cell leukemias, and on the Qa-1, Qa-2, and Qa-3 cell surface antigens, which control the expression of antigeneic determinants on different subpopulations of lymphocytes. On the same chromosome, there also are loci controlling embryonic differentiation (t complex), hair growth (tf and thf), a set of polymorphic enzymes (GLO-I, PgK-2, Ce-2, Ap1, Map-2), minor histocompatibility antigens (H-31, H-32, H-33), a blood group antigen (Ea-2), and the third component of the complement system (C3) (1).

The HLA genetic linkage group is composed of a series of genes very similar to those of the murine H-2 linkage group. HLA Class I–like cell surface antigens, which are not classic HLA-A, HLA-B, or HLA-C antigens, also have been identified. These antigens have been detected in human T cell leukemias and on thymocytes. One such lymphocyte differentiation antigen, CD1 (Thy, p 45–12) (5), was originally recognized by a murine monoclonal antibody NA1/34 (25). It is not presently known whether the CD1 (Thy, p 45–12) antigens are coded for by HLA linked genes. Also linked to HLA are several enzyme-encoding loci: SOD-2, PGM-3, ME-1, Pg, and GLO-I. Of particular interest is the gene for the enzyme glyoxalase I (GLO-I), which is located centromeric to HLA (see Figure 45–3).

Genetic Polymorphism

Polymorphism is the occurrence in a population of two or more genetically determined forms in such frequencies that the rarest of them could not be maintained by mutation alone. Mutations, or gene conversions, are the mechanism of polymorphism. Such changes in the genome can be neutral, occurring in a region of the molecule that does not affect function (neutral mutation) and therefore conferring no selective advantage or disadvantage. Other genetic changes affect the function of molecules that are encoded by genes, causing disease (deleterious mutation). In such individuals, selection forces operate by increasing

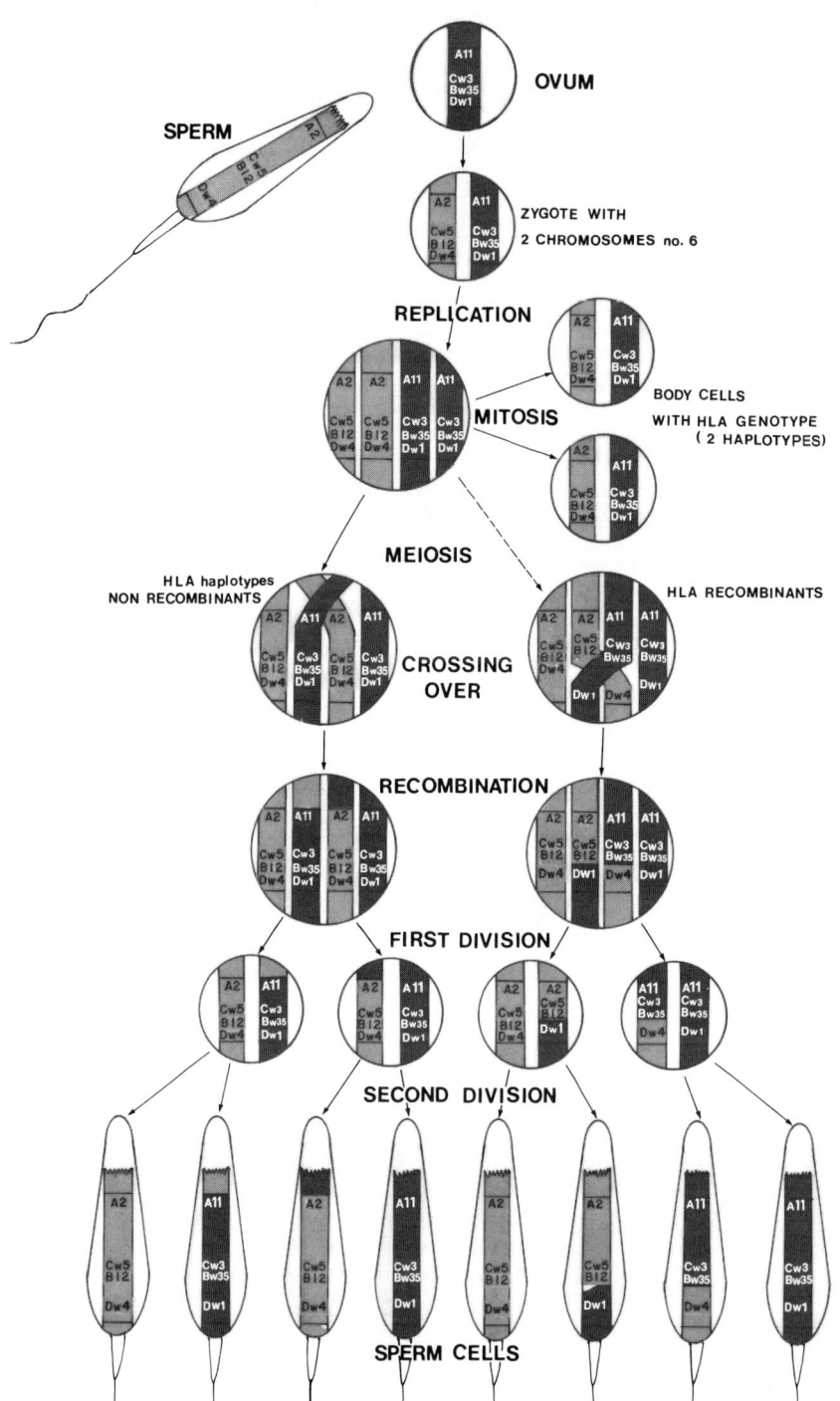

Figure 45–2. Mitosis and meiosis. Illustration of inheritance of HLA with examples of HLA haplotypes and intra-HLA recombination in chromosome 6. The diagram shows reshuffling of alleles during sexual reproduction. The germ cells are formed by meiosis or reduction division, during which the homologous chromosomes exchange genes (in this example, the HLA-D portion) by the process called recombination (modified from Scientific American 236:64, 1978).

or decreasing fitness. In the biologic sense, fitness is a measure of fertility and therefore of the contribution made by an individual to the genes of the succeeding generation. Selection may operate on a gene at any time from conception to adult life. A mutant gene is "lethal" when it interferes with embryogenesis, resulting in spontaneous abortion, or when it causes sterility.

In a state of equilibrium, the rate at which a detrimental trait is produced by new mutations is balanced by the rate at which the trait is removed from the population by selection forces; assuming that the mutation rate remains constant, one can deduce that genes conferring greater biologic fitness tend to increase in frequency, whereas those lowering biologic fitness tend to decrease.

In general, mutation rates tend to be constant and relatively low so that the gene frequencies of mutants are maintained in different proportions either by selective advantage in the heterozygote

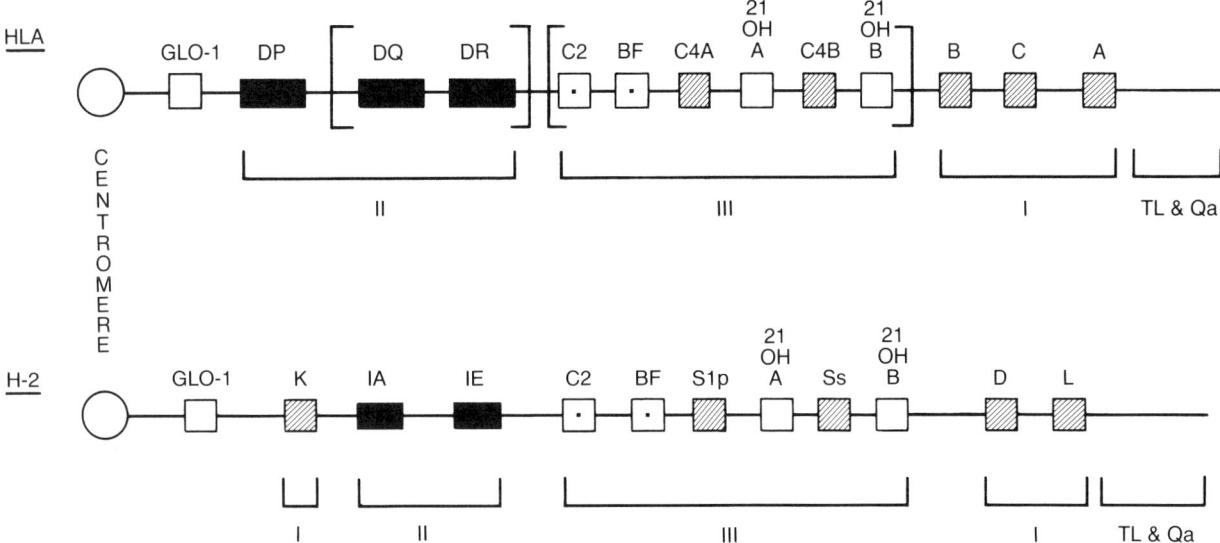

Figure 45–3. The brackets of the map indicate that the sequence of genes included is known but the orientation of the particular group could be the reverse. For example, C2 may be proximal or distal to HLA-B. Recently, the sequence of genes has been determined as being DP, DQ, DR.

or by nonselective forces such as genetic drift (i.e., the shift of gene frequency by chance or by gene migration). Genetic drift can occur either by diminution of alleles through the bottleneck effect (e.g., extinction of alleles during epidemic outbreaks of infections) or by an increase in the frequency of alleles via founder effects. The founder effect occurs when a new population is formed from a very small number of individuals whose gene pool differs by chance from that of the original population. Gene migration (or gene flow) occurs when there is a mixture of diverse populations with resultant exchange of genes. (Polymorphism can be maintained either by deleterious genes involving selection or by neutral mutations without the participation of selective mechanisms.) In humans, polymorphisms maintained by selection are balanced with two or more different genetic forms maintained by selective advantage. A good example is the sickle cell gene. In parts of Africa, up to 40 per cent of the population is affected by the sickle cell gene, and one person in three is a carrier. Sickle cell anemia is most frequent in regions in which *Plasmodium falciparum* malaria is epidemic. It has been found that carriers of the sickle cell gene are more resistant to infection by this organism than are normal persons (i.e., heterozygote erythrocytes parasitized by *P. falciparum* are removed more effectively from the circulation by phagocytes than those of normal individuals). In such geographic locations, the increased fertility of the heterozygotes balances the elimination of the sickle cell genes through affected homozygotes. Sickle cell polymorphism is transient in American blacks because lack of exposure to malaria has eliminated the selective advantages of sickle cell trait. In addition, blacks have increased resistance to "quartain" malaria due to *P. vivax* because they are usually Duffy blood group–negative and have red cells that are resistant to that infection (26).

The reasons for the extensive genetic polymorphism of the HLA loci are presently unknown. It has been suggested that HLA polymorphism has occurred through the mechanisms of gene conversion during meiosis in the female (27) and maintained by selective advantage of the heterozygotes (28). However, it is not understood why genes of the MHC show the most extensive polymorphisms in mammals. As will be discussed in the next section, many diseases involving autoimmune reactions are associated with certain alleles of HLA. This fact has led many to believe that MHC polymorphism protected the species during the course of evolution. The assumption made is that protection was exerted by certain MHC alleles during infancy and childhood prior to the individual's reaching reproductive age. It is possible that the protection is related to resistance to viral infection. The presently known HLA disease associations are, however, found for diseases that mostly occur in adult life, at a time when selective forces are not operating significantly.

HLA CLASS I

All the HLA Class I loci are highly polymorphic. The most polymorphic locus is HLA-B, with 47 known alleles, followed by HLA-A, which has 23 alleles. These two polymorphisms have been characterized to such a degree that it is possible to type for almost all alleles without the observation of "blanks" (i.e., undetectable alleles). The same is not true for HLA-C, for which only eight alleles have been described and the frequency of "blank" alleles is significant; this is probably because of the weak immunogenicity of the C locus antigens such that production occurs in only a few cases.

HLA terminology is designated by the IUIS/WHO Committee for HLA Nomenclature. International exchanges of typing reagents are organized every 2 to 4 years (International Histocompatibility Workshops) (16). Provisional assignments are designated by a "w" preceding the number. Table 45–1 shows the currently established HLA and workshop ("w") specificities. Alleles within each HLA locus are numbered not consecutively but, for historical reasons, according to the order of their initial identification. Following each workshop, several old specificities are "split" as the antigen definition becomes more accurate. The private (narrower, or less public) specificities are named subtypic, and the more public are called supertypic. For example, Bw54, Bw55, and Bw56 are subtypic specificities of the supertypic Bw22.

The numbers 4 and 6 are not used as designation for conventional alleles at the HLA-A or HLA-B loci because they were reserved for the supertypic specificities 4a and 4b, which were being investigated in 1967, when the original nomenclature system was developed. Now it is known that the 4a (Bw4) and 4b (Bw6) reside on a unique epitope on the HLA-B molecule, which is distinctly different from the epitope that expresses the HLA-B allospecificities. Each HLA-B molecule

Table 45–1. COMPLETE LIST OF RECOGNIZED HLA SPECIFICITIES*

A	B		C	D	DR	DQ	DP
A1	B5	Bw4	Cw1	Dw1	DR1	DQw1	DPw1
A2	B7	Bw6	Cw2	Dw2	DR2	DQw2	DPw2
A3	B8		Cw3	Dw3	DR3	DQw3	DPw3
A9	B12		Cw4	Dw4	DR4		DPw4
A10	B13		Cw5	Dw5	DR5		DPw5
A11	B14		Cw6	Dw6	DR6		DPw6
Aw19	B15		Cw7	Dw7	DR7		
A23 (9)	B16		Cw8	Dw8	DRw8		
A24 (9)	B17			Dw9	DRw9		
A25 (10)	B18			Dw10	DRw10		
A26 (10)	B21			Dw11 (w7)	DRw11 (5)		
A28	Bw22			Dw12	DRw12 (5)		
A29 (w19)	B27			Dw13	DRw13 (w6)		
A30 (w19)	B35			Dw14	DRw14 (w6)		
A31 (w19)	B37			Dw15			
A32 (w19)	B38 (16)			Dw16	DRw52		
Aw33 (w19)	B39 (16)			Dw17 (w7)	DRw53		
Aw34 (10)	B40			Dw18 (w6)			
Aw36	Bw41			Dw19 (w6)			
Aw43	Bw42						
Aw66 (10)	Bw44 (12)						
Aw68 (28)	B45 (12)						
Aw69 (28	Bw46						
	Bw47						
	Bw48						
	B49 (21)						
	Bw50 (21)						
	B51 (5)		Bw61 (40)				
	Bw52 (5)		Bw62 (15)				
	Bw53		Bw63 (15)				
	Bw54 (w22)		Bw64 (14)				
	Bw55 (w22)		Bw65 (14)				
	Bw56 (w22)		Bw67				
	Bw57 (17)		Bw70				
	Bw58 (17)		Bw71 (w70)				
	Bw59		Bw72 (w70)				
	Bw60 (40)		Bw73				

*Antigens followed by a number in parentheses are recognized as splits of the antigen in the parentheses (e.g., A23 is a split of A9).

therefore expresses either Bw4 or Bw6 in addition to the HLA-B private specificity.

The antibodies used to type HLA antigens are obtained from postpartum sera, from individuals immunized through blood transfusions, from patients who have been allotransplanted, and from individuals who have received a planned immunization. Because the HLA-A, HLA-B, and HLA-C alloantigens are expressed on most nucleated cells, they can be detected only by complement-dependent cytotoxicity tests on either T or B lymphocytes, whereas the Class II antigens are easily detectable only on B lymphocytes and some macrophages. In the presence of complement (e.g., rabbit serum), specific antibodies produce injury to the membrane of cells possessing the corresponding HLA antigen or antigens. Cell death is determined by the uptake of dye (trypan blue or eosin), which is excluded by living cells. Thus, positive serologic reactions define a particular HLA-A, HLA-B, HLA-C, or HLA-DR phenotype (Fig. 45–4) (29). There is extensive cross-reactivity among different alleles of both the HLA-A and the HLA-B loci. This may complicate the definition of HLA antigens, the selection of donors for transplantation, and the selection of platelets for transfusion. Some strong cross-reactivities include those of HLA-A2 with HLA-A28; HLA-A30 with HLA-A31; HLA-A23 with HLA-A24; HLA-A11 with HLA-A3; HLA-Aw34 with HLA-A25; HLA-A25 with HLA-A32 of the HLA-A locus; HLA-B5 with HLA-B35; HLA-B35 with HLA-Bw53; and HLA-B35 with HLA-Bw53 of the HLA-B locus. These are commonly referred to as cross-reactive groups (CREG).

HLA CLASS II

The cell surface antigens encoded for by the HLA-D region genes (i.e., DR, DQ, and DP) share two important features: (1) They consist of two glycoprotein chains (α chain and β chain), and (2) these antigens are expressed only on certain cells. These HLA Class II antigens are therefore called differentiation antigens. The cell types on which they are expressed include B lymphocytes, monocyte/macrophages, dendritic cells, and Langerhans cells of the skin.

The HLA-D region products were originally identified as encoded for by a genetic locus distinct from the HLA Class I loci by their capacity to induce T lymphocyte activation on the in vitro mixed lymphocyte culture (MLC) reaction (30). The HLA-D determinants are defined as the HLA-encoded determinants that can be recognized in the MLC test with HLA-D homozygous typing cells (HTC) (17). Between 1973 and 1980 it became evident, however, that HLA-D is a complex genetic region composed of many genetic loci and that the cellular in vitro response in MLC is a composite reaction due to the HLA-D region haplotype (31).

Serologic Identification of HLA Class II Antigens and HLA-DR Antigens. Allospecificities present on B but not T lymphocytes were described in the early 1970's (32). During the Seventh International Histocompatibility Workshop (1977), a large number of B cell–reactive antisera were tested against a panel of HLA-D–typed lymphocytes. On the basis of their reactivity, the resulting antiserum clusters against that panel were associated with, but not identical with, HLA-D of previously known allospecificities. Thus, the eight alleles of this B cell antigen system together were designated HLA-DR (D-related) (DR1 to DR8) (33). At present, 14 HLA-DR allospecificities can be recognized (see Table 45–1). Two additional serologically detectable Class II antigens appear to be encoded for by the HLA-DR region. The latter antigens are called DRw52 (formerly MT2) and DRw53 (formerly MT3). As shown in Figure 45–5, these two HLA-

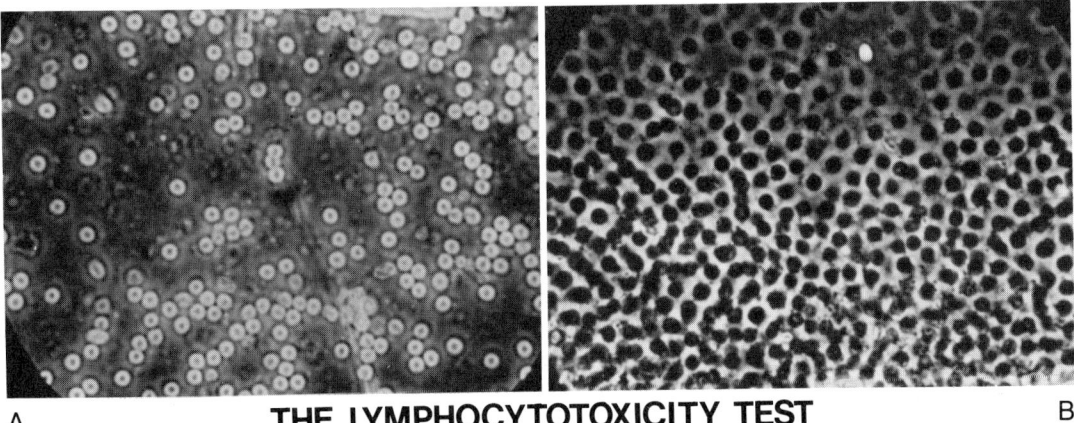

Figure 45–4. The complement-dependent microcytotoxicity test used for serologic HLA typing. *A,* Demonstration of a positive reaction and *B,* a negative reaction. The dead lymphocytes are the dark cells. The living cells are bright white and exclude the dye (eosin).

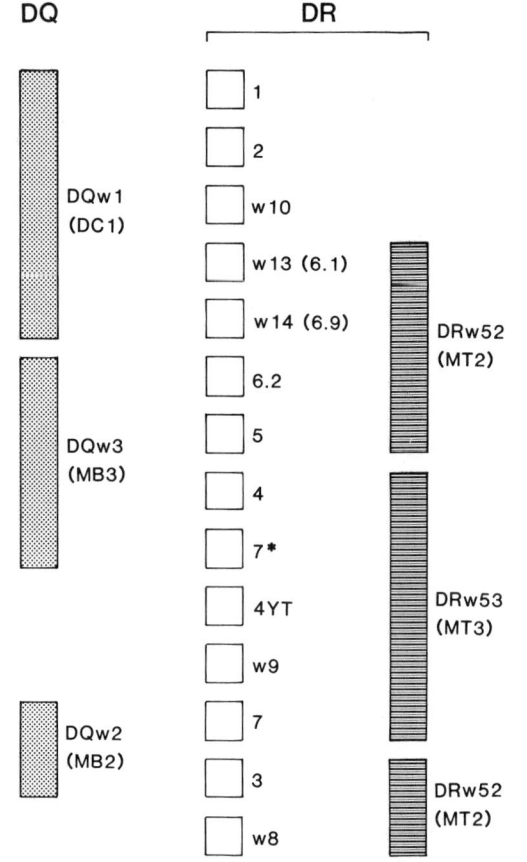

Figure 45–5. The block diagram shows the overlap of Class II allelic specificities. The DQ alleles appear to include several DR alleles. The DRw52 and DRw53 also overlap with several DR specificities.

DR antigens are shared by several different DR alleles.

HLA-DQ Antigens. A second series of HLA Class II antigens, which could be detected serologically or biochemically, was recognized in 1978 and 1979 (34, 35). This component of the HLA-D region has now been designated HLA-DQ (16). The presently recognized HLA-DQ specificities are listed in Table 45–1. As in the case of DRw52 and DRw53, DQw1 (previously DC1, MB1, MT1), DQw2 (previously MB2, DC3, Te24), and DQw3 (previously MB3, MT4, DC4, TB21) were considered during the Seventh and Eighth International Workshops to be cross-reacting specificities, including DR1, DR2, DRw6, and DRw10 for DQw1; DR3 and DR7 for DQw2; and DR4 and DR5 for DQw3. The fact that DQw1 and DRw6 are on different sets of gene products clearly indicates that DQw1 does not contribute to the definition of DRw6. The strong association between these and other analogous combinations of specificities can now be clearly seen to be due to strong positive genetic linkage disequilibrium between alleles at very closely linked loci coding for DR and DQ products (see Figure 45–5).

HLA-DP Determinants. HLA-DP specificities were previously known as SB determinants and were defined by an in vitro cellular assay for alloreactivity called primed lymphocytes test (PLT) (36, 37). Several investigators have demonstrated that cells could be primed in the in vitro MLC test for antigens other than HLA-D (38–40) and that their reactivities in secondary restimulated cultures were not associated with any known HLA specificities. In some families, priming of lymphocytes between two siblings who are identical for HLA-A, HLA-B, HLA-C, HLA-D, and HLA-DR has given positive stimulation (41); in one such study (42), the results were interpreted as being indicative of a recombination between the new determinant and the HLA-D region because there was D:GLOI recombination. Priming of donor pairs who were identical for HLA-A, HLA-B, HLA-C, and HLA-DR resulted in the development of typing reagents that could be used for the description of a new allelic system of HLA-related determinants (SB) (18). Six provisional DPw determinants were identified during the Ninth International Histocompatibility Workshop (see Table 45–1). Studies of B lymphoblastoid cell lines in which HLA-region deletions have been induced have confirmed that SB (i.e., DP) is a system of separate gene products that maps centromeric to HLA-D (43). The putative HLA-DP antigens have been biochemically identified as typical Class II antigens (by the use of monoclonal antibodies). Serologic detection of DP alloantigens has not been unequivocally established (44, 45).

GENETIC LINKAGE DISEQUILIBRIUM

Studies of HLA antigen frequencies have been performed in many different ethnic populations. It is well established that the antigen frequencies for a given HLA allele (e.g., HLA-B8) vary greatly among different ethnic groups and even within the same ethnic group of different geographic locations (46). The antigen phenotype frequency for a given HLA allele in a population can be converted to an estimation of the gene frequency in the population according to the following formula: $g = 1 - \sqrt{1-f}$, where g is the gene frequency and f is the antigen phenotype frequency. By calculating the gene frequency of, for example, the HLA-A1 allele (called p) and the HLA-B8 allele (called q), one can calculate the expected frequency (h) for the HLA-A1,B8 haplotype as $h = p \times q$. When such a calculation is performed for different combinations of HLA alleles from the different HLA loci, it is found that the expected HLA haplotype frequencies differ, in most instances, from the observed frequencies. The difference between the expected and observed haplotype frequencies (i.e., $h - pq = 0$) is called the delta value (Δ) and is due to the phenomena of genetic linkage disequilibrium (also called nonrandom gametic association). If Δ is greater than 0, the linkage disequilibrium is termed positive; if Δ is less than 0, it is termed negative. If Δ is positive for a particular haplotype, that HLA haplotype occurs in higher frequency in the population than expected from the gene frequencies of the alleles in the population. Similarly, if Δ is negative, the haplotype occurs less frequently than expected. Genetic linkage disequilibrium exists for the alleles of the HLA Class III region genes as well. Although the classic definition of linkage disequilibrium involves only alleles at two closely linked loci, it has been shown that certain combinations of alleles at the C2, BF, and C4 loci occur much more frequently than expected. The term complotypes has been coined to describe this phenomenon (47). Fourteen complotypes with frequencies in excess of 1 per cent occurred in one white population (47). The term extended haplotypes has been used to describe specific allelic combinations of the HLA-A, HLA-B, HLA-C segment, the complotype, and the HLA-D region determinants (48). In some instances, these extended haplotypes have included specific alleles at the GLOI locus (49). The chromosomal distribution of HLA-A, HLA-B, HLA-C, and HLA-DR and of the serum complement protein alleles (complotypes) was studied in normal white families. Eight combinations were found to occur in haplotypes at frequencies significantly higher than expected. In such combinations, which were defined as extended MHC haplotypes, HLA-A showed limited variation. Some extended haplotypes are more frequent than others (e.g., B8, DR3, F_1C30). There are two mechanisms that seem likely to produce long-term maintenance of linkage disequilibrium: (1) selection and (2) suppression of genetic recombination (50, 51). The mouse T/t complex appears to provide examples of selective suppression of recombination and of selection at the gametic level, with both resulting in the appearance of nonmendelian distributions of segregation ratios (i.e., male transmission bias) or nonrandom association of alleles. One extended HLA haplotype (i.e., HLA-B8, C4AQ0, B1, BfS, C2C, DR3, GLO2) was found to be transmitted from males to 83 per cent of their offspring, whereas the same haplotype with GLO1 had no transmission bias (48). It has been suggested that this GLO2-marked chromosome may be a human analogue of a murine t mutant. However, it is possible that most of the known extended haplotypes may occur as the result of nonrandom association resulting from gene migration or from founder effects.

HLA CLASS III

The four HLA-linked structural genes coding for the serum complement components C2, BF, C4A, and C4B are polymorphic genetic loci. Homozygous deficiencies for three of these gene products have been described (22, 24). Of these, complement C2 deficiency is a relatively uncommon condition that occurs with a frequency of less than one in 15,000. In contrast to this, C4A deficiency (i.e., lack of the red cell antigen Rodgers) and C4B deficiency (i.e., lack of the red cell antigen Chido) are relatively common, occurring in 2 per cent and 4 per cent of the population, respectively (52, 53). Complete deficiency for complement C4 (i.e., homozygous deficiency for both C4A and C4B) is very uncommon (54, 55). Homozygous deficiency for BF has not been identified. Structural variants of C2, BF, C4A, and C4B can be detected by immunoelectrophoresis. There are at least two alleles for C2, four alleles for BF, and at least seven C4A alleles and seven C4B alleles (56). The most common complotype that is cancerous is SC31 (BFS, C2C, C4AB, and C4B1), but complotypes that have C4 null alleles are relatively common and are designated C4AQ0 or C4BQ0— i.e., SC01 (BFS, C2C, C4AQ0, and C4B1).

Congenital adrenal hyperplasia due to adrenal 21-hydroxylase deficiency, an inborn error in biosynthesis of steroid hormones, is an autosomal recessive disease that segregates with HLA (24). It has been demonstrated that this disease occurs in several different forms ranging from severe, congenital deficiency of both cortisol and aldosterone production, to congenital deficiency of cortisol production alone, to cases with asymptomatic deficiency in cortisol production. These various disease manifestations are due to different combinations of defective allelic variants at one or both of the two 21-hydroxylase loci (57). Genetic polymorphism of normally functioning 21-hydroxylase alleles has not yet been identified.

TISSUE DISTRIBUTION, BIOCHEMISTRY, AND MOLECULAR GENETICS OF HLA

Tissue Distribution

The HLA Class I molecules are ubiquitous in somatic cells, occurring in relatively high concentration on cells of the immune system. Embryos have a lower content of these antigens, and tumors derived from early embryos (teratocarcinomas) are completely devoid of Class I molecules. The same seems to be true for the embryonic cells present between the fetus and the mother in the uterus (i.e., trophoblastic cells).

In contrast, HLA Class II molecules are differentiation antigens that are present only on certain somatic cells. Class II antigens are found on the surface of B lymphocytes, monocytes, macrophages, dendritic cells, and epidermal Landerhans cells. Although all the Class II antigens (i.e., DR, DQ, and DP) are expressed on B lymphocytes, some monocytes do not seem to express the DQ determinants (58). Studies in the mouse have demonstrated that the dendritic cells in the cortex of the thymus are unusual because they express extremely high levels of Class II antigens and very low levels, if any, of Class I antigens (59, 60). Human cortical dendritic cells also express HLA Class I antigens very weakly, if at all (61). Because of this phenomenon, the thymocytes will undergo exposure to very high concentrations of self–Class II antigens during their differentiation and maturation in the thymus. This process could be the mechanism by which autoreactive, autoaggressive immature thymocytes become activated and subsequently removed.

The MHC Class II antigens also are expressed on some of the hematopoietic progenitor cells at different stages of their differentiation in the bone marrow (reviewed by Broxmeyer and Dupont; see reference 62). The murine hematopoietic pluripotential stem cell does not express Class II antigens (63). A probable human pluripotential stem cell identified in long-term bone marrow culture also is negative for HLA Class II determinants (64). In contrast, the human multipotential colony-forming unit (CFU-GEMM), the erythroid burst-forming unit (BFU-E), the erythroid colony-forming unit (CFU-E), and granulocyte-macrophage (CFU-GM) progenitor cells are positive for HLA Class II antigens (65–70). Similarly, the murine CFU-GM cells have I-A and I-E on their cell surfaces (71). There is evidence that the human CFU-GEMM (66), BFU-E, and CFU-GM (70) and the murine CFU-GM (71) express increasing amounts of Class II antigens during the S-phase of the cell cycle. A differential expression of various HLA-Class II antigens between lymphoid cells and BFU-E and CFU-GM has been observed (72, 73).

HLA Class II antigens are also strongly expressed on activated T lymphocytes (74). This occurrence of the Class II antigens on functionally active, fully differentiated T cells is probably important for the effector functions of the cells.

The HLA Class II antigens are also expressed on malignant solid tumors and cell lines derived from such tumors. This was first observed for tumor cell lines derived from malignant melanoma (75, 76). It has been shown that many human tumor cell lines—as well as cell lines derived from normal tissues such as fibroblasts, endothelial cells (77), keratinocytes, and glial cells (78)—can express HLA Class II antigens following exposure to gamma interferon (77).

Biochemistry

The HLA cell surface antigens have been studied biochemically by techniques that in principle involve five steps: (1) radiolabeling of the cell surface antigens; (2) solubilization of the cell membranes by nonionic detergents; (3) purification of glycoproteins; (4) immunoprecipitation of the specific cell surface antigen with appropriate antibodies; and (5) polyacrylamide gel electrophoresis (PAGE) or gel filtration. These methods have provided isolated MHC molecules for further analysis.

HLA CLASS I MOLECULES

The MHC Class I antigens consist of one heavy chain and one light chain, called beta$_2$ microglobulin (β_2m). Only the heavy chain is encoded for by genes within the HLA region; genes for β_2m are located on chromosome 15 (79). The Class I heavy chain consists of three external domains (each about 90 amino acids long), a transmembrane region (40 residues), and a short internal cytoplasmic component (approximately 30 residues). The β_2m light chain is noncovalently associated with one of the three external heavy chain domains and is not attached to the membrane (Fig. 45–6). The HLA Class I antigens cannot be expressed on the cell surface except in association with β_2m. The molecular weight of the heavy chain is approximately 45 kD, of which about 3 kD are contributed by carbohydrate moities. The molecular weight of β_2m is 12 kD.

The degree of homology among different Class I heavy chains varies. The two heavy chains of two alleles may differ by as many as 40 to 50 residues or may be identical except for a single or a few amino acids. The HLA-A and HLA-B loci alleles share approximately 80 per cent of their amino acids, and a similar degree of homology exists between the murine K and D loci. This observation supports the idea that these loci arose by gene duplication from a common ancestral gene. Although the 20 per cent of differences between the products of the loci occur throughout the heavy chain, there are two hypervariable regions: one between residues 60 and 80 and another between 105 and 114. Additionally, human and murine Class I MHC molecules share approximately 70 to 75 per cent of their amino acids, a degree of homology somewhat less than that between two Class I loci of a single species. The murine K locus is more similar to the human A locus than it is to the human B locus (reviewed by Klein; see reference 1). A general description of the biochemistry of HLA Class I molecules has been provided by Parham and colleagues (see reference 80).

HLA CLASS II MOLECULES

HLA Class II molecules, like Class I molecules, are heterodimer (i.e., they are composed of two chains that are noncovalently associated). In contrast to the chains of Class I molecules, both the

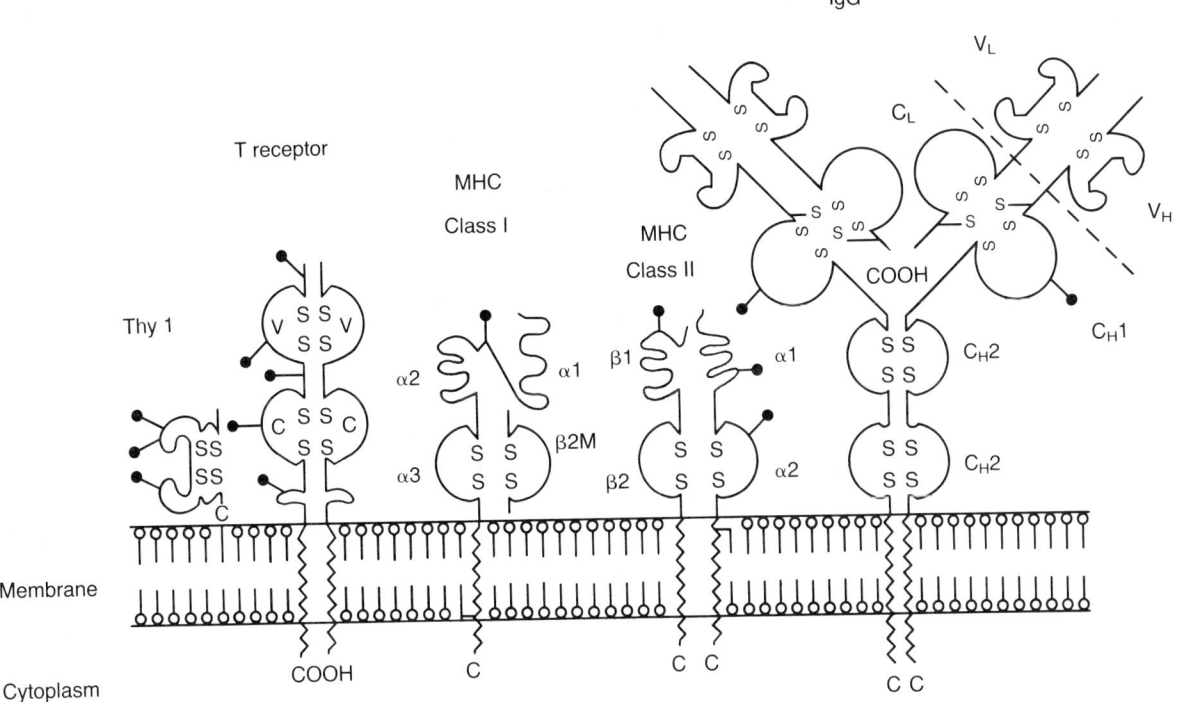

Figure 45–6. Models of membrane proteins with homology to immunoglobulin. The Class I and Class II MHC antigens each contain two immunoglobulin-like domains adjacent to the membrane.

chains of Class II molecules are encoded for by genes within the HLA region, and each chain is anchored in the cell membranes. The Class II molecules are glycoproteins; both the heavier alpha (MW, 31 to 33 kD) and the lighter beta (MW, 26 to 29 kD) have two external domains, a transmembrane component, and an intracytoplasmic region (Fig. 45–6) (81, 82). Amino acid sequence analysis as well as nucleotide sequence determinations have demonstrated that DR and probably DP molecules have substantial homology with murine I-E molecules, whereas DQ molecules are homologous with I-A molecules. There seems to be hypervariability in DR beta regions localized between residues 60 and 69.

Molecular Genetics

At first, studies concerning MHC genes involved the isolation and enrichment of mRNA from cells producing the appropriate MHC gene product. Examples include mRNA from B lymphoblastoid cell lines for the HLA Class I and II messages and, from liver cells, mRNA corresponding to the complement genes (Class III). From the total mRNA of the appropriate cell type, the particular mRNA was enriched, for example, by fractionation according to size. With the enzyme reverse transcriptase, the mRNA was then used to synthesize the complementary DNA (i.e., cDNA), which was inserted into a vector. The cloned cDNA (cDNA library) was then screened for the ability to bind the mRNA that directs MHC antigen synthesis. When an appropriate clone was deleted, the inserted DNA was excised and its sequence determined. (The DNA sequences within this sequence should correspond to the known protein sequence of the product.) Because the aforementioned procedure is cumbersome, one may instead use a DNA probe that cross-hybridizes with the desired product. A synthetic oligonucleotide, which corresponds to a portion of the known amino acid sequence of the antigen under study, is used as a primer in directing the synthesis of complementary DNA along mRNA molecules.

The details of transfer of information from genes to proteins have been accumulated with great rapidity in the past decade. Figure 45–7 illustrates the system in a highly simplified form.

STRUCTURE OF MHC GENES

Class I Genes. The structures of human and murine Class I genes are very similar. Starting at the 5' end, there is a noncoding region followed by the start signal peptide coding sequence. Three exons encoding the three extracellular domains are next, followed by one exon encoding the transmembrane region and two or three exons encoding the cytoplasmic domain. The first exon, which codes for a signal sequence, is cleaved from the protein during the passage through the membrane (Fig. 45–8). This organization of Class I genes coincides with the protein structure.

Within both HLA and H-2 there are numerous

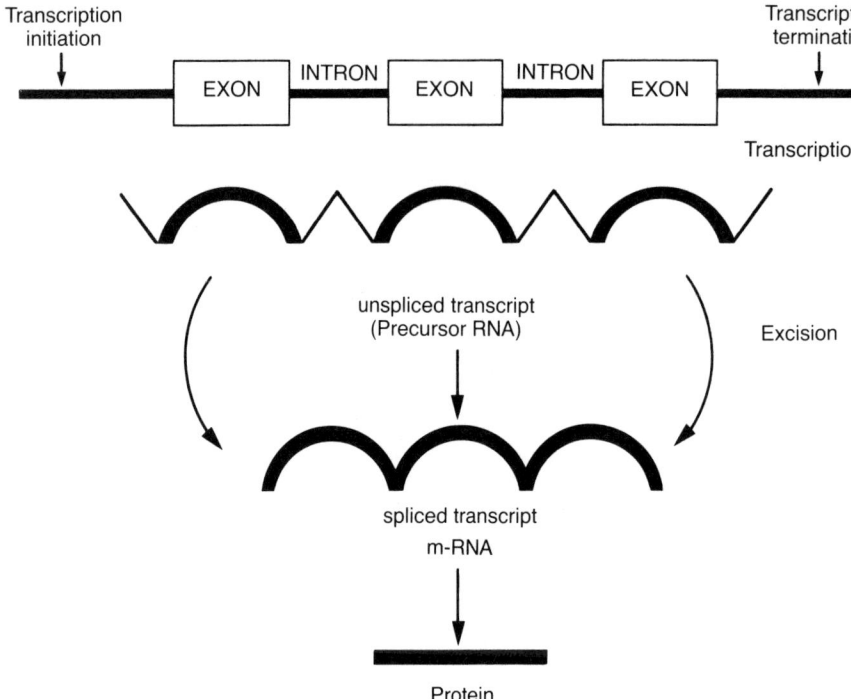

Figure 45–7. This figure depicts a simplified diagram of the main events that occur in the cell. The top shows a structural gene from initiation to termination. The diagram demonstrates the difference between exons and introns. Exons and introns are transcribed to precursor RNA, which is intranuclear. Then the introns are spliced out to produce mRNA transcript, this is transported to cytoplasm, where it is translated to produce a protein. (Modified from Emery, A. E. H.: Lancet 2:1406, 1981.)

Class I–like genes. Not all strains of inbred mice have the same number of Class I genes. For example, C57BL/10 has two genes in the H-2K region, two in the H-2DL region, 10 in the Qa region, and 11 in the TL region. In contrast, BALB/c has 31 genes in the Qa and TL regions (83). Similar studies of human genomic DNA with HLA Class I cDNA probes have demonstrated that a similar large number of Class I genes exist (84, 85). It is not presently known how many of these extra Class I genes are expressed, although it is possible that some are pseudogenes. These extra genes could also be involved in different stages of development. Another possibility is that aberrant expression during life could be involved in malignant transformation (86).

Nucleotide sequence comparison between Class I genes for various HLA alleles at different loci reveals a high degree of sequence homology among nonallelic genes. For example, it has been

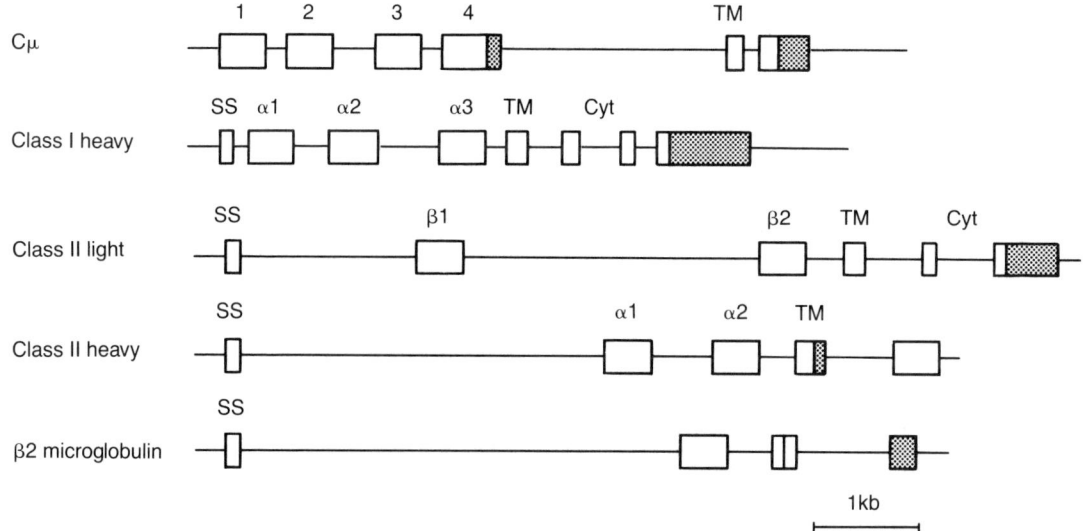

Figure 45–8. Genomic structures of six related genes (SS, signal sequence; TM, transmembrane region; cyt, cytoplasmic region; exons representing extracellular domains are so numbered). Shaded boxes denote 3' untranslated regions. Cμ represents the constant region of a Cμ heavy chain gene.

shown that an 82.9 per cent homology exists between the A3 and Cw3 gene sequences, and if the comparison is made with the known pseudogenes the percentage of homology is higher. In contrast, the degree of homology between human and murine Class I genes is considerably lower than that observed among nonallelic human genes, especially in the noncoding region. Comparison of nucleotide sequences for the different exons of the HLA Class I genes has demonstrated locus-specific sequences, particularly in the exons encoding for the intracytoplasmic segment. In contrast, allele-specific sequences for Class I genes are observed in regions of the exons coding for the first and second domains. The exon coding for the third external domain (α_3) is highly conserved compared with the other exons. This domain represents the region that interacts with β_2m. Both β_2m and the third domain exhibit homologies with constant domains of immunoglobulin molecules (87).

Class II Genes. The HLA-D Class II region is similar to the H-2I region in the mouse. At present, a few more genes have, however, been identified in man than in the mouse (Fig. 45–9). The reasons for this "expansion" of the Class II region in man or contraction of the Class II region in mouse are not known. At least two alpha and two beta genes have been identified in the HLA-DP subregion, two alpha and two beta genes in the DQ, and one alpha and three beta genes in the DR subregion. One additional alpha gene, called DZα, has been identified (88–92), as well as one additional β gene called DOβ. Recently the genomic organization of the human Class II region has been determined using pulse-field gel electrophoresis. The order of the HLA-D subregions centromeric to the telomeric is: DP/DZ–DO–DX/DQ–DR, and the size of the region is 1100 kilobases (92a). A tentative sequence of the Class II genes is shown in Figure 45–4. The alpha and beta genes of Class II antigens are encoded by three extracellular exons (starter signal and two exons for the extracellular domains), one transmembranous exon, and one intracytoplasmic exon (Fig. 45–8). Nucleotide sequence determinations of a limited number of Class II alpha and beta genes indicate that DRα, DPα, and DXα (i.e., one of the two DQα genes) have limited polymorphism, if any. In contrast, some of the beta genes are polymorphic, particularly those for the exons encoding the first external domain (β_1) (Fig. 45–6). The genes for which this polymorphism presently have been shown include one of the DRβ genes and at least one of the DPβ genes. Furthermore, the DQα gene is found to be highly polymorphic.

Class III Genes. The HLA Class III region is the component of the HLA complex that presently is

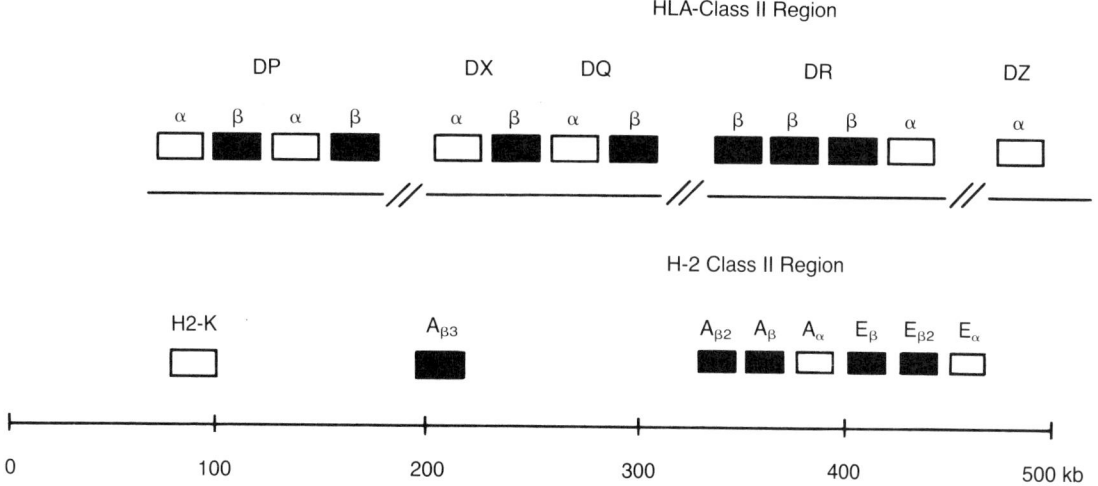

Figure 45–9. Comparative molecular map of the HLA and H-2 Class II genetic region. The β genes are shown as solid boxes; the α genes as open boxes. Nucleotide sequence data indicates that the I-A genes correspond to the DQ and DX genes, while the I-E genes have a high degree of homology with the DR genes. The nucleotide sequence data for the DP genes are very similar to those for the I-Aβ3 gene. The distance between the H-2 Class II genes as shown in this figure has been determined by overlapping cosmid clones from genomic DNA of the B10 and the BALB/C mouse. A similar series of overlapping cosmid clones has not yet been obtained for the complete HLA Class II region. This is indicated on the figure by the three interruptions in the HLA gene map. Recently the genomic organization of the human Class II region has been determined using pulse-field electrophoresis. The order of the HLA-D subregions centromeric to the telomeric is: DP/DZ–DO–DX/DQ–DR, and the size of the region is 1100 kilobases (92a).

most completely characterized. As shown in Figure 45–6, it has been demonstrated, by the use of overlapping cosmid clones, that the gene composition, gene orientation, and gene map are practically identical for the Class III region of H-2 and for HLA. The common gene map seen in both H-2 and HLA is C2:BF:C4A:21-OHA:C4B:21-OHB (in humans) and C2:BF:Slp:21-OHA:Ss:21-OHB (in mice) (93–102). At present, no overlapping clones connecting the MHC Class III region with the Class I or Class II region have been identified. It should be noted that the genes for C2 and BF seem, on the basis of nucleotide sequences, to belong to the same gene family. There also is extensive homology between the C4A and C4B genes, between Slp and Ss (i.e., murine complement C4), and between 21-OHA and 21-OHB. This implies that a series of tandem gene duplications in the ancestral Class III region genes occurred prior to mammalian speciation mouse-man, possibly several million years ago. Another interesting observation has been the demonstration that only one of the two 21-OH genes seems to be functional in each of the two species. In mice, the 21-OHA gene adjacent to the Slp gene is 25 times more effectively transcribed than the 21-OHB gene. In humans, the 21-OHB gene adjacent to the C4B gene is biologically functional, although there presently is no evidence that the 21-OHA gene is transcribed (102).

RESTRICTION FRAGMENT LENGTH POLYMORPHISMS (RFLPs)

Complementary DNA probes for MHC genes are presently being applied extensively in family and population studies of HLA. One uses the Southern blot technique (103) to determine possible correlations between HLA phenotypes and restriction fragment length polymorphisms (RFLPs). Restriction endonucleases are enzymes that recognize specific sequences in the DNA (every few hundred nucleotides on average for enzymes that cleave four nucleotide sites to every 10,000 or more nucleotides for those cleaving at rare six nucleotide sites). Essentially, it is possible, with the application of such enzymes, to find a discrete fragment on which a gene resides. DNA is digested by a restriction enzyme, subjected to electrophoresis so that fragments are separated by size, and transferred to a filter. The DNA is then hybridized with a radioactive cloned probe (cDNA or genomic probe), and the filter is washed (so that unhybridized probe is removed) and exposed to x-ray film. One to several bands may be visualized when the film is developed. These bands represent sequences identified in or homologous to those of the gene from which the probe was derived. RFLPs are those bands that vary in size between two individuals, reflecting polymorphisms (104–109).

GENE FAMILIES AND SUPERFAMILIES

As early as 1972 it became evident that the amino acid sequence of beta$_2$-microglobulin (β_2m) was structurally related to the CH$_3$ domain of IgG (110, 111). The amino acid homology between the two molecules was only 28 per cent, but strikingly, of the 11 positions at which all Ig-constant domains are identical, 10 were shared with β_2m. It was subsequently found that β_2m has substantial homology with the α_3 domain of HLA Class I heavy chains (112) (Fig. 45–6). Similar homologies have been observed between the α_2 and β_2 domains of MHC Class II molecules (Fig. 45–6). Most recently, sequence analysis of cDNA clones for the alpha and beta chains of the T cell receptors in both humans and mice have demonstrated the same kind of homology with Ig-constant domains (113–115). On the basis of these findings, it has been suggested that all these genes belong to the same supergene family and could have evolved from the same ancestral genes. It has been proposed that several additional molecules may belong to the same gene family; they include the gene for the thy-1 molecule and the poly Ig receptor of intestinal epithelium (see Figure 45–6). An alternative possibility is that the homology between these immunologically important molecules is an example of evolutionary convergence due to independent development of similar sequences in several unrelated molecules under the influence of similar selective processes.

CLINICAL HISTOCOMPATIBILITY TESTING

Tests that are important clinically for selection of transplantation donors will be discussed in this section. Laboratory tests related to rejection of grafts or to immunosuppression will, however, be covered in the sections dealing with problems of kidney and bone marrow transplantation, respectively.

The laboratory methods for histocompatibility testing (tissue typing) are used for identification or study of potential donors within a family member or an unrelated population (e.g., cadaver donors for kidney transplantation). Study of families is mandatory, especially in selection of donors for bone marrow transplantation and of living related donors for kidney transplantation. This discussion is divided into two parts: (1) problems of kidney transplantation, and (2) problems of allogeneic bone marrow transplantation.

Problems of Kidney Transplantation

Organ transplantation represents an alternative in the treatment of several diseases, especially those involving an irreversible loss of organ function. Kidney transplantation is the most common, but cornea, heart, liver, and pancreas transplants also are performed, although in a more limited number of patients and at few institutions.

Important factors in renal transplantation include the degree of histocompatibility between donor and recipient, the presence or absence of presensitization in the recipient, the recipient's blood transfusion history, and immunosuppression.

HISTOCOMPATIBILITY TESTING OF DONOR AND RECIPIENT

Although the value of HLA genotype matching in renal transplantation between related individuals is undisputed, the results of matching for HLA phenotypes in cadaver transplantation are still unclear. In kidney recipients who are receiving immunosuppressive therapy and transplants from related donors, the ranking of matches shows a significant decrease in graft survival when siblings with HLA that is genotypically identical with that of the recipient are compared with family donors differing with respect to one (HLA-haploidentical) or two HLA haplotypes (116–119). Nevertheless, 10 to 15 per cent of HLA-identical renal allografts are rejected, often within the first weeks following transplantation (120). It is likely, although unproven, that these failures represent states of prior sensitization to non-HLA antigens, such as antibodies against endothelial cells (120, 121). Because a number of patients receiving poorly matched grafts do quite well, it is apparent that HLA typing alone does not necessarily provide an absolute measure of incompatibility in a given case.

The outcome of cadaveric renal transplantation depends on many factors, including clinical care, immunosuppressive protocols, histocompatibility, crossmatching, and blood transfusion history. When the contribution of HLA matching in cadaveric transplantation was analyzed at different transplant centers with similar clinical protocols, a clear influence of the degree of HLA matching in graft survival was observed (122). For example, during the Ninth International Histocompatibility Workshop, more than 10,000 kidney allograft cases over a 2-year period were analyzed, and it was possible to compare several clinical protocols, especially the degree of HLA matching, effects of the number of blood transfusions, and the type of immunosuppression. Zero mismatches to four mismatches resulted in 11 per cent differences over 6 months. Equally, the effect of DR mismatches approximated the effect on survival of HLA-A and HLA-B mismatches. Combined analysis of HLA-A and HLA-DR loci showed the strongest effect on graft survival. Another factor that influenced the outcome of the kidney allografts was that DRw6-positive recipients are at increased risk of graft failure if transplanted with DRw6-negative kidney (123). In addition, cyclosporine has improved cadaveric kidney graft survival rates for the first 2 years to equal that for grafts from one haplotype–matched living related donors (124–126). This effect has been observed primarily in centers in which kidney transplantations have been performed with a success rate of approximately 60 per cent over 2 years.

The probability of finding a cadaveric kidney that is phenotypically and serotypically HLA-identical for a patient awaiting transplantation depends on the sizes of the donor pools and recipient pools. To maximize the chance of providing a "good" match whenever a cadaveric kidney becomes available, cooperative groups have been organized (e.g., Eurotransplant, Scandiatransplant).

Although not used routinely, other methods for the selection of donors for transplantation, especially in related haploidentical donors, have been the mixed lymphocyte culture and the cell-mediated lymphocytotoxicity test (127). In general, there is a better success rate for kidney transplantation in recipients with low MLR responses against lymphocytes of haploidentical donors than in cases transplanted with haploidentical donors with high MLR responses (128–130).

TESTS FOR PRESENSITIZATION

The most useful tests for presensitization are serologic. These include tests for the presence of preformed cytotoxic antibodies against the donor's lymphocytes (usually referred as the crossmatch) and for the presence of ABO isoagglutinins (131–134). However, the presence of preformed killer cells, detected by a cell-mediated cytotoxicity test, is not a predictor of graft failure (135), possibly because immunosuppression eliminates these reactive cells.

Tests for presensitization that are used so that hyperacute rejection of kidney allografts is avoided are tests for ABO compatibility and for the presence of antibodies against Class I histocompatibility antigens of the donor, as detected by the lymphocytotoxicity assay (133–135). Although the significance of the role played by antibodies against Class I histocompatibility antigens in rejection of an organ is well established, the importance of recipient alloantibodies against donor B lymphocytes (Class II alloantigens) is still being evaluated (136). Furthermore, successful transplantation can be accomplished in the presence of a positive crossmatch (serologic detection of antibodies present in the serum of a recipient against the tissues of the donor—i.e., lymphocytes) when the serum of the patient reacts with the lymphocytes obtained from his own blood as well (120). Additionally, there have been reports of successful kidney transplantation in recipients from whom sera collected weeks or months prior to transplantation contained antibodies against the donor's lymphocytes, but serum samples collected immediately prior to transplantation did not react with donor lymphocytes (137, 138). However, most transplant centers rule out a potential donor when the crossmatch test of the recipient has shown antibodies against the donor's lymphocytes in a sample of serum obtained from the patient days or even months prior to the day of the tentative transplant, even if serum taken on the day of the transplant does not demonstrate reactivity (139). A crossmatch method distinguishing harmful and nonharmful antibodies has not yet been discovered. When such a test is found, it will be able not only to discriminate among antibodies but also to explain how it is possible to produce different types of antibodies to HLA or other antigens and why some of these antibody responses vary in both their temporal response and their degree of tissue damage.

BLOOD TRANSFUSIONS

As already mentioned, an important factor in the outcome of renal cadaveric allograft is the patient's history of blood transfusions. The larger the number of transfusions, the better the rate of graft survival (122, 140, 141). Unfortunately, about 30 per cent of randomly transfused end stage renal disease patients develop cytotoxic antibodies. In the remaining patients, however, blood transfusion appears to induce nonresponsiveness, presumably by induction of suppressor cell systems or by production of enhancing antibodies. It is important to point out that the effect of transfusion is best demonstrated by comparison of patients without a history of transfusion with those who received up to five transfusions prior to transplantation.

Because both transfusions and HLA-DR matching have beneficial effects on cadaveric graft survival, patients receiving kidneys matched for one or two HLA-DR alleles have greater success than those receiving DR-mismatched kidneys. This effect was best demonstrated in patients with a transfusion history of 10 to 20 units of blood prior to transplantation and primarily in centers in which the success rate of kidney allografting was approximately 60 per cent over 2 years (120, 122, 140, 141).

Living-donor haploidentical grafts present strong histocompatibility barriers and, like cadaveric grafts, appear to benefit from blood transfusions. In particular, the use of donor-specific blood prior to transplantation results in superior graft survival in those 70 per cent of recipients who do not become sensitized. Again, the effect is one of negative selection of the nonresponders, in whom an additional degree of specific unresponsiveness may be induced. In these studies, the MLR high responders to lymphocytes from haploidentical donors receive the greatest benefits from transfusion, with success of engraftment increasing from an expected 60 per cent to approximately 90 per cent (140–141). Also increased with the number of transfusions was the success of kidney haploidentical grafts in centers with a low success rate (122).

IMMUNOLOGIC MONITORING OF RECIPIENTS

Rejection of a vascularized organ allograft is associated with a variety of pathologic and clinical patterns. This heterogeneity reflects the variable effects of the responsiveness of a given host to a given set of histocompatibility antigens, states of prior sensitization, and responsiveness to therapeutic manipulation.

All alloimmune responses are not harmful per se to an allograft, as evidenced by the apparent benefits of deliberate preimmunization with blood transfusion. Experimentally, such priming has been termed enhancement. For example, rat renal allografts can enjoy long-term successful function, even in the presence of infiltrating cytotoxic T cells, provided that the IgG antibodies to the vascular endothelium suppress their activity. Although a variety of cell types are present in rejection lesions, recovery of these cells and elution of antibodies bound to graft cells have shown that it is cytotoxic T cells and IgG antibodies that specifically accumulate in grafts. However, recruitment into rejecting grafts of very large numbers of B lymphocytes, null cells, and macrophages—as well as of cells capable of mediating antibody-dependent cell-mediated cytotoxicity (ADCC)—has been clearly documented, showing that final effector pathways may be multiple (120).

The following section describes a series of immunologic tests that have been employed in the assessment of graft rejection. Investigators have used these tests to evaluate samples obtained from peripheral blood of the patients, which may not reflect the immunologic reactivity in the transplanted organ. Although this information will be summarized, it needs to be emphasized that there is no single test capable of predicting at an early stage all cases of renal failure following kidney transplantation. Abnormalities in laboratory measurements of renal function, such as serum creatinine and blood urea nitrogen, definitively measure graft failure (142).

Two basic types of assays exist: (1) those that reflect specific host antidonor immune activity, and (2) those that reflect nonspecific host responses.

Specific Assays for Detection of Rejection. Between 4 and 5 days after renal transplantation in a host treated with azathioprine and steroids, cytotoxic T cells become detectable in the blood. The number of these cells initially peaks by the end of the first week, declines by the end of the second week, but reappears later in the circulation at levels that vary in relation to rejection severity (143).

Antibody-dependent cell-mediated cytotoxicity (ADCC) is a very sensitive assay for IgG antibodies directed against cell surface antigens. This method is able to detect both anti-HLA and non-HLA antibodies. A positive ADCC against donor cells is closely associated with acute rejection (144). Antidonor antibodies may induce lysis of donor target cells by complement activation (complement-dependent cytotoxicity, or CDC), an effect that is often detectable after transplantation and is associated with rejection (145).

Two other promising assays are (1) the study of MLR suppressor cells, which disappear during rejection (146, 147); and (2) the detection of anti-idiotype antibody, which is correlated with good graft function (148). Donor-specific anti–B cell antibodies have been shown to develop after transplantation in association with rejection. The continued presence of antidonor antibody in the circulation after treatment for rejection (ADCC, or anti–B cell antibody) is a poor prognostic sign (120).

Nonspecific Assays for Detection of Rejection. Several investigators have found a significant increase in DNA or RNA synthesis by peripheral blood lymphocytes either prior to or concomitant with clinical signs of early and late rejection (149). Several groups have found that administration of antithymocyte globulin (ATG) in the early posttransplant period produces a reduction in total T cells with decreased incidence of rejection. Preliminary results suggest that when the normal ratio of T helper cells to T cytotoxic/suppressor cells (2:1) is present, rejection is highly likely, despite immunosuppressive therapy (142). The measurement of interleukin-2 lymphocyte response, which is increased during rejection episodes (150), also may be useful in the confirmation of clinical rejection.

Thus, not all assays described are useful in predicting clinical rejection; donor-specific assays, however, may be most helpful in determining when the immune response has been adequately controlled by immunosuppressive treatment.

Chronic rejection is the usual cause of progressive late failure of long-surviving renal allografts. These rejections are usually associated with protracted humoral injury manifested by intimal fibro-obliterative arterial lesions. These intimal abnormalities are thought to represent repetitive cycles of chronic immune injury to vascular endothelium with focal thrombosis.

IMMUNOSUPPRESSION

Although tissue matching by tissue typing and a history of blood transfusion or antithymocyte globulin (ATG) administration improves the outcome of allotransplantation, the success of clinical transplantation is directly related, in part, to the development of good methods of immunosuppression. In general, it is known that patients receiving kidney transplants that are genotypically identical or haploidentical for HLA require less immunosuppression than patients given unrelated grafts. Most protocols consist of a combination of corticosteroids, azathioprine, and antilymphocyte serum (ALS). Immunosuppression is not antigen-specific; rather, it depresses the entire immune system including, preferentially, the thymus-dependent functions. Consequently, immunosuppressed patients not only are vulnerable to bacterial, viral, and fungal infections but also may have a higher risk of developing malignancy (151).

During the Ninth International Histocompatibility Workshop, it was possible to compare the effects of HLA matching, blood transfusion history, and immunosuppression either according to conventional protocol or by treatment with cyclosporine A (CyA) (122, 141), a cyclic peptide of fungal origin that blocks the secretion of interleukin-2 (IL-2) by $T4^+$ helper/inducer cells. Because suppressor T cells do not appear to depend on the presence of IL-2, CyA selectively blocks the effector response while allowing the suppressor response to proceed. Generally speaking, CyA is more effective in improving the success of kidney transplantation at centers with a low success of kidney allograft survival (122).

Prospective recipients with a suitable living related two-haplotype–matched donor do as well with conventional azathioprine immunosuppression as with CyA. Most investigators agree that transplants from one-haplotype–mismatched living related donors with D/DR compatibility result in a 1-year postgraft survival rate equal to that of the same category of transplants in patients receiving CyA treatment (152). Graft survival of the more common high-MLR, DR-mismatched living related recipient on azathioprine is equivalent to that of the CyA-treated patient (85 to 90 per cent at 1 year) only if the recipient is multiply transfused. This latter pretransplant treatment, however, carries with it a risk of sensitization ranging from 15 to 30 per cent, depending on whether random blood or donor-specific blood is given and on whether the recipient is concomitantly immunosuppressed with drugs. Current practice is to ensure that all recipients of haploidentical kidneys are D/DR-compatible with the donor, are recipients of donor-specific or multiple random transfusion, or are maintained on CyA. Cadaver allograft recipients on azathioprine do as well as CyA-treated patients only if they are similarly polytransfused (more than 10 transfusions) and are DR-compatible with the donor. The problem of possible sensitization and the rarity of a complete DR match sway the balance toward CyA treatment for most cadaver recipients. However, approximately 20 per cent of patients develop toxic kidney reactions that require modification of dosage and/or a combination of immunosuppressive agents using a lower dosage of CyA plus steroids (153–157).

Antilymphocyte globulin has been used with some success in the therapy of acute rejection episodes and in some centers has been used on a routine basis during the first 2 weeks after transplantation (158). Also, clinical trials aimed at treating acute rejection have been attempted, with at least three monoclonal antibodies against T cell surface antigens. These include T3 and T12 (both of which are expressed on virtually all resting, mature T cells) and CBL1 (which is an activation antigen expressed selectively on antigen-stimulated cells). For the present, however, the results of these treatments are inconclusive (159–160).

Problems of Allogeneic Bone Marrow Transplantation

Since the mid 1970's, marrow transplantation has been shown to provide an approach to the cure of a number of acquired hematopoietic malignancies and to the treatment of a number of lethal congenital diseases (161, 162). Marrow transplantation has become a very promising treatment of several forms of leukemia and is also the treatment of choice for most patients with aplastic anemia. With the exception of the rare situations in which a syngeneic bone marrow transplant can be obtained from an identical (monozygotic) twin donor, it is necessary to select an allogeneic marrow donor (163). Frequently, patients and sibling donors with HLA that is genotypically identical have sufficient histocompatibility to allow engraftment of allogeneic bone marrow without the development of fatal graft-versus-host disease (GVHD). Most recently, techniques for selective removal of T lymphocytes ex vivo from the bone marrow prior to transplantation have allowed extension of marrow transplantation to patients without HLA-identical siblings. Here both the major problems in clinical marrow transplantation and some of the approaches that presently are being used to overcome these problems are only briefly described. The details are provided in Chapter 6.

The major problems in bone marrow transplantation are GVHD, graft rejection, infection, and leukemic relapse. GVHD and posttransplantation infections are problems affecting all groups of marrow graft recipients. Although patients with leukemia only rarely reject the marrow graft, this problem is of particular concern in patients with aplastic anemia. It has been demonstrated that most instances of graft rejection in the latter patients can be ascribed to host lymphocytes previously sensitized to minor donor histocompatibility antigens through prior blood transfusion. This explains why the incidence of graft rejection among transfused aplastic anemia patients is significantly increased. In some cases, graft rejection or failure of engraftment may be due to abnormalities of the marrow microenvironment of the host.

GVHD develops in 30 to 70 per cent of patients receiving HLA-identical bone marrow and accounts for 20 to 40 per cent of transplant-related deaths (164, 165). The clinical presentations of acute graft-versus-host reactions are skin rash, liver involvement, and diarrhea. The risk factors for acute GVHD include high age of the recipient and marrow grafts from female donors. The mechanisms by which GVHD develops and the cells involved in the process are poorly understood at present. It is generally accepted, however, that engrafted alloreactive T lymphocytes initiate the process. A contribution to natural killer cells also is possible. Many patients with GVHD experience a spontaneous resolution of the disease; it is possible that the development of acquired graft-host tolerance is an active process that depends on the development of suppressor cells.

Chronic GVHD develops in approximately 15 to 40 per cent of transplanted patients (166–168). This disease is distinct from active GVHD, presenting with scleroderma-like skin changes, skin and joint contractions, biliary cirrhosis, and malabsorption. The mechanisms of development of this condition are presently unknown.

Infections as complications of marrow transplantation also are very common. Decontamination of patients with nonabsorbable antibiotics in leukemia and the use of prophylactic granulocyte transfusions have reduced the incidence of serious infections in the immediate posttransplant period. Interstitial pneumonia is a common complication during early engraftment and is particularly common in patients with acute GVHD.

Current treatment of interstitial pneumonia remains largely ineffective. Antiviral agents have been used. Particularly promising is the prophylactic administration of hyperimmunoglobulin or plasma for the prevention of cytomegalovirus infections (169).

DONORS WITH GENOTYPICALLY DIFFERENT HLA

The sibling with HLA that is genotypically identical with that of the patient is clearly preferred as the appropriate donor for allogeneic bone marrow transplantation. Because of the dominant mendelian inheritance of the HLA system, however, it is to be expected that only 35 per cent of potential candidates for allogeneic bone marrow transplantation will have an HLA-identical sibling donor (i.e., if an average of 2.5 siblings per patient is assumed). A large group of patients with aplastic anemia, acute leukemia, and severe combined immunodeficiency will thus not be able to receive allogeneic bone marrow grafts from such a donor.

Incentive to pursue the issue of bone marrow donor selection from individuals other than siblings with HLA that is genotypically identical with that of the patient came from the study of allogeneic bone marrow transplantation in severe combined immunodeficiency (SCID) (170, 171). The selection of allogeneic bone marrow donors for SCID patients lacking an HLA-identical sibling has been based on the assumption that compatibility between donor and recipient for the determinants responsible for stimulation in the mixed lymphocyte culture (MLC) plays a major role in prevention of severe GVHD. The subsequent selection of marrow donors for patients with aplastic anemia and leukemia who lack an HLA-identical sibling has been based on the additional assumption that compatibility for MLC-stimulating determinants plays a major role in the prevention of both graft rejection and GVHD. Feasibility of this approach was subsequently demonstrated in patients with SCID, aplastic anemia, and leukemia who received grafts from related donors with HLA that was genotypically nonidentical (172–174).

Marrow transplantation with HLA-nonidentical marrow grafts has now been performed in several transplant centers. The most substantial results have been reported from the Seattle Marrow Transplant Team (175). These investigators reported on 13 patients with aplastic anemia and 78 with leukemia. Eleven patients received grafts from phenotypically identical donors; the remainder received transplants from donors who were incompatible for at least one HLA antigen. The donor-recipient pairs were genotypically identical for one HLA haplotype, with the exception of one patient who received a marrow graft from an unrelated donor with phenotypically identical HLA. The results in patients with aplastic anemia treated with HLA-nonidentical marrow grafts were very discouraging, with only one of 13 patients becoming a long-term survivor. The results of marrow transplantation for leukemia patients receiving HLA-nonidentical marrow were much more encouraging. Overall survival for 36 patients who received transplants during remission was similar to that obtained in patients receiving a marrow transplant from a sibling with HLA that was genotypically identical. This study indicates that, in leukemia, a patient's incompatibility for a difference of one HLA antigen between donor and recipient can be tolerated as well as HLA-identical marrow grafts. Preliminary data on the outcome of marrow grafting with two HLA antigen incompatibilities are very limited, but the results are quite discouraging, at least with the conventional proven transplantation regimen.

EX VIVO T LYMPHOCYTE DEPLETION OF BONE MARROW GRAFTS PRIOR TO TRANSPLANTATION

Many different approaches to facilitation of the establishment of immunologic tolerance between donor and recipient have been attempted. The elimination of T lymphocytes ex vivo from allogeneic bone marrow or spleen cells before their use for immunologic and/or hematologic reconstitution of lethally irradiated recipients has been investigated in several experimental systems (176–178) and has been applied in clinical bone marrow transplantation (179, 180). It was originally demonstrated in a dog bone marrow transplantation model that GVHD can be prevented by in vitro T lymphocyte depletion of histocompatible bone marrow by use of antibodies with broad antilymphocyte activity. Subsequent studies in mice and monkeys have conclusively demonstrated that T cell depletion (TCD) ex vivo in bone marrow grafts can prevent GVHD. Therefore, many methods for TCD have been developed. The initial clinical trials with ex vivo TCD were performed by differential agglutination with soybean agglutinin (SBA) and sheep red blood cell rosette depletion (179, 180) or by elimination of T lymphocytes with complement-fixing monoclonal antibodies (181), immunotoxins (182, 183) or counterflow centrifugation. It has been demonstrated that TCD of bone marrow grafts ex vivo can dramatically reduce the incidence and severity of GVHD in marrow transplantation between HLA-identical siblings. Furthermore, TCD ex vivo does provide a method for marrow transplantation between related donors and recipients who differ for one complete HLA haplotype. Although TCD of bone marrow ex vivo presently provides the most encouraging prospects for GVHD prophylaxis and makes it possible to extend marrow transplantation to patients who lack HLA-identical siblings, these techniques present some still unresolved problems. Even though the incidence and severity of GVHD following marrow transplantation with TCD marrow have declined, an increased incidence of graft rejection has been observed. Development of methods for prevention of graft rejection is presently a topic of intensive investigation. They may involve the administration of T cell derived hematopoietic growth factors (see Chapter 6).

IMMUNOSUPPRESSION

It is necessary to eliminate the capacity of the allogeneic marrow graft recipient to reject the graft or resist its engraftment. Only marrow from a syngeneic donor (i.e., an identical twin) will be accepted without the ablation of host immunocompetence. Standard immunosuppression procedures depend on the nature of the disease for which the patient is being treated.

Patients with aplastic anemia are normally prepared for transplantation by 4 days of treatment with cyclophosphamide in a dose of 50 mg per kg. In patients with leukemia, this immunosuppressive conditioning regimen in preparation for marrow transplantation is combined with supralethal leukemia treatment by total-body irradiation. A number of modifications of these pretransplantation treatments have been introduced. In particular, more intensive leukemia treatment has been widely used, including combinations of chemotherapy with fractionated, total-body irradiation.

Treatment of acute GVHD normally involves administration of corticosteroids or antithymocyte globulin or both. Prophylactic administration of methotrexate during the first 100 days after transplantation was introduced on the basis of experimental data on GVHD prophylaxis in the dog. Shorter courses of methotrexate and more selective immunosuppressive agents, such as cyclosporine A, have shown promising GVHD prophylaxis. Multiply transfused aplastic marrow transplant recipients have a very high rate of graft rejection. Cyclosporine A prophylaxis in such patients seems to offer promising results, but in preliminary studies the accumulated experience regarding prevention of graft rejection suggests that selective methods should be applied, based on the status of the immune systems of donor and the host.

HLA-ASSOCIATED DISEASE

The MHC effect on disease susceptibility was first demonstrated in mice with virally induced leukemia (184). It is now well established that a variety of multifactorial diseases are associated with certain HLA determinants. Studies of HLA disease associations have provided new insights into genetic host factors involved in etiology and pathogenesis. It is impressive that many highly diverse diseases are, in fact, associated with HLA. However, no common denominator can be identified at present that would account for these associations (185). In fact, the apparent diversity among HLA-associated diseases indicates that no single mechanism is likely to be found that will provide a fundamental biologic explanation. However, one conclusion can be made. A number of different HLA-linked genes are involved in resistance or susceptibility of the host to the development of disease. Moreover, it is now possible to identify diseases in which at least one of the important genetic factors is HLA-linked. Major genetic components have previously been recognized in, for example, juvenile diabetes mellitus (JDM) and multiple sclerosis and it is now recognized that one of the genetic factors in each of these diseases is HLA-linked. This has provided new approaches to the continued study of pathogenic and etiologic factors in these diseases.

Diseases are the result of many factors, including the genetic composition of the individual and the environment. The majority of studies of HLA and disease have been performed on a population basis, involving conditions that generally do not occur in several members of a family. A detailed description of these conditions has been provided (186). Most of the studies are, therefore, reports of HLA disease "associations" based on comparison of antigen frequencies in a patient group with those of a normal control population. Statistical analysis is performed by calculation of the relative risk (RR) factor. As summarized in Table 45–2, most RR values for factors in HLA-associated diseases range from 3 to 15. For example, a relative risk of 5.5 among HLA-B8–positive individuals for developing one particular disease indicates that such people have a 5.5-fold higher risk for developing the disease than HLA-B8–negative individuals.

In a few cases, the HLA region has also served as a genetic marker for detection of possible disease genes in definite linkage with HLA or with nonrandom associated alleles of the MHC (56).

Linkage of Disease Genes to HLA

Theoretically, the simplest study of the linkage of disease genes to HLA involves monogenic disease. Two genes are genetically linked when they are located close together on the same chromosome and frequently segregate as a unit in families. Genetic linkage is detected in family studies. The standard method for linkage analysis is the Lod score analysis (187). Another approach is the SIB pair method, which compares expected and observed frequencies of haplotypes. For example, the incidence of an affected pair would be expected to be 25 per cent for recessive genes and 50 to 75 per cent for dominant genes.

In some cases, the HLA region has served as a genetic marker for recessive or dominant disease genes. At present, three dominantly inherited diseases have been studied in which genetic linkage to HLA has been suggested: Paget's disease of the bone (188), hereditary hemorrhagic telangiectasis (Osler-Weber-Rendu disease), and spinocerebellar ataxia (189).

Another condition that has been studied for linkage to HLA is idiopathic hemochromatosis. In the past, this disease was thought to be inherited as an autosomal dominant trait, with incomplete penetrance in females because of excessive blood loss during menstruation and pregnancy (190). It is now established, however, that the disease is inherited as an autosomal recessive trait (191). Studies of linkage to HLA in families with the disorder indicate either that two HLA-linked genes are probably involved in development of the disease or that the disease is simply autosomal

Table 45–2. EXAMPLES OF ASSOCIATION BETWEEN HLA AND DISEASE

Disease	HLA Antigen	Relative Risk (RR)*
Arthropathies		
Ankylosing spondylitis	B27	87.4
Reiter's syndrome	B27	37.0
Rheumatoid arthritis	DR4	4.2
Endocrine diseases		
Juvenile and/or insulin-dependent diabetes	D/DR3	3.3
	D/DR4	6.4
	D/DR2	0.2
Graves' disease	D/DR3	3.7
Idiopathic Addison's disease	D/DR3	6.3
Eye diseases		
Acute anterior uveitis	B27	10.4
Optic neuritis	D/DR2	2.4
Inflammatory disease		
Subacute thyroiditis	B35	13.7
Intestinal disease		
Celiac disease	D/DR3	10.8
Liver disease		
Chronic autoimmune hepatitis	B8	9.0
Neurologic disease		
Multiple sclerosis	D/DR2	4.1
Skin diseases		
Psoriasis vulgaris	Cw6	13.3
Pemphigus (Jews)	D/DR4	14.4
Dermatitis herpetiformis	D/DR3	15.4
Behçet's disease	B5	6.3
Systemic diseases		
Myasthenia gravis	D/DR3	2.5
	B8	2.7
Sjögren's (sicca) syndrome	D/DR3	9.7
Systemic lupus erythematosus	D/DR3	5.8
Idiopathic hemochromatosis	A3	8.2
	B14	4.7
Goodpasture's syndrome	D/DR2	15.9
Idiopathic membranous nephropathy	D/DR3	12.0

*Calculated by $\frac{a \times d}{b \times c}$, where a and b are the number of individuals with the character present or absent in the patients, and c and d are the characters present or absent in the control population.

recessive in character and controlled by a gene located 10 to 15 centimorgans outside the HLA complex (192). In either case, the studies demonstrate that the important gene or genes in iron metabolism are located close to the HLA complex. It also has been shown that the idiopathic hemochromatosis gene is in genetic linkage disequilibrium with the HLA determinants A3 and B14.

The most recent finding regarding HLA-linked disease genes is the discovery that the congenital adrenal hyperplasia 21-hydroxylase deficiency gene is possibly close to the HLA-B locus. The genes for 21-hydroxylase deficiency were separated by genetic recombination and by molecular genetic studies. The results demonstrate that genes coding for the biosynthesis of steroid hormones can be mapped within the HLA complex and near the two C4 genes, one near C4A and the other next to C4B (98–102).

The structural genes for isolated deficiency of serum complement C2 (56) and C4 (54) also are closely linked to HLA. They are located between the HLA-B and the HLA-D loci (193).

Genetic studies of patients with juvenile diabetes mellitus of the insulin-dependent type (JDM) have been controversial for many years. Here, the use of the HLA as a genetic marker system has provided new insights into the importance of genetic factors. Linkage analysis in JDM is complicated by the problems of age of onset of the disease and the degree of genetic penetrance. Some studies suggest that the JDM gene is recessive, with 50 per cent penetrance, and located close to the HLA complex (194, 195). Other studies suggest that two dominant HLA-linked genes with incomplete penetrance are involved (196).

Mechanisms in HLA-Associated Disease

The HLA and H-2 antigens appear to have an important biologic role in immune surveillance, since they can serve as substrates for viruses or chemicals that may subsequently alter these antigens by the production of an immune response. This immune response is restricted to cells bearing the same altered HLA or H-2 molecules (1–3).

The findings of absence of cell surface HLA-A and HLA-B substances in a few patients with combined immunodeficiency support the concept that HLA antigens have an immunologic role (197, 198).

Theoretically, an infectious or chemical agent can affect an individual because the inability of that individual to eliminate it due to lack of immune response. However, these agents may produce alterations of the HLA molecules, eliciting an immune reaction accompanied by elimination of altered cells. Any change in the process of elimination of the agents may be accompanied by immune dysregulation, with resulting disease (i.e., cancer or autoimmunity). The mechanisms proposed for explanation of HLA and disease association are of two general kinds: (1) the mimicry and receptor hypothesis, and (2) the Ir gene and linked locus hypothesis.

MIMICRY AND RECEPTOR HYPOTHESIS

The MHC antigens of an individual may be identical with or closely related to the structure of an antigen or antigens of an infectious agent, thus rendering the immune system unresponsive to the agent (mimicry hypothesis) (184, 198, 199).

Postinfectious arthropathy is one condition in which a high proportion of patients with HLA-B27 develop arthritis following infections with *Yersinia, Salmonella,* or *Shigella*. Because it has been found that the HLA molecule can serve as a receptor for viruses, it may be that the HLA-B27 group of diseases (ankylosing spondylitis, Reiter's syndrome, and anterior uveitis) share a common etiology in which an agent reacts either with the HLA-B27 antigen or with another HLA antigen immunologically cross-reactive with B27. Related to this hypothesis is the finding of a factor in *Klebsiella pneumoniae* that modifies HLA-B27 and that could produce a cross-reaction with some tissues (200).

IR GENE AND LINKED LOCUS HYPOTHESIS

Genes of the MHC region may be closely linked to genes whose products may or may not be involved with immune reactions but that nevertheless are involved in the pathogenesis of a disease. The associations seen between specific HLA phenotypes or an HLA haplotype and certain diseases might thus, in fact, be a reflection of linkage disequilibrium between HLA and the corresponding genes. Such associations may include monogenic disease (e.g., C2 deficiency) in which there is association to A25, B18, DR2, SCQ042, and 21-hydroxylase deficiency, in which there is association to Bw47, DR7, FC91,0 (56, 200a). The association can also be a single gene of polygenic diseases such as juvenile onset diabetes, in which there is association to B8 DR3 SC01, B18 DR3 F1C30, and/or B62 DR4 SC33 (201).

Interpretation of the MHC disease association is complicated by the fact that in almost all cases the causative agent is unknown. Most of the known associations are with determinants controlled by the HLA-B locus, but this fact also could be the result of a defective human immune response locus. For example, in Japanese patients, the haplotype Bw54, DYT, DR4 is associated with high responses to antigens, defects of suppressor cells, and susceptibility to juvenile onset diabetes and rheumatoid arthritis (202).

Difficulties of single mechanisms to explain most HLA disease associations are to be expected, since the development of a disease is a complex process influenced by many factors, environmental as well as genetic.

As described, molecular biology has provided both a new approach to the study of the genetics of MHC and the possibility of identifying susceptibility or resistance to diseases. For example, the use of several restriction endonucleases and MHC probes with the Southern blot technique should provide genetic information that will explain MHC and disease associations (203).

CONCLUSIONS

This chapter has reviewed the basic principles and present state of knowledge in the rapidly developing field of human immunogenetics and transplantation immunology. It has not attempted to offer a comprehensive review of this extensive area but should provide the reader with the necessary fundamental information, including references to original publications as well as references to comprehensive review articles covering particularly important areas.

The practical applications of immunogenetics to clinical medicine are at present limited to clinical transplantation, blood transfusion therapy, and certain diagnostic procedures for HLA-linked diseases. The elucidation of the genetic composition of the HLA region and of the role of the gene products in immunoregulation and disease susceptibility has provided significant insights into important regulatory functions in health and diseases. It is to be expected that application of molecular biology to the study of expression and regulation of the HLA genes will provide the tools necessary for further practical application of immunogenetics in clinical medicine.

Molecular biology of the MHC genes has also provided a new approach to the study of the defense mechanisms of the organism against foreign invaders. Restriction enzymes that digest the DNA molecules have already produced a large number of polymorphic fragments that carry HLA genes and possibly genes of susceptibility or resistance to diseases. It has become possible to redefine the known associations of these fragments with several diseases, and it is hoped that with this new technology new polymorphic markers (within or outside MHC) will be more closely associated with susceptibility or resistance to diseases. Furthermore, it will be possible with these tools to find new DNA polymorphisms that will be associated with diseases and thus to discover the interactions of genes of various susceptibilities which in turn will explain the genetic basis of polygenic diseases.

ACKNOWLEDGEMENTS

The authors thank Dr. Elizabeth Slater for her expert editing assistance, Mrs. Ada Watson for her assistance in drawing the figures, and also Mrs. Judy Boyer for her help in typing many drafts of the manuscript.

References

1. Klein, J.: The major histocompatibility complex. In *Immunology: The Science of Self and Non-Self Discrimination*. A Wiley-Inter-Science Publ., New York, John Wiley & Sons, 1982, p. 270.
2. Zinkernagel, R. M., and Doherty, P. C.: Restriction of in vitro T cell–mediated cytotoxicity in lymphocytic choriomeningitis within a syngeneic or semi-allogeneic system. Nature 248:701, 1974.
3. Zinkernagel, R. M., and Doherty, P. C.: MHC-restricted cytotoxic T cells: studies on the biological role of the polymorphic major transplantation antigens determining T-cell restriction-specificity, function and responsiveness. Adv. Immunol. 27:51, 1979.
4. Cantor, H., and Boyse, E. A.: Functional subclasses of T lymphocytes bearing different Ly antigens. II. Cooperation between subclasses of Ly and Ly+ cells in the generation of killer activity. J. Exp. Med. 141:1390, 1975.
5. Nomenclature Committee IUIS/WHO, Leukocyte Differentiation Antigens. In *Leukocyte Typing*. Barnard, A., Bounsell, L., et al. (eds.), Berlin, Springer-Verlag, 1984, p. 133.
6. Flomenberg, N., Naito, K., et al.: Allocytotoxic T cell clones: both Leu 2+3− and Leu 2−3+ T cells recognize class I histocompatibility antigens. Eur. J. Immunol. 13:905, 1983.
7. Levine, B. B., Ojeda, A., et al.: Studies on artificial antigens. III. The genetic control of the immune response to hapten poly-L-lysine conjugates in guinea pigs. J. Exp. Med. 118:953, 1963.
8. McDevitt, H. O., and Chinitz, A.: Genetic control of the antibody response: relationships between immune response and histocompatibility (H-2) type. Science 163:1207, 1969.
9. Dorf, M. E., and Benacerraf, B.: Suppressor cells and immunoregulation. Ann. Rev. Immunol. 2:127, 1984.
10. Gershon, K. K., and Kondo, K.: Cell interactions in the induction of tolerance: the role of thymic lymphocytes. Immunology 18:732, 1970.
11. Gorer, P. A.: The detection of antigenic differences in mouse erythrocytes by the employment of immune sera. Br. J. Exp. Pathol. 17:42, 1936.
12. Gorer, P. A., Lyman, S., et al.: Studies on the genetic and antigenic basis of tumor transplantation: linkage between a histocompatibility gene and "fused" genes in mice. Proc. R. Soc. 135:499, 1948.
13. Snell, G. D.: Methods for the study of histocompatibility genes. J. Genetics 49:87, 1948.
14. Shreffler, D. C., and David, C. S.: The H-2 major histocompatibility complex and the immune response region: genetic variation, function, and organization. Adv. Immunol. 20:125, 1975.
15. Francke, U., and Pellegrino, M. A.: Assignment of the major histocompatibility complex to a region of the short arm of chromosome 6. Proc. Natl. Acad. Sci. USA 74:1147, 1977.
16. WHO Committee, Bodmer, W. F., Albert, E., et al.: Nomenclature for factors of the HLA system. Vox Sang. 48:42, 1985.
17. Dupont, B., Hansen, J. A., et al.: Human mixed lymphocyte culture reaction: genetics, specificity and biological implications. Adv. Immunol. 23:107, 1976.
18. Shaw, S., Johnson, A. H., et al.: Evidence for a new segment series of B cell antigens that are encoded in the HLA-D region and that stimulate secondary allogeneic proliferation and cytotoxic responses. J. Exp. Med. 12:565, 1980.
19. Cepellini, R., Curtoni, E. S., et al.: Genetics of leukocyte antigens. A family study of segregation and linkage. In *Histocompatibility Testing 1967*. Curtoni, E. S., Mattiuz, P. L., et al. (eds.), Copenhagen, Munksgaard, 1967, p. 149.
20. Dausset, J., Colombani, J., et al.: Genetics of the HL-A system: deduction of 480 haplotypes. In *Histocompatibility Testing 1970*. Terasaki, P. I. (ed.), Copenhagen, Munksgaard, 1970, p. 53.
21. Allen, F. H., Jr.: Linkage of HL-A and GBG. Vox Sang. 27:382, 1974.
22. Fu, S. M., Kunkel, H. G., et al.: Evidence for linkage between HLA histocompatibility genes and those involved in the synthesis of the second component of complement. J. Exp. Med. 140:1108, 1974.
23. Rittner, C., Hauptman, G., et al.: Linkage between HLA and genes controlling the synthesis of the fourth component of complement. In *Histocompatibility Testing 1975*. Kissmeyer-Nielsen, F., (ed.), Copenhagen, Munksgaard, 1975, pp. 945–954.
24. Dupont, B., Oberfield, S. E., et al.: Close genetic linkage between HLA and congenital adrenal hyperplasia (21-hydroxylase deficiency). Lancet 2:1309, 1977.
25. McMichael, A. J., Pilch, J. R., et al.: A human thymocyte antigen defined by a hybrid myeloma monoclonal antibody. Eur. J. Immunol. 9:205, 1979.
26. Emery, A. E. H.: Elements of Medical Genetics, 6th ed. New York, Churchill Livingstone, 1983.
27. Loh, D. Y., and Baltimore D.: Sexual preference of apparent gene conversion events in MHC genes of mice. Nature 30:639, 1984.
28. Black, F. L., and Slazano, F. M.: Evidence for heterosis in the HLA system. Am. J. Hum. Genet. 33:894, 1981.
29. Terasaki, P. I., and McClelland, J. D.: Microdroplet assay of human serum cytotoxins. Nature 204:998, 1964.
30. Yunis, E. J., and Amos, D. B.: Three closely linked genetic systems relevant to transplantation. Proc. Natl. Acad. Sci. USA 68:3031, 1971.
31. Dupont, B., Jersild, C., et al.: Typing for MLC determinants by means of LD-homozygous and LD-heterozygous test cells. Transpl. Proc. 5:1543, 1973.
32. Van Leeuwen, A., Schuit, H. R. E., et al.: Typing for MLC (LD). II. The selection of nonstimulator cells by MLC inhibition tests using SD-identical stimulator cells (MISIS) and fluorescence antibody studies. Transpl. Proc. 5:1539, 1973.
33. Bodmer, W., Batchelor, J. R., et al. (eds.): Nomenclature for factors of the HLA system—1977. WHO-IUIS Terminology Committee in Histocompatibility Testing, Copenhagen, Munksgaard, 1978, p. 14.
34. Tosi, R., Tanigaki, N., et al.: Immunological dissection of human Ia molecules. J. Exp. Med. 148:1592, 1978.
35. Duquesnoy, R. J., Marrari, M., et al.: Identification of an HLA-DR associated system of B cell alloantigens. Transpl. Proc. 11:1757, 1979.
36. Fradelizi, D., and Dausset, J.: Mixed lymphocyte reactivity of human lymphocytes primed in vitro. I. Secondary

response to allogeneic lymphocytes. Eur. J. Immunol. 5:295, 1975.
37. Sheehy, J. J., Sondel, P. M., et al.: HLA-LD (lymphocyte defined) typing: a rapid assay using primed lymphocytes. Science 188:1308, 1975.
38. Mawas, C., Charmot, D., et al.: Secondary responses of in vitro primed human lymphocytes to allogenic cells. I. Role of the HLA antigens and mixed lymphocyte reaction stimulating determinants in secondary in vitro proliferative response. Immunogenetics 2:449, 1975.
39. Termijtelen, A., Van der Berge, S. J., et al.: LB-Q1 and LB-Q2. Two determinants defined in the primed lymphocyte test and independent of HLA/D/R, MB/LB-E or SB. Hum. Immunol. 8:11, 1983.
40. Wank, R., Schendel D. J., et al.: Two different HLA restimulating determinants separated by recombination and titration. Transpl. Proc. 9:1729, 1977.
41. Fuller, T. C., Einarson, M. E., et al.: Genetic evidence that HLA-DR (Ia) specificities include multiple HLA-D determinants on a single haplotype. Transpl. Proc. 10:781, 1978.
42. Robinson, M. A., Long, E. O., et al.: Recombination within the HLA-D region. J. Exp. Med. 160:222, 1984.
43. Roux-Desseta, M., Huffray, D., et al.: Genetic mapping of a human Class II antigen β-chain cDNA clone to the SB region of the HLA complex. Proc. Natl. Acad. Sci. USA 80:6036, 1983.
44. Nadler, L. M., Slashenko, P., et al.: Monoclonal antibody: identifies a new Ia-like (p 29, 34) polymorphic system linked to the HLA/DR region. Nature 290:591, 1981.
45. Hurley, C. K., Shaw, S., et al.: Alpha and beta chains of SB and DR antigens are structurally distinct. J. Exp. Med. 156:1557, 1982.
46. Bodmer, J. G., Rocques, P., et al.: Joint report of the Fifth International Histocompatibility Workshop. In Histocompatability Testing 1972. Dausset, J., and Colombani, J. (eds.), Copenhagen, Munksgaard, 1973, p. 619.
47. Alper, C. A., Raum, D., et al.: Serum complement "supergenes" on the major histocompatibility complex in man (complotypes). Vox Sang. 45:65, 1983.
48. Awdeh, Z. L., Raum, D., et al.: Extended HLA/complement allele haplotypes: evidence for T/t-like complex in man. Proc. Natl. Acad. Sci. USA 80:259, 1983.
49. Fleischnick, E., Awdeh, Z. L., et al.: Extended MHC haplotypes in 21-hydroxylase-deficiency cogenital adrenal hyperplasia: shared genotypes in unrelated patients. Lancet 1:152, 1983.
50. Dunn, L. C.: A test for genetic factors influencing abnormal segregation ratios in the house mouse. Genetics 28:29, 1943.
51. Bennett, D., Alton, A. K., et al.: Genetic analysis of transmission ratio distortion by T-haplotypes in the mouse. Genet. Res. 41:29, 1983.
52. O'Neill, G. J., Yang, S. Y., et al.: Chido and Rodgers blood groups are district antigenic components of human complement, C4. Nature (Lond.) 273:668, 1978.
53. Awdeh, Z. L., Raum, D. D., et al.: Genetic polymorphism of the fourth component of human complement: detection of heterozygotes. Nature (Lond.) 282:205, 1979.
54. Ochs, H. D., Rosenfeld, S. I., et al.: Linkage between the gene(s) controlling synthesis of the fourth component of complement (C4) and the major histocompatibility loci. New Engl. J. Med. 296:470, 1977.
55. Awdeh, Z. L., Ochs, H. D., et al.: Genetic analysis of C4 deficiency. J. Clin. Invest. 67:260, 1981.
56. Alper, C. A., Awdeh, Z. L., et al.: Complement genes of the human major histocompatibility complex: implications for linkage disequilibrium and disease associations. In Immunogenetics. Panayi, G. S., and David, C. S. (eds.), London, Butterworths, 1984, pp. 50–91.
57. New, M. I., Dupont, B., et al.: Congenital adrenal hyperplasia and related conditions. In The Metabolic Basis of Inherited Diseases, 5th ed. Stanbury, J. G., Wyngaarden, J. B., et al. (eds.), New York, McGraw-Hill, 1983, pp. 973–1000.
58. Nunez, G., Giles, R. C., et al.: Expression of HLA-DR, MB, MT and SB antigens on human mononuclear cells: identification of two phenotypically distinct monocyte populations. J. Immunol. 133:1300, 1984.
59. Rouse, R. V., Van Ewijk, W., et al.: Expression of MHC antigens by mouse thymic dendritic cells. J. Immunol. 122:2508, 1979.
60. Van Ewijk, W., Rouse, R. V., et al.: Distribution of H-2 micro-environments in the mouse thymus. J. Histochem. Cytochem. 28:1089, 1980.
61. Rouse, R. V., Parham, P., et al.: Expression of HLA antigens by human thymic epithelial cells. Hum. Immunol. 5:21, 1982.
62. Broxmeyer, H. E., and Dupont, B.: A role for Class II major histocompatibility complex antigens in the regulation of myelopoiesis. Prog. Allergy 36:203, 1985.
63. Basch, R. S., Janossy, G., et al.: Murine pluripotential stem cells lack Ia antigen. Nature (Lond.) 270:520, 1977.
64. Moore, M. A. S., Broxmeyer, H. E., et al.: Continuous human bone marrow culture: Ia antigen characterization of probable pluripotential stem cells. Blood 55:682, 1980.
65. Fitchen, J. H., Lefevre, C., et al.: Expression of Ia-like and HLA-A, B antigens on human multipotential hematopoietic progenitor cells. Blood 59:1880, 1982.
66. Lu, L., Broxmeyer, H. E., et al.: Association of cell cycle expression of Ia-like antigenic determinants on normal human multipotential (CFU-GEMM) and erythroid (BFU-E) progenitor cells with regulation in vitro by acidic isoferritins. Blood 61:250, 1983.
67. Winchester, R. J., Ross, G. D., et al.: Expression of Ia-like antigen molecules on human granulocytes during early phases of differentiation. Proc. Natl. Acad. Sci. USA 74:4012, 1977.
68. Janossy, G., Francis, G., et al.: Cell sorter analysis of leukemia-associated antigens on human myeloid precursors. Nature (Lond.) 276:176, 1978.
69. Winchester, R. J., Meyers, P. A., et al.: Inhibition of human erythropoietic colony formation by treatment with Ia antisera. J. Exp. Med. 148:613, 1978.
70. Broxmeyer, H. E.: Relationship of cell-cycle expression of Ia-like antigenic determinants on normal and leukemia human granulocyte-macrophage progenitor cells to regulation in vitro by acidic isoferritins. J. Clin. Invest. 69:632, 1982.
71. Broxmeyer, H. E.: Association of the sensitivity of mouse granulocyte-macrophage progenitor cells to inhibition by acidic isoferritins with expression of Ia antigens for I-A and I-E/C subregions during DNA synthesis. J. Immunol. 129:1002, 1982.
72. Torok-Storb, B., Nepom, G. T., et al.: HLA-DR antigens on lymphoid cells differ from those on myeloid cells. Nature (Lond.) 305:541, 1983.
73. Lipton, J. M., Nadler, L. M., et al.: Evidence for genetic restriction in the suppression in erythropoiesis by T lymphocytes in man. J. Clin. Invest. 72:649, 1983.
74. Evans, R. L., Faldetta, R. J., et al.: Peripheral human T cells sensitized in mixed lymphocyte culture synthesize and express Ia-like antigens. J. Exp. Med. 148:1440, 1978.
75. Wilson, B. S., Indiveri, F., et al.: DR (Ia-like) antigens on human melanoma cells. Serological detection and immunochemical characterization. J. Exp. Med. 149:658, 1979.
76. Winchester, R. J., Wang, C. Y., et al.: Expression of Ia-like antigens on cultured human malignant melanoma cell lines. Proc. Natl. Acad. Sci. USA 75:6235, 1978.
77. Pober, J. S., Collins, T., et al.: Lymphocytes recognize human vascular endothelial and dermal fibroblast Ia antigens induced by recombinant immune interferon. Nature 305:726, 1983.
78. Houghton, A. N., Thomson, T. M., et al.: Surface antigens on melanoma and melanocytes. Specificity of induc-

tion of Ia antigens by human interferon. J. Exp. Med. *160*:255, 1984.
79. Goodfellow, P. N., Jones, E. A., et al.: The β2 microglobulin gene is on chromosome 15 and not in the HLA region. Nature *254*:267, 1975.
80. Parham, P., Coppin, H., et al.: Biochemical approaches to understanding the structure and function of Class I MHC (HLA-A,B,C molecules). In *Lymphocyte Surface Antigens 1984*. ASHI Publication, Tenth Annual Meeting, pp. 1–34, 1984.
81. Humphreys, R. E., McCune, J. M., et al.: Isolation and immunologic characterization of a human B-lymphocyte-specific, cell surface antigen. J. Exp. Med. *144*:98, 1976.
82. Springer, T. A., Kaufman, J. F., et al.: Purification of HLA-linked B lymphocyte alloantigens in immunologically active form by preparative sodium dodicylsulfate-gel electrophoresis and studies on their subunit association. J. Biol. Chem. *252*:6201, 1977.
83. Hood, L., Steinmetz, M. et al.: Genes of the major histocompatibility complex of the mouse. Ann. Rev. Immunol. *1*:529, 1983.
84. Malissen, M., Damotte, M., et al.: HLA cosmid clones show complete, widely spaced human class I genes with occasional clusters. Gene *20*:485, 1982.
85. Malissen, M., Malissen, B., et al.: Exon/intron organization and complete nucleotide sequence of an HLA gene. Proc. Natl. Acad. Sci. USA *79*:893, 1982.
86. Brickell, P. M., Latchman, D. S., et al.: Activation of a Qa/TLa class I histocompatibility antigen gene is a general feature of oncogenes in the mouse. Nature *306*:756, 1983.
87. Orr, H. T., Lancet, D., et al.: The heavy chain of human histocompatibility antigen HLA-B7 contains an immunoglobulin-like region. Nature *282*:266, 1979.
88. Wake, C. T., Widera, G., et al.: Organization and expression of the murine MHC. In *Advances in Gene Technology: Molecular Biology of the Immune System*. ISU Short Reports, Vol. 2. Streilin, J. W., et al. (eds.), New York, Cambridge University Press, 1985, pp. 33–36.
89. Lee, J. S., Trosdale, J., et al.: Sequence of an HLA-DRα chain cDNA clone and intron-exon organization of the corresponding gene. Nature *299*:750, 1982.
90. Korman, A. J., Auffray, G., et al.: The amino acid sequence and gene organization of the heavy chain of the HLA-DR antigen: homology to immunoglobulins. Proc. Natl. Acad. Sci. USA *79*:6013, 1982.
91. Larhammar, D., Schenning, L., et al.: Complete amino acid sequence of an HLA DR antigen like β chain as predicted from the nucleotide sequence: similarities with immunoglobulins and HLA -A, -B, and -C antigens. Proc. Natl. Acad. Sci. USA *79*:3687, 1982.
92. Long, E. O., Wake, C. T., et al.: Complete sequence of an HLA-DR β chain genes. EMBO *2*:384, 1983.
92a. Hardy, D. A., Bell, J. I., et al.: Mapping of the class-II region of the human major histocompatibility complex by pulse-field gel electrophoresis. Nature *323*:453, 1986.
93. Carroll, M. C., and Porter, R. R.: Cloning of human complement component C4 gene. Proc. Natl. Acad. Sci. USA *80*:264, 1983.
94. Carroll, M. C., Campbell, R. D., et al.: A molecular map of the human major histocompatibility complex class III region linking complement genes C4, C2 and factor B. Nature *307*:237, 1984.
95. Chaplin, D. D., Woods, D. E., et al.: Molecular map of the murine S region. Proc. Natl. Acad. Sci. USA *80*:6947, 1983.
96. Carroll, M. C., Belt, T., et al.: Structure and organization of the C4 genes. Phil. Trans. R. Soc. Lond. *306*:379, 1984.
97. Belt, K. T., Carroll, M. C., et al.: The structural basis of the multiple forms of human complement component C4. Cell *36*:907, 1984.
98. White, P. C., New, M. I., et al.: Cloning and expression of cDNA encoding a bovine adrenal cytochrome P-450 specific for steroid 21-hydroxylation. Proc. Natl. Acad. Sci. USA *81*:1986, 1984.
99. White, P. C., New, M. I., et al.: HLA-linked congenital adrenal hyperplasia results from a defective gene encoding a cytochrome P-450. Proc. Natl. Acad. Sci. USA *81*:7505, 1984.
100. White, P. C., Chaplin, D. D., et al.: Two steroid 21-hydroxylase genes are located in the murine S region. Nature *312*:465, 1984.
101. Carroll, M. C., Campbell, R. D., et al.: Mapping of steroid 21-hydroxylase genes adjacent to complement component C4 genes in HLA, the major histocompatibility complex in man. Proc. Natl. Acad. Sci. USA *82*:521, 1985.
102. White, P. C., Grossberger, D., et al.: Two genes encoding steroid 21-hydroxylase and located near the genes encoding the fourth component of complement in man. Proc. Natl. Acad. Sci. USA *82*:1089, 1985.
103. Southern, E.: Detection of specific sequences among DNA fragments separated by gel electrophoresis. J. Mol. Biol. *98*:503, 1975.
104. Orr, H. T.: Use of Southern blotting to analyze the size and restriction fragment polymorphism of HLA class I DNA in the human population. Transpl. Proc. *15*:1900, 1983.
105. Cann, H. M., Ascanio, L., et al.: Polymorphic restriction endonuclease fragment segregates and correlates with the gene for HLA-B8. Proc. Natl. Acad. Sci. USA *80*:1665, 1983.
106. Cohen, D., Paul, P., et al.: Analysis of HLA class I genes with restriction endonuclease fragments: implications for polymorphism of the human major histocompatibility complex. Proc. Natl. Acad. Sci. USA *80*:6289, 1983.
107. Auffray, C., Lillie, J. W., et al.: Isotypic and allotypic variation of human class II histocompatibility antigen x-chain genes. Nature *308*:327, 1984.
108. Wake, C. T., Long, E. O., et al.: Allelic polymorphism and complexity of the genes for HLA-DR β-chains—direct analysis by DNA-DNA hybridization. Nature *300*:372, 1982.
109. Spielman, R. S., Lee, J. S., et al.: Six HLA-D regional alpha-chain genes on human chromosome 6: polymorphisms and associations of DC alpha-related sequences with DR types. Proc. Natl. Acad. Sci. USA *81*:3461, 1984.
110. Smithies, O., and Poulik, M. D.: Initiation of protein synthesis at an unusual position in an immunoglobulin gene? Science *175*:187, 1972.
111. Peterson, P. A., Cunningham, B. A., et al.: B2 immunoglobulin a free immunoglobulin domain. Proc. Natl. Acad. Sci. USA *69*:1697, 1972.
112. Strominger, J. L.: Structure of products of the major histocompatibility complex in man and mouse. Prog. Immunol. *4*:541, 1980.
113. Hendrick, S. M., Cohen, D. I., et al.: Isolation of cDNA clones encoding T cell–specific membrane-associated proteins. Nature *308*:149, 1984.
114. Yanagi, Y., Yasunobu, Y., et al.: A human T cell–specific cDNA clone encodes a protein having extensive homology to immunoglobulin chains. Nature *308*:145, 1984.
115. Saito, M., Dranz, D. M., et al.: A third rearranged and expressed gene in a clone of cytotoxic T lymphocytes. Nature *312*:36, 1984.
116. Opelz, G., Mickey, M. R., et al.: Calculations on long-term graft and patient survival in human kidney transplantation. Transpl. Proc. *9*:27, 1977.
117. Dausset, J., Hors, J., et al.: Serologically defined HL-A antigens and long-term survival of cadaver kidney transplants. New Engl. J. Med. *290*:979, 1974.
118. Scandiatransplant Report: HLA matching and kidney graft survival. Lancet *1*:240, 1975.
119. Simmons, R. I., Yunis, E. J., et al.: 115 patients with first cadaver kidney transplants followed two to seven and a

119. half years. A multifactorial analysis. Am. J. Med. 62:234, 1977.
120. Carpenter, C. B., and Milford, E. L.: Renal transplantation: immunology. In *The Kidney*, 2nd ed. Brenner, B., and Rector, F. (eds.), Philadelphia, W. B. Saunders Co., 1986.
121. Moraes, J. R., and Stasny, P. J.: A new antigen system expressed in human endothelial cells. J. Clin. Invest. 60:449, 1977.
122. Opelz, G.: Report of the International Collaborative Transplant Study. Ninth International Histocompatibility Workshop Renal Transplantation Study. In *Histocompatibility Testing, 1984*. Albert, E. D., Baur, M. P., et al. (eds.), New York, Springer-Verlag, 1984, pp. 342–347.
123. Hendricks, G. F. J., Persijn, G. G., et al.: HLA-DRw6 positive recipients are high responders in renal transplantation. Transplant. Proceed. 15:1136, 1983.
124. European Multicenter Trial Group: Cyclosporin A as sole immunosuppressive agent in recipients of renal allografts from cadaver donors. Preliminary results of a European Multicenter Trial. Lancet 2:57, 1982.
125. Canadian Transplant Study Group: A randomized clinical trial of cyclosporine in cadaveric renal transplantation. New Engl. J. Med. 309:809, 1983.
126. Tilney, N. L., Milford, E. L., et al.: Experience with cyclosporine and steroids in clinical renal transplantation. Ann. Surg. 200:605, 1984.
127. Harmon, W. E., Parkman, R., et al.: Comparison of cell-mediated lympholysis and mixed lymphocyte culture in the immunologic evaluation for renal transplantation. J. Immunol. 129:1573, 1982.
128. Cochrum, K. C., Perkins, M. A., et al.: The correlation of MLC with graft survival. Transplant. Proc. 5:391, 1973.
129. Opelz, G., and Terasaki, P. I.: Significance of mixed leukocyte culture testing in cadaver kidney transplantation. Transplantation 23:375, 1966.
130. Walker, J., Opelz, G., et al.: Correlation of MLC response with graft survival in cadaver and related donor kidney transplants. Transpl. Proc. 10:949, 1978.
131. Ceppellini, R., Curtoni, E. S., et al.: Survival of test skin graft in man. Effect of genetic relationship and of blood group incompatibility. Ann. NY Acad. Sci. 129:421, 1966.
132. Gleason, R. E., and Murray, J. E.: Analysis of variables in the function of human kidney transplants. I. Blood group compatibility and transplantation. Report from Kidney Transplant Registry 5:343, 1967.
133. Kissmeyer-Nielsen, F., Olsen, S., et al.: Hyperacute rejection of kidney allografts associated with pre-existing humoral antibodies against donor cells. Lancet 2:662, 1966.
134. Milgrom, F., Litvak, B. I., et al.: Humoral antibodies in renal homografts. J.A.M.A. 198:136, 1966.
135. Carpenter, C. B., and Morris, P. J.: The detection and measurement of pretransplant sensitization. Transpl. Proc. 10:509, 1978.
136. Garavoy, M. R., Colombe, B. W., et al.: Flow cytometry crossmatching for donor-specific transfusion recipients and cadaveric transplantation. Transpl. Proc. 17:673, 1975.
137. Cardella, C. J., Falk, J. A., et al.: Do repeated blood transfusions prevent successful transplantation in highly sensitized potential transplant recipients? Lancet 2:1240, 1982.
138. Falk, J. A., Cardella, C. J., et al.: Transplantation can be performed with positive (nonconcurrent) crossmatch. Transpl. Proc. 16:1533, 1985.
139. Thorsby, E.: On the antibody crossmatch controversies. Transpl. Proc. 16:1533, 1985.
140. Cochrum, K., Hanes, D., et al.: Improved graft survival with donor-specific transfusion pre-treatment. Transpl. Proc. 13:190, 1981.
141. Opelz, G.: For the collaborative transplant study. Current relevance of the transfusion effect in renal transplantation. Transpl. Proc. 10:1015, 1985.
142. Kahan, B.: Immunologic monitoring: utility and limitations. Transpl. Proc. 16:1537, 1985.
143. Kovithavongs, T., and Dossetor, J. B.: Lack of HLA restriction of immune events in HLA identical grafts: speculation on specificity of cytotoxic effector cells in peripheral blood. Transpl. Proc. 15:1804, 1983.
144. Gailiunas, P., Busch, G., et al.: Prediction of reversibility of renal allograft rejection. Transpl. Proc. 11:17, 1979.
145. Gailiunas, P., Suthanthiran, M., et al.: Immunologic monitoring in the diagnosis of renal allograft rejection. Transpl. Proc. 9:1823, 1977.
146. Charpentier, B. M., Bach, M., et al.: Expression of OKT8 antigen and Fc receptors by suppressor cells mediating specific unresponsiveness between recipient and donor on renal-allograft-tolerant patients. Transplantation 36:495, 1983.
147. Charpentier, B., Lang, P., et al.: Specific recipient-donor unresponsiveness mediated by a suppressor cell system in human kidney allograft tolerance. Transplantation 36:495, 1983.
148. Suciu-Foca, N., Rohowsky, C., et al.: MHC-specific idiotypes on alloactivated human T-cells: *in vivo* and *in vitro* studies. Transpl. Proc. 15:784, 1983.
149. Thomas, J. H., Pierce, G. E., et al.: Spontaneous blastogenesis as a monitor of renal allograft rejection. Transplant. Proc. 15:1823, 1983.
150. Lotze, M. T., Marquis, D. M., et al.: Two new assays for the early detection of transplant rejection: Il-2 response and PHA-augmented NK activity. Transpl. Proc. 15:1796, 1983.
151. Simmons, R. L., Kjellstrand, C. M., et al.: Kidney transplantation. In *Tissue Typing and Organ Transplantation*. Yunis, E. J., Gatti, R. A., et al. (eds.), New York, Academic Press, 1973, p. 165.
152. Milford, E. L.: Advance in kidney transplantation. Cyclosporin and T12.AKF. Nephrol. Let. 1:5, 1984.
153. Reeve, C. E., Harley, F., et al.: A randomized trial of cyclosporin in cadaveric renal transplantation. Canadian Multicenter Transplant Study Group. New Engl. J. Med. 309:809, 1983.
154. Harder, F., Loertscher, R., et al.: Cyclosporin in cadaveric renal transplantation: one year follow up of a multicenter trial. European Multicenter Trial Group. Lancet 2:986, 1983.
155. Illner, W. D., Land, W., et al.: Cyclosporine in combination with azathioprine and steroids in cadaveric renal transplantation. Transpl. Proc. 17:1181, 1985.
156. Morris, P. J., French, M. E., et al.: A controlled trial of cyclosporine in renal transplantation with conversion to azathioprine and prednisone after three months. Transplantation 36:273, 1983.
157. Calne, R. Y.: Clinical transplantation summary. Transpl. Proc. 16:1599, 1985.
158. Wechter, W. J., Morrell, R. M., et al.: Extended treatment with antithymocyte globulin (ATGAM) in renal allograft recipients. Transplantation 28:365, 1979.
159. Kirkman, R. L., Araujo, J. L., et al.: Treatment of acute renal allograft rejection with monoclonal anti-T12 antibody. Transplantation 36:620, 1983.
160. Cosimi, A. B., Burton, R. C., et al.: Treatment of acute renal allograft rejection with OKT3 monoclonal antibody. Transplantation 32:535, 1981.
161. Thomas, E. O.: Marrow transplantation for malignant diseases. J. Clin. Oncol. 1:517, 1983.
162. O'Reilly, R. J.: Allogeneic bone marrow transplantation: current status and future directions. Blood 62:941, 1983.
163. Fefer, A., Einstein, A. B., et al.: Bone marrow transplantation for hematologic neoplasia in 16 patients with identical twins. New Engl. J. Med. 290:1389, 1974.
164. Thomas, E. D., Buckner, C. D., et al.: One hundred patients with acute leukemia treated by chemotherapy, total body irradiation and allogeneic marrow transplantation. Blood 49:511, 1977.

165. Storb, R., Prentice, R. L., et al.: Treatment of aplastic anemia by marrow transplantation from HLA identical siblings. J. Clin. Invest. 59:625, 1977.
166. Simes, M. A., Johannsson, E., et al.: Scleroderma-like graft-versus-host disease as late consequences of bone marrow transplantation. Lancet 2:831, 1977.
167. Gratwohl, A. A., Moutsopoulos, H. M., et al.: Sjögren-type syndrome after allogeneic bone marrow transplantation. Ann. Intern. Med. 87:703, 1977.
168. Shulman, H. M., Sullivan, K. M., et al.: Chronic graft-versus-host syndrome in man: a clinico-pathological study of 20 long-term Seattle patients. Am. J. Med. 69:204, 1980.
169. O'Reilly, R. J., Reich, L., et al.: A randomized trial of intravenous hyperimmune globulin for the prevention of cytomegalovirus (CMV) infections following marrow transplantation. Preliminary results. Transpl. Proc. 15:1405, 1983.
170. Koch, C., Henriksen, K., et al.: Bone marrow transplantation from an HL-A non-identical but MLC identical donor. Lancet 1:1146, 1973.
171. O'Reilly, R. J., Dupont, B., et al.: Reconstitution in severe combined immunodeficiency by transplantation of marrow from an unrelated donor. New Engl. J. Med. 297:1311, 1977.
172. Dupont, B., O'Reilly, R. J., et al.: Use of HLA genotypically different donors in bone marrow transplantation. 7th International Conference of the Transplantation Society, Rome, 1978. Transpl. Proc. 11:219, 1979.
173. Clift, R. A., Hansen, J. A., et al.: Marrow transplantation from donors other than HLA-identical siblings. Transplantation 28:235, 1979.
174. Hansen, J. A., Clift, R. A., et al.: Marrow transplantation from donors other than HLA identical siblings. Hum. Immunol. 1:31, 1981.
175. Clift, R. A., and Hansen, J. A.: The role of HLA in clinical bone marrow transplantation. Blume, K. G., and Petz, L. D. (eds.), New York, Churchill Livingstone, 1983, pp. 313–329.
176. Rodt, H., Thierfelder, S., et al.: Anti-lymphocyte antibodies and marrow transplantation. Eur. J. Immunol. 4:25, 1974.
177. Rodt, H., Kolb, H., et al.: GVHD suppression by incubation of bone marrow grafts with anti-T-cell globulin: effect in the canine model and application to clinical bone marrow transplantation. Transpl. Proc. 11:962, 1979.
178. Vallera, D. A., Soderling, C., et al.: Bone marrow transplantation across major histocompatibility barriers in mice. Transplantation 31:218, 1981.
179. Reisner, Y., Kapoor, N., et al.: Transplantation for acute leukemia with HLA-A and B non-identical parental marrow cells fractionated with soybean agglutinin and sheep red blood cells. Lancet 2:327, 1981.
180. O'Reilly, R. J., Collins, N., et al.: Transplantation of HLA–non-identical marrow depleted of T-cells by soybean lectin agglutination and E-rosette depletion: possible major histocompatibility complex related graft resistance in leukemia transplant recipients. Transpl. Proc. 17:455, 1985.
181. Reinherz, E. L., Geha, R., et al.: Reconstitution after transplantation with T-lymphocyte–depleted HLA haplotype-mismatched bone marrow for severe combined immunodeficiency. Proc. Natl. Acad. Sci. USA 79:6047, 1982.
182. Vallera, D. A., Youle, R. J., et al.: Monoclonal antibody toxin conjugates for experimental graft-versus-host disease prophylaxis. Transplantation 36:73, 1983.
183. Filopovich, A. H., Vallera, D. A., et al.: Ex-vivo treatment of donor bone marrow with anti–T-cell immunotoxins for prevention of graft-versus-host disease. Lancet 1:469, 1984.
184. Lilly, F.: The inheritance of susceptibility to the gross leukemia virus in mice. Genetics 53:529, 1966.
185. Svejgaard, A.: HLA and disease. In *Manual of Clinical Immunology*, 3rd ed. Washington, D.C., American Society for Microbiology, 1986, pp. 912–920.
186. Svejgaard, A., and Ryder, L. P.: Association between HLA and disease. In *HLA and Disease*. Dausset, J., and Svejgaard, A. (eds.), Copenhagen, Munksgaard, 1977, pp. 46–53.
187. Maynard-Smith, S., Penrose, L. S., et al.: *Mathematical Tables for Research Workers in Human Genetics*. London, J. & A. Churchill, 1961, pp. 47–71.
188. Fotino, M., Haymovits, A., et al.: Evidence for linkage between HLA and Paget's disease. Transpl. Proc. 9:1867, 1977.
189. Jackson, J. F., Currier, R. D., et al.: Spinocerebellar ataxia and HLA linkage. New Engl. J. Med. 296:1138, 1977.
190. McKusick, V. A.: *Mendelian Inheritance in Man*, 4th edition. Baltimore, The Johns Hopkins University Press, 1975, p. 124.
191. Cartwright, G. E., Edwards, C. Q., et al.: Hereditary hemochromatosis: phenotypic expression of the disease. New Engl. J. Med. 301:175, 1979.
192. Simon, M., Bourel, M., et al.: Idiopathic hemochromatosis. Demonstration of recessive transmission and early detection by family HLA typing. New Engl. J. Med. 297:1017, 1977.
193. Yunis, E. J., Awdeh, Z., et al.: Complotype genetic loci segregate more frequently with HLA-DR than with HLA-B. Immunogenetics 21:25, 1985.
194. Barbosa, J., Chern, M. M., et al.: Analysis of linkage between the major histocompatibility system and juvenile insulin-dependent diabetes in multiplex families. J. Clin. Invest. 62:492, 1978.
195. Rubinstein, P., Suciu-Foca, N., et al.: Genetics of juvenile diabetes mellitus. A recessive gene closely linked to HLA-D and with 50 per cent penetrance. New Engl. J. Med. 297:1036, 1978.
196. Nerup, J., Cathelinean, C., et al.: HLA and endocrine diseases. In *HLA and Disease*. Dausset, J., and Svejgaard, A. (eds.), Copenhagen, Munksgaard, 1977, p. 150.
197. Touraine, J. L., Betuel, H., et al.: Combined immunodeficiency associated with absence of cell-surface HLA-A and -B antigens. J. Pediatr. 93:47, 1978.
198. Snell, G. D.: The H-2 locus of the mouse: observations and speculations concerning its comparative genetics and its polymorphism. Folia Biol. (Praha) 14:335, 1968.
199. Dupont, B.: Mechanisms for HLA and disease associations in the biology and function of the major histocompatibility complex. Arlington, VA, American Association of Blood Banks, 1980, pp. 61–79.
200. Geczi, A. F., Alexander, K., et al.: HLA-B27, Klebsiella and ankylosing spondilitis: biological and chemical studies. In *Immunological Reviews*. Moller, G. (ed.), Copenhagen, Munksgaard, 70:23–50, 1981.
200a. Schneider, P. M., Carroll, M. C., et al.: Polymorphism of the human complement C4 and steroid 21-hydroxylase genes. Restriction fragment length polymorphisms revealing structural deletions, homoduplications, and size variants. J. Clin. Invest. 78:650, 1986.
201. Raum, D., Awdeh, Z., et al.: Extended major histocompatibility complex haplotypes in type I diabetes mellitus. J. Clin. Invest. 74:449, 1984.
202. Sasasuki, T., Nishimura, Y., et al.: HLA linked genes controlling immune response and disease susceptibility. In *Immunological Reviews*. Moller, G., (ed.), Copenhagen, Munksgaard, 70:51, 1974.
203. Cohen, D., Cohen, O., et al.: HLA Class II DCβ DNA restriction fragments differentiate among HLA-DR2 individuals in insulin dependent diabetes and multiple sclerosis. Proc. Natl. Acad. Sci. USA 81:1774, 1984.

GENETICS

CHAPTER 46
Serum Proteins and Other Genetic Markers of the Blood

CHESTER A. ALPER
DAVID G. NATHAN

PLASMA PROTEINS 1550
Albumin
α_1-Antitrypsin
α_1-Acid Glycoprotein (Orosomucoid)
Haptoglobin
Ceruloplasmin
Gc-Globulin (Vitamin D–Binding Globulin)
Pseudocholinesterase
Transferrin
Lipoproteins
α_2-HS Glycoprotein
Transcobalamin II
Factor XIII
Plasminogen
β_2-Glycoprotein I
C3
C5
C6
C7
C8
Factor H (β_{1H}-Globulin)
C4BP (C4-Binding Protein)
CR1 (Complement Receptor 1, C3b Receptor)
Factor B
C2
C4
Complotypes
Extended Haplotypes
Immunoglobulins
Localization and Evolution of Genes for Some Plasma Proteins
RED CELL ENZYMES 1573
Red Cell Acid Phosphatase
Phosphoglucomutase
Red Cell Adenylate Kinase
Catalase
Galactose-1-Phosphate Uridyl Transferase

This chapter offers a summary of the important genetic markers in human blood other than those on cell surfaces. It emphasizes plasma proteins and erythrocyte enzymes. The most recent relevant reviews of the latter are those of Harris and of Harris and Hopkinson.*

Study of human allotypes is critically important both for clinical reasons and for the purpose of extending our knowledge of the human genome. The immediate clinical applications include blood cell transfusion, paternity exclusion, establishment of marrow and organ transplantation, and antenatal diagnosis. The ultimate clinical goal is effective treatment of severe inherited disease by gene replacement or modification either in utero or in early childhood. Although the latter goal is certainly distant, immensely valuable biologic data are being collected en route as assignment of particular genes to particular chromosomes is in progress.

This chapter is organized into two sections: The first deals with the major serum proteins in some detail; the second consists of a much briefer review of blood cell enzymes. The genetic nomenclature used is that proposed by an international committee and approved by the International Society for Human Genetics.†

PLASMA PROTEINS

Genetically controlled structural variation among human plasma proteins is the rule and not the exception. For the most part, this variation consists of single amino acid substitutions and is not usually attended by detectable alterations in function. The mutations that gave rise to the variant genes appear to have persisted, in the main, because their bearers have thrived and multiplied, rather than because of positive evolutionary selective pressure. It is clear that the extent of this genetic heterogeneity of all proteins and of their genes is far greater than the meager catalogue we have at present.

Electrophoresis is by far the most common technique for the detection of genetic structural variation in plasma proteins; serologic methods are used in a few instances. Rarely, structurally variant proteins can be detected, but not identified, by

---

*Harris, H.: *The Principles of Human Biochemical Genetics*, 3rd ed. Amsterdam, North-Holland, 1980; Harris, H., and Hopkinson, D. A.: *Handbook of Enzyme Electrophoresis in Human Genetics.* New York, Elsevier-North Holland, 1976.
†Shows, T. B., Alper, C. A., et al.: International system for human gene nomenclature (1979), ISGN (1979). Cytogenet. Cell Genet. 25:96, 1979.

abnormalities in their function or serum concentration. Electrophoresis detects variants that differ grossly in net surface charge owing to substitution of an amino acid by one of *different* charge. The introduction of isoelectric focusing in gels has permitted the detection of variants that differ by less than a whole net charge owing to substitution of an amino acid by one of *similar* charge. With the development of recombinant DNA technology, genes for a number of plasma proteins have been examined directly, and restriction fragment length polymorphisms (RFLPs) for several plasma protein genes have been identified.

The extent of variation of individual plasma proteins varies enormously from population to population and from protein to protein. For some proteins and populations, there is remarkable homogeneity and a very low incidence of variants, whereas for others there are two or more "common" types. Variation can be so extensive that no single variant is found in more than half the population. Arbitrary definitions requiring that, in order to qualify as genetic polymorphism, variants of a given protein must be found in more than some arbitrary percentage of some population somewhere have been proposed, but they are clearly not useful.

Albumin

Albumin is by far the most plentiful of the plasma proteins. Its concentration is approximately equal to that of the combined concentrations of all other proteins in plasma (3.5 to 4.5 g per dl). Albumin maintains the blood's colloid osmotic pressure, and a great variety of positively and negatively charged and hydrophobic substances bind to it (1). In certain instances (e.g., for pharmacologic agents), this affords a transport function for albumin. The human albumin gene is approximately 16.5 kb long. Each of the three homologous albumin domains is encoded by four exons. There is extensive sequence homology between albumin and alpha fetoprotein, and the two genes are less than 15 kb apart on chromosome 4 in humans (2), suggesting multiple tandem duplications by a series of common ancestral genes giving rise to the current genes for the two proteins.

The albumin molecule consists of three domains of homologous structure but of differing ability to bind specific substances. The presence of these domains suggests that present-day albumin evolved by gene triplication from a gene for a low-molecular-weight primordial protein (3).

Genetic variants of albumin are detected as single electrophoretic bands of a mobility either slower or faster than that of the usual protein, as is true of the usual variants of hemoglobin A (Fig. 46–1). All are relatively rare in most populations and occur with a frequency of less than 1 per cent. Rare exceptions have been found in certain American Indian populations in which rather high gene frequencies (up to 0.13) occur. This has been true in the Naskapi and Montagnais tribes of Quebec. There appear to be at least 25 electrophoretically detectable albumin variants described in addition to common albumin (4, 5). In all instances, the variants are found in concentrations equal to those of common albumin in heterozygotes, except in the case of an unusual albumin variant found in Sweden (6). In that case, the albumin zone was broadened in agarose gel electrophoresis and could be resolved into common albumin and a slower-moving variant of lower concentration. The variant tended to dimerize more readily than common albumin. This variant is of particular clinical interest because of its high incidence in orthopedic patients (5 per 1550) and the possibility that it might be associated with a defect in connective tissue leading to back pain, other bone and joint complaints, and impaired hearing.

The single amino acid substitutions responsible for several albumin variants are known. Albumin

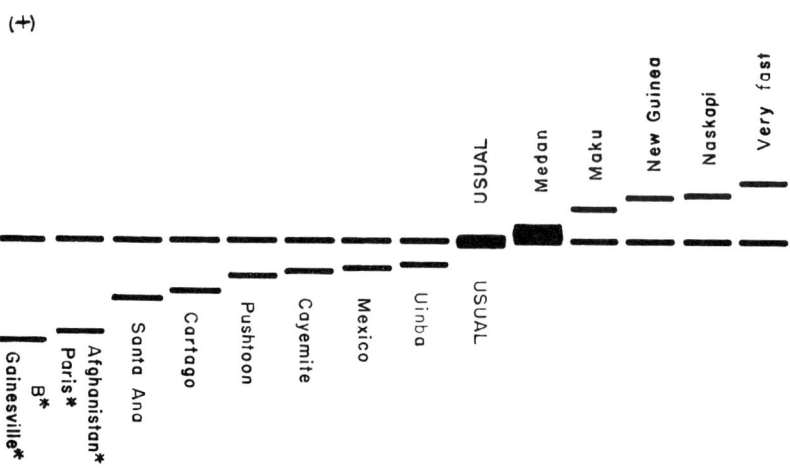

Figure 46–1. Diagram of albumin variants as they appear in electrophoresis (in starch or agarose gel) at pH 8.6. Variants marked with an asterisk have different mobilities from common albumin at other pH's. (Adapted from Schell, L. M., and Blumberg, B. S.: In *Albumin—Its Structure, Function and Uses in Man.* Rosenoer, V. M., Rothschild, M. A., et al. [eds.], London and New York, Pergamon Press, 1977.)

Christchurch (7) is an interesting variant six amino acids longer than usual albumin. In it there is a substitution of Glu for Arg such that the normal proteolytic cleavage between the profragment and mature albumin cannot occur.

At least eight different RFLPs are present in or near the albumin gene (8). Variants constitute seven different haplotypes (of 256 possible combinations). Some haplotypes are race specific, others occur in all humans, and one apparently antedates the separation of humans from the great apes.

Analbuminemia is a rare inherited disorder with virtually complete absence of albumin in serum (9). This characteristic is inherited as an autosomal recessive trait, and the parents of such individuals have normal albumin concentrations. Albumin concentrations in affected persons are not zero, but range from 10 to 40 mg per dl. Results of studies with isotopically labeled albumin conclusively demonstrate that the defect in this disorder is defective synthesis rather than increased catabolism of albumin. The albumin gene was present and grossly normal in one analbuminemic subject (10).

Nevertheless, most individuals with hereditary analbuminemia, particularly males, have only mild edema. Thus, hypoproteinemic edema (e.g., the anasarca of severely nephrotic patients) is not merely a reflection of the low serum albumin concentration; other processes must be operative as well. In addition, analbuminemic patients may have developed compensatory mechanisms that minimize edema.

α_1-Antitrypsin

The major inhibitor of trypsin in serum is a protein designated α_1-antitrypsin (11). It also inhibits chymotrypsin, collagenase, elastase, and leukocyte proteases. The mean concentration in the serum of normal individuals is about 250 mg per dl. Inherited deficiency of α_1-antitrypsin is associated with markedly increased susceptibility to lung and liver disease (12–14).

Although the great majority of individuals in most populations studied have a single major α_1-antitrypsin band on agarose gel electrophoresis at pH 8.6, some sera show variant bands (Fig. 46–2) (15, 16). With starch gel or acrylamide gel electrophoresis at an acidic pH (usually approximately 4.95), the common form and the variants are seen as a series of five major bands migrating ahead of the bulk of the serum proteins (17), as shown in Figure 46–3, in which only the two most prominent bands are shown. Specific identification of variants can be facilitated by crossed immunoelectrophoresis into agarose gel containing specific antibody to α_1-antitrypsin (18). Most of the microheterogeneity of α_1-antitrypsin seen in homozygotes is the result of differences in sialic acid content of each of the bands (19).

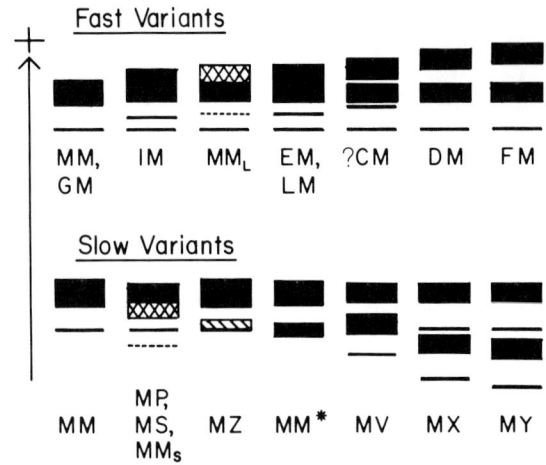

Figure 46–2. Diagram of some α_1-antitrypsin (PI) phenotypes observed in prolonged agarose gel electrophoresis at pH 8.6 and developed by immunofixation with specific antiserum. (Courtesy of Dr. A. Myron Johnson.)

The variants are inherited in autosomal codominant fashion. At present, there are at least 25 recognized alleles at the locus for α_1-antitrypsin, a locus called PI (protease inhibitor) (20). The common form of α_1-antitrypsin is called PI M. The rare variants have been given letter designations that run alphabetically from anode to cathode. Some of the variant gene products are shown in Figures 46–2 and 46–3.

Of particular importance because of the diseases with which they are associated are *PI∗Z* and *PI∗S*. The products of these genes are found in lower concentrations than those of the other alleles. The mean concentrations of α_1-antitrypsin of types PI ZZ, SZ, MZ, and MS are approximately 10 per cent, 30 per cent, 60 per cent, and 70 per cent of PI MM (12, 20). Other "hypomorphic" alleles exist, such as *PI∗P*, *PI∗W*, and one (*PI∗MMAL* [Malton]) whose product has the electrophoretic mobility of PI M at pH 8.6. An allele with no detectable product (*PI∗QO*) also has been identified (21). Individuals homozygous for *PI∗Z*, *PI∗QO*, or *PI∗MMAL* or heterozygous for these genes and other low concentration alleles, including *PI∗S*, are prone to develop neonatal hepatitis as infants, cirrhosis as children, and chronic obstructive pulmonary disease as adults.

Although the reason for the low serum concentration of PI Z and other "deficient" gene products is not fully understood, some clues are available. Alpha$_1$-antitrypsin can be detected in normal or supernormal amounts in hepatocytes in the liver of patients with severe α_1-antitrypsin deficiency. Electron microscopic studies have revealed inclusions in liver cells in such patients that represent α_1-antitrypsin. The *PI∗Z* gene expressed in *Xenopus* oocytes or human monocytes synthesizes pro-

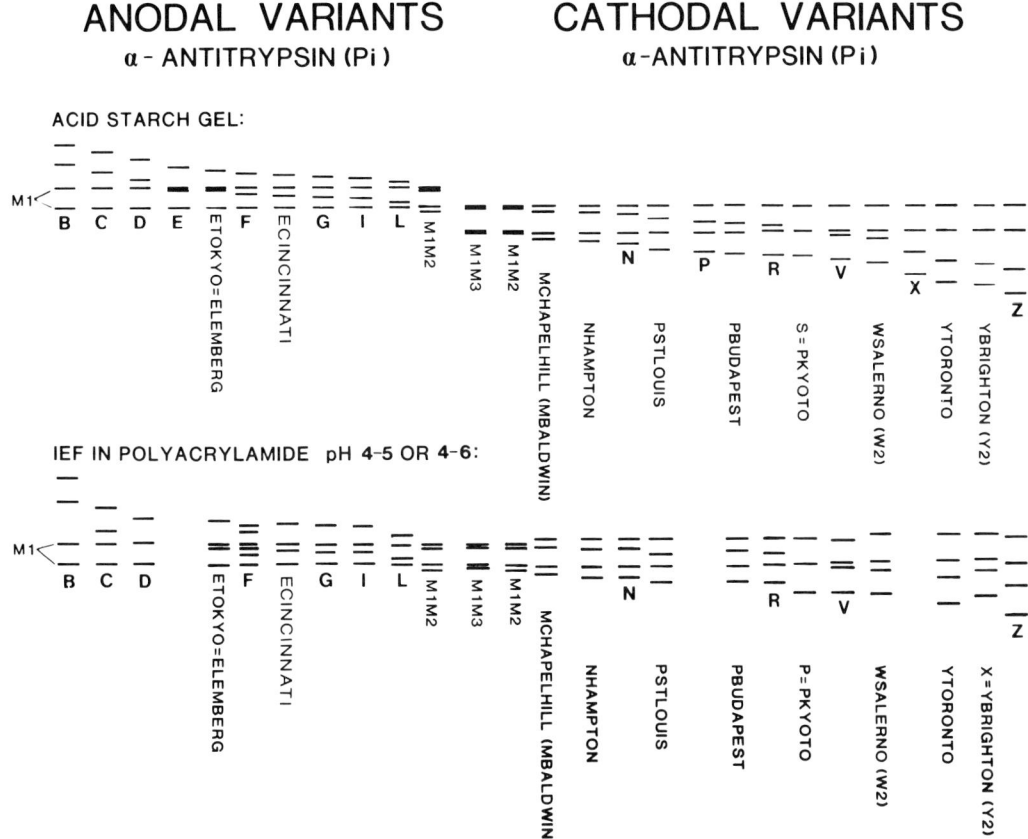

Figure 46–3. Alpha₁-antitrypsin (PI) variants as they appear in starch gel electrophoresis at pH 4.95 and isoelectric focusing at acid pH. Each variant gives rise to a pattern of eight bands, of which only the two major bands are shown in this diagram. (Based on information kindly supplied by Dr. Diane Cox.)

tein intracellularly at the same rate as does *PI∗M*. However, there is markedly delayed secretion and intracellular accumulation of underglycosylated PI Z (22).

It is likely that all the inherited α_1-antitrypsin structural variants discovered to date represent point mutations with single amino acid substitutions. This has been shown to be true of PI Z, in that a glutamate of PI M is replaced by a lysine, and of PI S, in that a different glutamate is replaced by a valine (23, 24). Both defects are the result of single nucleotide changes.

The introduction of isoelectric focusing in polyacrylamide gels for PI-typing has revealed subtypes of PI M (25). Of these, the most common in all populations studied has been designated PI M1. The frequency of the gene for the more basic PI M2 variant is approximately 0.02 in blacks, slightly higher in Orientals, and up to 0.20 in some European populations (Table 46–1).

The concentration of α_1-antitrypsin may be altered under various physiologic and pathophysiologic circumstances. Alpha₁-antitrypsin rises in concentration as part of the acute phase plasma protein response, during estrogen administration, and in pregnancy. There is a selective, although variable, fall in α_1-antitrypsin levels (and α_2-macroglobulin concentration) during severe neonatal respiratory distress syndrome. In experimental animals it has been shown that α_1-antitrypsin forms an important defense against the administration of proteolytic enzymes, such as trypsin and chymotrypsin. When the capacity of this protein (and that of other protease inhibitors) to complex with and inactivate these enzymes is exceeded, shock and death rapidly ensue.

Despite our ignorance of precise mechanisms leading to disease in α_1-antitrypsin deficiency, it seems possible that incompletely inhibited leukocyte proteases and gut proteases may digest lung parenchymal elastin and damage the liver.

There is a methionine at position 358 in the elastase-binding site of normal α_1-antitrypsin. This methionine is easily oxidized (e.g., by cigarette smoke), and the molecule loses its inhibitory capacity for elastase (26). This may contribute to tobacco-induced lung disease. A rare variant, PI PIT (Pittsburgh), has Arg in place of Met at position 358, and the molecule no longer inhibits elastase; however, remarkably, it does inhibit

Table 46–1. SOME *PI* GENE FREQUENCIES IN VARIOUS POPULATIONS

Population	PI*M1	PI*M2	PI*M3	PI*M4	PI*S	PI*Z	PI*F	PI*I	PI*V	PI*W
White										
France	0.626	0.092	0.104	0.037						
Sardinia	0.587	0.204	0.046	0.094	0.062	0.005				
Spain	----------------------0.866----------------------*				0.112	0.012	0.003	0.001	0.0026	0.0026
Norway	----------------------0.946----------------------*				0.023	0.016	0.013	0.001	0.0004	
Oriental										
China	0.765	0.173	0.051		----------------------------0.011----------------------------†					
Lapps	----------------------0.992----------------------*					0.008				

*PI M subtyping not done.
†All non-*PI*M alleles pooled.
(Abridged and updated from Fagerhol, M. K., and Laurell, C.-B.: Prog. Med. Genet. 7:96–111, 1970, by permission of Grune & Stratton.)

thrombin (normal α_1-antitrypsin does not), leading to a hemorrhagic tendency in patients who carry it (27).

The gene for α_1-antitrypsin has been cloned, is about 5 kb long, and contains three introns (28). There is some sequence homology with other proteinase inhibitors. A DNA probe specific for the PI Z mutation has been produced and provides the ability to diagnose the deficiency state in utero (29). For screening sera (including those from umbilical cord blood), a monoclonal antibody specific for PI Z (30) is available.

The α_1-antitrypsin cDNA has been modified by site-specific mutagenesis to yield a variant with Val in place of Met at position 358. This molecule, genetically engineered in microorganisms (31–33), is resistant to oxidation, is 10 times more potent as an elastase inhibitor than PI M in vitro, and thus may be useful in the treatment of inherited or acquired α_1-antitrypsin deficiency.

α_1-Acid Glycoprotein (Orosomucoid)

This protein is among the most highly glycosylated in serum. Its serum concentration is hormone-sensitive and falls during pregnancy and even more so during administration of oral estrogen-progesterone contraceptive medication. Alpha$_1$-acid glycoprotein is a marked acute phase reactant, and its level can increase up to five- or sixfold in the present of acute inflammation. The protein binds and transports a number of basic drugs, including local anesthetics and propranolol.

Alpha$_1$-acid glycoprotein exhibits genetic polymorphism of an unusual kind. This protein in native serum migrates as multiple bands on electrophoresis (34). If whole serum or purified protein is treated with neuraminidase to remove sialic acid, the electrophoretic behavior of the molecule is greatly simplified. Material from different individuals forms one of three patterns (Fig. 46–4): a

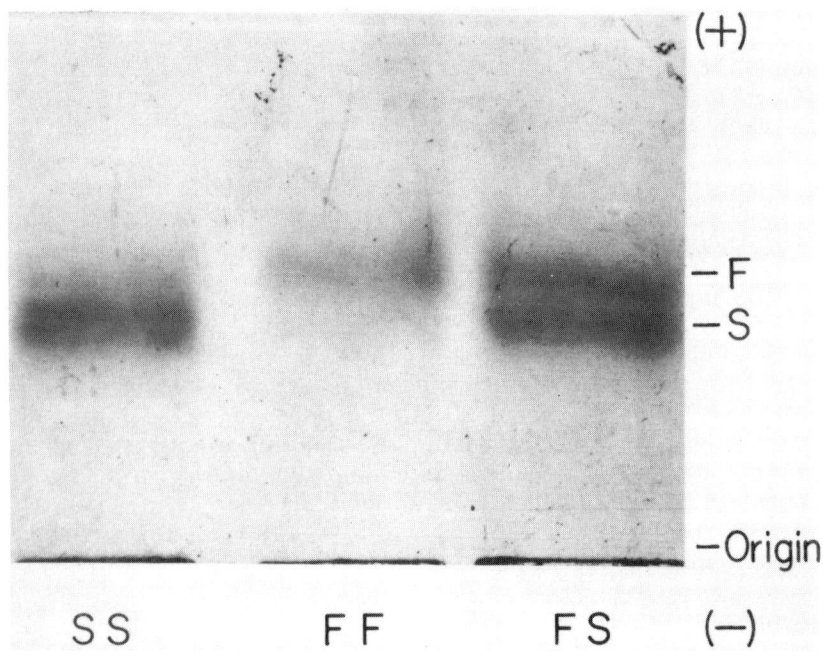

Figure 46–4. Orosomucoid (OR) patterns obtained with desialidated whole sera after electrophoresis at pH 8.6 and immunofixation with specific antiserum. (From Johnson, A. M., Schmid, K., et al.: J. Clin. Invest. *48*:2293, 1969.)

Table 46–2. SOME *OR* GENE FREQUENCIES IN VARIOUS POPULATIONS

Population	OR*S	OR*F
Bechuana	0.62	0.38
White American	0.36	0.64
Chinese	0.47	0.53
Congolese	0.47	0.53
Finnish	0.50	0.50
French	0.49	0.51
Indian	0.44	0.56
Amerindian	0.54	0.46
Japanese	0.27	0.73
Nigerian	0.41	0.59
Nyambian	0.44	0.56
Swedish	0.67	0.33
Zulu	0.37	0.63

(Abridged from Johnson, A. M., Schmid, K., et al.: J. Clin. Invest. *48*:2293, 1969.)

major fast band and a minor slow band, a major slow band and a minor fast band, or two bands of approximately equal concentrations (35). The corresponding genotypes are *OR*F/OR*F*, *OR*S/OR*S*, and *OR*F/OR*S*, in which F and S refer to fast and slow. Inheritance is autosomal codominant, but the genes appear to control the relative amounts of OR F and OR S in individuals, all of whom have the same structural genes. The protein is a single chain, and OR F contains glutamine at position 20, whereas OR S contains arginine at this position (36). *OR* gene frequencies are given in Table 46–2.

Haptoglobin

Haptoglobin is an α_2-glycoprotein occurring in normal serum at a concentration of 30 to 160 mg per dl (expressed as hemoglobin-binding capacity) Although there are strong homologies with the chymotrypsinogen family of serine proteases (37), haptoglobin also shows weak homologies with immunoglobulin light chain and concanavalin A. Its concentration rises within 1 to 2 days of the onset of acute inflammation or tissue necrosis as part of the acute-phase response. Elevated levels are also found in individuals treated with androgens. Only 10 per cent of newborns have detectable serum haptoglobin measured as hemoglobin-binding capacity. The level usually rises to the adult range after several months but may remain low in some otherwise healthy children.

The most striking property of haptoglobin is its ability to bind with hemoglobin to form a stable complex. Present evidence suggests that the binding site on hemoglobin is on the beta chain but that alpha chains also are required for the complex to form. Haptoglobin consists of two kinds of subunits (also designated alpha and beta) (39), and it is the haptoglobin beta chain that bears the globin-binding site. Formation of haptoglobin-hemoglobin (Hp-Hb) complexes occurs with half-molecules of hemoglobin ($\alpha\beta$), and saturated complexes consist of one molecule of haptoglobin and two hemoglobin half-molecules.

When the Hp-Hb complex forms in vivo as the result of hemolysis, it is rapidly cleared by the reticuloendothelial system (40). No stimulus to haptoglobin synthesis occurs in response to this removal, and therefore the concentration of serum haptoglobin falls to subnormal levels and may approach zero. In the presence of acute inflammation, because of increased haptoglobin synthesis, the serum level of haptoglobin may be normal or even elevated despite hemolysis in vivo (41). Its concentration will nevertheless be relatively lowered compared with those of other positive acute phase reactants such as α_1-antitrypsin, orosomucoid, or α_1-antichymotrypsin. Therefore, when using the measurement of serum haptoglobin as a guide to hemolysis, one must also measure one or two other positive acute-phase reactants.

Inherited molecular variation in human haptoglobin was one of the earliest understood of the genetic polymorphisms among the serum proteins, owing largely to the work of Smithies. Initially it was noted that when hemoglobin was added to sera from various individuals, the mixtures subjected to starch gel electrophoresis, and the resulting gels stained for peroxidase with a benzidine–hydrogen peroxide reagent, three strikingly different common patterns were seen (Fig. 46–5)

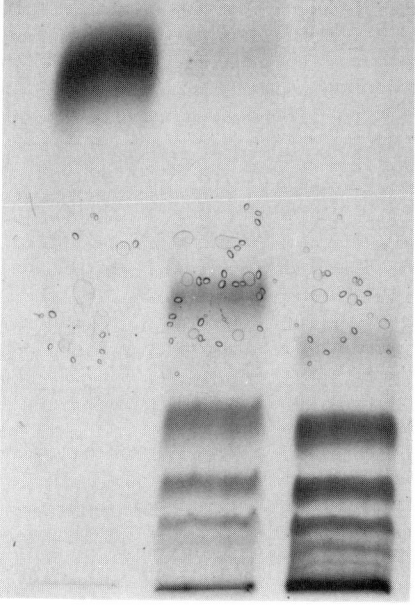

Figure 46–5. Common haptoglobin types in polyacrylamide gel electrophoresis at pH 8.0. Individual serum samples were saturated with hemoglobin, and patterns were developed by a benzidine–hydrogen peroxide reagent.

(42). It soon became evident that the patterns reflected polymorphism in haptoglobin and that the benzidine reagent detected the known peroxidase activity of the Hp-Hb complex. The patterns were named as shown in Figure 46–5, and the postulated codominant alleles for haptoglobin were designated *HP*1* and *HP*2*. Haptoglobin 1 occurs as a single molecular species with a molecular weight of about 85,000 daltons; haptoglobin 2-1 consists of some material identical with HP 1 in electrophoretic mobility and molecular size and heavier protein species, indicating the presence of heteropolymers. Haptoglobin 2 consists only of polymers. Because of the sieving action of starch gel during electrophoresis, the polymers are retarded in proportion to their size, so that forms seen are dimer, trimer, and so on.

When haptoglobin was purified from individual sera, resolved into its constituent polypeptide chains, and examined in starch gel electrophoresis (43), the original polymorphism was found in the alpha chains and, furthermore, the 1α chains showed polymorphism (Fig. 46–6). The two kinds of 1α chains were called 1F (fast electrophoretic mobility) and 1S (slow electrophoretic mobility), and the genes were designated *HPA*1F* and *HPA*1S*. Thus, three common alleles at the haptoglobin locus were defined that produced six common phenotypes. Gene frequencies in several populations are given in Table 46–3.

The structural and genetic bases for the haptoglobin polymorphism were further elucidated when the amino acid composition of HPA 1F was shown to differ from that of HPA 1S by a single amino acid, lysine, in place of asparagine or glutamine in HPA 1S (Fig. 46–7). This accounts for the charge difference between the two gene products. The differences between HPA 1 and HPA 2 proved to be more complex. First, molecular weight determinations of these isolated polypeptide chains indicate that HPA 2 is about twice the size of HPA 1F or HPA 1S. Analysis of peptides produced by partial digestion of the three types of chains reveals many similarities but sufficient differences between the 2α and 1α chains to exclude simple amino acid substitution as an explanation for the overall differences.

The amino and carboxyl terminal peptides found in both HPA 1F and HPA 1S are also found in HPA 2, whereas HPA 2 contains both peptides that distinguish HPA 1F from HPA 1S. In addition, HPA 2 contains a peptide not found in either HPA 1F or HPA 1S. The ingenious and most

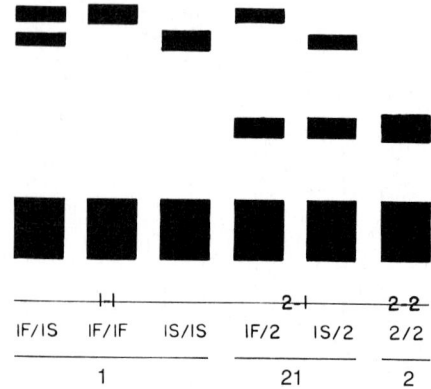

Figure 46–6. A diagram of the electrophoretic patterns of purified haptoglobin of various types in acid urea starch gels in the presence of reducing agent. Subunits are visualized, and the alpha chain is seen to be highly polymorphic.

Table 46–3. *HPA* GENE FREQUENCIES IN VARIOUS POPULATIONS*

Population	*HPA*1S*	*HPA*1F*	*HPA*2*
Nigerian	0.258	0.473	0.27
White			
Italy	0.252	0.118	0.63
India	0.104	0.046	0.85
Korean	0.321	0	0.68
Japanese	0.227	0.003	0.77
Chinese	0.341	0	0.66
Thai	0.236	0	0.76
Eskimo (Baffin Island)	0.239	0	0.76
Amerindian			
United States	0.374	0	0.63
Chile*	0.774	0	0.23

**HPA*2* frequency includes one *HPA*2FF* individual.
(Abridged from Shim, B. S., and Bearn, A. G.: Am. J. Hum. Genet. *16*:477–480, 1964, by permission of Grune & Stratton.)

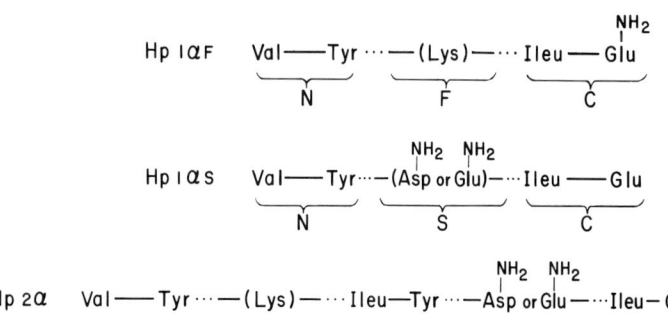

Figure 46–7. Outlines of structures of three common haptoglobin α-polypeptide chains based on studies of chymotryptic peptides. (Adapted from Smithies, O., Connell, G. E., et al.: Nature [Lond.] *196*:232, 1962.)

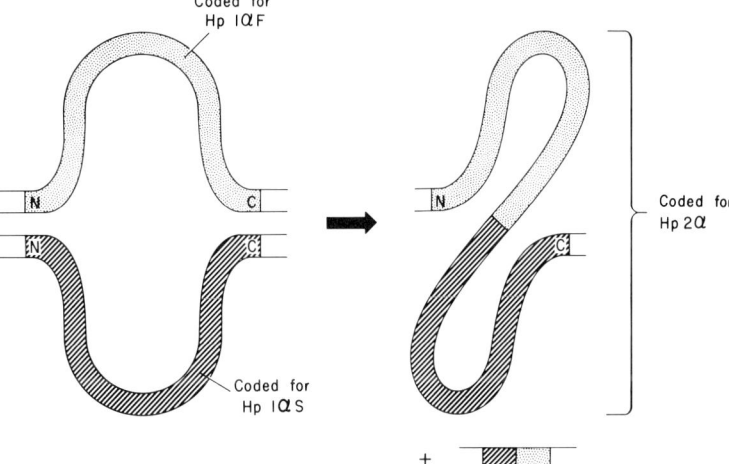

Figure 46–8. Possible mechanism by which *HPA*∗*2* gene arose by nonhomologous crossing-over in a heterozygote from *HPA*∗*1F* and *HPA*∗*1S*. (Adapted from Smithies, O., Connell, G. E., et al.: Nature [Lond.] *196*:232, 1962.)

reasonable explanation of these observations is shown in the postulated structure of the various kinds of HP α chains illustrated in Figure 46–7. It thus appears that HPA 2 is composed essentially of the HPA 1F chain joined via a junctional peptide to the HPA 1S chain. The most likely genetic mechanism to explain the formation of such a polypeptide chain from two different allelic genes is nonhomologous crossover of two chromosomes in a heterozygote *(HPA*∗*1F/HPA*∗*1S)*, with a resultant almost complete gene duplication and an almost complete gene deletion. The postulated genetic mechanism is illustrated in Figure 46–8.

The genetic event postulated in the origin of the *HPA*∗*2* gene must be a rare occurrence. Nevertheless, it was predicted that the same sort of genetic mechanism could, if it occurred in a homozygote *(HPA*∗*1F/HPA*∗*1F* or *HPA*∗*1S/HPA*∗*1S)*, lead to the establishment of two additional types of HPA 2 polypeptide chains. This prediction was confirmed (45) by the detection of individuals in isolated populations with *HPA*∗*2FF* instead of the usual *HPA*∗*2FS* (or *HPA*∗*2SF*, since the order of F and S was not then established). Evidence from DNA sequencing indicates that the nonhomologous crossover point in the generation of HPA 2FS was within different introns of the original *HPA*∗*1* genes (46) and that there are four nucleotide differences between the 1F and 1S domains of HPA 2.

In addition to the genetic variants of haptoglobin already described, rare types occur that reflect polymorphism at the beta chain locus, unequal production of 1α and 2α chains in an individual of type HPA 21, and further polymorphism at the alpha chain locus. Because available evidence suggests that the binding of hemoglobin by haptoglobin is via a site on the beta chain of haptoglobin, it is not too surprising that some beta chain variants should be detected by abnormalities in hemoglobin binding. An interesting case is HPB MAR (Marburg). This variant was first recognized because of its atypical reactivity with antiserum to haptoglobin. Antiserums to haptoglobin may distinguish the following kinds of antigenic determinants:

1. If the antiserum is made to HPA 22 or HPA 21, it may contain antibodies specific for the 2α chains as well as antibodies reacting with all the usual haptoglobin types (47).

2. Most antiserums against haptoglobin of any type react with an antigenic determinant present on free haptoglobin only, not on haptoglobin bound to hemoglobin (48). The latter site is presumably on the beta chain and appears to be rendered inaccessible when the complex with hemoglobin is formed. HPB MAR is immunologically similar to free haptoglobin, despite the addition of hemoglobin sufficient to saturate the haptoglobin in the serum in question. The most likely interpretation of this phenomenon is that HPB MAR is a beta chain variant with diminished hemoglobin-binding ability.

The genetic loci for HP alpha and beta chains *(HPA* and *HPB)* are immediately contiguous on the long arm of chromosome 16 (49). It is probable that haptoglobin is synthesized as a single chain precursor so that there is a single *HP* cistron rather than two.

Relative underproduction of HPA 2 in an individual who is HPA 21 results in a starch gel or acrylamide electrophoretic pattern termed HPA 21M. In this pattern, there is relatively more material with the mobility of HPA 1 and a paucity of polymer bands, which migrate more slowly than those that occur in the usual HPA 21 form. Such patterns are inheritable and occur in highest frequency among blacks. Genetically determined anhaptoglobinemia appears to be found in such families as a variant of HPA 21M. There is a spectrum of patterns between HPA 21 and HPA 21M that presumably reflects variable degrees of disproportion between production of 1α and 2α chains.

More rarely, variant haptoglobin patterns are encountered that show duplication of bands and resemble an artificial mixture of HPA 21 and HPA 2. These variants may represent a relative underproduction of 1α chains or, very rarely, true genetic mosaicisms in which some liver cells in a single individual presumably produce HPA 21 and other cells produce HPA 2.

Ceruloplasmin

The remarkably rich, deep, and heavenly blue color of this protein prompted Holmberg and Laurell, who were the first to purify and characterize it, to name it ceruloplasmin (50). Ceruloplasmin is a 7S α2-glycoprotein, with 7 per cent carbohydrate and approximately 132,000 daltons molecular weight. The ceruloplasmin molecule is a single polypeptide chain and probably contains 6 atoms of copper. It is the presence of the copper that determines the blue color of the protein, since if one removes the copper to produce apoceruloplasmin, all color disappears. About 90 per cent of the total serum copper is to be found in ceruloplasmin, and the remainder is largely bound to albumin. The copper in ceruloplasmin is not exchangeable in vivo, so that ceruloplasmin does not function as a transport protein for copper (51) (but albumin probably does). Ceruloplasmin is able to catalyze the oxidation of some amines, and p-phenylenediamine has been used as a convenient substrate for this enzymatic action (52). The concentration of ceruloplasmin in serum can thus be, and has been, measured by three different methods: as serum copper, as amine oxidase activity, and as the protein part of the molecule by means of specific antibodies.

The complete covalent structure of ceruloplasmin is known (53). The molecule shows evidence of internal homology, suggesting an internal triplication. There are regions of significant homology with other copper-containing proteins, such as the azurins, plastocyanins, cytochrome oxidase, and superoxide dismutase (54).

The concentration of ceruloplasmin in newborn serum is about one third that of normal adult serum and rises to the adult level within the first year of life. Its concentration is hormone-sensitive, and high serum levels are found in pregnant women and women on oral contraceptives. Elevation of serum ceruloplasmin levels occurs as part of the acute-phase plasma protein response, and if the ceruloplasmin content is sufficiently high, such serum may have a greenish tinge. After the first year of life, low ceruloplasmin concentration is almost always pathognomonic for Wilson's disease (55), provided that protein-losing states have been ruled out. Affected persons almost always (and carriers sometimes) have low serum ceruloplasmin concentrations. Although Wilson's disease clearly has a genetic basis, the depression of ceruloplasmin appears to be a secondary phenomenon. A rare primary genetic deficiency of ceruloplasmin without Wilson's disease has been reported (56).

Electrophoretic variants in ceruloplasmin were first detected in starch gel electrophoresis followed by staining for amine oxidase activity (57). Alternatively, variants can be tested for by prolonged agarose gel electrophoresis and immunofixation with specific anticeruloplasmin (58). Four common variants, A, B, BNH and C—as well as a number of rare variants (59)—have been identified, as shown in Figure 46–9. The lettering is from anode to cathode at alkaline pH, and BNH refers to a variant from New Haven. From the gene frequen-

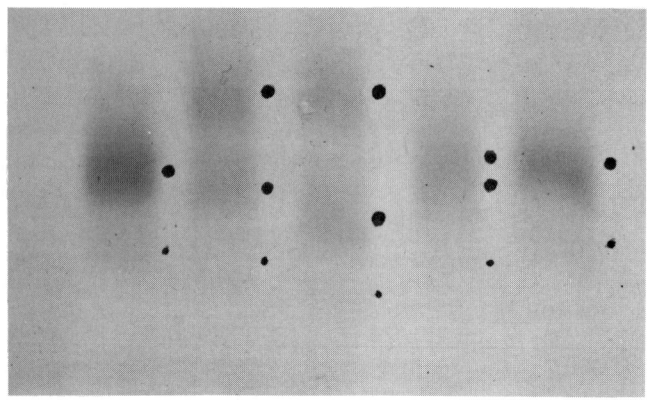

Figure 46–9. Patterns of ceruloplasmin variants obtained by prolonged agarose gel electrophoresis of serum at pH 8.6 and by immunofixation with specific antiserum. The ink marks indicate the bands.

Table 46–4. *CP* GENE FREQUENCIES IN VARIOUS POPULATIONS

Population	*CP*∗A	*CP*∗B	*CP*∗C	*CP*∗BNH
White				
Boston	0.010	0.983	0.003	0.003
Ann Arbor	0.006	0.988	—	—
Black				
Boston	0.052	0.914	0.017	0.017
Ann Arbor	0.053	0.943	0.003	—
Oriental (Boston)	—	1.000	—	—

(Adapted from Shreffler, D. C., Brewer, G. J., et al.: Biochem. Genet. *1*:101, 1967; and Alper, C. A., and Johnson, A. M.: Vox Sang. *17*:445, 1969.)

cies listed in Table 46–4, it is evident that *CP*∗B is the most common gene in all populations studied and that only blacks have high frequencies of other alleles. All the known variants have amine oxidase activity by virtue of the original method of detection and the failure to find additional variants by immunochemical means.

Gc-Globulin (Vitamin D–Binding Globulin)

The "group-specific component," or Gc-globulin, is an α_2-mobility protein in zone electrophoresis occurring in a concentration of about 75 mg per dl of normal serum. Its level falls in advanced liver disease and is elevated in pregnancy and during oral contraceptive therapy.

Gc-globulin has a molecular weight of about 51,000 daltons (60). It is the vitamin D transport protein of plasma (61).

Extensive genetic polymorphism in Gc-globulin was discovered in 1959 by Hirschfeld (62), who used immunoelectrophoresis for the detection of variants. The study of Gc polymorphism has been greatly aided by the use of crossed immunoelectrophoresis (63) and immunofixation electrophoresis (64). Figures 46–10 and 46–11 show the common patterns of GC 1, 21, and 2 in the two latter techniques. It is evident that GC 1 has two major bands (1A and 1C for anodal and cathodal) and at least one minor band anodal to 1A. GC 2, however, consists of a single major band and a corresponding minor band under a wide variety of electrophoresis conditions. In addition to these major common bands, over 30 inherited GC structural variants are known (Fig. 46–12). In the case of double-banded variants, including GC 1, there appears to be a spectrum of inherited variation reflected in differences in relative concentration of the two bands. The failure to recognize these relationships has led to multiple descriptions and designations of some of the variants and to the general impression that there are more structural variants than, in fact, exist. Thus, by the use of immunofixation electrophoresis and crossed immunoelectrophoresis, it was found that the re-

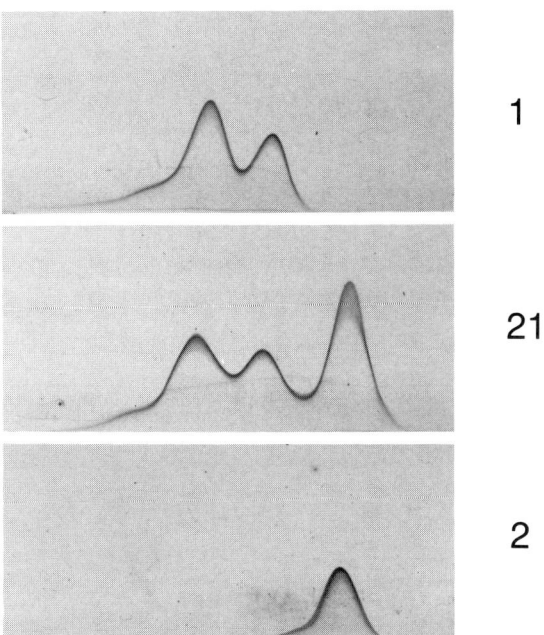

Figure 46–10. Crossed immunoelectrophoresis patterns of the three common GC phenotypes. The anode for the first separation was at the left, and for the second at the top. Both electrophoreses were carried out at pH 8.6.

ported variants GC AB (Aborigine) and GC Y were identical in electrophoretic appearance, as were GC D (Darmstadt) and GC ESK (Eskimo). GC D and GC J differ only in that both J bands appear to be hypomorphic compared with the common allele product in the same serum.

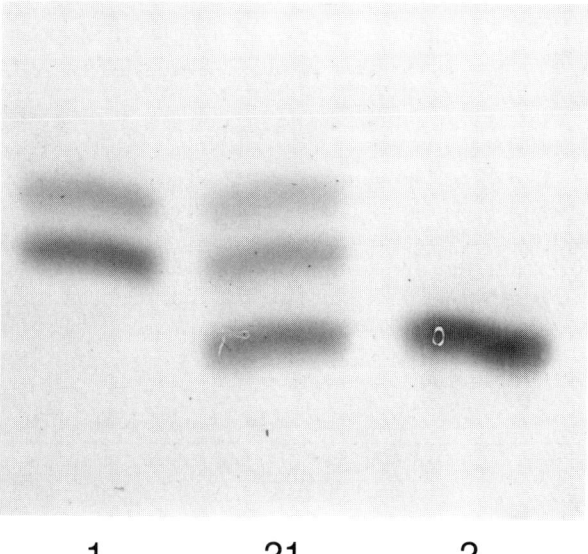

Figure 46–11. The common GC phenotypes, as developed by prolonged agarose gel electrophoresis at pH 8.6 and immunofixation. Minor components are evident (as they are also in Figure 46–10) anodal to the major bands.

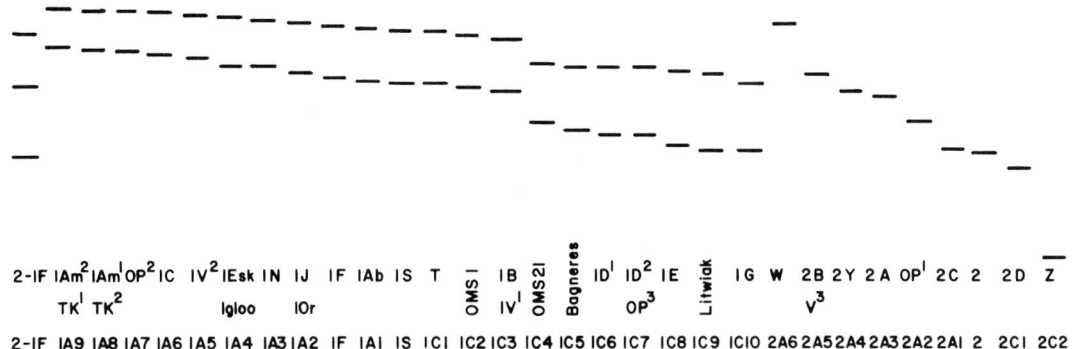

Figure 46–12. Diagrammatic representation of the common and rare GC variants as they appear in isoelectric focusing, with an attempt to relate their positions to the common forms.

Some structural work has been done on Gc-globulin. The evidence (65) suggests that the molecule consists of two polypeptide chains of similar size. GC 1A and 1C appear to differ by at least one amino acid, and at least one tryptic peptide is different when GC 1 and GC 2 are compared.

The introduction of isoelectric focusing (66) in the analysis of Gc-globulin types not only expanded the number of variants but revealed that there were two types of GC 1: 1F and 1S (see Figure 46–12). Frequencies of some of the more common alleles are given for several populations in Table 46–5. Considerable ethnic variation in GC allele frequencies is evident.

Pseudocholinesterase

Plasma contains a glycoprotein enzyme of 348,000-dalton molecular weight and α_2-mobility, which is capable of hydrolyzing acetylcholine (67, 68), among other substrates. This enzyme, acylcholine acylhydrolase, EC 3.1.1.8, or pseudocholinesterase, is of clinical importance because persons deficient in it are subject to apnea if they are given the muscle relaxant succinylcholine as an adjunct to anesthesia.

The physiologic function of pseudocholinesterase is unknown. The serum level is somewhat lower at birth than in later life, but adult levels are attained by 2 months of age (69, 70). The concentration is higher in childhood than in middle and old age. Serum levels may be depressed in severe hepatocellular disease, uremia, organic phosphate poisoning (the enzyme is irreversibly inhibited by organic phosphates), carcinoma of the large bowel, and malnutrition (71, 72). Increased serum levels are found in nephrosis (73). The rare individuals with inherited deficiency of pseudocholinesterase activity are healthy and have been recognized for some time (74). Extensive studies of serum from such persons, from their relatives, and from random populations have revealed that several mutant genes at a locus designated *CHE1* may be responsible for deficient enzymic activity (75–78). These studies have involved kinetics of inhibition, using various substrates and inhibitors. By this means, usual (U) and atypical (A) pseudocholinesterases could be defined. The atypical enzyme revealed by these studies is presumably a dysfunctional genetic variant, a product of *CHE1∗A*. In addition to these variants (CHE1 A, CHE1 U), CHE1 S (silent) with little or no immunoreactive protein, CHE1 J with approximately one-third normal activity, CHE1 K with approximately two-thirds normal activity, and CHE1 F with normal dibucaine number and markedly reduced fluoride number have been defined (79).

The *CHE1∗A* allele has a frequency of between 0.01 and 0.02 in most white populations studied (80), but frequencies as high as 0.051 have been observed in non-Ashkenazi Jews (81). The gene has an even lower frequency in most African, Asiatic, native American, and oceanic populations studied. The frequency of *CHE1∗F* heterozygotes

Table 46–5. GC GENE FREQUENCIES IN VARIOUS POPULATIONS

Population	*GC∗1F*	*GC∗1S*	*GC∗2*	*GC∗1A1*	*GC∗1A9*	*GC∗2A3*	*GC∗1A2*
White							
France	0.077	0.512	0.412				
Germany	0.125	0.603	0.272				
Oriental							
Bolivia (Amerindian)	0.231	0.636	0.122		0.009		
Japan	0.466	0.259	0.257				0.018
Black (Central African Republic)	0.584	0.191	0.064	0.054		0.107	

is about 1 per cent in Europeans. The *CHE1*S* (82) gene frequency is probably even lower than that of *CHE1*F*.

If starch gel electrophoresis of serum is performed at pH 5 to 6, pseudocholinesterase patterns show one (C4) or two (C4 and C5) bands (83). The presence or absence of the C5 band appears to be controlled by a gene at a locus distinct from *CHE1*, designated *CHE2*. This trait is probably inherited as an autosomal dominant characteristic, but there appears to be interaction with CHE1 expression. Persons who are C5+ (CHE2 QI [quantity increased]) have 30 per cent higher enzyme levels than those who are CHE2 QN (quantity normal). The C5+ phenotype is found in about 10 per cent of whites (84) and in a lower percentage of blacks.

Transferrin

Iron is transported in the serum by a 5S β-globulin called transferrin (85). The molecular weight of the molecule is about 75,000 daltons, and it contains 5.5 per cent carbohydrate. Each molecule has two binding sites for Fe^{3+}. The molecule is a single polypeptide chain with an internal duplication, suggesting evolution from a molecule half the current size with a single iron-binding site by tandem gene duplication. Iron-free transferrin is colorless, whereas the saturated molecule is salmon pink.

The concentration of transferrin in normal serum has a rather narrow range of 200 to 320 mg per dl, with a mean of 250 mg per dl. There is a direct correspondence between the total iron-binding capacity of serum and its transferrin concentration. On both theoretical and experimental grounds, it has been found that 1 mg of transferrin binds 1.25 μg of iron under full saturation (86). The metabolic behavior of transferrin is such that the apoprotein has a half-life of 7 to 10 days, but the iron half-life is on the order of 90 minutes (87), in keeping with the transport function of transferrin for iron.

Serum transferrin concentration rises in iron deficiency, in the latter portion of pregnancy, and in women on oral contraceptive medication. During any acute or chronic inflammatory state or in the presence of tissue necrosis, transferrin (like albumin) acts as a negative acute-phase reactant, and its serum concentration falls.

A very rare and probably inherited deficiency state for transferrin has been described (88, 89). This state is characterized by severe hypochromic microcytic anemia and death in childhood from excessive iron deposition in tissues, particularly the myocardium, liver, and spleen.

The common form of transferrin has been named TF C, but a large number of inherited variants have been recognized (90). These are distinguished by differences in electrophoretic mobility from TF C, the more anodal variants being designated B, with numerical or geographic modifiers, and the more cathodal variants named D, with modifiers. Figure 46–13 shows transferrin patterns containing these variants in association with TF C or other variants or in the homozygous state. These variants are inherited in mendelian autosomal codominant fashion. In all instances, such inheritance patterns suggest that the variants are controlled by mutant alleles at a single locus, *TF*.

These transferrin variants occur in low frequency in all populations, and individual alleles appear to occur in some geographic areas and populations but not others: *TF*B2* has a frequency of up to 0.015 in whites; *TF*D1*, *TF*D2*, and *TF*D3* are found in blacks; and *TF*B3* has been found among Japanese, for example. All the variants studied have had normal function in terms of iron-binding. Structural studies have indicated that the variants are mostly, if not exclusively, the products of single point mutations. For example, there is evidence that TF B2 differs from TF C in that it contains a glutamic acid residue at the site where TF C has a glycine (91). TF DCHI however, contains an arginine in place of a histidine in TF C (92). No immunochemical differences between TF variants have been uncovered.

When serum is subjected to isoelectric focusing and transferrin is examined, an inherited polymorphism in TF C is observed (93). There are

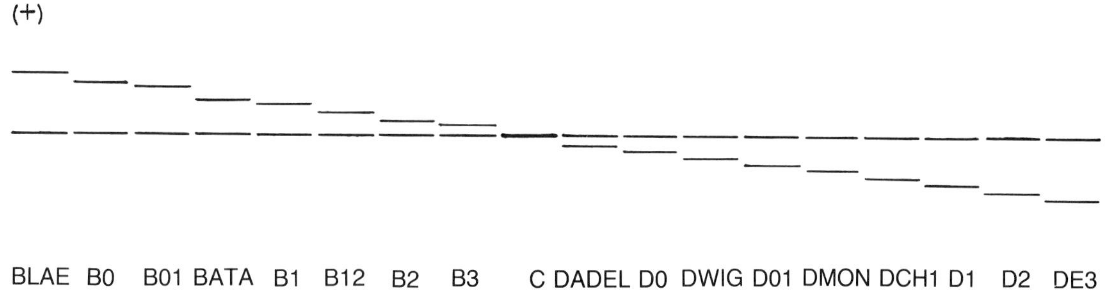

Figure 46–13. Diagram of variants of transferrin in relation to transferrin C, as seen in alkaline gel electrophoresis. (Adapted from Giblett, R. E.: *Genetic Markers in Human Blood*. Oxford, Blackwell Scientific Publications, 1969, p. 126.)

Table 46–6. *TF* GENE FREQUENCIES IN VARIOUS POPULATIONS

Population	*TF*C1	*TF*C2	*TF*C3	*TF*B2
White				
Germany	0.782	0.135	0.071	0.012
Italy	0.778	0.180	0.036	0.004
Nepal*	0.722	0.250	0.017	
Oriental (Japan)†	0.773	0.212		

*TF*CNEP* (C Nepal) or *TF*C9* has a frequency of 0.010 in this population.

†*TF*DCHI* has a frequency of 0.008 in this population.

more than 12 recognized subtypes of TF C of which only TF C1, 2, and 3 are common in whites. TF C4 is common in Amerindians, and TF C5 is common in black Americans. Table 46–6 gives the frequencies of common TF alleles in a number of populations.

Lipoproteins

The serum lipoproteins are divisible into two major groups according to their lipid content and apoprotein composition. The high-density lipoproteins (d = 1.093 to 1.149) have Sf values of 2 to 8, molecular weights of 200,000 to 400,000 daltons, and electrophoretic mobilities in the α_1-range. The low-density lipoproteins (d = <1.019 to 1.063) appear to be under separate genetic control and have different proportions of specific apoproteins, more lipid, and molecular weights in excess of 2×10^6. These low-density lipoproteins can be further subdivided into very-low-density (VLDL) with α_2- or pre β-mobility and low-density lipoproteins with β-mobility. The entire low-density lipoprotein group of molecules appears to function in the transport of lipids and lipid-soluble material.

The concentrations of the lipoproteins vary under certain pathophysiologic conditions. The α-lipoproteins (high-density lipoproteins) may be decreased in patients with chronic renal disease. In thyrotoxicosis there tends to be a decrease in the concentration of low-density lipoproteins, whereas in myxedema, their concentration increases. Increases in low-density lipoproteins are also seen in biliary obstruction and diabetic acidosis.

Hereditary deficiency of β-lipoprotein (94) is a rare disorder inherited as an autosomal recessive characteristic. Affected individuals, in addition to the absence of β-lipoprotein (low-density lipoprotein) from their serum, have neuromuscular disturbances with degenerative changes in the cerebellum and posterolateral columns of the spinal cord, retinitis pigmentosa, malabsorption, and spiculated erythrocytes (acanthocytes) associated with intermittent hemolytic anemia. The striking red cell deformity is at least partially reversible by transfer into normal plasma or by the intravenous administration of cottonseed oil. Thus, the abnormal red cell shape in this disorder is probably a secondary phenomenon. Inheritance of half-normal serum concentrations of β-lipoprotein as an autosomal dominant trait appears to be a condition different from classic abetalipoproteinemia. Affected individuals may be asymptomatic or have some of the clinical manifestations of abetalipoproteinemia.

Polymorphisms in the β-lipoproteins detectable by precipitation (or lack of precipitation) with certain antiserums can be classified into two groups, depending on the source of the antiserum. The AG determinants (95) are detected by antibodies found in the serum of some patients who have received large numbers of whole blood or plasma transfusions, particularly in such patients with thalassemia major. The lipoprotein determinants LP and LD are detected by antisera prepared in rabbits that have been immunized with whole serum or β-lipoprotein from a single individual (96).

There are 10 AG specificities (97, 98), designated X, Y, A1, D, C, G, T, Z, H, and I. These occur as antithetical pairs, the elements of which reflect haplotypes of alleles at five postulated genetic loci for apolipoprotein B. Fourteen specific *AG* haplotypes have been observed, of which some at least are population-specific. The relationship between the LP and AG systems is not clear. LP A occurs in approximately 35 per cent of whites and is found on pre–β-lipoproteins.

There is genetically determined polymorphism in apolipoprotein E detected by isoelectric focusing of purified apolipoprotein or VLDL (99, 100). Three common alleles control the variants; these are, from most acidic to most basic, *APOE*2*, *APOE*3*, and *APOE*4*. The amino acid substitutions involved are known, and the allele frequencies among whites are as follows: *APOE*2* = 0.15, *APOE*3* = 0.74, and *APOE*4* = 0.11. Homozygosity for *APOE*2* is associated with type III hyperlipoproteinemia. There is evidence that the amino acid substitution in APOE 2 interferes with receptor binding and utilization of apolipoprotein E, which accounts for its accumulation in homozygotes. There also is evidence that *APOE*4*, particularly in homozygotes, is associated with Type V hyperlipoproteinemia (101).

With isoelectric focusing and special pretreatment of serum, charge variants of apolipoproteins A-I and A-IV (102–104) have been detected, and A-II also has been visualized. In the case of apolipoprotein A-IV, the most common allele, *APOA4*1*, has an approximate frequency of 0.92 in whites, *APOA4*2* has a frequency of approximately 0.07, and a rare variant designated APOA4 MUE (Muenster) has been recognized with a frequency of approximately 0.0025 (104).

Nucleotide probes for a number of apolipoprotein genes have been produced, and progress in

Table 46-7. TC2 GENE FREQUENCIES IN VARIOUS POPULATIONS*

Population	TC2*1	TC2*2	TC2*3	TC2*4	TC2*5
Black					
United States	0.178		0.635	0.187	
White					
United States	0.450		0.531	0.015	0.004
Switzerland	0.406	0.010	0.578	0.004	0.002
Oriental					
United States	0.486		0.514		
Guatemala	0.236		0.764		

*The nomenclature proposed in reference 114 is used, in which alleles are named according to electrophoretic mobility at alkaline pH from cathode to anode. This is not the same as in reference 113.

elucidation of their structure, RFLPs, and chromosomal localization has been rapid. A number of associations between specific RFLP alleles and alterations in lipids or lipoproteins or both have been observed. For example, DNA polymorphisms in or near the apolipoprotein A-1 gene *(APOA1)* have been found to be associated with hypertriglyceridemia (105) and with premature atherosclerosis (106, 107).

The high-density α-lipoprotein is hereditarily absent from the serum of patients with Tangier disease (108). Such patients show deposition of cholesterol esters throughout the reticuloendothelial system. Their serum contains decreased cholesterol, decreased phospholipid, and normal or increased triglyceride concentrations. By appropriate techniques, very small amounts of abnormal high-density lipoprotein can be found in the serum of patients with Tangier disease. Individuals heterozygous for Tangier disease are asymptomatic but have decreased concentrations of α-lipoprotein. Synthesis of apolipoprotein A-1 is normal in Tangier disease despite very low serum levels, suggesting defective processing as the primary problem.

α_2-HS-Glycoprotein

Named for the two investigators who first independently described it, Heremans and Schmid (109, 110), α_2-HS-glycoprotein has an Mr of 49,000 and increases phagocytosis by both monocytes and neutrophils. Its serum concentration is approximately 60 mg per dl but falls as part of the plasma protein acute-phase response.

Polymorphism in this protein was found as the result of whole-serum screening by two-dimensional electrophoresis (111). There are two alleles with differing net surface charge. After removal of sialic acid, the charge difference disappears, but a small (1000 Da) difference between the sizes of the variants persists, suggesting that it is due to variations in neutral carbohydrate. The α_2-HS alleles have frequencies of 0.36 and 0.64 in whites and 0.27 and 0.73 in Japanese (112).

Transcobalamin II

This globulin, a transport protein for vitamin B_{12} (as its name implies), exhibits considerable genetic polymorphism (113, 114), which is detected by addition of radioisotopically labeled B_{12} to serum, isoelectric focusing, or electrophoresis and autoradiography. Four common variants are found in whites. Gene frequencies are given in Table 46-7.

Factor XIII

Factor XIII crosslinks fibrin in the evolving blood clot by a transglutaminase reaction. Each of the subunits of this protein exhibits genetic polymorphism, detected by gel electrophoresis and incorporation of a fluorescent label (dansyl cadaverine) into a casein overlay for Factor XIII A subunit after agarose gel electrophoresis (115) or by immunofixation with specific antiserum after agarose gel electrophoresis for the B subunit (116). Immunofixation can also be used for detection of the A subunit polymorphism. Gene frequencies for *F13A* and *F13B* in a number of populations are given in Tables 46-8 and 46-9.

Plasminogen

Plasminogen is the zymogen for the enzyme plasmin of the fibrinolytic system. Genetic poly-

Table 46-8. *F13A* GENE FREQUENCIES IN VARIOUS POPULATIONS

Population	F13A*1	F13A*2	F13A*4
Melanesian			
Fiji Islands	0.783	0.209	0.008
Loyalty Islands	0.768	0.232	
Polynesian			
Cook Islands	0.925	0.075	
Oriental			
Japan	0.900	0.100	
South America (Pima)	0.841	0.159	
White			
Denmark	0.817	0.177	0.003
Germany	0.797	0.203	

Table 46-9. *F13B* GENE FREQUENCIES IN TWO POPULATIONS

Population	F13B*1	F13B*2	F13B*3
White			
Australia	0.747	0.084	0.169
Germany	0.708	0.109	0.183

Table 46-10. *PLGN* GENE FREQUENCIES IN VARIOUS POPULATIONS

Population	PLGN*A	PLGN*B	PLGN*B3	Rare
White				
England	0.710	0.290		
United States	0.686	0.299		
Black				
United States	0.795	0.193		0.012
Gambia	0.860	0.140		
Oriental				
United States	0.964	0.029		0.007
Japan	0.958	0.020	0.022	

Note: There are differences in nomenclature, so the variant PLGN B3 in Japanese has other names and may not be the same as the European PLGN B3.

morphism in this molecule is detected on isoelectric focusing of native (117, 118) or neuraminidase-treated (119) plasma. Patterns are developed by immunofixation (or immunoblotting) with specific antiserum or by suitable substrate overlays containing casein or fibrin. Neuraminidase treatment in our hands results in far simpler and less ambiguous patterns. *PLGN* gene frequencies for several populations are given in Table 46-10.

β₂-Glycoprotein I

Genetic polymorphism in β₂-glycoprotein is unusual in that it is dependent not on a charge or molecular size difference in variants but on concentration (120). Individuals homozygous for a deficient allele have no detectable protein but are healthy. The deficient allele at the *BG* locus has a frequency of approximately 0.03 in whites. Heterozygotes have half-normal serum levels, and there is apparently no overlap with homozygotes for the normal gene in serum concentration of β₂-glycoprotein I.

C3

The third component of human complement has a critical role in the complement system and is discussed in Chapter 28. Many of the complement-mediated functions that contribute to the inflammatory response, such as chemotaxis, opsonization of bacteria, generation of anaphylatoxin, and bactericidal activity, require C3 directly or indirectly. Genetic defects affecting C3, when present in homozygous form, may result in markedly increased susceptibility to infection by pyogenic bacteria.

The serum concentration of C3 may be lowered in patients with systemic lupus erythematosus, membranoproliferative and acute glomerulonephritis, immune complex disease, and advanced chronic liver disease. Deposits of C3 are found in glomeruli in these conditions, usually accompanied by immunoglobulins. C3 concentrations are usually markedly elevated in biliary obstruction. Lesser elevations occur as part of the acute phase response. In newborns, the concentration of C3 is about 60 per cent that of adult serum and rises into the normal range within the first few months of life.

C3 exhibits extensive genetic polymorphism (121). Approximately 25 or more alleles have been identified, of which only two are common (122). The most common form is C3 S (for slow), and the second most common type is C3 F (for fast). These, and the rare variants, are identified by prolonged high-voltage electrophoresis of whole serum (Fig. 46-14). Because C3 is the most abundant of the complement components with a normal range of concentration in serum of 100 to 200 mg per dl, it can be seen directly on protein staining of electrophoretic patterns of serum. To facilitate this visualization, one adds Ca^{2+} (or Mg^{2+}) to the electrophoresis buffer to reduce the migration of C3 and separate it from transferrin and β-lipoprotein. Gene frequencies for the more common C3 alleles are given in Table 46-11.

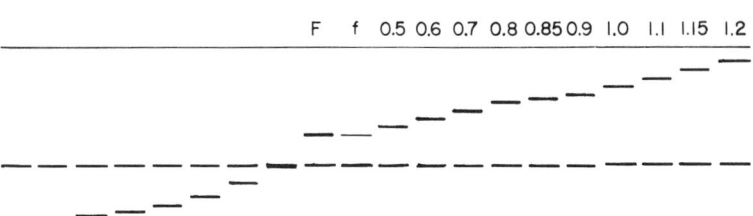

Figure 46-14. Diagram of variants of C3 in relation to C3 S in agarose gel electrophoresis at pH 8.6 with 0.0018 M calcium lactate present. (Adapted from Alper, C. A., Azen, E. A., et al.: Vox Sang. 25:18, 1973.)

Table 46–11. C3 GENE FREQUENCIES IN VARIOUS POPULATIONS

Population	C3*S	C3*F	C3*SO4
White			
United States	0.77	0.22	0.003
Norway	0.80	0.19	0.003
Germany	0.78	0.21	0.003
Black			
United States	0.92	0.07	—
Angola	0.95	0.05	0.001
Oriental			
United States	0.99	—	—
Tibet	1.00	—	—

The rare variants have been designated by numbers indicating their relative mobilities with respect to C3 S, with use of Ca^{2+} at 0.0018 M in the gel and electrophoresis buffers. One of the more rapid C3 variants was arbitrarily named C3 F1, and the distance from C3 S to C3 F1 is 1.0. Thus, C3 F0.85 migrates 85 per cent of the distance between C3 F1 and C3 S, and C3 S0.65 migrates 65 per cent of this unit distance, but toward the cathode. A number of the C3 variants have been studied functionally, and no abnormality has been found. A variant with the electrophoretic mobility of C3 F has been identified that is associated with about half the serum concentration of the other variants. This variant has been named C3 FQL and has been identified only in heterozygotes with C3 S. The total serum C3 concentration of such persons is normal.

A silent gene, C3*Q0, in heterozygotes results in half-normal serum levels (123). Complement-mediated functions are mildly abnormal in such sera, but these individuals are asymptomatic. The homozygous state for C3*Q0 (124), however, is associated with extreme deficiency of C3; serum complement-mediated functions are severely impaired, and there is a markedly increased susceptibility to infection by pyogenic bacteria. Homozygous C3 deficiency is rare, and only six such patients have been identified.

Low levels of serum C3 are associated with an inherited deficiency of Factor I (the C3b inactivator) (125). The latter protein is an enzyme that inhibits the hemolytic and other activities of activated C3 and functions as an inhibitor of the properdin or alternative pathway of complement activation. As a result, in homozygous Factor I deficiency (126–128) there is consumption and secondary serum deficiency of properdin Factor B (see next discussion) and C3. Most patients with this disorder have a markedly increased susceptibility to infection by pyogenic bacteria, much as patients homozygous for C3 deficiency and boys with agammaglobulinemia do.

C5

The fifth component of complement shows structural homology to C3 and C4, although it lacks the internal thiolester of the latter two proteins. Inherited structural polymorphism in C5 has thus far been recognized only in Melanesians and related populations (129).

C6

The sixth component of human complement shows considerable genetic polymorphism (130). Variants are most clearly detected by isoelectric focusing in gel of whole-serum samples followed by development of C6 patterns with an overlay containing properly sensitized sheep erythrocytes and C6-deficient animal serum (Fig. 46–15). Table 46–12 gives C6 gene frequencies for a variety of ethnic groups. A number of rare variants are recognized (131), and the alleles have been designated C6*B2, B3, B4, A1, A2, A3, M1, M2, and A21.

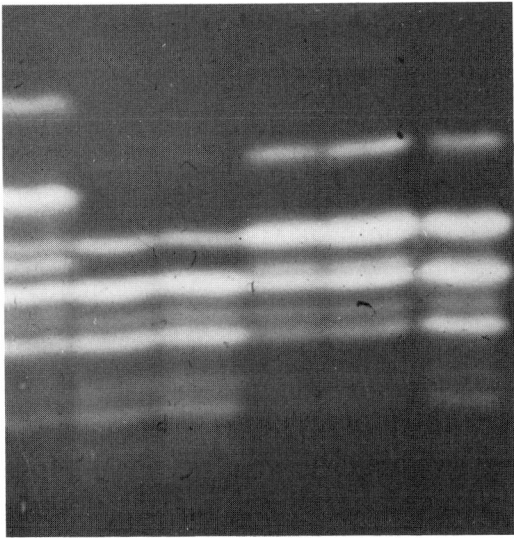

Figure 46–15. C6 patterns obtained by isoelectric focusing of serum and development of patterns of hemolysis. The cathode was at the top, and samples were applied near the anode. The patterns from left to right are C6 ABr, A, A, B, B, and AB.

Table 46–12. C6 GENE FREQUENCIES IN VARIOUS POPULATIONS

Population	C6*A	C6*B	C6*B2	C6*M
Oriental				
Japan	0.432	0.503	0.060	0.005
United States	0.590	0.350	-------0.050-------	
Black (United States)	0.560	0.380	-------0.060-------	
White				
United States	0.610	0.370	-------0.015-------	
Germany	0.613	0.379	-------0.008-------	

Note: All alleles other than C6*A and C6*B are pooled except in the Japanese.

Several individuals have been identified whose serum lacks detectable C6 (132, 133). These persons, like those with hereditary deficiency of C5, C7, or C8, have increased susceptibility to systemic infection with *Neisseria meningitidis* and *Neisseria gonorrhoeae* (134). As is true of sera deficient in these other late-acting components, hemolytic and bactericidal activities are grossly defective in C6 deficiency and are the only demonstrably compromised complement-mediated function in C6, C7, or C8 deficiency. Chemotaxis also is decreased in C5 deficiency. As for C3 deficiency (123), the genes producing C6 and C8 deficiency are silent or near-silent alleles of the structural genes (135, 136).

C7

With isoelectric focusing and a functional detection system, three alleles of C7 *(C7∗1, C7∗2,* and *C7∗3)* have been identified in whites (137), but the most common allele probably has a frequency of over 0.99. However, there is moderate polymorphism in Japanese (138), with allele frequencies as follows: *C7∗B,* 0.858; *C7∗M,* 0.096; and *C7∗A,* 0.046. In the latter study, electroblotting after isoelectric focusing was used to detect variants.

C8

The eighth component of human complement, C8, is a 151,000-Da molecule composed of three subunits (139, 140). The α-γ subunits are bound covalently through disulfide bonds, but the β subunit is associated via weaker, noncovalent bonds. Inherited C8 deficiency may affect either the α-γ or β chains (134, 141, 142); in either case, affected homozygotes have no C8 functional activity.

With appropriate C8-deficient serum used as a reagent to detect α-γ or β chains after isoelectric focusing in polyacrylamide gel electrophoresis, genetic polymorphism was defined in C8 α-γ–chains (the *C81* locus) (143) (Fig. 46–16) and C8 β-chains

Table 46–13. *C81* GENE FREQUENCIES IN VARIOUS POPULATIONS

Population	*C81∗A*	*C81∗B*	*C81∗A1*
Black			
Brazil	0.662	0.309	0.029
United States	0.700	0.246	0.054
White			
United States	0.649	0.348	0.003
Germany	0.554	0.429	0.018

(the *C82* locus) (142). Alternatively, one may detect the polymorphism in C81 by immunoblotting using anti-C8 (144). The incorporation of 3.1 M urea helps separate C8 α-γ from C8 β for optimal detection of both polymorphisms. Table 46–13 gives *C81* gene frequencies in several populations. There are two common alleles of *C82* in whites: *C82∗A* (for acidic), with a frequency of 0.952; and *C82∗B,* with a frequency of 0.044. A rare allele, *C82∗A1,* was found to have a frequency of 0.004 (142). There was no evidence of linkage between the two C8 loci.

Factor H (β_{1H}-Globulin)

This protein is a cofactor for the enzymatic control protein of the alternative complement pathway, Factor I, in its cleavage of C3b. Polymorphism has been detected by isoelectric focusing of dissociated immunoprecipitates made with serum and anti-H (145). Two common alleles, *FH∗1* and *FH∗2,* are found in whites with frequencies of 0.691 and 0.300, respectively. A rare allele, *FH∗3,* has a frequency of 0.006.

C4BP (C4-Binding Protein)

C4BP is a cofactor in the cleavage of C4b by I. Genetic polymorphism in this protein was detected by isoelectric focusing of immunoprecipitates of serum made with anti-C4BP (146). Two alleles,

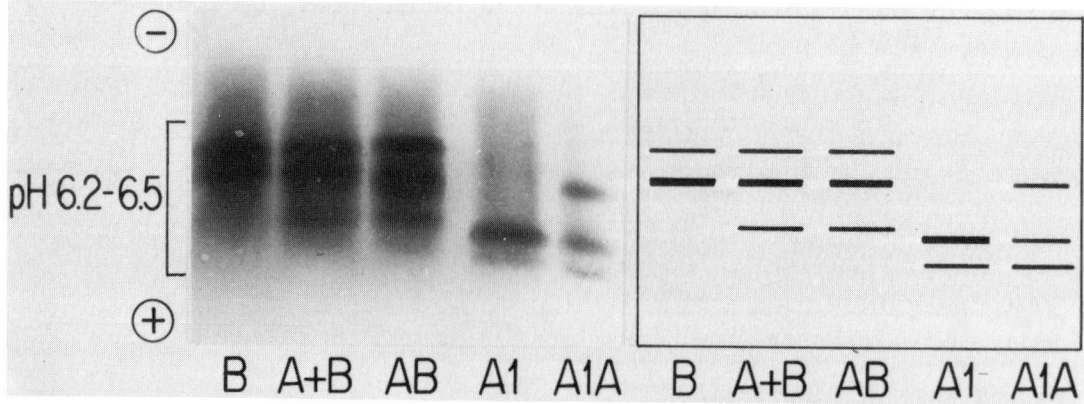

Figure 46–16. C81 patterns as bands of hemolysis after isoelectric focusing.

C4BP*1 and *C4BP*2*, have been found in whites, with frequencies of 0.98 and 0.02, respectively. Only C4BP 1 was found in samples from 30 South American Indians.

CR1 (Complement Receptor 1, C3b Receptor)

This protein is not, strictly speaking, a plasma protein; rather, it is found on cell membranes, where it binds specifically to the major activation fragments of C3 and C4, C3b and C4b. It also acts as cofactor in I-mediated cleavage of C3b. A molecular size difference under simple codominant genetic control is detected by SDS polyacrylamide gel electrophoresis (147, 148). Approximate gene frequencies in whites are 0.18 for the high-molecular-weight form, *C3BRM*S*, and 0.82 for the low-molecular-weight form, *C3BRM*F*. There is, in addition, evidence for genetic control of CR1 levels on red cell membranes at a locus unrelated to that controlling the structural polymorphism (149).

Factor B

Factor B of the alternative complement pathway is a 6S single polypeptide chain protein occurring in normal serum at a concentration of 12 to 56 mg per dl. On activation of the alternative pathway, Factor B is cleaved into two fragments, Ba (acidic) and Bb (basic). The complex between C3b and Bb constitutes the alternative pathway C3 (and C5) convertase, with its enzymatic site on Bb.

On electrophoresis of whole fresh serum or plasma and immunofixation with specific antiserum, Factor B forms multiple bands (Fig. 46–17). The specific patterns have been shown to be genetically determined by four common alleles at a genetic locus designated *BF* (150). The two most comon alleles in all populations studied are *BF*F* (fast) and *BF*S* (slow). The less common alleles are *BF*F1* and *BF*S1*. Many rare variants have been found (151, 152), and these are named, in analogy to the C3 system, BF F1.6, F0.85, F0.65, F0.55, S0.25, S0.3, and S0.45. It is of interest that the mobility variation of BF F and BF S is on the Ba fragment, whereas Bb carries the charge variation of the entire molecule for all other BF variants studied.

Gene frequencies for various populations are given in Table 46–14, and it can be seen that there are striking racial differences.

Low levels of Factor B in serum occur in patients with advanced chronic liver disease (along with low levels of C3). There is only modest and inconstant lowering of serum Factor B concentration in disease states characterized by complement activation in vivo. Although heterozygotes for Factor B deficiency have been identified (153), homozygous deficiency has yet to be described. The heterozygous B–deficient persons are asymptomatic and carry a null allele at the *BF* locus.

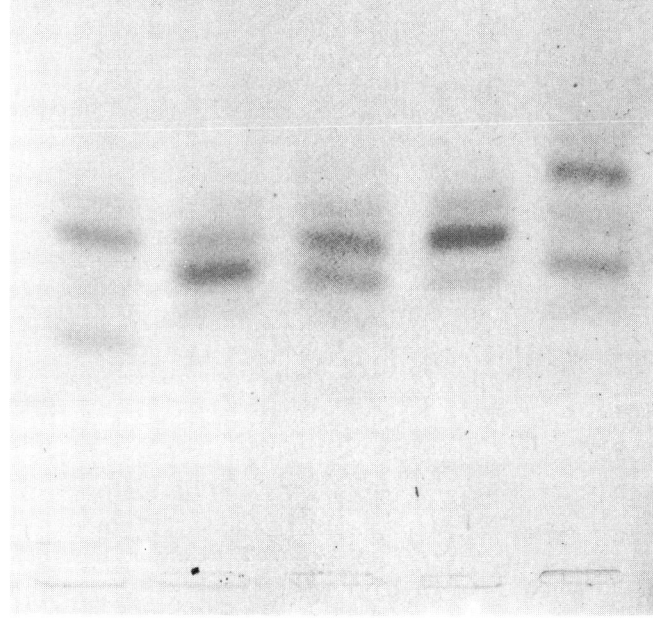

Figure 46–17. Prolonged agarose gel electrophoretic patterns of BF variants developed by immunofixation with specific antiserum.

Table 46-14. *BF* GENE FREQUENCIES IN VARIOUS POPULATIONS

Populations	*BF*F*	*BF*S*	*BF*F1*	*BF*S1*
Black				
Northeastern United States	0.512	0.437	0.051	
Southeastern United States	0.626	0.327	0.034	0.013
South Africa	0.655	0.282	0.034	0.025
White				
Northeastern United States	0.185	0.513	0.006	0.009
West Germany	0.177	0.800	0.008	0.016
France (Normans)	0.229	0.742	0.020	0.009
France (Basques)	0.305	0.562	0.124	0.008
Sardinia	0.219	0.578	0.198	0.005
Saudi Arabia	0.321	0.517		0.151
Oriental				
Norway (Lapps)	0.112	0.888		
Japan	0.198	0.801		
China	0.128	0.870		0.002

C2

There is limited structural polymorphism in C2 in whites (154, 155), with the most common allele, *C2*C*, having a frequency of approximately 0.96; an allele for a basic variant, *C2*B*, having a frequency of 0.026; and other rare alleles (including two for acidic proteins, *C2*A1* and *C2A*2*) having a combined frequency of less than 0.01. A null gene has a frequency of 0.005 to 0.01. In Japanese (156), *C2*C* has a frequency of 0.939, *C2*B* has a frequency of 0.022, an allele designated *C2*AT* has a frequency of 0.034, and rarer alleles have a combined frequency of 0.005. A number of RFLPs for C2 have been defined (157, 158) that show more polymorphism than the protein. They should therefore be useful in population genetic studies and other investigations of C2 genetically controlled variation.

C4

Human C4 is synthesized as a single polypeptide chain that undergoes postsynthetic processing to yield the mature disulfide-linked structure containing chains of 75 (beta), 95 (alpha), and 30 (gamma) kDa (159). Like α_2-macroglobulin and the complement protein C3, C4 has an internal thioester as part of its alpha chain (160, 161). On activation of the molecule, this chemical group splits and is transiently capable of acylating hydroxyl, amino, and similar moieties on soluble and cell-surface proteins and water.

There are two closely linked genetic loci for C4 (162), designated *C4A* and *C4B*. In general, products of *C4A* are more negatively charged, have lower hemolytic activity (163), and have alpha chains of slightly lower electrophoretic mobility in sodium dodecyl sulfate polyacrylamide gel (164) than the products of *C4B* have. In addition, C4A products usually carry Rodgers antigenic reactivity, whereas C4B products carry Chido reactivity (165). There is extensive genetic structural polymorphism at both C4 loci (163), best detected by agarose gel electrophoresis of desialated fresh plasma and immunofixation with anti-C4 (Fig. 46–18). In addition to showing some of the C4A and C4B genetic variants common in whites, Figure 46–18 illustrates the detection of half-null C4A-C4B haplotypes common in this racial group (162, 166). Electrophoretic variants at each locus are designated by arabic numerals, and the null alleles are named Q0 (for quantity zero) (163). It appears likely that at least some of the null alleles arose by unequal crossover during meiosis (see the discussion of alpha thalassemia in blacks in Chapter 22) (163). The same process would be expected to generate duplications of *C4A* or *C4B*, and C4 haplotypes with such duplications have been observed (167–169). From sequence analysis of C4A and C4B proteins (170, 171), six amino acid differences in the C4d fragment of the alpha chains have been detected. In addition to the relatively common variants C4A2, 3, 4, 6, Q0 and C4B 1, 2, 3, Q0 and the duplicated C4A 3,2 and C4B 1,2, there is a very large number of rare variants at both loci (172).

Nucleotide analysis of genomic DNA has revealed that the coding regions of *C4A* and *C4B* differ by 14 of over 4600 nucleotides (173), of which 12 are in the C4d region of the alpha chain and one each in the beta chain– and gamma chain–coding regions. Probes for this difference cluster involving codons 1101 to 1106 distinguish the two C4 genes. The nucleotide and amino acid differences between a number of C4A and C4B variants have been determined (174) and appear to represent point mutations. The *C4A* gene is approximately 22 kb; the *C4B* gene is usually 16 kb but is sometimes 22 kb. There are several RFLPs for the C4 genes (175–177), including one specific for *C4A*6* (175). It is of considerable interest that *C4A*Q0* is associated with a deletion

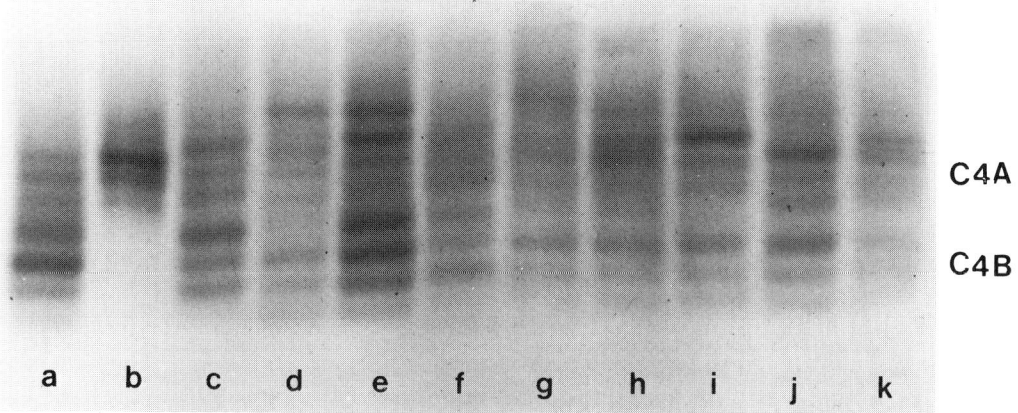

Figure 46–18. C4 patterns produced by electrophoresis of fresh desialated EDTA plasma in agarose gel electrophoresis at pH 8.8 and immunofixation with anti C4. The anode was at the top. Each gene product typically consists of three bands, the most anodal of which is usually the darkest. The C4A area is toward the anode, C4B toward the cathode. The C4 phenotypes of the patterns, from left to right, are: (a) C4A3,2 C4B2,1,1; (b) C4A3,3,2 C4BQ0,Q0; (c) C4A4,Q0 C4B2,2; (d) C4A6,3 C4B1,Q0; (e) C4A6,4 C4B2,1; (f) C4A4,3 C4B2,Q0; (g) C4A6,3,2 C4B1,Q0; (h) C4A3,2 C4B1,Q0; (i) C4A3,3 C4B1,Q0; (j) C4A2,2 C4B1,1; and (k) C4A3,2 C4B1,Q0. The presence of a single null gene (Q0) is detected by the ratio of protein in C4A to that in C4B. For example, in sample (c), C4B2 is about twice as abundant as C4A4, indicating the presence of a single C4AQ0. Homozygous Q0 is, of course, obvious from the absence of C4 bands in either C4A or C4B, as in pattern (b).

of *C4A* by nucleotide analysis in a number of instances (175).

Complotypes

From family studies, it was shown that *BF (176)*, *C2* (177, 154), and *C4A* and *C4B* (163, 178) were closely linked to HLA and other genes of the major histocompatibility complex (MHC) as well as to each other. These four complement genes were localized between HLA-B and HLA-DR, closer to HLA-DR (179). In many thousands of informative meioses, no crossovers among the four complement genes were noted, leading to the concept that the four genes formed a single genetic unit, or "complotype" (180). Complotypes are arbitrarily designated by their BF, C2, C4A, C4B variants with a shorthand notation in which Q0 is 0. Thus, *BF*S, C2*C, C4A*Q0, C4B*1* is written SC01. Table 46–15 gives complotypes in whites occurring with a frequency of more than about 0.01. It is clear that this four-gene complex is remarkably polymorphic; in fact, it is second in humans only to HLA-B in this regard.

DNA studies established that the order of genes is in fact *C2, BF, C4A, C4B* (181), and, surprisingly, immediately following the 3' end of each C4 gene was a gene for the adrenal enzyme, 21-hydroxylase (182, 183). A schematic representation of the region is shown in Figure 46–19. Because the entire coding regions of the MHC complement genes span only about 100 kb of genomic DNA, the physical basis for the rarity of crossovers between them is clear.

Extended Haplotypes

Linkage disequilibrium is the simultaneous occurrence of alleles on the same chromosome at closely linked genetic loci in members of a defined population at frequencies different from those predicted by the frequency of the individual alleles. The phenomenon is particularly striking and well known in the MHC. For example, both HLA-

Table 46–15. COMMON COMPLOTYPES IN WHITES*

Complotype†	Frequency
SC31	0.389
SC01	0.127
FC31	0.112
SC30	0.064
SC42	0.050
SC61	0.031
SC21	0.028
FC30	0.026
SC02	0.022
SC33	0.020
FC01	0.016
SB42	0.016

*Based on 643 normal haplotypes in white families.
†Complotypes are given in abbreviated form and arbitrary order as BF, C2, C4A, C4B types in which null (or Q0) alleles are designated "0."

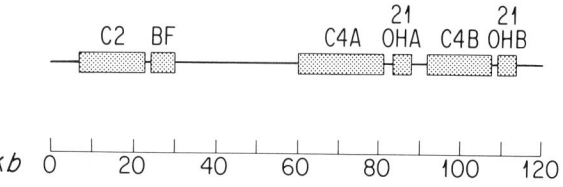

Figure 46–19. The complotype area on chromosome 6p.

B8 and HLA-DR3 have an allele frequency of approximately 0.12 in whites. One might therefore expect chromosomes carrying both HLA-B8 and DR3 together to have a frequency in this ethnic group of 0.12 × 0.12, or 0.014. In fact, the HLA-B8-DR3 haplotype has a frequency of 0.087 and therefore exhibits striking linkage disequilibrium. If one analyzes for linkage disequilibrium between complotypes, HLA-B alleles, and HLA-DR alleles, approximately a dozen exhibit significant linkage disequilibrium (184). These have been termed "extended haplotypes." They account for most of the linkage disequilibrium pairs of HLA alleles noted previously and for many of the MHC allele–disease associations previously reported (185). Extended haplotypes in whites with frequencies of approximately 0.01 or more are given in Table 46–16.

Immunoglobulins

Humoral antibody activity resides in a group of molecules of unique structural heterogeneity, the immunoglobulins (see Chapter 27). The basic structural units of these proteins consist of two kinds of chains, designated heavy and light, held together by disulfide bridges and by noncovalent forces (186). The arrangement of IgG1, the most plentiful of the immunoglobulins, serves as a model for this structure (Fig. 46–20). It should be noted that the molecule is symmetric and that the light chains and heavy chains about the axis of symmetry are identical in structure. The kind of heavy chain determines the immunoglobulin class: γ, α, μ, δ, and ϵ chains are found in IgG, IgA, IgM, IgD, and IgE, respectively. Subclasses have been identified in IgG (IgG1, 2, 3, and 4) and IgA (IgA1 and IgA2). The order on human chromosome 14 for the immunoglobulin heavy chain genes is $\gamma 3$, $\gamma 1$, $\psi\epsilon$, $\alpha 1$, $\psi\epsilon$, $\gamma 2$, $\gamma 4$, ϵ, $\alpha 2$ (187–189). The light chains in any immunoglobulin molecule are one of two types, designated κ and λ. The

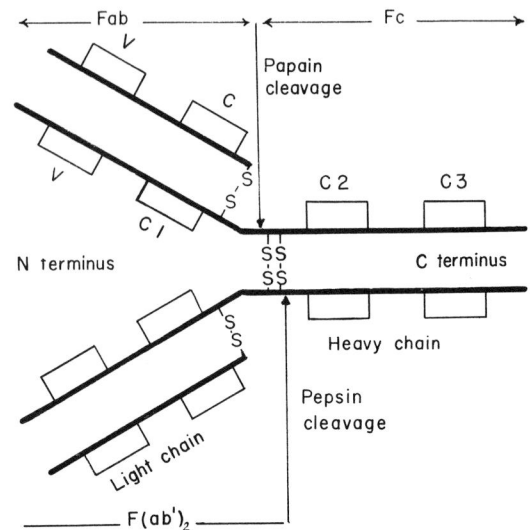

Figure 46–20. A simplified model of the IgG1 molecule.

amino acid sequences of two molecules of the same immunoglobulin subclass are found to be very similar in the C-terminal half of the light chain and the C-terminal three fourths of the heavy chain. These areas of the molecule have been called constant (C) regions, and the structural bases for the human genetic markers to be discussed are found here. The remaining N-terminal variable (V) regions of both heavy and light chains show marked differences in amino acid sequences from molecule to molecule, even within a single immunoglobulin subclass. This remarkable diversity is undoubtedly related to the specific antibody function of the immunoglobulins. The molecular bases for this diversity in immunoglobulin molecules have been elucidated by DNA studies of the structure and ontogeny of immunoglobulin genes. For a fuller description of the immunoglobulins and their structure and function and the genes involved, see Chapter 27.

The two major unlinked genetic systems are GM, controlling IgG C-region heavy chain synthesis, and INV, controlling the C-region of κ chains (190–191), and now called KM. The methods for detecting these markers are primarily serologic and require some detailed description. (See Chapter 28.)

The GM system was discovered by Grubb and Laurell (192), who were investigating the agglutination of red cells coated with gamma globulin (incomplete Rh antibodies) by serum from patients with rheumatoid arthritis. If the gamma globulin coats were from single individuals, certain of these rheumatoid agglutinins (Ragg's) agglutinated some coated red cells, but not others, and agglutination could be inhibited by the serum from certain normal individuals, but not others. It later became clear that similar and usually more specific agglutinins were found in serum from some nor-

Table 46–16. SOME COMMON EXTENDED HAPLOTYPES IN WHITES

HLA-B	Complotype	HLA-DR	Frequency	Δ/Δ Max* Corrected
8	SC01	DR3	0.076	0.65
7	SC31	DR2	0.070	0.54
12(44)	SC30	DR4	0.031	0.51
12(44)	FC31	DR7	0.030	0.29
17(57)	SC61	DR7	0.017	0.55
35	FC(3,2)0†	DR1	0.011	0.70
15(62)	SC33	DR4	0.011	0.55
14	SC2(1,2)‡	DR1	0.010	1.00

*A measure of linkage disequilibrium, corrected for pairwise linkage disequilibrium.
†*C4A* is duplicated in this complotype.
‡*C4B* is duplicated in this complotype.

mal subjects (SNagg's) (193). A third source of specific agglutinins is suitably absorbed animal antiserum to purified M-components (structurally homogeneous immunoglobulins from patients with multiple myeloma and related disorders) (194). The ability of some human serums to inhibit this kind of agglutination is inherited in mendelian fashion and resides in the immunoglobulins. A heavy chain genetic marker (AM) has been found on IgA2 subclass molecules (195).

In practice, two sources of IgG are used to coat human type O red cells for the detection of GM and KM factors. Incomplete anti-Rh (D) (see Chapters 15 and 44) is usually of the IgG1 or IgG3 subclass and renders Rh (D)-positive cells a useful indicator particle. Alternatively, purified M-components can be linked chemically to type O red cells to provide an indicator.

The various known GM, KM, and AM factors are listed in Table 46–17. Two major nomenclatures are in use, and some factors originally considered as separate are, in fact, very similar or identical. In our discussion, we will use the letter nomenclature and deal only with some major markers.

The markers on IgG1 include G1M A, Z, X, and F; those on IgG3 are G3M and the B group as well as C, S, and T, whereas a single marker, G2M N, is known for IgG2 (196). These markers, the genes for which are known to be very close to one another, are inherited as gene complexes in a manner analogous to the Rh antigens (see Chapter 44). These gene complexes vary among different ethnic groups (197). Table 46–18 lists the GM and AM gene complexes for the major races. Because their genes are contiguous and there are many areas of structural homology shared by the C-regions of the heavy chains of the IgG subclass molecules, it seems highly likely that the subclasses arose by gene duplication (187, 189). Natvig and associates (198) studied rare families with unusual gene complexes arising presumably from unequal homologous chromosomal crossover (similar to the origins of Lepore hemoglobin and HPA 2).

Intensive investigation of myeloma proteins has established the structural bases for many of the serologically detected genetic markers. Some of these findings are shown in Table 46–19. It will be noted that in some instances (e.g., G1M F and G1M Z), the markers are determined by the presence of one or another amino acid at the same position in the sequence. In other cases, an alternative sequence at a given position for a marker residue is not recognized as a marker by any specific serologic testing system. Furthermore, this alternative sequence is often shared by other IgG subclasses. The antigen in such cases is termed a "nonmarker." In all the examples given, the differences in sequence between markers or between markers and nonmarkers can be explained by point mutations consistent with the genetic code.

Because there is specific transport of maternal IgG of all subclasses across the placenta into the fetal circulation and some fetal blood leaks into the maternal circulation, particularly during the final trimester of pregnancy, it is not surprising that SNagg's arise in both the fetus and the pregnant woman (199) to different genetic markers on each other's immunoglobulins. These antibodies are for the most part transient and probably harmless. Most are IgM and, if they are maternal, do not cross the placenta. There is some suggestion, however, that the rare IgG SNagg produced by the mother during pregnancy may be responsible for the syndrome of transient hypogamma-

Table 46–17. NOMENCLATURE FOR IMMUNOGLOBULIN GENETIC MARKERS (ALLOTYPES)

WHO	Original	Intl. Soc. Hum. Genet.	
Gm(1)	a	G1M	A
Gm(2)	x	G1M	X
Gm(3) = Gm(4)	b^w, b^2	G3M	B2
Gm(4) = Gm(3)	f	G1M	F
Gm(5)	b, b^1	G3M	B
Gm(6)	c, like	G3M	C
Gm(7)	r		R
Gm(8)	e		E
Gm(9)	p		P
Gm(10)	b^α	G3M	BA
Gm(11)	b^β, b^O	G3M	B0
Gm(12)	b^γ	G3M	BG
Gm(13)	b3	G3M	B3
Gm(14)	b4	G3M	B4
Gm(15)	s	G3M	S
Gm(16)	t	G3M	T
Gm(17)	z	G1M	Z
Gm(18)	Rouen 2		Rou 2
Gm(19)	Rouen 3		Rou 3
Gm(20)	z (S.F.)	G1M	ZSF
Gm(21)	g	G3M	G
Gm(23)	n	G2M	N
Gm(24)	cs	G3M	CS
—	m		M
Km(1)	1	KM	1
Km(2)	a	KM	2
Km(3)	b	KM	3
A2M	1 or +	A2M	1

Table 46–18. MAJOR GENE COMPLEXES OF DIFFERENT POPULATIONS

Ethnic Group	A2M	G2M	G3M	G1M
White	+	N+	B	FNON-A
White	+	N−	B	FNON-A
White and Mongoloid	+	N−	G	Z A
White	+	N−	G	Z AX
Black	−	N−	B	Z A
Mongoloid	+	N+	B	F A
Mongoloid	−	N−	B	Z A

(Adapted from Natvig, J. B., and Kunkel, H. G.: Adv. Immunol. *16*:1, 1973.)

Table 46–19. AMINO ACID DIFFERENCES RELATED TO GENETIC MARKERS

Antigen	Chain	Papain Fragment	Sequence No.	Amino Acids
G1M A	γ1	Fc	356–358	Asp Glu Leu
NON-A	γ1, 2, 3	Fc	356–358	Glu Glu Met
G1M F	γ1	Fd	214	Arg
G1M Z	γ1	Fd	214	Lys
G3M G	γ3	Fc	296	Tyr
NON-G	γ2, 3	Fc	296	Phe
G3M B0	γ3	Fc	436	Phe
NON-B0	γ1, 2, 3	Fc	436*	Tyr
KM 1	κ	(Fab)	191	Leu
KM 2	κ	(Fab)	191	Val

*This position may be related to another G3M B marker.
(Adapted from Natvig, J. B., and Kunkel, H. G.: Adv. Immunol. 16:1, 1973.)

globulinemia. Although it may be that all infants who themselves lack maternal immunoglobulin genetic markers produce antibodies to these antigens during the latter part of the first year of life, these tend to disappear gradually over the next 2 or 3 years (200). Nevertheless, SNagg's can be found in 1 or 2 per cent of the healthy, untransfused normal population.

Localization and Evolution of Genes for Some Plasma Proteins

Chromosome assignment of human genes has proceeded at an accelerating rate. Information has been derived from studies of somatic cell hybrids that have retained only one or two human chromosomes, of families with chromosome translocations, of hybridization of DNA genetic probes to chromosomes in situ, and of classic linkage in families in which the chromosomal linkage of one of the loci is already known.

Albumin and α-fetoprotein show marked amino acid sequence homology, and their genes are closely linked (2). The gene for albumin is also linked to GC (201), with which it shares a function (ligand-binding). All three genetic loci are on chromosome 4 (202), as are the genes for the MNSs blood group and phosphoglucomutase 2, among others.

The genes for both transferrin and α_2-HS glycoprotein are on chromosome 3 (203, 204), as is the gene for the transferrin receptor. Because the loci for transferrin and ceruloplasmin (205) and transferrin and cholinesterase (206) have been reported to be linked, it may well be that these genes also are on chromosome 3. The gene for haptoglobin α and β chains is on chromosome 16 (207).

Chromosome 9 carries the gene for α_1-acid glycoprotein (204, 208) in addition to the genes for the ABH blood group system, adenylate kinase 1 and red cell δ-amino levulinic acid dehydrase. There is an extensive linkage group on chromosome 19, involving genes for C3 (209), for apolipoproteins E, CI, and CII (which also show linkage disequilibrium) (210), for the blood group systems Se, Lu, and H, and for myotonic dystrophy and peptidase D. Genes for apolipoproteins AI and CIII (211) are linked to the insulin gene on chromosome 11. The gene for apolipoprotein AII is on chromosome 1 (212).

The genes for immunoglobulin heavy chains are on chromosome 14 (213), linked to PI (α_1-antitrypsin) (214), whereas κ chains are encoded on chromosome 2, and λ chains are encoded on chromosome 22.

The complotype loci C2, BF, C4A, and C4B are between HLA-B and HLA-DR on the short arm of chromosome 6. C2 and BF show extensive sequence and functional homology at both the amino acid and nucleotide levels and probably arose by tandem gene duplication of a common ancestor. Both carry stretches of amino acid and nucleotide sequences characteristic of the serine protease family of proteins. Moreover, both have triple direct repeats involving about 60 amino acid residues (215) also found in C4-binding protein, Factor H, β_2-glycoprotein I, and CR1 (C3b/C4b receptor). Because all these proteins except β_2-glycoprotein I have binding affinity for C3b or C4b or both, the long repeats may be involved in this function. It is of great interest in this regard that the genes for CR1, Factor H, and C4-binding protein are linked (216, 217), with evidence (218) assigning them to chromosome 1, which carries the gene for the B chain of C1q as well (219).

The complement proteins C3, C4, and C5 show structural homologies in their N-terminal heavy chain regions (C3a, C4a, and C5a). The corresponding fragments have anaphylatoxin activity in common, suggesting a common origin (as does the thioester in C3d and C4d, but not C5). Nevertheless, these genes are not linked and are apparently encoded on different chromosomes. C6 and C7, however, are similar molecules and their genes are closely linked (220) but not yet assigned to a specific chromosome. Evidence suggests that C8l and perhaps *C82* are on chromosome 1 (221). The genes for coagulation Factors VII and X appear to be on the long arm of chromosome 13 (222). The localization of genes for Factors VIII and IX and for thyroxine-binding globulin to the X chromosome has been known for decades.

RED CELL ENZYMES

Chapters 18 and 19 describe the presently known clinical disorders associated with deficiencies in quality or quantity of blood cell enzymes. Two valuable monographs contain summaries of the blood cell enzymes that exhibit polymorphism (223, 224). Therefore, in this section of the chapter only selected examples of blood cell enzyme heterogeneity will be presented. For further details the reader should consult the references just cited.

Red Cell Acid Phosphatase

During his extensive studies of blood cell enzymes in human diseases, Valentine and co-workers (225) discovered that red cell acid phosphatase activity is higher in young cells (reticulocytes) than in an older cell population. Oski and associates (226) and Choremis and co-workers (227) reported that red cell acid phosphatase activity is decreased in whites with glucose-6-phosphate dehydrogenase (G6PD) deficiency, and it has been proposed that glutathione levels influence the activity of this enzyme in human cells. However, the relationship between G6PD and acid phosphatase activity has not been confirmed in subsequent studies (228).

Starch gel electrophoresis patterns of acid phosphatase activity (223) (zymograms) usually reveal six different phenotypes of varying frequency, one of which (CC) is extremely rare. The phenotypes are the result of heterozygosity for three alleles labeled A, B, and C. These alleles are responsible for differences in both activity and structure. For example, type BB individuals tend to have approximately 50 per cent more activity than type AA individuals, and type AB individuals have intermediate activity (164).

Rare acid phosphatase types also have been discovered that are due to combinations with other rare alleles seen mainly in black populations (224).

Phosphoglucomutase

The conversion of glucose-1-phosphate to glucose-6-phosphate, an important step in glycogen metabolism, is catalyzed by phosphoglucomutase (224). Glucose-1,6-diphosphate is an intermediate in the reaction. The enzyme is present in red cells, although glycogen is virtually absent in these cells. Two different *PGM* loci control the production of the common red cell PGM electrophoretogram (Fig. 46–21). The phenotypes are designated PGM1 1, 21, and 2 and are created by the products of two common alleles at the *PGM1* locus, termed *PGM1*∗1* and *PGM1*∗2*, as well as the products of the second *PGM* locus (*PGM2*), which has very little variation. Thus, the PGM1 1 phenotype represents homozygosity for the *PGM1*∗1* allele, PGM1 2 represents homozygosity for the *PGM1*∗2* allele, and PGM1 21 represents heterozygosity (*PGM1*∗1/PGM1*∗2*). Why each allele is represented by two enzyme bands (e.g., bands A and C of PGM1 1) is not clear but is certainly related to post-translational alteration of enzyme mobility. Some believe that the bands represent the phospho- and dephospho-enzymes.

Even more complexity has been introduced into PGM genetics by the finding of other uncommon alleles at the *PGM1* and *PGM2* loci and by the discovery of a third locus, *PGM3*. The potential complexity of a PGM zymogram is bewildering, and careful family studies are often necessary to decipher them. The *PGM3* locus (which contributes a very small fraction of total red cell PGM activity) was detected by examination of PGM zymograms from cells other than red cells that contain much more PGM activity. Placenta is an excellent source of PGM3, as are leukocytes. In fact, it is by linkage studies of leukocyte PGM3

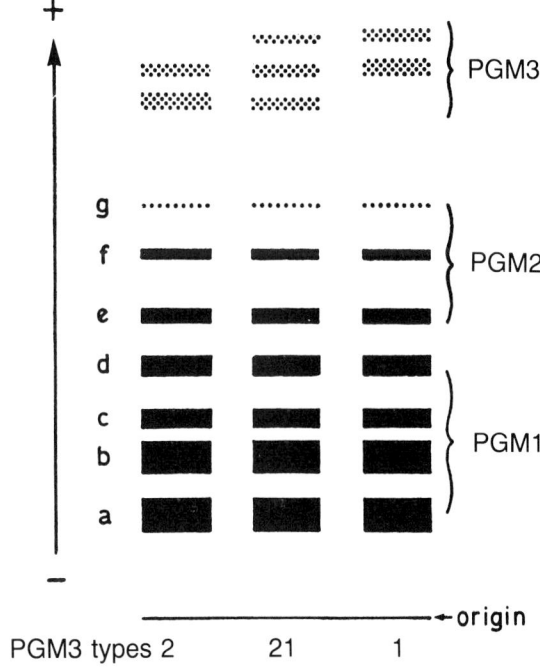

Figure 46–21. Diagram of three types of PGM3 isozymes, PGM3 1, PGM3 21, and PGM3 2, as seen in placental extracts. In each case the PGM1 isozymes are PGM1 21, and the PGM2 isozymes are PGM2 1. (From Harris, H: *Frontiers of Biology: The Principles of Human Biochemical Genetics*. Vol. 19, Neuberger, A., and Tatum, E. L. [eds.], Amsterdam, North-Holland Publishing Company, 1970, p. 50.)

that the HLA system has been traced to chromosome 6, where these histocompatibility loci are probably linked to *PGM3*.

Red Cell Adenylate Kinase

Adenylate kinase catalyzes 2 ADP ⇌ ATP + AMP and thereby contributes to the regulation of ATP metabolism. In muscle, the enzyme is known as myokinase. Deficiency of this enzyme has been associated with hemolytic anemia (229, 230).

As occurs in the case of PGM, zymograms of ADK activity from red cells are rendered somewhat confusing by post-translational increments in the number of enzyme bands produced by a single allele. Despite this source of difficulty, it has been possible to define four major ADK phenotypes, three of which conform to a relatively simple model, such as that which explains acid phosphatase zymograms. There is one *ADK* locus with two common alleles expressed in the red cell. The ADK 1 phenotype represents homozygosity for the *ADK*1* allele; the ADK 2 phenotype represents homozygosity for the *ADK*2* allele; and the ADK 21 phenotype is due to heterozygosity *ADK*1*/*ADK*2*. A fourth phenotype, ADK 41, is rare.

Catalase

Catalase is a heme enzyme that accelerates the breakdown of H_2O_2 to H_2O and O_2. As such, this activity should play an important role in the removal of unwanted H_2O_2 from the red cell. However, homozygous catalase deficiency (acatalasemia) is not associated with oxidative hemolysis, probably because H_2O_2 is mainly disposed of in red cells via the glutathione reductase hexose monophosphate shunt system (231). In some individuals with absent catalase, ulcerating lesions of the oral and nasal mucosa occur (232, 233).

There is no firm evidence for molecular heterozygosity in the catalase system (223). Multiple bands are observed in zymograms, but these represent post-translational artifacts. Aebi and Cantz (234) have shown that the enzyme is cell age–dependent, being much more active in reticulocytes. The deficiency state is similar to G6PD deficiency in that some catalase activity is observed in young cells, whereas none is present in old cells. Thus, the deficiency appears to be the result of the synthesis of an unstable enzyme protein (235).

Galactose-1-Phosphate Uridyl Transferase

This enzyme catalyzes the reaction Gal-1-P + UDPG → G-1-P + UDPGal. Deficiency of this enzyme and accumulation of Gal-1-P in tissues are responsible for hereditary galactosemia, a syndrome that, when severe, is characterized by anorexia, distention, diarrhea, vomiting, hypoglycemic attacks, jaundice, and chronic liver disease. Cataracts are common, as is mental deficiency in severe cases. The kidneys also are affected (236).

Deficiency of the enzyme appears to be due to a hypomorphic allele that is associated with decreased production of the normal protein, as is the case in beta thalassemia and pyruvate kinase deficiency. A convenient spot test for the enzyme in red cells makes it possible to screen newborns for the defect with relative ease (237).

One electrophoretic variant (the Duarte variant) has been described and appears to occur in about 10 per cent of the population (238).

References

1. Schultze, H. E., and Heremans, J. F.: *Molecular Biology of Human Proteins*, Vol. I. New York, Elsevier, 1966, p. 183.
2. Urano, Y., Sakai, M., et al.: Tandem arrangement of the albumin and alpha-fetoprotein genes in the human genome. Gene *32*:255, 1984.
3. Brown, J. R.: Structural origins of mammalian albumin. Fed. Proc. *35*:2141, 1976.
4. Scheurlen, P. G.: Über Serumeiweissenveränderungen beim Diabetes mellitus. Klin. Wochenschr. *33*:198, 1955.
5. Schell, L. M., and Blumberg, B. S.: The genetics of human serum albumin. In *Albumin—Its Structure, Function and Uses in Man*. Rosenoer, V. M., Rothschild, M. A., et al. (eds.), London and New York, Pergamon Press, 1977, p. 113.
6. Laurell, C.-B., and Niléhn, J. E.: A new type of inherited serum albumin anomaly. J. Clin. Invest. *45*:1935, 1966.
7. Brennan, S. O., and Carrell, R. W.: A circulating variant of human proalbumin. Nature (Lond.) *274*:908, 1978.
8. Murray, J. C., Mills, K. A., et al.: Linkage disequilibrium and evolutionary relationships of DNA variants (restriction enzyme fragment length polymorphisms) at the serum albumin locus. Proc. Natl. Acad. Sci. USA *81*:3486, 1984.
9. Bennhold, H., Peters, H., et al.: Über einen Fall von kompletter Analbuminämie ohne wesentliche klinische Krankheitzeichen. Verh. Dtsch. Ges. Inn. Med. *60*:630, 1954.
10. Murray, J. C., Demopolus, C. M., et al.: Molecular genetics of human serum albumin: restriction enzyme fragment length polymorphisms and analbuminemia. Proc. Natl. Acad. Sci. USA *80*:5951, 1983.
11. Schultze, H. E., Heide, K., et al.: α_1-Antitrypsin aus Humanserum. Klin. Wochenschr. *40*:427, 1962.
12. Eriksson, S., and Laurell, C.-B.: A new abnormal serum globulin α_1-antitrypsin. Acta Chem. Scand. *17*:5150, 1963.
13. Eriksson, S.: Pulmonary emphysema and alpha$_1$-antitrypsin deficiency. Acta Med. Scand. *175*:197, 1964.
14. Sharp, H. L., Bridges, R. A., et al.: Cirrhosis associated with alpha$_1$-antitrypsin deficiency. A previously unrecognized inherited disorder. J. Lab. Clin. Med. *73*:934, 1969.
15. Axelsson, U., and Laurell, C.-B.: Hereditary variants of serum α_1-antitrypsin. Am. J. Hum. Genet. *17*:466, 1965.
16. Laurell, C.-B., and Ericksson, S.: The electrophoretic α_1-globulin pattern of serum in α_1-antitrypsin deficiency. Scand. J. Clin. Lab. Invest. *15*:132, 1963.
17. Fagerhol, M. K., and Braend, M.: Serum prealbumins: polymorphism in man. Science *149*:986, 1965.
18. Fagerhol, M. K., and Laurell, C.-B.: The polymorphism of "prealbumins" and α_1-antitrypsin in human sera. Clin. Chim. Acta *16*:199, 1967.
19. Jeppsson, J.-O., Laurell, C.-B., et al.: Properties of isolated human α-1-antitrypsins of Pi types M, S and Z. Eur. J. Biochem. *83*:143, 1978.

20. Fagerhol, M. K., and Laurell, C.-B.: The Pi system—inherited variants of serum α_1-antitrypsin. Prog. Med. Genet. 7:96, 1970.
21. Talamo, R. C., Langley, C. E., et al.: Alpha-1-antitrypsin deficiency: a variant with no detectable alpha-1-antitrypsin. Science 181:70, 1973.
22. Perlmutter, D. H., Kay, R. M., et al.: The cellular defect in α_1 proteinase inhibitor (α_1 PI) deficiency is expressed in human monocytes and in *Xenopus* oocytes injected with human liver mRNA Proc. Natl. Acad. Sci. USA, 82:6918, 1985.
23. Jeppsson, J.-O.: Amino acid substitution—Glu leads to Lys alpha$_1$-antitrypsin PiZ. FEBS Lett. 65:195, 1976.
24. Owen, M. C., and Carrell, R. W.: Alpha-1-antitrypsin: molecular abnormality of S variant. Br. Med. J. 1:130, 1976.
25. Frants, R. R., and Ericksson, A. W.: α_1-antitrypsin: common subtypes in PiM. Hum. Hered. 26:435, 1976.
26. Carp, H., Miller, F., et al.: Potential mechanism of emphysema: α_1-proteinase inhibitor recovered from lungs of cigarette smokers contains oxidized methionine and has decreased elastase inhibitory capacity. Proc. Natl. Acad. Sci. USA 79:2041, 1982.
27. Owen, M. C., Brennan, S. O., et al.: Mutation of antitrypsin to antithrombin. α_1-antitrypsin Pittsburgh (358 Met → Arg), a fatal bleeding disorder. New Engl. J. Med. 309:694, 1983.
28. Long, G. L., Chandra, T., et al.: Complete sequence of the cDNA for human α_1-antitrypsin and the gene for the S variant. Biochemistry 23:4828, 1984.
29. Kidd, V. J., Wallace, R. B., et al.: α_1-antitrypsin deficiency: detection by direct analysis of the mutation in the gene. Nature 304:230, 1983.
30. Wallmark, A., Alm, R., et al.: Monoclonal antibody specific for the mutant *PiZ* α_1-antitrypsin and its application in an ELISA procedure for identification of *PiZ* gene carriers. Proc. Natl. Acad. Sci. USA 81:5690, 1984.
31. Rosenberg, S., Barr, P. J., et al.: Synthesis in yeast of a functional oxidation-resistant mutant of human α_1-antitrypsin. Nature 312:77, 1984.
32. George, P. M., Vissers, M. C., et al.: A genetically engineered mutant of α_1-antitrypsin protects connective tissue from neutrophil damage and may be useful in lung disease. Lancet 2:1426, 1984.
33. Courtney, M., Jallat, S., et al.: Synthesis in *E. coli* of α_1-antitrypsin variants of therapeutic potential for emphysema and thrombosis. Nature 313:149, 1985.
34. Schmid, K., Binette, J. P., et al.: The polymorphic forms of α_1-acid glycoprotein of normal Caucasian individuals. J. Clin. Invest. 43:2347, 1964.
35. Johnson, A. M., Schmid, K., et al.: Inheritance of human α_1-acid glycoprotein (orosomucoid) variants. J. Clin. Invest. 48:2293, 1969.
36. Nimberg, R., Motoyama, T., et al.: The amino acid substitutions found in genetic variants of α_1-acid glycoprotein. J. Biol. Chem. 246:5817, 1971.
37. Kurosky, A., Barnett, D. R., et al.: Covalent structure of human haptoglobin: A serine protease homolog. Proc. Natl. Acad. Sci. USA 77:3388, 1980.
38. Polonovski, M., and Jayle, M.-F.: Sur la preparation d'une nouvelle fraction des protéines plasmatiques, l'haptoglobine. C. R. Acad. Sci. (Paris) 211:517, 1940.
39. Smithies, O., Connell, G. E., et al.: Gene action in the human haptoglobins. I. Dissociation into constituent polypeptide chains. J. Mol. Biol. 21:213, 1966.
40. Laurell, C.-B., and Nyman, M.: Studies on the serum haptoglobin level in hemoglobinemia and its influence on renal excretion of hemoglobin. Blood 12:493, 1957.
41. Whitten, C. F.: Studies on serum haptoglobin: a functional inquiry. New Engl. J. Med. 266:529, 1962.
42. Smithies, O.: Zone electrophoresis in starch gels: group variations in the serum proteins of normal human adults. Biochem. J. 61:629, 1955.
43. Connell, G. E., Dixon, G. H., et al.: Subdivision of the three common haptoglobin types based on 'hidden' differences. Nature (Lond.) 193:505, 1962.
44. Smithies, O., Connell, G. E., et al.: Chromosomal rearrangements and evolution of haptoglobin genes. Nature (Lond.) 196:232, 1962.
45. Nance, W. E., and Smithies, O.: New haptoglobin alleles: a prediction confirmed. Nature (Lond.) 198:869, 1963.
46. Maeda, N., Yang, F., et al.: Duplication within the haptoglobin Hp2 gene. Nature (London) 309:131, 1984.
47. Korngold, L.: Antigenic differences among human haptoglobins. Int. Arch. Allergy, 23:268, 1963.
48. Korngold, L.: The effect of hemoglobin on the haptoglobin–anti-haptoglobin reaction. Immunochemistry 2:103, 1965.
49. McGill, J. R., Yang, F., et al.: Localization of the haptoglobin alpha and beta genes (HPA and HPB) to human chromosome 16q22 by in situ hybridization. Cytogenet. Cell. Genet. 38:155, 1984.
50. Holmberg, C. G., and Laurell, C.-B.: Investigations in serum copper. II. Isolation of the copper containing protein, and a description of some of its properties. Acta Chem. Scand. 2:550, 1948.
51. Gitlin, D., and Janeway, C. A.: Turnover of the copper and protein moieties of ceruloplasmin. Nature (Lond.) 185:693, 1960.
52. Holmberg, C. G., and Laurell, C.-B.: Oxidase reactions in human plasma caused by ceruloplasmin. Scand. J. Clin. Lab. Invest. 31:103, 1951.
53. Takahashi, N., Ortel, T. L., et al.: Single-chain structure of human ceruloplasmin: the complete amino acid sequence of the whole molecule. Proc. Natl. Acad. Sci. USA 81:390, 1984.
54. Takahashi, N., Bauman, R. A., et al.: Internal triplication in the structure of human ceruloplasmin. Proc. Natl. Acad. Sci. USA 80:115, 1983.
55. Scheinberg, I. H., and Gitlin, D.: Deficiency of ceruloplasmin in patients with hepatolenticular degeneration (Wilson's disease). Science 116:484, 1952.
56. Cox, D. W.: Factors influencing serum ceruloplasmin levels in normal individuals. J. Lab. Clin. Med. 68:893, 1966.
57. Shreffler, D.C., Brewer, G. J., et al.: Electrophoretic variation in human serum ceruloplasmin: a new genetic polymorphism. Biochem. Genet. 1:101, 1967.
58. Alper, C. A., and Johnson, A. M.: Immunofixation electrophoresis: a technique for the study of protein polymorphism. Vox Sang. 17:445, 1969.
59. Mohrenweiser, H. W., and Decker, R. S.: Identification of several electrophoretic variants of human ceruloplasmin including Cp Michigan, a new polymorphism. Hum. Hered. 32:369, 1982.
60. Cleve, H., Prunier, J. H., et al.: Isolation and partial characterization of the two principal inherited group-specific components of human serum. J. Exp. Med. 118:711, 1963.
61. Daiger, S. P., Schanfield, M. S., et al.: Group-specific component (Gc) proteins bind vitamin D and 25-hydroxyvitamin D. Proc. Nat. Acad. Sci. U. S. A. 72:2076, 1975.
62. Hirschfeld, J.: Immunoelectrophoretic demonstration of qualitative differences in normal human sera and their relation to the haptoglobins. Acta Pathol. Microbiol. Scand. 47:160, 1959.
63. Cleve, H., Kitchin, F. D., et al.: A faster migrating Gc-variant: Gc Darmstadt, Humangenetik 9:26, 1970.
64. Johnson, A. M., Cleve, H., et al.: Variants of the group-specific component system as demonstrated by immunofixation electrophoresis. Report of a new variant, Gc Boston (Gc B). Am. J. Hum. Genet. 27:728, 1975.
65. Bowman, B. H., and Bearn, A. G.: The presence of subunits in the inherited group-specific protein of human serum. Proc. Natl. Acad. Sci. USA 53:722, 1965.
66. Constans, J., and Viau, M.: Group-specific component:

evidence for two subtypes of the Gc¹ gene. Science 198:1070, 1977.
67. Surgenor, D. M., and Ellis, D.: Preparation and properties of serum and plasma proteins. Plasma cholinesterase. J. Am. Chem. Soc. 76:6049, 1954.
68. Haupt, H., Heide, K., et al.: Isolierung und physikalisch-chemische Charakterisierung der Cholinesterase aus Humanserum. Blut 14:65, 1966.
69. McCance, R. A., Hutchinson, A. O., et al.: The cholinesterase activity of the serum of newborn animals and of colostrum. Biochem. J. 45:493, 1949.
70. Lehmann, H., Cook, J., et al.: Pseudocholinesterase in early infancy. Proc. R. Soc. Med. 50:147, 1957.
71. Waterlow, J.: Liver choline-esterase in malnourished infants. Lancet 1:908, 1950.
72. Wetstone, H. J., LaMotta, R. V., et al.: Studies of cholinesterase activity. V. Serum cholinesterase in patients with carcinoma. Ann. Intern. Med. 52:102, 1960.
73. Kunkel, H. G., and Ward, S. M.: Plasma esterase activity in patients with liver disease and nephrotic syndrome. J. Exp. Med. 86:325, 1947.
74. Forbat, A., Lehmann, H., et al.: Prolonged apnoea following injection of succinyldicholine. Lancet 2:1067, 1953.
75. Davies, R. O., Marton, A. V., et al.: The action of normal and atypical cholinesterase of human serum upon a series of esters of choline. Can. J. Biochem. Physiol. 38:545, 1960.
76. Harris, H., and Whittaker, M.: Differential inhibition of human serum cholinesterase with fluoride. Recognition of two new phenotypes. Nature (Lond.) 191:496, 1961.
77. Bamford, K. F., and Harris, H.: Studies on "usual" and "atypical" serum cholinesterase using α-naphthyl acetate as substrate. Ann. Hum. Genet. 27:417, 1964.
78. Kalow, W., and Staron, N.: On distribution and inheritance of atypical forms of human serum cholinesterase, as indicated by dibucaine numbers. Can. J. Biochem. Physiol. 35:1305, 1957.
79. Evans, R. T., Iqbal, J., et al.: A family segregating for E_1^j and E_1^k at cholinesterase locus 1. J. Med. Genet. 17:464, 1980.
80. Giblett, E. R.: Genetic Markers in Human Blood. Oxford, Blackwell Scientific Publications, 1969, p. 208.
81. Szeinberg, A., Pipano, S., et al.: Frequency of atypical pseudocholinesterase in different population groups in Israel. Proc. Congr. Eur. Anaesthesiol., Copenhagen (Part 2). Acta Anaesthesiol. Suppl. 24:199, 1966.
82. Simpson, N. E., and Kalow, W.: The "silent" gene for serum cholinesterase. Am. J. Hum. Genet. 16:180, 1964.
83. Harris, H., Robson, E. B., et al.: Evidence for non-allelism between genes affecting human serum cholinesterase. Nature (Lond.) 200:1185, 1963.
84. Robson, E. B., and Harris, H.: Further data on the incidence of genetics of the serum cholinesterase phenotype C5+. Ann. Hum. Genet. 29:403, 1966.
85. Holmberg, C. G., and Laurell, C.-B.: Studies on the capacity of serum to bind iron. A contribution to our knowledge of the regulation mechanisms of serum iron. Acta Physiol. Scand. 10:307, 1945.
86. Schade, A., Reinhart, R., et al.: Carbon dioxide and oxygen in complex formation with iron and siderophilin, the iron-binding component of human plasma. Arch. Biochem. Biophys. 20:170, 1949.
87. Katz, J. H.: Iron and protein kinetics studied by means of doubly labeled human crystalline transferrin. J. Clin. Invest. 40:2143, 1961.
88. Heilmeyer, L., Keller, W., et al.: Kongenitale Atransferrinämie bei einem sieben Jahre alten Kind. Dtsch. Med. Wochenschr. 86:1745, 1961.
89. Goya, N., Miyazaki, S., et al.: A family of congenital atransferrinemia. Blood 40:239, 1972.
90. Giblett, E. R.: Genetic Markers in Human Blood. Oxford, Blackwell Scientific Publications, 1969, p. 126.
91. Wang, A. C., Sutton, H. E., et al.: A chemical difference between transferrins B_2 and C. Am. J. Hum. Genet. 18:454, 1966.
92. Wang, A. C., Sutton, H. E., et al.: Human transferrins C and D_{Chi}: an amino acid difference. Biochem. Genet. 1:55, 1967.
93. Kühnl, P., and Spielmann, W.: Transferrin: evidence for two common subtypes of the Tf^c allele. Hum. Genet. 43:91, 1978.
94. Salt, H. B., Wolff, O. H., et al.: On having no beta-lipoprotein: a syndrome comprising abeta-lipoproteinaemia, acanthocytosis, and steatorrhea. Lancet 2:325, 1960.
95. Allison, A. C., and Blumberg, B. S.: An isoprecipitation reaction distinguishing human serum protein types. Lancet 1:634, 1961.
96. Berg, K.: A new serum type system in man—the Lp system. Acta Pathol. Microbiol. Scand. 59:369, 1963.
97. Allison, A. C., and Blumberg, B. S.: An isoprecipitation reaction distinguishing human serum protein types. Lancet 1:634, 1961.
98. Bütler, R., Brunner, E., et al.: Contribution to the inheritance of the Ag groups: a population genetic study. Vox Sang. 26:485, 1974.
99. Utermann, G., Hees, M., et al.: Polymorphism of apolipoprotein E and occurrence of dysbetalipoproteinemia in man. Nature 269:604, 1977.
100. Zannis, V. I., Just, P. W., et al.: Human apolipoprotein E isoprotein subclasses are genetically determined. Am. J. Hum. Genet. 33:11, 1981.
101. Ghiselli, G., Gregg, R. E., et al.: Phenotype study of apolipoprotein E isoforms in hyperlipoproteinaemic patients. Lancet 2:405, 1982.
102. Utermann, G., Feussner, G., et al.: Genetic variants of group A lipoproteins. Rapid methods for screening and characterization without ultracentrifugation. J. Biol. Chem. 257:501, 1982.
103. Menzel, H.-J., Kladetzky, R. G., et al.: One-step screening method for the polymorphism of apolipoproteins A-I, A-II, and A-IV. J. Lipid Res. 23:915, 1982.
104. Menzel, H.-J., Kövary, P. M., et al.: Apolipoprotein A-IV polymorphism in man. Hum. Genet. 62:349, 1982.
105. Rees, A., Shoulders, C. C., et al.: DNA polymorphism adjacent to human apoprotein A-1 gene: relation to hypertriglyceridaemia. Lancet 1:444, 1983.
106. Norum, R. A., Lakier, J. B., et al.: Familial deficiency of apolipoproteins A-I and C-III and precocious coronary artery disease. New Engl. J. Med. 306:1513, 1982.
107. Karathanasis, S. K., Norum, R. A., et al.: An inherited polymorphism in the human apolipoprotein A-I gene locus related to the development of atherosclerosis. Nature 301:718, 1983.
108. Fredrickson, D. S., Altrocchi, P. H., et al.: Tangier disease: combined clinical staff conference at the National Institutes of Health. Ann. Intern. Med. 55:1016, 1961.
109. Heremans, J.: Les Globulines Sériques du Systéme Gamma. Brussels, Editions Arscia, 1960, p. 130.
110. Schmid, K., and Bürgi, W.: Preparation and properties of the human plasma Ba-$α_2$-glycoprotein. Biochim. Biophys. Acta 47:440, 1961.
111. Anderson, N. L., and Anderson, N. G.: Microheterogeneity of serum transferrin, haptoglobin and $α_2$HS glycoprotein examined by high resolution two-dimensional electrophoresis. Biochem. Biophys. Res. Comm. 88:258, 1977.
112. Umetsu, K., Kashumura, S., et al.: Classification of $α_2$HS glycoprotein ($α_2$HS) types by isoelectric focusing. Z. Rechtsmed. 91:33, 1983.
113. Daiger, S. P., Labowe, M. L., et al.: Detection of genetic variation with radioactive ligands. III. Genetic polymorphism of transcobalamin II in human plasma. Am. J. Hum. Genet. 30:202, 1978.
114. Fráter-Schröder, M., Hitzig, W. H., et al.: Studies on

transcobalamin. I. Detection of transcobalamin II isoproteins in human serum. Blood 53:193, 1979.
115. Board, P. G.: Genetic polymorphism of the A subunit of human coagulation Factor XIII. Am. J. Hum. Genet. 31:116, 1979.
116. Board, P. G.: Genetic polymorphism of the B subunit of human coagulation Factor XIII. Am. J. Hum. Genet. 32:348, 1980.
117. Raum, D., Marcus, D., et al.: Genetic control of human plasminogen (PLGN) (abstr). Clin. Res. 27:458A, 1979.
118. Hobart, M. J.: Genetic polymorphism of human plasminogen. Ann. Hum. Genet. 42:419, 1979.
119. Raum, D., Marcus, D., et al.: Genetic polymorphism of human plasminogen. Am. J. Hum. Genet. 32:681, 1980.
120. Cleve, H.: Genetic studies on the deficiency of β_2-glycoprotein I of human serum. Humangenetik 5:295, 1968.
121. Alper, C. A., and Propp, R. P.: Genetic polymorphism of the third component of human complement (C'3). J. Clin. Invest. 47:2181, 1968.
122. Alper, C. A., Azen, E. A., et al.: Statement of the polymorphism of the third component of complement in man (C3). Vox Sang. 25:18, 1973.
123. Alper, C. A., Propp, R. P., et al.: Inherited deficiency of the third component of human complement (C'3). J. Clin. Invest. 48:553, 1969.
124. Alper, C. A., Colten, H. R., et al.: Homozygous deficiency of C3 in a patient with repeated infections. Lancet 2:1179, 1972.
125. Abramson, N., Alper, C. A., et al.: Deficiency of the C3 inactivator in man. J. Immunol. 107:19, 1971.
126. Alper, C. A., Abramson, N., et al.: Increased susceptibility to infection associated with abnormalities of complement-mediated functions and of the third component of complement (C3). New Engl. J. Med. 282:349, 1970.
127. Alper, C. A., Abramson, N., et al.: Studies in vivo and in vitro on an abnormality in the metabolism of C3 in a patient with increased susceptibility to infection. J. Clin. Invest. 49:1975, 1970.
128. Alper, C. A., Rosen, F. S., et al.: Inactivator of the third component of complement as an inhibitor in the properdin pathway. Proc. Nat. Acad. Sci. 69:2910, 1972.
129. Hobart, M. J., Vaz-Guedes, M. A., et al.: Polymorphism of human C5. Ann. Hum. Genet. 45:1, 1981.
130. Hobart, M. J., Lachmann, P. J.: Polymorphism of human C6. Prot. Biol. Fluids 22:575, 1974.
131. Mauff, G., Alper, C. A., et al.: Statement of the nomenclature of human C6 polymorphism. Immunobiology 158:139, 1980.
132. Leddy, J. P., Frank, M., et al.: Hereditary deficiency of the sixth component of complement in man. I. Immunochemical, biologic, and family studies. J. Clin. Invest. 53:544, 1974.
133. Heusinkveld, R. S., Leddy, J. P., et al.: Hereditary deficiency of the sixth component of complement in man. II. Studies of hemostasis. J. Clin. Invest. 53:554, 1974.
134. Petersen, B. H., Lee, T. J., et al.: *Neisseria meningitidis* and *Neisseria gonorrhoeae* bacteremia in association with deficiency of a late acting complement component, C6, C7, or C8. Ann. Intern. Med. 90:917, 1979.
135. Glass, D., Raum, D., et al.: Inherited deficiency of the sixth component of complement: a silent or null gene. J. Immunol. 120:538, 1978.
136. Raum, D., Spence, M. A., et al.: Genetic control of the eighth component of complement. J. Clin. Invest. 64:858, 1979.
137. Hobart, M. J., Joysey, V., et al.: Inherited structural variation and linkage relationships of C7. J. Immunogenet. 5:157, 1978.
138. Nakamura, S., Ooue, O., et al.: Genetic polymorphism of the seventh component of complement in a Japanese population. Hum. Genet. 66:279, 1984.
139. Kolb, W. P., and Müller-Eberhard, H. J.: The membrane attack mechanism of complement: the three polypeptide chain structure of the eighth component. J. Exp. Med. 143:1131, 1976.
140. Steckel, E. W., York, R. G., et al.: The eighth component of human complement: purification and physiochemical characterization of its unusual subunit structure. J. Biol. Chem. 255:11997, 1980.
141. Tedesco, F., Densen, P., et al.: Two types of dysfunctional eighth component of complement (C8) molecules in C8 deficiency in man. Reconstitution of normal C8 from the mixture of two abnormal C8 molecules. J. Clin. Invest. 71:183, 1983.
142. Alper, C. A., Marcus, D., et al.: Genetic polymorphism in C8 β-chains. Evidence for two unlinked genetic loci for the eighth component of human complement (C8). J. Clin. Invest. 72:1526, 1983.
143. Raum, D., Spence, M. A., et al.: Genetic control of the eighth component of complement. J. Clin. Invest. 64:858, 1979.
144. Rittner, C., Hargesheimer, W., et al.: Population and formal genetics of the human C81 (α γ) polymorphism. Hum. Genet. 67:166, 1984.
145. Rodríguez de Córdoba, S., and Rubinstein, P.: Genetic polymorphism of human factor H (β1H). J. Immunol. 132:1906, 1984.
146. Rodríguez de Córdoba, S., Ferreira, A., et al.: Genetic polymorphism of human C4-binding protein. J. Immunol. 131:1565, 1983.
147. Dykman, T. R., Cole, J. L., et al.: Polymorphism of human erythrocyte C3b/C4b receptor. Proc. Natl. Acad. Sci. USA 80:1698, 1983.
148. Wong, W. W., Wilson, J. G., et al.: Genetic regulation of a structural polymorphism of human C3b receptor. J. Clin. Invest. 72:685, 1983.
149. Wilson, J. G., Wong, W. W., et al.: Mode of inheritance of decreased C3b receptor on erythrocytes of patients with systemic lupus erythematosus. New Engl. J. Med. 307:981, 1982.
150. Alper, C. A., Boenisch, T., et al.: Genetic polymorphism in human glycine-rich beta-glycoprotein. J. Exp. Med. 135:68, 1972.
151. Mauff, G.: Untersuchungen zum Komplement system des Menschen. Genetik und Biochemie der dritten und vierten Komponente des Komplementsystems sowie des Properdinfaktor B. Thesis, University of Cologne, 1977.
152. Hauptmann, G., Tongio, M. M., et al.: Bf polymorphism: study of a new variant (F 0.55). Hum. Genet. 33:275, 1976.
153. Weidinger, S., Schwarzfischer, F., et al.: Properdin factor B polymorphism. An indication for the existence of a Bf 0 allele. Z. Rechtsmed. 83:259, 1979.
154. Alper, C. A.: Inherited structural polymorphism in human C2: evidence for genetic linkage between C2 and Bf. J. Exp. Med. 144:1111, 1976.
155. Hobart, M. J., and Lachmann, P. J.: Allotypes of complement components in man. Transplant. Rev. 32:26, 1976.
156. Tokunaga, K., Araki, C., et al.: Genetic polymorphism of the complement C2 in Japanese. Hum. Genet. 58:213, 1981.
157. Woods, D. E., Edge, M. D., et al.: Isolation of a cDNA clone for the human complement protein C2 and its use in the identification of a restriction fragment length polymorphism. J. Clin. Invest. 74:634, 1984.
158. Bentley, D. R., and Campbell, R. D.: C2 and factor B: structure and genetics (abstr.) Biochem. Soc. Symp. 51:7, 1986.
159. Hall, R. E., and Colten, H.R.: Molecular size and subunit structure of the fourth component of guinea pig complement. J. Immunol. 118:1903, 1977.
160. Isenman, D., and Young, J. R.: The molecular basis for the difference in immune hemolysis activity of the Chido and Rodgers isotypes of the human complement component C4. J. Immunol. 132:3019, 1984.
161. Law, S. K. A., Dodds, A. W., et al.: A comparison of the

properties of two classes, C4A and C4B, of the human complement component C4. EMBO J. *3*:1819, 1984.
162. O'Neill, G. J., and Yang, S. Y.: Two *HLA*-linked loci controlling the fourth component of human complement. Proc. Natl. Acad. Sci. USA *75*:5165, 1978.
163. Awdeh, Z. L., and Alper, C. A.: Inherited structural polymorphism of the fourth component of human complement. Proc. Nat. Acad. Sci. U. S. A. *77*:3576, 1980.
164. Roos, M. H., Mollenhauer, E., et al.: A molecular basis for the two-locus model of human complement component C4. Nature (Lond.) *298*:854, 1982.
165. O'Neill, G. J., Yang, S. Y., et al.: Chido and Rodgers blood groups are distinct antigenic components of human C4. Nature (Lond.) *273*:668, 1978.
166. Awdeh, Z. L., Raum, D., et al.: Genetic polymorphism of human complement C4 and detection of heterozygotes. Nature (Lond.) *282*:205, 1979.
167. Bruun-Petersen, G., Lamm, L. U., et al.: Genetics of human complement C4. Two homoduplication haplotypes C4S,C4S and C4F;C4F in a family. Hum. Genet. *61*:36, 1982.
168. Raum, D., Awdeh, Z., et al.: Human C4 haplotypes with duplicated C4A or C4B. Am. J. Hum. Genet. *36*:72, 1984.
169. Uring-Lambert, B., Goetz, J.: C4 haplotypes with duplication at the C4A or C4B loci: frequency and associations with Bf, C2 and HLA-A, B, C, Dr alleles. Tissue Antigens *24*:70, 1984.
170. Hellman, U., Eggertsen, G., et al.: Primary sequence differences between Chido and Rodgers variants of tryptic C4d of the human complement system. FEBS Lett. *170*:254, 1984.
171. Chakravarti, D. N., Campbell, R. D., et al.: Amino acid sequence of a polymorphic segment from fragment C4d of human complement component C4. FEBS Lett. *154*:387, 1983.
172. Mauff, G., Alper, C. A., et al.: Statement of the nomenclature of human C4 allotypes. Immunobiology *164*:184, 1983.
173. Belt, K. T., Carroll, M. C., et al.: The structural basis of the multiple forms of the human complement component C4. Cell *36*:907, 1984.
174. Belt, K. T., Yu, C. Y., et al.: Polymorphism of human complement component C4. Immunogenetics *21*:173, 1985.
175. Carroll, M. C., Belt, K. T., et al.: Molecular genetics of the fourth component of human complement and steroid 21-hydroxylase. Immunol. Rev., *87*:39, 1985.
176. Allen, F. H., Jr.: Linkage of HL-A and GBG. Vox Sang. *27*:382, 1974.
177. Fu, S. M., Kunkel, H. G., et al.: Evidence for linkage between HL-A histocompatibility genes and those involved in the synthesis of the second component of complement. J. Exp. Med. *140*:1108, 1974.
178. Ochs, H. D., Rosenfeld, S. I., et al.: Linkage between the gene (or genes) controlling synthesis of the fourth component of complement and the major histocompatibility complex. New Engl. J. Med. *296*:470, 1977.
179. Yunis, E. J., Awdeh, Z., et al.: Complotype genetic loci segregate more frequently with HLA-DR than with HLA-B. Immunogenetics *21*:25, 1985.
180. Alper, C. A., Raum, D., et al.: Serum complement "supergenes" of the major histocompatibility complex in man (complotypes). Vox Sang. *45*:62, 1983.
181. Carroll, M. C., Campbell, R. D., et al.: A molecular map of the major histocompatibility complex class III region of man linking complement genes C4, C2 and factor B. Nature (London) *307*:237, 1984.
182. White, P. C., Chaplin, D. D., et al.: Two steroid 21-hydroxylase genes are located in the murine S region. Nature (London) *312*:465, 1984.
183. Carroll, M. C., Campbell, R. D., et al.: The mapping of 21-hydroxylase genes adjacent to complement component C4 genes in HLA, the major histocompatibility complex. Proc. Natl. Acad. Sci. USA *82*:521, 1985.
184. Awdeh, Z. L., Raum, D., et al.: Extended HLA/complement allele haplotypes: evidence for T/t-like complex in man. Proc. Natl. Acad. Sci. USA *80*:259, 1983.
185. Bodmer, W. F., and Bodmer, J. G.: Evolution and function of the HLA system. Br. Med. Bull. *34*:309, 1978.
186. Edelman, G. M., Cunningham, B. A., et al.: The covalent structure of an entire γG immunoglobulin molecule. Proc. Natl. Acad. Sci. USA *63*:78, 1969.
187. Flanagan, J. G., and Rabbitts, T. H.: Arrangement of human immunoglobulin heavy chain constant region genes implies evolutionary duplication of a segment containing γ, ε and α genes. Nature (Lond.) *300*:709, 1982.
188. Ellison, J., and Hood, J.: Linkage and sequence homology of two immunoglobulin γ heavy chain constant region genes. Proc. Natl. Acad. Sci. USA *79*:1984, 1982.
189. Takahashi, N., Ueda, S., et al.: Structure of human immunoglobulin γ genes: implications for evolution of a gene family. Cell *29*:671, 1982.
190. Natvig, J.B., and Kunkel, H. G.: Human immunoglobulins: classes, subclasses, genetic variants, and idiotypes. Adv. Immunol. *16*:1, 1973.
191. Pandey, J. P., and Whitten, H. D., et al.: Genetics of human immunoglobulins. In *Immunogenetics*. Panayi, G. S., and David, C. S. (eds.), London, Butterworths, 1984, p. 92.
192. Grubb, R., and Laurell, A. B.: Hereditary serological human serum groups. Acta Pathol. Microbiol. Scand. *39*:390, 1956.
193. Ropartz, C., Lenoir, J., et al.: Possible origins of the anti-Gm sera. Nature (Lond.) *188*:1120, 1960.
194. Litwin, S. D., and Kunkel, H. G.: Genetic factors of human gamma globulin detected by rabbit antisera. Transfusion *6*:140, 1966.
195. Kunkel, H. G., Smith, W. K., et al.: Genetic marker of the γA2 subgroup of γA immunoglobulins. Nature (Lond.) *223*:1247, 1969.
196. Kunkel, H. G., Yount, W. J., et al.: Genetically detected antigen of the Ne subgroup of gamma globulin: detection by precipitin analysis. Science *154*:1041, 1966.
197. Natvig, J. B., and Kunkel, H. G.: Genetic markers of human immunoglobulins. The Gm and Inv systems. Ser. Haematol. *1*:66, 1968.
198. Natvig, J.B., Kunkel, H. G., et al.: Genetic studies on the heavy chain subgroups of gamma G globulin. In *Gamma Globulins*. Killander, J. (ed.), Nobel Symp. 3. New York, Interscience Publishers, 1967, p. 313.
199. Fudenberg, H. H., and Fudenberg, B. R.: Antibody to hereditary human γ-globulin (Gm) factor resulting from maternal-fetal incompatibility. Science *145*:170, 1964.
200. Fudenberg, H. H., Pink, J. R. L., et al.: *Basic Immunogenetics*. New York, Oxford University Press, 1972, p. 48.
201. Weitkamp, L. R., Rucknagel, D. L., et al.: Genetic linkage between structural loci for albumin and group specific component. Am. J. Hum. Genet. *18*:559, 1966.
202. Mikkelsen, M., and Jacobsen, P.: Possible localization of Gc-system on chromosome 4. Loss of long arm 4 material associated with father-child incompatibility within the Gc-system. Hum. Hered. *27*:105, 1977.
203. Yang, F., Lum, J. B., et al.: Human transferrin: cDNA characterization and chromosomal localization. Proc. Natl. Acad. Sci. USA *81*:2752, 1984.
204. Cox, D. W., and Francke, U.: Direct assignment of orosomucoid to human chromosome 9 and α₂HS-glycoprotein to chromosome 3 using human fetal liver x rat hepatoma hybrids. Hum. Genet. *70*:109, 1985.
205. Weitkamp, L. R.: Evidence for linkage between the loci for transferrin and ceruloplasmin in man. Ann. Hum. Genet. *47*:293, 1983.
206. Robson, E. B., Sutherland, I., et al.: Evidence for linkage between the transferrin locus (Tf) and the serum cholin-

esterase locus (E_1) in man. Ann. Hum. Genet. 29:325, 1966.
207. Robson, E. B., Polani, P. E., et al.: Probable assignment of the alpha locus of haptoglobin to chromosome 16 in man. Nature (Lond.) 223:1163, 1969.
208. Eiberg, H., Mohr, J., et al.: Δ-Aminolevulinate-dehydrase: synteny with ABO-AKI-ORM (and assignment to chromosome 9). Clin. Genet. 23:150, 1983.
209. Whitehead, A. S., Solomon, E., et al.: Assignment of the structural gene for the third component of human complement to chromosome 19. Proc. Natl. Acad. Sci. USA 79:5021, 1982.
210. Olaisen, B., Teisberg, P., et al.: The locus for apolipoprotein E (apo E) is linked to the complement component C3 (C3) locus on chromosome 19 in man. Hum. Genet. 62:233, 1982.
211. Knott, T. J., Eddy, R. L., et al.: Chromosomal localization of the human apoprotein CI gene and of a polymorphic apoprotein AII gene. Biochem. Biophys. Res. Comm. 125:299, 1984.
212. Francke, U., Brown, M. S., et al.: Assignment of the human gene for the low density lipoprotein receptor to chromosome 19: synteny of a receptor, a ligand, and a genetic disease. Proc. Natl. Acad. Sci. USA 81:2826, 1984.
213. McBride, O. W., Battey, J., et al.: Localization of human variable and constant region immunoglobulin heavy chain genes on subtelomeric band of q32 of chromosome 14. Nucl. Acids Res. 10:8155, 1982.
214. Gedde-Dahl, T., Jr., Fagerhol, M. K., et al.: Autosomal linkage between the *Gm* and *Pi* loci in man. Ann. Hum. Genet. 35:393, 1972.
215. Bentley, D. R., and Campbell, R. D.: Primary structure of C2 and relationship to other components of the complement system (abstr.). Complement, 2:9, 1985.
216. Rodríguez de Córdoba, S., Dykman, T. R., et al.: Evidence of linkage between the loci coding for the binding protein for the fourth component of human complement (C4BP) and for the C3b/C4b receptor. Proc. Natl. Acad. Sci. USA 81:7890, 1984.
217. Rodríguez de Córdoba, S. R., Dykman, T. R., et al.: A new gene cluster controlling complement components (abstr.). Hum. Immunol. 12:105, 1985.
218. Klickstein, L. B., Wong, W. W., et al.: Identification of long homologous repeats in human CR1 (abstr). Complement, 2:44, 1985.
219. McAdam, R., Tenner, A., et al.: An abnormal Taq I restriction fragment in a C1q-deficient patient is caused by absence of a restriction site in the B chain coding region (abstr.) Complement 2:52, 1985.
220. Lachmann, P. J., and Hobart, M. J.: C6-C7: a further "complement supergene" (abstr.). J. Immunol. 120:1781, 1978.
221. Rogde, S., Olaisen, B., et al.: Complement component C8: genetic polymorphisms and linkage relationships (abstr.). Complement, p. 67, 1985.
222. de Grouchy, J., Dantzenberg, M.-D., et al.: Regional mapping of clotting Factors VII and X to 13q 34. Expression of Factor VII through chromosome 8. Hum. Genet. 66:230, 1984.
223. Giblett, E. R.: *Genetic Markers in Human Blood*. Oxford, Blackwell Scientific Publications, 1969.
224. Harris, H.: *The Principles of Human Biochemical Genetics*, 3rd ed. Amsterdam, North-Holland, 1980.
225. Valentine, W. N., Tanaka, K. R., et al.: Erythrocyte acid phosphatase in health and disease. Am. J. Clin. Pathol. 36:328, 1961.
226. Oski, F. A., Shahidi, N. T., et al.: Erythrocyte acid phosphomonoesterase and glucose-6-phosphatase dehydrogenase deficiency in Caucasians. Science 139:409, 1963.
227. Choremis, C., Kattamis, C., et al.: Erythrocyte acid phosphomonoesterase in glucose-6-phosphate dehydrogenase deficient Greeks. Lancet 1:108, 1964.
228. Scheltini, F., Meloni, T., et al.: Red cell acid phosphatase in normal and G6PD-deficient Sardinian subjects. Acta Haematol. (Basel) 33:230, 1965.
229. Boivin, P., Galand, C., et al.: Déficit congenital en adenylat-kinase erythrocitaire. Presse Med. 78:1443, 1970.
230. Szeinberg, A., Kahana, D., et al.: Hereditary deficiency of adenylate kinase in red blood cells. Acta Haematol. 42:111, 1969.
231. Jacob, H. S., Ingbar, S. H., et al.: Oxidative hemolysis and erythrocyte metabolism in hereditary acatalasia. J. Clin. Invest. 44:1187, 1965.
232. Büttner, R., Frei, J., et al.: Observations in two Swiss families with acatalasia. Enzymol. Biol. Clin. (Basel) 2:1, 1963.
233. Takahara, S.: Progressive oral gangrene probably due to lack of catalase in the blood (acatalasemia), report of nine cases. Lancet 2:1101, 1952.
234. Aebi, H., and Cantz, M.: Über die celluläre Verteilung der Katalase im Blut homozygoter und heterozygoter Defektträger (Akatalasie). Humangenetik 3:50, 1966.
235. Matsubara, S., Suter, H., et al.: Fractionation of erythrocyte catalase from normal, hypocatalatic and acatalatic humans. Humangenetik 4:29, 1967.
236. Bondy, P. K.: Disorders of carbohydrate metabolism. In *Duncan's Diseases of Metabolism*, 7th ed. Bondy, P. K., and Rosenberg, M. D. (eds.), Philadelphia, W. B. Saunders Co., 1974, p. 221.
237. Beutler, E., and Baluda, M. C.: A simple spot screening test for galactosemia. J. Lab. Clin. Med. 68:137, 1966.
238. Beutler, E., Balauda, M., et al.: The genetics of galactose-1-phosphate uridyl transferase deficiency. J. Lab. Clin. Med. 68:646, 1966.

TRANSFUSION THERAPY

CHAPTER 47
Red Cell Transfusion

MARTIN T. FOSBURG
SHERWIN V. KEVY

INTRODUCTION 1580
SURVIVAL OF TRANSFUSED CELLS 1580
INDICATIONS FOR TRANSFUSION 1581
Acute Blood Loss
Chronic Anemia
Congenital Enzymopathies
CHOICE OF A RED CELL PRODUCT 1582
SPECIAL SITUATIONS 1584
Neonatal Transfusion
Transfusion in the Immunocompromised Host
Massive Transfusion
Profound Anemia with Cardiac Compromise
ADVERSE EFFECTS OF TRANSFUSION 1585
Post-Transfusion Hepatitis
Cytomegalovirus (CMV)
Acquired Immune Deficiency Syndrome (AIDS)
Other Infections
Citrate Toxicity
Transfusion Reactions
Urticarial Reactions
Febrile Nonhemolytic Reactions
Hemolytic Transfusion Reactions
Delayed Transfusion Reactions

INTRODUCTION

From ancient times to the present, blood has played a central role in medical therapy. First thought to embody the characteristics of the human or animal donor from whom it was obtained (chiefly courage, wisdom, tranquillity, or sexual prowess), physicians prescribed it for those lacking in any of such virtues. By the mid-seventeenth century, advances in surgical technology allowed two physicians to perform the first intravenous transfusions. One of the patients, an elderly wealthy gentleman with a young, comely, and impatient wife, was a somewhat less than enthusiastic participant. As this case ended with the death of the patient, a malpractice suit against the physician, and a murder conviction of the wife, the enthusiasm of the medical community for the practice of transfusion was understandably diminished (1). Curiously, the potential utility of blood transfusion for treating patients with hemorrhage was not generally recognized until the late nineteenth century. Since that time, and greatly spurred on by the exigencies of two world wars, the capacity to draw, store, and then safely transfuse blood has been continuously refined. Reflecting the ubiquitous use of blood in present-day therapeutics, over 10 million transfusions were given in the United States in 1985. This chapter describes red cell transfusion and includes discussions concerning the storage of red cells, the variety of red cell products available to the clinician, indications and strategies for red cell transfusion, special situations requiring the use of blood transfusion, and potential side effects. For a comprehensive discussion of these topics, the reader is referred to Mollison's text "Blood Transfusion in Clinical Medicine" (2).

SURVIVAL OF TRANSFUSED CELLS

Once removed from the body, red blood cells undergo a progressive loss of viability, leading to a decline in post-transfusion survival—the so-called storage lesion(s). The two criteria for viability of stored red blood cells are (a) a mean of 75 per cent survival 24 hours post-transfusion, and (b) less than 1 per cent hemolysis in the red blood cell unit on the final day of storage (3). Over the past 75 years, multiple modifications have been made in anticoagulant solutions, blood product containers, and storage conditions (e.g., temperature), all designed to prolong in vitro red blood cell viability.

There is as yet no single lesion that accounts for this loss of viability. Structural changes in stored red blood cells include increased rigidity, vesiculation, loss of membrane lipid, loss of the discoid shape, and decreased osmotic fragility. The biochemical correlates of these membrane alterations include decreased levels of ATP and of 2,3-DPG, and transient loss of the Na/K pump, leading to cellular swelling (4). Of these biochemical changes, loss of ATP seems most important. There is a complex correlation among loss of ATP, morphologic changes in stored red blood cells, and decreased post-transfusion survival (5). Even when ATP levels fall to <20 per cent of normal and major red blood cell shape changes have occurred, incubation of the red blood cells with substrates designed to restore ATP leads to return of normal red blood cell morphology and 24-hour post-transfusion survival of >75 per cent (6).

Standard practice, at present, is to draw 450 ml of donor blood into a polyvinyl chloride (with a phthalate plasticizer) bag containing 64 ml of citrate-phosphate-dextrose-adenine solution (CPDA-1). This must be stored at between 1 and 6°C and has a shelf life of 35 days. Each 100 ml of CPDA-1 contains 2.63 g trisodium citrate, 0.327 g citric acid, 0.22 g sodium dihydrogen phosphate, 3.19 g dextrose, and 0.27 g adenine. This solution provides an anticoagulant (citrate), an energy substrate (dextrose), a nucleotide designed to maintain ATP levels (adenine), and a substrate for 2,3-DPG (sodium dihydrogen phosphate). The pH of the CPDA-1 blood mixture is 7.0, which is optimum for the enzymes of the glycolytic pathway.

As extended shelf life of red blood cells allows for greater efficiency in utilizing the limited blood supply, efforts are in progress to better define the storage lesion in order to modify storage conditions to further prolong the allowable storage period. This effort has lead to the development of crystalline preservative solutions containing saline, mannitol, adenine, and glucose. These, when added to packed red blood cells within 24 hours of collection, provide satisfactory post-transfusion survival following 42 days' storage.

INDICATIONS FOR TRANSFUSION

All too often blood is administered with little thought given to the indications for its use, the proper dose required, and potential adverse consequences. Leaving aside the issue of hypovolemia, there is only one indication for red cell transfusion—to provide a patient with sufficient red cells to prevent or reverse tissue hypoxia. There is surprisingly little information concerning the level of hematocrit that will accomplish this. Evidence obtained from observations on the effects of anemia on coronary sinus oxygen saturation in dogs (7) and surgical experience with sickle cell patients in Jamaica (8) suggest that otherwise healthy young individuals can tolerate a hematocrit of 20 without short-term adverse consequences. Routine transfusion of such patients is not indicated.

The appropriate hematocrit for very young or old patients, or for those with major organ dysfunction who must undergo the stress of surgery or medical illness, is more difficult to define. The conservative assumption is that the "sicker" a patient is, the closer he should be maintained to a normal hematocrit for age. It is common practice in intensive care units to use transfusions to maintain a hematocrit of 35 to 40 in children and one of 45 to 50 in neonates with cardiorespiratory compromise. In contrast, young, healthy individuals should not be transfused without a compelling reason to do so or until the hematocrit is quite low. Patients with cardiovascular compromise should not be allowed to develop severe anemia.

Acute Blood Loss

The lifesaving value of blood transfusion was first demonstrated in the treatment of hemorrhage encountered on the battlefield and in the maternity ward. The replacement of blood lost to bleeding remains the major role of transfusion today.

Diagnosis of the presence and degree of blood loss is, in practice, quite difficult, especially in a young and otherwise healthy child who may sustain a relatively large amount of hemorrhage with few external signs of distress. Signs of impending shock such as pallor, anxiety, and tachypnea are frequently subtle and easily overlooked or attributed to other causes. By the time signs of cardiovascular compromise become evident (i.e., pallor, stupor, tachycardia or bradycardia, hypotension, cool extremities, weak peripheral pulses, and decreased capillary filling), the patient has likely lost at least 25 per cent of his blood volume (9). Hypotension is one useful clinical sign of moderate to severe blood loss. Patients who have lost >25 per cent of their blood volume frequently have age-related systolic hypotension: <65 mm Hg (<4 years of age); <75 mm Hg (5–8 years); <85 mm Hg (9–12 years); and <95 mm Hg (adolescents and adults).

Acute blood loss of this degree may have three related but distinct components—anemia, hypovolemia, and coagulopathy. (A pre-existing coagulopathy may have caused the hemorrhage. In addition, if insufficient clotting factors and/or platelets are administered during replacement therapy, a secondary deficiency may develop.) Each of these blood components may be present to a different degree and will change in relation to one another and with time. The often repeated dictum that such blood loss should be treated isovolumetrically with whole (and preferably fresh) blood sounds simple but is difficult to implement.

The exception to this is blood loss during surgery, in which the timing and amount of bleeding is fairly predictable and for which blood products can be prepared in advance.

More frequently, a patient will be found in a state of shock in a situation in which the cause for and amount of blood loss are not immediately apparent. In such clinical situations, the extent of hemorrhage and the type and amount of blood products needed are best determined by measuring the arterial and central venous pressures (CVP), taking a hematocrit, and performing tests of coagulation. A CVP monitor is invaluable in managing patients with moderate to severe blood loss. It allows for rapid red cell and volume replacement while decreasing the attendant risks of overtransfusion and hypervolemia. In severe hemorrhage the pretransfusion CVP will be from 0 to 2. Blood and other fluids may be administered very rapidly until the CVP rises to between 6 and 7. At this point the circulation is restored and further transfusion may proceed at a more measured pace.

Since the purposes of transfusion in acute blood loss are to restore the red blood cell mass, correct hypovolemia, and correct any hemostatic defects, blood component therapy has major advantages over whole blood replacement, for the following reasons: (1) the supply of immediately available fresh whole blood is usually limited; (2) packed cells are more efficacious for raising the hematocrit; (3) fresh frozen plasma has higher levels of clotting factors; (4) crystalloid contains no citrate; (5) whole blood cannot supply viable platelets.

Minor amounts of blood loss (<10 per cent of the blood volume) rarely require transfusion unless the fall in blood volume or hematocrit causes symptoms or, for whatever reason, the bone marrow cannot be expected to produce sufficient red cells to make good the loss. Severe acute hemorrhage requires intensive monitoring and laboratory investigation to define the degree of red cell deficiency, volume loss, and coagulant deficiency, and to assess the effects of replacement therapy.

Chronic Anemia

In this instance, the body is deficient in red cells while the plasma volume is normal or increased; coagulopathy is present only if it is part of the underlying disease. Listed in Table 47–1 are the childhood anemias that are likely to require intermittent or long-term transfusion. When planning for chronic transfusions (months to years), several guidelines should be followed:

1. If at all possible, transfusion should be avoided or minimized by aggressive treatment of the underlying disorder (e.g., renal transplant).
2. Red cell phenotyping should be performed

Table 47–1. DISEASES REQUIRING INTERMITTENT OR CHRONIC RED CELL TRANSFUSIONS IN CHILDHOOD

1. Chronic renal failure	5. Leukemia
2. Thalassemia	6. Blackfan-Diamond anemia
3. Sickle cell disease	7. Transient erythroblastopenia
4. Aplastic anemia Constitutional Acquired	

prior to initiating transfusion. The transfusion should be done with antigen-matched red blood cells in order to avert sensitization to minor red cell antigens (see Table 47–2).

3. A plasma and leukocyte poor red cell product should be used to avert volume overload and sensitization to leukocyte and plasma protein alloantigens.
4. Sufficient red cells should be given to prevent symptomatic anemia and allow for normal growth.

Congenital Enzymopathies

Red cell transfusion has been used to deliver adenosine deaminase to infants with combined immunodeficiency due to lack of this enzyme. The results are not spectacular (9a). Such transfusions have also been used to suppress endogenous erythropoiesis in congenital erythropoietic prophyria, with salutary effect (9b).

CHOICE OF A RED CELL PRODUCT

The components of a freshly drawn unit of whole blood are listed in Table 47–3. Whole blood may be modified in several ways, all of which are designed to remove varying proportions of its non–red cell components. Listed in Table 47–4 are currently available red cell products, including the percentage of each non–red cell component that is retained following processing, and the likelihood of the more common transfusion-related side effects associated with each. A brief description of the usual indications for each product follows.

Whole Blood (<21 days' storage). There are limited indications for this product in pediatric

Table 47–2. MINOR RED BLOOD CELL ANTIGENS LIKELY TO PROVOKE SENSITIZATION AND DELAYED TRANSFUSION REACTIONS

System	Antigen
Rh-hr	C, c, D, e
Kell	K
MNS	M, S, s
Duffy	Fy^A, Fy^A
Kidd	Jk^A, Jk^B

Table 47-3. COMPOSITION OF WHOLE BLOOD STORED IN CPD ANTICOAGULANT*†

	Days of Storage				
	0	7	14	21	28
% viable cells (24-hr post transfusion)	100	98	85	80	75
Plasma pH (measured at 37°C)	7.20	7.00	6.89	6.84	6.78
ATP (% of initial value)	100	96	83	86	75
2,3-DPG (% of initial value)	100	99	80	44	35
Plasma Na (dl)	168	166	183	156	154
Plasma K (K)	3.9	11.9	17.2	21.0	22.5
Red blood cell Na (dl)	(3)	(7)	(14)	(18)	—
Red blood cell K (dl)	(90)	(73)	(65)	(62)	—
Plasma hemoglobin (mg/dl)	1.7	7.8	12.5	19.1	28.9
Plasma NH_3 (mg/dl)	(50)	(260)	(470)	(680)	—
Whole blood NH_3 (mg/dl)	282	300	447	500	705
Plasma dextrose (mg/dl)	345	312	282	231	230
Hematocrit	36.3	35.8	36.5	34.7	35.7
MCHC (Coulter counter)	33.5	33.1	32.6	—	32.8
Inorganic PO_4 (mM/liter)	3.6	3.6	4.2	4.9	5.5
WBC ($\times 10^3$)	4.9	4.1	4.1	3.2	2.9

*Figures in parentheses indicate blood drawn in ACD.
†From *Technical Manual of the American Association of Blood Banks,* 7th ed. Miller, W. V. (ed.), Washington D.C., American Association of Blood Banks, 1977, p. 55.

patients. It may be used in cases of acute blood loss if more suitable products are not immediately available.

Fresh Whole Blood (<72 hours' storage). This product has higher levels of coagulation factors and 2,3-DPG; and lower ammonia and potassium levels than does blood stored for longer periods, thus making it more suitable for exchange transfusion in neonates and to replace blood lost in acute hemorrhage.

Fresh Whole Blood (<4 hours' storage at room temperature). Leukocyte transfusions have been shown to improve the chances for survival in septic, neutropenic neonates. Leukocytes may be obtained by pheresis or harvested from whole blood. Alternatively, if fresh blood is administered via exchange transfusion, within 4 hours of drawing it can deliver the same number of viable leukocytes with considerably less preparation time and morbidity (10).

Packed Cells (35 days' storage). This product is similar in its cellular constituents to whole blood but with about 40 per cent of the plasma and citrate removed. It is the component of choice in cases of red cell loss or underproduction.

Washed Packed Cells. The washing process removes about 90 per cent of the white cells and more than 99 per cent of the plasma. Its main use is in patients with a history of nonhemolytic transfusion reactions and in other circumstances in which transfusion of leukocytes and plasma is contraindicated.

Frozen Deglycerolized Packed Cells. The processes of freezing and thawing red cells involve extensive washing with solutions of differing osmolalities, a process that removes over 95 per cent of the white cells. Only $1/10^6$ of the original plasma is retained. This is the red cell product most nearly free of non–red cell components and therefore is the product of choice for chronic transfusion.

Table 47-4. CURRENTLY AVAILABLE RED BLOOD CELL PRODUCTS

	Percentage of Non–Red Cell Components Remaining in Each Red Cell Product					Likelihood of Each Product to Produce Transfusion-Associated Side Effects*			
Product	Plasma	PMNs	Lymphocytes	Coagulation Factors	Platelets	Citrate Toxicity	Viral Infection	Febrile Reaction	Graft vs. Host Disease
Whole blood (<21 days)	100%	100%	100%	Decreased V, VIII, II, VII, IX, X	<1%	4+	4+	4+	4+
Whole blood (<48 hr)	100%	100%	100%	Decreased V, VIII	<1%	4+	4+	4+	4+
Whole blood (<4 hr)	100%	100%	100%	100%	>90%	4+	4+	4+	4+
Packed cells	20–50%	100%	100%	20–50%	<1%	2+	4+	4+	4+
Leukofiltered cells	10%	<5%	<5%	10%	<1%	2+	4+	1+	3+
Washed packed cells	<1%	10%	10%	<1%	<1%	1+	4+	1+	3+
Frozen deglycerolized cells	<1%	<5%	<5%	<1%	<1%	0	2+	1+	3+

*0 = No chance of a specific side effect.
4+ = Product most likely to produce a specific side effect.

Leukofiltered Blood. Passing blood diluted with saline through cotton wool fiber containing filters removes approximately as many white cells as does freezing or washing. Alternatively, passing citrated whole blood stored longer than 7 days through microaggregate blood filters removes much of the leukocyte and platelet debris (11). Either technique may be used to prepare leukocyte-poor blood when frozen blood is not available.

Irradiation of Red Cell Products. Irradiation of any blood product serves one purpose: to prevent lymphocytes in that product from proliferating when transfused into a host with congenital or acquired deficiency in cell-mediated immunity, which could cause transfusion-associated graft-versus-host disease (TAGVHD). TAGVHD may occur from 4 to 30 days after transfusion of blood products containing viable lymphocytes. Once acquired, there is no effective therapy. The mortality rate in TAGVHD is greater than 90 per cent. All blood products except fresh frozen plasma can cause TAGVHD. The minimum dose of lymphocytes needed to cause TAGVHD is about 1×10^7 per kg.

Lymphocytes in blood products may be inactivated by irradiation; either cesium 137 irradiators or cobalt 60 therapy machines may be used. Radiation in doses of up to 10,000 cGy has little or no effect on red cells; and up to 5000 cGy may be used without affecting granulocyte or platelet function and survival. The most common recommended dose is 1500 cGy, although 5000 cGy is used in the author's laboratory (12, 13).

SPECIAL SITUATIONS

Neonatal Transfusion

Neonates differ from older children and adults in several respects relevant to transfusion practice. They have small blood volumes, difficulty with temperature regulation, citrate intolerance, and immature immune systems. In addition, sick premature infants require frequent small-volume transfusions (14).

Initial compatibility testing for newborns should include ABO/Rh typing of neonatal and maternal red blood cells, antibody screening, and, if there is ABO incompatibility, tests for circulating anti-A/B. As the neonatal immune system is relatively unresponsive to red blood cell antigenic stimulation, repeated cross-matching and antibody screening are not necessary prior to each transfusion during the first 4 months of life. The exception to this is when antibody is detected in the initial newborn or maternal sample. In this case, compatibility testing and antibody screening must be done prior to each transfusion.

An intensively monitored sick premature infant may lose 10 to 15 per cent of its blood volume daily from blood sampling. Standard practice is to replace such losses isovolumetrically with packed red blood cells. Because of the need for daily small-volume transfusions, it is our practice to divide each donor red cell unit into five aseptically separated aliquots, with the hematocrit of each adjusted to >70. Aliquots are then issued daily or less often as needed. In order to prevent hypotension from hypocalcemia and/or hypothermia, neonates should receive red cells that are prewarmed and low in citrate. Finally, to avoid volume overload, repeated small volume transfusions (<10 per cent of the child's blood volume) are preferred. Reference 14 contains the formulas for calculating the volume of transfusion suitable for neonates.

Transfusion in the Immunocompromised Host

Transfusion poses three potential hazards to these patients—sensitization to alloantigens, induction of graft-versus-host disease, and transmission of cytomegalovirus infection (15). In order to prevent these problems, all blood products for these patients should be irradiated, white blood cell–poor red cell products (washed or frozen cells) should be used, and those patients without serologic evidence of prior exposure to cytomegalovirus should not receive blood products capable of carrying this infection.

Massive Transfusion

This is defined as the replacement of more than one blood volume. Such blood loss is usually associated with trauma, certain surgical procedures (e.g., liver transplant), or massive gastrointestinal hemorrhage. Four problems may result from such transfusion:

1. *Citrate Toxicity.* See under Adverse Effects of Transfusion, below.

2. *Alkalosis and Hypokalemia.* During massive transfusion, the potassium level of the recipient falls, owing to the alkalosis caused by the metabolism of citrate to bicarbonate. Each unit of whole blood contains 7.6 mmol of citrate, which generates 22.8 mEq of bicarbonate. Potassium moves into cells, and hydrogen ions leave in response to this bicarbonate load (16).

3. *Coagulopathy.* During a large rapid blood loss, the body is unable to produce more than a small fraction of the coagulation proteins and platelets lost to bleeding, which therefore must be supplied exogenously. This may be accomplished with fresh blood or alternatively with fresh frozen plasma, cryoprecipitate (for fibrinogen), and platelet concentrates. Moderate thrombocytopenia will invariably occur with massive transfusion with whole blood.

4. *Microaggregates.* Depending on the type and age of the red cell products transfused, a variable number of microaggregates (composed of leukocyte and platelet debris) are administered. These have been reported to cause deterioration of pulmonary function in adults. This is easily avoided by transfusing through a microaggregate filter.

Profound Anemia with Cardiac Compromise

There are a number of circumstances in which profound anemia due to bleeding, hemolysis, or red cell underproduction coexists with normo- or hypervolemia and cardiac compromise. Such patients need red cells but may not tolerate volume. In these circumstances the hematocrit can be raised rapidly and safely by either manual or automated exchange transfusion.

ADVERSE EFFECTS OF TRANSFUSION

Infection remains the most common lethal side effect of transfusion. Post-transfusion hepatitis, acquired immunodeficiency syndrome, and cytomegalovirus account for most serious transfusion-related infections.

Post-Transfusion Hepatitis

Hepatitis A. As there is no chronic carrier state associated with this virus, it is rarely, if ever, transmitted via transfusion.

Hepatitis B. Since the elimination of paid donors and the introduction of increasingly sensitive tests for detection of hepatitis B viral antigens, the incidence of transfusion-related hepatitis B has fallen to 1 per 1000. It is still possible for donors to transmit this infection if they donate blood during the incubation phase of the disease, when viremia is present, but prior to the appearance of serologic evidence of infection (17). It is our policy to administer hepatitis B vaccine to all patients at the outset of chronic transfusion therapy.

Non-A, Non-B Hepatitis (NANB). Current evidence suggests that there are at least two viruses responsible for transfusion-associated NANB hepatitis. The detection of reverse transcriptase in some of these patients suggests that one or more as yet unclassified retroviruses may be the causative agent(s). The incidence of NANB hepatitis is 6 per cent of patients receiving blood (18). About 70 per cent of these infections are initially asymptomatic. More disturbing are reports that 40 to 50 per cent of all patients with NANB hepatitis develop biopsy evidence of chronic active or persistent hepatitis. As yet, there is no direct serologic test to identify donors carrying this infection. Studies have shown that infected donors frequently have an elevated level of alanine aminotransferase (ALT, SGPT) and/or a positive test for antibody to the core antigen of the hepatitis B virus (19). Mandatory testing of blood donors for ALT and anti-HB_c was introduced in 1986.

Cytomegalovirus (CMV)

This virus is carried in and transmitted via lymphocytes. In a normal host, transfusion-associated CMV infection causes a mild "mononucleosis" type illness 3 to 4 weeks post transfusion. Transfusion of CMV-containing blood products to an immunocompromised host without serologic evidence of prior exposure to CMV can cause a lethal systemic infection. Therefore, patients with inherited or acquired immunodeficiency states (this includes all neonates) should receive frozen or washed red cells or any blood product from a CMV antibody–negative donor (20).

Acquired Immune Deficiency Syndrome (AIDS)

This infection, which is due to a retrovirus termed HTLV-III (human T cell leukemia virus Type III) was first documented in homosexual males in the late 1970's. As of February 1986, more than 16,000 cases had been reported in the United States and Western Europe. Of these, 2 per cent have been transmitted via blood transfusion. Once acquired, this virus is propagated in and eventually destroys helper/inducer T lymphocytes, leading to immunodeficiency with consequent opportunistic infections and/or malignancy. Once acquired, AIDS is invariably fatal.

Since 94 per cent of those with AIDS are found in so-called high-risk groups (homosexual or bisexual males, intravenous drug users, hemophiliacs, and the sexual partners of these individuals), steps were taken in 1984 to eliminate those in these groups from the donor pool. In April 1985, a serologic test for antibodies to HTLV-III was introduced nationwide. The presence of this antibody in a blood donor is taken as presumptive evidence of viral genetic material in the lymphocytes. All blood from antibody-positive donors is discarded. Although neither donor screening nor testing for HTLV-III antibody is by itself 100 per cent effective in identifying donors capable of transmitting AIDS, the use of both methods will likely prevent almost all future transfusion-related disease. The interval between the time of transfusion and the diagnosis of AIDS in children (mean 13.5 months) is much shorter than that for adults (mean 30 months). As AIDS may have an incubation phase of 5 years or more, transfusion-related cases will continue to be identified for several more years (21–23).

The knowledge that this lethal disease can be transmitted via blood products has had a profound impact on transfusion practices. Our patients and their parents, who in the past took transfusion for granted, are now quite fearful when they learn that blood products are to be administered. Perhaps the single beneficial effect of the AIDS epidemic is that it has forced physicians to acknowledge that blood transfusion may cause lethal, if rare, side effects and that decisions to transfuse should be made with care and blood products administered only when absolutely necessary.

Other Infections

EB virus, syphilis, malaria, Chagas disease, babesiosis, and filariasis are potentially transmissible via blood transfusion.

Citrate Toxicity

Blood products are anticoagulated by the addition of citrate, which prevents coagulation by lowering ionized calcium. When infused rapidly, citrate may cause symptomatic hypocalcemia. The only red cell product that contains large amounts of plasma (and hence citrate) is whole blood. Each milliliter of whole blood contains 2.5 mg of citrate ion. In normal hosts, the dose rate at which hypocalcemia may appear is 1 mg of citrate ion per kg per minute (24). A 30-kg child receiving whole blood at a dose rate of 12 ml per minute would be at this threshold. This rate of transfusion would not be unusual for a child with major bleeding. As hypotension is commonly found with major hemorrhage, an exacerbation of hypotension due to citrate toxicity could easily go unnoticed. The potential for citrate toxicity is the major drawback in using whole blood for rapid red cell and volume replacement during hemorrhage.

Transfusion Reactions

During a 22-year period at Children's Hospital in Boston, 2 to 3 per cent of 268,593 transfusions were associated with some form of reaction. Of these, 41 per cent were febrile nonhemolytic, 58 per cent were urticarial, and the remainder were delayed hemolytic reactions.

Urticarial Reactions

Unlike febrile nonhemolytic reactions, urticaria can be seen with the first transfusion a patient receives. If localized urticaria occurs, the transfusion is interrupted and an antihistamine is administered. Recipients who experience repeated urticarial reactions should receive washed or frozen red blood cells. If reactions persist, patients should be pretreated with an antihistamine or corticosteroid. The cause of these reactions is unknown. Allergy of a transfusion recipient to a soluble antigen in the donor plasma is often suspected but rarely proven.

Febrile Nonhemolytic Reactions

The occurrence of fever, chills, or diapheresis during blood transfusion is almost always due to a reaction between antibodies in the host and leukocyte or plasma protein alloantigens in the blood product. As the formation of these antibodies requires exposure to blood products, such reactions occur exclusively in patients with a history of prior transfusion or pregnancy. Many chronically transfused patients who receive red cell products containing white blood cells and plasma will develop such reactions. Such patients should receive washed or frozen cells from the outset or, if given standard packed cells, should be switched to such products if and when reactions occur. These reactions may be prevented, modified, or treated by some combination of antipyretics, antihistamines, or, if severe, corticosteroids.

Hemolytic Transfusion Reactions

These are most often due to donor-recipient ABO incompatibility. Such reactions are invariably due to "clerical" errors such as mislabeling of blood in the blood bank or giving the wrong blood to a patient. Hemolytic reactions are characterized by fever, chills, abdominal and lower back pain, tachycardia, hypotension, renal failure, and shock. Laboratory findings include anemia, spherocytosis, DIC, hemoglobinemia, hemoglobinuria, and the appearance of a positive Coombs test. The clinical and laboratory effects of hemolytic transfusion reactions are due to antibody-antigen interaction with consequent complement activation. Treatment is immediate cessation of transfusion and administration of steroids, fluid, mannitol, and pressors as needed to maintain the circulation and prevent oliguria.

Delayed Transfusion Reactions

Occasionally patients receiving fully compatible red cells will experience some or all of the symptoms of a hemolytic reaction 3 to 10 days post transfusion. Such patients have been sensitized to one or more "minor" blood group antigens during a prior transfusion. By the time a subsequent transfusion is given, their antibody titers have fallen to levels below the threshold necessary for detection. When they are reexposed to these antigens, an amnestic response occurs. When sufficient antibody is produced, hemolysis occurs. The clinical syndrome is generally milder than that associated with ABO incompatibility, but delayed transfusion reactions can produce profound anemia. Such a reaction should be suspected in multitransfused patients who develop unexplained anemia several days to a week following transfusion. As with immediate reactions, the diagnosis is confirmed by the presence of a positive Coombs test and identification of new red cell antibodies in the patient.

References

1. Diamond, L. K.: A history of blood transfusion. In *Blood, Pure and Eloquent*. Wintrobe, M. M. (ed.), New York, McGraw-Hill, 1980, p. 661.
2. Mollison, P. L.: *Blood Transfusion in Clinical Medicine*. Oxford, Blackwell Scientific Publications, 1983.
3. Code of Federal Regulations, Food and Drug Act #21, Parts 600 to 799, April 1, 1985.
4. Wolfe, L. W.: The red cell membrane and the storage lesion. Clin. Hematol., 14:259, 1985.
5. Haradin, A., Weed R., et al.: Changes in physical properties of stored red cells. Transfusion 9:229 1969.
6. Valeri, C. R., and Zaroulis, G. G.: Rejuvenation and freezing of outdated stored human red cells. New Engl. J. Med. 297:1307, 1972.
7. Case, R. B., Berglund, E., et al.: Ventricular function. VII. Changes in coronary resistance and ventricular function resulting from acutely induced anemia and the effect thereon of coronary stenosis. Am. J. Med., 18:397, 1955.
8. Homi, J., Reynolds, J., et al.: General anesthesia in sickle-cell disease. Br. Med. J. 1:1599, 1979.
9. Tovey, G. H., and Lennon, G. G.: Blood volume studies in accidental hemorrhage. J. Obstet. Gynaecol. Br. Comm. 5:749, 1962.
9a. Polmar, S. H., Wetzler, E. M., et al.: Restoration of in vitro lymphocyte responses with exogenous adenosine deaminase in a patient with severe combined immunodeficiency. Lancet 2:743, 1975.
9b. Piomelli, S., Poh-Fitzpatrick, M. B., et al.: Complete suppression of the symptoms of congenital erythropoietic porphyria by long-term treatment with high-level transfusions. New Engl. J. Med. 314:1029, 1986.
10. Christensen, R. D., Anstall, H. B., et al.: Use of whole blood exchange transfusion to supply neutrophils to septic, neutropenic neonates. Transfusion 22:504, 1982.
11. Hughes, A. S. B., and Brozovic, B.: Leukocyte depleted blood, an appraisal of available techniques. Br. J. Haematol. 50:381, 1982.
12. Button, L. W., DeWolf, W. C., et al.: The effect of irradiation on blood components. Transfusion 21:419, 1981.
13. Leitman, S. F., and Holland, P. V.: Irradiation of blood products; indications and guidelines. Transfusion 25:293, 1985.
14. Wolfe, L., Epstein, M., et al.: Blood transfusion for the neonatal patient. Hum. Pathol. 14:256, 1983.
15. Mollison, P. L.: *Blood Transfusion in Clinical Medicine*. Oxford, Blackwell Scientific Publications, 1983, p. 173.
16. Howland, W. S.: Calcium, potassium and pH changes during massive transfusion. In *Massive Transfusion Symposium*. Nusbacher, J. (ed.), Washington, D.C., American Association of Blood Banks, 1978, p. 17.
17. Alter, H. J., Holland, P. V., et al.: Post-transfusion hepatitis after exclusion of the commerical and hepatitis B antigen donor. Ann. Intern. Med. 77:681, 1972.
18. Stevens, C. E., Aach, R. D., et al.: Hepatitis B antibody in blood donors and the occurence of non-A, non-B hepatitis in transfusion recipients: an analysis of the transfusion transmitted virus study. Ann. Intern. Med. 101:733, 1984.
19. Aach, R. D., Szmuness, W., et al.: Serum alanine aminotransferase of donors in relation to the risk of non A, non B in recipients: the transfusion-transmitted viruses study. New Engl. J. Med. 304:989, 1981.
20. Adler, S. P.: Transfusion associated cytomegalovirus infections. Rev. Infect. Dis. 5:977, 1983.
21. Groopman, J. E., Zaki, S., et al.: Virologic studies in a case of transfusion associated AIDS. New Engl. J. Med. 311:1414, 1984.
22. Curran, J. W., Lawrence, D. W., et al.: Acquired immunodeficiency syndrome (AIDS) associated with transfusions. New Engl. J. Med., 310:69, 1984.
23. Fiorenc, P. M., Taffett, W., et al.: Transfusion associated acquired immunodeficiency syndrome: evidence for persistent infection in blood donors. New Engl. J. Med. 312:1293, 1985.
24. Perkins, H. A., Snyder, M., et al.: Calcium ion activity during roped exchange transfusion with citrated blood. Transfusion 11:204, 1971.

TRANSFUSION THERAPY

CHAPTER 48
Platelet Transfusion

RITCHARD G. CABLE

INTRODUCTION 1588
METHODS OF COLLECTION 1588
STORAGE OF PLATELETS 1589
Frozen Platelet Storage
PLATELET DOSE 1590
FACTORS INVOLVED IN POOR RESPONSE TO
 PLATELET TRANSFUSION 1590
CLINICAL USES OF PLATELETS 1591
Bone Marrow Failure
Accelerated Platelet Destruction
Massive Transfusion Situations—Surgery and Extracorporeal
 Circulation
Massive Transfusion Situations—Exchange Transfusion
Abnormal Platelet Function
Miscellaneous Uses
TECHNIQUE OF TRANSFUSION 1594
PLATELET TRANSFUSION REACTIONS 1594
PLATELET MATCHING 1594

INTRODUCTION

Platelet transfusions have been used in some form in clinical medicine for approximately 70 years, beginning with Duke's demonstration that the abnormal bleeding time of thrombocytopenic patients could be corrected with fresh blood transfusions (1). As the ability to anticoagulate, preserve, and separate blood into components has developed, platelet transfusions have evolved from use of fresh unanticoagulated blood; to use of fresh anticoagulated whole blood, employing mostly citrate-based anticoagulants; to use of platelet-rich plasma; and today to use of platelet concentrates. Recent developments have allowed separation of platelets in high yield from whole blood, their concentration in small volumes of donor plasma, and their successful storage for up to 7 days after collection. In addition, the development of pheresis procedures, both manual and automated, has allowed the production of multiple units of platelets from single donors. Finally, the development of successful centralized blood collection facilities and the interfacility sharing of blood and components have virtually eliminated shortages of platelets in most areas of the United States.

METHODS OF COLLECTION

Single units of platelets (platelet concentrates) can be prepared from multiple whole blood collections, or the equivalent yield of multiple-collection platelet concentrates can be prepared by a pheresis procedure from a single donor. Preparation of platelet concentrates is performed at room temperature from whole blood that is collected into a three-compartment closed plastic container (triple pack) and anticoagulated with acid citrate dextrose (ACD), citrate phosphate dextrose (CPD), or, more commonly, CPD–adenine, the anticoagulant-preservative most often used in blood collection today (2, 2a).

A slow-speed centrifugation of the whole blood separates packed red cells from platelet-rich plasma. The latter is expressed into the second bag of the triple pack and subjected to a faster centrifugation, which concentrates the platelets at the bottom of the bag. Sedimentation speeds and times vary from institution to institution, but guidelines for optimal recovery exist (3). Platelet-poor plasma is then expressed into the third bag of the triple pack. After 1 hour of undisturbed incubation at room temperature to allow the breakdown of released adenosine diphosphate (ADP) (4), the sedimented platelets are resuspended in a small volume of residual plasma to yield a platelet concentrate. This procedure requires that blood be collected into triple packs, be maintained at room temperature, and be completely processed within 6 hours of collection (5). These requirements, plus the 5- to 7-day dating period of platelet concentrates (6), necessitate close cooperation between physician, transfusion service, and collection facility to insure that platelet production is matched to platelet need on a day-to-day basis.

Platelets collected by pheresis entail the removal of whole blood from the donor; its separation into platelets, platelet-poor plasma, and red cells; and the return of the two latter components to the donor. This can be done manually by repetitive withdrawal of units of whole blood, with preparation of components and reinfusion of plasma and red cells between each cycle of donation (7), or it can be done using machines that remove blood from the donor, separate it into components by an integral centrifugation apparatus akin to a cream separator, and return the unwanted components to the donor. Because the latter method is more efficient and faster and eliminates the chance of reinfusion of the wrong blood product to the donor, it has become the preferred pheresis procedure for platelet collections. The available techniques include discontinuous and continuous flow centrifugation (8–11). These same machines have been used for removal of plasma and white cells either from donors for usable clinical products or from patients as a therapeutic modality.

Plateletpheresis procedures have several advantages: they allow platelet matching between donor and recipient by providing a usual adult therapeutic dose from a single donor; they diminish recipient exposure to hepatitis and AIDS and to soluble and cellular antigens; and they allow collection of large numbers of platelets in emergency situations without the need to recruit numerous whole blood donors. However, such procedures have disadvantages. They are more costly. They require more dedication and time from the donor and expose him to a greater (though small) risk than that associated with whole blood donations (12). They require special care to avoid donors who have functionally abnormal platelets or those who recently ingested aspirin or other platelet toxins. Finally, some collection processes require an open system, and consequently a higher bacterial contamination potential and a 24-hour outdating period.

STORAGE OF PLATELETS

Platelets can be stored at two different temperatures, 1 to 6°C ("cold" platelets) and 20 to 24°C ("warm" platelets) (Table 48–1). Viability and recovery of warm stored platelets remain nearly constant for from 5 (12a) to 7 days.

Storage temperature has been the subject of a lively debate in the past. However, platelet storage in the last several years has clearly been shown to be improved at 20 to 24°C (13). Previous claims of more immediate hemostatic effectiveness for platelets stored at 1 to 6°C (14–16) have been reversed (17), and two independent studies have shown the bleeding time of recipients to be as well controlled immediately following transfusion of "warm" platelets as of "cold" platelets (13, 17). Since all investigators agree that warm storage results in better post-transfusion intravascular survival, the earlier suggestions that both warm and cold platelets can be made available (warm platelets for prophylaxis, cold platelets for treatment of active bleeding) (18) seem inoperative.

All platelet producers in the United States have adopted routine 20 to 24°C storage, as its advantages have been demonstrated. There are, however, disadvantages to room temperature storage. Because platelets and contaminating white and red cells are metabolically active during room temperature storage, production of acid equivalents, in the form of lactic and other organic acids, requires plasma buffering to maintain the pH above 6.0, below which platelet viability is markedly impaired (19). The amount of plasma required when platelet recovery is optimized can be as high as 70 ml per unit (20). New plastic formulations for platelet containers, which have higher gas permeability than older formulations, have allowed more reliable maintenance of pH above 6.0 with smaller amounts of buffering plasma and with dating periods as long as 7 days (21a, 21b).

These high volumes can cause difficulties in transfusion of pediatric patients, particularly when out-of-group incompatible plasma is infused. Some transfusion services have the capability of concentrating pooled platelets to smaller volumes or resuspending platelets in AB plasma or electrolyte solutions (22). Another option is to use plateletpheresis products whose volumes can be regulated at the time of collection and whose donors can be easily selected to be ABO compatible.

Table 48–1. PLATELET STORAGE (21)

Factors	Cold	Warm
Temperature	1–6° C	20–24° C
Volume of plasma	20–30 ml	30–50 ml
Agitation required during storage	No	Yes
Minimum number of platelets	5.5×10^{10}	5.5×10^{10}
Minimum pH after storage	6.0	6.0
Maximum storage time	24 hours	5–7 days

A potential disadvantage of room temperature storage is bacterial contamination at collection with bacterial growth enhanced by the warm storage temperature. Early reports demonstrated a high incidence of contamination in pooled platelet concentrates, increasing with room temperature storage time (23). Other studies, however, have shown no contamination (24–26). More recently, a significant increase in contamination after 5 to 7 days of storage has been observed. As a result, platelet concentrate dating has been reduced to 5 days (26a, 26b). Clinical experience has, in general, confirmed the bacteriologic safety of room temperature storage. However, care must be taken in drawing and pooling platelet concentrates.

Finally, at least one plateletpheresis donor has been shown to have supplied contaminated platelets because of low-grade chronic bacteremia with *Salmonella choleraesuis* (27). Gram stains and culture of the unit transfused are indicated in the investigation of fever following use of any blood product.

Frozen Platelet Storage

Platelets can be frozen in either glycerol (28, 29) or dimethylsulfoxide (DMSO) (30, 31). Both techniques require meticulous attention to detail and have not been introduced into routine blood banking. DMSO has shown more promising results, but its potential for routine use is limited by its potential toxicity. Glycerol is already used in routine red cell cryopreservation and has no toxicity, being a metabolic intermediate.

Currently, use of frozen platelets is limited to research protocols in cancer centers. However, exciting results have been reported in the use of autologous platelets harvested during leukemia remission, frozen in DMSO, and reinfused during subsequent relapse and reinduction therapy (32, 33). This methodology has also been used to store HLA-matched platelets for subsequent use to meet the donor's convenience and avoid later difficulties in providing urgent pheresis of HLA-matched platelets (34).

Within the next 5 years, frozen platelets promise to be available in most major blood centers, although their exact role in hemotherapy requires more precise definition.

PLATELET DOSE

A unit of platelets contains at least 5.5×10^{10} platelets (35). Immediately after transfusion, between 50 and 70 per cent of the transfused platelets are recovered in the circulating blood (13, 36). This figure will be higher in a patient with a splenectomy and lower in a patient with splenomegaly.

The expected platelet increment can then be calculated as follows:

Platelet increment (per mm^3) =

$$\frac{5.5 \times 10^{10} \times (\text{number of units given}) \times 0.5}{(\text{total blood volume in ml}) \times 10^3}$$

If a dose of 0.1 unit per kg is given, the anticipated increment is about 40,000 cells per mm^3. Another rule of thumb is that one unit of platelets will raise a child's platelet count by 10,000 cells per mm^3 for each square meter of body surface area. It should be recognized that these considerations apply to a 1-hour post-transfusion increment. The in vivo half-life of platelets is about 4 days for cells stored 5 to 7 days at room temperature and is shorter for cold-stored platelets (20). The next day's platelet increment, 24 hours after infusion, will be significantly lower with cold-stored platelets, but nearly the same with room-temperature platelets.

FACTORS INVOLVED IN POOR RESPONSE TO PLATELET TRANSFUSION

The above guidelines for platelet dose make the assumption that platelet recovery and survival after transfusion will be normal. However, in many clinical situations this is not the case. Recovery is irregularly diminished because of splenomegaly (20a), and survival may be shortened by a consumptive or destructive process (Table 48–2).

Reasons for poor platelet response can be divided into immune and nonimmune causes. Immune causes include idiopathic thrombocytopenic purpura (ITP); drug-induced immune thrombocytopenia; alloimmunization to platelet antigens

Table 48–2. MECHANISMS INVOLVED IN POOR PLATELET RESPONSE

Immunologic Mechanisms:

Alloimmunization to platelet antigens:
    Multiple transfusions
    Pregnancy
    Organ transplantation
Idiopathic thrombocytopenic purpura
Drug-induced thrombocytopenia
Posttransfusion purpura
Isoimmune neonatal thrombocytopenia

Nonimmunologic Mechanisms:

Splenomegaly
Disseminated intravascular coagulation
Fever
Thrombotic thrombocytopenic purpura
Hemolytic-uremic syndrome
Active bleeding
Microangiopathic states

due to pregnancies or previous transfusions of red cells, platelets, or white cells; and passive transfer of platelet antibodies, as in isoimmune neonatal thrombocytopenia. Nonimmune causes for poor response to platelet transfusion include fever, sepsis, splenomegaly, disseminated intravascular coagulation (DIC), massive tumor burden, and active bleeding, including menses (which consumes platelets in the clot and shed blood). Recently, circulating immune complexes have been identified as coexisting with poor platelet responsiveness (36a, b).

In addition, variables in the product and its administration can influence results. Therefore, platelet yield in the concentrate, storage conditions, and pH values after storage are important. Finally, inappropriate transfusion practices (such as use of some microaggregate filters, failure to give platelets when ordered, or giving them to the wrong patient), as well as inaccurate platelet counts before and after transfusion, can influence the apparent results of platelet transfusion.

These considerations also apply to changes in hemostatic function after platelet transfusion. Because of disparities between platelet number and function (to be discussed), the desired transfusion effect, i.e., improved hemostasis, may not result from a response of the platelet count. Hemostasis may fail, despite an adequate quantitative transfusion response, because of qualitative defects in the transfused platelets. These may be caused by aspirin ingestion in the donor; platelet abnormalities induced by storage (36c); platelet disorders in the recipient (e.g., circulating substances inhibiting platelet function, as in uremia); or other factors.

Conversely, it might be argued that hemostasis may be achieved without a response in the platelet count. This question is frequently raised regarding prophylactic transfusions of platelets to patients in whom increments in platelet count cannot be achieved. Unfortunately, there is only suggestive evidence (37) to believe that this is the case, although arguments to justify such transfusions have proposed that transfused platelets "plug holes," maintain the vascular endothelium, and so forth.

Finally, failure to respond to platelet transfusion by achievement of hemostasis may reflect other factors contributing to or primarily responsible for bleeding, such as deficiencies in the coagulation cascade; local bleeding sites induced by trauma, tumor, or surgery; and others.

CLINICAL USES OF PLATELETS

The clinical use of platelets should not be based solely on the platelet count. In patients whose platelets function normally, there is a linear relationship between platelet count and bleeding time, with a normal bleeding time when the platelet count is above 100,000 cells per mm^3 and a bleeding time greater than 30 minutes when the count is below 10,000 cells per mm^3 (38) (Fig. 48–1).

In various clinical situations, however, this relationship can be altered. For example, patients who are uremic, have taken aspirin, or have von Willebrand's disease have bleeding times in excess of that predicted from their platelet count. Patients whose platelets are older than average (e.g., during a fall in platelet count after complete bone marrow suppression) have a longer bleeding time than predicted by platelet count alone. Patients whose platelets are younger than average (e.g., in ITP, in which a healthy bone marrow is rapidly producing new platelets to counter immune destruction, or in the recovery phase of bone marrow suppression from drugs or disease) have a shorter bleeding time than predicted by the platelet count. In addition to the platelet count and platelet function, vascular integrity, coexisting coagulopathies, and patient age and clinical status must all be assessed in determining the amount and frequency of platelet transfusions.

The clinical situations requiring platelet transfusion are outlined below.

Bone Marrow Failure

Patients with thrombocytopenia due to diminished platelet production are the most frequent users of platelets. These include patients with leukemia; aplastic anemia; certain congenital thrombocytopenias; and extensive bone marrow replacement by lymphoma, cancer, myelofibrosis, and so forth; as well as patients on cancer che-

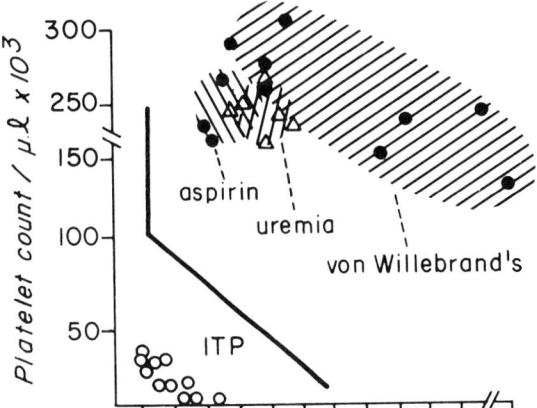

Figure 48–1. The relationship between bleeding time and platelet count. The bleeding time (in minutes) on the abscissa is plotted against platelet count (per µl. × 10^3) for normal platelet function (straight line) and for a variety of abnormalities. (Reprinted with permission from Harker, L. A.: *Hemostasis Manual.* Philadelphia, F. A. Davis Co., 1974.)

motherapy or those who have received other bone marrow toxins.

Significant spontaneous bleeding in these patients is rare when the platelet count is above 30,000 cells per mm^3. It has been shown, however (39), that the risk of spontaneous bleeding in adult and child leukemic patients increases markedly as the platelet count drops below 20,000 cells per mm.^{3} Most cancer treatment centers, therefore, transfuse platelets prophylactically to such patients when their platelet count drops below approximately 20,000 cells per mm^3. For prophylaxis, adult patients should receive 4 to 8 units of platelets per transfusion. Children should receive an equivalent dose depending on blood volume. In any event, no attempt should be made to raise their platelet count above 50,000 cells per mm^3 by transfusion, unless there is significant bleeding with a lower count.

Patients who have significant bleeding or extensive petechiae should be transfused more aggressively and with less attention to platelet count. However, as the bleeding time is ordinarily completely corrected at a platelet count of 100,000 cells per mm^3, there usually is no rationale for attempts to keep the count higher. In fact, in the absence of extensive trauma or surgery, it is seldom necessary to maintain the platelet count above 50,000 cells per mm^3 to allow near-normal hemostasis.

More recently, concerns have been expressed regarding the wisdom of prophylactic transfusion to the nonbleeding thrombocytopenic patient with leukemia or aplastic anemia. There are definite hazards of platelet transfusion, e.g., AIDS; hepatitis; bacterial infection; isoimmunization to platelet and white cell antigens, rendering subsequent needed transfusions useless; and predictable transfusion reactions to platelets in certain patients. In addition, long-term prophylactic platelet transfusion is extraordinarily expensive.

Prospective randomized controlled studies have confirmed the validity of prophylactic platelet transfusions in childhood and adult leukemia (37, 40). However, clinical events such as fever or sepsis, in addition to a low platelet count, were also related to bleeding episodes (37). In a more recent randomized study (41) there was little advantage of prophylactic transfusion over waiting for therapeutic transfusion for bleeding episodes. Further studies will be necessary to refine the indications for prophylactic platelet transfusions (41a). The availability of HLA-matched platelets in related or unrelated donors, the length of the anticipated period of thrombocytopenia, the ultimate disease prognosis, the predictability of bleeding episodes, and the effect of prophylactic transfusion on the community platelet resources are all factors that should impact on the decision to use platelets prophylactically in a given patient. An early study (42) did not demonstrate an advantage of high dose platelets (0.06 unit per pound) over low dose platelets (0.03 unit per pound) when used as prophylaxis. Thus, use of a smaller dose of platelets for prophylaxis would extend available platelet resources and diminish exposure to hepatitis, platelets and white cell antigens, and so forth. The decision to use prophylactic platelet transfusion should also be reviewed periodically, as the patient's clinical status and response to transfusion change.

Earlier clinical experience before the routine availability of platelets has indicated that severe thrombocytopenic bleeding in these patients is exacerbated by fever, sepsis, trauma, anemia, platelet inhibitors, hypertension, and drugs causing gastrointestinal toxicity. Bed rest, avoiding trauma and aspirin, control of hypertension and emesis, transfusion for severe anemia, prompt treatment of local infections, and, on occasion, the use of aminocaproic acid (42a, b) are all important adjuncts to platelet transfusion in the prevention of bleeding episodes.

Accelerated Platelet Destruction

Platelets can be rapidly destroyed after release from the bone marrow by immune mechanisms (ITP, many drug-induced thrombocytopenias) or nonimmune mechanisms (DIC, thrombotic thrombocytopenic purpura, hemolytic-uremia syndrome, extensive tumor vascular bed). Splenomegaly can cause both enhanced platelet sequestration and accelerated destruction.

In patients with immune platelet destruction, the bleeding time is shorter than predicted on the basis of their platelet count. These patients should seldom be transfused. They rarely have significant bleeding, even with platelet counts below 10,000 cells per mm^3. In addition, the benefits of platelet transfusion are short-lived because of rapid immune destruction. Transfusion of these patients should be reserved for life-threatening bleeding or during needed splenectomy. Even then, platelets must be given prudently, as one patient can deplete the entire platelet reserve of a community if attempts are made to significantly raise his platelet count. Platelets, when given, are probably more rationally administered in small multiple doses to extend the therapeutic effect. A dose of 50 units will be destroyed in these patients as rapidly as a dose of 5 units. The treatment of ITP is discussed in Chapter 42.

Isoimmune neonatal thrombocytopenia (43) occurs approximately once in every 5000 births. Maternal IgG platelet isoantibodies, induced by the current pregnancy or by previous pregnancy or transfusion, cross the placenta and destroy fetal platelets. Many of these antibodies have been shown to be directed against Pl^{A1}, a platelet-specific antigen found in 97 per cent of the normal population. Less commonly, other platelet antigen-antibody systems have been responsible for this clinical entity (44).

In these clinical situations the mother's platelets, which lack the corresponding antigen, are the most convenient source of compatible platelets (45, 46). These platelets should be washed free of maternal antibodies before transfusion.

Another interesting disease entity involving the Pl^{A1} antigen system is posttransfusion purpura. As this disorder has not been reported in pediatric practice the interested reader is referred elsewhere (47, 48).

Drug-induced thrombocytopenia is usually due to a mechanism involving peripheral destruction of platelets (see Chapter 42). Withdrawal of the drug is the most effective therapeutic maneuver. Because of their shortened life span, transfusion of platelets is ordinarily of little benefit and probably should be reserved for serious bleeding episodes. Successful transfusion therapy has been described, however (49).

Thrombocytopenia resulting from nonimmune peripheral destruction, utilization, or sequestration of platelets represents a wide spectrum of syndromes, many with multiple underlying etiologies. Therefore, the use of platelets in the treatment of clinical conditions such as DIC, thrombotic thrombocytopenic purpura (TTP), hemolytic-uremic syndrome, hypersplenism, and microangiopathic states has not been well studied. In general it can be concluded that platelet transfusion is of severely limited benefit in such conditions because of the often serious nature of the underlying disease, the markedly shortened platelet survival, the frequent coexistence of other defects in the coagulation mechanism, and the lack of effective specific therapy for the underlying condition.

Transfusion, therefore, should be given only for serious bleeding episodes rather than prophylactically for a given platelet count. The underlying disease should be aggressively treated, and other coagulation replacement therapy such as cryoprecipitate, fresh-frozen plasma (FFP), and coagulation factor concentrates should be given as indicated by appropriate laboratory testing.

Finally, massive platelet transfusion of the individual patient must be weighed against the necessity to conserve the community platelet resources. Often, effective replacement therapy, which may require up to 20 to 40 units of platelets per day, is very difficult. Therefore, the prognosis of the patient is important in this regard.

Massive Transfusion Situations—Surgery and Extracorporeal Circulation

Massive transfusion situations, i.e., those requiring greater than total blood volume replacement, cause a lowering of the platelet count. This is due to dilution of platelets with bank blood, which contains no viable platelets after 24 hours of storage, and with colloid and crystalloid solutions (50). Thrombocytopenia exacerbates the bleeding in massive transfusion more often than does deficiency of coagulation factors (50). Platelet transfusion is indicated in these situations, but attempts to raise the platelet count above 100,000 cells per mm^3 are not appropriate, as hemostasis is ordinarily entirely normal at that value (38). In fact, clinically satisfactory hemostasis is often maintained at a much lower platelet count. Unusual bleeding during or after surgery should not ordinarily be attributed to a platelet count over 100,000 cells per mm^3 and is unlikely to be due to a platelet count of 50,000 to 100,000 cells per mm^3. Other causes for the bleeding, such as deficient coagulation factors, other coagulopathies, or inadequate surgical hemostasis, should be considered.

Open heart surgery frequently involves dilutional thrombocytopenia due to volume replacement with bank blood. However, platelets are also sequestered and destroyed in the oxygenator and on other foreign surfaces. Therefore, the platelet count rapidly falls to approximately 100,000 cells per mm^3 upon initiation of extracorporeal circulation and often remains depressed for approximately 7 days following this procedure (51). There have been conflicting reports regarding the coexistence of a platelet function defect in extracorporeal circulation (52, 53). Clinical evaluation in these cases is complicated by preoperative platelet abnormalities, particularly in cyanotic heart disease; by intraoperative heparinization; and by the difficulty of evaluating whether bleeding is due to surgical or nonsurgical causes.

Massive Transfusion Situations—Exchange Transfusion

Unless blood is transfused within 24 hours of collection, dilutional thrombocytopenia will occur during exchange transfusion. The thrombocytopenia, however, will ordinarily be mild and usually does not cause clinical bleeding. The nadir of platelet count is seldom below 60,000 cells per mm^3, although the thrombocytopenia often persists for 7 to 10 days (54). In the presence of bleeding sites or a coexistent coagulopathy the thrombocytopenia may assume clinical importance. In these situations blood less than 24 hours old should be used for exchange, or platelets should be administered concurrently. The latter product is more likely to be readily available, particularly in emergency situations.

Abnormal Platelet Function

Patients with platelet function defects due to aspirin, other drugs, uremia, thrombasthenia, and so forth may have a significant bleeding defect despite a normal platelet count. This is often revealed at the time of surgery. Platelet transfusion may be useful in these situations, but clinical data and bleeding times, rather than the platelet count, must be used to guide the frequency and volume of platelet transfusion. If platelet function is inhibited by circulating platelet toxins (e.g., uremia), platelet transfusion will not be beneficial. Removing toxic substances by dialysis or similar methods is indicated if bleeding is on this basis. If the bleeding is due to von Willebrand's disease, cryoprecipitate, rather than platelet transfusion, will correct the abnormality.

Miscellaneous Uses

Platelets have recently been utilized in the treatment of ITP to deliver a therapeutic agent, vinblastine, presumably by enhancing the delivery of this agent to primed macrophages (55). Such innovative uses may greatly expand the scope of platelet transfusion. Platelet transfusion does not appear to enhance renal allograft survival (55a).

TECHNIQUE OF TRANSFUSION

Platelets should be administered through a standard 170-μ blood filter. The availability of microaggregate filters of 20- to 40-μ pore size in the operating room and surgical intensive care unit can lead to inappropriate use for platelet transfusion as well. Removal of platelets by passage through some varieties of these filters is often overlooked as a cause for poor platelet transfusion results. Unless small volumes are administered, the use of platelet administration sets with integral syringes is not warranted. If syringes are used, they should have an in-line 170-μ filter. Platelets can be hung one bag a time or can be pooled in the blood bank before transfusion. There is no need to change the blood filter with each bag. Electromechanical pumps can be used (55b).

PLATELET TRANSFUSION REACTIONS

Reactions to platelet transfusions are ordinarily of the febrile nonhemolytic type. These consist of fever, with or without chills, ordinarily starting 1 to 2 hours after transfusion. More severe reactions cause cough, dyspnea, and pulmonary infiltrates (56). These reactions are presumably caused by antibodies in the recipient's serum to white cells that inevitably contaminate the product (57). Usually these responses coexist with a negative or zero platelet increment. The patient's platelet count, and occasionally white cell count, can actually fall after transfusion, owing to a presumed "innocent bystander" destruction of his own white cells and platelets (58). This white cell destruction may initiate a septic episode in a compromised host. These reactions can be avoided by careful matching or by removal of most of the white blood cells from the platelet concentrate by a slow centrifugation (59).

Other risks of transfusion with platelets are the same as with whole blood transfusions except that hemolytic transfusion reactions ordinarily do not occur. These risks include bacterial contamination (59a, 59b), transmission of hepatitis, AIDS, and other infectious diseases, urticarial and anaphylactic reactions to plasma proteins, and immunization to platelets and to white cell and red cell antigens that invariably contaminate platelet concentrates.

PLATELET MATCHING

Random platelet concentrates can be matched for ABO and Rh antigens, although the necessity for doing so is not clear. ABO-compatible platelets may have a marginally better survival than ABO-incompatible platelets (60, 60a), but this is disputed by many (61–63). The logistics of platelet supply often render matching impossible. ABO-incompatible platelets clearly can be given safely and effectively. ABO-incompatible plasma can be more of a problem, especially when large numbers of platelet concentrates are transfused to infants or small children. Positive direct Coombs' tests occur fairly often in recipients of large numbers of out-of-group platelets. Occasionally there is some evidence of shortened red cell survival. The problem can be avoided by pooling the platelets and resuspending them in ABO-compatible plasma.

Rh matching is clearly not important for the survival and efficacy of platelet transfusions. However, small numbers of red cells invariably contaminate platelet concentrates and can immunize Rh-negative recipients to Rh-positive red cells. The risk of this is low in immunosuppressed patients on chemotherapy (64) but is probably higher in other patients. Rh-negative females of childbearing age should probably receive Rh-negative platelets or, if these are not available, should be protected with Rh-immune globulin against Rh sensitization.

Many patients receiving multiple platelet and other transfusions become immunologically refractory to subsequent platelet transfusions. Previous pregnancies also appear to immunize women to platelet antigens. The refractory state may occur as early as 2 weeks after the first exposure to platelet antigens, may wax and wane or progressively worsen, or may never occur despite multiple transfusions (65).

The refractory state correlates somewhat closely with the development of lymphocytotoxic antibodies, and these and other antibodies are thought responsible for poor platelet responses in most refractory patients. Most HLA antigens are expressed on platelets, although the degree of this expression varies from donor to donor and for different HLA antigens (see discussion in reference 63).

Other, i.e., platelet-specific, antigens have been described that may also have an important role in platelet transfusion in certain patients. Finally, the immune responsiveness of the patient, particularly one having an underlying disease or receiving cytotoxic therapy that inhibits immunologic functions, undoubtedly influences the development and maintenance of platelet antibodies.

The availability of large numbers of platelets from a single donor obtainable by pheresis has allowed attempts to match the HLA and other antigens of donor platelets with the recipient. HLA matching has been shown helpful in improving platelet responsiveness in the multi-transfused patient who is refractory to random platelet transfusions (61, 66). Close HLA matching, however, requires HLA testing of several thousand donors as a pool of unrelated potential candidates for platelet donations. Because siblings of a patient have a one in four chance of being HLA-antigen-identical, they frequently are a more effective source of close HLA matches. Other relatives are also worthy of testing.

Recent reports have suggested that close HLA matching of donors and recipients is not necessary for good results and that selected HLA-mismatched platelets may be successful (67). In addition, the HLA type of the recipient influences his tolerance of HLA-mismatched platelets (68). These findings are encouraging because they would allow matching procedures to be successful with a small pool of HLA-matched donors, within the capabilities of many blood centers or hospitals. However, another report disputes many of these findings (63).

In all studies to date, HLA matching has not been uniformly predictive of good platelet responses in the immunologically refractory recipient, presumably because of the involvement of other than HLA antigens and antibodies (68a–c). Additional crossmatching procedures that mix donor platelets with recipient sera have been employed, using a variety of methods (69–72b).

HLA matching, while of proven effectiveness for refractory patients, is of uncertain benefit for those patients who respond to pooled random platelet concentrates. Although theoretically desirable, the benefits of single-donor pheresis platelets, matched or unmatched, for patients who respond to pooled random platelet concentrates have not been clearly demonstrated. Policies vary from institution to institution, although randomly selected single-donor pheresis platelets have been justified on the basis of a diminished risk of hepatitis, AIDS, and alloimmunization (73). Large-scale use of HLA-matched platelets before the recipient becomes refractory to random platelets has not been attempted. Controlled studies will be necessary to judge the wisdom of these approaches. Treatment of such sensitized patients with high-dose immunoglobulin or splenectomy does not reduce the requirement for matched platelets (73a,b), though the value of immunoglobulin is disputed (73c).

References

1. Duke, W. W.: The relationship of blood platelets to hemorrhagic disease. J.A.M.A. 55:1185, 1910.
2. Simon, E. R.: The introduction of adenine-supplemented anticoagulant preservative solution into United States Blood Services. In *Red Cell Metabolism and Function*. Brewer, G. (ed.), New York, Alan R. Liss, 1977.
2a. Federal Register 45:27926, 1980.
3. Slichter, S. J., and Harker, L. A.: Preparation and storage of platelet concentrates. I. Factors influencing the harvest of viable platelets from whole blood. Br. J. Haematol. 34:395, 1976.
4. Mourad, N.: Studies on release of certain enzymes from human platelets. Transfusion 8:363, 1968.
5. Code of Federal Regulations, Title 21, 640.24.
6. Code of Federal Regulations, Title 21, 610.53.
7. Widmann, F. K. (ed.): *Hemapheresis*. Technical Manual, American Association of Blood Banks, 1985.
8. Szymanski, I. O., Patti, K., et al.: Efficacy of the Latham bowl processor to perform plateletpheresis. Transfusion 13:405, 1973.
9. Aisner, J., Schiffer, C. A., et al.: A standardized technique for efficient platelet and leukocyte collection using the Model 30 Blood Processor. Transfusion 16:437, 1976.
10. Nusbacher, J., Scher, M. L., et al.: Plateletpheresis using the Haemonetics Model 30 Cell Separator. Vox Sang. 33:9, 1977.
11. Hester, J. P., McCredie, K. B., et al.: The use of disposable plastic channels in an IBM Modified Separator for granulocyte and platelet collection. Transfusion 17:685, 1977 (Abstr.).
12. Nusbacher, J.: Controlling the leukopheresis process. In *Leukopheresis and Granulocyte Transfusions*. Washington, D.C., American Association of Blood Banks, 1975.
12a. Schiffer, C. A., Lee, E. J., et al.: Clinical evaluation of platelet concentrates stored for one to five days. Blood 67:1591, 1986.
13. Slichter, S. J., and Harker, L. A.: Preparation and storage of platelet concentrates. Br. J. Haematol. 34:403, 1976.
14. Becker, G. A., Tuccelli, M., et al.: Studies of platelet concentrates stored at 22°C and 4°C. Transfusion 13:61, 1973.
15. Valeri, C. R.: Hemostatic effectiveness of liquid-preserved and previously frozen human platelets. New Engl. J. Med. 290:353, 1974.
16. Valeri, C. R.: Circulation and hemostatic effectiveness of platelets stored at 4°C or 22°C: Studies in aspirin-treated normal volunteers. Transfusion 16:20, 1976.
17. Filip, D. J., and Aster, R. H.: Relative hemostatic effectiveness of human platelets stored at 4° and 22°C. J. Lab. Clin. Med. 91:618, 1978.
18. Kattlove, H. E.: Platelet preservation—what temperature? A rationale for strategy. Transfusion 14:328, 1974.
19. Murphy, S.: Platelet metabolism, morphology, and function during storage for transfusion. In *Platelet Physiology and Transfusion*. Washington, D.C., American Association of Blood Banks, 1978.
20. Slichter, S. J., and Harker, L. A.: Preparation and storage

of platelet concentrates. II. Storage variables influencing platelet viability and function. Br. J. Haematol. 34:403, 1976.
20a. Witzig, T. E., Ducatman, B. S., et al.: Platelet transfusion therapy in acute leukemia: lack of effect of splenomegaly on transfusion requirements and risk of hemorrhage. Am. J. Hematol. 18:345, 1985.
21. Code of Federal Regulations, Title 21, 620.24.
21a. Murphy, S., Kahn, R. A., et al.: Improved storage of platelets for transfusion in a new container. Blood 60:194, 1982.
21b. Murphy S., Holme, S., et al.: Paired comparison of the in vivo and in vitro results of storage of platelet concentrates in two containers. Transfusion 24:31, 1984.
22. Silvergleid, A. J., Hafleigh, E. B., et al.: Clinical value of washed-platelet concentrates in patients with non-hemolytic transfusion reactions. Transfusion 17:33, 1977.
23. Buchholz, D. H., Young, V. M., et al.: Bacterial proliferation in platelet products stored at room temperature. New Engl. J. Med. 285:429, 1971.
24. Mallin, W. S., Reuss, D. T., et al.: Bacteriological study of platelet concentrates stored at 22°C and 4°C. Transfusion 13:439, 1973.
25. Goddard, D., Jacobs, S. I., et al.: The bacteriological screening of platelet concentrates stored at 22°C. Transfusion 13:103, 1973.
26. Katz, A. J., and Tilton, R. C.: Sterility of platelet concentrates stored at 25°C. Transfusion 10:329, 1970.
26a. Heal, J. M., Singal, S., et al.: Bacterial proliferation in platelet concentrates. Transfusion 26:388, 1986.
26b. Braine, H. G., Kickler, T. S., et al.: Bacterial sepsis secondary to platelet transfusion: an adverse effect of extended storage at room temperature. Transfusion 26:391, 1986.
27. Rhame, F. S., Root, R. K., et al.: An epidemic of septicemia due to Salmonella cholera-suis var. Kunzerdorf. In *Eleventh Inter-Science Conference on Anti-Microbiological Agents and Chemotherapy*. Atlantic City, N.J., 1971.
28. Cohen, P., and Gardner, F. H.: Platelet preservation. IV. Preservation of human platelet concentrates by controlled slow freezing in a glycerol medium. New Engl. J. Med. 274:1400, 1966.
29. Dayian, G., Reich, L. M., et al.: Platelet preservation: Use of glycerol to preserve platelets suitable for transfusion. Cryobiology 2:563, 1974.
30. Djerassi, I., and Roy, A.: A method for preservation of viable platelets: Combined effects of sugars and dimethylsulfoxide. Blood 22:703, 1963.
31. Murphy, S., Sayar, S. N., et al.: Platelet preservation by freezing: Use of dimethylsulfoxide as cryoprotective agent. Transfusion 14:139, 1974.
32. Schiffer, C. A., Buchholz, D. H., et al.: Frozen autologous platelets in the supportive care of patients with leukemia. Transfusion 16:321, 1976.
33. Schiffer, C. A., Aisner, J., et al.: Frozen autologous platelet transfusion for patients with leukemia. New Engl. J. Med. 299:7, 1978.
34. Schiffer, C. A.: Future research in platelet transfusion. In *Platelet Physiology and Transfusion*. Washington, D.C., American Association of Blood Banks, 1978.
35. Code of Federal Regulations, Title 21, 620.24.
36. Hirsch, E. O., and Gardner, F. H.: The transfusion of human blood platelets. J. Lab. Clin. Med. 39:556, 1952.
36a. Kutti, J., Zaroulis, C. G., et al.: Evidence that circulating immune complexes remove transfused platelets from the circulation. Am. J. Hematol. 11:255, 1981.
36b. Safai-Kutti, S., Zaroulis, C. G., et al.: Platelet transfusion therapy and circulating immune complexes. Vox Sang 39:22, 1980.
36c. Rodgers, S. E., Lloyd, J. V., et al.: Platelet function in platelet concentrates and in whole blood. Anaesth. Intensive Care 13:355, 1985.

37. Higby, D. J., Cohen, E., et al.: The prophylactic treatment of thrombocytopenic leukemic patients with platelets: A double blind study. Transfusion 14:440, 1974.
38. Harker, L. A., and Slichter, S. J.: The bleeding time as a screening test for evaluation of platelet function. New Engl. J. Med. 287:155, 1972.
39. Gaydos, L. A., Freireich, E. J., et al.: The quantitative relation between platelet count and hemorrhage in patients with acute leukemia. New Engl. J. Med. 266:905, 1962.
40. Murphy, S., Koch, P. A., et al.: Randomized trial of prophylactic vs. therapeutic platelet transfusion in childhood acute leukemia. Clin. Res. 24:379a, 1976 (Abstr.).
41. Solomon, J., Beutler, E., et al.: Indications for the administration of platelet transfusions during remission-induction therapy of acute leukemia. Blood 50(Suppl.):210, 1977 (Abstr.).
41a. Aderka, D., Praff, G., et al.: Bleeding due to thrombocytopenia in acute leukemias and reevaluation of the prophylactic platelet transfusion policy. Am. J. Med. Sci. 291:147, 1986.
42. Roy, A. J., Jaffe, N., et al.: Prophylactic platelet transfusions in children: A dose response study. Transfusion 13:283, 1973.
42a. Woog, J. J., Dortzbach, R. K., et al.: The role of aminocaproic acid in lacrimal surgery in dyskeratosis congenita. Am. J. Ophthalmol. 100:728, 1985.
42b. Gardner, F. H., and Helmer, R. E.: Aminocaproic acid—use in control of hemorrhage in patients with amegakaryocytic thrombocytopenia. J.A.M.A. 243:35, 1980.
43. Pearson, H. A., Shulman, N. R., et al.: Isoimmune neonatal thrombocytopenic purpura: Clinical and therapeutic considerations. Blood 23:154, 1964.
44. Kostyu, D. D., and Amos, D. B.: Human leukocyte and platelet antigens and antibodies. In *Hematology*. Williams, W. J., et al. (eds.), New York, McGraw-Hill, 1977.
45. Adner, M. M., Fisch, G. R., et al.: Use of "compatible" platelet transfusions in treatment of congenital isoimmune neonatal thrombocytopenic purpura. New Engl. J. Med. 280:244, 1969.
46. McIntosh, S., O'Brien, R. T., et al.: Neonatal isoimmune purpura: Response to platelet infusions. J. Pediatr. 82:1020, 1973.
47. Shulman, N. R., Aster, R. H., et al.: Immunoreactions involving platelets. V. Post-transfusion purpura due to a complement-fixing antibody against a genetically controlled platelet antigen: A proposed mechanism for thrombocytopenia and its relevance in "autoimmunity." J. Clin. Invest. 40:1597, 1961.
48. Abramson, N., Eisenberg, P. D., et al.: Posttransfusion purpura: immunologic aspects and therapy. New Engl. J. Med. 291:1163, 1974.
49. Moss, R. A., and Castro, O.: Platelet transfusion for quinidine-induced thrombocytopenia. New Engl. J. Med. 288:522, 1973.
50. Sherman, L. A.: Alterations in hemostasis during massive transfusion. In *Massive Transfusion*. Washington, D.C., American Association of Blood Banks, 1978.
51. Moriau, M., Masure, R., et al.: Haemostasis disorders in open heart surgery with extracorporeal circulation. Vox Sang. 32:41, 1977.
52. McKenna, R., Bachmann, F., et al.: The hemostatic mechanism after open-heart surgery. II. Frequency of abnormal platelet functions during and after extracorporeal circulation. J. Thor. Cardiovasc. Surg. 70:298, 1975.
53. Umlas, J.: In vivo platelet function following cardiopulmonary bypass. Transfusion 15:596, 1975.
54. Hathaway, W. E., and Bonnar, J.: *Perinatal Coagulation*. New York, Grune and Stratton, 1978.
55. Ahn, Y. S., Byrnes, J. J., et al.: The treatment of idiopathic thrombocytopenia with vinblastine-loaded platelets. New Engl. J. Med. 298:1101, 1978.
55a. Chapman, J. R., Ting, A., et al.: Failure of platelet

transfusion to improve human renal allograft survival. Transplantation *41*:468, 1986.
55b. Snyder, E. L., Ferri, P. M., et al.: Use of an electromechanical infusion pump for transfusion of platelet concentrates. Transfusion *24*:524, 1984.
56. Wolf, C. F. W., and Canale, V. C.: Fatal pulmonary hypersensitivity reaction to HLA incompatible blood transfusion: Report of a case and review of the literature. Transfusion *16*:135, 1976.
57. Brittingham, T. E., and Chaplin, H., Jr.: Febrile transfusion reactions caused by sensitivity to donor leukocytes and platelets. J.A.M.A. *165*:819, 1957.
58. Herzig, R. H., Poplack, D. G., et al.: Prolonged granulocytopenia from incompatible platelet transfusions. New Engl. J. Med. *290*:1220, 1974.
59. Herzig, R. H., Herzig, G. P., et al.: Correction of poor platelet transfusion responses with leukocyte-poor HL-A-matched platelet concentrates. Blood *46*:743, 1975.
59a. Arnow, P. M., Weiss, L. M., et al.: Escherichia coli sepsis from contaminated platelet transfusion. Arch. Intern. Med. *146*:321, 1986.
59b. Van-Lierde, S., Fleischer, G. R., et al.: A case of platelet transfusion-related Serratia marcescens sepsis. Pediatr. Infect. Dis. *4*:293, 1985.
60. Tomasulo, P. A.: Management of the alloimmunized patient with HLA-matched platelets. In *Platelet Physiology and Transfusion*. Washington, D.C., American Association of Blood Banks, 1978.
60a. McElligott, M. C., McFarland, J. G., et al.: ABO incompatibility in HLA-matched platelet transfusions. Blood *64*(Suppl.):228a, 1984.
61. Lohrmann, H. P., Bull, M. I., et al.: Platelet transfusions from HLA-compatible unrelated donors to alloimmunized patients. Ann. Intern. Med. *80*:9, 1974.
62. Shulman, N. R.: Immunological consideration attending platelet transfusion. Transfusion *6*:39, 1966.
63. Tosato, G., Applebaum, F. R., et al.: HLA-matched platelet transfusion therapy of severe aplastic anemia. Blood *52*:846, 1978.
64. Goldfinger, D., and McGinniss, M.: Rh incompatible platelet transfusions—risk and consequences of sensitizing immunosuppressed patients. New Engl. J. Med. *284*:942, 1971.
65. Howard, J. E., and Perkins, H. A.: The natural history of alloimmunization to platelets. Transfusion *18*:496, 1978.
66. Yankee, R. A., Graff, K. S., et al.: Selection of unrelated compatible platelet donors by lymphocyte HLA-matching. New Engl. J. Med. *288*:760, 1973.
67. Duquesnoy, R. J., Filip, D. J., et al.: Successful transfusion of platelets "mismatched" for HLA antigens to alloimmunized thrombocytopenic patients. Am. J. Hematol. *2*:219, 1977.
68. Duquesnoy, R. J., Filip, D. J., et al.: Influence of HLA-A2 on the effectiveness of platelet transfusions in alloimmunized thrombocytopenic patients. Blood *50*:407, 1977.
68a. Peters, A. M., Porter, J. B., et al.: The kinetics of unmatched and HLA-matched ^{111}In-labeled homologous platelets in recipients with chronic marrow hypoplasia. Br. J. Haematol. *60*:117, 1985.
68b. Dunstan, R. A., Simpson, M. B., et al.: Presence of P blood group antigens on human platelets. Am. J. Clin. Pathol. *83*:731, 1985.
68c. Dunstan, R. A., Simpson, M. B., et al.: Le$_a$ blood group antigen on human platelets. Am. J. Clin. Pathol. *83*:90, 1985.
69. Mittal, K. K., Ruder, E. A., et al.: Matching of histocompatibility (HL-A) antigens for platelet transfusion. Blood *47*:31, 1976.
70. Wu, K. K., Hoak, J. C., et al.: Selection of compatible platelet donors: A prospective evaluation of three cross-matching techniques. Transfusion *17*:638, 1977.
71. Herzig, R. H., Terasaki, P. I., et al.: The relationship between donor-recipient lymphocytotoxicity and the transfusion response using HLA-matched platelet concentrates. Transfusion *17*:657, 1977.
71a. Kickler, T. S., Braine, H., et al.: The predictive value of crossmatching platelet transfusion for alloimmunized patients. Transfusion *25*:385, 1985.
72. Brand, A., Van Leeuwen, A., et al.: Platelet transfusion therapy. Optimal donor selection with a combination of lymphocytotoxicity and platelet fluorescence tests. Blood *51*:781, 1978.
72a. Ware, R., Reisner, E. G., et al.: The use of radiolabeled and fluorescein-labeled antiglobulins in assays to predict platelet transfusion outcome. Blood *63*:1245, 1984.
72b. Freedman, J., Hooi, C., et al.: Prospective platelet crossmatching for selection of compatible random donors. Br. J. Haematol. *56*:9, 1984.
73. Reiss, R. F., and Katz, A. J.: Statewide support of thrombocytopenic patients with ABO matched single donor platelets. Transfusion *16*:312, 1976.
73a. Schiffer, C. A., Hogge, D. E., et al.: High-dose intravenous gammaglobulin in alloimmunized platelet transfusion recipients. Blood *64*:937, 1984.
73b. Hogge, D. E., Dutcher, J. P., et al.: The ineffectiveness of random donor platelet transfusion in splenectomized, alloimmunized recipients. Blood *64*:253, 1984.
73c. Junghans, R. P., Ahn, Y. S.: High-dose intravenous gamma globulin to suppress alloimmune destruction of donor platelets. Am. J. Med. *76*:204, 1984.

TRANSFUSION THERAPY

CHAPTER 49
Granulocyte Transfusion

THOMAS J. ERVIN

INTRODUCTION 1598
LABORATORY STUDIES 1598
CLINICAL STUDIES 1599
GRANULOCYTE COLLECTION 1600
INDICATIONS 1601
Prophylactic Granulocyte Transfusion
Granulocyte Transfusion in Neonates
REACTIONS TO GRANULOCYTE TRANSFUSION 1602
GRANULOCYTE ADMINISTRATION AND STORAGE 1603

INTRODUCTION

Granulocyte transfusions have been widely used in the supportive care of patients with hematologic disorders that compromise defense against infection. The recipients are patients with aplastic anemia, immunologic disorders, acute and chronic leukemias, and other bone marrow failure states. The purpose of the procedure is to treat or, in some instances, to prevent bacterial or fungal infection. In patients with severe immunodeficiency states, lymphocyte transfusions have been used in an attempt to control overwhelming viral infections. Recent advances in technology have improved collection methods for granulocytes as well as other blood components. This chapter reviews the experience with and appropriate application of these methods. It must be emphasized at the outset that the value of these techniques remains controversial except in those unusual circumstances in which sufficient numbers of granulocytes can be administered.

LABORATORY STUDIES

As a result of improvements in platelet support, infection is now the major cause of morbidity and mortality for patients with bone marrow failure. Indeed, infection is the documented cause of death in 80 per cent of patients with unresolved hematologic malignancy or aplastic anemia and is often related to the presence of neutropenia (1). In contrast, the return of bone marrow function and circulating granulocytes is associated with recovery from serious bacterial infection.

Therapeutic trials in experimental animals have demonstrated that allogeneic granulocyte transfusions can serve as a means of controlling life-threatening infection in neutropenia. These studies have also provided important information concerning the limitations of this approach (2–11). Following experimentally induced granulocytopenia and sepsis, a single granulocyte transfusion (1×10^{10} granulocytes per m²) was shown to decrease circulating bacterial colony counts and transiently delay the appearance of secondary lethal bacteremic episodes. Repeated daily granulocyte transfusions administered to gentamycin-treated neutropenic dogs that had been inoculated with *Pseudomonas aeruginosa* offered prolonged survival to approximately 21 days (5). No such study comparing use of granulocytes plus optimal antibiotics versus antibiotics alone has yet been reported.

Response to granulocyte transfusions in neutropenic animals may be related to several factors. The presence of serum opsonin activity prior to granulocyte transfusion may improve survival (4). The addition of active immunization using type-specific *Pseudomonas* polysaccharide has improved survival in granulocytopenic dogs treated with granulocyte transfusion (12). Prior blood product sensitization with demonstration of anti-HLA antibodies has been shown to decrease post-transfusion granulocyte counts as well as tissue penetration by granulocytes (8).

The role of granulocyte transfusion in fungal infection is less well studied. Experimental models have, however, revealed a decrease in circulating fungal colony counts as well as tissue fungi counts following granulocyte transfusions (13).

It is clear from these observations that the management of sepsis and neutropenia involves cellular, hormonal, and immunologic factors. Such interacting factors complicate the spectrum of clinical illness defined by neutropenia and sepsis in humans. Analysis of these interacting factors in human infection would help to identify the potential role for granulocyte transfusions in such patients.

CLINICAL STUDIES

The role of granulocyte transfusions in neutropenic patients continues to be a subject of significant debate. As with the animal models, human illness, particularly in the setting of severe neutropenia, is complex and difficult to study. The impact of granulocyte transfusion on reversal of infection in neutropenic patients must be viewed in the context of such variables as antibiotic administration, underlying illness, immunologic suppression, and the severity of the infection in question. The decision to use granulocyte transfusions must include the analysis of such variables.

The most common clinical setting in which granulocyte transfusion is used is bacterial infection occurring in the presence of neutropenia. Multiple studies have documented the seriousness of this condition (14). In one study conducted at the National Cancer Institute between 1965 and 1971, the majority of the patients dying from hematologic malignancies succumbed to infection (19). More then 50 per cent of the organisms identified were bacterial. In aplastic anemia and drug-induced agranulocytosis, the most common cause of death is infection alone or infection in combination with hemorrhage (20). Bodey and associates (21) demonstrated a quantitative relationship between the absolute circulating granulocyte count and the incidence of infection in leukemic patients in remission and in relapse. Both the incidence and duration of infection increased markedly when circulating granulocyte counts were less than 500 cells per mm^3.

In an attempt to decrease the morbidity and mortality associated with infections that occur during neutropenia, several supportive care measures have been utilized. Prophylactic antibiotics given at the time that neutropenia occurs may decrease the incidence of microbiologically documented infections (22, 23). These trials do not, however, alter fungal infections, and they may lead to colonization by drug-resistant bacterial strains. Suppression of intestinal flora by means of absorbable (24) or nonabsorbable antibiotics (25) may decrease colonization by bacteria; however, antibiotics promote drug-resistance, and the nonabsorbable types may be poorly tolerated by the patient. Oral administration of antifungal agents such as ketoconazole may prevent fungal colonization in neutropenic patients (26). Providing a protective environment, including laminar air flow conditions, has also been shown to decrease infection rates in severely immunocompromised patients (27, 28, 29). In general, these supportive care procedures are implemented when the total granulocyte count falls below 1000 cells per mm^3. The prophylaxis is continued until the granulocyte nadir has occurred and the peripheral granulocyte count has returned to greater than 1000 cells per mm^3.

Despite such prophylactic maneuvers, a significant number of patients will develop infection when granulocyte counts fall below 1000 cells per mm^3. The absolute risk of infection is proportional to the severity and length of the neutropenic period. In general, 40 per cent of patients who present with fever and a WBC of less than 200 cells per mm^3 will have an identifiable infection (21). Additionally, almost all such patients followed without antibiotics will develop an infection within a 21-day observation period (21). Because of this high rate of established or potential infection in febrile neutropenic patients, broad-spectrum antibiotics are administered empirically in standard practice. The antibiotic choices may vary according to the clinical presentation and previous infectious history. Prompt administration of full-dose antibiotics is an essential feature of the initial management of the febrile neutropenic patient. The decision to add granulocyte transfusion therapy can then be made based on the severity of the clinical infection, culture results, initial response to antibiotics, and the overall progress.

Human studies of the effectiveness of granulocyte transfusions are heterogeneous. Indications for granulocyte transfusion, granulocyte transfusion dose, collection method, method of analysis, and clinical endpoint have varied from study to study. This variability coupled with the complex nature of severely ill immunocompromised patients has made it difficult to develop clear indications for the use of this expensive, labor-intensive, and potentially hazardous procedure. The lack of clear clinical indications is especially frustrating for directors of transfusion services who must apportion the efforts of a limited number of trained technologists and nurses to provide granulocyte concentrates.

GRANULOCYTE COLLECTION

Broad application of granulocyte transfusions has been hampered by the inability to harvest large numbers of granulocytes from normal volunteer donors. Human studies utilizing granulocytes harvested from chronic myelogenous leukemia (CML) donors clearly show a dose-response relationship between the number of transposed granulocytes and clinical response (30). Clinical improvement as defined by defervescence of fever was documented in 30 per cent of cases receiving 2×10^{10} granulocytes. This defervescense rate improved to 80 per cent in patients receiving up to 1×10^{11} granulocytes per dose. Infused CML granulocytes, while carrying the Philadelphia chromosome, will migrate to infected sites and can be shown to both phagocytose and kill bacteria in vivo (31). CML granulocytes may, however, be contaminated with unknown viruses capable of producing untoward effects in recipient patients. Despite the ability to avoid CML engraftment by irradiation of the CML granulocytes prior to infusion, CML patients are not routinely used as granulocyte donors.

Following the early use of CML donors, most transfusion services have used only normal volunteer donors as a source of granulocytes. At first, a series of uncontrolled trials documented feasibility and technique. Subsequent trials that attempted to assess efficacy have been published, and a short summary of the collection techniques is provided in Table 49–1. Table 49–1 shows that several significant differences in technique exist. In general, filtration leukopheresis provides the highest granulocyte yields. Filtration-derived granulocytes are, however, partially activated by their adherence to nylon fibers during the collection. Such activated granulocytes circulate poorly and may be associated with an increased rate of febrile reactions when transfused (41). Filtration procedures also require that the donor be systemically heparinized for the procedure. Centrifugation collection procedures, whether continuous or discontinuous, are less efficient. Granulocyte yields are lower when donors are not stimulated with corti-

Table 49–1. METHODS OF GRANULOCYTE PROCUREMENT

Method*	Trade Name	Donor Preparation	Granulocyte Yield	Comment
Gravity Centrifugation 32	—	None	3×10^8 per unit of whole blood	(a) 15–20 normal donors needed for transfusion (b) Increased infectious risk (c) No proven benefit unless CML donor used
Filtration 33, 34, 35, 36	Leuko-PAC (Fenwal)	Systemic heparin	$3-5 \times 10^{10}/3$ hr	(a) Donor systemically heparinized (b) High donor and recipient febrile reaction rate (c) Leukocytes show defective function in vitro
Intermittent Centrifugation 37, 38	Haemonetics M-50	Dexamethasone[1] + Methylprednisolone	$1 \times 10^{10}/3$ hr	(a) HES used[2] (b) Large extracorporeal blood volume needed (c) Platelets collected concurrently
Continuous Centrifugation 39, 40	IBM 2991 Fenwal CS 3000	Dexamethasone[1] + Methylprednisolone	$2 \times 10^{10}/3$ hr	(a) HES used[2] (b) Low platelet yield (c) Low extracorporeal volume needed (d) Closed system[3]

*Numbers indicate references at end of chapter.
[1]Optional stimulation of normal donors with *dexamethasone*, 10 mg PO, 12 hours prior to donation, or *methylprednisolone*, 0.5 mg/kg IV, 4 hours prior to donation, will increase granulocyte yields.
[2]HES = hydroxyethyl starch, a rouleau-inducing agent that may cause acute volume expansion and anaphylaxis.
[3]Fenwal CS 3000 only. A closed system may provide a means of long-term aseptic granulocyte storage if granulocyte preservation becomes feasible.

costeroid premedication. Such exposure to glucocorticoids may impair granulocyte function (42). To aid in the collection, centrifuge methods require the use of hydroxyethyl starch (HES) for better separation of white and red blood cell compartments. On repeated donation, HES may accumulate within the reticuloendothelial system and has been associated with hyperamylasemia. Repeated exposure to HES is not recommended but is necessary in cases in which only a few donors are available for granulocyte support.

Continuous centrifugation machines offer the advantage of maintaining a low extracorporeal volume, needed for centrifugation. Intermittent centrifugation machines have the advantage of allowing for simultaneous platelet collection and requiring only one arm for venous access. Despite these variabilities, no difference in overall clinical efficacy has been noted between centrifuge-derived and filtration-derived granulocyte transfusions administered in appropriate daily doses (43, 44).

INDICATIONS

Assuming that an appropriate number of granulocytes can be collected, one must decide on the clinical setting in which daily granulocyte transfusion may be of some benefit. Despite more than a dozen published reports, consensus on this problem is not complete. Generalizations that can be made from the large clinical experience with granulocyte transfusion (30, 41, 43–54) often require qualification. An outline of generally accepted criteria for granulocyte transfusion is given in Table 49–2.

In all granulocyte transfusion trials, transfusion is reserved for the neutropenic patient. Granulocytes are not appropriate treatment for patients with >1000 granulocytes per mm^3 unless functionally incompetent granulocytes, as seen in chronic granulomatous disease, are present (55). Although the degree of neutropenia below 1000 cells per mm^3 often varies among clinical studies, it is generally agreed that patients presenting with probable or documented infection and less than 200 granulocytes per mm^3 are at serious risk to fail despite optimal antibiotic therapy. These patients, when clinically infected, should be considered for granulocyte transfusion.

Granulocyte transfusion is usually begun when clinical infection and/or sepsis is documented. Several controlled trials have demonstrated no benefit of granulocyte transfusion for febrile neutropenic patients without a documented infectious source (43, 48, 51). Conversely, several controlled trials have documented a beneficial effect of granulocyte transfusions for patients with established infection and/or sepsis (41, 43, 48, 49, 51, 52). In these studies, the beneficial effect can be further stratified to *those patients who had documented infection but no early bone marrow recovery*. Clearly, patients with recovering bone marrow function rarely require granulocyte support. The absence of monocytosis, or a bone marrow aspirate showing no evidence of bone marrow function, supports the decision to administer granulocyte transfusion.

Response to granulocyte transfusion has been associated with the number of daily transfusions given. Patients who receive one or two granulocyte transfusions as a last chance rarely benefit, often because they are terminally ill at the time of treatment and have uncontrollable infection or underlying disease. Patients experiencing early bone marrow recovery also do not benefit. A serious effort to supply four or more daily transfusions in the correct clinical setting will often provide benefit. Patients receiving such treatment should have no evidence of early bone marrow recovery and should not have overwhelming sepsis at the initiation of granulocyte transfusion. It is important to remember that granulocyte transfusion is capable only of *stabilization* of the septic neutropenic patient and cannot be expected to reverse overwhelming septicemia in the presence of hypotension, severe disseminated intravascular coagulation, and respiratory failure. For this reason, the decision to use granulocytes should be made at the correct moment in the patient's course, so as to avoid, if possible, the use of this costly treatment as a heroic—and clinically useless—measure in dying patients.

Among published granulocyte trials, there is a wide range in the daily dose of granulocytes used. As mentioned in the CML studies, a daily dose of 10^{11} granulocytes per m^2 is needed to assure a good clinical response. Conventional granulocyte trials administer *daily* granulocyte doses of between 1×10^{10} granulocytes per m^2 and 3×10^{10} granulocytes per m^2. These doses are very low and, if at all compromised, can be expected to be ineffective. A *minimum effective daily* granulocyte dose is considered to be 1×10^{10} granulocytes per m^2. The granulocyte dose response is not confined to CML studies. Studies using normal donors (51, 54) have also showed an increase in clinical response as well as survival with increasing granulocyte dose. A recently published randomized trial

Table 49–2. GUIDELINES FOR THE DECISION TO ADMINISTER GRANULOCYTE TRANSFUSION

1. Granulocyte count of 200 cells per mm^3 in peripheral blood smear.
2. Documented or highly suspicious infection and/or sepsis.
3. Failure to respond to appropriate antibiotics for 24–48 hours.
4. Expected duration of neutropenia >7 days.
5. Expected bone marrow recovery if infection controlled.
6. Available donor.

using a daily dose of 2.5×10^9 granulocytes per m^2 suggests that there is no advantage to daily granulocyte transfusion (46). Given the extremely low dose of granulocytes administered, it seems premature to exclude benefit based on this study. Further controlled investigation (with granulocyte doses $>2.5 \times 10^9$ granulocytes per m^2 per day) might confirm or disprove this finding. This is of particular relevance in pediatric patients for whom adequate dosage is more likely to be achieved.

Prophylactic Granulocyte Transfusion

Because of the seriousness of established infection in the neutropenic patient and because of the marginal numbers of normal granulocytes available for daily granulocyte transfusion, it was hypothesized that daily granulocytes given to afebrile neutropenic patients might *prevent* the development of established infections in these patients. Several controlled trials have now been reported (57–60). In general, the trials have shown no overall advantage of prophylactic granulocyte transfusion when compared with oral nonabsorbable antibiotics in transplant patients (60) and with routine supportive care in patients undergoing chemotherapy for acute leukemia (56, 57). In one study (57), the incidence of sepsis, but not of overall infection, was decreased in the group receiving prophylactic granulocyte transfusions. There is no clear evidence that supports the use of prophylactic granulocyte transfusion during the neutropenia.

Granulocyte Transfusion in Neonates

Granulocyte transfusion, either as fresh whole blood exchange (60) or as a fresh buffy coat transfusion (62), has been found to be efficacious in treating neutropenia complicating sepsis in the newborn. Exhaustion of neutrophil production is a frequent concomitant of sepsis in the newborn period and may be heralded by a "left shift" of peripheral and marrow blood granulocytes (62a, 62b). Small clinical trials have suggested that granulocyte transfusions may decrease the mortality of neonatal sepsis in infants (62c, 62d) when exhaustion of granulocyte production is imminent. Neonatal nurseries should establish firm guidelines for the application of granulocyte support, since the risks of virus transmission may exceed benefits unless appropriate indications are strictly followed. All granulocyte transfusion products should be irradiated to prevent graft-versus-host disease. Granulocyte transfusion may also be useful in chronic granulomatous disease complicated by infection (55, 63).

REACTIONS TO GRANULOCYTE TRANSFUSION

While the disadvantages of granulocyte transfusions include their being both costly and time-consuming to prepare, a more important objection to their use is the potential for recipient toxicity. As with all blood products that contain a significant fraction of red cells (approximately 5 to 10 per cent), granulocyte transfusions must be ABO-compatible. Hepatitis, AIDS, and CMV transmission must also be considered. In addition to these standard problems, there are other potential problems that may occur.

A febrile reaction is common in patients who receive granulocyte transfusions. This reaction is often related to infusion rate and controlled by premedication with meperidine, 0.75 mg per kg IV, prior to the transfusion. Granulocyte transfusions may transmit cytomegalovirus (CMV) infection. An increased incidence of CMV infection was noted in patients receiving prophylactic and therapeutic transfusions (64). This increased incidence was seen only in initially seronegative recipients who received granulocyte transfusions from seropositive donors. This issue can be avoided by accepting only CMV seronegative donors for granulocyte transfusion to seronegative recipients.

Alloimmunization may occur with repeated granulocyte transfusions. This production of anti-HLA antibodies may make other blood component support more difficult. The incidence of alloimmunization is variable, with reported rates of between 20 and 60 per cent (53, 65). This problem, while usually manageable, must be taken into consideration, particularly in the light of future bone marrow transplant potential. The appearance of multispecific anti-HLA antibiotics is a relative contraindication for further granulocyte transfusion. Donors whose granulocytes exhibit a positive HLA crossmatch reaction with recipient serum should be avoided. Granulocyte transfusions administered despite documented HLA incompatibility may be complicated by febrile or pulmonary reactions (see below).

Patients receiving large numbers (usually greater than 50) of transfusions may develop leukoagglutinin antibodies. Such antibodies are unusual, but their appearance in the recipient or donor is an absolute contraindication to further granulocyte transfusion due to the possibility of pulmonary reactions (see below).

Because granulocyte transfusions contain 5 to 10 per cent red cells by volume, polycythemia may occur in children receiving granulocyte transfusion (53). As with any blood product containing viable lymphocytes, granulocyte transfusions may produce graft-versus-host disease when administered to a severely immunocompromised host (66,

67). This phenomenon most often occurs in pediatric patients or post-transplant patients. It can be avoided by routine irradiation of all granulocyte transfusions. A radiation dose of 5000 cGy administered over 2.7 minutes will effectively destroy the proliferative capacity of lymphocytes. Platelet, red cell, and granulocyte functions are preserved (68, 69).

The most serious reaction reported following granulocyte transfusion is that of pulmonary toxicity. The appearance of acute pulmonary infiltrates and/or respiratory failure has been associated with the procedure. This reaction may be related to leukoagglutinin production by the recipient (70). A recent publication has linked the appearance of pulmonary compromise to the concomitant use of amphotericin B in actively septic patients (71). In this study, patients already receiving granulocyte transfusions developed pulmonary compromise when amphotericin B was added. This association with amphotericin B has not been confirmed in other studies (52, 72), but it must be considered when granulocytes are administered. This pulmonary reaction is but one type of reaction that may occur in patients receiving granulocyte transfusions. Table 49–3 outlines a complete list of potential causes of pulmonary toxicities. Our experience suggests that patients receiving granulocyte transfusions may avoid pulmonary reactions by being administered a small dose of glucocorticoid, such as hydrocortisone, 1 mg per kg IV, given as a premedication to each daily granulocyte transfusion. Agglutination of transfused granulocytes in the pulmonary vasculature may be inhibited by steroid administration, which inhibits pulmonary complement activation as a mediating pathologic step (74).

GRANULOCYTE ADMINISTRATION AND STORAGE

Once collected, granulocyte concentrates should be administered as soon as possible. Overnight storage at 4°C or 40°F is acceptable, but granulocyte phagocytic and chemotactic functions rapidly diminish on further storage (74). In general, granulocytes should be administered within 24 hours of procurement. The collection should be ABO-compatible, HLA-compatible, and irradiated prior to administration.

Patients who receive granulocytes should be carefully evaluated for fluid status and pulmonary reserve. A baseline chest x-ray should be done prior to granulocyte administration. Premedication with meperidine, 0.75 mg per kg IV, or hydrocortisone, 1 mg per kg IV, may prevent chills and pulmonary reactions, respectively. Each collection should be administered slowly over 2 to 4 hours, using a routine blood infusion set. During the infusion, patients should be monitored twice hourly for temperature elevation or signs of pulmonary compromise. Small children receiving daily granulocytes must be watched carefully for fluid overload or polycythemia. Any adverse reaction should be reported promptly. In general, granulocyte transfusions should be continued on a daily basis until there is a return of granulocytes to a count of >500 cells per mm^3.

The role of granulocyte transfusions as a means of controlling infections in the neutropenic patient continues to be debated. In certain situations, patients clearly can benefit from the administration of daily full doses ($> 1 \times 10^{10}$ granulocytes per m^2 per day) of carefully matched granulocytes. Further studies employing larger or more frequent granulocyte doses are needed. Because of the cost and potential toxicities of granulocyte transfusion, it is mandatory to make a careful consideration of the clinical situation and the goals of therapy, as well as the means of collection and administration, before using this important blood product.

References

1. Levine, A. S., Schimpff, S. C., et al.: Hematologic malignancies and other marrow failure states: progress in the

Table 49–3. PULMONARY REACTIONS DURING THE COURSE OF GRANULOCYTE TRANSFUSION*

Type	Definition	Clinical Reactions
a. Leukoagglutination	Bilateral, severe interstitial, or alveolar infiltrates during or within minutes of completion of a granulocyte transfusion	1. Acute respiratory distress 2. Potentially fatal 3. May be increased when granulocytes administered with amphotericin B
b. Sequestration	Air space consolidation due to the "lighting up" of a previously unrecognized pulmonary infection	Acute respiratory distress
c. Unexplained	Apparently noninfectious infiltrates not present prior to the initiation of a granulocyte transfusion	Reactions varied from severe to asymptomatic
d. Fluid overload	Bilateral infiltrates with cardiomegaly and rapid response to diuretics	Reactions varied from mild congestive failure to pulmonary edema

*Adapted from Karp, D. D., et al.: Vox Sang. 42:57, 1982, with permission.

management of complicating infections. Semin. Hematol. 11:141, 1974.
2. Epstein, R. B., Clift, R. A., et al.: The effect of leukocyte transfusions on experimental bacteremia in the dog. Blood 34:782, 1969.
3. Appelbaum, F. R., Bowles, C. A., et al.: Granulocyte transfusion therapy of experimental pseudomonas septicemia: study of cell dose and collection technique. Blood 52:323, 1978.
4. Epstein, R. B. and Zander, A. R.: Granulocyte transfusions in leukopenic dogs. In *The Granulocyte: Function and Clinical Utilization*. Greenwalt, T. J., and Jamieson, G. H. (eds.), New York, A. R. Liss, 1977, p. 227.
5. Dale, D. C., Reynolds, H. Y., et al.: Granulocyte transfusion therapy of experimental pseudomonas pneumonia. J. Clin. Invest. 54:664, 1974.
6. Appelbaum, F R., Norton, L., et al.: Migration of transfused granulocytes in leukopenic dogs. Blood 49:483, 1977.
7. Boggs, D. R.: The effect of exposure of neutrophils to hydrocortisone on their movement into induced inflammatory exudates. Exp. Hematol. 7:211, 1979.
8. Appelbaum, F. R., Norton, L., et al.: The influence of cell collection techniques and prior alloimmunization on the migration of transfused granulocytes in leukopenia. Exp. Hematol. 7:241, 1979.
9. Price, T. H., and Dale, D. C.: Neutrophil transfusion: effect of storage and collection method on neutrophil blood kinetics. Blood 51:789, 1978.
10. Keusch, G. T., Ambinder, E. P., et al.: Role of opsonins in clinical response to granulocyte patients. Am. J. Med. 73:552, 1982.
11. Brecher, G., Wilbur, K. M., et al.: Transfusion of separated leukocytes into irradiated dogs with aplastic marrows. Proc. Soc. Exp. Biol. Med. 84:54, 1953.
12. Harvath, L., and Anderson, B. R.: Evaluation of type-specific and non–type-specific pseudomonas vaccine for treatment of pseudomonas sepsis during granulocytopenia. Inf. Immunol. 13:1139, 1976.
13. Ruthe, R. C., Anderson, B. R., et al.: Efficacy of granulocyte transfusions in the control of systemic candidiasis in the leukopenic host. Blood 52:493, 1978.
14. Bannatype, R. M., and Cheung, R.: Integrated management of bacteraemic shock in neutropenia. Anticancer Res. 3:233, 1984.
15. Schimpff, S. C.: Empiric antibiotic therapy for granulocytopenic patients. Bull. N.Y. Acad. Med. 58:750, 1982.
16. Pizzo, P. A., Robichaud, K. J., et al.: Empiric antibiotic and antifungal therapy for cancer patients with prolonged fever and granulocytopenia. Am. J. Med. 72:101, 1982.
17. Kramer, B. S., Pizzo, P. A., et al.: Role of serial microbiologic surveillance and clinical evaluation in the management of cancer patients with fever and granulocytopenia. Am. J. Med. 72:561, 1982.
18. Wade, J. C., Schimpff, S. C., et al.: A comparison of trimethoprim-sulfamethoxazole plus nystatin with gentamicin plus nystatin in the prevention of infections in acute leukemia. New Engl. J. Med. 304:1057, 1981.
19. Levine, A. S., Graw, R. G., et al.: Management of infections in patients with leukemia and lymphoma: current concepts and experimental approaches. Semin. Hematol. 9:141, 1972.
20. Williams, D. M., Lynch, R. E., et al.: Drug-induced aplastic anemia. Semin. Hematol. 10:195, 1973.
21. Bodey, G. P., Buckley, M., et al.: Qualitative relationships between circulating leukocytes and infections in patients with acute leukemia. Ann. Intern. Med. 64:328, 1966.
22. Gualtieri, R. J., Donowitz, G. R., et al.: Double-blind randomized study of prophylactic trimethoprim/sulfamethoxazole in granulocytopenic patients with hematologic malignancies. Am. J. Med. 74:934, 1983.
23. Kauffman, C. A., Liepman, M. K., et al.: Trimethoprim/sulfamethoxazole prophylaxis in neutropenic patients. Am. J. Med. 74:599, 1983.
24. Hargadon, M. T., Young, V. M., et al.: Selective suppression of alimentary tract microbial flora as prophylaxis during granulocytopenia. Antimicrob. Agents Chemother. 20:620, 1981.
25. Hahn, D. M., Schimpff, S. C., et al.: Infection in acute leukemia patients receiving oral non-absorbable antibiotics. Antimicrob. Agents Chemother. 13:958, 1978.
26. Meunier-Carpenter, F., Cruciani, M., et al.: Oral prophylaxis with miconazole or ketoconazole of invasive fungal disease in neutropenic cancer patients. J. Cancer Clin. Oncol. 19:43, 1983.
27. Levine, A. S., Siegel, S. E., et al.: Protected environments and prophylactic antibiotics: a prospective controlled study of their utility in the therapy of acute leukemia. New Engl. J. Med. 288:477, 1973.
28. Nauseef, W. M., and Maki, D. G.: A study of the value of simple protective isolation in patients with granulocytopenia. New Engl. J. Med. 304:448, 1981.
29. Ribas-Mundo, M., Granena, A., et al.: Evaluation of a protective environment of granulocytopenia patients: a comparative study. Cancer 48:419, 1981.
30. Morse, E. E., Freireich, E. J., et al.: The transfusion of leukocytes from donors with chronic myelocytic leukemia to patients with leukopenia. Transfusion 6:183, 1966.
31. Sohet, S. B.: Morphologic evidence for the *in vivo* activity of transfused chronic myelogenous leukemia cells in a case of massive staphylococcal septicemia. Blood 32:111, 1968.
32. Morse, E. E., Carbone, P. P., et al.: Repeated leukapheresis of donors with chronic myelocytic leukemia. Transfusion 6:175, 1966.
33. Djerassi, I., Kim, J. S., et al.: Continuous flow filtration-leukapheresis. Transfusion 12:75, 1972.
34. Rubins, J. M., MacPherson, J. L., et al.: Granulocyte kinetics in donors undergoing filtration leukapheresis. Transfusion 16:56, 1976.
35. Wright, D. G., Kauffmann, J. C., et al.: Functional abnormalities of human neutrophils collected by continuous flow filtration leukapheresis. Blood 46:901, 1975.
36. Wade, P. H., Shrabut, E. M., et al.: *In vitro* function of granulocytes isolated from blood of normal volunteers using continuous-flow centrifugation in the IBM-Aminco Celltrifuge and adhesion-filtration leukopenia using nylon fiber. Transfusion 17:136, 1977.
37. Tullis, J. L., and Eberle, W. G.: Plateletpheresis, description of a new technique. Transfusion 8:154, 1968.
38. Huetis, D. W., White, R. F., et al.: Use of hydroxyethyl starch to improve granulocyte collection in the Latham blood processor. Transfusion 15:559, 1975.
39. Freireich, E. J., Judson, G., et al.: Separation and collection of leukocytes. Cancer Res. 25:1516, 1965.
40. Ervin, T. J.: Personal communication, 1983.
41. Schiffer, C. A., Buchholz, D. H., et al.: Clinical experience with transfusion of granulocytes obtained by continuous flow filtration leukapheresis. Am. J. Med. 58:373, 1975.
42. Boggs, D. R., Athens, J. W., et al.: The effect of adrenal glucocorticosteroids upon the cellular composition of inflammatory exudates. Am. J. Pathol. 44:763, 1964.
43. Herzig, R. H., Herzig, G. P., et al.: Successful granulocyte transfusion therapy for gram-negative septicemia. A prospectively randomized controlled study. New Engl. J. Med. 296:701, 1977.
44. Morse, E. E., Katz, A. J., et al.: Clinical effectiveness of transfusion of granulocytes obtained by filtration or intermittent flow centrifugation. Cancer 47:974, 1981.
45. Ambinder, E. P., Button, G. R., et al.: Filtration versus gravity leukapheresis in febrile granulocytopenic patients: a randomized prospective trial. Blood 57:836, 1981.
46. Reiss, R. F., Pindyck, J., et al.: Transfusion of granulocyte rich buffy coats to neutropenic patients. Med. Pediatr. Oncol. 10:447, 1982.

47. Winston, D. J., Ho, W. G., et al.: Therapeutic granulocyte transfusions for documented infections. Ann. Intern. Med. 97:509, 1982.
48. Vogler, W. R., and Winton, E. F.: A controlled study of the efficacy of granulocyte transfusion in patients with neutropenia. Am. J. Med. 63:548, 1977.
49. Graw, R. G., Jr., Herzig, G., et al.: Normal granulocyte transfusion therapy. Treatment of septicemia due to gram-negative bacteria. New Engl. J. Med. 287:367, 1972.
50. Granena, A., Rozman, C., et al.: Granulocyte transfusion. Clinical evaluation of the results. Exp. Hematol. 7:369, 1979.
51. Alavi, J. B., Root, R. K., et al.: A randomized clinical trial of granulocyte transfusions for infection in acute leukemia. New Engl. J. Med. 296:706, 1977.
52. Higby, D. J., Burnett, D., et al.: Granulocyte transfusions: experience at Roswell Park Memorial Institute. In *The Granulocyte: Function and Clinical Utilization*. Greenwalt, T. J., Jamieson, G. A. (eds.), New York, A. R. Liss, 1977, p. 293.
53. Karp, D. D., Ervin, T. J., et al.: Pulmonary complications during granulocyte transfusions: incidence and clinical features. Vox Sang. 42:57, 1982.
54. Lowenthal, R. M., Golman, J. M., et al.: Granulocyte transfusions in the treatment of infections in patients with leukemia and aplastic anemia. Lancet 1:353, 1975.
55. Buecher, E. S., and Gallin, J. I.: Leukocyte transfusions in chronic granulomatous disease. New Engl. J. Med. 307:800, 1982.
56. The EORTC Int antimicrobial group. Three antibiotic regimens in the treatment of infection in febrile granulocytopenic patients with cancer. J. Infect. Dis. 137:14, 1978.
57. Strauss, R. G., Connett, J. E., et al.: A controlled trial of prophylactic granulocyte transfusions during initial induction chemotherapy for acute myelogenous leukemia. New Engl. J. Med. 305:597, 1981.
58. Winston, D. J., Ho, W. G., et al.: Prophylactic granulocyte transfusions during chemotherapy of acute nonlymphocytic leukemia. Ann. Intern. Med. 94:616, 1981.
59. Tobias, J. S., Brown, B. L., et al.: Prophylactic granulocyte support in experimental septicemia. Blood 47:473, 1976.
60. Winston, D. J., Ho, W. G., et al.: Prophylactic granulocyte transfusions during human bone marrow transportation. Am. J. Med. 68:893, 1980.
61. Christensen, R. D., Anstall, H. B., et al.: Use of whole blood exchange transfusion to supply neutrophils to septic, neutropenic neonates. Transfusion 22:504, 1982.
62. Christensen, R. D., Rothstein, G., et al.: Granulocyte transfusions in neonates with bacterial infection, neutropenia, and depletion of mature marrow neutrophils. Pediatrics 70:1, 1982.
62a. Christensen, R. D., Bradley, P. P., et al.: The leukocyte left shift in clinical and experimental neonatal sepsis. J. Pediatr. 98:101, 1981.
62b. Christensen, R. D., and Rothstein, G.: Brief clinical and laboratory observations: exhaustion of mature marrow neutrophils in neonates with sepsis. J. Pediatr. 96:316. 1980.
62c. Cairo, M. S., Rucker, R., et al.: Improved survival of newborns receiving leukocyte transfusions for sepsis. Pediatrics 74:887, 1984.
62d. Laurenti, F., Ferro, R., et al.: Polymorphonuclear leukocyte transfusion for the treatment of sepsis in the newborn infant. J. Pediatr. 98:18, 1981.
63. Yomiovian, R., Abramson, J., et al.: Granulocyte transfusion therapy in chronic granulomatous disease. Transfusion 21:739, 1980.
64. Hersman, J., Meyers, J. D., et al.: The effect of granulocyte transfusions on the incidence of cytomegalovirus infection after allogeneic marrow transplantation. Ann. Intern. Med. 96:149, 1982.
65. Mannoni, P., Rodet, M., et al.: Importance of antigens in granulocyte transfusions. Exp. Hematol. 7:302, 1979 (Abstr.).
66. Weiden, P. L., Zucherman, N., et al.: Fatal graft vs. host disease in a patient with lymphoblastic leukemia following normal granulocyte transfusions. Blood 57:328, 1981.
67. Ford, J. M., Lucey, J. J., et al.: Fatal graft-versus-host disease following transfusion of granulocytes from normal donors. Lancet 2:1167, 1975.
68. Zuck, T. F., and Brown, G. L.: Effects of *in vitro* irradiation on platelet function and lymphocyte viability. Transfusion 13:344, 1973.
69. Thomas, E. D., Stork, R., et al.: Bone marrow transplantation. New Engl. J. Med. 292:832, 1975.
70. Ward, H. N.: Pulmonary infiltrates associated with leukoagglutinin transfusion reactions. Ann. Intern. Med. 73:689, 1970.
71. Wright, D. G., Robichaud, K. J., et al.: Lethal pulmonary reactions with the combined use of amphotericin B and leukocyte transfusions. New Engl. J. Med. 304:1185, 1981.
72. Dana, B. W., Durle, B. G. M., et al.: Concomitant administration of granulocyte transfusions and amphotericin B in neutropenic patients: absence of significant pulmonary toxicity. Blood 57:90, 1981.
73. Craddock, P. R., Fehr, J., et al.: Complement and leukocyte-mediated pulmonary dysfunction in hemodialysis. New Engl. J. Med. 296:769, 1977.
74. McCullough, J., Carter, S. J., et al.: Effects of anticoagulants and storage on granulocyte function in bank blood. Blood 43:207, 1974.

TRANSFUSION THERAPY

CHAPTER 50
Coagulation Factors

GEORGE R. BUCHANAN

GENERAL PRINCIPLES OF TRANSFUSION THERAPY 1606
WHOLE PLASMA 1607
CRYOPRECIPITATE 1608
FACTOR VIII CONCENTRATES 1610
PROTHROMBIN COMPLEX CONCENTRATES 1611
  Activated Prothrombin Complex Concentrates for Patients with Circulating Inhibitors
OTHER PLASMA PRODUCTS 1613
USE OF PLASMA PRODUCTS IN THE MANAGEMENT OF SPECIFIC COAGULATION DISORDERS 1613
COMPLICATIONS OF PLASMA PRODUCT THERAPY 1613
  Transfusion Reactions
  Hepatitis
  Acquired Immune Deficiency Syndrome (AIDS)
  Other Viral Infections
  Hemolytic Anemia
  Other Immunologic Sequelae
  Miscellaneous Complications
THE FUTURE OF COAGULATION FACTOR THERAPY 1616

For nearly 5 decades whole plasma and its fractionated components have been used for volume replacement and for treatment of bleeding disorders caused by clotting factor deficiencies. Initially only whole blood and fresh or outdated banked plasma were widely available, but it was soon appreciated that fresh frozen plasma had several important advantages. After World War II the framework was laid for efficient fractionation of plasma (1, 2) and subsequently for the concentration of certain of its constituent coagulation proteins (3–7). A wide variety of plasma concentrates now exist for the prevention and treatment of hemorrhage in children and adults with hereditary and acquired disorders due to deficiencies of single or multiple factors (3–9).

GENERAL PRINCIPLES OF TRANSFUSION THERAPY

This chapter will discuss methods of preparation and storage, clinical uses, and specific advantages and side effects for each individual plasma product. However, certain general principles of replacement transfusion therapy apply for all preparations (5–9). The product being employed must contain adequate amounts of the deficient factor or factors. For example, cryoprecipitate, which is devoid of significant Factor IX activity, should never be given to a patient with Factor IX deficiency. Yet this error has unfortunately been made on numerous occasions (10). Moreover, the patient should receive an adequate initial dose and subsequent infusions at frequent enough intervals to achieve and maintain hemostasis. Both the first dose and the number and frequency of later infusions depend upon a number of variables unique to each clinical situation and to each plasma product (5, 7, 8, 11, 12). As indicated in Table 50–1 and discussed more fully in Chapters 39 and 41, the initial postinfusion recovery in the circulation varies somewhat with each protein and depends upon its diffusion into the extravascular space as well as nonspecific binding to platelets, endothelial cells, and other tissues. The circulating half-life varies tremendously among the clotting factors. This is due not only to the same variables that affect initial recovery but also to the true biologic half-life of the protein, i.e., its rate of catabolism (5, 8, 11) (Table 50–1).

The amount of material infused depends in great part on the minimum level of the deficient factor that is required for hemostasis (9). This

Table 50–1. CHARACTERISTICS OF PLASMA COAGULATION FACTORS RELEVANT TO REPLACEMENT TRANSFUSION THERAPY

Factor	Preferred Transfusion Product(s)*	Stability at 4°C	Recovery in Circulation Post-Infusion		Biologic Half-Life	Minimal Hemostatic Level
			% of Administered Dose	Increase in Plasma Level after Administration of 1 U/kg†		
Fibrinogen	C, P	Stable	50	3 mg/dl	4–5 days	75 mg/dl
Prothrombin (II)	P, PCC	Stable	40–80	1%	3 days	15–40%
V	P	Unstable	50–80	1.5%	12–36 hr.	10–15%
VII	P, PCC	Stable	70–100	1%	4–6 hr.	5–10%
VIII	C, P, FEC	Stable	50–80	2%	12–15 hr.	20–30%
IX	P, PCC	Unstable	25–50	1%	18–30 hr.	20–30%
X	P, PCC	Stable	50–100	1%	1½–2½ days	10–20%
XI	P	Stable	80–100	2%	1–3 days	10–30%
XII	None required	Stable	—	—	—	—
XIII	P	Stable	50–100	1–3%	3–10 days	1–5%

*Abbreviations: C = cryoprecipitate, P = fresh frozen plasma, PCC = prothrombin complex concentrate, and FEC = Factor eight concentrate.
†One unit is the amount of the clotting factor in 1 ml. of normal fresh pooled citrated plasma.
(The information in this table is taken in part from references 5, 7, 8, 9, and 11.)

critical "minimal hemostatic level" varies tremendously among the different factors (Table 50–1). For example, circulating levels of only 1 to 2 per cent of normal are usually necessary for Factor XIII (14), whereas experience dictates that levels of at least 20 per cent are required to achieve adequate hemostasis in individuals with Factor VIII or Factor IX deficiency (4). In addition, the amount administered depends upon the baseline level of the deficient factors in the patient and the degree of hemostasis that is required (6). For example, a child with Factor VIII deficiency who is having surgery needs normal factor levels for 7 to 14 days, but if only mild spontaneous soft tissue bleeding has occurred, a single dose to achieve a level of 10 to 20 per cent may suffice (4). Situations leading to accelerated consumption, such as circulating inhibitors or disseminated intravascular coagulation, require larger doses and more frequent treatments. Periodic laboratory monitoring of factor levels is sometimes advisable in the child with hemophilia or another bleeding disorder who is receiving multiple infusions.

In summary, a careful assessment of the clinical situation, an understanding of the biology of the clotting factor or factors to be replaced, and a familiarity with the plasma products being employed generally permit accurate replacement therapy.

WHOLE PLASMA

Freshly drawn plasma that is promptly separated from the red blood cells and buffy coat contains normal activity of its constituent clotting factors. However, obtaining fresh plasma for immediate transfusion is impractical. Single donor plasma separated from outdated banked whole blood contains sufficient amounts of Factor IX and most of the other stable factors but is markedly lacking in Factor V and Factor VIII (5, 15) and may contain potentially harmful fibrin degradation products (16), microaggregates (15), and excessive potassium content. Therefore, it too is rarely used in current practice (Table 50–2). Fresh or outdated freeze-dried plasma, prepared either as single units or pooled, is also infrequently used in the United States at present (Table 50–2).

In the late 1940's, fresh frozen plasma became the mainstay of plasma replacement therapy. Whole blood collected in citrate phosphate dextrose (CPD) or CPD-adenine from single donors or by plasmapheresis is separated by rapid centrifugation within 4 to 6 hours after collection. The supernatant plasma, diluted approximately 20 per cent by the anticoagulant, is then separated in a closed system, rapidly frozen, and stored at or below −30°C (15). It is stable, with minimal loss of activity of most clotting proteins, for up to 1 year. After thawing with constant mixing in a 37°C water bath, the plasma contains essentially normal levels of all factors except Factors V and VIII, which often lose some activity during several months of storage, even at temperatures of −30°C (11). Factor VIII levels are usually 0.6 to 0.7 units per ml (60 to 70 per cent) in the thawed material.

Fresh frozen plasma was once the preferred treatment for all patients with hemophilia A or B (4, 6). Despite the current availability of factor concentrates (to be discussed), plasma remains useful for patients with hemophilia and von Willebrand's disease in circumstances in which circulating levels of only 10 to 15 per cent above the baseline are transiently required (4) or if emer-

Table 50–2. UNFRACTIONATED PLASMA PREPARATIONS

Preparation	Storage Conditions	Shelf Life	Contents	Major Clinical Indications	Disadvantages and Side Effects
Fresh plasma	Used immediately	—	All clotting factors	All clotting factor deficiencies	Not readily available
Fresh frozen plasma	Less than −20°C Less than −40°C	6 mo 12 mo	All clotting factors (diminished Factors V and VIII after several months)	See text	See text
Fresh freeze dried plasma	Less than 25°C in dark	8 yr	All factors except V and VIII	Rarely used	
Plasma from outdated whole blood (single-donor plasma)	4°C	12 mo	All factors except V and VIII	Volume expansion,* Factor IX deficiency*	High potassium content, microaggregates, fibrin split products
Freeze dried outdated plasma	Less than 25°C in dark	8 yr	All factors except V and VIII	Volume expansion,* rarely used*	High potassium content, microaggregates
Freeze dried pooled outdated plasma	Less than 25°C in dark	8 yr	All factors except V and VIII	Rarely used	High potassium content, microaggregates

*Not the preferred therapy.

gency therapy is required when the patient's exact diagnosis is uncertain or when concentrates are unavailable (15). Moreover, plasma is the only known treatment for patients with the rare inherited deficiencies of Factor V, Factor XI, and Factor XIII (5, 8). It may also be of value for children with acquired bleeding disorders such as disseminated intravascular coagulation and hemorrhage secondary to liver disease (11, 17). When vitamin K deficiency is responsible for a hemorrhagic diathesis, parenteral vitamin K usually suffices, and factor replacement is generally not required except secondary to overdosage of coumarin anticoagulants. Reliance on vitamin K to promote rapid reversal of anticoagulant therapy results in inability to resume oral anticoagulation for a number of days (18). Fresh frozen plasma should *not* be used as a volume expander for patients with normal blood coagulation (19).

Fresh frozen plasma is usually administered immediately after thawing in the maximum tolerated dose, 10 to 15 ml per kg, at intervals of 8 to 24 hours. It should be compatible with the recipient's ABO blood type in order to avoid hemolytic reactions. Infusions of greater than 30 ml per kg per 24 hours for more than 2 or 3 days usually causes volume overload with resultant cardiorespiratory embarrassment, even in normal children. The major advantages of fresh frozen plasma are that it contains all known clotting factors and carries a relatively low risk of viral hepatitis and other blood-borne infections. Disadvantages include frequent bothersome transfusion reactions and inability to achieve factor levels greater than 20 per cent in excess of the baseline without risking pulmonary edema. Accordingly, patients with severe factor deficiencies cannot be adequately covered for surgical procedures with fresh frozen plasma, since circulating levels greater than 30 per cent are generally required for surgical hemostasis (see Chapter 41). In order to achieve higher levels, plasmapheresis with plasma exchange (20, 21) or the administration of fresh frozen plasma doses of greater than 15 ml per kg, along with vigorous diuretic therapy, may be attempted. Fresh frozen plasma is somewhat inconvenient and time-consuming to give, for the material must be thawed and a complete intravenous infusion set (support pole, plastic tubing, and other apparatus) is required (9). Consequently, use of plasma in hemophilia home treatment programs has been limited.

CRYOPRECIPITATE

One of the most important breakthroughs in the management of patients with hemophilia A was the development of preparations containing Factor VIII in a concentrated form. In 1959 Pool and Robinson (22) noted that Factor VIII was poorly soluble immediately after thawing of frozen plasma, and in 1964 these workers described a simple method of using normal plasma to obtain a "cryoprecipitate" that contained much of the Factor VIII present in the starting plasma (23, 24). These findings rapidly had profound implications for hemophiliacs throughout the world (see Chapter 41).

The capabilities for making cryoprecipitate are possessed by almost all blood banks. It is prepared from fresh plasma collected in either CPD, CPD-adenine, or heparin and separated from whole blood within 6 hours of procurement (25–28). The plasma is rapidly frozen at −70°C and is then slowly thawed at 2 to 4°C for 18 to 24 hours. The supernatant plasma is separated by rapid centrifugation from the newly formed precipitate. The resulting 3 to 10 ml of precipitate is re-frozen, sometimes with a small amount of plasma, in its original bag and stored at temperatures at or below $-18°C$ for 3 to 12 months. The supernatant plasma is used for other purposes, as it contains all clotting factors except Factor VIII and fibrinogen (6).

Cryoprecipitate consists of large quantities of antihemophilic factor (Factor VIII:C) (24); the ristocetin cofactor, or von Willebrand factor (VIIIR:CoF) (29, 30); Factor VIII-related antigen (VIIIR:Ag); fibrinogen (24, 31, 32); fibrinectin (cold insoluble globulin) (33); Factor XIII (34); trace amounts of other clotting factors; and variable quantities of certain other plasma proteins (8, 35). Factor IX is *not* present in clinically significant amounts (6). There is wide variability in the "potency" of cryoprecipitate from different blood banks and even among units collected from different donors by the same blood bank under carefully standardized conditions (25–27). The mean Factor VIII content per bag may vary widely, ranging between 40 and 160 units.* This variation appears to be due to differences in the techniques of centrifugation, freezing, thawing, and storage, and to variances in the time after phlebotomy before the plasma is separated and frozen (25–27, 36).

Current blood bank regulations dictate that 75 per cent of bags must contain no less than 80 units of Factor VIII per bag. It should never be assumed that more than 100 units per bag are actually present. At least 50 per cent of the Factor VIII:C is usually lost during the preparation process, primarily during freezing and thawing (26, 27). Certain technical modifications, however, may increase the yield appreciably (28, 36, 37).

There are only a few disorders in which cryoprecipitate should be used: hemophilia A, von Willebrand's disease, congenital afibrinogenemia, and, rarely, disseminated intravascular coagulation (4, 29, 31, 34, 38). With cryoprecipitate, normal factor levels can be achieved without danger of volume overload, and surgical procedures can be safely undertaken (4, 6). In a few areas of the United States, cryoprecipitate is less expensive than commercial factor VIII concentrates and remains widely used for patients with hemophilia A. It is the treatment of choice for children with von Willebrand's disease, since it contains both Factor VIII:C and the high molecular weight multimers of the von Willebrand factor, that are necessary for correcting the bleeding time by promoting platelet adhesion to subendothelium (see Chapters 37, 39) (29, 30).

Treatment always requires multiple bags of cryoprecipitate, since the average of 80 to 100 units in a single bag is less than would be administered for almost any therapeutic purpose. The infant who requires as little as 100 Factor VIII units is best treated with two bags to assure that an adequate dose is received. Otherwise, dosage of cryoprecipitate varies tremendously, depending upon the specific circumstances, and Chapter 41 should be consulted for further details. In most centers it is the practice to dissolve the precipitate in saline and pool it into a transfer pack prior to infusion.

Cryoprecipitate has certain advantages over fresh frozen plasma and the commercial Factor VIII concentrates (5, 11, 15). It contains approximately 20 times as much Factor VIII per unit volume as fresh frozen plasma, permitting extremely high levels to be achieved in vivo post-transfusion without risk of volume overload. Moreover, cryoprecipitate causes transfusion reactions less frequently than does plasma, probably because few foreign "immunogenic" proteins are cryoprecipitable. Both cryoprecipitate and fresh frozen plasma retain normal von Willebrand factor activity and are equally useful to prevent or treat hemorrhage in von Willebrand's disease (see Chapter 41). Finally, use of cryoprecipitate in patients with von Willebrand's disease and mild hemophilia may be associated with less risk of hepatitis and acquired immune deficiency syndrome (AIDS) than administration of Factor VIII concentrate (40, 41). This issue will be discussed further in the section on side effects, below.

Certain problems exist with the use of cryoprecipitate. To retain Factor VIII activity more than a few weeks it must be kept frozen at less than $-18°C$, a temperature not easily achievable in many home freezers. Cryoprecipitate is often extremely viscous, difficult to mix and pool, and quite time-consuming and laborious to administer (6, 11). Accordingly, its use in home infusion programs for hemophiliacs has been somewhat limited, and Factor VIII concentrates are currently preferred by most physicians caring for patients with severe hemophilia (9) who are over 4 years of age. Because of the variability in Factor VIII content from bag to bag and the inability to assay Factor VIII concentration in individual bags, one is never certain exactly how many Factor VIII units are being infused. The danger of hepatitis is much greater than with fresh frozen plasma, since multiple donor units are given; unlike Factor VIII concentrate, cryoprecipitate cannot be heat treated to eliminate contaminating viruses. Other less common side effects of cryoprecipitate, i.e., hemolytic anemia and paradoxical hemorrhage due to defective platelet function, are described later in this chapter.

---

*One unit equals that amount of clotting activity in 1 ml of fresh citrated pooled plasma.

As reviewed elsewhere (Chapter 41), these many side effects of cryoprecipitate may be avoided by using the vasopressin analog 1-deamino-8-D-arginine vasopressin (DDAVP) for bleeding complications in von Willebrand's disease and mild hemophilia A (42).

FACTOR VIII CONCENTRATES

In 1937 Patek and Taylor recognized that a specific protein, which they termed antihemophilic globulin, was deficient in the plasma of patients with hemophilia (43). An assay for the antihemophilic globulin, developed in 1953, helped lead to the production of highly concentrated forms of the protein, which was later designated Factor VIII (6). From the late 1940's through the early 1960's certain plasma fractions, including Cohn fraction I and fraction I-0 (44), were noted to contain sizable amounts of antihemophilic globulin, and such preparations were used in a few clinical trials (6). Animal Factor VIII concentrates were first produced in 1955 (45, 48), but it was only after the observations of Pool and co-workers regarding concentration of Factor VIII by cryoprecipitation (23, 24) that intensified efforts were undertaken commercially to produce human Factor VIII concentrates on a mass scale. The first successful and widely used lyophilized concentrate of Factor VIII became available by 1968 (47–49), and currently there are more than 20 preparations in use around the world, nearly a half dozen of them in the United States (13, 50) (see Table 50–3).

The exact production methods vary somewhat among manufacturers, but the basic principles are similar (6, 44). Large pools of fresh frozen plasma (often more than 1000 liters) are prepared by plasmapheresis from hundreds or even thousands of paid donors, and the Factor VIII is purified and concentrated by combinations of cryoprecipitation and precipitation with glycine, polyethylene glycol, or ethanol (5, 8, 15). The resulting insoluble material containing Factor VIII is further fractionated, freeze dried, and assayed for clotting activity.

In order to reduce the risk of hepatitis and acquired immune deficiency syndrome (see below), most manufacturers are now subjecting the plasma or dried concentrate to heat treatment at some stage during the production process (52). The exact heating techniques vary among the manufacturers. The issue of heat treatment is discussed in more detail in the section on side effects.

All currently available products, including those that have been heat treated (Table 47–3), have been intensively studied in vitro and have similar in vivo recoveries and circulating half-lives (9). Products are packaged in individual vials, which are labeled with the exact number of units of Factor VIII activity contained within. Factor VIII content per unit volume is 10 to 40 or more times greater than plasma (Table 50–3). Most manufacturers produce vials of several different sizes (usually 250 to 300, 500 to 600, and 900 to 1100 units) and make available packages containing lyophilized concentrate, saline or distilled water for reconstitution, filter needles, and all materials necessary for the venipuncture. Easy and prompt outpatient use is thus facilitated.

In addition to Factor VIII, these products contain a variable amount of fibrinogen and isohemagglutinins and small quantities of other proteins (53). Most, if not all, Factor VIII concentrates appear to contain a form of the von Willebrand factor molecule that has been altered and thereby rendered nonfunctional (29, 30, 54–56). This appears to be the result of loss of the Factor VIII von Willebrand antigen's high-molecular-weight multimers, which are most important in correcting the bleeding time in von Willebrand's disease (83).

The only patients for whom Factor VIII concentrates should be used are those with hemophilia A and, rarely, children with severe von Willebrand's disease, i.e., when the Factor VIII:C levels are less than 5 to 10 per cent of normal (29). The dose is extremely variable, depending upon the clinical circumstances discussed in Chapter 41. Children with mild or moderately severe von Willebrand's disease, whose bleeding is due more to lack of the von Willebrand factor than to Factor VIII:C deficiency, should receive plasma, cryoprecipitate, or 1-deamino-8-D-arginine vasopressin (DDAVP) instead.

The major advantages of the commercial Factor VIII concentrates compared with fresh frozen plasma and cryoprecipitate are their stability at 4°C (permitting storage in a home refrigerator), ease of reconstitution and administration by syringe, and extremely small volume (often 10 ml or less for 300 or more units), allowing rapid achievement of hemostatically effective levels (57). Concentrates can even be stored at room temperature for variable periods of time and after reconstitution the Factor VIII contained within is stable for many hours. Accordingly, continuous infusion of Factor VIII may be used in surgical patients, without the peaks and nadirs seen with intermittent dosing (58). Furthermore, transfusion reac-

Table 50–3. SOME OF THE FACTOR VIII CONCENTRATES MOST FREQUENTLY USED IN THE UNITED STATES

Name of Product*	Manufacturer
Profilate	Alpha
Factorate	Armour
Koate	Cutter
Hemofil	Hyland
Antihemophilic Factor	American Red Cross

*All products are currently heat-treated (see text).

tions are extremely uncommon with Factor VIII concentrates.

There are certain disadvantages, however. Since Factor VIII concentrates are prepared from large lots of pooled plasma, they carry a major risk of transmission of hepatitis (59, 60). Acquired immune deficiency syndrome also may result from concentrate infusions (see below), and the consequences may be fatal (61, 62). Isoimmune hemolytic anemia may occur secondary to the anti-A and anti-B isohemagglutinins (53, 63–65).

Factor VIII concentrates are extremely expensive. Their cost to the patient currently averages approximately 15 to 17 cents per unit, or $40 to $200 per infusion. In some areas of the United States cryoprecipitate is less expensive, although this cost differential varies widely (61, 66, 67). Unfortunately, the more complete purification processes result in lesser yields of Factor VIII (4, 9, 68), particularly following heat treatment. High-purity material, containing 50 to 100 units per ml has only 10 to 15 per cent of the Factor VIII present in the starting plasma.

Factor VIII concentrates prepared from bovine and porcine animal sources have not been licensed for use in the United States. However, there is a great deal of experience with their use abroad (4, 68, 69). They have been life-saving in a number of instances and proved extremely useful in the late 1950's and early 1960's for hemophiliacs undergoing major surgery, permitting achievement and maintenance of high Factor VIII levels (46). The limited use of a new purified porcine Factor VIII in patients with Factor VIII inhibitors (69–71) will probably continue until alternative forms of therapy for these patients are more uniformly successful (see Chapter 41 and later in this chapter). The materials are quite antigenic; therefore, allergic reactions may occur frequently after the second or third infusion (6, 15). Decreased yield and survival of animal Factor VIII may result from cross-reactivity with a patient's Factor VIII antibody, (70), a phenomenon that can be predicted by in vitro measurements (71).

Large-scale production of Factor VIII by means of recombinant DNA technology rather than fractionation from plasma has not yet been realized, but this may be an achievable goal within the next decade.

PROTHROMBIN COMPLEX CONCENTRATES

Until recently, plasma was the only transfusion product for patients with hemophilia B or with acquired disorders of the prothrombin complex. However, during the past 15 years, fractionation procedures have been developed that concentrate Factor IX and the other vitamin K-dependent factors from whole plasma (6, 72). The common physicochemical properties of these proteins allow their separation from plasma or cryoprecipitate supernate by barium sulfate precipitation and column chromatography using a variety of adsorbents (4, 8, 15). A number of commercial products have now been developed in the United States and abroad for use in patients deficient in one or more of these factors (73–78). A listing of some of these preparations is contained in Table 50–4. Like the Factor VIII concentrates, they are prepared from large lots of pooled plasma obtained from paid donors, lyophilized, packaged in individual vials, and labeled with the number of units of Factor IX (and sometimes the other factors) in each bottle. Heat-treated preparations (to reduce the risk of hepatitis) are also now commercially available. They can be stored at refrigerator temperatures for up to 2 years.

All prothrombin complex concentrates contain Factors II, IX, and X, and many have Factor VII and some Factor XI in addition (6, 79). The naturally occurring circulating anticoagulant Protein C, a vitamin K–dependent zymogen that inactivates Factors V and VIII, is also present (80, 81). Some preparations are practically devoid of Factor VII (73). Small amounts of heparin are sometimes added in order to stabilize the product and neutralize any activated clotting factors generated during production or storage (75). Nevertheless, trace amounts of thrombin, activated Factor X, activated Factor IX, and other poorly defined activated intermediates may be present in the reconstituted product (82–85). Recent production methods among various manufacturers have resulted in the presence of fewer of these activated factors (81, 86, 87), a development that has become a "mixed blessing" (see below).

The major use of the prothrombin complex concentrates is in patients with moderate and severe congenital Factor IX deficiency or hemophilia B (88, 89) or for those mildly affected children who require higher circulating levels than can be achieved by fresh frozen plasma treatment (e.g., prior to surgery or after major hemorrhage (6)). In addition, numerous uncontrolled observations

Table 50–4. SOME OF THE MOST FREQUENTLY USED STANDARD AND "ACTIVATED" PROTHROMBIN COMPLEX CONCENTRATES*

Name of Product	Manufacturer	Type of Product
Konyne	Cutter	Standard
Proplex SX	Hyland	Standard
Proplex	Hyland	Standard
Profilnine	Alpha	Standard
Prothar	Armour	Standard
Autoplex	Hyland	Activated
FEIBA (Factor Eight Bypassing Activity)	Immuno (Vienna)	Activated

*All products are currently or will soon be heat-treated (see text).

and two controlled studies have shown that the preparations are moderately successful in promoting hemostasis in patients with hemophilia who have developed high-titer inhibitors and who fail to respond to the usual methods of factor replacement (87–100). Prothrombin complex concentrates have also been used for the rare congenital deficiencies of Factors II, VII, and X and for some acquired bleeding disorders. They may also have utility in patients with thrombosis due to protein C deficiency (101).

Children with bleeding due to vitamin K deficiency are usually best treated with intravenous vitamin K and occasionally with fresh frozen plasma, but in life-threatening circumstances or when circulatory embarrassment contraindicates the volume of plasma, the prothrombin concentrates are of benefit (102). Their use in liver disease cannot currently be recommended, since contaminating activated clotting factors that may be present can promote thrombosis and disseminated intravascular coagulation (103–106). Patients with liver disease are often unable to clear these activated intermediates from the circulation (107). However, a "clean" product, containing few activated factors, has proved to be safe and useful for correcting abnormal clotting tests prior to liver biopsy if administered along with fresh frozen plasma (108, 109). Lack of fibrinogen and Factor V results in incomplete normalization of clotting studies after infusion of prothrombin complex preparations alone (102). These products are absolutely contraindicated in patients with disseminated intravascular coagulation, as a worsening of the thrombotic and hemorrhagic tendency nearly always occurs after their infusion in such circumstances (110, 111).

The merits and the side effects of prothrombin complex concentrates generally parallel those of the Factor VIII–containing products. They are also stored, reconstituted, and administered in a similar manner. Infusions must be given slowly in order to avoid headaches, flushing, and other mild reactions. Hepatitis is unfortunately extremely common, and the products are expensive, but immune hemolytic anemia has not yet been encountered. The risk of acquired immune deficiency syndrome (AIDS) associated with the prothrombin complex concentrates is not well defined at present. At the time of this writing, AIDS has been reported in only several hemophilia B patients (41), and altered T cell subset values appear to be less striking in hemophilia B patients receiving prothrombin complex concentrates than in patients with hemophilia A being treated with Factor VIII preparations (112).

The most serious risk of the prothrombin complex concentrates is one not shared by other blood products—acceleration of blood clotting with resultant localized or generalized thrombosis. Observations in the mid-1960's suggested that these preparations were potentially thrombogenic (113), but the real dangers of hypercoagulability were not widely appreciated until 1973 when Kasper reported postoperative thrombosis in 6 of 13 patients with hemophilia B who received infusions of Factor IX concentrates (114). Subsequently, numerous instances of serious and even fatal thrombosis or thromboembolism (104, 105, 110, 111, 115–119) have been described. A number of commercial products have been implicated, although some appear to be safer than others (82, 87, 89). Those preparations containing small amounts of heparin appear to have less in vivo and in vitro clot promoting activity than those without heparin (82). Both of the most widely used products manufactured in the United States, Proplex and Konyne, have been implicated as being thrombogenic. Superficial and deep thrombosis, either localized to the site of infusion or occurring elsewhere, have followed treatment with Konyne or Proplex in patients with a wide variety of underlying diseases, including hemophilia B, liver disease, and disseminated intravascular coagulation (89, 110, 118, 119). Nearly all patients are adults, many are recovering from surgery or are otherwise at risk of venous stasis, and most have ongoing hepatic disease or accelerated intravascular coagulation (110, 119). Otherwise healthy children and young adults with hemophilia B have suffered from thrombosis after receiving "routine" infusions (110, 119). Several cases of myocardial infarction immediately following Proplex or Konyne treatment have recently been reported (120, 121). In each instance, however, the dose and frequency of administration greatly exceeded those usually recommended (122) (Chapter 41). Overall, the concentrates' long record of safety in children with severe hemophilia B is unquestioned, and warnings that their use should be limited to life-threatening hemorrhage (123) are over-cautious.

Attempts to identify the substances in the concentrates causing thrombosis have consisted of in vitro measurements of procoagulants using nonspecific tests such as the partial thromboplastin time or identification of specific activated intermediates (81–83, 85, 90, 95). Thrombogenicity can also be assessed by infusing the material into experimental animals (82, 84, 125). Activated Factors IX and X, thrombin, and platelet coagulant activity have all been identified (82, 83, 91, 95, 126, 127). However, wide variability among the different commercial products currently exists, reflecting the multiple manufacturing techniques. Unfortunately, there is still no proven assay method available that permits the physician to gauge the risk of thrombosis (95). Therefore, the clinical indications must be carefully assessed, and the preparations should be avoided in patients in whom predisposing factors such as symptomatic liver disease or DIC are present (123) or in mild hemophilia B patients in whom fresh frozen plasma might suffice as therapy. Addition of extra heparin and plasma or anti-thrombin III should theoretically render these preparations safer by inactivating the serine proteases generated within the product, but in actual practice this has not been uniformly successful.

Activated Prothrombin Complex Concentrates for Patients with Circulating Inhibitors

During the past several years, two manufacturers have marketed "activated" prothrombin complex concentrates for specific use in patients with high titer inhibitors (90, 91, 95, 96, 100, 131–138) (Table 50–4). These purposefully activated products, Autoplex and FEIBA, differ from standard prothrombin complex concentrates in several ways. Initially they represented the most thrombogenic (and hence previously discarded) lots. However, specific activation procedures, monitored by quality control testing, are now used to prepare materials with a standard and known clot-promoting potential (95). The exact identity of the "Factor VIII bypassing activity" remains uncertain, but it is thought to represent activated Factor IX, activated Factor X, and/or minute amounts of thrombin (85, 90, 95, 131, 139). Unfortunately, the laboratory measurement of these substances is not well standardized and fails to correlate with clinical response. The arbitrarily defined "unit" of bypassing activity differs between the two products, making it difficult to compare them in terms of cost and efficacy (95).

Indications for the activated prothrombin concentrates remain extremely controversial (140) and are discussed at greater length in Chapter 41. The dose is empirical, since the amount and nature of the substances being infused are not well defined (95). In uncommon clinical situations in which standard prothrombin complex concentrates and/or other measures have failed to achieve hemostasis in inhibitor patients with life-threatening hemorrhage, the activated products have been effective (141). However, their routine use in patients with inhibitors cannot currently be recommended because of their great expense ($3000 to $5000 per dose) and their inability to always promote hemostasis (142). Moreover, several small but controlled studies have shown them to be no more effective than standard nonactivated preparations in achieving hemostasis following an acute hemarthrosis (100, 143).

OTHER PLASMA PRODUCTS

Purified dried human fibrinogen, prepared from pooled plasma, was introduced in the 1950's (7, 11, 144). These fibrinogen concentrates are not used today, however (15), since the high risk of hepatitis and the development of safer forms of therapy (such as cryoprecipitate for congenital afibrinogenemia and plasma with or without heparin for DIC) have resulted in a ban on production by the Food and Drug Administration (144, 145).

A concentrate of antithrombin III for the rare patient with hereditary antithrombin deficiency has been developed (146, 147) but is available only for investigational use in this country (146). A Factor XIII concentrate developed in Europe (14, 148) has not achieved wide use.

USE OF PLASMA PRODUCTS IN THE MANAGEMENT OF SPECIFIC COAGULATION DISORDERS

General principles of treating children with plasma and plasma products are discussed earlier in this chapter, as well as in Chapters 5 and 41 under each individual disease. In addition, Table 50–5 contains a summary of the plasma products of choice for the most commonly encountered hemorrhagic disorders in children. The physician must not forget important adjunctive measures such as avoidance of aspirin, vigorous management of any underlying systemic problems (such as anemia, volume depletion, or infection), and use of various mechanical devices such as pressure dressings and splints.

COMPLICATIONS OF PLASMA PRODUCT THERAPY

Transfusion Reactions

Patients who have previously received multiple transfusions with fresh frozen plasma frequently suffer mild transfusion reactions during subsequent treatments (9). These reactions also occur with cryoprecipitate (149), but are much less common with the Factor VIII and IX concentrates (150). Signs and symptoms include fever, hives, shaking chills, and abdominal pain (9). Angioneurotic edema and severe pulmonary reactions occur infrequently, but they are occasionally severe and several fatalities have been reported (149, 151). The pathogenesis of these episodes remains obscure, but they are thought to be due to circulating antibodies in the recipient directed against foreign proteins in the donor plasma. These reactions are managed by stopping the infusion and giving a dose of an antihistamine such as diphenhydramine. There is no need to be concerned about the

Table 50–5. USE OF PLASMA PRODUCTS IN PATIENTS WITH CONGENITAL AND ACQUIRED FACTOR DEFICIENCIES

Disorder	Treatment of Choice*	Other Plasma Products Available	Additional Measures
Hemophilia A:			
Mild	P, C, FEC	—	DDAVP
Moderate or severe	C, FEC	P	
Hemophilia B:			
Mild	P	PCC, OBP	
Moderate or severe	PCC	P, OBP	
Hemophilia A or B with inhibitor:			
Low titer	As in patients without inhibitor		Steroids, episilon-amino caproic acid, splints, and so forth (consult Chapter 41 for further details)
High titer	Standard or activated PCC		
von Willebrand's disease	C	P	DDAVP
Factor II, VII, or X deficiency	P, PCC		
Factor V, XI, or XIII deficiency	P		
Congenital afibrinogenemia	C	P	
Vitamin K deficiency	—	P, PCC	Vitamin K†
Liver disease	P	PCC rarely	
Disseminated intravascular coagulation	P, Pl	C	Treat underlying disease, heparin, exchange transfusion

*Abbreviations: P = fresh frozen plasma, C = cryoprecipitate, PCC = prothrombin complex concentrate, Pl = platelet concentrate, FEC = factor eight concentrate, and OBP = outdated banked plasma.
†Except when imminent resumption of therapeutic oral anticoagulation is desired.
Chapter 41 should be consulted for more details about blood product replacement for each specific disorder.

theoretical effects of the administered antihistamines on platelet function (152–154). Patients who have a history of frequent reactions are best treated prophylactically with an oral antihistamine prior to infusion. In rare circumstances parenteral epinephrine is required to treat the more severe reactions.

Hepatitis

Hepatitis remains a common side effect of transfusion therapy. The hepatitis B virus was formerly a frequent offender, but the number of its clinically apparent infections is decreasing as a result of greater reliance on volunteer donors and the careful screening of all blood donations for hepatitis B surface antigen (HBsAg) by radioimmunoassay or enzyme-linked immunoassay (155). Manufacturers of concentrates are required to screen each donor for hepatitis B prior to inclusion of his or her plasma into large pools. Still, high rates of subclinical infection have occurred in multi-transfused patients (156–163), because the screening tests are somewhat insensitive and so many donors are used to prepare a batch of concentrate (164).

Despite the infrequency of clinically apparent hepatitis, most multi-transfused hemophiliacs have mildly abnormal liver function tests, particularly intermittent or sustained elevations in serum alanine aminotransferase (ALT) and/or aspartate aminotransferase (AST). Most have detectable antibody against HBsAg (157, 158), and a small number of patients are chronic HBsAg carriers (157, 165). Biopsy-proved chronic active or persistent hepatitis has been demonstrated in a disturbingly large number of these patients (156–170).

Currently the most common cause of acute hepatitis in multi-transfused hemophiliacs is non-A, non-B hepatitis, which has a variable incubation period and usually causes mild disease (60, 171, 172). It is not usually caused by cytomegalovirus (156, 173) and is probably heterogenous, as evidenced by multiple separate episodes of acute hepatitis (not due to hepatitis B) in certain patients (174).

Among the many risk factors for the development of hepatitis, the most important are the transfusion history of the recipient and the number of blood donors to whom the recipient is exposed (40). Infection rates are greatest in mildly affected patients who have received few infusions and who are thus less likely to have developed a spectrum of protective antibodies (60, 165). Fresh frozen plasma and cryoprecipitate are associated with less risk than concentrate. Yet, even administration of cryoprecipitate prepared from a volunteer donor pool results in a significant risk of subclinical hepatitis (175, 176).

The sequelae of mild chronic hepatitis in multi-transfused patients are uncertain (177), and careful monitoring of liver function in all patients receiving transfusions of plasma products is essential. Hepatitis B vaccine became commercially available in 1982 and is strongly recommended in these high-risk patients (178, 179). A recent study has shown the vaccine to be highly immunogenic in children with hemophilia and other conditions characterized by high blood transfusion requirements (180). Widespread use of the vaccine should result in reduced numbers of infections due to this viral pathogen in the future.

Heat-treated concentrates (181) were introduced several years ago as a means of reducing the hepatitis risk. In vitro studies by a number of manufacturers have shown that concentrate that is "spiked" with viruses (such as cytomegalovirus and Sindbis virus) and then heat treated is rendered free of viral particles thereafter. Moreover, infusion of heat-treated material into chimpanzees (the only applicable animal model of viral hepatitis) may be less likely to induce seroconversion and/or rise in ALT than concentrate that has not been heated. Yet the ability of heated concentrate to prevent or markedly reduce the frequency of hepatitis in hemophiliacs has not been proved. Preliminary information suggests that hepatitis may still occur despite exclusive use of heated material. Concern has also been expressed about the unforeseen complications of heat-treated concentrate (such as alteration of the coagulation proteins contained within, possibly resulting in an increased risk of inhibitors), as well as their added cost. Despite these many uncertainties, heat-treated factor VIII and prothrombin complex concentrates are now being increasingly used.

Acquired Immune Deficiency Syndrome (AIDS)

In 1981 a syndrome of opportunistic infection, usually *Pneumocystis carinii* pneumonia, with or without Kaposi's sarcoma, was reported in previously healthy homosexual males (62). This often fatal illness, quickly designated acquired immune deficiency syndrome (AIDS), reached epidemic proportions in the homosexual community within 2 years (62). Other high-risk groups include heroin addicts and hemophiliacs (182). Since 1982, *P. carinii* pneumonia, unusual fungal infections, Burkitt's lymphoma, idiopathic thrombocytopenic purpura, and a syndrome of lymphadenopathy, fever, diarrhea, and wasting (considered by some to be a prodrome of AIDS) have been reported with increasing frequency in hemophiliacs (41, 183). All of these patients had received multiple transfusions of blood products, usually obtained from paid donors. In addition, numerous individuals without hemophilia have also developed AIDS as a probable consequence of receiving one or more blood transfusions (61, 184).

The same groups that are frequently infected by hepatitis B are also at risk of AIDS (62). Although the cause of AIDS is currently not known for certain, evidence is mounting that it is due to retrovirus infection transmitted by blood products and body secretions such as saliva or semen. This agent (or group of related agents) has several names but has been most frequently designated HTLV-III (human T-cell leukemia virus) (185). Chronic immunologic stimulation by multiple antigens may also be a component of its pathogenesis. The discovery, investigation, and public arousal about the AIDS epidemic has been one of the major medical issues of the mid-1980's. Review articles more fully summarize the various aspects of the illness (62). As of November 1986, nearly 200 cases of AIDS, half of them fatal, have been reported in patients with hemophilia. Most of these individuals had received multiple infusions of Factor VIII or Factor IX concentrate, and some had been treated with other blood products in addition. Evidence that AIDS is transmitted by blood transfusion now seems incontrovertable. Fortunately, however, it still remains an uncommon infectious complication of transfusion therapy (61).

The vast majority of patients with AIDS possess a disordered immune system affecting both T and B lymphocytes. Typically, such patients have a marked reduction of helper T cells and an excess of suppressor T lymphocytes, resulting in a reduction of the T helper/T suppressor ratio (62). Many patients with hemophilia, without clinical evidence of AIDS, also possess these laboratory abnormalities (112, 186–189). Their identification and analysis has been a high priority in comprehensive hemophilia programs during the past several years, but the clinical significance of these alterations is uncertain.

Recent studies in the United States have shown that 60 to 90 per cent of severe multi-transfused hemophiliacs have in their serum antibody against the retrovirus HTLV-III (190–192). The significance of this observation, particularly how many of these individuals will ultimately develop AIDS, is unknown. Currently procedures are under way to screen all prospective blood donors for antibody against HTLV-III in order to attempt to reduce the spread of this putative AIDS virus (61).

Since heat treatment of factor concentrates destroys HTLV-III (193), there is hope that hemophiliacs in the future will not be exposed to the potential devastating effects of this viral agent. A preliminary study of young hemophiliacs receiving only heat-treated concentrate shows no seroconversion to HTLV-III despite up to 18 months of intensive infusion therapy (194).

Other Viral Infections

Not surprisingly, factor concentrates derived from thousands of paid donors contain diverse infectious agents other than hepatitis B and non-

A, non-B viruses. Subclinical cytomegalovirus and Epstein-Barr virus infection occur with great frequency in hemophiliacs (187), as evidenced by the findings of serum antibody against cytomegalovirus in 40 per cent of multi-transfused patients and the serologic profile of acute or reactive Epstein-Barr virus infection in up to 70 per cent of affected subjects (195). In addition, antibody against the human parvovirus, which induces aplastic crises in patients with chronic hemolytic anemia (196), is present in far larger numbers of hemophiliacs than in controls (197). It appears that heat treatment may destroy all of these pathogens, thus reducing their potential risk in subjects receiving the newer heat-treated preparations.

Hemolytic Anemia

All Factor VIII concentrates contain appreciable quantities of the major isohemagglutinins, anti-A and anti-B. Seeler and co-workers (53) have detected titers of 1:1,024 or more in some commercial preparations. When large volumes of Factor VIII concentrates or pooled cryoprecipitate are given to a hemophilic recipient after a surgical procedure, clinically apparent immune hemolytic anemia may result if the patient has A, B, or AB red blood cells. Such patients are noted to have a falling hematocrit level, microspherocytes on the peripheral blood smear, and a positive indirect and direct antiglobulin test (53, 63–65). Management consists of transfusions with type O packed red blood cells, use of corticosteroids, and, if possible, administration of ABO type-specific cryoprecipitate or a commercial preparation that has a lower concentration of antibody (63, 64). Fortunately, this complication appears to be uncommon, yet declines in serum haptoglobin have been reported in many hemophiliacs (198, 199). Hemolysis has not yet been reported following use of Factor IX concentrates (53). Fresh frozen plasma used in replacement therapy should always be of a compatible ABO type. Otherwise, isoimmune hemolysis may occur as well.

Other Immunologic Sequelae

It is not surprising that patients who receive multiple infusions of plasma products may have a variety of immunologic abnormalities (discussed above in conjunction with AIDS), since they receive dozens or even hundreds of foreign antigens with each transfusion. Circulating immune complexes are frequently present in such patients (200, 201). Some instances of hematuria in patients with hemophilia may be associated with intraglomerular immune complex deposition (202). Moreover, amyloidosis has been reported in several adult hemophiliacs (174, 203). Alloimmunization to red cell antigens (204), alterations in serum immunoglobulins (205), and immune-mediated thrombocytopenia (188, 206) have also been noted in multi-transfused patients. Lymphadenopathy and/or splenomegaly occurs in many hemophiliacs, perhaps secondary to chronic antigenic stimulation (156, 163).

It is uncertain how many of these immunologic alterations are related to specific viral agents like HTLV-III (see above) or, alternatively, are nonspecific sequelae of antigenic "overload" (201).

Miscellaneous Complications

Administration of large volumes of cryoprecipitate or Factor VIII concentrate has been reported to result in hemorrhage due to defective platelet function, possibly caused by deleterious effects of the accompanying fibrinogen or its degradation products (50, 207–209). However, alterations in primary hemostasis cannot be uniformly demonstrated and may be present even in hemophiliacs who have not recently received blood products (210, 211). Thus, their importance to the clinician remains uncertain.

Although it has been feared that a more vigorous approach to infusion of foreign clotting proteins into patients lacking these substances might result in an increased frequency of circulating anticoagulants or inhibitors, several extensive studies indicate that the incidence of inhibitors is the same now as it was approximately 20 years ago (66, 212).

Despite all of these complications, the benefits from plasma and plasma concentrates in patients with severe bleeding disorders usually vastly outweigh the potential risks, and the majority of children have few clinically obvious troublesome side effects despite years of replacement therapy.

THE FUTURE OF COAGULATION FACTOR THERAPY

At present, all blood coagulation factors administered to patients with hemorrhagic disorders are derived from blood plasma. In the near future, there is promise for successfully utilizing the techniques of recombinant DNA technology to make available for clinical use synthetic Factor VIII. The genes on the X chromosome that encode Factor VIII and Factor IX have already been successfully cloned (213, 214). The cloned DNA has been manipulated in vitro to allow for characterization of human Factor VIII (215) and for production of a functional Factor VIII molecule that has shortened the clotting time of hemophilic plasma (216). Several pharmaceutical manufacturers, in collaboration with corporations specializing in recombinant DNA methodology, are devoting much effort to refining techniques to allow for production of the protein on a much larger scale. It is hoped that within several years clinical testing can begin in order to ascertain the efficacy and safety of the bacterially derived product. All physicians treating patients with bleeding disorders hope that a preparation that is safe, inexpensive, and effective will be available by the end of this decade.

References

1. Cohn, E. J.: The separation of blood into fractions of therapeutic value. Ann. Intern. Med. 26:341, 1947.
2. Cohn, E. J., Strong, L. E., et al.: Preparation and properties of serum and plasma proteins. IV. A system for the separation into fractions of the protein and lipoprotein components of biological tissues and fluids. J. Am. Chem. Soc. 68:459, 1946.
3. Minot, G. R., Davidson, C. S., et al.: The coagulation defect in hemophilia: the effect, in hemophilia, of the parenteral administration of a fraction of the plasma globulins rich in fibrinogen. J. Clin. Invest. 24:704, 1945.
4. Biggs, R. (ed.): *The Treatment of Haemophilia A and B and von Willebrand's Disease.* Oxford, Blackwell Scientific Publications, 1978.
5. Johnson, A. J., Aronson, D. L., et al.: Preparation and clinical use of plasma and plasma fractions. In *Hematology,* 3rd ed. Williams, W. J., Beutler, E., et al. (eds.), New York, McGraw-Hill, 1983, pp. 1563–1583.
6. Biggs, R., and Rizza, C. R. (eds.): *Human Blood Coagulation, Haemostasis and Thrombosis,* 3rd. ed. Oxford, Blackwell Scientific Publications, 1984.
7. Cash, J.: Blood replacement therapy. In *Haemostasis and Thrombosis.* Bloom, A. L., and Thomas, D. P. (eds.), Edinburgh, Churchill Livingstone, 1981, pp. 472–490.
8. Levine, P. H.: The clinical manifestations and therapy of hemophilias A and B. In *Hemostasis and Thrombosis: Basic Principles and Clinical Practice.* Colman, R. W., Hirsh, J., et al. (eds.), Philadelphia, J. B. Lippincott Co., 1982, pp. 75–90.
9. Rizza, C. R.: Coagulation factor therapy. Clin. Haematol. 5:113, 1976.
10. Hensley, M. J.: Use and misuse of cryoprecipitate. New Engl. J. Med. 292:1299, 1975.
11. Urbaniak, S. J., and Cash, J. D.: Blood replacement therapy. Br. Med. Bull. 33:273, 1977.
12. Wallace, J.: Preparation of blood and blood products for the management of coagulation defects. Clin. Haematol. 2:129, 1973.
13. Agle, D. P., Hilgartner, M. W., et al.: *Home Therapy for Hemophilia. A Manual for Physicians.* New York, National Hemophilia Foundation, 1977.
14. Losowsky, M., and Miloszewski, K. J. A.: Factor XIII. Br. J. Haematol. 37:1, 1977.
15. Wallace, J.: Blood Transfusion for Clinicians. Edinburgh, Churchill Livingstone, 1977.
16. Honig, G. R., Abildgaard, C. F., et al.: Some properties of the anticoagulant factor of aged pooled plasma. Thrombos. Diath. Haemorrh. 22:151, 1969.
17. Roberts, H. R., and Cederbaum, A. I.: The liver and blood coagulation: physiology and pathology. Gastroenterology 63:297, 1972.
18. Brozovic, M.: Oral anticoagulants in clinical practice. Semin. Hematol. 15:27, 1978.
19. Oberman, H. A.: Inappropriate use of fresh-frozen plasma. J.A.M.A. 253:556, 1985.
20. Perkins, H. A.: Plasmapheresis of the patient as a method for achieving effective levels of plasma coagulation factors, using fresh frozen plasma. Transfusion 6:293, 1966.
21. Laningham, J. E. T.: Partial plasma exchange, an adjunct in therapy to complex clinical problems. Transfusion 17:547, 1977.
22. Pool, J. G., and Robinson, J.: Observations of plasma banking and transfusion procedures for haemophilia patients using a quantitative assay for antihaemophilic globulin (AHG). Br. J. Haematol. 5:24, 1959.
23. Pool, J. G., Hershgold, E. F., et al.: High-potency antihaemophilic factor concentrate prepared from cryoglobulin precipitate. Nature (Lond.) 203:312, 1964.
24. Pool, J. G., and Shannon, A. E.: Production of high-potency concentrates of antihemophilic globulin in a closed-bag system. New Engl. J. Med. 273:1443, 1965.
25. Burka, E. R., Harker, L. A., et al.: A protocol for cryoprecipitate production Transfusion 15:307, 1975.
26. Slichter, S. J., Counts, R. B., et al.: Preparation of cryoprecipitated factor VIII concentrates. Transfusion 16:616, 1976.
27. Kasper, C. K., Myhre, B. A., et al.: Determinants of factor VIII recovery in cryoprecipitate. Transfusion 15:312, 1975.
28. Rock, G., Smiley, R. K., et al.: In vivo effectiveness of a high-yield factor VIII concentrate prepared in a blood bank. New Engl. J. Med. 311:310, 1984.
29. Zimmerman, T. S., and Ruggeri, Z. M.: von Willebrand's disease. Clin. Haematol. 12:185, 1983.
30. Green, D., and Potter, E. V.: Failure of AHF concentrate to control bleeding in von Willebrand's disease. Am. J. Med. 60:357, 1976.
31. Hattersley, P. G., and Dimick, M. L.: Cryoprecipitates in treatment of congenital fibrinogen deficiency. Transfusion 9:261, 1969.
32. Ness, P. M., and Perkins, H. A.: Cryoprecipitate as a reliable source of fibrinogen replacement. J.A.M.A. 241:1690, 1979.
33. Mazurier, C., Samor, B., et al.: The role of fibronectin in factor VIII/von Willebrand factor cryoprecipitation. Thrombos. Res. 37:651, 1985.
34. Amris, C. J., and Hilden, M.: Treatment of factor XIII deficiency with cryoprecipitate. Thrombos. Diath. Haemorrh. 20:528, 1968.
35. American Association of Blood Banks: *Physician's Handbook for Blood Component Therapy.* Chicago, American Association of Blood Banks, 1969.
36. Mason, E. C.: Thaw-siphon technique for production of cryoprecipitate concentrate of factor VIII. Lancet 2:15, 1978.
37. McLeod, B. C., and Scott, J. P.: Use of "single donor" factor VIII from plasma exchange donation. J.A.M.A. 252:2726, 1984.
38. Hattersley, P. G., and Kunkel, M.: Cryoprecipitates as a source of fibrinogen in treatment of disseminated intravascular coagulation (DIC). Transfusion 16:641, 1976.
39. Dallmann, P. R., and Pool, J. G.: Treatment of hemophilia with factor VIII concentrates. New Engl. J. Med. 278:199, 1968.
40. Cedarbaum, A. I., Blatt, P. M., et al.: Abnormal serum transaminase levels in patients with hemophilia A. Arch. Intern. Med. 142:481, 1982.
41. Evatt, B. L., Ramsey, R. B., et al.: The acquired immunodeficiency syndrome in patients with hemophilia. Ann. Intern. Med. 100:499, 1984.
42. Warrier, A. I., and Lusher, J. M.: DDAVP: a useful alternative to blood components in moderate hemophilia A and von Willebrand disease. J. Pediatr. 102:228, 1983.
43. Patek, A. J., Jr., and Taylor, F. H. L.: Hemophilia. II. Some properties of a substance obtained from normal human plasma effective in accelerating the coagulation of hemophilic blood. J. Clin. Invest. 16:113, 1937.
44. Blomback, M., and Nilsson, I. M.: Treatment of hemophilia A with human antihemophilic globulin. Acta Med. Scand. 161:301, 1958.
45. Bidwell, E.: The purification of bovine antihaemophilic globulin. Br. J. Haematol. 1:35, 1955.
46. MacFarlane, R. G., Mallam, P. C., et al.: Surgery in haemophilia. The use of animal antihaemophilic globulin and human plasma in thirteen cases. Lancet 2:251, 1957.

47. Webster, W. P., Roberts, H. R., et al.: Clinical use of a new glycine-precipitated antihemophilic fraction. Am. J. Med. Sci. 250:643, 1965.
48. Brinkhous, K. M., Shanbrom, E., et al.: A new high-potency glycine-precipitated antihemophilic factor (AHF) concentrate. J.A.M.A. 205:613, 1968.
49. Wagner, R. H., McLester, W. D., et al.: Purification of antihemophilic factor (factor VIII) by amino acid precipitation. Thrombos. Diath. Haemorrh. 11:64, 1964.
50. Hilgartner, M.: Current therapy. In *Hemophilia in Children*. Hilgartner, M. W., (ed.), Littleton, MA, Publishing Sciences Group, Inc. 1976, pp. 151–170.
51. Johnson, A. J., Karpatkin, M. H., et al.: Clinical investigation of intermediate- and high-purity antihaemophilic factor (factor VIII) concentrates. Br. J. Haematol. 21:21, 1971.
52. Allain, J. P.: Transfusion support for haemophiliacs. Clin. Haematol. 13:99, 1984.
53. Seeler, R. A., Telischi, M., et al.: Comparison of anti-A and anti-B titers in factor VIII and IX concentrates. J. Pediatr. 89:87, 1976.
54. Blatt, P. M., Brinkhous, K. M., et al.: Antihemophilic factor concentrate therapy in von Willebrand disease. Dissociation of bleeding-time factor and Ristocetin-cofactor activities. J.A.M.A. 236:2770, 1976.
55. Perkins, H. A.: Correction of the hemostatic defects in von Willebrand's disease. Blood 30:375, 1967.
56. Chediak, J. R., Telfer, M. C., et al.: Platelet function and immunologic parameters in von Willebrand's disease following cryoprecipitate and factor VIII concentrate infusion. Am. J. Med. 62:369, 1977.
57. Le Quesne, B., Maragaki, C., et al.: Home treatment for patients with haemophilia. Lancet 2:507, 1974.
58. Hathaway, W. E., Christian, M. J., et al.: Comparison of continuous and intermittent factor VIII concentrate therapy in hemophilia A. Am. J. Hematol. 17:85, 1984.
59. Craske, J., Dilling, N., et al.: An outbreak of hepatitis associated with intravenous injection of factor-VIII concentrate. Lancet 2:221, 1975.
60. Fletcher, M. L., Trowell, J. M., et al.: Non-A non-B hepatitis after transfusion of factor VIII in infrequently treated patients. Br. Med. J. 287:1754, 1983.
61. Editorial: Blood transfusion, haemophilia, and AIDS. Lancet 2:1433, 1984.
62. Fauci, A. S., Macher, A. M., et al.: Acquired immunodeficiency syndrome: epidemiologic, clinical, immunologic, and therapeutic considerations. Ann. Intern. Med. 100:92, 1984.
63. Ashenhurst, J. B., Langehenning, P. A., et al.: Hemolytic anemia due to anti-B in antihemophilic factor concentrates. J. Pediatr. 88:258, 1976.
64. Orringer, E. P., Koury, M. J., et al.: Hemolysis caused by factor VIII concentrates. Arch. Intern. Med. 136:1018, 1976.
65. Rosati, L. A., Barnes, B., et al.: Hemolytic anemia due to anti-A in concentrated antihemophilic factor preparations. Transfusion 10:139, 1970.
66. Rabiner, S. F., and Lazerson, J.: Home management and prophylaxis of hemophilia. Prog. Hematol. 8:223, 1973.
67. Hilgartner, M. W.: Home care for hemophilia: current state of the art. Scand. J. Haematol. 30(Suppl.):58, 1977.
68. Smith, J. K., and Bidwell, E.: Therapeutic materials used in the treatment of coagulation defects. Clin. Haematol. 8:183, 1979.
69. Rubin, R., Niemetz, J., et al.: Use of animal AHG concentrates (factor VIII) in the treatment of life-threatening hemorrhage in patients with factor VIII antibodies. Ann. NY Acad. Sci. 240:362, 1975.
70. Kernoff, P. B. A., Thomas, N. D., et al.: Clinical experience with polyelectrolyte-fractionated porcine factor VIII concentrate in the treatment of hemophiliacs with antibodies to factor VIII. Blood 63:31, 1984.
71. Ciavarella, N., Antoncecchi, S., et al.: Efficacy of porcine factor VIII in the management of haemophiliacs with inhibitors. Br. J. Haematol. 58:641, 1984.
72. Didisheim, P., Loeb, J., et al.: Preparation of a human plasma fraction rish in prothrombin, proconvertin, Stuart Factor, and PTC and a study of its activity and toxicity in rabbits and man. J. Lab. Clin. Med. 53:322, 1959.
73. Dike, G. W. R., Bidwell, E., et al.: The preparation and clinical use of a new concentrate containing factor IX, prothrombin and factor X and of a separate concentrate containing factor VII. Br. J. Haematol. 22:469, 1972.
74. Hoag, M. S., Johnson, F. F., et al.: Treatment of hemophilia B with a new clotting-factor concentrate. New Engl. J. Med. 280:581, 1969.
75. Gilchrist, G. S., Ekert, H., et al.: Evaluation of a new concentrate for the treatment of factor IX deficiency. New Engl. J. Med. 280:291, 1969.
76. Gunay, U., Choi, H. S., et al.: Commercial preparations of prothrombin complex. A clinical comparison. Am. J. Dis. Child. 126:775, 1973.
77. Zauber, N. P., and Levin, J.: Factor IX levels in patients with hemophilia B (Christmas disease) following transfusion with concentrates of factor IX or fresh frozen plasma (FFP). Medicine 56:213, 1977.
78. Breen, F. A., and Tullis, J. L.: Prothrombin concentrates in treatment of Christmas disease and allied disorders. J.A.M.A. 208:1848, 1969.
79. Bick, R. L., Adams, T., et al.: Surgical hemostasis with a factor XI-containing concentrate. J.A.M.A. 229:163, 1974.
80. Seghatchian, M. J.: Protein C in clinical factor IX concentrates. Lancet 1:1047, 1983.
81. Menache, D., Behra, H. E., et al.: Coagulation factor IX concentrate: method of preparation and assessment of potential in vivo thrombogenicity in animal models. Blood 64:1220, 1984.
82. Kingdon, H. S., Lundblad, R. L., et al.: Potentially thrombogenic materials in factor IX concentrates. Thrombos. Diath. Haemorrh. 33:617, 1975.
83. White, G. C., Roberts, H. R., et al.: Prothrombin complex concentrates: potentially thrombogenic materials and clues to the mechanism of thrombosis in vivo. Blood 49:159, 1977.
84. Cash, J. D., Dalton, R. G., et al.: Studies on the thrombogenicity of Scottish factor IX concentrates in dogs. Thrombos. Diath. Haemorrh. 33:632, 1975.
85. Tishkoff, G. H.: Prothrombin complex to treat factor VIII inhibition. New Engl. J. Med. 292:754, 1975.
86. Kelly, P., and Penner, J. A.: Antihemophilic factor inhibitors. Management with prothrombin complex concentrates. J.A.M.A. 236:2061, 1976.
87. Chandra, S., and Wickerhauser, M.: Large scale preparation of nonthrombogenic prothrombin complex. Thrombos. Res. 12:571, 1978.
88. Lane, J. L., Rizza, C. R., et al.: A five year experience of the use of factor IX type DE(I) concentrate for the treatment of Christmas disease at Oxford. Br. J. Haematol. 30:435, 1975.
89. Editorial: Clinical concentrates of clotting-factor IX. Lancet 2:855, 1975.
90. Kurczynski, E. M., and Penner, J. A.: Activated prothrombin concentrate for patients with factor VIII inhibitors. New Engl. J. Med. 291:164, 1974.
91. Sonoda, T., Solomon, A., et al.: Use of prothrombin complex concentrates in the treatment of a hemophilic patient with an inhibitor of factor VIII. Blood 47:983, 1976.
92. Abildgaard, C. F., Britton, M., et al.: Prothrombin complex concentrate (Konyne) in the treatment of hemophilic patients with factor VIII inhibitors. J. Pediatr. 88:200, 1976.
93. Pearson, H. A.: Treatment of hemophilic children who have factor VIII inhibitors. J. Pediatr. 88:367, 1976.

94. Yolken, R. H., and Hilgartner, M. W.: Prothrombin complex concentrates. Use in treatment of hemophiliacs with factor VIII inhibitors. Am. J. Dis. Child. *132:*291, 1978.
95. Buchanan, G. R., and Kevy, S. V.: Use of prothrombin complex concentrates in hemophiliacs with inhibitors: clinical and laboratory studies. Pediatrics *62:*767, 1978.
96. Penner, J. A., and Kelly, P. E.: Management of patients with factor VIII or IX inhibitors. Semin. Thrombos. Hemostas. *1:*386, 1975.
97. Bloom, A. L.: Clotting factor concentrates for resistant haemophilia. Br. J. Haematol. *40:*21, 1978.
98. Ekert, H., Price, D. A., et al.: A randomized study of factor VIII or prothrombin complex concentrate infusions in children with haemophilia and antibodies to factor VIII. Aust. N.Z. J. Med. *9:*241, 1979.
99. Lusher, J. M., Shapiro, S. S., et al.: Efficacy of prothrombin-complex concentrates in hemophiliacs with antibodies to factor VIII. A multicenter therapeutic trial. New Engl. J. Med. *303:*421, 1980.
100. Sjamsoedin, L. J. M., Heijnen, L., et al.: The effect of activated prothrombin-complex concentrate (FEIBA) on joint and muscle bleeding in patients with hemophilia A and antibodies to factor VIII. A double-blind clinical trial. New Engl. J. Med. *305:*717, 1981.
101. Sills, R. H., Marlar, R. A., et al.: Severe homozygous protein C deficiency. J. Pediatr. *105:*409, 1984.
102. Sandler, S. G., Rath, C. E., et al.: Prothrombin complex concentrates in acquired hypoprothrombinemia. Ann. Intern. Med. *79:*485, 1973.
103. Gazzard, B. J., Lewis, M. L., et al.: Coagulation factor concentrate in the treatment of the haemorrhagic diathesis of fulminant hepatic failure. Gut *15:*993, 1974.
104. Davey, R. J., Shashaty, G. G., et al.: Acute coagulopathy following infusion of prothrombin complex concentrates. Am. J. Med. *60:*719, 1976.
105. Blatt, P. M., Lundblad, R. L., et al.: Thrombogenic materials in prothrombin complex concentrates. Ann. Intern. Med. *81:*766, 1974.
106. Marassi, A., Manzullo, V., et al.: Thromboembolism following prothrombin complex concentrates in major surgery in severe liver disease. Thrombos. Haemostas. *39:*248, 1978.
107. Deykin, D.: The role of the liver in serum-induced hypercoagulability. J. Clin. Invest. *45:*256, 1966.
108. Mannucci, P. M., Franchi, F., et al.: Correction of abnormal coagulation in chronic liver disease by combined use of fresh-frozen plasma and prothrombin complex concentrates. Lancet *2:*542, 1976.
109. Green, G., Dymock, I. W., et al.: Use of factor-VII-rich prothrombin complex concentrate in liver disease. Lancet *1:*1311, 1975.
110. Kasper, C. K.: Thromboembolic complications. Thrombos. Diath. Haemorrh. *33:*640, 1975.
111. Bick, R. L., Schmalhorst, W. R., et al.: Disseminated intravascular coagulation and blood component therapy. Transfusion *16:*361, 1976.
112. Ragni, M. V., Lewis, J. H., et al.: Decreased helper/suppressor cell ratios after treatment with factor VIII and IX concentrates and fresh frozen plasma. Am. J. Med. *76:*206, 1984.
113. Tullis, J. L., Melin, M., et al.: Clinical use of human prothrombin complexes. New Engl. J. Med. *273:*667, 1965.
114. Kasper, C. K.: Postoperative thrombosis in hemophilia B. New Engl. J. Med. *289:*160, 1973.
115. Edson, J. R.: Prothrombin-complex concentrates and thromboses. New Engl. J. Med. *290:*403, 1974.
116. Steinberg, M. H., and Dreiling, B. J.: Vascular lesions in hemophilia B. New Engl. J. Med. *289:*592, 1973.
117. Schimpf, K., Zimmerman, K., et al.: DIC and postoperative wound bleeding under factor IX substitution therapy in a case of hemophilia B; successful treatment with heparin. Thrombos. Res. *8:*65, 1976.
118. Aledort, L. M.: Factor IX and thrombosis. Scand. J. Haematol. *30*(Suppl.):40, 1977.
119. Kasper, C. K.: Blood—its derivates and its problems—factor IX. Ann. N. Y. Acad. Sci. *240:*172, 1975.
120. Sullivan, D. W., Purdy, L. J., et al.: Fatal myocardial infarction following therapy with prothrombin complex concentrates in a young man with hemophilia A. Pediatrics *74:*279, 1984.
121. Gruppo, R. A., Bove, K. E., and Donaldson, V. H.: Fatal myocardial necrosis associated with prothrombin-complex–concentrate therapy in hemophilia A. New Engl. J. Med. *309:*242, 1983.
122. Lusher, J. M.: Myocardial necrosis after therapy with prothrombin-complex concentrate. New Engl. J. Med. *310:*464, 1984.
123. Ratnoff, O. D.: Prothrombin complex preparations: a cautionary note. Ann. Intern. Med. *81:*852, 1974.
124. Hultin, M. B.: Studies of factor IX concentrate therapy in hemophilia. Blood *62:*677, 1983.
125. Kingdon, H. S., and Hassell, T. M.: Hemophilic dog model for evaluating therapeutic effectiveness of plasma protein fractions. Blood *58:*868, 1981.
126. Sas, G., Owens, R. E., et al.: In vitro spontaneous thrombin generation in human factor-IX concentrates. Br. J. Haematol. *31:*25, 1975.
127. Vermylen, J., Schetz, J., et al.: Evidence that "activated' prothrombin concentrates enhance platelet coagulant activity. Br. J. Haematol. *38:*235, 1978.
128. Gobel, U., von Voss, H., et al.: Use of heparin in combination with factor-VII-rich prothrombin complex concentrate. Lancet *2:*279, 1975.
129. Campbell, E. W., Neff, S., et al.: Therapy with factor IX concentrate resulting in DIC and thromboembolic phenomena. Transfusion *18:*94, 1978.
130. Hedner, U., Nilsson, I. M., et al.: Various prothrombin complex concentrates and their effect on coagulation and fibrinolysis in vivo. Thrombos. Haemostas. *35:*386, 1976.
131. English, P. J., Sheppard, E. M., et al.: Factor VIII inhibitor bypassing activity. Lancet *2:*207, 1976.
132. English, P. J., Sheppard, E. M., et al.: Traumatic rupture of the liver in a haemophiliac patient with factor-VIII inhibitors. Lancet *1:*1299, 1976.
133. Lewis, J. H., and Oskins, P. B.: Discussion paper: treatment of the hemophiliac with anti-VIII. Ann. N.Y. Acad. Sci. *240:*407, 1975.
134. Sultan, Y., Brouet, J. C., et al.: Treatment of inhibitors to factor VIII with activated prothrombin concentrate. New Engl. J. Med. *291:*1087, 1974.
135. Ekert, H., and McVeagh, P.: Activated PPSB in the treatment of a patient with haemophilia and antibodies to factor VIII. Med. J. Aust. *2:*675, 1975.
136. Hilgartner, M. W., Knatterud, G. L., et al.: The use of factor eight inhibitor by-passing activity (FEIBA Immuno) product for treatment of bleeding episodes in hemophiliacs with inhibitors. Blood *61:*36, 1983.
137. Hutchinson, R. J., Penner, J. A., et al.: Anti-inhibitor coagulant complex (Autoplex) in hemophilia inhibitor patients undergoing synovectomy. Pediatrics *71:*631, 1983.
138. Aronstam, A., McLellan, D. S., et al.: The use of an activated factor IX complex (Autoplex) in the management of haemarthroses in haemophiliacs with antibodies to factor VIII. Clin. Lab. Haematol. *4:*231, 1982.
139. Vinazzer, H.: Comparison between two concentrates with factor VIII inhibitor bypassing activity. Thromb. Res. *26:*21, 1982.
140. Deykin, D.: Factor VIII inhibitors. New Engl. J. Med. *291:*205, 1974.
141. Heisel, M. A., Gomperts, E. D., et al.: Use of activated prothrombin complex concentrate over multiple surgical

episodes in a hemophilic child with an inhibitor. J. Pediatr. *102*:951, 1983.
142. Blatt, P. M., White, G. C., et al.: Failure of activated prothrombin complex concentrates in a hemophiliac with an anti-factor VIII antibody. J.A.M.A. *251*:67, 1984.
143. Lusher, J. M., Blatt, P. M., et al.: Autoplex versus Proplex: a controlled, double-blind study of effectiveness in acute hemarthroses in hemophiliacs with inhibitors to factor VIII. Blood *62*:1135, 1983.
144. Bove, J. R.: Fibrinogen—is the benefit worth the risk? Transfusion *18*:129, 1978.
145. Revocation of fibrinogen licenses. FDA Drug Bulletin *8*:15, 1978.
146. Schipper, H. G., Jenkins, C. S. P., et al.: Antithrombin-III transfusion in disseminated intravascular coagulation. Lancet *1*:854, 1978.
147. Mannucci, P. M., Boyer, C., et al.: Treatment of congenital antithrombin III deficiency with concentrates. Br. J. Haematol. *50*:531, 1982.
148. Fear, J. D., Miloszewski, K. J. A., et al.: The half life of factor XIII in the management of inherited deficiency. Thromb. Haemostas. *49*:102, 1983.
149. Reese, E. P., Jr., McCullough, J. J., et al.: An adverse pulmonary reaction to cryoprecipitate in a hemophiliac. Transfusion *15*:583, 1975.
150. Eyster, M. E., Bowman, H. S., et al.: Adverse reactions to factor VIII infusions. Ann. Intern. Med. *87*:248, 1977.
151. Kernoff, P. B. A., Durrant, I. J., et al.: Severe allergic pulmonary oedema after plasma transfusion. Br. J. Haematol. *23*:777, 1972.
152. Champion, L. A. A., Schwartz, A. D., et al.: The effects of four commonly used drugs on platelet function. J. Pediatr. *89*:653, 1976.
153. Buchanan, G. R., Martin, V., et al.: The effects of "antiplatelet" drugs on bleeding time and platelet aggregation in normal human subjects. Am. J. Clin. Pathol. *68*:355, 1977.
154. Buchanan, G. R., and Handin, R. I.: Impairment of hemostasis in patients with severe hemophilia. Failure of diphenhydramine, chlorpromazine, and guaifenesin. J.A.M.A. *240*:2173, 1978.
155. Prince, A. M.: Can the blood-transmitted hepatitis problem be solved? Ann. N.Y. Acad. Sci. *240*:192, 1975.
156. Levine, P. H., McVerry, B. A., et al.: Health of the intensively treated hemophiliac, with special reference to abnormal liver chemistries and splenomegaly. Blood *50*:1, 1977.
157. Mannucci, P. M., Capitanio, A., et al.: Asymptomatic liver disease in haemophiliacs. J. Clin. Pathol. *28*:620, 1975.
158. Seeff, L. B., and Hoofnagle, J.: Chronic hepatitis in hemophilia. Ann. Intern. Med. *86*:818, 1977.
159. Hilgartner, M. W., and Giardina, P.: Liver dysfunction in patients with hemophilia A, B, and von Willebrand's disease. Transfusion *17*:495, 1977.
160. Holsteen, V., Skinhøj, P., et al.: Hepatitis, Type B, in haemophiliacs. Relationship to the source of clotting factor concentrates. Scand. J. Haematol. *18*:214, 1977.
161. McVerry, B. A., Voke, J., et al.: Immune complexes and abnormal liver function in haemophilia. J. Clin. Pathol. *39*:1142, 1977.
162. Gomperts, E. D., Lazerson, J., et al.: Hepatocellular enzyme patterns and hepatitis B virus exposure in multitransfused young and very young hemophilia patients. Am. J. Hematol. *11*:55, 1981.
163. Meyer, W. H., Levin, J., et al.: Abnormalities of the spleen and liver in patients with hemophilia. Am. J. Hematol. *14*:235, 1983.
164. Stirling, M. L., Murray, J. A., et al.: Incidence of infection with hepatitis B virus in 56 patients with haemophilia A, 1971–1979. J. Clin. Pathol. *36*:577, 1983.
165. Kasper, C. K., and Kipnis, S. A.: Hepatitis and clotting-factor concentrates. J.A.M.A. *221*:510, 1972.
166. Lesesne, H. R., Morgan, J. E., et al.: Liver biopsy in hemophilia A. Ann Intern. Med. *86*:703, 1977.
167. Spero, J. A., Lewis, J. H., et al.: Asymptomatic structural liver disease in hemophilia. New Engl. J. Med. *298*:1373, 1978.
168. Spero, J. A., Lewis, J. H., et al.: The high risk of chronic liver disease in multitransfused juvenile hemophiliac patients. J. Pediatr. *94*:875, 1979.
169. Preston, F. E., Underwood, J. C. E., et al.: Percutaneous liver biopsy and chronic liver disease in haemophiliacs. Lancet *2*:592, 1978.
170. White, G. C., II, Zeitler, K. D., et al.: Chronic hepatitis in patients with hemophilia A: histologic studies in patients with intermittently abnormal liver function tests. Blood *60*:1259, 1982.
171. Hoofnagle, J. H., Gerety, R. J., et al.: Transmission of non-A, non-B hepatitis. Ann. Intern. Med. *87*:14, 1977.
172. Alter, H. J., Purcell, R. H., et al.: Transmissible agent in non-A, non-B hepatitis. Lancet *1*:459, 1978.
173. Feinstone, S. M., Kapikian, A. Z., et al.: Transfusion-associated hepatitis not due to viral hepatitis type A or B. New Engl. J. Med. *292*:767, 1975.
174. Myers, T. J., Tembrevilla-Zubiri, C. L., et al.: Recurrent acute hepatitis following the use of factor VIII concentrates. Blood *55*:748, 1980.
175. Gralnick, H. R., Coller, B. S., et al.: Factor VIII. Ann. Intern. Med. *86*:598, 1977.
176. Rickard, K. A., Batey, R. G., et al.: Hepatitis and haemophilia therapy in Australia. Lancet *2*:146, 1982.
177. Mannucci, P. M., Colombo, M., and Rizzetto, M.: Non-progressive course of non-A, non-B chronic hepatitis in multitransfused hemophiliacs. Blood *60*:655, 1982.
178. Centers for Disease Control: Inactivated hepatitis B virus vaccine. Recommendation of the Immunization Practices Advisory Committee. Ann. Intern. Med. *97*:379, 1982.
179. Health and Public Policy Committee, American College of Physicians: Hepatitis B vaccine. Ann. Intern. Med. *100*:149, 1984.
180. Buchanan, G. R., Richards, N., et al.: Serologic response to hepatitis B vaccine in children receiving multiple blood transfusions. Pediatr. Infect. Dis. *5*:68, 1986.
181. Dolana, G., Tse, D., et al.: Hepatitis risk reduction in hemophilia: a heated factor VIII preparation. Blood *60*(Suppl. 1):210a, 1982.
182. Ragni, M. V., Lewis, J. H., et al.: Acquired-immunodeficiency-like syndrome in two haemophiliacs. Lancet *1*:213, 1983.
183. Gordon, E. M., Berkowitz, R. J., et al.: Burkitt lymphoma in a patient with classic hemophilia receiving factor VIII concentrates. J. Pediatr. *103*:75, 1983.
184. Curran, J. W., Lawrence, D. N., et al.: Acquired immunodeficiency syndrome (AIDS) associated with transfusions. New Engl. J. Med. *310*:69, 1984.
185. Broder, S., and Gallo, R. C.: A pathogenic retrovirus (HTLV-III) linked to AIDS. New Engl. J. Med. *311*:1292, 1984.
186. Luban, N. L. C., Kelleher, J. F., Jr., et al.: Altered distribution of T-lymphocyte subpopulations in children and adolescents with haemophilia. Lancet *1*:530, 1983.
187. Weintrub, P. S., Koerper, M. A., et al.: Immunologic abnormalities in patients with hemophilia A. J. Pediatr. *103*:692, 1983.
188. Menitove, J. E., Aster, R. H., et al.: T-lymphocyte subpopulations in patients with classic hemophilia treated with cryoprecipitate and lyophilized concentrates. New Engl. J. Med. *308*:83, 1983.
189. Gill, J. C., Menitove, J. E., et al.: Generalized lymphadenopathy and T cell abnormalities in hemophilia A. J. Pediatr. *103*:18, 1983.
190. Evatt, B. L., Gomperts, E. D., et al.: Coincidental appearance of LAV/HTLV-III antibodies in hemophiliacs and the onset of the AIDS epidemic. New Engl. J. Med. *312*:483, 1985.

191. Kitchen, L. W., Barin, F., et al.: Aetiology of AIDS—antibodies to human T-cell leukaemia virus (type III) in haemophiliacs. Nature *312*:367, 1984.
192. Eyster, M. E., Goedert, J. J., et al.: Development and early natural history of HTLV-III antibodies in persons with hemophilia. J.A.M.A. *253*:2219, 1985.
193. Levy, J. A., Mitro, G., and Mozen, M. M.: Recovery and inactivation of infectious retroviruses from factor VIII concentrates. Lancet *2*:722, 1984.
194. Rouzioux, C., Chamaret, S., et al.: Absence of antibodies to AIDS virus in haemophiliacs treated with heat-treated factor VIII concentrate. Lancet *1*:271, 1985.
195. Cheeseman, S. H., Sullivan, J. L., et al.: Analysis of cytomegalovirus and Epstein-Barr virus antibody responses in treated hemophiliacs. Implications for the study of acquired immune deficiency syndrome. J.A.M.A. *252*:83, 1984.
196. Blacklock, H. A., and Mortimer, P. P.: Aplastic crisis and other effects of the human parvovirus infection. Clin. Haematol. *13*:679, 1984.
197. Mortimer, P. P., Luban, N. L. C., et al.: Transmission of serum parvovirus-like virus by clotting-factor concentrates. Lancet *2*:482, 1983.
198. Egberg, N., and Blomback, M.: High frequency of low plasma haptoglobin values found in hemophilia A patients on prophylactic treatment with factor VIII concentrates—a sign of hemolysis? Thrombos. Haemostas. *46*:554, 1981.
199. Shulman, G., Ballard, J. O., et al.: Changes in plasma haptoglobin and alpha-2-macroglobulin in hemophiliacs receiving factor replacement therapy. Am. J. Hematol. *18*:223, 1985.
200. Gomperts, E. D., Jordan, S., et al.: Circulating immune complexes pre and post clotting factor infusion in hemophilia. Thromb. Haemostas. *46*:694, 1981.
201. Ceuppens, J. L., Vermylen, J., et al.: Immunological alterations in haemophiliacs treated with lyophilized factor VIII cryoprecipitate from volunteer donors. Thromb. Haemostas. *2*:207, 1984.
202. Lazerson, J.: Renal disease in hemophilia. In *Hemophilia in Children*. Hilgartner, M. W. (ed.), Littleton, MA, Publishing Sciences Group, 1976, pp. 71–78.
203. Prentice, C. R. M., Izatt, M. M., et al.: Amyloidosis associated with the nephrotic syndrome and transfusion reactions in a haemophiliac. Br. J. Haematol. *21*:305, 1971.
204. Louizou, C., Panayotopoulou, C., et al.: Isoimmunization in haemophiliacs. Scand. J. Haematol. *30*(Suppl.):51, 1977.
205. Enck, R. E., and Condemi, J. J.: Immunologic survey of a multitransfused population. Clin. Res. *25*:307, 1976.
206. Ratnoff, O. D., Menitove, J. E., et al.: Coincident classic hemophilia and "idiopathic" thrombocytopenic purpura in patients under treatment with concentrates of antihemophilic factor (factor VIII). New Engl. J. Med. *308*:439, 1983.
207. Sutor, A. H., Jesdinsky-Buscher, C., et al.: Alteration of primary hemostasis in hemophiliacs after treatment with lyophilized antihemophilic globulin. Scand. J. Haematol. *30*(Suppl.):33, 1977.
208. Hathaway, W. E., Mahasandana, C., et al.: Paradoxical bleeding in intensively transfused hemophiliacs: alteration of platelet function. Transfusion *13*:6, 1973.
209. Sutor, A. H., and Jesdinsky-Buscher, C.: Blutungszeitveranderung bei hamophiliebehandlung mit lyophilisiertem antihamophilem globulin (AHG). Deutsch. Med. Wochenchr. *101*:1715, 1976.
210. Buchanan, G. R., and Holtkamp, C. A.: Prolonged bleeding time in children and young adults with hemophilia. Pediatrics *66*:951, 1980.
211. Eyster, M. E., Gordon, R. A., et al.: The bleeding time is longer than normal in hemophilia. Blood *58*:719, 1981.
212. Biggs, R.: Jaundice and antibodies directed against factors VIII and IX in patients treated for haemophilia or Christmas disease in the United Kingdom. Br. J. Haematol. *26*:313, 1974.
213. Gitschier, J., Wood, W. I., et al.: Characterization of the human factor VIII gene. Nature *312*:326, 1984.
214. Toole, J. J., Knopf, J. L., et al.: Molecular cloning of a cDNA encoding human antihaemophilic factor. Nature *312*:342, 1984.
215. Vehar, G. A., Keyt, B., et al.: Structure of human factor VIII. Nature *312*:337, 1984.
216. Wood, W. I., Capon, D. J., et al.: Expression of active human factor VIII from recombinant DNA clones. Nature *312*:330, 1984.

TRANSFUSION THERAPY

CHAPTER 51
Therapeutic Plasma Exchange and Cytapheresis

MARTIN FOSBURG

INTRODUCTION 1622
TYPES OF SEPARATORS 1622
VASCULAR ACCESS 1623
BLOOD VOLUME AND HEMATOCRIT 1623
CONSIDERATIONS IN CRITICALLY ILL PATIENTS 1623
ANTICOAGULATION 1624
REPLACEMENT SOLUTIONS 1624
DOSE AND SCHEDULE 1625
PLASMAPHERESIS AS IMMUNOTHERAPY 1625
ILLNESSES TREATED BY PLASMAPHERESIS 1625
LYMPHOCYTAPHERESIS 1626
ERYTHROCYTAPHERESIS 1626
Polycythemia Due to Cyanotic Congenital Heart Disease
Technical Considerations
RED CELL EXCHANGE IN SICKLE CELL DISEASE 1628
Technical Considerations
LEUKAPHERESIS IN LEUKEMIA 1628
Technical Considerations
CONCLUSIONS AND FUTURE DIRECTIONS 1629

INTRODUCTION

Blood-letting, or apheresis (Greek, *aphairesis*, forcible removal), is among the oldest medical therapies, having been practiced in many diverse cultures for several thousand years (1). After a brief period of disfavor from the early 1800's through the mid 1900's, it has once again emerged as a widely used therapeutic tool.

Since the sixth century B.C., Western medicine has defined health as a state of perfect equilibrium among a number of innate "factors." In this framework, disease is characterized as a disturbance of balance (dyscrasia) (2). The symptoms of any particular disorder depend on the nature of the factor that is in excess. Blood-letting, by removing excess factor, was thought to re-establish equilibrium and thus to restore health. Over the ensuing 2500 years, the characterization of these factors has changed but the underlying principle and thus the rationale for apheresis has remained the same since the age of Hippocrates.

The modern era of apheresis began in the early 1960's with the development of machinery that could separate blood into its component parts and permit their selective removal (3). Presented in this chapter are the therapeutic applications of removal of plasma (plasmapheresis, or plasma exchange), lymphocytes (lymphocytapheresis), red cells (erythrocytapheresis), and leukocytes (leukocytapheresis), with particular reference to the technical modifications necessary for treatment of infants and children. It should be emphasized that despite its ancient lineage, therapeutic apheresis is in its infancy and its ultimate role in the treatment of many of the diseases in which it is currently used remains to be determined.

TYPES OF SEPARATORS

Blood can be separated into its component parts by filtration or centrifugation (4). In centrifugal machines, anticoagulated blood enters a spinning bowl or disposable channel, where its components separate according to density, yielding plasma, buffy coat, and red cell layers. Because the components of the buffy coat and red cell layers also have density differences, more or less distinct bands of platelets, mononuclear and PMN cells, and large buoyant as well as small dense red cells are produced. The machines can be adjusted so that an entire band or one of its components can be harvested. Because of this flexibility, centrifugation apparatus can be used for both plasmapheresis and cytapheresis.

In a filtration apparatus, anticoagulated blood is passed through hollow fibers or between flat plate membranes having pore sizes small enough to prevent the passage of platelets and larger cells. Separation is a function of membrane composition, pore size, and transmembrane pressure. These machines separate plasma from whole blood but cannot isolate its various cellular components. Both types of apparatus can be equally adapted for use in pediatric patients.

VASCULAR ACCESS

The difficulties associated with the placement and maintenance of vascular access are the major sources of morbidity in pediatric apheresis (5). Indeed, the decision to treat a child is most often based on the benefit of apheresis versus the morbidity of line placement. Unfortunately, peripheral veins of children rarely accommodate needles large enough to sustain the minimal flow rates necessary for apheresis (20 to 40 ml per minute). Alternative modes of access are arteriovenous connections and central venous catheters (6). Arteriovenous connections may be either internal (fistula or graft) or external (shunt). Because both require technically demanding vascular surgery they are usually reserved for those patients who need chronic therapy. In this writer's experience, shunts are preferable to fistulas in children largely because clotted shunts can be embolectomized at the bedside, whereas fistulas, once clotted, require operative reconstruction.

Central venous catheters are more suitable for brief periods of treatment. Ideally, catheters used for apheresis should be stiff so that they do not collapse when negative pressure is applied and should have multiple orifices so that a single clot or adherence of a portion of the catheter tip to a vessel wall will not ablate flow. Standard intracaths and silicone catheters designed for hyperalimentation collapse at low flow rates. There are catheters with the requisite qualities, designed for short-term hemodialysis, that, when placed in the subclavian or femoral veins, give excellent and sustained flow (7).

The chief complications of access are clotting and infection (8). Systemic infection with methicillin-resistant staphylococci and thrombosis at the catheter tip are frequent occurrences in central venous lines (9, 10). Although these lines may remain patent for purposes of infusion and blood sampling for many months, the capacity to draw blood through them at high flow rates is much shorter-lived. Even though clotting and infection occur in arteriovenous connections as well, these remain the most consistently successful long-term modes of access in dialysis and apheresis (6). It is the practice of this writer to treat patients who have shunts with aspirin and dipyridamole to inhibit clotting (11), although the efficacy of this therapy has not been proved.

BLOOD VOLUME AND HEMATOCRIT

Maintenance of a constant blood volume and red cell distribution is the single most important aspect of safe apheresis in infants and children. The extracorporeal volumes of apheresis apparatus range from 40 to 400 ml, which can represent a significant portion of a child's blood volume. As the machines are primed with saline, the child's hematocrit will be diluted by

$$\frac{\text{extracorporeal volume of machine}}{\text{patient blood volume}}$$

at the beginning of the exchange. The smaller the child, the less the ability to tolerate such perturbations.

The technique we have developed to prevent rapid fluctuations in blood volume and hematocrit was borrowed from that used in cardiac bypass—namely, to prime the extracorporeal circuits of the machines with packed red cells diluted with saline to yield a hematocrit equal to the patient's starting hematocrit. (For full details of the pediatric apheresis technique, see reference 5). With this procedure, a child of any size can be treated on any continuous flow apparatus, regardless of priming volume.

At the end of a procedure, the blood in the machine is left in situ, and thus the child has the same blood volume and hematocrit as found prior to treatment. This priming procedure is used when the extracorporeal volume of the machine is 12 per cent or more of the blood volume and in patients who are severely anemic or hemodynamically unstable.

During aphersis, it is possible to alter independently the blood volume and hematocrit; one can accomplish the former by returning a greater or lesser amount of replacement solution than the amount of plasma removed and the latter by priming the apparatus with blood having a hematocrit greater than the patient's and/or by using packed cells as part of the replacement solution.

CONSIDERATIONS IN CRITICALLY ILL PATIENTS

The capacity to alter blood volume and hematocrit can be an invaluable tool in clinical situations characterized by profound anemia and borderline to severe congestive heart failure. Such situations, familiar to hematology services, include patients with thalassemia and iron-induced cardiomyopathy, chronic hemolytic anemia during an aplastic crisis, severe allo- or autoimmune hemolytic anemia, and acute leukemia at presentation. In each instance, improved cardiac performance necessitates a higher hematocrit, yet the patient cannot tolerate volume. In these situations, the cell separator is primed with packed cells having a hematocrit 20 to 30 per cent higher than the patient's starting value. The exchange then proceeds very slowly, with removal of 1 to 2 ml per minute more in plasma than is replaced in red cells until the desired hematocrit and blood volume (measured by central venous pressure) are achieved. This slow, controlled manipulation of volume and red cell mass greatly improves cardiac performance and can be lifesaving in desperately ill children refractory to inotropic agents and diuretics. Naturally, such procedures are carried out in the intensive care unit with appropriate monitoring.

ANTICOAGULATION

Patients must be kept anticoagulated during apheresis so that clotting in the machinery is prevented. This can be done with citrate or heparin or both (12). For teenagers and adults with normal pretreatment coagulation status, any regimen consistent with the manufacturer's recommendation for a particular apparatus is acceptable. For children and all patients with coagulopathy, modifications in dosage and schedule must be made. In the latter group, the correct regimen is the minimal amount of anticoagulant that will prevent clotting.

Heparin. Our standard regimen for adults treated on centrifugal machines is a bolus of 2500 units followed by a constant infusion of 40 units per minute during treatment. In high-risk patients, we titrate the heparin dose by utilizing bedside-activated clotting times (normal values are ≤90 seconds). We start with a bolus of 0 to 40 units per kg (the dosage depends on pretreatment clotting time) to achieve a value of 150 to 180 seconds. Then, during the treatment, clotting times are repeated every 20 to 30 minutes and additional boluses of 0 to 20 units per kg are administered so that clotting time is maintained in the aforementioned therapeutic range. The side-effect of overheparinization is increased risk of bleeding.

Citrate. Citrate prevents clotting by reducing ionized calcium. The side-effect of excessive citrate is symptomatic hypocalcemia. Patients at high risk for citrate intoxication are those in shock, renal failure, or hepatic failure (14); those receiving citrated blood products as replacement solutions (15); and small children (5). We have observed toxicity in children with no other risk factors who were receiving minute doses of citrate. The symptom complex of citrate intoxication in children is, in temporal sequence, acute abdominal pain (with or without emesis) and pallor followed in minutes by bradycardia and hypotension. If any of these symptoms appear in a child receiving citrate, the procedure should be stopped and calcium administered. In small infants and critically ill, semiconscious patients, hypotension and bradycardia may be the first signs of citrate intoxication and should be assumed to be due to citrate until proven otherwise. Because citrate toxicity is the most common side-effect of apheresis (16), we use heparin exclusively when possible. When citrate is required (as in certain types of apparatus), we use the lowest possible dose.

Surprisingly, despite the necessity of anticoagulating patients who may have a high risk for bleeding because of pre-existing coagulopathy, serious bleeding is an infrequent complication of apheresis (16).

REPLACEMENT SOLUTIONS

The basic requirement for any replacement solution is that its volume, electrolyte composition, and protein oncotic pressure be equivalent to that of the plasma being removed. Beyond these considerations, the choice depends on both the beneficial and the adverse effects of the various solutions: fresh frozen plasma, albumin, plasma protein fraction, and, in situations in which 10 per cent or less of the blood volume is removed, saline (17).

Fresh Frozen Plasma. Plasma has a range of both immediate and long-term toxicities. These include transmission of viral infections, sensitization to alloantigens, citrate toxicity, hypernatremia, and acute allergic reactions (18). Because of these toxicities, plasma should be reserved for situations in which it is absolutely necessary. The major indications are treatment of thrombotic thrombocytopenic purpura (19) and the coagulopathy of liver failure. Situations in which its use is not indicated are routine replacement of coagulation factors removed during apheresis and replacement of immunoglobulins. A single 1.5-volume exchange (or the same dose on an alternate day schedule) will not remove sufficient factors to provoke bleeding in a patient with normal pretreatment coagulation status (20). In situations in which a very large volume of plasma is removed (> 2 plasma volumes) or in which daily treatment is necessary, the appropriate dose of plasma is the minimal amount that will largely correct the posttreatment PT, PTT, and fibrinogen. For replacement of immunoglobulin depleted by chronic apheresis, a safe and effective alternative to plasma is intravenous gammaglobulin (21).

Albumin. Albumin is largely free of plasma's side-effects because it does not transmit viral infections, does not contain citrate, does not cause allergic reactions, and has a normal sodium content. If the clinical situation warrants, the albumin concentration may be adjusted to increase, decrease, or maintain the patient's pretreatment plasma oncotic pressure. The sole disadvantage of albumin is its substantial cost. Plasma protein fraction shares many of these attributes but can cause hypotensive reactions (22).

DOSE AND SCHEDULE

There is no single correct dose (i.e., amount of plasma removed) or schedule for plasmapheresis. The correct dose and schedule for a particular disease consist of the minimal amount required to stop ongoing tissue damage. In most illnesses, treatment is initiated as outlined in Table 51–1. For illnesses with known mediators (antibody, immune complexes), the effect of a given dose and schedule on both mediator concentration and clinical symptoms should be determined. Further therapy is then based on these observations. The change in mediator concentration by itself is not sufficient to guide therapy because there may be poor correlations between particular antibody titers and disease activities (23).

In illnesses without known serum markers, plasmapheresis is usually investigational (i.e., does not have proven benefit). In order to develop a coherent body of experience in such situations, investigators should record the dose and schedule of each treatment and note the effect on clinical symptoms as well as a marker protein (e.g., IgG).

The effect of various treatment dosages and schedules on the concentrations of normal serum proteins is discussed in Chopek and McCullough's 1980 article (see reference 20). Most serum proteins fall 40 to 50 per cent per plasma volume exchanged. Because there is great variation in serum protein kinetics among individuals, changes in important proteins (i.e., those related to treatment side-effects) should be determined for each patient.

PLASMAPHERESIS AS IMMUNOTHERAPY

Because plasmapheresis is relatively new, there are few controlled trials comparing its benefits and side-effects with those of alternative forms of immune modulation. Various lists of illnesses treated by plasmapheresis include virtually all diseases known or thought to be mediated by the immune system (17, 24–26). It has been difficult to assess any type of treatment in patients with these illnesses because they tend to have frequent and unpredictable relapses and remissions. Ideally, the efficacy of plasmapheresis should be determined by double-blind studies comparing "sham" versus true apheresis alone or added to standard therapy. Although several such studies have been completed or are underway (27, 28), they will be unavailable for most diseases because of the considerable cost and complexity of such trials. In the absence of controlled trials, the decision to use apheresis should be based on an understanding of the type of immunosuppression produced by this technique.

Table 51–1. PLASMAPHERESIS DOSE SCHEDULE FOR AUTOIMMUNE DISEASE

1. Acute life or organ threatening complications: 1.5 to 3 plasma volumes daily until there is evidence of either clinical remission or worsening; generally 3 to 5 (+) treatments.
2. Acute exacerbation or initial presentation: 1.3 to 1.5 plasma volumes on alternate days for 3 to 5 treatments.
3. Maintenance therapy: From twice a week to biweekly.

Note: In most instances apheresis is combined with corticosteroids and/or cytotoxic drugs.

The single unique quality of plasmapheresis is its ability to reduce substantially and rapidly levels of preformed antibody, immune complexes, and various mediators of the inflammatory response. Table 51–2 shows the effect of a single apheresis on levels of immunoglobulins, complement, and acute-phase reactants. A single apheresis can reduce all serum proteins to a small fraction of their initial levels in a matter of hours. In this respect apheresis contrasts with chemotherapy, which can require weeks to reduce antibody levels by suppressing production, and with anti-inflammatory agents, which can take days to achieve maximal effect (29). In general, plasmapheresis will be most effective during periods of acute inflammation. Once fixed tissue damage has occurred, suppression of the immune and inflammatory responses is unlikely to be beneficial.

Plasmapheresis should be considered possible therapy for immune-mediated diseases in which there is an acute life- or organ-threatening complication. It may also be useful in less emergent situations in which symptoms must be controlled rapidly, thus limiting the duration of high-dose chemotherapy and shortening hospitalization.

The usefulness of plasmapheresis in chronic situations is much more limited. Owing to the side-effects of vascular access and to cost, apheresis is not first-line maintenance therapy. It may be appropriate when drugs alone cannot maintain remission or when the dosages of drugs necessary for clinical benefit cause unacceptable side-effects.

ILLNESSES TREATED BY PLASMAPHERESIS

There are several broad categories of illnesses that may be amenable to plasma exchange (26). These are characterized by an excess of a normal plasma constituent; the lack of a normal plasma constituent; the presence of pathogenic allo- or autoantibody and/or immune complexes; and the

Table 51–2. EFFECT OF A SINGLE LARGE-VOLUME PLASMA EXCHANGE ON MULTIPLE SERUM PROTEINS IN A PATIENT WITH SEPTICEMIA AND SEVERE DELAYED TRANSFUSION REACTION*

Plasma Volume Exchanged (%)	Alpha$_1$-Antitrypsin (%nl)	Haptoglobin (mg/dl)	Transferrin (mg/dl)	Orosomucoid (%nl)	C4 (%nl)	C3 (mg/dl)	IgG (mg/dl)	IgA (mg/dl)	IgM (mg/dl)	Properdin Factor B (mg/dl)	Beta-Lipoprotein (mg/dl)
0	206	48	155	232	62	138	800	85	124	37	92
15	160	34	115	178	26	108	620	70	98	35	60
35	142	32	80	150	12	88	440	65	90	31	44
50	126	28	80	136	6	70	360	55	84	23	40
100	84	22	50	86	2	40	160	40	52	13	22
170	34	16	30	22	≤5	26	60	20	30	9	15
250	8	12	30	12	≤5	20	40	15	24	7	6
270	8	12	20	0	0	14	≤10	≤10	15	7	6

*All starting values are normal except for increased alpha$_1$-antitrypsin and orosomucoid and decreased transferrin.

presence of toxin. Listed in Table 51–3 are examples drawn from each of these categories.

It is beyond the scope of this chapter to discuss, in detail, the numerous illnesses treated by plasmapheresis. Reference 30, an up-to-date compendium of these illnesses, includes indications for exchange, evidence for efficacy, doses, schedules, adjunctive chemotherapy, and references. Another general reference (31) includes a more complete discussion of a number of these entities.

LYMPHOCYTAPHERESIS

Although plasmapheresis dampens immune-mediated tissue damage by removing preformed antibody, antigen antibody complexes, and mediators of inflammation, it has no direct effect on their production, a process controlled by T and B lymphocytes (32). Attempts to modify the immune response by physical removal of lymphocytes either by surgical drainage of the throracic duct or by utilization of cell separators have met with limited success in small numbers of patients with rheumatoid arthritis and multiple sclerosis (33–36). The appeal of lymphocytapheresis lies in its potential capacity to produce lymphopenia without the side-effects of cytotoxic drugs or radiation.

Each lymphocytapheresis will remove about 5 × 10^9 lymphocytes in 300 to 500 ml of plasma. On a schedule of 2 to 3 treatments each week, the peripheral lymphocyte count will fall by about 30 and 60 per cent after 3 and 7 weeks, respectively, and may remain depressed for several more months. T cells decline more than B and null cells, although the ratio between helper and suppressor T cells does not change in any consistent fashion (33, 37).

Disadvantages of a several-week course of repeated lymphocytapheresis include high cost, frequent need for surgical procedures to obtain vascular access, and anemia. Lymphocytapheresis is thus a very expensive and cumbersome way of producing several months of relative lymphopenia. Furthermore, evidence for its efficacy as a single agent in immune disease is not convincing.

Long-term lymphocytapheresis should thus be reserved for those situations in which alternative forms of immunotherapy are not effective or are contraindicated. Its major use at present is in harvesting lymphocytes for research.

The development of monoclonal antibodies to specific T cell subpopulations may alter this picture. Attempts are underway to place such antibodies on columns through which whole blood or buffy coat–rich plasma could be passed and then reinfused into the patient. This technique has the potential of depleting specific subpopulations of T lymphocytes and thus would have obvious research and clinical applications.

ERYTHROCYTAPHERESIS

Polycythemia Due to Cyanotic Congenital Heart Disease

In the absence of hyperproteinemia, the chief determinant of whole blood viscosity is hematocrit (38). Patients with cyanotic congenital heart disease have varying degrees of polycythemia due to tissue hypoxia (39). In some patients, the rise in hematocrit is sufficient to cause a hyperviscosity state wherein blood flow to the microcirculation is compromised. The clinical correlates of hyperviscosity are headache, increased cyanosis, decreased exercise tolerance, and, in extreme cases, stroke (40). Absent a surgically correctable lesion, the only treatment for this polycythemia is phlebotomy. Traditionally, this has been done by admitting patients overnight and repeatedly removing aliquots of blood (usually without simultaneous volume replacement) until the desired hematocrit is obtained.

We have used outpatient erythrocytapheresis on the IBM cell separator as an alternative to manual phlebotomy (41). Our indications for treatment are symptoms of hyperviscosity with hematocrit greater than 60; incidental finding of a hematocrit greater than 75; and prophylactic treatment to keep the hematocrit less than 65 in patients with a history of stroke associated with polycythemia.

Table 51–3. SELECTED ILLNESSES TREATED BY PLASMA EXCHANGE

Disease	Category*	Serum Factor(s)	Adjunctive Therapy	Efficacy	Dose/Schedule	Comment	References
Familial hypercholesterolemia	A	Low density lipoprotein	Nicotinic acid	Definitely effective	1.5 PV† every 10–14 days	Mean of pre- and post-treatment cholesterol <250 mg%	55
Paraproteinemia	A	Mono- or polyclonal immunoglobulin	Cytotoxic drugs	Definitely effective	See Table 51-1	For relief of symptoms caused by paraprotein (hyperviscosity, hypervolemia)	56–58
ABO-incompatible marrow transplant	C	Isohemagglutinins	None	Definitely effective	1.5–2 PV every other day for 3–4 exchanges	Start 7–10 days before transplant; final titer ≤1:4	59–61
Thrombotic thrombocytopenic purpura	A, B	? Inhibitor to prostocycline production or absence of prostocycline precursor	Steroids, splenectomy, plasma, antiplatelet agents	Probably effective	1.5–3 PV daily	Replacement solutions should be largely plasma	62, 63
Hepatic failure (acute)	A, B, C	Multiple	Supportive	Effective in some cases	Large (2–3 [+]) PV exchanges daily	Replacement solution should be largely plasma, started as soon as diagnosis is made, and continued until remission	64
Multiple sclerosis	?C	Unknown	Steroids, cytotoxic drugs	Some benefit in acute and chronic cases	See Table 51-1	Both apheresis and cytotoxic drugs can be efficacious	65, 66
Myasthenia gravis	?C	Antibody to acetylcholine receptor	Cytotoxic drugs, steroids, anticholinesterase drugs	Frequently beneficial	See Table 51-1	Major use is in crisis to facilitate drug control	67, 68
Guillain-Barré syndrome	?C	Presumed antibody ? specificity	Acute: none Chronic: cytotoxic drugs, steroids	Frequently beneficial	See Table 51-1	Major indication is to prevent need for mechanical ventilation in those with a rapid downhill course	69
Mushroom poisoning	D	Amanitine	Supportive	Effective if begun early	2–3 PV, 1–3 exchanges	May work by temporary support of hepatic failure or removal of hepatotoxin or both	70
Consumption coagulopathy	A, B, C, D	Fibrin, degradation products, ? others	Treatment of infection, shock, acidosis, hypoxia	May be effective	2–3 PV exchanges daily	For cases not responsive to factor replacement alone	

*A = increased amount of normal plasma constituent; B = lack of a normal plasma constituent; C = presence of allo- or autoimmune antibody and/or immune complexes; D = presence of external toxin.
†PV = plasma volume.

Technical Considerations

1. One determines hematocrit by spinning the patient's blood in microhematocrit tubes for 5 minutes. On the average, Coulter hematocrits are 4 to 5 per cent lower than spun hematocrits in patients with cyanotic congenital heart disease and thus, the degree of polycythemia may be seriously underestimated with the former.

2. Treatments are designed to lower the hematocrit by 10 to 15 per cent.

3. Exchange volume is calculated by the following equation:

$$\text{Ml of RBC to be removed} = \frac{(WT[KG] \times 80)(HCT\ initial - HCT\ desired)}{0.9^*}$$

4. Patients receive the priming volume of the machine (250 ml of saline) as their blood enters the extracorporeal circuit so that volume contraction is avoided during treatment. During the exchange, the volume of red cells removed is continuously replaced by an equal volume of saline or 5 per cent albumin.

To date, we have performed 140 procedures on 32 patients without any serious morbidity. The intervals between therapy for an individual range from 4 weeks to 6 months. Those patients with mild to moderate iron deficiency tend to have lower hematocrits and therefore require less frequent treatment.

Outpatient erythrocytapheresis has numerous advantages over manual phlebotomy. The most important is that hematocrit is reduced while normovolemia is maintained. In patients with compromised flow to the microcirculation due to hyperviscosity, volume contraction could produce the very result that phlebotomy is designed to prevent (40). Other advantages are that outpatient erythrocytapheresis can be done in an hour and is performed under controlled circumstances with appropriate monitoring.

RED CELL EXCHANGE IN SICKLE CELL DISEASE

There are several clinical situations in sickle cell disease in which it may be desirable to remove the patient's red cells and replace them with those of a normal donor (Table 51–4) (42). Because sickle cells are denser than normal red cells, one can remove them rapidly and with great efficiency from a mixed red cell population using a cell separator (43). Since it is difficult to distinguish those complications that require exchange from those amenable to simple transfusion, it is our policy to utilize exchange in those situations in which immediate restoration of circulation is vital to preserving life or maintaining organ function. Also, red cell exchange is commonly performed prior to major surgery in sickle cell patients, although the risk of complications from perioperative sickling is small (44).

Table 51–4. INDICATIONS FOR RED CELL EXCHANGE IN SICKLE CELL DISEASE

Stroke
Priapism
Acute chest syndrome
Preparation for general anesthesia
Bacterial septicemia (up to 5 years of age)

Technical Considerations

1. Patients with sickle cell disease should receive antigen-matched frozen cells, preferably drawn from a black donor pool.

2. A single red cell volume exchange will remove between 70 and 80 per cent of the patient's cells. Because the hematocrit of the removed cells is 90 per cent and that of the replacement packed cells is 70 per cent, the patient's hematocrit will decline by about 20 per cent during the red cell exchange. After one red cell volume is exchanged, packed cells are exchanged for plasma so that the hematocrit is raised to the desired level.

a. Red cell volume = (WT [KG] × 80) (HCT)

b. Volume of packed* cells required to raise Hct by X%
$$= \frac{(WT [KG] \times 80)(X)}{\text{Hct of packed cells}}$$

In nonacute situations, in which chronic suppression of endogenous erythropoiesis is necessary (e.g., in early pregnancy) (45), one can utilize exchange at the onset to remove sickle cells and raise the hematocrit and then maintain the patients on a transfusion program. One can accomplish the same goal, albeit more slowly, by starting patients on a transfusion program without initial exchange. Finally, neither exchange nor simple transfusion has any place in the management of a vaso-occlusive crisis.

LEUKAPHERESIS IN LEUKEMIA

Leukapheresis by cell separator is not standard remission induction or maintenance therapy for any type of leukemia. That said, there may be situations in slowly proliferating leukemias in which, owing to side-effects from or resistance to

---

*HCT of the removed RBC.

*When packed cells are exchanged for plasma.

chemotherapy, chronic leukapheresis can be used to control symptoms due to a high number of circulating blasts (46, 47).

The major use of leukapheresis is in the acute management of the hyperviscosity state caused by extreme leukocytosis. With peripheral blast counts of 100,000 to 500,000 per mm^3, the packed leukocyte volume can be as high as 25 per cent, which, when added to packed red cell volume, may result in dramatically increased whole blood viscosity (48).

The two organ systems most susceptible to toxic effects of extreme leukocytosis are the lungs (49) and central nervous system (50). Pulmonary symptoms range from tachypnea to pulmonary failure; leukostasis in the nervous system can lead to hemorrhage or infarct or both. The presence of neurologic or pulmonary symptoms in a patient with extreme leukocytosis due to leukemia is a medical emergency.

The object of therapy is to reduce the white count as quickly as possible and to prevent it from rising. Treatment includes chemotherapy with S-phase–specific agents (commonly hydroxyurea or cytosine arabinoside) and leukapheresis (48, 51, 52).

Technical Considerations

1. As in polycythemia, normo- or hypervolemia should be maintained during the exchange.
2. Because patients with heavy tumor burdens are already prone to hypocalcemia, heparin is the preferable anticoagulant.
3. The replacement solution will be some combination of plasma, albumin, and possibly red cells, depending on the volume of exchange, starting hematocrit, and need for coagulation factors.
4. The goals of therapy are as follows:
    a. Relief of symptoms.
    b. Achievement of a WBC of less than 100,000 or a decrease of 50 to 60 per cent).
    c. Minimalization of performance time—4 to 6 hours of exchange is the most that the majority of patients can tolerate.
5. Daily therapy continues until the WBC is down and the symptoms are resolved.

CONCLUSIONS AND FUTURE DIRECTIONS

Despite its many limitations, plasmapheresis has proved a valuable and frequently lifesaving tool in situations refractory to other forms of therapy. The future applications of plasma- and cytapheresis will be determined by improvements designed to make therapy less expensive and more specific.

At present, the major cost is that of the albumin replacement solution. Mass production of albumin by genetic engineering techniques, a possibility for the future, may one day alleviate this problem. Side-effects of vascular access are not so easily reduced, especially in children, although more effective antithrombotic and thrombolytic agents would be a major step forward.

The development of columns containing monoclonal antibody and of other technologies that would allow for removal of specific proteins would greatly enhance treatment and reduce side-effects (53, 54). Much research and development will be required before such tools will be generally available. These devices will have to be highly efficient in order to remove the same amount of a pathologic substance as can be removed by the discarding of plasma in its entirety. The cost would have to be less than that of standard albumin replacement. Finally, the binding of a target protein to bound antibody must not release substances (e.g., activated complement) that would be harmful when reinfused to the patient.

Perhaps the most exciting immediate application of columns designed to remove antibodies, immune complexes, and subpopulations of lymphocytes is in research—namely, efforts to define more precisely the role that such proteins and cells play in the pathophysiology of immune disease.

References

1. Sigerest, H. E.: *A History of Medicine*, Vol. 1. New York, Oxford University Press, 1951, p. 202.
2. Sigerest, H. E.: *Civilization and Disease*. Ithaca, Cornell University Press, 1943, p. 150.
3. Judson, G., Jones, A., et al.: Closed continuous flow centrifuge. Nature (Lond.) *217*:816, 1968.
4. Mollison, P. L.: *Blood Transfusion in Clinical Medicine*, 7th ed. Oxford, Blackwell Scientific Publications, 1983, pp. 216–217.
5. Fosburg, M., Dolan, M., et al.: Intensive plasma exchange in small and critically ill pediatric patients: techniques and clinical outcome. J. Clin. Apheresis *1*:215, 1983.
6. Wilson, S. E., Stable, B. E., et al.: Current status of vascular access techniques. Surg. Clin. North Am. *62*:531, 1982.
7. Shaldon Polyethylene Catheter. Surgimed Inc., Summerville, SC.
8. Pollack, P. F., Kadden, M., et al.: 100 patient years experience with the broviac silastic catheter for central venous nutrition. J.P.E.N. *5*:32, 1981.
9. Lowry, F. D., and Hammer, S. M.: Staphylococcus epidermidis infections. Ann. Intern. Med. *99*:834, 1983.
10. Bambauer, R., and Jutzler, G. A.: Transcutaneous insertion of the Shaldon catheter through the internal jugular vein as access for acute hemodialysis. Transplant. *11*:766, 1982.
11. Hathaway, W. E.: Use of antiplatelet agents in pediatric hypercoagulable states. Am. J. Dis. Child. *138*:301, 1984.
12. Mollison, P. L.: *Blood Transfusion in Clinical Medicine*, 7th ed. Oxford, Blackwell Scientific Publications, 1983, pp. 32–33.
13. Sorrell, M., and Irosen, J.: Ionized calcium serum values during symptomatic hypocalcemia. J. Pediatr. *87*:67, 1975.
14. Bunker, J. P., Stetson, J. B., et al.: Citric acid intoxication. J.A.M.A. *157*:1361, 1955.

15. Collins, J. A.: Problems associated with the massive transfusion of stored blood. Surgery 75:274, 1974.
16. Anonymous: Hazards of apheresis. Lancet 2:1205, 1982.
17. McCullough, J., Bussell, A., et al.: What are the established clinical indications for therapeutic plasma exchange and how important is the choice of replacement fluid? Vox Sang. 43:270, 1982.
18. Mollison, P. L.: *Blood Transfusion in Clinical Medicine,* 7th ed. Oxford, Blackwell Scientific Publications, 1983, pp. 738–78.
19. Bulowski, R. M., Hewlett, J. S., et al.: Therapy of thrombotic thrombocytopenic purpura: an overview. Semin. Thromb. Hemost. 7:1, 1981.
20. Chopek, M., and McCullough, J.: Protein and biochemical changes during plasma exchange. Therapeutic Hemapheresis: Technical Workshop (AABB), 1980, pp. 13–52.
21. Morell, A., Schurch, B., et al.: In vivo behavior of gamma globulin preparations. Vox Sang. 38:272, 1980.
22. Alung, B. M., and Mojuma, Y.: Hypotension associated with prekallikrein (Hageman factor fragments) in plasma protein fraction. New Engl. J. Med. 299:66, 1978.
23. Lenzhofer, R., Graninger, W., et al.: Plasmapheresis in the treatment of myasthenia gravis. Wien. Klin. Wochenschr. 95:266, 1983.
24. Kennedy, M. S., and Domen, R. E.: Therapeutic apheresis: applications and future directions. Vox Sang. 45:261, 1983.
25. Verrier-Jones, J., Clough, J. D., et al.: The role of therapeutic plasmapheresis in the rheumatic diseases. J. Lab. Clin. Med. 97:589, 1981.
26. Shumak, K. H., and Rock, G. A.: Therapeutic plasma exchange. New Engl. J. Med. 310:762, 1984.
27. Schulz, S. C., Van-Kammen, D. P., et al.: Double blind evaluation of plasmapheresis in schizophrenic patients: A pilot study. Artif. Organs 7:317, 1983.
28. Weiner, H. L., Dall, P., et al.: Plasma exchange in acute multiple sclerosis: design of a cooperative study. Arch. Neurol. 40:691, 1983.
29. Hersh, E. M., and Bodey, G. P. (eds.): Symposium on clinical immunosuppression. Transplant. Proc. 5:1155, 1937.
30. Dau, P. C. (ed.): *Therapeutic Plasma Exchange Disease Compendium.* Lakewood, CO, Cobe Laboratories, 1983.
31. Tindall, R. S. A. (ed.): *Therapeutic Apheresis and Plasma Perfusion.* New York, A. R. Liss, 1982.
32. Paul, W. E.: Lymphocyte biology. In *Clinical Immunology.* Parker, C. W. (ed.), Philadelphia, W. B. Saunders Co., 1980, pp. 19–48.
33. Hauser, S. L., Fosburg, M., et al.: Lymphocytapheresis in chronic progressive multiple sclerosis: immunologic and clinical effects. Neurology 34:922, 1984.
34. Tilney, N. L., and Murray, J. E.: Chronic thoracic duct fistula: operative techniques and physiologic effects in man. Ann. Surg. 167:1, 1968.
35. Karsh, J., Klippel, J. H., et al.: Lymphocytapheresis in rheumatoid arthritis: a randomized trial. Arthritis Rheum. 24:867, 1981.
36. Giordano, G. F., Masland, W., et al.: An investigation of lymphocytapheresis in multiple sclerosis. Plasma Ther. Transfusion Technol. 3:417, 1982.
37. Wright, D. G., Karsh, J., et al.: Lymphocyte depletion and immunosuppression with repeated leukapheresis by continuous flow centrifugation. Blood 58:451, 1981.
38. Pearson, T. C., Humphrey, D. J., et al.: Hematocrit, blood viscosity, cerebral blood flow, and vascular occlusion. In Clinical Aspects of Blood Viscosity and Cell Deformability. Lowe, G. D. O., Barbenel, et al. (eds.), Berlin, Springer-Verlag, 1981, pp. 97–107.
39. Rudolph, A. M., Nadas, A. S., et al.: Hematologic adjustments to cyanotic congenital heart disease. Pediatrics 11:454, 1983.
40. Rosenthal, A., Nathan, D. G., et al.: Acute hemodynamic effects of red cell volume reduction in polycythemia of cyanotic congenital heart disease. Circulation. 42:287, 1970.
41. Fosburg, M., Jacobson, M., et al.: Red cell exchange for polycythemia in congenital heart disease: techniques and the effect of iron status on hematocrit and blood viscosity. Procedures of the International Society of Blood Transfusion, Munich, 1984, p. 132.
42. Charache, S., Lubin, B., et al.: Management and therapy of sickle cell disease. National Institutes of Health Publication No. 84-2117, 1984, p. 17.
43. Kernoff, L. M., Botha, M. C., et al.: Exchange transfusion in sickle cell disease using a continuous flow cell separator. Transfusion 17:269, 1977.
44. Homi, J., Reynolds, J., et al.: General anesthesia in sickle cell disease. Br. J. Med. 1:1599, 1979.
45. Key, T. C., Horger, E. O., et al.: Automated erythrocytapheresis for sickle cell anemia during pregnancy. Am. J. Obstet. Gynecol. 138:73, 1980.
46. Lowenthal, R. M.: Chronic leukemias—treatment by leukapheresis. Exp. Hematol. 5:73, 1977.
47. Meyer, R. J., Cuttner, J., et al.: Therapeutic leukapheresis of acute myelomonocytic leukemia in pregnancy. Med. Pediatr. Oncol. 4:77, 1978.
48. Lichtman, M. A., and Rowe, J. M.: Hyperleukocytic leukemias: rheological, clinical and therapeutic considerations. Blood 60:279, 1982.
49. Frost, T., Isbister, J. P., et al.: Respiratory failure due to leukostasis in leukemia. Med. J. Aust. 68:94, 1981.
50. Freireich, E. J., Thomas, L. B., et al.: A distinctive type of intracerebral hemorrhage associated with "Basic Crisis" in patients with leukemia. Cancer 13:146, 1960.
51. Lane, T. A.: Continuous flow leukapheresis for rapid cytoreduction in leukemia. Transfusion 20:455, 1980.
52. Carpentieri, U., Patten, E. V., et al.: Leukapheresis in a 3 year old child with lymphoma in leukemic transformation. J. Pediatr. 94:919, 1979.
53. Pinead, A. A.: Methods for selective removal of plasma constituents. In *Therapeutic Apheresis and Plasma Perfusion.* Tindall, R. S. A. (ed.), New York, A. R. Liss, 1982, pp. 361–373.
54. Saal, S. D., and Gordon, B. R.: Extracorporeal modification of plasma and whole blood. In *Therapeutic Apheresis and Plasma Perfusion.* Tindall, R. S. A. (ed.), New York, A. R. Liss, 1982, pp. 375–384.
55. Harvell, R. J., and Kane, J. P.: Therapy of hyperlipidemic states. Ann. Rev. Med. 33:417–433, 1982.
56. Thomas, E. L., Olk, R. J., et al.: Irreversible visual loss in Waldenstrom's macro-globulinaemia. Br. J. Ophthalmol. 67:102, 1983.
57. Ginder, P. A., Middendorf, D. F., et al.: Pancytopenia with mixed cryoglobulinemia: Evidence for antiprecursor cell activity of cryoglobulin—effects of plasmapheresis. J. Clin. Immunol. 2:55, 1982.
58. Russell, J. A., Toy, J. L., et al.: Plasma exchange in malignant paraproteinemias. Exp. Hematol. 5:105, 1977.
59. Buckner, C. D., Clift, R. A., et al.: ABO incompatible marrow transplants. Transplantation 26:233, 1978.
60. Bensinger, W. I., Buckner, C. D., et al.: ABO incompatible marrow transplants. Transplantation 33:427, 1982.
61. Slapak, M., Naik, R., et al.: Renal transplant in a patient with major donor-recipient blood group incompatibility: reversal of acute rejection by the use of modified plasmapheresis. Transplantation 31:4, 1981.
62. Machin, S. J.: Clinical annotation. Thrombotic thrombocytopenia purpura. Br. J. Haematol. 56:191, 1984.
63. Bukowski, R. M., Hewlett, J. S., et al.: Therapy of thrombotic thrombocytopenic purpura: an overview. Semin. Thromb. Hemostas. 7:1, 1981.
64. Brunner, G.: Therapeutic plasma exchange in liver disease. In *Therapeutic Plasma Exchange Disease Compendium.* Dau, P.

(ed.), Lakewood, CO, Cobe Laboratories, 1983, pp. 160–164.
65. Hauser, S. L., Dawson, D. M., et al.: Intensive immunosuppression in progressive multiple sclerosis. New Engl. J. Med. *308*:173, 1983.
66. Hauser, S. L., Fosburg, M., et al.: Plasmapheresis, lymphocytapheresis and immunosuppressive drug therapy in multiple sclerosis. In *Therapeutic Apheresis and Plasma Perfusion*. Tindall, S. A. (ed.), New York, A. R. Liss, 1982, pp. 239–254.
67. Lenzhoffer, R., Graninger, W., et al.: Plasmapheresis in the treatment of myasthenia gravis. Wien. Klin. Wochenschr. *95*:266, 1983.
68. Dall, P. C.: Plasmapheresis in myasthenia gravis. Prog. Clin. Biol. Res. *88*:265, 1982.
69. Osterman, P. O., Fragius, J., et al.: Beneficial effects of plasma exchange in acute inflammatory polyradiculoneuropathy. Lancet *2*:1296, 1984.
70. Mercuriali, F., and Sirchia, G.: Plasma exchange for mushroom poisoning. Transfusion *17*:644, 1977.

CHAPTER 52
Hematologic Manifestations of Systemic Diseases

JAMES A. STOCKMAN III

INTRODUCTION 1632
CARDIAC DISEASE 1632
Hemolysis
Coagulation Abnormalities
Platelet Abnormalities
Treatment
Miscellaneous Hematologic Manifestations of Heart Disease
GASTROINTESTINAL DISEASE 1635
Diseases of the Upper Gastrointestinal Tract
Diseases of the Lower Gastrointestinal Tract
PANCREATIC DISEASE 1636
LIVER DISEASE 1636
Red Blood Cell Disturbances in Liver Disease
Coagulation Abnormalities in Liver Disease
Disseminated Intravascular Coagulation in Liver Disease
RENAL DISEASE 1638
The Red Blood Cell in Renal Disease
The White Blood Cell in Renal Disease
Coagulation Abnormalities in Renal Disease
Platelet Abnormalities in Renal Disease
ENDOCRINE DISORDERS 1641
Thyroid
Adrenal Gland
Testes and Ovaries
Pituitary
PULMONARY DISEASE 1644
Idiopathic Pulmonary Hemosiderosis (IPH)
Pulmonary Hemosiderosis from Other Causes
Hematologic Findings in Other Pulmonary Disorders
COLLAGEN VASCULAR DISEASES AND THE ANEMIA OF CHRONIC DISORDERS 1645
Hematologic Aspects of Collagen Vascular Disease
INFECTIONS 1649
General Hematologic Signs of Infection
Hematologic Aspects of Selected Specific Infections
Infectious Mononucleosis
METABOLIC DISEASES 1658
Diabetes Mellitus
Abnormalities of Lipid Metabolism
Other Metabolic Disorders
NEUROLOGIC AND PSYCHIATRIC DISORDERS 1659
Muscular Dystrophy
Myasthenia Gravis
Lesch-Nyhan Syndrome
Brain Trauma
Anorexia Nervosa
SKIN DISEASES 1660
Eczema and Psoriasis
Dermatitis Herpetiformis
Dyskeratosis Congenita
Hereditary Hemorrhagic Telangiectasias
Ehlers-Danlos Syndrome and Other Connective Tissue Disorders
Mast Cell Disease
LEUKOCYTE VARIATIONS IN DISEASE STATES 1661
Nuclear Changes
Hereditary Constitutional Hypersegmentation of Neutrophils
Hereditary Constitutional Hypersegmentation of Eosinophils
Hereditary Giant Neutrophils
Hereditary Prevalence of Nuclear Appendages
Cytoplasmic Abnormalities
Eosinopenia and Eosinophilia
Basophilia
Monocytosis
Lymphocytosis

INTRODUCTION

A chapter on the hematologic manifestations of systemic diseases must overlap other sections of this book. The approach here is different in that organ system diseases are reviewed and the hematologic findings peculiar to these problems are discussed. In a sense, then, this is an "inside-out" version of the rest of the book. Because it is impossible to review all the specific details of hematologic complications of systemic disease within a single chapter, the reader is referred to other chapters and to a comprehensive text* for additional information.

CARDIAC DISEASE

This section will deal primarily with the three major hematologic complications of cardiac disease—hemolytic anemia, coagulopathy, and increased platelet turnover.

Hemolysis

A number of instances of continuing hemolysis and progressive anemia have been reported following the insertion of prosthetic valves, particularly in the aortic area (1, 2). This may also occur postoperatively when intracardiac patches have been placed (the "Waring blender" syndrome). The mechanism of such erythrocyte destruction has been related to failure of endothelialization of patches, thrombosis or perforation of prosthetic valves, and improper placement of prosthetic valves, especially when insufficiency develops at the suture lines. Erythrocyte destruction and ensuing hemolysis, however, have been described in the absence of these complications and have been attributed to red blood cell mechanical trauma associated with apparently normal function of the prosthetic valve (3, 4).

Available evidence makes it most unlikely that any of the patients who have developed cardiac hemolytic anemia have had an intrinsic abnormality of the red cells. Red cell survival studies have

---

*Israels, M. G. G., and Delamore, I. W.: *Haematological Aspects of Systemic Disease.* London, W. B. Saunders Company, Ltd., 1976.

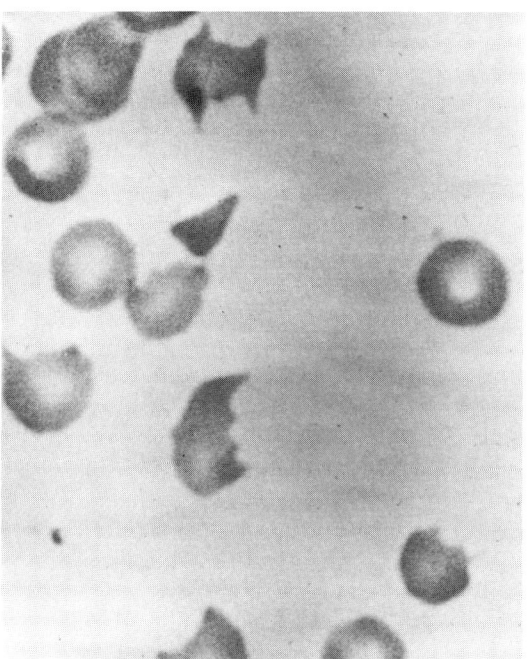

Figure 52–1. Microangiopathic red cell alterations in a patient with a prosthetic heart valve. The peripheral blood smear often reveals fragmented red blood cells with helmet forms and polychromasia.

clearly shown that the abnormality is due to an extracorpuscular defect (5). In general, hemolytic anemia results from fragmentation of the red cells as they are mechanically "battered" against a distorted vascular surface (6) (Fig. 52–1). In some cases, it has been postulated that the red cell fragmentation may be caused by contact with fibrin deposited in the small blood vessels as a result of localized intravascular coagulation (7). In most cases, however, hemolysis is the result of direct mechanical trauma. Nevaril and associates have demonstrated that a shearing stress of 300 dynes per cm^2 causes hemolysis in vitro, whereas lesser stresses may result in deformed red cells morphologically similar in appearance to cells in cardiac hemolytic anemias and microangiopathic hemolytic anemias (6).

The consequence of this process is a hemolytic anemia of the intravascular type associated with hemoglobinemia and often hemoglobinuria. Patients with this disorder quickly become iron-deficient as a result of an increased loss of body iron in the form of hemosiderin, which is shed within renal tubular cells into the urine (8, 9). The onset of iron deficiency may be of clinical importance. In iron deficiency, the microcytic hypochromic cell is more rigid, leading to an accelerated rate of hemolysis from mechanical shearing in the microvasculature (9). Plasma haptoglobin and hemopexin levels fall. Large quantities of red cell lactate dehydrogenase (LDH) are released into the serum (10). A close correlation exists between the logarithm of serum LDH and the half-life of Cr-labeled erythrocytes (Fig. 52–2). The rate of hemolysis may or may not result in anemia. If surgical correction of the defect causing hemolysis is not possible, the patient should be treated with both iron and folate as well as a red cell transfusion. The last is intended to correct anemia, reduce stroke volume, and presumably reduce the shear forces. Sears and Crosby have observed that the severity of hemolysis is directly related to physical activity (11). This has been used as a test to determine whether the hemolysis is cardiac in origin, since, if it is, rest also will diminish the rate of hemolysis.

The mechanical injury to red cells may result in loss of pieces of cell membrane, with or without a loss of hemoglobin. This will cause the formation of spherocytes. Consequently, in many patients with heart valve hemolysis, the red cell osmotic fragility test may be abnormal (8).

Occasionally, autoimmune hemolytic anemia is observed following cardiac surgery with the placement of foreign material within the vascular system (12). This may also occur in association with subacute bacterial endocarditis.

Coagulation Abnormalities

Many investigations have suggested that a coagulopathy exists in some patients with cyanotic congenital heart disease. Thrombocytopenia, low plasma fibrinogen levels, defective clot retraction, hypoprothrombinemia, Factors V and VIII deficiency, and evidence of fibrin degradation products in the serum have been reported (13–17).

Dennis and associates first reported five patients

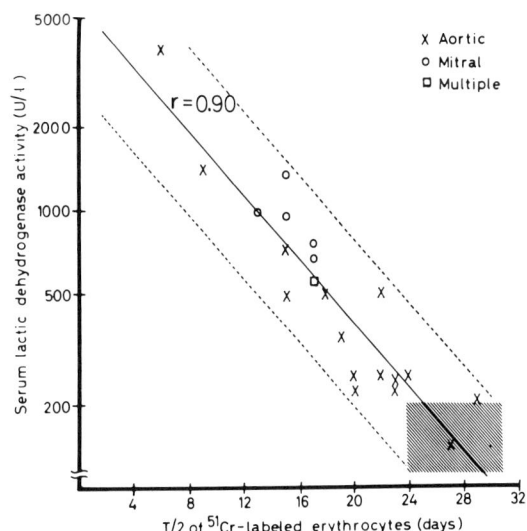

Figure 52–2. Serum LDH levels in patients with aortic and mitral valve dysfunction causing intravascular hemolysis. The hatched area represents the normal ranges. (From Myhre, E., Rasmussen, K., et al.: Am. Heart J. *80*:463, 1970.)

with cyanotic congenital heart disease associated with coagulation abnormalities correctable by heparin. Consumptive coagulopathy was thought responsible (18). These early reports have been criticized, however, because of failure to reduce the amount of anticoagulant in the tubes of blood samples collected from such patients (19).

It is now generally thought that the presence of coagulation abnormalities correlates best with the extent of polycythemia. The exact mechanism producing the coagulopathy, when present, is not known.

Hyperviscosity may lead to tissue hypoxemia, which then triggers a consumptive process (22). Conflicting data suggest that the coagulation defects associated with cyanotic congenital heart disease must be multifactorial in origin. Therefore, each child should be studied individually.

Platelet Abnormalities

Quantitative and qualitative platelet abnormalities are commonly associated with cardiac disease. In one series, the mean platelet count for cyanotic patients with arterial oxygen saturations of less than 60 per cent was 185,000 cells per mm^3, compared with a value of 315,000 cells per mm^3 for patients with a saturation greater than 60 per cent (23). Examination of the bone marrow has failed to demonstrate any quantitative changes in the megakaryocytes to account for these platelet differences (23). This, together with the finding of shortened platelet survival in many cases, has suggested that the mechanism of the thrombocytopenia is a destructive one. Some patients, especially those with minimal cyanosis, may have elevated platelet counts. It should be noted that although iron deficiency is common in association with cyanotic congenital heart disease, the quantitative platelet abnormalities are not related to iron status.

Qualitative platelet defects associated with cyanotic congenital heart disease may include prolonged bleeding times and abnormal aggregation in response to adenosine diphosphate, epinephrine, and collagen (24). In as many as 70 per cent of patients, both a delayed or absent second wave of platelet aggregation and disaggregation are observed (25). These platelet functional abnormalities appear to be due to a defective platelet release mechanism because diminished release of ^{14}C-serotonin occurs in response to adenosine diphosphate, whereas uptake of ^{14}C-serotonin is normal (26). Platelet release abnormalities are more common in patients over 4 years of age, in those with hematocrit concentrations greater than 60 per cent, and in those with platelet counts less than 175,000 cells per mm^3. There is no correlation between abnormalities of platelet aggregation and release and the abnormal bleeding time.

Treatment

The management of these hemostatic defects is unsettled. It is agreed that they may predispose to postoperative hemorrhage, but they are rarely associated with preoperative clinical bleeding tendencies. Suggested management procedures have included the use of heparin (18) to lower viscosity, erythrocytopheresis with plasma exchange (22, 22a), and ϵ-aminocaproic acid to inhibit fibrinolysis (27). Whether any of these modalities is indicated and indeed whether they might be uniformly effective are speculative. If erythrocytopheresis is chosen, the procedure should be done with great care in cyanotic patients. Withdrawal of red cells must be accompanied by an equal volume of fresh frozen plasma. Simple removal of red cells without volume replacement in polycythemic individuals may cause an acute increase in viscosity, vascular collapse, seizures, and even strokes (27a). Because of the high incidence of cerebrovascular accidents in children with cyanotic congenital heart disease, some workers have felt that a "hypercoagulable" state exists. Hyperviscosity alone may account for some ischemic infarctions. The clinician should be alert to the possibility of iron deficiency predisposing to stroke in the presence of polycythemia. Several children have been described who have developed neurologic deficits following the onset of iron deficiency in the presence of polycythemia (28, 29). Card and Weintraub have shown that red blood cells from animals with iron deficiency have decreased deformability (30). Altered deformability in the presence of increased blood viscosity theoretically could result in vascular ischemia.

Shortening of platelet survival with or without thrombocytopenia has been observed in both children and adults with prosthetic heart valves (31). The increased platelet turnover may result from a combination of mechanical damage to the platelet or adhesion to the foreign material. The use of antiplatelet aggregating agents may correct this shortened survival, although the clinical benefit of the use of this class of drugs is not established. Drugs such as acetylsalicylic acid, dipyridamole, and sulfinpyrazone have been used either singly or in combination (32–34).

Miscellaneous Hematologic Manifestations of Heart Disease

Subacute bacterial endocarditis may be associated with a variety of hematologic manifestations. Anemia is often present and is usually the result of chronic infection. The white blood cell count is usually normal, although marked leukocytosis or leukopenia may occur. Pancytopenia has been reported (34a). Thrombocytopenia has been noted in a few patients (34b).

Congestive heart failure may result in sufficient hypoxia to cause nucleated red blood cells to appear in the peripheral blood in association with a mild reticulocytosis (34c). Thrombocytopenia may be noted but is almost exclusively the result of hypersplenism (34d).

Cyanotic heart disease may result in poor perfusion of the spleen, causing a functional hyposplenia, manifested by Howell-Jolly bodies in the peripheral blood (34e). This finding is likely to lead to the mistaken conclusion that a child may have the asplenia syndrome (absence of the spleen, cardiovascular malformations, abdominal situs inversus, and other anatomic malformations) with its associated poor prognosis.

GASTROINTESTINAL DISEASE

Hematologic complications of gastrointestinal disease appear in a large number of disorders. This section will not deal with the wide range of situations in which blood loss occurs from the gastrointestinal tract but rather will focus on specific diseases and their hematologic complications.

Diseases of the Upper Gastrointestinal Tract

Esophagus. The Plummer-Vinson syndrome (dysphagia, postcricoid webs, and iron deficiency) (35) occurs in older individuals. It is very infrequent in young adults. Iron deficiency anemia may be the only manifestation of gastroesophageal reflux that stresses the importance of endoscopy in evaluating unexplained iron deficiency anemia (35a).

Stomach. The gastric mucosa is important in both vitamin B_{12} and iron absorption, and disorders of the gastric mucosa may cause defective absorption of either of these nutrients.

Chronic atrophic gastritis is usually a disorder of older adults but occasionally is seen in the young adult. Accompanying iron deficiency is a result of a combination of blood loss and iron malabsorption secondary to achlorhydria (36). Vitamin B_{12} absorption defects may occur in association with chronic atrophic gastritis (37).

Gastric resection also may result in iron or vitamin B_{12} deficiency—the former from bleeding at the sites of anastomosis and the latter, years later, because of lack of intrinsic factor. A macrocytic, megaloblastic anemia resulting from vitamin B_{12} deficiency has been reported in association with gastric trichobezoars (37a). It is presumed that this results from bacterial overgrowth of the upper gastrointestinal tract.

In congenital intrinsic factor deficiency, the gastric biopsy is normal, and no antibodies to parietal cells or intrinsic factor are present (38).

The Zollinger-Ellison syndrome is a disorder associated with increased parietal cell production of hydrochloric acid. This may cause iron deficiency from mucosal ulceration. Carcinoid syndrome may cause a similar problem. In both conditions, vitamin B_{12} malabsorption may occur because of reduced pH in the ileum.

Small Bowel. Celiac disease may cause a panmalabsorption syndrome. Isolated iron deficiency results from blood loss due to ulcerations at the origins of the loop, and vitamin B_{12} deficiency may be caused by consumption of this vitamin by stagnant intestinal bacteria (39). Blind loops created surgically for treatment of obesity have been reported to cause an unusual autoimmune disorder in young adults (40), characterized by immune intravascular hemolysis, neutropenia, and thrombocytopenia. Immune complex–mediated complement activation apparently accounts for the blood cell destruction, perhaps owing to bacterial antigens that enter the blood and initiate the immune complex formation. Carcinomas and lymphomas are found with increased frequency in adult patients with celiac disease (40a).

Ileal resection may cause vitamin B_{12} deficiency if the receptors for the vitamin B_{12} intrinsic factor complex have been removed.

Regional enteritis may cause iron deficiency from blood loss and vitamin B_{12} deficiency from inflammatory disease of the terminal ileum or from the development of the blind loop syndrome as small bowel fistulas form.

Disorders such as tropical sprue, dermatitis herpetiformis, bowel lymphoma, amyloidosis, and connective tissue disturbances (including the Ehlers-Danlos syndrome and pseudoxanthoma elasticum) may produce pan- or selective malabsorption. Certain disorders such as intestinal lymphangiectasia may cause protein losses of sufficient magnitude to impair globin chain synthesis. This may also be associated with a selective loss of thymic-dependent (T) lymphocytes into the bowel lumen, causing lymphopenia and altered delayed-type hypersensitivity.

Eosinophilic gastroenteritis is a disorder most often characterized by recurrent bouts of abdominal pain, nausea, vomiting, diarrhea, and an elevated peripheral blood eosinophil count for which there is no other explanation (40b). The gut wall may be infiltrated by eosinophils.

Diseases of the Lower Gastrointestinal Tract

Ulcerative colitis is often associated with iron deficiency anemia from blood loss. Immune hemolytic anemia is also observed. Occasionally, vitamin B_{12} deficiency will occur after many years if a "backwash" ileitis is present. A polymorphonuclear leukocytosis is common. Occasionally, an increase in plasma fibrinolytic activity will be observed. Some clinicians have treated this complication with ε-aminocaproic acid (41). Platelet functional abnormalities may exist and are discussed elsewhere.

Constipation has been reported to cause a rise in sulfmethemoglobin levels (42). It has been suggested that there may be an excess nitrite absorption from the gut in some patients as a result of abnormal bowel function (43).

The symptoms of Peutz-Jeghers syndrome (gastrointestinal polyposis and mucocutaneous pigmentation) may present in early childhood (43a). The increased risk of intestinal cancer associated with this syndrome also may be manifested in childhood (43b).

Hereditary hemorrhagic telangectasia (Osler-Weber-Rendu disease) may result in iron deficiency from gastrointestinal bleeding. Alterations of hemostasis (disseminated intravascular coagulation, platelet dysfunction, and Factor XI deficiency have been reported) (43c). An association between this disorder and von Willebrand's disease may exist (43d).

PANCREATIC DISEASE

Acute hemorrhagic pancreatitis may cause an acute anemia during the first week of the illness, which may result from hemodilution, intravascular coagulation, and blood losses (44). Leukocytosis with neutrophilia is a usual finding. Markedly elevated levels of fibrin split products usually suggest that a consumptive coagulopathy is present. A concomitant fall in platelet count also is common (45). High levels of methemalbumin are common in the ascitic fluid of individuals with hemorrhagic pancreatitis (46) and can be used to distinguish this disorder from nonhemorrhagic pancreatitis.

Cystic fibrosis may cause malabsorption, which produces the expected hematologic abnormalities. A specific pattern of anemia in association with edema and hypoproteinemia may be observed in some children with cystic fibrosis. This is found most commonly in children who have a low dietary nitrogen intake, such as patients who receive their protein primarily from breast milk or soybean formula (42b). The edema is secondary to hypoalbuminemia. The anemia responds to adequate dietary protein enrichment and pancreatic enzyme supplementation, but not to iron adminstration. Cystic fibrosis may also be associated with malabsorption of fat-soluble vitamins and consequent coagulopathy related to vitamin K deficiency. Vitamin E deficiency also may occur. This is manifested by a mild hemolytic anemia and abnormal red cell peroxide hemolysis as well as by hyperaggregation of platelets (42c).

LIVER DISEASE

Red Blood Cell Disturbances in Liver Disease

Anemia is common in acute and chronic liver disease and is apparently of diverse etiology (47).

The red blood cells in liver disease are frequently macrocytic, with mean corpuscular volumes often in the range of 100 to 110 μ^3. Target cells and acanthocytes or spur cells are frequently observed (48, 49). Stomatocytosis has been reported in alcoholic liver disease (50). These morphologic abnormalities appear to be in direct proportion to the increase in red cell membrane phospholipid and cholesterol that may accompany liver disease whenever any obstructive component is present (51–52a). Such membrane lipid alterations result in an increase in red cell membrane area, which accounts for the target cells and spur cells. Increased osmotic resistance is a consequence of this increased surface area.

A shortened red cell survival may be observed in some patients without evidence of blood loss (53, 53a). Acute hemolysis also has been observed in patients with acute liver disease who have glucose-6-phosphate dehydrogenase deficiency as well.

The exact mechanism by which red blood cell (RBC) survival is shortened is unclear. Erythrocytes from patients with active liver disease have an increased tendency toward Heinz body formation following incubation with an oxidant chemical such as acetylphenylhydrazine or sodium ascorbate. This increase in Heinz body formation is associated with increased instability of red cell–reduced glutathione, decreased hexose monophosphate shunt activity, and decreased glucose recycling through the hexose monophosphate shunt (54). It has not been possible to demonstrate any decreased activity of red cell glutathione reductase, glutathione peroxidase, glucose-6-phosphate dehydrogenase, 6-phosphogluconate dehydrogenase, or transketolase (55).

The exact significance of these metabolic alterations is speculative. Normal red cell metabolism appears to return within a few weeks following an insult to the liver. All the metabolic consequences of liver disease can be reproduced in normal intact red cells by their prolonged incubation in plasma from patients with active liver disease.

In patients with active liver disease, it may be wise to withhold any drug that potentially may represent an oxidant challenge to the RBC. Similar acquired abnormalities of hexose monophosphate shunt activity have been associated with drug-induced hemolysis in patients with uremia. Yawata and associates have reported that primaquine will result in an acceleration of hemolysis in such patients (56).

Coagulation Abnormalities in Liver Disease

Because the liver is involved to some extent in the synthesis of most of the coagulation factors, it is not unexpected that liver dysfunction would be associated with the presence of abnormal clotting studies (Table 52–1). In most instances, these abnormalities are a laboratory finding only. Less commonly, severe aberrations of clotting are seen, which result in a serious risk of bleeding.

Factor I (Fibrinogen). Fibrinogen levels are usually normal in liver disease. This may be accounted for by the fact that although fibrinogen synthesis has been demonstrated in liver cells, it is also produced in extrahepatic sites (57).

Low levels of fibrinogen may be observed in fulminant acute liver failure. Under these circumstances, it has been speculated that intravascular coagulation contributes to the coagulation disturbance by depletion of some of the clotting factors.

An increased catabolic rate of labeled fibrinogen has been noted in acute and chronic active hepatitis despite normal levels of plasma fibrinogen (58). In chronic active hepatitis, the rate of fibrinogen catabolism appears to correlate with the activity of the disease as assessed by variations in the plasma aminotransferase levels (58). This situation is less clear in acute hepatitis. Altered rates of fibrinogen catabolism may be the result of primary fibrinogenolysis or intravascular coagulation. In 1949, Ratnoff documented primary fibrinolysis in cirrhosis of the liver (59), although more recent studies have failed to note this finding consistently. Disseminated intravascular coagulation in liver disease is a complex and controversial area that is discussed later.

High levels of fibrinogen are occasionally observed in liver disease, mainly because fibrinogen is an acute phase reactant. Elevated levels of fibrinogen are commonly observed in obstructive jaundice, biliary cirrhosis, and hepatoma (60).

An abnormal fibrin monomer aggregate has been described in a number of patients with liver dysfunction (61). The appearance of clotting defects involving a prolongation of reptilase and thrombin clotting times, despite a normal fibrinogen concentration, should suggest that dysfibrinogenemia is present. An examination by SDS polyacrylamide gel electrophoresis of isolated fibrins from patients with liver disease has failed to detect any molecular or structural defect associated with the polypeptide chains of fibrinogen (62). An increase of sialic acid in the carbohydrate moiety of fibrinogen has been noted (63).

Factors II, VII, IX, and X (Vitamin K–Dependent Factors). The levels of vitamin K–dependent factors are frequently reduced in patients with liver disease (64). This appears to result primarily from impaired synthesis. When hepatocellular damage is minimal (e.g., in mild acute or chronic hepatitis, obstructive jaundice, or biliary cirrhosis), these factors may be normal or increased (65, 66).

In acute and chronic liver disease, Factor VII activity is generally reduced first and Factor IX activity last (67).

Of all the factors that may reflect hepatocellular damage, Factor VII appears to be the most sensitive. Factor VII is synthesized almost exclusively in the liver and has the most rapid half-life (about 2 hours) of all the liver-dependent factors. In a study of patients with acute liver failure, it appeared that all those with a Factor VII activity exceeding 8 per cent survived, whereas the others

Table 52–1. COAGULATION CHANGES IN ACUTE LIVER DISEASE*

Laboratory Test	Acute Infectious Hepatitis without Liver Failure	Acute Liver Failure Due to Infectious Hepatitis
Prothrombin time	Prolonged in 40 to 60% of patients	Greatly prolonged in all patients
Partial thromboplastin time	Prolonged in 10% of patients	Prolonged in all patients
Factors II, V, VII, and X	Mild to moderate reduction in 40% of patients	Rapid parallel decrease to very low values
Factor IX	Reduced in 15% of patients	Moderately reduced
Fibrinogen	Reduced in 15% of patients	Variable
Factor VIII	Normal	Greatly increased
Factor VIII antigen	Increased, returning to normal within 22 weeks in uncomplicated cases	Greatly increased
Factor XIII	Reduced in 25% of adult patients and in most children	Greatly reduced
Antithrombin III	Moderately reduced, with functional assay giving lower values than immunoassay	Heparin cofactor activity greatly reduced
Thrombin time	Slightly prolonged in 25% of patients	Greatly prolonged

*Modified from Lechner, K., Niessner, H., et al.: Coagulation abnormalities in liver disease. Semin. Thromb. Hemostas. 4:40, 1977.

died (75). Unfortunately, direct Factor VII assay is not available in many clinical laboratories, although some indication of Factor VII activity is implied from the prothrombin time.

Factor V. Factor V activity usually parallels the activity of Factors II and X in liver disease when the defect appears to be solely one of hepatic synthesis (68). If disseminated intravascular coagulation occurs in association with liver disease, the Factor V level may be significantly depressed. Markedly elevated levels of Factor V may be seen in obstructive liver disease, again as an acute phase–reactant phenomenon (65).

Factor VIII. Factor VIII procoagulant activity is generally normal or elevated in liver disease of all types (69). Factor VIII antigen activity follows a similar pattern except that antigenic activity will often exceed procoagulant activity by severalfold (70). The explanation for this finding is not known.

Factors XI and XII. Factor XI activity is usually normal in hepatocellular disease but may be decreased (71). The same is true of Factor XII activity. Both these factors may be elevated when the primary insult is obstructive (65).

Factor XIII (Fibrin-Stabilizing Factor). There are conflicting reports concerning Factor XIII levels in liver disease. Reports of low activity have been based primarily on results of clot solubility tests (72); however, when immunologic or radioisotopic techniques are used, more variable results are found (73).

Plasminogen. Plasminogen levels are commonly decreased in liver disease. In one study, such levels were depressed in 45 per cent of patients with liver disease but without hepatic failure, whereas all patients with hepatic failure demonstrated diminished plasminogen levels (68).

Antithrombin III. Antithrombin III levels are frequently decreased in patients with acute and chronic liver disease, whereas elevations may be observed in those with obstructive disease (65, 74).

Alpha$_2$-Macroglobulin. This inhibitor of thrombin and plasmin has been found to be elevated in liver cirrhosis.

Tests for Coagulation Disturbances. Screening tests for coagulation disturbances often fail to give any indication that liver dysfunction exists. Both the prothrombin time and partial thromboplastin time vary markedly from laboratory to laboratory with respect to their sensitivity in detecting mild to moderate depressions of factor levels.

Although most studies have failed to show good correlations between clotting tests and cholesterol, transaminase, or gamma globulin levels, the prothrombin time still appears to be the most convenient clotting test for monitoring liver function.

As noted earlier, Factor VIII antigen activity rises to very high levels with hepatocellular dysfunction. The level of Factor VIII antigen can, therefore, be used to determine whether chronic active hepatitis is present, since in uncomplicated acute hepatitis, antigen activity returns to normal within a few months.

Disseminated Intravascular Coagulation in Liver Disease

Patients with liver disease commonly manifest a spectrum of coagulation abnormalities that are highly suggestive of disseminated intravascular coagulation (DIC) (76). Findings consistent with DIC include hypofibrinogenemia, thrombocytopenia, increased fibrinogen catabolism, increased levels of fibrin degradation products, and depressed levels of other coagulation factors. This pattern of abnormalities is not specific for disseminated intravascular coagulation and may simply reflect the severity of the hepatocellular disease process. For example, fibrinogen levels may be depressed on a synthetic basis alone. Increased catabolism of fibrinogen may reflect distribution in extravascular spaces, such as formation of ascitic fluid or proteolysis by enzymes other than thrombin. Thrombocytopenia may occur for a variety of reasons and often is not present when other signs of DIC are present. Changes in the levels of Factors V and VIII are very variable and nonspecific. Because fibrin degradation products are cleared by the liver, severe liver dysfunction itself may cause elevations of these products without implicating DIC. Studies that report that heparin corrects DIC in liver disease also are open to some criticism because there is no evidence that the patients studied were in a steady state at the time of heparin therapy.

Whether true disseminated intravascular coagulation occurs in liver disease will most probably remain controversial for some time to come. As yet, no general recommendation for the use of heparin can be made. In the only controlled trial of heparin therapy in acute hepatic necrosis to date, there was no difference in the recovery rates with or without heparin (77). Fresh frozen plasma factor concentrates and platelet transfusions remain the treatments of choice. Care must be exerted when factor concentrates are used because, if contaminated by activated Factor X, they may cause diffuse thrombosis (78).

RENAL DISEASE

Renal disease may produce disturbances of red cells, white cells, platelets, and the coagulation factors. In many cases, the abnormalities that are found do not parallel the status of the renal function but rather reflect the activity of the disease process that results in renal dysfunction.

The Red Blood Cell in Renal Disease

ANEMIA

Anemia is a common finding in renal disease. The erythrocytes of patients with renal diseases are generally normochromic and normocytic without any distinguishing morphologic characteristics. Occasionally, scalloped or burr cells are observed, usually in association with uremia due to specific causes or related to specific syndrome complexes such as the hemolytic-uremic syndrome. In diseases associated with microangiopathic hemolytic anemia, red cell fragmentation is common. This may be observed in patients with malignant hypertension, renal cortical necrosis, polyarteritis nodosa, the hemolytic-uremic syndrome, systemic lupus erythematosus, and thrombotic thrombocytopenic purpura.

The anemia of renal disease can have many causes, including a decreased rate of red blood cell production (the "anemia of chronic disorders"), a shortened red blood survival, and nutritional factors.

In renal disease, unlike many other chronic disease states, there is a close correlation between erythrocyte mass and erythrocyte survival (79). This implies that shortening of red cell survival has an important role in the development of anemia in these patients. About 70 per cent of patients with renal disease have a shortened red cell survival related to a host of potential alterations. These cells demonstrate increased mechanical fragility, autohemolysis, diminished deformability, and a variety of metabolic defects (80, 81).

Decreased red cell production is, however, the major cause of the anemia of chronic renal failure. A deficiency of erythropoietin production is probably the primary cause (81a, 81b), but the toxic suppression of hematopoiesis also is certainly a contributing factor. Patients with acute or chronic renal failure due to nephrectomy can maintain normal or even increased erythropoietin production (81c).

The red cells of patients with uremia have been found to have either a normal or an increased rate of glucose utilization. The increased glycolytic rate appears to be primarily the result of the associated hyperphosphatemia because inorganic phosphorus is a well-recognized stimulant of red cell glucose utilization (82).

In uremic states, Hb A_1 is elevated (82a). The increased Hb A_1 level in uremia correlates with the level of BUN and results from the carbamylation of hemoglobin by urea-derived cyanate. Most interestingly, the carbamylated hemoglobin level integrates the average BUN levels—a situation analogous to that seen in glycosylation of hemoglobin in diabetes (82a).

A circulating inhibitor of red cell metabolism accumulates in some, but not all, uremic patients. This inhibitor diminishes recycling of glucose through the hexose monophosphate shunt (80), a defect that may be clinically important. There are several reports of severe hemolytic disease in uremic patients given sulfa drugs. In patients with renal disease who have undergone splenectomy, Heinz bodies are commonly observed. Because of this problem, caution in the use of oxidant drugs is advised in those with azotemia (83). This decreased shunt activity may be secondary to a metabolic defect within the shunt itself or to a block within the main glycolytic pathway. When erythrocytes from patients with renal insufficiency are stressed with oxidant compounds such as sodium ascorbate, glucose consumption and lactate formation are abnormally increased, whereas lactate:pyruvate ratios are abnormally diminished. Red cell glycolytic intermediates—including fructose-1,6-diphosphate, glyceraldehyde-3-phosphate, 3-phosphoglycerate, phosphoenol pyruvate, and pyruvate—markedly accumulate. No increase in 2-phosphoglycerate occurs, suggesting that inefficient phosphoglyceromutase activity may underlie this defective glucose reutilization (80).

Adenosine triphosphate (ATP) levels are significantly increased in uremic red blood cells. This may not result solely from elevated serum phosphorus levels because red cells from uremic patients incubated in artificially low phosphate medium demonstrate an increased ATP synthetic activity (84). Pyruvate kinase activities are significantly increased in uremic, as opposed to normal, red cells, suggesting the presence of a younger red blood cell population (84).

Red blood cell 2,3-diphosphoglycerate levels are increased as well for similar reasons (85). This results in a significant shift to the right in the hemoglobin oxygen dissociation curve, favoring oxygen release. Following dialysis with correction of acidosis and hyperphosphatemia, there is a sharp rise in arterial pH and a fall in red cell 2,3-diphosphoglycerate levels. Both these changes result in an acute change in the oxygen dissociation characteristics of the red cells. Whether this produces any physiologic impairment following dialysis is unclear (84).

Other incidental causes of hemolysis may be observed during hemodialysis. It has been demonstrated that contaminants such as copper, nitrate, and chloramines in hemodialysis baths may cause varying degrees of hemolysis (86–88).

Anemia associated with megaloblastic changes in the bone marrow is not uncommon in chronic renal failure. This is usually due to folate deficiency (89) caused by poor dietary intake, hemodialysis, peritoneal dialysis, or the effects of immunosuppressive drugs. In addition, defective protein-mediated folate transport may be present (90). Uremic serum may contain an increased folic acid–binding protein (90). Folate deficiency is usually suspected when large numbers of macro-ovalocytes are seen in association with hypersegmentation of polymorphonuclear leukocytes on the peripheral blood smear.

Treatment may or may not be needed for the anemia associated with renal disease. In chronic renal disease, anemia is partially compensated for by improved oxygen unloading as a result of the high red cell content of 2,3-diphosphoglycerate. Androgenic steroids may cause an increase in hemoglobin concentration by increasing the rate of erythropoiesis (91). The response, however, may be in part erythropoietin-mediated because little rise in hemoglobin concentration occurs in anephric patients undergoing androgen treatment (92). The possible benefits of androgen therapy must be weighed against the side effects of this class of drugs.

POLYCYTHEMIA

Erythrocytosis is a well-recognized complication of hydronephrosis (93) and has occasionally been noted in association with chronic glomerulonephritis, pyelonephritis, nephrosclerosis, and the nephrotic syndrome in adults (94). The cause of the elevation of red cell mass in most patients appears to be erythropoietin-mediated.

The White Blood Cell in Renal Disease

Azotemia and uremia, per se, appear to have relatively little effect on white blood cell function. Granulocytopenia is common during hemodialysis (95) and appears to be due to a transient sequestration of granulocytes in the pulmonary vascular bed followed by a later release back into the circulation. Following hemodialysis there is a transient augmentation of granulocyte adherence that coincides with the time of pulmonary vascular bed sequestration (96). The adherence augmenting factor in the plasma of dialyzed patients is heat-stable. Craddock and co-workers feel that this factor is complement-activated by contact with the dialysis coil (97). It should be noted, however, that the use of 5-hydroxy-indole-3-acetic acid, a complement inhibitor, fails to block the granulocytopenia of dialysis (98).

Neutropenia as a result of folate deficiency may be present in patients with renal failure. The cause of neutrophil nuclear hypersegmentation associated with uremia is unknown and need not be ascribed to folate deficiency.

Coagulation Abnormalities in Renal Disease

Patients with uremia may have variable changes in certain of the coagulation factors. Among the most common abnormalities observed are mild to moderate depressions of Factors V, VII, IX, and X (99, 100). These are related to the high incidence of hepatic dysfunction in patients with uremia or vitamin K deficiency (24). The level of fibrinogen is regularly elevated because it is an acute phase reactant (101–103). Increased fibrinogen turnover has been demonstrated in experimental models (104), and excessive fibrin degradation products have been found in the urine and serum of uremic patients (105). When a decrease in one or more consumable clotting factors (Factors I, II, V, or VIII) also is present, this may signify the existence of consumptive coagulopathy (99–100a). Because fibrin deposition may occur in the absence of such a coagulopathy, it is often helpful to determine whether high-molecular-weight fibrin degradation products are present in the urine and serum. If found only in the urine, such products are probably derived from the dissolution of fibrin deposits in the kidneys. If demonstrable simultaneously in the urine and serum, their presence indicates renal injury because such degradation products cannot be demonstrated in the urine of patients with streptokinase-induced fibrinolysis who have no renal disease (106, 106a). Fibrin degradation products in the urine and serum usually indicate active renal disease, although patients with renal disease may have other reasons for this finding. Fibrin degradation products may also result from concomitant liver disease or from an external shunt used for hemodialysis (30). Urinary fibrinolytic activity has been found to be either diminished or absent in renal failure, and inhibitors of urokinase-induced plasminogen activation are demonstrable (106).

The nephrotic syndrome is often accompanied by changes in a number of coagulation factors (107). Increased levels of fibrinogen, Factor VIII, and the Factors VII–X complex are commonly present (108). A prolonged partial thromboplastin time is frequently observed and is usually due to a decrease in the plasma level of Factor IX (109). Factor IX is consistently found in urine containing more than 10 g of protein per 24 hours in patients with the nephrotic syndrome (110). Plasma levels of Factor IX rarely fall below 10 per cent, and clinical bleeding is unusual. With clearing of proteinuria on corticosteroid therapy, the levels of Factor IX rise. Factors II and VII also have been identified in considerable quantities in the urine of patients with the nephrotic syndrome, despite the finding of normal levels of these factors in the plasma (111). This suggests that the loss of some coagulation factors into the urine can be fully compensated for by an increased rate of synthesis. A prolonged partial thromboplastin time may also be due to a low level of Hageman factor (Factor XII) (112). Hageman factor has a molecular weight of approximately 75,000 daltons, similar to that of albumin, and losses into the urine are to be expected (113). Although Factor XII levels may decrease below 10 per cent, as with the congenital deficiency of this factor, bleeding is not a problem. Patients with the nephrotic syndrome appear to have a substantially higher risk of thromboembolic complications (106), although the exact reasons for this are still mainly unknown. Enhanced platelet function characterized by hyperaggregability has been observed (114). An identical defect is seen in diabetics (115) and in many patients with advanced cirrhosis of the liver (116). Such changes may relate to alterations in plasma lipid fractions and are discussed in detail in the chapter on platelet abnormalities (see Chapter 42). The coagulation defects associated with the nephrotic syndrome have been reviewed by Kaufmann and colleagues (428).

Whether therapy directed toward prevention of fibrin deposition within the kidney is of benefit to patients with certain forms of glomerulonephritis remains uncertain. Kincaid-Smith has employed a combination of an anticoagulant, dipyridamole, and cyclophosphamide in a series of patients with membranoproliferative glomerulonephritis (117, 118). A similar approach was reported by Robson and associates, substituting azathioprine for cyclophosphamide (119). In both studies it was suggested that these therapies produced improvement in the patients' clinical course. The concept of anticoagulation therapy for these disorders has been reviewed (120). The pathophysiology and management of the hemolytic-uremic syndrome are discussed in Chapters 16 and 42.

Platelet Abnormalities in Renal Disease

Mild thrombocytopenia occurs in approximately 25 per cent of patients with acute renal failure and 10 per cent of those with chronic renal disease (121). The thrombocytopenia is most likely due to impaired production because platelet life span in uremia is generally normal (102). Platelet function is abnormal in patients with renal failure. The standardized Ivy bleeding time is usually prolonged and generally correlates with the clinical tendency to bleeding in these patients (122). Platelet adhesion and platelet factor 3 availability are diminished in acute and chronic uremia (123). Impaired aggregation of platelet-rich plasma in the presence of adenosine diphosphate (124), epinephrine (125), thrombin (125), and collagen (125) has been observed by various workers.

Platelet functional abnormalities have not been shown to be due to an intrinsic platelet defect, as dialysis quickly reverses these changes, and incubation of normal platelets in uremic plasma promptly induces functional aberrations. Rather, platelet dysfunction appears to be due to the interaction of intrinsically normal platelets with various abnormal dialyzable metabolites found in the plasma of the uremic patient (126). Urea and creatinine, when elevated, can reproduce some of these findings (126). Phenols (101) and guanidinosuccinic acid (127), which accumulate in the plasma of uremic patients, can also account for platelet functional abnormalities. These findings are discussed in detail in Chapter 42.

Several hereditary disorders have been reported in which quantitative or qualitative platelet abnormalities have been observed in association with nephritis. In 1972, Epstein and associates described a family with hereditary macrothrombopathia, nephritis, and deafness (128). The renal pathologic findings are identical with those described in patients with classic hereditary nephritis and nerve deafness (Alport's syndrome) and consist of a sclerosing and proliferative glomerulonephritis and interstitial nephritis with fibrosis. Members of these families have large platelets, prolonged bleeding times, defective platelet factor 3 activity, and defective platelet aggregation to adenosine diphosphate, collagen, and epinephrine. Thrombocytopenia also is present in this autosomal dominant disorder (128a). A similar disorder, but with normal platelet function, has been described by Eckstein and associates (129). In these families, platelet survival studies have been normal.

ENDOCRINE DISORDERS

Disturbances in endocrine balance tend to produce real but relatively mild hematologic abnormalities. The most thoroughly evaluated of these abnormalities are those caused by thyroid disorders.

Thyroid

Thyroid hormone appears to exhibit many hematologic effects (Table 52–2), with the most impressive being the effect on erythropoiesis. Although thyroid hormones slightly stimulate erythropoiesis in vitro (130), the anemia due to thyroid hormone deficiency is a secondary finding. Most workers have correlated the erythropoietic effects of thyroid hormones with their calorigenic properties. Thyroid hormone increases oxygen consumption, which results in increased renal production of erythropoietin and stimulation of erythropoiesis. However, the erythropoietic stimulatory effect may, in fact, occur independently of erythropoietin. The administration of triiodothyronine (T_3) and thyroxine (T_4) to nephrectomized rats produces an increase in bone marrow erythroid precursors (131).

The anemia of hypothyroidism is usually normochromic and normocytic and occasionally is mildly macrocytic (131a). Small numbers of irreg-

Table 52–2. HEMATOLOGIC EFFECTS OF THYROID HORMONE

↑ Thyroid Hormone	↓ Thyroid Hormone
↑ PRBC* volume	↓ PRBC volume
Variable effect on RBCs:	↑ Or normal MCV; spiculated RBCs
↑ Glucose utilization and hexose monophosphate shunt activity	↑ O₂ affinity
↓ Levels RBC glutathione, reduced	↓ 2,3-Diphosphoglycerate
↑ Red cell 2,3-diphosphoglycerate	↓ RBC Na⁺
↓ O₂ affinity	↓ Platelet adhesion
↑ Diphosphoglycerate mutase activity	↓ (Slight) platelet aggregability
↑ Glyceraldehyde-3-phosphate dehydrogenase	↓ Factor VIII activity
↑ Glucose-6-phosphate activity	↑ Fibrinolytic activity
↓ RBC carbonic anhydrase	↑ Plasminogen
↓ RBC zinc	↑ Plasminogen activation
↑ RBC Na⁺⁺	↓ Plasminogen activation
↑ (Slight) platelet turnover	↓ Capillary fragility
↑ Platelet adhesion	↓ Factors VIII, VII, IX, XI activity
↑ Platelet aggregability	
↑ Factor VIII activity	
↓ Plasminogen activation	
↑ Capillary fragility	

*Packed red blood cell

ularly contracted red blood cells may be noted on the peripheral blood smear (Fig. 52–3) (132). Red cell survival is normal, and ferrokinetic studies demonstrate a decreased rate of iron clearance. In adults with hypothyroidism, an unusually high incidence of iron deficiency (133) and pernicious anemia is found (134). A single confounding case of erythrocytosis in association with hypothyroidism has been described (135).

Somewhat opposite findings are noted in uncomplicated hyperthyroidism. Anemia is rare, and red blood cell indices are normal. There is usually an increase in red blood cell mass, which does not result in significant rises in hemoglobin concentration because a similar elevation of plasma volume also occurs (136). Erythrocyte survival is normal or mildly diminished, especially in thyrotoxic children (137). Peripheral blood and bone marrow lymphocyte counts may be increased.

Thyroid hormone may play some role in the regulation of red cell metabolism. Thyroxine has been reported to increase red cell glycolysis (138). Hexose monophosphate shunt activity may increase in the presence of triiodothyronine (139). The activity of glucose-6-phosphate dehydrogenase is consistently elevated in thyrotoxicosis, whereas normal levels are found in most cases of mild hyperthyroidism (140). Glutathione levels are usually depressed in hyperthyroidism. Thyroid hormone may affect the activities of several other red cell enzymes. This hormone stimulates diphosphoglycerate mutase and glyceraldehyde-3-phosphate dehydrogenase (141). These effects may be the cause of the elevated levels of red cell

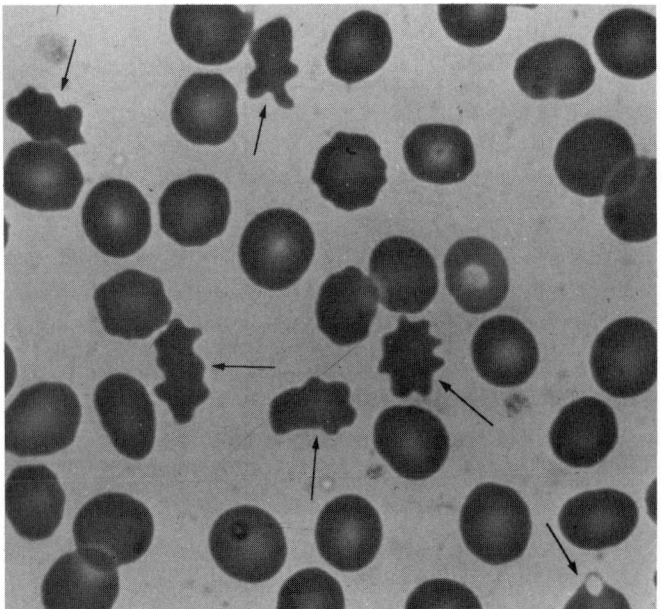

Figure 52–3. Red blood cell morphology in hypothyroidism. (From Wardrop, C., and Hutchinson, H. E.: Lancet 2:1243, 1969.)

2,3-diphosphoglycerate that are seen in patients with hyperthyroidism and that result in a decreased whole blood oxygen affinity and a shift to the right in the hemoglobin oxygen dissociation curve (142). Opposite effects are seen in hypothyroidism. Carbonic anhydrase activity of erythrocytes is diminished in hyperthyroidism and increased in hypothyroidism. Because red cell zinc is almost exclusively contained in carbonic anhydrase, hyperthyroidism will result in a decrease in total red cell zinc levels (143).

The red blood cells of patients with hyperthyroidism may have increased osmotic resistance (144). Red cell sodium concentration is significantly increased in hyperthyroidism, and decreased sodium pump activity may be present (145).

Neutropenia may be present in approximately 5 per cent of children with hyperthyroidism (145a). The mechanism of this is unclear, although some patients will demonstrate antineutrophil antibodies (145b).

Multiple effects on platelets and blood coagulation factors may occur in thyroid disease states. Marked hyperthyroidism may reduce platelet survival (146). Egeberg reported a patient with hypothyroidism who had a prolonged bleeding time and a low Factor VIII activity, similar to findings in von Willebrand's disease (147).

Simone and associates reported patients with hypothyroidism who had multiple coagulation factor deficiencies (148). A diminished platelet responsiveness to epinephrine and a low platelet adhesiveness may be present as well (149). Impressively low levels of Factor VIII occasionally occur, with milder depressions of Factors VII, IX, and XI being found either singly or in combination (149). In hypothyroidism, increased plasma fibrinolytic activity may result from an elevation in plasma plasminogen and a decrease in an inhibitor of plasminogen activation (150, 150a). This may account for the mild to moderate rise in fibrinogen and fibrin split products occasionally found in patients with hypothyroidism (149).

Adrenal Gland

Adrenal cortical steroid hormones appear to have a stimulatory effect on erythropoiesis. In Addison's disease, the adrenal insufficiency may cause mild to moderate anemia, probably secondary to reduced basal metabolism. In most cases, a decrease in plasma volume masks the decreased red cell mass. Following treatment of adrenal insufficiency, the plasma volume corrects quickly, whereas the red cell mass responds over several weeks. The usual effect of treatment is therefore a prompt fall in hemoglobin concentration followed by a gradual rise (151).

Erythrocytosis may occur in Cushing's syndrome, but in most cases the reported increase has been slight.

A variety of effects on leukocytes occur following steroid administration or endogenous overproduction of a steroid. These include granulocytosis, reduced lymphocyte count, involution of lymphatic tissue, and a decrease in peripheral blood eosinophils and monocytes. In Addison's disease, neutropenia, eosinophilia, and lymphocytosis appear (152).

Glucocorticosteroids affect lymphoid cells in many ways. The effects, however, are species-specific. The mouse, rat, hamster, and rabbit are steroid-sensitive; many of their lymphoid cells are easily lysed by steroids, and in these species, steroids inhibit antibody production. Human, simian, and guinea pig lymphoid cells are not easily lysed by steroids; in these species, it is difficult to demonstrate profound steroid inhibition of antibody production (153). Cellular metabolism, including nucleic acid synthesis and glucose uptake, is inhibited.

The mechanism by which endogenous or exogenous steroids lower the number of circulating eosinophils is unknown.

Testes and Ovaries

Hematologic abnormalities are rare in association with gonadal dysfunction. This does not mean that the gonadal hormones play no role in hematopoiesis. Androgens stimulate erythropoiesis, whereas estrogens, in general, depress red cell production. Castration of the adult male results in a definite decrease in the red cell mass (154). In disorders associated with androgen excess, such as Cushing's syndrome and congenital adrenal hyperplasia, the hemoglobin concentration may exceed normal values. Exogenous androgen administration may cause polycythemia and may also increase red cell 2,3-diphosphoglycerate (155). Androgens appear to stimulate erythropoiesis by increasing erythropoietin production as well as by having a direct effect on the bone marrow stem cells.

The normal menstrual cycle is associated with hematologic variations. Deliveria-Papadopoulos and associates described cyclic variations in endogenous carbon monoxide production during the menstrual cycle of fertile women and suggested that heme catabolism was increased during the progesterone phase (156). It has been known for some time that reticulocyte counts are increased during the late progestational phase (157). A cyclic variation in erythrocyte deformability also occurs during the menstrual cycle (158). The relationship between decreased red cell deformability, reticulocytosis, and increased heme catabolism is speculative. A similar decrease in deformability occurs during the last trimester of pregnancy and with the use of oral contraceptives (159, 160).

Pregnancy causes a rise in several of the coagulation factors, including Factors I, VII, VIII, IX, and X (161). Carriers of classic hemophilia and von Willebrand's disease may have significantly increased Factor VIII activity during pregnancy (161). Plasma fibrinolytic activity diminishes during pregnancy.

Pituitary

The hematologic effects of pituitary disease are usually the consequence of the action of the trophic hormone on target endocrine organ function. For example, anemia is common in patients with hypopituitarism (161a). This normochromic, normocytic anemia is associated with findings of lymphocytosis and eosinophilia, which indicate that this effect of hypopituitarism results from adrenal insufficiency. Erythropoietin production may be diminished as a consequence of a lower metabolic rate.

Growth hormone may play an important role in erythropoiesis. This hormone simulates erythropoiesis directly and indirectly by increased production of erythropoietin. The red cell count may fall with isolated growth hormone deficiency (162). Erythrocyte glucose-6-phosphate dehyrogenase activity is low in hypopituitarism and rises with growth hormone administration (163). Growth hormone depresses erythrocyte glycolysis (164).

PULMONARY DISEASE

Hypoxia may result from a wide variety of pulmonary disorders. This, in turn, results in a form of secondary polycythemia and compensatory shifts in the hemoglobin oxygen dissociation curve due to an increase in the red cell content of 2,3-diphosphoglycerate. Rarely, the polycythemia results in a state of extreme hyperviscosity and decreased tissue blood flow. Other than polycythemia, the hematologic findings of specific pulmonary disorders tend to be unique to those disorders.

Idiopathic Pulmonary Hemosiderosis (IPH)

This is an uncommon chronic disease usually affecting children and young adults. However, the age of onset may be as early as the newborn period (165). IPH is characterized by recurrent intrapulmonary hemorrhages and may result in hemoptysis and pulmonary insufficiency. The hematologic manifestation of this disorder is iron deficiency anemia.

The etiology of IPH is not known. A hereditary or familial tendency has been suggested. An immunologic cause seems likely because other findings that are occasionally found include a positive Coombs' test, the presence of cold agglutinins, and an increased number of mast and plasma cells in the lungs. Various etiologic hypotheses such as congenital weakness or fragility of the capillaries, milk allergy, and abnormal growth and function of the alveolar epithelial cells all have been suggested (166).

The most helpful clinical signs of IPH are iron deficiency anemia and recurrent or chronic cough, hemoptysis, dyspnea, wheezing, and often cyanosis. Any single feature may be present without the others. For example, the only clinical sign on occasion is iron deficiency anemia (167). Pulmonary symptoms may be present without radiologic findings and vice versa. When pulmonary symptoms are predominant, there may be associated fever, tachycardia, tachypnea, leukocytosis, an elevated sedimentation rate, and, occasionally, abdominal pain (168). Roentgenographic abnormalities vary from minimal transient infiltrates to massive parenchymal involvement with atelectasis, emphysema, and hilar adenopathy (169, 170).

The anemia reflects an iron deficiency state, as a result of excessive accumulation of iron in the lungs. This iron is usually sequestered in alveolar macrophages and is largely unavailable for new red cell formation. With time, however, the iron is eventually lost from the lungs (171). In some patients, iron administration fails to correct the anemia. This is usually a reflection of inadequate heme synthesis as a result of the anemia of chronic disease. Immune hemolytic anemia may occur, and cold agglutinins are frequently present. Eosinophilia is found in 15 to 20 per cent of children with idiopathic pulmonary hemosiderosis.

A diagnosis of IPH may be made by the finding of siderophages in the gastric aspirate. Siderophages will stain positive with the Prussian-blue reaction. If the diagnosis of IPH is seriously being considered, it may be necessary to perform a lung biopsy. Typical findings include alveolar epithelial hyperplasia, degeneration with excessive shedding of cells, large numbers of siderocytes, varying amounts of interstitial fibrosis and mast cell accumulation, elastic fiber degeneration, and sclerotic vascular changes (172). Electron microscopy has been reported to show no evidence of subendothelial deposits or basement membrane lesions (173). No evidence for localization of IgG, IgM, B_{1c}, C1q, or fibrinogen has been found (173). Needle aspiration or needle biopsy also may provide a diagnosis (174), although some workers have considered these to be hazardous.

The treatment of IPH continues to be controversial. Steroid therapy will sometimes produce a remission of disease activity (175). Immunosuppressive therapy may be useful, but the results of such treatment are unpredictable (176). In 1962, Heiner and associates reported the presence of precipitating antibodies to a small number of cow's milk antigens in the sera of several children with IPH (177). Reversal of symptoms followed withdrawal of cow's milk, and recurrence was noted with reinstitution of dietary cow's milk. Although many, if not most, children with IPH fail to show these responses, a trial of removal of cow's milk from the diet is appropriate in most instances (178). This should be continued for 2 to 3 months.

Pulmonary Hemosiderosis from Other Causes

Clinical findings of hypochromic and microcytic anemia and pulmonary infiltrates may be seen in association with glomerulonephritis (Goodpasture's syndrome), collagen vascular disease (especially periarteritis nodosa), Wegener's granulomatosis, and occasionally systemic lupus erythematosus (179–182). A similar presentation in association with anaphylactoid purpura has been noted.

Hematologic Findings in Other Pulmonary Disorders

Sarcoidosis usually does not cause specific hematologic disturbances, although a higher than average incidence of blood group antigen A has been reported in this disorder (183, 194). The significance of this is not known, but the altered immune response of these patients (184a) and an association of sarcoidosis and hemolytic anemia (185) and immune thrombocytopenia (186–186b) suggest that sarcoidosis represents a generalized autoimmune disorder and that it may be related to abnormal balance of T cell subset production. Severe thrombocytopenia may occur in subjects with sarcoidosis (186c).

Eosinophilia may be observed in a variety of pulmonary disorders including asthma, Löffler's syndrome, tropical pulmonary eosinophilia, polyarteritis nodosa, and sarcoidosis.

Patients with cystic fibrosis demonstrate a significant impairment in erythropoietic response to hypoxemia (186d). There is neither an appropriate increase in hemoglobin level nor an adequate shift in the red cell oxygen affinity curve. Disturbances in erythropoietin regulation as in the anemia of chronic disease and iron deficiency appear to be the principle causes of the relative anemia in children with cystic fibrosis (186e).

COLLAGEN VASCULAR DISEASES AND THE ANEMIA OF CHRONIC DISORDERS

The "anemia of chronic disorders" and its concomitant reticuloendothelial siderosis are associated with a wide variety of illnesses, including cancer, lymphoma, collagen vascular disease, severe tissue injuries, renal failure, and infectious processes (187). Unfortunately, each of these disorders may be associated with multiple sources of anemia, including blood loss, hemolysis, and drug suppression. A diagnosis of the anemia of chronic disorders should not be made without consideration of other potential causes.

The anemia of chronic disorders is usually mild in degree. It is characterized by decreased plasma iron levels, decreased total iron-binding capacity of the plasma, decreased saturation of transferrin by iron, decreased numbers of bone marrow sideroblasts, and normal or increased levels of reticuloendothelial iron (188) (Table 52–3).

The anemia, when it occurs, develops slowly over a month or more until a plateau is reached. The hematocrit concentration rarely falls below 30 per cent in adults and the low 20 per cent range in children. The anemia is most frequently normochromic and normocytic, with a low or normal percentage of reticulocytes. Occasionally, hypochromic and normocytic anemia is observed, and, less frequently, hypochromia and microcytosis are found (187). In contrast to the situation in iron deficiency anemia, the infrequent microcytosis of chronic disorders is rarely proportional to the degree of anemia associated with these disorders.

The pathophysiologic processes that cause the anemia of chronic disorders are complex. At least three factors are commonly operative: shortened red cell survival, impaired marrow response to anemia, and impaired flow of iron from reticuloendothelial cells to the bone marrow.

The shortening of red cell survival is certainly not seen in the anemia of all chronic disorders (189). The autologous survival may be mildly shortened, but when the red blood cells of an affected individual are transfused into normal recipients, the survival is normal (190). The nature of the extracorpuscular defect has not been defined.

The bone marrow fails to develop an erythropoietic response to the anemia. Although normal bone marrow can increase red blood cell produc-

Table 52–3. FINDINGS IN THE ANEMIA OF CHRONIC DISORDERS AND IRON DEFICIENCY

Factor	Chronic Disease	Iron Deficiency
Plasma iron	↓	↓
Iron binding capacity	↓	↑
Transferrin saturation	↓	↓
Marrow sideroblasts	↓	↓
Reticuloendothelial iron	Normal or ↑	↓
Free erythrocyte protoporphyrin	↑	↑
Serum ferritin	Normal	↓

tion six- to eightfold, the maximum response in the anemia of chronic disorders is one to two times normal.

Studies of the release of erythropoietin have produced conflicting results. In some cases, there appears to be defective production or release of erythropoietin (191).

A response to erythropoietin has been noted in rats having chronic inflammatory reactions (192). Cobalt, which acts via the production of cellular hypoxia and release of erythropoietin, improves the anemia of infection in dogs and humans (193, 194). It should be noted, however, that some resistance to the effects of erythropoietin is seen and probably relates to the block of iron release to transferrin (195).

An impairment of iron release from the reticuloendothelial system accounts for the iron-deficient type of erythropoiesis seen in these disorders. This block in iron utilization is most easily demonstrated by iron kinetic studies in which plasma iron clearance is normal but the presence of iron in circulating red blood cells (utilization) is markedly diminished (196, 196a). The consequences of this are a fall in plasma iron levels, a decrease in marrow sideroblasts, and a rise in red cell protoporphyrin concentration, all in the presence of normal or increased reticuloendothelial iron.

Iron absorption in the anemia of chronic disorders may be either normal or diminished. Diminished absorption is not due to defective uptake of iron into intestinal cells but rather results from an inability to release intracellular iron (197). In any event, sufficient iron is absorbed to maintain adequate reticuloendothelial stores.

The reduced levels of plasma transferrin so commonly noted may be due to diminished production or to increased binding to iron-overloaded reticuloendothelial cells (187). The latter cause may, in fact, be more important because transferrin levels tend to increase in the anemia of chronic disorders if iron deficiency develops.

There has been a common clinical impression that the degree of anemia associated with inflammation may vary with the specific cause of the inflammation. If the cause of the inflammation is infectious, this may not be true. Subjects with meningitis, cellulitis, mastoiditis, septic arthritis, osteomyelitis, bacterial endocarditis, and streptococcal pharyngitis all experience a mean fall in hemoglobin concentration of 1.8 g per dl during active inflammation over a 6-day period (197a).

Diagnosis of the anemia of chronic disorders is based on the typical findings of a low plasma iron level, low plasma transferrin concentration, and a low percentage of marrow sideroblasts despite normal or increased reticuloendothelial iron levels (see Table 52–4). A bone marrow examination is not critical in establishing the diagnosis if a serum ferritin determination is obtained because the serum ferritin level is normal or increased in the anemia of chronic disorders (198), even in the presence of hypoferremia. Plasma copper levels are usually increased.

There is no specific therapy for this anemia other than treatment of the basic disease. Iron therapy is of no value, since when given either orally or by intramuscular injection, the iron is first cleared in the reticuloendothelial system. Intravenous iron infusions would most probably improve marrow iron delivery but are neither practical nor therapeutically indicated for this problem. Occasionally, a patient with the anemia of chronic disorders is also iron-deficient, particularly one with rheumatoid arthritis (199), in whom gastrointestinal bleeding secondary to aspirin therapy is common. Such a patient may respond partially to iron therapy.

The reader who is interested in a comprehensive review of the anemia of chronic disorders is referred to Hansen's 1983 report (199a).

Hematologic Aspects of Collagen Vascular Disease

Many of the hematologic manifestations of the various collagen vascular diseases are similar. However, the characteristics that are unique to each syndrome will be emphasized in this section.

RHEUMATOID ARTHRITIS

The most common causes of anemia in rheumatoid arthritis are the anemia of chronic disorders and iron deficiency. These two causes can be difficult to distinguish because of overlap in many of the laboratory findings. In both cases, the serum iron level is depressed, and free erythrocyte protoporphyrin levels are elevated. The serum ferritin level may be normal in the iron deficiency associated with rheumatoid arthritis (199).

A high incidence of iron deficiency is seen in children with rheumatoid arthritis. This may be due to the ingestion of large quantities of aspirin or in part to defective iron absorption. Koerper and associates found that a serum ferritin concentration below 25 ng per ml was useful in predicting a response to oral iron, but a value above 25 ng per ml did not preclude a response (199). Because laboratory tests often fail to distinguish between iron deficiency and the anemia of chronic disorders, a clinical trial of iron may be necessary.

Occasionally, patients with juvenile rheumatoid arthritis develop macrocytic anemia (200). Although abnormal vitamin B_{12} metabolism has been suggested as a cause, this is not seen in children. Folate metabolism may, however, be abnormal. Some children with rheumatoid arthritis have diminished plasma and red cell folate levels (201). Increased folic acid plasma clearance and reduced protein binding also have been observed (202).

A few patients have had mild shortening of red cell survival as a result of an extracorpuscular defect (203). More severe hemolytic anemia is much less common than in other collagen vascular diseases. Erythroid aplasia has been reported in a child with juvenile rheumatoid arthritis (203a) that was responsive to steroids. Circulating inhibitors of erythropoiesis also have been noted (203b).

Leukocytosis and neutrophilia are common during acute flare-ups of juvenile rheumatoid arthritis; however, this is uncommon in the adult form of the disorder. Neutrophil chemotaxis may be mildly diminished (204). Phagocytosis is normal or mildly impaired (205). Nitroblue tetrazolium (NBT) dye reduction may be increased during active phases of this disease (206). These minimal alterations of white cell function do not produce any clinical disturbances. Wound healing, for example, is normal even after surgery in patients who have not been receiving high-dose corticosteroids (207). A peripheral blood eosinophil count greater than 5 per cent has been noted in slightly over 50 per cent of children with juvenile rheumatoid arthritis (207a). Some will also demonstrate basophilia and plasmacytoid lymphocytes (207b, 207c).

The symptoms and signs of rheumatoid arthritis can be very similar to those of acute lymphatic leukemia, including fever, joint pain, and anemia. Therefore, the diagnosis of acute lymphatic leukemia should be excluded before treatment of rheumatoid arthritis is instituted.

Elevated platelet counts are seen in many patients with juvenile rheumatoid arthritis. No consistent functional defects have been described.

FELTY'S SYNDROME

Felty originally described the triad of rheumatoid arthritis, splenomegaly, and neutropenia in 1924 (208). Whether cases of Felty's syndrome occur with juvenile rheumatoid arthritis is unclear. Splenomegaly is seen in about 20 per cent of all children with rheumatoid arthritis, especially in those with the acute extra-articular exacerbations of this disease. However, this alone is not suggestive of Felty's syndrome.

The neutropenia of Felty's syndrome is not a consequence of hypersplenism per se because only 60 per cent of adults who undergo splenectomy experience resolution of their neutropenia (209). In some cases, the bone marrow demonstrates granulocyte arrest. Lower than normal levels of granulocyte colony–stimulating activity have been reported infrequently (210). The neutropenia of Felty's serum may represent, in part, an immunologic phenomenon because IgG antibodies directed against neutrophils have been observed in the sera of patients with rheumatoid arthritis (211).

The neutropenia may be associated with serious infections. Splenectomy may be indicated under these circumstances because a favorable response may be observed. This response is variable. The most consistent result is a reduction of serum granulocyte–binding immunoglobulin (211a). An alternative to splenectomy is the use of lithium carbonate. Some patients will exhibit increased peripheral granulocyte counts with the administration of lithium carbonate in sufficient doses to raise the serum lithium concentration above 0.5 mg per liter (212, 213).

SYSTEMIC LUPUS ERYTHEMATOSUS

Anemia is the most common hematologic abnormality in lupus erythematosus (214, 215). The causes of anemia in this disease are multiple, although the anemia of chronic disorders is probably most common.

Acquired immune hemolytic anemia may greatly precede the onset of active lupus. Although a positive antiglobulin test is common (either to gamma globulin, complement, or both), true hemolysis seen is less than 10 per cent of patients (216).

Aplastic anemia has been reported in association with lupus but appears to be more common in scleroderma (217).

A reduction in the total white cell count is seen in most patients but is more common in adults than in children. The leukopenia is usually a combination of decreased numbers of granulocytes as well as lymphocytes (218). Antibodies to granulocytes have been proposed as one mechanism for the granulocytopenia. Granulocyte antibodies and peripheral granulocyte destruction have been observed (219). Bone marrow depression of granulocyte formation also may exist. Sera from patients with systemic lupus erythematosus can inhibit mouse bone marrow colony forming units (220). Qualitative abnormalities of granulocyte function also have been noted. Although several investigators have found no abnormalities of chemotaxis (221, 222), others have observed abnormal migration by the skin window technique and diminished in vitro phagocytosis (223, 224). These defects parallel the observed complement depressions. The qualitative defects of granulocyte function may be the result of altered humoral factors rather than defects in the phagocytic cells themselves.

Lymphopenia may be severe in lupus (225), sometimes due to IgG or IgM antilymphocyte antibodies (233–235). In contrast to the depression of T and B cells, the percentage and absolute numbers of null cells increase (226). The magnitude of T cell reduction parallels disease activity and is associated with defects in cellular immunity as measured by skin tests of delayed hypersensitivity, blast transformation in response to mitogen (phytohemagglutinin and concanavalin A), and macrophage-inhibiting factor production (225, 227). Unlike T cell function, B cell function is increased despite the decrease in absolute number of B cells (228, 229). There is actually an increase in IgG-synthesizing peripheral blood lymphocytes as well as elevated numbers of cells capable of binding native DNA and elevated numbers of IgM- and IgG-producing cells with antibody specificity against DNA antigen (230, 231). These changes in peripheral blood lymphocytes are associated with certain morphologic alterations. A strongly basophilic cytoplasm and a high nuclear:cytoplasmic ratio are noted in many lymphocytes thought to be "immunoblasts" (232). On electron microscopy, inclusions are identified within lymphocytes that appear as undulating tubules characteristically associated with the endoplasmic reticulum.

The platelet survival is shortened, and there are increased numbers of bone marrow megakaryocytes. The platelet antibody is an IgG, which has a molecular weight of 150,000 to 330,000 daltons and binds complement (237). The latter feature distinguishes the immune thrombocytopenia of systemic lupus erythematosus from that of idiopathic thrombocytopenic purpura (238). Danazol may have several serologic effects in patients with systemic lupus erythematosus, including a decrease in DNA antibodies and antiplatelet antibodies. This drug has shown some therapeutic effectiveness in patients with this disease who have immune-mediated thrombocytopenia (238a). A qualitative defect of platelet function also may be present (239). Patients with systemic lupus erythematosus may have a serum inhibitor of platelet aggregation (240).

Patients with systemic lupus erythematosus may also have a circulating anticoagulant in their plasma (241). The incidence of this in children is unknown, but the anticoagulant is seen in 5 to 10 per cent of adults with this disease (242). The anticoagulant inhibits the interaction between the prothrombin activator (Factor V, Factor Xa, phospholipid, calcium complex) and prothrombin, but the exact molecular substrate against which it is directed is not known (243). Most investigators have reported that the lupus anticoagulant is an immunoglubulin that may be of the IgG, IgM, or mixed IgG-IgM classes (244–247). In addition to the inhibitor itself, a cofactor in normal plasma is necessary for maximal action of the lupus anticoagulant. This cofactor, which may be a gamma globulin, potentiates the inhibitory action of the lupus anticoagulant (248).

The partial thromboplastin time is invariably prolonged in patients with the lupus anticoagulant and is considered to be the most sensitive screening test (242). The inhibitor is suspected when the addition of normal plasma to the patient's plasma fails to correct the defect (244).

The prothrombin time in patients with the lupus anticoagulant is often normal or minimally prolonged, owing to the influence of the inhibitor. True prothrombin deficiency may occur in patients with the inhibitor, but this is rare (249, 250).

Prolonged thrombin times in the absence of elevated levels of fibrin split products may occasionally be seen (251). The exact significance of this finding is unclear.

The lupus anticoagulant is usually found coincidentally on routine coagulation screening (251a). Bleeding is a rare manifestation, and patients have undergone surgery without unusual postoperative bleeding (252). In fact, some patients with the lupus anticoagulant may manifest thrombotic events, a situation observed with other inhibitors (253), particularly if the inhibitor has activity against antithrombin III.

Because bleeding is rarely a problem as a consequence of the presence of the inhibitor, specific therapy is not usually indicated.

POLYARTERITIS NODOSA

Anemia resulting from a chronic disease state is seen occasionally in patients with polyarteritis nodosa. A more common occurrence is microangiopathic hemolytic anemia in association with renal disease or hypertensive crises. The hemolytic process in these circumstances parallels disease activity.

Neutrophilia and eosinophilia are common. The eosinophilia may be extensive, often reaching levels suggestive of eosinophilic leukemia or Löffler's endocarditis. Marked eosinophilia is usually restricted to patients with clinically apparent pulmonary involvement.

WEGENER'S GRANULOMATOSIS

This disorder, characterized by a necrotizing vasculitis (particularly in the lungs and kidneys), is rare but can affect children (253a, 253b). The disease can also present in the newborn period (253c). The course is marked by fever, cough, hemoptysis, epistaxis, nasal discharge, obliteration of the nasal sinuses, and nodular pulmonary infiltrates. Renal failure may occur. As with most chronic disease states, a normochromic, normocytic anemia develops (253d). The peripheral smear may demonstrate anisocytosis, poikilocytosis, and marked fragmentation reflective of a microangiopathic process secondary to vasculitis (253e). A Coombs'-negative hemolytic anemia with splenomegaly may be present (253d). The white blood cell count is elevated, and eosinophilia can occur (253f). The disease is characterized by a marked thrombocytosis (253d). Various immunosuppressive therapies have been attempted. Cyclophosphamide is occasionally effective in the management of children with Wegener's granulomatosis (253g).

OTHER COLLAGEN VASCULAR DISEASES

The hematologic manifestations of these disorders are relatively nonspecific. No consistent hematologic abnormalities are recorded in polymyositis and dermatomyositis. Scleroderma may result in malabsorption of vitamin B_{12}, but this disease is rare in children.

INFECTIONS

General Hematologic Signs of Infection

RED CELL DISTURBANCES

The pathophysiologic findings of the anemia of chronic infection are similar to those of the anemia of chronic disorders. Although some infections, particularly viral infections, cause transient bone marrow aplasia or selective erythroid aplasia, anemia on this basis is rare because of the long life span of the red blood cell. In contrast, patients with hemolytic anemia may experience a rapid fall in hemoglobin concentration during viral and some bacterial infections. This is especially common in association with infectious episodes caused by parvovirus (253h). Such infections should be considered in any child with a congenital hemolytic anemia who experiences an "aplastic" crisis.

Even common childhood infections, especially those associated with inflammation, will cause a decline in hemoglobin concentration. During active inflammation, the hemoglobin concentration has been shown to decline about 13 per cent, usually within 1 week, followed by a rise of nearly 25 per cent during the resolution of active inflammation (197a).

Severe hemolytic anemia may be observed in certain types of infections. Clostridial infections may result in a high titer of hemolysins and cause severe anemia with hemoglobinemia and hemoglobinuria (254). A similar severe anemia may result from sepsis related to other bacterial organisms, including staphylococci, streptococci, pneumococci, and *Haemophilus influenzae* (255). Immune hemolytic anemia mediated by a cold agglutinin may be observed with *Listeria* and *Mycoplasma* infections (256) and occasionally with infections due to other organisms such as the Epstein-Barr virus.

Many viral illnesses may be associated with what appears to be a mild hemolytic anemia for which no pathologic mechanism has been defined. The most common morphologic finding under these circumstances is poikilocytosis. Certain viruses, such as most strains of influenza, contain neuraminidase activity, which is at least theoretically capable of affecting the sialic acid content of the red cell membrane. Whether this plays any significant role in the hemolysis associated with some viral diseases is not known.

Many congenital infections, including cytomegalovirus, herpes simplex, rubella, toxoplasmosis, and syphilis, produce a profound hemolytic anemia in the newborn period, even though these same agents may not significantly alter red cell survival at other times of life. The explanation for this also is unclear.

Finally, anemia may result from blood loss associated with intestinal parasitic infestation.

WHITE CELL DISTURBANCES

The white cell count may be normal, low, or high with infection. Viral illnesses may be associated with leukocyte counts below 5000 cells per mm^3, although bacterial diseases of certain types or overwhelming sepsis of any type may also cause leukopenia. The most common viral illnesses associated with leukopenia are infectious hepatitis, infectious mononucleosis, rubella, measles, and occasionally influenza. Of the bacterial infections, shigellosis may produce leukopenia with a marked increase in band forms. Sepsis caused by meningococci, pneumococci, staphylococci, and a few other bacterial pathogens also may cause leukopenia.

Neutrophilia, with or without an increase in band count, is a frequent result of bacterial infection. Occasionally, viral illness will also initially present with a neutrophilia. A variety of morphologic changes may appear in the neutrophils of patients with infection. Döhle bodies, pale blue cystlike inclusion bodies usually located in the periphery of the cytoplasm of neutrophils, may appear in bacterial infections (257). They are occasionally associated with viral illness but are also commonly seen in patients with burns, massive trauma, and cancer as well as in pregnancy and following the use of cyclophosphamide (257). Döhle bodies are also seen in the May-Hegglin anomaly (258). Increased size of neutrophil granules ("toxic granulation") may be seen in both bacterial and viral illnesses as well as in many of the other disorders associated with the presence of Döhle bodies. Vacuolization of the cytoplasm of neutrophils is the next most common morphologic abnormality of neutrophils in patients with significant bacteremias. In a study of neutrophils of patients with bacteremia, Zipursky and associates found toxic granulation, Döhle bodies, and vacuolization in 75 per cent, 29 per cent, and 24 per cent, respectively, of the patients studied (259).

Increased neutrophil alkaline phosphatase activity and nitroblue tetrazolium dye reduction also may occur (260, 261), but neither of these characteristics is specific for bacterial infection. Infections may be associated with the development of the Pelger-Huët anomaly, in which the granulocytes and eosinophils have one or two lobes per nucleus and assume a round, dumbbell, or peanut shape (262). This is most commonly observed with tuberculosis. The Pelger-Huët anomaly is seen in one in 6000 people as an autosomal disorder and is also observed occasionally in patients with preleukemia, leukemia, and other cancers and in those taking colchicine and sulfonamide medications (262).

Newborn infants, especially those born prematurely, may fail to demonstrate a rise in total white cell or mature neutrophil counts in the presence of infection. In fact, a fall in the neutrophil count often occurs. The most helpful signs of septicemia in this age group are a rise in the band count and the presence of toxic granulations and Döhle bodies (259, 263).

Leukocytosis may result from a lymphocytosis. The most common infections producing the greatest rise in lymphocyte counts are infectious mononucleosis, cat scratch disease, "acute infectious lymphocytosis of childhood," and pertussis. Many other viral illnesses such as cytomegalovirus, rubella, mumps, and hepatitis also may cause a rise in the lymphocyte count.

Eosinophilia may reflect the presence of parasitic infections. In the United States, the most common cause of marked elevations of eosinophil counts is *Toxocara* infestation, an infection often accompanied by high titers of isohemagglutinins. Other parasites commonly causing eosinophilia include organisms belonging to the genera *Trichinella, Echinococcus, Filaria, Strongyloides, Schistosoma, Enterobius, Ancylostoma,* and tapeworms other than *Echinococcus.* Allergic sensitization to mites may cause eosinophilia as well as fungal infections, especially aspergillosis (264). Eosinophilia is, of course, not specific for infestation. Marked degrees of eosinophilia may occur in association with prematurity. An absolute eosinophilia may be expected in about 75 per cent of low-birth-weight infants (264a). In some, the eosinophilia is marked (>3000 cells per mm^3), and the maximal rise seems to occur about the time birth weight is regained, although this is not true in all cases (264b).

Monocytosis is occasionally seen with specific infections, especially tuberculosis, syphilis, and subacute bacterial endocarditis. Monocytosis is often noted early in the course of many infections and again on recovery, especially in cases associated with granulocytopenia.

Basophilia is rarely seen in infection but has been reported with tuberculosis, influenza, and hookworm infestation (265).

CLOTTING ABNORMALITIES AND THROMBOCYTOPENIA

Disseminated intravascular coagulation may be triggered by infectious processes. Of the infectious causes, gram-negative septicemias are probably most frequent. *Meningococcus, Escherichia coli, Proteus, Pseudomonas, Aerobacter,* and *Klebsiella* are among the most common etiologic agents recovered from the blood stream (266, 267). Gram-positive septicemia can cause a similar picture. The most frequent offender is *Diplococcus pneumoniae*, especially in asplenic individuals. Other gram-positive agents causing disseminated intravascular coagulation include *Staphylococcus aureus, Streptococcus,* and *Clostridia*. A wide range of viral infections may cause a consumptive coagulopathy, often leading to purpura fulminans. Among the most common agents are those that cause infectious hepatitis, measles, rubella, varicella, and infectious mononucleosis. Less common causes of disseminated intravascular coagulation are severe mycoplasmal, rickettsial, and malarial infections.

Thrombocytopenia occurring separately from a true disseminated consumptive process is quite common in many infectious processes, especially in association with infectious mononucleosis, cytomegalovirus infection, rubella, measles, gram-negative bacteria, and rickettsial diseases. Congenital viral infections and congenital syphilis and toxoplasmosis, if clinically apparent, almost invariably are associated with an increased platelet turnover with or without thrombocytopenia. Thrombocytopenia may occur after immunization with live viral vaccines, especially measles vaccines (268). Corrigan has found that thrombocytopenia without a consumptive coagulopathy is an extremely common finding in infants and children with septicemias (269). In contrast, thrombocytosis is often present during the active phases of infectious processes.

Hematologic Aspects of Selected Specific Infections

Certain infectious processes are associated with specific or unique hematologic findings distinct from those described in the preceding section. These infections include *Bordetella pertussis* (pertussis, or whooping cough), *Salmonella typhosa* (typhoid fever), *Mycobacterium tuberculosis* (tuberculosis), *Plasmodium malariae* (malaria), *Clostridium perfringens, Bartonella bacilliformis* (bartonellosis, or Carrión's disease).

Typhoid fever produces a remarkable leukopenia and neutropenia early in the course of the illness. Bone marrow precursors are increased. A high white cell count in this disease usually is suggestive of a secondary bacterial infection. The leukopenia of typhoid fever is often associated with thrombocytopenia. Shigellosis may also be associated with leukopenia. The hallmark of *Shigella* infection, however, is a sharp rise in the band cell count.

Clostridium perfringens infections in the pediatric age group are most common among adolescent females who have undergone septic abortions. This organism has a potent exotoxin, a lecithinase, that disrupts cell membranes, liberating hemolytic materials such as lysolecithins. This may result in a fatal intravascular hemolytic anemia with spherocytosis (254).

Pertussis may cause a marked rise in the white cell count, with elevations to 40,000 cells per mm^3 or more, most of which is due to a rise in the lymphocyte count.

Tuberculosis produces a variety of hematologic abnormalities. Leukemoid reactions mimicking myeloproliferative disorders are frequent (270). Bone marrow involvement in miliary tuberculosis may result in a myelophthistic pattern on the peripheral blood smear (271). In this respect, tuberculosis is similar in its presentation to some cases of sarcoidosis. A bone marrow biopsy may show evidence of granulomas. Monocytosis is common, and thrombocytopenia and pancytopenia have been reported (272).

Bartonellosis is a disease transmitted by the sandfly and is associated with a potentially severe hemolytic anemia. This was first recognized in 1885 when a medical student inoculated himself with the *Bartonella* organism. The student, Daniel Carrión, died of a severe hemolytic anemia. For this reason, human bartonellosis, caused by *Bartonella bacilliformis*, is still called Carrión's disease (273). This organism will infect red blood cells, coating them (Fig. 52–4) and causing them to be rapidly removed from the circulation. Unlike malarial organisms, *Bartonella* organisms do not invade the red blood cell (274).

Hemolysis is common in malaria, especially with infection caused by *Plasmodium falciparum* (275). This disease, transmitted by *Anopheles* mosquitoes, results in parasitization with organisms at the merozoite stage within the red cell. The parasitization causes an altered permeability and an increased osmotic fragility (276). The presence of the organism within the cell is also reflected in a defect of red cell membrane shape. Hemolysis in malaria has been attributed to direct damage to the red cell by the parasite, to autoimmune destruction, to hypersplenism, to splenic pitting with formation of microspherocytes, and to loss of the cell surface negative charge secondary to alteration of the cell's metabolic functions by the parasite (277–278a). In addition to destroying infected cells, the spleen may merely remove the offending organisms, leaving membrane pits or cavities that may be seen on scanning electron microscopy (279). A particularly severe form of hemolysis called blackwater fever may occur with *Plasmodium falciparum* infection. The basis of the massive hemolysis is unknown.

Many hematologic abnormalities are seen in association with acquired immunodeficiency syndrome (AIDS), which is thought to be related to the human T cell leukemia virus. Among these findings are anemia, leukopenia, thrombocytopenia, a left shift in the granulocyte series, lymphopenia, atypical lymphocytes, vacuolated monocytes, marrow necrosis or aplasia, and a high incidence of myelofibrosis (279a).

Infectious Mononucleosis

There is unequivocal evidence that links this disease to the Epstein-Barr (EB) virus. Before etiologic evidence became established, the diagnosis of infectious mononucleosis was based on a triad of (1) a classic clinical picture, (2) atypical lymphocytosis, and (3) a positive heterophile test (280). It was maintained that the absence of any one of these three would negate the diagnosis. Serologic testing for the EB virus has helped explain certain puzzling diagnostic features. For example, it was previously not recognized that children under the age of 5 years frequently contract infectious mononucleosis. The heterophile test is usually negative in this age group, but antibody to the EB virus is positive. This specific serologic test also explains some cases in adults who seem to have a typical clinical picture of infectious mononucleosis and demonstrate atypical

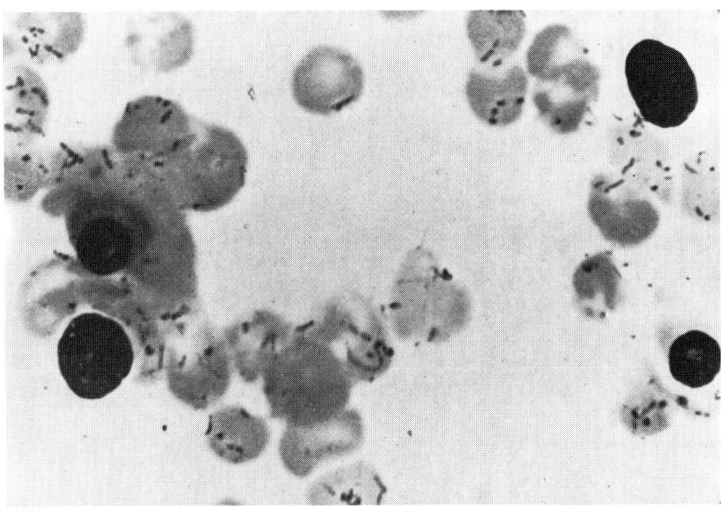

Figure 52–4. Parasitism of red blood cells in human *Bartonella* infection. (From Ricketts, W. E.: Blood 3:1025, 1948.)

lymphocytosis but whose heterophile test is negative. The masquerading disease is cytomegalovirus infection in most cases.

HISTORY

The major landmarks in diagnosing infectious mononucleosis have occurred in three areas. The first was the emergence of this disease as a separate clinical entity. The second was the establishment of a diagnostic test, the heterophile antibody test, and the third was the identification of the EB virus as an etiologic agent.

The history spans about 100 years. The earliest clinical descriptions are found in writings of Filatov (281) in 1885 and Pfeiffer (282) in 1889. The disease was initially termed "glandular fever" until 1920, when Sprunt and Evans, appreciating the presence of the now well-known atypical lymphocytosis, coined the name "infectious mononucleosis" (283).

The serendipitous discovery of the heterophile antibody is surpassed only by that of the EB virus as an etiologic agent. By the 1920's, the occurrence of sheep cell antibodies in serum sickness was well known. Because of the similarities in symptomatologies of serum sickness and rheumatic fever, Paul began to look for these antibodies in patients with rheumatic fever (284). Needless to say, little came of the primary purpose of this study, but one day, as part of this investigation, Paul and Bunnell found that a control serum had an extraordinarily high titer of heterophile antibody (285). This control serum was from a medical student who had typical infectious mononucleosis. Davidsohn completed this phase of the story in 1937 when he organized the differential absorption procedures (286).

The etiologic agent of infectious mononucleosis eluded investigators for half a century. In 1958, Burkitt described African children with the lymphoma now bearing his name (287). Because the distribution pattern of the disease coincided with the African mosquito belt, many investigators felt that a viral agent might be the cause of this lymphoma. Following the successful culturing of this tumor tissue in 1964, Epstein and Barr noted herpes-like virus particles in the tissues of patients with this lymphoma (288). By 1966, the Henles had developed an indirect immunofluorescence test to detect this viral particle, which was already called the Epstein-Barr virus (289, 290). With this test, EB viral antibody was found to be present in many healthy American children. A fortunate chance occurrence was observed when a technician in the Henles' laboratory developed infectious mononucleosis. Her white cells, which previously could not be grown in culture, now grew in continuous culture, and demonstrable EB viral antibody was noted. With sera that had been previously obtained from Yale University students, a correlation was then established that clearly linked the EB virus with the clinical appearance of infectious mononucleosis (291).

EPIDEMIOLOGY

EB virus infections are acquired at an early age in lower socioeconomic groups. In economically privileged children, infection is often delayed until adolescence and young adulthood. About 40 per cent of American children are seropositive by age 5 years (292–294). In a report from the United States Military Academy at West Point, 63.5 per cent of entering cadets had EB virus antibody, indicative of prior infection (295). During the college years, the infection rate among susceptible individuals is 12 to 15 per cent per year. The pattern of infection among different groups of susceptible persons is probably best explained by transmission of this virus in throat secretions. Low titers of infectious virus in throat specimens account for the moderate contagiousness of this infection and the requirement of intimate contact for transmission. Thus, infection might be more common at younger ages in lower socioeconomic groups because of a greater oral or oral/fecal transmission opportunity.

Another possible route of transmission of EB virus is transfusion. The EB virus is carried in circulating white blood cells. In 1942, Wising suggested that infectious mononucleosis could be transferred via blood transfusions (296). Subsequently, it was demonstrated that approximately 8 per cent of individuals undergoing cardiopulmonary bypass developed EB virus antibody in the postoperative period (297). EB virus does not appear, however, to be the cause of the postperfusion syndrome, which is most likely due to cytomegalovirus. Except for a rare case in which clinical infectious mononucleosis appears following transfusion of blood from a donor with this disorder, clinical disease from transfusion-transmitted EB virus is largely unknown.

The EB virus is present in saliva in most patients with infectious mononucleosis, in up to 20 per cent of healthy EB virus antibody–positive persons and in 50 per cent or more of seropositive patients receiving immunosuppressive drugs. The ease with which EB virus is recovered from oral secretions of persons with primary or reactivated EB viral infections suggests that a cell type freely permissive of EB virus replication exists in the oropharynx. It has been demonstrated that the oropharyngeal epithelial cell may be the target cell type that is productively infected in infectious mononucleosis (297a). Transmission requires intimate contact, so there is no significant spread of EB virus in the school setting. Intrafamilial spread, however, does frequently occur, and in this setting an incubation period of 4 to 6 weeks has been demonstrated (297b).

It has been suggested that EB virus infection may be transmitted congenitally (297c, 297d). A fatal illness in a 2-week-old infant diagnosed by detection of EB virus genomes from a lymph node biopsy has been described (297e). Such occurrences, if representative of true congenital EB virus infection, must be rare. A study of 4063 pregnant women showed that only 1.1 per cent were susceptible to infection early in gestation and less than 0.1 per cent showed seroconversion. Two of three infants born of seroconverted women were normal, but one had tricuspid atresia. None of the infants could be demonstrated to be actively infected (297f, 297g). Similar findings have been found by others (297h).

The relationship of infectious mononucleosis to other disorders known to be associated with EB virus infection or virus isolation is unclear. This includes nasopharyngeal carcinoma in addition to Burkitt's African lymphoma (298). A higher than anticipated association of EB virus with sarcoidosis (299), leprosy (300), and systemic lupus erythematosus (301) has been observed, although any specific relationship to these disorders remains as yet speculative (302).

In patients who undergo renal transplantation, a spectrum of lymphoproliferative diseases may occur as a result of activation of EB virus. These may vary from an infectious mononucleosis–like polyclonal B cell proliferation to a monoclonal B cell lymphoma. Therapeutic approaches to this problem usually fail (302a). Acyclovir may be helpful early in the course of illness. When frank malignancy has developed, chemotherapy is suggested.

CLINICAL PRESENTATION

The classic clinical presentation of infectious mononucleosis is seen generally only in adolescents and young adults. Younger children rarely present with a typical picture of this disease and most commonly demonstrate only a mild viral respiratory illness (292–294).

The onset of typical illness usually begins with a subtle prodrome consisting of fatigue, malaise, sweating, feverishness, and anorexia. As with infectious hepatitis, a distaste for cigarettes is common. Headache, nausea, and vomiting are not infrequent. The most common symptom during this period is a sore throat, which begins slowly and increases in intensity over a 1-week period. The usual findings of infectious mononucleosis then follow (Table 52–4). Fever often follows a specific pattern, with no temperature elevation in the morning but daily afternoon or evening peaks of 38.3°C to 39.4°C (101°F to 103°F). Occasionally, higher temperatures are observed. Fever usually lasts about 2 weeks.

Lymphadenopathy is seen in all cases. Symmetric, moderately enlarged, discrete, slightly tender nodes, especially in the posterior cervical region, are most characteristic. Adenopathy is common in the axillary, epitrochlear, and inguinal areas. The nodes are not matted and fail to show signs of heat, redness, or fluctuation. Rarely, enlargement of the mediastinal glands constitutes the only evidence of adenopathy and may be confused with a lymphomatous process.

Splenomegaly is seen in more than 50 per cent of patients with infectious mononucleosis. The spleen is usually just barely palpable but on rare occasions may be quite large. It is smooth, soft to firm, and sometimes slightly tender. In a few patients, splenomegaly persists for months, but the most common situation is resolution by 2 to 3 weeks from the onset of the illness.

Hepatomegaly occurs in about 20 per cent of patients, and clinical jaundice presents in 10 per

Table 52–4. INFECTIOUS MONONUCLEOSIS—APPROXIMATE FREQUENCY OF VARIOUS SIGNS AND SYMPTOMS IN YOUNG ADULTS*

Symptom or Sign	%	Symptom or Sign	%
Adenopathy	100	Myalgia	12–30
Malaise and fatigue	90–100	Hepatomegaly	15–25
Fever	80–95	Rhinitis	10–25
Sweats	80–95	Ocular muscle pain	10–20
Sore throat, dysphagia	80–95	Chest pain	5–20
Pharyngitis	65–85	Jaundice	5–10
Anorexia	50–80	Arthralgia	5–10
Nausea	50–70	Diarrhea or soft stools	5–10
Splenomegaly	50–60	Photophobia	5–10
Headache	40–70	Skin rash	3–6
Chills	40–60	Conjunctivitis	5
Bradycardia	35–50	Abdominal pain	5
Cough	30–50	Gingivitis	3
Periorbital edema	25–40	Pneumonitis	3
Palatal enanthem	25–35	Epistaxis	3
Liver or splenic tenderness	15–30		

*From Finch, S. C.: Clinical symptoms and signs of infectious mononucleosis. In *Infectious Mononucleosis*. Carter, R. L., and Penman, H. G. (eds.), Oxford, Blackwell Scientific Publications, 1969, p. 35.

cent of patients. The jaundice is invariably mild. Despite the low frequency of apparent hepatic dysfunction, virtually all patients with infectious mononucleosis demonstrate abnormal liver enzyme levels. Except in rare cases of acute liver failure, the hepatitis associated with this illness is self-limited. There is no evidence that chronic liver disease or cirrhosis results from infectious mononucleosis. A case of Reye's syndrome in a child with infectious mononucleosis has been reported (303).

Rashes occur occasionally and follow no particular pattern. The rash may be a diffuse, faint erythematous, or maculopapular eruption or it may be urticarial, scarlatiniform, petechial, or herpetiform. In general, the skin rashes of infectious mononucleosis have no unique features and are of little or no diagnostic help. Circulating immune complex and complement sequence activation occur only when rashes are present (304). If ampicillin is administered to patients with infectious mononucleosis, 69 to 100 per cent will develop a rash (305). Other penicillins may cause this response, but less frequently. This rash is not a reagin-mediated allergic reaction, and these antibiotics may be administered subsequently without ill effects.

Only a few patients with infectious mononucleosis have no pharyngitis. Almost all demonstrate hyperplasia of the pharyngeal lymphoid follicles. An exudate is common, and membrane formation often occurs. The inflammation may be so severe as to cause respiratory obstruction. Peritonsillar abscesses may complicate the course of illness (306a). A palatal enanthem is seen in about one third of patients, which consists of crops of sharply circumscribed petechiae, symmetrically distributed at the junction of the soft palate. Unfortunately, such petechiae are not specific for infectious mononucleosis and have been described in rubella and other viral disorders. In fact, the entire pharyngeal picture of infectious mononucleosis is clinically indistinguishable from streptococcal disease.

Periorbital edema is not rare and occasionally leads to the erroneous suspicion that renal disease or hypoproteinemia is present. The edema is self-limited, lasting only a few days.

COMPLICATIONS

Much attention is paid to the complications associated with infectious mononucleosis, although their overall occurrence is low (Table 52–5).

The neurologic complications listed vary in incidence from 0.37 to 7.3 per cent, depending on the reported series. A not rare occurrence in adolescence is the "Alice in Wonderland" phenomenon in which objects are visualized in a very distorted fashion, with exaggerations in size, being either too large or too small (306). A transverse myelopathy characterized by sudden onset of profound weakness of the lower extremities and urinary retention may complicate the clinical course of infectious mononucleosis (306b). An outline of the neurologic complications appears in Table 52–5.

Cardiac complications are infrequent, occurring in 1 to 6 per cent of reported series, and usually consist only of nonspecific T wave changes or minor conduction abnormalities. Myocarditis and pericarditis are infrequent.

Liver function abnormalities are rarely severe, although enzyme changes are frequent. Primary

Table 52–5. INFECTIOUS MONONUCLEOSIS—REPORTED COMPLICATIONS*

Type of Complication	Diagnosis or Description of Abnormality
Neurologic	Bell's palsy, cerebellar syndrome, encephalitis, encephalomyelitis, encephalomyelopathy, Guillain-Barré syndrome, meningitis, meningoencephalitis, myelitis, optic neuritis, peripheral neuritis, psychosis, radiculoneuritis Ataxia, positive Babinski sign, coma, convulsions, diplopia, extraocular palsy, facial diplegia, hemiplegia, hyperesthesia, meningismus, mental confusion, nystagmus, papilledema, psychotic reaction, ptosis, respiratory paralysis, positive Romberg sign, seizure, status epilepticus, scotomata
Cardiac	Electrocardiographic changes, myocarditis, pericarditis
Ocular	Conjunctivitis, diplopia, cyclic edema, hemianopia, lacrimal pericyclitis, nystagmus, optic neuritis, ptosis, retinal edema, retinal hemorrhage, retro-orbital pain, scotomata, uveitis
Respiratory	Laryngeal obstruction, peritonsillar abscess, pharyngeal edema, pleural effusion, pleuritis, pneumonitis
Hematologic	Acquired hemolytic anemia, agranulocytosis, eosinophilia, fibrinolysis, pancytopenia, splenic rupture, thrombocytopenia
Digestive	Esophageal varices, gingivitis, hepatic dysfunction, hepatic necrosis, jaundice, melena
Renal	Hematuria, hemoglobinuria, nephritis, nephrotic syndrome, porphyrinuria, proteinuria
Other	Bullous myringitis, endocervicitis, orchitis, otitis media, pancreatitis, porphyria, skin rashes

*From Finch, S. C.: Clinical symptoms and signs of infectious mononucleosis. In *Infectious Mononucleosis.* Carter, R. L., and Penman, H. G., (eds.), Oxford, Blackwell Scientific Publications, 1969, p. 35.

EB virus infection has been associated with a Reye's syndrome–like illness (306c). Spontaneous rupture of the spleen may occur (306d). Respiratory difficulties usually consist of upper airway obstruction. Transient interstitial infiltrations, some with effusions, have been recorded. Renal complications of infectious mononucleosis usually consist of hematuria associated with a picture of mild nephritis. Not all cases have been clearly separated from poststreptococcal glomerulonephritis. Eye findings in infectious mononucleosis are unusual but may be significant when they do occur. Hematologic complications of infectious mononucleosis include disturbances resulting in anemia, granulocytopenia, thrombocytopenia, and occasional coagulation defects.

Anemia is infrequent. Approximately 3 per cent of West Point cadets with infectious mononucleosis developed anemia of the immune hemolytic type (295). When it does occur, hemolysis usually begins 1 to 2 weeks into the course of the illness. The majority of cases terminate in less than 1 month, and chronic hemolysis is rare. Although usually mild, hemolysis is occasionally brisk and can then result in severe anemia. Jenkins and associates in 1965 reported the first case of hemolytic anemia in infectious mononucleosis that was mediated by the temporary induction of a high thermal amplitude cold agglutinin of anti-i specificity (307). Since then, several series have verified the high frequency of anti-i antibody as the cause of hemolysis in infectious mononucleosis. It should be noted that although hemolysis is not frequent in infectious mononucleosis, the presence of anti-i in the serum occurs in as many as 50 per cent of all cases. Not all immune hemolysis in infectious mononucleosis is caused by anti-i antibodies. Anti-N antibodies also have been reported, and in some cases the nature of the antibody has not been identified (308).

Aplastic anemia has been reported to follow the onset of infectious mononucleosis (309).

Granulocytopenia is common during the acute phase of infectious mononucleosis. It is rarely severe but on occasion is a cause of secondary bacterial infection (310). Spontaneous resolution is the rule.

Immune thrombocytopenia occurs infrequently in infectious mononucleosis. The peak age of incidence is between 10 and 30 years, with a preponderance of males. Most cases of thrombocytopenia are mild (311). Severe cases are similar in presentation to idiopathic thrombocytopenic purpura, except that in infectious mononucleosis hemorrhagic bullae of the mouth may occur. This is a rare finding in idiopathic thrombocytopenic purpura. The usual duration of thrombocytopenia is 4 to 8 weeks. Severe hemorrhagic complications are rare (312).

The thrombocytopenia of infectious mononucleosis appears to be immune in nature and has been associated with the presence of antiplatelet antibodies in several cases.

Treatment of the thrombocytopenia of infectious mononucleosis should be expectant. Severe cases may be treated with steroids, which generally promptly raise the platelet count (313). The frequency with which these hematologic abnormalities are found is shown in Table 52–6.

LABORATORY DIAGNOSIS (Fig. 52–5)

Atypical lymphocytosis is the hallmark of infectious mononucleosis. Several attempts have been made to classify these abnormal cells on morphologic grounds, the best known method being that of Downey and McKinlay (314). However, it is clear that atypical lymphocytes cannot be so easily classified into separate categories and that a spectrum of cell types exists. Undue emphasis on minor morphologic detail in stained films is not very rewarding. In general, the atypical lymphocytes of infectious mononucleosis are large but vary considerably in size. Their outlines are irregular, and many cells show a characteristic tendency to flow around adjacent erythrocytes. Nuclei are large and are usually eccentrically located and pleomorphic, with abundant coarse chromatin and occasional nucleoli. The cytoplasm is usually abundant and typically basophilic. Cytoplasmic vacuoles may be seen. These types of cells are not specific morphologically for infectious mononucleosis. Similar morphologic characteristics may be seen secondary to infections such as cytomegalovirus, infectious hepatitis, rubella, rubeola, and herpes simplex after the administration of certain drugs such as phenytoin (diphenylhydantoin) and para-aminosalicylic acid and following a number of chemical intoxications (315).

Table 52–6. INFECTIOUS MONONUCLEOSIS—LABORATORY FEATURES

Findings	% Positive
Lymphocytosis, relative and absolute	100
Atypical lymphocytosis, definite*	100
Epstein-Barr (EB) virus antibody in serum	100
Heterophile antibody	80–100
Liver enzyme abnormalities	80–100
Leukocytosis	60–80
Neutropenia	60–80
Hyperbilirubinemia	30–50
Bone marrow granulomas	50
Slight thrombocytopenia	25–50
Increased cold agglutinins	10–50
Occult hemolysis	20–40
Hyperuricemia	15–20
Leukopenia	10–20
Severe thrombocytopenia with bleeding	Rare
Positive direct Coombs' test	Rare
Significant anemia (usually due to hemolysis)	Rare

*Twenty per cent or more of white blood cells in peripheral blood.

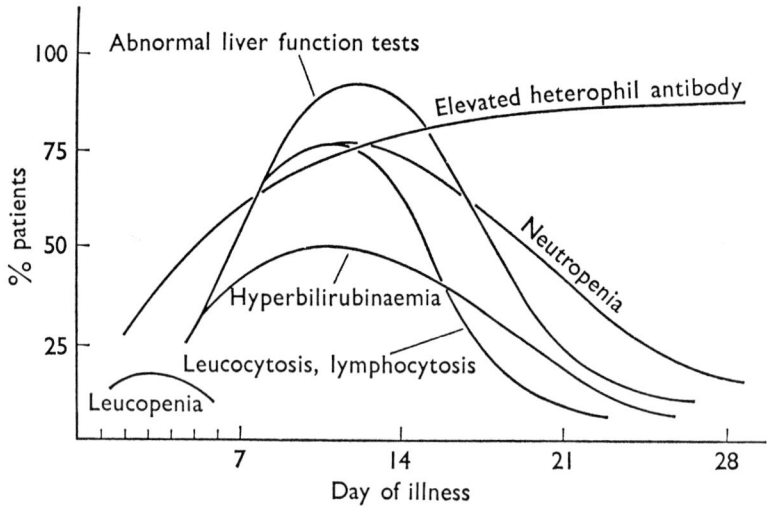

Figure 52–5. Major laboratory findings in infectious mononucleosis (From Finch, S. C.: Laboratory findings in infectious mononucleosis. In *Infectious Mononucleosis.* Carter, R. L., and Penman, H. C. (eds.): Oxford, Blackwell Scientific Publications, 1969, p. 47.)

The vast majority of atypical lymphocytes from patients with infectious mononucleosis are thymus-derived (316, 317). These atypical cells possess human T lymphocyte–specific antigens as well as sheep erythrocyte receptors (316). T lymphocytes appear to lack receptors for the EB virus, and it would appear that only the B lymphocyte is infected by this virus (317, 318). A possible unifying interpretation of the role of T lymphocytes is that these cells represent an immune reaction that protects against this potentially oncogenic virus. Increased numbers of B cells are found during the first week of illness and decline to normal levels in 3 weeks. T lymphocytes reach their peak later, usually 10 to 14 days after the onset of symptoms, and remain elevated for 5 weeks (319). There may be an early reversal of the ratio of T to B lymphocytes, with a subsequent increase in the percentage of T cells during the second through the fifth weeks of illness. It is possible that both T and B cells may be "transformed" into atypical lymphocytes—the B cells by infection with the EB virus and the T cells by an immunologic response to viral antigen itself, or the B cells may respond to altered antigens on their surface. EB virus–infected B lymphocytes account for only a minority of the atypical lymphocytes found in the peripheral blood. In the very early stages of symptomatic illness, however, nearly 20 per cent of all B cells in the circulation may be infected with the virus. The majority of atypical lymphocytes are T lymphocytes. Natural killer cell activity has been shown to be present during the acute phase of infectious mononucleosis. Interferons, which are inducers of natural killer cell activity, may have an inhibitory effect on the outgrowth of EB virus–infected B lymphocytes in vitro. Significant anergy and diminished lymphocyte responsiveness in vitro to mitogens and antigens exist during the first week of illness. These lymphocyte changes are reflected in a great increase in uric acid turnover, with 55 per cent of infected patients having serum uric acid levels of 8 mg per dl or higher (320).

Patients with infectious mononucleosis have lymph node pathologic findings that are easily confused with lymphoma. The nodal architecture is distorted by large, dark lymphoid cells, and the capsule may be infiltrated. Reed-Sternberg cells have been reported on several occasions (321, 322). Pathologic changes are not confined to lymphoid tissue, however. Perivascular cuffing of the brain vasculature, inflammation of the liver, and inflammatory infiltration of the kidney and bone marrow have been repeatedly observed.

The heterophil antibody is so named because the antigen to which the antibody reacts is found in more than one species. The antibody, like anti-i, is an IgM macroglobulin. It agglutinates sheep red cells and can be removed completely from serum by preincubation with beef red cells but not by guinea-pig kidney. Heterophil antibody titers usually rise after the third day of illness, peak at 2 weeks, and may remain positive for several months, ultimately becoming negative (unlike antibody specific for EB virus) (323). This traditional Paul-Bunnell serologic agglutination method has been largely replaced for screening purposes by the spot test, in which finely ground guinea-pig kidney or beef red cell stroma is added to serum on a slide, followed by a drop of horse cells (324). The test is considered positive if agglutination occurs in the presence of guinea-pig kidney (which absorbs out Forssman antibody but not heterophil antibody) but is negative with beef red cell stroma. The spot test requires only 2 minutes and is stated to be 96 to 99 per cent accurate. Both the Paul-Bunnell test and the spot test are usually negative in pre–school-aged children in whom heterophil antibody production is limited (325). This age group does produce diagnostic levels of EB virus–specific antibody.

The EB virus is a herpes-like DNA virus. This

is a relatively complex virus, and a variety of virus-associated antigens have been described (326). Antibodies to viral capsid antigen (VCA) and early antigen (EA) are detected early after the onset of EB virus–associated infectious mononucleosis (327). Antibodies to VCA reach their peak at about 3 weeks after the onset of clinical illness. They decline somewhat thereafter but remain for life (328). Antibodies to EA usually last 2 to 4 months. EA has two components that are differentiated by their immunofluorescent staining: "D" for diffuse and "R" for restricted staining. A technique for determining EB virus–specific IgM has been described (329). EB virus–specific IgM almost always occurs in the acute phase of infectious mononucleosis. It rarely persists more than 2 to 3 months. During this period, virus shedding from the oropharynx is easily demonstrable (330).

Figure 52–6 shows the characteristic antibody patterns observed in young adults experiencing EB virus–induced infectious mononucleosis. Prior to infection, no antibodies are present. During the acute phase of illness, high titers of IgM and IgG antibodies to VCA are seen. IgM antibodies are transient and disappear after 1 to 2 months. Antibodies appearing against the early antigens disappear after a few weeks to months. Antibodies against Epstein-Barr nuclear antigen (EBNA) are the last to appear 1 to 2 months following the illness. In young infants, VCA–IgM is found in only 60 per cent of cases, and EA antibody is discovered in only 50 per cent. The only persistent antibody response should be VCA–IgG and antibodies to EBNA.

X-LINKED LYMPHOPROLIFERATIVE SYNDROME

In 1974 and 1975, three families were described in which fatal infectious mononucleosis to EB virus occurred in young male members of these kindreds (331–331b). Acquired immunodeficiency and lymphoproliferative disorders occur with a higher than expected frequency in susceptible males. Of males who become affected, approximately 70 per cent succumb to fatal infectious mononucleosis. Of those surviving the initial infection, up to 40 per cent will develop a lymphoproliferative disorder. Virtually all survivors are immunocompromised. Sullivan and colleagues have found that those with common varied immunodeficiency demonstrate hypogammaglobulinemia and abnormal immune responses to in vivo immunization with various phage types of *Staphylococcus* (331c). Natural killer cell activity is diminished and unresponsive to interferon. This presumably leaves affected individuals with little defense against lymphoproliferative disorders characterized by multiplication of malignant cells containing the EB virus genome. Eighty per cent of males surviving the initial infection have absent or abnormal humoral immune responses to EB virus (331d). Prior to EB virus infection, susceptible males usually have no history of recurrent infections or difficulty in limiting infections.

Recognition of the X-linked lymphoproliferative syndrome has led to a wider understanding of the effect of EB virus infection with its immunologic consequences in other states. Transient immunodeficiency during asymptomatic EB virus infection

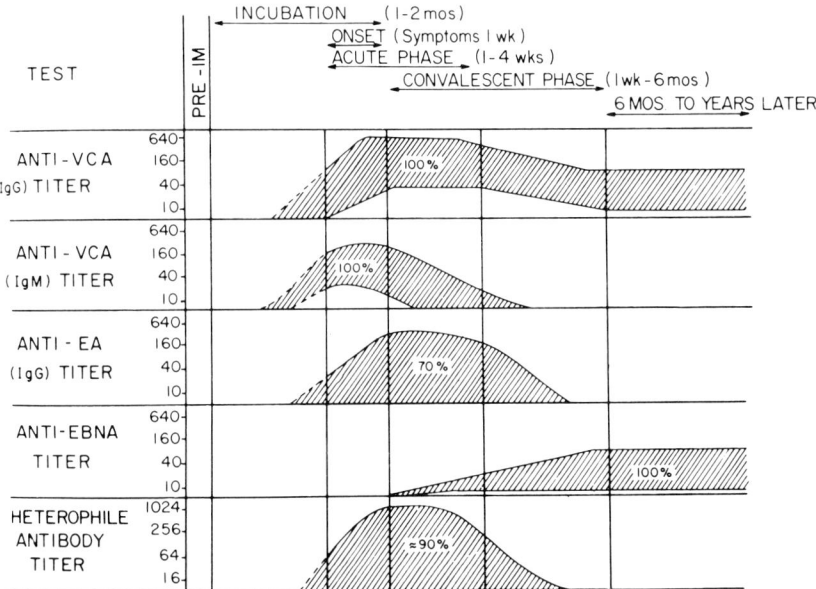

Figure 52–6. Characteristic Epstein-Barr specific antibody responses observed in young adults with acute infectious mononucleosis. (Adapted from references 330a and 330b.)

may occur in otherwise healthy children (331e). A non–X-linked susceptibility to severe EB virus infection has now been described (331f, 331g).

As noted, the outcome of the infection in susceptible individuals is extremely guarded (331h). Acyclovir treatment of two subjects with life-threatening infections with EB virus (one of whom had the X-linked lymphoproliferative syndrome) produced no apparent improvement (331i). Interferon trials are under way.

MANAGEMENT

There is no evidence that bedrest or rest in general shortens the course of illness from infectious mononucleosis. Patients will determine their own level of activity. The most significant risk during the acute illness is splenic rupture, but the incidence of this is extremely low.

Corticosteroids are frequently used in the treatment of infectious mononucleosis. Although steroids may produce improvement of symptoms, enhancement of general well-being, and reduction of fever, their use for these purposes should be restricted (331). Less controversial is the use of steroids for patients with airway obstruction from tonsillar hypertrophy, with severe hemolytic anemia, and with hemorrhagic thrombocytopenia (332).*

METABOLIC DISEASES

This section will be restricted to the hematologic consequences of diabetes mellitus, certain of the lipid disorders of metabolic origin, and methylmalonic and orotic acidurias.

Diabetes Mellitus

That diabetics are prone to anemia (333), infection (334), and thrombotic episodes with macrovascular and microvascular sequelae (335) has long been appreciated.

An unusual hemoglobin component in hemolysates prepared from the blood of certain diabetic patients was first noted by Rahbor and associates (336). A component that migrated near the position of fetal hemoglobin was described on agar gel electrophoresis at pH 6.2 in citrate buffers. This hemoglobin is present in normal individuals, constituting 5 to 7 per cent of the total hemoglobin (337), and is called Hb A_{Ic}. Rahbor's group observed a twofold increase of this hemoglobin fraction in some diabetics (338). Structurally, Hb A_{Ic} is a condensation product, via a Schiff base, between one molecule of Hb A and one molecule of an aldehyde or ketone, linked at the N-terminals of β-chains. The aldehyde or ketone group appears to be one or more hexoses, making Hb A_{Ic} a glycohemoglobin. Bunn and Briehl have shown that the oxygen affinity of Hb A_{Ic} is little affected by the addition of 2,3-diphosphoglycerate, which leads to a decreased oxygen affinity when added to Hb A (339). Although an early study failed to demonstrate a correlation between the degree of elevation of Hb A_{Ic} and clinical parameters of disease activity (337), more recent investigations have shown highly significant relationships between the percentage of Hb A_{Ic} and the response to an oral glucose tolerance test and overall diabetic control, as reflected in quantitative urinary glucose determinations (340, 341). In this sense, measurement of the glycohemoglobin provides an insight into diabetic control over many days. Although Hb A_{Ic} is a glycohemoglobin and an unusual glycoprotein has been found in the basement membrane material of kidneys of diabetic patients, a correlation between these has yet to be found (340).

Red cell survival, as measured by ^{51}Cr-labeling, may be mildly impaired during periods of poor diabetic control (mean erythrocyte half-life of 27 days). With improvement of diabetic control, the red cell survival will increase (mean half-life of 31 days) (342). During episodes of ketoacidosis, rapid shifts in the oxygen affinity of hemoglobin also may occur. A fall in pH causes a shift to the right with an increase in oxygen unloading. Very rapid correction of pH may impede oxygen delivery. A prompt fall in red cell 2,3-diphosphoglycerate levels occurs at these times (343). This is probably compensatory, an attempt to correct the oxygen affinity disturbances caused by the acidosis. A fall in red cell 2,3-diphosphoglycerate levels may also result from hypophosphatemia, should this occur during insulin treatment.

Anemia in diabetes is more often than not an example of the anemia of chronic disorders (discussed earlier). Adult diabetics have a higher incidence than normal individuals of pernicious anemia.

Polymorphonuclear cell function may be disturbed in diabetics. Leukocyte adherence is diminished in patients with poor control of diabetes, as is phagocytic capacity (344). Chemotaxis also may be abnormal, but this does not correlate with the status of the diabetic control (345). Impaired cellular metabolism and DNA synthesis have been

---

*Ed. comment: Young adolescents with persistent but non–life-threatening viral infections may present with symptoms and signs suggesting serious systemic diseases, such as tuberculosis or lymphoma. The symptoms may persist for weeks and include sweating, weight loss, fatigue, anorexia, low-grade fever, lymphadenopathy, and splenomegaly. There may be mild microcytic anemia, particularly in young women. Thrombocytosis and an elevated sedimentation rate and rare lymphoblasts with basophilic cytoplasm may be detected in the peripheral blood, particularly in smokers.

It may be difficult to resist the urge to perform lymph node biopsies or abdominal explorations in such patients. Most of them should be treated expectantly with simple home remedies, such as white meat of chicken or chicken soup (332a).

reported in the lymphocytes of some patients with diabetes (346).

A variety of coagulation and platelet abnormalities have been described in diabetics. A state of hypercoagulability associated with changes in clotting factors and platelet function has been postulated to be important in the increased thrombotic complications in diabetics. Ketoacidosis may be associated with disseminated intravascular coagulation (347). Altered levels of Factors V and VIII and diminished fibrinolytic activity have been reported in a few patients (348).

Many studies have emphasized the abnormalities of platelet adhesion and aggregation in patients with diabetes. The finding that enhanced platelet aggregation occurs before clinical evidence of diabetic vascular disease suggested that this defect may be acquired early in the natural history of diabetes and could underlie the vascular disease (349). Platelet aggregation in the diabetic is characterized by a shortened adenosine diphosphate–induced aggregation time (350). Increased platelet adhesiveness and platelet factor 3 and platelet factor 4 activities also occur (342, 351). Normal platelets incubated in the plasma of diabetics will become abnormal. This aggregation-enhancing activity is present in both plasma and serum and is nondialyzable and heat-resistant (350). In patients with this plasma factor, activity of von Willebrand's factor also is increased, suggesting that the two are related (352). The enhanced in vitro responsiveness of platelets from diabetics can be decreased by the prostaglandin synthetase inhibitors (349, 353). Platelets from diabetics demonstrate increased activity of the prostaglandin synthetase system, which results in increased synthesis of prostaglandin endoperoxides and, therefore, of prostaglandin E_2 (354). A lower prevalence and severity of diabetic retinopathy have been observed in a group of diabetic patients with concurrent rheumatoid arthritis who were taking high doses of aspirin. This finding suggests that inhibition of platelet aggregation and prostaglandin synthesis may be desirable in the management of the diabetic (355).

The hematologic consequences of diabetes also extend to the infant born of a diabetic mother. An increased incidence of thrombosis or thromboembolic phenomena is well recognized in these infants (356). Complications such as renal vein thrombosis, peripheral gangrene secondary to vascular occlusion, and cerebral thrombosis may occur (357).

Abnormalities of Lipid Metabolism

Abetalipoproteinemia is an autosomal recessive disorder that results in abnormalities of plasma lipids. Plasma levels of triglycerides, cholesterol, and phospholipids are diminished (358). These findings are associated with the presence of acanthocytic red blood cells. The cholesterol content of the red cell is normal or slightly increased, whereas the phospholipid content reflects that of the serum (358). Autohemolysis (359) and peroxidative hemolysis (360) may be increased, but osmotic fragility (359) and rates of glycolysis (359) are normal. Anemia, if present, is mild.

Patients with familial hyperbetalipoproteinemia (Type II hyperlipoproteinemia) have abnormal platelet function (361) characterized by increased sensitivity to aggregating agents and a release of increased amounts of nucleotides in response to aggregating agents. These findings suggest the possibility that platelet function may be involved in the thrombotic complications of familial hyperbetalipoproteinemia.

Essential fatty acid deficiency will result in a variety of characteristic changes in plasma lipids. Decreased prostaglandin formation in in vitro platelet studies involving animals with essential fatty acid deficiency has been reported (362). This results in a thrombocytopathy with impaired platelet aggregation and may reflect a deficiency of arachidonic acid necessary for the formation of thromboxane A_2 (362). Clinically, essential fatty acid deficiency is being recognized more frequently as a result of prolonged fat-free parenteral nutrition. Several infants have been described with hemorrhagic complications from this disorder (362).

Other Metabolic Disorders

A single infant with methylmalonic aciduria was found to have neutropenia (364). The mechanism of neutropenia in this child is unclear. More commonly, excessive urinary excretion of methylmalonic acid occurs as a result of vitamin B_{12} deficiency (365).

Infants and children with orotic aciduria, hyperglycinemia, and hyperglycinuria may have neutropenia (366). Patients with orotic aciduria may exhibit megaloblastic changes in the bone marrow and have macrocytic indices.

NEUROLOGIC AND PSYCHIATRIC DISORDERS

Muscular Dystrophy

Roses and Appel have reported decreased levels of red cell membrane protein phosphorylation in patients with myotonic muscular dystrophy (367). As a further example of the usefulness of red cells as biopsy tissue and also as possible additional evidence for the clinical importance of membrane protein phosphorylation, it also has been reported that increased phosphorylation of red cell spectrin occurs in patients with Duchenne's muscular dystrophy (368). These observations have prompted the hypothesis that the muscular defects in dystrophic patients may represent specific manifestations of a generalized membrane disorder (369). In addition, the red cells of patients with muscular dystrophy may demonstrate decreased deformability (370, 371). Almost 85 per cent of patients have an increased osmotic fragility (371a). The Pelger-Hüet anomaly has been associated with the autosomal dominant form of muscular dystrophy in one family (371b), as has Jordan's anomaly (371c). All these findings are subtle and require careful evaluation and confirmation.

Myasthenia Gravis

Because both myasthenia gravis and acquired pure red cell aplasia have been associated with the presence of thymoma, occasional reports of patients with myasthenia gravis and concomitant pure red cell aplasia have appeared (372). Pancytopenia may also occur. These occurrences in children are rare. In addition, there is a higher than average incidence of autoimmune hemolytic anemia in patients with myasthenia gravis (373).

Lesch-Nyhan Syndrome

The Lesch-Nyhan syndrome is an X-linked recessive disorder characterized by mental retardation, choreoathetosis, hyperuricemia, and self-mutilation. Cells from the affected individuals are unable to convert hypoxanthine and quanine to the corresponding nucleotides because of an inactive phosphoribosyl transferase. A patient with this syndrome has been described who developed a megaloblastic anemia, presumably as a result of deficient nucleic acid synthesis, because the administration of large amounts of adenine reversed the process (374). The enzyme is present in red cells, but its deficiency does not generally alter the function or survival of the mature red cell (375).

Rivard and associates have shown that patients with the Lesch-Nyhan syndrome cannot incorporate radioactive hypoxanthine into their platelet nucleotides (376). This results in a significantly lower ATP platelet content. Despite this, platelet function and number are normal in the Lesch-Nyhan syndrome.

Brain Trauma

Brain tissue from all mammalian species is rich in thromboplastin activity. Severe injury to the brain that disrupts brain architecture may release this material into the circulation. This most commonly occurs after gunshot wounds or crush injury to the head and has resulted in a picture of acute disseminated intravascular coagulation.

Anorexia Nervosa

Patients with anorexia nervosa may demonstrate many of the hematologic manifestations of severe malnutrition. In one patient with anorexia nervosa, the total amount of red cell lipids was normal, but there was an increased proportion of the long-chain polyunsaturated fatty acids associated with starvation (377). Small numbers of irregularly shaped red blood cells are frequently seen (378). The sedimentation rate is low. About one third of subjects will have a normochromic, normocytic anemia (378a). Slight to moderate leukopenia and neutropenia develop in about half the patients who are severely malnourished. The bone marrow may become hypoplastic and filled with gelatinous material and fat (378b). Leukocyte response to bacterial infection may be suboptimal. The white cell abnormalities of anorexia nervosa may require several months to resolve following adequate caloric intake. Platelet counts are usually normal, but mild depressions and occasionally severe depressions are observed (378c). A marked increase in platelet hyperaggregability may be found (378d).

SKIN DISEASES

Skin diseases are only rarely the direct cause of hematologic disturbances. More often than not, the hematologic alterations reflect a simultaneous disturbance in more than one developmental system, such as skin and blood. Certain disorders that affect the hematologic system in a major way, such as the Wiskott-Aldrich syndrome, are described in Chapter 28.

Eczema and Psoriasis

Patients with extensive eczema or psoriasis commonly have a mild anemia (379). This is usually normochromic and normocytic, although microcytosis may occur. More often than not, this anemia is associated with a low serum iron level and normal or decreased iron-binding capacity. Because bone marrow iron is not diminished, the anemia is best classified as an anemia of chronic disorders (379). Some individuals with extensive rashes will have a great expansion of whole blood and plasma volumes, which may result in a dilutional anemia (380, 381). A rare patient with eczema or psoriasis may develop long-standing steatorrhea, which causes folate malabsorption and macrocytic anemia (382).

Dermatitis Herpetiformis

Anemia may result from the malabsorption syndrome found in many individuals with this disease. This usually causes a megaloblastic anemia (383).

Splenic hypofunction and atrophy also may occur (384) and are detectable by the presence of Howell-Jolly bodies on the peripheral blood smear. This lymphoreticular dysfunction most probably relates to the high incidence of celiac disease found in association with dermatitis herpetiformis. Hyposplenism is also common in children and adults with celiac disease (385).

Dyskeratosis Congenita

An illness resembling Fanconi's aplastic anemia may occur in patients with this disorder (385a). Before the onset of the skin problem, thrombocytopenia, macrocytosis, and elevations of fetal hemoglobin concentrations may be seen (385b).

Hereditary Hemorrhagic Telangiectasias

This is an inherited structural abnormality of the vasculature characterized by the localized dilatation and convolution of venules and capillaries, giving rise to mucocutaneous telangiectasias. It is an autosomal dominant disorder that results in a bleeding tendency because of the friable blood vessels. The telangiectasias predominate on the lips, buccal mucosa, gingivae, palate, tongue, and skin of the face and upper parts of the body and may be present in visceral organs as well. Pulmonary arteriovenous fistulas are not rare but tend to appear later in life. Easy bruisability, epistaxis, and respiratory and gastrointestinal bleeding may be caused by these telangiectasias.

Ehlers-Danlos Syndrome and Other Connective Tissue Disorders

The elastic tissue defects of Ehlers-Danlos syndrome may result in an increased bleeding tendency. A somewhat similar problem occurs in association with pseudoxanthoma elasticum and Marfan's syndrome. Platelet dysfunction in the form of reduced aggregation to ADP, collagen, and norepinephrine has been described in both Ehlers-Danlos syndrome and Marfan's syndrome. A defective fibronectin has been proposed as the cause of the hypermobility and platelet dysfunction (385c).

Mast Cell Disease

In this disorder, large numbers of mast cells are found, often diffusely located in the skin or in the gastrointestinal tract (386). These cells periodically release histamine and heparin-like substances (386, 387). Trauma to involved areas may trigger this release and may also cause urticaria and blistering of affected parts of the body. A coagulation defect is the hematologic manifestation of mast cell disease. Laboratory testing demonstrates a heparin-like effect. Because fatal hemorrhage may result from this excessive anticoagulant effect, treatment may be necessary in the form of protamine sulfate.

Urticaria pigmentosa is one form of mast cell disease. On rare occasions, mast cell disease and urticaria pigmentosa precede the onset of a mast cell leukemia (388).

LEUKOCYTE VARIATIONS IN DISEASE STATES

Since the recognition by Huët in 1931 that a nuclear segmentation defect, now called the Pelger-Huët anomaly, was inherited, a wide variety of morphologic variations in leukocytes has been found (389). Many of these alterations are discussed in detail in other chapters.

Nuclear Changes

PELGER-HUËT ANOMALY

In this anomaly, there is a limitation of segmentation of the lobing in the neutrophilic leukocytes (Fig. 52–7). The anomaly was described first by Pelger in 1928, who thought that the finding was a manifestation of tuberculosis (390). Huët recognized that this appeared to be inherited as an autosomal dominant trait (389). Individuals with this disorder rarely have neutrophils or eosinophils with more than two lobes. In heterozygotes the neutrophils are unsegmented, dumbbell-shaped, or bilobed in the nuclei. In homozygotes, the vast majority of neutrophils have round nuclei.

This anomaly affects one in 6000 individuals. Although neutrophil migration may be minimally impaired, granulocyte function is otherwise nor-

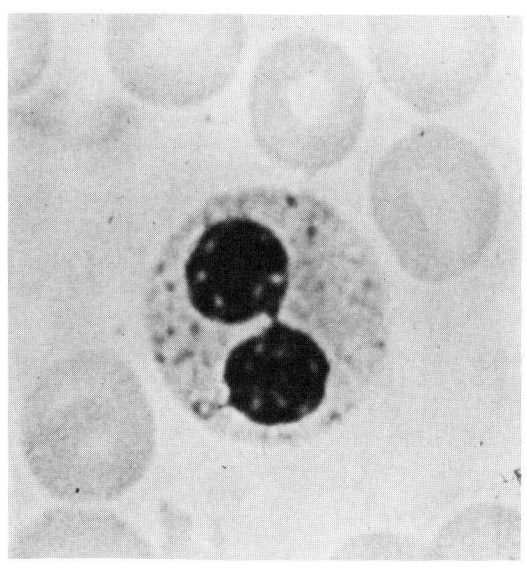

Figure 52–7. Pelger-Hüet anomaly.

mal, and individuals with this inherited anomaly suffer no adverse effects.

A Pelger-Huët–like change in granulocyte morphology may occur as an acquired condition in several disease states, such as chronic infections of the bowel, glandular fever, malaria, leukemia, and diffuse metastatic disease (391, 392). This same finding may be produced by toxins and certain drugs such as colchicine (393). Bilobed nuclei are common in many other animal species, most notably the rabbit.

Hereditary Constitutional Hypersegmentation of Neutrophils

In this autosomal dominant condition, the mean number of neutrophil nuclear lobes is approximately four, as opposed to approximately three lobes found in normal neutrophils (394). This hereditary form of neutrophil hypersegmentation is not associated with any adverse effects and appears to be more common than previously thought. It must be distinguished from more significant disorders such as vitamin B_{12} and folate deficiencies and myeloproliferative states.

Hereditary Constitutional Hypersegmentation of Eosinophils

This is probably an autosomal disorder in which the mean lobe count of eosinophils is between three and four, unlike the mean lobe count of normal eosinophils, which is 2.3. Affected individuals are otherwise normal (395).

Hereditary Giant Neutrophils

Normal neutrophils have an average cell size of 12.7 μ. In this hereditary autosomal dominant disorder, the neutrophil diameter is about 17 μ, which represents an approximate doubling of the white cell size (396). There are usually 6 to 10 nuclear lobes. Actually, only relatively few neutrophils demonstrate these morphologic abnormalities in affected individuals, but they are clearly distinguished from the normal population because these findings never occur otherwise.

Hereditary Prevalence of Nuclear Appendages

In general, threadlike and other small projections from the nucleus of neutrophils are relatively nonspecific. Excessive numbers of projections may be seen in various forms of carcinoma, in trisomy 13–15, and as a hereditary phenomenon (397) (Fig. 52–8).

These disorders must be distinguished from those that increase the number of neutrophil drumsticks, which are female-specific nuclear ap-

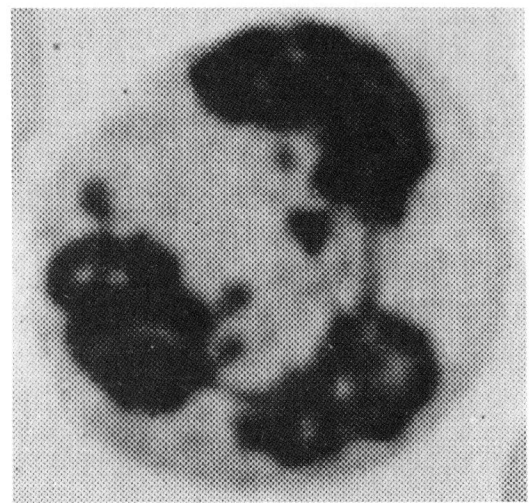

Figure 52–8. Increased nuclear appendages in a neutrophil of a patient with trisomy 13–15. (From Raymond, L. A., and Tew, J.: J. Neurol. Neurosurg. Psychiatry 41:83, 1978.)

pendages. In normal women, drumsticks are present in 2 to 10 per cent of mature neutrophils (398). At least six drumsticks per 500 neutrophils must be present for the sex to be determined as female. Pseudodrumsticks in the male generally occur, if at all, in fewer than six of 500 neutrophils. The drumstick number is increased in any condition with a raised average number of lobes per cell—for example, in the hypersegmentation anomaly, when there are multiple X chromosomes in the karyotype, and when there is an isochromosome of the long arms of an X chromosome (X-iso X). The presence of a Y chromosome reduces the drumstick number when there are supernumerary X chromosomes (XXY, XXXY, or XXXXY). The normal drumstick head is 1.5 μ in diameter. This increases in females with a long-arm isochromosome.

Cytoplasmic Abnormalities

GRANULATION DISTURBANCES

Alder-Reilly Anomaly. This anomaly, described independently by Alder and Reilly, is discussed in detail in Chapter 38 (399). It is a hematologic manifestation of Hurler's syndrome in which prominent granules (often called Reilly bodies) are found in neutrophils that stain positively with metachromatic stains (Fig. 52–9). Increased numbers of dense cytoplasmic granules may also be seen in other mucopolysaccharidoses. Lymphocytes, monocytes, and plasma cells also may be affected.

May-Hegglin Anomaly. This is a rare autosomal dominant disorder in which large (up to 5 μ) pale blue–staining inclusions are found in the cytoplasm of neutrophils, eosinophils, basophils, and monocytes (400). Thrombocytopenia and giant

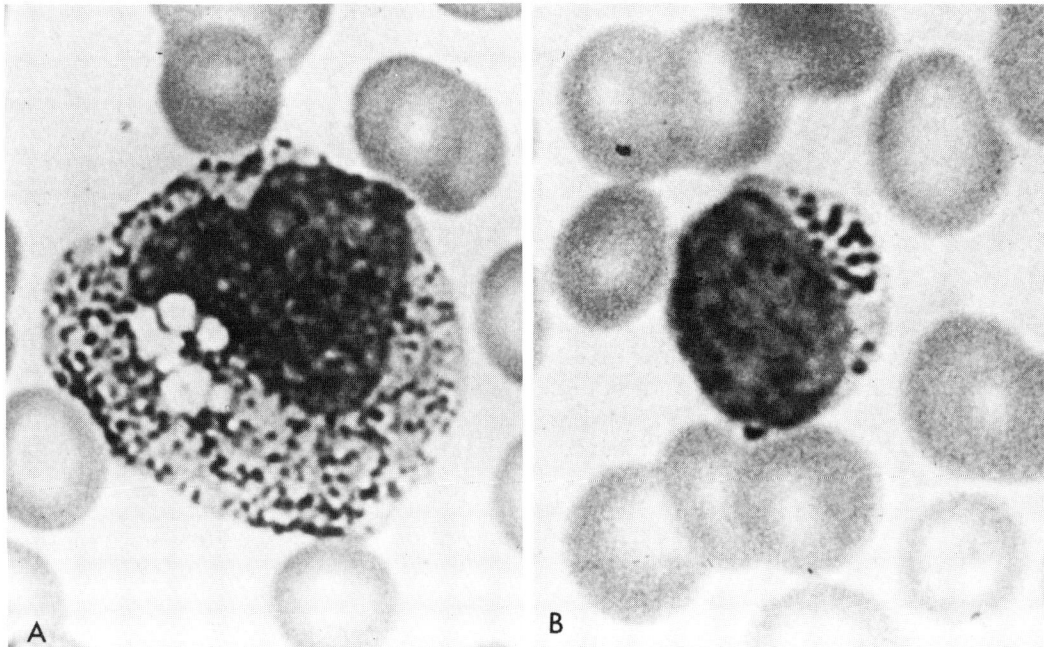

Figure 52–9. Reilly bodies in the cytoplasms of neutrophils (A) and lymphocytes (B) of a patient with Hurler's syndrome. Vacuoles are also present in the cytoplasm of the neutrophil.

platelets also are observed. The inclusions consist of material derived from endoplasmic reticulum and are similar to Döhle bodies in gross appearance.

Chédiak-Higashi Syndrome. This disorder is discussed in detail in Chapter 25. Giant granules give the cytoplasm of the neutrophil a bizarre appearance.

Batten-Spielmeyer-Vogt Disease. This degenerative neurologic disease was noted by Strouth and colleagues in 1966 to be associated with coarse azurophilic granulation in the neutrophils (401). Because these granules do not exhibit metachromasia, they can be easily differentiated from those observed in the mucopolysaccharidoses.

Hereditary Dense Granulation of Neutrophils. It should be emphasized that several normal individuals have been described who demonstrate dense granulation of neutrophils.

Hermansky-Pudlak Syndrome. This rare familial disorder is characterized by albinism, a bleeding problem related to platelet dysfunction and accumulation of ceroid-like pigment in bone marrow macrophages, and the presence of lipopigment bodies as well as other dense inclusions (402, 403).

VACUOLIZATION

Small vacuoles are not uncommonly associated with the granules in the cytoplasm of normal lymphocytes. Large vacuoles in both lymphocytes and neutrophils develop rapidly in specimens collected in anticoagulants, especially in ethylenediamine tetra-acetic acid. Cytoplasmic vacuolization may occur in response to certain stresses, such as burns and infections. Vacuolization of lymphocytes is noted in a variety of inherited disorders, including Tay-Sachs disease, Niemann-Pick disease, and some cases of Hurler's syndrome, possibly following the disappearance of specific granules (404–406). Some patients with Type II glycogen storage disease (Pompe's disease) have vacuolated lymphocytes. In this disease, a high percentage of the vacuoles stain with the periodic acid–Schiff reaction.

A familial vacuolization of leukocytes (Jordan's anomaly) has been described in which vacuoles are present in the cytoplasm of granulocytes, monocytes, and occasionally in lymphocytes and plasma cells (407). These vacuoles are lipid-containing and range in size from 2 to 5 µ. Members of some affected families have had ichthyosis, whereas others have had a progressive muscular dystrophy (408).

Eosinopenia and Eosinophilia

The lowest normal eosinophil counts are found in the immediate newborn period, following which the values in infants, children, and adults are remarkably similar (409). The mean absolute eosinophil count of children and adults is 150 cells per mm^3, with a range up to 700 cells per mm^3 (410). A diurnal variation in the eosinophil count exists, with the highest number being seen in the evening. These changes probably reflect varying activity in production of adrenal corticosteroids. Premature infants commonly demonstrate eosinophilia (264a, 264b).

Eosinopenia may occur as a result of adrenocortical hyperfunction or following the administration of pharmacologic doses of corticosteroids (411). Some children with Down's syndrome also have eosinopenia.

There are many causes of eosinophilia (Table 52–7). In the United States, allergy is the single most common cause of this finding. All types of allergy may result in eosinophilia, including asthma, hay fever, urticaria, eczema, serum sickness, and angioneurotic edema.

Drug exposure is an extremely frequent cause of eosinophilia. In most cases, no specific signs of drug allergy are present, and eosinophilia is noted coincidentally. Although some drugs are associated with a higher frequency of associated eosinophilia, any drug may potentially be a cause of this finding.

Parasitic infections are the most common cause of eosinophilia on a worldwide basis. A general rule is that whereas helminthic infections frequently cause eosinophilia, protozoal infections (with the exception of malaria) do not. Of the helminthic infections, those associated with tissue invasion, as opposed to those remaining within the bowel lumen, cause the greatest degree of eosinophilia. Among the infectious causes of eosinophilia, visceral larva migrans produces the most profound elevations of eosinophil counts, with white cell counts in excess of 100,000 cells per mm^3 not being uncommon. Parasitic infection as a cause of eosinophilia cannot be excluded by failure to demonstrate larvae or eggs in the feces. In children with blood groups other than type AB, a marked rise in isohemagglutinin titers is highly suggestive of infection with *Toxocara* organisms.

The hypereosinophilic syndrome, which is characterized by pulmonary infiltrates, cardiomegaly, congestive heart failure, and elevated eosinophil count, is a well-described but poorly understood entity (412). Eosinophilia in this disorder is marked. The hypereosinophilic syndrome is a term that encompasses disorders such as Löffler's syndrome, eosinophilic leukemoid reaction, endocarditis parietalis fibroplastica, pulmonary infiltrates with eosinophilia (PIE), disseminated eosinophilic collagen disease, and eosinophilic leukemia. The etiology of these syndromes is a source of controversy, and the possibility exists that these disorders represent a spectrum of a similar pathologic process. Eosinophilia has been noted in association with acute lymphoblastic leukemia (413). In several of the described cases, an illness similar to Löffler's syndrome preceded the onset of the leukemia (414). These cases are an interesting finding because eosinophilia is thought to be mediated by a stimulatory factor released by thymus-dependent lymphocytes (415, 416).

There are numerous other causes of eosinophilia, including collagen vascular disease, malignancy, cirrhosis, and certain skin disorders. Eosinophilia may also be observed as an autosomal dominant familial trait in some families (417).

Basophilia

Basophilia is usually said to occur when the basophil count exceeds 100 to 150 cells per mm^3 (418). Adrenocorticosteroids, infection, hyperthy-

Table 52–7. CAUSES OF EOSINOPHILIA

1. Allergic disorders: Asthma, urticaria, hay fever, angioneurotic edema, occasional drug sensitivity or simple exposure
2. Parasitic infections: Usual in invasive helminthic infections such as *Toxocara* infections, trichinosis, echinococcal infections, ascariasis, and less common in intestinal parasitism; rare in protozoal infection except for malaria
3. Skin disorders: Pemphigus, dermatitis herpetiformis
4. Hematologic and oncologic disorders: Hodgkin's disease, acute lymphatic leukemia, chronic myelogenous leukemia, pernicious anemia, postsplenectomy, immunodeficiency syndromes, polycythemia vera and other chronic myeloproliferative states, some solid tumors.
5. Infectious disorders other than parasitism: Scarlet fever, chorea, erythema multiforme, chlamydial infections
6. Inherited eosinophilia
7. Miscellaneous disorders: Rheumatoid arthritis, periarteritis nodosa, sarcoidosis, radiation therapy, peritoneal dialysis, cirrhosis, Löffler's syndrome (including pulmonary infiltration with eosinophilia [PIE] syndrome)

Table 52–8. CAUSES OF BASOPHILIA

1. Hematologic and oncologic disorders: Some hemolytic anemias, Hodgkin's disease, many chronic myeloproliferative disorders, including chronic myelogenous leukemia and polycythemia vera
2. Infections: Chronic sinusitis, smallpox, varicella
3. Endocrine: Hypothyroidism, ovulation, pregnancy
4. Drugs: Estrogens, antithyroid medications
5. Miscellaneous: Stress, nephrosis, radiation (may also decrease the basophil count)

Table 52–9. CAUSES OF MONOCYTOSIS

1. Bacterial infections: Syphilis, tuberculosis, subacute bacterial endocarditis, brucellosis
2. Nonbacterial infections: Rocky Mountain spotted fever, typhus, malaria, kala-azar, trypanosomiasis
3. Hematologic and oncologic disorders: Hodgkin's disease, preleukemia, leukemia, non-Hodgkin's lymphomas, myeloproliferative disorders, congenital and acquired neutropenias, some hemolytic anemias, metastatic solid tumors, postsplenectomy
4. Collagen vascular diseases: Systemic lupus erythematosus, rheumatoid arthritis, polyarteritis nodosa
5. Miscellaneous: Ulcerative colitis, regional enteritis, sarcoidosis, tetrachlorethane poisoning, Hand-Schüller-Christian syndrome

Table 52–10. CAUSES OF LYMPHOCYTOSIS

1. Infection: Pertussis, infectious mononucleosis, infectious lymphocytosis, infectious hepatitis, cytomegalovirus (including the postperfusion syndrome), toxoplasmosis, syphilis, brucellosis, many common viral illnesses
2. Hematologic disorders: Lymphocytic leukemias, neutropenias (a relative lymphocytosis)
3. Miscellaneous: Thyrotoxicosis, Addison's disease (a relative lymphocytosis)

roidism, and irradiation will decrease the basophil count. A wide variety of disorders may increase the basophil count, including ulcerative colitis, smallpox, varicella, and some cases of nephrosis (419). Basophilia is extremely common in association with myeloproliferative disorders such as chronic myelogenous leukemia, polycythemia vera, and myeloid metaplasia (420). Basophilia is occasionally seen in Hodgkin's disease and some hemolytic anemias (Table 52–8) (421).

Although urticaria pigmentosa and mast cell disease demonstrate increased numbers of basophils in the bone marrow and certain other tissues, the blood basophils are usually not increased.

Monocytosis

Monocytosis is common in many protozoal and rickettsial infections and is one of the hematologic hallmarks of certain bacterial infections, especially tuberculosis, subacute bacterial endocarditis, and syphilis (422). In any process that is associated with granulocytopenia, monocytosis will usually precede and herald recovery. Monocytosis will parallel disease activity in some cases of systemic lupus erythematosus and rheumatoid arthritis (423). Several hematologic malignancies may be associated with a peripheral blood monocytosis (Table 52–9).

Lymphocytosis

Except for pertussis, acute bacterial infections are rarely associated with lymphocytosis. Lymphocytosis should not be expected to be uniformly

Table 52–11. CAUSES OF LYMPHOCYTOPENIA

1. Infection: Active tuberculosis, malaria (some cases)
2. Collagen vascular disease: Systemic lupus erythematosus, regional enteritis
3. Certain immunodeficiency syndromes
4. Endocrine disorders: Hyperadrenalism and adrenal corticosteroid administration
5. Hematologic and oncologic disorders: Hodgkin's disease, solid tumors (some), aplastic anemia
6. Excessive losses: Thoracic duct drainage, intestinal lymphangiectasias

present in infants less than 6 months of age who have pertussis (424). Only 25 per cent of these infants will have an elevated lymphocyte count suggestive of pertussis. Chronic bacterial infections such as tuberculosis and brucellosis may cause a sustained lymphocytosis. Although many nonspecific viral infections may cause a mild lymphocytosis with the presence of transient atypical lymphocytes, infectious mononucleosis and cytomegalovirus infections are the only likely causes of persistent atypical lymphocytosis. Thyrotoxicosis in both children and adults also will cause a lymphocytosis (Table 52–10) (425).

The causes of lymphocytopenia are summarized in Table 52–11.

References

1. Dale, J., and Myhre, R.: Mechanical fragility of erythrocytes in normals and patients with heart valve prostheses. Acta Med. Scand. *190*:127, 1971.
2. Indeglia, R. A., Shea, M. A., et al.: Erythrocyte destruction by prosthetic heart valves. Circulation *37*(Suppl. 2):86, 1968.
3. Kaster, J. A., Akbarian, M., et al.: Paravalvular leaks and haemolytic anaemia following insertion of Starr-Edwards aortic and mitral valves. J. Thorac. Cardiovasc. Surg. *56*:279, 1968.
4. Baird, R. J., Lipton, I. H., et al.: An evaluation of the late results of aortic valve repair. J. Thorac. Cardiovasc. Surg. *49*:562, 1965.
5. Brodeur, M. T. H., Sutherland, D. W., et al.: Red blood cell survival in patients with aortic valvular disease and ball valve prosthesis. Circulation *32*:510, 1965.
6. Nevaril, G. G., Lynd, E. C., et al.: Erythrocyte damage and destruction induced by shearing stress. J. Lab. Clin. Med. *71*:784, 1968.
7. Steele, P., Weitz, H., et al.: Platelet survival time following aortic valve replacement. Circulation *51*:358, 1975.
8. Eyster, E., Rothchild, J., et al.: Chronic intravascular hemolysis after aortic valve replacement. Long-term study comparing different types of ball valve prosthesis. Circulation *44*:657, 1971.
9. Slater, S. D., and Fell, G. S.: Intravascular hemolysis and urinary iron losses after replacement of heart valves by a prosthesis. Clin. Sci. *42*:545, 1972.
9a. Linderkamp, O., Klose, H. J., et al.: Increased blood viscosity in patients with cyanotic congenital heart disease and iron deficiency. J. Pediatr. *95*:567, 1979.
10. Myhre, E., Rasmussen, K., et al.: Serum LDH activity in patients with prosthetic heart valves: a parameter of intravascular hemolysis. Am. Heart J. *80*:463, 1970.
11. Sears, D. A., and Crosby, W. H.: Intravascular hemolysis due to intracardiac prosthetic devices. Am. J. Med. *39*:341, 1965.
12. Pirofsky, B., Sutherland, D. W., et al.: Haemolytic anemia complicating aortic valve surgery. An autoimmune syndrome. New Engl. J. Med. *272*:235, 1965.
13. Bahnson, H. T., and Siegler, R. F.: A consideration of the causes of death following operation for congenital heart disease of the cyanotic type. Surg. Gynecol. Obstet. *90*:60, 1950.
14. Hartmann, R. C.: A hemorrhagic disorder occurring in patients with cyanotic congenital heart disease. Bull. Johns Hopkins Hosp. *91*:49, 1952.
15. Kontras, S. B., Sirak, H. D., et al.: Hematologic abnormalities in children with congenital heart disease. J.A.M.A. *195*:611, 1966.

16. Ekert, H., and Gilchrest, G. S.: Coagulation studies in congenital heart disease. Lancet 2:280, 1968.
17. Ekert, H., Gilchrest, G. S., et al.: Hematostasis and cyanotic congenital heart disease. J. Pediatr. 76:221, 1970.
18. Dennis, L. H., Stewart, J. L, et al.: Heparin treatment of hemorrhagic diathesis in cyanotic congenital heart disease. Lancet 1:1088, 1967.
19. Johnson, C. A., Abelgaard, C. F., et al.: Absence of coagulation abnormalities in children with cyanotic congenital heart disease. Lancet 2:660, 1968.
20. Ekert, H., Gilchrist, G. S., et al.: Hemostasis in cyanotic congenital heart disease. J. Pediatr. 76:221, 1970.
21. Komp, D. M., and Sparrow, A. W.: Polycythemia in cyanotic heart disease—a study of altered coagulation. J. Pediatr. 76:231, 1970.
22. Kontras, S. B., Bodenbender, J. G., et al.: Hyperviscosity in congenital heart disease. J. Pediatr. 76:214, 1970.
22a. Rosenthal, A., Nathan, D. G., et al.: Acute hemodynamic effects of red cell volume reduction in polycythemia of cyanotic congenital heart disease. Circulation 13:297, 1970.
23. Gross, S., Keefer, V., et al.: The platelet in cyanotic congenital heart disease. Pediatrics 42:651, 1968.
24. Mauer, H. M., McCue, C. M., et al.: Impairment in platelet aggregation in congenital heart disease. Blood 40:207, 1972.
25. Ekert, H., and Sheers, M.: Preoperative and postoperative platelet function in cyanotic congenital heart disease. J. Thorac. Cardiovasc. Surg. 67:184, 1974.
26. Ekert, H., and Dowling, G.: Platelet release abnormality and reduced prothrombin levels in children with cyanotic congenital heart disease. Aust. Paediatr. J. 13:17, 1977.
27. Gralnick, H. R.: ε-Aminocaproic acid in preoperative correction of hemostatic defect in cyanotic congenital heart disease. Lancet 1:1204, 1970.
27a. Maurer, H. M.: Hematologic effects of cardiac disease. Pediatr. Clin. North Am. 19:1083, 1972.
28. Martelle, R. R., and Linde, L. M.: Cerebrovascular accidents with tetrology of Fallot. Am. J. Dis. Child. 101:98, 1961.
29. Cottrell, C. M., and Kaplan, S.: Cerebrovascular accidents in cyanotic congenital heart disease. Am. J. Dis. Child. 125:484, 1973.
30. Card, R. T., and Weintraub, L. R.: Metabolic abnormalities of erythrocytes in severe iron deficiency. Blood 37:725, 1971.
31. Stuart, R. K., McDonald, J. W., et al.: Platelet survival times in patients with prosthetic heart valves. Am. J. Cardiol. 33:840, 1974.
32. Stiele, P., Weitz, H., et al.: Platelet survival time following aortic valve replacement. Circulation 51:358, 1975.
33. Bonchek, L. I., and Starr, A.: Ball valve prostheses: current appraisal of late results. Am. J. Cardiol. 35:843, 1975.
34. Harker, L. A., and Slichter, S. J.: Studies of platelet and fibrinogen kinetics in patients with prosthetic heart valves. New Engl. J. Med. 283:1302, 1970.
34a. Weinstein, L.: Infective endocarditis in the antibiotic era. New Engl. J. Med. 274:199, 1966.
34b. Mandell, G. L., Douglas, R. G., et al.: *Principles and Practice of Infectious Diseases.* New York, John Wiley & Sons, 1979.
34c. Ward, H. P., and Holman, J.: The association of nucleated red cells in the peripheral smear with hypoxemia. Ann. Intern. Med. 67:1190, 1967.
34d. Palva, I. P., Salokannel, S. J., et al.: Thrombocytopenia in heart failure: preliminary report. Acta Med. Scand. 187:429, 1970.
34e. Pearson, H. A., Schiebler, G. L., et al.: Functional hyposplenia in cyanotic congenital heart disease. Pediatrics 48:277, 1971.
35. Chisholm, M.: Iron deficiency and auto-immunity in postcricoid webs. Quart. J. Med. 40:427, 1971.
35a. Fisher, M., Katz, S., et al.: Silent erosive esophagitis with severe iron deficiency anemia. NY State J. Med. 1:1740, 1980.
36. Delamore, I. W., and Shearman, D. J. C.: Chronic iron deficiency anemia and atrophic gastritis. Lancet 1:889, 1965.
37. Wood, I. J., Ralston, M., et al.: Vitamin B_{12} deficiency in chronic gastritis. Gut 5:27, 1964.
37a. Bernstein, L. H., Gutstein, S., et al.: Trichobezoar: an unusual cause of megaloblastic anemia and hypoproteinemia in childhood. Digest. Dis. 18:67, 1973.
38. McIntyre, O. R., Sullivan, L. W., et al.: Pernicious anemia in childhood. New Engl. J. Med. 272:981, 1965.
39. Grady, M.: Intestinal absorption in the contaminated small bowel syndrome. Gut 12:403, 1971.
40. Moake, J. L., Kageler, W. V., et al.: Intravascular hemolysis, thrombocytopenia, leukopenia and circulatory immune complexes after jejunal ileal bypass surgery. Ann. Intern. Med. 86:576, 1977.
40a. Katz, A. J., and Falchuk, Z. M.: Current concepts in gluten sensitive enteropathy (celiac sprue). Pediatr. Clin. North Am. 22:767, 1975.
40b. Kravis, L. P., South, M. A., et al.: Eosinophilic gastroenteritis in the pediatric patient. Clin. Pediatr. 21:713, 1982.
41. Salter, R. H., and Read, A. E.: Epsilon aminocaproic acid therapy in ulcerative colitis. Gut 11:585, 1970.
42. Discombe, G.: Sulphaemoglobinemia and gluathione. Lancet 2:371, 1962.
43. Finch, C. A.: Methemoglobinemia and sulfhemoglobinemia. New Engl. J. Med. 239:470, 1948.
43a. Yosoivitz, P., Hobson, R., et al.: Sporadic Peutz-Jeghers syndrome in early childhood: a diagnostic dilemma. Am. J. Dis. Child. 128:709, 1974.
43b. Reid, J. D.: Intestinal carcinoma in the Peutz-Jeghers syndrome. J. A. M. A. 229:833, 1974.
43c. Bick, R. L., and Fekete, L. F.: Hereditary hemorrhagic telangiectasia and associated thrombohemorrhagic defects. Abstr. Am. Soc. Hematol. p. 101, 1979.
43d. Conlon, C. L., Weinger, R. S., et al.: Telangiectasia and von Willebrand's disease in two families. Ann. Intern. Med. 89:321, 1978.
44. Murphy, D., Jmrie, C. W., et al.: Haematological abnormalities in acute pancreatitis. A prospective study. Postgrad. Med. 53:310, 1977.
45. Shinowara, G. Y., Stutman, L. J., et al.: Hypercoagulability in acute pancreatitis. Am. J. Surg. 105:714, 1963.
46. Geokas, M. C., Rinderknecht, H., et al.: Methemalbumin in the diagnosis of acute hemorrhagic pancreatitis. Ann. Intern. Med. 81:483, 1974.
47. Kimber, C., Deller, D. J., et al.: The mechanism of anemia in chronic liver disease. Quart. J. Med. 34:33, 1965.
48. Smith, J. A., Lonergan, E. T., et al.: Spur cell anemia with red cells resembling acanthocytes in alcohol cirrhosis. New Engl. J. Med. 275:639, 1966.
49. Silber, R., Amorosi, E., et al.: Spur-shaped erythrocytes in Laennec's cirrhosis. New Engl. J. Med. 275:639, 1966.
50. Douglass, C. C., and Tivomey, J. J.: Transient stomatocytosis with hemolysis: a previously unrecognized complication of alcoholism. Ann. Intern. Med. 72:159, 1970.
51. Neerhout, R. C.: Abnormalities of erythrocyte stromal lipids in hepatic disease. J. Lab. Clin. Med. 71:438, 1968.
52. Cooper, R. A., Diloy-Purray, M., et al.: An analysis of lipoproteins, bile acids and red cell membranes associated with target cells and spur cells in patients with liver disease. J. Clin. Invest. 51:3182, 1972.
52a. Balistreri, W. F., Leslie, M. H., et al.: Increased cholesterol and decreased fluidity of red cell membranes (spur cell anemia) in progressive intrahepatic cholestasis. Pediatrics 67:461, 1981.
53. Jandl, J. H.: The anemia of liver disease—observations on its mechanisms. J. Clin. Invest. 34:390, 1953.
53a. Cooper, R. A.: Hemolytic syndromes and red cell mem-

54. Smith, J. R., Kay, N. E., et al.: Abnormal erythrocyte metabolism in hepatic disease. Blood 46:955, 1975.
55. Yawata, Y., Kitajima, K., et al.: Abnormal red cell metabolism in patients with hepato-biliary disorders: increased susceptibility to oxidative stress. Acta Haematol. Jap. 40:9, 1977.
56. Yamata, Y., Howe, R., et al.: Abnormal red cell metabolism causing hemolysis in uremia. Ann. Intern. Med. 79:362, 1973.
57. Deutsch, E.: Blood coagulation changes in liver disease. In *Progress in Liver Disease.* Popper, H., and Schaffner, F. (eds.), New York, Grune and Stratton, 1965, pp. 69–83.
58. Clark, R. D., Gazzard, B. G., et al.: Fibrinogen metabolism in acute hepatitis and active chronic hepatitis. Br. J. Haematol. 30:95, 1975.
59. Ratnoff, O. D.: Studies on proteolytic enzyme in human plasma; rate of lysis in normal and diseased individuals with particular reference to hepatic disease. Bull. Johns Hopkins Hosp. 84:29, 1949.
60. Jedrychowski, A., Hillenbrand, P., et al.: Fibrinolysis in cholestatic jaundice. Br. Med. J. 1:640, 1973.
61. Lane, D. A., Scully, M. F., et al.: Acquired dysfibrinogenemia in acute and chronic liver disease. Br. J. Haematol. 35:301, 1977.
62. Mester, L., and Szabados, L.: Structure defectueuse et biosynthese des fractions glucidiques dans les variantes pathologiques du fibrinogene. Nouv. Rev. Fr. Hematol. 10:679, 1970.
63. Mester, L., Szabados, J., et al.: Les modification de la composition glucidique du fibrinogene dans les cas de dysfibrinogenemie acquise. C. R. Acad. Sci. (Paris) 271:1813, 1970.
64. Rapaport, S. I., Ames, S. B., et al.: Plasma clotting factors in chronic hepatocellular disease. New Engl. J. Med. 263:278, 1960.
65. Cederblad, G.: Observations of increased levels of blood coagulation factors and other plasma proteins in cholestatic liver disease. Scand. J. Gastroenterol. 11:391, 1976.
66. Ganrot, P. O., and Nilehn, J. E.: Synthesis of an abnormal prothrombin in malnutrition and biliary obstruction and during dicumarol treatment. Scand. J. Clin. Lab. Invest. 28:245, 1971.
67. Leckner, K., Niessner, H., et al.: Coagulation abnormalities in liver disease. Semin. Thromb. Hemostas. 4:40, 1977.
68. Gallus, A. S., Lucas, C. R., et al.: Coagulation studies in patients with acute infectious hepatitis. Br. J. Haematol. 22:761, 1972.
69. Kupfer, H. G., Gee, W., et al.: Statistical correlation of liver function tests with coagulation factor deficiencies in Laennec's cirrhosis. Thromb. Diath. Haemorrh. 10:317, 1964.
70. Green, A. J., and Ratnoff, O. D.: Elevated antihemophiliac factor (factor VIII) procoagulant activity and AHF-like antigen in alcoholic cirrhosis of the liver. J. Lab. Clin. Med. 83:189, 1974.
71. Rapaport, S. I.: Plasma thromboplastin antecedent levels in patients receiving coumarin anticoagulants and in patients with Laennec's cirrhosis. Proc. Soc. Exp. Biol. Med. 108:115, 1961.
72. Gerhold, W. M., Tiongson, T., et al.: Studies of fibrin stabilizing factor. Fed. Proc. 25:446, 1966.
73. Hedner, U., Henriksson, P., et al.: Factor XIII in a clinical material. Scand. J. Haematol. 14:114, 1975.
74. Abildgaard, U., Fagerhol, M. K., et al.: Comparison of progressive antithrombin activity and the concentrations of three thrombin inhibitors in human plasma. Scand. J. Clin. Lab. Invest. 26:349, 1970.
75. Dymock, I. W., Tucker, J. S., et al.: Coagulation studies as a prognostic index in acute liver failure. Br. J. Haematol. 29:385, 1974.
76. Straub, P. W.: Diffuse intravascular coagulation in liver disease. Semin. Thromb. Hemostas. 4:29, 1977.
77. Gazzard, B. G., Clark, R., et al.: A controlled trial of heparin therapy in the coagulation defect of paracetamol-induced hepatic necrosis. Gut 15:89, 1974.
78. Marassi, A., Manzullo, U., et al.: Thromboembolism following prothrombin complex concentrates in major surgery in severe liver disease. Thromb. Haemostas. 39:248, 1978.
79. Rosenmund, A., Binswanger, U., et al.: Oxidative injury to erythrocytes, cell rigidity and splenic hemolysis in hemodialyzed uremic patients. Ann. Intern. Med. 82:460, 1975.
80. Yawata, Y., and Jacob, H. S.: Abnormal red cell metabolism in patients with chronic uremia. Nature of the defect and its persistence despite adequate hemodialysis. Blood 45:231, 1975.
81. Forman, S., Bischel, M., et al.: Erythrocyte deformability in uremic hemodialyzed patients. Ann. Intern. Med. 79:841, 1973.
81a. Anagnostou, A., Vercellotti, G., et al.: Factors which affect erythropoiesis in partially nephrectomized and sham-operated rats. Blood 48:425, 1976.
81b. Anagnostou, A., Barone, J., et al.: Effect of erythropoietin therapy on the red cell volume of uraemic and non-uraemic rats. Br. J. Haematol. 37:85, 1977.
81c. Nathan, D. G., Schupak, E., et al.: Erythropoiesis in anephric man. J. Clin. Invest. 43:2158, 1964.
82. Lichtman, M. A., and Miller, D. R.: Erythrocyte glycolysis, 2,3 diphosphoglycerate, and adenosine triphosphate concentration in uremic subjects: Relationship to extracellular phosphate concentration. J. Lab. Clin. Med. 76:267, 1970.
82a. Fluckiger, R., Harmon, W., et al.: Hemoglobin carbamylation in uremia. New Engl. J. Med. 304:823, 1981.
83. Yawata, Y., Howe, R., et al.: Abnormal red cell metabolism during hemolysis in uremia. A defect potentiated by tap water hemodialysis. Ann. Intern. Med. 79:362, 1973.
84. Chillar, R. K., and Desferges, J. F.: Red cell organic phosphates in patients with chronic renal failure on maintenance hemodialysis. Br. J. Haematol. 26:549, 1974.
85. Hurt, G. A., and Chanutin, A.: Organic phosphate compounds of erythrocytes from individuals with uremia. J. Lab. Clin. Med. 64:675, 1964.
86. Malter, B. J., Pederson, J., et al.: Lethal copper intoxication in hemodialysis. Trans. Am. Soc. Artif. Intern. Org. 15:309, 1969.
87. Carlson, D. J., and Shapiro, F. L.: Methemoglobin from well water nitrates. A complication of hemodialysis. Ann. Intern. Med. 73:757, 1970.
88. Eaton, J. W., Kolpin, C. F., et al.: Chlorinated urban water. A cause of dialysis-induced hemolytic anemia. Science 181:463, 1973.
89. Retief, F. P., Heyns, A. DuP., et al.: Aspects of folate metabolism in renal failure. Br. J. Haematol. 36:405, 1977.
90. Waxman, S., and Schreiber, C.: Characteristics of folic acid-binding protein in folate deficient serum. Blood 42:291, 1973.
91. Richardson, J. R., and Weinstein, M. B.: Erythropoietic response of dialyzed patients to testosterone administration. Ann. Intern. Med. 73:403, 1970.
92. Fried, W., Jonasson, O., et al.: The hematologic effect of androgen in uremic patients. Study of packed cell volume and erythropoietin responses. Ann. Intern. Med. 79:823, 1973.
93. Ways, P., Huff, J. W., et al.: Polycythemia and histologically proven renal disease. Arch. Intern. Med. 107:154, 1961.
94. Hoppin, E. C., Depner, T., et al.: Erythrocytosis associated with diffuse parenchymal lesions of the kidney. Br. J. Haematol. 32:557, 1976.

95. Kaplow, L. S., and Goffinit, J. A.: Profound neutropenia during the early phase of hemodialysis. J.A.M.A. 203:1135, 1968.
96. MacGregor, R. R.: Granulocyte adherence changes induced by hemodialysis, endotoxin, epinephrine, and glucocorticoids. Ann. Intern. Med. 86:35, 1977.
97. Craddock, P. R., Fehr, J., et al.: Hemodialysis leukopenia. Pulmonary vascular leukostasis resulting from complement activation by dialyzer cellophane membranes. J. Clin. Invest. 59:879, 1977.
98. Woodward, J., and Brubaker, L. H.: Production of neutropenia-over-shoot cycle in sheep by reinfusion of cellophane exposed blood. Clin. Res. 21:56, 1973 (Abstr.).
99. Lewis, J. H., Tucker, M. B., et al.: Bleeding tendency in uremia. Blood 11:1073, 1956.
100. Singh, G., Hussain, S. K., et al.: Hemostatic mechanism in uremia. Ind. J. Med. Sci. 23:387, 1969.
100a. Vaziri, N. D., Branson, H. E., et al.: Changes of coagulation factors IX, VIII, VII, X, V in nephrotic syndrome. Am. J. Med. Sci. 280:167, 1980.
101. Rabiner, S. F.: Bleeding in uremia. Med. Clin. North Am. 56:221, 1972.
102. Kendall, A. G., Lowenstein, L., et al.: The hemorrhagic diathesis in renal disease (with special reference to acute uremia). Can. Med. Assoc. J. 85:405, 1961.
103. Wardle, E. N., and Taylor, G.: Fibrin breakdown products and fibrinolysis in renal disease. J. Clin. Pathol. 21:140, 1968.
104. Galasinski, W., Worowski, K., et al.: Turnover of ^{131}I-fibrinogen in mercury chloride intoxicated dogs. Thromb. Diath. Haemorrh. 18:268, 1967.
105. Larsson, S. O.: On coagulation and fibrinolysis in renal failure. Scand. J. Haematol. Suppl. 15, 1971.
106. Bouma, B. M., Hedner, U., et al.: Typing of fibrinogen degradation products in urine in various clinical disorders. Scand. J. Clin. Lab. Invest. 27:331, 1971.
106a. Salem, H. H., Whitworth, J. A., et al.: Hypercoagulation in glomerulonephritis. Br. Med. J. 282:2083, 1981.
107. Erickson, R. V., Williams, M., et al.: A true hypercoagulability state in patients on chronic hemodialysis. Trans. Am. Soc. Artif. Intern. Org. 12:205, 1966.
108. Dossetor, J. B., Gutelius, J. R., et al.: The thromboembolic potential of the nephrotic syndrome. International Congress of Nephrology. Proceedings, p. 184, 1966 (Abstr.).
109. Handley, D. A., and Lawrence, J. R.: Factor IX deficiency in the nephrotic syndrome. Lancet 1:1079, 1967.
110. Natelson, E., Lynch, E. C., et al.: Acquired factor IX deficiency in the nephrotic syndrome. Ann. Intern. Med. 73:373, 1970.
111. Lewis, J. H.: Separation and molecular weight estimation of coagulation and fibrinolytic proteins by sephadex gel filtration. Proc. Soc. Exp. Biol. Med. 116:120, 1964.
112. Honig, G. R., and Lindley, A.: Deficiency of Hageman factor (factor XIII) in patients with the nephrotic syndrome. J. Pediatr. 78:633, 1971.
113. Donaldson, V. H., and Ratnoff, O. D.: Hageman factor: alterations in physical properties during activation. Science 150:754, 1965.
114. Bang, N. U., Trygstad, C. W., et al.: Enhanced platelet function in glomerular renal disease. J. Lab. Clin. Med. 81:651, 1973.
115. Kwaan, H. C., Colwell, J. A., et al.: Increased platelet aggregation in diabetes mellitus. J. Lab. Clin. Med. 80:236, 1972.
116. Thomas, D. P.: Abnormalities of platelet aggregation in cirrhosis. Ann. N.Y. Acad. Sci. 201:243, 1972.
117. Kincaid-Smith, P.: The natural history and treatment of mesangiocapillary glomerulonephritis. In Glomerulonephritis: Morphology, Natural History and Treatment. Kincaid-Smith, P., Matthew, T. H., et al. (Eds.), New York, John Wiley & Sons, Inc., 1973, p. 515.
118. Kincaid-Smith, P.: The treatment of chronic mesangiocapillary (membranoproliferative) glomerulonephritis with impaired renal function. Med. J. Aust. 2:587, 1972.
119. Robson, A. M., Cole, B. R., et al.: Severe glomerulonephritis complicated by coagulopathy: treatment with anticoagulant and immunosuppressive drugs. J. Pediatr. 90:881, 1978.
120. West, C. D.: Anticoagulant and immunosuppressive drugs in the treatment of severe glomerulonephritis with coagulopathy. J. Pediatr. 90:1051, 1978.
121. Stewart, J. H.: Platelet numbers and lifespan in acute and chronic renal failure. Thromb. Diath. Haemorrh. 17:532, 1967.
122. Willoughby, M. C. N., and Crouch, S. J.: An investigation of the hemorrhagic tendency in renal failure. Br. J. Haematol. 7:315, 1961.
123. Salzman, E. W., and Neri, L. L.: Adhesiveness of blood platelets in uremia. Thromb. Diath. Haemorrh. 15:84, 1966.
124. Custaldi, P. A., Rozenberg, M. C., et al.: The bleeding disorder of uremia. A qualitative platelet defect. Lancet 2:66, 1966.
125. Joist, H. H., Pechan, J., et al.: Studies on the nature and etiology of uremic thrombocytopathy. Verh. Dtsch. Ges. Inn. Med. 75:476, 1969.
126. Hellem, A. J., Odegaard, A. E., et al.: Platelet adhesiveness in chronic renal failure. Xth Congress International Society of Haematology, Stockholm K:1, 1964 (Abstr.).
127. Horowitz, H. I.: Uremic toxins and platelet function. Arch. Intern. Med. 126:823, 1970.
128. Epstein, C. J., Sahud, M. A., et al.: Hereditary macrothrombocytopathia, nephritis, and deafness. Am. J. Med. 52:299, 1972.
128a. Gubler, M., Levy, M., et al.: Alport's syndrome: a report of 58 cases and a review of the literature. Am. J. Med. 70:493, 1981.
129. Eckstein, J. D., Filip, D. J., et al.: Hereditary thrombocytopenia, deafness and renal disease. Ann. Intern. Med. 82:639, 1975.
130. Golde, D. W., Bersch, N., et al.: Thyroid hormones stimulate erythropoiesis in vitro. Br. J. Haematol. 37:173, 1977.
131. Malgor, L. A., Blanc, C. C., et al.: Direct effects of thyroid hormones on bone marrow erythroid cells of rats. Blood 45:671, 1975.
131a. Chu, Y., Monteleone, J. A., et al.: Anemia in children and adolescents with hypothyroidism. Clin. Pediatr. 20:696, 1981.
132. Wardrop, C., and Hutchinson, H. E.: Red cell shape in hypothyroidism. Lancet 2:1243, 1969.
133. Tudhope, G. R., and Wilson, G. M.: Anemia in hypothyroidism. Quart. J. Med. 29:513, 1960.
134. Tudhope, G. R., and Wilson, G. M.: Deficiency of vitamin B_{12} in hypothyroidism. Lancet 1:703, 1962.
135. Falko, J. M., and Cohen, J. R.: Erythrocytosis and hypothyroidism. Ann. Intern. Med. 84:446, 1976.
136. Das, K. C., Mukherjee, M., et al.: Erythropoiesis and erythropoietin in hypo- and hyperthryroidism. J. Clin. Endocrinol. 40:211, 1975.
137. Rodman, G. P., and Jensen, W. N.: A study of red blood cell survival in hypo- and hyperthyroidism. Clin. Res. Proc. 5:8, 1957.
138. Macho, L.: The effect of thyroid hormone on the glycolytic activity of blood. Clin. Chim. Acta 2:345, 1957.
139. Necheles, T. F., and Beutler, E.: The effect of triiodothyronine on the oxidative metabolism of erythrocytes. I. Cellular studies. J. Clin. Invest. 38:797, 1959.
140. Pearson, H. A., and Druyan, R.: Erythrocyte glucose-6-phosphate dehydrogenase activity related to thyroid activity. J. Lab. Clin. Med. 57:343, 1961.
141. Pangaro, J. A., Weinstein, M., et al.: Red cell zinc and red cell zinc metalloenzymes in hyperthyroidism. Acta Endocrinol. 76:645, 1974.

142. Synder, L. M., and Reddy, W. J.: Mechanism of action of thyroid hormones on erythrocyte 2,3 diphosphoglycerate. J. Clin. Invest. *49*:1993, 1970.
143. Lie Injo, L. E., Lopey, C. G., et al.: Erythrocyte carbonic anhydrase activity in health and disease. Clin. Chim. Acta *29*:541, 1970.
144. Matsuda, Y.: Studies on osmotic abnormalities of erythrocytes in thyrotoxicosis. Acta Haematol. Jap. *29*:717, 1966.
145. Goolden, A. W. G., Bateman, D., et al.: Red cell sodium in hyperthyroidism. Br. Med. J. *2*:552, 1971.
145a. Barnes, H. V., and Blizzard, R. M.: Antithyroid drug therapy for toxic diffuse goiter (Graves' disease): 30 years' experience in children and adolescents. J. Pediatr. *91*:313, 1977.
145b. Lightsey, A. L., Chapman, R. M., et al.: Immune neutropenia. Ann. Intern. Med. *86*:60, 1977.
146. Lamberg, B. A., Kwikangas, V., et al.: Thrombocytopenia and decreased life span of thrombocytes in hyperthyroidism. Ann. Clin. Res. *3*:98, 1971.
147. Egeberg, O.: Thyroid function and hemostasis. Scand. J. Clin. Lab. Invest. *16*:511, 1964.
148. Simone, J. V., Abildgaard, C. T., et al.: Blood coagulation in thyroid dysfunction. New Engl. J. Med. *27*:1057, 1965.
149. Edson, J. R., Fecher, D. R., et al.: Low platelet adhesiveness and other hemostatic abnormalities in hypothyroidism. Ann. Intern. Med. *82*:342, 1975.
150. Hume, R.: Fibrinolytic activity and thyroid function. Br. Med. J. *1*:686, 1965.
150a. Ardeman, S., Boralessa, H., et al.: Coagulation inhibitor in hypothyroidism. Br. Med. J. *282*:1508, 1981.
151. BoezVillasenor, J., Ruth, C. E., et al.: The blood picture in Addison's disease. Blood *3*:769, 1948.
152. Plotz, C. M., Knowlton, A. I., et al.: The natural history of Cushing's syndrome. Am. J. Med. *13*:597, 1952.
153. Claman, H. N.: Corticosteroids and lymphoid cells. New Engl. J. Med. *287*:388, 1972.
154. VanDyke, D. C., Contopoulos, A. N., et al.: Hormonal factors influencing erythropoiesis. Acta Haematol. *11*:203, 1954.
155. Parker, J. P., Beirne, G. J., et al.: Androgen-induced increase in red cell 2,3 diphosphoglycerate. New Engl. J. Med. *287*:381, 1972.
156. Delivoria-Papadopoulos, M., Coburn, C. F., et al.: Cyclic variations of rate of carbon monoxide production in normal women. J. Appl. Physiol. *36*:49, 1974.
157. Berlin, R.: Red cell survival studies in normal and leukemic subjects. Acta Med. Scand. *252* (Suppl.):42, 1951.
158. Mercke, C., and Lundh, B.: Erythrocyte filterability and heme catabolism during the menstrual cycle. Ann. Intern. Med. *85*:322, 1976.
159. Durocher, J. R., Weir, M. S., et al.: Effect of oral contraceptives and pregnancy on red cell deformability and surface charge. Proc. Soc. Exp. Biol. Med. *150*:368, 1975.
160. Oski, F. A., Lubin, B., et al.: Reduced red cell filterability with oral contraceptive agents. Ann. Intern. Med. *77*:417, 1972.
161. Pechet, L., and Alexander, B.: Increased clotting factors in pregnancy. New Engl. J. Med. *265*:1093, 1961.
161a. Escamilla, R. F., and Lisser, V. H.: Simmond's disease. J. Clin. Endocrinol. *2*:65, 1942.
162. Rodriguez, J. M., and Shahidi, N. T.: Red cell 2,3 DPG in adaptive red-cell volume deficiency. New Engl. J. Med. *285*:479, 1971.
163. Root, A. W., Oski, F. A., et al.: Red cell G-6-PD activity in children with hypothyroidism and hypopituitarism. J. Pediatr. *70*:369, 1967.
164. Oski, F. A., Root, A. W., et al.: In vitro inhibition of RBC glucose consumption by human growth hormone. Nature *215*:81, 1967.
165. Livingstone, C. S., and Boezarow, B.: Idiopathic pulmonary hemosiderosis in a newborn. Arch. Dis. Child. *42*:543, 1967.
166. Soergel, K. M., and Sommers, S. C.: Idiopathic pulmonary hemosiderosis and related syndromes. Am. J. Med. *32*:499, 1962.
167. Gilman, P. A., and Zinkham, W. H.: Severe idiopathic pulmonary hemosiderosis in the absence of clinical or radiologic evidence of pulmonary disease. J. Pediatr. *75*:118, 1969.
168. Matsaniotis, N., Karpouzas, J., et al.: Idiopathic pulmonary hemosiderosis in children. Arch. Dis. Child. *43*:307, 1968.
169. Elgenmark, O., and Kjellberg, S. R.: Hemosiderosis of the lungs—Typical roentgenological findings. Acta Radiol. *29*:32, 1948.
170. Fleischner, F. G., and Berenberg, A. L.: Idiopathic pulmonary hemosiderosis. Radiology *62*:522, 1954.
171. Hammond, D., and Crane, J.: Sequestration of iron in the lungs in idiopathic pulmonary hemosiderosis. Am. J. Dis. Child. *96*:503, 1958 (Abstr.).
172. Hyatt, R. W., Edelstein, E. R., et al.: Ultrastructure of the lung in idiopathic pulmonary hemosiderosis. Am. J. Med. *52*:822, 1972.
173. Irwin, R. S., Cottrell, T. S., et al.: Idiopathic pulmonary hemosiderosis: An electron microscopic and immunofluorescent study. Chest *65*:41, 1974.
174. Gellis, S. S., Reinhold, P. I. D., et al.: Use of aspiration lung puncture in diagnosis of idiopathic pulmonary hemosiderosis. Am. J. Dis. Child. *85*:303, 1953.
175. Halvorsen, S.: Cortisone treatment of idiopathic pulmonary hemosiderosis. Acta Paediatr. *45*:139, 1956.
176. Byrd, R. B., and Gracey, D. R.: Immunosuppressive treatment of idiopathic pulmonary hemosiderosis. J.A.M.A. *226*:458, 1973.
177. Heiner, D. C., Sears, J. W., et al.: Multiple precipitins to cow's milk in chronic respiratory disease. A syndrome including poor growth, gastrointestinal symptoms, evidence of allergy, iron deficiency anemia and pulmonary hemosiderosis. Am. J. Dis. Child. *103*:634, 1962.
178. Matthews, T. S., and Soothill, J. F.: Complement activation after milk feeding in children with cow's milk allergy. Lancet *2*:893, 1970.
179. Rose, G. A., and Spencer, H.: Polyarteritis nodosa. Quart. J. Med. *26*:43, 1957.
180. DeGowin, R. I., Oda, Y., et al.: Nephritis and lung hemorrhage. Goodpasture's syndrome. Arch. Intern. Med. *111*:16, 1963.
181. Byrd, R. B., and Trunk, G.: Systemic lupus erythematosus presenting as pulmonary hemosiderosis. Chest *64*:129, 1973.
182. Thomas, A. M.: A case of Wegener's granulomatosis. J. Clin. Pathol. *11*:146, 1958.
183. Jorgensen, G., and Wurm, K.: The ABO blood group in sarcoidosis. Proceedings of the International Conference on Sarcoidosis, Stockholm, 1963.
184. Lewis, J. G., and Woods, A. C.: The ABO and rhesus blood groups in patients with respiratory disease. Tubercle *42*:362, 1961.
185. Hirschman, R. J., and Johns, C. J.: Hemoglobin studies in sarcoidosis. Ann. Intern. Med. *62*:129, 1965.
186. Edwards, M. H., Wagner, J. A., et al.: Sarcoidosis with thrombocytopenia. Ann. Intern. Med. *37*:803, 1952.
186a. Scully, R. E., Galdabini, J. J., et al.: Case records of the Massachusetts General Hospital. New Engl. J. Med. *299*:765, 1978.
186b. Dickerman, J. D., Holbrook, P. R., et al.: Etiology and therapy of thrombocytopenia associated with sarcoidosis. J. Pediatr. *81*:758, 1972.
186c. Knodel, A. R., and Beekman, R. F.: Severe thrombocytopenia in sarcoidosis. J. A. M. A. *243*:258, 1980.
186d. Vichinsky, E. P., Pennathur-Das, R., et al.: Inadequate erythroid response to hypoxia in cystic fibrosis. J. Pediatr. *105*:15, 1984.
186e. Ater, J. L., Herbst, J. J., et al.: Relative anemia and iron deficiency in cystic fibrosis. Pediatrics *71*:810, 1983.

187. Cartwright, G. E.: The anemia of chronic disorders. Semin. Hematol. 3:351, 1966.
188. Cartwright, G. E., and Wintrobe, M. M.: The anemia of infection. In *Advances in Internal Medicine*, Vol. 5. Dock, W., and Snapper, J. (eds.), Chicago, Year Book Medical Publishers, 1952, p. 165.
189. Freireich, E. J., Ross, J. F., et al.: Radioactive iron metabolisms and erythrocyte survival studies of the mechanisms of the anemia associated with rheumatoid arthritis. J. Clin. Invest. 36:1043, 1951.
190. Ebaugh, F. G.: The anemia of rheumatoid arthritis. In *Iron in Clinical Medicine*. Wallerstein, M., and Methier, G. (eds.), Berkeley, University of California Press, 1958, p. 261.
191. Ward, H. P., Kurnick, J. E., et al.: Serum level of erythropoietin in anemias associated with chronic infection, malignancies and hematopoietic disease. J. Clin. Invest. 50:332, 1971.
192. Lukens, J. N.: Control of erythropoiesis in rats with adjuvant-induced chronic inflammation. Blood 41:37, 1973.
193. Wintrobe, M. M., Grinstein, M., et al.: The anemia of infection. VI. The influence of cobalt on the anemia associated with inflammation. Blood 2:323, 1947.
194. Robinson, J. C., James, G. W., III, et al.: The effect of oral therapy with cobaltous chloride on the blood of patients suffering with chronic suppurative infection. New Engl. J. Med. 240:749, 1949.
195. Hillman, R. A., and Henderson, D. A.: The control of marrow production by the level of iron supply. J. Clin. Invest. 48:454, 1969.
196. Hurani, F. I., Burke, W., et al.: Defective reutilization of iron in the anemia of inflammation. J. Lab. Clin. Med. 65:560, 1965.
197. Shade, S. G.: Normal incorporation of iron into intestinal ferritin in inflammation. Proc. Soc. Exp. Biol. Med. 139:620, 1972.
197a. Abshire, T. C., and Reeves, J. D.: Anemia of inflammation in children. J. Pediatr. 103:868, 1983.
198. Lipschitz, D. A., Cook, J. D., et al.: A clinical evaluation of serum ferritin as an index of iron stores. New Engl. J. Med. 290:1213, 1974.
199. Koerper, M. A., Stempel, D. A., et al.: Anemia in patients with juvenile rheumatoid arthritis. J. Pediatr. 92:930, 1978.
199a. Hansen, N. E.: The anaemia of chronic disorders: a bag of unsolved questions. Scand. J. Haematol. 31:397, 1983.
200. Partridge, R. E. H., and Duthie, J. J. R.: Incidence of macrocytic anemia in rheumatoid arthritis. Br. Med. J. 1:89, 1963.
201. Omer, A., and Mowat, A. G.: Nature of anemia in rheumatoid arthritis. IX. Folate metabolism in patients with rheumatoid arthritis. Ann. Rheum. Dis. 27:414, 1968.
202. Alter, H. J., Zvaifler, N. J., et al.: Interrelationship of rheumatoid arthritis, folic acid and aspirin. Blood 38:405, 1971.
203. Richmond, J., Alexander, W. R. M., et al.: Nature of anemia in rheumatoid arthritis. V. Red cell survival measured by radioactive chromium. Ann. Rheum. Dis. 20:133, 1961.
203a. Rubin, R. N., Walker, B. K., et al.: Erythroid aplasia in juvenile rheumatoid arthritis. Am. J. Dis. Child. 132:760, 1978.
203b. Dainiak, N., Hardin, J., et al.: Humoral suppression of erythropoiesis in SLE and rheumatoid arthritis. Am. J. Med. 69:537, 1980.
204. Mowat, A. G., and Baum, J.: Chemotaxis of polymorphonuclear leukocytes from patients with rheumatoid arthritis. J. Clin. Invest. 50:2541, 1971.
205. Turner, R. A., Schumacker, H. R., et al.: Phagocytic function of polymorphonuclear leukocytes in rheumatic diseases. J. Clin. Invest. 52:1632, 1973.
206. Segal, A. W.: Nitroblue-tetrazolium tests. Lancet 2:1248, 1974.
207. Garner, R. W., Mowat, A. G., et al.: Wound healing after operations on patients with rheumatoid arthritis. J. Bone Joint Surg. 55B:134, 1973.
207a. Brewer, E. J., Jr.: *Juvenile Rheumatoid Arthritis*. Philadelphia, W. B. Saunders Co., 1980.
207b. Athreya, B. H., Moser, G., et al.: Increased circulating basophils in juvenile rheumatoid arthritis: a preliminary report. Am. J. Dis. Child. 129:935, 1975.
207c. Debarre, F., LeGo, A., et al.: Hyperbasophilic immunoblasts in circulating blood in chronic inflammatory, rheumatic and collagen diseases. Ann. Rheum. Dis. 34:422, 1975.
208. Felty, A. R.: Chronic arthritis in the adult associated with splenomegaly and leukopenia. Bull. Johns Hopkins Hosp. 35:16, 1924.
209. Collier, R. L., and Brush, B. E.: Hematologic disorders in Felty's syndrome: Prolonged benefits of splenectomy. Am. J. Surg. 112:869, 1966.
210. Gupta, R. C., Robinson, W. A., et al.: Granulopoietic activity in Felty's syndrome. Ann. Rheum. Dis. 34:156, 1975.
211. Rosenthal, F. D., Beeley, J. M., et al.: White cell antibodies and the etiology of Felty's syndrome. Quart. J. Med. 43:189, 1974.
211a. Blumfelder, T. M., Logue, G. L., et al.: Felty's syndrome: effects of splenectomy upon granulocyte count and granulocyte-associated IgG. Ann. Intern. Med. 94:623, 1981.
212. Gupta, R. C., Robinson, W. A., et al.: Efficacy of lithium in rheumatoid arthritis with granulocytopenia (Felty's syndrome): A preliminary report. Arthritis Rheum. 18:179, 1975.
213. Harker, G. W., Rothstein, G., et al.: Stimulation of neutrophil production by lithium. Clin. Res. 23:103A, 1975.
214. DuBois, E. Z., and Tuffanelli, D. L.: Clinical manifestations of systemic lupus erythematosus. Computer analysis of 520 cases. J.A.M.A. 190:104, 1964.
215. Fries, J. F., and Holman, H. H.: *Systemic Lupus Erythematosus, Clinical Analyses*. Philadelphia, W. B. Saunders Co., 1975, p. 79.
216. Weens, J. H., and Schwartz, R. S.: Etiologic factors in hemolytic anemia. Semin. Hematol. 7:303, 1974.
217. Westerman, M. P., Martinez, R. C., et al.: Anemia and scleroderma. Frequency, causes, marrow findings. Arch. Intern. Med. 122:39, 1968.
218. Michael, S. R., Vural, I. L., et al.: The hematological aspects of systemic lupus erythematosus. Blood 6:1059, 1951.
219. Boxer, L. A., Greenberg, M. S., et al.: Autoimmune neutropenia. New Engl. J. Med. 293:748, 1975.
220. Duckham, D. J., Rhyne, R. L., et al.: Retardation of colony growth of in vitro bone marrow culture using sera from patients with Felty's syndrome, disseminated lupus erythematosus (SLE), rheumatoid arthritis, and other disease states. Arthritis Rheum. 18:323, 1975.
221. Mowat, A. G., and Baum, J.: Chemotaxis of polymorphonuclear leukocytes from patients with rheumatoid arthritis. J. Clin. Invest. 50:2541, 1971.
222. Zivkovic, M., and Baum, J.: Chemotaxis of polymorphonuclear leukocytes from patients with systemic lupus erythematosus and Felty's syndrome. Immunol. Commun. 1:39, 1972.
223. Gewurz, H., Page, A. R., et al.: Complement activation and inflammatory neutrophil exudation in man. Int. Arch. Allerg. Appl. Immunol. 32:64, 1974.
224. Orozco, J. H., Jasin, H. E., et al.: Defective phagocytosis in patients with systemic lupus erythematosus (SLE). Arthritis Rheum. 13:342, 1970 (Abstr.).
225. Messener, R. P., Lindstrom, F. D., et al.: Peripheral blood lymphocyte cell surface markers during the course of systemic lupus erythematosus. J. Clin. Invest. 52:3046, 1973.

226. Glinski, W., Gershwin, M. E., et al.: Fractionation of cells on a discontinuous ficoll gradient. Study of peripheral blood lymphocyte subpopulations in normal humans and patients with systemic lupus erythematosus. J. Clin. Invest. 57:604, 1976.
227. Lockshin, M. D., Eisenhauer, A. C., et al.: Cell-mediated immunity in rheumatic diseases. II. Mitogen responses in systemic lupus erythematosus and other illnesses: correlation with T and B lymphocyte populations. Arthritis Rheum. 18:245, 1975.
228. Jasen, H. E., and Ziff, M.: Immunoglobulin synthesis by peripheral blood cells in systemic lupus erythematosus. Arthritis Rheum. 18:219, 1975.
229. Vaughan, J. H., and Chihara, T.: Lymphocyte function in rheumatic disorders. Arch. Intern. Med. 135:1324, 1975.
230. Bankhurst, A. D., and Williams, R. C., Jr.: Identification of DNA binding lymphocytes in patients with systemic lupus erythematosus. J. Clin. Invest. 56:1378, 1975.
231. Bell, D. A., Clark, C., et al.: Anti DNA antibody production by lymphoid cells of NZB/W mice and human systemic lupus erythematosus (SLE). Clin. Immunol. Immunopathol. 1:293, 1973.
232. Delbarre, F., Go, A. L., et al.: Hyperbasophilic immunoblasts in the circulating blood in chronic inflammatory rheumatic and collagen diseases. Ann. Rheum. Dis. 34:422, 1975.
233. Winfield, J. B., Winchester, R. J., et al.: Different types of antilymphocyte antibodies in the sera of systemic lupus erythematosus (SLE) patients. Clin. Res. 22:432A, 1974 (Abstr.).
234. Williams, R. C., Jr., Emmons, J. D., et al.: Studies of human sera with cytotoxic activity. J. Clin. Invest. 50:1514, 1971.
235. Stastny, P., and Ziff, M.: Lymphocyte and platelet autoantibodies in SLE. Lancet 1:1239, 1971 (Letter).
236. Rabinowitz, Y., and Dameshek, W.: Systemic lupus erythematosus after idiopathic thrombocytopenia purpura. Ann. Intern. Med. 52:1, 1960.
237. Karpatkin, S., Strick, N., et al.: Cumulative experience in the detection of antiplatelet antibody in 234 patients with idiopathic thrombocytopenic purpura, systemic lupus erythematosus and other clinical disorders. Am. J. Med. 52:776, 1972.
238. Dixon, R., Rosse, W., et al.: Quantitative determination of antibody in idiopathic thrombocytopenic purpura. Correlation of serum and platelet bound antibody with clinical response. New Engl. J. Med. 292:230, 1975.
238a. Agnello, V., Pariser, K., et al.: Preliminary observations on danazol therapy of systemic lupus erythematosus: effects on DNA antibodies, thrombocytopenia and complement. J. Rheumatol. 10:682, 1983.
239. Clancy, R., Jenkins, E., et al.: Qualitative platelet abnormalities in idiopathic thrombocytopenic purpura. New Engl. J. Med. 286:622, 1972.
240. Karpatkin, S., and Lackner, H. L.: Association of antiplatelet antibody with functional platelet disorders. Am. J. Med. 59:599, 1975.
241. Conley, C. L., and Hartman, R. C.: A haemorrhagic disorder caused by circulating anticoagulant in patients with disseminated lupus erythematosus. J. Clin. Invest. 31:621, 1952.
242. Feinstein, D. I., and Rapaport, S. I.: Acquired inhibitors of blood coagulation. Prog. Hemostas. Thromb. 1:75, 1972.
243. Lechner, K.: Acquired inhibitors in nonhemophiliac patients. Haemostosis 3:65, 1974.
244. Lechner, K.: A new type of coagulation inhibitor. Thromb. Diath. Haemorrh. 21:482, 1969.
245. Regan, M. G., Lachner, H., et al.: Platelet function and coagulation profile in lupus erythematosus. Studies in 50 patients. Ann. Intern. Med. 81:462, 1974.
246. Green, D.: Circulating anticoagulants. Med. Clin. North. Am. 56:145, 1972.
247. Gonyea, L., Herdman, R., et al.: The coagulation abnormalities in systemic lupus erythematosus. Thromb. Diath. Haemorrh. 20:455, 1968.
248. Rivard, G. E., Schiffman, S., et al.: Co-factor of the lupus anticoagulant. Thromb. Diath. Haemorrh. 32:554, 1974.
249. Corrigan, J., Patterson, J. H., et al.: Incoagulability of the blood in systemic lupus erythematosus. Am. J. Dis. Child. 119:365, 1970.
250. Rapaport, S. I., Ames, S. B., et al.: A plasma coagulation defect in systemic lupus erythematosus arising from hypoprothrombinemia combined with anti-prothrombinase activity. Blood 15:212, 1960.
251. Ratnoff, O. D.: An accelerating property of plasma for the coagulation of fibrinogen by thrombin. J. Clin. Invest. 33:1175, 1954.
251a. Editorial comment: Lupus anticoagulant. Lancet 1:1157, 1984.
252. Veltkamp, J. J., Kerkhoven, P., et al.: Circulating anticoagulant in disseminated lupus erythematosus. Haemostasis 2:253, 1973/4.
253. Green, D., and Rezza, C. R.: Myocardial infarction in a patient with a circulating anticoagulant. Lancet 2:434, 1967.
253a. Chyu, J. Y., Hagstrom, W. J., et al.: Wegener's granulomatosis in childhood: cutaneous manifestations as the presenting signs. J. Am. Acad. Dermatol. 10:341, 1984.
253b. Hansen, L. P., Jacobsen, J., et al.: Wegener's granulomatosis in a child. Eur. J. Respir. Dis. 64:620, 1983.
253c. Teiselkotter, W., and Muller, K. M.: Infantile Wegener's granulomatosis. Arch. Anat. Cytol. Pathol. 25:273, 1977.
253d. Fauci, A. S., and Wolff, S. M.: Wegener's granulomatosis: studies in eighteen patients and a review of the literature. Medicine 52:535, 1973.
253e. Crummy, C. S., Perlin, E., et al.: Microangiopathic hemolytic anemia in Wegener's granulomatosis. Am. J. Med. 51:544, 1971.
253f. DeRemee, R. A., McDonald, T. J., et al.: Wegener's granulomatosis: anatomic correlates, a proposed classification. Mayo Clin. Proc. 51:777, 1976.
253g. Moorthy, A. Y., Chesney, R. W., et al.: Wegener granulomatosis in childhood: prolonged survival following cytotoxic therapy. J. Pediatr. 91:616, 1977.
253h. Kelleher, J. F., Luban, N. L. C., Mortimer, P. P., et al.: Human serum "Parvovirus:" A specific cause of aplastic crisis in children with hereditary spherocytosis. J. Pediatr. 102:720, 1983.
254. Mahn, H. E., and Dantuono, L. M.: Postabortal septicotoxemia due to clostridium welchii. Am. J. Obstet. Gynecol. 70:604, 1955.
255. Neter, E.: Bacterial hemagglutination and hemolysis. Bacteriol. Rev. 20:166, 1956.
256. Rytel, M. W.: Primary atypical pneumonia—current concepts. Am. J. Med. Sci. 247:84, 1964.
257. Itoga, T., and Laszlo, J.: Dohle bodies and other granulocytic alterations with cyclophosphamide. Blood 20:668, 1962.
258. Jordan, S. W., and Larsen, W. E.: Ultrastructure studies of the May-Hegglin anomaly. Blood 250:921, 1965.
259. Zipursky, A., Palko, J., et al.: The hematology of bacterial infections in premature infants. Pediatrics 57:839, 1976.
260. Segal, A. W.: Nitrotetrazolium tests. Lancet 2:1248, 1974.
261. Steigbigel, R. T., Johnson, P. K., et al.: The nitrotetrazolium blue test versus conventional hematology in the diagnosis of bacterial infections. New Engl. J. Med. 290:235, 1974.
262. Dorr, A. D., and Moloney, W. C.: Acquired pseudo-Pelger anomaly of granulocytic leukocytes. New Engl. J. Med. 261:742, 1959.
263. Faden, H. S.: Early diagnosis of neonatal bacteremia by buffy coat examination. J. Pediatr. 88:1032, 1976.

264. Crofton, J. W., Livingstone, J. L., et al.: Pulmonary eosinophilia. Thorax 7:1, 1952.
264a. Gibson, E. L., Vaucher, Y., et al.: Eosinophilia in premature infants: relationship to weight gain. J. Pediatr. 95:99, 1979.
264b. Bhat, A. M., and Scanlon, J. W.: The pattern of eosinophilia in premature infants. J. Pediatr. 98:612, 1981.
265. Paar, J. A., Steinman, M. M., et al.: Disseminated nonreactive tuberculosis with basophilia, leukemoid reaction and terminal pancytopenia. New Engl. J. Med. 274:335, 1966.
266. Corrigan, J. J., and Jordan, C. M.: Heparin therapy in septicemia with disseminated intravascular coagulation. New Engl. J. Med. 233:778, 1970.
267. Corrigan, J. J., Walker, L. R., et al.: Changes in the blood coagulation system associated with septicemia. New Engl. J. Med. 279:851, 1968.
268. Oski, F. A., and Naiman, J. L.: Effect of live measles vaccine on the platelet count. New Engl. J. Med. 275:352, 1966.
269. Corrigan, J. J., Jr.: Thrombocytopenia: a laboratory sign of septicemia in infants and children. J. Pediatr. 85:219, 1974.
270. Proudfoot, A. T.: Cryptic disseminated tuberculosis. Br. J. Hosp. Med. 5:773, 1971.
271. Glasser, R. M., Walker, R. I., et al.: The significance of hematologic abnormalities in patients with tuberculosis. Arch. Intern. Med. 125:691, 1970.
272. Medd, W. E., and Hayhoe, F. G. J.: Tuberculous miliary necrosis with pancytopenia. Quart. J. Med. 24:351, 1955.
273. Ricketts, W. E.: Bartonella bacilliformis anemia (Oroya fever): a study of thirty cases. Blood 3:1025, 1948.
274. Clark, K. G. A.: A basophilic, micro-organism infecting human red cells. Br. J. Haematol. 29:301, 1975.
275. George, J. N., Wicker, D. J., et al.: Erythrocytic abnormalities in experimental malaria. Soc. Exp. Biol. Med. 124:1086, 1967.
276. Overman, R. R.: Reversible cellular permeability alterations in disease: In vivo studies on sodium, potassium and chloride concentrations in erythrocytes of the malarious monkey. Am. J. Physiol. 152:113, 1948.
277. George, J. N., Stokes, E. F., et al.: Studies of the mechanism of hemolysis in experimental malaria. Milit. Med. 131:1217, 1966.
278. Conrad, M. E.: Pathophysiology of malaria. Hematologic observation in human and animal studies. Ann. Intern. Med. 70:134, 1969.
278a. Woodruff, A. W., Ansdell, V. E., et al.: Cause of anaemia in malaria. Lancet 2:1055, 1979.
279. Balcerzak, S. P., Arnold, J. D., et al.: Anatomy of red cell damage by plasmodium falciparum in man. Blood 40:98, 1972.
279a. Spivak, J. L., Bender, B. S., et al.: Hematologic abnormalities in the acquired immunodeficiency syndrome. Am. J. Med. 77:224, 1984.
280. Hoagland, R. J.: *Infectious Mononucleosis*. New York, Grune & Stratton, 1967, p. 3.
281. Filatov, N. F.: *Lektuse ob Ostrikj Infektsion, Nikh Lolieznyak.* (*Lectures on Acute Infectious Diseases of Children*). Moscow, U. Dietel, 1885.
282. Pfeiffer, E.: Drusenfieber, Jahrb. Kinderheilk. 29:257, 1889.
283. Sprunt, T. P., and Evans, F. A.: Mononucleosis leukocytosis in reaction to acute infections (infectious mononucleosis). Bull. Johns Hopkins Hosp. 31:409, 1920.
284. Paul, J. R.: From the notebook of John Rodman Paul. In *Virology and Epidemiology.* Horstman, D. M. (ed.), Hamden, Conn. Archon Books, 1971, pp. 2–20.
285. Paul, J. R., and Bunnell, W. W.: The presence of heterophile antibodies in infectious mononucleosis. Am. J. Med. Sci. 183:91, 1932.
286. Davidsohn, I. and Lee, C.: The laboratory diagnosis of infectious mononucleosis. Med. Clin. North Am. 46:225, 1962.
287. Burkitt, D.: A sarcoma involving the jaws in African children. Br. J. Surg. 46:218, 1958.
288. Epstein, M. A., Achong, B. G., et al.: Virus particles in cultured lymphoblasts from Burkitt's lymphoma. Lancet 1:702, 1964.
289. Henle, G., and Henle, W.: Immunofluorescence in cells derived from Burkitt's lymphoma. J. Bacteriol. 91:1248, 1966.
290. Henle, G., Henle, W., et al.: Antibodies to Epstein-Barr virus in Burkitt's lymphoma and control groups. J. Nat. Cancer Inst. 43:1147, 1969.
291. Niederman, J. C., McCollum, R. W., et al.: Infectious mononucleosis. Clinical manifestations in relation to EB virus antibodies. J.A.M.A. 203:205, 1968.
292. Pereira, M. S., Blake, J. M., et al.: EB virus antibody at different ages. Br. Med. J. 4:526, 1969.
293. Joncas, J. H., Boucher, J., et al.: Epstein-Barr virus infection in the neonatal period and in childhood. Can. Med. Assoc. J. 110:33, 1974.
294. Shapiro, L. R., Hirshaut, Y., et al.: Epstein-Barr virus in infancy. J. Pediatr. 80:1025, 1972.
295. Hallee, T. J., Evans, A. S., et al.: Infectious mononucleosis at the United States Military Academy. A prospective study of a single class over four years. Yale J. Biol. Med. 3:182, 1974.
296. Wising, P. J.: A study of infectious mononucleosis (Pfeiffer's disease) from the etiological point of view. Acta Med. Scand. 133(Suppl.):1, 1942.
297. Henle, W., Henle, G. E., et al.: Antibody responses to Epstein-Barr virus and cytomegaloviruses after open-heart and other surgery. New Engl. J. Med. 282:1068, 1970.
297a. Sixby, J. W., Nedrud, J. G., et al.: Epstein-Barr virus replication in oropharyngeal epithelial cells. New Engl. J. Med. 310:1225, 1984.
297b. Fleisher, G. R., Pasquariello, P. S., et al.: Intrafamilial transmission of Epstein-Barr virus infections. J. Pediatr. 98:16, 1981.
297c. Joncas, J. H., Alfieri, C., et al.: Simultaneous congenital infection with Epstein-Barr virus and cytomegalovirus. New Engl. J. Med. 304:1399, 1981.
297d. Goldberg, G. N., Fulginiti, V. A., et al.: In utero Epstein-Barr virus (infectious mononucleosis) infection. J. A. M. A. 246:1579, 1981.
297e. Horowitz, C. A., McClain, K., et al.: Fatal illness in a 2-week-old infant: diagnosis by detection of Epstein-Barr virus genomes from a lymph node biopsy. J. Pediatr. 103:752, 1983.
297f. Fleisher, G., and Bolognese, R.: Epstein-Barr virus infections in pregnancy: a prospective study. J. Pediatr. 104:374, 1984.
297g. Fleisher, G., and Bolognese, R.: Infectious mononucleosis during gestation: report of three women and their infants studied prospectively. Pediatr. Infect. Dis. 3:308, 1984.
297h. Le, C. T., Shihman, R., et al.: Epstein-Barr virus infections during pregnancy. Am. J. Dis. Child. 137:466, 1983.
298. Henle, W., Ho, H. C., et al.: Antibodies to EBV-related antigens in nasopharyngeal carcinoma. Comparison of active cases with long-term survivors. J. Nat. Cancer Inst. 510:361, 1973.
299. Hirshaut, Y., Glade, P., et al.: Sarcoidosis, another disease associated with serologic evidence for herpes-like virus infection. New Engl. J. Med. 283:502, 1970.
300. Papageorgiou, P. S., Sorokin, C., et al.: Herpes-like virus in leprosy. Nature (Lond.) 231:47, 1971.
301. Evans, A. S., Rothfield, N. F., et al.: Raised antibody titres to EB virus in systemic lupus erythematosus. Lancet 1:167, 1971.
302. Evans, A. S.: Clinical syndromes associated with EB virus infection. Adv. Intern. Med. 18:77, 1972.

302a. Hanto, D. W., Gajl-Peczalska, K. J., et al.: Epstein-Barr virus (E.B.V.) induced polyclonal and monoclonal B-cell lymphoproliferative diseases occurring after renal transplantation. Ann. Surg. *198:*356, 1983.
303. Rahal, J. J., Jr., and Henle, G.: Infectious mononucleosis and Reye's syndrome. A fatal case with studies for Epstein-Barr virus. Pediatrics *46:*776, 1970.
304. Wands, J. R., Perrotto, J. L., et al.: Circulating immune complexes and complement sequence activation in infectious mononucleosis. Am. J. Med. *60:*269, 1976.
305. Kerns, D. L., Shira, J. E., et al.: Ampicillin rash in children. Relationship to penicillin allergy and infectious mononucleosis. Am. J. Dis. Child. *125:*187, 1973.
306. Copperman, D. A.: "Alice in Wonderland' syndrome as a presenting symptom of infectious mononucleosis in children: a description of three affected young people. Clin. Pediatr. *16:*143, 1977.
306a. Portman, M., Ingall, D., et al.: Peritonsillar abscess complicating infectious mononucleosis. J. Pediatr. *101:*712, 1984.
306b. Silber, M. H.: Acute transverse myelopathy in Epstein-Barr virus infection. S. A. Mediese Tydskrif *64:*753, 1983.
306c. Fleisher, G., and Schwartz, J.: Primary Epstein-Barr virus infection in association with Reye syndrome. J. Pediatr. *97:*935, 1980.
306d. Johnson, M. A.: Spontaneous rupture of the spleen in infectious mononucleosis. Am. J. Roentgenol. *136:*111, 1981.
307. Jenkins, W. J., Koster, H. G., et al.: Infectious mononucleosis: An unsuspected source of anti-i. Br. J. Haematol. *11:*480, 1965.
308. Wilkinson, L. S., Petz, L. D., et al.: Preappraisal of the role of anti-i in haemolytic anemia in infectious mononucleosis. Br. J. Haematol. *25:*715, 1973.
309. Mir, M. A., and Delamore, I. W.: Aplastic anemia complicating infectious mononucleosis. Scand. J. Haematol. *11:*314, 1973.
310. Neel, E. U.: Infectious mononucleosis. Death due to agranulocytosis and pneumonia. J.A.M.A. *236:*1493, 1976.
311. Radel, E. G., and Schorr, J. B.: Thrombocytopenic purpura with infectious mononucleosis. J. Pediatr. *63:*46, 1963.
312. Carter, R. L., and Penman, H. G.: *Infectious Mononucleosis.* Oxford, Blackwell Scientific Publications, 1969.
313. Carter, R. L.: Platelet levels in infectious mononucleosis. Blood *25:*817, 1965.
314. Downey, H., and McKinlay, C. A.: Acute lymphadenosis compared with acute lymphatic leukemia. Arch. Intern. Med. *32:*82, 1923.
315. Litwins, J., and Leibowitz, S.: Abnormal lymphocytes (virocytes) in virus diseases other than infectious mononucleosis. Acta Haematol. *5:*223, 1951.
316. Pattengale, P. K., Smith, R. W., et al.: Atypical lymphocytes in acute infectious mononucleosis. Identification by multiple T and B lymphocyte markers. New Engl. J. Med. *291:*1145, 1974.
317. Enberg, R. N., Eberle, B. J., et al.: T and B cells in peripheral blood during infectious mononucleosis. J. Infect. Dis. *130:*104, 1974.
318. Pattengale, P. K., Smith, R. W., et al.: B-cell characteristics of human peripheral and cord blood lymphocytes transformed by Epstein-Barr virus. J. Nat. Cancer Inst. *52:*1081, 1974.
319. Mangi, R. J., Neiderman, J. C., et al.: Depression of cell-mediated immunity during acute infectious mononucleosis. New Engl. J. Med. *291:*1149, 1974.
320. Nessan, V. J., Geerken, R. C., et al.: Uric acid excretion in infectious mononucleosis: A function of increased purine turnover. J. Clin. Endocrinol. Metab. *38:*652, 1974.
321. Lukes, R. J., Tindle, B. H., et al.: Reed-Sternberg-like cells in infectious mononucleosis. Lancet *2:*1003, 1969.
322. Agliozzo, C. M., and Rheingold, I. M.: Infectious mononucleosis simulating Hodgkin's disease. Am. J. Clin. Pathol. *56:*730, 1971.
323. Hoagland, R. J.: Infectious mononucleosis. Am. J. Med. *13:*158, 1952.
324. Lee, C. L., Davidsohn, I., et al.: Horse agglutinins in infectious mononucleosis. II. The spot test. Am. J. Clin. Pathol. *49:*12, 1968.
325. Tamir, D., Benderly, A., et al.: Infectious mononucleosis and Epstein-Barr virus in childhood. Pediatrics *53:*330, 1974.
326. Henle, W., Henle, G. E., et al.: Epstein-Barr virus specific diagnostic tests in infectious mononucleosis. Hum. Pathol. *5:*551, 1974.
327. Sumaya, C. V.: Primary Epstein-Barr virus infections in children. Pediatrics *59:*16, 1977.
328. Tischendorf, P., Shramek, G. J., et al.: Development and persistence of immunity to Epstein-Barr virus in man. J. Infect. Dis. *122:*401, 1970.
329. Schmitz, H., and Scherer, M.: IgM antibodies to Epstein-Barr virus in infections. Arch. Gesamte. Virus Forsch. *37:*332, 1972.
330. Miller, G., Niederman, J. C., et al.: Prolonged oropharyngeal excretion of Epstein-Barr virus after infectious mononucleosis. New Engl. J. Med. *288:*229, 1973.
330a. Sullivan, J. L.: Epstein-Barr virus and the X-linked lymphoproliferative syndrome. In *Advances in Pediatrics,* Vol. 30. Barness, L. (ed.), Chicago, Year Book Medical Publishers, 1984, pp. 365–399.
330b. Henle, W., Henle, G. E., et al.: Epstein-Barr virus specific diagnostic tests in infectious mononucleosis. Hum. Pathol. *5:*551, 1974.
331. Purtilo, D. T., DeFlorio, D., et al.: Variable phenotypic expression of an X-linked recessive lymphoproliferative syndrome. New Engl. J. Med. *297:*1077, 1977.
331a. Bar, R. S., Delor, C. J., et al.: Fatal infectious mononucleosis in a family. New Engl. J. Med. *290:*363, 1974.
331b. Provisor, A. J., Iacuone, J. J., et al.: Acquired agammaglobulinemia after a life-threatening illness with clinical and laboratory features of infectious mononucleosis in three related male children. New Engl. J. Med. *243:*62, 1975.
331c. Sullivan, J. L., Byron, K. S., et al.: Deficient natural killer cell activity in the X-linked lymphoproliferative syndrome. Science *105:*543, 1980.
331d. Sakamoto, K., Freed, H., et al.: Antibody responses to Epstein-Barr virus in families with the X-linked lymphoproliferative syndrome. J. Immunol. *125:*921, 1980.
331e. Bowen, T. J., Wedgwood, R. J., et al.: Transient immunodeficiency during asymptomatic Epstein-Barr virus infection. Pediatrics *71:*964, 1983.
331f. Purtilo, D. T., Sakamoto, K., et al.: Epstein-Barr virus induced diseases in boys with the X-linked lymphoproliferative syndrome (XLP): update on studies of the registry. Am. J. Med. *73:*49, 1982.
331g. Fleisher, G., Starr, S., et al.: A non–X-linked syndrome with susceptibility to severe Epstein-Barr virus infections. J. Pediatr. *100:*727, 1982.
331h. Sullivan, J. L., Byron, K. S., et al.: X-linked lymphoproliferative syndrome. J. Clin. Invest. *71:*1765, 1983.
331i. Sullivan, J. L., Byron, K. S., et al.: Treatment of life-threatening Epstein-Barr infections with acyclovir. Am. J. Med. *73*(1A):262, 1982.
332. Muthuswamy, K., Lee, C. K., et al.: Infectious mononucleosis and severe thrombocytopenia. Am. J. Med. Sci. *272:*221, 1976.
332a. Caroline, N. H., and Schwartz, H.: Chicken soup rebound and relapse of pneumonia: Report of a case. Chest *67:*215, 1975.
333. Goldstein, H. H.: Disorders of the blood. In *Joslin's Diabetes Mellitus.* Marble, A., White, P., et al. (eds.), Philadelphia, Lea & Febiger, 1971, pp. 637–652.
334. Westlund, K.: *Mortality of Diabetes Life Insurance Companies*

Institute for Medical Statistics at the Oslo City Hosp. Report 13. Oslo, Univeritelsforlaget, 1969.
335. Bensoussan, D., Levy-Toledano, S., et al.: Platelets hyperaggregation and increased plasma level of von Willebrand's factor in diabetics with retinopathy. Diabetologia *11*:307, 1975.
336. Rahbor, S.: An abnormal hemoglobin in red cells of diabetics. Clin. Chem. Acta *22*:296, 1968.
337. Trivelli, L. A., Ranney, H. M., et al.: Hemoglobin components in patients with diabetes mellitus. New Engl. J. Med. *284*:353, 1971.
338. Rahbar, S., Blumenfeld, O., et al.: Studies of an unusual hemoglobin in patients with diabetes mellitus. Biochem. Biophys. Res. Commun. *36*:838, 1969.
339. Bunn, H. F., and Briehl, R. W.: The interaction of 2,3 diphosphoglycerate with various human hemoglobins. J. Clin. Invest. *49*:1088, 1970.
340. Koenig, R. J., Peterson, C. M., et al.: Hemoglobin A_{1c} as an indicator of the degree of glucose intolerance in diabetes. Diabetes *25*:230, 1976.
341. Lanoe, R., Thibult, N., et al.: Glycosylated haemoglobin concentrations and Clinitest results in insulin-dependent diabetes. Lancet *1*:1156, 1977.
342. Peterson, C. M., Jones, R. L., et al.: Reversible hematologic sequelae of diabetes mellitus. Ann. Intern. Med. *86*:425, 1977.
343. Alberti, K. G. M., Darley, J. H., et al.: 2,3 Diphosphoglycerate and tissue oxygenation in uncontrolled diabetes mellitus. Lancet *2*:391, 1972.
344. Bybee, J. D., and Rodgers, D. E.: The phagocytic activity of polymorphonuclear leukocytes obtained from patients with diabetes mellitus. J. Lab. Clin. Med. *64*:1, 1964.
345. Miller, M. E., and Baker, L.: Leukocyte functions in juvenile diabetes mellitus: Humoral and cellular aspects. J. Pediatr. *81*:979, 1972.
346. Brody, J. I., and Marlee, K.: Metabolic and biosynthetic features of lymphocytes from patients with diabetes mellitus: similarities to lymphocytes in chronic lymphocytic leukemia. Br. J. Haematol. *19*:193, 1970.
347. Egebart, O.: The blood coagulability in diabetic patients. Scand. J. Clin. Lab. Invest. *15*:533, 1963.
348. Mayne, E. E., Bridges, J. M., et al.: Platelet adhesiveness, plasma fibrinogen and factor VIII level in diabetes mellitus. Diabetologia *6*:436, 1970.
349. Sagel, J., Colwell, J. A., et al.: Increased platelet aggregation in early diabetes mellitus. Ann. Intern. Med. *82*:733, 1975.
350. Kwaan, H. C., Colwell, J. A., et al.: Increased platelet aggregation in diabetes mellitus. J. Lab. Clin. Med. *80*:236, 1972.
351. Nordoy, A., and Rodset, J. M.: Platelet phospholipids and their function in patients with juvenile diabetes mellitus. Diabetes *19*:698, 1970.
352. Colwell, J. A., Halushka, P. V., et al.: Altered platelet function in diabetes mellitus. Diabetes *25*(Suppl. 2):826, 1976.
353. Born, G. V. R.: Aggregation of blood platelets by adenosine diphosphate and its reversal. Nature *194*:927, 1962.
354. Halushka, P. V., Lurie, D., et al.: Increased synthesis of prostaglandin-E-like material by platelets from patients with diabetes mellitus. New Engl. J. Med. *297*:1306, 1977.
355. Powell, E. D. U., and Field, R. A.: Diabetic retinopathy and rheumatoid arthritis. Lancet *2*:17, 1964.
356. Grupe, W.: Renal vascular thrombosis. In *Diseases of the Newborn*. Schaffer, A. J., and Avery, M. E. (eds.), Philadelphia, W. B. Saunders Co., 1977, p. 456.
357. Ward, T. F.: Multiple thromboses in an infant of a diabetic mother. J. Pediatr. *90*:982, 1977.
358. Ways, P., Reed, C. F., et al.: Red cell and plasma lipids in acanthocytosis. J. Clin. Invest. *42*:1248, 1963.
359. Simon, E. R., and Ways, R.: Incubation hemolysis and red cell metabolism in acanthocytosis. J. Clin. Invest. *43*:1311, 1964.
360. Dodge, J. T., Cohen, G., et al.: Peroxidative hemolysis of red blood cells from patients with abetalipoproteinemia (acanthocytosis). J. Clin. Invest. *46*:357, 1967.
361. Carvalho, A. C. A., Coleman, R. W., et al.: Platelet function in hyperlipoproteinemia. New Engl. J. Med. *290*:434, 1974.
362. Friedman, Z., Lamberth, E. L., et al.: Platelet dysfunction in the neonate with essential fatty acid deficiency. J. Pediatr. *90*:439, 1977.
363. Vincent, J. E., Melai, A., et al.: Comparison of the effect of prostaglandin E on platelet aggregation in normal and essential fatty acid deficient rats. Prostaglandins *5*:369, 1974.
364. Rosenberg, L. E., Lilljeqvist, A., et al.: Methylmalonic aciduria: an inborn error leading to metabolic-acidosis, long chain ketonuria and intermittent hyperglycinemia. New Engl. J. Med. *278*:1319, 1968.
365. Cox, E. V., and White, A. M.: Methylmalonic acid excretion: a sensitive indicator of B_{12} deficiency in man. Lancet *2*:853, 1962.
366. Huguley, C. M., Bain, J. A., et al.: Refractory megaloblastic anemia associated with excretion of orotic acid. Blood *14*:615, 1959.
367. Roses, A. D., and Appel, S. H.: Protein kinase activity in erythrocyte ghosts of patients with myotonic muscular dystrophy. Proc. Nat. Acad. Sci. USA *70*:1855, 1973.
368. Roses, A. D., Herbstreith, M. H., et al.: Membrane protein kinase alteration in Duchenne muscular dystrophy. Nature *254*:350, 1975.
369. Shohet, S. B., and Layzer, R. B.: The "muscle" of the red cell. New Engl. J. Med. *294*:221, 1976.
370. Matheson, D. W., and Howland, J. L.: Erythrocyte deformation in human muscular dystrophy. Science *184*:165, 1974.
371. Percy, A. K., and Miller, M. E.: Reduced deformability of erythrocyte membranes from patients with Duchenne muscular dystrophy. Nature *258*:147, 1975.
371a. Kim, H. D., Luthra, M. G., et al.: Factors influencing osmotic fragility of red blood cells in Duchenne muscular dystrophy. Neurology *30*:726, 1980.
371b. Scheneiderman, L. J., Sampson, W. I., et al.: Genetic studies of a family with two unusual autosomal conditions: Muscular dystrophy and Pelger-Huët anomaly. Am. J. Med. *46*:380, 1969.
371c. Jordans, G. H. W.: The familial occurrence of fat-containing vacuoles in the leukocytes diagnosed in two brothers suffering from dystrophia musculorum progressiva (ERB). Acta Med. Scand. *145*:419, 1953.
372. Schmid, J. R., Kiely, J. M., et al.: Thymoma associated with pure red cell agenesis. Review of the literature and report of 4 cases. Cancer *18*:216, 1965.
373. Cohen, S. M., and Waxman, S.: Myasthenia gravis, chronic lymphocytic leukemia and autoimmune hemolytic anemia. Arch. Intern. Med. *110*:717, 1967.
374. van der Zee, S. P. M.: Megaloblastic anemia in the Lesch-Nyhan syndrome. Lancet *1*:1427, 1968.
375. Seegmiller, J. E., Rosenbloom, F. M., et al.: An enzyme defect associated with a sex-linked human neurological disorder and excessive purine synthesis. Science *155*:1682, 1967.
376. Rivard, G. F., Izadi, P., et al.: Functional and metabolic studies of platelets from patients with Lesch-Nyhan syndrome. Br. J. Haematol. *31*:245, 1975.
377. Cooper, R. A., and Jandl, J. H.: Acanthocytosis. In *Hematology*. W. J. Williams (ed.), New York, McGraw Hill Book Co., 1977, p. 464.
378. Mant, M. J., and Faragher, B. S.: The hematology of anorexia nervosa. Br. J. Haematol. *23*:737, 1972.
378a. Kay, J., and Strickler, R. B.: Hematologic and immunologic abnormalities in anorexia nervosa. South. Med. J. *76*:1008, 1983.
378b. Pearson, H. A.: Marrow hypoplasia in anorexia nervosa. J. Pediatr. *71*:211, 1967.

378c. Amrein, P. C., Friedman, R., et al.: Hematologic changes in anorexia nervosa. J. A. M. A. *241:*2190, 1979.
378d. Luck, P., Mikhailidis, D. P., et al.: Platelet hyperaggregability and increased adrenoceptor density in anorexia nervosa. J. Clin. Endocrinol. Metabol. *57:*911, 1983.
379. Marks, J., and Shuster, S.: Iron metabolism and skin disease. Arch. Dermatol. *98:*469, 1968.
380. Fox, R. H., Shuster, S., et al.: Cardiovascular metabolic and thermoregulatory disturbances in patients with erythrodermic skin diseases. Br. Med. J. *1:*619, 1965.
381. Marks, J., and Shuster, S.: Method for measuring capillary permeability and its use in patients with skin disease. Br. Med. J. *2:*88, 1966.
382. Summerly, R., and Giles, C.: Question of psoriatic enteropathy. Arch. Dermatol. *103:*678, 1971.
383. Fry, L., Kier, P., et al.: Small intestinal structure and function and haematological manifestations of dermatitis herpetiformis. Lancet *1:*557, 1968.
384. Petit, J. E., Hoffbrand, A. V., et al.: Splenic atrophy in dermatitis herpetiformis. Br. Med. J. *2:*438, 1972.
385. McCarthy, C. F., Fraser, I. D., et al.: Lymphoreticular dysfunction in idiopathic steatorrhea. Gut *7:*140, 1966.
385a. Trowbridge, A. A., Sirinavin, C., et al.: Dyskeratosis congenita: hematologic evaluation of a sibship and review of the literature. Am. J. Hematol. *3:*143, 1977.
385b. DeBoeck, K., Degreef, H., et al.: Thrombocytopenia: first symptom in a patient with dyskeratosis congenita. Pediatrics *67:*898, 1981.
385c. Arneson, M. A., Hammerschmidt, D. E., et al.: A new form of Ehlers-Danlos syndrome: fibronectin corrects platelet dysfunction. J.A.M.A. *244:*144, 1980.
386. Brett, E. M., Ong, B. H., et al.: Mast-cell disease in children. Br. J. Dermatol. *79:*197, 1967.
387. Griffith, G. C., Nichols, G., et al.: Heparin osteoporosis. J.A.M.A. *193:*85, 1965.
388. Waters, W. J., and Lacson, P. S.: Mast cell leukemia presenting as urticaria pigmentosa. Pediatrics *19:*1033, 1957.
389. Huet, G. J.: Familial anomaly of leukocytes. Discuss. Med. Tijdschr. Geneesk. *75:*5956, 1931.
390. Pelger, K.: Demonstratie van een paar zeldzaam voorkomende typhen van bloedlichaampjes en bespreking der patienten. Discuss. Med. Tijdschr. Geneesk *72:*1178, 1928.
391. Door, A. D., and Moloney, W. C.: Acquired pseudo-Pelger anomaly of granulocytic leukocytes. New Engl. J. Med. *261:*742, 1959.
392. Linman, J. W., and Saarni, M. I.: The preleukemic syndrome. Semin. Hematol. *11:*93, 1974.
393. Laszlo, J., and Rundles, R. W.: Morphology of granulocytes and their precursors. In *Hematology.* Williams, W. J., Beutler, E., et al.: (eds.), New York, McGraw-Hill Book Co., 1977, p. 665.
394. Undritz, V. E.: Eine neve Sippe mit erblichkonstitutioneller hochsegmentierung der Neutrophilenkerne. Schweiz. Med. Wochenschr. *88:*1000, 1958.
395. Presently, B.: A new anomaly of eosinophilic granulocytes. Am. J. Clin. Pathol. *49:*887, 1968.
396. Davidson, W. M., Milner, R. D. G., et al.: Giant neutrophil leucocytes: An inherited anomaly. Br. J. Haematol. *6:*339, 1960.
397. Huehns, E. R., Lutzner, M., et al.: Nuclear abnormalities of the neutrophils in D (13–15) trisomy syndrome. Lancet *1:*589, 1964.
398. Davidson, W. M.: Sexing the blood leucocytes in abnormalities of the sex chromosomes. Minerva Pediatr. *17:*585, 1965.
399. Reilly, W. A.: The granules in the leukocytes in gargoylism. Am. J. Dis. Child. *62:*489, 1941.
400. Davidson, W. M.: Inherited variations in leukocytes. Br. Med. Bull. *17:*190, 1960.
401. Strouth, J. C., Zeman, W., et al.: Leukocyte abnormalities in familial amaurotic idiocy. New Engl. J. Med. *274:*36, 1966.
402. Halon, P. J., and Mitus, W. J.: Ceroid storage in albinism. XIII Congress, International Society of Hematology, Munich, 1970, p. 322 (Abstr.).
403. White, J. G.: The Hermansky-Pudlak syndrome: Inclusions in circulating leucocytes. Br. J. Haematol. *24:*761, 1973.
404. Plum, C. M.: Lymphocyte degeneration in amaurotic familial idiocy. Dan. Med. Bull. *4:*156, 1957.
405. Mittwock, U.: Nuclear segmentation of the neutrophils in heterozygous carriers of gargoylism. Nature (Lond.) *193:*1209, 1962.
406. Bowman, J. E., Mittwoch, U., et al.: Persistence of mucopolysaccharide inclusions in culture of lymphocytes from patients with gargoylism. Nature (Lond.) *195:*612, 1962.
407. Jordan, G. H.: The familial occurrence of fat-containing vacuoles in leukocytes. Acta Med. Scand. *145:*419, 1953.
408. Rozenszajn, L.: Jordan's anomaly in the white blood cells. Blood *28:*258, 1966.
409. Lukens, J. N.: Eosinophilia in children. Pediatr. Clin. North Am. *19:*969, 1972.
410. Orfanakis, N. G., Ostlund, R. E., et al.: Normal blood leukocyte concentration values. Am. J. Clin. Pathol. *53:*647, 1970.
411. Archer, R. K.: Regulatory mechanisms in eosinophil leukocyte production, release and distribution. In *Regulation of Hematopoiesis.* Vol. II. New York, Appleton-Century-Crofts, 1972.
412. Hardy, W. R., and Anderson, R. E.: The hypereosinophilic syndromes. Ann. Intern. Med. *68:*1120, 1968.
413. Nelken, R. P., and Stockman, J. A., III: The hypereosinophilic syndrome in association with acute lymphoblastic leukemia. J. Pediatr. *89:*771, 1976.
414. Spitzer, G., and Garson, O. M.: Lymphoblastic leukemia with marked eosinophilia: A report of two cases. Blood *42:*377, 1973.
415. Basten, A., Boyer, M. H., et al.: Mechanisms of eosinophilia. I. J. Exp. Med. *131:*1271, 1970.
416. Basten, A., and Beeson, P. B.: Mechanism of eosinophilia. II. J. Exp. Med. *131:*1288, 1970.
417. Naiman, J. L., Oski, F. A., et al.: Hereditary eosinophilia: Report of a family and review of the literature. Am. J. Hum. Genet. *16:*195, 1964.
418. Braunsteiner, H., and Thumb, N.: Quantitative Veranderungen der Blutbasophilen und ihre klinische Bedeutung. Acta Haematol. *20:*339, 1958.
419. Dvorak, H. F., and Mihm, M. C.: Basophilic leukocytes in allergic contact dermatitis. J. Exp. Med. *135:*235, 1972.
420. Juhlin, L.: Basophilic leukocyte differential in blood and bone marrow. Acta Haematol. *29:*89, 1963.
421. Mitchell, R. G.: Basophilic leukocytes in children in health and disease. Arch. Dis. Child. *33:*193, 1958.
422. Hill, R. W., and Bayrd, E. D.: Phagocytic reticuloendothelial cells in subacute bacterial endocarditis with negative cultures. Ann. Intern. Med. *52:*310, 1960.
423. Michael, S. R., Vural, I. L., et al.: The hematological aspects of disseminated (systemic) lupus erythematosus: Review of the literature and clinical analysis of 138 cases. Medicine *33:*291, 1954.
424. Lagergren, J.: The white blood cell count and the erythrocyte sedimentation rate of pertussis. Acta Pediatr. *52:*405, 1963.
425. Daughaday, W. H., Williams, R. H., et al.: The effect of endocrinopathies on the blood. Blood *3:*1342, 1948.
426. Bass, H. N., and Miller, A. A.: Cystic fibrosis presenting with anemia and hypoproteinemia in identical twins. J. Pediatr. *59:*126, 1977.
427. Farrell, P. M., Bieri, J. G., et al.: The occurrence and effects of human vitamin E deficiency. A study in patients with cystic fibrosis. J. Clin. Invest. *60:*233, 1972.
428. Kaufmann, R. H., Veltkamp, J. J., et al.: Acquired antithrombin III deficiency and thrombosis in the nephrotic syndrome. Am. J. Med. *65:*607, 1978.

APPENDIX

Reference Values in Infancy and Childhood

BERTRAM H. LUBIN

INTRODUCTION 1677
THE NORMAL CORD BLOOD HEMOGLOBIN 1678
NORMAL HEMATOLOGIC VALUES DURING THE FIRST 2 WEEKS OF LIFE IN THE TERM INFANT 1678
NORMAL VALUES OF HEMOGLOBIN (g/dl), HEMATOCRIT (%), ERYTHROCYTE COUNT (10^{12}/liter), MEAN CORPUSCULAR HEMOGLOBIN (pg), MEAN CORPUSCULAR VOLUME (fl), AND MEAN CORPUSCULAR HEMOGLOBIN CONCENTRATION (g/dl) 1679
HEMOGLOBIN CONCENTRATIONS (g/dl) FOR IRON-SUFFICIENT PRETERM INFANTS 1679
RED BLOOD CELL VALUES AT VARIOUS AGES: MEAN AND LOWER LIMIT OF NORMAL (-2 SD) 1680
HEMOGLOBIN AND MCV PERCENTILE CURVES FOR GIRLS AND BOYS 1680
HEMOGLOBIN CONCENTRATION IN WHITE, BLACK, AND ORIENTAL CHILDREN 1681
HUMAN ERYTHROCYTE ENZYMES IN NORMAL ADULTS 1681
HUMAN ERYTHROCYTE INTERMEDIATE METABOLITES IN NORMAL ADULTS 1682
RED CELL ENZYME ACTIVITY IN ADULTS AND TERM INFANTS 1682
RED CELL GLYCOLYTIC INTERMEDIATES IN NORMAL ADULTS, TERM INFANTS, AND PREMATURE INFANTS 1682
RELATIVE CONCENTRATION OF Hb F IN INFANTS AND ITS VARIATION WITH AGE 1683
PERCENTAGE OF HEMOGLOBINS F AND A2 IN THE NEWBORN AND ADULT 1683
METHEMOGLOBIN LEVELS IN NORMAL CHILDREN 1684
VALUES OF SERUM IRON (SI), TOTAL IRON-BINDING CAPACITY (TIBC), AND TRANSFERRIN SATURATION (S%) FROM INFANTS DURING THE FIRST YEAR OF LIFE 1684
NORMAL VALUES FOR SERUM IRON AND TRANSFERRIN SATURATION 1685
NORMAL RANGES FOR FOLATE ASSAYS AND FIGLU TEST 1686
NORMAL SERUM FOLIC ACID LEVELS (ng/ml) 1686
NORMAL SERUM VITAMIN E LEVELS (mg/dl) IN NEWBORNS 1686
PLASMA CONCENTRATION OF HEMOPEXIN AND HAPTOGLOBIN IN TERM AND PREMATURE INFANTS ON FIRST DAY OF LIFE 1687
ESTIMATED BLOOD VOLUMES 1687
NORMAL LEUKOCYTE COUNTS 1688
POLYMORPHONUCLEAR LEUKOCYTE AND BAND COUNTS IN THE NEWBORN DURING THE FIRST 2 DAYS OF LIFE 1688
ASSESSMENT OF LEUKOCYTE FUNCTION 1689
BONE MARROW CELL POPULATIONS OF NORMAL INFANTS 1690
COAGULATION FACTOR ASSAYS (MEAN ± 1 SD) AND SCREENING TESTS IN THE FETUS AND NEONATE 1692
VASCULAR-PLATELET INTERACTIONS IN THE FETUS AND NEONATE 1692
RELATION OF SERUM PROTEIN LEVELS TO AGE 1693
SERUM IMMUNOGLOBULIN LEVELS IN NORMAL INDIVIDUALS 1693
SERUM IgM LEVELS IN HEALTHY NEONATES 1694
SERUM IgE LEVELS IN INFANTS AND CHILDREN 1694
SERUM IgD CONCENTRATIONS IN INFANTS, CHILDREN, AND ADULTS 1694
RELATION OF IMMUNOGLOBULIN AND ISOHEMAGGLUTININ (IHA) LEVELS TO AGE 1695
PERCENTAGE OF B LYMPHOCYTES IN NORMAL CHILDREN 1695
AGE-RELATED VARIATION IN THE PROPORTION OF CIRCULATING T CELLS 1696
SEDIMENTATION RATE IN THE NEWBORN PERIOD 1696

INTRODUCTION

The normal range for most hematologic parameters in infancy and childhood is quite different from that in adults. Dramatic changes occur in hematologic values during the first few weeks of life and continue throughout the child's growth and development. Nutritional intake exerts a critical effect during periods of rapid growth. Since hematologic measurements are frequently used as screening procedures to detect abnormalities within a population, recognition of these variables in the pediatric age group will prevent needless medical and laboratory investigation.

The criteria for establishing normality are based upon either a random sample of an entire population without excluding values of abnormal individuals or a sampling of a population in which all subjects have been removed who have evidence of common abnormalities or adverse environmental circumstances that might be expected to bias the data (1). In this chapter, normal hematologic values have been collected from a variety of sources that utilized one or the other of these approaches. Detailed information on the newborn period and during the first year of life has been collected. Technical variations among laboratories may result in slightly different values. Biologic variations are now being recognized as factors that may affect the normal range. For example, racial factors may regulate the range for normal hemoglobin (2) and white blood cell count (3). As understanding of factors that determine the normal range expands and technologic advances are made, adjustments and modifications in these normal values will have to be made.

THE NORMAL CORD BLOOD HEMOGLOBIN*

Authors	Mean Hemoglobin (g/dl)	Range (g/dl)	Number of Observations
Mollison	16.6		134
Dochain et al.	17.9	14.4–2.16	40
Walker et al.	16.5		145
Marks et al.	16.9	12.3–22.0	221
Guest et al.	17.1	13.0–25.0	59
McKay	17.4		60
Rooth et al.	16.7	11.2–26.6	414
Mean	16.8		

*Approximately 95 per cent of all cord blood hemoglobin values fall between 13.7 and 20.1 g/dl. In the presence of a normal reticulocyte and nucleated red cell count, a value of 13.6 g/dl may be considered the lower limit of normal.

The time of cord blood clamping, the site from which the blood has been obtained, and the infant's age affect the hemoglobin concentration in the newborn. Late cord blood clamping can increase the blood volume by 60 per cent. Poorly obtained capillary blood samples may have a hemoglobin concentration 12 per cent greater than venous samples. Fluid volume shifts within the first few hours after birth may increase the hemoglobin concentration as much as 6 g/dl. Interpretation of values on each patient must take these factors into consideration.

(From Oski, F. A., and Naiman, J. L.: *Hematologic Problems in the Newborn*, 2nd ed. Philadelphia, W. B. Saunders Co., 1972, p. 11.)

NORMAL HEMATOLOGIC VALUES DURING THE FIRST 2 WEEKS OF LIFE IN THE TERM INFANT*

Value†	Cord Blood	Day 1	Day 3	Day 7	Day 14
Hb (g/dl)	16.8	18.4	17.8	17.0	16.8
Hematocrit (%)	53.0	58.0	55.0	54.0	52.0
Red cells (mm^3)	5.25	5.8	5.6	5.2	5.1
MCV (fl)	107	108	99.0	98.0	96.0
MCH (pg)	34	35	33	32.5	31.5
MCHC (g/dl)	31.7	32.5	33	33	33
Reticulocytes (%)	3–7	3–7	1–3	0–1	0–1
Nuc. RBC/(mm^3)	500	200	0–5	0	0
Platelets (1000's/mm^3)	290	192	213	248	252

*During the first 2 weeks of life a venous hemoglobin below 13.0 g/dl or a capillary hemoglobin below 14.5 g/dl should be regarded as anemia.

†MCV = mean corpuscular volume, MCH = mean corpuscular hemoglobin, MCHC = mean corpuscular hemoglobin concentration, and Nuc. RBC = nucleated red blood cells.

(From Oski, F. A., and Naiman, J. L.: *Hematologic Problems in the Newborn*, 2nd ed. Philadelphia, W. B. Saunders Co., 1972, p. 13.)

NORMAL VALUES OF HEMOGLOBIN (g/dl), HEMATOCRIT (%), ERYTHROCYTE COUNT (10^{12}/liter), MEAN CORPUSCULAR HEMOGLOBIN (pg), MEAN CORPUSCULAR VOLUME (fl), AND MEAN CORPUSCULAR HEMOGLOBIN CONCENTRATION (g/dl)*

	Age (mo)						
n	0.5 (N = 232)	1 (N = 240)	2 (N = 241)	4 (N = 52)	6 (N = 52)	9 (N = 56)	12 (N = 56)
Hb (mean ± SE)	16.6 ± 0.11	13.9 ± 0.10	11.2 ± 0.06	12.2 ± 0.14	12.6 ± 0.10	12.7 ± 0.09	12.7 ± 0.09
−2 SD	13.4	10.7	9.4	10.3	11.1	11.4	11.3
Hct (mean ± SE)	53 ± 0.4	44 ± 0.3	35 ± 0.2	38 ± 0.4	36 ± 0.3	36 ± 0.3	37 ± 0.3
−2 SD	41	33	28	32	31	32	33
RBC count (mean ± SE)	4.9 ± 0.03	4.3 ± 0.03	3.7 ± 0.02	4.3 ± 0.06	4.7 ± 0.05	4.7 ± 0.04	4.7 ± 0.04
−2 SD + 2 SD	3.9–5.9	3.3–5.3	3.1–4.3	3.5–5.1	3.9–5.5	4.0–5.3	4.1–5.3
MCH (mean ± SE)	33.6 ± 0.1	32.5 ± 0.1	30.4 ± 0.1	28.6 ± 0.2	26.8 ± 0.2	27.3 ± 0.2	26.8 ± 0.2
−2 SD	30	29	27	25	24	25	24
MCV (mean ± SE)	105.3 ± 0.6	101.3 ± 0.3	94.8 ± 0.3	86.7 ± 0.8	76.3 ± 0.6	77.7 ± 0.5	77.7 ± 0.5
−2 SD	88	91	84	76	68	70	71
MCHC (mean ± SE)	314 ± 1.1	318 ± 1.2	318 ± 1.1	327 ± 2.7	350 ± 1.7	349 ± 1.6	343 ± 1.5
−2 SD	281	281	283	288	327	324	321

*These values were obtained from a selected group of 256 healthy term infants followed at the Helsinki University Central Hospital who were receiving continuous iron supplementation and who had normal values for transferrin saturation and serum ferritin.

Values at the ages of 0.5, 1, and 2 months were obtained from the entire group, and those at the later ages from the iron-supplemented infant group after exclusion of iron deficiency. (From Saarien, U. M., and Siimes, M. A.: J. Pediatr. 92:414, 1978.)

HEMOGLOBIN CONCENTRATIONS (g/dl) FOR IRON-SUFFICIENT PRETERM INFANTS*

		Birth Weight	
Age	No.	1000–1500 g	1501–2000 g
2 wk	17, 39	16.3 (11.7–18.4)	14.8 (11.8–19.6)
1 mo	15, 42	10.9 (8.7–15.2)	11.5 (8.2–15.0)
2 mo	17, 47	8.8 (7.1–11.5)	9.4 (8.0–11.4)
3 mo	16, 41	9.8 (8.9–11.2)	10.2 (9.3–11.8)
4 mo	13, 37	11.3 (9.1–13.1)	11.3 (9.1–13.1)
5 mo	8, 21	11.6 (10.2–14.3)	11.8 (10.4–13.0)
6 mo	9, 21	12.0 (9.4–13.8)	11.8 (10.7–12.6)

*These infants were admitted to the Helsinki Children's Hospital during a 15-month period. None had a complicated course during the first 2 weeks of life or had undergone an exchange transfusion. All infants were iron sufficient, as indicated by a serum ferritin ≥ 10 ng/ml. (From Lundstrom, U., Siimes, M. A., et al.: J. Pediatr. 91:882, 1977.)

RED BLOOD CELL VALUES AT VARIOUS AGES: MEAN AND LOWER LIMIT OF NORMAL (−2 SD)*

Age	Hemoglobin (g/dl)		Hematocrit (%)		Red Cell Count (10^12/liter)		MCV (fl)		MCH (pg)		MCHC (g/dl)	
	Mean	−2 SD	Mean	−2 SD	Mean	−2 SD	Mean	−2 SD	Mean	−2 SD	Mean	−2 SD
Birth (cord blood)	16.5	13.5	51	42	4.7	3.9	108	98	34	31	33	30
1 to 3 days (capillary)	18.5	14.5	56	45	5.3	4.0	108	95	34	31	33	29
1 week	17.5	13.5	54	42	5.1	3.9	107	88	34	28	33	28
2 weeks	16.5	12.5	51	39	4.9	3.6	105	86	34	28	33	28
1 month	14.0	10.0	43	31	4.2	3.0	104	85	34	28	33	29
2 months	11.5	9.0	35	28	3.8	2.7	96	77	30	26	33	29
3 to 6 months	11.5	9.5	35	29	3.8	3.1	91	74	30	25	33	30
0.5 to 2 years	12.0	10.5	36	33	4.5	3.7	78	70	27	23	33	30
2 to 6 years	12.5	11.5	37	34	4.6	3.9	81	75	27	24	34	31
6 to 12 years	13.5	11.5	40	35	4.6	4.0	86	77	29	25	34	31
12 to 18 years—female	14.0	12.0	41	36	4.6	4.1	90	78	30	25	34	31
male	14.5	13.0	43	37	4.9	4.5	88	78	30	25	34	31
18 to 49 years—female	14.0	12.0	41	36	4.6	4.0	90	80	30	26	34	31
male	15.5	13.5	47	41	5.2	4.5	90	80	30	26	34	31

*These data have been compiled from several sources. Emphasis is given to recent studies employing electronic counters and to the selection of populations that are likely to exclude individuals with iron deficiency. The mean ± 2 SD can be expected to include 95 per cent of the observations in a normal population. (From Dallman, P. R.: In *Pediatrics,* 16th ed. Rudolph, A. [ed.], New York, Appleton-Century-Crofts, 1977, p. 1111.)

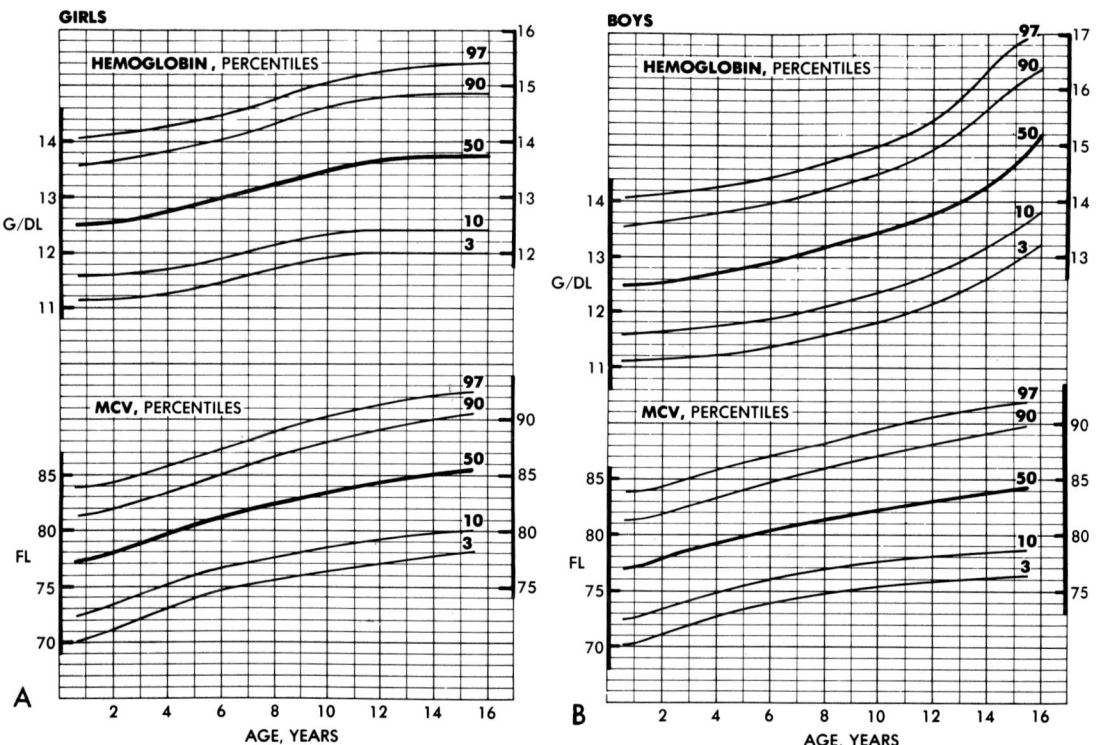

A, Hemoglobin and MCV percentile curves for girls; and *B,* hemoglobin and MCV percentile curves for boys. These figures were obtained from populations of nonindigent white children residing in either Northern California or Finland. Hemoglobin values were derived from a total of 9946 children and MCV values from 2314 children. The reference population excluded subjects with laboratory evidence of iron deficiency, thalassemia minor, and/or hemoglobinopathy. (From Dallman, P. R., and Siimes, M. A.: J. Pediatr. *94:*28, 1979.)

HEMOGLOBIN CONCENTRATION IN WHITE, BLACK, AND ORIENTAL CHILDREN*

	Males			Females		
Age	No.	Median	2.5 to 97.5 Percentile Range	No.	Median	2.5 to 97.5 Percentile Range
5 to 9 years						
White	305	13.0	11.6–14.3	291	12.9	11.5–14.4
Black	87	12.6	11.1–14.1	104	12.5	11.2–13.6
Oriental	50	13.1	11.9–14.4	64	13.0	11.6–14.2
10 to 14 weeks						
White	447	13.7	12.3–15.5	484	13.4	12.0–14.9
Black	143	13.1	11.5–15.2	150	12.9	11.2–14.3
Oriental	87	13.7	12.1–15.6	79	13.5	12.2–14.7

*Hemoglobin concentration in subjects with hemoglobin AA, normal glucose-6-phosphate-dehydrogenase screen, and mean corpuscular volume 95 per cent or more of median value for whites of same age and sex. The data strengthen the impression that blacks normally have a concentration of hemoglobin, averaging about 0.5 g/dl less than whites. (From Dallman, P. R., Barr, G. D., et al.: Am. J. Clin. Nutr. *31*:379, 1978.)

HUMAN ERYTHROCYTE ENZYMES IN NORMAL ADULTS*

Enzyme (Synonym)	Enzyme Activity (IU/g hemoglobin)	Enzyme (Synonym)	Enzyme Activity (IU/g hemoglobin)
1. Acetylcholinesterase	36.9 ± 3.83	14. Glutathione reductase (NAD(P)H)	7.18 ± 1.09
2. Adenosine deaminase	1.11 ± 0.23	15. Glutathione synthetase	0.19 ± 0.03
3. Adenylate kinase	258 ± 29.3	16. Hexokinase	1.16 ± 0.17
4. Bisphosphoglyceromutase (2,3,-diphosphoglyceromutase)	4.78 ± 0.65	17. Hypoxanthine phosphoribosyl-transferase (hypoxanthine guanosine-phosphoribosyltransferase)	1.72 ± 0.3
5. Catalase	15.3 ± 2.39 × 10^4	18. Methemoglobin reductase	2.60 ± 0.71
6. Fructose-bisphosphate aldolase (aldolase)	3.19 ± 0.86	19. 6-Phosphofructokinase	11.0 ± 2.33
7. Galactokinase	0.079 ± 0.006	20. Phosphogluconate dehydrogenase (decarboxylating)	8.78 ± 0.78
8.	0.029 ± 0.006		
9. Galactose-1-phosphate uridylyl-transferase	28.4 ± 6.94	21. Phosphoglycerate kinase	320 ± 36.1
		22. Pyrimidine 5'-nucleotidase	0.11 ± 0.03
10. Glucose-6-phosphate dehydrogenase	8.34 ± 1.59	23. Pyruvate kinase	15.0 ± 1.96
		24. Triosephosphate isomerase	2111 ± 397
11. Glucose phosphate isomerase (phosphoglucose isomerase)	60.8 ± 11.0	25. Uroporphyrinogen I synthase	2.52
12. γ-Glutamyl-cysteine synthetase	0.43 ± 0.04		
13. Glutathione peroxidase [1.11.1.9]	31.4 ± 2.97		

*From Beutler, E., and Blume, K. G.: In *Human Health and Disease*, II. Altman, P. L., and Dittmer, D. S. (eds.), Bethesda, Md., Federation of American Societies for Experimental Biology, 1977, p. 156.

HUMAN ERYTHROCYTE INTERMEDIATE METABOLITES IN NORMAL ADULTS*

Intermediate Metabolite (Synonym)	Concentration (μ moles/liter erythrocytes)
1. Adenosine 5'-diphosphate	635 ± 105
2. Adenosine 5'-monophosphate	62 ± 10
3. Adenosine 5'-triphosphate	1200 ± 102
4.	1438 ± 99
5. Dihydroxyacetone phosphate	9.4 ± 2.8
6. 2,3-Diphosphoglycerate	4171 ± 636
7. Fructose 1,6-bisphosphate (fructose 1,6-diphosphate)	1.9 ± 0.6
8. Fructose 6-phosphate	9.3 ± 2.0
9. Glucose 1,6-biphosphate (glucose 1,6-diphosphate)	180–300
10. Glucose 6-phosphate	27.8 ± 7.5
11. Glutathione, oxidized	4.2 ± 1.5
12. reduced	2234 ± 354
13. Lactate	748.6 ± 63.7
14. Mannose 1,6-bisphosphate (mannose 1,6-diphosphate)	150
15. Phosphoenolpyruvate	12.2 ± 2.2
16. 2-Phosphoglyceric acid	7.3 ± 2.5
17. 3-Phosphoglyceric acid	44.9 ± 5.1
18. Pyruvate	67.7 ± 7.8

*From Beutler, E., and Blume, K. G.: In *Human Health and Disease*, II. Altman, P. L., and Dittmer, D. S. (eds.), Bethesda, Md., Federation of American Societies for Experimental Biology, 1977, p. 156.

RED CELL ENZYME ACTIVITY IN ADULTS AND TERM INFANTS*

Enzyme	Adults (20)	Infants (10)
Hexokinase	12.9 ± 2.1	34.0 ± 6.0
Phosphoglucose isomerase	406 ± 37	560 ± 112
Phosphofructokinase	148 ± 24.5	84.5 ± 24
Aldolase	24.5 ± 3.7	42.0 ± 10.0
Glyceraldehyde-3-phosphate dehydrogenase	885 ± 127	884 ± 245
Triosephosphate isomerase	26,323 ± 3240	29,111 ± 4100
Phosphoglycerate kinase	2795 ± 144	3926 ± 528
Phosphoglycerate mutase	751 ± 99	1049 ± 160
Enolase	252 ± 54	517 ± 121
Pyruvate kinase	179 ± 16	256 ± 50
Lactic dehydrogenase	2033 ± 287	2756 ± 425
Glucose-6-phosphate dehydrogenase	215 ± 18	328 ± 40

*Infant samples were obtained from babies weighing more than 2800 g whose gestational age was 39 weeks or greater. Blood was drawn within 24 hours of birth. All the infants were clinically healthy. Adult samples were obtained from healthy, normal volunteers. (From Oski, F. A.: Pediatrics 44:89, 1969. Copyright, American Academy of Pediatrics, 1969.)

RED CELL GLYCOLYTIC INTERMEDIATES IN NORMAL ADULTS, TERM INFANTS, AND PREMATURE INFANTS*

Intermediate	Normal Adults (10)	Term Infants (10)	Premature Infants (11)	Normals (5)
Glucose-6-phosphate	24.8 ± 9.8	45.2 ± 8.7	66.8 ± 34.8	27 ± 2.4
Fructose-6-phosphate	5.4 ± 1.0	9.9 ± 2.3	20.5 ± 8.9	11 ± 2.5
Fructose,1,6-diphosphate	4.6 ± 1.0	3.8 ± 0.7	3.6 ± 0.8	5 ± 0.9
Dihydroxyacetone phosphate	4.9 ± 3.5	11.9 ± 5.0	18.6 ± 10.7	12 ± 3.7
Glyceraldehyde-3-phosphate	2.6 ± 0.7	1.9 ± 1.6	6.5 ± 3.2	4 ± 1.5
3-Phosphoglycerate	61.6 ± 12.4	58.2 ± 14.4	47.5 ± 14.2	48 ± 16.1
2-Phosphoglycerate	4.3 ± 1.8	4.9 ± 1.6	4.4 ± 2.5	7 ± 1.7
Phosphoenolpyruvate	8.8 ± 2.6	7.6 ± 2.9	7.4 ± 3.0	12 ± 0.9
Pyruvate	73.5 ± 33.1	70.4 ± 32.3	78.4 ± 4.15	71 ± 17.7
2,3-Diphosphoglycerate	4423 ± 1907	3609 ± 800	3152 ± 2133	4000

*Samples from normal adults and term infants were identical to those described in the preceding table. Premature infants had birth weights below 2200 g and gestational age less than 37 weeks. These premature infants were healthy at the time of investigation. (From Oski, F. A.: Pediatrics 44:87, 1969. Copyright, American Academy of Pediatrics, 1969.)

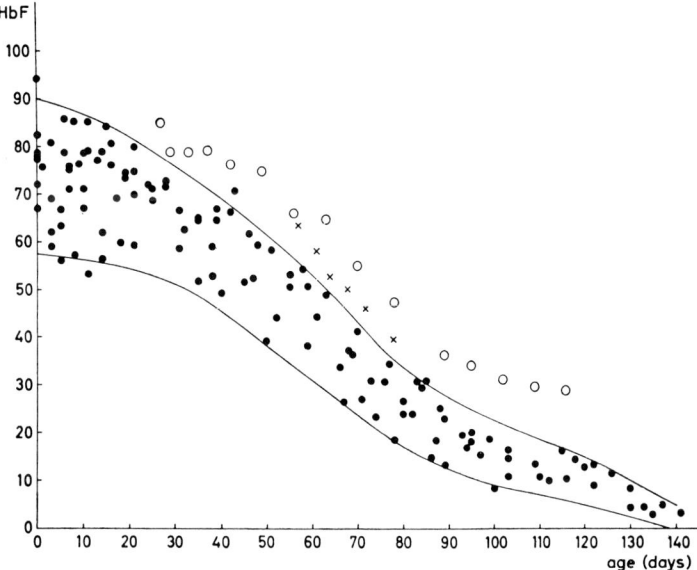

The relative concentration of Hb F in infants and its variation with age. The region between the curved lines contains 120 observations in 17 normal children. (From Garby, L., and Sjolin, S.: Acta Paediatr. *51*:245, 1962.)

PERCENTAGE OF HEMOGLOBINS F AND A2 IN THE NEWBORN AND ADULT*

	% Hb F (Gα:Aα ratio)	% Hb A2
Newborn	60–90 (3:1)	<1.0
Adult	<1.0 (2:3)	1.6–3.5

*The α chains of fetal hemoglobin contain either a glycyl residue or an alanyl residue at position 136. The Gα:Aα ratio in the newborn undergoes a considerable change between the third and fourth months of life, at which time it approximates that of the Hb F of adults (ref. 16). (From Charache, S.: In *Human Health and Disease,* II. Altman, P. L., and Dittmer, D. S. [eds.], Bethesda, Md., Federation of American Societies for Experimental Biology, 1977, p. 159.)

METHEMOGLOBIN LEVELS IN NORMAL CHILDREN*

	No. Cases	No. Det.	Methemoglobin (g/dl)			No. Cases	No. Det.	Methemoglobin as Per Cent of Total Hemoglobin		
			Mean	*Range*	*Standard Dev.*			*Mean*	*Range*	*Standard Dev.*
Premature (birth–7 days)	29	34	0.43	(0.02–0.83)	±0.07	24	28	2.3	(0.08–4.4)	±1.26
Prematures (7–72 days)	21	29	0.31	(0.02–0.78)	±0.19	18	23	2.2	(0.02–4.7)	±1.07
Prematures (total)	50	63	0.38	(0.02–0.83)	±0.10	42	51	2.2	(0.08–4.7)	±1.10
Cook County Hospital, prematures (1–14 days)	8	8	0.52	(0.18–0.83)	±0.08	—	—	—	—	—
Newborns (1–10 days)	39	39	0.22	(0.00–0.58)	±0.17	25	30	1.5	(0.00–2.8)	±0.81
Infants (1 month–1 year)	8	8	0.14	(0.02–0.29)	±0.09	8	8	1.2	(0.17–2.4)	±0.78
Children (1–14 years)	35	35	0.11	(0.00–0.33)	±0.09	35	35	0.79	(0.00–2.4)	±0.62
Adults (14–78 years)	30	30	0.11	(0.00–0.28)	±0.09	27	27	0.82	(0.00–1.9)	±0.63

*The premature and full-term infants were free of known disease. None had respiratory distress or cyanosis. Analysis of milk and water ingested by these infants revealed the nitrate level less than 0.027 ppm. The premature infants routinely received vitamin C orally each day from the seventh day of life. (From Kravitz, H., Elegant, L. D., et al.: J. Dis. Child. *91*:2, 1956, Copyright 1956, American Medical Association.)

VALUES OF SERUM IRON (SI), TOTAL IRON-BINDING CAPACITY (TIBC), AND TRANSFERRIN SATURATION (S%) FROM INFANTS DURING THE FIRST YEAR OF LIFE*

			Age (mo)						
			0.5	1	2	4	6	9	12
SI	Median 95% range	μmol/liter	22 11–36	22 10–31	16 3–29	15 3–29	14 5–24	15 6–24	14 6–28
		μg/dl	120 63–201	125 58–172	87 15–159	84 18–164	77 28–135	84 34–135	78 35–155
TIBC (mean ± SD)		μmol/liter	34 ± 8	36 ± 8	44 ± 10	54 ± 7	58 ± 9	61 ± 7	64 ± 7
		μg/dl	191 ± 43	199 ± 43	246 ± 55	300 ± 39	321 ± 51	341 ± 42	358 ± 38
S%	Median 95% range		68 30–99	63 35–94	34 21–63	27 7–53	23 10–43	25 10–39	23 10–47

*These data were obtained from a group of healthy, full-term infants who were born at the Helsinki University Central Hospital. Infants received iron supplementation in formula and cereal throughout the 12-month period. Infants with hemoglobin below 110 g/dl, mean corpuscular volume of red blood cells below 71 μ^3, or serum ferritin below 10 ng/ml were excluded from the study. The 95 per cent range of the transferrin saturation values indicates that the lower limit of normal is about 10 per cent after 4 months of age. (From Saarien, U. M., and Siimes, M. A.: J. Pediatr. *91*:876, 1977.)

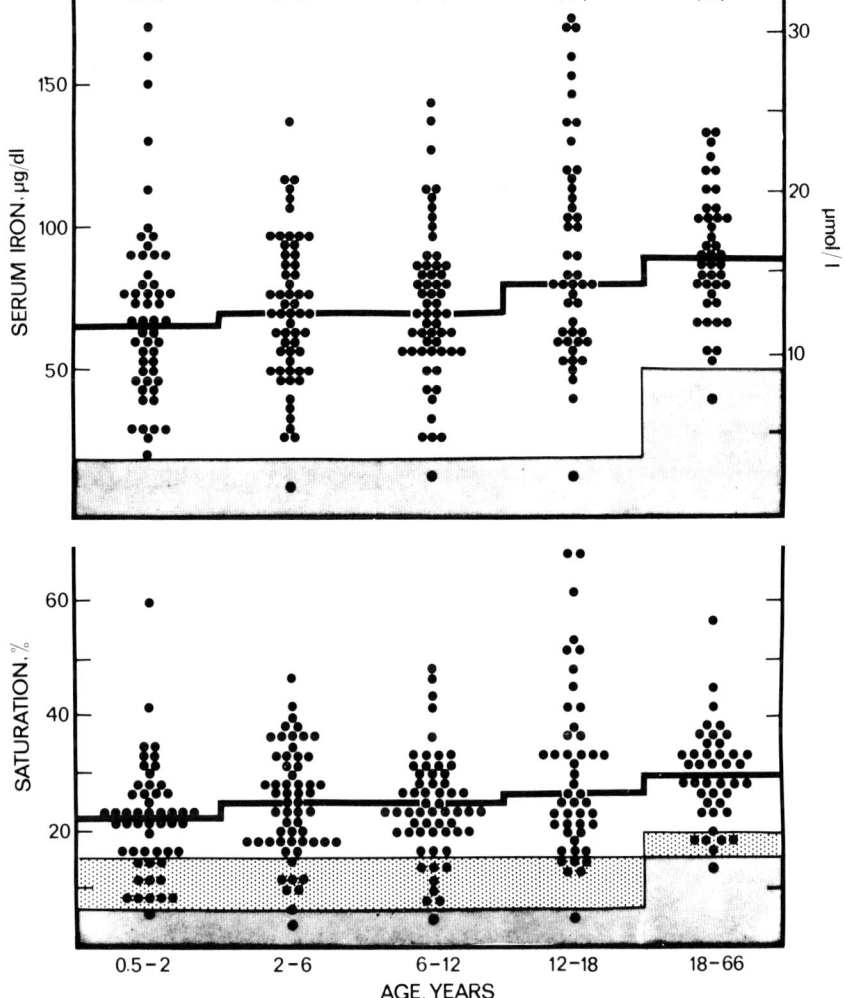

Normal values for serum iron and transferrin saturation in subjects who met the criteria for normal values of hemoglobin, mean corpuscular volume, free erythrocyte protoporphyrin, and serum ferritin. (From Koerper, M. A., and Dallman, P.: J. Pediatr. 91:871, 1977.)

NORMAL RANGES FOR FOLATE ASSAYS AND FIGLU TEST*

L. casei activity expressed as ng/ml

Serum Folate	Range	Mean	Author
Adults	6.0–18.6	9.7	Hoffbrand et al.
Children 1 year	3.0–35	9.3	Vanier and Tyas
Children 1–6 years	4.1–21.2	11.4	Shojania and Gross
Children 1–10 years	6.5–16.5	10.3	Dormandy et al.
Red Cell Folate			
Adults	160–640	316	Hoffbrand et al.
Infants <1 year	74–995	277	Vanier and Tyas
Children 1–11 years	96–364	215	McNeish and Willoughby
Whole Blood Folate			
Adults	50–150	89	Izak et al.
Adults	60–400	195	Vanier and Tyas
Infants <1 year	20–160	87	Kende et al.
Infants 1 year	31–400	86	Vanier and Tyas
Infants 2–24 months	35–160	96†	Grossowicz et al.
Children up to 11 years	52–164	97	McNeish and Willoughby

FIGLU Excretion	Histidine Load	Collection Period	Total mg FIGLU	
Adults	15 g	0–8 hours	up to 17 mg	Chanarin and Bennett
Infants	100–300 mg/kg	0–6 hours	up to 6 mg	Vanier and Tyas
Children	0.12 g/lb	0–24 hours	up to 30 mg	Luhby and Cooperman

*Serum folate levels (fasting) below 3.0, red cell folate below 100, or whole blood folate below 60 can be regarded as abnormal.
†Derived after correction for a packed cell volume of 45 per cent.
(From Willoughby, M. L. N.: *Pediatric Haematology*. New York, Churchill Livingstone, 1977, p. 17.)

NORMAL SERUM FOLIC ACID LEVELS (ng/ml)*

Age	Range	Mean ± SD
Normal Premature Infants		
1–4 days	7.17–52.00	29.54 ± 0.98
2–3 weeks	4.12–15.62	8.61 ± 0.55
1–2 months	2.81–11.25	5.84 ± 0.35
2–3 months	3.56–11.82	6.95 ± 0.50
3–5 months	3.85–16.50	8.92 ± 0.86
5–7 months	6.00–12.25	9.02 ± 0.74
Normal Children		
1–6 years	4.12–21.15	11.37 ± 0.82
Normal Adults		
20–45 years	4.50–28.00	10.29 ± 1.14

*From Shojania, A., and Gross, S.: J. Pediatr. 64:323, 1964.

NORMAL SERUM VITAMIN E LEVELS (mg/dl) IN NEWBORNS*

Weeks	1	2	3	4	5	6	7	8	9	10
<1500 g	0.40	0.30	0.25	0.25	0.25	0.25	0.25	0.25	0.35	0.45
28–32 weeks	[0.05]	[0.04]	[0.03]	[0.03]	[0.03]	[0.03]	[0.03]	[0.03]	[0.04]	[0.05]
1500–2000 g	0.45	0.04	0.40	0.45	0.45	0.45	0.50	0.50	0.60	0.70
32–36 weeks	[0.05]	[0.05]	[0.05]	[0.05]	[0.05]	[0.05]	[0.05]	[0.05]	[0.06]	[0.06]
2000–2500 g	0.50	0.45	0.50	0.60	0.70	0.75	0.75	0.75	0.75	0.80
36–40 weeks	[0.05]	[0.05]	[0.05]	[0.06]	[0.06]	[0.06]	[0.60]	[0.60]	[0.60]	[0.70]
>2500 g	0.55	0.55	0.55	0.60	0.75	0.80	0.85	0.85	0.85	0.85
Term	[0.60]	[0.60]	[0.60]	[0.60]	[0.70]	[0.70]	[0.80]	[0.80]	[0.80]	[0.80]

*Mean ± [1 SD]. (From Klaus, M., and Fanaroff, A.: *Care of the High Risk Neonate*. Philadelphia, W. B. Saunders Co., 1973, p. 343.)

The plasma concentration of hemopexin and haptoglobin in 39 term and 27 premature infants on the first day of life. The means ± are indicated to the right of the hemopexin results. (From Lundh, B., Oski, F. A., et al.: Acta Paediatr. Scand. 59:121, 1970.)

ESTIMATED BLOOD VOLUMES*

Age	Plasma Volume (ml/kg) (PV)	Red Cell Mass (ml/kg) (RCM)	Total Blood Volume (ml/kg)	
			(From PV)	(From RCM)
Newborn	41.3	43.1	82.1	86.1
	46.0			84.7
			78.0	
1–7 days	51–54		82–86	
		37.9		77.8
1–12 months	46.1		78.1	
		25.5		72.8
1–3 years	44.4		73.8	
	47.2		81.8	
		24.9		69.1
4–6 years	48.5		80.0	
	49.6		85.6	
		25.5		67.5
7–9 years	52.2		87.6	
	49.0		86.1	
		24.3		67.5
10–12 years	51.9		87.6	
	46.2		83.2	
		26.3		67.4
13–15 years	51.2		88.3	
16–18 years	50.1		90.2	
Adults	39–44	25–30	68–88	55–75

*From Price, D. C., and Ries, C.: In *Nuclear Medicine in Clinical Pediatrics.* Handmaker, H., and Lowenstein, J. M. (eds.), New York, Society of Nuclear Medicine, 1975, p. 279.

NORMAL LEUKOCYTE COUNTS*

Age	Total Leukocytes		Neutrophils			Lymphocytes			Monocytes		Eosinophils	
	Mean	(Range)	Mean	(Range)	%	Mean	(Range)	%	Mean	%	Mean	%
Birth	18.1	(9.0–30.0)	11.0	(6.0–26.0)	61	5.5	(2.0–11.0)	31	1.1	6	0.4	2
12 hours	22.8	(13.0–38.0)	15.5	(6.0–28.0)	68	5.5	(2.0–11.0)	24	1.2	5	0.5	2
24 hours	18.9	(9.4–34.0)	11.5	(5.0–21.0)	61	5.8	(2.0–11.5)	31	1.1	6	0.5	2
1 week	12.2	(5.0–21.0)	5.5	(1.5–10.0)	45	5.0	(2.0–17.0)	41	1.1	9	0.5	4
2 weeks	11.4	(5.0–20.0)	4.5	(1.0–9.5)	40	5.5	(2.0–17.0)	48	1.0	9	0.4	3
1 month	10.8	(5.0–19.5)	3.8	(1.0–9.0)	35	6.0	(2.5–16.5)	56	0.7	7	0.3	3
6 months	11.9	(6.0–17.5)	3.8	(1.0–8.5)	32	7.3	(4.0–13.5)	61	0.6	5	0.3	3
1 year	11.4	(6.0–17.5)	3.5	(1.5–8.5)	31	7.0	(4.0–10.5)	61	0.6	5	0.3	3
2 years	10.6	(6.0–17.0)	3.5	(1.5–8.5)	33	6.3	(3.0–9.5)	59	0.5	5	0.3	3
4 years	9.1	(5.5–15.5)	3.8	(1.5–8.5)	42	4.5	(2.0–8.0)	50	0.5	5	0.3	3
6 years	8.5	(5.0–14.5)	4.3	(1.5–8.0)	51	3.5	(1.5–7.0)	42	0.4	5	0.2	3
8 years	8.3	(4.5–13.5)	4.4	(1.5–8.0)	53	3.3	(1.5–6.8)	39	0.4	4	0.2	2
10 years	8.1	(4.5–13.5)	4.4	(1.8–8.0)	54	3.1	(1.5–6.5)	38	0.4	4	0.2	2
16 years	7.8	(4.5–13.0)	4.4	(1.8–8.0)	57	2.8	(1.2–5.2)	35	0.4	5	0.2	3
21 years	7.4	(4.5–11.0)	4.4	(1.8–7.7)	59	2.5	(1.0–4.8)	34	0.3	4	0.2	3

*Numbers of leukocytes are in thousands per mm^3, ranges are estimates of 95 per cent confidence limits, and percentages refer to differential counts. Neutrophils include band cells at all ages and a small number of metamyelocytes and myelocytes in the first few days of life. (From Dallman, P. R.: In *Pediatrics*, 16th ed. Rudolph, A. M. (ed.), New York, Appleton-Century-Crofts, 1977, p. 1178.)

POLYMORPHONUCLEAR LEUKOCYTE AND BAND COUNTS IN THE NEWBORN DURING THE FIRST 2 DAYS OF LIFE*

Age (hours)	Absolute Neutrophil Count (mm^3)	Absolute Band Count (mm^3)	B/N Ratio
0	3500–6000	1300	0.14
12	8000–15,000	1300	0.14
24	7000–13,000	1300	0.14
36	5000–9000	700	0.11
48	3500–5200	700	0.11

*Normal values were obtained from the assessment of 3100 separate white blood cell counts obtained from 965 infants; 513 counts were from infants considered to be completely normal at the time the count was obtained and for the preceding and subsequent 48 hours. There was no difference in the normal ranges when infants were compared by either birth weight (> or <2500 g) or gestational age. (From Manroe, B. L., Browne, R., et al.: Pediatr. Res. *10*:428, 1976.)

ASSESSMENT OF LEUKOCYTE FUNCTION*

Test Name	Normal Values	Test Name	Normal Values
Bacterial killing	Less than 10% of most bacterial species remain viable after 60 min. at 37° C incubation with an equal number of PMN	Chemiluminescence	$142.5 \pm 64 \times 10^3$ counts/min per 13 min per 10^7 PMN
Oxygen consumption	Rst: 7.4 ± 3.8 µl O_2 consumed per hour per 10^7 cells; Phg: 37.6 ± 22.5 µl O_2 consumed per hour per 10^7 cells	Nitroblue tetrazolium (NBT) reduction	Rst: 0.088 ± 0.040 OD_{515} per 15 min. per 10^7 cells; Phg: 0.319 ± 0.112 OD_{515} per min. per 10^7 cells
^{14}C-glucose oxidation	Rst: 62.6 ± 10 nmoles glucose oxidized per 30 min per 5×10^6 cells; Phg: 169 ± 28 nmoles glucose oxidized per 30 min per 5×10^6 cells	Phagocytic uptake of oil red O particles	0.138(0.121–0.157) mg liquid petrolatum taken up per min per 10^7 cells
^{14}C-formate oxidation	Rst: 0.6(0.2–1.1) nmoles formate oxidized per hour per mg protein; Phg: 2.8(1.1–5.9) nmoles formate oxidized per hour per mg protein	Chemotaxis assay	Chemotactic index: 13 ± 5 (without chemotactic factor); 67 ± 16 (with chemotactic factor)
Hydrogen peroxide release	Rst: 0.012 ± 0.003 nmole H_2O_2 released per min per 2.5×10^6 cells; Phg: 0.445 ± 0.064 nmole H_2O_2 released per min per 2.5×10^6 cells	Rebuck skin window	3 h: PMN; 6 h: PMN + monocytes; 12 h: monocytes
Iodination of ingested particles	Rst: 0.04 ± 0.03 nmole iodide consumed per hour per 10^7 cells; Phg: 3.95 ± 0.82 nmoles iodide consumed per hour per 10^7 cells	Endotoxin stimulation	Mean increase of PMN/µl: 6060 ± 880
Superoxide production	Rst: 0.50 nmole O_2^- per 15 min per 10^7 cells; Phg: 1.0 nmole per 15 min per 10^7 cells	Hydrocortisone stimulation	Mean increase of PMN/µl: 4220 ± 320
		Epinephrine stimulation	Twofold increase of PMN/µl compared with pre-injection value

*Absolute values for these tests vary among laboratories, depending on the specific conditions of the assay. All tests must be run parallel with control samples, or normal control values must be established prior to testing. Abbreviation: PMN = polymorphonuclear leukocyte(s), Rst = resting, Phg = phagocytic, OD_{515} = optical density at 515 nm, values in parentheses are ranges. (From Baehner, R. L.: In *Human Health and Disease*. II. Altman, P. L., and Dittmer, D. A. [eds.], Bethesda, Md., Federation of American Societies for Experimental Biology, 1977, pp. 62–64.)

BONE MARROW CELL POPULATIONS OF NORMAL INFANTS*

Cell Type	Month				
	0(n = 57)†	1(n = 71)	2(n = 48)	3(n = 24)	4(n = 19)
Small lymphocytes	14.42 ± 5.54	47.05 ± 9.24	42.68 ± 7.90	43.63 ± 11.83	47.06 ± 8.77
Transitional cells	1.18 ± 1.13	1.95 ± 0.94	2.38 ± 1.35	2.17 ± 1.64	1.64 ± 1.01
Proerythroblasts	0.02 ± 0.06	0.10 ± 0.14	0.13 ± 0.19	0.10 ± 0.13	0.05 ± 0.10
Basophilic erythroblasts	0.24 ± 0.25	0.34 ± 0.33	0.57 ± 0.41	0.40 ± 0.33	0.24 ± 0.24
Early erythroblasts	0.27 ± 0.26	0.44 ± 0.42	0.71 ± 0.51	0.50 ± 0.38	0.28 ± 0.30
Polychromatic erythroblasts	13.06 ± 6.78	6.90 ± 4.45	13.06 ± 3.48	10.51 ± 3.39	6.84 ± 2.58
Orthochromatic erythroblasts	0.69 ± 0.73	0.54 ± 1.88	0.66 ± 0.82	0.70 ± 0.87	0.34 ± 0.30
Extruded nuclei	0.47 ± 0.46	0.16 ± 0.17	0.26 ± 0.22	0.19 ± 0.12	0.16 ± 0.17
Late erythroblasts	14.22 ± 7.14	7.60 ± 4.84	13.99 ± 3.82	11.40 ± 3.43	7.34 ± 2.54
Early/late erythroblasts ratio‡	1:50	1:15	1:18	1:22	1:23
Fetal erythroblasts	14.48 ± 7.24	8.04 ± 5.00	14.70 ± 3.86	11.90 ± 3.52	7.62 ± 2.56
Blood reticulocytes	4.18 ± 1.46	1.06 ± 1.13	3.39 ± 1.22	2.90 ± 0.91	1.65 ± 0.73
Neutrophils					
Promyelocytes	0.79 ± 0.91	0.76 ± 0.65	0.78 ± 0.68	0.76 ± 0.80	0.59 ± 0.51
Myelocytes	3.95 ± 2.93	2.50 ± 1.48	2.03 ± 1.14	2.24 ± 1.70	2.32 ± 1.59
Early neutrophils	4.74 ± 3.43	3.27 ± 1.94	2.81 ± 1.62	3.00 ± 2.18	2.91 ± 2.01
Metamyelocytes	19.37 ± 4.84	11.34 ± 3.59	11.27 ± 3.38	11.93 ± 13.09	6.04 ± 3.63
Bands	28.89 ± 7.56	14.10 ± 4.63	13.15 ± 4.71	14.60 ± 7.54	13.93 ± 6.13
Mature neutrophils	7.37 ± 4.64	3.64 ± 2.97	3.07 ± 2.45	3.48 ± 1.62	4.27 ± 2.69
Late neutrophils	55.63 ± 7.98	29.08 ± 6.79	27.50 ± 6.88	31.00 ± 11.17	31.30 ± 7.80
Early/late neutrophil ratio	1:12	1:9	1:9	1:9	1:11
Total neutrophils	60.37 ± 8.66	32.35 ± 7.68	30.31 ± 7.27	34.01 ± 11.95	34.21 ± 8.61
Total eosinophils	2.70 ± 1.27	2.61 ± 1.40	2.50 ± 1.22	2.54 ± 1.46	2.37 ± 4.13
Total basophils	0.12 ± 0.20	0.07 ± 0.16	0.08 ± 0.10	0.09 ± 0.09	0.11 ± 0.14
Total myeloid cells	63.19 ± 9.10	35.03 ± 8.09	32.90 ± 7.85	36.64 ± 12.26	36.69 ± 8.91
Monocytes	0.88 ± 0.85	1.01 ± 0.89	0.91 ± 0.83	0.68 ± 0.56	0.75 ± 0.75
Miscellaneous					
Megakaryocytes	0.06 ± 0.15	0.05 ± 0.09	0.10 ± 0.13	0.06 ± 0.09	0.06 ± 0.06
Plasma cells	0.00 ± 0.02	0.02 ± 0.06	0.02 ± 0.05	0.00 ± 0.02	0.01 ± 0.03
Unknown blasts	0.31 ± 0.31	0.62 ± 0.50	0.58 ± 0.50	0.63 ± 0.60	0.56 ± 0.53
Unknown cells	0.22 ± 0.34	0.21 ± 0.25	0.16 ± 0.24	0.19 ± 0.21	0.23 ± 0.25
Damaged cells	5.79 ± 2.78	5.50 ± 2.46	5.09 ± 1.78	4.75 ± 2.30	4.80 ± 2.29
Total	6.38 ± 2.84	6.39 ± 2.63	5.94 ± 1.94	5.63 ± 2.36	5.66 ± 2.30

*Percentages of cell types (means ± Standard Deviation) in tibial bone marrow of infants from birth to 18 months of age. Data were obtained from normal American infants of black, white, and Asian racial origin. The changes in the marrow during the first 18 months of postnatal life are based on differential counts of 1000 cells classified on stained smears on each of 10 serial marrow samples aspirated from the same population of infants. Criteria for including bone marrow data in this study consisted of absence of any clinical evidence of disease, normal rate of growth, and normal serum proteins and transferrin saturations.

†n = number of infants studied at each stage.

‡Expressed in round figures for facilitating comparison. Means ± SD were calculated from values obtained in individual infants, and statistical comparisons were performed.

(From Rosse, C., Kraemer, M. J., et al.: J. Lab. Clin. Med. 89:1228, 1977.)

BONE MARROW CELL POPULATIONS OF NORMAL INFANTS* Continued

5(n = 22)	6(n = 22)	9(n = 16)	12(n = 18)	15(n = 12)	18(n = 19)
47.19 ± 9.93	47.55 ± 7.88	48.76 ± 8.11	47.11 ± 11.32	42.77 ± 8.94	43.55 ± 8.56
1.83 ± 0.89	2.31 ± 1.16	1.92 ± 1.39	2.32 ± 1.90	1.70 ± 0.82	1.99 ± 1.00
0.07 ± 0.10	0.09 ± 0.12	0.07 ± 0.09	0.02 ± 0.04	0.07 ± 0.12	0.08 ± 0.13
0.47 ± 0.33	0.32 ± 0.24	0.31 ± 0.24	0.30 ± 0.25	0.38 ± 0.37	0.50 ± 0.34
0.55 ± 0.36	0.41 ± 0.30	0.39 ± 0.28	0.39 ± 0.27	0.46 ± 0.36	0.59 ± 0.34
7.55 ± 2.35	7.30 ± 3.60	7.73 ± 3.39	6.83 ± 3.75	6.04 ± 1.56	6.97 ± 3.56
0.46 ± 0.51	0.38 ± 0.56	0.39 ± 0.48	0.37 ± 0.51	0.50 ± 0.65	0.44 ± 0.49
0.14 ± 0.11	0.16 ± 0.22	0.22 ± 0.25	0.23 ± 0.25	0.17 ± 0.12	0.21 ± 0.19
8.16 ± 2.58	7.85 ± 4.11	8.34 ± 3.31	7.42 ± 4.11	6.72 ± 1.80	7.62 ± 3.63
1:15	1:17	1:19	1:17	1:15	1:10
8.70 ± 2.69	8.25 ± 4.31	8.72 ± 3.34	7.81 ± 4.26	7.18 ± 1.95	8.21 ± 37.1
1.38 ± 0.65	1.74 ± 0.80	1.67 ± 0.52	1.79 ± 0.79	2.10 ± 0.91	1.84 ± 0.46
0.87 ± 0.80	0.67 ± 0.66	0.41 ± 0.34	0.69 ± 0.71	0.67 ± 0.58	0.64 ± 0.59
2.73 ± 1.82	2.22 ± 1.25	2.07 ± 1.20	2.32 ± 1.14	2.48 ± 0.94	2.49 ± 1.39
3.60 ± 2.50	2.89 ± 1.71	2.48 ± 1.46	3.02 ± 1.52	3.16 ± 1.19	3.14 ± 1.75
11.89 ± 3.24	11.02 ± 3.12	11.80 ± 3.90	11.10 ± 3.82	12.48 ± 7.45	12.42 ± 4.15
14.07 ± 5.48	14.00 ± 4.58	14.08 ± 4.53	14.02 ± 4.88	15.17 ± 4.20	14.20 ± 5.23
3.77 ± 2.44	4.85 ± 2.69	3.97 ± 2.29	5.65 ± 3.92	6.94 ± 3.88	6.31 ± 3.91
29.73 ± 7.19	29.86 ± 6.74	29.86 ± 7.36	30.77 ± 8.69	34.60 ± 7.35	32.93 ± 7.01
1:8	1:10	1:12	1:10	1:10	1:10
33.12 ± 8.34	32.75 ± 7.03	32.33 ± 7.75	33.79 ± 8.76	37.76 ± 7.32	36.06 ± 7.40
1.98 ± 0.86	2.08 ± 1.16	1.74 ± 1.08	1.92 ± 1.09	3.39 ± 1.93	2.70 ± 2.16
0.09 ± 0.13	0.10 ± 0.13	0.11 ± 0.13	0.13 ± 0.15	0.27 ± 0.37	0.10 ± 0.12
35.40 ± 8.54	34.93 ± 7.52	34.18 ± 8.13	35.83 ± 8.84	41.42 ± 7.43	38.86 ± 7.92
1.29 ± 1.06	1.21 ± 1.01	1.17 ± 0.97	1.46 ± 1.52	1.68 ± 1.09	2.12 ± 1.59
0.08 ± 0.09	0.04 ± 0.07	0.09 ± 0.12	0.05 ± 0.08	0.00 ± 0.00	0.07 ± 0.12
0.05 ± 0.11	0.03 ± 0.07	0.01 ± 0.03	0.03 ± 0.07	0.07 ± 0.12	0.06 ± 0.08
0.50 ± 0.37	0.56 ± 0.48	0.42 ± 0.50	0.37 ± 0.33	0.46 ± 0.32	0.43 ± 0.45
0.17 ± 0.22	0.10 ± 0.15	0.14 ± 0.17	0.11 ± 0.14	0.13 ± 0.18	0.20 ± 0.23
4.86 ± 1.25	5.04 ± 1.08	4.89 ± 1.60	5.34 ± 2.19	4.99 ± 1.96	5.05 ± 2.15
5.66 ± 1.41	5.78 ± 1.16	5.55 ± 1.74	5.90 ± 2.03	5.65 ± 2.02	5.81 ± 2.16

COAGULATION FACTOR ASSAYS (MEAN ± 1 SD) AND SCREENING TESTS IN THE FETUS AND NEONATE*

Assays of Coagulation Factors	Normal Adult Values	28 to 31 Weeks' Gestation	32 to 36 Weeks' Gestation	Term	Time at Which Values Attain Adult Norms
Fibrinogen (mg/dl)	150–400	215 ± 28(SE)	226 ± 23(SE)	246 ± 18(SE)	†
		270 ± 85	244 ± 55	246 ± 55	
II (%)	100	30 ± 10	35 ± 12	45 ± 15	2–12 months
V (%)	100	76 ± 7(SE)	84 ± 9(SE)	100 ± 5(SE)	†
		90 ± 26	72 ± 23	98 ± 40	
VII and X (%)	100	38 ± 14	40 ± 15	56 ± 16	2–12 months
VIII (%)	100	90 ± 15(SE)	140 ± 10(SE)	168 ± 12(SE)	†
		70 ± 30	98 ± 40	105 ± 34	
IX (%)	100	27 ± 10	NA	28 ± 8	3–9 months
XI (%)	100	5–18	NA	29–70	1–2 months
XII (%)	100	NA	30 ±	51(25–70)	9–14 days
XIII	100				†
Bioassay (%)		100	100	100	
Quantitative (units/ml)	21 ± 5.6	5 ± 3.5	NA	11 ± 3.4	3 weeks
Prothrombin time (sec)‡	12–14	23 ±	17(12–21)	16(13–20)	1 week
Activated partial thromboplastin time (sec)‡	44	NA	70 ±	55 ± 10	2–9 months
Thrombin time (sec)‡	10	16–28	14(11–17)	12(10–16)	few days

*Assays quoted are biologic, unless otherwise specified. SE = standard error; NA = not available.
†Adult levels attained prenatally.
‡Values vary between laboratories depending on reagents employed.
(From Hathaway, W. E.: Semin. Hematol. *12*:175, 1975, by permission of Grune & Stratton; and from Gross, S. J., and Stuart, M. J.: Clin. Perinatol. *4*:260, 1977.)

VASCULAR-PLATELET INTERACTIONS IN THE FETUS AND NEONATE*

Vascular-Platelet Interactions	Normal Adult Values	27 to 31 Weeks' Gestation	32 to 36 Weeks' Gestation	Term	Term Infant >1 to 2 Months
Capillary fragility	N	Increased	N	N	N
Platelet count (10^3 per mm^3)	300 ± 50	275 ± 60	290 ± 70	310 ± 68	280 ± 56
Platelet retention (%)	N	NA	NA	N or decreased	N
Platelet aggregation with ADP, epinephrine collagen	N	Abn	Abn	Abn	
Platelet aggregation with ristocetin	N	NA	NA	N or increased	N
Platelet release I (adenine nucleotides)	N	Abn	Abn	Abn	
Platelet factor 3	N	Abn	Abn	Abn	
Platelet factor 4	N	NA	NA	N	N
Bleeding time (min)	4.0 ± 1.5		4 ± 1.5	4 ± 1.5	N

*N = normal; Abn = abnormal; NA = not available. (From Hathaway, W. E.: Semin. Hematol. *12*:175, 1975, by permission of Grune & Stratton; and from Gross, S. J., and Stuart, M. J.: Clin. Perinatol. *4*:260, 1977.)

RELATION OF SERUM PROTEIN LEVELS TO AGE*

	Total Proteins (g/dl) Mean ± 1 SD and Range	Albumin (g/dl) Mean ± 1 SD and Range	Alpha-1 (g/dl) Mean ± 1 SD and Range	Alpha-2 (g/dl) Mean ± 1 SD and Range	Beta (g/dl) Mean ± 1 SD and Range	Gamma (g/dl) Mean ± 1 SD and Range
Cord blood	6.22 ± 1.21 (4.78–8.04)	3.23 ± 0.82 (2.17–4.04)	0.41 ± 0.10 (0.25–0.66)	0.68 ± 0.14 (0.44–0.94)	0.74 ± 0.30 (0.42–1.56)	1.28 ± 0.23 (0.81–1.16)
1–3 months	5.64 ± 1.04 (3.64–7.38)	3.41 ± 0.72 (2.05–4.46)	0.24 ± 0.09 (0.08–0.43)	0.74 ± 0.24 (0.40–1.13)	0.59 ± 0.20 (0.39–1.14)	0.66 ± 0.24 (0.25–1.05)
4–6 months	5.43 ± 0.84 (4.29–6.10)	3.46 ± 0.36 (3.17–3.88)	0.17 ± 0.04 (0.12–0.25)	0.67 ± 0.11 (0.52–0.84)	0.61 ± 0.14 (0.44–0.76)	0.61 ± 0.26 (0.24–0.90)
7–12 months	6.54 ± 0.76 (5.10–7.31)	3.62 ± 0.60 (3.22–4.31)	0.35 ± 0.15 (0.15–0.55)	0.99 ± 0.30 (0.78–1.46)	0.79 ± 0.16 (0.63–0.91)	0.84 ± 0.36 (0.32–1.18)
13–24 months	6.66 ± 0.93 (3.69–7.50)	3.63 ± 0.80 (1.89–5.03)	0.31 ± 0.15 (0.09–0.58)	0.88 ± 0.42 (0.41–1.36)	0.77 ± 0.31 (0.36–1.41)	1.09 ± 0.32 (0.36–1.62)
25–36 months	6.98 ± 0.66 (6.38–8.06)	4.11 + 0.78 (3.57–5.50)	0.23 ± 0.09 (0.19–0.26)	0.89 ± 0.14 (0.68–1.09)	0.67 ± 0.14 (0.47–0.91)	1.08± 0.28 (0.73–1.46)
3–5 years	6.65 ± 0.85 (4.88–8.06)	3.95 ± 0.57 (2.93–5.21)	0.21 ± 0.08 (0.08–0.40)	0.70 ± 0.15 (0.43–0.99)	0.67 ± 0.11 (0.47–1.01)	1.13 ± 0.31 (0.54–1.66)
6–8 years	6.95 ± 0.55 (5.97–7.94)	4.03 ± 0.45 (3.26–4.95)	0.22 ± 0.09 (0.09–0.45)	0.67 ± 0.10 (0.50–0.83)	0.72 ± 0.11 (0.45–0.93)	1.21 ± 0.32 (0.70–1.95)
9–11 years	7.43 ± 0.84 (6.32–9.00)	4.24 ± 0.79 (3.16–4.97)	0.30 ± 0.07 (0.12–0.38)	0.75 ± 0.27 (0.67–0.87)	0.84 ± 0.16 (0.63–1.02)	1.46 ± 0.41 (0.79–2.03)
12–16 years	7.25 ± 0.85 (6.25–8.75)	4.26 ± 0.64 (3.19–5.13)	0.19 ± 0.07 (0.09–0.32)	0.71 ± 0.15 (0.50–0.97)	0.68± 0.15 (0.48–0.88)	1.40 ± 0.31 (1.08–1.96)
Adult	7.41 ± 0.96 (6.44–8.32)	4.31 ± 0.59 (3.46–4.78)	0.23 ± 0.06 (0.16–0.30)	0.61 ± 0.14 (0.51–0.86)	0.81 ± 0.22 (0.59–1.06)	1.45 ± 0.46 (0.68–2.11)

*From Park, B. H., and Ellis, E. F.: In *Children Are Different: Developmental Physiology*, 2nd ed. Johnson, T. R., and Moore, W. M. (eds.), Columbus, Ohio, Ross Laboratories, 1978, p. 188.

SERUM IMMUNOGLOBULIN LEVELS IN NORMAL INDIVIDUALS*

Subjects		IgG		IgA		IgM	
Age	No.	mg/dl	% of Adult Level	mg/dl	% of Adult Level	mg/dl	% of Adult Level
Newborn	20	1004(598–1672)	95	<5(0–<5)	<2	9(6–15)	12
1–3 months	10	365(218–610)	34	32(20–53)	12	24(11–51)	32
4–6 months	12	381(228–636)	36	44(27–72)	17	38(25–60)	50
7–9 months	10	488(292–816)	46	44(27–73)	17	47(18–124)	62
10–18 months	13	640(383–1070)	60	67(27–169)	25	56(28–113)	74
2 years	8	708(423–1184)	67	89(35–222)	33	65(32–131)	86
3 years	6	798(477–1334)	75	100(40–251)	38	57(28–116)	75
4 years	8	906(542–1515)	85	120(48–301)	45	41(20–82)	54
5 years	5	901(539–1506)	85	134(53–336)	50	52(26–106)	68
6 years	11	954(571–1597)	90	131(52–329)	49	57(28–115)	75
7 years	11	1066(638–1783)	100	223(89–559)	84	48(24–98)	63
8 years	8	976(583–1631)	92	213(85–535)	80	55(27–112)	72
9 years	7	1006(599–1673)	95	230(92–578)	86	56(28–113)	74
10 years	7	991(593–1657)	93	188(75–472)	71	60(29–120)	79
11 years	7	989(586–1637)	93	257(102–644)	97	56(28–113)	74
12 years	7	855(511–1430)	81	232(92–581)	87	55(27–111)	72
13 years	13	961(575–1607)	91	235(94–588)	88	52(26–105)	68
14 years	8	940(562–1571)	89	217(86–544)	82	67(33–135)	88
Adult	30	106(635–177)	100	266(106–668)	100	76(37–154)	100

*Geometric means are presented for each immunoglobulin at every age. The bounds, given in parentheses, are obtained by taking the mean logarithm ± twice the pooled standard deviations of the mean logarithms, and then taking the antilogs of the results. In the case of IgA, the first four age groups have a pooled standard deviation separate from the other ages. In the case of IgM, the bounds of the first four age groups are ± twice the individual group standard deviations. (From Buckley, R. H., Dees, S. C., et al.: Pediatrics 41:600, 1968. Copyright, American Academy of Pediatrics, 1968.)

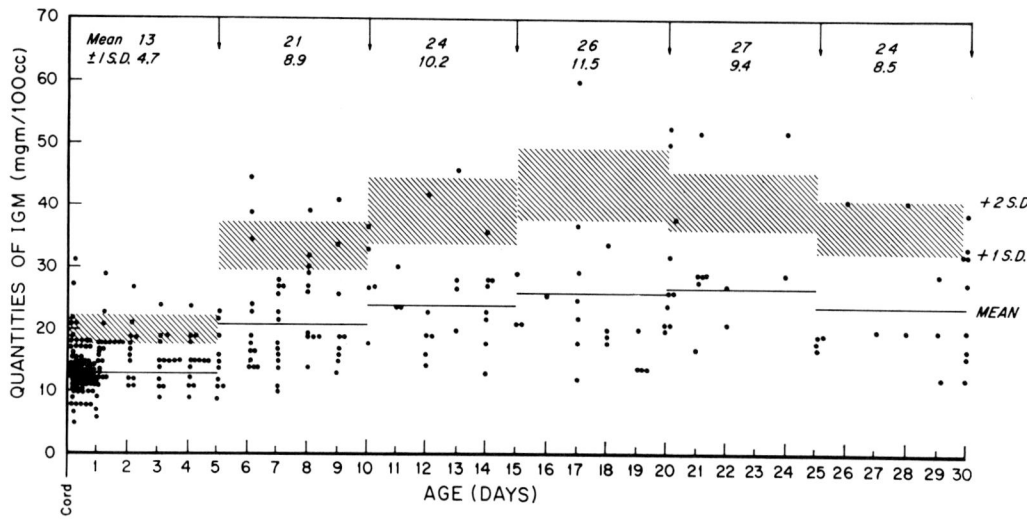

Serum IgM globulin in healthy neonates. Mean values (first and second standard deviation limits) of serum IgM in an uninfected population of neonates are indicated. The average amounts shown here were compiled from determination of IgM globulin quantities in 400 specimens of sera collected from 176 neonates at various intervals in the month following delivery. In all these cases, attempts were made to exclude infection. (From Blankenship, W., Willard, J., et al.: J. Pediatr. 75:1271, 1969.)

SERUM IgE LEVELS IN INFANTS AND CHILDREN*

Age	N	Range	Geometric Mean	Geometric Mean ± 2SD
Birth	24	<0.1–1.5	0.22	0.04– 1.28
6 weeks	17	<0.1–2.8	0.69	0.08– 6.12
3 months	15	0.3–3.1	0.82	0.18– 3.76
6 months	15	0.9–28.0	2.68	0.44– 16.25
9 months	16	0.7–8.1	2.36	0.76– 7.31
1 year	12	1.1–10.2	3.49	0.80– 15.22
2 years	18	1.1–49.0	3.03	0.31– 29.48
3 years	6	0.5–7.7	1.80	0.19– 16.86
4 years	7	2.4–34.8	8.58	1.07– 68.86
7 years	18	1.6–60.0	12.89	1.03–161.32
10 years	17	0.3–215	23.66	0.98–570.61
14 years	19	1.9–159	20.07	2.06–195.18

*From Park, B. H., and Ellis, E. F.: *Children Are Different: Developmental Physiology*, 2nd ed. Johnson, T. R., and Moore, W. M. (eds.), Columbus, Ohio, Ross Laboratories, 1978, p. 188.

SERUM IgD CONCENTRATIONS IN INFANTS, CHILDREN, AND ADULTS*

Group	Number	Ages	Range	Geom. Mean	P Value (t Test)	Median	P Value (Mann-Whitney)
Normal infants	23	(6 weeks–19 months)	(<1–1.6)	0.1 (0–0.6)*	—	0.1	—
Normal children	105	(3–14 years)	(<1–36)	1.6 (0–70)*	—	3.0	—
Normal adults	57	(21–55 years)	(<1–11.2)	2.4 (0–61)*	—	4.6	—

*95 per cent confidence interval.
(From Buckley, R. H., and Fiscus, S. A.: J. Clin. Invest. 55:157, 1975.)

RELATION OF IMMUNOGLOBULIN AND ISOHEMAGGLUTININ (IHA) LEVELS TO AGE

	IgG* (mg/dl) Mean ± 1 SD and Range	IgA* (mg/dl) Mean ± 1 SD and Range	IgM* (mg/dl) Mean ± 1 SD and Range	IHA Titer Mean and Range
Cord blood	1086 ± 290 (740–1374)	2 ± 2 (0–15)	14 ± 6 (0–22)	0[a]
1–3 months	512 ± 152 (280–950)	16 ± 10 (4–36)	28 ± 14 (15–86)	1:5[b] 0–1:10
4–6 months	520 ± 180 (240–884)	22 ± 14 (11–52)	26 ± 18 (21–74)	1:10[b] 0–1:160
7–12 months	742 ± 226 (281–1280)	54 ± 17 (22–112)	76 ± 27 (36–150)	1:80[c] 0–1:640
13–24 months	945 ± 270 (290–1300)	67 ± 19 (9–143)	88 ± 36 (18–210)	1:80[c] 0–1:640
25–36 months	1030 ± 152 (546–1562)	89 ± 34 (21–196)	94 ± 23 (43–115)	1:160[d] 1:10–1:640
3–5 years	1150 ± 244 (546–1760)	126 ± 31 (56–284)	87 ± 24 (26–121)	1:80 1:5–1:640
6–8 years	1187 ± 289 (596–1744)	147 ± 35 (56–330)	108 ± 37 (54–260)	1:80 1:5–1:640
9–11 years	1217 ± 261 (744–1719)	146 ± 38 (44–208)	104 ± 46 (27–215)	1:160 1:20–1:640
12–16 years	1248 ± 221 (796–1647)	168 ± 54 (64–290)	96 ± 31 (60–140)	1:160 1:10–1:320
Adult	1274 ± 280 (664–1825)	227 ± 53 (59–311)	127 ± 46 (45–205)	1:160 1:10–1:640

*Immunochemical.
[a]Isohemagglutinin activity is rarely detectable in cord blood.
[b]50 per cent of normal infants will not have isohemagglutinins at this age.
[c]10 per cent of normal infants will not have isohemagglutinins at this age.
[d]Beyond this age all normal individuals (except blood type AB) have isohemagglutinins.
(From Ellis, E. F., and Robbins, J. B.: In *Children Are Different: Developmental Physiology*, 2nd ed. Johnson, T. R., and Moore, W. M. (eds.), Columbus, Ohio, 1978, p. 189.)

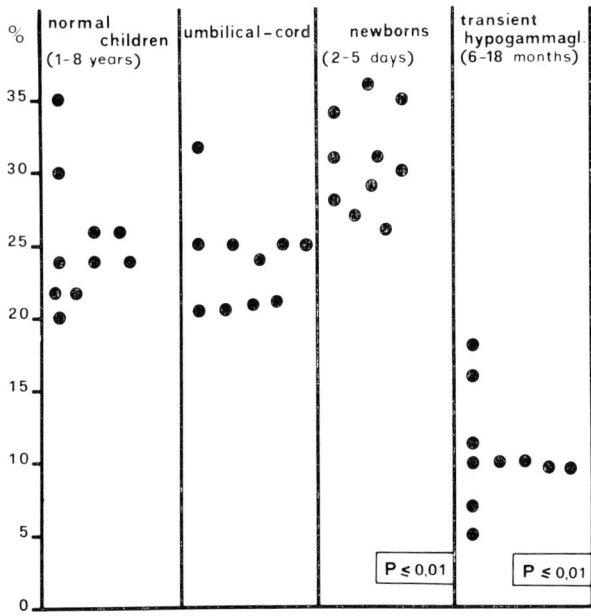

Percentage of B lymphocytes in normal children. (From Moscatelli, P., et al.: Helv. Paediatr. Acta *28*:553, 1973, with permission of S. Karger AG, Basel.)

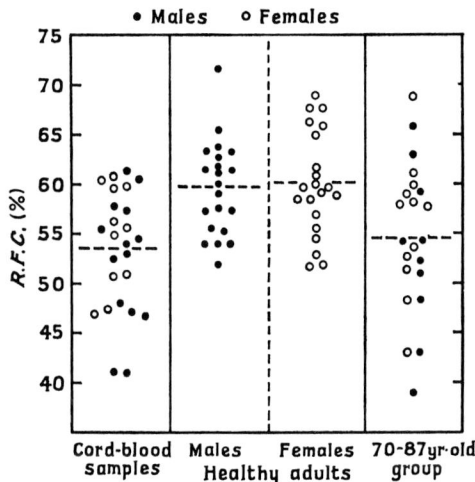

Age-related variation in the proportion of circulating T cells. The percentage of rosette-forming cells (R.F.C.) among circulating mononuclear cells is shown for each of the three groups. The mean for each group is also shown. (From Smith, M. D., Evans, J., et al.: Lancet 2:923, 1974.)

Sedimentation rate in the newborn period. The erythrocyte sedimentation rate was measured in capillary blood in healthy full-term and low-birth-weight newborn infants. Normal values ranged from 1 mm/1 hr at 12 hours of age to 17 mm/1 hr at 14 days of age. All values of neonates with hematocrit values less than 40 per cent were corrected to 40 per cent. (From Adler, S. M., and Denton, R. L.: J. Pediatr. 86:942, 1975.)

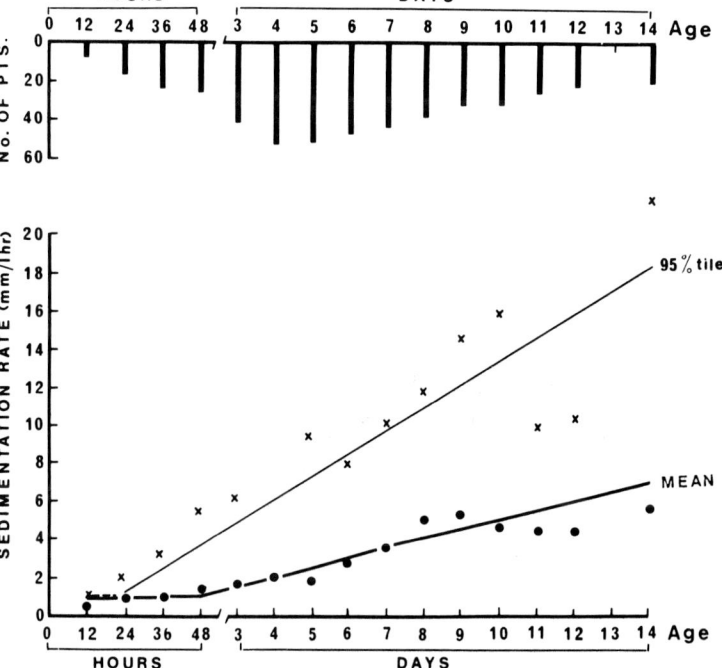

References

1. Galen, R. S., and Gambino, S. R.: *Beyond Normality: The Predictive Value of Efficiency of Medical Diagnoses.* New York, John Wiley & Sons, 1975.
2. Dallman, P. R., Barr, G. D., et al.: Hemoglobin concentration in white, black and Oriental children: is there a need for separate criteria in screening for anemia? Am. J. Clin. Nutr. *31*:379, 1978.
3. Shaper, A. G., and Lewis, P.: Genetic neutropenia in people of African origin. Lancet *2*:1021, 1971.
4. Oski, F. A., and Naiman, J. L.: *Hematologic Problems in the Newborn,* 2nd ed. Philadelphia, W. B. Saunders Co., 1972, p. 11.
5. Saarien, U. M., and Siimes, M. A.: Developmental changes in red blood cell counts and indices of infants after exclusion or iron deficiency by laboratory criteria and continuous iron supplementation. J. Pediatr. *92*:414, 1978.
6. Lundstrom, U., Siimes, M. A., et al.: At what age does iron supplementation become necessary in low birth weight infants? J. Pediatr. *91*:882, 1977.
7. Dallman, P. R.: Blood and blood forming tissues. In *Pediatrics,* 16th ed. Rudolph, A. (ed.), New York, Appleton-Century-Crofts, 1977, pp. 1111, 1178.
8. Dallman, P. R., and Siimes, M. A.: Percentile curves for hemoglobin and red cell volume in infancy and childhood. J. Pediatr. *94*:28, 1979.
9. Beutler, E., and Blume, K. G.: In *Human Health and Disease,* II. Altman, P. L., and Dittmer, D. S. (eds.), Bethesda, Md., Federation of American Societies for Experimental Biology, 1977, pp. 154–156.
10. Oski, F. A.: Red cell metabolism in the newborn infant. V. Glycolytic intermediates and glycolytic enzymes. Pediatrics *44*:87, 1969.
11. Garby, L., and Sjolin, S.: Development of erythropoiesis. Acta Paediatr. *51*:245, 1962.
12. Charache, S.: In *Human Health and Disease,* II. Altman, P. L., and Dittmer, D. S. (eds.), Bethesda, Md., Federation of American Societies for Experimental Biology, 1977, p. 159.
13. Schroeder, W. A., et al.: Postnatal changes in the chemical heterogeneity of human fetal hemoglobin. Pediatr. Res. *5*:493, 1971.
14. Kravitz, H., Elegant, L. D., et al.: Methemoglobin values in premature and mature infants and children. J. Dis. Child. *91*:2, 1956.
15. Saarien, U. M., and Siimes, M. A.: Serum iron and transferrin in iron deficiency. J. Pediatr. *91*:876, 1977.
16. Koerper, M. A., and Dallman, P.: Serum iron concentration and transferrin saturation in the diagnosis of iron deficiency in children: normal developmental changes. J. Pediatr. *91*:871, 1977.
17. Willoughby, M. L. N.: *Pediatric Haematology.* New York, Churchill Livingstone, 1977, p. 17.
18. Shojania, A., and Gross, S.: Folic acid deficiency and prematurity. J. Pediatr. *64*:323, 1964.
19. Klaus, M., and Farnaroff, A.: *Care of the High Risk Neonate.* Philadelphia, W. B. Saunders Co., 1973, p. 343.
20. Lundh, B., Oski, F. A., et al.: Plasma hemopexin and haptoglobin in hemolytic diseases of the newborn. Acta Paediatr. Scand. *59*:121, 1970.
21. Price, D. C., and Ries, C.: In *Nuclear Medicine in Clinical Pediatrics.* Handmaker, H., and Lowenstein, J. M. (eds.), New York, Society of Nuclear Medicine, 1975, p. 279.
22. Manroe, B. L., Browne, R., et al.: Normal leukocyte (WBC) values in neonates. Pediatr. Res. *10*:428, 1976.
23. Baehner, R. L.: In *Human Health and Disease,* II. Altman, P. L., and Dittmer, D. A. (eds.), Bethesda, Md., Federation of American Societies for Experimental Biology, 1977, pp. 63, 64.
24. Rosse, C., Kraemer, M. J., et al.: Bone marrow cell populations of normal infants: the predominance of lymphocytes. J. Lab. Clin. Med. *89*:1228, 1977.
25. Hathaway, W. E.: The bleeding newborn. Semin. Hematol. *12*:175, 1975.
26. Gross, S. J., and Stuart, M. J.: Hemostasis in the premature infant. Clin. Perinatol. *4*:260, 1977.
27. Park, B. H., and Ellis, E. F.: In *Children Are Different: Developmental Physiology,* 2nd ed. Johnson, T. R., and Moore, W. M. (eds.), Columbus, Ohio, Ross Laboratories, 1978, p. 188.
28. Buckley, R. H., Dees, S. C., et al.: Serum immunoglobulins: I. Levels in normal children and in uncomplicated childhood allergy. Pediatrics, *41*:600, 1968.
29. Blankenship, W., Cassady, G., et al.: Serum gamma-M globulin responses in acute neonatal infections and their diagnostic significance. J. Pediatr. *75*:1271, 1969.
30. Buckley, R. H., and Fiscus, S. A.: Serum IgD and IgE concentrations in immunodeficiency diseases. J. Clin. Invest. *55*:157, 1975.
31. Ellis, E. F., and Robbins, J. B.: In *Children Are Different: Developmental Physiology,* 2nd ed. Johnson, T. R., and Moore, W. M. (eds.), Columbus, Ohio, Ross Laboratories, 1978, p. 189.
32. Moscatelli, P., Dagna Bricarelli, F., et al.: Immunoglobulins on the surface of lymphocytes, their distribution in cord blood, newborns and infants affected by transient hypogammaglobulinaemia. Helv. Paediatr. Acta *28*:553, 1973.
33. Smith, M. D., Evans, J., et al.: Age-related variation in proportion of circulating T-cells. Lancet *2*:923, 1974.
34. Adler, S. M., and Denton, R. L.: The erythrocyte sedimentation rate in the newborn period. J. Pediatr. *86*:942, 1975.

GLOSSARY OF ABBREVIATIONS AND SYMBOLS

A (1) blood group A; (2) adenine; (3) actinomycin-D (dactinomycin); (4) factor in the alternate pathway of activation of complement (properdin factor); (5) antibody
a activated (factor)
α alpha heavy chain
Å angstrom
AA arachidonic acid
AAA adenosine-adenosine-adenosine
Ab-MLV a replication defective virus
ABVD chemotherapy regimen: Adriamycin/bleomycin/vinblastine/dacarbazine
ACD acid citrate dextrose
ACEH acid cholesteryl ester hydrolase
ACOP+ chemotherapy regimen: Adriamycin/cyclophosphamide/vincristine/methotrexate/prednisone
ACT activated clotting time
ACTH adrenocorticotropic hormone
ADA adenosine deaminase activity
ADCC antibody-dependent cell-mediated cytolysis
ADH antidiuretic hormone
ADK adenylate kinase
ADM Adriamycin
AdoCbl 5′-adenosylcobalamin
ADP adenosine diphosphate
AEV avian erythroblastosis virus
AFP alpha-fetoprotein
$α_H$ heavy chain of IgA molecule
AHA autoimmune hemolytic anemia
AHF antihemophilic factor (Factor VIII)
AIDS acquired immune deficiency syndrome
AIP acute intermittent porphyria
AK adenylate kinase
AKR lymphoma AKR strain of murine lymphoma
ALA aminolevulinic acid
ALAD aminolevulinic acid dehydratase
ALG antilymphocyte globulin
ALS antilymphocyte serum
ALT alanine aminotransferase
ALV avian leukosis virus
AMA acute myelogenous anemia
AML acute myelogenous leukemia
AMM agnogenic myeloid metaplasia
AMML acute myelomonocytic leukemia
AMP adenosine monophosphate
AMV avian myeloblastosis virus
Ank ankyrin
ANLL acute nonlymphocytic leukemia
APCC activated prothrombin complex concentrates
APO (1) apolipoprotein; (2) chemotherapy regimen: Adriamycin/prednisone/vincristine
APRT adenosinephosphoribosyl transferase
APTT activated partial thromboplastin time
AR ascorbate reductase
ara-C cytosine arabinoside (cytarabine)
ARDS adult respiratory distress syndrome
AS adult and sickle hemoglobin; sickle cell trait
ASA acetylsalicylic acid
AST aspartate aminotransferase
AT antithrombin
ATG antithymocyte globulin
ATL (1) adult T cell leukemia; (2) adult T cell lymphoma
ATP adenosine triphosphate
ATPase adenosine triphosphatase
ATS antithymocyte serum
AUL acute undifferentiated leukemia
B (1) blood group B; (2) factor in the alternate pathway of activation of complement (properdin factor); (3) derived from the bursa of Fabricus in avian species
β beta heavy chain
BaEV baboon endogenous virus
BAL British anti-lewisite (2,3-dimercaptopropanol)
BAT brain adjacent tumor
BCD chemotherapy regimen: bleomycin/Cytoxan/actinomycin
BCDF B cell differentiation factor
B cell bursal-derived cell
BCG *bacillus Calmette-Guérin*
BCGF B cell growth factors
BCNU 1,3-*Bis*(2-chloroethyl)-1-nitrosourea
B lymphocyte bursal-derived lymphocyte
BFU-E erythroid burst forming unit
BPA burst promoting activity
C (1) centigrade; (2) complement; (3) cytosine; (4) constant region
Ca calcium
$C_α$ constant region of alpha heavy chain sequence

CAA constitutional aplastic anemia
CALLA common acute lymphocytic leukemic antigen
cAMP cyclic adenosine monophosphate
CaNaEDTA calcium-disodium ethylenediaminetetraacetic acid
CB Coomassie blue
Cbl cobalamin (vitamin B_{12})
CCNU nitrosourea
CCSG Children's Cancer Study Group
C_δ constant region of delta heavy chain sequence
CDA congenital dyserythropoietic anemia
CDC Centers for Disease Control
cDNA complementary deoxyribonucleic acid
C_ϵ constant region of epsilon heavy chain sequence
CFU-C colony-forming unit in culture
CFU-E erythroid colony-forming unit
CFU-Eos eosinophil colony-forming unit
CFU-G granulocyte colony-forming unit
CFU-GEMM granulocyte-macrophage, erythroid, megakaryocyte (multipotential) colony-forming unit
CFU-GM granulocyte-macrophage colony-forming unit
CFU-L lymphoid colony-forming unit
CFU-M megakaryocyte colony-forming unit
CFU-Meg megakaryocyte colony-forming unit
CFU-S colony-forming unit in spleen
C_γ constant region of gamma heavy chain sequence
CGD chronic granulomatous disease
CGP circulatory gene pool
cGy centi-Gray/absorbed radiation measurement
CHBA congenital Heinz body hemolytic anemia
CHD congenital heart disease
CHE pseudocholinesterase
CH$_3$H$_4$PteGlu methyltetrahydrofolic acid
CH$_4$ methane
ChlVPP chemotherapy regimen: chlorambucil/vinblastine/procarbazine/prednisone
cis (Latin): on the same side
CISCA$_{II}$/VB$_{IV}$ chemotherapy regimen: Cytoxan/Adriamycin/*cis*-platinum/vinblastine/bleomycin
C_κ constant region of kappa light chain sequence
Cl chlorine
C_λ constant region of lambda light chain sequence
CLL chronic lymphocytic leukemia
C_μ constant region of mu heavy chain sequence
CML (1) cell-mediated lysis; (2) chronic myelogenous leukemia
CMML chronic myelomonocytic leukemia
CMV cytomegalovirus
Cn-Cbl cyanocobalamin
CNS central nervous system
CNSHA congenital nonspherocytic hemolytic anemia
CO cobalt
CO (1) carbon monoxide; (2) chemotherapy regimen: cyclophosphamide/vincristine
CO$_2$ carbon dioxide
^{14}CO$_2$ carbon-14 labeled carbon dioxide
^{57}2CO Co^{57}-labeled cyanocobalamin
CoA coenzyme A
COAP chemotherapy regimen: cyclophosphamide/cytosine arabinoside/vincristine/prednisone
c-*onc* cellular oncogene
COMP chemotherapy regimen: cyclophosphamide/vincristine/methotrexate/prednisone
COP chemotherapy regimen: cyclophosphamide/Oncovin/procarbazine
COPAD chemotherapy regimen: cyclophosphamide/vincristine/Adriamycin/prednosine/cytarabine/asparaginase/intrathecal methotrexate
COPP chemotherapy regimen: COP + prednisone
COPRO coproporphyrin
CPD citrate phosphate dextrose
CPDA-1 citrate phosphate dextrose adenine
CR complete response
^{51}Cr chromium-51
CrRT cranial radiotherapy
CS clinical state
CSA colony-stimulating activity
CSF (1) colony-stimulating factor; (2) cerebrospinal fluid
CT computed tomography
CTX; CTY cyclophosphamide (Cytoxan)
CUG cytidine-uridine-guanidine
CVA common variable agammaglobulinemia
CVP (1) central venous pressure; (2) chemotherapy regimen: cyclophosphamide/vinblastine/prednisone
CyA cyclosporin A
D (1) diaphorase; (2) diversity region
δ delta heavy chain
DAF decay accelerating factor
DAG diacylglycerol
DCIP dichlorophenolindophenol
DCT direct Coombs' test
DDAVP 1-deamino-8-D-arginine vasopressin
DES diethylstilbestrol
DFP^{32} diisofluorophosphate
DFS disease-free survival
D_H diversity region of heavy chain
$δ_H$ heavy chain of IgD molecule
DHA dihydroxyacetone
DHAP dihydroxyacetone phosphate
DIC disseminated intravascular coagulation
DIDS 4,4′-diisothiocyanostilbene-2,2-disulfonate
dl (1) deciliter; (2) equimolecular mixture of the dextrorotatory/levorotatory enantiomorphs: the sign ± is currently used
DMSO dimethylsulfoxide
DNA deoxyribonucleic acid
2,3 DPG 2,3-diphosphoglycerate
2,3 DPGM 2,3-diphosphoglycerate mutase

GLOSSARY OF ABBREVIATIONS AND SYMBOLS

DTIC chemotherapy regimen: diethyl-triazeno-imidazole-carboxamide
dTMP deoxythyminide monophosphate
dU deoxyuridine
dUMP deoxyuridine monophosphate
DWM pokeweed mitogen
E (1) extralymphatic involvement in Hodgkin's disease; (2) pseudocholinesterase; (3) sheep erythrocytes
ϵ epislon heavy chain
EA early antigen
EACA epsilon aminocaproic acid
EBNC Epstein-Barr nasopharyngeal carcinoma
EBV Epstein-Barr virus
ECF-A eosinophil chemotactic factor of anaphylaxis
E. coli Escherichia coli
EDTA ethylenediaminetetraacetic acid
EEG electroencephalogram
EF extended field
EGF epidermal growth factor
ϵ_H heavy chain of IgE molecule
E rosette receptor ethyl hepatobiliary iminodiacetic acid
eIf$_2$ erythrocyte initiation factor
EP erythrocyte protoporphyrin
EPA erythroid potentiating activity
ESR electron spin resonance
ET essential thrombocythemia
F fast (electrophoretically fast variant of C3)
FAB French-American-British cooperative group
FABP fatty acid–binding protein
Factor I fibrinogen
Factor II prothrombin
Factor III thromboplastin
Factor IV calcium
Factor V proaccelerin
Factor VI not currently assigned a name or function
Factor VII proSPCA (pro–serum prothrombin converting activity)
Factor VIII antihemophilic factor
Factor IX Christmas factor, plasma thromboplastin component
Factor X Stuart factor
Factor XI plasma thromboplastin antecedent
Factor XII Hageman factor
Factor XIII fibrin-stabilizing factor
Factor B a complement component C3 proactivator
Factor D an acting serine esterase that splits Factor B from C3B
Factor H biotin
Factor I pyridoxine
FAD flavin adenine dinucleotide
F( ):C Factor ( ) coagulant activity
F cells fetal hemoglobin-containing erythrocyte
Fc component fragment, crystallizable, of IgG molecule
FDP (1) fibrin degradation products; (2) fructose diphosphate
Fe iron
Fe^{+2} ferrous iron
Fe^{+3} ferri(met)-iron
^{59}Fe iron-59
FeCl$_3$ ferric chloride
FECU Factor VIII correctional unit
Fe^{+2}Hgb ferrohemoglobin
Fe^{+3}Hgb ferri(met)-hemoglobin
FEL familial erythrophagocytic lymphohistiocytosis
FeLV feline leukemia virus
FEP free erythrocyte protoporphyrin
FFA free fatty acid
FFP fresh frozen plasma
FIGLU formiminoglutamic acid
F( )R:Ag Factor ( ) related antigen
F( )R:C Factor ( ) related cofactor activity
FSBA fluorosulfonylbenzoyladenosine
FSH follicle-stimulating hormone
G (1) globular; (2) glycogen; (3) guanidine
γ gamma heavy chain
GABA gamma-amino butyric acid
Gal galactose
Gal-1-P galactose-1-phosphate
GBG glycine-rich beta-glycoprotein
Gd gadolinium
Ge$^-$ Gerbich negative
GL glycolipid
GL-4 glycosphingolipid
GLO glyoxalase I
G/M granulocyte/macrophage
GM-CSA granulocyte-macrophage colony-stimulating activity
GM-CSF granulocyte-macrophage colony-stimulating factor
GMP guanosine monophosphate
GP glycophorin
Gp glycoprotein
GPA glycophorin A
GPA$_2$ dimer of glycophorin A
GPB glycophorin B
GPB$_2$ dimer of glycophorin B
GPA-GPB heterodimer of GPA
GPC glycophorin C (glycoconnectin)
G6P glucose-6-phosphate
G6PD glucose-6-phosphate dehydrogenase
G3PD glyceraldehyde-3-phosphate-dehydrogenase
GPI glucose phosphate isomerase
GR glutathione reductase
GSH L-α-glutamyl-L-cysteinyl-glycine (glutathione, reduced)
GSH-Px glutathione peroxidase
GSR generalized Shwartzman reaction
GSSG glutathione, oxidized
GSSG-R glutathione reductase
GTP guanosine triphosphate
GVH graft-versus-host

GVHD   graft-versus-host disease
Ha-MSV   Harvey murine sarcoma virus
HAT   hypoxanthine-aminopterin-thymidine
Hb   hemoglobin (also: Hg, Hbg)
HBABA   hydroxybenzeneazobenzoic acid
Hb F   fetal hemoglobin
HB$_s$AG   hepatitis B surface antigen
HCG   human chorionic gonadotropin
HCT   hemocrit
H   heavy chain
HCO$_3$ the bicarbonate radical
HD   Hodgkin's disease
^{3}H-DFP   tritiated diisopropyl-flourophosphorate
HDL   high density lipoprotein
HDMTX   high-dose methotrexate
HE   hereditary elliptocytosis
HE$_s$ stomocytic hereditary elliptocytosis
HE$_c$ common hereditary elliptocytosis
HEMPAS   hereditary erythroblastic multinuclearity with a positive acidified serum test
HETE   12-L-hydroxy-eicosatetraenoic acid (12-OH fatty acid)
Hg   (1) mercury; (2) hemoglobin
Hgb   hemoglobin
HGPRT   hypoxanthine guanine phosphoriboxyl transferase
HHT   12-L-hydroxy-heptadecatrienoic acid
HIDA   iminodiacetic acid, oxidized
H. influenza   *Haemophilus influenza*
HIV   human immunodeficiency virus
HJ   Howell-Jolly
HK   hexokinase
HLA   (1) human leukocyte antigen; 82) histocompatibility antigen
HLF   heat-labile factor
HLV   hamster leukosis virus
HMW   high molecular weight
HMWK   high-molecular-weight kininogen
H$_2$O$_2$ hydrogen peroxide
HOS   human osteogenic sarcoma
Hp   haptoglobin
H$_4$PteGlu   tetrahydrofolic acid
HPETE   12-hydroperoxy-eicosatetraenoic acid
HPFH   hereditary persistence of fetal hemoglobin
HPLC   high performance liquid chromatography
HPP   hereditary pyropoikilocytosis
HPRT   hypoxanthine phosphoribosyl transferase
HS   hereditary spherocytosis
HSR   homogeneously staining region
HSV   herpes simplex virus
^{3}HT   tritiated thymidine
HTC   homozygous typing cells
HTLV   human T cell lymphotropic virus
HUS   hemolytic-uremic syndrome
HVA   homovanillic acid
ICH   intracranial hemorrhage
ICT   indirect Coombs' test
IDP   idiopathic pulmonary hemosiderosis
IESS   Intergroup Ewing's Sarcoma Study
IF   (1) interferon; (2) involved field; (3) intrinsic factor
IFRT   involved field radiotherapy
Ig   immunoglobulin
IGA   infantile genetic agranulocytosis
IL   interleukin
ILS   increase in life span
IMP   intramembranous particles
^{111}InCl   indium-111 chloride
IOV   inside-out vesicles
IP$_3$ inositol triphosphate
IPH   idiopathic pulmonary hemosiderosis
IRS   Intergroup Rhabdomyosarcoma Study
ISC   irreversibly sickled cell
ISG   immune serum globulin
ITMTX   intrathecal methotrexate
ITP   (1) immune thrombocytopenia; (2) idiopathic thrombocytopenic purpura
IU   immunizing unit
IVIC syndrome   Instituto Venezolano de Investigaciones Cienticicas syndrome
IV   intravenous
IVP   intravenous pyelogram
IVS   intervening sequence
J   joining region
JCML   juvenile chronic myelogenous leukemia
JDM   juvenile diabetes mellitus
J$_H$ joining region of heavy chain
J$_\kappa$ joining region of kappa light chain sequence
J$_\lambda$ joining region of lambda light chain sequence
JRA   juvenile rheumatoid arthritis
K   potassium
κ   kappa light chain
kD   kilodaltons
kg   kilogram
Km   Michaelis constant: substrate concentration of half maximal velocity of reaction
K-MSV   Kirsten murine sarcoma virus
L   leader sequence
λ   lambda light chain
LAK   lymphokine-activated killer
LAP   leukocyte alkaline phosphate activity
L-ASP   L-asparaginase
L. casei   *Lactobacillus casei*
LCAT   lecithin: cholesterol acyltransferase
$^{L-14}$C-histidine   carbon-14 labeled histidine
LDH   lactate dehydrogenase
LDL   low density lipoprotein
LH   luteinizing hormone
LHRF   luteinizing hormone releasing factor
LLV   lymphoid leukosis virus
LMB   leukomethylene blue, reduced
LORF   long open reading frame
LPC   lysophosphatidylcholine
LPE   lysophosphatidylethanolamine
LP-X   abnormal low density lipoprotein
LSA$_2$L$_2$ chemotherapy regimen: cyclophosphamide/vincristine/methotrexate/daunomycin/prednisone/cytarabine/thioguanine/asparaginase/carmustine/hydroxyurea with IT MTX

LTR (1) location *trans*activating region; (2) long terminal repeat sequences
LW a blood group antigen
Lyso-PC lysophosphatidyl phosphatidylcholine
M (1) methyl; (2) mitochondria; (3) mitosis; (4) molar
μ (1) micron; (2) mu heavy chain
MAC-1 stumptail monkey virus
MB methylene blue, oxidized
MBS myeloblastic syndrome
MCH mean corpuscular hemoglobin
M-CSF macrophage colony-stimulating factor
MCT oil medium chain triglyceride oil
MeCbl methylcobalamin
Meg-CSA megakaryocyte colony-stimulating activity
methyl-CCNU a nitrosourea
5,10-methylene-THF 5,10 methylene tetrahydrofolic acid
Mg magnesium
μg (1) microgram; (2) immunoglobulin chain
MGC minimum gelling concentration
MGP marginating granulocyte pool
MH malignant histiocytosis
μ$_H$ heavy chain of IgM molecule
MHC major histocompatibility complex
MHPG 3-methoxy-4-hydroxyphenylethylene glycol
MHR (1) major histocompatibility region; (2) methemoglobin reductase
MIF migration inhibition factor
MLC mixed lymphocyte culture
MLR mixed lymphocyte culture reaction
μM millimole
mm millimeter
MMTV mouse mammary tumor virus
ml milliliter
μl microliter
MLC mixed lymphocyte culture
MM mediastinal mass
μM micromole
Mn manganese
MNNG *N*-methyl-*N*′-nitro-*N*-nitrosoguanidine
Mo-MLV Moloney murine leukemia virus
MOPP chemotherapy regimen: nitrogen mustard/vincristine/procarbazine/prednisone
6-MP 6-mercaptopurine
MPGM monophosphoglycerate mutase
MPMV Mason-Pfizer monkey virus
MPO myeloperoxide deficiency
mRNA messenger ribonucleic acid
MS multiple sclerosis
MSH melanocyte-stimulating hormone
MSV murine sarcoma virus
MTT methyl tetrazolium
MTV mammary tumor virus
MTX methotrexate (formerly amethopterin)
Multi-CSF multi–colony-stimulating factor
M.W. molecular weight
N a blood group antigen
n Hill constant: an index of heme-heme interaction
Na sodium
(Na$^+$ + K$^+$)ATPase sodium and potassium activated ouabain inhibitable adenosine triphosphatase
NaCl sodium chloride
NAD nicotinamide adenine dinucleotide
NADH nicotinamide-adenine dinucleotide, reduced
NADP$^+$ nicotinamide-adenine dinucleotide phosphates, oxidized
NADPH nicotinamide-adenine dinucleotide phosphate, reduced
NANB non-A, non-B
NBT nitroblue tetrazolium
NCI National Cancer Institute
N-DSK N-terminal disulfide knot
ng nanograms
NH$_3$ ammonia
NH$_4$ ammonium
NHANES National Health and Nutrition Survey
NHL non-Hodgkin's lymphoma
NIH National Institutes of Health
NK cells natural killer cells
nm nanometer
N^5-methyl-H$_4$PteGlu N^5-methyltetrahydrofolic acid
NMR nuclear magnetic resonance
NP nucleoside phosphorylase
NPD Niemann-Pick disease
NR no response
NSE neuron-specific enolase
NWTS National Wilms' Tumor Study
O (1) oxygen; (2) blood group O
O$_2$ diatomic form of oxygen
OAF osteoclast-activating factor
OAG oleylacylglycerol
OF osmotic fragility
OH-Cbl hydroxycobalamin
OPPA chemotherapy regimen: vincristine/procarbazine/prednisone/Adriamycin
OR orosomucoid (α$_1$-acid glycoprotein)
p short arm of chromosome
P (1) propionic; (2) a red cell antigen
P$_{50}$ partial pressure of oxygen at 50% saturation
^{32}P radioactive phosphorus
PA (1) phosphatidic acid; (2) pernicious anemia
PAGE polyacrylamide gel electrophoresis
PAIgG platelet-associated immunoglobulin G
PALA *N*-(phosphonacetyl)-L-aspartate
PAS (1) periodic acid–Schiff; (2) para-aminosalicylic acid
Pb lead
PBG prophobilinogen
PC phosphatidylcholine
PCC prothrombin complex concentrate
PCMB parachloromercuribenzoate
pCO$_2$ partial pressure of carbon dioxide
PCT porphyria cutanea tarda

PCV packed cell volume
PDGF platelet-derived growth factor
PDW platelet distribution width
PE phosphatidylethanolamine
PEP phosphoenolpyruvate
PEP C peptidose C
P. falciparum *Plasmodium falciparum*
PFK phosphofructokinase
PG prostaglandin
PGA pteroylmonoglutamic acid
6PGAD 6-phosphogluconic acid dehydrogenase
PGB prophobilinogen
PGF prostaglandin factor
PGI prostacyclin
PGI$_2$ vascular prostaglandin (prostacyclin)
PGK phosphoglycerate kinase
PGM phosphoglucomutase
Ph^1 Philadelphia chromosome
pH hydrogen ion concentration
PHA phytohemagglutinin
PI phosphatidylinositol
Pi protease inhibitor
P$_i$ inorganic phosphate
PIP$_2$ phosphoinositol-4,5-biphosphate
PI-P phosphatidylinositol-4-phosphate
PIPIDA *p*-isopropylacetanilido HIDA
PI-PP phosphatidylinositol-4,5-biphosphate
PK pyruvate kinase
Pl^{A1} platelet antigen A1
PLM per cent labeled mitoses
PLT primed lymphocyte testing
PMN polymorphonuclear
P-5'-N pyrimidine-5'-nucleotidase
PNET primitive neuroectodermal tumor
PNH paroxysmal nocturnal hemoglobinuria
***p*-NO$_2$** *p*-nitrosochloramphenicol
pO$_2$ partial pressure of oxygen
PPP pluripotent progenitor
PPT activated partial thromboplastin time
PR partial response
PRCA pure red cell aplasia, acquired
PROTO protoporphyrin
PRPP phosphoribosyl pyrophosphate
PS (1) pathologic state; (2) phosphatidyl serine
PSP phenolsulfonphthalein
PT prothrombin time
PTC plasma thromboplastin component (Factor IX/Christmas factor)
PteGlu pteroylglutamic acid
PTH parathyroid hormone
PTT partial thromboplastin time
PV polycythemia vera
PVeBy chemotherapy regimen: *cis*-platinum/vincristine/bleomycin/VP-16
PVP polyvinylpyrrolidone
q long arm of chromosome
RA refractory anemia
rad radiation absorbed unit
RAEB refractory anemia with excess blasts

RAEBIT refractory anemia with excess blasts in transformation
RARS refractory anemia with ringed sideroblasts
RAV Rous-associated virus
Rb rubidium
RBC red blood cell
RCV red cell volume
RD114 feline endogenous virus
RDW red cell distribution width
RE retriculoendothelial
RER rough endoplasmic reticulum
RES reticuloendothelial system
RFLP restriction endonuclease fragment length polymorphism
Rh (1) symbol for Rhesus factor; (2) chemical symbol for rhodium
RNA ribonucleic acid
R5P ribose-5-phosphate
RPI reticulocyte production index
RPK ribosephosphate kinase
RR relative response
RR factor relative risk factor
RSC reversible sickled cell
RSV Rous sarcoma virus
RT radiotherapy
S (1) slow (electrophoretically slow variant of C3); (2) sulfate; (3) DNA synthesis; (4) sickle; (5) spectrin (also: Sp)
S% transferrin saturation
SBA soybean agglutinin
SCC small cell lung cancer
SCE sister chromatid exchange
SCID severe combined immunodeficiency
SD (1) standard deviation; (2) serum-defined antigen; (3) spectrin dimers (also: Sp-D)
sDNA synthetic deoxyribonucleic acid
SDS sodium dodecyl sulfate
SDS-PAGE sodium dodecyl sulfate-polyacrylamide gel electrophoresis
SEER Surveillance, Epidemiology, and End Results Program of the National Cancer Institute
SFC soluble fibrin-fibrinogen complexes
SGF sarcoma growth factor
SGOT serum glutamic-oxaloacetic transaminase
SGPT serum glutamic-pyruvate transaminase
SHMC sinus histiocytosis with massive lymphadenopathy
SI serum iron
SIOP International Society of Pediatric Oncology
Sl/Sl$_d$ Steel mouse
SLE systemic lupus erythematosus
SM sphingomyelin
SNagg's agglutinins for gamma globulin found in normal serum
SO spectrin oligomers (also: Sp-O)
^{35}SO$_4$ sulphate labeled with sulfur-35
Sp spectrin (also: S)
SP spectrin alpha chain

S phase DNA synthetic phase of cell cycle
SRS simple repeat sequence
SS homozygous sickle cell anemia
ST spectrin tetramers (also: Sp-T)
SV40 simian virus 40
T (1) thymidine; (2) thymus-derived
T$_3$ triiodothyronine
T$_4$ thyroxine
t translocation
T-2 chemotherapy regimen: vicristine/Adriamycin/actinomycin
T activation T cell activation
TAGVHD transfusion-associated graft-versus-host disease
T-ALL T cell acute lymphoblastic anemia
T antigen tumor-associated antigen
TAR (1) thrombocytopenia with absent radii; (2) *trans*acting factor responsive sequence
TBI total body irradiation
TC transcobalamin
TC I transcobalamin I (an alpha globulin/glycoprotein)
TC II transcobalamin II (a beta globulin)
TC III transcobalamin III (an alpha globulin/glycoprotein—leukocyte derived)
TCD T cell depletion
T cell thymus-derived cell
Td-CIA T cell–derived colony-inhibiting activity
TEC transient erythroblastopenia of childhood
TEM intra-arterial triethylenemalamine
TF transferrin
Tf C transferrin, common form
T-helper cell thymus-derived helper cell
THF tetrahydrofolic acid
THI transient hypogammaglobulinemia of infancy
TIBC total iron-binding capacity
T-lymphocytes thymus-derived lymphocytes
TNI total nodal irradiation
T-NHL T cell–derived non-Hodgkin's leukemia
TPN total parenteral nutrition
TPO triose phosphate isomerase
TRF thyroid-releasing factor
tRNA transfer ribonucleic acid
TSH thyroid-stimulating hormone
TTP thrombotic thrombocytopenia purpura
UDP uridine diphosphate
UDPGA uridine diphosphoglucuronic acid
UF unknown factor
V (1) vinyl; (2) variable region
VA chemotherapy regimen: vincristin/adriamycin
VAB-6 chemotherapy regimen: vincristine/actinomycin/bleomycin/*cis*-platinum/Cytoxan
VAC chemotherapy regimen: vincristine/Adriamycin D/cyclophosphamide
VAHS virus-associated hemophagocytic syndrome
VAMP chemotherapy regimen: vincristine/methotrexate/6-mercaptopurine/prednisone
Vbl vinblastine
VCR vincristine (Oncovin)
V$_H$ variable region of heavy chain
V$_\kappa$ variable region of kappa light chain sequence
V$_\lambda$ variable region of lambda light chain sequence
VHDL very high density lipoproteins
VLB vinblastine (Velban)
VLDL very low density lipoproteins
VMA vanillylmandelic acid
V$_{max}$ maximal enzyme velocity
VPB chemotherapy regimen: vincristine/bleomycin/*cis*-platinum
VP16 epipodophyllotoxin
VWD von Willebrand's disease
vWF von Willebrand factor
VZV varicella zoster virus
WAS Wiskott-Aldrich syndrome
WBC white blood cell
WBCT whole blood clotting time
WT syndrome disorder resembling Fanconi's anemia but with an autosomal dominant inheritance pattern; named after the initials of the two families
W/W^v a mouse strain with anemia
XLP X-linked lymphoproliferative syndrome
Y (1) hepatic Y protein, which binds and transfers bilirubin; (2) Hill equation: the fractional saturation of hemoglobin with oxygen
Z hepatic Z protein, which binds and transfers bilirubin

INDEX

Note: Page numbers that are *italic* indicate figures; numbers followed by (t) indicate tables.

cis-AB blood group, 1505
Abdomen, germ cell tumors of, 1179
  pain in, in sickle cell disease, 672
Abelson oncogene, in chronic myelogenous leukemia, 1481, *1481*
Abetalipoproteinemia, 1659
  hemolytic anemia and, 505–506
ABO antigen, 1505
ABO blood group, 1504–1505, *1505*
  erythrocyte compatibility in, in bone marrow transplantation, 244
  incompatibility in, vs hereditary spherocytosis, 485
  matching in platelet transfusion, 1594
ABO erythroblastosis, hyperbilirubinemia with, 84
ABO hemolytic disease of newborn, 66–68
  hyperbilirubinemia with, 84
Abortion, in Rh-negative women, 57
ABVD regimen, for chemotherapy of Hodgkin's disease, 1110, 1110(t)
Acanthocytes, vs echinocytes, in hemolytic anemia, 505, *505*
Acanthocytosis, abetalipoproteinemia and, 505–506
  with neurologic disease and normal lipoproteins, 506
Acetaminophen, neutropenia with, 806
Acetylcholinesterase, 454
Acetylsalicylic acid. See *Aspirin*.
Acid-elution technique, Kleihauer-Betke, 30, 58, *200*
α_1-Acid glycoprotein, genetic polymorphism of, 1554–1555, *1554*, 1555(t)
Acid lipase deficiency, 1240–1241
Acid phosphatase, red cell, variants of, 1573
Acidosis, kernicterus risk and, 90
Aciduria, methylmalonic, and homocystinuria, 352
  treatment of, 357
  vitamin B_{12} nonresponsive, 351–352
  vitamin B_{12} responsive, 351
  orotic, 357–358
Aconitase, 277
Acquired immune deficiency syndrome. See *AIDS*.
Actin, filaments of, in phagocytes, 779, *781*
  in platelet activation, 1276
  neutrophil dysfunction of, 825
  proteins associated with, 460–461
  red cell membrane, 459
Actinomycin-D (Dactinomycin), 1003(t)
Actinomyosin, in red cell shape maintenance, 468
Activated clotting time test, 1297
Activated partial thromboplastin time test, 1297, *1298*
Acyclovir, for infections with bone marrow transplantation, 249
  in X-linked lymphoproliferative syndrome, 1125

Adenine diphosphate, deficiency of, in platelet dense granule deficiency, 1438
Adenine nucleotides, platelet, defective metabolism of, 1440
  granule bound, deficiency of, 1438
  in indirect platelet measurement, 1400
  in neonates, 1444
Adenosine deaminase deficiency, hemolytic anemia and, 572
  in severe combined immunodeficiency, 884–885
  platelet abnormalities in, 1441
Adenosine diphosphate (ADP), in platelet aggregation, 1283–1284
  in platelet signal transduction, 1345
Adenosine triphosphate, deficiency of, in platelet dense granule deficiency, 1438
  in hereditary spherocytosis, 479–481, *480*
  in pyruvate kinase deficient red cells, 565
  in RNA splicing, 712
  in uremic red cells, 1639
  in xerocytosis, 517
  metabolic abnormalities of, hemolytic anemia with, 569–570
  red cell, in screening for glycolytic enzymopathy, 547
  red cell shape and, 468
Adenosylcobalamin deficiency, methylcobalamin deficiency and, 352
  vitamin B_{12} deficiency and, 351
Adenovirus, oncogenic potential of, 946
Adenylate cyclase, neutrophil dysfunction and, 825, 833
Adenylate kinase, deficiency of, hemolytic anemia and, 571–572
  red cell, phenotypes of, 1574
ADM. See *Adriamycin*.
Adolescence, folate levels in, 320
  function of, in beta thalassemia, 747
  21-hydroxylase in, HLA complex and, 1525, 1531
β-Adrenergic blockers, for acute intermittent porphyria, 380
Adriamycin (ADM), for liver tumors, 1181
  for Wilms' tumor, 1149–1150
  properties of, 1002(t)
Afibrinogenemia, congenital, 1320–1321
Aflatoxin, liver tumors and, 1180
Africa, G6PD mutants in, 592
  sickle genes in, 655–656
Agammaglobulinemia, common variable, immunoglobulin gene rearrangement in, 874
  T-cell regulation of B-cell function and, 853, 853(t)
  congenital, 880–882. See also *Agammaglobulinemia, X-linked*.
  "nonsecretory," 874
  Swiss-type, 884. See also *Immunodeficiency, severe combined*.

Agammaglobulinemia *(Continued)*
  X-linked, 880–882
    immunoglobulin gene rearrangement in, 866–867, 874
Age, developmental, malnutrition diagnosis and, 308
  graft versus host disease and, 247
  iron compounds and, 279
  of children with cancer, 918
Agglutinins, saline reactive, 1497
AIDS, blood transfusions and, 1585–1586, 1615
  Factor VIII concentrates and, 1301
  hematologic abnormalities in, 1651
  pediatric, 890–892, 891(t)
AIDS-related complex (ARC), 890
  pediatric, 891(t)
Air, lead in, 389–390
  and blood levels of lead, 390, *390*
ALA. See *δ-Aminolevulinic acid.*
Albers-Schonberg disease, *213*, 214–215. See also *Osteopetrosis.*
Albumin, bilirubin and, 76–77
  in Rh hemolytic disease, 55–57, *55*
  kernicterus and, 89–90
  phototherapy effects on, 91
  for blood replacement, 1624–1625
  in exchange transfusion, 62
  genetic variants of, 1551–1552, *1551*
Alcohol, cirrhosis due to, spur cell anemia with, 506–507
  folate deficiency with, 328
  lead intoxication and, 398
  platelet function and, 1454
  sideroblastic anemia and, 372
  stomatocytosis and, 516
  thrombocytopenia and, 1394
Alder-Reilly bodies, 1216, 1231, 1662
Aldolase deficiency, hemolytic anemia and, 555
Alkaline phosphatase, in leukocytes, in chronic myelogenous leukemia, 1066
Alkylating agents, cancer risk and, 922
  complications of, 173
  for autoimmune hemolytic anemia, 422–423
Allergy, eosinopenia with, 1664
  eosinophilia with, 814
  pure red cell aplasia and, 196
  thrombocytopenia with, 1382
Alloantibodies, 1498
Alloimmunization, with granulocyte transfusion, 1602
Alphafetoprotein, 1171, 1171(t), 1180
Alpha-thal-1 trait, 730, 732, 733
Alpha-thal-2 gene, 730, 733
Alport's syndrome, 1641
Alymphocytosis, 884. See also *Immunodeficiency, severe combined.*
AM system, of immunoglobulins, 1571
Amegakaryocyte thrombocytopenia, aplastic anemia and, 192–193, *193*
Amethopterin (methotrexate), 1000(t)
Amicar (epsilon-aminocaproic acid; EACA), for platelet dysfunction, 1443. See also *Epsilon-aminocaproic acid (EACA).*
Amino acid differences, genetic markers and, 1572(t)
ε-Aminocaproic acid (EACA). See *Epsilon-aminocaproic acid (EACA).*
Aminoimidazolecarboxamide excretion, in vitamin B_{12} deficiency, 354
δ-Aminolevulinic acid, acute intermittent porphyria and, 376, 378–380

δ-Aminolevulinic acid *(Continued)*
  in heme synthesis, 363
  in lead poisoning, 399
  urinary, blood levels and, 393, *394*
δ-Aminolevulinic acid dehydratase, effects of lead on, 393–394
  in lead poisoning screening, 393, 407
δ-Aminolevulinic acid synthetase, in acute intermittent porphyria, 379–380
  heme effects on, 363–364
  in heme synthesis, 363
  lead effects on, 398
  in porphyria, 375
  in sideroblastic anemia, 371–373
Amniocentesis, in Rh hemolytic disease, 59–60, *60*
Amniotic fluid, bilirubin and, 55, 59–60, *60*
Amphotericin B, for infections with bone marrow transplantation, 249
  neutrophil aggregation and, 821
Amputation, for osteosarcoma, 1163
Amyloidosis, coagulation defects with, 1329–1330
Analgesia, in sickle cell disease, 682
Anaphylatoxins, 894
Anaphylaxis, thrombocytopenia and, 1382
Androgens, effect on red cells, 1643
  therapy with, complications of, 173
  for aplastic anemia, 172–173
  for Fanconi's anemia, *182*, 183, *183*, 184
Anemia, aplastic. See *Aplastic anemia.*
  blood loss and, 1581. See also *Blood loss.*
  chronic, red cell transfusions for, 1582
  chronic aregenerative. See *Diamond-Blackfan syndrome.*
  chronic congenital aregenerative. See *Diamond-Blackfan syndrome.*
  classification of, 266, 266(t), 267(t)
  congenital dyserythropoietic, 207–210, 207(t), 358
  congenital hypoplastic. See *Diamond-Blackfan syndrome.*
  definition of, 265, 266(t)
  diagnosis of, 267–273, 267(t)–272(t)
    blood film for, 270(t), 271, 272(t), 273
    differential diagnosis of, 265–273
    electronic cell counting in, 267, 269, 269(t), 271
    physical findings in, 268(t)
  Diamond-Blackfan, 197–205. See also *Diamond-Blackfan syndrome.*
  erythroblastic, 3
  etiology of, 267(t), 268(t)
  evaluation of patient with, 267–273, 267(t), 272(t)
  exchange transfusion indicated by, 63
  Fanconi's. See *Fanconi's anemia.*
  fetal, in Rh hemolytic disease, 54
  following exchange transfusion, 65
  genetic aspects of, 3
  hemolytic. See *Hemolytic anemia.*
  hemolytic process, in neonates and, 33–36, 33(t)
  hypochromic, hemoglobin synthesis in, 370–371
  hypochromic microcytic, iron deficiency with, 303
    thalassemia trait diagnosis and, 737–738, 737(t)
  hypoplastic, 160
  iron deficiency. See *Iron deficiency anemia.*
  in infancy, historical aspects of, 2–3

Anemia *(Continued)*
  in myelodysplasia, 1075–1076
  in protein-calorie malnutrition, 305–306, *306*
  in renal disease, 1639–1640
  in rheumatoid arthritis, 1646–1647
  in systemic lupus erythematosus, 1647
  macrocytic, in congenital dyserythropoietic anemia, 208
  megaloblastic. See *Megaloblastic anemia.*
  methemoglobinemia and, 647
  neonatal, blood loss causing, 28–32, 29(t)
    internal hemorrhage, 31–32
    malformations of placenta and cord, 31
    obstetric accidents, 31
    occult hemorrhage prior to birth, 29–31
    diagnosis of, 37–40, *38*
    in fetal to maternal hemorrhage, 30
  nutritional, classification of, 274–275
    differential diagnosis of, 275
    masked, 275–276
    mixed, 275
  of chronic disorders, 1645, 1645(t)
  of lead poisoning, 399–400
  pernicious, congenital, 345–346, 346(t)
    juvenile (autoimmune), 346, 346(t)
      with endocrinopathies, 346–347, 346(t)
      with IgA deficiency, 346(t), 347
    Schilling test and, 342
    vitamin B_{12} deficiency and, 342
  physiologic, of prematurity, 37, 39–40
  pure red cell. See *Pure red cell aplasia.*
  pyridoxine-responsive, 358
  refractory, 218
  severe, in Rh hemolytic disease, 64
  spur cell, 506–508
  stress erythropoiesis in, 139
  systemic disease manifested by, 276
  transient erythroblastopenia of childhood, 205–207
  von Jaksch's, 2–3
  with copper deficiency, 304–305
Angioid streaks, 486
Angioneurotic edema, hereditary, complement deficiency in, 894–895
Anions, polyvalent red cell, in membrane skeleton, 462
  influence on red cell osmotic properties, 462–463
  permeability and transport of, 465
  protein 3 and, 452–454
Aniridia-Wilms' tumor syndrome, 1154
Ankyrin, binding site of, 452–453
  defective binding by protein 3, 502
  defective binding to spectrin, 500
  nonerythroid, 468
  red cell membrane, integral membrane protein mobility and, 466
  structure and function of, 458–459
Ann Arbor staging system, for Hodgkin's disease, 1107, 1107(t)
Anodic stripping voltometry, 406
Anorexia nervosa, 506, 1660
Antibiotics, for aplastic anemia, 171–172
  for febrile neutropenia patients, 1599
  neutropenia with, 806
  platelet dysfunction and, 1453
Antibody(ies). See also *Immunoglobulins* and specific antibodies.
  agglutinating antineutrophil specific, 805
  anti-idiotype, 1539, 1655
  blood group. See *Blood group antibodies.*

Antibody(ies) *(Continued)*
  classes of, 861
  complete, 1497
  defective, in primary immunodeficiency disease, 879(t)
  diversity of, gene transcription and translation and, 866–868
    mechanisms for generating and regulating, 862–863
    theories of, 860–863
  heterophil, in infectious mononucleosis, 1656
  I, 1512
  in Epstein-Barr virus–induced infectious mononucleosis, 1657, *1657*
  incomplete, 1497
  leukoagglutinating, 804–805
  maternal, in ABO hemolytic disease, 66
  monoclonal, for graft versus host disease treatment, 248
  opsonic activity of, 786–787
  Sp_1, 1512
  splenic, 908
Antibody deficiency syndrome, 879
  molecular bases of, 874–875
Antibody-dependent cell-mediated cytotoxicity, for IgG antibodies against cell surface antigens, 1539
Anticoagulant(s), acquired, 1330
  lupus, 1648
  protein calcium as, 1256–1257
Anticoagulation, during apheresis, 1624
Anticonvulsants, maternal, vitamin K deficiency in neonates and, 118
Antifibrinolytics, 1304
  for von Willebrand's disease, 1319
Antigen(s), acquired changes in, blood groups and, 1500–1501
  blood group, characteristics and distribution of, 1501
    non–red cell, 1501, 1501(t)
    on glycophorins, 451–452
  cell surface, in HLA complex regions, 1524, 1529
  common acute lymphoblastic leukemia (CALLA), 1034
  Epstein-Barr virus, 1657
  Fy, 1512–1513
  Ia, in T cell activation, 849–850
  Js^a, 1510
  neonatal deficiency of, 1500
  neutrophil-specific, 804, 805
  Pl^{A1}, in isoimmune neonatal thrombocytopenia, 111–113
  related to Kell blood group system, 1509–1510, 1510(t)
  related to Lutheran blood group system, 1509(t)
  Rh, 1507–1508
  Rh(D), 1507
  T, 945
  T cell recognition of, 849
  Tj^a, 1507
Antigen-presenting cells, 1119
Antigenicity, of Rh-positive erythrocyte, 45–46, *45*
Antiglobulin (Coombs') test, 1498. See also *Coombs' test.*
Anti-idiotypes, in spleen, 428
Antilymphocytic globulin, bone marrow colony growth and, 169
  for aplastic anemia, 174–175, 174(t)

Antilymphocytic globulin *(Continued)*
  mechanism of action of, 175
  side effects of, 174–175
Antimetabolite therapy, folate deficiency with, 328
Antiplasmin, fibrinolytic regulation and, 1261, 1265
α_2-Antiplasmin deficiency, 1325
Antiplatelet agents, for treatment of hemolytic uremic syndrome, 438
  platelet-mediated thrombotic disorders and, 1452–1453
Antirheumatic drugs, 806
Antithrombin, inhibition of coagulation cascade by, 1263–1265
Antithrombin III, concentrate of, 1613
  in disseminated intravascular coagulation treatment, 1335
  uses of, 1303
  deficiency of, 1325–1326
  in liver disease, 1638
  measurement of, 1300
Antithymocyte globulin, for aplastic anemia, 174–175, 174(t)
  in kidney transplantation, 1539
Antithyroid drugs, 806
α_1-Antitrypsin, deficiency of, conjugated hyperbilirubinemia and, 95–96
  genetic variants of, 1552–1554, *1552, 1553*
Apheresis, 1622. See also *Lymphocytapheresis; Erythrocytapheresis*, etc.
  anticoagulation during, 1624
  blood volume during, 1623
  hematocrit in, 1623
  in critically ill patients, 1623–1624
  replacement solutions for, 1624–1625
  vascular access for, 1623
Aplastic anemia, 159–193
  acquired, 160–176
    causes of, 161–165, 161(t), 162(t)
    clinical appearance of, 160–161
    epidemiology of, 160–161
    incidence of, 160
    laboratory findings in, 165–166
    pathophysiology of, 166–170, 167(t)
    prognosis of, 170
    therapy and outcome of, 170–176
  amegakaryocytic thrombocytopenia, 192–193, *193*
  as autoimmune disorder, 168, 251
  bone marrow transplantation for, 251
    graft rejection in, 246, 1540
  childhood red cell, 205(t)
  chloramphenicol-hepatitis syndrome of, 163
  classification of, 160(t)
  constitutional, 176–193. See also *Fanconi's anemia.*
    age at diagnosis, *176*
    incidence of, 176
    types of, 176
  definition of, 159
  dyskeratosis congenita, 188–190, 188(t), *189*
  familial, 186–188, 186(t)
  familial marrow dysfunction in, 186–188, 186(t)
  idiosyncratic, 162–163
  immune deficiencies and, 187
  preceding acute leukemia, 216–217, *217*
  pure red cell, 194–210
    acquired, 195–197
    congenital, 197–205
  reticular dysgenesis, 193

Aplastic anemia *(Continued)*
  Shwachman-Diamond syndrome, 190–192, *192*
  therapy for, androgens, 172–173
    immunotherapy, 173–176
    lithium, 172
    supportive care, 171–172
  thrombocytopenia due to, 1393
  type 2 constitutional, 113
  vs acute leukemia, 1041
  with hypocellular marrow, 358
Aplastic crisis, in hemolytic anemia, 194–195
  in hereditary spherocytosis, 486–487, *487, 488*
  in sickle cell anemia, 674
Apoferritin, in iron loading in beta thalassemia, 744
  uptake of Fe(II) by, 370
Apolipoproteins, polyorphism in, 1562
Apotransferrin, in iron uptake, 367–368
Apt test, 119(t)
Ara-C (cytosine arabinoside), 1002(t)
Arachidonate, 780
Arachidonic acid, metabolism in platelets, *1284*, 1285–1287, 1432, 1448
  deficiency of, platelet dysfunction and, 14
  in neonatal platelets, 1444–1445
  inherited defects of, 1438–1440, *1439*
ARDS, neutrophil adherence and, 821
Arias syndrome, 85–86
Arterial hypoxemia, decreased oxygen affinity and, 622–623, *623*
  in beta thalassemia, 748
Arterial thrombosis, 1377
Arteriovenous shunts, 1453
Arthritis, juvenile, vs acute leukemia, 1041
Ascorbate cyanide test, 561, 564
Ascorbic acid, absorption of non-heme iron and, 282, *282*
  folic acid and, 320
  for Chédiak-Higashi syndrome, 827
  for methemoglobinemia, 644, 650
  in iron overload, 753
  in neutrophils, 833
  iron absorption and, 299
L-Asparaginase, 1004(t)
Aspartylglucosaminuria, 1240
Aspirin, bleeding time test and, 1296–1297
  blood loss due to, iron deficiency anemia and, 292, 301
  dose effects of, 1449
  for Kawasaki syndrome, 1458
  for rheumatoid arthritis, 293
  gastrointestinal bleeding with, 285, 1450
  iron deficiency anemia and, 292–293, 301
  maternal ingestion of, neonatal hemorrhage and, 114
  mode of action of, 1448–1450
  myocardial infarction and, 1452
  neonatal hemostasis and, 114, 1450
  neutropenia with, 806
  platelet function and, 1286, 1304–1305, 1448–1450
  substitutes for, 1450
Asplenia, congenital, 902–903
  functional, in sickle cell disease, 674
  neutrophilia with, 811
  syndrome of, 901–903
Astrocytoma, cerebellar, 1190–1191
  cerebral, 1189–1190
  hypothalamic, 1190
Ataxia-pancytopenia syndrome, 187

Ataxia-telangiectasia, immunodeficiency with, 887–888
  premalignancy with, 216
Atherosclerosis, 676
Atransferrinemia, congenital, 370
Autoantibodies, cold reactive, 1515
  in acquired autoimmune hemolytic anemia, 1515–1516
  to pluripotent stem cells, 168
Autohemolysis, 484, 515–516
  test for, 484, 545–546
Autoimmune hemolytic anemia, 417–423, 417(t). See also *Hemolytic anemia, autoimmune.*
Autoimmunity, aplastic anemia and, 168–169, 251
  following idiopathic thrombocytopenic purpura of childhood, 1354
  hyposplenism and, 909
  in juvenile pernicious anemia, 346, 346(t)
  plasmapheresis dose schedule for, 1625(t)
Autoplex, 1303, 1613
  for inhibitor hemophiliacs, 1314
5-Azacytidine, 756–757, *756*
Azathioprine, for autoimmune hemolytic anemia, 422
  for childhood ITP refractory to splenectomy, 1370
  in kidney transplantation, 1539

B cell(s), activation of, T-cell regulation of, 851–855, *852*, 853(t)
  deficiencies of, primary, 825, 878–879
  differentiation of, 146, 851
  function of, 851
  growth factors influencing, 851
  immune response of, vs T cell immune response, 1523
  in acute lymphoblastic leukemia, 1487–1489, *1488*
  in antibody deficiency diseases, 874–875
  in Burkitt's lymphoma, 1095
  in chronic myelogenous leukemia, 1067
  in infectious mononucleosis, 1656
  in non-T, non-B acute lymphoblastic leukemia, 869–870
  in spleen, 428
  in viral infection, 1120
  interaction with T cells, 854–856
  lymphocytapheresis and, 1626
  molecular generation and differentiation of, 862, *862*
  normal levels of, *1695*
  terminal differentiation of, 868
Bacterial infection. See *Infection, bacterial.*
BAL, for lead poisoning, 402, 403(t), *403*, 404
Bartonellosis, 1651, *1651*
Bartter's syndrome, 1441
Basophil(s), morphology and function of, 816
  vs mast cells, 816
Basophilia, 1664–1665
  causes of, 1664(t)
  disorders associated with, 816–817, 816(t)
Basophilic stippling, in congenital nonspherocytic hemolytic anemia, 546
  in lead intoxication, 399
  in unstable hemoglobinopathies, 633
Basophilopenia, 816–817
Bassen-Kornzweig syndrome (abetalipoproteinemia), 505–506

Batten-Spielmeyer-Vogt disease, 1663
Baty, J. M., 9
Bayley Scale of Infant Development, 298
BCNU, properties of, 1005(t)
Benzene, aplastic anemia and, 163
Bernard-Soulier syndrome, 1280, 1281, 1433, 1436
  thrombocytopenia in, 1391
Beta:alpha biosynthetic globin ratio, 731, 734–735
Bile, bilirubin in, 78
  pigment structure in, *364*
Biliary atresia, conjugated hyperbilirubinemia and, 93–94
  vs causes of cholestasis, 94
  vs idiopathic neonatal giant cell hepatitis, 94
Bilirubin, absorption of, in newborn, 79–81
  albumin binding to, 76–77
    in Rh hemolytic disease, 55–57, *55*
  blood-brain barrier for, kernicterus and, 89–90
  conjugation of, 77–78
    acquired defects in, 86–88
    inherited defects in, 85–86
    in newborn, 81, 85–88
  direct-reacting, kernicterus risk and, 90
    vs indirect-reacting, 82–83
  encephalopathy due to, 89–90. See also *Kernicterus.*
  enterohepatic circulation of, breast milk jaundice and, 87
  exchange transfusion and, 62–63, 89, 89(t)
  excretion of, 78–79
    in newborn, 80
  hepatic uptake of, 77
    in physiologic jaundice of newborn, 81
  in amniotic fluid, 59–60, *60*
  in phototherapy, 92
  in physiologic jaundice of newborn, 81
  in Rh hemolytic disease, 55–57
    cord concentration of, exchange transfusion and, 63
  in sickle cell disease, 677
  metabolism and transport of, in newborn, abnormal, 82–83
    unconjugated hyperbilirubinemia, 84–88
    normal, 79–82
  removal in exchange transfusion, 62
  reticuloendothelial function and, 431
  serum concentration of, exchange transfusion and, 89, 89(t)
  structure of, 76, *76*
  synthesis of, 74–76, *75*
    in newborn, 79–80
  toxicity of, 89–92
    prevention of, 90–92
  transport in plasma, *75*, 76–77
  unconjugated, absorbed from bowel, 79
    conjugation of, 77–78
    free, estimation of, 56–57
    hepatic uptake of, 77
    in newborn, 79–81
    intestinal concentration of, in newborn, 80–81
    reabsorption of, 79
    transport in plasma, 76–77
Bilirubin IX, 76, *76*, 78
Biliverdin reductase, 76
Birbeck granules, 1119, *1119*
Birth defects, cancer risk and, 927
BK virus, 946

Blacks, G6PD deficiency in, 603, 656
  sickle cell disease incidence in, 655–656
Blackwater fever, 1651
Bladder, rhabdomyosarcoma of, 1158
Blast cells, in acute leukemia, 1040
Blast crisis, in chronic myelogenous leukemia, 1068
  chromosomal abnormalities in, 1482
Blastema, nodular renal, Wilms' tumor and, 1146
Bleeding. See also *Blood loss; Hemorrhage; Coagulation disorders.*
  coagulation tests for, 1297–1300
  history of, 1293–1294
  in Gaucher's disease, 1226
  in hemophilia A, 1309–1310
  in hemostatic disease, 1347, 1347(t)
  in idiopathic thrombocytopenic purpura of childhood, 1364
  intraventricular, in premature infants, 117
  neonatal, diagnostic approach to, 107, *107*
    laboratory evaluation of, 105(t), 108, *109*, 109(t)
  platelet function tests and, 1296–1297
Bleeding diathesis, generalized, neonatal, 119
Bleeding time, in Bernard-Soulier syndrome, 1433
  in neonates, 1445
  in uremia, 1445–1446
  methods of testing for, 1296
  platelet count and, 1591
  significance of, 1429
Bleomycin, iron reactivity and, 367
Blind loop syndrome, 349
Blindness, sickle cell disease and, 678
Blood, circulation of, in bone marrow, 133, *133*
  peripheral, progenitor cells in, 135
  splenic, 901
  cord, normal hemoglobin values in, 27, 27(t)
  lead levels in, 392
    erythrocyte protoporphyrin and, 397–398, *397*
    heme synthesis and, *394*
    for lead poisoning screening, 401, 406
    normal, 389
    "safe," 402
  peripheral, in folate deficiency, 330
    in myelodysplastic syndromes, 1075(t)
    in storage disease, 1216–1217
    in vitamin B_{12} deficiency, 353, 354, *353*
  separation into components of, 1622–1623. See also *Blood components.*
  stored, 2,3 diphosphoglycerate in, 623
  used in exchange transfusion, 63–64
Blood-brain barrier, brain tumor chemotherapy and, 1188–1189
  for bilirubin, kernicterus and, 89–90
Blood components. See also specific components (e.g., *Plasma; Red cells; Neutrophil(s)*, etc.).
  removed in exchange transfusion, 62
  separation of, 1622–1623
  therapy with, 1300–1304. See also *Transfusion.*
Blood dyscrasia, megaloblastic anemia with, 358
Blood film, 271, 273
Blood flow, splenic, 481(t)
Blood group(s). See also names of specific blood groups.
  clinical importance of, 1500–1501
  definition of, 1499

Blood group(s) *(Continued)*
  disease and, 1502–1504
  frequency of, disease and, 1504
  genetics of, 1499–1500, 1499(t)
  maturation of, 1500
  recognition of, 1498–1499
  routine studies for, 1498
  technical procedures relating to, 1497–1498
  tests for disputed paternity and, 1516
Blood group antibodies, anti-A, ABO hemolytic disease and, 66
  anti-B, ABO hemolytic disease and, 66
  anti-D, complement fixation of, 47–48
    destruction of fetal erythrocytes by, 51–54
    detection of, 47
    immunoglobulins of, 47
    in exchange transfusion, 62
    in experimental subjects, 48–49, 48(t), 49(t), *49*
    in gamma globulin for Rh immunization prevention in mothers, 57–58, 57(t), 58(t)
    in Rh negative women, 59
    mechanism of action of, 47
    naturally occurring, 47, 50
    nature of, 46
    placental transfer of, 48
    serologic reactions of, 47
  minor, causing hemolytic disease of newborn, 68–69
  routine testing for, 1498
Blood lakes (peliosis hepatis), with androgen therapy, 173
Blood letting, 1622–1631. See also *Apheresis.*
Blood loss. See also *Hemorrhage; Blood volume; Pallor.*
  acute, red cell transfusion for, 1581–1582
  aspirin induced, iron deficiency anemia due to, 292
  from laboratory tests, 300
  gastrointestinal, in acute leukemia, 1038
    iron deficiency and, 284–285
  hemodialysis induced, 292
  neonatal, acute and chronic, 30(t)
  neonatal anemia and, 28–32, 29(t)
    internal hemorrhage, 31–32
    malformations of placenta and cord, 31
    obstetric accidents, 31
    occult hemorrhage prior to birth and, 29–31
    recognition of, 32–33, 32(t)
  occult, iron deficiency and, 285
Blood transfusion. See *Transfusion.*
Blood vessels, in neonates, 104–105
Blood volume. Se also *Blood loss.*
  at birth, with cord clamping, 26–27
  in apheresis, 1623
Bloom's syndrome, 215–216
B-lymphocyte(s). See *B cell(s).*
Bodian-Shwachman syndrome. See *Shwachman-Diamond syndrome.*
Bohr effect, 618, *618*, 622, 623
Bone changes, in acute leukemia, 1038
  in Gaucher's disease, 1226
  in severe beta thalassemia, 742, *743*
Bone infarction, of sickle cell disease, vs osteomyelitis, 669, 671
Bone marrow. See also *Erythropoiesis; Hematopoiesis.*
  anatomy of, 131–133, *132, 133*
    circulation in, 133, *133*
    microenvironment of, 131, *132*, 167–168

Bone marrow *(Continued)*
  aplasia of, neonatal thrombocytopenia and, 113–114
  aspiration of, in leukemia diagnosis, 1040
    of donor bone marrow, 245
  early studies in, 7–8
  examination of, in aplastic anemia, 165–166, *166*
    in hereditary spherocytosis, 484
    in idiopathic thrombocytopenia of childhood, 1353
    in thrombopoiesis, 147–148
  familial dysfunction of, 186–188, 186(t)
  hypocellular, megaloblastosis with, 358
  in chronic neutropenia, 802
  in drug-induced neutropenia, 807
  in folate deficiency, 330
  in megaloblastic anemia, 354, *354*
    folate deficiency in skin disease and, 325
  in sideroblastic anemia, 374
  in storage disease, 1217
  infiltration of, thrombocytopenia due to, 1393
  macrophage distribution in, 785
  normal cell populations in infants, 1690(t)–1691(t)
  release of cells from, 133, *134*
  stem cell replication in, 167–168
Bone marrow failure, 159–241, 220(t). See also *Aplastic anemia; Cytopenia; Leukoerythroblastosis; Preleukemia.*
  characteristics of, 159
  chloramphenicol and, 161–163, 162(t)
  constitutional, 220(t)
  in myelodysplastic syndromes, 1075, 1975(t)
  platelet transfusion for, 1591–1592
  preleukemic, 215(t). See also *Preleukemia.*
  prenatal diagnosis of, 219
  single cytopenias in, 193–213
  treatment of, 219
Bone marrow transplantation, allogeneic, 243, 253, 1540–1542
  antilymphocyte globulin therapy and, 175
  autoimmune neutropenia and, 806
  autologous, 256–257
  chemoradiation preparation for, 244–245
  complications of, 246–250
  diseases utilized in, 250–256
  donor selection for, 243–244, 1540–1541
  haploidentical, 243, 244, 246, 250
  history of, 242–243
  immunosuppression with, 1541–1542
  for acute lymphoblastic leukemia, relapsed, 1047–1048
  for acute myelogenous leukemia, 1049
  for adult chronic myelogenous leukemia, 1069
  for aplastic anemia, 167, 219, 251
  for beta thalassemia, 755–756
  for chronic granulomatous disease, 830
  for Diamond-Blackfan syndrome, 204, 254
  for erythroid disorders, 254
  for Ewing's sarcoma, 1169
  for Fanconi's anemia, 183
  for Gaucher's disease, 255–256
  for granulocyte disorders, 254
  for Kostmann's disease, 803
  for leukemia, 251–253
  for lipidoses, 256
  for mucopolysaccharidoses, 256
  for neuroblastoma, 1144
  for osteopetrosis, 214, 254
  for platelet disorders, 254, 1443

Bone marrow transplantation *(Continued)*
  for severe combined immunodeficiency, 250, 886, *887, 888*
  for sickle cell anemia, 254
  for storage disease, 1223
  for thalassemia, 254–255
  for Wiskott-Aldrich syndrome, 253–254, 889
  historical aspects of, 7
  inherited hematopoietic disorders and, 253–256
  leukemia risk and, 253, 928
  marrow procurement and engraftment in, 245–246
  patient selection in, 243
  syngeneic, 243, 245
  T-lymphocyte depletion from grafts prior to transplantation and, 1541
  thrombocytopenia with, 1383
  types of, 243
Bone pain, in sickle cell disease, 669, *670,* 671–672
Bone tumors, 1161–1169. See also names of specific tumors.
Bordetella pertussis infection, phagocyte dysfunction with, 825, 883
Bowel, small, disease of, 1635
Boyden chamber assay, 822, 823
Brain, bilirubin toxicity and, 89. See also *Kernicterus.*
  in protein calorie malnutrition, 307
  mitochondria of, hyperbilirubinemia and, 56
Brain trauma, 1660
Brain tumors, anatomic distribution of, *1186*
  brainstem glioma, 1191–1192
  cerebellar astrocytoma, 1190–1191
  cerebral astrocytoma, 1189–1190
  choroid plexus papilloma, 1194
  clinical manifestations of, 1186–1187
  craniopharyngioma, 1196
  ependymoma, 1193–1194
  histologic classification of, 1186(t)
  hypothalamic astrocytoma, 1190
  medulloblastoma, 1192–1193
  metastases of, 1187
  oligodendroglioma, 1194
  optic glioma, 1190
  pineal tumors, 1194–1195
  primitive neuroectodermal, 1193
  prognosis of, 1187, *1188*
  treatment of, 1187–1189
Brainstem glioma, 1191–1192
Breast feeding, breast milk iron and, 280, 281
  breast milk jaundice and, 86–88
Breast milk, 86–88, 280–281
  iron absorption from, 281, 299
  vitamin B_{12} in, 344
  vitamin K deficiency and, 117
Breast milk jaundice, 86–88
Bronze baby syndrome, 91
Bruton's disease, 880–882. See also *Agammaglobulinemia, X-linked.*
Burkitt's lymphoma, chromosomal rearrangements in, 873, 1487
  diagnosis of, 1094–1095
  epidemiologic data on, 928–929
  Epstein-Barr virus and, 947
  histology of, 1094–1095
  immunoglobulin gene rearrangements in, 947
Burns, hemolytic anemia with, 435, 503
Burst-forming units–erythroid, differentiation of, 139
  in Diamond-Blackfan syndrome, 202

Burst-forming units–erythroid *(Continued)*
   in erythroid differentiation, 145–146
   in peripheral blood, 145
   production of, 138–139
   proliferation and differentiation of, 139
Burst-promoting activity, 139, 145–146
Busulfan, for bone marrow transplantation preparation, 245

Calcium, in hereditary spherocytosis, 476
   in phagocytosis, 788
   in sickle cells, 664–665
   metabolism of, in leukemia treatment, 1042
   mobilization of, in platelets, 1440
   permeability and transport in, red cells of, 464–465, *465*
Calcium disodium ethylenediaminic acid (CaNaEDTA), for lead poisoning, 402, 403(t), *403*, 404–405, 405(t)
   mobilization test with, 404–405
Calcium gluconate, in exchange transfusion, 63
Calcium pump, in red cell, 464, 465, *465*
   in sickle cells, 664
Calmodulin, 464, 788
CaNaEDTA, 402, 403(t), *403*, 404–405, 405(t)
Cancer. See also *Malignancy; Tumor(s);* and *Preleukemia,* as well as names of specific tumors (e.g., *Neuroblastoma*).
   cellular oncogenes and, 960, 965
   clinical case studies of, 919–920
   clusters of, 919
   demographic characteristics of, 918–920, 919(t)
   dyskeratosis congenita and, 190
   epidemiologic data on, 918–941
   familial, risk of, 927
   Fanconi's anemia and, 184–186
   general features of, 1136–1137
   growth rate of, response to chemotherapy and, 988–997. See also *Cancer chemotherapy.*
   in children, 933–934
   incidence in children, 918–921, 919(t), 1136, 1137(t)
   maps of, 919, *920*
   mortality data for, 934, 1136
   neutropenia with, 803
   risk factors for, 921–927
      birth defects, 927
      chemical carcinogens, 922–923
      chromosomal disorders, 926–927, 925(t)–926(t)
      drugs, 922, 923(t)
      familial cancers, 925(t), 926(t), 927
      infectious agents, 923–924
      ionizing radiation, 921–922
      single gene disorders, 924, 925(t)–926(t)
   Shwachman-Diamond syndrome and, 191
   treatment of, 1137–1138. See also *Cancer chemotherapy; Radiation therapy.*
   types of, 1136, *1137*
Cancer chemotherapy. See also names of specific drugs and types of drugs (e.g., *Alkylating agents*).
   alternating non-crossresistent programs in, 1006–1008
   clinical pharmacokinetics in, 987
   clinical trials of, 983–985, 983(t)
   combination, 998, 998(t), 1006

Cancer chemotherapy *(Continued)*
   combination, drug interactions in, 998, 1006, 1006(t)
      for acute leukemia, 1043
      for Hodgkin's disease, 1108, 1109(t), 1110–1111, 1112
      principles of, 998(t)
   drugs used in, development and testing of, 982–985
      clinical trials, 983–985, 983(t)
      screening systems for, 982–983
   first order kinetics of, 987, 991–992
   interactions of, 987–988, 988(t)
   most common, 997–1009, 999(t)–1005(t)
   new, 982–958, 1008
   resistance to, 1006–1008
   thrombocytopenia related to, 1393
   for brain and CNS tumors, 1188–1189
      brainstem glioma, 1191–1192
      cerebral astrocytoma, 1190
      ependymoma, 1194
      medulloblastoma, 1192–1193
      pineal tumors, 1195
   for Ewing's sarcoma, 1167–1168
   for liver tumors, 1181
   for microscopic disease, 993–994
   for neuroblastoma, 1142–1143
   for non-Hodgkin's lymphoma, 1098, 1099(t), 1100
   for osteosarcoma, 1164–1166, *1165*
   for retinoblastoma, 1185–1186
   for rhabdomyosarcoma, 1155–1158
   for testicular tumors, 1176–1177
   for Wilms' tumor, 1149–1150, 1150(t)
   general features of, 981–982
   Gompertzian kinetics and protocol design in, 992–993, *993*
   historical aspects of, 982
   indications for, 932(t)
   kinetics and protocol design in, 991–993, *993*
   limitations of, 982(t)
   nutritional support in, 987
   passive immunotherapy in, 1008
   radiation interaction in, 1023
   response to, adjuvant preoperative, 994
      cell cycle–dependent cytotoxicity and, 996
      cell kinetics and, 997
      cell recruitment and, 997
      cell synchronization and, 996–997
      drug responsiveness based on tumor stem cell assays, 995–996
      tumor growth rate and, 988–997
         cell cycle and, 994–995
         kinetics of microscopic disease and, 993–994
         protocol design and, 991–993, *993*
         volume doubling time and, 988–990, *989, 990*
      tumor stem cells and, 995–996
   therapeutic index of, 986
   therapeutic strategy in, 1008
   toxicity control in, 986–987
   treatment considerations in, 985–988, 1008
Carbamino formation, in hemoglobin function, 619
Carbamylation, for sickle cell disease, 667
Carbohydrates, complex, metabolism of, diseases relating to, 1235–1241
Carbon dioxide, effect on hemoglobin, 619
   generated by pentose pathway, 584, *586*

Carbon monoxide, bilirubin synthesis and, 75–76
  in Rh hemolytic disease, 54
  intoxication with, abnormal hemoglobin function and, 635–636
  production of, heme degradation and, 80
Carbon monoxide technique, for determining red cell survival, 20
Carboxyhemoglobin, 80, 635–636
Cardiac abnormalities, hemolytic anemia with, 433–434
  in beta thalassemia, 745–746, 746(t)
  in leukemia, 1039
  in sickle cell disease, 675–676
  platelet dysfunction with, 1446
Cardiac function, noninvasive studies of, 745–746, 746(t)
Cardiopulmonary bypass, hemostatic defects with, 1328
  platelet dysfunction with, 1446
  thrombocytopenia due to, 1383–1384
Carrion's disease, 1651
Cartilage-hair hypoplasia, in Shwachman-Diamond syndrome, 191
  neutropenia with, 803
Castleman's disease, 1089–1090
Catalase, 1574
Catheters, thrombocytopenia due to, 1383–1384
Cations, monovalent, red cell membrane, in hereditary spherocytosis, 475
    influence on red cell oncotic pressure of, 463, *463*
    permeability and transport of, 463–464, *464*
    red cell hydration and 465, *465*
  permeability of, in pyruvate kinase deficient red cells, 565
  in sickle cells, 664
Celiac disease, 1635
  iron deficiency with, 301–302
  vitamin B_{12} malabsorption with, 348
Cell(s), aging of, 2,3-DPG and, 622
  HL-60, 1031
  hybridization of, X chromosome mapping and, 593
  in hematopoiesis, aplastic anemia and, 168–170
  in malnutrition, 307
  inhibitors of, in Diamond-Blackfan syndrome, 201–202
  lead effects on, 398–399
  leukemic blast, 1031
  radiation survival curve of, 1020–1021, *1021*, 1023
  repair of radiation damage to, 1021
  sickling of, 662–664, *663*
  tumor stem, 995–996
  virus transformed, 944(t)
Cell cycle, cancer chemotherapeutic response and, 994–995
  labeling techniques of, 994–995
  radiation sensitivity of, 1021–1022, *1022*
  synchronization of cancer drugs with, 996–997
Central nervous system, in acute lymphoblastic leukemia, 1051
    relapse and, 1046–1047
    treatment of, 1044
  in acute myelogenous leukemia, 1049

Central nervous system *(Continued)*
  in cobalamin deficiency, 343
  in iron deficiency anemia, 297–298
  in leukemia, 1036–1037
  in lysosomal storage diseases, 1215
  in sickle cell disease, 672–673, 679
  tumors of, 1186–1196
    clinical manifestations of, 1186–1187
    epidemiology of, 930
    prognosis of, 1187, *1188*
    treatment of, 1187–1189
Central venous catheters, for apheresis, 1623
Cephalosporins, platelet dyfunction and, 1453
Ceramides, in Farber's disease, 1229
  in sphingolipidoses, 1224, *1224*
Cereals, infant, iron fortified, 299, 300
Cerebral astrocytoma, 1189–1190
Cerebrovascular accident, in sickle cell disease, 672
Cerebrovascular disease, antiplatelet agents and, 1453
  sickling in, exchange transfusion for, 673
Ceroid-lipofuscinosis, neuronal, 1241–1242
Ceruloplasmin, 1558–1559
CFU-E. See *Colony-forming unit-erythroid.*
CFU-GEMM. See *Colony-forming unit–granulocyte-macrophage, erythroid, megakaryocyte.*
CFU-GM. See *Colony-forming unit–granulocyte-macrophage.*
CFU-S. See *Colony-forming unit in spleen.*
Chédiak-Higashi syndrome, 826–828, 826(t), *827*, 1663
  abnormal neutrophil chemotaxis in, 823
  hematologic manifestations in, 826(t), *827*
Chelation therapy, for beta thalassemia, 751–753
  for lead poisoning, 402, *403*, 403(t), 404–405
  for thalassemia intermedia, 755
  iron removal from cells and, 367
Chemicals, aplastic anemia and, 163–164
  cancer risk and, 922
  oxidant, methemoglobinemia and, 647, 648, 648(t), 649(t)
Chemoradiation therapy, 243
  in bone marrow transplantation recipients, 244–245, 249, 251
Chemotactic factors, inactivators of, 822
  regulating movements of phagocytes, 782–783, 783(t)
Chemotactic receptors, down regulation of, 823
Chemotaxis, 821
  in Chédiak-Higashi syndrome, 826
  in neutrophils, 821–824, 821(t), 828
Chemotherapy, cancer. See *Cancer chemotherapy.*
Cherry-red myoclonus syndrome, 1235–1236
Chest, pain in, in sickle cell disease, 671–672
Chlorambucil, for autoimmune hemolytic anemia, 422
Chloramphenicol, aplastic anemia and, 161–163, 162(t)
  for Kostmann's disease, 803
  sideroblastic anemia and, 372
  thrombocytopenia and, 1393
Chloride-bicarbonate exchange, protein 3 and, 452
Chlorosis, iron deficiency anemia and, 5
Chlorpromazine, for acute intermittent porphyria, 380

Cholecystitis, in sickle cell disease, 672
Cholestasis. See also *Hyperbilirubinemia, conjugated, in newborn.*
  definition of, 78, 93
  in hereditary spherocytosis, 487
  with paucity of bile ducts, 95
Cholesterol, in macrophage membranes, 782
  in platelet membranes, 1279
  in red cell membrane, intercalation with phospholipids, 446–447
    organization of, 445
    renewal pathways of, 447–448, *447*
  in spur cell anemia, 507–508, *507*
Cholesterol ester storage disease, 1240–1241
Chondroitin-6-sulfate, in Morquio's disease, *1232*
Choriocarcinoma, 1170
Choroid plexus papilloma, 1194
Christmas disease. See *Hemophilia B.*
Christmas factor, 1251. See also *Factor IX/IXa.*
Chromium-51, in platelet kinetic studies, 1274–1275, *1275*
  in red cell survival studies, 20, 20(t)
Chromosome(s). See also *DNA; Gene(s); RNA.*
  abnormalities of, cancer risk and, 926
    consistent, 1492–1494, *1493*
    critical recombinations in, 1493–1494, *1493*
    deletions of, 1480
    fragile sites and, 1479–1480
    in acute lymphoblastic leukemia, 1487–1490
    in acute nonlymphoblastic leukemia, 1483–1487
    in ataxia telangiectasia, 887
    in Burkitt's lymphoma, 873, 1095
    in children vs adults, 1486, 1486(t)
    in chronic myelogenous leukemia, 1480–1483
    in Diamond-Blackfan syndrome, 201
    in Ewing's sarcoma, 1492
    in Fanconi's anemia, 180, 182
    in leukemia, survival and, 1487
    in myelodysplasia, 218, 1077
    in neuroblastoma, 1138, 1492
    in retinoblastoma, 1182, 1490–1491
    in tumors, 1479–1496
    in Wilms' tumor, 1491–1492
    inversions, 1480
    methods of study of, 1480
    terminology used in, 1480
    time of occurrence of, 1492–1493
    translocations, 1480
      in activation of proto-oncogenes, 963
      in lymphoid neoplasma, 874(t)
      mediation of by immunoglobulin gene loci, 873–874
    types of, 1480
  band 13q14 of, retinoblastoma and, 1182
  haplotypes of, in prenatal diagnosis of beta thalassemia, 761
  mutation 6p(iso6p), retinoblastoma and, 1182
  Philadelphia, 870, *871.* See also *Philadelphia chromosome.*
Chronic disorders, anemia of, 1645, 1645(t)
Cigarette smoking, cancer risk and, 923
Cimetidine, aplastic anemia and, 163
Circumcision, 119
Cirrhosis, spur cell anemia with, 506–507
Cis activity, in thalassemia, 704
Cis asymmetry, of phospholipids in red cell membrane, 446

Citrate, for anticoagulation during apheresis, 1624
  toxicity of, post-transfusion, 1586
Citrate phosphate dextrose, in stored blood, 623
Clathrin, 789
Clear-cell sarcoma, 1146
Clostridium, septicemia due to, 504, 1650
Clot retraction inhibition, in indirect platelet measurement, 1400
Clotting factors. See *Coagulation factors.*
CNSHA. See *Hemolytic anemia, congenital nonspherocytic.*
Coagulation. See also *Hemostasis; Coagulation disorders.*
  common pathway of, interaction with coagulation cascades, 1255–1256
    tests showing disorder in, 1297
  disseminated intravascular. See *Disseminated intravascular coagulation.*
  fibrin clot formation in, 1257–1258
  fibrinolytic mechanism in, 1258–1262
  fluid phase, 1248–1270. See also *Thrombin, generation of.*
  disorders of, 1293–1342. See also *Coagulation disorders.*
  inhibition of, 1263–1265
    in neonate, 106–107, 118–119
  inhibitors of, activated prothrombin complex concentrates for, 1615
    protease (new), 1266
    tests for, 1299
  limiting reactions in, 1262–1266
  platelet function in, 1271–1292
  proteins needed for, in neonates, 105–106
Coagulation cascade, antithrombin inhibition of, 1263–1265, *1264*
  extrinsic, 1253
    common pathway and, kinetic relationships among, 1255–1256
    defects of, vs intrinsic pathway disorders, 1297, *1298*
  intrinsic, 1249–1253
    common pathway and, kinetic relationship among, 1255–1256
Coagulation disorders, acquired, 1326–1336
  amyloidosis and, 1329–1330
  anticoagulant acquisition and, 1330
  cardiac disease and, 1328–1329, 1633–1634
  disseminated intravascular coagulation, 1330–1336. See also *Disseminated intravascular coagulation.*
  infections and, 1650
  liver disease and, 1326–1327, 1637–1638
  renal disease and, 1329, 1640
  snakebite and, 1336
  vitamin K deficiency and, 1327–1328
  blood loss and, 1581
  classification of, 1295(t)
  consumption, miscellaneous causes of, 1388
  diagnosis of, 1293–1300
    history in, 1293–1294
    laboratory tests for, 1296–1300
    physical examination in, 1294, 1296
  hereditary, 1305–1326
    frequency and mode of transmission in, 1320(t)
    neonatal hemorrhage due to, 118–119
  sickle cell disease and, 682–683
  tests for, 1297–1300, 1638
    in idiopathic thrombocytopenic purpura of childhood, 1353

Coagulation disorders *(Continued)*
    tests for, screening tests, 1297, *1298*, 1299
        in neonates, 105(t), 108, *109*, 109(t)
        normal values for, 105(t)
        specific assays, 1299–1300
    treatment of, 1300–1305
    vs platelet defects, 1347(t)
Coagulation factors. See also under *Factor(s)*.
    disseminated intravascular coagulation and, 116
    in fetus and neonate, 1692(t)
    in hemolytic uremic syndrome, 436
    in neonates, 106
    in pregnancy, 1644
    in thyroid disease, 1643
    plasma, characteristics relevant to transfusion therapy, 1607(t)
    platelet interaction with, 1432
    transfusion therapy with, 1606–1621. See also *Plasma products*.
    future of, 1616–1617
Cobalamin. See also *Vitamin B_{12}*.
    deficiency of, 342–343
Cobalophilins, 341
Cold agglutinins, Ii blood group and, 1512
    titer of, for diagnosis of cold hemagglutinin disease, 421
Cold exposure, cold hemagglutinin disease and, 417–418
Cold hemagglutinin disease, anemia in, 417–418
    pathophysiology of, 418–419
    therapy for, 422–423
Cold reactive autoantibodies, red cell autoimmune states and, 1515
Collagen, interaction with platelets, 1282–1283, 1345, 1432
Collagen vascular disease, 1646–1649
Colony-forming unit in culture, in granulopoiesis, 142
Colony-forming unit in spleen (CFU-s), 136–137
    in hematopoiesis, 135–137
    self-replication of, 137
Colony-forming unit–erythroid (CFU-E), humoral inhibition of, in transient erythroblastopenia of childhood, 206
    inhibition of, in Diamond-Blackfan syndrome, 201–202
    production of, 138–139
    pure red cell aplasia and, 196
Colony-forming unit–granulocyte-macrophage (CFU-GM), 141–145, 798, 1118
    in aplastic anemia, 169
    in neutropenic states, 809(t)
    vs pluripotent stem cell, 142
Colony-forming unit–granulocyte-macrophage-erythroid-megakaryocyte (CFU-GEMM), 139
Colony-forming unit–megakaryocyte (CFU-M), 1395
    differentiation and proliferation of, 1272
    in thrombocytopenia, 148
    thrombocytosis and, 1395
Colony-stimulating activity, granulocyte-macrophage, 798
    in erythroid differentiation, 145
    in thrombopoiesis regulation, 148, *149*
Colony-stimulating factors, functions of, 143–144, 144(t)
    purified human, 144(t)
Complement system, 892–897
    acquired defects of, 896–897

Complement system *(Continued)*
    activation of, 892–893
        down regulation of, 893
    alternative pathway of, 892
        deficiencies of, 896
    cell membrane and, 425
    classic pathway of, 892
        in autoimmune hemolytic anemia, 418
        in clearance of IgG coated erythrocytes, 414, *414*
    components of, biosynthesis of, 894
        C1, acquired INH deficiency of, 895
            receptor for, 1567
        C2, 1525
            deficiency of, HLA complex and, 1531
            polymorphism of, 1568
        C3, deficiency of, 895–897
            pyogenic infections with, 825
            vs primary B cell deficiency, 879
            excessive binding to blood cells of, in paroxysmal nocturnal hemoglobinuria, 424, 425
            gene frequencies of, 1565(t)
            genetic polymorphism of, 1564–1565
            in Coombs' test for autoimmune hemolytic anemia, 420–421
            opsonic activity of, 786–787
            serum concentration of, 1564
        C3b, in paroxysmal nocturnal hemoglobinuria, 424, 425
            receptor for, 1567
            reticuloendothelial opsonization and, 431
        C3bi, in congenital plasma membrane glycoprotein deficiency, 819
            receptor for, in opsonization disorders, 824–825
            on granulocyte-macrophage progenitor cells, 798
        C4, 1525
            binding protein of, 1566–1567
            deficiency of, HLA complex and, 1531
            polymorphism of, 1568–1569, *1569*
        C5, 1565
        C5a, neutrophil adhesiveness and, 821
        C6, 1565, 1565(t), 1566
        C7, 1566
        C8, genetic polymorphism of, 1566, 1566(t)
        early acting, deficiencies of, 895
        late acting, deficiencies of, 896
        serum, 1525
    defective, impaired neutrophil chemotaxis and, 822
    deficiency of, opsonization disorders and, 825
    genetic deficiencies of, 894–896
    genetics of, 894
    in neutrophil recognition of target cells and, 824
    in paroxysmal nocturnal hemoglobinuria, 424–425
    inflammation and, 893–894
    platelet-associated, 1400–1402, *1401*, *1402*, 1405
    proteins of, in movement of phagocytes, 783, 783(t)
    reticuloendothelial opsonization and, 431
    role in clearance of antibody-coated erythrocytes from circulation, 414–416, *414*, *415*
    terminal phase of, 893
Complement-dependent cytotoxicity test, 1524, 1529, *1529*

Complement-fixation, 892–894
  in indirect platelet measurement, 1399
  of anti-D antibody, 47–48
Complotypes, 1569, 1569(t)
Computed tomography, for staging of Hodgkin's disease, 1105–1106
Connective tissue disorders, 1441
Constipation, 1636
Convulsions, in lead poisoning, 402
Cooley, Thomas B., 3–4
Cooley's anemia. See *Thalassemia, beta, severe.*
Coombs' test, in ABO hemolytic disease, 66, 68
  in autoimmune hemolytic anemia, 420–421
  negative, hemolytic anemia with, vs hereditary spherocytosis, 486
  technique of, 1498
Copper, deficiency of, anemia with, 304–305
    definition of, 275
    diagnosis and treatment of, 305
    pathogenesis of, 304
    vs Menkes' syndrome, 304–305
  metabolism of, 304
  toxicity of, hemolytic anemia with, 518
COPRO, in porphyria cutanea tarda, 381
COPRO III, excretion of, in coproporphyria, 381
    variegate porphyria and, 380
COPROgen, in heme biosynthesis, 364, 366
Coproporphyria, 381
Coproporphyrinogen decarboxylase, lead effects on, 398
Coproporphyrinogen oxidase, in sideroblastic anemia, 372
Coronary artery abnormalities, in Kawasaki syndrome, 1458
Corticosteroids. See also *Prednisone* and names of other drugs.
  effect on leukocytes, 810(t), 1643
  effect on neutrophil adherence, 820
  for acute graft versus host disease, 247
  for aplastic anemia, 175
  for autoimmune hemolytic anemia, 421
  for Diamond-Blackfan syndrome, 202–204
  for idiopathic thrombocytopenic purpura of childhood, 1356, 1358(t)–1359(t), 1360–1362, 1371
    in pregnant patients, 1373
  for Kasabach Merritt syndrome, 1387
  for neutropenia, 809
  for platelet dysfunction, 1443
  high-dose, for hemolytic uremic syndrome, 438
  in clearance of antibody-coated erythrocytes, 416, 417
Coulter Counter, 269
Coumarin compounds, vitamin K deficiency with, 118, 1328
Craniopharyngioma, 1196
Creatinine height index, 308
Crigler-Najjar syndrome, 85–86
Crohn's disease, folic acid deficiency and, 324
  vitamin B_{12} deficiency with, 348
Cryohydrocytosis, 515–516
Cryoprecipitate, advantages and disadvantages of, 1609
  components of, 1609
  disorders used for, 1301, 1609
  for bleeding in uremia, 1445–1446
  for congenital storage pool deficiency, 1443
  for hemophilia A, 1307
  for von Willebrand's disease, 1318–1319
  transfusion therapy with, 1608–1610
Cryotherapy, for retinoblastoma, 1185

Crystalluria, 357
Cyanosis, in methemoglobinemia, 647
  M hemoglobins with, 634–635
  sulfhemoglobinemia and, 650–651
Cyclic AMP, 1285
  effect on neutrophil adherence, 820
Cyclo-oxygenase, aspirin inhibition of, 1448
  indomethacin and, 1450–1451
  platelet, in aggregation and release, 1285–1286
    in arachidonic acid metabolism, 1448
    defects of, 1439
  sulfinpyrazine and, 1451
Cyclophosphamide (Cytoxan), 1003(t)–1004(t)
  for aplastic anemia, 173–174
  for autoimmune hemolytic anemia, 422
  for bone marrow transplantation preparation, 244
  for childhood ITP refractory to splenectomy, 1370
  for Fanconi's anemia, 183
  in immunosuppression for bone marrow transplantation, 1542
  toxicity to, 249
Cyclosporine, for acute graft versus host disease, 247
  for aplastic anemia, 175
  in kidney transplantation, 1539
Cyst(s), splenic, 903
Cystathionine-B-synthetase deficiency, homocystinuria and, 1457
Cystic fibrosis, 1636, 1645
  conjugated hyperbilirubinemia and, 96
  iron deficiency with, 301
Cytochrome(s), function and distribution of, 276–277
Cytochrome b, neutrophilic, in chronic granulomatous disease, 831
Cytochrome b_5, 277
  in methemoglobin reduction, 645, *645*, 647, 648
    deficiency of, acquired methemoglobinemia and, 635
Cytochrome c, 276–277
  iron deficiency and, 296–297, *297*
Cytochrome P-450, 277
  intestinal, iron deficiency and, 299
  lead toxicity and, 399
Cytogenetic analysis, of tumors, 1479–1496. See also *Chromosome(s), abnormalities of.*
Cytomegalovirus infection, bone marrow transplantation and, 248–249
  granulocyte transfusion and, 1602
  intrauterine, thrombocytopenia and, 113
  lymphoreticular response to, 1120–1121
  post-transfusion, 1585
Cytopenia, in preleukemic myelodysplasic syndromes, 218
  single, 193–213
    classification of, 160(t)
Cytosine arabinoside (Ara-C), properties of, 1002(t)
Cytoxan (cyclophosphamide), 1003(t)–1004(t). See also *Cyclophosphamide.*

D antigen, on Rh-positive erythrocytes, 45–46
  sites on erythrocytes of different genotypes, 46(t)
  vs Rh-negative cells, 46
Dactinomycin (actinomycin-D), 1003(t)

Danazol, for antithrombin III deficiency, 1326
　for autoimmune hemolytic anemia, 423
　for chronic idiopathic thrombocytopenic purpura, 1371
　for hemophilia, 1311
　for lupus erythematosus, 1648
　uses of, 1304
Darrow, Ruth, 10
DDAVP. See *Desmopressin.*
Dearing, B. F., 2
Decay accelerating factor (DAF), 425
Deferoxamine, for beta thalassemia, 751–753
　for liver pathology in beta thalassemia, 746
　for thalassemia intermedia, 755
Degranulation, by phagocytes, 789–790
　definition of, 786
Delivery, traumatic, neonatal anemia and, 31–32
Delves cup technique, for measuring blood lead levels, 406
Dendritic cells, structure and function of, 1119–1120
Dental bleeding, in hemophilia A, 1309–1310
Deoxygenation, molecular sickling and, 656, *657, 658*
　of sickled cells, reversible and irreversible, 663, *663*
Deoxyhemoglobin, 2,3-DPG binding to, 619–620, *620*
　oxygen affinity of, 617–618
　structure of, *617*
Deoxyhemoglobin S, polymer formation of, 659–661, *660–661*
　delay time concept in, 660–662, *662*
Deoxythymidine monophosphate, methylated from deoxyuridine monophosphate, 318
Deoxyuridine suppression test, for folate deficiency diagnosis, 331–332
Dermatan sulfate, mucopolysaccharidoses and, *1231*
Dermatitis, atopic, T cell activity in, 853, 855, 856
　erythematous, with hereditary spherocytosis, 488
　in congenital erythropoietic porphyria, 376
Dermatitis herpetiformis, 1660–1661
Dermatologic manifestations, in acute graft versus host disease, 247
　in congenital erythropoietic protoporphyria, 377
　in dyskeratosis congenita, 188
　in porphyria cutanea tarda, 381
1-Desamino-8-D-arginine vasopressin. See *Desmopressin.*
Desmopressin, advantages and side effects of, 1319(t)
　effects on test of hemostasis, 1319(t)
　for bleeding in liver disease, 1446
　for bleeding in uremia, 1445–1446
　for mild hemophilia, 1311
　for platelet dysfunction, 1443
　for von Willebrand's disease, 1317(t), 1319, 1319(t)
　persons likely to benefit from, 1319(t)
　uses of, 1304
Dextran, platelet function and, 1454
Diabetes mellitus, hematologic complications of, 1658–1659
　HLA linkage in, 1543
　hypercoagulability and, 1456–1457
　in beta thalassemia, 747–748
　maternal, neonatal hyperbilirubinemia and, 89

Diacylglycerol, in platelet signal transduction, 1284
　in protein 4.1 binding, 460, *461*
cis-Diamminodichloroplatinum, properties of, 1005(t)
Diamond, L.K., 9–10
Diamond-Blackfan syndrome, 197–205
　bone marrow transplantation for, 254
　causes of death in, 204
　chromosomes in, 201
　description of, 197–199, 220(t)
　diagnostic criteria for, 197
　inheritance of, 198
　laboratory features of, 199–201
　neonatal, 36
　pathophysiology of, 201–203
　physical abnormalities in, 198(t)
　pregnancy and, 198
　prognosis for, 204–205
　purine metabolism in, 201
　pyrimidine metabolism in, 201
　therapy and outcome of, 203–205, *204*
　vs transient erythroblastopenia of childhood, 205, 205(t), 206
Diarrhea, folic acid malabsorption and, 323–324
　infective, hemolytic uremic syndrome and, 435
　phototherapy and, 91
Diego blood group, 1515, 1515(t)
Diet, cancer chemotherapy and, 987
　cobalamin deficiency and, 344
　deficient, lead absorption and, 391
　folate deficient, 322, 324
　folate requirements in, 318–319
　iron content of, 280–282, 284
　　in infants vs adults, *285*
　　iron deficiency and, 284, 290–291, 299
　　iron requirements and, 284
　　iron supplementation for, 299–300
　lead in, 390–391
　nitrate in, in neonatal methemoglobinemia, 648
　nutritional anemia and, 275
Diethylstilbestrol, cancer risk and, 922
DiGeorge's syndrome, 889
Dihydrofolate reductase deficiency, 325–326
　folate deficiency and, 325
Dihydropteridine reductase deficiency, folate metabolic errors with, 329
Dilantin, folate deficiency with, 324
Dimercaptopropanol (BAL), for lead poisoning, 402, 403(t), *403*, 404
Dimercaptosuccinic acid, for lead poisoning, *403*, 405
2,3-Diphosphoglycerate, binding of, in erythrocyte hexokinase deficiency, 549
　in hemoglobin function, 619–620
　in hypoxic states, 621–622, *621–622*
　in metabolic acidosis, oxygen affinity and, 623
　in neonatal erythrocytes, 24
　in pyruvate kinase deficient red cells, 564–565
　in stored blood, 623
　in uremic red cells, 1639
　postnatal rise in, 624
　red cell osmotic properties and, 462–463
　reduced synthesis of, in 2,3-diphosphoglycerate mutase deficiency, 560
　structure of, 619, *619*
2,3-Diphosphoglycerate mutase deficiency, hemolytic anemia with, 560–561

Diphyllobothrium latum infestation, vitamin B_{12} deficiency with, 349
Diplococcus pneumoniae, postsplenectomy sepsis with, 912
Dipyridamole, platelet function and, 1451
Disseminated intravascular coagulation, causes of, 1330–1332, 1330(t), 1386(t)
  diagnosis of, 1332–1333, 1333(t)
  hemolytic anemia with, 439
  in acute promyelocytic leukemia, 1050
  in infections, 1380, 1650
  in liver disease, 1327, 1638
  in neonates, 115–117, 115(t)
    thrombocytopenia and, 113
  red cell fragmentation in, 433
  risk of, with use of prothrombin complex concentrates, 1302
  schistocytic hemolytic anemia and, 433
  thrombocytopenia and, 113–114, 1385–1386, 1386(t)
    infection-induced, 1380
Diuresis, in lead poisoning, 402
Diuretics, thiazide, thrombocytopenia and, 1394
DNA, analysis of, for identifying linkage between thalassemia mutations and chromosomal haplotypes, 718–721
  of fetal red cells, for prenatal diagnosis of beta thalassemia, 760–762
  defect in, in Fanconi's anemia, 181
  endoreduplication of, in megakaryocyte maturation, 150
  Factor VIII concentrates prepared from clones of, 1303
  fetal, restriction endonuclease analysis of, for sickle cell disease diagnosis, 667
  human tumor, transforming activity of, 960(t)
  information flow gene to protein in, 705–707, *705*, *706*
  radiation effects on, 1020
  rearrangement of, heavy chain class switch and, 865–866
    in B-cell development, 862–863
    in light chain genes, in B-cell leukemia and lymphoma, 864–865, *865*
    in T-cell antigen-specific receptor genes, 872
  repaired defects in, in immunodeficiency with ataxia telangiectasia, 887
  synthesis of, bone marrow, chloramphenicol inhibition of, 163
    relation to oncogenes and growth factors, 966–967
  transfection of, 958
    for examination of relation between cancer and cellular oncogenes, 960–965, 962(t)
DNA tumor viruses, 943–948
  vs RNA tumor viruses, 943
Dohle bodies, in infections, 1649
  in May-Hegglin anomaly, 1391
Donath-Landsteiner cold hemolysis, 420
Down's syndrome, leukemia risk and, 928
  platelet disorders in, 1441
  vs congenital leukemia, 1052–1053
Drugs. See also *Cancer chemotherapy*; and names of specific drugs.
  acute intermittent porphyria due to, 379, 380
  antiplatelet, neonatal hemorrhage and, 114
  antisickling, for sickle cell disease, 667

Drugs *(Continued)*
  antituberculous, sideroblastic anemia and, 371–372
  aplastic anemia associated with, 161–163, 161(t)
  cancer risk and, 922, 923(t)
  eosinopenia with, 1664
  hemolysis due to, in G6PD deficiency, 597–598, 599(t)
    in pregnant women, neonatal jaundice and, 600
  hyperbilirubinemia and, 88
  in bleeding disorders, 1294
  interactions of, in cancer chemotherapy, 987–988, 988(t), 998, 1006, 1006(t)
  megaloblastosis due to, 353(t), 358–359
  membrane-active, platelet dysfunction with, 1453
  neutropenia due to, 806–807
  oxidant, methemoglobinemia and, 647–648, 648(t), 649(t)
  pharmacokinetics of, 987
  platelet dysfunction and, 1447–1455, 1455(t)
  pure red cell aplasia due to, 194, 194(t)
  resistance to, in cancer chemotherapy, 1006–1008
    mechanisms of, 1007–1008
    pleiotropic, 1007
  thrombocytopenia due to, 1373–1379, 1378(t)
    marrow suppression and, 1393
    platelet-associated IgG measurements for, 1406
    platelet-specific suppression and, 1393–1394
  variegate porphyria due to, 380
Duchenne's muscular dystrophy, 1441, 1659–1660
Duffy antigen, 656
Duffy blood group system, 1512–1513, 1513(t)
  malaria resistance and, 1502, 1527
Duke method, of testing bleeding time, 1296
Dust, lead in, 391
Dyserythropoietic anemia, congenital, 207–210, 358
  Type I, 207–208
  Type II, 208–210
  Type III, 210
  with hereditary elliptocytosis, 496
Dysfibrinogenemia, congenital, 1321
Dysgammaglobulinemia, (hyperimmunoglobulin M syndrome), 801, 874–875
Dysgenesis, reticular, 800
Dysgerminoma, ovarian, 1173
Dyskeratosis congenita, 1661
  aplastic anemia and, 188–190, 188(t), *189*
  Fanconi's anemia and, 188(t), 189
  general features of, 220(t)
  neutropenia with, 803
  survival curve in, 190, *190*
Dysprothrombinemia, congenital, 1321–1322

E rosette receptor-negative, γ-Fc receptor-positive cells, in erythropoiesis, 146
EACA. See *Epsilon-aminocaproic acid*.
Ears, in sickle cell disease, 678
Ecchymoses, hyperbilirubinemia and, in newborn, 84
Echinocytes, vs acanthocytes, in hemolytic anemia, 505, *505*

Echinocytosis, 467
Eczema, 1660
  immunodeficiency with, 888–889. See also *Wiskott-Aldrich syndrome.*
EDTA, in direct assays of platelets, 1403
  platelet clumping due to, 1346
Ehlers-Danlos syndrome, 1661
Electronic cell counting, 267, 269, 269(t), 271
  in screening tests for iron deficiency anemia, 289, 290
Elliptocytosis, hereditary, 490–503
  clinical subtypes of, 491–497, 492(t)
    common, 491, *493*, 496–497
      Melanesian (stomatocytic), 497
      spherocytic, 497
  effects of heat on red cells in, *493*
  etiology and pathogenesis of, 497–502, *498–499, 501*
  genetics of, 490
  hereditary pyropoikilocytosis, 496
  history of, 490
  homozygous, 496
  mild, 491
  neonatal, 36
  pathophysiology of, 502–503
  peripheral blood morphology in, *493*
  prevalence of, 490–491
  silent carrier state in, 491
  with chronic hemolysis, 496
  with dyserythropoiesis, 496
  with infantile poikilocytosis, 491, 496
Embden-Meyerhof pathway, 21, 23, *546*
  enzymes of, in fetal erythrocytes, 21, 23
Emboli, from prosthetic heart valves, antiplatelet agents and, 1453
Embryonal carcinoma, 1169
  of testes, 1176–1177
Embryonic hemoglobins, 624–625, *625*
Embryonic tumors, chromosomal changes in, 1490–1492
En blood group system, 1514
Encephalopathy, bilirubin. See *Kernicterus.*
  lead poisoning and, clinical aspects of, 400–401
    heme synthesis damage and, 399
Endocarditis, subacute bacterial, 1634
Endocrine disorders, hematologic complications in, 1641–1644
  in iron overload in beta thalassemia, 746–748
  in juvenile pernicious anemia, 346–347, 346(t)
  in leukemia survivors, 1052
Endocytosis, by phagocytes, 788–789
  receptor mediated, 455, 789
    definition of, 786, *786*
Endodermal sinus (yolk sac) tumor, 1170, 1174
  of testis, 1176
Endothelial cells, arachidonic acid transformation in, platelet function and, 1285–1287
  platelet interactions with, 1278–1279
Enolase, deficiency of, hemolytic anemia with, 561
  in neonatal red cells, 21, 24
Enzyme(s), assays for, in diagnosis of methemoglobinemia, 649
  erythrocyte, glycolytic mechanism and, 573
    in adults, 1681(t), 1682(t)
  G6PD. See *Glucose-6-phosphate dehydrogenase.*
  genetic heterogeneity of 1573–1574
  hereditary deficiencies of, 36

Enzyme(s) *(Continued)*
  lead sensitive, 392
  lysosomal, function of, 1213–1214
    genes coding for, 1214, 1214(t)
    in storage disease diagnosis, 1220, 1222
    replacement therapy with, 1222–1223
  of Embden-Meyerhof pathway, in fetal erythrocyte, 21, 23
  proteins of, mutant, 546(t)
Enzymopathies, acquired, 573–574
  congenital. See also *Hemolytic anemia, congenital nonspherocytic.*
    red cell transfusion for, 1582
    early investigations of, 12–13
  glycolytic, hemolytic anemia and, 545–572. See also *Hemolytic anemia, congenital nonspherocytic.*
Eosinopenia, 815, 1663–1664
Eosinophil(s), altered numbers of, clinical states associated with, 812–815
  function of, 813–814, 813(t)
  hereditary constitutional hypersegmentation of, 1662
  in acute myelomonocytic leukemia, 1485, *1485*
  kinetics of, 812
  normal levels of, 812
  production of, 812
  stimulation of, 812
  structure of, 812–813
Eosinophil progenitor, vs granulocyte macrophage progenitor, 142
Eosinophilia, 1663–1664
  causes of, 814–815, 814(t), 1664(t)
  in infections, 1650
  in pulmonary disease, 1645
Eosinophilic gastroenteritis, 1635
Eosinophilic granuloma, in histiocytosis X, 1129, 1130, *1130*
Eosinophilic leukemia, 815
Ependymoma, 1193–1194
Epinephrine, neutrophil adherence and, 820
  neutrophilia with, 811
Epithelial tissues, in malnutrition, 308
Epsilon-aminocaproic acid (EACA), for oral bleeding in hemophilia A, 1310, 1311
  for platelet dysfunction, 1443
  uses of, 1304
Epstein-Barr virus, antigens of, 1657
  aplastic anemia and, 164, 187
  Burkitt's lymphoma and, 929, 1094
  diseases associated with, 946–947
  for B cell function assays, 851
  infectious mononucleosis and, 1651–1652
  lymphoreticular response to, 1120–1121
  pediatric AIDS and, 891, *891*
  transmission of, 1652–1653
  unusual response to, immunodeficiency with, 889
  virus-associated hemophagocytic syndrome and, 1127
  X-linked immunodeficiency to, 1122–1126
Epstein syndrome, 1441
Erythroblast(s), dyserythropoietic, 207–208
  globin gene expression in, 130–131
Erythroblastopenia, chronic idiopathic with aplastic anemia. See *Diamond-Blackfan syndrome.*
  transient of childhood, 205–207
    vs Diamond-Blackfan syndrome, 205, 205(t), 206

Erythroblastosis fetalis, 9–10
  pure red cell aplasia and, 194
  thrombocytopenia with, 1389
Erythrocytapheresis, 1626, 1628, 1634
Erythrocytes. See *Red cell(s); Red cell membrane.*
Erythrocytosis, in renal disease, 1640
  with hemoglobin variants, 633–634
Erythrodontia, 376
Erythrogenesis imperfecta. See *Diamond-Blackfan syndrome.*
Erythroid burst-forming units (BFU-E). See *Burst-forming units–erythroid.*
Erythroid cells, development of, in Diamond-Blackfan syndrome, 199, 200, 201
  differentiation of, burst-promoting activity and, 145–146
  hyperplasia of, in congenital dyserythropoietic anemia, 208
    in sideroblastic anemia, 374
  hyperproduction of, in hereditary spherocytosis, 484
  iron uptake in, 369–370
  maturation of, 140–141, *140*
  precursors of, proliferation of, 137–139
  progenitor cells of, 138–139
  stem cells of, in Diamond-Blackfan syndrome, 202
    in HEMPAS, 210
Erythroid colonies, formation of, in Diamond-Blackfan syndrome, 201–202
  growth of, in pure red cell aplasia, 196
Erythroid colony-forming units (CFU-E). See *Colony-forming unit-erythroid.*
Erythroid disorders, bone marrow transplantation for, 254
Erythroid failure. See *Aplastic crisis.*
Erythroid potentiating activity (EPA), in humoral control of hematopoiesis, 143
Erythron, 140
Erythrophagocytosis, in hereditary spherocytosis, 482
Erythropoiesis, 137–141. See also *Red cell(s).*
  adrenal gland disorders and, 1643
  development of, in neonate, 16–19
  differentiation in, 138–139
  disorders of. See also specific types of anemia and names of specific disorders (e.g., *Porphyrias(s); Copper, deficiency of; Lead poisoning,* etc.).
    in anemia classification, 266(t)
    neonatal, 36
  fetal, 18, 129–131, *130*
    progenitors of, 17
  growth hormone and, 1644
  in chronic disorders, 1646
  in Fanconi's anemia, 180
  ineffective, 275. See also *Dyserythropoietic anemia.*
    classification of, 266(t)
    in beta thalassemia, 739–740
    in hemolytic anemia, folate deficiency and, 324–325
    in lead intoxication, 400
    in megaloblastic anemia, 316
    in sideroblastic anemia, 374
    in vitamin B_{12} deficiency, 355
    reticulendothelial system function and, 431
  inhibition of, in Diamond-Blackfan syndrome, 201
  iron deficiency, syndromes associated with, 302–303
  megaloblastic, in embryo, 16

Erythropoiesis *(Continued)*
  neonatal, 37, 39
    development of, 16–19, 278–279, *278, 279, 703*
    impaired, 36
  normoblastic, in embryo, 16
  precursor differentiation of, 140–141
  progenitors of, 137–139
    morphology of, 140–141, *140*
  radioactive patterns in, 141, *141*
  rate of, during development, 278–279, *278, 279*
  regulation of, 144–147
  sites of, during development, *703*
  stress. See *Stress erythropoiesis.*
  thyroid hormone effect on, 1641
Erythropoietic porphyria, congenital, 376–377
Erythropoietic protoporphyria, congenital, 377–378
Erythropoietin, CFU-E production and, 138
  in aplastic anemia, 168
  in chronic disorders, 1646
  in Diamond-Blackfan syndrome, 202, 203
  in erythrocyte production, 138
  in erythroid differentiation, 139
  in erythropoiesis regulation, in fetus, 18
  sites of, 144–145
  in Rh hemolytic disease, 54
  in stress erythropoiesis, 139
  in thrombopoiesis, 148
  neonatal, 37, 39
Erythrostases, hereditary spherocytosis pathology and, 478–479, *480*
Escherichia coli, 436, 1503
Esophagus, disease of, 1635
Estradiol, in clearance of IgG-coated erythrocytes, 416
Estren-Damshek familial aplasia, 178, 179, 186
Estrogens, acute intermittent porphyria and, 379
  thrombocytopenia and, 1394
Ethanol gel test, 1300
Etiocholanolone, for Fanconi's anemia, 183, *183*
Euglobulin clot lysis time test, 1300
Evans' syndrome, 423–424
Ewing's sarcoma, 1166–1169
  chromosomal changes in, 1492
  extraosseous, 1161, 1166
  of soft tissue, 1161
Exchange transfusion, anemia following, 65
  bilirubin concentration and, in neonates, 89, 89(t)
  blood loss and, iron deficiency and, 285
  for autoimmune hemolytic anemia, 423
  for Crigler-Najjar syndrome, 85
  for disseminated intravascular coagulation, 116–117
  for G6PD deficient jaundiced newborn, 600
  for hyperbilirubinemia with Rh erythroblastosis, 83–84
  for Rh hemolytic disease, 61–65
  for sickle cell disease, 683
  neonatal thrombocytopenia and, 114
  platelet transfusion for, 1593
  thrombocytopenia following, 1389–1390
Exons, vs introns, *1534*
Extremities, rhabdomyosarcoma of, 1158
Eyes. See also *Retinoblastoma.*
  abnormalities of, in sickle cell disease, 677–678
  enucleation of, in retinoblastoma, 1184
  in acute leukemia, 1039

F cells, in stress erythropoiesis, 139
Fabry's disease, 1224, 1226
Factor(s), vitamin K dependent, in liver disease, 1637
Factor B, gene frequencies of, 1568(t)
 genetic polymorphism of, 1567, *1567*
Factor H (P$_{1H}$-globulin), 1566
Factor I. See *Fibrinogen.*
Factor II. See *Prothrombin.*
Factor V/Va, activation of, 1255, *1255*
 deficiency of, 1322
 in liver disease, 1638
 in platelets, 1432
 in thrombin generation, 1254–1255
 sensitivity to action of protein Ca, 1256–1257
Factor VII, deficiency of, 1322
 in coagulation cascade, 1253
 in conversion of Factor IX to Factor IXa, 1255
 in liver disease, 1327
 proteolysis by Factor XIIa and, 1256
Factor VIII, assays measuring, 1299
 complexed to von Willebrand's factor, 1252
  hemolytic uremic syndrome and, 436
  in platelet adhesion, 1344
  in thrombotic thrombocytopenic purpura, 438
  properties and nomenclature of, 1316(t)
 concentrates of. See also *Cryoprecipitate.*
  advantages and disadvantages of, 1610–1611
  commercially prepared, 1301
  dosage of for hemophilia A, 1307, 1308(t)
  for hemophiliac inhibitors, 1313–1314
  from cloned DNA, 1303
  heat-treated, 1301
  porcine, 1302, 1611
   for hemophiliac inhibitors, 1313–1314
  preparation of, 1610
  transfusion therapy with, 1610–1611, 1610(t)
  uses of, in coagulation disorders, 1301–1302
 control mechanism governing, 1255
 deficiency of. See also *Hemophilia A.*
  in screening tests for bleeding, 1296
  vs von Willebrand's disease, 1253
 in coagulation cascade, 1251–1252
 in cryoprecipitate, 1608. See also *Cryoprecipitate.*
 in liver disease, 1638
 in neonates, 106
 inhibitor of, acquired, 1330
  measurement of, 1299
 structure of, *1252*
Factor IX/IXa (Christmas factor), antithrombin action and, 1264
 concentrates of, 1303
 deficiency of. See *Hemophilia B.*
 for hemophilia B, dosage of, 1312(t)
 in coagulation cascade, 1251, *1251*, 1253
 in nephrotic syndrome, 1640
Factor X/Xa, antithrombin action of, 1264
 conversion of Factor X to Xa, 1249–1253
  control mechanisms governing, 1255
 deficiency of, 1322–1323
 in coagulation cascade, 1251, 1253
 in thrombin generation, 1251, 1254
 interaction with Factor Va in conversion of prothrombin to thrombin, 1255
 interaction with Factor IX, control mechanisms governing, 1255

Factor XI/XIa, antithrombin action and, 1264
 deficiency of, 1323–1324
 in coagulation cascade, 1250
 in liver disease, 1638
Factor XII/XIIa, antithrombin action and, 1264
 deficiency of, 1324
 in conversion of plasminogen to plasmin, 1260
 in disseminated intravascular coagulation, 1331, 1385
 in intrinsic coagulation cascade, 1249–1250, *1250*
 in liver disease, 1638
 in nephrotic syndrome, 1640–1641
Factor XIII/XIIIa, 1563
 deficiency of, 1299, 1323
 gene frequencies of, 1563(t), 1564(t)
 in formation of crosslinked fibrin clot, 1258, *1259*
 in liver disease, 1638
Failure to thrive, in vitamin B$_{12}$ malabsorption, 348
Familial erythrophagocytic lymphohistiocytosis, 1121–1122, *1122*
Familial hemophagocytic reticulosis, 1121–1122
Familial hyperbetalipoproteinemia, 1659
Fanconi, Guido, 8
Fanconi's anemia, age at diagnosis, *177*
 Bloom's syndrome and, 215–216
 bone marrow transplantation for, 251
 complications of, 184-186, 184(t)
 cytogenetic findings in, 180–182, *181*
 diagnosis of, 181
 dyskeratosis congenita and, 188(t), 189
 erythrocyte hexokinase deficiency and, 547
 general features of, 176–179, 220(t)
 genetic characteristics of, 178–180
 laboratory findings in, 179–181
 neutropenia with, 803
 oncogenic sensitivity in, 180
 pathophysiology of, 181–182
 physical findings in, 177(t), 178–179, 178(t)
 pluripotent stem cells in, aplastic anemia and, 167
 prognosis for, 182–183
 therapy and outcome of, androgen therapy, *182*, 183, *183*
  supportive care, 183
 thrombocytopenia with, 1391
 vs thrombocytopenia absent radii syndrome, 113, 211–212, 212(t)
 with lead encephalopathy, 400
Farber, Sidney, 11–12
Farber's disease, 1229
Fatty acid–binding protein, 77
Fatty acid deficiency, 1659
Fatty acids, long chain unesterified, breast milk jaundice and, 87
 of red cell membrane phospholipids, acylation pathway of, 448
 motion of, 446
 thrombocytopenia associated with, 1390
Fava beans, 599
Fc fragment, of IgG, in clearance of IgG-coated erythrocytes, 414, 416
 in opsonic expression of IgG, 787
 on granulocyte-macrophage progenitor cells, 798
 receptors of, in autoimmune hemolytic anemia, 419, 421

Fc fragment *(Continued)*
  receptors of, in neutrophils, 824
    in phagocytes, 430
    reticuloendothelial function and, 1349–1351
Febrile nonhemolytic reaction, 1586
FEIBA, 1303, 1613
  for inhibitor hemophiliacs, 1314
Felty's syndrome, 1647
  autoimmune neutropenia with, 806
Femoral head, aseptic necrosis, in sickle cell anemia, 678
Ferris hydroxides, formation of, 366
Ferritin, function and distribution of, 277
  in erythrocyte destruction in Rh hemolytic disease, 53–54
  in iron metabolism, 370
  serum, for familial hemochromatosis diagnosis, 303
    for iron deficiency diagnosis, 286, 286(t), 291, 291(t)
    vs chronic inflammatory disease, 293–294
  in iron loading in beta thalassemia, 744
Ferrochelatase, effects of lead on, 394, *395, 396*
  in congenital erythropoietic protoporphyria, 377
  in heme synthesis, 364, 366
  in sideroblastic anemia, 372–373
  in variegate porphyria, 380–381
Ferrokinetic studies, of aplastic anemia, 165–166
Ferrous sulfate, for iron deficiency, 295
Fetus. See also *Red cell(s), fetal.*
  anemia of, in Rh hemolytic disease, 54
  bilirubin metabolism in, 55, 81–82
  coagulation factors in, 1692(t)
  cobalamin deficiency in, 344
  development of, iron compounds during, 278–279
  erythropoiesis in, 129–131, *130*
    in Fanconi's anemia, 180
  fetal to fetal hemorrhage in, 31
  fetal to maternal hemorrhage in, 29–31, 30(t)
  hematopoiesis in, 16–19
  hemoglobin of. See *Hemoglobin, fetal.*
  iron requirements of, 368
  liver of, used in bone marrow transplantation, 244
  Rh hemolytic disease in, anemia from, 54
    prevention of death from, 58–61
    response to erythrocyte destruction in, 54–55
    treatment of, 60–61
  scalp platelet count in, in chronic idiopathic thrombocytogenic purpura, 1373
  sickle cell disease diagnosis in, 667
  vascular-platelet interactions in, 1692(t)
Fibrin, dissolution of, by fibrinolytic mechanism, 1258–1262
  polymerization of, 1258, *1259*
Fibrin clots, degradation of by plasmin products, 1261–1262
  formation of, 1257–1258, *1259*
Fibrin degradation products, in uremia, 1640
  tests for, 1300
Fibrin monomers, in liver disease, 1637
  tests for, 1300
Fibrinogen, congenital abnormalities of, 1320–1321
  consumption of, thrombocytopenia with, 1385–1388

Fibrinogen *(Continued)*
  conversion to fibrin, 1257–1258
  degradation of, by plasmin, 1261, *1261, 1262*
  in liver disease, 1637, 1640
  in neonates, normal values for, 105(t), 108
  in platelet aggregation, 1430–1431
  in platelet granules, 1432
  measurement of, 1299
  platelet binding of, 1281, *1283*
  purified dried, 1613
  structure of, 1257, *1259*
Fibrinogen degradation products, in liver disease, 1446
Fibrinolamellar carcinoma, 1179
Fibrinolysis, agents inhibiting, 304
  antiplasmin, 1265
  in neonates, 106–107
  measurement of, 1300
  mechanism of, 1258–1262
  regulation of, 1261
  therapy using, for hemolytic uremic syndrome, 438
Fibrinonectin, 431
  in platelets, 1281–1282, 1432
Fibrinopeptide A, in conversion of fibrinogen to fibrin, 1257
  in fibrinogen proteolysis, 1261
  in thrombus formation, 1262
Fibrin-stabilizing factor (Factor XIII), deficiency of, 1323
Fibrosarcoma, 1159–1160
FIGLU. See *Formiminoglutamic acid.*
Fisher Autocytometer, 269
Fitzgerald-Williams-Flaujeac factor, 1250
Fletcher factor (prekallikrein), in coagulation cascade, 1249
  deficiency of, 1324
Flipase, 445
Fluid and electrolyte therapy, for malnutrition, 309
Foam cells, in storage diseases, 1217, 1217(t), *1218*
Folate. See also *Megaloblastic anemia.*
  absorption of, 317–318, 319(t)
  analogs of, folate deficiency with, 328
  biochemistry of, 317–320
  clearance test for, 332
  deficiency of. See *Folate deficiency.*
  depletion in humans, 318
  developmental changes affecting serum levels of, 320
  dietary requirements for, 318–319
  dietary sources of, 318–319, 320(t)
  excretion of, 318
  for folate deficiency, 333–334
  for vitamin B_{12} deficiency, 357
  in antimetabolite therapy, 11–12
  in sideroblastic anemia, 374–375
  interconversion of, defective, 325–326
  malabsorption of, acquired disorders of, 323–324
    congenital disorders of, 322–323
  megaloblastic anemia of infancy and, 7
  metabolism of, 317–318, 319(t)
    inborn errors affecting, 325–330, 325(t)
  red cell, 331, 33(t)
  serum, 331, 331(t), 355
  utilization of, defective, 326–328
Folate deficiency, causes of, 321–329
  defective absorption, 322–324, *323,* 323(t)
  inadequate intake, 321–322
  increased excretion, 328–329

Folate deficiency (Continued)
  causes of, increased requirements, 324–325
    metabolic disorders, 325–328
  clinical manifestations of, 330
  diagnosis of, 333
    therapeutic trial in, 332–333
  in anemia with kidney diseases, 1639–1640
  in beta thalassemia, 754
  iron deficiency and, 294
  laboratory findings in, 330–333
  treatment of, 333–334
  vitamin B_{12} deficiency and, 333, 343
Folic acid. See Folate.
Food, folate content in, 320(t)
  lead in, 390–391
Formiminoglutamic acid, excretion test with, 332, 332
Formiminotransferase deficiency, folate deficiency with, 326–327, 327(t)
Fructose-6-phosphate, in pentose pathway, 584
Fructosemia, conjugated hyperbilirubinemia and, 96
Fucosidosis, 1238–1239
Fungal infections, with bone marrow transplantation, 248
Fy antigen, 1512–1513

Galactose-1-phosphate uridyl transferase, 1574
Galactosemia, conjugated hyperbilirubinemia and, 96
Galactosialidosis, 1236–1237
Gallbladder disease, in hereditary spherocytosis, 487–489
Gallstones, in hereditary spherocytosis, 487
Gamma globulin, anti-D, 57–58, 57(t), 58(t)
  for autoimmune hemolytic anemia, 423
  for X-linked agammaglobulinemia, 882
Gamma glutamyl carboxypeptidase, 317
Gamma interferon, monocyte-macrophage activation of, 1121
  T-cell use of, 856
Ganglioneuroblastoma, 1138
Ganglioneuroma, 1138
Gangliosidoses, G_{M1}, 1229–1230
  G_{M2}. See also Tay-Sachs disease.
    Sandhoff variant, 1230
Gardos phenomenon, 465, 465, 479, 480
  in sickle cells, 664–665
Gasser, Conrad, 8
Gastrectomy, total, 347
Gastric mucosal disease, intrinsic factor deficiency with, 347
Gastric resection, 1635
Gastritis, chronic atrophic, 1635
Gastroenteritis, eosinophilic, 1635
Gastrointestinal bleeding, aspirin ingestion and, 1450
Gastrointestinal disorders, eosinophilia and, 814
  hematologic complications with, 1635–1636
  in acute leukemia, 1038–1039
  in graft versus host disease, 247
  iron deficiency anemia and, 298–299
Gastrointestinal tract, hemorrhage in, in neonate, 119
  iron absorption by, in beta thalassemia, 743–745
    transfusion therapy and, 749
Gaucher cell, 1218–1219, 1218
Gaucher's disease, 1226–1227
  bone marrow transplantation for, 255–256
  conjugated hyperbilirubinemia and, 96

Gc-globulin, genetic polymorphism of, 1559–1560, 1559, 1560
Gel electrophoresis, for study of platelet membrane glycoproteins, 1461
Gelsolin, actin assembly in platelets and, 1276
  in phagocytes, 788–789
Gene(s). See also DNA; Chromosome(s); Oncogenes; RNA.
  antigen-specific T-cell receptor, DNA rearrangements in, 872
  c-myc, 947
    translocation of, in Burkitt's lymphoma, 873
  exons of, 705, 707
  expression of, enhancer sequences and, 728
  families and superfamilies of, 1536
  for blood groups, 1499
  for hemoglobin, 701–702
  for lysosomal enzyme activities, 1214, 1214(t)
  for plasma proteins, localization and evolution for, 1572–1573
  globin. See Globin genes.
  HLA complex, 1524–1525
    polymorphism of, 1525–1531
  HLA linkage group, 1525
  HLA-linked, 1542–1543
  immunoglobulin, 861–862, 866
    heavy chain locus in, 862, 862, 865–866
      molecular basis of disorders of, 868–869
    heavy chain rearrangement in, 867–868
      in B-cell precursor acute lymphoblastic leukemia, 869–870, 869
    light chain locus of, DNA rearrangements in B-cell leukemia and lymphoma, 864–865, 865
      kappa, 863–864, 863
      lambda, 864, 865
    mediation of chromosomal translocations by, 873–874
    sequence joining of, 866–867
  information flow to protein from, 705–707, 705, 706
  introns of, 705, 707
  major histocompatibility complex, in MHC linkage group, 1525
    molecular structure of, 1533–1535
  mapping of, 1517, 1522
  migration of, 1527
  mutations of causing thalassemia, 707, 708(t)–711(t), 714–715. See also Thalassemia mutations.
  nature of, 707, 707, 710
  PI, variants of, 1552–1554, 1554(t)
  RNA transcription of, 706
  sickle cell, polymorphism of, 1527
  v-onc, 950, 954
Gene therapy, for beta thalassemia, 757–758
Genetic disorders, cancer risk in children and, 924–927, 925(t)–926(t)
Genetic drift, 1527
Genetic linkage disequilibrium, 1530–1531
Genetic markers, amino acid differences and, 1572(t)
  blood group tests and, 1516
  cell surface, 1499–1500, 1522–1523. See also HLA complex, genetics of.
  in acute lymphoblastic leukemia, 1034–1035
  in Hodgkin's disease, 1092
  other than cell surface, 1550–1572
Genetics, molecular, cellular events in, 1534
  of HLA complex, 1533–1536
  of alpha thalassemia, 733–734
  of beta thalassemia, 740–742

Genetics *(Continued)*
   of G6PD deficiency, 583–584, 588–593
   of lysosomal storage diseases, 1214–1215, 1214(t)
   of methemoglobinemia, 646–647
   of retinoblastoma, 1181–1182
Genital tract, female, rhabdomyosarcoma of, 1158
Genitourinary tract, in acute leukemia, 1037–1038
Gerbich blood group, 1514
Germ cell tumors, 1169–1179
   anatomic distribution of, 1171–1179, 1171(t)
   head and neck, 1178–1179
   histologic variants of, 1169–1171
   intra-abdominal, 1179
   mediastinal, 1178
   no-germ malignancies in, 1170–1171
   ovarian, 1172–1174
   retroperitoneal, 1179
   sacrococcygeal, 1171–1172
   testicular, 1175–1179
   tumor markers of, 1171, 1171(t)
Germinoma, 1169
   mediastinal, 1178
Ghosts, red cell membrane, 443, 444(t), *498*
Gilbert's syndrome, Arias syndrome and, 85–86
   hyperbilirubinemia and, 84
   vs congenital dyserythropoietic anemia, 210
GL-4, red cell membrane, 443, *444*
Glanzmann's thrombasthenia, 114, 1282, 1436–1437
Glioma, brainstem, 1191–1192
   optic, 1190
Globin. See also *Hemoglobin.*
   beta:alpha biosynthetic ratio, in beta thalassemia trait, 734–735
     in severe beta thalassemia, 739, *739*, 740
   biosynthesis of, during development, 702, *703*
     in prenatal diagnosis of beta thalassemia, 760
   crossover, 724, 726, *726*
   delta synthesis of, in beta thalassemia trait, 735–736
   gamma, in hereditary persistence of fetal hemoglobin, 712
     increased synthesis of, in treatment of beta thalassemia, 756–757
   polypeptide chains of, 613–614
     alpha, 614–616, *614*
     beta, 614–616, *615*
   stability of, mutations affecting, 717–718
   structural variants of, interaction with thalassemia and, 758–759
Globin genes, alpha, 701–702, *702*
   deletion mutations in, 721–723, *722*
   effect on beta thalassemia trait, 741–742, 741(t)
   elongated, 730, 731
   in hemoglobin H disease, 729
   in silent carrier alpha thalassemia, 730
   mutations affecting, 703
   physicochemical properties of, 700
   terminator codon mutations in, 716–717, *717*
   beta, 701–702, *702*
     biosynthetic imbalance in, in severe thalassemia, 739–740
     frameworks of, 720, *720*
     in beta thalassemia, 703

Globin genes *(Continued)*
   beta, mutations affecting fetal hemoglobin synthesis, 723–729
     physicochemical properties of, 700
     premature termination mutations in, 716
     promoter of, mutations of causing thalassemia, 710, *710*, 712
     restriction endonuclease fragment length polymorphism in, 718–720, *719*, *720*
   chromosomal organization of, 701–702, *702*
   expression of, in fetal switch of hemoglobin synthesis, 130–131
     molecular events during, *705*
   functional elements of, *707*
   linkage to mutations causing thalassemia, 704
   structure of, 707, *707*, 710
   synthesis of, disorders of. See also *Sickle cell disease; Thalassemia.*
     effects of lead on, 398
Globulin, Gc, 1559–1560, *1559–1560*
   B_{1H} (Factor H), 1566
   vitamin D–binding, 1559–1560, *1559–1560*
Glomerular disease, thrombocytopenia in, 1388
   C3 deficiency in, 896
Glossitis, 343
Glucocorticoid administration, neutrophilia with, 811
Glucose, biosynthesis of, in hexokinase deficiency cells, 549
   consumption of. See also *Glycolysis.*
     in neonatal erythrocytes, 24
   metabolism of, in pentose pathway, G6PD role in, 587–588
Glucose-6-phosphate, affinity of G6PD for, 587, 595–596
   in erythrocyte glycolysis, 584–588
   in G6PD deficiency, 506
Glucose-6-phosphate dehydrogenase, activity level in tissues, 594
   characteristics and structure of, 587
   dosage compensation effect and, 588
   function of, 584–588, *585*
   in chronic myelogenous leukemia, 1066–1067
   instability of, 594
   mutants of, 589, 591
     congenital nonspherocytic hemolytic anemia associated, 595–596, 601–602, *603*
     Gd^{A-}, 591, 593–594
       activity in leukocytes, 594
       acute hemolysis and, 593–594, *594*
       hemolytic crisis in, 597–598
       in steady state, 597
       sickle cell anemia and, 600
       vs $Gd^{Mediterranean}$, 598(t)
     Gd^{A+}, 591, 597
     Gd^{B}, 591
     $Gd^{Mediterranean}$, 591, 597
       favism in, 599
       hemolytic crisis in, 597, 598
       thalassemia trait and, 601
       vs Gd^{A-}, 598(t)
     in Africa, 592
   pentose pathway and, 584, *586*, 587
   purification of, 587
   red cell age and, 593–594
   regulatory role of, 587–588
Glucose-6-phosphate dehydrogenase deficiency, biochemistry of, 593–596
   chronic hemolysis and, 601–602, *603*
   clinical effects of, 596–601

Glucose-6-phosphate dehydrogenese deficiency *(Continued)*
  congenital nonspherocytic hemolytic anemia and, 595–596, 601–602, *603*
  diagnosis of, 601–604
    detection of heterozygote in, 602
    in patients with sickle cell anemia, 600
    methods of, 601
    screening for, 602–604
  discovery of, 583–584
  early investigation of, 13
  favism and, 599
  frequency of, 592
  genetic heterogeneity of, 589, 591
  genetic polymorphism of, 583–584
  genetics of, 588–593
  genotypes in, 588, 588(t)
  hemolytic crisis in, 594–595, 597–599
  in neutrophilia, 832
  in steady state, 596–597
  malarial hypothesis and, 591–592
  methemoglobin elution test for, *590*
  neonatal jaundice and, 599–600
  of erythrocytes, hyperbilirubinemia and, 84
  racial distribution of, 591–592
  sickle cell anemia and, 600–601, 655–656
  thalassemia trait and, 601
  treatment of, 604
  X linkage of, 592–593
Glucose phosphate isomerase, hemolytic anemia and, 550–553, 551(t)
Glucose transport protein, 454–455
Glucosylceramide lipidoses, 1226–1227
β-Glucuronidase deficiency, 1234
Glucuronyl transferase, bilirubin metabolism in newborn, 56, 81
  breast milk jaundice in, 86–87
  deficiency of, type I inherited, 85
    type II inherited, 85–86
      vs type I glucuronyl transferase deficiency, 86
  pyloric stenosis and, 88
  uridine diphosphate and, 78
Glutamate formiminotransferase deficiency, folate deficiency and, 326–327, 327(t)
Glutamyl-cysteine synthetase deficiency, 604
Glutathione, biosynthesis of, *605*
  defective cycle of, 833
  for methemoglobinemia, 644
  instability of, in neonatal erythrocytes, 25
  metabolism of, abnormalities of, 604–606
  stability test of, for G6PD deficiency, 602
Glutathione peroxidase deficiency, 606, 834, 836
Glutathione peroxidase-glutathione reductase, in hemolytic crisis, is G6PD deficiency, 594–595, *595*
Glutathione reductase deficiency, 606, 833–834
Glutathione synthetase deficiency, 834
  with 5-oxoprolinuria, 605–606, *605*
  without 5-oxoprolinuria, 604
Glyceraldehyde-3-phosphate, in methemoglobin reduction, 643
  in pentose pathway, 584
Glyceraldehyde-3-phosphate dehydrogenase deficiency, hemolytic anemia with, 556–557
Glyceryl guaiacolate, platelet function and, 1454
Glycine metabolism, defective, folate deficiency with, 329
Glycocalin, thrombin-binding function of, 1281, 1430

Glycogenosis type IV, conjugated hyperbilirubinemia and, 96
Glycolipids, in polymorphonuclear leukocytes, 780
  red cell membrane, 443, *444*
  organization of, 445
Glycolysis, defects of, platelet function and, 1278
  erythrocyte, acquired disorders of, 572–574
    glucose-6-phosphate in, 584–588
    in fetal erythrocytes, 21, 23–25
    in pyruvate kinase-deficient erythrocytes, 564
  G6PD function and, 584–588
  in polymorphonuclear leukocytes, 780
  inhibition of, in methemoglobin reduction, 643–644
  intermediates in, in normal red cells in adults, 1682(t)
    in pyruvate kinase–deficient red cells, 564, *564*
Glycophorin(s), red cell membrane, malaria and, 452, 1502–1503
Glycophorin A, function of, 451
  protein 4.1 binding to, 460
  structure of, 449–451, *450*
  variants of, 451–452
Glycophorin B, function of, 451
  structure of, 451
  variants of, 451–452
Glycophorin C, deficiency of, 502
  function of, 451
  hereditary defects of, 494(t)–495(t), *501*, 502
  structure of, 451
  variants of, 451–452
β$_2$-Glycoprotein I, 1564
Glycoprotein(s), α$_1$-acid, genetic polymorphism of, 1554–1555, *1554*, 1555(t)
  growth factors of, hematopoietic, 143
  LFA-1, function of, 819, 820(t)
  Mol, abnormal chemotaxis and, 823
    function of, 819, 820(t)
  of granulocyte plasma membrane, congenital deficiency of, 819–820, 820(t)
  p150,95, function of, 819, 820(t)
  platelet membrane, inherited disorders of, Bernard-Soulier syndrome, 1433, 1436
    Glanzmann's thrombasthenia, 1436–1437
    Ib, 1280–1281, *1280*, *1283*
      deficiency of, in Bernard-Soulier syndrome, 1433, 1436
      in platelet adhesion, 1344
      structure and function of, 1430, *1430*
    IIb/IIIa complex, 1281–1282, *1283*
      in Glanzmann's thrombasthenia, 1436–1437
      in platelet aggregation, 1345, 1430–1431, *1431*
    V, function of, 1431
    IX, function of, 1431
      relation with glycoprotein Ib, 1430, *1430*
    techniques used to study, 1461–1463
Goat's milk, folate intake and, 311–322
Gompertzian growth pattern of tumors, 990–991
  protocol design and, 992–993, *993*
Gonadal dysfunction, with bone marrow transplantation, 249
Gonadoblastoma, 1170

Goodpasture's syndrome, iron deficiency with, 302
Gout, with hereditary spherocytosis, 488
Graft rejection, in bone marrow transplantation, 246, 251, 1540
  major histocompatibility complex system and, 1523
Graft versus host disease. See also *Bone marrow transplantation.*
  acute, 248
  acute vs chronic, 247
  chronic, 247, 249, 251, 853, 853(t)
  donor selection and, 243, 244
  in bone marrow transplantation, 242–243, 246–248, 251, 256, 1540–1541
  leukemia relapse and, 253
  modification of, 243
  T-cell control of B-cell function and, 853, 853(t)
  transfusion associated, 1584
  with bone marrow transplantation for aplastic anemia, 251
  with granulocyte transfusion, 1602
Graft versus leukemia effect, 253
Granulation disturbances, in leukocytes, 1662–1663
Granules, platelet, 1277
Granulocyte(s), circulating, in megaloblastic anemia, 316
  disorders of, bone marrow transplantation for, 254
    quantitative, basophilic disorders, 816–817, 816(t)
      eosinophil number alteration, 812–815
      monocyte disorders, 817–818
      neutropenia, 799–810, 810(t). See also *Neutropenia.*
      neutrophilia, 810–812, 810(t)
  function of, disorders of, 818–836
    disorders of chemotaxis and cell movement, 821–824
    disorders of degranulation, 826–828
    disorders of margination and adherence, 819–821
    disorders of oxidant removal, 833–835
    disorders of oxidative metabolism, 828–833
    disorders of recognition and ingestion, 824–825
  in lupus, 1647
  hyperplasia of, in chronic myelogenous leukemia, 1065
  life span of, 135
  regulation of, 141, 142
  storage of, 1603
Granulocyte colony-stimulating factor (G-CSF), 143
  humoral control of hematopoiesis and, 143
Granulocyte-macrophage colony-forming unit (CFU-GM). See *Colony-forming unit-granulocyte-macrophage.*
Granulocyte-macrophage progenitor cells, development of, 798–799
  surface characteristics of, 798
  T cell macrophage activity in differentiation of, 145–146
Granulocyte-macrophage system, development of, 141–144, 798–799
Granulocyte transfusions, 1598–1605
  administration of, 1603
  collection of for transfusion, 1600–1601, 1600(t)
  dose of, 1601

Granulocyte transfusions *(Continued)*
  in neonates, 1602
  indications for, 1601–1602, 1601(t)
  prophylactic, 171, 1602
  reactions to, 1602–1603
  response to, 1601
Granulocytopenia, in renal disease, 1640
  with bone marrow transplantation, 248
Granulomatosis, lymphomatoid, 1128
Granulomatous disease, chronic, 829(t), 830–831
  biochemical defect in, 830
  genetic aspects of, 509
  pathogenesis of, 831
  pathology of, 830–831
Granulopoiesis, colony assays for, 142
  ineffective, 803–804
Gray platelet syndrome, 1437–1438
Growth and development, in sickle cell disease, 679–680, *680, 681*
  iron deficiency and, 284
  retarded, estimation of, 308
    in beta thalassemia, 746–747
    in protein-calorie malnutrition, 306
    radiation-induced, 1025
Growth factors, cellular oncogenes and DNA synthesis and, 956–957, 966–967
  platelet-derived, 1277
Growth hormone, erythropoiesis and, 1644
  in Fanconi's anemia, 180
Guest, George, 4–5
GVHD. See *Graft versus host disease.*

Hageman factor (Factor XII), deficiency of, 1324
  in coagulation cascade, 1249–1250, *1250*
Haltia-Santavuori syndrome, 1241
Ham's acidified serum test, 424, 425, 897
Hand-foot syndrome, in sickle cell disease, 669, *670*
Hand-Schüller-Christian disease, in histiocytosis X, 1129–1131
Haplotypes, extended, 1569–1570, 1570(t)
Haptoglobin, genetic polymorphism of, 1555–1558
  properties and variants of, 1555–1558, *1555–1557*
Head and neck, germ cell tumors of, 1178–1179
  injury to, in hemophilia A, 1309
  rhabdomyosarcoma of, 1157
Hearing loss, in sickle cell disease, 678
Heart disease, acquired, thrombocytopenia secondary to, 1385
  congenital, eosinophilia and, 814
    hemostatic abnormalities with, 1328–1329
    iron deficiency with, 301–302
    platelet defects in, 1634
    thrombocytopenia secondary to, 1384–1385
  cyanotic, 301, 1634–1635
  folate deficiency with, 328
  hematologic complications with, 1632–1635
  hemolytic anemia and, 433–434
Heart surgery, 433–434
Heart valves, prosthetic, cardiac hemolytic anemia and, 433–434
  embolization from, 1453
  hypercoagulability and, 1456
  platelet survival with, 1634
Heavy chain disease, molecular genetic basis of, 868–869. See also *Gene(s), immunoglobulin, heavy chain locus of.*

Heinz bodies, formation of, 25, 631
  test for, for diagnosis of G6PD deficiency, 602
  in congenital Heinz body hemolytic anemia, 630–633
  in drug-induced hemolysis, 597–598, *597*
  in hemolytic crisis, 595
  in liver disease, 1636
Hemangioma, cavernous, hemolytic anemia with, 438
  thrombocytopenia with, 1386–1388
Hemarthroses, acute, in hemophilia A, 1307–1309
Hematocrit, and hemoglobin, for iron deficiency screening, 288–290, 289(t)
  at birth, capillary venous ratio of, 26
  in apheresis, 1623
  lowering of, by erythrocytapheresis, 1626, 1628
  normal values of, 266(t), 1679(t)
Hematofluorometer, for lead poisoning screening, 406
Hematologic values, at birth, 25–27
  in normal term infant, 27(t), 28(t), 1678(t)
Hematomas, blood progenitor functions in, 133–135, *136*
  hyperbilirubinemia and, in newborn, 84
Hematopoiesis. See also *Bone marrow; Erythropoiesis; Granulopoiesis.*
  anatomy and physiology of, 128–158
  aplastic anemia and, 166–170, 167(t)
  bone marrow anatomy and, 131–133, *132, 133*
  bone marrow transplantation and, 244–245, 253–256
  glycoprotein growth factors in, 143
  hepatic, 17, *17*
  history of, 128–129
  humoral control of, 134, 143–144, 144(t), 168, 206
  in embryo and fetus, 16–19, *17, 19*
  in Fanconi's anemia, 182
  ineffective, 159
  inherited disorders of, bone marrow transplantation and, 253–256
  megaloblastic, 16–17
  myeloid, 17–18
  ontogeny of, 129–131
  phagocyte development in, 141–144
  phylogeny of, 129
  pluripotent stem cell in, 135–137
    in bone marrow transplantation rejection, 246
  precursor cells of, defective, cyclic neutropenia and, 801
  progenitors of, functions of, 133–135, *136*
  regulation of, 133–135, *136*
    by reticuloendothelial system, 431
  splenic control of, 905–907
  transfer of cells from marrow into sinus, 133, *134*
Hematuria, in hemophilia A, 1310
  in sickle cell disease, 676
Heme, bilirubin synthesis and, 53–54, 74–75, 80
  biosynthesis of, disorders of, 370–382. See also *Sideroblastic anemia; Porphyria(s).*
  effects of lead on, 393–399, *394–396*
    neurotoxic, 399
    nonerythropoietic, 398–399
  in congenital erythropoietic porphyria, 376

Heme *(Continued)*
  biosynthesis of, in congenital erythropoietic protoporphyria, 377
    in porphyria, 375
    in variegate porphyria, 380–381
    normal pathways of, 363–370, *365*
      iron in, 366–370
      porphyrins in, 363–366
    other factors affecting, 398
  degradation of, in Rh hemolytic disease of newborn, 53–54
  displacement of, unstable hemoglobin formation and, 631
  effects of ALA synthetase, 363–364
Heme-heme interaction, 617–618
Heme oxygenase, bilirubin synthesis and, 53–54, 75
Heme proteins, age-related changes in, 279
  depressed production of, with iron deficiency anemia, 296–297, *297*
  dietary iron in, 281
  function and distribution of, 276–277
  synthesis and turnover of, 278
Hemochromatosis, folate deficiency with, 328
  hereditary, diagnosis of, 303–304
    iron overload with, 303–304
  idiopathic, HLA linkage to, 1542–1543
    iron absorption in, 369
  in sideroblastic anemia, 374, 375
  with hereditary spherocytosis, 488
Hemodialysis, blood loss with, iron deficiency and, 292, 301
  eosinophilia and, 814
  folate deficiency with, 328
Hemoglobin. See also *Globin.*
  and hematocrit, for iron deficiency screening, 288–290, 289(t)
  at birth, site of sampling and, 25–26, *26*
  by race, 1681(t)
  by sex, *1680*
  chains of, 18(t), *130*
    alpha chain, 614–616, *614*
    beta chain, 615–616, *615*
      unstable, 631, *632*
      variants of, 629–630, *630*
    gamma chain, 626, 631
  components of, 624–628, 624(t)
  concentration of, cord clamping and, 27(t)
    in cord, exchange transfusion and, 63
    in infections, 1649
    maintained in transfusion therapy for beta thalassemia, 748–749
    needed in low-birth-weight infants, 40(t)
  deletion mutations of, 727–728
  disorders of. See *Hemoglobinopathy(ies); Thalassemia.*
  during development, 18(t), 278–279, *279*
  embryonic, 624–625, *625*
  erythrocyte protoporphyrin binding to, in lead intoxication, 395–397
  fetal. See also *Hemoglobin F.*
    beta globin mutations affecting synthesis of, 723–729
    by age, *1683*
    hereditary persistence of. See *Hereditary persistence of fetal hemoglobin.*
    in Diamond-Blackfan syndrome, 199, *200*
    in myelodysplastic syndromes, 1076
    in newborn and adult, 1683(t)
    in sickle cell disease, 685–686
    in stress erythropoiesis, 139
    synthesis of, 729

Hemoglobin (Continued)
   function and distribution of, 276, 617–624
      acquired abnormalities of, 635–636
   genes for, 701–702
   glucose adducts of, 627
   in Diamond-Blackfan syndrome, 199
   in iron-sufficient preterm infant, 1679(t)
   iron deficiency and, 297, *297*
   ligand binding to, 616, *616, 617*, 618
   normal values for, 266(t), 1679(t)
      in screening tests for iron deficiency, 289(t)
   oxygenation of, 618–620, *618*. See also *Oxygenation.*
   plasma, in Rh hemolytic disease, 54
   posttranslational changes in, 627–628
   red cell membrane, in hereditary spherocytosis, 475
   red cell osmotic properties and, 462–463
   structure of, 613–617
      acquired abnormalities of, 635–636
      defective, in neonates, 33–35
      primary and secondary, 614–616, *614–616*
      quaternary, 616–617, *616, 617*
      tertiary, 616
   switching of, 727–728
   synthesis and turnover of, 277–278
      after birth, 19–20, *20*
      at birth, 19, *19*
      defective, neonatal, 35–36
      fetal switch and, 129–131
         globin gene expression in, 130–131
   unstable, 630–633
      beta chain mutants of, 631, *632*
   values of, in neonatal fetal to maternal hemorrhage, 30
      in newborn, historical aspects of, 1–2, 5
      in normal cord blood, 27, 27(t), 1678(t)
      in premature infants, 27, *29*
      in term infants, 27, *29*
   variants of, 628–635. See also names of specific hemoglobins (e.g., *Hemoglobin Constant Spring*).
      assembly of, 629–630
      clinically important, 629(t)
      congenital Heinz body hemolytic anemia, 630–633
      M hemoglobins, 634–635
      molecular bases of, 628(t)
      unstable, 630–633
      with abnormal oxygen binding, 633–634
Hemoglobin A, 701
   interaction with hemoglobins S and F, 662, *662*
Hemoglobin A_1, 627, *627*
   in uremia, 1639
Hemoglobin A_{1c}, 627, *627*
   in diabetes, 1658
Hemoglobin A_2, 626–627, 701
   in beta thalassemia trait classification, 736–737
   in delta thalassemia, 735–736
   in newborn and adult, 1683(t)
   in various disorders, 626(t)
Hemoglobin Bart's, 627
   in alpha thalassemia, 35, 731
   in hemoglobin H disease, 35, 732
   in hydrops fetalis, 35, 733
Hemoglobin C-beta thalassemia, 759
Hemoglobin C disease, homozygous, 686–687
Hemoglobin C_{Harlem} disease, 685
Hemoglobin Chesapeake, 633–634
Hemoglobin-coated charcoal radioassay, for measuring serum vitamin B_{12}, 355
Hemoglobin Constant Spring, mutations causing, 717, *717*
Hemoglobin E-beta thalassemia, 758–759
Hemoglobin E disease, 759
Hemoglobin F, 625–626, 701. See also *Hemoglobin, fetal.*
   in beta thalassemia trait, 736–737
   in newborn, 626, *626*
   in sickle cell disease, 666, 685–686
   interactions of thalassemia mutations with, 741
   interactions with hemoglobins S and F, 662, *662*
   synthesis of, in erythroid maturation in thalassemia, 741
      pharmacologic manipulation of, for treatment of beta thalassemia, 756–757
Hemoglobin Gower I, 701
Hemoglobin H, 627
   in hydrops fetalis, 733
Hemoglobin H ($beta_4$), 700
Hemoglobin H disease. See also *Thalassemia, alpha.*
   acquired, 733
   alpha globin genes in, 729
   clinical features of, 732
   hemoglobin pattern in, 731
   mental retardation with, 732–733
   pathophysiological features of, 731–732, *732*
   neonatal, 35
   therapy for, 732
Hemoglobin Hammersmith, 631
Hemoglobin Hasharon, 34
Hemoglobin Indianapolis, 718
Hemoglobin Kenya, 724, *726*
Hemoglobin Köln, 631
Hemoglobin Korle Bu sickle disease, 685
Hemoglobin Lepore, 724, *726*
   anti-Lepore, 724, *726*
Hemoglobin M, 634–635, 634(t)
Hemoglobin Portland, in hydrops fetalis, 733
Hemoglobin Q-alpha thalassemia, 759
Hemoglobin S, deoxygenated, polymer formation of, 659–661, *660–661*
   delay time concept in, 660–662, *662*
   fiber of, 656, *659*
   for sickle cell disease treatment, 666–667
   interaction with hemoglobins A and F, 662, *662*
   polymerization of, 659–662, *660–662*
      hemolytic severity of sickle syndromes and, 663–664
      irreversible, 663
      molecular sickling and, 656, *657–659*
      reversible, 603
      rheologic properties of, 661–662
   red cell membrane damage and, 666
Hemoglobin SC alpha thalassemia, 685
Hemoglobin SC disease $\alpha_2\beta_2$, 684–685
Hemoglobin SD sickle disease, 685
Hemoglobin SO Arab sickle disease, 685
Hemoglobin Zurich, 631, 633
Hemoglobinopathy(ies), alpha chain, 33–34
   beta chain, 34
   early research on, 12
   gamma chain, 34–35, 34(t)
   methemoglobinemia, 641–654. See also *Methemoglobinemia.*

Hemoglobinopathy(ies) *(Continued)*
  neonatal, 33–36
  sickle cell, 34
  thalassemia, 759. See also *Thalassemia.*
Hemoglobin-oxygen dissociation curve, in preterm infants, 39–40
Hemoglobinuria, march, 435
Hemolysis. See also *Hemolytic anemia.*
  chronic, biochemical defect in, 595–596
    folate requirements in, 319
    G6PD deficiency and, 601–602, *603*
    hyperbilirubinemia with, in newborn, 84
    with hereditary elliptocytosis, 496
  definition of, 443
  drug-induced, G6PD activity and, 593–594, *594*
    in pregnant women, neonatal jaundice and, 600
  erythrocyte hexokinase deficiency and, 548–549
  extravascular, by spleen, 51–53, *52*
    in ABO hemolytic disease, 67
  haptoglobin concentration and, 1555
  immune, blood groups and, 1500
  in cold hemagglutinin disease, 417–418
  in thalassemias, 699–700
  intravascular, iron deficiency and, 302
    in G6PD deficiency, 597–598, *597, 598*
    in Rh hemolytic disease, 54
    in schistocytic hemolytic anemia, 432, 433
  oxidant, 517–518
  phototherapy effects on, 91
  unstable hemoglobins and, 631, 633
Hemolytic anemia. See also *Hemolysis.*
  ABO. See *ABO hemolytic disease of newborn.*
  adenosine deaminase deficiency and, 572
  adenosine triphosphate metabolism and, 569–570
  adenylate kinase deficiency and, 571–572
  aldolase deficiency and, 555
  aplastic crisis in, 194–195
  autoimmune, 413–426, 417(t)
    clinical features of, 420–421
    diseases associated with, 417–418, 418(t)
    experimental model of, 413–417
    globin biosynthesis in, vs that in beta thalassemia, 739, *739*
    laboratory features of, 420–421
    mortality from, 420
    natural history of, 419–420
    pathophysiology of, 418–419
    therapy for, 421–423
    with thrombocytopenia, 423–424
  burns with, 435
  C3 deficiency, in, 897
  cardiac, 433–434, 1632–1633
  chronic. See *Hemolysis, chronic.*
  classification by predominant morphology, 270(t)
  congenital, vs thalassemia major, 742
  congenital Heinz body, 630–633
  congenital nonspherocytic, 545–572
    adenosine deaminase deficiency, 572
    adenylate kinase deficiency, 571–572
    aldolase deficiency, 555
    ATP metabolic disorders, 569–570
    2,3-diphosphoglycerate mutase deficiency, 560–561
    enolase deficiency, 561
    glucose-6-phosphate dehydrogenase deficiency, 594–596, 601–602, *603*

Hemolytic anemia *(Continued)*
  congenital nonspherocytic, glucose phosphate isomerase deficiency, 550–553
    glyceraldehyde-3-phosphate dehydrogenase deficiency, 556–557
    hexokinase deficiency, 547–550
    lactate dehydrogenase deficiency, 569
    phosphofructokinase deficiency, 553–555
    phosphoglycerate kinase deficiency, 557–560
    pyrimidine-5'-nucleotidase deficiency, 571
    pyruvate kinase deficiency, 561–569
    triose phosphate isomerase deficiency, 555–556
    vs hereditary spherocytosis, 545
  Coombs' negative, vs hereditary spherocytosis, 486
    Wilson's disease and, 518
  Coombs' positive, 504
  copper-induced, 518
  2,3-diphosphoglycerate mutase deficiency and, 560–561
  Factor VIII concentrate transfusion and, 1616
  folate requirements in, 319, 324–325
  Gasser's contributions to, 8–9
  G6PD deficiency and, 13, 594–596, 601–602, *603*
  hypophosphatemia and, 504
  immune, 417–425, 417(t)
    acquired, in lupus, 1647
    immune adherence and, 503
    IgM-induced, 417. See also *Cold hemagglutinin disease.*
  in infections, 1649
  in infectious mononucleosis, 1655
  in liver disease, 506–508, *507–508*
  in lupus erythematosus, 1647
  in McLeod's blood group, 509
  infantile pyknosis with, 508–509
  inherited disorders of red cell cation permeability and volume and, 511–517, 512(t), *513–514*
  intravascular, in cardiac disease, 1633
  microangiopathic, thrombocytopenia with, 1383
  paroxysmal nocturnal hemoglobinuria, 424–425
  red cell cation permeability and volume, inherited disorders of, 511–517, 512(t), *513–514*
  red cell membrane and, decreased surface, 470–503
    increased surface, 510–511
    mechanical injury to, 504
    spiculated cells, 505–510
    thermal injury to, 503–504
    various disorders, 517–518
  Rh. See *Rh hemolytic disease.*
  schistocytic, 432–438
    chronic relapsing, and thrombocytopenia of childhood, 438
    disorders associated with, 432, 433(t)
    disseminated intravascular coagulation and, 433
    malignant hypertension with, 434–435
    with hemolytic uremic syndrome, 436–437
    with mild thrombocytopenia, 433–435
    with normal platelet count, 433–435
    with severe thrombocytopenia, 435–438
  splenic hypertrophy and, 431

Hemolytic anemia *(Continued)*
  toxins and venoms and, 504–505
  uremia with, 509
  venoms and, 504
  vitamin E deficiency with, 508
Hemolytic crisis, in G6PD deficiency, 594–595
  drug-induced, 597–599
  with hereditary spherocytosis, 486
Hemolytic disease of newborn, due to minor blood group antibodies, 68–69
  historical aspects of, 10–11
  unconjugated hyperbilirubinemia and, 83–84
Hemolytic process, causing neonatal anemia, 33–36, 33(t)
Hemolytic transfusion reactions, 1586
Hemolytic uremic syndrome, 435–438
  adult, 438
  bacterial infections with, 435–438
  clinical features of, 435
  epidemiology of, 435
  incidence of, 435
  laboratory features of, 436–437
  therapy of, 437–438
  viral infections with, 436
Hemophagocytic syndrome, virus-associated, *1126–1127*
Hemophilia(s), 1305–1315
  carrier detection in, 1314–1315
  clinical manifestations of, 1305–1306, *1306*
  diagnosis of, 1305
  heterogeneity of, 1305
  inhibitor development in, 1312–1313
    classification of, 1313
    detection and quantitation of, 1313
    management of, 1313–1314
  neonatal hemorrhage and, 118–119
  prenatal diagnosis of, 1315
  treatment of, 1306–1311
    hemophilia A, 1307–1311
    hemophilia B, 1311
    home care, 1307
    regional comprehensive care, 1306–1307
Hemophilia A, characteristics of, 1305
  cryoprecipitate for, 1608–1609
  Factor VIII concentrates for, 1610
  hematuria in, 1310
  surgical procedures in, 1310
    oral surgery, 1311
  treatment of, 1307–1311
    for acute hemarthroses, 1307–1309
    Factor VIII dosage, 1307, 1308(t), 1610
    for head injury, 1309
    for muscle hemorrhage, 1309
    oral bleeding, 1309–1310
Hemophilia B, 1305
  treatment of, 1311, 1611
Hemophilus influenzae infection, in sickle cell disease, 675
Hemorrhage. See also *Blood loss; Bleeding; Coagulation disorders.*
  fetal to fetal, 31
  fetal to maternal, 29–31, 30(t)
  in acute leukemia, 1050–1051
  in Rh hemolytic disease, 64–65
  in sickle cell disease, 673
  intracranial, in idiopathic thrombocytopenic purpura of childhood, 1354, 1356, 1357(t)
  intraventricular, in premature infants, 117
  neonatal, 104–127
    diagnostic approach to, 107, *107*

Hemorrhage *(Continued)*
  neonatal, due to inherited disorders of coagulation, 118–119
    laboratory evaluation of, 105(t), 108, *109*, 109(t)
    miscellaneous causes of, 31–32, 64–65, 119–120
    occult, prior to birth, 29–31
    platelet dysfunction and, 114–115
    vitamin K deficiency-induced and, 118
  with transfusion therapy, 1616
Hemosiderin, function and distribution of, 277
Hemosiderosis, idiopathic pulmonary, 1644–1645
  iron deficiency erythropoiesis with, 302
  pulmonary, due to other causes, 1645
Hemostasis. See also *Coagulation.*
  abnormalities of, screening tests for, 105(t), 108, *109*, 109(t)
    treatment of, 1300–1305
  inhibitors of, activated prothrombin complex concentrates for, 1303
  mechanism of, 1250(t), *1294*
    limiting reactions in, 1262–1266
    transformations in, 1248–1249, *1249*
  normal neonatal, 104–107
  platelet function in, 1344
  primary, 1272
  secondary, 1272
HEMPAS (hereditary erythroblastosis multinuclearity with a positive acidified serum test), 207, 208–210
  Ham's test for, 424
Henoch-Schönlein purpura, 1459–1461, *1460*
Heparan sulfate, *1231*
Heparin, antithrombin function and, 1263–1264, *1264*
  for anticoagulation during apheresis, 1624
  for disseminated intravascular coagulation treatment, 116, 1333, 1335–1336
  for intravascular coagulation in Rh hemolytic disease, 65
  for Kasabach-Merritt syndrome, 1387
  mechanism of action of, 1263, *1264*
  platelet function and, 1454
  tests for presence of, 1300
  thrombocytopenia induced by, 1377, 1379
Hepatic dysfunction. See also *Hepatitis.*
  in graft versus host disease, 247
Hepatic tumors, hepatitis B and, 932
  with androgen therapy for aplastic anemia, 173
Hepatitis, coagulation disorders with, 1327
  conjugated hyperbilirubinemia in newborn and, 95
  Factor VIII concentrates and, 1301
  idiopathic neonatal giant cell, 94–95
  in bone marrow transplantation recipients, 249
  in infectious mononucleosis, 1654
  infectious, coagulation changes with, 1637(t)
  neonatal, vs biliary atresia, 94
  post-transfusion, 1585, 1614–1615
  toxic, cholesterol and, 96
  type B, congenital, 95
  oncongenic potential of, 932–933, 948, 1180
  viral, aplastic anemia and, 164
    pure red cell aplasia and, 194
Hepatobiliary system, in sickle cell disease, 677
Hepatoblastoma, 1179–1181
Hepatocellular carcinoma, 1179–1181

Hereditary elliptocytosis. See *Elliptocytosis, hereditary.*
Hereditary erythroblastic multinuclearity with a positive acidified serum test (HEMPAS), 207–210
Hereditary hemorrhagic telangiectasia, 1636, 1661
Hereditary persistence of fetal hemoglobin, 758
  mutations causing, 712, 727–729, 728(t)
Hereditary spherocytosis. See *Spherocytosis, hereditary.*
Hermansky-Pudlak syndrome, 1663
Herpesvirus infection, 946
  lymphoreticular response to, 1120–1121
  oncogenic potential of, 946
Heterophil antibody, in infectious mononucleosis, 1656
Hexachlorobenzene, acquired porphyria and, 382
Hexokinase, deficiency of, hemolytic anemia and, 547–550, 548, 548(t)
  glucose-6-phosphate function and, 584
  in neonatal red cells, 23–24
  in pentose pathway, 584–588, 585–586
  properties of, 548(t)
Hexosaminidase, deficiency in G_{M2}-gangliosidosis, 1230
Hexose monophosphate shunt, in triose phosphate isomerase deficiency, 556
  methemoglobin reduction and, 643, *643*
High performance liquid chromatography, 1220
Histidine, in FIGLU excretion test for folic acid deficiency, 332, *332*
Histiocytes, function of, 1119
  in bone marrow in storage disease, 1217, 1217(t), *1218*
  in familial erythrophagocytic lymphohistiocytosis, 1121
Histiocytic medullary reticulosis, 1131–1133. See also *Histiocytosis, malignant.*
Histiocytosis, Langerhans cell, 1129–1131. See also *Histiocytosis X.*
  malignant, 1131–1133, *1132*
    differential diagnosis of, 1133
    vs virus-associated hemophagocytic syndrome, 1126–1127
  sinus, with massive lymphadenopathy, 1127–1128
Histiocytosis X, 1129–1131
  lymphadenopathy and, 1090
  vs malignant histiocytosis, 1133
Histocompatibility, in bone marrow transplantation for severe combined immunodeficiency, 250. See also *HLA complex.*
Historical aspects, of pediatric hematology, 1–13
HLA complex, antigens of, bone marrow transplantation and, 242
  class I, 1524–1525
    antibodies against, testing for, in kidney transplantation, 1537–1538
    molecular structure of, 1532
  class II, molecular structure of, 1532–1533
    polymorphism of, 1529–1530
    serologic identification of, 1529–1530
    tissue distribution of, 1532
  class III, molecular genetics of, 1535–1536
    polymorphism of, 1531
  genetic linkage disequilibrium and, 1530–1531

HLA complex *(Continued)*
  antigens of, HLA-B27 antigen, disease linkage with, 1544
    resistance to platelet transfusion and, in aplastic anemia, 171
  biochemistry of, 1532–1533
  class I loci of, 1524–1525
    polymorphism of, 1528–1529
  class II genes in, 1524–1525
    molecular genetics of, 1535, *1535*
  class III genes in, 1525
  clinical histocompatibility testing in, 1536–1542
    early work with, 242
    in bone marrow transplantation, 243, 1540–1541
    in treatment for platelet function disorders, 1443–1444, 1595
    isoimmune neonatal thrombocytopenia due to incompatibility, 112
  disease genes linkage to, 1542–1543, 1543(t)
    mechanisms in, 1543–1544
  gene map of, 1525, *1527*
  genetics of, 1524–1531
    molecular genetics, 1533–1536
    polymorphism of, 1525–1531·
      and restriction fragment length polymorphism, 1536
  specificities of, 1528, 1528(t)
  terminology of, 1528
  tissue distribution of, 1531–1532
HLA-A region, antigens coded for in, 1524
  cross-reactivity with HLA-B, 1529
  polymorphism of, 1528
HLA-B region, antigens coded for in, 1524
  cross-reactivity with HLA-A, 1529
  polymorphism of, 1528
HLA-C region, antigens coded for in, 1524
  polymorphism of, 1528
HLA-D region, antigens coded for in, 1524, 1529
  in T-cell activation, 849–850
  molecular map of, 1535, *1535*
  polymorphism of, 1529–1530
HLA-DP region, 1530
HLA-DQ region, antigens coded for by, 1530, *1530*
HLA-DR region, antigens of, on macrophages, 1119
  class II, coded for by, 1529–1530
  kidneys matched for in kidney transplantation, 1538
  on dendritic cells, 119
HLA genotype, 1524, *1525*
HLA haplotype, 1524, *1525, 1526*
HLA linkage group, 1525, *1527*
HLA phenotype, 1524, *1524, 1525*
Hodgkin's disease, 1101–1112
  cellular origins of, 1101–1104, *1102–1103*
  classification of, 1102, *1102–1103*, 1104
  clinical presentation of, 1104
  definition of, 1101
  epidemiology of, 929
  histopathology of, 1101–1104, *1102–1103*
  immune status in, 1101, 1101(t)
  laboratory findings in, 1104–1105
  staging of, 1105–1107, 1105(t)
    Ann Arbor system, 1107, 1107(t)
  treatment of, 1108, 1110–1111
    combined modality, 1110–1112
    results of, 1109(t), 1111

Homocystinuria, folate deficiency with, 329
  hypercoagulability with, 1457–1458
  pyridoxine treatment for, folate deficiency with, 328
  with methylmalonic aciduria, 352
Host factors, cancer risk and, 924–927, 925(t)–926(t)
  splenic function in, 907–908
Howell-Jolly bodies, 316, 902, 906
β_2-HS-Glycoprotein, 1563
HTLV virus, 953–954
  AIDS and, 1615
Human chorionic gonadotropin, as marker of germ cell tumors, 1171, 1171(t)
Human immunodeficiency virus (HIV), in pediatric AIDS, 890–892
Human papovaviruses, 945–946
Human T cell lymphotropic virus (HTLV), 953–954
  AIDS and, 1615
Hunter's disease, 1233
Hurler's disease, 1231–1233
Hurler-Scheie compound, 1231–1233
Hyate:C, for inhibitor hemophiliacs, 1313–1314
Hydantoin, lymphadenopathy with, 1089
Hydrocytes, 513
Hydrocytosis, hereditary, 513–514
Hydrogen peroxide, produced by NADPH oxidase, removal of, 833–834
  produced by neutrophils in chronic granulomatous disease, 830
  produced by phagocytes, 790–791
12-Hydroperoxy-eicosatetraenoic acid (HPETE), 1448
Hydrops fetalis, 35, 733
  in Rh hemolytic disease, 54, 61, 64
12L-Hydroxy-eicosatetraenoic acid (HETE), 1448
Hydroxyethyl starch, in granulocyte collection, 1601
21-Hydroxylase deficiency, in congenital adrenal hyperplasia, HLA linkage to, 1543
Hydroxyurea, for beta thalassemia, 756–757
Hyperbilirubinemia. See also *Jaundice*.
  bilirubin conjugation defects and, 86–88
  conjugated (direct-reacting), biliary atresia and, 93–94
    bronze baby syndrome and, 91
    cholestasis with paucity of bile ducts and, 95
    hepatitis due to infectious agents and, 95
    idiopathic neonatal giant cell hepatitis and, 94–95
    in newborn, 82, 92–97, 93(t), 599
    metabolic disorders and, 95–96
    Rh erythroblastosis and, 83
  G6PD deficiency and, 599
  in ABO hemolytic disease, 68
  in newborn, 79–89, 92–97, 599
    in premature infants, 82
    in pyruvate kinase deficiency, 561
    prevention of, 61–66
  in Rh hemolytic disease of newborn, 56–57, 83
  in sickle cell disease, 677
  rebound, after exchange transfusion, 64
  transient familial neonatal, 88
  unconjugated, congenital hypothyroidism and, 89
    diseases associated with, 83–89
    disordered hepatic bilirubin metabolism and, 84–88

Hyperbilirubinemia *(Continued)*
  unconjugated, exaggerated jaundice of undetermined mechanism, 88–89
    hemolytic disorders and, 83–84
    maternal diabetes and, 89
Hypercoagulability, 1455–1459
  diseases associated with, 1456(t)
  in diabetes, 1659
Hypereosinophilia, in acute leukemia, 1040
Hypereosinophilic syndrome, 815, 1664
Hyperglycinemia, 329
Hyperimmunoglobulin E syndrome, 824
Hyperimmunoglobulin M syndrome *(dysgammaglobulinemia)*, 801, 874–875
Hyperkalemia, 1042
Hyperleukocytosis, 1042
Hypernephroma, 1151–1152
Hyperphosphatemia, 1042
Hypersplenism, 510, 1394
Hypertension, malignant, hemolytic anemia with, 434–435
Hyperthyroidism, 1642–1643
Hypertransfusion, for beta thalassemia, 748–749
Hyperuricemia, 1042
Hyperviscosity, 1626, 1629
Hyphema, sickle cell disease and, 678
Hypocalcemia, phototherapy and, 91
Hypochromia, in sideroblastic anemia, 374
  in thalassemia, 699
Hypogammaglobulinemia, acquired, 883–884
  secondary, 890
  transient, of infancy, 879–880
    T-cell control of B-cell function in, 852–853, 853(t)
Hypoglycemia, in Rh hemolytic disease, 65
Hypophosphatemia, 2,3-DPG deficiency in, 623
  erythrocyte glycolysis and, 572–573
  hemolytic anemia and, 504
  impaired neutrophil chemotaxis in, 823
Hypoprothrombinemia, congenital, 1321–1322
Hyposplenism, 431–432, 909
Hyposthenuria, with sickle cell disease, 676
Hypotension, in disseminated intravascular coagulation, 1331
Hypothermia, sideroblastic anemia and, 372
  thrombocytopenia and, 1395
Hypothyroidism, anemia of, 1641–1642, *1642*
  in beta thalassemia, 747
  neonatal hyperbilirubinemia and, 89
Hypovolemia, 1581
Hypoxanthine-guanine-phosphoribosyltransferase, in detection of G6PD deficiency, 592, 602
Hypoxemia, arterial, decreased oxygen affinity and, 622–623, *623*
  in beta thalassemia, 748
Hypoxia, blood oxygen affinity and, 621–624, *621, 622*
  in sickle cell anemia, 672
  with pulmonary disease, 1644

i antigen, in HEMPAS, 209
Ia antigen, 798, 856
I-cell disease, 1237
Icterus, bilirubin and, 74
Icterus praecox, 68. See also *ABO hemolytic disease of newborn.*
Idiopathic thrombocytopenic purpura. See *Thrombocytopenic purpura, idiopathic.*

α-Iduronidase activity, in Scheie and Hurler-Scheie diseases, 1231
α-L-Iduronidase deficiency, 1231–1233
Ii blood group, 1512
Ileum, function of, Schilling test for, 356
　resection of, 348, 1635
　vitamin B_{12} malabsorption and, 348–349
Imferon (iron dextran), for iron deficiency anemia, 295
Immune neutropenia, 804–806
Immune pancytopenia, 423–424
Immune response, drug-induced thrombocytopenia and, 1373–1375
　in reticuloendothelial system, 428
　phases of, 848–849, *848*
　regulation of, MHC gene products and, 1523–1524
　T-cell control of, 848–859
　　major histocompatibility complex and, 1522–1524
　to neuroblastoma, 1140
Immune system, eosinophils related to, 813–814
　spleen in, 430–431, 907–908
Immune thrombocytopenia, 1348–1383. See also *Thrombocytopenia, immune.*
　neonatal, 109–110, 1382
Immunity, cellular. See *T cell(s).*
　hemolytic anemia and, 417–425, 417(t)
　iron deficiency anemia and, 298
　sideroblastic anemia and, 370
Immunoblot technique, 1462–1463, *1463*
Immunocompromised host, red cell transfusion in, 1584
Immunodeficiency, acquired syndrome of. See *AIDS.*
　aplastic anemia and, 187
　associated with other major defects, 881(t)
　combined, classification of, 880(t)
　common variable, 883–884
　eosinophilia and, 814
　following splenectomy, 890
　in ataxia telangiectasia, 887–888
　in megaloblastic anemia, 316
　primary, classification of, 879(t)–881(t)
　severe combined, 884–887, *885–888*
　　bone marrow transplantation in, 250, 1541
　　variants of, 886–887
　unclassified, 883–884
　with normal or increased immunoglobulins, 883
　with thrombocytopenia and eczema, 888–889, *888*. See also *Wiskott-Aldrich syndrome.*
　with unusual response to Epstein-Barr virus, 889
　X-linked, with increased IgM, 882–883
Immunoglobulin(s). See also *Antibody(ies).*
　AM system of, 1571
　characteristics of, 861, 861(t)
　deficiency of, selective, 883
　genes of, 861–862, 866
　　expression of, 866
　　light chain locus in, 863–864, *863, 865*
　　　gene rearrangement in, in B cell leukemia and lymphoma, 864–865, *865*
　　heavy chain gene loci in, 862, *862*, 865–866
　　　gene rearrangement in, 867–868
　　　　in B cell precursor acute lymphoblastic leukemia, 869–870, *869*
　　　　molecular basis of disorders of, 868–869

Immunoglobulin(s) *(Continued)*
　genes of, mediation of chromosomal translocations by, 873–874
　　rearrangements of. See also *Chromosome(s); DNA; RNA.*
　　　as B-cell associated clonal markers in lymphoid neoplasms, 870–872
　　　heavy chain rearrangement in, 867–868
　　　in lymphoid blast crisis of chronic myelogenous leukemia, 870
　　　light chain loci of, 863–864, *863, 865*
　　sequence joining of, 866–867
　　transcription of, 867
　genetic markers of, 1570–1572
　GM system of, 1570–1571
　in aplastic anemia, 166
　in sickle cell disease, 675
　intravenous, for idiopathic thrombocytopenic purpura of childhood, 1362–1364
　isotypes of, 861
　KM system of, 1571
　molecular composition of, 861, *861*
　normal levels of, by age, 1695(t)
　opsonization function of, 786
　production of, disorders in, due to abnormal T-cell regulation of B cell function, 852–854, 853(t)
　splenic, 908
　T-cell control of, 851–854, 853(t)
　serum, normal levels of, 1693(t)
　structure of, 1570
Immunoglobulin A, deficiency of, 346, 347, 883
　general features of, 878
　in Henoch-Schönlein purpura, 1461
　secretory, selective deficiency of, 883
Immunoglobulin D, serum, in infants, children, and adults, 1694(t)
Immunoglobulin E, binding factors of, in T-cell regulation of immunoglobulin synthesis, 854
　general features of, 878
　in hyperimmunoglobulin E syndrome, 824
　serum, in infants, children, and adults, 1694(t)
Immunoglobulin G, ABO hemolytic disease and, 66–67
　as immune suppressant for idiopathic thrombocytopenic purpura of childhood, 1362–1365
　as inhibitors of Factor VIII in hemophilia, 1312–1313
　classes of, 430
　erythrocyte coated by, clearance of, 414–417, *414*
　Fab terminus of, 1349
　　in drug-induced immune thrombocytopenia, 1375–1376
　Fc fragment of, 52–53, *53*
　general features of, 878
　genetic markers on, 1571
　in autoimmune hemolytic anemia, 417, 419
　in Coombs' test for autoimmune hemolytic anemia, 420–421
　in drug-induced idiosyncratic immune thrombocytopenia, 1375–1376, *1375*
　in immune hemolysis, 1500
　in immune thrombocytopenia, 1348–1349
　in red cell agglutination, 1497–1498
　in red cell clearance, 431
　in Rh disease pathogenesis, 46
　in transient hypogammaglobulinemia of infancy, 880

Immunoglobulin G *(Continued)*
  intravenous, for chronic idiopathic thrombocytopenic purpura, 1367, 1368(t), 1373
  molecular structure of, 1348–1349
  opsonic activity of, 767
  plasma, reticuloendothelial opsonization and, 430–431
  platelet-associated, 1348–1350
    and platelet size, 1403
    assays for, other uses of, 1405–1406
    controversies concerning measurement of, 1402–1404
    in idiopathic thrombocytopenic purpura of childhood, 1353
    in infection-induced thrombocytopenia, 1380
    in normals, 1404
      measurements of, for ITP diagnosis, 1404–1405, 1405(t)
    platelet-bound, 1350–1351, *1351*
      direct measurement of, 1400–1402, *1401–1402*
  selective deficiency of, 883
Immunoglobulin M, erythrocytes coated by, clearance of, 415–416, *415*
  in chronic idiopathic thrombocytopenic purpura, 1366
  in cold hemagglutinin disease, 417–418
  in neonates, *1694*
  in red cell agglutination, 1497
  in Rh disease pathogenesis, 46
  in X-linked immunodeficiency, 882–883
  opsonic activity of, 777
  platelet associated, measurements of, 1405
  response to cell-bound antigen, spleen and, 428
  subnormal levels of, splenectomy and, 432
Immunohemolytic anemia, blood groups and, 1500
  causing spherocytosis, 503
Immunologic abnormalities, in hemolytic uremia syndrome, 437
  in plasma product transfusion, 1616
  in X-linked lymphoproliferative syndrome, 1125, 1125(t)
Immunologic reconstitution, in bone marrow transplantation, 245
Immunologic tests, for graft rejection in kidney transplantation, 1538–1539
Immunology, of fetal red cell membrane, 21
Immunosuppression, in bone marrow transplantation, 244, 248, 1541–1542
  graft rejection and, 246
  in kidney transplantation, 1539–1540
Immunosuppressive therapy, for autoimmune hemolytic anemia, 422–423
  nonsteroidal, for chronic idiopathic thrombocytopenic purpura, 1370
Immunotherapy, for aplastic anemia, 169–170, 173–176
  for bone marrow failure syndromes, 219
  for Fanconi's anemia, 184
  for leukemia in remission, 1045
  for osteosarcoma, 1166
  passive, for cancer, 1008
  plasmapheresis as, 1625
  response to, 175–176
Indomethacin, platelet dysfunction and, 114, 1450–1451
Infantile genetic agranulocytosis (IGA), 210–211

Infants. See also *Neonates; Premature infants.*
  bone marrow cell populations in, 1690(t)–1691(t)
  iron supplements for, 299–300
  low birth weight, phototherapy in, 91
  term, erythrocyte morphology of, 21, *22*
    normal hematologic values in first 2 months in, 1678(t)
    red cell enzyme activity in, 1682(t)
    red cell glycolytic intermediates in, 1682(t)
  vitamin B_{12} deficiency in, 344
Infection. See also *Inflammation; Virus(es).*
  acute, vs iron deficiency anemia, 293
  autoimmune hemolytic anemia and, 418(t), 420
  bacterial, hemolytic uremic syndrome and, 435–436
    hyperbilirubinemia and, 84
    neutropenia with, 799, 804
      granulocyte transfusion for, 1599
    splenectomy and, 431–432
  cutaneous, neutropenia with, 804
  folate-deficient megaloblastic anemia with, 325
  fungal, in acute leukemia, 1051
  hematologic signs of, 1649–1650
  hyperbilirubinemia and, in newborn, 84, 96
  in acute leukemia, 1051
  in Chédiak-Higashi syndrome, 826
  in Kostmann's disease, 803
  in neonates, 84, 96, 113
  in severe combined immunodeficiency, 886
  in sickle cell diseases, 671(t), 674–675
  iron deficiency anemia and, 298
  neutropenia with, 799, 800, 804
    treatment of, 809, 1599
  opportunistic, in acute leukemia, 1051
    in AIDS, 890
    in bone marrow transplantation, 248–249
  parasitic, eosinopenia with, 1664
    eosinophilia and, 814–815
  postsplenectomy, 750–757, 910–913, *912*
  pure red cell aplasia due to, 194
  pyogenic bacterial, B cell deficiency and, 878–879
    C3 deficiency and, 825
    in X-linked agammaglobulinemia, 880–881
    with neutropenia, 799
  recurrent, B-cell deficiency and, 878–879
    in chronic granulomatous disease, 829
    work-up for, *835*
  respiratory, cold hemagglutinin disease and, 420
  thrombocytopenia induced by, 1380–1382
  viral, hemolytic uremic syndrome and, 436
    neutropenia with, 804
  with bone marrow transplantation, 1540
  with impaired neutrophil chemotaxis, 822
Infectious agents, aplastic anemia and, 164
  cancer risk and, 923–924
Infectious mononucleosis, 1651–1658
  aplastic anemia and, 164
  clinical signs of, 1653–1654, 1653(t)
  complications of, 1654–1655, 1654(t)
  epidemiology of, 1652
  Epstein-Barr virus and, 1651–1652
  etiology of, 1652
  laboratory diagnosis of, 1655–1657, 1655(t), *1656*
  lymphadenopathy in, 1089

Infectious mononucleosis *(Continued)*
  lymphoreticular responses to, 1120–1121
  vs acute leukemia, 1041
Inflammation, anemia with, 1646
  complement activation and, 893–904
  due to phagocytes, 792(t)
  iron absorption and, 300
  vs iron deficiency anemia, 293–294
Inosine, in blood storage medium, 623
  metabolism of, in red cells, 460, *461*
Inositol triphosphate, in platelet signal transduction, 1284
Insecticides, associated with aplastic anemia, 161(t)
Interleukin-1, in T-cell activation, 850
Interleukin-2, in T-cell activation, 850
Interleukin-3, 143
  in T-cell control of monocyte macrophages, 856
Interferon, aplastic anemia and, 168
  for X-linked lymphoproliferative syndrome, 1126
Intestines, bilirubin absorption in, 79–81
  blood loss in, iron deficiency and, 284
  iron transport in, 368–369
  obstruction of, hyperbilirubinemia and, 88
  phototherapy and, 91
  vitamin B_{12} malabsorption in, 347–349
Intralipid, 1390
Intramembranous particles, or red cell membrane proteins, 454, *454*
Intrapulmonary hemorrhage, neonatal, 119
Intravascular coagulation, in Rh hemolytic disease, 65
Intrinsic factor, binding vitamin B_{12}, 341
  failure to secrete, 345–347
  in congenital vitamin B_{12} malabsorption, 347
  in Schilling test, 355–356
Introns, vs exons, *1534*
Ions, as signals in phagocytosis, 787–788
Iron, absorption of, gastrointestinal, 281–283, *281–283*
  in anemia of chronic disease, 1646
  in beta thalassemia, 743–744, 749
  in infants, 283
  in inflammatory disease, 300
  as redox intermediate, 366
  dietary, 280–282, 284
    in infants vs adults, *285*
    iron deficiency and, 284
    requirements for, 284
  ferric, in iron transport, 366
    in methemoglobinemia, 642
    uptake of, 369
  ferrokinetic studies of, in aplastic anemia, 165–166
  ferrous, in iron transport, 366
    in iron uptake and release by ferritin, 370
    interconversion of, to ferric iron, vitamin C and, 753
    uptake of, 369
  free serum, in iron overloading in beta thalassemia, 744
  heme proteins of, depressed production of in tissues, 296–297
    dietary, 281
    in methemoglobinemia, 642, *642*
    in oxygen binding, 642, *642*
    transport of, 368
  in heme biosynthesis, 366–370
  inorganic, transport of, 368

Iron *(Continued)*
  intramuscular, administration of, for iron deficiency anemia, 295
  intravenous administration of, for iron deficiency anemia, 295
  iron deficiency anemia of infancy and, 5–6
  losses of, 283–284
  non-heme, absorption of, 282, *282*
    in diet, 280–281
  reactivity of, 367
  released from transferrin in erythroid cells, 367, 369–370
  required by cells, 368
  required by various tissues, 368–370
  serum, for confirmation of iron deficiency, 292
    normal values for, 1684(t), *1685*
  stored, disorders of, iron deficiency anemia with, 303
    during development, 278–279
    functions and distribution of, 277
    in hypochromic anemia, 370–371
    in iron overload in beta thalassemia, methods of measuring, 745
    in sideroblastic anemia, 374
  serum ferritin and, 291
  synthesis and turnover of, 278
  supplementation of, 299–300
  transport of, cellular mechanisms of, 368–370
    diseases of, 370
    effects of lead on, 394, *395*
    in erythroid cells, 369–370
    in heme synthesis, 366–370
    in intestines, 368–369
    in macrophages, 369
    in mitochondria, 370
    in placenta, 368
    in red cell precursors, 366–370
    transferrin receptor and, 455
Iron chelating agents, for sideroblastic anemia, 374
Iron compounds. See also *Hemoglobin; Myoglobin; Cytochromes,* etc.
  distribution of, 276–277
  during development, 278–279
  function of, 276–277
  synthesis and turnover of, 277–278
Iron deficiency anemia, 274, 276–300
  behavior and, 298
  causes of, 284–285
  diagnosis of, 285–295
    confirmatory tests for, 291–293, 291(t)
    differential, 293–295
    laboratory tests for, 285–296, 286(t), *287, 288, 293*
    therapeutic trial for, 290–291
  erythrocyte glycolysis and, 573
  erythrocyte protoporphyrin levels in, 407–408
  erythropoiesis in, syndromes associated with, 302–303
  hemoglobin synthesis in, 370–371
  hereditary spherocytosis and, 488
  historical aspects of, 5–6
  in blacks, 289
  in cardiac hemolytic anemia, 1633
  in developing countries, 300
  in gastrointestinal disease, 1635
  in protein-calorie malnutrition, 306, *306*
  in rheumatic arthritis, 1646

Iron deficiency anemia (Continued)
  latent, 287
  lead intoxication and, 400
  masked, 275
  metabolism and pathogenesis of, 276–285
  mild, diagnosis of, 286, 287, 290, 291
  prevalence of, 299
  prevention of, 299–300
    related to diagnostic criteria in screening tests, 289
  screening tests for, 288–290, 289(t)
    abnormal findings in, 290
  stages of, 286–287, 287
  steady-state, 287–288
  systemic abnormalities associated with, 296–299
  treatment of, 295–296
    response to, 296
  vs copper deficiency, 304
  vs thalassemia trait, 737(t)
  with other illnesses, 300–302
Iron deposition, cardiac, 745–746, 746(t)
Iron dextran (Imferon), for iron deficiency anemia, 295
Iron enzymes, 277
Iron loading, in porphyria cutanea tarda, 382
  in sideroblastic anemia, 374
Iron metabolism, 280–284
  spleen and, 428
Iron overload, in beta thalassemia, cardiac abnormalities in, 745–746, 746(t)
    endocrine abnormalities in, 746–748
    hepatic abnormalities in, 746
    in severe disease, 743–748
    measure of stored iron in, 745
    toxic mechanisms in, 743–745
  in hereditary hemochromatosis, 303–394
  in thalassemia intermedia, 754–755
  source of chelated iron in, 751
  vitamin C and, 753
  vitamin E supplementation and, 754
Iron salts, oral, for iron deficiency treatment, 295
Iron-sufficient preterm infant, hemoglobin values in, 1679(t)
Iron-sulfur proteins, 277
Isocoproporphyrin, in porphyrin cutanea tarda, 381
Isohemagglutinin, normal levels of, by age, 1695(t)
Isoimmune neonatal thrombocytopenia, 111–113
Isomerase enzyme, 364
Isotypes, defined, 861
Isovaleric acidemia, thrombocytopenia with, 1390
IVIC syndrome, 186
Ivy method, of testing bleeding time, 1296

Jansky-Bielschowsky syndrome, 1242
Jaundice. See also *Hyperbilirubinemia.*
  in hereditary spherocytosis, 482–483
  neonatal, bilirubin and, 74
    breast feeding-related, 87–88
    breast milk, 86–88
    ethnic factors and, 88–89
    G6PD deficiency and, 599–600
    phototherapy for, 90–92, 92(t)
    physiologic, 79–82
      historical aspects of, 2
      vs pathophysiologic jaundice, 82–83

Jaundice (Continued)
  obstructive. See also *Cholestasis.*
    hereditary spherocytosis and, 488
    in Rh hemolytic disease, 65
JC virus, 945
Job's syndrome, 824
Joints, acute bleeding into, in hemophilia A, 1306
  treatment of, 1307–1309
  in Henoch-Schönlein purpura, 1460
Josephs, Hugh, 6
Ja^a (Sutter), antigen, 1510
Juvenile rheumatoid arthritis, suppressor T-cell activity in, 853

Kallikrein, in coagulation cascade, 1250
Kasabach-Merritt syndrome, 1386–1388
Kato, Katsuki, 8
Kawasaki syndrome, hypercoagulability in, 1458–1459
  T-cell regulation of B-cell function and, 853, 853(t)
Kell blood group system, 1509–1510, 1510(t)
  chronic granulomatous disease and, 1503–1504
Keratan sulfate, in Morquio's disease, *1232*
Kernicterus, 89
  determining factors for, 56–57
  direct-reacting bilirubin and, 83
  hyperbilirubinemia and, 56
    with Rh erythroblastosis, 83
  in Crigler-Najjar syndrome, 85
  pathogenesis of, 89–90
  prevention of, 90–92
  risk of, in newborn period, 89, 89(t), 90
Ketoacidosis, with adenosylcobalamin deficiency, 351
Kidd blood group, 1513
Kidney transplantation, cadaveric, 1537
  histocompatibility testing for, 1536–1540
    blood transfusion and, 1538
    donor and recipient, 1537
    immunologic monitoring of recipients, 1538–1539
    presensitization, 1537–1538
  immunosuppression methods in, 1539–1540
Kininogen, high-molecular-weight, deficiency of, 1324–1325
  in coagulation cascade, 1249–1250
  in platelets, 1432
Kinky hair syndrome, vs copper deficiency, 304–305
Kleihauer-Betke acid elution test, 30, 58, *200*
KM system, of immunoglobulins, 1571
Kostmann's disease, 210–211, 220(t), 803
Kufs' disease, 1242
Kwashiorkor, 305, 322

Labor, premature induction of, 60
Lactate dehydrogenase, deficiency of, 569
  in schistocytic hemolytic anemia, 433, 434
Lactobacillus casei, folate measurement and, 331
Lactoferrin, in iron uptake process, 367
Laetrile, 1008–1009
Langerhans cell(s), structure and function of, 1119–1120
  histiocytosis of, 1129–1131. See also *Histiocytosis X.*
Laparotomy and splenectomy, for staging of Hodgkin's disease, 1106, 1107(t)

Lazy leukocyte syndrome, 823
Lead, blood levels of, 392
    encephalopathy in children due to, 401
    heme synthesis of, *394*
    in screening for lead poisoning, 406
    normal, 389
    "safe," 402
  effects on δ-aminolevulinic acid dehydratase, 393–394
  effects on erythrocyte function, 399–400
  effects on heme synthesis, 393–399, *394*
    neurotoxic, 399
    nonerythropoietic, 398–399
  hematologic effects of, 392–402
    biochemical, 392–393
    on erythrocyte function, 399–400
    on heme synthesis, 393–399, *394*
  low-level exposure to, 401–402
  neurologic effects of, 401
  sources of, 389–392, 390(t)
    additivity of, 392
    air, 389–390
      and lead in blood, 390, *390*
    dust, 391
    food, 390–391
    miscellaneous, 391–392
    paint, 391
    water, 390–391
Lead encephalopathy, damage to heme synthetic pathway in, 399
  sequelae of, 400–401
Lead poisoning, 389–412
  abnormal hemoglobin function in, 636
  anemia of, 399–400
  clinical aspects of, 400–402
  erythrocyte protoporphyrin value and, 292
  in adults, 401
  in asymptomatic children, 406–407, 407(t)
  in children, 392
  mild, 401–402
  model of, 399
  prevention of, 407
  pyrimidine-5′-nucleotidase deficiency and, 571
  screening for, 405–407
  severe, 400–401
  sideroblastic anemia and, 372–373
  treatment of, 400–405
Lecithin-cholesterol acyltransferase (LCAT), deficiency of, familial, 510–511
  in abetalipoproteinemia, 505
  in conversion of cholesterol to esterified cholesterol, 447
Left ventricular dysfunction, in sickle cell disease, 676
Leg ulcers, with hereditary spherocytosis, 488
  in sickle cell disease, 678
Legionnaires' disease, 833
Lehndorff, Heinrich, 1
Lesch-Nyhan syndrome, 358, 1660
  folate deficiency with, 329
Letterer-Siwe disease, in histiocytosis X, 1129, 1131
Leucine, interconversion of using leucine aminomutase, 340
Leucine aminomutase, in interconversion of α- and β-leucine, 340
Leukapheresis, in leukemia, 1628–1629
Leukemia. See also *Preleukemia.*
  acute, bone and joint manifestations in, 1038
    cardiac manifestations in, 1039
    central nervous system manifestations in, 1036–1037, 1046–1047

Leukemia *(Continued)*
  acute, classification of, 1028–1030, *1032–1033*, 1034(t)
    clinical manifestations of, 1035–1040
    death from, 1054
    diagnosis of, 1040–1041
    differential diagnosis of, 1040–1041
    emotional aspects of, 1053–1054
    extramedullary, 1036–1040
    findings at diagnosis of, 1035–1036, 1036(t)
    gastrointestinal manifestations of, 1038–1039
    genitourinary tract manifestations of, 1037–1038
    laboratory findings in, 1040
    leukapheresis in, 1628–1629
    leukemic infiltrates in, treatment of, 1042
    miscellaneous manifestations of, 1039–1040
    ocular manifestations of, 1039
    oral manifestations of, 1039
    pathophysiology of, 1030–1031, 1034–1035
      cellular heterogeneity in, 1034–1035
      clonal expansion theory in, 1031
      progenitors and precursors of, 1030–1031
    platelet function disorders in, 1447
    protean nature of, 1036
    pulmonary manifestations of, 1039
    survival from, 1051–1052
    treatment of, 1042–1043, 1050–1051
      for acute lymphoblastic leukemia, 1043–1048
      for acute myelogenous leukemia, 1040–1050
    historical aspects of, 11–12
  acute lymphoblastic, B-cell, 1034
    chromosomal changes in, 1487–1489, *1488*
    light chain gene rearrangement in, 864–865, *965*
  bone marrow transplantation for, 252
  central nervous system relapse in, 1046–1047
  cessation of therapy and, 1046
  chromosomal changes in, 1487–1490
    1:19 translocation in, 1489
    4:11 translocation in, 1488
    8:14 translocation in, 1487–1488
    Ph¹ chromosome, 1488–1489
  chromosomal gain in, 1490
  cytoplasmic markers in, 1035
    surface immunologic, 1034–1035
  monoclonal antibody reactivity in, 1034–1035, 1034(t)
  near haploid, chromosomal changes in, 1490
  non T, non B, 869–879, *869*, *1488*, 1490
  prognosis for, 1048, 1048(t)
  relapsed, treatment for, 1046–1047
  T-cell, 1034
    chromosomal changes in, 1489–1490, *1490*
  testicular relapse in, 1047
  treatment of, 1043–1048
    cessation of therapy and, 1045–1046
    CNS prophylaxis, 1044
    other extramedullary prophylaxis, 1044–1045
    remission induction, 1043–1044
    treatment in remission, 1045

Leukemia (Continued)
  acute monocytic, chromosomal structural alterations of 11q in, 1486
  acute myeloblastic, 8:21 chromosomal translocation in, 1484
    surface markers in, 1035
  acute myelogenous, bone marrow transplantation for, 252
    prognosis for, 1049–1050
    sideroblastic anemia and, 372
    treatment of, 1048–1050
  acute myelomonocytic, chromosomal changes in, del(160) in, 1485
    inv(16) in, 1485, *1485*
    sideroblastic anemia and, 372
  acute nonlymphoblastic, bone marrow transplantation for, 252
  acute promyelocytic, 1050
    15:17 chromosomal translocation in, 1484–1485
  aplastic anemia and, 165
  B-cell, 1034
    chromosomal changes in, 1487–1489, *1488*
    light chain gene rearrangement in, 864–865, *865*
  blast cells in, 1031
  bone marrow transplantation for, 251–253
  cellular heterogeneity in, 1034–1035
  central nervous system, 1036–1037, 1046–1047
    treatment of, 1042, 1044
  chromosomal abnormalities in, 1481(t). See also under specific types of leukemia.
    in children vs adults, 1486, 1486(t)
    survival and, 1487
  chronic granulocytic, bone marrow transplantation for, 252–253
  chronic myelogenous, adult type, 1064–1066
    clinical characteristics of, 1065–1066, 1065(t)
    clinical course of, 1067–1068
    clonal nature of, 1066
    differential diagnosis of, 1067
    etiology of, 1066
    treatment of, 1068–1069
    chromosomal abnormalities in, 1480–1483
    juvenile, 1069–1070
    pathophysiology of, 1066–1067
    progenitor cells in, 1066
  congenital, 1052–1053
  eosinophilic, 815
  epidemiologic data on, 927–928
  Fanconi's anemia and, 184
  in Kostmann's disease, 803
  lymphoblasts vs myeloblasts in, 1029–1030, *1032–1033*
  meningeal, 1036–1037
  ocular, treatment of, 1042
  pre-B cell, 1034
  relapsed, 1046–1047
    following bone marrow transplantation, 253
  testicular, 1037–1038, 1047
Leukemic hiatus, 213
Leukemoid reaction. See also *Neutrophilia*.
  differentiation of, 811–812
  in thrombocytopenia with absent radii syndrome, 212
  vs acute leukemia, 1041
  vs leukoerythroblastosis, 213
Leukoagglutinin antibodies, with granulocyte transfusion, 1602

Leukocyte(s), alkaline phosphatase activity in, in chronic myelogenous leukemia, 1066
  blood group antigens of, 1501
  corticosteroid effects on, 810(t)
  cytoplasmic abnormalities of, 1662–1663
  in infections, 1649–1650
  in iron deficiency anemia, 298
  in megaloblastic anemia, 353
  in renal disease, 1640
  in sickle cell disease, 675
  infusions of, in lysosomal storage disease, 1222–1223
  life span of, 135
  nuclear changes in, 1661–1662
  phagocytosis of, in indirect platelet measurement, 1399
  polymorphonuclear, chemotactic factors regulating movement of, 783
    distribution of, 782–784
    factors influencing movement of, 783(t)
    in megaloblastic anemia, 316
    life cycle of, in humans, 782(t)
    metabolism of, 779–780
    morphology and structure of, 779–780
    secretory products of, 780(t)
  splenic destruction of, 907
  variation in disease states, 1661–1665
Leukocytosis, in thrombocytopenia with absent radii syndrome, 211–212
  postsplenectomy, 907
Leukoerythroblastosis, 213–215, *213*, 213(t)
Leukopenia, in infections, 1640
  in lupus, 1647
Leukostasis, in chronic myelogenous leukemia, 1065
Leukotrienes, in polymorphonuclear lipid metabolism, 780
Levamisole, in hyperimmunoglobulin E syndrome, 824
Levine, P., 10–11
Lewis blood group system, 1510–1512, 1511(t)
Lipid(s), in macrophage membranes, 782
  in polymorphonuclear leukocytes, 780
  in target cells, 510
  metabolism of, abnormalities of, 1659
  red cell membrane, asymmetry of, 467
    composition of, 443–445, 444(t)
    in hereditary spherocytosis, 475
    in sickle cell anemia, 665
    organization of, 445–448
Lipid bilayer, of red cell, 467–468
  in abetalipoproteinemia, 505
Lipidoses, bone marrow transplantation for, 256
Lipogranulomatosis (Farber's disease), 1229
Lipoprotein(s), beta, 1562
  low density, in abetalipoproteinemia, 505
  LP-X, 510, 511
  normal, acanthocytosis with, 506
  serum, concentrations of, 1562
    genetic polymorphism of, 1562–1563
  very low density, in abetalipoproteinemia, 505
Ligand binding, to hemoglobin, 616, *616, 617,* 618
Ligandin, bilirubin metabolism in newborn and, 56, 77
  physiologic jaundice of newborn and, 81
Limb salvage procedures, for osteosarcoma, 1163–1164
Linear accelerators, 1019
Listeria infection, hepatitis due to, 95
  phagocyte function in, 833

Lithium, for aplastic anemia, 172
    for Fanconi's anemia, 184
    for neutropenia, 809–810
Liver, abnormalities of, in iron overload in beta thalassemia, 746
    in sickle cell disease, 677
    as organ of hematopoiesis, 17, *17*
    bilirubin metabolism in, in newborn, 55–56, 77
        breast milk jaundice and, 87
        physiologic jaundice and, 81
        unconjugated hyperbilirubinemia and, 84–88
    biopsy of, percutaneous, for differential diagnosis of biliary atresia, 94
    clearance of IgM-coated cells in, 415, *415*, 418
    coagulation factors produced in, 1299(t)
    fetal, for bone marrow transplantation, 244
    in congenital erythropoietic protoporphyria, 37
    in storage diseases, 1217(t), 1219
    macrophage distribution in, 785
    rupture of, neonatal anemia and, 32
Liver disease, Fanconi's anemia and, 185
    hematologic complications with, 1636–1638
    hemolytic anemia with, 506–508, *507–508*
    hemostatic defects with, 1326–1327
    iron deficiency with, serum ferritin value and, 291
    platelet function in, 1446
    target cells in, 510
    veno-occlusive, in bone marrow transplantation recipients, 249
Liver transplant, in storage disease, 1223
Liver tumors, 1179–1181
    epidemiology of, 932–933
Lucas, William Palmer, 2
Lumbar puncture, in CNS leukemia, 1044
Lungs, abnormalities of, in sickle cell disease, 679
    macrophage distribution in, 785
Lutheran blood group system, 1508–1509, 1509(t)
Lymph node, anatomy of, 1087–1088, *1088*
    evaluation in rhabdomyosarcoma, 1155
    giant hyperplasia of, 1089–1090
    in infectious mononucleosis, 1656
    in X-linked lymphoproliferative syndrome, 1123, *1123*
    macrophage distribution in, 785
    reactive hyperplasia of, 1089
Lymphadenopathy, 1087–1090
    anatomy relating to, 1087–1088
    causes of, 1089, 1089(t)
    approach to patient with, 1088–1089
    differential diagnosis of, 1089–1090
    mediastinal masses and, 1090, 1090(t)
    non-neoplastic enlargement of, 1088–1090
    sinus histiocytosis with, 1127–1128
    vs malignant lymphoma, 1086
Lymphoblasts, vs myeloblasts, 1029–1030, *1032–1033*
Lymphocytapheresis, 1626
Lymphocytes, B-. See *B cell(s)*.
    deoxyuridine suppression test with folate status and, 332
    in aplastic anemia, bone marrow inhibition by, 169
    in bone marrow transplantation, 245
    in plasma membrane glycoprotein deficiency, 820
    life span of, 135

Lymphocytes *(Continued)*
    T-. See *T cell(s)*.
    transformation of, in indirect measurement of platelets, 1399
    vacuolization of, 1663
    in storage disease, 1216
Lymphocytopenia, causes of, 1665(t)
Lymphocytosis, 1665, 1665(t)
    atypical, in infectious mononucleosis, 1655
    chronic T cell, pure red cell aplasia and, 196
    in infections, 1650
Lymphography, for staging in Hodgkin's disease, 1105
Lymphohistiocytic disorders, 1118–1135
Lymphohistiocytosis, generalized, of infancy, 1121–1122
    reactive, differential diagnosis of, 1128–1129, 1129(t)
    familial erythrophagocytic lymphohistiocytosis, 1121–1122, *1122*
    lymphomatoid granulomatosis, 1128
    sinus histiocytosis with massive lymphadenopathy, 1127–1128
    virus-associated hemophagocytic syndrome, 1126–1127, *1126–1127*
    X-linked lymphoproliferative syndrome, 1122–1126
Lymphoid neoplasms, B-cell associated clonal markers in, immunoglobulin gene rearrangements as, 870–872
    chromosomal translocations in, 874(t)
Lymphoid system, anatomy and physiology of, 1087–1088
    in bone marrow transplantation, 245
Lymphokines, defined, 849
    T-cell, function of, 856, *856*
Lymphoma(s), B-cell, light chain rearrangements in, 864–865, *865*
    controversies in management of, 1111–1112
    epidemiologic data on, 928–930
    immunoblastic, 1095
    malignant, vs lymphadenopathy, 1086
    noncleaved follicular center, 1095
    non-Hodgkin's, 1091–1101
        cell marker identification in, 1092
        cellular lymphoid origins of, 1091–1092
        classification of, 1091–1095, 1091(t), *1092–1094*
        clinical presentation of, 1095–1096
        clonal origin of, 1091
        definition of, 1091
        epidemiology of, 929–930
        "histiocytic," 1095
        immunohistopathology of, 1091–1095, *1092–1094*
        laboratory findings in, 1096
        large cell, 1095
        lymphoblastic, 1092–1094, *1092*
        staging, 1096–1097, 1097(t)
        treatment of, 1097–1098, 1099(t), 1100
            complications of, 1100–1101
        undifferentiated, Burkitt's type, *1093*, 1094–1095
Lymphomatoid granulomatosis, 1128
Lymphopenia, in lupus, 1647
Lymphoproliferative syndrome, X-linked, 1122–1126, 1122(t), *1123–1124*, 1124(t), 1657
Lymphoreticular responses, to viral infections, 1120–1121
Lysophosphatides, in phospholipid renewal, 448
Lysosomal storage disease. See *Storage diseases*.

Lysosomes, enzymes in, 1213–1214
  in Chédiak-Higashi syndrome, 826
  morphology and physiology of, 1213–1214

M hemoglobins, 634–635, 634(t)
Macrocytosis, in Diamond-Blackfan syndrome, 199, *199*
  with megaloblastic anemia, 353
α$_2$-Macroglobulins, in liver disease, 1638
  neutralization of proteolytic enzymes by, 1265–1266
Macrophage(s). See also *Monocytes*.
  erythrophagocytosis by, 52–53
  function of, 817–818, 1119
    T-cell control of, 856
  in erythropoiesis, 146
  influence on red cells, in hereditary spherocytosis, 481
  in granulocyte progenitor differentiation, 145
  interaction with T cells, 850–851, 856
  iron transport in, 369
  maturation of, 782
  receptors of (Fc and C3), in antibody-coated erythrocyte clearance, 414–416, *414–415*
    in autoimmune hemolytic anemia, 418–419, 421
  structure of, 781, 1119
  tissue, 817–818
    in bone marrow transplant recipients, 245–246
Macrophage colony stimulating factor, 143
Macrothrombocytopathia, 1441
Magnesium deficiency, erythrocyte glycolysis and, 573
Major histocompatibility complex (MHC), 1522
  disease association with, 1544
  genes in, structure and functions of, 1523–1524, 1533–1535
  immune response regulation and, 1522–1524
  polymorphism of, 1527–1528
  T-cell activation and, 849, 855
Major histocompatibility complex linkage group, 1525, *1527*
Malabsorption, 1636
  folate deficiency and, 324
  hematologic complications with, 1635
  in Shwachman-Diamond syndrome, 191
  of vitamin B$_{12}$, failure of small intestines to absorb, 347–349
    failure to secrete intrinsic factor, 345–347
    intestinal disease causing, 348–349
    vitamin B$_{12}$ deficiency and, 342
Malaria, Duffy blood group and, 1502, 1512–1513, 1527
  G6PD deficiency and, 591–592
  glycophorins and, 452
  hemolysis in, 1651
  sickle cell disease and, 655–656
  thalassemia and, 704
  thrombocytopenia with, 1381–1382
Malignancy, hemolytic anemia with, 418, 438
  folic acid deficiency in, 325
Malnutrition. See *Protein-calorie malnutrition*.
Mannose, phagocytosis and, 767
Mannosidosis, 1239–1240
Marasmus, 305
Marble bone disease, *213*, 214–215, 255. See also *Osteopetrosis*.

March hemoglobinuria, 435
Maroteaux-Lamy syndrome, 1234
Mast cell, disease of, 1661
  vs. basophils, 816
May-Hegglin anomaly, 1391–1392, 1441, 1662
McLeod phenotype, of Kell blood group, 1510
  chronic granulomatous disease and, 1503
  hemolytic anemia with, 509
Mean corpuscular hemoglobin concentration (MCHC), in hereditary spherocytosis, 483–484
  in megaloblastic anemia, 316
  in screening tests for iron deficiency anemia, 290
  in sickle cell disease, 663–664, 666–667
  normal, 1679(t)
  oxygen affinity and, 620
Mean corpuscular volume (MCV), for iron deficiency diagnosis, 286, 286(t)
  in girls and boys, *1680*
  in megaloblastic anemia, 316
  in screening tests for iron deficiency anemia, 290
  normal values for, 266(t), 1679(t)
  red cell distribution width in disease and, 269, 269(t)
Mean platelet volume, 1347, 1352
Meckel's diverticulum, iron deficiency and, 285
Mediastinal germ cell tumor, 1178
Mediastinal masses, differential diagnosis of, 1090, 1090(t)
  in lymphoblastic lymphoma, 1093
Mediterranean stomatocytosis, 517
Medulloblastoma, 1192–1193, 1192(t)
Megakaryocyte(s), aplasia of, neonatal thrombocytopenia and, 113
  defective, hematologic disorders involving, 1274
  fragmentation of, 151
  hypoplasia of, congenital thrombocytopenia with, 1391
  maturation of, 149–151, *149, 150, 151*, 1272–1276, *1273*
    cytologic characteristics of, 149(t)
  platelet morphology and function and, 147–151, 1273–1274, *1273*
  potentiator of, 1272
Megakaryocyte colony stimulating activity, thrombocytosis and, 1395
Megakaryocyte colony stimulating factor, 1272
  in thrombopoiesis regulation, 147, 148
Megakaryocytopoiesis, 1395
Megaloblast(s), definition of, 16–17, 315, *316*
Megaloblastic anemia. See also *Folate deficiency; Vitamin B$_{12}$, deficiency of*.
  approach to patient with, 356
  causes of, 315, 317(t)
  congenital familial, 358
  definition of, 315
  diagnosis of, 332–333
    Schilling test for, 355–356
  erythrokinetic abnormalities in, 316
  hematologic changes in, *316*
  hypersegmentation in, *316*
  megaloblastic change in, 354
  not caused by folate or vitamin B$_{12}$ deficiency, 357–359
  of infancy, nutrition and, 320
  refractory, 358
  thiamine-responsive, 358
  with cobalamin deficiency, 345
Megaloblastic crises, with hereditary spherocytosis, 487

Megaloblastosis, drugs producing, 353(t)
Megathrombocytes, 1274
Melanesian hereditary elliptocytosis, 497
Militten, 504
Meningococcemia, disseminated intravascular coagulation and, 1331, *1332*
Menkes' kinky hair syndrome, vs copper deficiency, 304–305
Menstrual cycle, hematologic variations with, 1643–1644
  iron losses and, 284
Mental retardation, in hemoglobin H disease, 732–733
  in methemoglobinemia, 646–647
Mentzer index, 294, 737, 737(t)
6-Mercaptopurine, 1001(t)
  for autoimmune hematologic anemia, 422
Mesenchymoma, malignant, 1179
Mesoblastic nephroma, Wilms' tumor and, 1146
Metabolic acidosis, due to 5-oxoproline, 834
  oxygen affinity and, 623
Metabolic disorders, congenital, defective folate interconversion and, 325–326
  defective folate utilization and, 326–328
  conjugated hyperbilirubinemia in newborn and, 95–96
  folate deficiency due to, 325–328
    acquired, 328
    congenital, 325–328
  hematologic complications of, 1658–1659
  in leukemia treatment, 1042
  in sideroblastic anemia, 372–373
  inherited, thrombocytopenia with, 1390
  vitamin B_{12} deficiency with, 351–352
Metabolism, abnormal, neutropenia with, 802
  as signal in phagocytosis, 788
  folate, inborn errors affecting, 329–330
Metabolites, intermediate red cell, in adults, 1682(t)
Metalloflavoproteins, 277
Metaplasia, agnogenic myeloid, 1073–1075
Metastases, in osteosarcoma, 1163
  of neuroblastoma, 1139
  tumor stem cells and, 996
Methemalbumin, in Rh hemolytic disease, 54
Methemoglobin, normal levels of, 1684(t)
Methemoglobin elution test, 602
  for G6PD deficiency, *590*, 593
Methemoglobin reductase, 644–645, 647–648
Methemoglobin reduction test, for G6PD deficiency, 602
Methemoglobinemia, 641–654
  acquired, abnormal hemoglobin structure and function and, 635
  biochemistry of, 642–646
  clinical correlations of, 645–646
  congenital, due to M hemoglobin, 634–635
  diagnosis of, 647–649
  differentiation from other forms of cyanosis, 649
  genetic aspects of, 646–647
  history of, 642
  in neonatal erythrocytes, 25
  management of, 649–650, 650(t)
Methionine, in cobalamin deficiency, 343
Methionine adenosyltransferase deficiency, 329
Methotrexate, 1000(t)
  for osteosarcoma, 1164–1165
Methylcobalamin deficiency, 351
  with adenosylcobalamin deficiency, 352
Methylene blue, for glucose phosphate isomerase deficiency, 553

Methylene blue *(Continued)*
  for methemoglobinemia diagnosis and treatment, 644, 649, 650
Methylene-THF reductase deficiency, folate deficiency and, 326
  folate metabolism errors and, 330
Methylmalonic acid excretion, in vitamin B_{12} deficiency, 354
Methylmalonic aciduria, 1659
L-Methylmalonyl CoA, conversion to succinyl CoA, cobalamin and, 339–340
Methylmalonyl-CoA mutase, vitamin B_{12} deficiency and, 351–352
Methylmalonyl-CoA mutase apoenzyme formation deficiency, vitamin B_{12} deficiency and, 351–352
Methylprednisolone, for aplastic anemia, 175
N^5-Methyltetrahydrofolate, 317
N^5-Methyltetrahydrofolate homocysteine methyl-transferase, deficiency of, 327–328, 352
  vitamin B_{12} deficiency and, 351–352
Methyltransferase reaction, cobalamin and, 340–341
Microcirculation, disorders of, schistocytic hemolytic anemia and, 432, 433(t)
Microcytosis, in iron deficiency, erythrocyte protoporphyrins and, 408
Micropherocytosis, in ABO hemolytic disease, 67
Microtubules, in movement of polymorphonuclear leukocytes, 784
Milk, boiled, folate deficiency and, 321, 324
  breast, iron in, 280, 281
    vitamin B_{12} in, 344
  cow's, folate deficiency and, 321
    iron deficiency anemia and, 280, 281, 284, 299, 300
  goat's, folate deficiency and, 321–322
  powdered, folate deficiency and, 324
Mineral supplements, in malnutrition treatment, 309
Mithramycin, platelet function and, 1454
Mitochondria, iron transport into, 370
  lead effects on, 392–393, 394, *395*
  sideroblastic anemia and, 373
Mixed lymphocyte culture, in donor selection for bone marrow transplantation, 1541
Miyasato's disease, 1325
MN blood group, 1505–1506, 1506(t)
Molecular sickling, 656, *657–659*
Monoclonal antibodies, for graft versus host disease, 248
  for leukemia in remission, 1045
  for osteosarcoma, 1166
  in bone marrow transplantation for severe combined immunodeficiency, 250
  OKT9, 455
  reactivity in acute leukemia, 1034–1035, 1034(t)
  to specific T cell subpopulations, 1626, 1629
Monocytes. See also *Macrophages.*
  erythrophagocytosis by, 52–53
  function of, 817–818
    T cell control of, 856
  in chronic neutropenia, 799
  structure and function of, 780–782, 1118–1119
Monocytopenia, disorders associated with, 818, 818(t)
Monocytosis, 1664(t), 1665
  disorders associated with, 818, 818(t), 1650
Monoglutamates, 317

Mononuclear phagocyte system, 785, 1118–1121. See also *Phagocyte(s), mononuclear; Monocytes; Macrophage(s)*.
Monosomy 7, in myelodysplasia, 1078
Monosomy 16, retinoblastoma and, 1182
Montreal platelet syndrome, 1441
MOPP regimen, for Hodgkin's disease, 1108, 1110, 1110(t)
Morquio's syndrome, *1232*, 1233–1234
Mouth, bleeding into, in hemophilia A, 1309–1310
MTX (methotrexate), 1000(t)
Mucolipidoses, 1235–1241
Mucolipidosis II, 1237
Mucolipidosis, III, 1238
Mucolipidosis IV, 1238
Mucopolysaccharidoses, bone marrow transplantation for, 256
  characteristics of, 1230–1231, *1231*, 1232(t)
Mucosulfatidosis, 1234
Multi-colony stimulating factor, humoral control of hematopoiesis and, 143
Mus musculus, hereditary spherocytosis hemolytic anemia in, 472–473
Muscle, hemorrhage into, in hemophilia A, 1309
  striated, dysfunction with iron deficiency anemia, 297
Muscular dystrophy, 1659
Myasthenia gravis, 1660
Mycoplasma pneumonia, cold hemagglutinin disease and, 417, 420
Myeloblasts, vs lymphoblasts, 1029–1030, *1032–1033*
Myelodysplasia, 1077–1078
Myelodysplastic syndromes, 1075–1078
  clinical presentation of, 1075–1076
  differential diagnosis of, 1077
  pathophysiology of, 1076–1077
  preleukemia, 217–219
Myelofibrosis, in agnogenic myeloid metaplasia, 1073–1075
Myelokathexis, 802
Myeloma, multiple, 488
Myeloperoxidase deficiency, of neutrophils, 832–833
Myelophthisis, in osteopetrosis, 214
Myelopoiesis, regulation of, 141–142
  cell-cell interactions in, 144–147
Myeloproliferative disorders, chronic, 1064–1075, 1482–1483
  adult type chronic myelogenous leukemia, 1064–1069
  agnogenic myeloid metaplasia/myelofibrosis, 1073–1075
  essential thrombocythemia, 1072–1073
  juvenile chronic myelogenous leukemia, 1069–1070
  neutrophilia and, 811
  platelet dysfunction with, 1398, 1446–1447, 1447(t)
  polycythemia vera, 1070–1072
  vs acute leukemia, 1041
  vs congenital leukemia, 1052
Myocardial dysfunction, in sickle cell disease, 676
Myocardial infarction, antiplatelet agents and, 1452–1453
  risk with use of prothrombin complex concentrates, 1302
Myoclonus, in type I sialidosis, 1235
Myoglobin, function and distribution of, 276
  iron deficiency and, 296–297, *297*

Myopathy, in phosphofructokinase deficiency, 553–554
Myosin, red cell membrane, 461

NADH, in methemoglobin reduction, 642–643
NADH-diaphorase I, 644–645
NADH-diaphorase II, 644
NADP, G6PD and, 587, 596
  in pentose pathway, 584–588, *585–586*
NADP/NADPH ratio, G6PD regulatory role in, 587–588, 596
NADPH, generated by pentose pathway, 584, *586*, 587. See also *Pentose-phosphate shunt*.
  in diagnosis of G6PD deficiency, 601, 832
  in congenital nonspherocytic hemolytic anemia, 596
NADPH diaphorase, deficiency of, 606
  methemoglobin reduction and, 644–645
  variants of, 646
NADPH oxidase, in chronic granulomatous disease, 830–832
  in removal of oxidant products in neutrophilic function, 833–835
Nasopharyngeal carcinoma, Epstein-Barr virus and, 947
Neel, James V., 12
Neonates. See also *Infants; Premature infants*.
  anemia in, 27–33
    as result of hemolytic process, 33–36
    diagnostic approach to, 37–40
    from hemolytic process, 33–36, 33(t)
  aspirin ingestion in, 1450
  bilirubin metabolism in, 55–56, 79–82
    abnormal, 82–83
  bleeding in, 107, *107*
    laboratory evaluation of, 105(t), 108, *109*, 109(t)
  coagulation factors in, 1692(t)
  defective chemotaxis in, 823
  disseminated intravascular coagulation in, 115–117
  eosinopenia in, 1663
  erythrocyte sedimentation rate in, *1696*
  erythrocytes in, 16–25
    in ABO hemolytic disease, 66–67, 67(t)
  granulocyte transfusion in, 1602
  hematologic values at birth, 25–27
  hematology of, historical aspects of, 1–13
  hemolytic disease of, due to minor blood group antibodies, 68–69
    hyperbilirubinemia with, 83–84
  hemorrhage in, due to inherited disorders of coagulation, 118–119
    miscellaneous causes of, 119–120
    secondary to platelet dysfunction in, 114–115
  hemorrhagic diseases in, 104–127
  hemostasis in, 104–107
  hereditary spherocytosis in, 484–485
  hyperbilirubinemia in, 79–82
    conjugated, 92–97
    from Rh hemolytic disease, 61–66
    unconjugated, diseases associated with, 83–89
  immune thrombocytopenia in, 1382
  iron compounds in, 278–279
  jaundice in, 2
    G6PD deficiency and, 599–600
  platelet function in, 1444–1445
  red cell enzyme deficiencies in, 36

Neonates *(Continued)*
  red cell membrane, hereditary disorders of, 36
  red cell production in, impaired, 36
  red cell transfusion in, 1584
  sickle cell disease in, 667
  thrombocytopenia in, 108–114, 1389–1390
  thrombosis in, accelerated, 117
  vascular-platelet interactions in, 1692(t)
  vitamin K deficiency in, 117–118
Nephroblastomatosis, related to Wilms' tumor, 1146
Nephroma, malignant mesenchymal, 1147
  mesoblastic, 1146
Nephrotic syndrome, 1640–1641
  hypercoagulability and, 1458
Neural origin, of soft tissue tumors, 1160–1161
Neuroblastoma, 1138–1145
  biochemical features of, 1139
  biologic behavior of, 1139–1140
  cervical, 1143–1144
  chromosomal changes in, 1492
  clinical features of, 1138–1139
  cytogenetics of, 1138
  epidemiology of, 930
  immune response to, 1140
  intraspinal, 1144
  management of, 1142–1143
    newer techniques of, 1144–1145
  metastases of, 1139
  pathology of, 1138
  prognosis of, 1141–1142, *1143*
  regression of, 1140
  staging of, 1140–1141, 1141(t)
  thoracic, 1144
  vs acute leukemia, 1041
Neuroectodermal tumors, primitive, 1193
Neurofibromatosis, leukemia risk and, 928
Neurologic disorders, acanthocytosis with, normal lipoproteins and, 506
  in acute bone marrow transplantation for mucopolysaccharidoses, 256
  in Chédiak-Higashi syndrome, 826
  in gangliosidoses, 1229–1230
  in Gaucher's disease, 1227
  in lead exposure, 401
  in lysosomal storage disease, 1215
  in Niemann-Pick disease, 1228
  in sickle cell disease, 679
  in vitamin B$_{12}$ deficiency, 343
Neuronal ceroid-lipofuscinosis, 1241–1242
Neuropathy, peripheral, in lead poisoning in adults, 401
  with vitamin B$_{12}$ deficiency, 353
Neurotoxicity, lead intoxication and, 399
Neutropenia, 210–211
  autoimmune, 804–806
  benign, with metabolic disturbances, 802
  C5a, 804
  chronic, 801–802, 810
  classification of, 799–800
  congenital, severe, 210–211, 220(t), 803
  cyclic, 800–801, *800*
  defined, 799
  drug-induced, 806–807
  evaluation of patients with, 807, 808(t), 809
  granulocyte transfusion for, 1598–1599, 1601
  immune, 804–806
  in Felty's syndrome, 1647
  in hyperthyroidism, 1643
  in megaloblastic anemia, 316

Neutropenia *(Continued)*
  in renal disease, 1640
  in Shwachman-Diamond syndrome, 190–191
  laboratory tests for, 807, 808(t), 809
  neonatal, autoimmune, 804
  sepsis induced, vs acute leukemia, 1041
  therapy of, 809–810
  with disorders of proliferation of committed myeloid stem cells, 801–802
  with disorders of proliferation of committed stem cells, 800–801
  with phenotypic abnormalities, 802–803
  with T and B lymphocyte abnormalities, 801
Neutrophil(s), actin dysfunction syndrome of, 825
  blood group antigens of, 1501
  characteristics of, 797–798
  degranulation function of, in Chédiak-Higashi syndrome, 826–827
  G6PD deficiency in, 832
  granulated, in storage diseases, 1216–1217
  hereditary constitutional hypersegmentation of, 1662
  hereditary dense granulation of, 1663
  hereditary giant, 1662
  hereditary prevalence of nuclear appendages of, 1662, *1662*
  hypersegmentation of, in folate deficiency, 330–331
  impaired chemotaxis of, conditions associated with, 821–824, 821(t)
  in congenital plasma membrane glycoprotein deficiency, 819
  in infections, 1649
  in Pelger-Huet anomaly, 1073, *1073*, 1661–1662, *1661*
  iron deficiency anemia and, 298
  production of, 144, *145*
  respiratory burst of, in acquired disorders, 833
    in chronic granulomatous disease, 828–831
    in G6PD deficiency of neutrophils, 832
    in myeloperoxidase deficiency, 832
  specific granule deficiency, 828
  survival of, disorders of, neutropenia with, 804–807
Neutrophilia, 810–812, 810(t)
Neutrophil-releasing activity, 799
Niemann-Pick disease, 1227–1229
  conjugated hyperbilirubinemia and, 96
  subtypes of, 1228–1229
Nitrates, dietary neonatal methemoglobinemia and, 648
Nitroblue tetrazolium test, for chronic granulomatous disease, 829–830
Nitrofurantoin, platelet function and, 1454
Nonsteroidal anti-inflammatory agents. See also *Aspirin.*
  platelet function and, 1448–1451
Norepinephrine, urinary, iron deficiency anemia and, 298
Nosebleeds, 1293–1294
Nuclear magnetic resonance, for brain tumor evaluation, 1187
Nucleic acid synthesis, in monocyte maturation, 782
Nucleoside phosphorylase, deficiency of, in severe combined immunodeficiency, 885, *886*
Nutrition, counseling in, for iron deficiency anemia treatment, 296

Nutrition *(Continued)*
  deficiency in. See also *Protein-calorie malnutrition.*
    combined with iron deficiency, 294–295
    thrombocytopenia with, 1394
    pure red cell aplasia and, 194
Nutritional support, in cancer chemotherapy, 987

Obstetric accidents, 31
OKT9, 455
Oligodendroglioma, 1194
Oligonucleotide probes, for detecting thalassemia mutations, 721, *721*
  for prenatal diagnosis of beta thalassemia, 762
Oligosaccharides, in mucolipidoses, 1235
Oncogenes, 957–968
  cellular, 923–924, 942–957, 943(t)
    cancer and, 960–965
    cellular growth factors and, 942
    characteristics of, 955(t), 958–960
    clinical applications of, 967–968
    cooperation of, in oncogenesis, 965
    c-fgr, 947
    c-myc, Burkitt's lymphoma and, 873
    growth factor and DNA synthesis and, 966–967
    hybridization analysis of, 960–961, *960*
    in nonviral tumors, 957–958
    inappropriate, 942
    myc, associated with cancer, 961
    N-*myc*, 963–964
    molecular biology of, 958–960
    proteins encoded by, 958–960
    ras, gene products of, 958–960
    relation to cancer, 961
    role in normal cell, 965–967, *966*
    tissue specificity and, 965
    vs viral oncogenes, 958
  growth factors and, 956–957
  RNA viral, cell transformation by, 954, 956–957
  products of, 954, 956–957
Oncovin, 999(t)
Opsonins, neutrophil function and, 797
  serum, in sickle cell disease, 675
  splenic, 430
Opsonization, cellular disorders of, 825
  definition of, 786
  humoral disorders of, 825
  in neutrophil disorders, 824
Optic glioma, 1190
Oral bleeding, in hemophilia A, 1309–1310
Oral lesions, in acute leukemia, 1039
  in aplastic anemia, 171
Oral surgery, in hemophilia A, 1311
Orbit, rhabdomyosarcoma of, 1156
Organelles, subcellular, in protein-calorie malnutrition, 307
Orosomucoid, genetic polymorphism of, 1554–1555, *1554*, 1555(t)
Orotic aciduria, 357–358, 1659
Orotidylic decarboxylase, 357
Orotidylic pyrophosphorylase, 357
Osler-Weber-Rendu syndrome, 1636
Osmotic fragility, of erythrocytes, in lead poisoning, 399
  of spherocytes, in hereditary spherocytosis, 477–478, *479*

Osmotic fragility test, in hereditary spherocytosis, 484
Osteoclasts, in osteopetrosis, 214
Osteomyelitis, vs bone infarction, of sickle cell disease, 669, 671
Osteopetrosis, bone marrow transplantation for, 254–255
  juvenile, 818
  malignant, 213, 214–215
Osteosarcoma, 1161–1163
  treatment of, 994, 1163–1166
Ovaries, cancer of, epidemiology of, 933
  disease of, hematologic abnormalities with, 1643
  germ cell tumors of, 1172–1174
  in leukemia, 1038
Ovotransferrin, in iron uptake process, 367
Oxidant drugs and chemicals, methemoglobinemia and, 647–648, 648(t), 649(t)
Oxidant hemolysis, 517–518
Oxidant-induced injury, neonatal erythrocyte response to, 25
Oxidative metabolism, 584. See also *Pentose-phosphate shunt.*
  disorders of, 828–833
    acquired, 833
5-Oxoproline, metabolic acidosis due to, in glutathione synthetase deficiency, 834
Oxygen, transport across placenta, blood oxygen affinity and, 624, 625
Oxygen affinity, of hemoglobin, 617–618
  alterations, in, 620–624, *621–624*
  Bohr effect and, 618, *618*
  2,3-diphosphoglycerate and, 619
  hemoglobin variants with, 633–634
  in fetal blood, 623–625
  index of, 617
  oxygen delivery to tissues and, 620–624
  in preterm infants, 39
Oxygen binding, heme iron in, in methemoglobinemia, 642, *642*
Oxygen effect, radiation damage and, 1022
Oxygen metabolism, of phagocytes, 790–792
Oxygenation, of hemoglobin, 617–624. See also *Deoxygenation.*
  oxygen cooperativity in, 617–618
Oxyhemoglobin, structure of, *617*
Oxyhemoglobin dissociation curve, *617*, 618, 622
  displacement in various disorders, 621(t)
  factors influencing, 620, 621(t)
  in carbon monoxide intoxication, 636
  in methemoglobinemia, 635
  in sulfhemoglobinemia, 651
  in unstable hemoglobinopathies, 633
  oxygen affinity of, 617–618
Oxymetholone, for Fanconi's anemia, 183
Oxytocin, breast feeding-related jaundice and, 88

P antigen, 1503
P blood group, 1506–1507
  phenotypes in, 1507(t)
Pain, in sickle cell crises, abdominal, 673
  bone, 670, *671*
  central nervous system, 673–674
  chest, 671–672
  priapism, 674
  management of, 682–683
Paint, lead in, 391

Pallor. See also *Blood loss.*
  differential diagnosis of, 32(t)
  in autoimmune hemolytic anemia, 420
  in transient erythroblastopenia of childhood, 205
Pancreas, disease of, hematologic complications with, 1636
  function of, in beta thalassemia, 747–748
    in Shwachman-Diamond syndrome, 190–191
Pancreatitis, acute hemorrhagic, 1636
  chronic, vitamin B_{12} malabsorption with, 348
Pancytopenia, immune, 423–424
  in dyskeratosis congenita, 189
  in Fanconi's anemia, 179–180, *179*, 182, 185–186
  serum humoral inhibitors of, aplastic anemia and, 168
  with bone marrow failure, 159. See also *Bone marrow failure.*
Papillary necrosis, in sickle cell disease, 676, *677*
Papillomavirus, 944–945
Papovavirus, 944–946
Pappenheimer bodies, in sideroblastic anemia, 372
Parahemophilia, 1322
Parasitic infections, eosinophilia and, 814–815
Parathyroid function, in iron overload in beta thalassemia, 748
Parathyroid hormone, hemolytic anemia in advanced renal failure, 509
Paresthesia, with vitamin B_{12} deficiency, 353
Paroxysmal nocturnal hemoglobinuria, 424–425
  aplastic anemia and, 165
  autoimmune neutropenia and, 806
  bone marrow transplantation for, 251
  tests for, 897
Parsons, Leonard, 9
Partial thromboplastin time (PTT), in neonates, normal values for, 105(t), 108, 109(t)
Parvovirus infection, aplastic anemia and, 164, 194–195, 674
Passavoy effect, 1325
Pauling, Linus, 12
PBG. See *Porphobilinogen.*
Pelger-Huet anomaly, 1073, *1073*, 1649–1650, 1661–1662, *1661*
Peliosis hepatis, with androgen therapy, 173
Penicillamine, for lead poisoning, *403*, 405
Penicillin, for postsplenectomy sepsis, 912, 1370
Penicillin derivatives, platelet dysfunction and, 1453
Pentamidine, for bone marrow transplantation, 249
Pentose-phosphate shunt, defects of, 604–606
  G6PD deficiency and, 584, *586*, 587
  glucose metabolism in, 587–588
  in glucose phosphate isomerase deficiency, 552
  in neonatal erythrocytes, 25
  trigger of, 587–588
Perinatal aspiration syndromes, 1389
Perineal area, rhabdomyosarcoma of, 1158
Pernicious anemia, vitamin B_{12} deficiency and, 342
Pertussis, 1651
Petechiae, in neonatal thrombocytopenia secondary to maternal ITP, 110
  platelet defects and, 1347

Peutz-Jeghers syndrome, 1636
PFK. See *Phosphofructokinase.*
PGK. See *Phosphoglycerate kinase.*
pH, oxygen affinity and, 620
Phagocyte(s), classification of, 779
  cytocidal and digestive activity of, 790–792
    control of, 792–793
  defined, 779
  development of, 798–799
  distribution of, 782–785
  factors influencing movement of, 783(t)
  functions of, 785–793
    degranulation, 789–790
    endocytosis, 788–789
    recognition, 785–787
    recognition-response coupling, 787–768
  granulocyte function disorders and, 818–836
  granulopoietic disorders and, 797, 818
  life cycle in humans, 782(t)
  metabolism of, 779–782
  mononuclear, 1118–1121
    distribution of, 784–785
    filtering function of, 784–785
    metabolism of, 781–785
    structure of, 780–782
  morphology of, 779–782
  oxygen-dependent toxicity of, 790–791
  oxygen-independent toxicity of, 791–792
  secretory products of, 780(t)
  structure of, 779–782
Phagocytosis, antibody-induced, 430
  definition of, 786
  in malignant histiocytosis, 1132
  mechanism of, 787–788
  spherocytosis and, 503
  splenic, 905–906
Phagosomes, formation of, 797
Pharyngitis, in infectious mononucleosis, 1654
Phenobarbital, bilirubin metabolism and synthesis and, 56, 75
  for neonatal jaundice, 81, 600
  for prevention of kernicterus, 90
  for type II glucuronyl transferase deficiency, 86
  megaloblastic anemia with, 328
Phenothiazines, neutropenia and, 806–807
Phenylalanine, folate deficiency and, 329
Phenylbutazone, neutropenia with, 806
Phenytoin, folate deficiency and, 324
  megaloblastic anemia with, 328
Pheresis, for platelet collection, 1589
Philadelphia chromosome, 963
  in acute lymphoblastic leukemia, 1488–1489
  in chronic myelogenous leukemia, 1065–1066, 1068, 1480–1482, *1482*
  as tumor marker, 870, *871*
  time of occurrence of, 1492–1493
Phlebotomy, erythrocytapheresis as alternative to, 1626
  for polycythemia vera, 1072
Phorbol esters, in phagocytosis, 788
Phosphate, inorganic, acquired erythrocyte glycolytic disorders and, 572, 572(t)
Phosphatidyl choline, structure of, *444*, 444(t), 445
  xerocytosis and, 516
Phosphatidyl ethanolamine, structure of, *444*, 444(t), 445, 665
Phosphatidyl serine, 665
  macrophage binding to, in hereditary spherocytotic red cells, 476
  structure of, *444*, 444(t), 445
Phosphatidylinositol-4,5-biphosphate, 460, *460*

INDEX

Phosphoenolpyruvate, 563
  in hereditary spherocytosis, 476
Phosphofructokinase, hemolytic anemia and, 553–555, 554(t)
  in neonate, 23–24
Phosphoglucomutase, red cell, phenotypes of, 1573–1574
6-Phosphogluconate dehydrogenase deficiency, 604
Phosphoglycerate kinase, *558*, 559
  deficiency of, hemolytic anemia with, 557–560, 558(t), *558*
  in neonatal red cells, 21
  X linkage of, 593
Phosphokinase C, in T cell activation, 850
Phospholipase, in phagocytosis, 788
  in platelet signal transduction, 1284
  in venoms, 504
Phospholipids, acidic, in phagocytosis, 788
  flip-flop, 445
  in platelet membrane, 1279
  in polymorphonuclear leukocytes, 780
  red cell membrane, 443, *444*
    asymmetry of, 445–446, 467
    in sickle cell disease, 665
    intercalation with cholesterol, 446–447
    lateral diffusion of, 447
    motions of, 446–447
    organization of, 445
    renewal pathways of, 447–448
Phosphorylated sugars, phagocytosis and, 787
Phosphorylation, of red cell membrane proteins, in hereditary spherocytosis, 476
  in red cell membrane skeleton, 462
  red cell shape and, 468
  protein modification by, in retroviruses, 954, 956
Photobilirubin, 92
Photodegradation, 92
Photoisomerization, in phototherapy, 92
Photosensitivity, in congenital erythropoietic porphyria, 376
  in congenital erythropoietic protoporphyria, 378
  in lead intoxication, 396
Phototherapy, complications of, 90–91
  direct-reacting bilirubin and, 83
  for hyperbilirubinemia of newborn, 56
  for hyperbilirubinemia with Rh erythroblastosis, 83
  for neonatal jaundice, 90–92, 92(t)
  for retinoblastoma, 1185
  in Crigler-Najjar syndrome, 85
  indications for, 91–92, 92(t)
  mechanism of action of, 92
  platelet dysfunction and, 114
  thrombocytopenia with, 1389
Physical therapy, for hemophilia A, 1309
Phytonadione, for prevention of hemorrhagic disease of newborn, 117–118
PI gene variants, 1552–1554, 1554(t)
Pica, lead poisoning and, 391
Pincer cells, in hemolytic crisis of G6PD deficiency, 597–598, *598*
Pineal tumors, 1194–1195
Pinocytosis, 786–788
Pituitary disease, hematologic effects of, 1644
PiZZ genotype, of α_1-antitrypsin deficiency, 96
PK. See *Pyruvate kinase.*
PL^{A1} antigen, 1382, 1405, 1431
Placenta, abnormalities of, neonatal anemia and, 31

Placenta *(Continued)*
  anti-D antibodies transferred through, 48
  bilirubin transport through, in Rh hemolytic disease, 55
  iron uptake by, 368
  oxygen transport across, 624, 625
Plasma, bilirubin transport in, *75*, 76–77
  clotting tests done on, 1297
  fresh frozen, 1607–1624
    uses in coagulation disorders, 1300–1301
  other products of, 1613
  removed from citrated blood for exchange transfusion, 64
  whole, transfusion therapy with, 1607–1608, 1608(t)
Plasma exchange, in treatment of hemolytic uremic syndrome, 437
Plasma infusion, for chronic idiopathic thrombocytopenic purpura, 1371
Plasma membrane glycoprotein deficiency, congenital, 819–820, 820(t)
Plasma products. See also *Cryoprecipitate; Factor VIII, concentrates of; Prothrombin complex concentrates.*
  heat-treated concentrates of, hepatitis risk and, 1615
  transfusion therapy with, complications of, 1613–1616
  future developments in, 1616–1617
  uses of, 1613, 1614(t)
Plasmapheresis, as immunotherapy, dose and schedule for, 1625, 1625(t)
  for autoimmune hemolytic anemia, 423
  for chronic idiopathic thrombocytopenic purpura, 1371
  for hemolytic uremic syndrome, 437
  illness treated by, 1625–1626,1627(t)
  of Rh-negative women, for treatment of Rh hemolytic disease in fetus, 61
  replacement solutions used in, 1624–1625
Plasmin, conversion from plasminogen, 1259–1260, *1260*
  degradation of fibrin clots by, 1261–1262
  degradation of fibrinogen by, 1261, *1261*, 1262
  in coagulation cascade, 1251
  in scission of B-beta chain of fibrin I monomer, 1262
Plasminogen, 1563–1564
  activation of, 1260
  conversion to plasmin, 1259–1260, *1260*
  in coagulation cascade, 1250–1251
  in fibrinolytic mechanism, 1258–1261, *1260*
  in liver disease, 1638
  levels of, in neonates, 106
Plasmodium falciparum malaria. See also *Malaria.*
  Duffy blood group and, 1527
  G6PD deficiency and, 591–592
  hemolysis in, 1651
  membrane glycoproteins and, 452, 1502–1503
Plasmodium vivax, Duffy blood group and, 1502, 1527
Platelet(s). See also *Thrombocytopenia.*
  adhesion of, 1344–1345, 1430
    to subendothelium, 1283
  aggregation of, 1281, 1283–1284, *1284*, 1344, *1345*, 1430–1432
    abnormalities in, to epinephrine as stimulus, 1444
    antibody-induced, indirect assays of, 1400
    in diabetes, 1659

Platelet(s) *(Continued)*
   aggregation of, in Glanzmann's thrombasthenia, 1436
      pathways of, 1431
   alloantigens of, 1281–1282
   antibodies of, indirect assays of, 1399–1400, *1399*
   arachidonic acid metabolism in, inherited defects of, 1438–1440, *1439*
   assays of, direct, 1400–1402, *1401, 1402*
      controversies concerning, 1402–1404
      indirect, 1399–1400, *1399*
   circulating, functions of, 1271
      in thrombocytopenia, 147
   coagulant activity of, 1287, *1287*
   cold agglutinins of, 1346
   collagen, interactions with, 1282–1283, 1344, *1345*
   complement bound to, measurement of, 1405
   consumption of, thrombocytopenia with, 1385–1388
   count of. See *Platelet count.*
   crossmatching of, 1594–1595
      by platelet-associated IgG measurements, 1406
   destruction of, accelerated, platelet transfusions for, 1592–1593
      indirect assay of, 1400
      mechanical, neonatal thrombocytopenia due to, 113
      splenic, 907
   development and kinetics of, 1272–1276, *1273*
   disorders of. See *Platelet disorders.*
   electronic counting of, pseudothrombocytopenia and, 1345
   energy metabolism of, 1277–1278
   factor 3 release, in indirect platelet measurement, 1400
   Fc receptor, function of, 1431
   fragments of, in platelet-associated IgG direct assays, 1403
   frozen, 1590
   function of. See *Platelet function.*
   glycoproteins of. See also *Glycoproteins.*
      inherited disorders of, Bernard-Soulier syndrome, 1433, 1436
         Glanzmann's thrombasthenia, 1436–1437
   granules of, 1276–1277, *1276–1277*, 1431–1432
      α-granules, coagulation factors in, 1432
      inherited disorders of, 1437–1438
   IgG bound to, direct assays of, 1400–1402, *1401, 1402*
      controversies concerning, 1402–1404
      uses of, 1405–1406
      in pathogenesis of immune thrombocytopenia, 1348–1351
      indirect assays of, 1399–1400
   IgM bound to, measurements of, 1405
   in exchange transfusion, 62
   in hemostasis, 1344
   interaction with coagulation proteins, 1432
   isotope labeling of, 1274–1276
   maternal transfusion, for isoimmune neonatal thrombocytopenia, 111–112, *112*
   membrane of, structure and function of, 1279–1282
   membrane proteins, 1271
   morphology of, 1276–1277

Platelet(s) *(Continued)*
   pheresis procedure for, 1589
   plug formation by, reactions involved in, 1272
   precursors of, 149–151, 149(t), *149, 150*
   progenitors of, 148–149, *149, 150*
   production of, 147–151
   refractory, in acute leukemia, 1050
   satellitism of, 1346
   secretion defects in, congenital, 1440
   secretory products of, 1272
   signal transduction in, 1284–1285, 1345
   size and age relationships of, 1347
      platelet-associated IgG and, 1403
   splenic sequestration of, 1275
      thrombocytopenia due to, 1394–1395
   structure and function relationships of, 1344, 1429–1432
   surface of, function in coagulation activities, 1271–1272
   survival of, 135, 1275
      autologous, 1348
      in idiopathic thrombocytopenic purpura of childhood, 1353
   thrombotic disorders mediated by, antiplatelet agents and, 1452–1453
Platelet count, 1347
   bleeding time and, 1591
   fetal scalp, 1373
   in chronic idiopathic thrombocytopenic purpura, 1352, 1364, 1366–1367, 1373
   in isoimmune neonatal thrombocytopenia, 111–112
   neonatal, 108–109
Platelet-derived growth factor, 1277
Platelet disorders, acquired, 1445–1447, 1448(t)
   bone marrow transplantation for, 254
   congenital, 1432–1444, 1434(t), 1435(t)
      diagnosis and management of, 1429(t), 1441–1444, 1442(t)
      miscellaneous, 1441
   drugs causing, 1302–1305
   hemorrhage secondary to, in neonates, 114–115
   in cardiac disease, 1634
   in essential thrombocythemia, 1072
   in hemolytic uremic syndrome, 436
   in lupus erythematosus, 1648
   in megaloblastic anemia, 316
   in myeloproliferative disease, 1398
   in pseudo von Willebrand's disease, 1319
   in renal disease, 1641
   in thyroid disease, 1643
   physiologic qualitative, 1444–1445
   platelet transfusion for, 1593–1594
   quantitative, pseudothrombocytosis, 1345–1346
      thrombocytopenia, 1346–1383. See also *Thrombocytopenia.*
   vs plasma coagulation defects, 1347(t)
Platelet function, 1344, 1429–1432
   alcohol and, 1454
   drug ingestion and, 1447–1455
      antibiotics, 1453
      antiplatelet agents, 1451–1452
      dextran, 1454
      glyceryl guaiacolate and, 1454
      heparin and, 1454
      membrane-active drugs, 1453–1454
      miscellaneous, 1454
      nitrofurantoin, 1454

Platelet function *(Continued)*
  drug ingestion and, nonsteroidal anti-inflammatory agents, 1448–1451
    sodium valproate, 1454
    thrombocytopenia, due to, treatment of, 1454–1455
    vinca alkaloids, 1454
  drugs inhibiting, 1455(t)
  endothelial cell function interaction with, 1278–1279, 1285–1286
  in circulation, 1271
  in coagulation, 1271–1292
  in diabetes, 1456–1457
  in homocystinuria, 1458
  in Kawasaki syndrome, 1458
  in leukemia and preleukemia, 1447
  in liver disease, 1446
  in myeloproliferative disorders, 1446–1447, 1447(t)
  in nephrotic syndrome, 1458
  in renal disease, 1641
  in uremia, 1445–1446
  inhibited, indirect assays of, 1400
  neonatal, 104–105, 1444–1445
  structure and, 1429–1432
  tests of, 1296–1297
  with cardiac defects, 1446
  with cardiopulmonary bypass, 1446
Platelet migration inhibition, in indirect platelet measurement, 1400
Platelet matching, 1594–1595
Platelet storage pool defects, neonatal, 1444
Platelet transfusion, 1588–1597
  clinical uses of, 1591–1594
  concentrates for, 1442–1443
    preparation of, 1588–1589
  dose of, 1590
  for aplastic anemia, 171
  for thrombocytopenia absent radii syndrome, 212
  platelet storage for, 1589–1590
  poor response to, 1590(t), 1591
  prophylactic, 1592
  reactions to, 1594
  refractory state with, 1594–1595
  technique of, 1594
Platelet-vascular interactions, in fetus and neonate, 1692(t)
Pluripotent stem cell, in aplastic anemia, 167–168
  in bone marrow transplantation rejection, 246
  in hematopoiesis, 135–137
  in reticular dysgenesis, 193
  of spleen vs that of granulocyte-macrophage, 142
Pluripoietin, 143
Plummer-Vinson syndrome, 1635
Pneumococcal pneumonia, conjugated hyperbilirubinemia and, 96
Pneumococcal sepsis, in sickle cell disease, 674–675
  vaccination and, 432, 489–490, 1369
Pneumococcal vaccine, for prevention of postsplenectomy sepsis, 432, 489–490, 912–913, 1369
Pneumocystis carinii pneumonia, in acute leukemia, 1051
  in bone marrow transplantation, 248–249
Pneumonia, bacterial, in sickle cell disease, 672
  interstitial, with bone marrow transplantation, 248

Pneumonia *(Continued)*
  pneumococcal, conjugated hyperbilirubinemia and, 96
  Pneumocystis carinii, in acute leukemia, 1051
Pneumonitis, chronic, pediatric AIDS and, 890, *891*
Pokeweed mitogen, 851
Poland's syndrome, preleukemia and, 216
Polyacrylamide gel electrophoresis in sodium dodecyl sulfate (SDS-PAGE), 449–451, 457, 1461
Polyagglutination, 1501
Polyanions. See *Anions, polyvalent red cell.*
Polyarteritis nodosa, 1648
Polyclonal immunoglobulin synthesis, T-cell control of, 851–854
Polycythemia, classification of, 1070(t)
  due to cyanotic congenital heart disease, erythrocytapheresis for, 1626, 1628
  in renal disease, 1640
  neonatal, 1390
  secondary, iron deficiency and, 301
  with cyanotic congenital heart disease, 1328
Polycythemia vera, 1070–1072, 1447
Polyglutamates, 317
Polygonal cell tumor with fibrous stoma, 1179
Polymerization, hemolytic severity of sickle cell syndromes and, 663–664
  in hemoglobin SC disease, 685
  of deoxy-hemoglobin S, 659–661, *660–661*
    delay time concept in, 660–662, *662*
Polyoma virus, 945
Polyphosphoinositides, in red cell shape maintenance, 468
Polysplenia syndrome, congenital, 903
Porphobilinogen, acute intermittent porphyria and, 376, 378–380
  in heme synthesis, 364
  urinary, screening test for, 379
Porphobilinogen deaminase, in acute intermittent porphyria, 379
Porphyria(s), 375–382
  acquired, 382
  acute intermittent, 378–380, 378(t)
  characteristics of, 375
  classification of, 375–376, 376(t)
  congenital erythropoietic, 376–377
    hyperbilirubinemia and, 84
  hepatic, 378–382
  hepatoerythropoietic, 382
  types of, 376
  variegate (mixed), 380–381
Porphyria cutanea tarda, 381–382
Porphyrins, 364–365, *364*
  overproduction of, 376
  precursors of, in acute intermittent porphyria, 378–380
  vs porphyrinogens, 364–365, 364(t)
Porphyrinogens, 363, *364*, 365
  vs porphyrins, 364–365, 364(t)
Porphyrinuria, 382
Postsplenectomy, target cells in, 511
  septicemia in, 432, 489–490, 674–675, 910–913, *912*, 1369
Post-transfusion purpura, 1382
Potassium, metabolism of, in leukemia treatment, 1042
  permeability of, in hereditary hydrocytosis, 513
    in hereditary xerocytosis, 514
  transport of, in sickle cells, 664

pp60, viral, 954, 956
  cellular, 958
Prednisone, for autoimmune hemolytic anemia, 421
  for cancer, 999(t)–1000(t)
  for Diamond-Blackfan syndrome, 203–204
  for Henoch-Schönlein purpura, 1461
  for paroxysmal nocturnal hemoglobinuria, 424
  for pure red cell aplasia, 197
  with azathioprine, for chronic graft versus host disease, 247
  with vincristine, 1043
Preeclampsia, thrombocytopenia in, 1388–1389
Pregnancy, aplastic anemia and, 164
  coagulation factors in, 1644
  Diamond-Blackfan syndrome and, 198
  folate requirements in, 319–320, 324
  in chronic idiopathic thrombocytopenia purpura, 1372–1373
  in sickle cell disease, 683 684
  iron losses and, 284
  Rh immunization during, 50, 50, 51
  toxemia of, hydrops fetalis and, 733
  vitamin B_{12} deficiency in, 344
Pregnane-3a,20β-diol, breast milk jaundice and, 87
Prekallidrein, deficiency of, 1324
  in coagulation cascade, 1249
Preleukemia. See also Leukemia; Myelodysplastic syndromes.
  ataxia-telangiectasia and, 216
  Bloom's syndrome and, 215–216
  bone marrow failure syndromes and, 215–219
  childhood, comparison of, 218(t)
  chromosome pattern in, 1482
  definition of, 1028
  hypoplastic, 216–217
  in myelodysplastic syndromes, 217–219, 1077
  neutropenia with, 803
  platelet function disorders in, 1447
  Poland's syndrome and, 216
  refractory sideroblastic anemia as, 372
Premalignancy, amegakaryocytic thrombocytopenia and, 193
  dyskeratosis congenita and, 190
  Fanconi's anemia and, 184–186
  Shwachman-Diamond syndrome and, 191
Premature infants, bilirubin concentration in, 79, 80
  blood coagulation screening tests in, normal values for, 105(t), 108, 109, 109(t)
  blood transfusions in, 40, 40(t)
  blood volume at birth, 27
  disseminated intravascular coagulation in, 115–117
  erythrocyte morphology in, 21, 22
  folate deficiency in, 324
  folate intake in, 321
  hemoglobin values in, 27, 29
  hemoglobin-oxygen dissociation curve in, 39–40
  hemostasis in, 104–105
  hyperbilirubinemia in, 82
  intravascular hemorrhage in, 117
  iron balance and erythropoiesis in, 278–279, 278
  iron-sufficient, hemoglobin values in, 1679(t)
  iron supplementation in, 280
  phototherapy in, 91
  physiologic anemia of, 37, 39–40

Premature infants (Continued)
  physiologic jaundice in, 81
  red cell glycolytic intermediates in, 1682(t)
  serum folate in, 320
  thrombocytopenia in, 1389
  tissue oxygenation in, 39
  transfusions in, 40
  vitamin E deficiency in, 508
  with respiratory problems, increased oxygen affinity and, 624
Prenatal diagnosis, of Bloom's syndrome, 216
  of bone marrow failure syndromes, 219
  of Fanconi's anemia, 181
  of hemophilia, 1315
  of lysosomal storage disease, 1223–1224
  of thrombocytopenia absent radii syndrome, 213
  of thalassemia, 760–762
Priapism, in leukemia, 1938
  in sickle cell disease, 673
Primidone, megaloblastic anemia with, 328
Progenitor cells. See also under Colony-forming unit.
  bone marrow failure and, 159
  erythroid, classes of, 139
    in Diamond-Blackfan syndrome, 202, 202
  functions of, 133–135, 136
  hematopoietic, MHC class II antigens on, 1532
  in aplastic anemia, 167
  in Fanconi's anemia, 182
  in chronic myelogenous leukemia, 1066
  in leukemia, 1030–1031
  in peripheral circulation, 135
Promethazine, maternal ingestion of, neonatal hemorrhage and, 114
Prostacyclin, in platelet aggregation and secretion, 1448
  synthesis of, aspirin inhibition of, 1449
    in diabetes, 1457
Prostaglandin(s), in platelet arachidonic acid metabolism, 1448
  synthesis of, aspirin inhibition of, 1449
Prostaglandin G_2, in platelet aggregation and release, 1285–1286
Prostaglandin I_2. See also Prostacyclin.
  in hemolytic uremic syndrome, 437
  platelet aggregation and, 1286
Prostaglandin synthetase system, in diabetes, 1659
Prostate, rhabdomyosarcoma of, 1158
Prostheses, thrombocytopenia due to, 1383–1384
Prosthetic devices, in circulation, hypercoagulability and, 1456
Protamine precipitation test, 1300
Protease inhibitiors, of coagulation system, 1266
Protein(s). See also Glycoproteins; Lipoproteins.
  coagulation, neonatal, 105–106, 105(t)
  complement, 783, 783(t)
  contact activation, deficiency of, 1323–1324
  contractile, in actin gel of phagocytes, 784
    in platelet activation, 1276–1277
  deficiency of, definition of, 305
    pure red cell aplasia and, 194
  fatty acid-binding (FABP), 77
  G regulatory, 853
  genetic information influencing, 705–707, 705–706
  GTP dependent, in platelet aggregation and secretion, 1285
  heme. See Heme proteins.

Protein(s) *(Continued)*
  in malnutrition, 307, 308(t)
  in platelet granules, 1277
  in platelet membrane phospholipid bilayer, 1279–1282, *1280*
  mutant enzyme, 546(t)
  of red cell membrane. See *Red cell membrane, proteins of.*
  plasma. See also names of specific proteins (e.g., *Albumin; Transferrin;* etc.).
    as genetic markers, 1550–1572
    genes for, localization and evolution of, 1572–1573
    serum, by age, 1693(t)
    plasmapheresis effect on, 1625, 1626(t)
  synthesis of, 707
    in macrophage maturation, 782
    in protein-calorie malnutrition, 307–308
  Y, 77
  Z, 77
Protein C/Ca, activation of, 1256–1257, *1256*
  congenital deficiency of, 1326
  thrombomodulin mechanism and, in coagulation, 1256–1257, *1256*
Protein-calorie malnutrition, 275, 305
  clinical and laboratory findings in, 305(t)
  diagnosis of, 308–309
  masked anemias with, 275
  treatment of, 309
  types of, 305
  with iron deficiency, 294
Protein kinase, phosphorylation of membrane skeletal proteins by, 462
Protein kinase C, 788, 1284
Protein S, 1257, 1326
Proteinuria, in abnormal ileal uptake of vitamin B_{12}, 347
Prothrombin, congenital deficiency and abnormalities of, 1321–1322
  conversion to thrombin, 1249, 1253–1255
  structure of, 1253
Prothrombin complex, coagulation factors in, 1299(t)
  concentrates of, activated, 1303
    for coagulation defects in liver disease, 1327
    for inhibitor hemophiliacs, 1314
    heat-treated, 1303
    risks of, 1302–1303
    transfusion therapy with, 1611–1613, 1611(t)
    uses of, 1302
Prothrombin time (PT), 1297, *1298*
  coagulation factors measured by, 1299(t)
PROTO IX, fecal excretion of, in variegate porphyria, 380
PROTOgen, in heme biosynthesis, 364, 366
PROTOgen oxidase, in variegate porphyria, 381
Proto-oncogenes, 957–958
  activation of, 961, 963–965
Protoporphyria, erythropoietic, congenital, 377–378
  protoporphyrin accumulation in, vs that in lead intoxication, 396
Protoporphyrin, in erythrocytes, accumulation of, 394–398, *395*
  correlation with blood lead levels in lead intoxication, 397–398, *397*
  in iron deficiency, 407–408
  measurements of, 402, 406
  in sideroblastic anemia, 374

Protoporphyrin IX, in congenital erythropoietic protoporphyria, 377–378
Pseudocholinesterase, genetic polymorphism of, 1560–1561
Pseudogenes, 702, *702*
Pseudo-Hurler polydystrophy, 1238
Pseudoleukemia, in infants, 2–3
Pseudomosaicism, 593
Pseudothrombocytopenia, 1345–1346
Psoriasis, 1660
Psychologic aspects, of acute leukemia, 1053–1054
  of sickle cell disease, 680–681
Pteroyglutamic acid, biochemistry of, 317–320. See also *Folate.*
  defect in, 322
Puberty, delayed, 747
Puerto Rican isoenzyme, methemoglobinemia and, 646
Pulmonary disease, 1644–1645
  in histiocytosis X, 1130
  in leukemia, 1039
Pulmonary hypertension, in perineal aspiration syndromes, 1389
Pulmonary metastases, of osteosarcoma, 1166
  of Wilms' tumor, 1151
Pulmonary toxicity, with granulocyte transfusion, 1603, 1603(t)
Pure red cell aplasia, 194–210
  acquired, 195–197
  causes of, 194–195
  congenital, 197–205. See also *Diamond-Blackfan syndrome.*
Purine metabolism, in Diamond-Blackfan syndrome, 201
Purine nucleoside phosphorylase deficiency, in severe combined immunodeficiency, 885, *886*
Purpura, allergic (Schönlein-Henoch purpura), 1459–1461, *1460*
  idiopathic thrombocytopenic. See *Thrombocytopenic purpura, idiopathic.*
  post-transfusion, 1382
  thrombotic thrombocytopenic, 438
  causes of, 1459(t)
  vascular, 1459–1461
Purpura fulminans, disseminated intravascular coagulation and, 1333, *1334*
Pyknocytosis, infantile, hemolytic anemia with, 508–509
Pyloric stenosis, 88
Pyridine nucleotides, in methemoglobin reduction, 642–643, *643*
Pyridoxine, for homocystinuria, 328
  sideroblastic anemia and, 371, 375
    aminolevulinac acid synthetase and, 372–373
Pyridoxine/folic acid-responsive formiminotransferase deficiency, 327
Pyridoxine-responsive anemia, megaloblastic marrow with, 358
Pyrimidine metabolism, folate deficiency with, 329
  in Diamond-Blackfan syndrome, 201
Pyrimidine-5'-nucleotidase, deficiency of, hemolytic anemia with, 570–571
  lead effects on, 399
Pyropoikilocytosis, hereditary, 496–497, *499*
Pyrrole ring, *364*
Pyruvate, in methemoglobin reduction, 643
Pyruvate kinase, deficiency of, hemolytic anemia with, 13, 561–569

Pyruvate kinase *(Continued)*
  mutants of, 567–568, 568(t)
  regulatory influences on, 563–564
  subunits of, 562

R binders, of cobalamin, 341
Race, in statistics of children with cancer, 919
  thalassemia and, 704
Radiation. See also *Radiation therapy*.
  absorption by matter, 1020
  aplastic anemia and, 164
  biologic principles of, 1020–1024
  cancer risk and, 921–922
  cell cycle sensitivity to, 1021–1022, *1022*
  damage due to, cell repair of, 1021, 1023
    cell survival curve and, 1020–1021, *1021*, 1023
    mechanisms and site of action of, 1020
    methods of cell killing by, 1020
    oxygen effects and, 1022
    protection from, 1022–1023
  leukemia risk and, 928
  particulate, 1020
  physical properties of, 1019
  thrombocytopenia due to, 1393
Radiation therapy. See also *Radiation*.
  clinical principles of, 1024–1026
  complications of, 1024–1025
  dose of, 1019, *1020*
  dose-rate effect of, 1023–1024
  for ataxia telangiectasia, 887
  for brain tumors, 1187–1188
  for brainstem glioma, 1191
  for cerebellar astrocytoma, 1191
  for cerebral astrocytoma, 1189
  for craniopharyngioma, 1196
  for ependymoma, 1194
  for Ewing's sarcoma, 1167
  for Hodgkin's disease, 1108, 1110, 1112
  for liver tumors, 1181
  for medulloblastoma, 1192
  for neuroblastoma, 1142–1144
  for non-Hodgkin's lymphoma, 1098, 1099(t)
  for osteosarcoma, 1161, 1164
  for retinoblastoma, 1184–1185
  for rhabdomyosarcoma, 1155–1157
  for seminoma, 1177–1178
  for Wilms' tumor, 1148–1149, 1150
  interaction with cancer chemotherapeutic agents, 1023
  late effects of, 1024–1025
  physical principles of, 1019–1020, *1019*
  therapeutic index of, 1024
  total body, for bone marrow transplantation preparation, 244–245, 249
    for Ewing's sarcoma, 1168–1169
  tumor localization for, 1026
Radioimmunoprecipitation, for study of platelet glycoprotein, 1461–1462, *1462*
Radioisotopic imaging, for differential diagnosis of biliary atresia, 94
Radiologic examination, for lead poisoning diagnosis, 42
Rapoport-Luebering cycle, 622, *622*
Raynaud's phenomenon, in cold hemagglutinin disease, 417
Rebuck skin window, 817, 819, 822, 826
Receptors, complement, 894
  on monocytes and macrophages, 781
  on phagocytes, 783

Receptors *(Continued)*
  on polymorphonuclear leukocytes, 780
  on red cell membrane, 455–456
Receptor-mediated endocytosis, 786, *786*
Red cell(s). See also *Erythropoiesis; Red cell membrane*.
  A sites on, 67(t)
  abnormalities of, phototherapy and, 91
    splenic function and, 906
  acid phosphatase of, 1573
  adenylate kinase of, 571–572, 1574
  age of, G6PD activity and, 593–594
    glucose phosphate isomerase deficiency and, 552
  antibody-coated, autoimmunity to, 413–417. See also *Hemolytic anemia, autoimmune*.
    in Diamond-Blackfan syndrome, 201
  antigens of, transfusion reactions with, 1582(t)
  bilirubin stored in, 77
  calcium permeability and transport in, 464–465, *465*
  complement coated, autoimmunity to, 413–417. See also *Hemolytic anemia, autoimmune*.
  deformability of, diseases associated with, 430(t)
    splenic filtering of, 428, *430*
  destruction of, by reticuloendothelial system, 431
    by spleen, 905
    by vasculature and reticuloendothelial system, 427–442
  development of, 129–131, *130*
  early investigations of, 13
  electronic cell counting of, 267, 269, 269(t), 271
  enzymes of, glycolytic mechanism and, 573
    genetic heterogeneity of, 1573–1574
    hereditary deficiencies of, 36
    in adults, 1681(t), 1682(t)
    in fetal cell, 21, 23
  exchanged in sickle cell disease, 1628
  fetal, 16–25
    anti-D antibody and, 51–54
    Rh immunization pathogenesis and, 49–50
    vs adult, 130
  folate levels in, 33, 331, 331(t)
  fragmentation of, complicating disseminated intravascular coagulation, 433
    hereditary spherocytosis and, 472
    in beta thalassemia, 739
  G6PD deficiency in. See *Glucose-6-phosphate dehydrogenase deficiency*.
  Gerbich-negative, Leach phenotype of, 502
  glycolytic disorders of, 545–582. See also *Glycolysis*.
    acquired, 572–574
    congenital. See *Hemolytic anemia, congenital nonspherocytic*.
  glycolytic intermediates of, in adults, 1682(t)
  hemolytic disorders of. See *Hemolysis; Hemolytic anemia*.
  hydration of, disorders of, 511–517, 512(t), *513, 514*
    red cell metabolism and cation transport and, 465, *465*
    spleen and, 463
  hydrocytosis-xerocytosis syndromes in, 512(t), *513, 514*
    intermediate syndromes, 515–516
  hypoplasia of, transcobalamin deficiency with, vitamin B_{12} deficiency and, 350

Red cell(s) *(Continued)*
  immunoglobulin G coated, clearance of, 414–417, *414*
  immunoglobulin M coated, clearance of, 415–416, *415*
  in ABO hemolytic disease, 66–68
  in Diamond-Blackfan syndrome, 206
  in exchange transfusion, 62
  in fetus and neonate, 16–25
  in HEMPAS, 209
  in hereditary elliptocytosis, 498, *498*
  in infections, 1649
  in iron deficiency anemia, 296
  in lead poisoning, 373, 399–400
  in liver disease, 1636
  in megaloblastic anemia, 353, *353*
  in marrow regenerative states, vs fetal and adult cells, 130
  in pure red cell aplasia, 194
  in renal disease, 1639–1640
  in Rh hemolytic disease, 54–55
  in thalassemia, 699–700
  in transient erythroblastopenia of childhood, 206
  inclusions of, 271(t)
    in beta thalassemia, 739–740
    in hemoglobin H disease, 732, *732*
    in thalassemia, 700, *701*
  indices of, at birth, 27, 28(t)
    in hereditary spherocytosis, 483
  intermediate metabolites of, in adults, 1682(t)
  life span of, 20–21, 135
  leukofiltered, 1584
  mechanical injury to, 504, 1633
  metabolism of, cation transport and red cell hydration and, 464, *464*
    G6PD in, 584–588, 596
    hereditary enzyme deficiency of, 36
    in neonate, 21, 23–25, 23(t)
    phosphofructokinase in, 554
    thyroid hormone and, 1624
  monovalent cations in, influence on ionic environment and hydration, 463–465, *465*
  morphology of, 21, *22*
  neonatal, after birth, 19–20
    development of erythropoiesis in, 16–19
    in ABO hemolytic disease, 66–67, 67(t)
    life span of, 20–21
    metabolism of, 21, 23–25, 23(t)
    morphology of, 21, *22*
    red cell membrane of, 21, *22*
    unique characteristics of, 21–25
  number of, at birth, 27, 28(t)
  old, in transfusion therapy for beta thalassemia, 750
  osmotic properties of, 462–463
  packed, 1583
    frozen deglycerolized, 1583
  permeability of, disorders of, 511–517, 512(t), *513–514*
    intermediate syndromes of, 515–516
  phagocyte interactions with, 503
  physiologic removal by reticuloendothelial cells, 431
  pocked, 21
  polyvalent anions in, influence on ionic environment and hydration, 463–465
  precursors of, globin gene expression in, 130–131
  products of, 1582–1583, 1584(t)

Red cell(s) *(Continued)*
  protoporphyrin in, accumulation of, 394–398, *395*
    blood lead levels of, in lead intoxication, 397–398, *397*
    measurement of, 395
    in iron deficiency, 291(t), 292, 286, 286(t), 407–408
    in lead poisoning, 402, 406
  pyruvate kinase deficient, 564
  reductive pathways in, for methemoglobin reduction, 642–644
  Rh-positive, 45–46
    antigenicity of, 48
  size of, in anemia classification, 267, 269, 269(t), 271
    in screening tests for iron deficiency, 290
  spiculated, 505–510
  splenic interaction with, in hereditary spherocytosis, 479–482, 481(t)
  structural abnormalities of, hyperbilirubinemia and, 84
  surface to volume ratio of, 469–470
  survival of. See also *Hemolytic anemia; Hemolysis.*
    after removal from body, 1580–1581
    in diabetes, 1658
    in G6PD deficiency, 596
    in lead intoxication, 400
    in vitamin B_{12} deficiency, 355
  thermal injury to, 503–504
  thermal lability of, in G6PD deficiency, 552
  transfusions of, 1580–1587
    adverse effects of, 1585–1587
    choice of red cell product for, 1582–1584, 1583(t)
    components vs whole blood, 1582
    in anemia with cardiac compromise, 1585
    in beta thalassemia, 749–750
    in immunocompromised host, 1584
    in neonates, 1584
    indications for, 1581–1582
    massive, 1584–1585
    storage of, for transfusion, 1580–1581
  unincubated osmotic fragility test of, 470
  values of, at various ages, 1680(t)
  volume of, disorders of, 511–517, 512(t), *513–514*
    in polycythemia vera, 1071
    in sickle cells, 664
  whole blood, 1582–1583
Red cell count, normal, 1679(t)
Red cell distribution width, 290
  and mean corpuscular volume in disease, 269, 269(t)
Red cell membrane. See also *Red cell(s).*
  abnormalities of, 469–470, *470*
  classification of, 471(t)
  adult vs fetal, 469
  analysis of, *448*, 449, 449(t)
  antigenicity of, 45–46, *45*
  composition of, 444(t)
  development and aging of, 468–469
  durability of, 465–466
  endocytosis and fusion in, 467
  fetal, 469
  flexibility of, 465–466
  fluidity of, 446–447
  glycophorins of. See also *Glycophorins.*
    malaria and, 1502–1503
  hydration of, 462–465

Red cell membrane *(Continued)*
  in ABO hemolytic disease, 67–68
  in beta thalassemia, 740
  in hereditary elliptocytosis, *498*
  in hereditary spherocytosis, 475–477
    leakiness of vs fragility, 479–482, 481(t)
  in iron deficiency anemia, 296
  in neonate, 21, *22*
  in paroxysmal nocturnal hemoglobinuria, 424–425
  in sickle cell disease, 664–666
  ionic environment control in, 462–465
    in sickle cell disease, 665
  lipid structure of, 443–448
  lipids of, asymmetry of, 467
    in hereditary spherocytosis, 475
    in sickle cell anemia, 665
  mechanical injury to, 504
  miscellaneous defects of, 518
  normal anatomy of, 443
  normal physiology of, 462–469
    in fetus, 409
  proteins of, anion exchange, 452–454, *453*
    composition of, 448–449, *448*, 449(t)
    hereditary defects of, 36, 494(t)–495(t), 497–498, 500–502
    in hereditary spherocytosis, 475
    in nonerythroid cells, 468
    in Rh$_{null}$ disease, 516–517
    integral, 449–456
      acetylcholinesterase, 454
      distribution and mobility of, 466–467
      glucose transport protein, 454–455
      glycophorins, 449–452, *450*. See also *Glycophorins.*
      intramembranous particles, 454, *454*
      protein 3, 452–454, *453*
        defective binding of ankyrin by, 502
        hereditary defects of, 494(t)–495(t), 502
        structure and function of, 452–454, *453*
      protein 4.1, binding site of, 453
        brain, 468
        hereditary defects of, 494(t)–495(t), 500–502, *501*
        integral protein mobility and, 466
        lipid asymmetry and, 467
        structure and function of, 459–460, *458*, *460*
        spectrin binding defect and, 474
      protein 4.2, binding of, 453
        in hereditary spherocytosis, 475
        target cells and, 510
      protein 4.9, 460
        role in endocytosis and fusion of skeleton, 467
      transferrin receptor, 455
      sodium-potassium-ATPase, 455
      various receptors of, 455–456
    of membrane skeleton, 456–461, *456–458*, *460*
      defects of, 494(t)–495(t), 497–498, 500–502
    peripheral, 449, 456–462
    phosphorylation of, in hereditary spherocytosis, 476
    structure of, 448–462, 502
  proteolytic artifacts and, 518
  shape of, *466*, 467–468
  skeleton of, functions of, 465–468
    in hereditary elliptocytosis, 502–503
    in hereditary spherocytosis, 476

Red cell membrane *(Continued)*
  skeleton of, in sickle cell disease, 666
    inherited disorders of, 470–503
    modulation of skeletal structure and, 462
    normal functions of, 465–468
    organization of, 461–462, *461*, *462*
    proteins of, 456–461, *456–458*, *460*
      hereditary defects of, 494(t)–495(t), 497–498, 500–502
  surface area of, decreased, due to inherited disorders of membrane skeleton, 470–503. See also *Ellipotocytosis, hereditary; Spherocytosis, hereditary.*
    due to other causes, 503–510
      hypersplenism, 510
      hypophosphatemia, 504
      immune adherence, 503
      mechanical injury, 504
      spiculated red cells, 505–510
      thermal injury, 503–504
      toxins and venoms, 504–505
    increased, 510–511
  surface to volume ratio, in hereditary spherocytosis, 477, *480*
  transport in, protein 3 and, 452–454
Red cell sedimentation rate, in neonates, *1696*
Redox stress, 594, 596
Reed-Sternberg cell, *1087*, 1101
Regional enteritis, 1635
Renal blastema/nephroblastomatosis, Wilms' tumor and, 1146
Renal cell carcinoma, 1151–1152
Renal disease, hematologic abnormalities with, 1638–1641
  in acute leukemia, 1038
  in Henoch-Schönlein purpura, 1460
  in sickle cell disease, 676–677
Renal failure, hemostatic abnormalities in, 1329
  in hemolytic uremic syndrome, 436, 437
Renal tumors, Wilms' tumor and, 1146
Reptilase time, 1300
Restriction endonuclease mapping, of thalassemia mutations, 718–719, *719–720*
Restriction fragment length polymorphism, for molecular mapping of X chromosome, 593
  for prenatal diagnosis of beta thalassemia, 760–761
  HLA phenotype and, 1536
  in alpha globin gene cluster, 723, *723*
  in beta globin gene cluster, 718–720, *719*, *720*
Reticular dysgenesis, 800
  in aplastic anemia, 193
Reticulocyte(s), destruction of, in glucose phosphate isomerase deficiency, 552
  in hereditary spherocytosis, 483
  in neonatal anemia diagnosis, 37, *38*
  in pyruvate kinase deficiency, 561–562
Reticulocytopenia, in autoimmune hemolytic anemia, 420
  in Diamond-Blackfan syndrome, 201
Reticuloendothelial cells, definition of, 427
  function of, 427–428
  in red cell destruction, 431
  sequestration of, immune neutropenia with, 806
Reticuloendothelial system, 785
  immune response generation in, 428
  in hemolytic anemia, 431
  in pathogenesis of immune thrombocytopenia, 1349–1351

Reticuloendothelial system (Continued)
  splenic function and, 428–431, 429, 430
  storage diseases of. See Storage diseases.
  structure and function of, 427–432
Reticulum cell sarcoma, 1095
Retinal changes, with phototherapy, 91
Retinoblastoma, 1181–1186
  chromosomal changes in, 1490–1491
  clinical features of, 1182–1183
  epidemiology of, 932
  genetics of, 1181
  metastases of, 1183
  prognosis of, 1183–1184, 1183(t)
  staging of, 1183, 1183(t)
  treatment of, 1184–1186
Retinopathy, in sickle cell disease, 677–678
Retroperitoneum, germ cell tumors of, 1179
Retrovirus. See also RNA viruses.
  classification of, 948, 949(t)
  diseases associated with, 950
  host range of, 950
  life cycle of, 950, 950
  oncogenic potential of, 950–954, 951
  slow, 952–954
  transduction by, 956
  transforming genes and products of, 954, 956–957, 956
  types of, 950–954
  vectors of, used in gene therapy for beta thalassemia, 757–758
Reverse transcriptase, in RNA viruses, 948
Rh antibody, 46–48
Rh antigens, 1508(t)
  historical aspects of, 10–11
  in autoimmune hemolytic anemia, 417
  matched, in platelet transfusion, 1594
  terminology of, 45
Rh blood group system, 1507–1508
Rh hemolytic disease, bilirubin metabolism in, 56–57
  hyperbilirubinemia and, 83–84
  destruction of fetal erythrocytes by anti-D antibody in, 51–54
  fetal response to erythrocyte destruction, 54–55
  incidence of, 44, 44(t)
  intravascular hemolysis in, 54
  nature of positive erythrocyte, 45–46
  pathogenesis of, 45–48
    Rh immunization in Rh-negative women, 48–50
  prevention and treatment of, in fetus, 58–61
    in mother, 57–58
    in neonate, 61–66
    special problems in, 64–66
  prognosis for, 45
  spleen in, 53
  thrombocytopenia with, 1389
Rh immunization, in Rh-negative women, 48–50
  mechanism during pregnancy, 50, 50, 51
  prevention of, in mother at risk, 57–58, 57(t), 58(t)
Rh-negative cells, definition of individual with, 45
  differentiation from D antigen of low reactivity, 46
  Rh immunization in women with, 48–50
    prevention of, 57(t), 58(t)
Rh$_{null}$ disease, 1502, 1508, 516–517
Rh-positive erythrocytes, antigenicity of, 48
Rhabdoid sarcoma, 1146

Rhabdomyosarcoma, classification of, 1153
  clinical manifestations of, 1153
  epidemiology of, 931
  pathology of, 1153
  prognosis of, 1154
  sites affected by, 1156–1159
  staging of, 1154(t)
  treatment of, 1155–1156
Rheumatoid arthritis, 1646–1647
  complement deficiency in, 897
Rho(D) antigen, in Rh$_{null}$ disease, 516
Riboflavin deficiency, phototherapy and, 90
Ristocetin, cofactor of, 1299
  in von Willebrand's disease, 1315, 1317, 1318
  platelet aggregation to, in Bernard-Soulier syndrome, 1433, 1436
RNA, intranuclear processing of, 706–707
  messenger, 705
    defects of, early investigation of, 12
    deficiency of, due to premature termination mutations, 716
    delta, in delta thalassemia, 735–736
    splicing function and, 713
    translation into protein, 707
      mutations affecting, 716–717
  splicing function of, 712–715, 713
RNA viruses, 948
  human, 953–954
  molecular biology of, 948–954
  pathogenesis of, 948, 950–953
  replication of, 948
  structure of, 948, 949
  taxonomy of, 948
Roux sarcoma virus, 951
  gene products of, 954
Rubella, intrauterine infection with, 113

Salicylates. See also Aspirin.
  bilirubin estimation in, 57
  in pyruvate kinase deficiency, 569
Saline agglutination test, 1497
Salmonella, causing osteomyelitis in sickle cell disease, 671
Sandhoff's disease, 1230
Sanfilippo's disease, 1233
Sarcoma, clear cell, 1146
  Ewing's. See Ewing's sarcoma.
  rhabdoid, 1146
  skeletal, epidemiology of, 931
  soft tissue, 1152–1161
    classification of, 1153
    epidemiology of, 931
    Ewing's sarcoma, 1161
    fibrosarcoma, 1159–1160
    neural origin of, 1160–1161
    rhabdomyosarcoma, 1152–1159
    synovial sarcoma, 1160
  undifferentiated, 1179
  synovial, 1160
Sarcoidosis, 1645
  lymphadenopathy in, 1089
Scheie's disease, 1231–1233
Schilling test, 342, 342, 355–356
Schistocytic hemolytic anemia, 432–438. See also Hemolytic anemia, schistocytic.
Schönlein-Henoch purpura, 1459–1461, 1460
Schumm's test, 355
Scianna blood group, 1515

Scintigraphy, bone marrow, in aplastic anemia, 165–166
Scoliosis, idiopathic, platelet abnormalities in, 1441
Sedatives, neutropenia with, 806
Selenomethionine, in platelet kinetic studies, 1274
Seminoma, 1177–1178
Sepsis, hemolytic anemia with, 439
  neutropenia with, 804
    vs acute leukemia, 1041
  postsplenectomy, 432, 489–490
Serine protease, 1248–1249, *1249*
Serotonin release, in indirect measurement of platelets, 1400
Serum immunoglobulins, in sickle cell disease, 675
Sexual development, in beta thalassemia, 747
  in sickle cell disease, 680, *681*
Shigella infections, 435
Shock, bacterial septic, disseminated intravascular coagulation and, 1331, *1332*
  red cell transfusion and, 1582
Shwachman-Diamond syndrome, 190–192, *192*, 220(t)
  neutropenia in, 802–803
Sialidosis, 1235–1237
  dysmorphic, 1236–1237
  type I, 1235–1236
  type II, 1236–1237
Sialyloligosaccharide, in mucolipidoses, 1235
Sickle beta thalassemia, 686
Sickle cell(s), adherence to endothelial cells, 467, 665, 667
  deformability of, 666
  irreversible, causing xerocytosis, 517
    red cell membrane abnormalities and, 664, *665*
  reversible, red cell membrane in, *665*
Sickle cell crisis, 669–674
  acute sequestration, 673–674
  aplastic, 674
  management of, 682–683
  vaso-occlusive, 669–673
Sickle cell disease, alpha thalassemia with, 686
  approach to therapy for, 666–667
  bone marrow transplantation for, 254
  cardiovascular abnormalities in, 675–676
  cell deformability in, 666
  clinical manifestations of, 668–681
  death in, 684
  diagnosis of, 667–668, 668(t)
  early discoveries in, 12
  eye abnormalities in, 677–678
  fetal hemoglobin levels in, 729
  functional hyposplenism in, 909
  G6PD deficiency in, 600–601, 655–656
  gene replacement in, 666
  growth and development in, 679–680, *680*, *681*
  hearing loss in, 678
  hemoglobin F production in, 666
  hepatobiliary abnormalities in, 677
  history of, 655
  incidence of, 655–656
  infections in, 671(t), 674–675
  iron deficiency with, 302
  lung abnormalities in, 679
  malaria and, 665–656
  mortality in, 684
  neonatal, 34
  neurologic abnormalities in, 679

Sickle cell disease *(Continued)*
  pregnancy in, 683–684
  psychologic aspects of, 680
  red cell exchange for, 1628
  red cell membrane abnormalities and, 664–666
  renal abnormalities in, 676–677
  routine health maintenance in, 681–682
  sexual development in, 680, *681*
  skeletal abnormalities in, 678
  treatment of, 681–684
Sickle cell gene, polymorphism of, 1527
Sickle cell trait, 684
Sickle syndromes, 684–687
Sickling, cellular, 662–664, *663*
  molecular, 656, *657–659*
Sideroblastic anemia, 370–375
  characteristics of, 371
  classification of, 371–372, 371(t)
  clinical and laboratory features of, 373–374, 373(t)
  course and therapy of, 374–375
  etiology of, 371–372, 371(t)
  metabolic defects in, 372–373
  pyridoxine responsive, 371, 372–373
  refractory, 372
  with lead toxicity, 373
Sideroblasts, ringed, 372–374
Simian virus, 40, 945
Sinus histiocytosis, lymphadenopathy in, 1090
  massive, 1127–1228
    vs malignant histiocytosis, 1133
Skeleton, in sickle cell disease, 678
Skin disorders, eosinophilia and, 814
  folate deficiency and, 325
  hematologic complications of, 1660–1661
  in Henoch-Schönlein purpura, 1460
  in infectious mononucleosis, 1654
  in prophyria cutanea tarda, 381
  in sickle cell disease, 678
  in storage diseases, 1217(t), 1219
Skin fibroblasts, in diagnosis of storage disease, 1220
Skin puncture, for iron deficiency screening, 288
Skull, in thalassemia major, 742, *743*
Smith, Carl, 10
Snakebite, coagulation disorders with, 1336
  hemolytic anemia and, 504
Sodium, leak of, in hereditary spherocytosis, 475–476
  red cell permeability to, in hereditary hydrocytosis, 513
  in hereditary spherocytosis, 478–479, *480*
Sodium bicarbonate, in exchange transfusion, 63
Sodium-potassium ATPase, of red cell membrane, 455
Sodium-potassium pump, in sickle cells, 664
  red cell cation transport and, 464, 465, *465*
Sodium valproate, platelet function and, 1454
Soft tissue sarcoma, 1152–1161
  classification of, *1153*
  Ewing's sarcoma, 1161
  fibrosarcoma, 1159–1161
  neural origin of, 1160
  rhabdomyosarcoma, 1152–1159
  synovial sarcoma, 1160
Solvents, associated with aplastic anemia, 161(t)
South Africa, porphyria cutanea tarda in, 381
  variegate porphyria in, 380

Southern blot analysis, for prenatal diagnosis of beta thalassemia, 761
  for correlation between HLA phenotype and restriction fragment length polymorphism, 1536. See also *Restriction fragment length polymorphism.*
Sp₁ antibody, 1512
Spectrin, binding properties of, 549
  defective, in hereditary spherocytosis, 473–474
  deficiency of, 466, *466*
    in hereditary spherocytosis, 472–475, *473–475*, 482
  distribution of, 458
  domains of, 457, *458*
  hereditary defects of, 472–475, *473–475*, 482, 494(t)–495(t), 497–498, *499*, 500–502, *500*
    involving alpha chain, 497–498, *499*, 400
    involving beta chain, 500, *500*
    involving binding to ankyrin, 500
  in hereditary pyropoikilocytosis, *499*
  in hereditary spherocytosis, 472–475, 482
  in red cell membrane skeleton, 461, *461*
  inextractable, 474
  nonerythroid, 468
  phospholipid asymmetry and, 445, 467
  properties of, 458
  structure and function of, 456–458, *457, 458*
Spectrophotometric methods, for diagnosis of G6PD deficiency, 601
Spherocytes, in ABO hemolytic disease, 67
  osmotic fragility of, in hereditary spherocytosis, 477–478, *479*
  spleen and, in hereditary spherocytosis, 477–478, *478–479*, 482
Spherocytic hereditary elliptocytosis, 497
Spherocytosis, hereditary, 470–490
    atypical, 486
    clinical features of, 482–483
    complications of, 486–488
    diagnosis of, 488–489
    early history of, 470–472
    etiology of, 472–477
    genetics of, 472
    laboratory features of, 483–484
    mild, 485–486
    neonatal, 36, 484–485
    pathophysiology of, 477–482, *480*
    prevalence of, 472
    severe, 485
    vs congenital nonspherocytic hemolytic anemia, 545
  immunohemolytic anemia and, 503
  snake venoms and, 504–505
  spectrin deficiency and, 466, *466*
  splenic filtering function and, 428
Sphingoglycolipids, in storage diseases, 1220, 1221(t)
  metabolism of, 1224, *1225*
Sphingolipidoses, Farber's disease, 1229
  gangliosidosis, 1229–1230
  Gaucher's disease, 1226–1227
  mechanism of disease in, 1224, *1225*, 1226
  Niemann-Pick disease, 1227–1229
Sphingomyelin lipidoses (Niemann-Pick disease), 1227–1229
Spiders, hemolytic anemia due to bite of, 504
Spielmeyer-Sjögren syndrome, 1242
Spinal cord, disease of, hereditary spherocytosis and, 486
Spinal cord tumors, 1196

Spinal puncture, in lead poisoning diagnosis, 402
Spleen, accessory, 903
  anatomy of, *478*, 901, *902*
  atrophy of, 904–905, 905(t)
  in beta thalassemia, 750
  blood flow in, 481(t)
  circulation in, 901
  clearance function of, 428–431, *429, 430*
    filtering, 428, *430*, 430(t)
    immune, 430–431
  cysts of, 903, *904*
  embryology of, 901
  erythrocyte clearance and, 414, *414*, 416, 419
  erythrocyte destruction by, 51–53, *52*
  function of, development aspects of, 908–909
    historical aspects of, 900–901
    normal, 905–908, 905(t)
  glucose metabolism in, hexokinase deficiency and, 549
  histology of, 901, *902*
  hypoplasia of, 904–905, 905(t)
  immune surveillance of, 428
  in Rh hemolytic disease of newborn, 53
  infected, in sickle cell disease, 674–675
  macrophage distribution in, 785
  platelet sequestration by, 1275
  polysplenia syndromes involving, 903
  pyruvate kinase deficiency and, 566–567
  red cell hydration and, 463
  red cell interaction with, in hereditary spherocytosis, 479–482, 481(t)
  reticuloendothelial cells in, platelet clearance and, 1349–1351
  rupture of, neonatal anemia and, 32
  spherocytes and, in hereditary spherocytosis, 477–478, *478–479*, 482
  surface remodeling in, 511
  tumors of, 903, *904*
  Wiskott-Aldrich syndrome and, 1392
Splenectomy, 910–913
  for autoimmune hemolytic anemia, 422
  for chronic idiopathic thrombocytopenic purpura, 1367, 1369–1370
  for congenital dysfunction, 1443
  for Diamond-Blackfan syndrome, 203
  for Fanconi's anemia, 184
  for Gaucher's disease, 1226
  for glucose phosphate isomerase deficiency, 553
  for hereditary spherocytosis, 489–490
  for idiopathic thrombocytopenic purpura of childhood, 1364
  for neutropenia, 810
  for pyruvate kinase deficiency, 568–569
  for severe beta thalassemia, 750–751
  for thalassemia intermedia, 755
  for Wiskott-Aldrich syndrome, 889
  hazards of, 431–432
  historical aspects of, 900
  immunodeficiency following, 890
  in children, 912–913
  in clearance of antibody- and complement-coated erythrocytes, 416
  indications for, 910, 911(t)
    for staging of Hodgkin's disease, 1106, 1107(t)
  in hemolytic anemia, 428, 430(t)
  prophylactic measures with, 912–913
  septicemia and, 432. See also *Postsplenectomy.*
  side effects of, 422

Splenic sequestration crisis, in sickle cell anemia, 673–674
Splenomegaly, 909–910
  causes of, 910(t)
  in infectious mononucleosis, 1653
  massive, neonatal thrombocytopenia and, 114
Splenosis, 903–904
Spur cell anemia, 506–508, *507–508*
Staphylococcus aureus, chronic granulomatous disease and, 829
  infection by, in hyperimmunoglobulin E syndrome, 824
  neutrophil aggregation and, 821
Starvation, breast feeding-related jaundice and, 87
Stem cell(s), acquired disorders of, neutropenia with, 803
  committed, antibodies to, aplastic anemia and, 168
  committed myeloid, disorders of proliferations of, neutropenia with, 801–802
  multipotent, clonal diseases involving, 1065(t)
Steroids. See *Corticosteroids.*
Stillbirth, from Rh hemolytic disease, 58–61
Stomach, disease of, 1635
Stomatocytic disorders, 516–517
Stomatocytic hereditary elliptocytosis, 497
Stomatocytic xerocytosis, 516
Stomatocytosis, 467, 513–514. See also *Hydrocytosis, hereditary.*
  acquired, 516
  hereditary, neonatal, 36
  Mediterranean, 517
Storage diseases, age at onset, 1216(t)
  bone marrow transplantation for, 1213
  diagnosis of, 1215–1516, 1216(t)
  general concepts of, 1213–1224
  genetics of, 1214–1215, 1214(t)
  hematologic aspects of, 1212–1213
  laboratory findings in, biochemical, 1219–1220, 1221(t), 1222
    morphological, 1216–1219, 1217(t)
  lysosomes and, 1213–1214
  pathogenesis of, 1214
  phenotypic heterogeneity of, 1213
  prenatal diagnosis of, 1223–1224
  presenting signs of, 1216(t)
  prevention of, 1223–1224
  substances accumulating in, 1219–1220, 1221(t)
  treatment of, 1222–1223
Storage pool deficiency, of granule-bound nucleotides, 1438
  neonatal, 1444
Streptococcus pneumoniae, vaccination against, with splenectomy, 432
Streptokinase, vs urokinase, 1260
Stress erythropoiesis, congenital dyserythropoietic anemia and, 207
  in Fanconi's anemia, 180
  in preleukemic myelodysplastic syndromes, 218
  in transient erythroblastopenia of childhood, 206
  morphology of, 140–141
Stroke, in sickle cell disease, 673
Sturgeon, Philip, 10
Subendothelium, platelet adhesion to, 1282–1283
Succinyl CoA, converted from L-methylmalonyl CoA cobalamin and, 339–340

Sulfhemoglobinemia, 650–651
Sulfhydryl compounds, as radioprotector, 1022–1023
  lead affinity for, 392, 393
Sulfhydryl reagents, for pyruvate kinase deficiency, 569
Sulfinpyrazone, with myocardial infarction, 1452
  platelet function with, 1451
Superoxide, produced by NADPH oxidase removal of, 833–834
  produced by neutrophils in chronic granulomatous disease, 830
  produced by phagocytes, 790–791
Supertransfusion, for beta thalassemia, 748–749
Surgery, in hemophilia, 1310–1311
  in sickle cell disease patients, 683
SV40, 945
Synovial sarcoma, 1160
Synovitis, with hemophilia A, 1308
Systemic lupus erythematosus, 1647–1648
  acquired anticoagulant with, 1330
  autoimmune neutropenia with, antineutrophil autoantibodies and, 805
  suppressor T cell activity in, 853

T antigens, 945
  polyoma virus, tumorigenesis and, 945, 954, 965
  red cell, in autoimmune hemolytic anemia, 418
T cell(s), activation of, 848, 851, *849*
  by blood groups, 1501
    HLA class II antigens expressed on, 1532
    signals needed for, 850, *850*
  antigen presentation to, by B cells, 854–855, *855–856*
  antigen-specific receptor genes, DNA rearrangements in, 872
  B cell differentiation and, 146
  B cells, interaction with, 851–856
  clonal marker associated, for T cell malignancies, 872
  clones specific for Ia antigens, 851
  control of polyclonal immunoglobulin synthesis by, 851–854
  cytotoxic, 855
  cytotoxic/suppressor, glycoprotein defining, 1523
    in herpesvirus infection, 1120–1121
  deficiencies of, primary, 884–892
    severe combined immunodeficiency, 884–887, *885–888*
  depletion of, from bone marrow grafts prior to transplantation, 243, 244, 1541
    graft versus host disease and, 246, 248
    in severe combined immunodeficiency, 250
  helper, activation of, 850, *850*
    glycoprotein defining, 1523
    T4 cells, in polyclonal immunoglobulin synthesis, 851–853
    MHC antigens and, 1523
  helper-suppressor ratio of, in common variable immunodeficiency, 884
  hematopoietic differentiation and, 146
  immune response by, control of, 848–859
    major histocompatibility complex and, 1522–1524
    vs B cell immune response, 1523

T cell(s) *(Continued)*
  in acute lymphoblastic leukemia, chromosomal changes in, 1489–1490, *1490*
  in chronic myelogenous leukemia, 1067
  in Diamond-Blackfan syndrome, 202
  in erythroid differentiation, 146
  in granulocyte progenitor differentiation, 145
  in Hodgkin's disease, 1101–1102
  in infectious mononucleosis, 1656
  in iron deficiency anemia, 298
  in lymphoblastic lymphoma, 1093–1094
  in pure red cell aplasia, 196
  in spleen, 428
  in Wiskott-Aldrich syndrome, 889
  in X-linked lymphoproliferative syndrome, 1125
  inducer, in erythropoiesis, 146
  isotype switch, 854
  lymphocytapheresis and, 1626
  macrophage interaction with, 850–851
  nonimmune cells, interaction with, 856–857
  normal levels of, by age, *1696*
  receptor of, 850
  regulatory function of, B cell activation and, 851–855, *852*, 853(t)
    antigen-specific regulation, 854–855
    isotype-specific regulation, 854
    regulation of polyclonal immunoglobulin production, 851–854
    of immunoglobulin synthesis, 854
    of monocyte/macrophage function, 856
    of other immune cells, 855
    of signals derived from, 849
  subsets of, monoclonal antibodies to, 1626, 1629
    T4, 851–852, 855
    T8, 851–852, 855
  suppressor, 851
    antigen-specific, 854–855
    in aplastic anemia, 169
    in erythropoiesis, 146
    in polyclonal immunoglobulin synthesis, 851–853
    major histocompatibility complex and, 1523
    pure red cell aplasia and, 196
    splenic source of, 428
Tangier disease, 1563
TAR. See *Thrombocytopenia with absent radii syndrome.*
Target cells, disorders associated with, 510
Tay-Sachs disease, 1224, 1230
Technicon Autoanalysers, 269
Teratomas, 1169–1170
  immature, mediastinal, 1178
  ovarian, 1173–1174
  testicular, 1176–1177
Testes, disease of, hematologic abnormalities with, 1643
  in acute leukemia, 1037–1038
  in acute lymphoblastic leukemia, 1044, 1047
Testicular germ cell tumor, 1175–1178
Testicular sarcoma, 1159
Testicular tumors, classification of, 1175
  epidemiology of, 933
  management of, 1176–1178
  metastases, 1175
  staging of, 1175–1176
Tetrazolium salts, 601

Thalassemia, alpha. See also *Hemoglobin H disease.*
  alpha thalassemia trait in, 730–731
  distribution of, 699, *700*
  genetics of, 733–734
  hemoglobin Constant Spring and, 730, *731*
  hydrops fetalis and, 733
  neonatal, 35
  polyadenylation mutations causing, 715
  silent carrier, 729–730, *731*
  syndromes of, 704(t)
  with sickle cell anemia, 686
alpha-beta globin biosynthesis ratio in, *700*
aminoacid sequencing of, early studies in, 12
beta, distribution of, 699, *700*
  mild, 734–737
    silent carrier state in, 729, 734
  neonatal, 35–36
  Sardinian, 741
  severe, 738–758
    cardiac abnormalities in, 745–746
    chelation therapy for, 751–753
    clinical features of, 742
    endocrine abnormalities in, 746–748
    genetic heterogeneity of, 740–742
    hepatic abnormalities in, 746
    history of, 738
    iron deposition in, 743–748
    laboratory values in, 742
    new treatment approaches, 755–758
    pathophysiology of, 739–740
    radiologic changes in, 742–743, *743*
    sickle cell anemia with, 686
    splenectomy for, 750–751
    transfusion therapy for, 748–750
    transfusion-dependent, 736, 737
    vitamin supplementation for, 753–754
bone marrow transplantation for, 254
classification of, 12, 702–704, 703(t)
clinical heterogeneity of, 729
Cooley's discovery of, 3
delta, 735–736
delta-beta, 755
gamma, neonatal, 36
gamma delta beta, 758
genetic heterogeneity of, 762
geographic distribution of, 718–721
hemoglobin synthesis in, 371
interaction with globin structural variants in, 758–759
malaria and, 704
neonatal, 35–36
nondeletion delta-beta, 728
prenatal diagnosis of, 760–762
race and, 704
Thalassemia intermedia, 736, 740, 742, 754–755, *754*
  delta-beta form of, 755
Thalassemia major. See *Thalassemia, beta, severe.*
Thalassemia minor. See *Thalassemia, beta, mild.*
Thalassemia mutations, 704–718, 708(t)-711(t)
  clinical heterogeneity of, diversity of mutations and, 729
  detected by oligonucleotide probes, 721, *721*
  in alpha globin gene cluster, deletion mutations, 721–723, *722*
    interaction with beta thalassemia mutations, 741–742
  in alpha thalassemia, 733–734
  in beta globin gene cluster, affecting fetal hemoglobin synthesis, 723–729
    deletion mutations, 724, *725*, 726–728

Thalassemia mutations *(Continued)*
  in beta globin gene cluster, deletion mutations, beta°, 726
    crossover globins, 724, 726
    delta-beta, 726–727
    gamma delta beta, 727
    ᴬgamma delta beta, 727
    hemoglobin switching, 727–728
    hereditary persistence of fetal hemoglobin, 727
    Sicilian type, 726
  frequency of, 718–721
  interaction with alpha mutations, 741–742
  nondeletion delta-beta mutations, 728
  nondeletion hereditary persistence of fetal hemoglobin mutations, 728–729, 728(t)
  racial distribution of, 718–721
  in beta thalassemia, 740–742
  in beta thalassemia trait, 736–737
  initiation codon mutations, 716
  interaction with globin variants, 758–759
  linkage to chromosomal haplotypes, 719–720, *719*
  point mutations, 762
    mutations affecting globin stability, 717–718
    mutations affecting mRNA translation, 716–717, *717*
    polyadenylation mutations, 715–716
    promoter mutations, 710, *710*, 712, 728
    splicing mutations, 712–715
  restriction endonuclease mapping of, 718–721
  terminator codon mutations, 716–717, *717*
  transacting, 729
Thalassemia trait, beta, classification of, 736–737
  clinical features of, 734
  delta, 736
  delta globin synthesis in, 735–736
  effect of alpha gene deletions on hematologic parameters, 741(t)
  genetics of, 736–737
  globin biosynthetic ratio in, 734–735
  high Hb A$_2$, 736
  high Hb A$_2$ high F, 736–737
  normal Hb A$_2$, 737
  peripheral blood smear in, 734, *735*
  differential diagnosis of, 737–738, 737(t)
  G6PD deficiency and, 601
  microcytosis with high protoporphyrin levels and, 408
  vs iron deficiency, hematologic parameters in, 737(t)
Thalassemic hemoglobinopathies, 759
Theta positive cells, hematopoiesis and, 146
Thiamine-responsive megaloblastic anemia, 358
Thiamphenicol, 163
Thiazide diuretics, thrombocytopenia and, 1394
Thioguanine, for autoimmune hemolytic anemia, 422
Thiophosphate derivatives, as radioprotectors, 1022–1023
Thorax, neuroblastoma of, 1144
  rhabdomyosarcoma of, 1157–1158
Thrombin, as platelet aggregating agent, 1345
  as platelet agonist, 1432
  conversion of protein C to protein Ca and, 1256
  conversion to, from prothrombin, 1253–1255

Thrombin *(Continued)*
  generation of, 1249–1257. See also *Coagulation*.
    coagulation cascades in, kinetic relationships with common pathway in, 1255–1256
    coagulation common pathway in, 1253–1255
  glycoprotein Ib binding of, 1281
  in scission of B-beta chain of fibrin I monomer, 1262
Thrombin time, heparin detection by, 1300
Thrombocytopenia, 1346–1383. See also under *Platelets*.
  acquired, 1393–1394
  alcohol and, 1394
  allergy and anaphylaxis and, 1382
  amegakaryocytic, 113, 192–193, *193*, 211, 220(t)
  aplastic anemia and, 192–193, *193*, 1393
  cardiopulmonary bypass and, 1383–1384
  catheters and, 1383
  circulating platelets in, 147
  congenital, 211–213
    with megakaryocyte hypoplasia, 1391
  congenital and hereditary, due to impaired production, 1390–1393
  destructive, 1348
    miscellaneous causes of, 1388–1390
    with nonimmunologic microangiopathic processes, 1383–1385
    with platelet and fibrinogen consumption, 1385–1388
  diagnostic approach to, 1346–1347, 1395, *1396*
  differential diagnosis of, 1397(t)–1398(t)
  dilutional, platelet transfusion for, 1593
  drug-induced, 1373–1379
    idiosyncratic immune, 1373, 1375, 1376–1377
      drugs causing, 1378(t)
      heparin induced, 1377, 1379
      treatment of, 1379
      valproic acid induced, 1379
    pathogenesis of, 1374(t), 1374–1376
    platelet-associated IgG measurements for, 1406
    treatment of, 1454–1455
    with marrow suppression, 1393
    with platelet-specific suppression, 1393–1394
  essential, 1072–1073
  estrogens and, 1394
  fatty acid-induced, 1390
  Glanzmann's, 114, 1282, 1436–1437
  immune, 1348–1383
    difficulty of developing tests for, 1400
    idiopathic thrombocytopenic purpura of childhood, 1351–1364. See also *Thrombocytopenic purpura, idiopathic, of childhood*.
    in infectious mononucleosis, 1655
    pathogenesis of, 1348–1351, *1348–1349*
    problems of direct platelet assays in, 1403–1404
    with various disorders, 1383
  immunodeficiency with, 888–889. See also *Wiskott-Aldrich syndrome*.
  in cardiac disease, 1634
  in infections, 1380–1382, *1381*
  in preeclampsia, 1388–1389
  in renal disease, 437, 1388, 1641
  in Rh hemolytic disease, 65
  inherited, 1393

Thrombocytopenia *(Continued)*
  marrow infiltration causing, 1393
  neonatal, 108–114, 1389–1390
    alloimmune, platelet-associated IgG assays for, 1405–1406
    due to decreased platelet production, 113–114
    due to increased mechanical platelet destruction, 113
    exchange transfusion and, 114
    immune-mediated, 109–110, 1382
    isoimmune, 111–113, 1592
    secondary to maternal idiopathic thrombocytopenic purpura, 110–111
    splenomegaly and, 114
    Wiskott-Aldrich syndrome and, 114
  platelet sequestration and, 1394–1395
  platelet transfusion for, 1591–1592
  postsplenectomy, 907
  post-transfusion, 1382
  prostheses and, 1383–1384
  schistocytic hemolytic anemia and, 433–435
  secondary to heart disease, 1384–1385
  severe, schistocytic hemolytic anemia with, 435–438
  spurious, 1345–1346
  thiazide diuretics and, 1394
  transplant rejection and, 1382–1383
  types of, 1347
  with autoimmune hemolytic anemia, 423–424
  with giant cavernous hemangioma, 1386–1388
  with malaria, 1381–1382
  with microangiopathic hemolytic anemia, 1383
  with nutritional deficiency, 1394
  with schistocytic hemolytic anemia, 438
Thrombocytopenia with absent radii (TAR) syndrome, 113, 211–213, 220(t), 1390–1391
Thrombocytopenic purpura, idiopathic, characteristics of, 1351
  chronic, 1364–1375
    diagnosis of, 1366
    in pregnant adolescents, 1372–1373
    long-term follow-up care in, 1372
    management of, 1366–1371
    natural history of, 1371
    pathogenesis of, 1365–1366
    recurrent, 1371–1372
  clinical features of, 1351–1352, 1352(t)
  differential diagnosis of, 1352–1354
  intracranial hemorrhage in, 1354, 1356, 1357(t)
  laboratory evaluation in, 1352–1354
  management of, 1356, 1358(t)–1359(t), 1360–1364
  maternal, neonatal thrombocytopenia secondary to, 110–111
  natural history of, 1354, 1355(t), 1356
  of childhood, 1351–1364
  platelet fragments in, 1403–1404
  platelet-associated IgG measurement in, 1404–1405, 1405(t)
  prognosis for, 1354–1356
  thrombotic, 438
Thrombocytosis, 1395, 1398–1399, 1398(t)
  postsplenectomy, 910
  spurious, 1345–1346
Thromboembolic disease, associated with antithrombin III deficiency, 1325

Thrombogenicity, risk of, with use of prothrombin complex concentrates, 1302
Thrombomodulin-protein C mechanism, in coagulation, 1256–1257, *1256*
Thrombopoiesis, regulation of, 147–151, *149–151*
Thrombopoietin, in thrombopoiesis regulation, 147–148, *149*, 150
  megakaryocyte development and, 1272
Thrombosis, arterial, with heparin-induced thrombocytopenia, 1377
  etiologic factors with, 1455–1459, 1456(t)
  in nephrotic syndrome, 1458
  neonatal, 106–107, 117
  protein C deficiency and, 1326
  prothrombin complex concentrates and, 1612
  venous, in paroxysmal nocturnal hemoglobinuria, 424–425
Thrombospondin, in platelets, 1432
Thrombotic disorders, platelet mediated, 1452–1453
  protein deficiency associated with, 1325–1326
Thrombotic thrombocytopenic purpura, 438
Thromboxane A_2, platelet, 1286, 1449
  deficits of, 1439–1440
  in aggregation and release, 1283, 1285–1286, 1432
  in arachidonic acid metabolism, 1448
  production of, in diabetes, 1456–1457
  in neonates, 1445
Thrombus(i), arterial vs venous, antiplatelet agents and, 1452
  in infants of diabetic mothers, 1457
Thumb anomalies, in Diamond-Blackfan anemia, 199
  in Fanconi's anemia, 178
  in thrombocytopenia with absent radii syndrome, 211
Thymectomy, for pure red cell aplasia with thymoma, 197
Thymic alymphoplasia, 884. See also *Immunodeficiency, severe combined.*
Thymic aplasia, congenital, 889.
Thymic carcinoma, Epstein-Barr virus and, 947
Thymidylate synthetase, 318
Thymoma, aplastic anemia and, 165
  differential diagnosis of, 1090
  pure red cell aplasia and, 195–197
Thymostimulin, for aplastic anemia, 175
Thymus, in immunodeficiency with ataxia telangiectasia, 887
  in severe combined immunodeficiency, 884, *885*
  Thymus-derived cells, hematopoietic role of, 134
Thyroid gland, disorders of, 1641–1642
  function of, in beta thalassemia, 747
Thyroid hormone, hematologic effects of, 1642(t)
Ticlopidine, platelet function and, 1451
Tissue(s), in protein-calorie malnutrition, 307
  iron requirement of, 368–370
Tissue factor, in coagulation, 1253
  in conversion of Factor IX to Factor IXa, control mechanisms governing, 1255
Tissue-type plasminogen activator, 1260
Tj^a antigen, 1507
T-lymphocyte(s). See *T cell(s).*
Total iron-binding capacity, for confirmation of iron deficiency, 292–293

Total iron-binding capacity *(Continued)*
  in hypochromic anemia, 370–371
  normal values for, 1684(t), *1685*
Total parenteral nutrition, cholestasis, 96
Toxemia of pregnancy, hydrops fetalis and, 733
Toxicity, in cancer chemotherapy, 986–987
Toxins, aplastic anemia and, 161(t), 163–164
  hemolytic anemia and, 504
Trace metals, in beta thalassemia, 754
Transcobalamin I, binding vitamin B_{12}, 341
  deficiency of, 351
Transcobalamin II, 1563
  deficiency of, 349–351, 357, 883
Transferrin, deficiency of, 302–303
  function and distribution of, 277
  genetic polymorphism of, 1561–1562, *1561*
  in intestinal absorption of iron, 282, *283*
  in iron loading in beta thalassemia, 744
  in iron uptake, 367, 369–370
    receptor of, 367–368
      on granulocyte-macrophage progenitor cells, 798
      on red cell membrane, 455
  plasma, in anemia of chronic disease, 1646
  saturation of, for confirmation of iron deficiency, 291(t), 292
    in hereditary hemochromatosis, 303
    in iron overloading in beta thalassemia, 744
  normal values for, 1684(t), *1685*
Transfusion, autoimmune neutropenia and, 806
  blood groups and, 1500
  compatibility tests for, 1498
  Epstein-Barr virus transmission with, 652
  exchange. See *Exchange transfusion.*
  for aplastic anemia, 169
  for autoimmune hemolytic anemia, 423
  for beta thalassemia, 738, 748–750
    iron overload with, 743–745
  for Diamond-Blackfan syndrome, 203
  for disseminated intravascular coagulation, 116
  for iron deficiency anemia, 296
  for sickle cell disease, 673, 683
  for thalassemia, intermediate, 755
  general principles of, 1606–1607
  granulocyte, 1598–1605
    clinical studies of, 1599–1600
    for chronic granulomatous disease, 830
    in neonates, 1602
    indications for, 1600–1602
    laboratory studies of, 1598–1599
    prophylactic, 171, 1602
    reactions to, 1602–1603
  in kidney transplantation, 1538
  in premature infants, 40, 40(t)
  intrauterine, for Rh hemolytic disease in fetus, 60–61
  pediatric, historical aspects of, 6–7
  placental, effects on neonatal blood volume, 26–27
  platelet, 1588–1597
    for aplastic anemia, 171
    for bone marrow failure, 1591–1592
    for disseminated intravascular coagulation, 116, 1591–1592
    for thrombocytopenia, 1591–1592
    massive, 1593
    maternal, for isoimmune neonatal thrombocytopenia, 111–112, *112*
    prophylactic, 1050

Transfusion *(Continued)*
  platelet, reactions to, 1590–1591, 1594
    storage of platelets for, 1589–1590
    uses of, 1591–1594
  purpura associated with, 1382
  reactions to, 1585–1587, 1590–1591, 1594, 1602–1603, 1613–1614
    delayed, plasmapheresis effect on, 1626(t)
  red cell, 1580–1587
    choice of product for, 1582–1584, 1583(t)
    for aplastic anemia, 171
    in immunocompromised host, 1584
    in neonates, 1584
    indications for, 1581–1582
    massive, 1584–1585
    reactions to, 1585–1587
    storage of, for transfusion, 1580–1581
Transient hypogammaglobulinemia of infancy, T cell control of B cell function in, 852–853, 853(t)
Transplant rejection, thrombocytopenia associated with, 1382–1383
Transplantation. See also *Bone marrow transplantation.*
  histocompatibility testing for, 1536–1542
  major histocompatibility complex system and, 1523
Trauma, cancer risk and, 923
  disseminated intravascular coagulation following, 1331, 1335
Treponema, hepatitis due to, conjugated hyperbilirubinemia and, 95
Trichobezoar, vitamin B_{12} deficiency with, 349
Triethylenemelamine, for retinoblastoma, 1185
Trimethoprim-sulfamethoxazole, for bone marrow transplantation infections, 249
  for chronic granulomatous disease, 830
Triose phosphate isomerase deficiency, hemolytic anemia and, 555–556
Trisomy 21, phosphofructokinase activity in, 555
Tropomyosin, red cell membrane, 460–461
Trunk, rhabdomyosarcoma of, 1157
Tryptophan pyrrolase, 277
Tuberculosis, 1651
Tuftsin, 431, 908
Tumor(s). See also *Cancer* and names of specific tumors.
  cell cycle of, drug classification according to cytotoxicity of, 996
  chromosomal changes in, 1479–1496
  embryonic, chromosomal changes in, 1490–1492
  growth rate of, cell cycle and, 994–995
    cell kinetics and, 997
    cell recruitment and, 997
    cell synchronization and, 996–997
    exponential, 990–991
    Gompertzian, 990–991
    response to chemotherapy and, 988–997
    protocol design in, 991–993, *993*
    stem cell in, drug resistance and, 995–996, 1006–1007
    volume doubling time of, 993–994, 988–990, *989*, *990*
  malignant solid. See also names of specific tumors.
    incidence of, *1137*, 1137(t)
    HLA class II antigen expression and, 1532
    presentation of, 1136–1137
    treatment of, 1137–1138
  splenic, 903, *904*

Tumor markers, for CNS tumors, 1187
　for germ cell tumors, 1171, 1171(t)
　in chronic myelogenous leukemia, 870, *871*
TW260/240 protein, 468
Twins, bone marrow transplantation in, 243, 251
　　leukemic relapse in, 253
　　monozygotic, fetal to fetal hemorrhage before birth in, 31
Typhilitis, 1039
Typhoid fever, 435, 1650
Tyrosine phosphorylation, in virus transformation of cells, 954
Tyrosinemia, conjugated hyperbilirubinemia and, 96

Ulcer(s), leg, 488, 678
Ulcerative colitis, 1635
Umbilical cord, abnormalities of, neonatal anemia and, 31
　clamped, blood volume and, 26–27
　　hemoglobin concentration and, 27(t)
　　normal hemoglobin values in, 27, 27(t), 1678(t)
　vessels of, at birth, 26–27
Uremia, coagulation factors in, 1640
　hemolytic anemia with, 509
　platelet function in, 1445–1446
　red cells in, 1639
　sickle cell disease and, 676–677
Uric acid, in leukemia treatment, 1042
Uridine diphosphate, bilirubin conjugation and, 77–78
Uridine diphosphate glucuronic acid (UDPGA), 2
Uridine diphosphate glucuronyl transferase, bilirubin conjugation and, 78
Urinary α-ALA, blood lead levels and, 393, *394*
Urinary screening test, for orotic aciduria, 358
　for porphobilinogen, 379
Urinary tract infection, 96
Urobilinoids, 79
URO, in porphyria cutanea tarda, 381
URO I, in congenital erythropoietic porphyria, 376
Urocanic acid, folate deficiency diagnosis and, 352
UROgen, in heme biosynthesis, 364, 366
UROgen decarboxylase, in acquired porphyria, 382
　in porphyria cutanea tarda, 381–382
UROgen I, 364, *365*
UROgen I synthetase, 379, 380
UROgen III, 364, *365*
UROgen III cosynthetase, in congenital erythropoietic porphyria, 376
Urokinase, in plasminogen activation, 1260
Uroporphyrinogen synthetase, lead effects on, 398
Urticaria, solar, 377
Urticarial transfusion reaction, 1586
Uterine sarcoma, 1159

Vaccine(s), pneumococcal, for postsplenectomy sepsis, 432, 489–490, 912–913, 1369
　in sickle cell disease, 675
Vaginal sarcoma, 1158–1159
Valproic acid, causing thrombocytopenia, 1379
Van den Bergh technique, of bilirubin concentration, 78, 82
Vascular purpura, 1459–1461
　causes of, 1459(t)
Vascular-platelet interactions, in fetus and neonate, 1692(t)
Vaso-occlusive sickle crises, 669–673
Vegetarianism, maternal cobalamin deficiency and, 344
Velban (vinblastine), 999(t)
Veno-occlusive disease, of liver, in bone marrow transplant recipients, 249
Venous blood sampling, for iron deficiency screening, 288
Vertebrae, codfish, 678, *679*
Ventricular function, in sickle cell disease, 676
Ventriculojugular shunts, 1453, 1456
Vinblastine, 999(t)
Vinca alkaloids, for childhood ITP refractory to splenectomy, 1370
　platelet function and, 1454
Vincristine, 999(t)
　for hemolytic uremic syndrome, 438
　with prednisone, for acute lymphoblastic leukemia, 1043
Viral hepatitis, aplastic anemia and, 164
　pure red cell aplasia and, 194
Viral infections, cancer risk and, 923–924
　hemolytic anemia with, 1649
　neutropenia with, 804
　suppressive T cell activity in, 853
　transient erythroblastopenia of childhood and, 206
　vs acute leukemia, 1041
　with bone marrow transplantation, 248
　with transfusion therapy, 1615–1616
Virus(es), Abelson, 950–951
　acute leukemia, 950–951
　avian erythroblastosis, 951
　avian lymphoid leukosis, 952, *952*
　avian myeloblastosis, 951
　cells transformed by, properties of, 944(t)
　DNA tumor, 943–948
　　adenovirus, 946
　　herpesvirus, 946–948
　　hepatitis B virus, 948
　　papovavirus, 944–946
　　vs RNA tumor, 943
　feline leukemia, 953
　hepatitis due to, conjugated hyperbilirubinemia and, 95
　human T cell lymphotropic (HTLV), 953–954
　　AIDS and, 1615
　mouse mammary tumor, 953
　murine leukemia, 953
　myelocytomatosis, 951
　oncogenic, 923–924, 942–957, 943(t). See also *Oncogenes, cellular.*
　recombinant, in therapy for beta thalassemia, 757–758
　RNA human, 953–954
　RNA tumor, 948–957
　sarcoma, 951–952
Virus-associated hemophagocytic syndrome, 1126–1127, *1126–1127*
　vs malignant histiocytosis, 1133
Vitamin(s), deficiency of, iron deficiency anemia and, 295
　supplements of, for beta thalassemia, 753–754
　for malnutrition, 309

Vitamin B$_{12}$, absorption of, 341
  absorption tests of, 355–356
  binders of, 341
  biochemistry of, 339–343
  cobalamin binders and, 341
  competition for, 349
  congenital defects in, folate metabolic errors with, 329
  daily requirements of, 341–342
  deficiency of, biochemical basis for, 342–343
    causes of, 344–352, 345(t)
      competition for vitamin B$_{12}$, 349
      defective absorption, 345–349, 346(t)
        drugs producing, 353(t)
        Schilling test for, 355–356
      defective transport, 349–350
      inadequate intake, 344
      metabolic disorders, 351–352
    clinical manifestations of, 352–353
    diagnosis of, 355–356
    dietary, 344
    in children, 344
    in gastrointestinal disease, 1635
    laboratory findings in, 353–355
    prevention of, 356
    treatment of, 356–357
    with iron deficiency, 294–295
  excretion of, 341
  folate deficiency and, 333
  metabolic function of, 339–341
    lead intoxication and, 399
  serum, in vitamin B$_{12}$ deficiency, 355
    tests of, 355
  sources of, 341–342
  structure of, 339, *340*
  synthesis of, 339, *340*
Vitamin C, for beta thalassemia, 753
Vitamin D-binding globulin, genetic polymorphism of, 1559–1560, *1559*, *1560*
Vitamin E, deficiency of, hemolytic anemia with, 508
  in abetalipoproteinemia, 505–506
  for beta thalassemia, 740, 744, 753–754
Vitamin K, coagulation factors and, 105–106, 105(t)
  in liver disease, 1327, 1637
  in prothrombin complex concentrates, 1299(t), 1302
  deficiency of, coagulation disorders with, 1327–1328
    in neonates, 106, 117–118, 118(t)
  for disseminated intravascular coagulation, 117
Vitamin K oxide, administration of, 117–118
Von Jaksch's anemia, of infants, 2–3
Von Recklinghausen's neurofibromatosis, leukemia risk and, 928
Von Willebrand's disease, 1315–1319, 1609
  abnormalities in, vs Factor VIII deficiency, 1253
  acquired, 1330
  assays helpful in, 1299
  characteristics of, 1315
  classification of, 1316–1317, 1317(t), *1318*
  clinical expression of, 1318
  cryoprecipitates for, 1301
  diagnosis of, 1315, 1316
  history of, 1315
  incidence of, 1318
  inheritance of, 1318
  pseudo (platelet-type), 1319, 1437
  treatment of, 1318–1319

Von Willebrand factor, function in platelet adhesion, 1252, 1283, *1283*, 1430, 1432
  glycoprotein Ib as receptor for, 1280–1281

Warts, due to papilloma virus, 944–945
Water, lead in, 390–391
Watson-Schwartz test, for acute intermittent porphyria, 379
Wegener's granulomatosis, 1648
Western blot technique, 1462–1463, *1463*
Wiener, Alexander, 11
Wilms' tumor, 1145–1152
  anaplastic, 1145
  bilateral, 1150–1151
  chromosomal changes in, 1491–1492
  clinical features of, 1147
  epidemiology of, 931–932
  genetics of, 1145
  management of, 1147–1151
    chemotherapy, 1149–1150, 1150(t)
    preoperative, 1147–1148
    radiotherapy, 1148–1149, 1150
    surgical approach to, 1148
  metastatic spread, 1147, 1151, *1152*
  oncogenesis and, 964
  pathology of, 1145–1147
  renal tumors related to, 1146–1147, 1151–1152
  staging of, 1148(t)
Wilson's disease, hemolysis in, 518
Wiskott-Aldrich syndrome, 888–889, *888*
  bone marrow transplantation for, 253–254
  eosinophilia and, 814
  impaired neutrophil chemotaxis in, 823
  neonatal thrombocytopenia and, 114
  postsplenectomy infection in, 911
  thrombocytopenia in, 1392–1393
Wolman's disease, 1240
Woronet's trait, 510
WT syndrome, 186

X chromosome, diseases linked to, agammaglobulinemia, 880–882
    gene rearrangement in, 866–867, 874
    neutropenia and, 801
  dyskeratosis congenita, 188, 190
  immunodeficiency with increased IgM concentration, 882–883
  lymphoproliferative syndrome, 187, 1122–1126, 1122(t), *1123–1124*, 1124(t), 1657
  McLeod phenotype of Kell blood group and, 1503
  of G6PD deficiency, 592–593, 583, 588–589, *590*
    mapping of, 592–593
  Xg^a blood group, 1513–1514
  dosage compensation effect and, 588
Xerocytosis, hereditary, 514–515, *514*
  neonatal, 36
  stomatocytic, 516
  various causes of, 517
  with high phosphatidylcholine, 516
Xg blood group, 1513–1514
X-porphyria, in variegate porphyria, 380

Y protein, bilirubin bound to, 77

Z protein, bilirubin bound to, 77
Zieve's syndrome, 508
Zinc, -ALAD activity and, 393–394
Zinc protoporphyrin, in erythropoietic protophyria, 396
   in lead toxicity, 394, *395*, 396, *396*, 397
Zinsser-Cole-Engman syndrome, 188–190, 188(t), *189*. See also *Dyskeratosis congenita*.
Zymogen, activation of, in hemostatic mechanism, 1248–1249, *1249*
Zollinger-Ellison syndrome, 1635